Temperature equivalents

Celsius	Fahrenheit	Celsius	Fahrenheit
34.0	93.2	38.6	101.4
34.2	93.6	38.8	101.8
34.4	93.9	39.0	102.2
34.6	94.3	39.2	102.5
34.8	94.6	39.4	102.9
35.0	95.0	39.6	103.2
35.2	95.4	39.8	103.6
35.4	95.7	40.0	104.0
35.6	96.1	40.2	104.3
35.8	96.4	40.4	104.7
36.0	96.8	40.6	105.1
36.2	97.1	40.8	105.4
36.4	97.5	41.0	105.8
36.6	97.8	41.2	106.1
36.8	98.2	41.4	106.5
37.0	98.6	41.6	106.8
37.2	98.9	41.8	107.2
37.4	99.3	42.0	107.6
37.6	99.6	42.4	108.0
37.8	100.0	42.4	108.3
38.0	100.4	42.6	108.7
38.2	100.7	42.8	109.0
38.4	101.1	43.0	109.4

TO CONVERT FAHRENHEIT TO CELSIUS:
(Temperature minus 32) $\times \frac{5}{9}$
EXAMPLE: To convert 98.6 degrees Fahrenheit to Celsius:
$98.6 - 32 = 66.6 \times \frac{5}{9} = 37$ degrees

TO CONVERT CELSIUS TO FAHRENHEIT:
$\frac{9}{5} \times$ temperature $+ 32$
EXAMPLE: To convert 40 degrees Celsius to Fahrenheit:
$\frac{9}{5} \times 40 = 72 + 32 = 104$ degrees

Essentials of
Maternity Nursing

THE NURSE AND
THE CHILDBEARING FAMILY

Essentials of Maternity Nursing

THE NURSE AND THE CHILDBEARING FAMILY

IRENE M. BOBAK, R.N., M.S., Ph.D

Professor, San Francisco State University,
San Francisco, California

MARGARET DUNCAN JENSEN, R.N., M.S.

Professor Emeritus, San Jose State University,
San Jose, California

SECOND EDITION

THE C. V. MOSBY COMPANY

ST. LOUIS • WASHINGTON, D.C. • TORONTO   1987

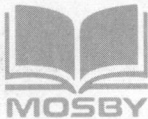

MOSBY

A TRADITION OF PUBLISHING EXCELLENCE

Developmental Editors: **Susan R. Epstein, Rhonda Kumm**
Assistant Editor: **June Schaffer Heath**
Design: **Diane M. Beasley**
Production: **Jean Genz, Ginny Douglas, Judy Bamert, Maureen Hayes**

SECOND EDITION

Copyright © 1987 by The C.V. Mosby Company

Previous edition copyrighted 1983.

Printed in the United States of America

The C.V. Mosby Company
11830 Westline Industrial Drive, St. Louis, Missouri 63146

Library of Congress Cataloging-in-Publication Data

Bobak, Irene M.
  Essentials of maternity nursing.

  Includes bibliographies and index.
  1. Obstetrical nursing.   I. Jensen, Margaret
Duncan. II. Title. [DNLM: 1. Obstetrical
Nursing. 2. Perinatology—nurses' instruction.
WY 157 B663e]
RG951.B66 1987   610.73'678   86-23591
ISBN 0-8016-0717-5

C/VH/VH 9 8 7 6 5 4 3 2 1   02/A/246

Contributors

PRESENT EDITION

BEVERLY GAGLIONE, R.N., M.A.

Chairperson, Director of Nursing, Professor of Parent
Child Nursing, East Stroudsburg University, East
Stroudsburg, Pennsylvania; Ph.D. Candidate,
Anthropology, Rutger's University, Newark, New Jersey

CHERYL HARRIS, R.N., B.S.

Staff Nurse, Neonatal Intensive Care Unit, Childrens Mercy
Hospital, Kansas City, Missouri

ROSEMARY MANN, C.N.M., Esq.

Attorney at Law; Director, Women's Health Care Training
Project, Stanford University, Stanford, California

FIRST EDITION

JEANNE DeJOSEPH, Ph.D., C.N.M., F.A.A.N.

Assistant Professor, University of California, San Francisco,
California; Lecturer, Department of Family, Community
and Preventive Medicine, Stanford University Medical
School, Stanford, California; Affiliated Faculty Member,
Center for Research on Women, Stanford University

JOAN EDELSTEIN, R.N., P.N.P., Dr.P.H.

Associate Professor, San Jose State University, San Jose,
California

BEVERLY HORN, R.N., Ph D

Associate Professor, School of Nursing, University of
Washington, Seattle, Washington

BARBARA PETREE, R.N., M.A.

Nurse Educator for Midcostal California Outreach Perinatal
Program, Department of Obstetrics and Gynecology,
Stanford University Medical Center, Stanford, California

CELESTE PHILLIPS, R.N., Ed.D.

Maternity Instructor, Cabrillo College, Aptos, California;
Director of Professional Relations, Borning Corporation,
Spokane, Washington

SUSAN TUCKER, R.N., B.S.N., P.H.N.

Assistant Director of Nursing, Kaiser-Permanente Medical
Center, Panorama City, California

LUCILLE WHALEY, R.N., M.S.

Professor Emeritus, San Jose State University, San Jose,
California

**BONNIE WORTHINGTON-ROBERTS,
Ph.D.**

Professor, Director of Nutritional Sciences and Chief
Nutritionist, Child Development Center, University of
Washington, Seattle, Washington

MARIANNE K. ZALAR, R.N., Ed.D.

Formerly, Assistant Director of Nursing, Department of
Nursing Research, Stanford University Hospital and
Medical Center, Stanford, California; Associate Clinical
Professor, Department of Family Health Care Nursing,
University of California, San Francisco, California;
President, ZBS Research Associates, San Mateo, California

To the following members of our families who, by virtue of their belief in us, prompted the courage and motivation to complete this book:

Marianne K. Zalar
Albert B. Bobak
Irene L. Bobak
Stephen J. Bobak
Veronica Bobak
Sister Mary Eleanor, V.S.C.

IRENE M. BOBAK

Russ Duncan
John F. Duncan
Marjory Jensen
Carlo Jensen
And to the memory of my sister:
Doreen Elizabeth Duncan

MARGARET DUNCAN JENSEN

Preface

Professional nursing practice continues to evolve and adapt to the changing health care needs of society. Childbearing has significance for parents, extended families, and society as a whole. Birth is an intense physical and emotional experience that creates new life and potential for society. Nothing is more wondrous than the creation of another human being. Every culture establishes acceptable behavior for pregnancy, the birth process, and care of the newborn. The maternity nurse is challenged to acquire a sound knowledge base in order to provide sensitive quality care to individual clients and their families.

Essentials of Maternity Nursing: The Nurse and the Childbearing Family has been revised and redesigned to focus on the *basics* of providing safe nursing care to the childbearing family. The nursing process continues to be the primary organizational feature of the text. It serves as a systematic approach to providing quality nursing care. Nursing actions are derived from the nursing assessment and diagnoses and are evaluated for their effectiveness in meeting the clearly defined goals. *Essentials of Maternity Nursing: The Nurse and the Childbearing Family* emphasizes the role of the nurse as support person, teacher/counselor/advocate, and technician. Knowledge of vital information places the nurse in a key position for providing health care teaching that encourages client and family participation in the childbearing experience. This second edition presents current, accurate, and theoretically sound content for the delivery of safe, comprehensive, and holistic care of the childbearing family.

APPROACH

Educators in maternal-newborn nursing courses are faced with the challenge of providing students with extensive knowledge within a limited timeframe. *Essentials of Maternity Nursing: The Nurse and the Childbearing Family* is designed to emphasize the normal childbirth experience and the nurse's role in health promotion and self-care. For this reason, deviations from normal are presented in a separate unit at the end of the text. Throughout, emphasis on both physical and psychosocial content is presented as the foundation for providing scientific holistic nursing care. Culturally sensitive care is woven into the text with examples provided to assist the learner in recognizing the uniqueness of each client.

Special attention has been given to the reading level of the text to provide clear and concise wording and presentation. A two-color format has been incorporated in the design of the text to enhance its readability. As with the first edition, numerous charts, tables, and illustrations augment and support the text and provide quick reference information.

Detailed chapter outlines in the table of contents afford the reader an opportunity to review a chapter's material at a glance. Each chapter introduces the reader to the content and ends with a summary highlighting the chapter's key concepts. Extensive references and bibliographies offer areas for further exploration. The 12 appendixes provide resource information for students and practitioners alike. The detailed index is an invaluable aid in assisting readers in finding information logically and quickly.

Several new features have been developed to meet the specific needs of the learner. They facilitate the narrative and enhance the usefulness of the text as a practical resource. The *summaries of nursing actions* offer comprehensive reviews of the essential components of nursing care. The summaries serve as future references for the practicing nurse, clearly stating nursing goals, priorities for care, and outcome criteria for evaluation. The evaluation serves as a basis for adapting care plans to changing conditions. General summaries assist the nurse in developing individualized care plans using the nursing process format. Summaries are placed strategically throughout the text in order to assist the reader in grasping the key concepts that are necessary to planning care.

The *applications of the nursing process* serve as examples of adapting the content presented in the chapters to the individualized needs of specific clients. The care plans so developed use functional health patterns as guides to developing a systematic approach to nursing assessment. The assessment leads to nursing diagnoses that direct the plan of care. Evaluation is based on measurable criteria that reflect the client's response to curative or rehabilitative therapy.

Guidelines for client teaching illustrate strategies for organizing and relating health care content to the childbearing family. Goals for teaching are gleaned from the nursing diagnoses and the client's health care needs. Content and teaching actions are designed to meet the desired goals. References and teaching aids serve as further resources for developing teaching plans for clients. Sample teaching strategies encourage the nurse to develop individualized teaching plans.

Procedures supply the knowledge necessary to provide competent technical skills to the maternity client and her newborn. Equipment lists allow the nurse to approach the procedure in an organized, systematic fashion. Specific step-by-step nursing actions and their rationales assure that technical expertise can be obtained. In addition to care of the mother, procedures help to describe the technical care of the high-risk neonate in Unit 7, as well as care of the normal newborn.

Two additional features have been designed specifically with the learner's needs in mind. First, *drug cards* provide essential pertinent drug information for commonly used maternal and newborn drugs. Easily transported, the cards are designed for use in the clinical setting and serve as a quick reference. They supplement the use of a pharmacology text and hospital formulary.

Second, a *cervical dilation teaching guide* is printed on the inside back cover of the text. It assists the novice maternity nurse in visualizing different phases of cervical dilation in the childbearing client. It can be used as a teaching aid when describing the birth process to the client. All the features unique to *Essentials of Maternity Nursing: The Nurse and the Childbearing Family* have been designed to meet the specific learning needs of the maternity nurse.

ORGANIZATION

The text is comprised of seven units organized to enhance learning. The first six units focus on normal content, with Unit 7 discussing deviations from normal. Unit 1, "The Childbearing Family: A Unit of Care," provides the theoretic basis for family-centered holistic maternity nursing care. An overview of the breadth of maternity nursing practice is presented. The special

features of the text are further described in the introductory chapters to assist the learner in understanding their broad application to nursing practice. The unit examines the family, its structure, and its supportive roles. A separate chapter on legal and ethical aspects of family-centered maternity nursing provides an understanding of the issues faced by today's maternity nurse.

Unit 2, "Basic Concepts of Human Sexuality," presents the fundamental concepts of human sexuality and reproduction. The biologic and psychologic aspects of reproduction are emphasized as the foundation for care before, during, and after pregnancy. Infertility, fertility, control of fertility, and surgical interruption of pregnancy are discussed in considerable detail.

Unit 3, "Normal Pregnancy," progresses from conception through family preparation for the birth of the newborn. Nursing care during pregnancy requires knowledge of fetal development, as well as an understanding of the childbearing family's adaptation to the biopsychosocial realities of pregnancy. Separate chapters on maternal and fetal nutrition and family preparation for the birth of a child reflect the growing body of knowledge in maternity nursing practice. The nurse plays an important role in emphasizing and encouraging early client education and involvement in health care, thus promoting family wellness and self-care. Numerous procedures are found in Unit 3 to assist the nurse in providing competent technical care to the childbearing family.

Unit 4, "Normal Childbirth," begins with the essential factors and processes that influence the outcome of childbirth. Each stage of labor is presented separately using the nursing process as the organizing feature. Family participation is emphasized to include the support person, spouse, grandparents, and siblings. The nurse's role related to pharmacologic control of discomfort and fetal monitoring is discussed in a separate chapter.

Unit 5, "The Normal Newborn," includes content on both the biologic and behavioral characteristics of the healthy neonate at term. The nursing process is used as an organizational base for the chapter on the care of the normal newborn. Nursing roles of teacher/counselor/advocate, support person, and technician are discussed fully. Content is presented in narrative form, procedures, and teaching guides for parents. A Summary of Nursing Actions and Application of the Nursing Process are included. The nutritional needs of the newborn and the nursing care associated with breast or bottle feeding of the infant are presented in a separate chapter.

Unit 6, "Normal Postpartum Period," is devoted to nursing care of the new mother and her family. There is extensive development of the sections on maternal physiology and on the psychologic impact of parenthood on the mother and family members. This provides the basis for the selection of nursing strategies appropriate for individualized care.

Unit 7, "The High-risk Family," describes populations at high risk and necessary alterations in the plans of care for the high-risk childbearing family. Selected risk factors are presented in considerable depth in a framework of biologic and psychosocial dysfunction. This format facilitates a conceptual approach to common symptoms and therapies (preventive, curative, rehabilitative), as well as study of the distinctive characteristics of specific disorders.

The major maternal and fetal-neonatal complications—PIH, infection, and hemorrhage—are presented in separate chapters for ease of teaching and learning. Separate chapters on loss and grief and adolescent pregnancy highlight some special considerations in providing nursing care to the high-risk client. Summaries of nursing actions, procedures, guidelines for client teaching, and applications of the nursing process can be found throughout the content in Unit 7. Emphasis is placed on keeping the family's childbearing experience in focus, rather than concentrating solely on the risk factors.

TEACHING AND LEARNING PACKAGE

To facilitate the teaching-learning process and help instructors and students in using the text to its fullest potential, three supplements are offered: an instructor's manual, a test bank, and an overhead transparency set.

1. The *Instructor's Manual* includes 31 chapters, each keyed to one chapter in the text. Each chapter includes the goals for learning, an overview of content presented, a list of key terms introduced in the chapter, a chapter outline, and suggestions for clinically based activities.

2. The *Test Bank* includes over 500 questions directly related to the student learning objectives. Answer key and page references for the questions are also included.

3. An overhead transparency set includes 50 two-color illustrations from this new text.

We are fully aware of the increasingly important contribution men are making to the nursing profession as well as the growing number of women entering the medical profession. We hope this trend will continue. The construction of the English language, however, sometimes makes it awkward to totally eliminate the feminine and masculine pronouns. Therefore, to present material clearly and smoothly we have generally used the feminine pronoun to refer to the nurse.

Over the years we have received many comments and suggestions regarding our maternity nursing texts. Some of these comments provided the impetus for writing *Essentials of Maternity Nursing: The Nurse and the Childbearing Family,* and we have incorporated many of these suggestions in the organization and development of this text. We welcome comments from instructors, students, and practitioners who use this text so that we may continue to be responsive to the needs of the profession.

Irene M. Bobak
Margaret Duncan Jensen

Acknowledgments

We wish to thank those whose comments and suggestions enhanced this collaborative effort. In alphabetical order they are Melanie R. Ashworth, RN, Stanford, California; Marcia Biggs, RN, NNP, Fountain Valley, California; Priscilla Ebersole, RN, PhD, San Francisco, California; Alison Driessen, RN, Fountain Valley, California; Jo Ann Hattner, RD, MPH, Palo Alto, California; Barbara Hayes, Nurse Midwife, Melbourne, Australia; Sheldon B. Korones, MD, Memphis, Tennessee; Jack Kundin, MD, San Mateo, California; Rosemary J. Mann, CNM, JD, Stanford, California; Susan Smith Noyes, RN, MSN, Wilmington, Delaware; Helen Pyne, RN, MSN, Bethesda, Maryland; M. Colleen Stainton, RN, DNS, Calgary, Alberta, Canada; Ellen J. Stein, MD, Stanford, California; Vivian Wahlberg, RN, CM, DrMedSc, Stockholm, Sweden; Deborah Y. Ward, RN, MS, Arnold, Maryland; Lucille F. Whaley, RN, MS, San Jose, California; Marianne K. Zalar, RN, EdD, San Mateo, California.

We would like to thank the following photographers: Judith Bamber, San Jose, California; Joan Edelstein, San Jose, California; Nanci Newell, Fountain Valley, California; and M. Colleen Stainton, Calgary, Alberta, Canada. A special thank you goes to Marjorie Pyle, RNC, Lifecircle, Costa Mesa, California. Marjorie Pyle is the official photographer for this text and for *Maternity and Gynecologic Care: the Nurse and the Family*.

Several families in addition to our own have made unique contributions to the original photographs in this text. We are indebted to these families, who embody the philosophical basis for our text—family centered nursing care.

To the staffs of Stanford University Medical Center, Stanford, California; Kaiser-Permanente Hospital and Santa Clara Valley Medical Center, Santa Clara, California; St. Luke's Hospital, Kansas City, Missouri; Jewish Hospital and Barnes Hospital, St. Louis, Missouri; Mills Memorial Hospital, San Mateo, California; and the Woman's Hospital of Texas, Houston, Texas, we offer thanks for their shared expertise and photographs.

We are indebted to our typists Shirley Knutzen, Barbara Liston, and Mindy Bobak for their willing and tireless efforts. This edition contains artwork by George Wassilchenko, Oral Roberts University, Tulsa, Oklahoma, whose precise, detailed anatomic drawings have made a substantial contribution to facilitating the study of complex theory. We look forward to a continuing association with this outstanding medical illustrator.

Special words of gratitude are extended to David P. Carroll, Rhonda Kumm, Suzi Epstein, Mary Espenschied, and June S. Heath, The C.V. Mosby Company, St. Louis, Missouri, for their encouragement, inspiration, and assistance in the preparation and production of this text. We acknowledge the assistance of our families, both concrete and supportive, and we thank each other for the stimulation, support, and mutual respect generated by this collaboration.

Irene M. Bobak
Margaret Duncan Jensen

Contents

UNIT 3
NORMAL PREGNANCY

Guidelines for Client Teaching

Summaries of Nursing Action

Procedures

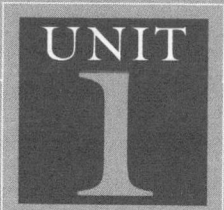

UNIT 1

The Childbearing Family: A Unit of Care

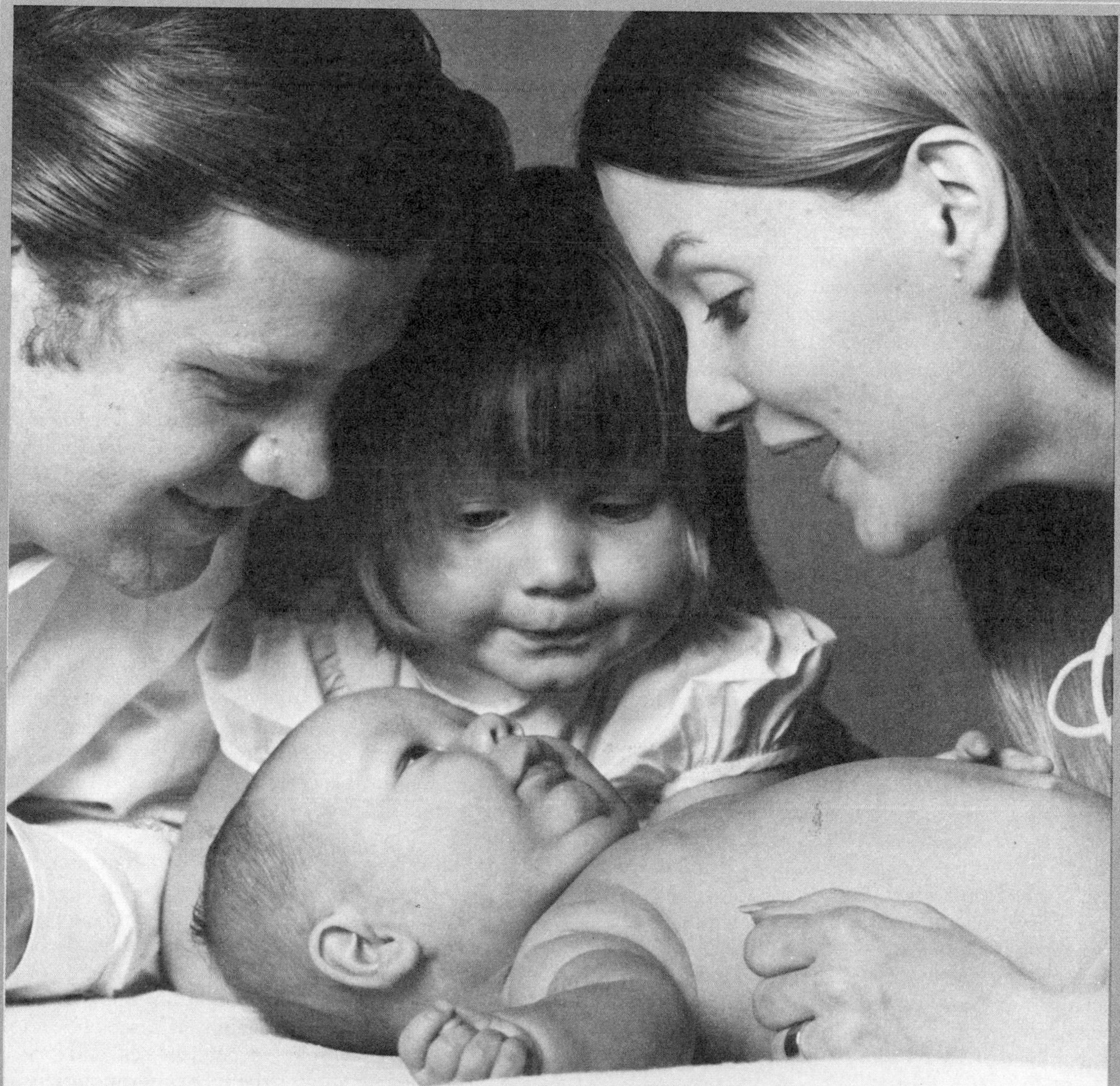

The Childbearing Family

I was a mother and looked into his eyes so clear; fell into his eyes, and in love" (Lang, 1972).

Since recorded time, birth has occasioned such emotions. It is one of the dramatic episodes in life—a moment when the past merges with the present and the present holds all the potential for a future. Wonder and excitement, awe and reverence are stirred by evidence of creation of another human. Creation that began with conception, moved through an orderly process of biologic development, and culminated in birth. Each culture, concerned as it must be with the care and rearing of future generations, develops patterns of behavior associated with the birth process and describes the social roles of the participants—mother, father, and infant—and the persons designated to offer assistance.

Being born, being cared for by parents, and in turn caring for others in a like manner are events shared by all of us. They form part of life's continuum and are universal experiences.

Childbearing has significance for parents, extended family, and society as a whole (Fig. 1.1). Complex meanings that vary cross-culturally underlie each aspect of the process, from conception until recognition of attainment of adult status. Because of the importance of childbearing to society, each society develops social groups that assume major responsibility for the introduction and socialization of the children. The most important of these groups is the family. The family is recognized as the fundamental social unit because most people have more continuous contact with this social group than with any other. The family forms a social network that acts as a potent support system for its members.

Definitions

Families are defined in many ways. Definitions of the family involve delineation of family structure, functions, composition, and affectional ties. The United Nations (1969, p. 20) describes the family as "those members of the household who are related, to a specific degree, through blood, adoption or marriage." Helvie (1981) defines the family as "a primary group of people living in a household in consistent proximity and intimate relationships." Because the concept of a family varies, the concept of *household* is sometimes substituted for that of the family. The term *household* is used to cover a number of family styles and refers to a group of people who share a common dwelling. Usually persons united by marriage, blood, or adoption form the core of the household; however, a household also may consist of a person or an unrelated group of people sharing the customary living arrangements of a family group. The concept of household encompasses not only traditional forms of family structure but also recently designated groups: (1) the never-married, (2) one parent and children living together as a one-parent family, (3) two homosexuals living together in a stable union, and (4) stable consensual unions, with or without children (WHO, 1978, p. 78). Despite the difficulty of defining the family precisely, members of a family can readily describe its composition, who is kin and who is not, how the family has affected their lives, and what family style they believe in.

However the family is defined, the *family unit* is incomplete without an adult. From an adult's perspective the family can comprise persons of any age or sex bound by a blood or love relationship or both. From the child's perspective, the family is a set of relationships between the child's dependent self and one or more protective adults, as the following quotations indicate:

Fig. 1.1
Four-generation family. (Courtesy Marjorie Pyle, RNC, Lifecircle, Costa Mesa, California.)

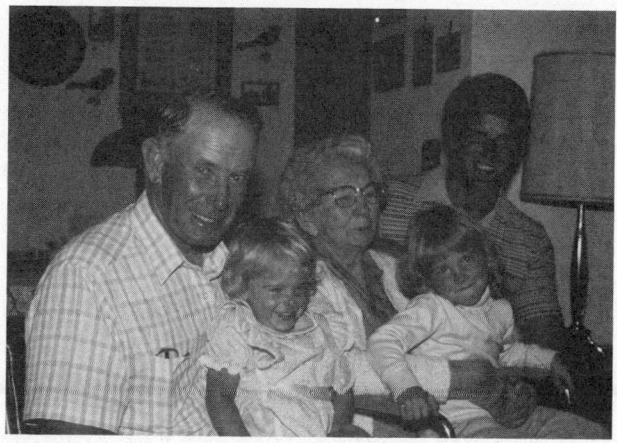

"God and me, Mommie, Daddy, and J.R., Nana and Grandpa, Grandma and Grandpa, and Great Nana—people who love you and you have fun together." (Stacie, age 5)

"A family is where everybody shares and cares for each other. A family is where there is love in the home. A family is where they go on vacations together. A family is where everybody shares with the work." (Robert, age 15)

Implications for Nursing

Because the family acts as a primary force in generating support for clients, an understanding of this unit is essential to the formulation of a nursing care plan. Many disciplines, such as nursing, history, anthropology, sociology, and economics, have become involved in the study of the relationships between the family and society. As a result we are increasingly aware of the effects of social change on the family and the contribution and responsiveness of the family to social transformation. This knowledge has led to an understanding of the importance of the family unit for personal health conditions and the health care system. Family patterns, attitudes, and responses to change play a determining part in the health of individual members and their use of health services.

Key factors in family health. Certain factors have proved important in determining the quality of family health:

1. Culture patterning in areas such as childbearing, child rearing, or use of health services determines many health-related responses.
2. Family dynamics, which encompass coordination of intrafamilial roles, distribution of power in the fam-

ily, and the process of decision making, affects the use of health services.
3. Family responses to crisis, including coping behaviors and the quality of personal responses and mutual concern, affect the level of support afforded family members.
4. Family socioeconomic characteristics are important. Social class affects expectations, obligations, and rewards, all of which affect use of health services. In addition the family acts as the primary economic unit in which incomes may be pooled, expenditure decisions taken jointly, and services rendered internally.

Family Functions

As the family progresses through its life cycle, beginning with the commitment of two people to share a life and ending with the dissolution of the family through death or other separations, it carries out certain *functions* for the well-being of its members. The functions extend over five basic areas: biologic, economic, educational, psychologic, and sociocultural (WHO, 1978). The interdependent functions are dependent on the physical and mental health of family members. As a supportive structure for these functions, each family develops certain common *beliefs, values* and *sentiments* that are used as criteria in the choice of alternative actions.

Biologic functions. Biologic functions include reproduction, care and rearing of children, nutrition, maintenance of health, and recreation. The ability to carry out such functions implies certain prerequisites: a healthy genetic inheritance, family planning, care during the maternity cycle, good dietary behavior, intelligent use of health services, companionship, and nurturing of the elderly.

Economic functions. Economic functions include making enough money to carry out the other functions, determining the allocation of resources, and ensuring the financial security of family members. To accomplish these tasks the family must have the necessary skills, opportunities, and knowledge.

Educational functions. Educational functions include the teaching of skills, attitudes, and knowledge relating to the other functions. To be able to do this, family members must have the necessary levels of intelligence and the necessary knowledge, skills, and experience.

Psychologic functions. The family is expected to provide an environment that promotes the natural development of personality, offers optimum psychologic protection, and promotes the ability to form relationships with people outside the family circle. These tasks require stable emotional health, common bonds of affection between individuals, and the ability to be mutually supportive, to tolerate stress, and to cope with crises.

Sociocultural functions. Sociocultural functions are associated with the socialization of children. The socialization of children includes the transfer of values relating to behavior, tradition, language, and prevailing or previous social mores. It results in the conditioning of family members to a variety of behavior norms appropriate to all stages of adult life. To be able to do this, the family must possess accepted standards and be sensitive to the varying social needs of children according to their ages. It must also accept and exemplify behavioral norms and be willing to explain, defend, and promote them. Although certain functions are relegated to or emphasized more in one phase of the family's life cycle than another, (for example, the care and socialization of children are part of the childbearing and child rearing phase of the cycle), many of the functions are continuous for the survival and progress of the family.

Family Dynamics

Families work cooperatively to accomplish family functions. To do this, family members assume appropriate social roles. Social roles are learned in the family, the first social group, and are learned in pairs, for example, mother-father, parent-child, and brother-sister. A social role does not exist by itself but is designed to mesh with that of a role partner. Pairing of roles enables social interactions to take place in an orderly, predictable manner—the roles are said to be complementary. Some families maintain a traditional pairing of roles, whereas other families have changed the behavior patterns to suit a change in family life-style. The process by which paired roles are brought into a new alignment is known as *negotiation*. Negotiation is essential if family equilibrium is to be maintained.

From the time it is formed, the family sets up *boundaries* between itself and the outside. People are extremely conscious of those considered members of their family and those who rank as outsiders—those who do not have kinship status. Some families isolate themselves from the community. Others have a wide community network to help in times of stress. Although boundaries exist for every family, family members set up *channels* through which they mediate external forces and attempt to protect the family from disturbances. The channels also ensure that the family receives its share of social resources.

Ideally the family provides a safe, intimate environment for the biopsychosocial development of children and its adult members. The family provides for the *nurturing* of the newborn and the gradual *socialization* of the growing child. It is the source of first relationships with others. The relationships children form with parents (or parenting persons) are the earliest and closest and persist throughout a lifetime. For better or worse, parent-child relationships influence a person's concepts of self-worth and ability to form later relationships. The family also interprets and mediates the child's perceptions of the complex outside world. The family provides the growing child with an identity that possesses both a past and a sense of the future. The family transmits cultural values and rituals from one generation to the next (Friedman, 1981).

Through everyday interactions the family develops and uses its own patterns of verbal and nonverbal *communication*. These patterns give insight into the feeling exchange within a family and act as reliable indicators of interpersonal functioning. Family members not only react to the communication or actions of other family members but also interpret and define them.

When assessing a family, nurses examine what is happening and who is doing what to whom. They also note how people perceive what is being done, what it means to them, and how this meaning is expressed. A baby cries to draw the attention of his or her mother, but the mother may interpret the crying as the baby's way of saying she is not a good mother.

Over time the family develops protocols for *problem solving,* particularly regarding decisions deemed important to the family, such as having a baby, buying a house, or sending only sons to college. The criteria used in making decisions are based on *family values* and *attitudes* concerning the appropriateness of the behavior of its various members and the moral, social, political, and economic events of the wider social system. The *power* to make critical decisions is conferred on a family member through tradition or negotiation. This power may be overt or covert and reflects the family's concepts of male or female dominance and cultural practices, social customs, and community norms. As a result family members are positioned into certain *statuses* or *hierarchies* and play out these statuses by assuming various *roles*. Most families have a member who "takes charge" or "is supportive" or "can't be expected to do anything."

Family Theories

Many academic disciplines have studied the family and have developed theories that provide differing perspectives for assessing it. Knowledge of these theories provides the nurse with guides to understanding family functioning. They provide a basis for planning the day-to-day care of families and help predict certain future events that may necessitate a modification of care.

Structural-functional theory. The structural-functional theory originated with the work of social anthropologists Malinowski (1945) and Radcliffe-Brown (1952), who documented the interrelatedness and interdependence of the national social system and all subsocial systems. According to this theory the family is a social system with components (family members) with specific roles and role behaviors, such as father role or mother role. Family dynamics are directed toward maintaining *equilibrium* between complementary roles to permit family functioning. Family structure is culturally determined. The United States represents a pluralistic culture in which varying family forms are recognized and accepted in differing degrees. Classification of families according to their structure provides insight into stresses that families may experience as they differ from the normative structures supported by the society.

Nuclear family. The nuclear family is the form considered "normal" in contemporary Western society

(Figs. 1.2 and 1.3). Despite talk of new life-styles, it still represents 73% of all households (U.S. National Center for Health Statistics, 1982). This family group consists of parents and their still-dependent children. The family lives apart from either the husband's or wife's family of orientation and is usually economically independent.

The percentage of families with two wage earners rose dramatically during the last decade. In 1979 no fewer than 59.1% of married women with children ages 6 to 17 were in the labor force. According to Harris (1982) this change was caused by the fact that by the early 1960s families were "finding it increasingly difficult to achieve or hold onto middle-class standards of consumption for themselves and their children."

Parents in the nuclear family are expected to play complementary roles of husband-wife and father-mother in giving emotional and physical support to each other and their children. Ideally the nuclear family provides for the care and socialization of children and social control for its members. It is held together by strong social bonds. It remains flexible enough to survive in an industrial world. The nuclear family can be perceived as "existing to fulfill the cultural dictates of its society as that society seeks to perpetuate itself"

Fig. 1.2
Nuclear family in the 1920s.

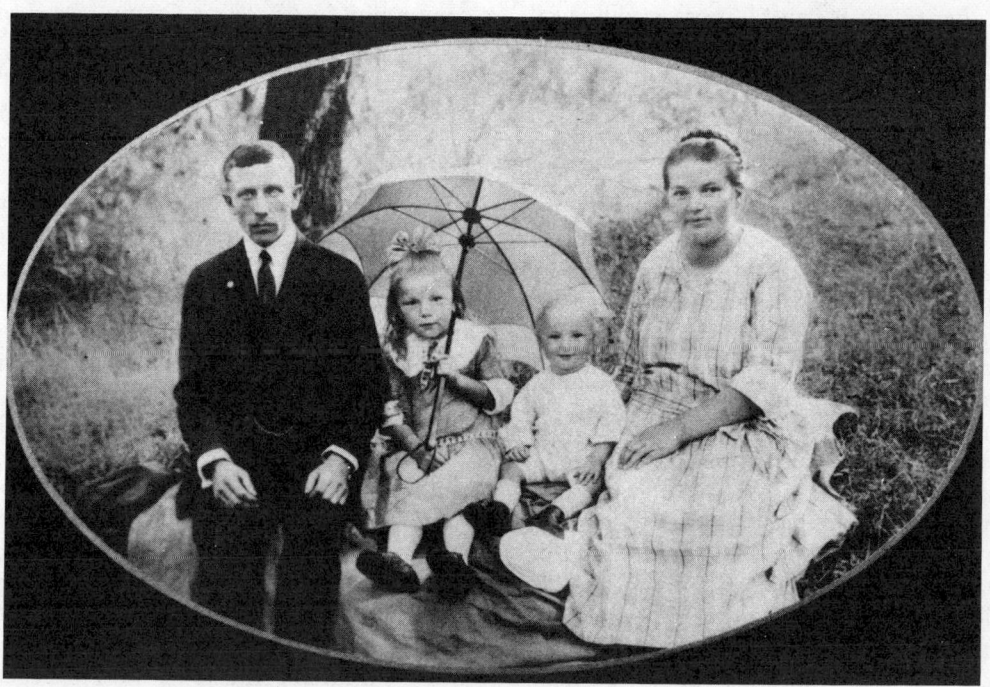

Fig. 1.3
Nuclear family in the 1980s. (Courtesy Marjorie Pyle, RNC, Lifecircle, Costa Mesa, California.)

Fig. 1.4
Extended family.

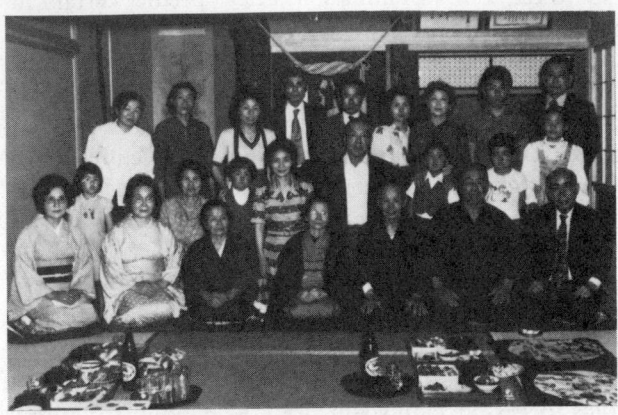

(Anderson and Carter, 1974). During times of crisis the family can become an important area for social change.

The nuclear family has been described as isolated, but there is increasing evidence that kinship ties to previous family structures are not broken. Sons and daughters frequently remain in the same community as their families of orientation, although they establish their own nuclear families. Visiting relatives is part of their social life. The increased mobility of all segments of population means that grandparents, sisters, uncles, cousins, and other relatives can be more readily available to the isolated family. We often hear new mothers say, "My mother is going to fly in to help me for a week or so." In addition, friends and social groups from church or work provide support for the nuclear family and act in the role of absent families.

Extended family. By definition the extended family (Fig. 1.4) includes three generations. It is family centered, its members live together as a group, and through its kinship network it provides supportive functions to all members. This family structure serves to prescribe the responsibilities and actions of family members. Some people believe the extended family impedes the mobility necessary in an industrialized society with its economic demands.

With an influx of new citizens from Southeast Asia, the Caribbean, and Mexico, the extended family is again playing an important role. The family provides the primary source of identity by maintaining language and cultural identification; it provides economic support by "taking in" needy relatives and sharing food, shelter, and jobs; it gives emotional support by maintaining kinship ties.

People who have experienced such a family may chafe at the bonds it creates, but when they leave, they may regret the absence of a wider sense of acceptance and recognition such a family provides. In changing to a more socially functional group, members of such "old-fashioned" families may need help in recognizing social institutions as an alternative family to which they can legitimately turn for help and sustenance in times of stress.

Communal family. Communal family groupings vary from the highly formalized structure of the Amish community in Lancaster County, Pennsylvania, to the loosely knit groups found in the Santa Cruz Mountains near Boulder Creek, California. These latter communities are formed for specific ideologic or societal purposes. They are considered an alternative life-style for people who feel alienated from a predominantly economically oriented society. Some communes consist of nuclear groups living in an extended or expanded family community and are envisioned as persisting over time. Others may provide temporary shelter. In some communes all parents participate in caretaking activities for all children. In many of these groups the combination is fluid; individuals and families are free to come and go as their needs dictate.

The effect of such communities with regard to the children has yet to be determined. Groups that lack some permanence may perpetuate the difficulties associated with the highly mobile nuclear family seeking stability and continuity in social contacts. Communes composed solely of young adults and their children may be reproducing the ghettolike aspects of suburbia, with its limited contacts with diverse age, cultural, and economic groups.

Single-parent family. The single-parent family is becoming an increasingly recognized structure in our society. The single-parent family may result from loss of a spouse by death, divorce, separation, or desertion; from the out-of-wedlock birth of a child; or from the adoption of a child. The 1984 U.S. Bureau of the Census reveals that 25.7% of all children 17 years old or younger live in a family with a single parent, another relative, or a nonrelative. This was the situation for 20% of white children and 59% of black children. As many as 85% of babies born to young unmarried mothers were kept by their mothers; 7% were given to other family members, leaving only 8% for adoption. Of the single parents, 95% are women, most commonly under 25 years of age and in a low-income bracket. Of the group with children under 6 years of age, almost 55% of the single parents are working; in the group with school-age children, about 65% are working mothers.

The single-parent family tends to be vulnerable economically and socially. Unless buttressed by a concerned society, it may create an unstable and deprived environment for the growth potential of children (Norton and Glick, 1986). Nutrition may be haphazard, communication and overt displays of affection curtailed, and discipline inconsistent (Hetherington, Cox, and Cox, 1977). For many of the adults involved this family structure represents a lonely existence in which decision making and other family tasks depend on a single adult (McLanahan, Wedemeyer, and Adelberg, 1981). Public policy is beginning to reflect recognition that a pluralistic society necessarily produces pluralistic forms of the family and that high levels of marital instability are probably to be expected in modern society. As with people who have broken away from the support of extended families, adults in single-parent families may need help in learning how to use community resources in developing or maintaining a satisfactory family life.

For other adults the single-parent family is a chosen life-style that provides a free and open system for development of parents and children. In these families, decision making and communication are seen as joint commitments between parent and child, and the parent-child relationship is considered a major source of life fulfillment.

Blended family. The blended family includes stepparents and stepchildren. Separation, divorce, and remarriage are common phenomena in our society, in which approximately 40% of marriages end in divorce. Divorce and remarriage may occur at any time in the family life cycle and therefore will have different impacts on family function. Whatever the timing, effort is required to restabilize old family groups and consti-

tute and stabilize new family groups. This emotional work must be accomplished before family and individual development can proceed.

Homosexual family. Homosexual families are being recognized increasingly in Western society. Children in such families may be the offspring of previous heterosexual unions of the homosexual parent or be conceived by one member of a lesbian couple through artificial insemination. Lesbian couples have the same biologic and psychologic needs as do heterosexual couples. They seek quality care for themselves and their unborn and newborn child.

Implications for nursing. Insights gained from the structural-functional approach can help the nurse become aware of family relationships. First the nurse can recognize the family's *relationship to the larger social system*. Some families establish rigid boundaries, outsiders are kept at a distance, and input from the community is curtailed. Other families are isolated, and when crisis strikes, they often find their inner resources inadequate as coping mechanisms. A third group of families maintains open boundaries through work, school, or community involvement. Energy can flow in both directions, and assistance often is given and accepted.

Second, noting the *internal relationships* of the family may reveal sources of strength or weakness. Frequently the socially conceptualized roles, such as husband and wife, may not fit reality. Hence people establishing or attempting to maintain the so-called normal family roles often face frustration. The interplay of traditionally designed complementary roles may be a source of role conflict. In many families today the husband's and wife's roles are interchangeable; that is, the wife assumes some instrumental functions (earning an income) and the husband assumes some expressive functions (caring for an infant). The ability to negotiate such exchanges is necessary to maintain equilibrium.

Third, the nurse needs to be aware of the development of *reciprocal relationships* within a family that can stunt a person's growth. Some families mold a family member to act as scapegoat; others designate a member to be forever dependent. As an example of the latter, some mothers of teenage parents use the situation to perpetuate the mother-daughter dominance.

The major drawback of the structural-functional theory is that its rigid adherence to roles and associated tasks requires a constant updating of the tasks assigned. In addition, this approach tends to "freeze the family in time."

Developmental theory. The developmental theoretic approach to the study of the family incorporates ideas from a number of theoretic and conceptual approaches to the study of society and the individual (social systems approach, structural-functional approach, life cycle concepts of developmental needs and tasks, and concepts of interacting personalities). Familiar proponents of the life cycle concept are Duvall (1977) and Wright and Leahey (1984). The central theme in the developmental theory is noting "the changes in the process of internal development with the dimension of time as central" (Bower and Jacobson, 1978). The family is described as a *small group, semiclosed* system that engages in interactive behavior within the larger cultural social system. The significant unit in this theory is the *person* rather than the role. The family process is one of *interaction* over the *life cycle* of the family.

Family members pass through phases of growth, from dependence through active independence to ultimate decay. The family also demonstrates variations in structure and function over time. Together these constitute the *family life cycle*. Stages and tasks of the family life cycle adapted from the developmental category of the Calgary Family Assessment Model (CFAM) (Wright and Leahey, 1984) are given at right.

Implications for nursing. The developmental theory has provided many useful insights into family functioning. Knowledge of types of problems, identified during certain phases of the life cycle, can assist nurses in providing anticipatory guidance for families. For example, helping families prepare for changing family relationships as school-age children become adolescents may minimize the development of crisis situations.

Because the family as a group and the family as individuals are simultaneously engaged in developmental tasks (Duvall, 1977; Erikson, 1968), disharmony (dissonance) is possible if the developmental task of the family is not synchronous with the developmental task of the person. There are many examples of such dissonance. The adolescent father grappling with his need to break from his family ties is expected to establish monetary and other support for the new family he has created. The mother of the pregnant adolescent, a woman who is ready to move from family involvement in the care of her own children to community involvement, may resent having to assume responsibility for her daughter's child. As parents grow older, the original parent-child relationship may undergo role reversal. Some children find it difficult to accept their parents as dependent, and, conversely, some parents resent the "interference" of children in their affairs. Awareness of the implications of situations such as these can be useful in helping the family develop appropriate coping mechanisms.

The developmental approach presents a concept of family that is fluid and changing and thus more in tune with reality. It is less difficult to plot the phases of the

Stages and Tasks of Family Life Cycle

1. Marriage: the joining of families
   a. Establishment of couple identity
   b. Realignment of relationships with extended family
   c. Decisions about parenthood
2. Families with infants
   a. Integration of infants into family unit
   b. Accommodation of new parenting and grandparenting roles
   c. Maintenance of marital bond
3. Families with preschoolers
   a. Socialization of children
   b. Adjustment to separation by parents and children
4. Families with schoolchildren
   a. Development of peer relations by children
   b. Family adaptation to peers and school influences
5. Families with teenagers
   a. Development of increasing autonomy
   b. Refocus on midlife marital and career issues
   c. Beginning shift toward concern for older generation
6. Families as launching centers
   a. Establishment of independent identities
   b. Renegotiation of marital relationship
7. Middle-aged families
   a. Reinvestment in couple identity
   b. Realignment to include in-laws and grandchildren
   c. Dealing with disabilities of older generation
8. Aging families
   a. Shift to retirement
   b. Maintenance of couple and individual functioning

life cycle in the nuclear family than in an extended family. The extended family may involve many generations. Sometimes it is difficult to document the life cycle of a family; often we can only catch glimpses of it. It changes or disintegrates before we can grasp its significance.

Interactional theory. Burgess (1926) first postulated the idea that the family could be perceived within an interactional framework. Mead (1934) presented the first concepts; Hill and Hansen (1960), Rose (1962), and Stryker (1959) made later additions.

The major theme of the interactional theory, also known as action theory or role theory, conceives of the family as a *unit of interacting personalities,* not bound necessarily by legal or contractual agreements, that exists as long as the interaction is taking place. The significant unit is *the individual.* The family process is one of *role taking.* This process is dynamic: family members are constantly testing the concept they have of the role of another and adjusting their own self-concept. The process is accomplished through *symbolic communication,* and all family behaviors stem from family members' playing their many roles.

Implications for nursing. The interactional theory is

particularly useful as a basis for nurse-family interactions. It is broad enough and inclusive enough to encompass various insights into human nature. It transcends family configuration and cultural, ethnic, or social class boundaries of families, such as nuclear family or extended family, and emphasizes *communication* as a central process (Schvaneveldt, 1966). It helps the nurse understand the implications of family dynamics rather than always taking family actions at face value.

Family theories lend themselves to the systematic study of the family through research. Nurses also use the knowledge from family theories to assist in establishing working relationships with families. When nurses question "who is doing what work," they are using knowledge from the structural-functional theory. When they ask about the significance of events such as birth, children leaving home, or death, they are using family developmental approach. When they assess the effect the birth of a child may have on a husband-wife relationship, they are using interactional family theory.

Family and Crisis

No family exists in a nonstress environment. For the family system, stress can arise internally or externally. Although many families cope with stress, the situation may become acute and take on the characteristics of a crisis. Crisis may be defined as a disturbance of habit: a disruption in a family's or an individual's usual means of maintaining control over a situation. If faced with a crisis, the family or person attempts to resolve the crisis using customary values and behaviors.

One of the goals of crisis intervention is to help the client learn new ways of dealing with conflicts or problems. Although the client may seek help for a specific problem, the strategies learned may be applied to future difficulties. The crises families or people experience can be centered around maturational or situational events.

Maturational crisis. Maturational crises develop as a result of normal growth and development. They characteristically evolve over time and involve *role* and *status* changes. They include events such as birth, infancy, childhood, adolescence, adulthood, and old age. Each phase of the family life cycle produces characteristic crises or events capable of creating stress of such severity that it can affect the health of one or more family members.

The birth of a child represents one of the most important events in the life of a family. Births and the subsequent care of the children require parental, intellectual, and psychologic maturity, and this may account for periods of crisis in a family.

Nurses assist with the birth of children and can provide support as the adults undertake active parenting roles. Nurses can provide knowledge of human psychosocial development, which will help parents both to see their children realistically and to establish appropriate criteria for children's behavior. Nurses may use this unique relationship with a family to promote birth as a family-centered happening with great potential for growth for all participants.

Situational crisis. Situational crises include such events as preterm birth, mental or physical illness, loss of financial or social support, experience of violence, divorce, death, and grief. These crises involve a threat to a person's sense of integrity, or loss or deprivation of some kind. Anxiety or depression are characteristic responses. If the situational crisis causes severe strain, it can result in impairment of health.

Response to crisis. In both maturational and situational crises the family plays a critical role in the alleviation of distress, successful adaptation, and healthy rehabilitation. The nurse's knowledge of a family's reactions to crisis prompts a more rational assessment of the family's ability to withstand the stress. The nurse can help the family mobilize its problem-solving abilities to deal with the problem.

Aguilera and Messick (1986) have devised a stratagem for assessing a family's or an individual's potential or actual response to a crisis. They maintain that three key areas or components act as balancing factors affecting equilibrium: (1) the client's perception of the crisis event, (2) the client's coping mechanisms, and (3) the client's support system. The interplay between these three areas is critical for the outcome or resolution of a problem. A brief discussion of each of the three areas follows.

Perception of event. What one person considers a crisis may or may not be perceived as a crisis by someone else. A factor such as *age* and *prior experience* can alter perception. For example, an event viewed as a crisis by an adolescent may not be seen as a crisis by a 30-year-old adult. *Emotional states, anxiety,* or *hostility* may color a person's perception. The highly anxious young mother of a firstborn child may become disorganized by her infant's crying, whereas a mother of four may accept the crying as normal.

Nursing intervention relative to a client's perception of a crisis-provoking event may be limited to helping the client state "what the problem is." However, if the event can have a negative effect on the client, the infant, or the family, more intervention is required as indicated in the following example.

In some cultures pregnancy is seen as such a natural event that no medical or nursing supervision is considered necessary. As complications of pregnancy can arise with detrimental effects for mother and child the nurse would encourage the family to participate in ongoing health care. The nurse could act as nurturer, information giver, or organizer.

Coping mechanisms. Coping mechanisms can be defined as patterns of behavior that people or families have developed for dealing with threats to their sense of well-being (Stuart and Sundeen, 1983). Coping mechanisms may be constructive or destructive. *Constructive coping mechanisms* lead to a resolution of a problem. They vary with the level of anxiety being experienced. For mild anxiety the individual may resort to crying, sleeping, eating, exercise, or smoking and drinking. In interpersonal situations, avoiding eye contact or limiting close relationships to those who cause no anxiety may be successful.

If the threat and consequent level of anxiety become severe, people will resort to the use of task-oriented reactions, ego-oriented reactions or psychologic or physiologic conversions. Task-oriented behaviors are aimed at relieving the stress situations. They are consciously directed and have been objectively appraised by the person using them. Ego-oriented reactions are also known as ego-defense mechanisms. They include repression, projection, and displacement. These reactions protect the person from feelings of inadequacy and worthlessness. However, such responses can be used to the person's detriment. They can distort reality, interfere with interpersonal relationships, and limit working ability. If misused they become *destructive coping mechanisms.* Such habitual responses may be incorporated into the unconscious, and considerable effort may be required to bring such responses into conscious focus to enable the person to change or adapt them.

Psychologic or physiologic conversions are exaggerated or inappropriate coping mechanisms. Fear of crowds, of being alone and of being in closed spaces are examples of psychologic conversions. An individual who reacts to stress with hypertension and eventual damage to the cardiovascular system is using physiologic conversion.

Nurses use knowledge of human coping mechanisms to assess the type of defense mechanism the person or family uses and the success of the mechanism in ameliorating problems. Attempts are made to substitute more beneficial behaviors if the defense is recognized as destructive. However, coping mechanisms, whether constructive or destructive, appear to be essential for all individuals and groups if they are to maintain emotional stability.

Support systems. Support systems refer to the support that people may expect from others in their environment during a time of crisis. Caplan (1959), one of the developers of crisis intervention, maintains that the successful resolution of a crisis often depends on the client's support system. If a client's support system is strong, only minimal intervention may be necessary to resolve a crisis and help the client recover. If the client's support system is not strong, disorganization may occur and the client may not recover.

A client's support system may include family, friends, and significant others in the environment. Other people who function as part of support systems are health personnel, or "community caretakers" (Caplan, 1959). Community caretakers are people in the various agencies that represent the organized health resources of a community. These individuals are knowledgeable and experienced. They may be able to assist those who are unable to handle crises on their own or with the help of family and friends. The assistance may take the form of teaching or counseling, or it may involve helping the client learn the procedures for enlisting the aid of other community agencies.

Client education and support are now essential parts of all medical and nursing practice. Nurses have developed *parent education programs* to provide women and men with mechanisms for coping with the stress of labor. These programs also help parents learn about their infants' needs and about child-care activities, so that the parents are better able to cope with the changing needs of a growing child.

In addition to professionally led groups, *peer support groups* are now available to clients. Peer groups encourage interactions between people with similar problems. The groups promote interaction, encourage acceptance and support among members, and serve as a resource. Nurses and social workers have been leaders in originating such groups, in the hospital and in the community. They have worked with others in planning and establishing the groups.

Cultural Context of the Family

The relationship of cultural patterns to the childbearing process is a central concern in nursing. The reproductive beliefs and practices of a culture are embedded in its economic, religious, kinship, and political structures. Childbearing concepts focus on four components of a cultural system: (1) the moral and value system, (2) the kinship system, (3) the knowledge and belief system, and (4) the ceremonial and ritual system. Nurses are becoming increasingly aware of the need to focus on cultural variations in childbearing because of cultural pluralism in the United States and the rapid expansion of international nursing. Clients have a right to expect that their cultural needs relative to reproduction will be met, as well as their physiologic and psychologic needs. Newton (1972) suggested that health professionals distinguish between health practices based on necessity and those based on social custom. Those social customs that help to comfort or make more meaningful the events of pregnancy and birth need to be maintained and supported.

Definitions. *Culture* has many definitions. Spradley (1981) defines culture as the "acquired knowledge people use to interpret experience and generate behavior." Each cultural group passes this knowledge to its members from generation to generation. Cultural knowledge includes beliefs and values about each facet of life from birth to death. A person's worldview results from his or her cultural knowledge and provides rules for interaction with others, with nature, and with the supernatural (Powers, 1982). These rules have been tested over time and relate to food, language, religion, art, health and healing practices, kinship relationships, and all other systems of behavior.

Subculture refers to a group existing within a larger cultural system that retains its own characteristics; individuals identify themselves as members of the group. A subculture may be an ethnic group or a group organized in other ways. For example, there is a subculture of nursing and a subculture of medicine.

Each subculture has rich and complex traditions regarding health practices that have proven effective over time. These traditions vary from group to group. Furthermore, nurses must always recognize that a wide range of diversity may exist within a group. Assessment of the beliefs and practices of a group and those within the group is essential for the health care provider striving to plan culturally sensitive health care.

Acculturation refers to changes that take place in one or both groups when people from different cultures come in contact with one another. People may retain some of their own culture and also reformulate cultural elements. Acculturation is contrasted with *assimilation,* in which a cultural group loses its identity and becomes a part of the dominant culture. An example of acculturation would be the adoption of food practices of ethnic groups in the United States. The original recipe for pizza, which is of Italian origin, has been accepted and adapted by many other groups.

Ethnocentrism is "being centered in one's own ethnic or cultural system, judging the world in general by the standards established in that particular system" (Downs, 1971). Socialization into the profession of nursing occurs within the framework of the Western health-care system. This system emphasizes the biomedical model, which in the United States is based primarily on the white, middle-class value system. The biomedical model presents pregnancy and childbirth as

phenomena with inherent risks, most appropriately managed through specific knowledge and technology. The nurse encountering behavior in women incongruent with this model may become perplexed and label the women's behavior inappropriate and in conflict with good health practices. If the Western health-care system provides the only standards for judging, the behavior of the nurse is termed ethnocentric.

Cultural relativism, the opposite of ethnocentrism, involves learning about and applying the standards of another person's culture to activities within that culture. To be culturally relativistic means the nurse recognizes that people from different cultural backgrounds actually see the same objects and situations differently. There are reasons why people behave the way they do, and these reasons are for the most part culturally determined.

Cultural relativism does not require nurses to accept the beliefs and values of another culture; rather, nurses recognize that the behavior of others may be based on a system of logic different from their own. Cultural relativism is an affirmation of the uniqueness and value of every culture.

Childbearing in various cultures. Childbearing represents one facet of health that is related to all aspects of a woman's life. Although most cultures do not regard pregnancy or childbirth as illnesses, the conditions are considered times of heightened susceptibility to dangerous elements. Stern and coworkers (1980) noted that "pregnant women seek security measures and court benevolent gods with ritualized behavior, whether anointing their abdomens with herbal oils in an African village or practicing daily yoga in California." Perception of the time of greatest vulnerability varies among cultures, with some groups placing greatest emphasis on the prenatal stage and others on labor and delivery or the puerperium. Western health care culture places the greatest emphasis on the prenatal and labor and delivery stages and least on the postpartum stage.

Childbearing in all cultures is complete with norms and behavioral expectations for each stage of the perinatal cycle. All relate to each culture's view of how a person maintains health and prevents illness. Health practices reflect theories of balance and harmony among opposing forces. The intrinsic factors influencing balance and harmony include heat and cold. The extrinsic factors include air and water, food and drink, sleep and wakefulness, movement, exercise and rest, evacuation and retention, and passions of the spirits, or emotions. Thus for pregnant women of many cultures, maintenance of health during childbearing implies a balance and harmony in each woman's relationship to her physical, social, and spiritual environment.

The American family. American culture is focused around a nuclear family that includes married parents and children. Extended family relationships are recognized as existing, but their influence varies. Each nuclear family is considered a self-sufficient unit and ultimately responsible for its own functioning, especially child rearing.

Children in the American family are desirable, but parents do not define themselves in terms of being parents only. If a couple cannot or chooses not to have children, they are accepted as being whole people and not incomplete in some way. Value is also placed on delaying the arrival of the first child until the married couple has adjusted to each other and until they are financially able to support a family. The desirable number of children in the American family is small, usually two or three.

Infants are immediately accepted as members of the society into which they are born. Children are regarded as individuals with certain rights. They are not considered miniature adults, and they are allowed to engage in some behaviors that do not necessarily prepare them for adulthood, play is valued for its own sake. On the other hand, early independence is encouraged.

Parents are the primary disciplinarians, and in the nuclear family they retain this function during the entire childhood. Parents may resent interference by others in the discipline of their child, even if the other person is a grandparent, aunt, or uncle. Discipline exists in the school system, but it is seen as a temporary extension of the parents' rights to discipline.

Parents are the major caretakers, with the mother assuming primary responsibility. Johnston (1980) points out that in the United States, parenting is not necessarily seen as intrinsically rewarding and enjoyable, but rather as a series of difficult, hygienic, and unrewarding activities. Children are enjoyed only when parental activities result in a child who gains weight, learns to walk and talk, or is toilet trained. Although recently father and mother are sharing more responsibility for care, in early infancy the father is often working and the mother remains at home to care for the infant. Other caretakers are used, but they are usually not kin. They may be baby-sitters or day-care workers. These caretakers are paid for their services, usually by the hour.

Cultural variations. Differences between the dominant culture of the United States and other cultures in general are reflected in how the roles of parents are expressed and how children are viewed. In contrast to the dominant American value system, some cultures regard becoming a parent as the major way individuals define themselves as whole persons. Mormons believe the highest place in heaven can be reached only through marriage and childbearing. The greater the number of children, the higher the place in heaven (Stark, 1982). The Navajo woman's role is defined to a large extent in reproductive terms (Wright, 1982). For many blacks, pregnancy is necessary for a man and woman to be seen as whole persons (Carrington, 1978). Puerto Rican couples have their first child as soon as possible to indicate to themselves and the community that the husband is virile and the woman fertile (Murillo-Rohde, 1978). Among the Gadsup (Leininger, 1979) a woman becomes a woman and a man a man when each is married and has at least one child. For Mexican-Americans, childbearing is a privilege and an obligation of married women, and they are encouraged to have children as often as they can (Enriquez, 1982). Thus, in many cultural groups parenthood is an ascribed status, and women have no social role without a family.

The importance of children within the family is part of the value system of many traditional cultures. Children are expected to contribute to the economic well-being of the family and to support the parents in their old age. They are regarded as "carriers of the culture." A family without children is abnormal, and a woman's failure to bear children is accepted as grounds for dissolution of a marriage.

Summary

The family represents a primary social group that influences and is influenced by other people and institutions. Regardless of the form it assumes or the society in which it is found, the family possesses enduring characteristics that have far-reaching personal and societal effects. According to Blehar (1979):

Despite disagreement about the state of the family and its definition, a consensus might be reached on three points: (1) the family is currently in a state of flux precipitated by economic and social pressures; (2) imperfect though it may be, it is difficult to imagine substituting an alternative that could perform all its functions as well; and (3) it is more desirable to bolster families than to attempt to supplant them with untried structures.

References

Aguilera, D.C., and Messick, J.M.: Crisis intervention: theory and methodology, ed. 4, St. Louis, 1986, The C.V. Mosby Co.

Blehar, M.C.: Families and public policy. In Corfman, E., editor: Families today, vol. 2, National Institute of Mental Health, Division of Scientific and Public Information, Science Monograph No. 1, Washington, D.C., 1979, U.S. Government Printing Office.

Bower, F., and Jacobson, M.: Family theories: frameworks for nursing practice. In Archer, S., and Fleshman, R., editors: Community health nursing: patterns and practice, N. Scituate, Mass., 1978, Duxbury Press.

Burgess, E.W.: The family as a unit of interacting personalities, Family 7:3, March, 1926.

Caplan, G.: Concepts of mental health and consultation, Children's Bureau, U.S. Department of Health, Education and Welfare, Washington, D.C., 1959, U.S. Government Printing Office.

Carrington, B.W.: The Afro-American. In Clark, A.L., editor: Culture/childbearing/health professionals, Philadelphia, 1978, F.A. Davis Co.

Downs, J.F.: Cultures in crisis, Beverly Hills, Calif., 1971, Glencoe Press.

Duvall, E.R.: Marriage and family development, ed. 5, Philadelphia, 1977, J.B. Lippincott Co.

Enriquez, M.G.: Studying maternal-infant attachment: a Mexican-American example. In Kay, M.A., editor: Anthropology of human birth, Philadelphia, 1982, F.A. Davis Co.

Erikson, E.H.: Identity: youth and crisis, New York, 1968, W.W. Norton & Co., Inc., Publishers.

Friedman, M.M.: Family nursing theory and assessment, New York, 1981, Appleton-Century-Crofts.

Harris, M.: America now: the anthropology of a changing culture, New York, 1982, Simon & Schuster.

Helvie, C.: Community health nursing: theory and process, New York, 1981, Harper & Row.

Hetherington, E.M., Cox, M., and Cox, R.: Beyond father absence: conceptualizations of the effects of divorce. In Hetherington, E.M., and Parke, R., editors: Contemporary readings in child psychology, New York, 1977, McGraw-Hill Book Co.

Hills, R., and Hansen, D.: The identification of conceptual frameworks used in family study, Marriage Fam. Living 22:311, 1960.

Johnston, M.: Cultural variations in professional and parenting patterns, J.O.G.N. Nurs. 9:9, 1980.

Lang, R.: Birth book, Ben Lomond, Calif., 1972, Genesis Press.

Leininger, M.: The Gadsup of New Guinea and early childcaring behaviors with nursing implications. In Leininger, M., editor: Transcultural nursing '79, New York, 1979, Masson Publishing U.S.A., Inc.

Malinowski, B.: The dynamics of cultural change, New Haven, Conn. 1945, Yale University Press.

McLanahan, S.S., Wedemeyer, N.V., and Adelberg, T.: Network structure, social support, and psychological well-being in the single-parent family, J. Marriage Fam. 43:601, Aug., 1981.

Mead, G.H.: Mind, self and society, Chicago, 1934, The University of Chicago Press.

Murillo-Rohde, I.: The Puerto Rican: Part II. In Clark, A., editor: Culture/childbearing/health professionals, Philadelphia, 1978, F.A. Davis Co.

National Center for Health Statistics: Annual summary of births, deaths and marriages and divorces, Monthly Vital Statistics Report 31(13), 1985.

Newton, M.: Cross-cultural perspectives. In Clark, A., and Alfonso, D., editors: Childbearing, a nursing perspective, Philadelphia, 1980, F.A. Davis Co.

Newton, N.: Childbearing in broad perspective: pregnancy, birth and the newborn baby, Boston, 1972, Delacorte Press.

Norton, A., and Glick, P.: One parent families: a social and economic profile, Family Relations 35(1):9, 1986.

Powers, B.A.: The use of orthodox and Black-American folk medicine, Adv. Nurs. Sci. 4:35, 1982.

Radcliffe-Brown, A.: Structure and function in a primitive society, New York, 1952, The Free Press.

Rose, A.: Human behaviors and social processes: an interactional approach, Boston, 1962, Houghton Mifflin Co.

Schvaneveldt, J.: The international framework in the study of the family. In Nye, F.A., and Bernardo, F.M., editors: Emerging conceptual frameworks in family analysis, New York, 1966, Macmillan Publishing Co.

Spradley, B.W.: Community health nursing, Boston, 1981, Little, Brown & Co.

Stark, S.: Mormon childbearing. In Kay, M.A., editor: Anthropology of human birth, Philadelphia, 1982, F.A. Davis Co.

Stern, P.N., and others: Culturally-induced stress during childbearing: the Filipino-American experience, Issues Health Care Women 2(3-4):67, 1980.

Stryker, S.: Symbolic interaction as an approach to family research, Marriage Fam. Living 21:111, May, 1959.

Stuart, G.W., and Sundeen, S.J.: Principles and practice of psychiatric nursing, ed. 2, St. Louis, 1983, The C.V. Mosby Co.

United Nations: Principles and recommendations for the 1970 population census, New York, 1969.

U.S. Bureau of the Census: Household and family characteristics, Population Reports Series P-20, No. 398, Washington, D.C., March, 1984, U.S. Government Printing Office.

U.S. Bureau of the Census: Marital status and living arrangements, Current Population Reports Series P-20, No. 365, Washington, D.C. Oct. 1981, U.S. Government Printing Office.

U.S. Bureau of the Census: Money income and poverty status of families and persons, Current Population Reports Series P-60, No. 146, Washington, D.C., 1983, U.S. Government Printing Office.

U.S. National Center for Health Statistics, U.S. Bureau of the Census, U.S. Department of Commerce, Washington, D.C., 1982, The Center.

Wright, A.: Attitudes toward childbearing and menstruation among the Navajo. In Kay, M.A., editor: Anthropology of human birth, Philadelphia, 1982, F.A. Davis Co.

Wright, L.M., and Leahey, M.: Nurses and families: a guide to family assessment and intervention, Philadelphia, 1984, F.A. Davis Co.

World Health Organization: Health and the family: studies in the demography of family life cycles and their health implication, Geneva, 1978, The Organization.

Bibliography

Affonso, D.D.: The Filipino American. In Clark, A.L., editor: Culture/childbearing/health professionals, Philadelphia, 1978, F.A. Davis Co.

Campbell, T., and Chang, B.: Health care of the Chinese in America, Nurs. Outlook 21:245, 1973.

Carrington, B.W.: The Afro-American. In Clark, A.L., editor: Culture/childbearing/health professionals, Philadelphia, 1978, F.A. Davis Co.

Chao, Y.: The family in Taiwan, School of Nursing, University of California, San Francisco.

Chung, J.J.: Understanding the Oriental maternity patient, Nurs. Clin. North Am. 12:67, 1977.

Clark, A.L., and Howland, I.H.: The American Samoan. In Clark, A.L., editor: Culture/childbearing/health professionals, Philadelphia, 1978, F.A. Davis Co.

Clark, M.: Health in the Mexican-American culture: a community study, Berkeley, 1970, University of California Press.

Cosminsky, S.: Knowledge and body concepts of Guatemalan midwives. In Kay, M.A., editor: Anthropology of human birth, Philadelphia, 1982, F.A. Davis Co.

Coughlin, R.: Pregnancy and birth in Vietnam. In Hart, D., and others, editors: Southeast Asian birth customs: three studies in human reproduction, New Haven, Conn., 1965, Human Relations Area Files.

Currier, R.L.: The hot-cold syndrome and symbolic balance in Mexican and Spanish-American folk medicine. In Martinez, R.A., editor: Hispanic culture and health care: fact, fiction, folklore, St. Louis, 1978, The C.V. Mosby Co.

Doherty, W.: Family interventions in health care. Family Relations 34(1):129, 1985.

Griffith, S.: Childbearing and the concept of culture, J.O.G.N. Nurs. 11:181, 1982.

Grosso, C., and others: The Vietnamese American Family . . . and grandma makes three, M.C.N. 6:177, 1981.

Hollingsworth, A.O., and others: The refugees and childbearing: what to expect, RN 43:45, 1980.

Horn, B.M.: Northwest coast Indians: the Muckleshoot. In Kay, M.A., editor: Anthropology of human birth, Philadelphia, 1982, F.A. Davis Co.

Kay, M.A., editor: Anthropology of human birth, Philadelphia, 1982, F.A. Davis Co.

Kendall, K.: Maternal and child care in an Iranian village. In Leininger, M., editor: Transcultural nursing '79, New York, 1979, Masson Publishing U.S.A.

Leininger, M.: Cultural diversities of health and nursing care, Nurs. Clin. North Am. 12:5, 1977.

McCay, E.: Childhood through the ages, Parents, New York, 1981, Raines & Raines.

McGoldrick, M.: Normal families: an ethnic perspective. In Walsh, F., editor: Normal family processes, New York, 1982, The Guilford Press.

Meleis, A.I., and Sorrell, L.: Bridging cultures: Arab American women and their birth experiences, M.C.N. 6:171, 1981.

Monroe, P., Garand, J., and Price, S.: Family health plan choices: the health maintenance organization option, Family Relations, 34(1):71, 1985.

Orque, M.S., and others: Ethnic nursing care: a multicultural approach, St. Louis, 1983, The C.V. Mosby Co.

Perry, D.S.: The umbilical cord: transcultural care and customs, J. Nurse Midwife 27(4):25, 1982.

Pillsbury, B.L.K.: "Doing the month": confinement and convalescence of Chinese women after childbirth, Soc. Sci. Med. 12:11, 1978.

The Single Parent Family, Special issue of Family Relations, Family Relations 35:1, Jan., 1982.

Zepeda, M.: Selected maternal infant care practices of Spanish-speaking women, J.O.G.N. Nurs. 11:371, 1982.

Maternity Client, Maternity Nurse, and the Nursing Process

Birth rituals vary widely throughout the world (Aamodt, 1978). In some cultures the birth ritual separates the mother from her infant; in other cultures, family and friends share in the process. In some cases the father is excluded from the birth; in other cases he plays an intimate role. In societies such as those in North America the cosmopolitan makeup of peoples and changing life-styles produce considerable variety in role expectations and procedures, even within the small community. This chapter is intended to help a nurse provide maternity care to many different kinds of people. The chapter discusses the maternity client, the maternity nurse with a range of competence and roles, and the nursing process. The four models of helping and coping and the teaching-learning process enhance the nurse's skill in caring for maternity clients and their families through the nursing process.

Maternity Client

Motivation. Although reproduction is almost entirely a function of human sexuality, each person involved may perceive its components—intercourse, pregnancy, birth, and parenthood—separately, and endow each with a special meaning. The meaning attached to any one component can profoundly affect the outcome of the total process for woman, man, and child.

Intercourse. Both men and women may use intercourse or related sexual acts in a variety of ways. In a positive sense, it expresses tenderness and love, assuages loneliness, and provides physical relief of sexual tension; in a negative sense, it becomes a weapon to belittle or demean a partner through refusal, giving grudgingly of oneself, or taking another by force (rape). Some people have intercourse to demonstrate their sexual desirability to a peer group, hoping to enhance their social acceptance. It may form part of the

experimenting process in moving toward adult sexuality. Increases in premarital intercourse and the less conventional practice of sharing partners appears to testify to the complex meaning that can be attached to the biologic act of intercourse.

Pregnancy can result from vaginal intercourse, regardless of either partner's purpose. A pregnancy may or may not be wanted or accepted. Being accountable and responsible for the consequences of the sexual act demonstrate one facet of adulthood in the sexual sense.

Pregnancy. Pregnancy may represent a period of great creativity for a woman. She becomes aware of feelings and sensations she never knew before. She may feel a sense of fulfillment. She may see pregnancy as making her a complete woman. For most women the close relationship of mother and fetus is felt deeply.

Birth. The birth of a child often unifies a family. Many partners insist on sharing this important event by actively participating in the pregnancy and labor. For some people the sharing extends beyond the immediate participants; other family members, friends, and community members are included.

Parenthood. Parenthood, beginning as it does with the excitement of pregnancy and birth, can serve many human purposes. To some it is a life-fulfilling state, a chance to help their children become the adults of the future. Children born to such parents are wanted children, whose dependency is recognized and accepted. The children's achievements bring much pleasure to their parents, their failures are also accepted, and love and support are forthcoming.

Some parents want children primarily for their own satisfaction. Such parents will expect their children to support the parents' self-concepts and need for love, acceptance, and success. But a young child is unable to live up to such expectations, so disappointment and frustration soon follow. Consequently the child may become a victim of neglect or even abuse.

Other children are born as a result of their parents' sexuality, but the resultant parenthood is neither planned nor desired. These children may suffer parental and material deprivation. Edwards (1973) contends that one of the greatest needs such children have is parents who have learned the art of "gentle socialization of children," of creating a nurturing environment peopled with interested, concerned, and loving adults.

Unlike other manifestations of human sexuality, parenthood can be both a biologic and psychologic entity, or it can be entirely psychologic as in adoption. After a child is born, the parent by substitution or adoption can fulfill this socially and personally important role. These parents need the same preparation and support as biologic parents.

Statistical picture and definitions. Potentially all sexually mature people are candidates for reproductive care. They come from all racial, ethnic, economic, and social groups. Approximately 70% are white, and 30% are nonwhite. They or their forebears were native-born Indians or Eskimos or came to this continent mainly from Europe, Africa, or Asia. Their age groups will vary from fetus and neonate, to the adolescent, to the young adult, and to individuals approaching middle age. Many, both men and women, will seek assistance concerning methods of contraception. Approximately 15% of all couples of childbearing age will seek help for infertility problems.

Approximately 3.9 million women, ranging in age from 12 to 52 years, give birth each year. Some of them will have the support of family, husbands, parents, children, and friends. Others will be alone. Some will be overjoyed by their pregnancies; others will be angry, defensive, or apathetic about their state. Most will be physically healthy; others, at least 500,000 a year, will be designated at *high risk* for either maternal, fetal, or familial reasons. Some of this latter group, through ignorance of American concepts of health care, will not seek medical attention until their or their infant's life is threatened.

The *fertility rate* is the number of births per 1,000 women between the ages of 15 and 44 years (inclusive) calculated on a yearly basis. It is a more accurate means of comparing different population groups than the birthrate. The U.S. National Center for Health Statistics (1982) noted the fertility rate in 1980 was 68.4 births per 1,000 women of childbearing age. The fertility rate among American women rose by 2% in 1980 to its highest level in 7 years but probably declined 1% in 1981.

The *birthrate,* the number of live births per 1,000 population, was 15.9 babies per 1,000 persons in 1980. It rose by 2% overall in 1980 and probably held steady in 1981. The largest increase in the birthrate

was among women age 30 to 34. More than 115,000 births in 1979 were to mothers in their thirties having their first child. This is 70% more than in 1975 (67,578 births) and more than twice as many as in 1970 (54,108 births). From 1974 to 1978, 9.5% of older women were having their first child; by 1982, 14.7% were first-time mothers (*USA Today,* Jan. 4, 1986).

A total of 665,747 babies, or 18.4% of those born in 1980, were born to unwed women. This was an increase of 11.4% from the previous year, although new methods of calculation accounted for a third of the increase. If the method had not changed, the 1980 rate would have been 645,000 births, up 7.9% from 1979. The increase in the rate of childbearing among unmarried women was attributed to "the substantial rise in the rate for unmarried white women," which rose by 18.1%, while the rate for unwed black women fell slightly.

The sharpest rise in births to unmarried women occurred in the 20- to 24-year-old age range, while the rate declined slightly for 15- to 19-year-old women. Although 9.4% of all white births, compared to 55% of all black births, were to unmarried women, the actual *increase* in out-of-wedlock births was 5% higher for white births.

Infant mortality is the yearly ratio of the number of deaths of infants before their first birthday per 1,000 live births. The mortality rate nationwide is currently 10.6 deaths per 1,000 live births, down by almost half from 1970.

Maternal mortality shows the number of maternal deaths per 100,000 live births. A *maternal death* is the death of a woman from *any* cause during pregnancy or within 42 days of the termination of pregnancy, regardless of the duration or site of the pregnancy. Maternal mortality has shown a remarkable decline. In 1930, 700 deaths occurred per 100,000 live births; in 1982 the rate was 7.9 per 100,000 live births. The mortality rate for women over 35 has also declined. In the years 1974 through 1978 there were 47.5 deaths per 100,000 live births to women over 35 years; in 1982 the rate was down to 24.2. The mortality rates included deaths from abortions.

A combination of factors stimulated this decline (WHO, 1976a; WHO, 1976b; WHO, 1977): availability of antimicrobial drugs for controlling infections, availability of blood and blood substitutes for treatment of hemorrhage, and formation of hospital and community committees to investigate causes and circumstances of each maternal death and to assign responsibility. In the over 35 category researchers suggested that the decline could be attributed to the higher socioeconomic status of such women having babies in recent years (*San Francisco Chronicle,* Jan. 2, 1986). The drop in maternal mortality also reflects the decrease in maternal deaths from abortion as states legalized the abortion procedure and safer techniques were employed.

Despite these efforts, mortality rates, both infant and maternal, for different segments of the population and different socioeconomic groups still show inequities (Naeye, 1979; Brook, 1980). Differences remain between white and nonwhite maternal mortality; the young and poor of any racial group also are vulnerable to maternity complications and maternal death. Many women still do not receive adequate prenatal care, and many women categorized as high risk are still without specialized treatment. Only 61.6% of black women and 79.1% of white women were receiving prenatal care during the first trimester. Almost 20% of women under the age of 15 years received no prenatal care or delayed prenatal care. This delay in prenatal care and the large number of black low-birth-weight infants may have resulted in the finding that black infants were twice as likely to receive low Apgar scores at 1 minute and 5 minutes as white infants. The percentage of black low-birth-weight infants was twice as high as the percentage of white low-birth-weight infants.

Infant neonatal mortality has been a traditional indicator of environmental influences. In the 1960s, professionals, local communities, and state and federal agencies identified factors that cause a higher mortality for the poor and designed programs to combat the problems. The major contributing factor to a higher mortality for the poor was *inadequate nutrition.* A second factor was the *lack of prenatal care* because the poor did not realize the importance of early and continuous prenatal care, they could not afford care, private providers limited or excluded them from their practice, and impersonal treatment was delivered in overcrowded public clinics (Slatin, 1971; Sprague and Taylor, 1979).

A third factor is related to the *availability of contraceptive techniques.* Contraceptive techniques are preventing many unwanted pregnancies; however, a large number of people are still not reached (Barnes, 1978). More than 3.5 million low- and marginal-income women and almost 2.5 million sexually active adolescents still lack family planning services. Even among married couples some births continue to be unwanted and mistimed.

More equal distribution and use of health resources among all citizens will be necessary to effect a beneficial change in maternal and child mortality and morbidity.

Human responses. Maternity clients and their families face biologic or psychologic events that center on reproductive processes. These events elicit human responses that cluster around the tasks of decision making, adaptation, or participation in a critical life event. Underlying these tasks is the theme of perceived locus of control or power.

Decision making. The Patient's Bill of Rights* takes a firm position on the right of each person to be informed. Each client is entitled to information that covers every facet of his or her health needs, proposed care, anticipated outcome, and available alternatives. This right to know forms the legal basis of informed consent (Chapter 3). Holistic health concepts place emphasis on education and self-care rather than on dependence. Possession of information closes the competence gap between the client and the health care provider. Collaboration between care provider and recipient assumes "that individuals have the *capability to make decisions* about their health and that they ultimately have *control of their own health* by virtue of the choices they make" (Fogel and Woods, 1981).

Both client and nurse bring to the interaction a highly personal definition of health. In a collaborative relationship, "information is freely exchanged with clients and informed decision-making is ideally the client's domain." The nurse, in conjunction with the client, identifies the health care practices the client currently engages in. The nurse and client collaborate to identify the client's assets and deficits. A nursing diagnosis is formulated. Finally, the nurse *and* the client set the goals of care before the nursing care is implemented. In the absence of collaboration, knowledge deficits, noncompliance, ineffective individual or family coping, or other concerns may arise.

Adaptation. The response of a woman and her family to the biologic reality of pregnancy is both physiologic and psychologic and can be adaptive or maladaptive. The physiologic processes involved are the adaptation of the newborn to extrauterine existence and the adaptation of both organisms to preexisting or presently existing physical and genetic insult. Psychologically the assumption of parental roles may overtax the coping mechanisms that each parent believed he or she developed. Anxiety about the ability to master new tasks, behaviors, attitudes, and sentiments inherent in the role may precipitate a crisis.

Without a nurturing environment there is potential for alterations in family processes or parenting or in health maintenance or for disturbance of self-concept. Anxiety and fear can result from lack of psychologic

---

*The Patient's Bill of Rights must be posted in a prominent place in each hospital. Many hospitals include it in the packet of information given to each person admitted.

preparation. Properly timed teaching is a nursing care skill that can provide psychologic preparation and facilitate adaptation.

Participation. Generally every person, regardless of level of income or social esteem, wishes to function in the best possible manner when confronted with a life event that has great personal implications. Many factors determine a person's ability to participate wholeheartedly in situations causing growth, joy, and pleasure to the self and others and, conversely, to face pain, separation, disability, or death adequately and well. Factors that influence a person's ability to cope with maturational and situational events include (1) the feelings a person has about his or her ability to maintain control, (2) the sharing of these critical life events with those who care, and (3) the nurturing provided by others in the environment.

Locus of control. Powerlessness can be experienced by anyone, of any age, educational background, profession, or marital status. Powerlessness is defined as a state in which a person *perceives* a loss of or a lack of personal control. The maternity client may feel powerless related to being pregnant. She may rejoice in the pregnancy but feel powerless relative to the events surrounding the child's birth. A sense of powerlessness can arise from many sources (Johnson, 1967; Beck, 1982), such as lack of knowledge about available resources or choices, cultural or social limitations, or alterations in plans for meeting personal goals. Responses to perceived powerlessness vary and may include apathy, anxiety, anger, or depression.

While a person feels powerless, positive adaptation and readiness to learn is impaired. However, a person with internal locus of control feels she can affect outcome. She is freer to participate in decision making, learning, or in manipulating herself or her environment. Nurses can help people increase their control by providing information and by helping them learn how to solve problems. Sharing the pregnancy, labor, and delivery with people who care can contribute to a sense of control. Nurturing provided by others—nurses, physicians, family, friends—can help a woman gain internal locus of control.

Maternity Nurse

Maternity nurses are in a unique position to effect change in the care women receive during their childbearing years. Maternity nurses have early, frequent, and continuing contact with the gravida and her family. The maternity nurse acts in a variety of roles to bring comprehensive health care to people during the childbearing years. As *clinicians,* nurses act as teachers, counselors, technicians, advocates, managers, and researchers. The degree to which nurses fulfill these roles depends on their level of competence.

Development of competence. People solve problems in a number of ways, depending on the situation and their knowledge and experience. Benner's work (1983, 1984) describes how a body of practical knowledge is developed as the nurse acquires expertise. Implementation of the nursing process may be accomplished on several levels, depending on the practitioner's competence. Benner (1984) identifies the following five levels.

Novice. Novices are beginners who have no experience in the nursing care of the woman (family) during the childbearing years. They may feel intimidated and be unable to see what nursing care they can provide. Benner (1984) states that novices "have little understanding of the contextual meaning of the recently learned textbook terms" (p. 21). The novice begins by learning rules for guiding practice. Yet even on the first day, unable to answer questions or determine the next course of action, the student has several years' experience in communicating with people, expressing concern, providing comfort, and seeking assistance. The presence of a caring human being is in itself valuable during a trying time.

Nursing students are not the only novices. The nurse who is new to a clinical area of practice or who is returning to nursing may also fall into this category. Highly competent practitioners in their first teaching experience are novice instructors.

Advanced beginner. Once students have had some experience with clients under the guidance of instructors and preceptors, they can begin to synthesize clinical findings. This synthesis, rather than rules alone, provides the basis to guide nursing actions.

Competent nurse. Nurses who have had experience working full time are able to more quickly establish priorities of need among their clients. Their organizational ability enables them to detect subtle cues in client behavior. These nurses have a feeling of mastery over situations likely to arise and can impart this feeling to clients and their families.

Proficient nurse. Nurses with many years of experience can pick out the key components of a situation. They grasp the heart of the matter and can move forward and backward to focus on providing holistic care. Benner (1984) describes the proficient nurse as one who "learns from experience what typical events to expect in a given situation and how plans need to be modified in response to these events" (p. 28).

Expert nurse. Benner (1984) describes the expert nurse as one who "with an enormous background of experience, now has an intuitive grasp of each situation and zeroes in on the accurate region of the problem without wasteful consideration of a large range of unfruitful, alternative diagnoses and solutions" (p. 32).

Teacher and counselor. Maternity nursing emphasizes the preventive aspects of health care. Much of this is accomplished through teaching and counseling clients. As a teacher or counselor the nurse tries to help clients learn how to make the best possible health care decisions for themselves or their children. The nurse provides a nonjudgmental environment in which these decisions can take place and helps clients evaluate their efforts realistically. The nurse acts as a role model for the technical care of clients or their infants. With supportive teaching the nurse can help even the most anxious or uninformed client learn to provide safe care.

Technician. Technical skills are required for every stage of the nursing process. Such skills help nurses assess health status, create a safe, comfortable environment for clients and others, initiate therapeutic nursing actions, and efficiently use time, energy, and materials. The nursing profession has developed standards for nursing practice that provide criteria for evaluating the degree of competence a nurse has attained. A competent nurse inspires confidence in clients. This confidence is an important part of the supportive care clients require. This concept is illustrated by an excerpt from a letter written by the husband of a woman, 8 months pregnant, who was admitted to the hospital with a massive vaginal hemorrhage:

> We would like to thank all those who helped my wife and myself during this difficult time. . . . The nurses were particularly helpful. They were skilled in the emergency care they gave my wife and at all times were kind to her and to myself. We felt we were in safe hands. It was very reassuring.

Advocate. As health care becomes more complex, someone must act as liaison or advocate between the client and other personnel or health agencies. The maternity nurse encourages clients to become aware of their health care rights and responsibilities. The nurse is committed to a holistic view of health care and therefore often knows more about clients than do other health workers. The nurse is in a position to explain, interpret, defend, or protect clients' rights. As an advocate the nurse attempts to modify health services on a local or national level so they reflect a humanitarian approach to health care. Therefore participation in professional organizations and politics (such as health-related legislation) is an important feature of nursing's commitment to ensuring health care for all (Archer and Goehner, 1982; Wilson, 1981).

Manager. Nurse managers coordinate and facilitate the many services required in the health care of clients

(Etheredge, 1985). Team leaders or charge nurses are examples of nurse managers since they direct the care of groups of clients and nursing personnel. They need to be knowledgeable about client care and able to communicate effectively with various types of health workers.

Researcher. Research has had an invaluable effect on shaping nursing practice and developing ideas for further inquiry that will keep our future practice alive. All nurses have the responsibility of adding knowledge through descriptive studies, the validation of knowledge using research design, and publication of results in professional literature. The idea of scientific research in nursing is as old as Florence Nightingale. She admonished nurses to develop the habit of systematically making and recording correct observations and then contemplating their meaning. Observations should not be for curious facts but rather as the only means for discovering and verifying knowledge useful for saving lives. Nurses need to evaluate the effectiveness of establishing methods of clinical nursing by measuring the outcomes in the health status of clients. Current research findings need to be evaluated for relevance to practice. Modification of practice needs to be based on scientific data to ensure quality care.

Expanding roles. The increasing health care needs of the public have necessitated an expansion in the responsibilities nurses have assumed and resulted in the development of new nursing roles (Arbeiter, 1984; Lewis, 1984; Bibb, 1979).

Such roles as obstetric-gynecologic nurse practitioner and nurse-midwife illustrate two of the more visible changes in the expanding responsibilities of nurses. These roles present practice options for a nurse's professional and personal growth.

Obstetric-gynecologic nurse practitioner. In 1979 the American College of Obstetrics and Gynecology (ACOG) and the Nurses' Association of the American College of Obstetrics and Gynecology (NAACOG) jointly defined the obstetric-gynecologic nurse practitioner as follows:

> A registered nurse who has satisfactorily completed a formal and accredited Obstetric-Gynecologic Nurse Practitioner educational program. The Obstetric-Gynecologic Nurse Practitioner will thus have been provided with special knowledge and skills in health maintenance, disease prevention, psychosocial and physical assessment, and management of health-illness needs in the primary care of women. This care is predominantly provided in an ambulatory setting. The Obstetric-Gynecologic Nurse Practitioner will provide such care interdependently with the physician and other members of the health care team.

In 1981 the NAACOG Certification Cooperation (NCC) instituted a certification program for the in-

Fig. 2.1
Obstetric-gynecologic nurse practitioner helps a husband listen to the fetal heartbeat during a prenatal examination. (Courtesy Stanford University Hospital.)

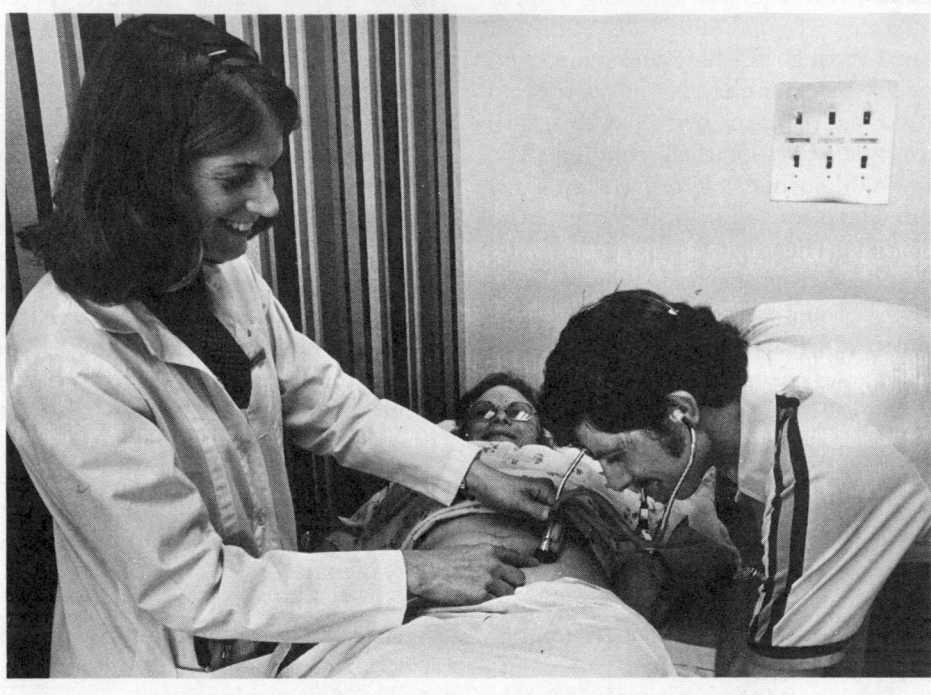

hospital obstetric nurse and for the obstetric-gynecologic nurse practitioner (Nurses' Association of the American College of Obstetrics and Gynecology, 1982). This program requires a candidate to meet eligibility criteria based on educational or practice requirements and to successfully complete a 200-item multiple choice examination. Nurses who achieve certification are entitled to use RNC (registered nurse certified) after their name. Beginning with the 1983 examination, all nurses taking the examination for the obstetric-gynecologic nurse practitioner certification are required to be graduates from a nurse-practitioner program acceptable to the NCC (Fig. 2.1). Also, since 1983 a neonatal nurse clinician/practitioner certification examination has been offered.

Starting in 1986 the two primary certifying agencies, the American Nurses' Association (ANA) and the National Association of Pediatric Nurse Associates and Practitioners, will require a minimum of a baccalaureate degree to become a nurse practitioner; by 1990 a master's degree probably will be required (Waters and Arbeiter, 1985).

Nurse-midwife. Certified nurse-midwives are registered nurses who have additional knowledge and skill gained through an organized program of study and clinical experience recognized by the American College of Nurse Midwives (ACNM). Certification for entry into practice includes successful passage of a 6-hour essay examination and meeting other ACNM criteria. If certified as a nurse-midwife, participants may use the designation CNM after their names. They can perform tasks and care for the client in the same way as obstetric-gynecologic nurse practitioners. The primary focus of the CNM is in the area of management and care of mothers and babies throughout the maternity cycle (including delivery), so long as maternal progress meets criteria accepted as normal. The nurse-midwife is prepared to teach, interpret, and provide support as an integral part of services (Haire, 1981; Burst, 1980; Beebe, 1980; Olsen, 1979; Roush, 1979).

The issue of who should deliver the low-risk client does not arise out of clients' nonacceptance of the nurse-midwife or because of questionable competency but rather because legislative controls limit the practice. Some states have not yet changed their laws or codes to legitimize the nurse-midwife's practice and third-party payers such as Blue Cross do not cover the services.

In 1970 the ACOG, the NAACOG, and the ACNM issued a joint statement that in "medically directed teams, qualified nurse-midwives may assume responsibility for the complete care and management of uncomplicated maternity patients." This position has opened the door to the increased use of nurse-midwives in North America. In a number of states in the United States that have not permitted the full functioning of these nurses, legislative bills are pending that will provide the necessary license to practice.

The professional role of the midwife as defined by the World Health Organization (1976b) and amended by the Working Party on Midwifery Training in European Countries is as follows:

A midwife is a person who is qualified to practice midwifery. She is trained to give the necessary care and advice to women during pregnancy, labor and the postnatal period, to conduct normal deliveries on her own responsibility and to care for the newly born infant. At all times she must be able to recognize the warning signs of abnormal or potentially abnormal conditions which necessitate referral to a doctor and to carry out emergency measures in the absence of a doctor. She may practice in hospitals, health units or domiciliary services. In any one of these situations she has an important task in health education with the family and the community.

Models of Helping and Coping

Nurses' helping effectiveness is influenced by their orientation to models of helping and coping. Nurses and the public they serve function in light of their assumptions about who is to blame for a problem and who is responsible for solving it. Four models are possible when assigning responsibility for both the problem and its solution, as shown below (Cronenwett and Brickman, 1983):

Client responsible for problem

		YES	NO
Client responsible for solution	YES	Moral	Compensatory
	NO	Enlightenment	Medical

Moral model. In the moral model of helping and coping, clients are seen as responsible for both the creation of and the solution to their own problems. One underlying assumption is that basically life is just; therefore people deserve what happens to them. The moral model is used by the couple who make the choice of having their baby at home among their family and friends (Cronenwett, 1980). If a complication occurs, the couple may perceive themselves as inferior, inadequate, or incompetent (Gross, 1979; Fischer and Nadler, 1974). Impairment to self-concept and potential for alterations in family processes or parenting, feeling of powerlessness, and spiritual distress may result. The nurse who also operates within the moral model may see the couple as responsible and may respond to them in a punitive nontherapeutic manner.

Compensatory model. In the compensatory model of helping and coping the client is not held responsible for the problem but is expected to solve it with the help of others (Cronenwett, 1983). Clients see themselves and are seen as deprived through failure of the environment to provide them with goods and services to which they are entitled. Clients must be assertive and may need training to help them deal more effectively with their environment (Redman, 1984).

Helpers mobilize resources that compensate for the deficiencies in the environment. With deficiencies removed the client's competence is increased. The International Childbirth Education Association (ICEA) was formed to mobilize resources and create an environment that helps clients experience childbirth in a manner best suited to their priorities (Cronenwett and Brickman, 1983). The strength of this model is that it allows people to direct their energies outward without berating themselves (Redman, 1984). Operating within this model, clients in labor are not as apt to suffer the alteration in self-concept or spiritual distress that can accompany unexpected problems or outcomes.

The weak point of this model is that people can see themselves as continually solving problems they do not create. They find themselves constantly striving to overcome barriers (such as protocols established by the hospital staff) and may become bitter toward those they consider the source of their problem or discomfiture.

Medical model. Health care providers are generally most familiar with this model. The medical model extends to all situations in which people are thought to be subject to forces such as disease that were and will continue to be beyond their control (Redman, 1984). Clients are seen as beings in need of treatment from the experts. The experts also prescribe the therapy and define what is a successful outcome. Input from clients is often not requested or heard (Cronenwett and Brickman, 1983). The helper's needs, rather than those of the client, are central to this model (Cronenwett and Brickman, 1983). The power lies with the helper.

According to Cronenwett and Brickman (1983) the majority of disagreements over policies affecting childbearing families in recent years originated between clients who favor a compensatory model and health care providers who function within the medical model. For most families, pregnancy remains a normal process. Therefore unless the client prefers it, the medical model may be dysfunctional.

The strength of the medical over the compensatory model lies in the freedom it provides to clients to accept help for unexpected problems during the childbearing or parenting experience. This model does allow people to claim help without blame for weakness; its deficiency is that it fosters dependency (Brickman and others, 1982; Redman, 1984).

Enlightenment model. The central emphasis is on enlightening participants to the true nature of their problem; since their impulses are out of control, they must submit to discipline by agents of the community. The solution can be maintained only so long as this relationship is maintained. These assumptions can be a basis for coping whenever people are unable to control what they experience as undesirable behavior on their part. Its deficiency is that it can lead to fanatic concern with certain problems and can reconstruct people's lives around the behaviors and relationships in the model. It puts tremendous power in the hands of agents who control what participants believe is their ability to cope with their lives (Brickman and others, 1982; Redman, 1984).

Examples of external authorities are such agencies as Overeaters or Alcoholics Anonymous. Early natural childbirth movements often operated within the enlightenment model. That is, it was thought that women would be tempted by the medicated experience the physicians offered, and they needed an external force to help them resist this temptation. The early movement for breast-feeding at any cost is another example. Some teachers developed a fanatic attachment to the system for its own sake, rather than for the ultimate goal of a healthy mother and baby (Ewy and Ewy, 1970; Cronenwett and Brickman, 1983). Nurses must remain vigilant to prevent the "natural" (nonmedicated) childbirth or the breast-feeding itself from becoming the *goal;* these goals are inappropriate if they induce tremendous guilt or give rise to anxiety. Insistence on an inappropriate goal can lead to potential for alterations in parenting or family processes, potential for powerlessness, spiritual distress, or ineffective individual or family coping.

Use of models in the real world.* Real-world settings often contain a mixture of assumptions that characterize these models. Several points can be made about these models:
1. Problems between helpers and recipients can arise when each is operating on a different model. Indeed, we may have the wrong models in place in a number of areas.
2. There are some data to support the hypothesis that models in which people are held responsible for so-

lutions are more likely to increase their competence.
3. The authors (Brickman and others, 1982) indicate a preference for the compensatory model, noting that it is the only one that justifies the act of helping (since the recipient is not responsible for problems) but still leaves clients with an active sense of control over their lives (since they have to use the help to find a solution).
4. Many questions remain. Are some helping models better than others or only for some clients? Has there been historic evolution of dominant models applied to different populations? There is now an emergence of the compensatory model in childbearing situations, over the previously predominant medical model.

The compensatory model is probably most congruent with the teaching approach advocated here—one with mutual participation by client and practitioner.

The Nursing Process

The term *nursing process* was introduced in an address by Lydia Hall in 1955 and in nursing literature by Orlando in 1961 (de la Cuesta, 1983). This step-by-step problem-solving process is derived from the scientific method of drawing conclusions from logical analysis of data systematically collected through the senses (Yura and Walsh, 1983; Roper, 1983; Hase, 1983; Bower, 1981). Although the phrase "nursing process" focuses on the nurse, both client and nurse should be sharing their thinking and problem solving together.

The nursing process is usually described in five separate stages: assessment, diagnosis, planning, implementation, and evaluation. Each stage has phases within it. The rate of progression through the phases depends on the nature of the health problem, the setting, the available resources, and the nurse's level of knowledge and skill.

Stage 1: assessment. Assessment begins when the nurse is alerted to a client's need. The stimulus itself forms part of the data base. It may be the way the client walks into the clinic, the client's opening comment, a change in color, a raised temperature, or increased activity. The assessment stage involves at least two phases: data collection and formulation of inferences or hypotheses from the data.

Data collection. Once alerted, the nurse attends to the client and begins the essential first phase in the assessment stage, the collection of sufficient accurate data to formulate a nursing diagnosis. Data is collected through interview, physical examination, and from

---

*From Redman, K.B.: The process of patient education, ed. 5, St. Louis, 1984, The C.V. Mosby Co., pp. 129-130.

laboratory tests. Sources of data collection include the client, her family and friends (if this is acceptable to the client or when the client is unable to provide essential information), and health care records.

Formulation of inferences. An inference is a nurse's judgment or interpretation of the data collected. Inferences are subjective. The nurse's knowledge, skill, experience, values, and beliefs influence the formulation of inferences. See the discussion on models of helping and coping, values clarification, and cultural aspects of care for examples of factors that may influence the nurse's subjective judgments.

Stage 2: nursing diagnosis. A nursing diagnosis is a summary statement of the analyzed data (Kim and Moritz, 1981; Gordon, 1982; Newman, 1984; Fadden, 1984; Tartaglia, 1985). The nursing diagnosis is a two-part statement (Carpenito, 1983). The first part consists of the diagnostic title, for example, parenting, alterations in, or coping, ineffective individual. The second part specifies the related etiologic or contributing factors. Following are two examples of nursing diagnoses: parenting, alterations in, related to breastfeeding difficulties; and, coping, ineffective individual, related to knowledge deficit about parenting.

Nursing diagnoses are organized within the Functional Health Framework developed by Gordon (1982).* The framework provides a means for organizing nursing assessment and standardizing data collection. The list of nursing diagnoses are grouped under functional health patterns in Table 2.1.

The nursing diagnosis statement indicates the nature and extent of the client's health problem. The second part of the statement gives direction to the nursing interventions and falls within the boundaries of nursing practice as stated in the nurse practice act. The diagnosis must also meet the standards of practice as set forth by the professional association.

The accuracy of the diagnosis depends on the *comprehensiveness of the data*. Three phases in processing the data are required to achieve accurate and meaningful nursing diagnosis: analysis, synthesis, and validation. *Analysis* is concerned with establishing categories of concerns or needs. *Synthesis* of the data is concerned with looking for relationships and patterns. *Validation* can be done in three ways: (1) with the client, for relevance and completeness, (2) with others on the nursing team, so the diagnosis fits the data available, and (3) with a member or members of the client's interpersonal system.

*Once the nursing diagnoses are established, the nurse takes time to explore the personal value judgments about the family that may affect and impede nursing interventions. The nursing diagnosis is crucial because it guides the selection and implementation of effective nursing interventions (Tartaglia, 1985).

Stage 3: planning of care. Each diagnosis stimulates the nurse to generate nursing actions. It is important to ask the client and family members how the client has coped with similar health problems or situations in the past. The client's self-care patterns should be incorporated into the nursing care plan as much as possible. Three essential phases in planning are (1) setting the goals in client-centered terms, (2) prioritizing the goals, and (3) selecting nursing actions that will help the client meet the goals.

Setting the goals. Determination of the goal or goals is done with the client if possible. On some occasions this is not possible; for example, if the client is a newborn, unconscious, or too ill. In some cases the nurse assumes responsibility for clarifying the objectives of care with family members or through peer review in health care conferences. At times the nursing care plan is developed in conjunction with other health team members' plans so that the client's care is designed in a coordinated fashion. Attention is given to such factors as the client's time commitment, fatiguing factors, and child care considerations. Clients whose life-style and other responsibilities are considered in planning will be more likely to participate actively in their own health care plan.

Prioritizing the goals. Prioritizing the goals is done on the basis of the immediacy of the problem (its life-threatening components) or the client's and nurse's preference. The nurse's preference is determined by the resources available, commitments to other clients, and the need for further data or plans of other health team members.

Once the goal is established, criteria used to measure progress toward the goal are selected. These outcome criteria are stated as objectively, specifically, and realistically as possible so they can be used both to direct nursing actions and as *outcome criteria*. For example, "Between 8 AM and 4 PM the client will drink between 800 and 1,000 ml of fluids." This objective considers the client's waking time and provides for less intake of fluids after 4 PM to reduce possible interference with sleep from increased elimination.

Selecting nursing actions. Nursing actions that will help the client meet the goals may be developed by the nurse from a repertoire of known nursing interventions, from the literature, and by consulting with other nurses and the client. As the nurse's personal knowledge increases, an expanding repertoire of nursing

Table 2.1
Functional Health Patterns* and Related Nursing Diagnoses

Functional Health Pattern	Nursing Diagnoses	Functional Health Pattern	Nursing Diagnoses

Health perception–health management	Altered growth and development
	Alteration in health maintenance
	Noncompliance
	Potential for infection
	Potential for injury
			Alteration in tissue perfusion
			  Cerebral
			  Cardiopulmonary
			  Renal
			  Gastrointestinal
			  Peripheral

Nutritional-metabolic	Altered growth and development
	Fluid volume deficit
	Alteration in fluid volume: excess
	Hyperthermia
	Hypothermia
	Alteration in nutrition: less than body requirements
	Alteration in nutrition: more than body requirements
	Alteration in oral mucous membrane
	Impairment of skin integrity
	Impaired swallowing
	Impaired tissue integrity
	Ineffective thermoregulation
	Potential alteration in body temperature
		Sleep-rest
		
		Cognitive-perceptual
			Altered growth and development
			Sleep pattern disturbance
			Alteration in comfort:
			  Pain
			  Chronic pain
			Altered growth and development
			Knowledge deficit (specify)
			Unilateral neglect
			Sensory-perceptual alteration:
			  Visual
			  Auditory
			  Kinesthetic
			  Gustatory
			  Tactile
			  Olfactory

Elimination	Alteration in bowel elimination:
	  Constipation
	  Diarrhea
	  Incontinence
	Altered growth and development
	Functional incontinence
	Reflex incontinence
	Stress incontinence
	Total incontinence
	Urge incontinence
	Alteration in patterns of urinary elimination
	Urinary retention
		Self-perception–self-concept	Alteration in thought processes
			Anxiety
			Fear
			Altered growth and development
			Hopelessness
			Powerlessness
			Disturbance in self-concept

Activity-exercise	Activity intolerance
	Ineffective airway clearance
	Ineffective breathing pattern
	Alteration in cardiac output: decreased
	Diversional activity deficit
	Impaired gas exchange
	Altered growth and development
	Impaired home maintenance management
	Impaired physical mobility
	Alterations in respiratory function†
	Self-care deficit:
	  Total†
	  Feeding
	  Bathing/hygiene
	  Dressing/grooming
	  Toileting
		Role-relationship
		
		Sexuality-reproductive
		
		Coping–stress tolerance
		
		Value-belief
			Impaired verbal communication
			Alteration in family process
			Grieving:
			  Anticipatory
			  Dysfunctional
			Altered growth and development
			Alteration in parenting
			Impaired social interaction
			Social isolation
			Potential for violence: self-directed or directed at others
			Altered growth and development
			Rape trauma syndrome
			Sexual dysfunction
			Altered sexuality patterns
			Impaired adjustment
			Ineffective family coping
			Ineffective individual coping
			Altered growth and development
			Post trauma response
			Altered growth and development
			Spiritual distress

*The functional health patterns were identified by M. Gordon in *Nursing Diagnosis: Process and Application* (New York, McGraw-Hill, 1982), with some minor changes by the authors. This nursing diagnosis list reflects the authors' adoption of the North American Nursing Diagnosis Association (NANDA) approved list from the Seventh National Conference (1986). The authors have deleted the listing of *actual* and *potential* next to a diagnostic category, since most diagnoses can be utilized as an actual or potential label.
†Diagnosis not included by NANDA, 1986.

skills enables him or her to make choices that finely tune the nursing actions to the client's needs and preferences.

Stage 4: implementation of care. Nursing actions are selected on the basis of anticipated effectiveness; the goals and outcome criteria desired by client and nurse; the amount of risk involved for the client; the availability of resources, facilities, and personnel; and the client's ability to comply with the proposed care (Glass, 1983). The implementation phase includes referral to other team members. The coordination of care given by the various members is also an important consideration during this phase.

The overall management of the health care setting is an essential, indeed critical, aspect of the implementation phase. *Each nurse contributes to the setting by supporting colleagues through review of nursing care plans, willing consultation and assistance in client care, and appropriate praise.*

Stage 5: evaluation. Evaluation is a joint process between nurse and family (Bloch, 1975). This phase involves assessing the client's progress toward or attainment of the goals using outcome criteria (Barba and others, 1978). The outcome of the evaluation phase determines the need for revision of goals, additional data, or modification of nursing actions (Fig. 2.2).

Tool: summary of nursing actions. Many forms have been devised to help nurses with the nursing process. These forms have spaces for each stage of the process. Nurses are provided with a guide to guard against omission of any part of the process.

Recording/charting. Each clinical setting has its own method of recording or charting. All pertinent information obtained at each contact with the client is recorded to ensure that each member of the health team contributes to the achievement of the goals and maintenance of continuity of care. The client who sees the team as working with her toward understood and mutually accepted goals is in a better position to mobilize her energy for resolving the health problem. In some settings clients have the right to full disclosure of the records documenting their care.

Written records for clients with similar health problems provide a rich source of data for review, discussion, and evaluation of care given to alleviate a health problem. These records are kept and periodically analyzed and audited for the standards of nursing practice in the particular setting (quality assurance) and also for nursing research. Careful records can be used as the basis for determining the amount of nursing care needed for each health problem. This information is needed for the present medically oriented DRGs and may be helpful in defining nursing-oriented DRGs. Three major recording systems—Kardex, nursing care

Fig. 2.2
Five stages of the nursing process.

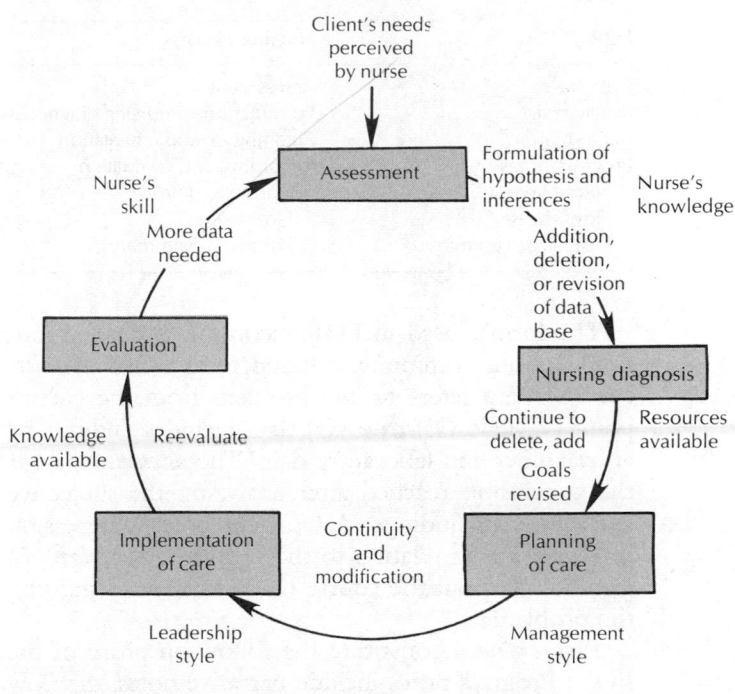

plan, and problem-oriented record—will be reviewed briefly here.

Kardex. One system for quick reference is the Kardex. A flip file, usually kept in pencil, is the most common format. Pertinent, current information about the client is kept updated. The Kardex does not have legal status as a record and is often discarded when the client is discharged.

Nursing care plan. The nursing care plan reflects the nursing process. The goal of this plan is to ensure consistency and continuity in the care given the client. Space is available for recording data collected—assessment, nursing diagnoses, prioritized goals, outcome criteria, and the planning, implementation, and evaluation of nursing care. To be effective, nursing care plans must be kept up-to-date and accessible to all those caring for the client (Rich, 1985; Sanborn, 1984).

Problem-oriented record. The problem-oriented record (POR) is essentially the same problem-solving format as the nursing process used for nursing care plans. The management of care is based on a succinct list of client problems and nursing diagnoses derived from a data base. The components of the POR are the data base, problem list or nursing diagnoses, initial plan, and progress notes. These components are analogous to those in the nursing process (Table 2.2).

Table 2.2
Comparison of Components of POR and the Nursing Process

POR	Nursing Process
Data base	Assessment
Problem list	Formulation of nursing diagnoses
Initial plan	Planning or implementation
Progress notes	Recording and evaluation
Narrative notes	Narrative notes
Flow sheets	Flow sheets
Discharge summary	Discharge summary

The format used in POR recording is divided into four sections commonly referred to as SOAP. *Subjective* (S) data refers to the problem from the client's point of view. *Objective* (O) data includes findings by an examiner and laboratory data. The *assessment* (A) is the conclusion reached after analyzing the subjective and objective findings. Assessment notes progression or regression in relation to the problem. The *plan* (P) signifies in detail the course to be followed regarding the problem.

Progress notes constitute the follow-up phase of the POR. Progress notes include narrative notes, the flow sheet, and the discharge summary. Each narrative note refers directly to a problem and is titled accordingly. The narrative note describes the progress of the client in relation to a specific problem and represents the evaluative phase of the nursing process.

The problem-oriented system also serves as a tool for quality control of medical and nursing care. Documentary proof regarding client problems is readily available. Health personnel become directly accountable to the client for the quality of care rendered.

The *discharge summary* focuses on providing for continuity of care and an overall assessment of accomplishments of the care given. The discharge summary includes proposed follow-up; any prescribed regimen is spelled out in detail. Consultations are requested on specific problems, but it is essential that the consultant be aware of all the client's problems so as to avoid treatment out of context.

The SOAP format is used to record the care given in the following case presentation. Note the similarity to the stages and phases of the nursing process.

■ Mary, age 21, pregnant for the first time, attends the prenatal clinic at the local hospital. Mary's pregnancy was confirmed 2 weeks ago. She is now in the eighth week of pregnancy. Mary's husband, Tim, brings her to the prenatal clinic, where she makes the following complaint: "I'm sick when I get up in the morning. It is even worse at night. I can't stand the smell of cooking."

Problem 1: Nausea and Vomiting of Early Pregnancy
Initial Plan

S   "I'm sick when I get up in the morning. It is even worse at night. I can't stand the smell of cooking."

O
1. Pregnancy of 8 weeks' duration.
2. No history of flu or contact with people with stomach upsets.
3. Episodes occur daily and are intermittent.
4. Temperature normal
5. Pulse: 80/min.
6. Blood pressure: 110/80.
7. No proteinuria or glycosuria.

A   Potential alterations in nutrition related to nausea and vomiting of early pregnancy.

P   Instruct woman concerning the following:
1. Probable cause: normal response to pregnancy; may be expected to last about 4 more weeks.
2. Diet: small frequent feedings, some carbohydrates (such as salt-free crackers and milk) before rising and as afternoon snack to prevent an empty stomach.
3. Motion: Discuss ways of rising slowly to minimize sudden hypotension.
4. Telephone progress report in 1 week's time.

Following Mary's next prenatal visit the nurse charts the following:

Problem 1: Nausea and Vomiting of Early Pregnancy
Progress Notes

S   "I haven't been sick to my stomach for 10 days. I feel really good now."

O
1. Pregnancy of 12 weeks' duration.
2. Appearance healthy: skin has good turgor.
3. Temperature: 96.6° F (37° C).
4. Pulse: 78/min.
5. Blood pressure: 105/76.
6. No proteinuria or glycosuria.

A   Recovered from nausea and vomiting of early pregnancy.

     Problem resolved.

P   No further action needed.

Teaching-Learning Process: the Nurse and the Family

Nursing leaders and client education. Early English leaders in nursing in the middle and late nineteenth century saw the importance of teaching families about sanitation, cleanliness, and care of the sick. Since much of the care of the sick at that time was done by the family, nurse's efforts to teach represented a way of extending their services (Redman, 1984).

Statements by the National League of Nursing Education reflect the concern during this century with preparing nurses for their teaching tasks. The following comment shows such a concern as early as 1918:

Another limitation of the ordinary training is that it deals only or mainly with disease, neglecting almost entirely the preventive and educational factors which are such an essential element in the many new branches of public health work, such as school and visiting nursing, infant welfare, industrial welfare, and hospital social service (National League of Nursing Education, 1918, p. 6).

The 1937 curriculum guide commented. "The nurse is essentially a teacher and an agent of health in whatever field [the nurse] may be working" (National League of Nursing Education, 1937).

The centrality of client teaching varies with formal philosophies of nursing (Redman, 1984). Kreuter (1957) identified teaching of self-care and counseling on health matters as nursing operations needed to provide care. Sister Olivia (1948) saw teaching as one of the tools of the nurse with the objective of promoting spiritual, mental, and physical health. Henderson (1964), Lambertsen (1964), and Peplau (1952) characterized nursing as an educative process and an educative instrument. Peplau (1977) sees a shift in emphasis from traditional mother-surrogate activities to more educative-nurturing ones. Hall (1964) saw some of the tenets of teaching as central to her philosophy of nurse-client interaction. Travelbee (1971) indicated that both the client and the nurse learn as a result of the interactive process and that if changes do not occur in either or both of the participants, a relationship has not been established.

King (1981) says one of the three fundamental health needs of human beings is usable health information at a time they need and can use it. Johnson (1980) (Behavioral System Model for nursing) sees teaching as one way to help people find new or better ways of behaving, contributing to an enlargement of choices. Kinlein's description of her practice, based on Orem's theory (self-care concept of nursing), provides a view of a truly nursing focus for client education (1977a). Kinlein proposes a health care system in which people are the primary givers of care to themselves—by virtue of choosing the health professional the person thinks would be most helpful at the time. Nursing's skills and strengths are teaching and counseling (Watters and Arbeiter, 1985).

Nursing is helping people in self-care practices with regard to their state of health (Redman, 1984). Instead of a practice focused on support of medical goals, the nursing focus in practice involves the use of nursing knowledge to help achieve the client's health

goals (Kinlein, 1977b; Redman, 1984). Indeed, the client's knowledge, skills, and problem-solving ability form a self-care asset worth developing in and of itself.

Both teaching and nursing involve a helping relationship that has development of independence in the subject as the main objective. Teaching is one nursing action that can help the client toward self-care, with both the nurse and the client assuming responsibility toward that goal (Redman, 1984).

High priority of health education. A number of factors have converged to bring health teaching into prominence (Redman, 1984):
1. A change in emphasis from treatment of disease to the maintenance of health.
2. Emphasis on self-care and the individual's values, preferences, and personal definition of health (Redman, 1984).
3. A trend toward holistic health care (Gordon, 1981). The emphasis in holistic health is on education and self-care rather than on treatment or dependence. In addition, holistic health incorporates the view that the setting where health care takes place is a place for education. The holistic health care movement is part of a broad movement to create humane, democratic alternatives to large, impersonal, unresponsive services and institutions (Gordon, 1981; Redman, 1984).
4. The consumerist movement to narrow the competence gap between helper and help recipient (Haug and Lavin, 1981).
5. Shortened hospitals stays including same-day surgery.
6. A Patient's Bill of Rights, American Hospital Association (1975). Of the 12 rights listed, seven are explicit about having information needs met.
7. Principles of medical ethics, American Medical Association, House of Delegates, 1980. This new version includes the statement, "A physician shall make relevant information available to patients and the public."

Definition of teaching. Teaching is the process through which a teacher helps a student learn. Teaching is communication specially structured and sequenced to promote learning (Redman, 1984). All interaction between health care providers and clients contributes to the process and objectives of teaching-learning (Taylor, 1984). Nurses also communicate nonverbally and by example about such topics as health and good hygiene practice (Redman, 1984).

General goals of teaching. The goal of health education is teaching people to live life in the healthiest way possible. It is possible to prevent, promote, maintain, or modify a number of health-related behaviors through teaching (Redman, 1984). Following are some goals for the client to achieve as a result of the teaching-learning process:

1. Participation in management of the problem, decision making, self-care, treatment, and follow-through.
2. Integration of the illness into her or his life experience.
3. Self-strengthening through strengthening role performance in childbearing and parenting.
4. Acquisition of correct information as a basis for decision making and assurance.
5. Education of society to gain support for health-related legislation and environmental controls.

The goals of learning have been classified into three domains: cognitive (understanding), affective (attitudes), and psychomotor (motor skills) (Bobak and Jensen, 1983; Redman, 1984; Bloom, 1956). Each of these domains responds best to a particular method of learning. Facts and concepts are taught by written materials, audiovisual aids, lectures, and discussions. Attitudes can be examined and perhaps changed if necessary by discussion that provides insight into affective behavior. Motor skills are best learned through a demonstration of the skills, with subsequent practice until they are perfected (Redman, 1984).

The teaching process. The teaching process uses the same steps as those of the nursing process (Fig. 2.3).

Stage 1: assessment. Need to learn. The first step is to identify the client's need for teaching. An individual may request information or express a desire to learn a task. The requested information may be about promoting health, preventing or treating a problem, or about a health facility and its services. Consumer groups, formed in response to needs perceived as unmet, define information to be shared with the public in general as well as with involved clients. Health care providers recognize areas of learning commonly associated with various problems.

Readiness to learn. Learning requires *motivation.* People who are not convinced they need to learn will resist efforts to teach them. Several conditions affect motivation, one being the value systems that vary by cultural group and socioeconomic class (Redman, 1984). People vary in their *readiness* for health learning because of their intellectual capability, general educational background, and attitude toward responsibility (Redman, 1984; Loughrey, 1983; Taylor, 1984). According to Redman (1984), "There are two facets of readiness to learn: One is emotional readiness, or motivation, which determines the individual's willingness to put forth the effort necessary to learn. A second facet is experiential readiness, the individual's background of experiences, skills, and attitudes and his or her ability to learn that which is considered desirable" (Redman, 1984:21). A pattern of response receiving considerable attention is the theory of *learned helplessness* (Redman, 1984). Learned helplessness decreases motivation to learn. If the outcome is supposed to be independence, fear and inability to cope may be the unexpected result.

Some people feel that nothing they do can affect their environment or what happens to them. These people are described as having no *internal locus of control* or internal motivation.

Timing is another factor that affects a person's ability to learn. The person must feel an unmet need and yet be comfortable (physically and in that environment) and therefore able to learn (McHatton, 1985; Miller, 1985; Redman, 1984).

Stage 2: diagnostic statement and setting of objectives. A nursing diagnosis can identify the existence of a knowledge deficit, for example, parenting, potential alterations in—related to knowledge deficit in physical care of the newborn. However, a well-stated learning objective is needed to specify exactly what a person is to learn. One such objective is "to give the baby a shampoo." The nurse validates the treatment with the parent. Subobjectives are present: (1) uses a safe method of holding the newborn, (2) protects the eyes from water and shampoo, (3) cleans the hair and scalp, (4) dries the hair, and (5) completes the shampoo without exposing the newborn to cold stress.

Stages 3 and 4: planning and implementation. Once the objective is known and validated, taking the woman's cultural or ethnic values and beliefs into consideration, the teaching method is chosen (Holden, 1985). The nurse plans teaching methods to cover all the domains. A discussion of giving a baby a shampoo identifies and helps the mother work through her attitudes (affective) about the activity. A discussion and

Fig. 2.3
The teaching process. (From Redman, B.K: The process of patient education, ed. 5, St. Louis, 1984, The C.V. Mosby Co.)

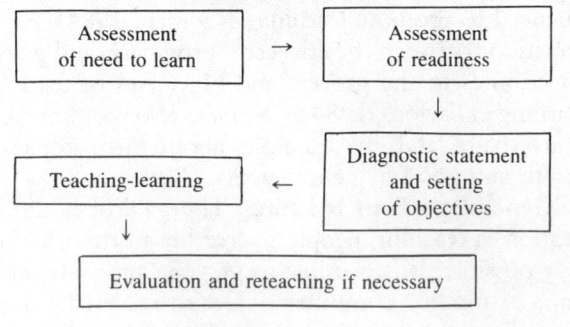

demonstration presented at the woman's intellectual and educational level help her understand (cognitive). Giving the baby a shampoo with supervision helps the parent develop necessary motor skills (psychomotor). *The teaching is offered when the mother is comfortable and rested and has asked to learn the activity.* Most women tire easily in the early postpartum period, so the session should be limited by the woman's tolerance.

Stage 5: evaluation. The nurse evaluates the effectiveness of teaching in several ways. For example, teaching is effective if:

1. The woman can shampoo the baby's hair, meeting each of the subobjectives.
2. The woman says she feels comfortable while giving the shampoo.
3. The woman says she understands related information.

If evaluation shows teaching was ineffective, the entire process is repeated beginning with assessment.

Teaching tools. Teaching tools can be developed to help nurses present information. An example of a teaching tool to be used in this text is the guidelines for client teaching format found in the clinical chapters. The nurse changes the teaching tool as knowledge is built from interactions with clients.

Summary

Maternity care is a direct service to women and their families during childbearing and the childbearing phases of the life cycle. This service provides care, based on the nursing process, that is preventive, curative and rehabilitative. Teaching is a central component of nursing care. Maternity nurses assume both traditional and new, expanded roles as they carry out the greater responsibilities such care engenders.

References

Aamodt, A.A.: Culture. In Clark, A.L., editor: Culture/childbearing/health professionals, Philadelphia, 1978, F.A. Davis Co.

American Hospital Association: A patient's bill of rights, Chicago, 1975, The Association.

American Medical Association: Principles of medical ethics, Chicago, 1980, The Association.

Arbeiter, J.S.: The big shift to home health nursing, RN 47:38, 1984.

Archer, S.E., and Goehner, P.A.: Nurses: a political force, Belmont, Calif., 1982, Wadsworth Publishing Co.

Barba, M., and others: The evaluation of patient care through use of ANA's standards of nursing practice, Superv. Nurse 9:42, 1978.

Barnes, F.E.F.: Ambulatory maternal health care and family planning services, Washington, D.C., 1978, American Public Health Association.

Beck, C.T.: The conceptualization of power, Adv. Nurs. Sci. 4(2):1, 1982.

Beebe, J.E.: NERCEN: a prototype of regional education efforts in nurse-midwifery (education exchange), J.O.G.N. Nurs. 25(3):22, 1980.

Benner, P.E.: From novice to expert: excellence and power in clinical nursing practice, Menlo Park, Calif., 1984, Addison-Wesley Publishing Co.

Benner, P.E.: Uncovering the knowledge embedded in clinical practice, Image 15(2):36, 1983.

Bibb, B.N.: The effectiveness of nonphysician as providers of family planning services, J.O.G.N. Nurs. 88:137, 1979.

Bloch, D.: Evaluation of nursing care in terms of process and outcome: issues in research quality assurance, Nurs. Res. 24:256, 1975.

Bloom, B.S., editor: Taxonomy of educational objectives: the classification of educational goals. Handbook I: cognitive domain, New York, 1956, David McKay Co.

Bobak, I.M., and Jensen, M.D.: A modular study guide to maternity care, St. Louis, 1983, The C.V. Mosby Co.

Bower, F.: The process of planning nursing care, ed. 3, St. Louis, 1981, The C.V. Mosby Co.

Brickman, P., and others: An attributional analysis of helping behavior. In Berkowitz, L., editor: Advances in experimental social psychology, vol. 15, New York, 1982, Academic Press.

Brook, C.: Social, economic and biologic correlates of infant mortality in city neighborhoods, J. Health Soc. Behav. 21(1), March 1980.

Burst, H.: The American College of Nurse Midwives: a professional organization, J. Nurse Midwife 25(1): Jan.-Feb. 1980.

Carpenito, L.J.: Nursing diagnosis: application to clinical practice, Philadelphia, 1983, J.B. Lippincott Co.

Cronenwett, L.R.: Helping and nursing models, Nurs. Res. 32(6):342, 1983.

Cronenwett, L.R.: Elements and outcomes of a postpartum support group program, Res. Nurs. Health 3(3):33, 1980.

Cronenwett, L., and Brickman, P.: Models of helping and coping in childbirth, Nurs. Res. 32(2):84, 1983.

de la Cuesta, C.: The nursing process: from development to implementation, J. Adv. Nurs. 8:365, 1983.

Edwards, M.: Communications: dimensions in childbirth education, Pacific Grove, Calif., 1973, M. Edwards.

Etheredge, M.L.: Nurse-manager . . . try that title on for size, Nurs. '85 15(8):26, 1985.

Ewy, D., and Ewy, R.: Preparation for childbirth: a Lamaze guide, New York, 1970, Signet.

Fadden, T.C., and Seiser, G.K.: Nursing diagnosis—a matter of form, Am. J. Nurs. 84(4):470, 1984.

Fischer, J.D., and Nadler, A.: The effect of similarity between donor and recipient on recipient's reactions to aid, J. Applied Soc. Psychology, 1974.

Fogel, C.I., and Woods, N.F.: Health care of women: a nursing perspective, St. Louis, 1981, The C.V. Mosby Co.

Glass, H.: Interventions in nursing: goal- or task-oriented? Int. Nurs. Rev. 30(2):53, 1983.

Gordon, J.S.: Holistic health centers, J. Holistic Med. 3(1):72, 1981.

Gordon, M.: Historical perspective: The National Group for classification of nursing diagnoses. In Kim, M.J., and

Moritz, D.S., editors: Classification of nursing diagnoses, New York, 1981, McGraw-Hill Book Co.

Gordon, M.: Nursing diagnosis: process and application, New York, 1982, McGraw-Hill Book Co.

Groos, A.E., and others: Reactance, attribution, equity, and the help recipient, J. Applied Soc. Psychology 9:297, 1979.

Haire, D.: Improving the outcome of pregnancy through increased utilization of midwives, J.O.G.N. Nurs. 26(11):5, 1981.

Hall, L.E.: Nursing—what is it? Can. Nurse 60:150, 1964.

Hase, S.: The nursing process: is it idol worhip? Aust. Nurses J. 13:39, 1983.

Haug, M.R., and Lavin, B.: Practitioner or patient—who's in charge? J. Health Soc. Behav. 22:212, 1981.

Henderson, V.: The nature of nursing, Am. J. Nurs. 64:62, 1964.

Holden, J.E.: Don't just tell your patients—*teach* them, RN 48(7):29, 1985.

Johnson, D.E.: The behavioral system model for nursing. In Riehl, J., and Roy, C., editors: Conceptual models for nursing practice, ed. 2, New York, 1980, Appleton-Century-Crofts.

Johnson, D.E.: Powerlessness: a significant determinant in patient behavior? J. Nurs. Educ. 6:39, 1967.

Kim, M., and Moritz, D., editors: Proceedings of the 3rd and 4th national conferences, classification of nursing diagnoses, New York, 1981, McGraw-Hill Book Co.

Kim, M.J., McFarland, G.K., and McLane, A.M.: Pocket guide to nursing diagnosis, St. Louis, 1984, The C.V. Mosby Co.

King, I.M.: A theory for nursing: systems, concepts, process, New York, 1981, John Wiley & Sons.

Kinlein, M.L.: Independent nursing practice with clients, Philadelphia, 1977a, J.B. Lippincott Co.

Kinlein, M.L.: The self-care concept, Am. J. Nurs. 77:598, 1977b.

Kreuter, F.R.: What is good nursing care? Nurs. Outlook 5:302, 1957.

Lambertsen, E.C.: Nursing definition and philosophy precede nursing goal development, Mod. Hosp. 103:136, 1964.

Lewis, H.R.: Specialism: the best career path? RN 47(6):40, 1984.

Loughrey, L.: Dealing with an illiterate patient . . . you can't read him like a book, Nurs. '83 13(1):65, 1983.

McHatton, M.: A theory of timely teaching, Am. J. Nurs. 85(7):798, 1985.

Miller, A.: When is the time ripe for teaching? Am. J. Nurs. 85(7):801, 1985.

Naeye, R.L.: Causes of fetal and neonatal mortality by race in a selected U.S. population, Am. J. Pub. Health 69:857, 1979.

National League of Nursing Education: Standard curriculum for schools of nursing, Baltimore, 1918, The Waverly Press.

National League of Nursing Education: A curriculum guide for schools of nursing, New York, 1937, The League.

Newman, M.A.: Nursing diagnosis: looking at the whole, Am. J. Nurs. 84(12):1496, 1984.

Nurses' Association of the American College of Obstetricians and Gynecologists: Standards for obstetric, gynecologic and neonatal nursing. The Nurses' Association of the American College of Obstetricians and Gynecologists, ed. 2, 1981.

Nurses' Association of the American College of Obstetricians and Gynecologists: Certification's role in nursing (part 1), NAACOG Newsletter 9(3), May/June 1982.

Olivia, Sister M.: Aims of nursing administration, Washington, D.C., 1947, The Catholic University of American Press. Cited by Brown, E.L.: Nursing for the future, New York, 1948, Russell Sage Foundation.

Olsen, L.: Portrait of nurse-midwifery patients in a private practice, J. Nurs. Midwife 24(4):10, July-Aug. 1979.

Peplau, H.E.: The changing view of nursing, Int. Nurs. Rev. 24(2):43, 1977.

Peplau, H.E.: Interpersonal relations in nursing, New York, 1952, G.P. Putnam's Sons.

Redman, B.K.: The process of patient education, ed. 5, St. Louis, 1984, The C.V. Mosby Co.

Rich, P.L.: With this flow sheet, less is more, Nurs. '85 15(7):25, 1985.

Roper, N., and others: Unity—with diversity: use of the nursing process, Nurs. Mirror 156(26):35, 1983.

Rousch, R.: The development of midwifery—male and female, yesterday and today, J.O.G.N. Nurs. 24(3):27, 1979.

San Francisco Chronicle, January 2, 1986.

Sanborn, W.W., and Blount, M.: Standard care plans, Am. J. Nurs. 84(11):1394, 1984.

Slatin, M.: Why mothers bypass prenatal care, Am. J. Nurs. 71:1388, 1971.

Sprague, H.A., and Taylor, J.R.: The health impact of maternity and infant care programs. Report of Michigan Public Health Service, 1979.

Tartaglia, M.J.: Nursing diagnosis: keystone of your care plan. Nurs. '85 15(3):34, 1985.

Taylor, J.A.: Are you missing what your patients can teach you? RN 47(6):63, 1984.

Travelbee, J.: Interpersonal aspects of nursing, ed. 2, Philadelphia, 1971, F.A. Davis Co.

USA Today, January 4, 1986.

U.S. National Center for Health Statistics, U.S. Bureau of the Census, U.S. Department of Commerce, 1982.

Waters, S., and Arbeiter, J.: Nurse practitioners: how are they doing now? RN 48(10):38, 1985.

Wilson, J.B.: Nurses and politics, Can. Nurse 77:40, 1981.

World Health Organization: Improvement in infant and perinatal mortality in the United States, 1965-1973, Washington, D.C., 1976a, U.S. Department of Health, Education and Welfare.

World Health Organization: Technical report series no. 331, Geneva, 1976b, The Organization.

World Health Organization: Population statistics, household and family characteristics, March 1977, Washington, D.C., 1977, U.S. Bureau of the Census, U.S. Department of Commerce.

World Health Organization: The obstetric-gynecologic nurse practitioner, ACOG and NAACOG, Geneva, 1979, The Organization.

Yura, H., and Walsh, M.B.: The nursing process: assessing, planning, implementing, evaluating, ed. 4, New York, 1983, Appleton-Century-Crofts.

Bibliography

American Nurses' Association: Nursing: a social policy statement, 1982. The Association.

American Nurses' Association: Standards of maternal and

child health nursing practice, Kansas City, Mo., 1973, The Association.

Beernink, H.E.: Choice of childbirth, Birth 10(3):182, 1983.

Bloch, D.: Some crucial terms in nursing: what do they really mean? Nurs. Outlook 22:689, 1974.

Brody, D.S.: The patient's role in clinical decision-making, Ann. Intern. Med. 93:718, 1980.

Dale, M.L.: "Helping" and the concept of individualization in perinatal care, J. Perinat. 5(1):6, Winter, 1985.

Edwards, M.E.: Unattended home birth, Am. J. Nurs. 73:1332, 1973.

Ellis, J.: What to choose in childbirth? Birth 10(3):183, 1983.

Field, L., and Winslow, E.H.: Moving to a nursing model, Am. J. Nurs. 85:1098, 1985.

Klein, M.: Some complexities of choice and trust in obstetrics, Birth 10(3):182, 1983.

Lubic, R.W.: Evidence that the childbearing center has influenced hospital maternity practice, Birth 10(3):179, 1983.

Norton, K.: Beyond "choice" in childbirth, Birth 19(3):179, 1983.

Simkin, P.: The birth plan: vehicle for trust and communication, Birth 10(3):184, 1983.

Legal and Ethical Aspects of Family-centered Maternity Nursing

The field of maternity and newborn care—in which birth and death, life and the capacity to make life are encountered on a daily basis—perhaps offers more legal and ethical challenges to the professional nurse than does any other area of nursing.

This chapter introduces the nurse to basic legal and ethical issues that currently influence women's health care and suggests nursing practices that promote quality professional care. The chapter contains three major divisions: (1) *legal issues,* a broad overview of the legal duties assumed by the maternity and newborn nurse as well as the ensuing potential liabilities, (2) *risk management,* a perspective on nursing behavior designed to minimize the risk of legal liability, and (3) *ethical issues,* an analysis of three major ethical issues encountered on the field of maternity and newborn care. Reading material suggested for further investigation is listed in the bibliography.

Legal Issues

Rosemary Mann

Laws affect nursing in many ways. Activities imposed upon the nurse by law include eye prophylaxis for the newborn and the reporting of venereal disease and child abuse. Criminal law affects nursing when the professional nurse exceeds the scope of the nursing domain and practices medicine without a license or aids and abets an unlicensed individual to practice medicine without a license. This discussion, however, is concerned with civil law that seeks to compensate parties who have been injured or damaged by the negligence of a professional nurse. This civil law has been called the law of torts. A tort is a civil offense.

NOTE: This chapter's content relates only to the United States.

Professional negligence is a tort. The logical sequence of events preceding a legal claim for damages caused by negligence is as follows:

1. The state licenses a professional nurse to practice nursing in a manner that is denied to an unlicensed person.
2. A member of the general public enters into a relationship with a professional nurse in which the nurse offers and delivers health care services.
3. By virtue of the license to practice and the special relationship created between the nurse and the client, duties and obligations are imposed upon the nurse. These duties and obligations are called the standards of care.
4. By some act or *failure* to act the professional nurse breaches a standard of care. The nurse fails to fulfill the duties and obligations imposed upon her. The nurse need not *intend* to do harm. Harm may be inflicted unintentionally through negligence.
5. As a direct or indirect but foreseeable result of that breach, an actual injury is sustained. The injury must be actual rather than potential or "at risk for" injury. Actual injury includes both physical harm and emotional distress.
6. The client may be compensated for the injury by monetary damages assessed against the nurse. "General damages" include the cost of health care and rehabilitation, income lost from absence from work, and income lost from the impaired ability to work. "Special damages" include pain and suffering experienced by the injured party.

Duty: the standard of care. The conduct of all legally competent individuals is held to a standard of care. The standard of care for an adult in today's society is that degree of care exercised by a reasonably prudent person under similar circumstances (Black, 1979). The standard of care for a professional nurse is that average degree of skill, care, and diligence exercised under similar circumstances by the reasonably prudent nurse with similar background, training, and experience (Black, 1979). To be successful in a lawsuit against a nurse the plaintiff-client must first define the nurse's duty or standard of care and then must prove that the nurse failed to conform to that standard of care.

The standard of care is an external code of behavior established by the nursing profession in relation to other health professions. It is measured and applied by the courts in the form of verdicts in lawsuits or settlements.

There are actually many standards of care, and they may be inconsistent or in conflict with each other. The legal system influences or determines nursing behavior by resolving those conflicts. For example, consider a hypothetical case involving electronic fetal monitoring for a normal woman in labor. The plaintiff-client may present expert witnesses who testify that the standard of care is electronic fetal monitoring for *all* women in labor. The defendant-nurse may present expert witnesses who testify that for women during normal labor fetal heart rates may be monitored by frequent auscultation. If the court were to decide that the nurse conformed to the standard of care by frequent auscultation of the fetal heart rate, that decision might establish a standard of care for nurses caring for women in normal labor. In subsequent cases concerned with the same or similar circumstances, courts would apply the standard of care established by previous court decisions. In other words, subsequent courts would find the standard of care to be auscultation of the fetal heart. Adherence to previous decisions is based on the legal principle of *stare decisis,* which means "let the decision stand." Its purpose is to promote consistency in legal decisions by making previous decisions binding in subsequent cases involving the same circumstances.

To determine the standard of care for professional nursing, the appropriate starting point is the Nurse Practice Act and the state regulations pertaining to nursing practice. These laws and regulations define the scope of nursing practice, standards for nursing education, and the point of articulation between the profession of nursing and the profession of medicine. To exceed the legal base of nursing practice is, by definition, to violate the standard of care and to be negligent. For instance, if a particular state declares it illegal for the nurse to dispense medication and the professional nurse hands the woman a month's supply of birth control pills without a physician's order, that action is a violation of the standard of care. If there are no policies or procedures to permit such nursing interventions, the nurse's actions are negligent no matter how safely done.

Standards of care are determined by the nursing profession in its definition of nursing practice, policies and protocols for nursing practice, standards of nursing education, and proscription of activities considered outside of nursing. Standards of care are further delineated by nursing specialist organizations and joint boards of medicine and nursing who define appropriate behavior in special and specific circumstances. An example of the professional nursing standard of care is the American Nurses' Association's Definition of Nursing and Standards for Nursing Practice, (ANA, 1973). An example of a specialist standard of care is the Nurses' Association of the American College of Obstetricians and Gynecologists' Standards for Obstetric, Gynecologic, and Neonatal Nursing (NAACOG, 1981). An example of a standard of care established by a joint board is the Joint Statement on Maternity Care issued by the American College of Nurse-Midwives, the American College of Obstetricians and Gynecologists, and the Nurses' Association of the American College of Obstetricians and Gynecologists (ACNM, 1982) (see Appendix B).

Other standards of care established by the profession are the policies and protocols governing nursing practice in a particular agency or unit of an institution. These policies and protocols define behavior expected of all professionals within their domain. They may act to expand behavior expected in a particular situation beyond the customary practice of nursing and into the practice of medicine. For instance, special or standardized procedures may permit a nurse in an intensive care unit to initiate drug therapy if a client displays a particular symptom. They may also permit a nurse to dispense birth control pills under special circumstances where otherwise that behavior would be illegal (Calif. Bus. and Prof. Code).

Professional nurses have a legal obligation to know and understand the standard of care or duty imposed upon them. Ignorance of a policy or protocol will not be accepted as an excuse for failure to follow it. This is one reason why it is critical for nurses to keep current in their specialties.

Some recent cases have established the duty of the nurse to oversee the behavior of other professionals, and to report situations in which other professionals' behavior fails to conform with the established standard of care (Cushing, 1985). For instance, when a physician writes an erroneous drug order, the nurse has a duty to report the error and obtain a corrected order (Annas, Glantz, and Katz, 1981). When the client is exposed to danger as a result of action by other professionals, the nurse has a duty to protect that client. That duty extends beyond mere reporting of the incident and requires the nurse to follow up on reporting until the client is returned to safety (Darling, 1982). Labor and delivery room nurses occasionally deal with this situation when they call for physician assistance and fail to get it. They must continue to ask for physician assistance until they do get it. The nurse's responsibility extends beyond the care of clients directly assigned to him or her and encompasses the behavior of other professionals functioning in the same area.

Breach: failure to conform to the standard of care. In a court of law the standard of care is established by the testimony of expert witnesses who generally are leaders in their field. Their credentials include administrative responsibiity, teaching, and research in addition to clinical competence. These expert witnesses are presented with the actual situation or with a hypothetical situation that is an exact duplicate of the case under consideration. They are then asked to state what behavior is required of the nurse and what behavior would fail to conform to the standard of care. The judge or jury makes the final determination regarding whether the defendant-nurse in the actual situation had breached the standard of care.

When the standard of care is breached and that breach is a cause of injury to the client, the nurse may be guilty of professional malpractice. The legal definition of malpractice is "professional misconduct, improper discharge of professional duties, or failure to meet the standard of care of a professional which resulted in harm to another" (Black, 1979). Professional malpractice is a form of negligence. The legal definition of negligence is "carelessness, failure to act as an ordinary, prudent person, or action contrary to what a reasonable person would have done" (Black, 1979). These definitions state the three ways in which a nurse might commit professional malpractice:

1. By performing a duty carelessly or improperly
2. By failing to perform a duty when it is indicated
3. By performing an unauthorized act

Liability and causation. Professional nurses are liable for the consequences of their actions. The best synonym for *liable* is *responsible*. Nurses are responsible for both the direct and indirect results caused by their actions. If a client falls out of bed as a consequence of the nurse's failure to put up the side rails, the nurse is responsible for the harm to the client directly caused by that failure to act. If the nurse fails to report the improper behavior of another and a client is injured by that other person, the nurse is responsible for that injury indirectly caused by the failure to act.

Until the last 10 years, courts rarely found nurses to be independently liable for their actions (Fiesta, 1983). Most courts found that nurses acted on the basis of orders given and were not autonomous or independent providers of services. The nurse functioned ei-

ther as an agent of the physician, in which case the physician assumed all liability, or as an employee of the hospital, in which case the hospital assumed all liability. The legal doctrine that assigns liability for the entity controlling the nurse is *respondeat superior* (Black, 1979). It literally means "let the master answer" and assigns liability for nursing action to the employer of the nurse. This sort of liability of the hospital and physician is called vicarious liability.

Within the last 10 years, however, a change in the legal perspective of nursing practice has occurred. Increasingly, nurses are viewed as autonomous health care providers who practice independently in certain clearly defined situations. Recent cases have found nurses to be independently liable and did not assign the liability to physicians and hospitals where nurses were acting outside of the direction of physicians and hospitals (Black, 1979).

It is important for the professional nurse to understand the distinction between the dependent practice of nursing, which is the implementation of the physician-directed management of care, and the independent practice of nursing. Based on the California Nurse Practice Act the California Nurses' Association's definition of the independent practice of nursing is:

1. Direct and indirect client care services that ensure the safety, comfort, personal hygiene, and protection of clients and the performance of disease prevention and restorative measures.
2. The performance of skin tests and immunization techniques and the withdrawal of human blood from veins and arteries.
3. The observation of signs and symptoms, reactions to treatment, and general behavior or physical condition and the determination of whether such observations exhibit abnormal findings and the appropriate reporting and referral of such abnormalities (Calif. Bus. and Prof. Code).

The independent practice of nursing encompasses those decisions and actions taken by the nurse based on nursing judgment and a nursing management plan rather than on a management plan directed by the physician. The independent practice of nursing may theoretically become the basis for future independent liability of the nurse.

Risk Management

Rosemary Mann

Risk management is an evolving concept stemming directly from the large losses sustained by hospitals, physicians, nurses, and professional liability insurance carriers. These losses result from lawsuits for malpractice. The concept seeks to minimize losses by establishing preventive practices, appropriate reporting practices, and discovery procedures for managing a lawsuit once it has been filed. The nurse should be familiar with the concepts of risk management and their implications for nursing practice. Effective risk management enhances the quality of care and minimizes the risk of a lawsuit against the nurse.

Preventive practices

Quality assurance. Quality assurance is an umbrella term used to encompass those activities that review and evaluate actual client care and institute remedial actions to bring client care into conformity with the standard of care (ACOG, 1980). Quality assurance includes chart review, chart audit, peer review, and performance evaluations.

The first step in quality assurance is to establish the acceptable standard of care. For example, one standard might be the taking and recording of vital signs once during every 8-hour shift. Another example might be the requirement of a minimum of graduate level nursing education for a clinical nurse specialist. A third example might be a rate statement, such as no more than 10 minutes' delay in administering a timed medication. These standards often take the form of policies and protocols.

The second step in quality assurance is to construct a test of the standard. Examples of testing procedures include the following:

1. Review of case management of all clients who develop decubiti
2. Chart review of all women admitted to labor and delivery room for adequacy of nursing history
3. Chart audit of random sample of charts of postpartum women to determine frequency of entry of vital signs
4. Quarterly performance evaluation of all labor and delivery nursing personnel using the job description as a standard of performance

After the test has been constructed and administered, its results are reviewed and compared to the standard of care. If the test results show a failure to conform to the standard of care, remedial action is defined, and a repeat test or evaluation is scheduled. The goal of quality assurance is to establish that all professional conduct meets the applicable standard of care.

Informed consent. The concept of informed consent is also a form of risk management. The concept of informed consent originates with the right of persons to consent to all forms of touching. Violation of that right is called battery. Informed consent is established by law and includes the right to consent to diagnostic and therapeutic measures and to refuse them (Calif. Adm. Code). Informed consent includes the provision of information about the procedure, its risks, its anticipated results, and any alternatives to it. It is usually the responsibility of the person performing the procedure to obtain informed consent.

Many problems have arisen from the process of informed consent (Chasing, 1984). The major problem for providers is that the only test for informed consent is the client's assertion that he understands and agrees. If at a later date the client denies that he understood, the provider may have to prove that the consent process was adequate. Unfortunately the only documentation of the procedure may be a short "informed consent obtained" statement on the chart.

The professional nurse should be aware of these issues regarding informed consent:

1. Responsibility for obtaining informed consent rests with the person performing the procedure and is usually not delegated to the nurse. The nurse may, however, contribute to the education process by providing background information about the procedure or by witnessing the signature process.
2. Consent must be obtained from a competent individual. The client must not be a minor and must be in a state of mind unaffected by drugs or injury. There are exceptions to the informed consent rules that apply to emergencies and to minors.
3. The information process must be geared to the client's level of understanding. It must be done in the language and with the words that the client is capable of understanding.
4. Blanket consents (I consent to everything) and blanket releases (I release everyone from liability) are traditionally disregarded by the courts. They may be seen as an effort to misinform or deceive the client.
5. The consent is only as good as its documentation. The best documentation is by the client in her or his own handwriting included in the chart. Oral consents are also legal and binding. They are, however, difficult to prove several years later in the process of a lawsuit.
6. Client's refusal should be carefully documented and thereafter respected.

Professional liability insurance. Professional liability insurance is a risk management concept because it may prevent nurses from incurring large losses that result from a legal settlement or judgment against them. Insurance is provided by contract based on the periodic payment of a premium. Coverage is limited by a ceiling amount per lawsuit or settlement and by an aggregate total per year. For example, with $1 million/$3 million coverage the company will pay up to $1 million per suit and no more than $3 million per contract period (usually one year). The insurance policy should be investigated carefully for the type of coverage, limits of coverage, and exceptions to coverage. Some policies do not cover nurses in expanded roles. Others do not cover independent nurses or self-employed nurses.

Employed nurses are confronted with the issue of whether to carry insurance in addition to the protection offered by their employers. The main argument against such coverage is that it adds to the cost of litigation because it involves an additional insurance company who will hire more lawyers and perhaps delay the proceedings. The main argument for carrying added coverage is to supplement coverage offered by the employer. It allows the nurse as an individual to find legal representation. Personal insurance will cover the nurse for activities outside the scope of employment. It will ensure that the nurse's interests as well as the interests of the hospital and the physician are represented.

Professional competency and currency. Maintaining professional competency and currency is a critical issue in risk management and in prevention of liability risk. The standard care for a professional is conduct required of the average member of the profession with a similar background under similar circumstances. The average member of the profession maintains a level of competency that does not incorporate ignorance of the standard of care. When expert witnesses establish the standard of care, it is inferred that the average professional is informed and competent in that standard. Ignorance may not be claimed as a defense.

Occasionally nurses are placed in situations in which their professional competency is impeded by an outside factor. Two common situations are "short staffing" and "floating." Professional nurses have a duty to report situations in which the standard of care is breached by circumstances inherent in the situation (Horsley, 1981). The duty extends to the point that communication is clearly given to a person who has the power to remedy the situation. The duty may require the nurse to ask for assistance, supervision, and orientation. Ultimately the nurse may have to try to reject the assignment. Unfortunately the professional nurse may be caught in a conflict with another professional duty, that of not abandoning the client. In trying to resolve this situation the nurse should make these points clear:

1. The breach of the standard of care was reported to a supervisor who was potentially able to remedy the situation.
2. Rejection of the assignment would have placed the client in greater danger from **abandonment.**

Quality of nurse-client relationship. A final concept of prevention is the **quality of the relationship** between the nurse and the client. It has been clearly documented that clients who feel angry, frustrated, and depersonalized by their health care are more likely to sue when an injury occurs (Wecht, 1982). It is also clear that anger and frustration are common accompaniments to illness and adjustment to the post-illness state. No nurse can make every client happy all of the time, but every nurse possesses the judgment and skill necessary to support a client through illness to recovery. It is helpful to identify early those situations in which the client seems unusually upset and in which that upset is directed toward the staff. Involvement of the client in the management plan, special attention to comfort measures, and perhaps changes in nursing assignments may help the client to feel less victimized and more in control of the situation.

Reporting practices. A major aspect of risk management is appropriate **documentation of client care** and effective communication of those incidents that may give rise to a malpractice suit. Documentation of client care is accomplished by charting occurrences and observations on the client record. Communication of problem situations is accomplished by incident reports. It is critical to be aware of the differences between the client record and incident reports.

The two main purposes for keeping client records are (1) to produce a clear and accurate history of the client in relation to the illness or problem and the management plan and (2) to enhance communication between the many health care providers who may provide services in any given situation. Therefore charting must be accurate, objective, and comprehensive.

Errors. A major issue in accuracy is how to deal with **errors.** There are some guidelines to follow:
1. *Never* change someone else's charting. If it is clearly inaccurate, place a note in the chart signed by you with the correct information. Do not state that "Ms. X charted in error." Merely make the correct observation. Bring the inaccuracy to the attention of the professional who made it so that the needed correction may be made.
2. To change an error in your own charting, draw one line clearly through the error and write ERROR over it. Do not obliterate the error. Make the necessary correction and sign and date it in a separate notice that is *legibly* written.
3. Never make accusations of error directly in the chart. The appropriate place for those notations may be in an incident report.
4. Always sign your full professional name and title.

Objectivity. Objectivity in charting may be problematic when conclusions rather than observations are charted. The most troublesome conclusions are those that cast aspersions on the character or reputation of the client such as alcoholism, substance abuse, violent nature, or irresponsibility. Those conclusions may be appropriate in charting when they represent a confirmed diagnosis or when they are items in a differential diagnosis. Otherwise it is far more accurate and objective to chart the actual behavior observed. Those observations are then available to support a subsequent diagnosis should it be appropriate. For instance, instead of charting that the client was drunk, chart that the client was unsteady, unable to walk, and had an odor of alcohol on his breath.

Comprehensiveness. No nurse completes client assignments with charts tucked under one arm for immediate recording. There is delay in virtually all charting. Delay may contribute to gaps and omissions in charting with the result that the charting is not comprehensive. There are some guidelines to follow:

1. Never chart out of time sequence or try to squeeze a note in between two other notes. Place the accurate time and date next to the note currently being made and chart the circumstances accounting for delay in the charting.
2. Chart significant observations or changes immediately. Make sure the time and date are accurate.
3. Never chart that something is done before it is done, especially with medications.
4. When the nurse is too involved with client care to chart, such as in emergency situations, have a recorder note events and changes. This should include accurate times and names of persons giving care. The recorder should not be a member of the family or a casual observer but rather a person with professional responsibility for charting.
5. Omissions in charting may be interpreted to mean that the care did not occur. When vital signs are not charted and the client claims the vital signs were not taken, there is no evidence that they actually were taken (Cushing, 1982). Therefore it is critical to chart all observations in order to avoid omitting essential information.

In the event of a lawsuit the client record is the only piece of evidence created at the time of the event that documents the actual circumstances and chain of happenings. Because the chart is compiled by health care providers, inaccuracies such as lack of comprehensiveness or objectivity in the chart would infer defects in the quality of care given. Health care providers can only fall back on their recollections of the event, which may be hazy or absent with the passage of time. Providers' allegations of quality care tend to sound self-serving on the witness stand when their recollections are contested by the word of the injured client. There is simply no substitute for a careful, accurate, objective client record.

Incident reports. Incident reports document situations in which the health care professional and the institution may incur liability. These reports are submitted only to hospital or agency administrators, specifically to risk managers and insurance claims agents. They may document errors or omissions in care that breach the standard of care, irresponsible or negligent professional behavior, and unfortunate outcomes in client care such as injury, disability, or death.

Incident reports are considered to be confidential communication between the institution's staff and administration. They are *not* included in the client's chart. If an incident report is found in the client's chart, that report may be used by the plaintiff-client against the hospital and nurse. Incident reports may be found to be privileged. If written as confidential documents between the institution's attorney and the client-institution, they are protected from disclosure by attorney-client privilege. The confidential and privileged nature of the incident report makes it the preferred vehicle for documentation of breach of the standard of care. It is the means by which effective change can take place within the institution to remedy situations exposing it to liability.

There are some guidelines for the use of incident reports (Cushing, 1985):

1. Never write "An incident report has been filed" in the client's record or place a copy of the report in the client's record.
2. The report should be written accurately and clearly, giving all the essential facts. Accusations and admissions should be avoided.
3. The report should be submitted to the appropriate member of the hospital administration. The more copies distributed, the weaker the assertion that the report is confidential and privileged.

Discovery and privileged communication. Discovery occurs after a lawsuit has been filed. It is the process by which both the plaintiff and the defendant attempt to "discover" everything they can about the event in dispute. Contrary to how it is done in "Perry Mason," both sides in the lawsuit attempt to bring every fact in the dispute into play. Both sides are wary of surprises. There is a legally required exchange of information between the plaintiff and the defendant so that each side has a reasonable opportunity to develop a fair case.

All records, conversations, and events are discoverable unless they are privileged. Attorney-client privilege may protect the incident report from disclosure. The physician-client relationships is ordinarily privileged except when the client makes it an object under dispute. Then all relevant aspects of the relationship are discoverable by the other side.

There are some guidelines to follow in relation to the process of discovery:

1. All unprivileged documents are discoverable, in-

cluding private journals. If the nurse has made a private record of the event and her participating in the event, the other side may require its disclosure. Records of the nurse's participation in the event should be in the form of an incident report submitted to the appropriate member of the administration. This is protected from disclosure by the attorney-client privilege.

2. Conversations are discoverable. No outside discussion of the event should occur without the consent of a representative of the institution's attorney (i.e., the risk manager or claims agent). This prohibition includes discussions with the client, the client's family, the client's attorney and colleagues, and friends of the nurse. If, however, the incident is discussed in a recognized peer review/quality assurance activity, that discussion may be privileged under a special legal exception. If asked to participate in such a discussion, the nurse should inquire whether the discussion is privileged before participating.

3. If the nurse has received an official request for information from the plaintiff-client, full cooperation should be given to comply with the request in good faith. Compliance with the request for information should be reviewed by the institution's attorney before material is submitted.

4. All communication with the client and the client's attorneys and investigators should be made in the presence of the institution's attorney or the nurse's representative with his or her knowledge and consent.

5. Nurses should be aware of their rights to hire an attorney on their own to represent their interests. However, the hospital has the obligation to defend its employees and should provide an attorney to be present during all contacts with the client and the client's attorneys after a lawsuit has been filed.

Ethical Issues

Cheryl Harris

Three ethical issues faced by the nurse in maternity and newborn care are presented. In vitro fertilization represents the wave of the future and can be expected to raise questions involving laboratory creation of human life. Abortion issues represent past considerations about creation of human life. Neonatal intensive care units (NICUs) and Baby Doe issues represent considerations about human life once born in contrast to human life prior to birth. Ethical issues need to be carefully evaluated and considered in providing nursing care. These examples will help nurses in their consideration of ethical issues that may confront them in the future.

In vitro fertilization and embryo transplantation. A recent ethical dilemma brought to focus by modern obstetrics is the technique of in vitro fertilization with subsequent embryo transplantation, the results of which are known as test-tube babies. Since the first live birth with this technique in 1978, numerous infants have been born as a result of this procedure.

In March 1979, the Ethics Advisory Board of the Department of Health, Education, and Welfare recommended to the Secretary that in vitro fertilization be considered not only ethically acceptable but also an inevitable treatment for infertility. Several questions were raised concerning the possible disrespect for human life, for example, regarding fertilized eggs that are discarded. Steinfels (1979) suggests that the developed eggs can be discarded at 14 days or less after fertilization because normal uterine implantation will have occurred by that time.

Whether the personnel and agency performing the procedure are legally liable for defects if the child conceived by in vitro fertilization is born with physical or mental handicaps is questionable. Because of the ethical issues of working with fertilized human eggs as experimental tissue, only minimal medical research has been done. Therefore the legal risks this technique may carry are unknown (Culliton, 1978).

Another ethical question raised by Smith (1982) concerns the relative cost of in vitro fertilization. In countries with limited medical resources available, decisions need to be made regarding how funds should be spent. Should they be allocated for renal dialysis for an adult who requires this accepted and proven method of treatment or for relief of the infertility problem faced by a couple who has been attempting to have a child for years?

The issue of in vitro fertilization is legally, ethically, and morally significant. As the use of this technique proliferates, questions will probably increase.

Abortion. "Pro-life" and "pro-choice" public groups have dramatically focused ethical and legal attention on the issue of abortion. Fromer (1982) reminds us that, like it or not, nurses are very much involved in abortion issues. Nurses may assist as an abortion is performed or may refuse to do so. Nurses are asked to give advice about abortions and to provide information about where a client may obtain one. To provide service to a client seeking an abortion, nurses must understand their personal ethical position on abortion (Thompson, 1981). Following is a review of legal proceedings and court cases to provide information about the legal aspects of this issue.

Supreme Court decision. As a result of the U.S. Supreme Court decision of January 1973 *(Roe* v. *Wade),* which was reaffirmed in June 1983 and June 1986, abortion is legal anywhere in the United States (Annas, 1983b). In their momentous original seven-to-two decision, the Court declared the following:

1. During the first trimester, the state cannot bar any woman from obtaining an abortion from a licensed physician.
2. In the second trimester, the state can regulate the performance of an abortion if such regulation relates to protection of the woman's health.
3. In the third trimester, the state can regulate and even prohibit abortions, except those deemed necessary to protect the woman's life and health, and the state may impose safeguards for the fetus.

The essence of the Court's decision is that existing state abortion control laws were found to be unconstitutional on the basis that they invaded the privacy of the mother. One of the major problems with the decision is that the Court did not decide the issue of when life begins. The court reasoned that since physicians, theologians, and philosophers were unable to decide this issue, neither could the judiciary. However, the Court did define viability as the point of development at which the fetus can survive outside the uterus (perhaps with artificial aid): about 22 to 23 weeks of gestation. The decision also included the concept that the fetus is not a person, for purposes of protection under the Fourteenth Amendment. Neither the woman's spouse nor the father of the fetus has any right to prevent an abortion.

The Supreme Court decision did not provide for abortion on demand; the physician still has the right and obligation to exercise professional judgment. Moreover, the decision did not mention pregnant minors. In some states, minors can obtain an abortion without consent of their parents. However, in 1981, the Court upheld as constitutional a Utah law requiring a physician to inform parents of their minor's seeking an abortion (Fromer, 1982).

Most state laws have provisions termed *conscience clauses.* These stipulations allow physicians, institutions, nurses, and other hospital personnel to refuse to assist in abortions. Providers may refuse if participation is against their moral, ethical, or religious principles, without fear of reprisal. Recent court decisions continue to uphold these conscience clauses. Nonetheless, public (city, county, and state) hospitals must permit their facilities to be used for abortions, since they are supported by public funds.

Congressional amendment. In December 1978, Congress passed the Hyde Amendment, which severely restricts the use of federal funds for abortions.

This law allows Medicaid funds to be used for abortions under three conditions only: (1) if the woman's life is endangered by carrying the fetus to term, (2) if two physicians have determined that the pregnancy would cause severe and long-lasting physical damage to the woman, or (3) if the pregnancy was a result of rape or incest and was reported promptly to a law enforcement or public health agency.

Fromer (1982) laments the fact that the result of the Hyde Amendment is discrimination against poor women. They may be unable to afford an abortion other than through public assistance. In response to the Hyde Amendment, a class action suit was filed in federal court, but the law's constitutionality was upheld. In July 1980 the U.S. Supreme Court upheld the Hyde Amendment.

Annas (1983b) reports another attempt to legislate against abortions by an Akron, Ohio, city ordinance. One of the provisions in this ordinance dealt with the "informed consent" of women seeking an abortion. The ordinance required physicians to describe the anatomy and physiologic functions of the fetus at its stage of development, including tactile sensitivity and reaction to pain. Physicians were also required to inform the woman that serious complications and severe emotional problems might result from an abortion. They were supposed to explain to her that various agencies were available to help her after the birth of her infant if she chose not to have the abortion. The Supreme Court rejected this ordinance as unconstitutional on the grounds that the ordinance was not designed to further inform the woman regarding her consent but rather to persuade her to not grant consent.

Ethical considerations. From an ethical perspective, abortion is essentially the removal of the woman's support from the fetus. This leads to fetal death, since the fetus cannot sustain its life without the mother. Bok (1978) suggests that if an abortion is performed after the diagnosis of a fetal defect, the parents have consented to remove support from that particular fetus. This raises the issue of abortion for the fetus's sake

Camenisch (1976) concludes that one does not have the right to inflict the pain and tragic consequences of certain detectable serious diseases on an innocent infant. In his view, this argument for abortion is not offered to mask other motives such as the economic and psychologic difficulties parents of such an infant would face. Rather the abortion alleviates the suffering of the child. By this reasoning, the fetus receives "nothingness" rather than abnormality and therefore no suffering because of its own malformations. He further suggests that if we could, we would choose health, normalcy, and lack of suffering for ourselves, so why not for another? If a damaged fetus is aborted, there is more room for a normal one. This line of thought raises the issue of who should determine the definition of normal and healthy.

Summarizing the abortion controversy is difficult, but basically the pro-choice proponents believe that the mother's rights take precedence and that she should have freedom of choice and privacy. Many pro-choice advocates believe that abortions should be used only as a last resort, with contraception and adoption being other alternatives. Most pro-life proponents believe that the fetus is human from the moment of conception and as such should be protected from abortion, which ends life.

Neonatal intensive care. Hundreds of neonatal intensive care units (NICUs) are available throughout the United States. They are confronted with difficult ethical questions and legal problems of all types.

Some of the ethical dilemmas in decision making are ironically caused by the dramatic advances in neonatal-perinatal care. The medical and nursing knowledge base has increased rapidly in a relatively short time. Infants who would have automatically died 10 years ago now have a good chance to survive with few undesirable consequences. In essence, the joint disciplines of perinatology and neonatology have pushed back the point of viability to unimagined degrees. A premature infant of less than 1500 g (3 lb, 5 oz) had a slim chance of survival in 1965. Whereas an infant of 1000 g (2 lb, 3 oz) has a good chance today. The advances in neonatal surgery have significantly improved the outcome for many infants born with heart defects or other congenital anomalies. This section will explore some of the issues faced by nurses who work in a NICU.

Costs of treatment. One ethical problem that arises not only in the NICU but in all areas of perinatal care involves societal pressures about money. Newborn intensive care and fetal surgery are costly. Considering the dwindling public funds available for health care, many persons question the appropriateness of diverting monies from preventive programs (such as immunization programs for the poor) to the care of one critically ill infant. The hospitalization cost for one NICU baby can easily exceed $100,000. Federal, state, and local funds used for this type of care will not be available for other health care programs.

Unpredictable prognoses. Many infants who receive care in the NICU have an unpredictable prognosis, which present ethical dilemmas for all personnel. For example, neonatal asphyxia has a variable outcome depending on the severity of the original episode. If the infant suffers a subsequent cardiac arrest, the appropriate care might be in question. Is resuscitation of the

infant ethically correct? How long should resuscitation efforts be continued? Is there an ethical imperative to save all infants?

The NICU is designed to facilitate diagnosis and treatment of infants with immediate and acute but essentially life-threatening problems, such as aspiration pneumonia or RDS. Proper care can result in a dramatic reduction in morbidity and mortality in these infants. However, an ethical question arises as to whether it is appropriate to use equipment and intensive care skills to keep an infant with a poor prognosis alive while "neglecting" an infant with a better prognosis.

Cohen (1977) discusses violation of the ethical principle of aiding one client while harming another. He suggests that if one assumes the obligation to provide intensive care to a client, terminating this care later because another client has a higher potential for survival violates the original obligation. However, he recognizes the difficult dilemma that intensive care personnel face when they do not want to sustain infants who are beyond salvage (e.g., an infant who has suffered a massive intracranial hemorrhage). Persons who care for these infants have difficulty deciding which infant would be better served if allowed to die.

Steinfels (1978) poses the question of whether the emphasis on neonatal intensive care for smaller and smaller premature infants has resulted in decreased efforts in the prevention of prematurity. Although a birth weight of 1000 g was formerly the lower limit of saving premature infants, many NICUs now use heroic efforts to save infants weighing as little as 600 to 700 g. Steinfels also suggests that more attention be paid to the impact on the family of the premature infant who is saved but severely impaired.

Silverman (1981) suggests that many parents may believe that producing an infant with severe handicapping conditions is worse than having an infant who dies. Furthermore, he deplores the "rescuer" role of many health professionals. In this role providers make unrestrained heroic efforts to prolong even the most fragile life with no concern for the parents' wishes. Silverman asserts that because parents will have the day-to-day responsibilities for consequences of neonatal intensive care, they should be among the primary decision makers regarding the care of their infant.

Baby Doe regulations. The first Baby Doe regulation was issued by the Secretary of the Department of Health and Human Services (DHHS) in March 1983. It was in response to the report of an infant with Down's syndrome who had died in Indiana because of uncorrected esophageal atresia. In the original regulation, any institution receiving federal funding was required to exhibit a poster-size notice that stated: "Discriminatory failure to feed or care for handicapped infants in this facility is prohibited by federal law." A 24-hour, toll-free telephone hotline number was listed to be used by anyone to report suspected hospital failures as enumerated in the notice. When calls were placed, the number was answered with "Infant Doe hotline."

The initial regulation caused major disruptions (Strains, 1983). Two calls to the hotline resulted in the dispatch of two different "Baby Doe squads," one to Strong Memorial Hospital and one to Vanderbilt University Hospital. In both instances, great amounts of nursing and physician time were wasted as these professionals assisted investigators. Client care was severely disrupted because charts were unavailable for posting orders or laboratory results. One infant remained in the pediatric intensive care unit for additional unnecessary time because his chart was being reviewed by the investigators. Several parents of infants in the NICUs became alarmed and questioned the hospital administration about the care their children were receiving. One family moved their seriously ill child from Strong Memorial Hospital before his treatment had been completed because they feared the institution was intentionally harming children. The final reports at both institutions showed that exemplary care was being given in both units and that the investigation had been completely unwarranted.

The American Academy of Pediatrics and others sought a court injunction against the regulation. Although this was denied, the court ordered that the regulation needed to be reissued after prescribed waiting periods to allow for public comment on the rule. Many spoke out vehemently against the Baby Doe regulation, including Annas (1983a), who objected to the essence of the regulation, which he believes labels physicians and parents as "child abusers." He views the objectors' anger as justified because physicians treat abused children and attempt to protect them from further harm.

Annas describes the reissuance of the Baby Doe regulation in September 1983, with few changes from the original. One change was that the hotline notice was to be posted only in nurses' stations. Annas cites that in her confirmation hearing DHHS Secretary Heckler stated that the Baby Doe regulation was necessary because nurses were afraid to report cases of child neglect to proper authorities. Annas deplores this assessment of current nursing practice as demeaning and unworthy of nurses as team members in the specialized units under scrutiny.

In January 1984, final rules pertaining to handicapped infants were issued by the office of the Secretary of DHHS ("Nondiscrimination on the Basis of Handicap," 1984). Hospitals are now required to post a notice regarding the legal rights of handicapped infants. The state protective service agencies are required to establish procedures protecting children from medical neglect. Hospitals are encouraged to set up infant care review committees to review all infants who might be denied care because of handicapped conditions. The final rules do not require NICUs to provide futile treatments that prolong the act of dying.

Berseth (1983) enumerates basic ethical concerns about original Baby Doe regulations. First, she believes such rulings interject an unwelcome participant in the middle of the physician-client relationship. The decisions regarding severely impaired infants are made within the realm of privacy of that relationship. Decisions such as the ones involved in Baby Doe cases are difficult to make under the best of circumstances. Berseth asserts that families are the primary social unit with a responsibility to their infant. Since family members will be involved with the long-term care of their baby, they earn the right to be primary decision makers regarding care for their infant with problems.

If the Baby Doe regulations are inappropriate, how should decisions regarding these infants be made? Many authorities have suggested that an ethics committee composed of clergy, ethicists, lawyers, physicians, nurses, and lay persons could review each case. Watchko (1983) recommends a model in which the physician and parent would make the original decision and then review their decision with an ethics committee. If disputes resulted about what was correct, the courts would be asked to intervene. In this solution, the parents represent a noninstitutional perspective and are subject to review by other family members, social agencies, such as churches, and close friends. The physician, who represents an institutional viewpoint, is subject to peer review. The hospital-based committee serves as a consultant. If the courts are involved, they assume the primary authority.

Summary

A wide variety of ethical and legal issues arise in maternity and newborn nursing. This chapter presents a review of current ethical and legal positions involved in the care of clients. Many of the ethical dilemmas are a result of the rapid advances taking place in all specialties. The new medical technology and expanded roles for nurses have increased the chances of survival for normal infants and improved the care for all newborns. Because family-centered maternity health care raises ethical and legal questions of monumental proportions, it is essential for all nurses who care for women, new mothers, and their infants to understand these issues.

References

American College of Nurse-Midwives, American College of Obstetricians and Gynecologists, Nurses Association of the American College of Obstetricians and Gynecologists: Joint statement on maternity care, 1971. Statement superseded by joint statement on practice relationships between obstetrician/ gynecologists and certified nurse-midwives, 1982.

American College of Obstetricians and Gynecologists: Quality assurance in obstetrics and gynecology. Washington, D.C., 1980, The College.

American Nurses Association: Standards of nursing practice, Kansas City, 1973, The Association.

Annas, G., Glantz, L., and Katz, B.: The rights of doctors, nurses and allied health professionals, Cambridge, Mass., 1981, Ballinger Publishing Co., p. 35.

Annas, G.J.: Baby Doe redux: doctors as child abusers, Hastings Center Rep. 13(5), 1983a.

Annas, G.J.: *Roe* vs. *Wade* reaffirmed, Hastings Center Rep. 13(4):21, 1983b.

Bellig, L.L., and Tumasulo-Roborecky, F.: The expanded neonatal nursing role and the high-risk family, Neonatal Network 2(3):9, 1983.

Berseth, C.L.: A neonatologist looks at the Baby Doe rule: ethical decisions by edict, Pediatrics 72(3):428, 1983.

Black, H.C.: Black's law dictionary, St. Paul, 1979, West Publishing Co., p. 1260.

Bok, S.: Ethical problems of abortion, Hastings Center Rep. 19(4):19, 1978.

California Administrative Code, Section 70707.

California Business and Professions Code, section 2725. California Administrative Code, section 1470 et seq.

Camenisch, P.F.: Abortion of the fetus' own sake, Hastings Center Rep. 6(2):38, 1976.

Cohen, C.V.: Ethical problems of intensive care, Anesthesiology 47:217, 1977.

Culliton, B.E.: Ethics Advisory Board confronts conception in the test tube, Science 202:4364, 1978.

Cushing, M.: Gaps in documentation, Am. J. Nurs. 82:1899, Dec., 1982.

Cushing, M.: Incidents reports: for your eyes only, Am. J. Nurs. 85:873, Aug., 1985.

Cushing, M.: Informed consent—an MD responsibility? Am. J. Nurs. 84:437, April, 1984.

Cushing, M.: Lesions from history: the picket-guard nurse. Am. J. Nurs. 85:1073, Oct., 1985.

Darling v. Charleston Community Memorial Hospital, 211 N.E. 2nd 253 (IL 1965).

Fiesta, J.: The law and liability: a guide for nurses, New York, 1983, John Wiley & Sons, Inc.

Fromer, M.J.: Abortion ethics, Nursing Outlook 30(4):234, 1982.

Horsley, J.E.: Short-staffing means increased liability for you, R.N. 44(2):73, 1981.

Nondiscrimination on the basis of handicap: procedures and guidelines relating to health care for handicapped infants, Fed. Register 49(8):1622, 1984.

Nurses Association of the American College of Obstetricians and Gynecologists: Standards for obstetric, gynecologic,and neonatal nursing, ed. 2, Washington, D.C., 1981, The Association.

Silverman, W.A.: Mismatched attitudes about neonatal death, Hastings Center Rep. 11(6):12, 1981.

Smith, P.K.: Ethics and in-vitro fertilization, Br. Med. J. 284:1287, 1982.

Steinfels, M.: New childbirth technology: a clash of values, Hastings Center Rep. 8:9, Feb., 1978.

Steinfels, M.: In vitro fertilization: "ethically acceptable" research, Hastings Center Rep. 9:5, June, 1979.

Strains, J.E.: The American Academy of Pediatrics comments on the "Baby Doe II" regulations, N. Engl. J. Med. 309:443, 1983.

Thompson, J.B., and Thompson, H.O.: Ethics in nursing, New York, 1981, Macmillan Publishing Co., Inc.

Watchko, J.F.: Decision making on critically ill infants by parents, Am. J. Dis. Child. 137:795, 1983.

Wecht, C., editor: Legal medicine 1982, Philadelphia, 1982, W.B. Saunders Co.

Bibliography

Alton, W.: Malpractice, Boston, 1977, Little, Brown & Co.

Buley, D.D.: When the burden of proof falls on you, Nurs. 86 16:41, Feb., 1986.

Bullough, B.: The law and the expanding role of the nurse, New York, 1981, Appleton-Century-Crofts.

Creighton, H.: Law every nurse should know. Philadelphia, 1981, W.B. Saunders Co.

Creighton, H.: Liability of nurse floated to another unit, Nurs. Management 13(3):54, 1982.

Cushing, M.: Verbal No-Code orders, Am. J. Nurs. 81:1215, June, 1981.

Cushing, M.: Failure to communicate, Am. J. Nurs. 82:1597, Oct. 1982.

Cushing, M.: Legal side: first, anticipate the harm . . . , Am. J. Nurs. 85:137, Feb., 1985.

Cushing, M.: Legal side: how a suit starts, Am. J. Nurs. 85:655, June, 1985.

Cushing, M.: Legal side: how courts look at nursing practice acts, Am. J. Nurs. 86:131, Feb., 1986.

Duke Univeristy Hospital Nursing Services: Quality assurance, guidelines for nursing, Philadelphia, 1980, J.B. Lippincott Co.

Eggland, E.: Charting: how and why to document your care daily and fully, Nurs. '80 10:(12):38-43, 1980.

Elias, S., and Annas, G.J.: Perspectives on fetal surgery, Am. J. Obstet. Gynecol. 145:807, 1983.

Freebairn, J., and Gwinup, K.: Ethics, values, and health, Irvine, Calif., 1980, Concept Media.

Fromer, M.J.: Ethical issues in sexuality and reproduction, St. Louis, 1983, The C.V. Mosby Co.

Huttman, B.R.: Dilemmas: not murder—just nothing, Am. J. Nurs. 85:959, Sept., 1985.

Isil, O.A.: Legal risks and perinatal health care. NAACOG update series, lesson 13, vol. 1, 1984.

LaBar, C.: Filling in the blanks on prescription writing, Am. J. Nurs. 86:30, Jan., 1986.

LaRocco, S.A.: Dilemmas in practice: a case of patient abuse, Am. J. Nurs. 85:1233, Nov., 1985.

Murchison, I., Nichols, T., and Hanson, R.: Legal accountability in the nursing process, ed. 2, St. Louis, 1982, The C.V. Mosby Co.

Penticuff, J.H.: Ethics in obstetric and gynecologic nursing, NAACOG update series, lesson 26, vol. 1, 1984.

Regan, W.A.: Nursing malpractice: a giant leap on damages, R.N. 44(12):69, 1981.

Rhodes, A., and Miller, R.: Nursing and the law, ed. 4, Rockville, Md., 1984, Aspen Publishing Co., p. 200 et seq.

Rocreto, L., and Maleski, C.: The legal dimensions of nursing practice, New York, 1982, Springer Publishing Co.

Shaffer, M.K., and Pfeiffer, I.L.: Dilemmas in practice: nursing research and patients' rights, Am. J. Nurs. 86:23, Jan., 1986.

Smith, S.J., and Davis, A.J.: Ethical dilemmas: conflict among rights, duties, and obligations, Am. J. Nurs. 80:1463, Aug., 1980.

Susina, S.V.: When drugs are used for unapproved indications, Legal Aspects of Pharm. Pract. 2(7):1, 1980.

Nursing Care of the Childbearing Family

Maternity nursing is initiated in response to women and other members of the childbearing family seeking help for actual or potential health problems. Maternity nursing today is a complex health service. Nursing activities range across the health-illness continuum from promotion of health to client rehabilitation. The greater scope and more sophisticated nature of the care offered the pregnant woman and her family today have mandated a collaborative, team approach to maternity care, involving the woman, her family, nurses, physicians, nutritionists, and other health professionals. No one group of health practitioners possesses either the competence or the time to act as the sole dispenser of health care—full utilization of all groups is needed.

This chapter includes an overview of the beliefs that serve as a basis for maternity nursing, a description of the range and organization of nursing services offered, and a discussion of the core of maternity nursing—the nurse-client relationship. A plan of care for the childbearing family is outlined to demonstrate one way of putting the content in this unit together.

Beliefs

Maternity nursing has as its basis the beliefs* common to all nursing, as well as specific beliefs that relate directly to the childbearing family. The specific beliefs outlined below serve as guidelines to the development of health services on national and local levels and for the selection of pertinent nursing strategies for maternity clients, their offspring, and their families.

1. *Childbearing is family centered.* The family is recognized by nursing and medical groups as the major

---

*For a more detailed discussion of beliefs about nursing see Styles, M.: On nursing: toward a new endowment, St. Louis, 1982, The C.V. Mosby Co.

support system for the pregnant woman and her infant.

2. *Childbearing is in essence a normal physiologic function.* For most women and their offspring, pregnancy and birth represent a physically and emotionally safe process.

3. *The childbearing process has cultural significance.* Some cultural expectations may introduce elements capable of producing crisis situations for women and their families.

4. *Continuity of care is essential to the health of the pregnant woman and her infant.* Maintenance of the biopsychosocial well-being of the gravida and her developing baby requires constant vigilance and timely intervention when appropriate.

5. *Parenthood is a responsible role.* Availability of different methods of birth control to an increasingly large number of people within our society means that parenthood is becoming more of a voluntary state.

6. *Children have a right to be "well-born" and to be provided with opportunities to realize their potential.* Care and socialization of children are recognized and accepted as functional prerequisites of any society.

These beliefs are subscribed to by professional nursing groups. Each nurse also will have personal beliefs about childbearing and the role the nurse will play in it. Personal beliefs can either support or undermine professional beliefs. Nurses need to be aware of this potential source of conflict.

Nature and Scope of Maternity Nursing

Maternity nursing involves actions that can be designated as preventive, curative, or rehabilitative in nature (Table 4.1). It spans the lifetime of an individual from preconceptional planning of children through pregnancy and birth and the early adjustment of the family

Table 4.1
Nature and Scope of Maternity Nursing

Goal	Examples of Nursing Actions
Prevention	Health education of people: nutrition, general hygiene (rest, exercise, stress management, cleanliness), signs and symptoms of illness, community resources (clinics, etc.), environmental agents to avoid (drugs/chemicals, communicable disease, x rays)* Encouragement for women to keep scheduled appointments Development of a caring and trusting relationship with each client and her family Following assessment for level of knowledge and readiness to learn, health education regarding expected physical and psychologic changes and expected duration of those changes
Cure	Identification of family history or personal history of biophysical (e.g., genetic disorder), psychologic (e.g., recurrent depression), or social (e.g., poverty) risk factors Continuous assessment for detection of risk factors whenever nurse is in contact with childbearing family Education of childbearing family, supplemented by written information, regarding signs and symptoms of complications (e.g., visual disturbances, vaginal bleeding) and emergency telephone numbers Maintenance of client records

Rehabilitation	Rapid notification of appropriate health team member (e.g., physician, nutritionist, social worker)
	 Assisting physician to
	      Explain (and re-explain) problem and its management to woman and family
	      Carry out prescribed therapy
	      Encourage client cooperation during therapy and follow-up
	      Maintain records
	 Maintenance of a trusting and caring relationship with woman and family
	 Assisting woman and family to cope with grief associated with being termed *high risk* (a term that some people see as a stigma) or having her fetus considered to be at risk; careful assessment of perceptions, coping mechanisms, and support systems permits nurse to use crisis theory (see Chapter 1) as a format for care (see Chapter 26 for details)

*In the broader sense, each nurse participates in prevention through working for legislation and with community efforts to reduce hazards in the environment and to educate the public regarding health maintenance.

to a newborn child. These activities may be carried out in the home, clinic, or hospital.

Preventive actions. The preventive aspects of maternity care include health promotion and prevention of disease states. Efforts are made to increase and strengthen the individual's ability to withstand the stress of everyday living. Nursing actions associated with these efforts represent many of the nurse's independent functions. They occur wherever nurse and client meet, whether the client is directly under the care of a physician or not. The nurse who teaches good nutrition, personal hygiene, and beneficial exercises to a pregnant woman is promoting the health of the woman and her developing fetus. The nurse who encourages a teenager to seek care for pregnancy or who discusses sexual adjustment with pregnant couples is acting to promote health and to prevent possible complications.

Curative actions. The early detection of physical and emotional disabilities in the mother or infant and initiation of corrective measures are essential components of maternity nursing. The checkpoints in prenatal evaluation correspond to the times during pregnancy when difficulties are known to occur. Women with diseases complicating pregnancy may be confined to a hospital for continuous evaluation and treatment.

Cesarean birth may be chosen to safeguard mother or child.

Rehabilitative actions. Rehabilitative activities are directed toward returning an individual to his or her previous state with an equal or greater ability to function. The care given a pregnant teenager illustrates the rehabilitative aspects of maternity care. Nurses hope that through the physical and emotional support provided these young people they will be able to complete their development toward responsible adulthood. Nurses have provided the impetus to founding teenage clinics, high school programs for pregnant teenagers, and follow-up care to help teenagers give their children the mothering needed.

■ ■ ■

Nursing actions—preventive, curative, and rehabilitative—often overlap as nurses give care to any one client. The nurse responsible for the care of a premature infant in a neonatal intensive care unit makes continuous assessments of the infant's condition and modifies care to maintain an optimal state (curative). The nurse promotes the infants' future welfare by educating the parents regarding their child's care following discharge (preventive). Weaning the infant from oxygen therapy and respirators is essential prior to discharge (rehabilitative).

Regionalization of Health Care Services

Diagnostic and therapeutic advances during the past decade have resulted in the evolution of new types of facilities for the care of gravidas and newborns at high risk. Newly acquired understanding of pathophysiology of pregnancy-induced conditions and intercurrent disorders as well as of fetal and neonatal problems and the capacity to apply this knowledge clinically required an appropriate setting in which severely ill clients could be managed. Simultaneously, developments in electronics, biochemistry, genetics, and surgical procedures have resulted in the availability of practical methods of identification and monitoring of risk factors. These advances and developments have revolutionized the care of clients at high risk. The need was created for new facilities, reorganization of services, and specially trained personnel in several disciplines who must function collaboratively for lives to be saved.

There is excellent evidence that mortality decreases when high risk is identified and intensive care applied. In addition, follow-up studies have shown that serious residual handicaps (physical and mental) of surviving infants have been dramatically reduced.

It is neither feasible nor reasonable for each hospital to develop and maintain the full spectrum of medical and nursing specialists, laboratory capabilities, and facilities with equipment. As a consequence, care is being regionalized. That is, all levels of care will be available within a given area, but facilities will be organized to provide different levels of care. A coordinated system within a region first requires the designation of certain hospitals for provision of levels of care based on their capacity to provide the care required. To provide appropriate services and continuity of care for each client, an effective pattern of communication for consultation and for transport of clients is mandatory. Fundamental to all these activities is a regional program for continuing education of personnel.

Ideally, a regionalized system includes primary care and three levels of facilities within a designated geographic area. Level I facilities have three main functions: (1) the management of normal pregnancy, labor, and delivery, (2) the earliest possible identification of high-risk pregnancy and high-risk newborns, and (3) the provision of competent care in the event of unanticipated obstetric or neonatal emergencies.

Level II facilities provide care for a number of maternal and neonatal complications as well as offer a full range of maternity and neonatal care in uncomplicated cases.

Level III facilities, the *regional centers,* have the capacity to manage uncomplicated maternity and neonatal cases and the most complex disorders. In addition, the regional centers provide outreach services, for example, consultation and continuing education for obstetricians, pediatricians, and nurses within the region.

Nurse-Client Relationships

The nurse-client relationship is an essential ingredient in nursing care because it assists the client in identifying and attaining desired goals. The nurse's interpersonal skills and the ability to communicate are basic to establishing and maintaining an effective nurse-client relationship. With practice the nurse can develop a repertoire of communication techniques that facilitate the interchange. Contributing to the nurse's success as a communicator is the ability to establish a trusting relationship, empathize with the client, and develop mutually acceptable goals and therapy for care. The nurse, aware that personal values and beliefs affect performance, is in a key position to help clients make logical decisions concerning health matters.

The nurse-client relationship is a dynamic *process* that evolves sequentially through four phases: preparation, initiation, consolidation and growth, and termination. Each phase accomplishes certain tasks and builds on a previous phase or phases.

PROCESS

Much of nursing takes place during interactions between two individuals: the client and the nurse. These interactions may be described as ones in which one person has "the intent of promoting the growth, development, maturity, improved functioning, and improved coping with the life of the other" (Rodgers, 1961). The process of developing a relationship is the same regardless of the time frame (short or long term) in which it takes place.

Preparation phase. Before the first meeting with a client the nurse gathers as much data as possible and plans the first interaction. For example, reviewing the prenatal record prior to admission for labor alerts the nurse to prenatal client problems and allows the nurse to personalize the routines of admission.

Initiation phase. The first meeting of client and nurse tends to set the stage for future contacts. The nurse attempts to establish a climate of trust, open communication, mutual understanding, and acceptance. The provision of *privacy* for the interview or ex-amination encourages client to retain a sense of control and dignity. Clients vary in the amount of privacy they deem essential. For some the gynecologic examination is embarrassing as well as frightening. Some may pre-fer female medical or nursing personnel rather than male.

One nurse reported that in a clinic in Texas the women and their families did not appear to want privacy during in-terviews. They would initiate conversations concerning their ailments in the waiting room. However, the bathrooms, originally designed with doors opening into the lobby, had to be moved down a hallway because no client would enter them in view of others.

It is probably better to err on the side of providing too much privacy. Then, based on cues from clients, an appropriate level of privacy can be provided.

The dialogue begins with an exchange of names. The client determines which name preference she pre-fers: Mrs., Ms., Miss, or given name. With some clients, using a given name tends to set them at ease, while others may view this practice as presumptuous.

During the initiation phase the nurse gathers bio-graphic and physical data. As information is elicited about support persons the woman wishes to include in her pregnancy and delivery, the gravida and her hus-band need to be made aware of agency policies that outline the extent to which family members may par-ticipate in care. If the couple is uncomfortable with the agency's policies, they may contact another agency for care. In addition to gathering and compiling data, the nurse has the following additional tasks to complete.

Contract for care. The nurse establishes a contract for care based on client participation and mutual goal setting. In establishing a contract for care, the nurse might introduce the topic by saying, "Let me tell you what to expect." The care as outlined by the nurse is then compared to the client's expectations, and any conflicts are resolved. The contract is not a formal one in the legal sense. Through discussion of expectations of nurse and client, conflict can be minimized and the client's sense of security increased.

Mutual goal setting. Determining appropriate nursing care for a particular client is largely the respon-sibility of the nurse. The extent to which the client accepts the therapy and complies with the recom-mended health regimen is an essential element in the success of the process. Formerly there was a tendency for medical and nursing personnel to dictate the form of therapy and the client's participation. Today many clients expect to share in planning their care and to make informed choices concerning therapy.

Nurse and client review the goals for care to arrive

at mutual goals. Then they discuss the client behavior needed to achieve those goals.

EXAMPLE
Goal: Maintain the client's hemoglobin and hematocrit within normal limits.
Client actions:
1. Select an adequate diet that reflects client's likes, dislikes, and availability of nutrients.
2. Eat prescribed diet daily.
3. Take iron supplements as directed.

During discussion innovative solutions to client dif-ficulties are often determined. Involving clients in the nursing care process increases their awareness of their responsibility for health. During the process of ther-apy, nurse and client mutually make periodic evalua-tions. At times, because of work related pressures, it is easy to resume old patterns of relationships (i.e., the all-knowing nurse and the dependent client). A con-scious effort has to be made to maintain a partnership.

Compliance with care. Once mutual goals have been established, the nurse may use various techniques to prompt compliance with the care. The atmosphere in which care is provided can be instrumental in the success of the therapy. Making clinics and hospitals more homelike can have a beneficial effect. A relaxed atmosphere encourages voicing of client needs and ex-change of ideas.

In a small rural community the nurses in the maternity clinic were concerned about the inadequate diets of their clients. To improve their clients' diets they instituted "morn-ing breaks" at the clinic; nurses and clients contributed re-freshments. Only healthful drinks were served (e.g., milk, fruit juice), and the food was prepared using natural ingre-dients. The women swapped recipes along with other helpful knowledge about pregnancy and child rearing. The health workers felt this approach to attain the goal of improved nutrition was one of the most successful in their health pro-gram.

Another effective technique to encourage compli-ance with care is to ensure client understanding of therapy (Table 4.2). Barriers to understanding can arise in various ways. Cultural differences can preclude understanding. Language differences may necessitate an interpreter. High anxiety levels can make it impos-sible for the client to "take in" the meaning of pre-scribed treatment. The nurse needs to repeat the teach-ing or counseling as often as it is needed.

Noncompliance with care may have serious conse-quences. Much of maternity care is preventive in na-ture. Preventive care depends on maintaining the health of mother and fetus, the prompt detection of disease, and the institution of remedial measures. Collaboration between nurse and client is essential for success. Client and nurse share accountability for successful health

Table 4.2
Examples of Client Noncompliance

Example	Reason for Noncompliance
I didn't take the iron pills; they made me constipated so I felt if they did that they couldn't be helping me.	Noncompliance related to negative side effects of prescribed treatment and knowledge deficit.
Client sent home and told to be on strict bed rest with bathroom privileges. Client has four children under 6 years of age, no help, husband at work from 6 AM to 7 PM.	Noncompliance related to family demands.
Client advised she was underweight and anemic; a special diet and iron supplementation were ordered.	Noncompliance related to health beliefs that run counter to professional advice.

care. Each needs to participate in a responsible way in decisions about care.

Confidentiality. Confidentiality is a legal right of clients (Chapter 3). If a client volunteers information that the nurse feels must be shared with other medical personnel, the nurse must make this clear to the client. In some instances a client may not wish her obstetric history reviewed openly with her husband. She may have had an infant out of wedlock or an elective abortion of which her husband is not aware. The knowledge is relevant to her obstetric care, but otherwise such information is treated confidentially. The client needs assurance that personal data will be recorded and stored for future use in such a way that it is not available to the general public. Confidentiality engenders trust between client and nurse and is therefore a key element in communication.

During the initiation phase the nurse and client lay the groundwork for an individualized plan of care. Development of that plan occurs during the next phase.

Consolidation and growth phase. Throughout the consolidation and growth phase the nurse and client clarify goals, plan care, and put the plans into action. It is a phase based on mutual trust, growing insight into the reasons behind behaviors, and a working together for the client's benefit. Two important aspects of this phase are the closeness between the nurse and client and client dependency.

Closeness. Caplan (1961) noted that nurses can be adept at bridging distances between themselves and the client. The ability to become close to the client is an advantage in their roles as counselors. Closeness is demonstrated in many ways.

Psychosocial closeness. Nurses, through their involvement with clients and family members, are able to develop trusting relationships and act as emotional supports. Because clients see nurses as less remote than physicians, they feel freer to speak openly with them about their feelings and to ask questions.

Closeness of space. Nurses touch clients; they stand close to them and seek eye contact. Nurses often comfort clients by putting an arm around them, stroking their hair, holding their hands. Closeness in space engenders feelings of safety in a client, much as parental closeness engenders feelings of safety in a child.

Closeness in time. Nurses are present with clients in times of stress and crisis. They participate in the birth process with families and are there when clients face grief or despair. Nurses are also present to share the joy of birth and recovery from illness. Families' memories of important events often include their feelings about their nurses' support and concern.

Client dependency. A certain amount of client dependency may be observed during the consolidation and growth phase. As long as dependency does not interfere with the client's ability to participate in care, it serves to cement the relationship. It is as though the client were saying, "If I need you, I know you will be there." As the nurse establishes a "safe" environment, the client becomes free to express anxieties or doubts openly, confident she will be heard by an understanding person. Dependency acts as a basis for future independent action as the client develops a feeling of self-esteem and respect for her own judgment.

Most of the care given to clients takes place during the consolidation and growth phase of the interpersonal relationship. During this phase the care given includes the following:

- Discussion of ongoing client problems and identification of stressors
- Evaluation of methods used by the client and her family to cope with present or potential crises and suggestions of alternatives as necessary
- Exploration of family and community support systems and plans for assistance in the care of other children as well as the new baby

Gradually both client and nurse reveal more of their true feelings and perceptions and share their concepts of the purposes of therapy and the responsibilities of client and professional worker. Part of the nurse's functions will relate to the process of evaluation of client progress and consequent restructuring of plans.

Termination phase. The termination phase serves as a summary for all that has gone before. Nurse and client review the goals they have accomplished and plan for future health care. This phase of the nurse-client relationship leaves a final impression of the health care system with the client. A positive impression can affect the client's future health maintenance.

Satisfied clients are more likely to return for health care that is preventive rather than just curative.

PERSONAL CHARACTERISTICS

Certain personal characteristics of the nurse have a positive effect on the nurse-client relationship. The nurse's ability to trust and be trusted, to empathize, and to work with the client toward mutually acceptable goals facilitates the interpersonal process.

Trust. When individuals trust each other they feel secure. Travelbee (1971) has defined trust as "the assured belief that other individuals are capable of assisting in times of distress and will probably do so."

Certain descriptive terms occur again and again when people are asked to describe someone they would trust. These include *consistent, reliable, genuine, sincerely interested,* and *accepting.* Nurses can give care without trusting or being trusted; however, the level of care tends to be more mechanical because the focus is limited to physical aspects.

Empathy. Empathy, the ability "to sense the client's private world *as if* it were your own but without losing the *'as if'* quality" (Rodgers, 1961), is an important component of the intrapersonal process. An empathetic individual is sensitive to another's thoughts and feelings. Care is taken to communicate this awareness while retaining one's own identity. Sympathy differs from empathy. Sympathy includes a feeling *for* another person—"I feel sorry for her." Empathy implies getting *inside* another person, feeling what that person is feeling—"I sensed in her (the client) an awful loneliness."

The uniqueness of each individual precludes our complete understanding of another. Yet the potential for understanding grows with life experiences and with increased self-awareness. The ability "to walk in another's shoes" describes the important aspect of empathy.

DECISION MAKING

Many of the individuals who seek nurses' help will be concerned about making major *decisions* that will affect their lives and those of others. Sexually mature adults make many decisions concerning their sexuality. If a couple decides to have intercourse, they must decide whether the woman is to become pregnant or not. If the woman becomes pregnant, the woman or couple must decide to abort the fetus, become a parent, or give up a child for adoption. To maintain health, sexually mature adults make decisions about living health-sustaining life-styles, attaining the use of health facilities or engaging the supervision of health professionals.

The values, beliefs, and attitudes of the individuals are factors in the decision-making process. Some persons make decisions based on carefully gathered information and consideration of consequences. Others make decisions without thought for the future, based on ignorance, prejudice, or myth.

Nurses may assist clients with decision making in a number of ways.

Collection of data. Sufficient valid data is needed as a basis for problem solving. The nurse can provide advanced and technical information at a level appropriate for client understanding, when the client is ready to hear it. The clinical significance of the information as it relates to the health of the mother, fetus, or newborn is shared with the client. Clients are referred to other resources for specialized information when the nurse is unable to provide it (e.g., genetic counseling, social services).

Consideration of alternative actions. The nurse can review with the client the risks and consequences of each action and the responsibilities each choice involves. A number of alternatives is discussed with the client. For instance, choices related to infant feeding are introduced early if possible. The parents therefore have ample time to discuss the advantages and disadvantages of breast and bottle feeding for their infant and themselves.

Formulation of outcome criteria for evaluation. The nurse and client can consider reasonable standards for the behavior of the client, newborn child, or family members. Rigid adherence to impossible standards can be destructive to self-concept. The nurse needs to be aware of the tendency to consider the standards as correct and appropriate and the individual's performance a failure. Such a response to a change in expectations may be seen as a result of incidents occurring during labor:

- Janice and Peter O. had attended prenatal classes and were planning a "natural birth" without analgesia or anesthesia. Everything progressed as planned until just before delivery. The fetal heart rate slowed to 90 (normal rate: 120 to 160). The physician decided to use outlet forceps to hasten the infant's birth. Anesthesia was used to numb the vagina and perineum; forceps were applied; and the infant was delivered. The cord was wrapped three times around the infant's neck and was considered the probable cause of the slowing of the heart rate. In spite of the fact that Janice could not have foreseen or controlled the event, she and Peter were depressed by her inability to deliver their infant as planned.

Nurses teaching prenatal or other classes need to discuss what can happen. Such interactions with the childbearing family can help eliminate unrealistic expectations. Role playing "what if . . ." can be used as an effective learning technique.

Problem solving and decision making. The nurse can encourage participation in decisions affecting an individual's welfare. Participation prompts a feeling of control over one's destiny, and self-esteem is increased. Therefore, when possible, the *locus* or place of decision making is with the client. Once the client assumes responsibility for a decision, accountability for the outcome rests with the client. If a decision is considered to be detrimental to the well-being of the mother or child, every effort is made to have the client modify the decision.

■ At 5 PM (1700) a woman phoned the delivery room at the hospital and reported that her membranes had ruptured, her contractions were coming every 5 minutes and were regular, and that she had considerable bloody mucus discharge. The nurse replied, "You sound as though you are in active labor. Because this is your third baby, you need to come to the hospital right away." The woman said she would wait until the other children had had their dinner. The nurse replied that she should come at once.

The mother persisted with preparing the children's dinner. At 6 PM (1800) her contractions became very strong. She delivered her baby at home at 6:15 PM (1815).

In this instance the mother made the decision not to go to the hospital when instructed (the *locus* of decision making was with the client), and the outcome (home birth) rested with her. In some instances, because of knowledge and expertise, the professional care giver assumes responsibility for decisions. The nursing care of critically ill infants illustrates the decision-making responsibilities of the nurse-clinician. The nurse must decide when the infant needs assistance with respiration or other therapy. The nurse assumes responsibility for decisions because the *locus* of decision making is with the care giver.

ESSENTIAL FACTORS

Communication. Communication is central to the nurse-client relationship. The communication process includes verbal (spoken or written) as well as nonverbal behavior. Every aspect of our lives conveys information about ourselves to others. The onlooker interprets and makes value judgments about such things as the way people dress, where they were born, their accents, or their church affiliations. Each culture sets up behavior and speech patterns appropriate to different

situations. These are known as normative patterns. Knowledge of these patterns is acquired by members of that culture as a result of mingling with various social groups and informally learning these patterns. The failure on the part of a stranger to that culture to recognize these communication patterns and operate within their context can lead to misunderstandings and the inability to carry on meaningful exchanges.

The use of language (verbal or written communication) and of space, time, touch and eye contact (nonverbal communication) can affect the quality of data nurses give to or obtain from clients. An understanding of these elements enables the nurse to carry on meaningful communication with clients.

Verbal communication

Language. The social or lay language of any culture contains elements that are known and recognized by all who speak it. Each subgroup in the culture, however, develops a language of its own. Subgroups may be determined by ethnic origin, age, or profession. The nurse learns a professional language as part of being initiated into the nursing group. For transactions between colleagues, a professional language facilitates precise, meaningful exchange of information.

Many clients in maternity nursing, however, are not familiar with medical terminology. Language that is not clear to both the sender and the receiver of communication will result in unmet goals. The nurse may have to translate terms such as dilation and effacement of the cervix or involution of the uterus. Information must be given in familiar language with feedback for mutual understanding. Otherwise, much of what is said is either unclear or lost.

Language may also be used defensively. Nurses who maintain a joking relationship with clients regardless of the seriousness of the client's condition may be acting to defend themselves against the hurt and weight of involvement in the pain of others. Using language as a defense mechanism is often an unconscious act; the nurse is unaware of why she or he behaves in such a manner. According to Luft (1970), "The individual, like the group of which he is a part, has limited awareness of the sources of his own behavior and the effects of his behavior on others."

Techniques. Certain communication techniques have proven successful as tools for strengthening therapeutic relationships. To become skilled in their use requires considerable practice. At first they may seem cumbersome or obvious. Gradually, however, they become part of the nurse's communication pattern and as such are useful in establishing the *meaning* of what one hears or says. Most of the techniques presented here are used together to elicit the information sought.

1. *Listening* is an active not a passive activity. It takes effort to hear what another says and to interpret and analyze its meaning. Nurses have to concentrate on the speaker, not on themselves, in an unbiased manner. A client may say something that triggers the listener's own values, reminding the nurse of personal concerns. Only practice will help the nurse cope with these interruptions to true listening. Listening is a sign of respect for another and acts as a powerful reinforcer.

2. *Broad opening statements* give the client an opportunity to select the topic for discussion. "What" questions can be helpful; for example, "What are you thinking about?" or "What were you able to do about . . . ?" "Why" questions tend to make a client defensive; for example, "Why did you miss last week's appointment?" This question might be more appropriately worded "I noticed you were not here for your appointment last week."

Closed questions that can be answered "yes" or "no" are to be avoided if the nurse is trying to find out what something means to a client. To gather demographic data the nurse would ask, "Are you single, married, or divorced?" A simple "yes" or "no" to these questions is sufficient. If the nurse is trying to discover how the client feels about not having a support person, a question such as "It must be hard to be on your own just now; how are you managing?" would be more effective. The nurse needs to be sensitive to a client's reluctance to discuss certain ideals or feelings and respect the need for privacy. The nurse can return to the topic when the bond between nurse and client is stronger.

3. *Focusing* assists the client in identifying and expanding an area of importance. The nurse can encourage the client to describe how she perceives an event. The client might be asked to compare a present response with a similar past experience. The nurse can bring the primary problem into focus by developing a time frame for a sequence of events. The following example illustrates this technique:

■ Patricia L., aged 14 years, came to the nurse in the clinic because she thought she was pregnant. During the interview with the nurse, Patricia gave a rambling report about how she loved her boyfriend, about her parents' angry divorce, and how they blamed everything on her. The nurse said, "Let me see if I can get the time frame worked out. Your parents got a divorce, and you feel they blame you. You have a loving boyfriend, you had intercourse, and now you feel you are pregnant. Let's talk about the possibility of your being pregnant first, and then we will go back to the others."

The nurse focused attention on the primary problem through identifying and analyzing the client's concerns.

4. *Clarification* occurs when the nurse attempts to elicit the *meaning* of what the client is saying. Often the client will find it difficult to express emotional responses in other than a hesitant or fragmentary manner. The nurse needs to help the client clarify feelings as a first step in the client's recognition of the correlation between thought and action. Statements such as "Did you mean . . . ?" or "I can't quite follow you. Are you saying . . . ?" are helpful.

5. *Restating* is the repetition of a client's main thought or concern. Restating can bring attention to a thought that may otherwise be treated as trivial. It indicates also that the nurse is listening attentively. The following example illustrates this technique:

■ Marie talked to the nurse about her concerns over taking care of the baby. She said she had no experience with children as she had been an only child. Her mother found the care of one child enough and had not had any more. Marie said she was like her mother in so many ways, people often thought they were sisters. She wanted the home care nurse to come and check on how she was doing.

The nurse commented, 'You said you were like your mother [restating]. Did you mean like your mother in finding the care of a baby difficult [clarification]?''

---

6. *Validation* of what is said and its meaning to the client conveys the nurse's understanding of not just content but also the feelings the client has about the content. If the nurse can reflect this accurately, the client senses the nurse's empathy, interest, and respect.

EXAMPLE

Client: I hate having to wear maternity clothes. It makes it so obvious you are pregnant. People treat you so differently, as though you weren't attractive anymore, just a dowdy old housewife.

Nurse: It is hard to see one's figure change—hard to get used to it can make a person feel quite different about herself [validation].

The information the nurse gains from interviews or discussions with clients forms an important part of the data used to plan nursing care. The professional nurse assumes responsibility for obtaining data that is pertinent and verifiable. The techniques discussed above help the nurse attain this end.

Nonverbal communication

Space. Hall's study (1966) of man's use of space showed that middle-class North Americans use space

Table 4.3
Examples of Topics Discussed and Use of Communication—Space, Voice, Touch, and Eye Contact—and Common Violations

Topic	Space	Tone of Voice	Touch and Eye Contact	Common Violations
Secret or sensitive information exchanged with client (e.g., positive VDRL); comforting parents whose infant has a defect; emotional responses of parents as they hold and admire child and express their love for child or each other	Intimate (3-18 in) Message: I accept you; I want to help you; I love you	Low, soft murmur	Nurse establishes eye contact with client; sits close to client in *en face* position; touches client (e.g., puts arm around shoulder); parents stroke, caress, kiss infant or each other	Condition of infant reported while nurse is standing at foot of mother's bed; sensitive information given out in loud voice during report at change of shift; healthy infants separated from parents before intimacy can take place
Report of health status; coaching during labor; assisting with feeding an infant; explanations of care; reports to other staff	Personal (1½-4 ft) Message: concern, warmth, friendliness	Soft, clear, concise	Eye contact maintained; nurse leans toward client; client discusses care with family; touch is with relaxed hand, gentle sure movements	Walks away from client while giving instructions; hurried, abrupt movements; voice loud, can be overhead by other clients, scolding tone; touch jerky, with flat of hand, poking with fingertips, grasps too firmly
Small group teaching of health care topics; discussions with parents in shared accommodation	Social (4-12 ft) Message: I like you; let us share this time	Louder, more definite, more formal	May stand or sit; eye contact maintained while talking; body gestures expansive, more formalized	Mumbling explanations; talking to one of a group only; gestures too unrestrained, "comes on too strong"; shouts instructions, greetings
Lecture topics; sanitation, health insurance	Public (over 12 ft) Message: I have information for you	Loud, clear; may be used dramatically	Gestures exaggerated to be seen (e.g., arms flung out); eye contact moves over whole audience	Use of models, charts, etc. that can be seen only by those in the front row; ignoring questions; staff shouting to each other in hospital corridors

between communicators in definite ways. There are distances used to connote varying interpersonal relationships. Voice range and tone, the topic discussed, and body language employed are specific for each range. Hall described four distances as follows: *intimate*, 3 to 18 inches; *personal*, 1½ to 4 feet; *social*, 4 to 12 feet; and *public*, beyond 12 feet. Voice tones progress from a murmur to a loud voice; topics discussed change from top secret to information considered in the public domain; and body language changes from caresses, stroking, and eye contact to exaggerated gestures and change in body stance (Table 4.3).

Personal involvement and concern are conveyed by interactions carried on within the intimate distance. The nurse can act as a model for personal involvement by showing an apprehensive new father how to enfold his infant in his arms and hold the baby close. At other times the nurse wishes to convey only professional concern even though the activities takes place in the intimate distance. The nurse can use various techniques to indicate the professional versus the personal nature of an activity. When performing a vaginal examination, for example, the nurse begins by giving the purpose of the procedure. She then assumes a definite body set: face becomes impassive and preoccupied, the touch firm but gentle and precise, and the eyes directed away from the client's eyes. By acting in this manner, the nurse changes the connotation from personal to professional. She thereby minimizes client embarrassment. In addition to enhancing the nurse-client relationship, the body set accomplishes another objective. It permits the nurse to concentrate thought processes on what is being palpated by eliminating distracting stimuli.

At times the nurse consciously or unconsciously prevents true communication with clients by using space inappropriately. The nurse pauses at a client's doorway and calls, "How are you?" The reply is usually noncommittal. An individual is unable to discuss personal matters in a public distance range and may feel frustrated at being placed in this unsuitable position.

Another example of the use of space is the procedure adopted in a physician's or midwife's office. Once an examination is completed, the woman is given time to dress and is then seated in a chair by the practitioner's desk. A pattern of personal distance is established. Personal matters may be discussed in a soft voice while maintaining eye contact. A feeling that the practitioner has a warm and friendly interest in the client, as well as a professional one, is conveyed.

Another aspect of space is the concept of territoriality. This has been called *personal space* (Sommers, 1959). It moves with the individual, with the body as its center. Violations of personal space arouse defensive responses, either covert or overt. Some of the difficulty experienced by those anxious to replace traditional hospital maternity units with family-centered ones relates to the concept of personal space. Nurses and physicians had to share or give up space that was formerly theirs. Fathers, grandparents and siblings now occupy it. Until new patterns of space assignments are accepted, rules are used to soften the impact (e.g., visiting hours).

A final aspect of space is the way it is utilized. In North America we arrange furniture in a room in definite ways (normative pattern). The outer areas of a room are traditionally used for sitting, leaving the center clear for activity. The pattern is often found in clinic waiting rooms. From a psychologic point of view, grouping of chairs or even single chairs would better answer the client's need to group together or to be alone. If clients change the chair arrangement of their own accord, the personnel often becomes uneasy

and make comments regarding the liberties some will take—the message against nonconformity has been communicated.

Time. Another element in nonverbal communication is time, its meaning and use. Many aspects of North American culture are related to time. Appointments are made at definite times. Although a little leeway is allowed, the person is expected to be on time and, conversely, does not expect to be kept waiting. To be kept waiting is interpreted as a slight, an indication that one is of an inferior status. This can be particularly enraging if individuals suspect that there may be reasons to assume others are downgrading their status. One might see such reactions in government-sponsored health clinics. If clients are required to wait, they may suspect that the staff is looking down on them.

Clients who do not keep appointments are assumed to be shiftless and unconcerned. One of us (M.J.) visited an Indian village on the west coast of British Columbia to carry out a previously planned immunization program. Only a few older residents were found there; the others had left because the salmon were running. No offense was intended—one project could wait; the other could not. Being guided by the timing of natural events rather than by hours, days, weeks, months, or any other division of time seems incomprehensible to many North Americans. Communication can break down on such provocation.

Touch. Touch is another important nonverbal component of communication. On a social level people use touch to convey various messages about liking or disliking another person. Most people respect a firm handshake but are angered by a crushing one. People may hug friends but are offended if strangers press against them in an elevator. Mothers who are observed caring for their firstborn begin by using a tentative fingertip touch. As they become more secure in their role, they use the whole hand to support or manipulate the infant.

In person-to-person contacts with clients, nurses can use touch therapeutically. Massaging the back of a client confined to bed relieves muscle fatigue and contributes to client comfort. Even though the nurse may not speak a client's language she can express concern by holding the client's hand or stroking her brow.

Nurses must be aware of the importance of touch as means of nonverbal communication. Failure to touch or the way in which one touches can convey distaste for another. Nurses may avoid touching people they dislike or touch them as little as possible. When giving them nursing care, the nurse holds her hand stiffly or uses abrasive pressure rather than a caress. The recipients readily interpret the message, "I am distasteful to this person; she does not wish to be near me." These messages can interfere with the therapy being given.

Voice. Tone or rate, rhythm, and intensity of the voice are critical elements in communicating with others. Parents croon to their infants, mothers and fathers talk in high-pitched voices when alerting a newborn, and a nurse repeats instructions in a calm, gentle tone. These uses of voice tone convey love and acceptance. Conversely, talking loudly, mumbling, or speaking rapidly or hesitantly convey negative messages. Sometimes nurses will unconsciously raise the tone of their voice when speaking to clients who do not speak English. Unfortunately, not only do they not help the client comprehend, but they appear angry as well as incomprehensible to the client. The following nurse's report illustrates this concept.

As I was in the neighborhood, I called at the Tam's house to let them know of changes in times the community clinic would be available. Mr. Tam, who acted as interpreter for the family, was not at home. I attempted to give the information to Mrs. Tam, whose English was limited. I suddenly realized that Mrs. Tam had moved away from me. She kept repeating, "Mr. Tam talk." I noticed I was talking very loudly as well as slowly. Once I realized what I was doing, I felt foolish. I wrote a note to Mr. Tam, thanked Mrs. Tam, and left.

Eye contact. The manner in which people use eye contact is another important facet of every culture's nonverbal communication patterns. Ethnic groups vary considerably in the way eye contact is initiated and maintained. Some ethnic groups expect eye contact on first being introduced to another person and feel it is to be maintained during an ensuing conversation. If eye contact is avoided, uneasiness develops. The avoidance may be interpreted in a number of ways; for example, "She's not telling me the truth" or "I'm not worth being looked at." Other ethnic groups may avert their eyes when introduced as a token of respect. For some people, looking at a new baby is avoided unless they are also able to touch the child. They believe that if the child is not touched while being looked at, misfortune may befall that child. This belief is termed the "evil eye."

A more detailed discussion on how North Americans use eye contact in establishing parent-child relationships is given in Chapter 23. As nurses we need to clarify our concepts of eye contact and validate the concepts with members of differing ethnic groups.

Nurses are becoming increasingly conscious of the significance of communication behaviors in establishing relationships with clients and members of the health team. An important first step in becoming skilled in interpersonal communication is to be able to recognize one's own thoughts and feelings—to become more self-aware. Self-awareness does not come easily; however, it is basic to becoming skilled in establishing meaningful relationships with clients.

Self-awareness
Value systems. "Why did I say that?" and "Why did I do that?" are questions that all of us ask ourselves. Part of the answer to such questions lies in becoming aware of the effect values have on actions. Values as defined by Uustal (1978) are "general guides to behavior, standards of conduct that one endorses and tries to live up to or maintain."

Personal values arise as individuals concern themselves with establishing self-identity and attaining chosen life roles within their society and culture. Certain areas of life are "value rich." These include health, personal habits, male-female roles, sex, love, family, friends, and religion. While other areas such as money and politics are also value laden, the first areas mentioned are of particular importance to maternity nursing. It is within these areas that much of maternity nursing takes place.

Nurses hold values that are both personal and professional. The professional values are derived as the individual becomes part of a professional group and subscribes to and supports the standards of the group (e.g., American Nurses' Association nursing standards). The more the values are in agreement, the fewer the possibilities of value conflict. However, to expect perfect harmony between sets of values is unrealistic. Each nurse needs to recognize value conflict when it occurs and how to go about resolving it.

We are aware of some of the values that guide our behaviors. Nurses openly support efforts to include the family in maternity care because they believe the family acts as an important support system for mother and infant. On the other hand, some values that affect actions are not consciously held. Persons often behave in certain ways "because that is the way it should be." Many of the values that influence actions stem from concepts of *social roles* and of *the self.* A brief review of these two concepts precedes the discussion of the process of values clarification.

Social role. Social roles may be defined as socially prescribed patterns for behavior. Persons who share common attitudes and beliefs and assume responsibilities for certain tasks are performing a social role. These roles are learned in the process of social interaction, which begins at birth and continues throughout life. Individuals' concepts of a role (role expectations) govern how they expect others to act and how they expect to act. Every society sets up cultural norms for essential roles that serve as models for individuals to emulate in developing their personalized versions.

Awareness of role comes from a myriad of sources. Individuals use all their senses (hearing, seeing, touching, tasting, and smelling) as well as their cognitive powers (assessing, planning, and evaluating). Once a person is committed to the idea of a role, it is incorporated into the self, and *values* are assigned to it.

The value nurses place on certain aspects of their role can prove of great benefit to a client. The following situation as reported by a student is an example.

■ One of the infants in the nursery developed suspicious facial lesions. The mother had a history of herpes simplex II infection. The baby roomed-in with the mother. All infants in the nursery were considered as potentially infected and were isolated in the "B" room. The incoming babies were admitted to "A" room. I realized maintaining medical asepsis was vital to the babies' well-being and knew the problem would be enforcement. During report I noticed two doctors coming from "B" room and going into "A" room without changing gowns or scrubbing. I took it on myself to confront this "traffic" and afterwards set up a routine for everyone to follow. I found it nerve-racking to stop doctors but realized the implications for the babies.

The student accepted the responsibility of acting as an advocate for her clients because she felt strongly (valued) that being an advocate was an important component of the nursing role. As a result her clients were protected from harm. As individuals come to value their concepts of social roles (role expectations) they may resist attempt to change the roles. Only minor modifications in attitudes, beliefs, and responsibilities are permitted. The role becomes traditional or stereotyped.

The traditional role of mother falls into the stereotyped category. In the traditional role the mother is expected to behave in a motherly fashion, that is, willingly give children love, attention, and physical care, even though she is simultaneously acting as career woman, lover, or wife. A nurse who expects a woman to function in the traditional role of mother can be upset if the client does not live up to the nurse's expectations. As a result the nurse may consciously or unconsciously withhold supportive care, for example, be abrupt in contacts, avoid touching the client, or teach the client as little as possible. The following incident is illustrative of this.

■ Laura P., a new mother, was a senior partner in a law firm. She announced she should be returning to work immediately and had hired a nurse to care for the baby. She did not appear for the informal discussion on baby

---

care. When her nurse was questioned as to why L.P. had not come, the nurse replied, "I did not tell her about it. I figured she's not interested. She's not going to be looking after the baby."

In this instance the nurse assumed the mother was not interested in her new baby because the mother did not conform to stereotyped mother-role behavior. The nurse's value judgment about the behavior prevented the nurse from functioning adequately in her role as a nurse.

The concept of a life role, with its various responsibilities and relationships, is not static. Change is inevitable as new life situations occur. If the initial adaptation to change results in a satisfactory outcome, subsequent alteration in role structure comes with less stress. Individuals can trust their ability to adjust, modify, or enlarge role commitments. The foundation for growth in the role is thereby established. The maternity nurse is in a unique position to assist women and men to adapt to the role of parent. Teaching classes such as preparation for parenthood during the prenatal period, encouraging participation by the father during birth, and instructing parents in the care of the newborn are examples of strategies the maternity nurse uses. As parents become proficient in the role, a favorable *self-concept* ensues.

Self-concept. The *self* has been variously defined since studies of the self began in the late 1800's. It still defies precise definition, although it is recognized as the core of an individual's personality. Through the self each person perceives and evaluates the world. The idea of the self develops slowly and has physical and social dimensions. Infants begin the process of awareness of their physical attributes and potential by defining the physical boundaries of themselves as they manipulate their bodies. The child and adult continue the process as they learn how to use their bodies effectively. The social concept of self develops through the assumption of social roles. Role taking continues through life. Two important components of self-concept are body image and self-esteem.

A subjective picture of one's physical appearance derived from one's own observations and by noting the response of others is known as *body image*. It represents the "sum of the conscious and unconscious attitudes the individual has toward his body. It includes present and past perceptions, as well as feelings about size, function, appearance, and potential" (Stuart and Sundeen, 1983). This picture is constantly changing as new perceptions and experiences occur. Adolescents become particularly conscious of their physical bodies as the body undergoes rapid change. Value judgments made about physical size, hair styles, and skin can be a source of pleasure or pain to the young person. The pregnant woman's body also reflects rapid change, and for some women this change can be disturbing.

The liking and disliking of the self is called *self-esteem*. Self-esteem develops as people attempt to master social roles (Satir, 1967).

Children begin to act as they observe others acting. They play at social roles, e.g., mother, father, teacher, nurse, and thereby practice role behaviors. As they grow older the social roles they adopt become more than play. They become part of their development toward adulthood. In some instances the process of role taking is formalized; the role taker becomes a student (nursing student). In other instances the actual role is assumed without a concerted social effort to prepare the participants. Until recently parenthood came into this latter category.

If individuals play out social roles well, they are applauded (rewarded) by people important to them (significant others) and as a result develop *high self-esteem*. If their efforts are not considered successful, the significant others may ignore them, criticize them, blame them. As a result of these responses the person develops *low self-esteem*. Sullivan (1963) called this process "learning about the self from the mirror of other people." How individuals view themselves (self-esteem) conditions their responses to their world. Some people feel masterful; others are afraid. Some develop methods of coping with crisis, others "go to pieces" if their daily routines are interrupted. Some become part of a social group that acts as a support system, others remain alone.

There are happenings in the lives of all of us that have great meaning to us personally. Assuming the role of parent is one of these important times. It will have an effect on us and others for all our lives. It can be called a crucial life experience. How individuals function during this time has an important effect on self-esteem. People need to share these times with others who care and to be helped by the nurturing of others in the environment. Clients often turn to nurses to help them develop the behaviors, attitudes, and responsibilities that are part of the role of parent.

Low self-esteem has an important impact on maternity nursing. Research has indicated that low self-esteem may be a determining factor in a person's consistent use of health facilities (Bullough and Bullough, 1982). Sustained contact between nurse and client is necessary to ensure a healthy outcome of pregnancy for mother, child, and family.

Values clarification. Values clarification is the process of identifying one's own values and beliefs. Once identified and recognized, the nurse can explore the ways values and beliefs can affect each phase of the nursing process. Hawley and Hawley (1975) noted that decisions were based largely on the values held by the decision maker. Decision making is a key component in the nursing process. Therefore nurses need to become aware of values, either their own or their clients, that can add to or detract from their efforts to make decisions congruent with therapeutic goals.

Uustal (1978) adapted the process of values clarification for nursing. Three major activities are involved in the process. They include choosing, prizing, and acting.

Choosing: Making choices about our values after consideration of alternatives.

EXAMPLE: I've thought and thought about going back to school just now, and I've come to the conclusion that I need to be with the kids at their ages. I have to put first things first. I talked it over with John, and he agrees. I can always go back to school later. After all, the kids will only be young once.

Prizing: Assigning a "value" to values, arranging our values in rank order, and acknowledging them publicly when appropriate.

EXAMPLE: Some principles I feel very strongly about, others I can adjust to circumstances. I try to let others know how I feel about certain things so they are forewarned about how I'll react if they try to make me change.

Acting: Behaving in a manner that is consistent with the individual's values. Through repetitious actions, a pattern of behavior can be discerned.

EXAMPLE: I could have said nothing about giving Mrs. S. the Tylenol instead of aspirin. They are both stock drugs so they wouldn't be missed and physically they wouldn't hurt her. But I felt I had to be honest and report the error or I couldn't stand myself. In some things such as medications, even small differences could have adverse effects. I feel better that I acted according to my beliefs.

In the three examples cited above the individuals were making decisions and acting on the basis of professed values. Values clarification is part of everyday living. However, it can be used in a formal sense to assist in recognizing the effect values have on action. The following example illustrates how a student used the values clarification process after a conflict in nurse-client values prevented her from providing therapeutic care.

■ Before beginning M.M.'s care, I reviewed her record and found the following history. She was 20 years old and unmarried. She had had an abortion at 16 and again at 17. She had a baby at 19 and kept the baby.

She was going to keep the baby from this pregnancy also. My reaction was one of shock. I felt resentment toward her and felt uncomfortable knowing I would have to interact with her. I remembered all I'd read and learned about unwed mothers and decided to accept this challenge. I did not want to let my feelings get in the way. My feelings stem from the fact that, as a result of a strict Catholic upbringing, I am fiercely against abortion. I consider it an act of murder. I was adopted. I am extremely sensitive to the fact that unwed girls are not giving their babies up for adoption, but rather bringing them home to an incomplete family.

After getting home I reflected on my behavior toward M.M. I failed in reaching my goal. I talked to M.M. only when it was necessary. When I did talk to her, I kept it brief in order to be able to ignore her situation. I did not want to explore her home situation—if she had an adequate income or a significant other for emotional support, for fear of what I would learn. When I did ask her about future contraceptive plans, she said she had never used any and felt there was no need to. It tore me apart inside to think she may possibly bring more children into her insufficient family. In essence, I wanted as little to do with her as possible.

I now realize how much my personal views prevented me from performing therapeutic nursing care. I definitely want to work on this. I know it will be difficult to overcome my feelings.

In an effort to work through the value conflicts the student sorted the data as follows:

My Values	Client's Values as Assumed by the Nurse
Abortion is morally wrong	Abortion is an acceptable means of birth control
Family should consist of a wedded mother and father with children	Family without a father is all right
Methods of birth control (other than abortion) should be used if a person is sexually active to prevent birth of children	Birth control other than abortion is not necessary

As a result of the conflict in values, the nurse had the following responses:

1. Shock and disbelief but desire to give good care.
2. Inability to set up therapeutic nurse-client relationship:
   "I talked to M.M. only when it was necessary. I wanted as little to do with her as possible."
3. Inadequate collection of data:
   "When I did talk to her, I kept it brief in order to be able to ignore her situation."

"I did not want to explore her home situation if she had an adequate income or a significant other for emotional support—for fear of what I would learn."

"When I did ask her about future contraceptive plans, she said she had never used any (abortion?) and felt there was no need to."
4. Feeling of guilt and anxiety over care given to client:
   "I now realize how much my personal views prevented me from performing therapeutic nursing care."
5. Desire to change approach to care:
   "I definitely want to work on this one. I know it will be difficult to overcome my feelings."

Once the data has been organized, the student used the values clarification process to help her with growth in the professional role. Table 4.4 illustrates how this student used values clarification to help her care for her clients more effectively in the future.

Nurse-client responsibility is at the heart of providing nursing care. Although all human relationships have characteristics in common, the nurse-client relationship is initiated by the nurse for the benefit of the client. Nurse-client relationships take place wherever the nurse and client meet. They may be of long or short duration. The nurse employs professional skills in communication and decision making to facilitate the process. The nurse's responsive dimensions, trust and empathetic understanding, are necessary ingredients of the nurse's role in therapeutic relationships. Awareness of client and nurse value systems contributes to acceptance of and progress toward mutually defined goals.

The family is a crucial support system for the client. All of the components of the nurse and individual client relationship are utilized when the client-family unit is the focus of care. A model for a family care plan follows.

Family Care Plan

Assessment. To plan for the care of a family or particular family member, the nurse must remember that a family operates as a system. That is, no one family member has a problem—the whole family has a problem. Solutions to problems can evolve only through family participation.

Data collection

Process. The *process* of an assessment in planning family care is often more difficult and complicated than that involved in assessing the physical health of clients. It requires skill in communication and the ability to establish a trusting relationship. In every family group,

Table 4.4
Example of Values Clarification Process Implemented by a Nursing Student

Choosing Values	Prizing	Acting
Abortion morally wrong.	Part of my religious and moral beliefs.	Would request another client assignment and give reasons for my request. If client asked for information about abortions, would find client another resource person (for legally accepted actions, see Chapter 3).
Sexually active adults need to assume responsible attitude toward possible pregnancy (through use of acceptable birth control, not abortion).	Part of my belief about being a responsible citizen.	Would include teaching and counseling about family planning in my care.
I feel every child should have a caring adult, social and economic support, and a place in society. A family should be formed through marriage and consist of a mother, father, and children.	I still feel the traditional family is the best. However, through reading and discussion, I can accept other family forms more readily.	I could work with single parents; I am going to act as volunteer this summer at "Center for Life," where counseling is given to pregnant women. The emphasis is on adoption, but community support systems for single parent families are explored if adoption alternative is not chosen.

areas of openness and privacy exist, and all groups resent interrogation by an outsider. The reasons for obtaining information must be explained to the client in a clear manner.

Information such as the address, marital status, and family members' ages can be obtained readily because it is generally given freely. Other information is attained by (1) *observing* and noting relationships, attitudes, and stress responses (who is doing what), (2) *listening* to conversation about community and family involvements or hopes and aspirations, and (3) *being aware* of matters such as why persons have missed appointments or refused to use existing health care facilities.

Cultural considerations. Cross-cultural variations in reproductive practices occur with respect to interpersonal relationships, family and kinship relationships, and folk practices. Clients have a right to expect that their cultural needs relative to reproduction will be met, as well as their physiologic and psychologic needs. A culture's reproductive beliefs and practices are embedded in that culture's social system and can truly be understood only as they related to that group's economic, religious, kinship, and political structures. To expect the nurse to have this kind of knowledge for each cultural group is unrealistic. How, then, can information presented in this chapter be used effectively by the nurse?

Stern (1981) developed a model for improving communication between individuals and families from a variety of ethnic and cultural backgrounds and Western health care providers. Identified in this model are barriers in communication that exist on three levels: approach, custom, and language. Such a model, if generalized to other cultures, is useful for nurses.

Approach includes numerous factors one considers in interpersonal relationships. The American approach to most issues in health care is to address the problem directly. With many cultures (Stern, 1981) engaging in small talk is vital before a serious discussion. Commenting on flowers or pictures and having tea or a cold drink are equated with showing respect. To begin talking to an expectant mother about the need for prenatal care before commenting on the other children, the pretty chair, or the weather might set up an atmosphere of distrust. In some cultures, women prefer a caregiver of the same sex. Therefore it is critical that the initial encounter be with a woman. Showing respect and patience are essential in building trust and effecting cultural change.

Custom includes practices and behaviors characteristic of a culture. Understanding that a cultural reason exists for all behaviors and making a sincere effort to ascertain the person's rationale for behavior are important steps in establishing trust. The clients themselves may be the most helpful in assisting the nurse to understand their cultural logic and individual differences. Assessment of health beliefs and practices is essential for the health care professional who is striving to achieve a holistic approach to care. For the client, adherence to a particular cultural custom provides a sense of constancy with one's cultural heritage.

Language is an important factor. Stern (1981) emphasizes the use of clear, jargon-free English. An interpreter, either a family member or a member of the same cultural group, may be used. When an interpreter is being used, it is important to address questions and responses to the client and not to the interpreter.

The following questions illustrate ways to elicit cultural explanations regarding childbearing:

1. What do you and your family think you should do to keep healthy during pregnancy?
2. What are the things you can do or not do to affect your health and the health of your baby?
3. Who are the persons you want with you during your labor and delivery?
4. What are considered abnormal signs during pregnancy?
5. What things or actions are important to you and your family to do after the baby is born?
6. What do you and your family expect from the nurse or nurses caring for you?
7. What are ways the nurse might help you and your family?
8. How will family members participate in your pregnancy, childbirth, and parenting?

A nurse cannot be expected to know all there is to know about every culture and subculture, as well as their many life-styles. Understanding one's own culture is necessary to come to a better realization of why we believe as we do. Understanding clients' cultures, through interview, study, contact, and a demonstrated sincere interest, is invaluable. This understanding enables nurses to render culturally sensitive and relevant nursing care.

Model for data collection. Following is an assessment model based on a guide developed by faculty members of San Jose State University Department of Nursing in 1982:

I. Family identification
   A. *Composition.* Who are the family members currently living in the household? Are they kin or nonkin? What are their ages?
   B. *Social history.* What is the social background of each member regarding education, income, occupation, marital status, ethnicity, and culture?
   C. *Community and neighborhood.* What is the general tone of the neighborhood? Are resources such as water, electricity, and sewers available? Is the area one of affluence or poverty? What are the residents of the neighborhood like (e.g., friendly, noncommittal)?
II. Individual and family data
   A. *Health history.* What is the family's health history? What actions has the family used in the past when one of its members was ill? What are the family's present reasons for seeking care?
   B. *Family dynamics.* How well does family work together to accomplish family functions? What social roles does each family member

assume? How are roles within the family negotiated? What are the family's boundaries? What channels do family members use to interface with the community? What communication patterns are employed? What are the family's protocols for problem solving? What are the family's values and attitudes as reflected in problem solving and decision making; for example, who has the power? What aspects of family theories are represented by this family: structural-functional, developmental, or interactional?

1. *Techniques* used in assessing individual and family dynamics include interviewing and observation. Robbins and Schacht (1982) have devised four basic steps nurses can use in observing communication behavior and inferring hierarchies within families.
   a. Observe the interactions of the entire family and remember that an observer has a part in the interactions.
   b. Outline the interactions just as a camera would record them, without inferred meaning. This outline may be written on paper.
   c. Review the interactions: who spoke first, who spoke with whom, and when, who summed up, who spoke or acted for whom, and who followed whose advice.
   d. Proceed with the appropriate intervention, exchanging information within the family's communication system.
2. *Recording* the assessment data under the following headings can reveal patterns that provide guidelines to planning nursing care:
   a. Communication patterns: direct or indirect, open or closed?
   b. Leadership: patriarchial, matriarchial, egalatarian, democratic?
   c. Hierarchies: who possesses the power and over what areas?
   d. Roles and relationships: who is the breadwinner, decision maker, leader, nurturer?
   e. Values: are values based on materialism, importance of family, religion, ethnic or cultural patterns?
   f. Beliefs regarding health and illness: do the beliefs reflect myths, old wives' tales, cultural influences?
   g. Priorities: are the priorities housing, jobs, food, other?

III. Family strengths: following is a checklist to assist the nurse in identifying present and potential family strengths and weaknesses based on health history and family dynamics:

A. Ability to maintain a healthy life style and general health status.

B. Ability to provide for the family's physical, emotional, spiritual, and cultural needs:
   1. Physical: providing adequate space, equipment, material goods, food, etc.
   2. Emotional: helping family members recognize and develop their capacity for sensitivity to each other's needs.
   3. Spiritual: sharing of basic beliefs and spiritual or religious values.
   4. Cultural: sharing of basic beliefs and cultural values.

C. Child-rearing practices and discipline:
   1. Capability of both parents to respect each other's views and decisions on child-rearing practices.
   2. If a single parent, capacity of the parent to be consistent and effective in raising the child or children.

D. Communication: ability to communicate and express a wide range of emotions and feelings both verbally and nonverbally.

E. Support, security, and encouragement:
   1. Capacity of the family to provide its members with feelings of security and encouragement.
   2. Ability to achieve balance in the pattern of family activities.

F. Growth-producing relationships: family's ability to maintain and build friendships and relationships in the neighborhood.

G. Responsible community relationships: capacity of the family members to assume responsibility through participation in social, cultural, or community activities.

H. Growing with and through children: capacity of parents to recognize that children may be a force for growth in the parents' lives.

I. Self-help and accepting help: family members' ability to seek and accept help when *they* think they need it.

J. Flexibility of family functions and roles: family members' ability to "fill in" for one another during times of illness or when needed.

K. Crisis as a means of growth: family members' ability to unite and become supportive during a crisis or traumatic experience.

L. Family unity, loyalty, and intrafamily cooperation: family members' ability to recognize and use family traditions and rituals that promote unity and pride.

Analysis, synthesis, validation. Following the data-gathering phase the nurse analyzes and synthesizes the findings. Inferences about the data are formulated. Because inferences are subjective and based not only on the nurse's competence level but also on individual values and beliefs, the nurse needs to validate the interpretation of the data with the client. Validation of inferences is followed by the development of nursing diagnoses.

Nursing diagnoses. Nursing diagnoses are formulated to reflect the family's perception of its needs as well as the nurse's perception. *It is important to determine the family's perception of its nursing care needs rather than that of any one family member.*

Once the nursing diagnoses are established, the nurse takes time to explore personal value judgments about the family that may affect and impede nursing interventions. It is also essential for the nurse to validate the diagnoses. In addition to direct validation with the family, a review of the literature, an analysis of norms, and discussion with other persons involved in the family are means of validation.

Planning

Setting goals. The next step is to set goals and outcome criteria related to each diagnosis. These are established as a joint enterprise between nurse and family. They are evaluated for realism and acceptance by family members. Goals for care are both short and long range. Once agreed on, the goals are assessed to determine priority. Certain health needs require immediate attention, for example, unexplained vaginal bleeding. Other health needs require more time to resolve, for example, anger over birth of a child of undesired sex.

Selecting nursing actions. Working with the available data, the nursing diagnoses, and the health goals, the nurse proceeds to organize a plan for implementing the most appropriate interventions. The nurse identifies the nursing role, that is, whether the role is teacher, direct care provider, or referrer. The nurse plans for the best use of resources available to the family, both internal and community support systems. The nurse must determine whether the resources are appropriate and whether the family is able or willing to use them.

Implementation. The selected nursing actions are implemented. Nursing actions that are preventive, curative, or rehabilitative in nature are tailored to the individual needs of the family and its members.

Evaluation. Evaluation is a joint process between nurse and family. Mutually determined goals and out-

Application of the Nursing Process

NURSING PROCESS WITH A FAMILY: MARIA AND JUAN

Mr. and Mrs. Gonzales are a young couple who recently moved to the United States from Mexico. Nineteen-year-old Maria is 8 weeks into her first pregnancy. Juan has accompanied his wife to the clinic because he is able to speak some English. He is 20 years old. Maria seems reluctant to obtain a urine specimen in the bathroom that is next to the waiting room. With considerable difficulty finding the "right" English words, Juan states he is worried because Maria cannot eat all the suggested diet for pregnant women. Juan says the foods are strange to her and she does not know how to prepare them. In addition, her mother, aunt, and grandmother, all of whom live nearby, have told her not to eat some of the foods on the diet she was given.

FUNCTIONAL HEALTH PATTERN: ASSESSMENT	NURSING DIAGNOSIS	RATIONALE: PLAN/ IMPLEMENTATION	EVALUATION
ROLE-RELATIONSHIP ■ Maria is unable to speak English. ■ Juan has minimal command of English.	Impaired verbal communication related to foreign language barrier.	*To facilitate communication:* ■ Obtain a fluent translator. ■ Use flash cards with pictures and words. ■ Watch nonverbal cues indicating their understanding.	M. and J. express understanding. M. and J. follow through on directions, keep appointments.
HEALTH PERCEPTION–HEALTH MAINTENANCE ■ M. seems reluctant to obtain urine specimen.	Alteration in health maintenance related to lack of privacy.	*To provide privacy:* ■ Escort M. to bathroom down the hall from the waiting area.	M. obtains a urine specimen.
NUTRITIONAL-METABOLIC ■ M. finds it difficult to prepare and eat foods that are strange to her. ■ Extended family is guiding her food intake.	Potential alteration in nutrition (less or more than requirement) related to knowledge deficit or cultural influences.	*To ensure adequate nutrition:* ■ Obtain a fluent translator to identify preferred diet, to develop a diet to meet her nutritional and cultural needs, and to determine if there is need for financial assistance for food.	Total weight gain and pattern of weight gain are appropriate for week of gestation. M.'s blood values (hemoglobin/hematocrit) remain within normal limits. M. and J. are happy with the prescribed diet and indicate that their "family" also approves the diet.

come criteria need to be stated precisely so that the degree to which goals are met can be determined. The criteria need to be realistic and flexible enough to permit modification as circumstances change.

References

Blehar, M.C.: Families and public policy. In Corfman, E., editor: Families today, vol. 2, National Institute of Mental Health, Division of Scientific and Public Information, Science Monograph 1, Washington, D.C., 1979, U.S. Government Printing Office.

Bullough, B., and Bullough, V.: Poverty, ethnic identity and health care, New York, 1972, Appleton-Century-Crofts.

Caplan, G.: An approach to community health, New York, 1961, Grune & Stratton.

Hall, E.: Hidden dimensions, Garden City, N.Y., 1966, Doubleday & Co.

Hawley, R.C., and Hawley, I.L.: Human values in the classroom: a handbook for teachers, New York, 1975, Hart Publishing Co.

Luft, J.: Group processes: an introduction to group dynamics, ed. 2, Palo Alto, Calif., 1970, National Press Books.

Rodgers, C.: On becoming a person, Boston, 1961, Houghton & Mifflin Co.

Satir, V.: Conjoint family therapy, Palo Alto, Calif., 1967, Science & Behavior Books.

Sommer, R.: Studies in personal space, Sociometry 20:247, 1959.

Stern, P.N.: Solving problems of cross-cultural health teaching: the Filipino childbearing family, Image 13:47, 1981.

Stuart, G., and Sundeen, S.: Principles and practice of psychiatric nursing, ed. 2, St. Louis, 1983, The C.V. Mosby Co.

Sullivan, H.S.: The interpersonal theory of psychiatry, New York, 1963, W.W. Norton & Co., Inc., Publishers.

Travelbee, J.: Interpersonal aspects of nursing, Philadelphia, 1971, F.A. Davis Co.

Uustal, D.B.: Values clarification in nursing application to practice, Am. J. Nurs. 78:2058, Dec. 1978.

Bibliography

American Nurses' Association: Nursing: a social policy statement, Kansas City, 1982, The Association.

Bailey, J.T., and Claus, K.E.: Decision making in nursing: tools for change, St. Louis, 1975, The C.V. Mosby Co.

Bentz, J.M.: Missed meanings in nurse/patient communication, M.C.N. 5:55, Jan./Feb., 1980.

Bloch, D.: Some crucial terms in nursing: what do they mean? Nurs. Outlook 22:689, 1974.

Bower, F.L.: Nursing process: roles and functions of the nurse. In Bower, F.L., and Bevis, E.O.: Fundamentals of nursing practice: concepts, roles, and functions, St. Louis, 1979, The C.V. Mosby Co.

Carpenito, L.J.: Nursing diagnosis: application of clinical practice, Philadelphia, 1983, J.B. Lippincott Co.

Forsyth, D.M.: Looking good to communicate better with patients, Nurs. '83 13:34, July, 1983.

Freebairn, J., and Gwinup, K.: Ethics, values, and health, Irvine, Calif., 1980, Concept Media.

Gordon, M.: Historical perspective: The national group of classification of nursing diagnoses. In Kim, M.J., and Moritz, D.A., editors: Classification of nursing diagnoses, New York, 1982, McGraw-Hill Book Co.

Hines, J.: Only five minutes—nurse-patient communications, M.C.N. 5:240, July/Aug., 1980.

Kalisch, B.: What is empathy? Am. J. Nurs. 73:1548, Sept. 1973.

Marieskind, H.I.: Women in the health system: patients, providers, and programs, St. Louis, 1980, The C.V. Mosby Co.

Maslow, A.H.: Motivation and personality, ed. 2, New York, 1970, Harper & Row, Publishers.

Norton, M.A.: Daring to care, Am. J. Nurs. 85:1098, Oct., 1985.

Orlando, I.J.: The dynamic nurse-patient relationship, New York, 1961, G.P. Putnam's Sons.

Peplau, H.E.: Interpersonal relations in nursing, New York, 1952, G.P. Putnam's Sons.

Richardson, J.I., and Berline-Nauman, D.: In the face of anger, Nurs. '84 14:66, Feb., 1984.

Sandelowski, M.: Women, health, and choice, Englewood Cliffs, N.J., 1981, Prentice-Hall.

Schaefer, J.: the interrelatedness of decision making and the nursing process, Am. J. Nurs. 74:1852, Oct., 1974.

Simon, S.B., and others: Value clarification: a handbook of practical strategies for teachers and students, rev. ed., New York, 1978, Hart Publishing Co.

Styles, M.M.: On nursing: toward a new endowment, St. Louis, 1982, The C.V. Mosby Co.

The Nursing Theories Conference Group: Nursing theories: a base for professional nursing, Englewood Cliffs, N.J., 1980, Prentice-Hall.

Walke, M.: When a patient needs to unburden his feelings, Am. J. Nurs. 77:1164, July, 1977.

UNIT 2

Basic Concepts of Human Sexuality

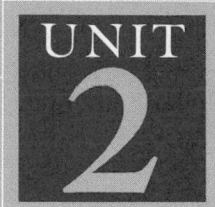

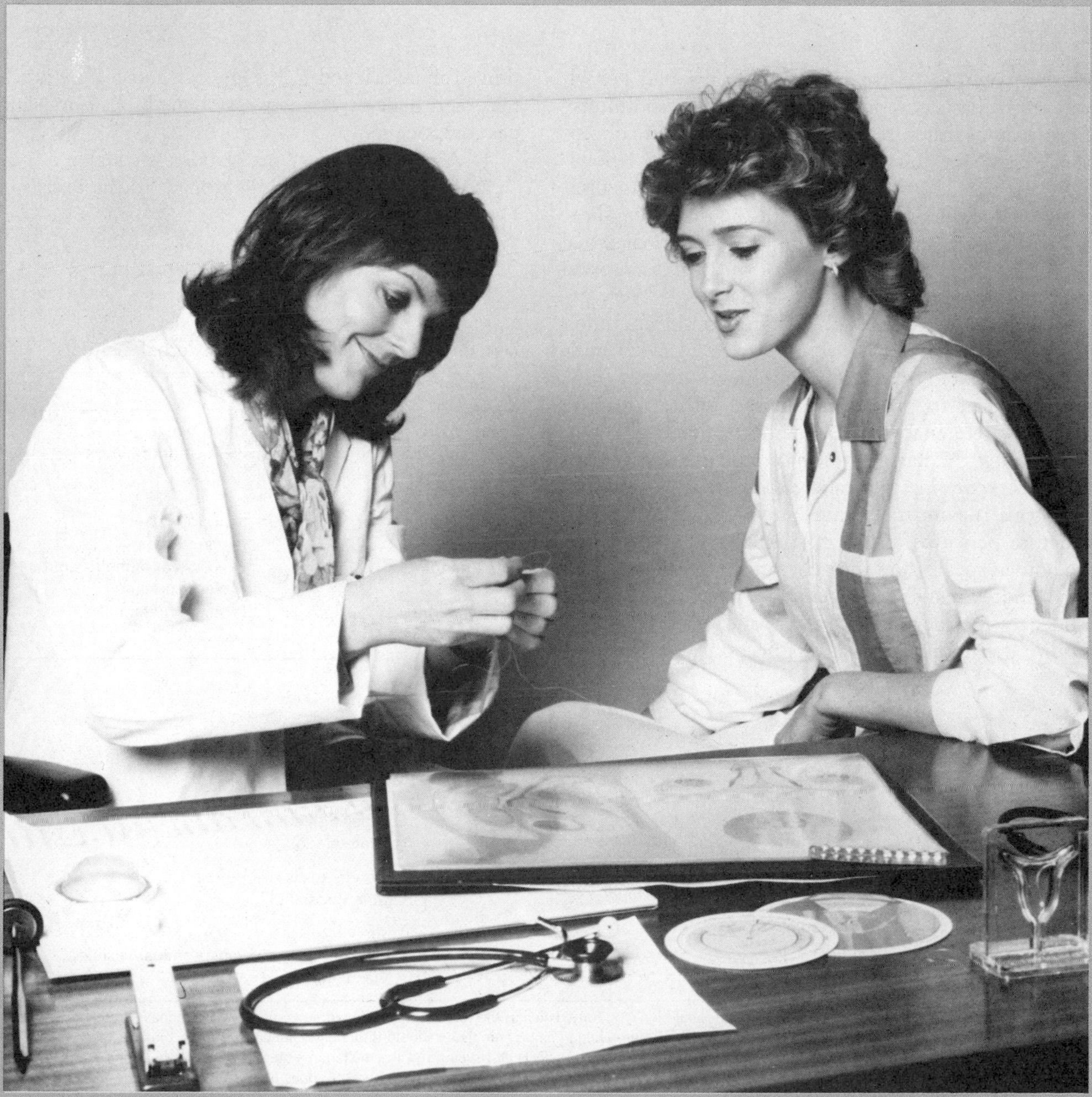

Anatomy and Physiology of Human Sexuality

The maternity nurse begins with a sound knowledge of the basic components of life and its continuity: the anatomic structures and their functions in conception, pregnancy, birth, and the puerperium. Knowledge of the anatomy and physiology is basic to utilization of the nursing process with the maternity client and her family. An understanding of the normal sexual response cycle provides the information for sexual counseling during pregnancy and the postdelivery period. The chapter ends with a discussion of immunology. Because of its importance today, considerable space is devoted to basic concepts of immunology. This is meant to provide the nurse with a ready resource for reference, not for memorization.

Although the female and male reproductive systems differ markedly in appearance, their structures are homologous (having the same embryonic origin). Each structure performs a vital role in the continuation of the human species and the generation and maintenance of secondary sexual characteristics. Through hormonal influences the reproductive tracts and accessory glands acquire the unique adaptations necessary to reproduction (Tables 5.1 and 5.2; Figs. 5.1 and 5.2). Both female and male reproductive systems have four principal components:

1. A pair of primary sex glands (gonads)
2. Ducts leading from the gonads to the body's exterior
3. External genitalia
4. Secondary (accessory) sex glands

Table 5.1
Female and Male Homologues: External Genitals

Female	Male
Glans clitoris	Glans penis
Prepuce (identifiable only by microscopic histologic examination	Prepuce (foreskin)
Corpus clitoris	Shaft (body)
Vestibule	Penile urethra
Labia minora	Penoscrotal raphe (seam that closes urethra)
Entire urethra	Prostatic urethra
Labia majora	Scrotum

Table 5.2
Female and Male Homologues: Internal Structures*

Female		Male	
Bartholin's glands		Cowper's glands	
Paraurethral glands		Prostate gland	
Uterine tubes			
Uterus	Müllerian ducts	Appendix testis	
Upper four fifths of vagina		Utricle (prostatic)	
Ovary		Testis	
Scattered vestigial (trace) remnants	Mesonephric ducts	Epididymis, vas deferens, seminal vesicles, ejaculatory duct	

*In the genetic *female* the müllerian embryonic tissue should develop fully, whereas the mesonephric embryonic tissue should disappear. In the genetic *male* the structures of mesonephric origin should develop fully, and the müllerian embryonic tissue should disappear. *Clinical significance:* drugs taken by the mother affect certain embryonic tissue; for example, diethylstilbestrol (DES) affects all structures of the müllerian system, leading to the syndrome called "DES daughter." In the male if the müllerian system does not degenerate or in the female if the mesonephric system does not degenerate, various abnormalities occur, for example, pseudohermaphroditism.

Fig. 5.1
Homologues of external genitals.

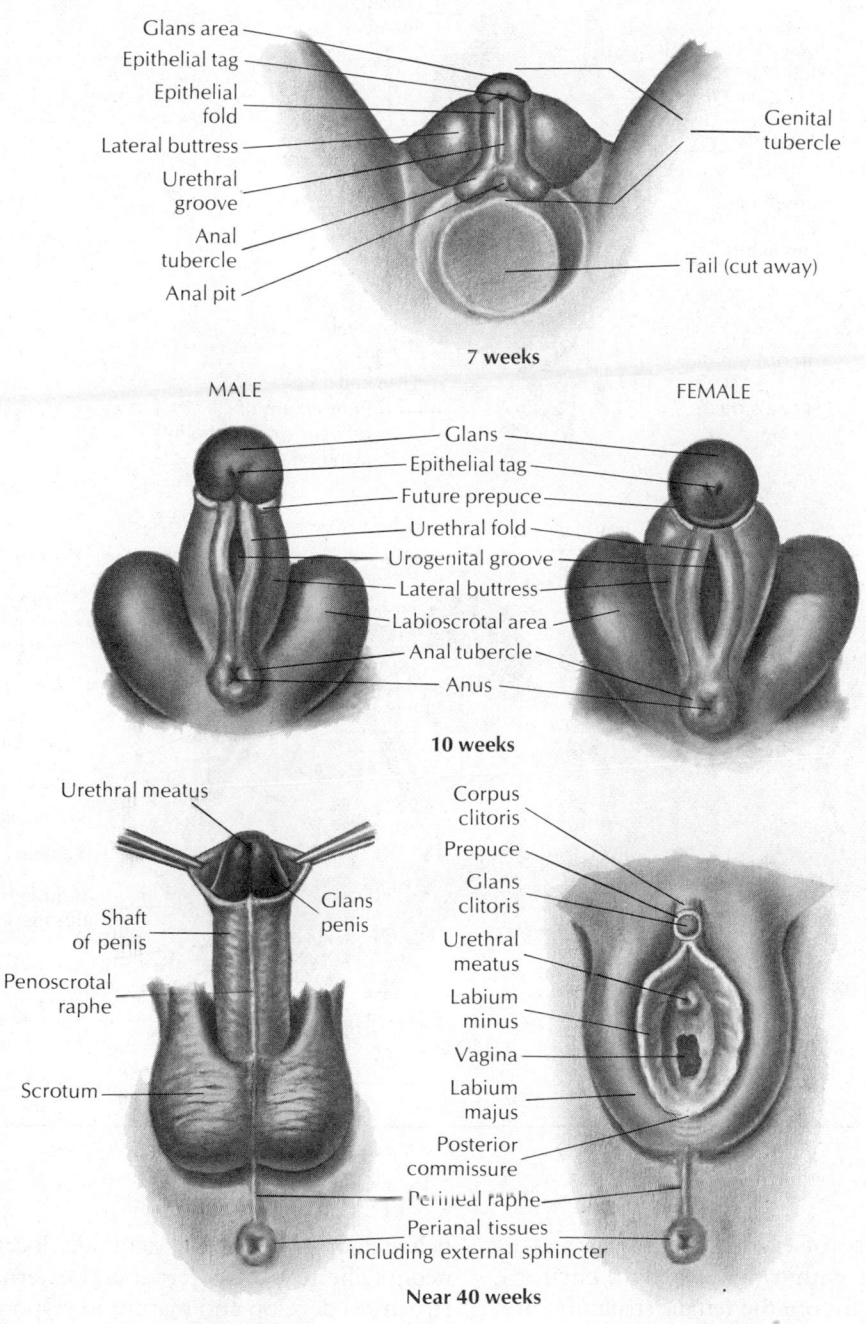

UNDIFFERENTIATED

Glans area
Epithelial tag
Epithelial fold
Lateral buttress
Urethral groove
Anal tubercle
Anal pit
Genital tubercle
Tail (cut away)

7 weeks

MALE   FEMALE

Glans
Epithelial tag
Future prepuce
Urethral fold
Urogenital groove
Lateral buttress
Labioscrotal area
Anal tubercle
Anus

10 weeks

Urethral meatus
Glans penis
Shaft of penis
Penoscrotal raphe
Scrotum

Corpus clitoris
Prepuce
Glans clitoris
Urethral meatus
Labium minus
Vagina
Labium majus
Posterior commissure
Perineal raphe
Perianal tissues including external sphincter

Near 40 weeks

G. J. Wassilchenko

Fig. 5.2
Homologues of internal genitals.

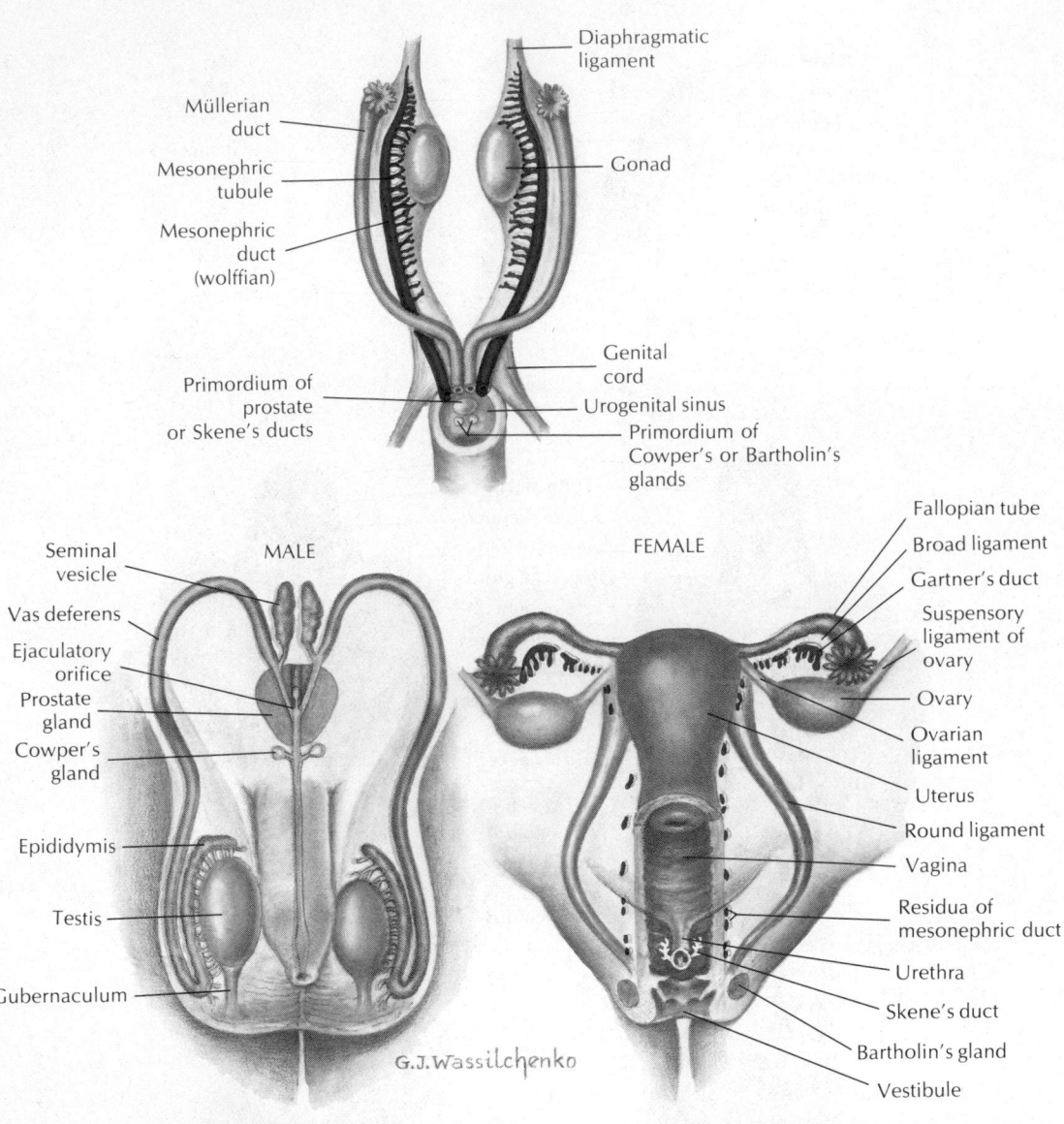

In the normal course of events, life begins and is sustained for 9 months within the protective environment of the female. Therefore the female structures are considered first.

Female Structures

The female reproductive system consists of internal organs, located in the pelvic cavity and supported by the pelvic floor, and external genitalia, located in the perineum. The female's internal and external reproductive structures develop and mature in response to estrogens and progesterones, starting in fetal life and continuing through puberty and throughout the childbearing years. The reproductive structures atrophy (decrease in size) with age or a drop in ovarian hormone production. An extensive and complex innervation and a generous blood supply support the functions of these structures. The appearance of the external genitalia

Fig. 5.3
Adult female pelvis. **A,** Anterior view. **B,** The three embryonic parts of the left innominate bone (pink tone). **C,** External view of right innominate bone (fused).

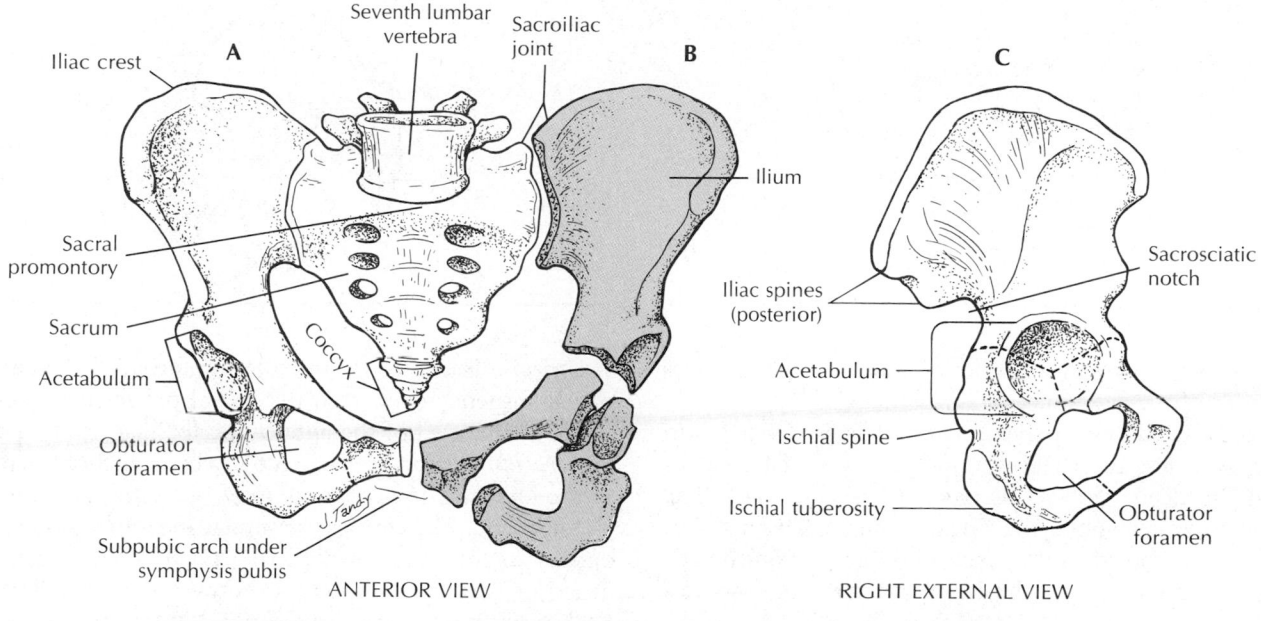

ANTERIOR VIEW   RIGHT EXTERNAL VIEW

varies greatly from woman to woman, since the size, shape, and color are determined by heredity, age, and race and the number of children a woman has borne.

THE BONY PELVIS

The nurse needs to be thoroughly familiar with the bony pelvis to understand the female reproductive tract and perineum. The pelvis serves three primary purposes: (1) Its bony cavity produces a protective cradle for pelvic structures. (2) Its architecture is of special importance in accommodating a growing fetus throughout pregnancy and during the birth process. (3) Its strength provides stable anchorage for the attachment of supportive muscles, fascia, and ligaments.

Bony structures. In a study of the bony pelvis the following structures and *landmarks* are especially important (Fig. 5.3):
1. Iliac crest and superior, anterior iliac spine
2. Sacral promontory
3. Sacrum
4. Coccyx
5. Symphysis pubis
6. Subpubic arch
7. Sacrosciatic notch
8. Ischial spines
9. Ischial tuberosities

The pelvis (Fig. 5.3, *A*) is made up of four bones: (1) and (2) the right and left innominate bones, each of which is made up of the right or left pubic bone, ilium, and ischium, which fuse after puberty (Fig. 5.3, *B*); (3) the sacrum; and (4) the coccyx. The two *innominate bones* (hip bones) form the sides and front of the bony passage, and the *sacrum* and *coccyx* form the back.

Below the *ilium* is the *ischium*, a heavy bone terminating posteriorly in the rounded protuberances known as the *ischial tuberosities* (Fig. 5.3, *C*). The tuberosities bear the body's weight in the sitting position. The *ischial spines*, the sharp projections from the posterior border of the ischium into the pelvic cavity, may be blunt or prominent.

The *pubis*, forming the front portion of the pelvic cavity, is located beneath the mons. In the midline the two pubic bones are joined by strong ligaments and a thick cartilage to form the joint called the symphysis pubis. In the female the angle formed by the subpubic arch optimally measures slightly more than 90 degrees.

The *sacrum* is formed by five fused vertebrae. The upper anterior portion of the body of the first sacral vertebra, the promontory, forms the posterior margin of the pelvic brim.

The *coccyx* (tailbone), composed of three to five fused vertebrae, articulates with the sacrum. The coc-

Fig. 5.4
Female pelvis: false pelvis is shallow basin above inlet; true pelvis is deeper cavity below inlet.

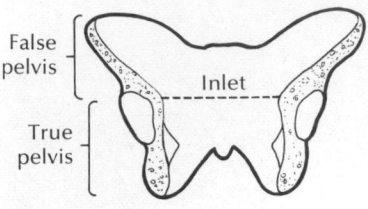

Fig. 5.5
Female pelvis: cavity of true pelvis is an irregularly curved canal.

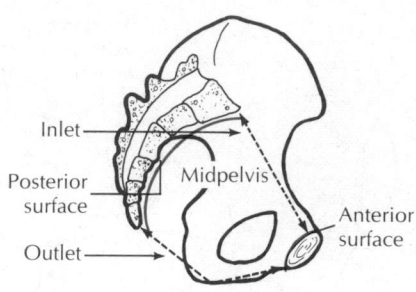

cyx projects downward and forward from the lower border of the sacrum.

False and true pelves. The pelvis is divided into two sections, the shallow upper basin, or false pelvis, and the deeper lower, or true, pelvis (Fig. 5.4). The *false pelvis* lies above the linea terminalis (brim, inlet) and varies considerably in size in different women. The *true pelvis* consists of the brim, or inlet, and the area below.

Pelvic planes. Pelvic planes include those of the *inlet,* the mid pelvis, and the *outlet.* The cavity of the mid true pelvis resembles an irregularly curved canal (Fig. 5.5) with unequal anterior and posterior surfaces. The anterior surface is formed by the length of the symphysis (4.5 cm). The posterior surface is formed by the length of the sacrum (12 cm).

Pelvic variations. Age, sex, and race are responsible for the greatest variations in pelvic shape and size. There is considerable change in the pelvis during growth and development. Pelvic ossification is complete at about 20 years of age or slightly later. Smaller people have smaller, lighter bones than larger people.

INTERNAL STRUCTURES

The internal reproductive organs are discussed in the order that reflects the path of the ovum. Supportive tissues are discussed along with the internal reproductive organs they support. The ureters are mentioned because of their proximity to the reproductive tract. Female pelvic structures are illustrated in Figs. 5.6 to 5.8. Segments of these figures accompany content discussion. Internal organs include the ovaries, uterine tubes, uterus, and vagina.

Ovaries: female gonads
Location and support. One ovary is located on each side of the uterus, below and behind the uterine tubes. The ovaries are held in place by two ligaments, the

mesovarian portions of the uterine broad ligament, which suspend them from the lateral pelvic side walls at about the level of the anterosuperior iliac crest, and the *ovarian* ligaments (Fig. 5.6), which anchor them to the uterus. The ovaries are movable with palpation.

Structure. The ovaries are similar in origin (homologous) to the testes in the male. Each ovary is composed of two layers around a central zone (Fig. 5.9). Each ovary resembles a large almond in size and shape. Each is whitish and rounded but flattened, weighes about 3 g, and measures approximately $3 \times 2 \times 1$ cm. At the time of ovulation, ovarian size may double temporarily. The oval-shaped ovaries are firm in consistency and slightly tender. The surface of the ovary is smooth before menarche. After sexual maturity, scarring from repeated ruptures of follicles and ovulation roughens the nodular surface.

Blood vessels and lymphatics. Ovarian arteries carry a rich blood supply from the aorta to the ovaries. The left ovarian vein empties into the left renal vein, but the right drains into the inferior vena cava. The ovarian lymphatics drain into the iliac and periaortic nodes.

Innervation. The nerve supply to the ovary is through T10 to L1, together with fibers of the pelvic sympathetic nervous system.

Functions. The two functions of the ovary are ovulation and hormone production. At birth the normal female's ovaries contain countless thousands of primordial (primitive) ova. At intervals during the reproductive life (generally monthly), one or more ova mature and undergo ovulation. The ovary is also the major site of production of steroid sex hormones (estrogens, progesterone, and androgens) in amounts required for normal female growth, development, and function.

Uterine tubes (oviducts)
Location and support. The paired uterine (fallopian) tubes are attached to the uterine fundus (Fig. 5.10).

Fig. 5.6
Uterus and adnexa, posterior view.

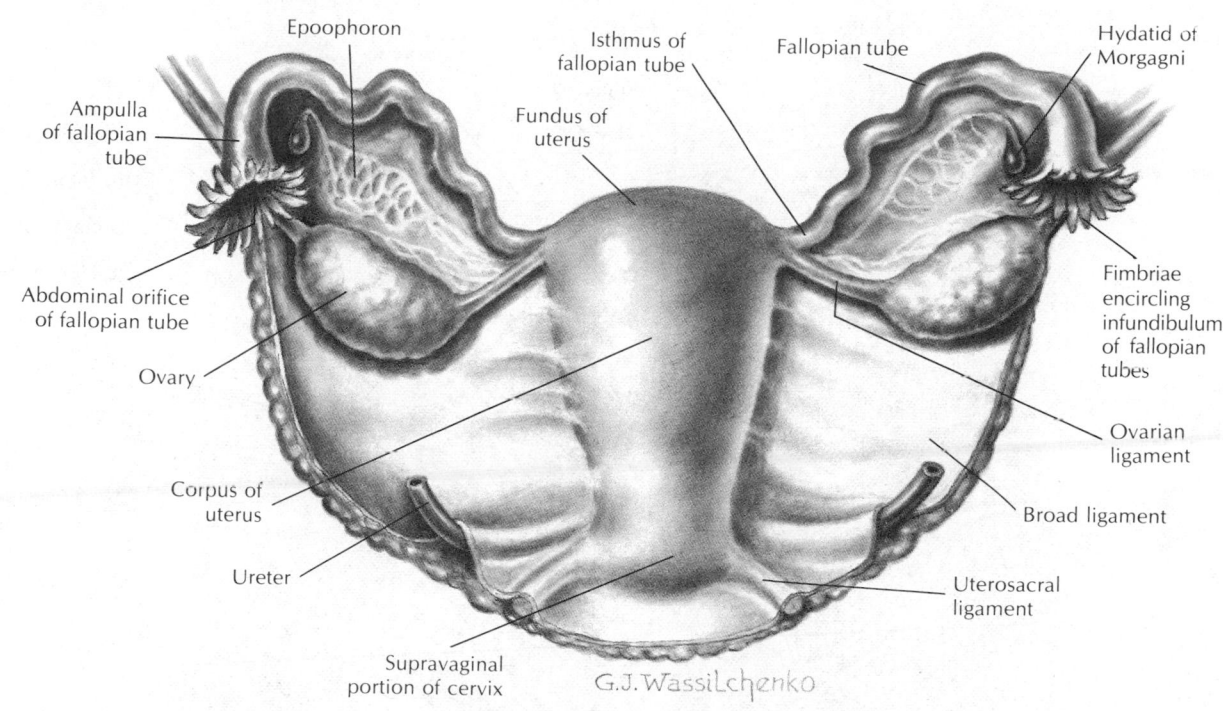

Fig. 5.7
Cross section of uterus, adnexa, and upper vagina.

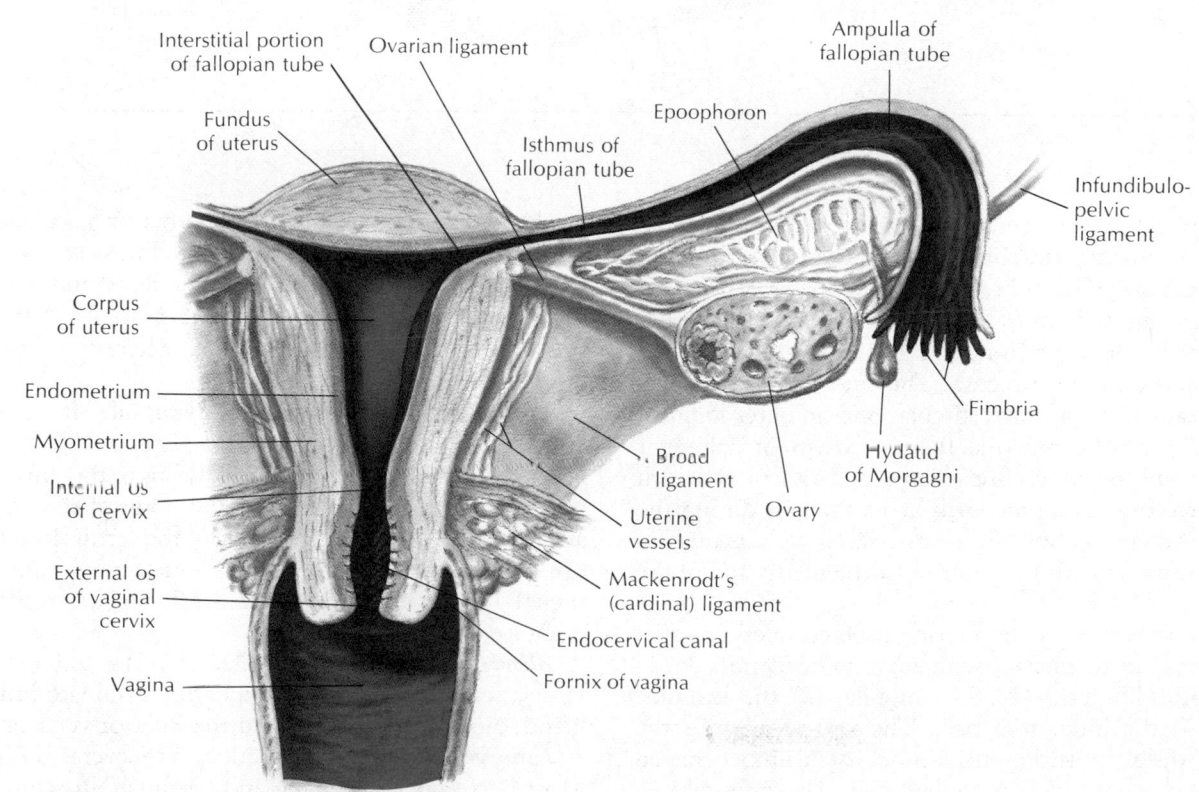

Fig. 5.8
Midsagittal view of female pelvic organs, with woman lying supine.

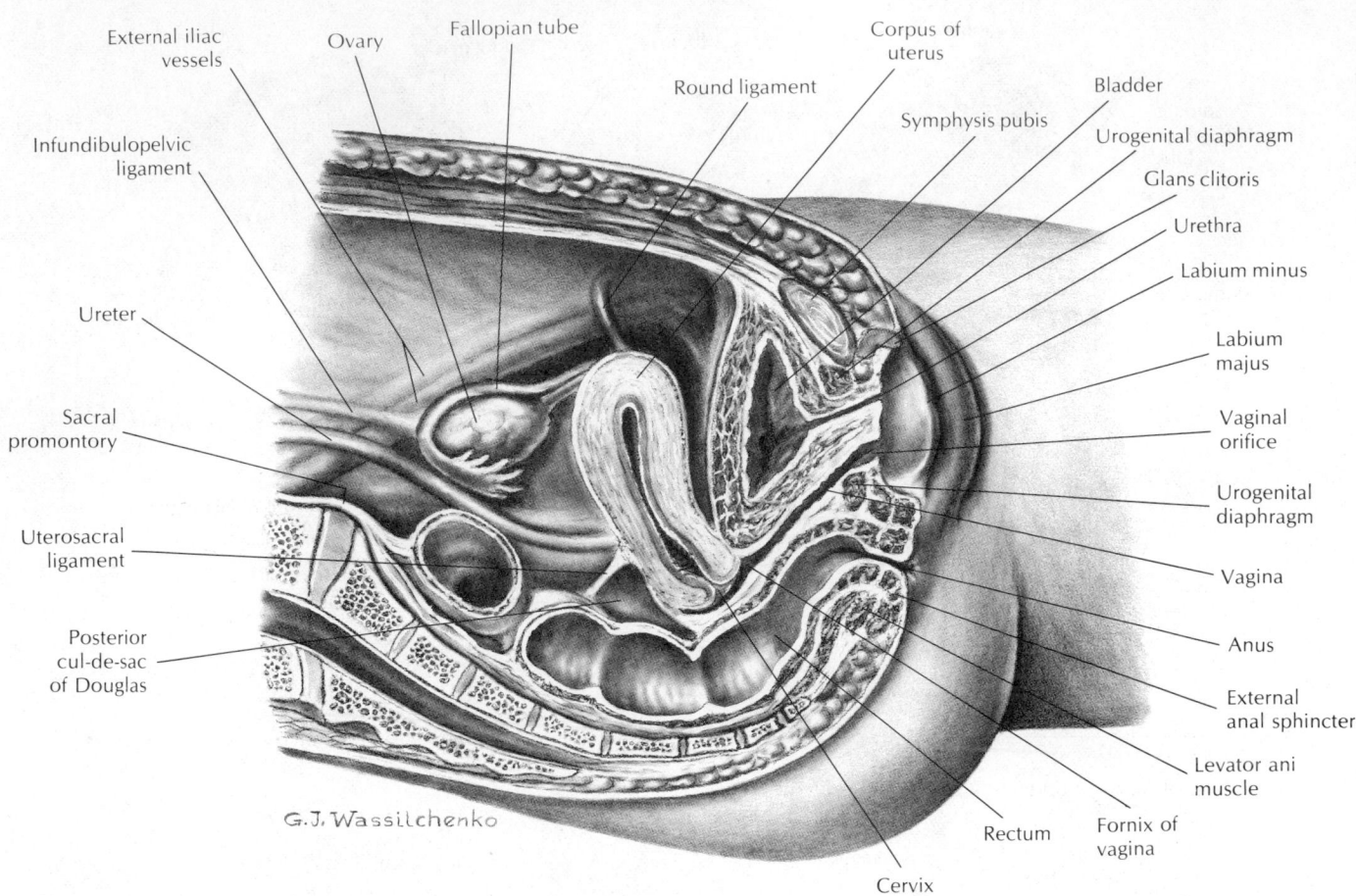

The tubes extend laterally, enter the free ends of the broad ligament, and curl around each ovary.

Structure. The tubes are approximately 10 cm (4 in) long and 0.6 cm (¼ in) in diameter. Each tube has an outer coat of peritoneum, a middle, thin muscular coat, and an inner mucosa. The smooth muscle fibers are arranged in an inner circular and an outer longitudinal layer. The mucosal lining consists of columnar cells, some of which are ciliated and others of which are secretory. The mucosa is at its thinnest during the time of menstruation. Each tube along with its mucosa is continuous with the mucosa of the uterus and of the vagina.

The structure of the uterine tube changes along its length. Four distinctive segments can be identified: (1) the infundibulum, (2) the ampulla, (3) the isthmus, and (4) the interstitial part. The *infundibulum* is the most distal portion. Its funnel or trumpet-shaped opening is encircled with fimbriae. The infundiblum

has been described as a ruffled petunia or a sea anemone. The fimbriae become swollen, almost erectile, at ovulation. The *ampulla* makes up the distal and middle segment of the tube. It is in the ampulla that the sperm and the ovum meet, that is, where fertilization occurs.

The *isthmus* is proximal to the ampulla. It is small and firm, much like the round ligament. The *interstitial* (or intramural) portion passes through the myometrium between the fundus and the body of the uterus and has the smallest lumen. Before the fertilized ovum can pass through this lumen or tunnel, measuring less then 1 mm in diameter, it has to discard its crown of granulosa cells.

Blood vessels and lymphatics. Ovarian and uterine vessels service the tubes. Lymphatics terminate in two glands alongside the aorta and the inferior vena cava.

Innervation. The nerve supply has several sources. Most nerve fibers originate and terminate in segments

Fig. 5.9
Cross section of ovary.

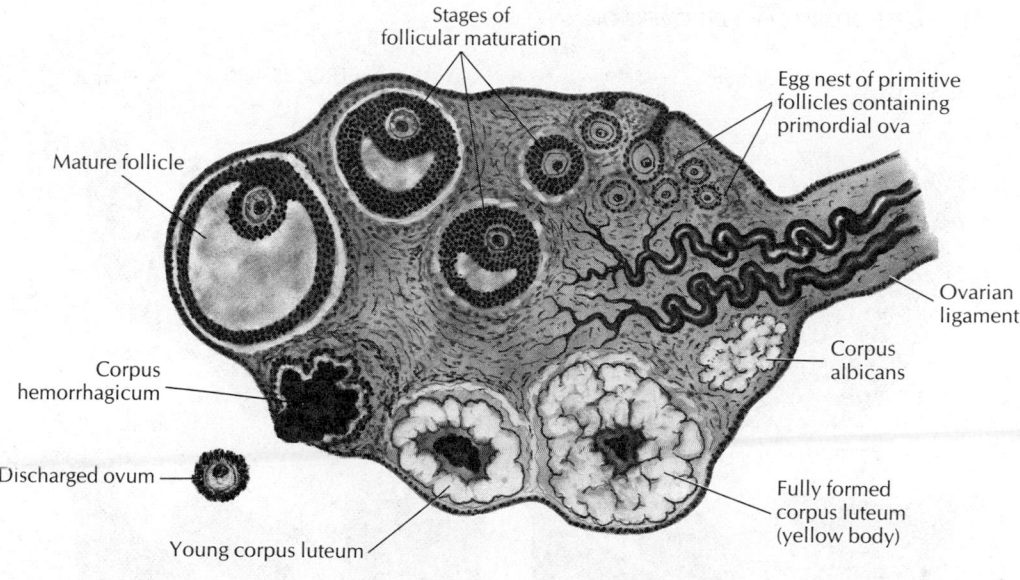

Stages of
follicular maturation

Egg nest of primitive
follicles containing
primordial ova

Mature follicle

Ovarian
ligament

Corpus
albicans

Corpus
hemorrhagicum

Discharged ovum

Fully formed
corpus luteum
(yellow body)

Young corpus luteum

Fig. 5.10
Structure of uterine tube. The ovum travels past the fimbria *(1)*, into the infundibulum *(2)*, and through the ampulla, *(3)*, isthmus *(4)*, and interstitial portion *(5)* into the uterine canal.

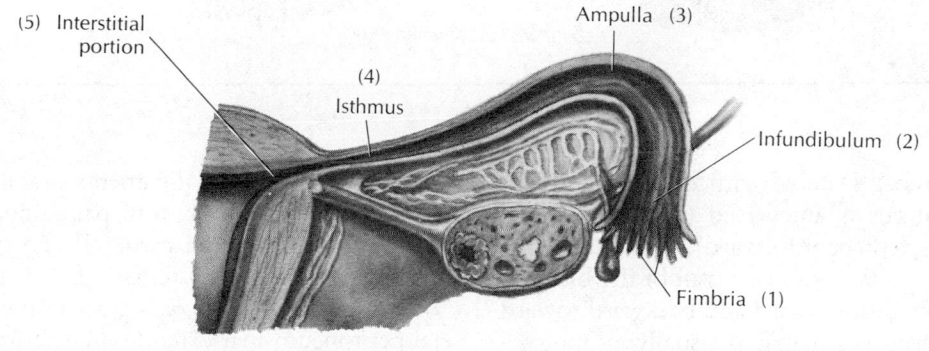

(5) Interstitial
portion

Ampulla (3)

(4)

Isthmus

Infundibulum (2)

Fimbria (1)

T10-L1. The exact role of this diversified innervation is not understood.

Functions. The uterine tubes provide a passageway for the ovum. The fingerlike projections (fimbriae) of the infundibulum pull the ovum into the tube with wavelike beckoning motions. The ovum is propelled along the tube, partially by the cilia but primarily by the peristaltic movements of the muscular coat, toward the uterine cavity. Peristaltic motion is influenced by estrogen and prostaglandins. Peristaltic activity of the uterine tubes and the secretory function of their mucosal lining are greatest at the time of ovulation. The columnar cells secrete a nutrient to sustain the ovum while it is in the tube.

Ureters. Although the ureters are not part of the reproductive tract, they are discussed here because of their anatomic proximity to the reproductive organs (see Figs. 5.6 and 5.8). As the ureters leave the kidney, they pass just behind the ovarian blood vessels close to the uterine tubes and in front of the uterine blood vessels.

Uterus
Location. Between birth and puberty the uterus descends gradually into the true pelvis from the lower abdomen. After puberty the uterus is usually located in the midline in the true pelvis behind the symphysis pubis and urinary bladder and in front of the rectum.

Fig. 5.11
Uterine positions.

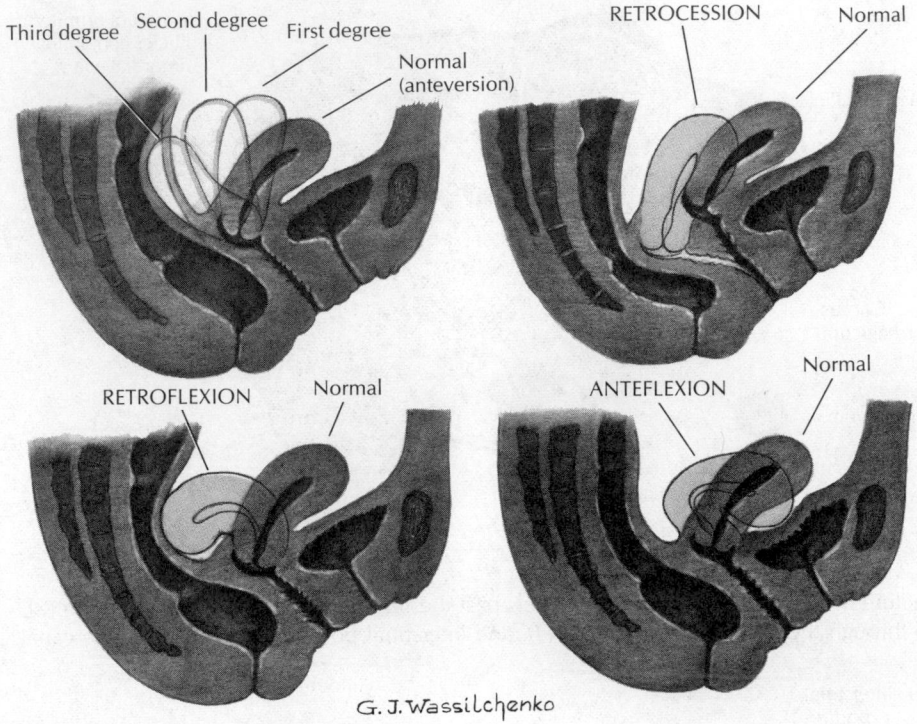

THE THREE DEGREES OF RETROVERSION

G. J. Wassilchenko

Position. For most women, with the urinary bladder empty, the uterus is anteverted (tipped forward) and slightly anteflexed (bent forward), with the corpus lying over the top of the posterior wall of the bladder. The cervix is directed downward and backward toward the tip of the sacrum so that it is usually at approximately a right angle to the plane of the vagina. For other women the uterus may be in the midposition or tipped backward (retroverted) (Fig. 5.11). The uterus that is bent more than usual so that the fundus is closer to the cervix is said to be anteflexed, or retroflexed (Fig. 5.11).

A full bladder pushes the uterus back toward the rectum, while a full rectum moves the uterus forward against the bladder. Uterine position also changes, depending on the woman's position (e.g., lying supine, prone, on her side, or standing), her age, and pregnancy.

The free mobility permits the uterus to rise slightly during the sexual response cycle so that the cervix is placed in a position to increase the likelihood of fertilization.

Support. The uterus is supported by ligaments and by muscles of the pelvic floor, including the perineal

body. A total of 10 ligaments stabilize the uterus within the pelvic cavity: four paired ligaments (broad, round, uterosacral, and cardinal) and two single ligaments (anterior and posterior) (Fig. 5.12).

The paired *broad ligaments* are double folds of parietal peritoneum that extend winglike from the sides of the uterus to the pelvic walls. These ligaments divide the pelvic cavity into anterior and posterior components. In the upper portion of the broad ligaments are suspended the uterine tubes, ovaries, round ligaments, and ovarian ligaments. This upper portion consists of loose connective tissue that does *not* influence uterine position.

The two *round ligaments* are composed of smooth muscle and connective tissue. The round ligaments extend from the upper outer angles formed where the uterine tubes join the uterine corpus (at the cornua), through the inguinal canals, and end in the labia majora. In the nonpregnant state it is a lax cord; in pregnancy it is stretched and increases in diameter (see discussion of discomforts of pregnancy, Chapter 11).

The single *anterior* (uterovesical or pubocervical) *ligament* is a continuation of parietal peritoneum that forms the anterior fold of the broad ligament, extend-

Fig. 5.12
Uterine support. **A,** Right posterior view. **B,** Left anterior view. **C,** Midsagittal view with woman lying supine.

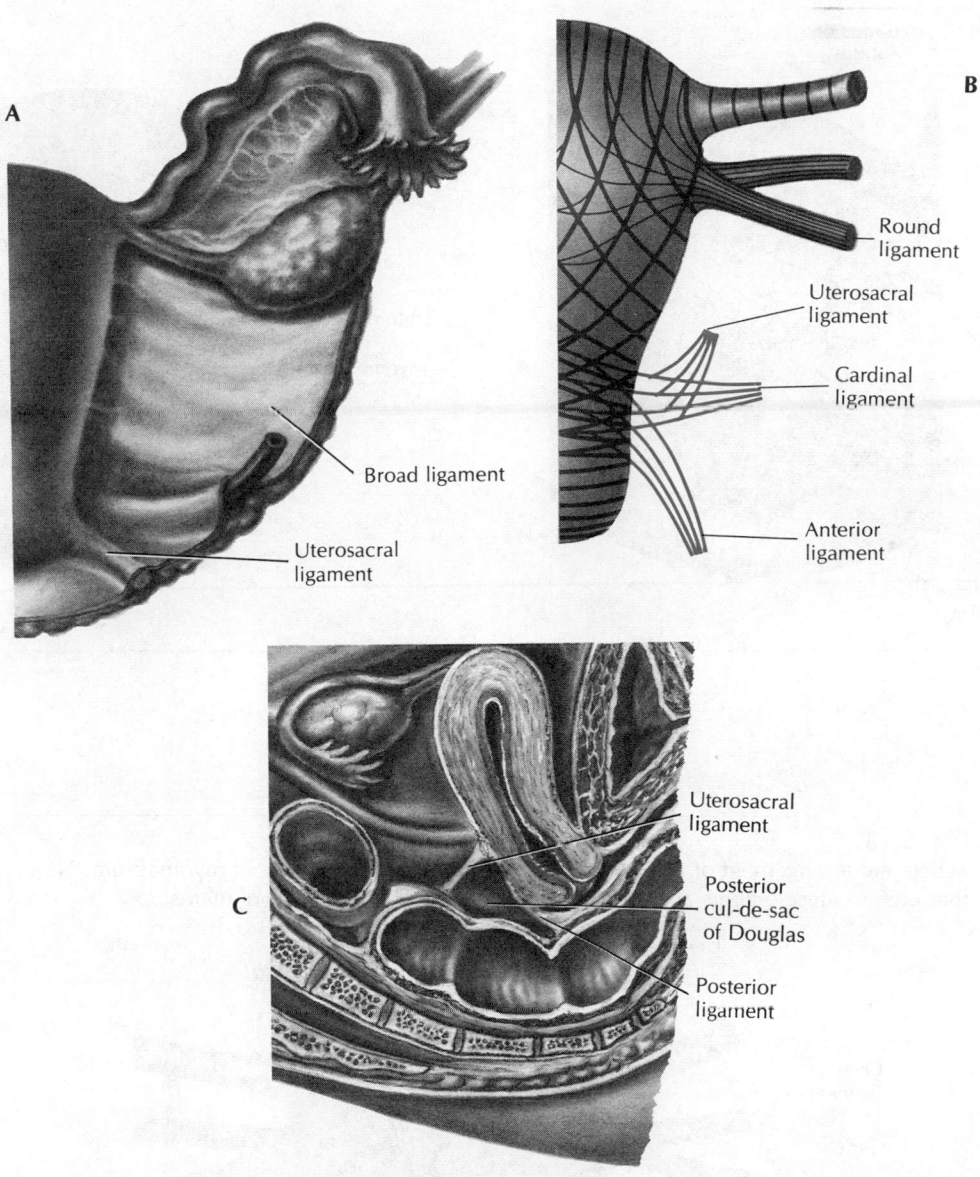

ing from the anterior surface of the supravaginal cervix of the uterus to the posterior surface of the bladder. The pouch formed by the fold of peritoneum is less deep than the posterior pouch.

The denser connective tissue of the lower portion of the broad ligaments is sometimes known as the *cardinal, transverse,* or *Mackenrodt's ligaments.* The uterine blood vessels and the ureters are enclosed within the cardinal ligaments, where they are connected to the lateral margin of the uterus. The cardinal ligaments form the upper portion of the posterior ligament.

The single *posterior* (or rectovaginal) *ligament* is a

continuation of parietal peritoneum (posterior fold of broad ligament) extending from the posterior surface of the uterus to the rectum. The posterior ligament forms the deep rectouterine pouch also known as the *cul-de-sac of Douglas.*

The two *uterosacral ligaments* are cordlike folds of peritoneum extending from the supravaginal cervical portion of the uterus to the fascia over the second and third sacral vertebrae and passing on each side of the rectum. These ligaments hold the uterus in position by maintaining traction on the cervix.

In summary the main uterine supports are the liga-

Fig. 5.13
Uterine fundus, corpus (body), and isthmus (lower uterine segment during pregnancy).

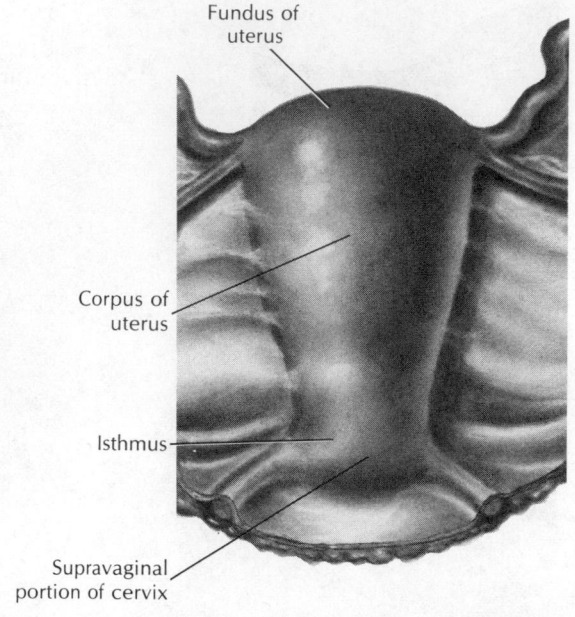

Fig. 5.14
Uterine wall: endometrium, myometrium, parietal peritoneum.

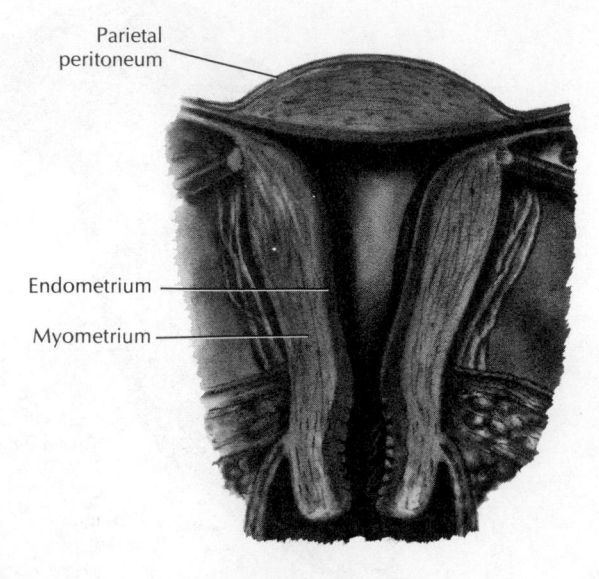

Fig. 5.15
Schematic arrangement of directions of muscle fibers of three layers of myometrium. Note that uterine muscle fibers are continuous with supportive ligaments of uterus.

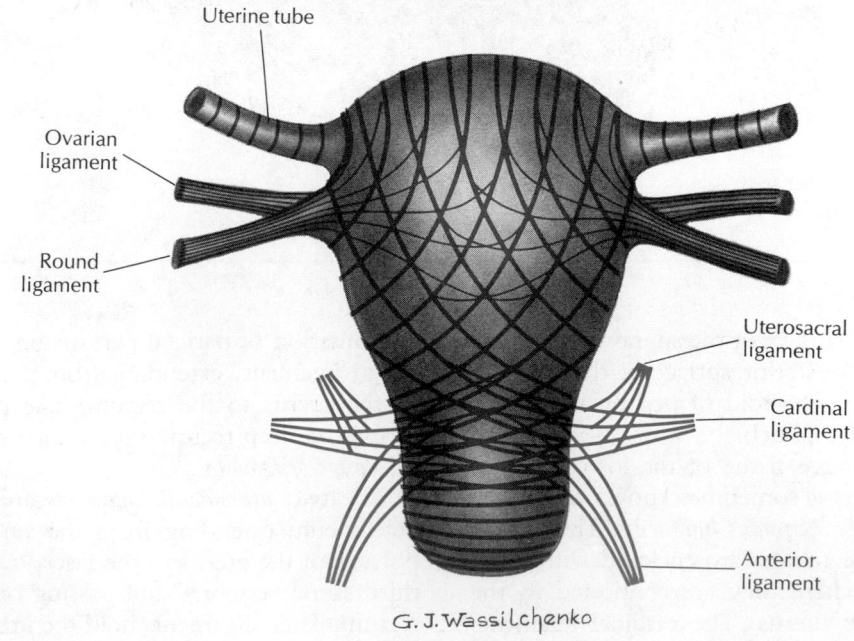

ments surrounding the supravaginal cervix:

1. Anterior (pubocervical)
2. Cardinal (transverse, Mackenrodt's)
3. Posterior (rectovaginal)
4. Uterosacral

Structure, Shape, size, and divisions. The uterus is a flattened, hollow, muscular, thick-walled organ that looks somewhat like an upside-down pear (Fig. 5.13). Its length, width, and thickness vary, averaging about 7.5 × 3.5 × 2 cm (3 × 1½ × ¾ in.). In the adult woman who has never been pregnant the uterus weighs 60 g (2 oz). The uterus normally is symmetric in shape and nontender, smooth, and firm to the touch. The degree of firmness varies with several factors; for example, it is spongier during the secretory phase of the menstrual cycle, softer during pregnancy, and firmer after menopause.

The uterus has three parts: the *fundus,* the upper, rounded prominence above the insertion of the uterine tubes; the *corpus,* or main portion, encircling the intrauterine cavity; and the *isthmus,* the slightly constricted portion that joins the corpus to the cervix and is known as the lower uterine segment during pregnancy.

Wall. The wall of the uterus is made up of three layers: the endometrium, the myometrium, and a partial outer layer of parietal peritoneum (Fig. 5.14).

The highly vascular *endometrium* is a lining of mucous membrane composed of three layers: a compact surface layer, a spongy middle layer of loose connective tissue, and a dense inner layer that attaches the endometrium to the myometrium. (The upper two layers are also referred to as the functional layer; and the inner layer, as the basal layer.) During menstruation and following delivery the compact surface and middle spongy layers slough off. Just after menstrual flow ends, the endometrium is 0.5 mm thick; near the end of the endometrial cycle, just before menstruation begins again, it is about 5.0 mm (less than ¼ in) thick.

Layers of smooth muscle fibers that extend in three directions (longitudinal, transverse, and oblique) make up the thick *myometrium* (Fig. 5.15). The smooth muscle fibers interlace with elastic and connective tissues and blood vessels throughout the uterine wall and blend with the dense inner layer of the endometrium. The myometrium is particularly thick in the fundus, thins out as it nears the isthmus, and is thinnest in the cervix.

The *outer* myometrial layer, found mostly in the fundus, is made up of longitudinal fibers and is therefore well suited for expelling the fetus during the birth process. In the thick *middle* myometrial layer the interlaced muscle fibers form a figure-of-eight pattern encircling large blood vessels. Contraction of the middle layer produces a hemostatic action. Only a few circular fibers of the *inner* myometrial layer are found in the fundus. Most of the circular fibers are concentrated in the cornua, the place where the uterine tubes join the uterine body, and around the internal os. The sphincter action of this layer prevents the regurgitation of menstrual blood out of the uterine tubes during menstruation. Their sphincter action around the internal cervical os helps to retain the uterine contents during pregnancy. Injury to this sphincter can weaken the internal os and result in an incompetent internal cervical os (see Chapter 29).

For clarity and interest, each muscle layer and its function were described individually. It must be remembered that the myometrium works as a whole. The structure of the myometrium, which gives strength and elasticity, presents an example of adaptation to function:

1. To thin out, pull up, and open the cervix and to push the fetus out of the uterus, the fundus must contract with the most force.
2. Contraction of interlacing smooth muscle fibers that surround the blood vessels controls blood loss after abortion and childbirth. Because of their ability to close off (ligate) blood vessels between them, the smooth muscle fibers of the uterus are referred to as the **living ligature** (Fig. 5.16).

Muscle fibers of the uterine myometrium are continuous with the muscle layers in the uterine tubes and vagina and with muscle fibers in the ovarian, round, and cardinal ligaments; they are minimally continuous with those in the uterosacral ligaments.

The *parietal peritoneum,* a serous membrane, coats all the uterine corpus except for the lower one fourth of the anterior surface, where the bladder is attached, and the cervix. Because parietal peritoneum does not completely cover this organ, it is possible for diagnostic tests and surgery involving the uterus to be performed without entering the abdominal cavity.

Cervix. The lowermost portion of the uterus is the cervix, or neck (Fig. 5.17). The attachment site of the uterine cervix to the vaginal vault divides the cervix into the longer supravaginal (above the vagina) portion and the shorter vaginal portion. The length of the cervix is about 2.5 to 3 cm, of which about 1 cm protrudes into the vagina in the nongravid woman.

The cervix is composed primarily of fibrous connective tissue with some muscle fibers and elastic tissue. The cervix of the nulliparous woman is rounded, almost conical, rather firm, spindle-shaped body approximately 2 to 2.5 cm in external diameter. The narrowed opening between the uterine cavity and the endocervical (canal inside the cervix that connects the uterine cavity with the vagina) canal is the internal os.

Fig. 5.16
The living ligature: interlacing smooth muscle fibers of the thick middle myometrium. Red denotes blood vessels. **A,** Relaxed muscle fibers. **B,** Contracted muscle fibers ligating the blood vessels.

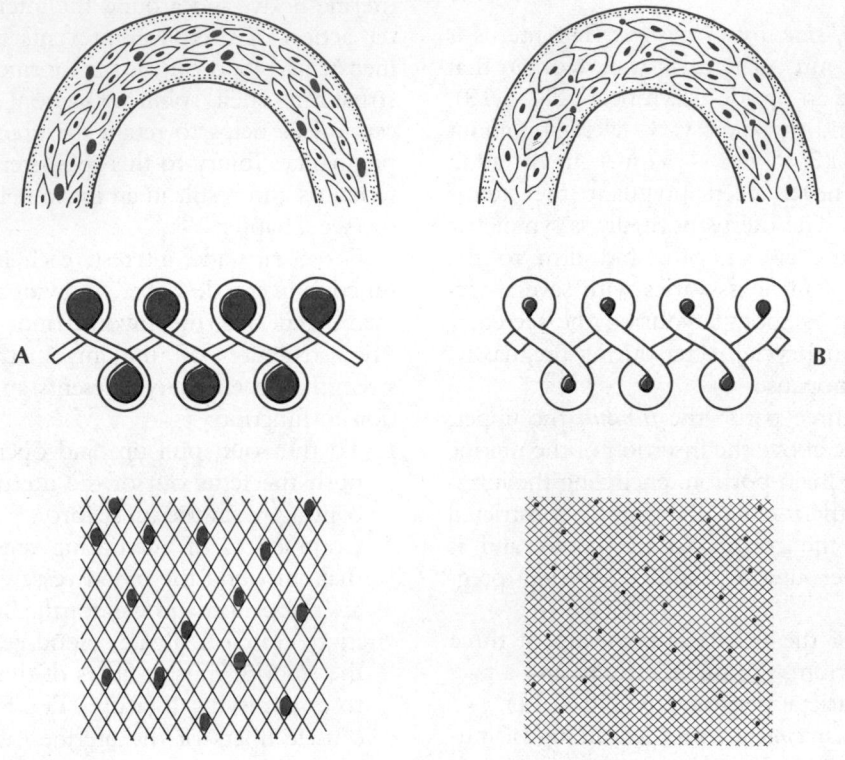

Fig. 5.17
Cervix. **A,** Intraabdominal posterior view of supravaginal portion of cervix. **B,** Cross section of supravaginal cervix and vaginal portion of cervix surrounded by the fornix.

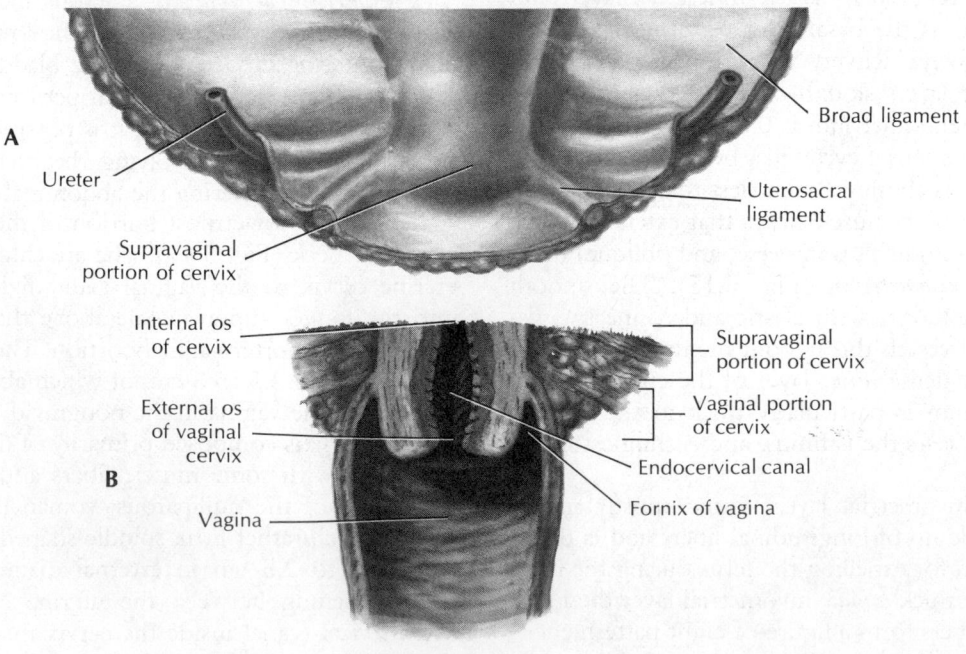

Fig. 5.18
External cervical os as seen through speculum.
A, Nonparous cervix. **B,** Parous cervix.

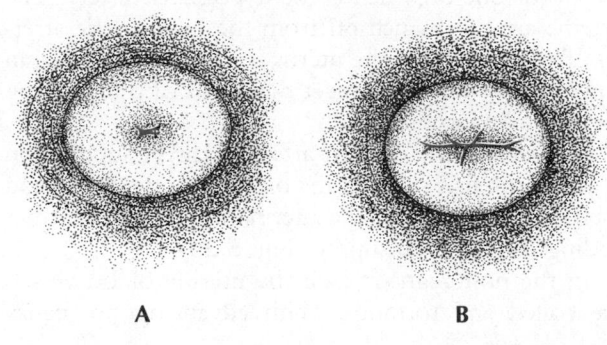

A   B

The narrowed opening between the endocervix and the vagina is the external os. The external os is a small circular opening in women who have not borne children. Childbirth changes the circular os to a small transverse opening dividing the cervix into an anterior and a posterior lip (Fig. 5.18).

When the woman is not ovulating or pregnant, the tip of the cervix feels firm much like the end of one's nose, with a dimple in the center. The dimple marks the site of the external os.

The most significant characteristic of the cervix is its ability to stretch during vaginal childbirth. Several factors contribute to cervical elasticity: high connective tissue and elastic fiber content, numerous infoldings in the endocervical lining, and a muscle fiber content of about 10%.

Canals. There are two cavities within the uterus, which are known as the uterine and cervical canals (Fig. 5.19). The uterine canal in the nonpregnant state is compressed by thick muscular walls so that it is only a potential space, flat and triangular in shape. The base of the triangle is formed by the fundus. The uterine tubes open into either end of the base. The apex of the triangle points downward and forms the internal os (opening) of the cervical canal.

The endocervical canal with its many infoldings has a surface layer of tall, columnar, mucus-producing cells (Fig. 5.19). *Columnar epithelium* is beefy red, deeper, and rougher looking than the epithelial outer covering of the cervix. After menarche (the start of menstruation) *squamous epithelium* covers the outside of the cervix (ectocervix). This external covering of flat cells gives a glistening pink color to the cervix. A deeper

Fig. 5.19
Uterine and cervical canals and the squamocolumnar junction.

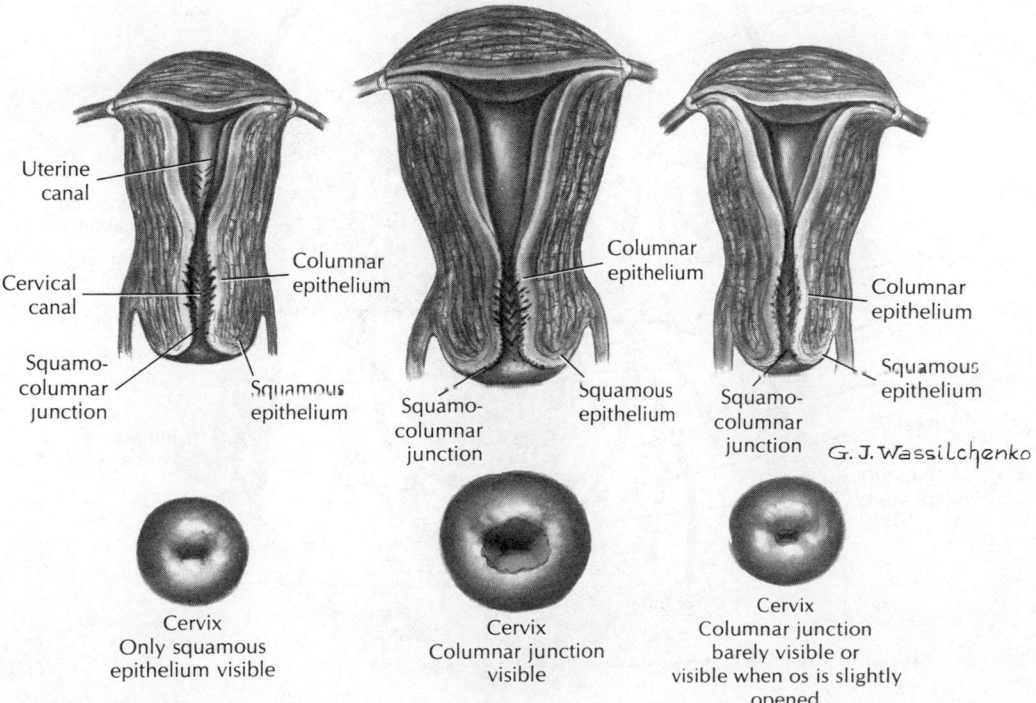

Uterine canal

Cervical canal

Columnar epithelium

Squamo-columnar junction

Squamous epithelium

Columnar epithelium

Squamous epithelium

Squamo-columnar junction

Columnar epithelium

Squamous epithelium

Squamo-columnar junction

G. J. Wassilchenko

Cervix
Only squamous epithelium visible

Cervix
Columnar junction visible

Cervix
Columnar junction barely visible or visible when os is slightly opened

bluish red color is seen when the woman is ovulating or pregnant. A reddened (hyperemic) cervix may indicate inflammation.

The two types of epithelium meet at the *squamocolumnar junction* (Fig. 5.19). This junction line is usually just inside the external cervical os but may be found on the ectocervix in some women. The squamocolumnar junction is the most common site of neoplastic cellular changes. Therefore cells for cytologic study, the Papanicolaou smear, are scraped from this junction.

The columnar epithelial cells produce odorless and nonirritating mucus in response to ovarian endocrine hormones—estrogen and progesterone.

Blood vessels. The abdominal aorta divides at about the level of the umbilicus and forms the two iliac arteries. Each iliac artery divides to form two arteries, the major one of which is the hypogastric artery. The uterine arteries branch off from the hypogastric arteries. The closeness of the uterus to the aorta ensures an ample blood supply to meet the needs of the growing uterus and conceptus.

In addition the ovarian artery, a direct subdivision of the aorta, first supplies the ovary with the blood and then proceeds to join the uterine artery, thus further adding to the blood supply (Fig. 5.20).

In the nonpregnant state the uterine blood vessels are coiled and tortuous. With advancing pregnancy

Fig. 5.20
A, Pelvic blood supply.

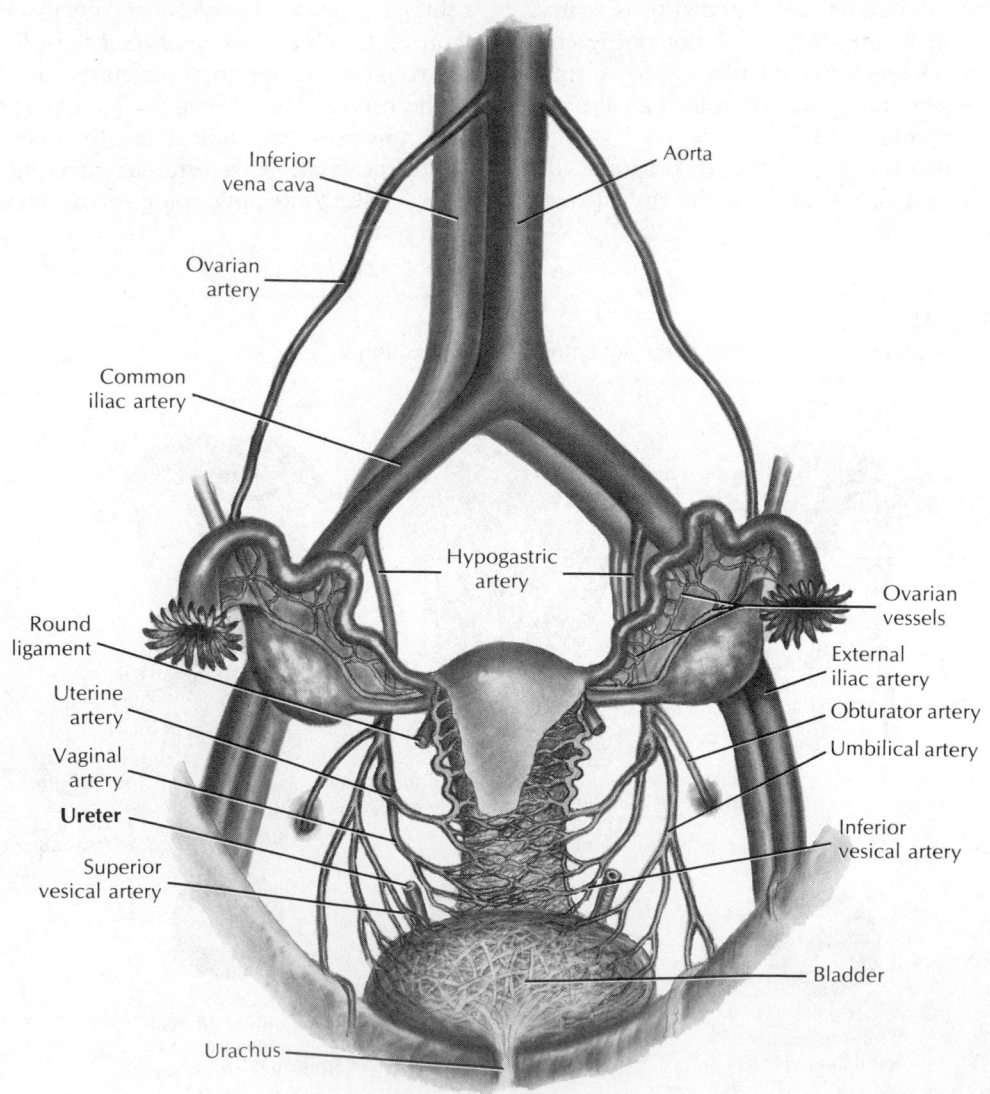

and an enlarging uterus, these blood vessels straighten out. The uterine veins follow along the arteries and empty into the internal iliac veins.

Lymphatics. The lymphatics of the uterus are extensive. They are contained in three networks: at the base of the endometrium, within the myometrium, and just under the peritoneal coat of the uterus. There are *no* lymphatics in the more superficial layers of the endometrium. Lymphatic drainage occurs mainly at the isthmus along the uterine vessels. Near the uterine fundus, drainage joins that of the ovarian and tubal lymphatics to nodes around the aorta. Some lymphatics may drain into femoral, iliac, and hypogastric nodes.

Innervation. The internal genitalia have a rich supply of afferent and efferent autonomic nerves, both motor and sensory.

Motor nerves. Parasympathetic fibers from the sacral nerves are probably responsible for producing vasodilation and inhibiting muscular contraction. Efferent sympathetic motor nerves arise from the ganglia of T5 (thoracic 5) to T10, come together over the sacrum, and reach the uterus through ganglia that lie near the base of the uterosacral ligaments. These efferent sympathetic motor nerves are believed to cause vasoconstriction and muscular contraction. The autonomic nerves just described (parasympathetic and efferent sympathetic motor) regulate the action of the uterus, but the uterus has an intrinsic motility (i.e., it can contract and relax even if the nerves to it are cut). This means that even if a woman suffers an accident that injures the spinal cord at or above T5, she may still be able to have uterine contractions sufficient to deliver an infant vaginally.

Sensory nerves. Sensory fibers, carrying pain sensation from the uterus, come together in the paracervical areas and proceed upward to pass just below the division (bifurcation) of the aorta, and then travel to the spinal cord at the level of T11 and T12. Because of this arrangement, pain that originates in the ovary or in the ureters may mimic pain that originates in the uterus, any of which may be felt in the flank and down to the inguinal and vulvar areas.

Fig. 5.20, cont'd
B, Blood supply of perineum and uterus.

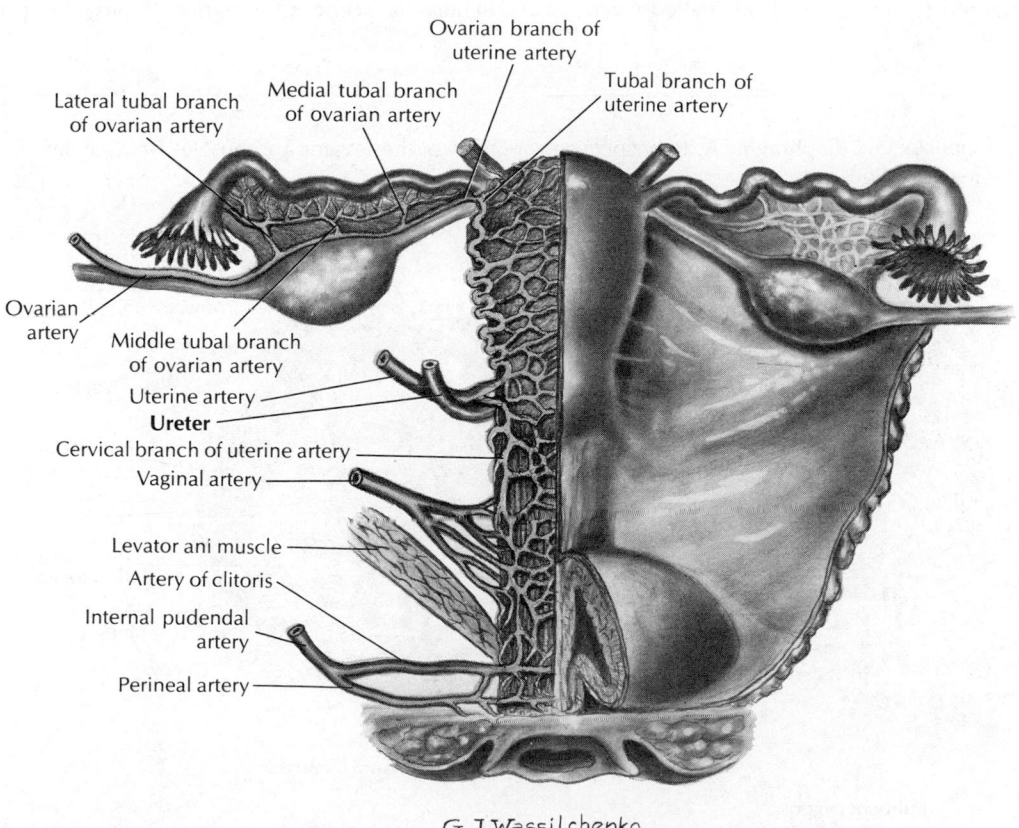

Ovarian branch of
uterine artery

Lateral tubal branch
of ovarian artery

Medial tubal branch
of ovarian artery

Tubal branch of
uterine artery

Ovarian
artery

Middle tubal branch
of ovarian artery

Uterine artery

Ureter

Cervical branch of uterine artery

Vaginal artery

Levator ani muscle

Artery of clitoris

Internal pudendal
artery

Perineal artery

G. J. Wassilchenko

Functions. The three functions of the uterus are essential for the survival of the species but not for the individual. These functions include cyclic menstruation with rejuvenation of the endometrium, pregnancy, and labor.

Vagina

Location and support. The vagina is a tubular structure located in front of the rectum and behind the bladder and urethra. The vagina extends from the introitus, the external opening in the vestibule between the labia minora of the vulva, to the cervix. When the woman is standing, the vagina slants backward and upward. It is supported mainly by its attachments to the pelvic floor musculature and fascia.

Structure. The vagina is a thin-walled, collapsible tube capable of great distention. Because of the way the cervix protrudes into the uppermost portion of the vagina, the length of the anterior wall of the vagina is only about 7 to 8 cm, while that of the posterior wall is about 10 cm. The recesses formed all around the protruding cervix are called fornices: right, left, anterior, and posterior. The posterior fornix is deeper than the other three.

The smooth muscle walls are lined with glandular mucous membrane. During the reproductive years this mucosa is arranged in transverse folds called *rugae.*

The vaginal mucosa responds promptly to estrogen and progesterone stimulation. Cells are lost from the mucosa, especially during the menstrual cycle and pregnancy. Cells scraped from the vaginal mucosa can be used to estimate steroid sex hormone levels.

Vaginal fluid. Vaginal fluid is derived from the lower or upper genital tract. The continuous flow of fluid from the vagina maintains relative cleanliness of the vagina. Therefore, vaginal douching in normal circumstances is not necessary. A spread of vaginal mucus from the posterior vaginal fornix and a scraping from the squamocolumnar junction of the cervix, fixed in ethyl ether and alcohol and then treated with trichrome nucleocytoplasmic stain, constitute the *Papanicolaou (Pap) smear* used throughout the world for gynecologic cancer detection.

Blood vessels and lymphatics. The copious blood supply to the vagina is derived from the descending branches of the uterine artery, the vaginal artery, and the internal pudendal arteries. The venous return of vaginal blood is through the pudendal, vaginal, and uterine veins. The lymphatics of the upper vagina drain to the rectovaginal, septal, presacral, external iliac, and hypogastric nodes. The lower vaginal lymphatics are directed to the superficial inguinal nodes.

Innervation. The vagina is relatively insensitive. There is some innervation from the pudendal and

---

Fig. 5.21
Upper pelvic diaphragm. **A,** Pubococcygeus portion of the levator ani muscles, midsagittal view. **B,** View from above.

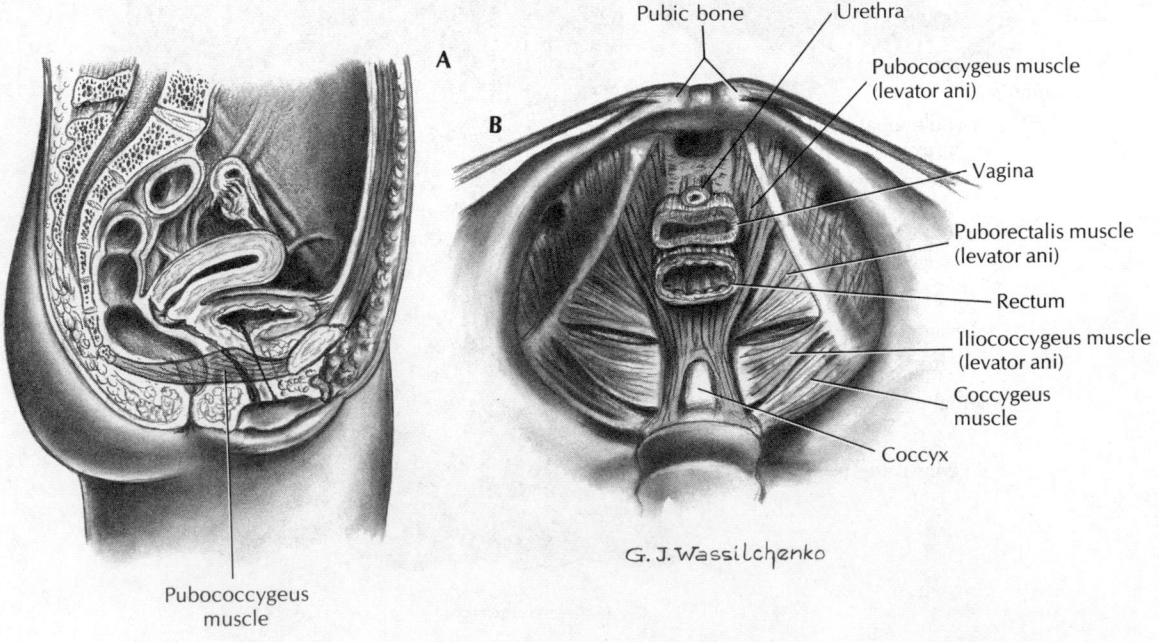

Pubic bone

Urethra

Pubococcygeus muscle
(levator ani)

Vagina

Puborectalis muscle
(levator ani)

Rectum

Iliococcygeus muscle
(levator ani)

Coccygeus
muscle

Coccyx

Pubococcygeus
muscle

G. J. Wassilchenko

hemorrhoidal nerves to the lowest one third. Because of this minimal innervation and no special nerve endings the vagina is the source of little sensation during sexual excitement and coitus and less pain during the second stage of labor than if this tissue were well supplied with nerve endings. The nerve supply is mainly autonomic. Sensations arising in the vagina terminate at the level of S2, S3, and S4.

Functions. The vagina functions as the organ for copulation (coitus) and as the birth canal.

PELVIC FLOOR AND PERINEUM

The pelvic floor and perineum are composed of the pelvic diaphragm, the urogenital diaphragm or triangle, and the muscles of the external genitalia and anus. The perineum is sometimes defined as including all the muscles, fascia, and ligaments of the upper (pelvic) and lower (urogenital) diaphragms. The perineal body adds strength to these structures.

Upper pelvic diaphragm. The upper pelvic diaphragm, composed of muscles and their fascia and ligaments, extends across the lowest part of the pelvic cavity like a hammock (Fig. 5.21). The largest and most significant portion of the diaphragm is formed by the pair of broad, thin *levator ani muscles* that extend sheetlike between the ischial spines and coccyx, and the sacrum. The levator ani group of muscles is made up of three muscle pairs: puborectalis, iliococcygeus, and pubococcygeus muscles. The pubococcygeus muscle is particularly significant for women. It plays a role in sexual sensory function, in bladder control, in controlling perineal relaxation during labor, and in expulsion of the fetus during birth.

The second paired muscles of the upper pelvic diaphragm are the closely joined *coccygeus muscles.* These

Fig. 5.22
Levator ani muscles of upper pelvic diaphragm and urogenital (lower pelvic) diaphragm, anterior view.

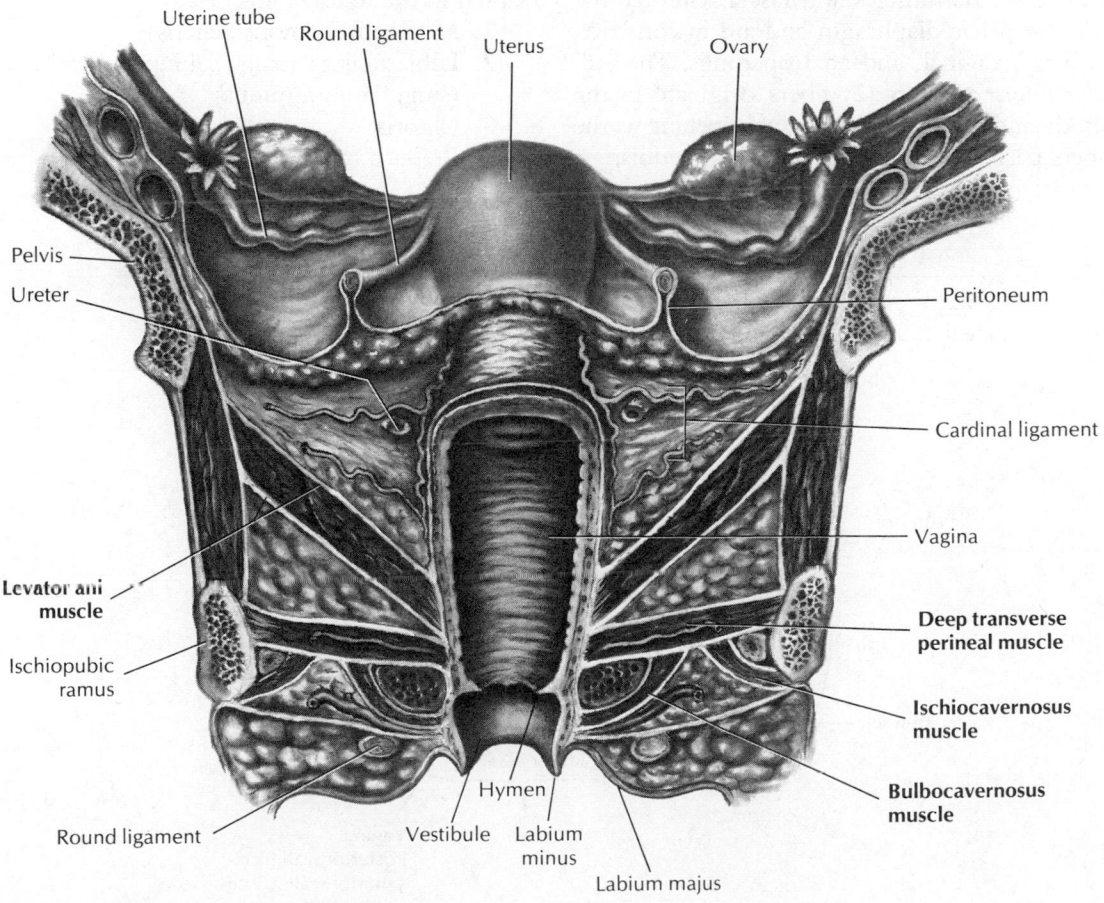

muscles extend from the ischial spines to the coccyx and lower sacrum. The several parts of the pelvic diaphragm provide a slinglike support to abdominal and pelvic viscera.

The strength and resilience of this sling are derived from the way in which the layered parts of this sling are interwoven and interlaced. The layers are not fixed; that is, they slide over each other. This unique arrangement strengthens the supportive capacity of the pelvic diaphragm, allows for dilation of the vagina during the birth process and for its closure after delivery, and assists with constriction of the urethra, vagina, and anal canal, which pass through the diaphragm.

Lower pelvic (urogenital) diaphragm. The lower pelvic diaphragm is located in the hollow of the pubic arch and consists of the transverse perineal muscles. The transverse perineal muscles originate at the ischial tuberosities and insert into the perineal body. The strong muscle fibers provide support to the anal canal during defecation and to the lower vagina during delivery. The deep transverse perineal muscles join to form a central seam or raphe. Some of their fibers encircle the urinary meatus and vaginal sphincters.

The *perineum* is located below the upper and lower pelvic diaphragm. Its muscles and fascia reinforce the strength of the pelvic diaphragm and aid in constricting the urinary, vaginal, and anal openings. The *bulbocavernosus muscle* (Fig. 5.22) fibers originate in the perineal body and surround the vaginal opening as the muscle fibers pass forward to insert into the pubis.

The *ischiocavernosus muscles* originate in the tuberosities of the ischium and continue at an angle to insert next to the bulbocavernosus muscles. These muscle fibers contract to cause erection of the clitoris.

Anal sphincter muscle fibers originate at the coccyx, separate to pass on either side of the anus, fuse, and then insert into the transverse perineal muscles.

The bulbocavernosus, transverse perineal, and anal sphincter muscle fibers can be strenghtened through Kegel exercises (see Chapter 11).

Perineal body. The *perineal body,* the wedge-shaped mass between the vaginal and anal openings, serves as an anchor point for the muscles, fascia, and ligaments of the upper and lower pelvic diaphragms (Fig. 5.23). The skin-covered base of the body is known as the perineum. The perineal body, about 4 cm wide by 4 cm deep, is continuous with the septum between the rectum and vagina. This tissue is flattened and stretched as the fetus moves through the birth canal.

EXTERNAL STRUCTURES

The external female genitalia (vulva, pudenda) are located in the perineum. The external structures are presented in the following order:
1. Mons pubis (mons veneris)
2. Labia majora (sing., labium majus) and minora (sing., labium minus)
3. Clitoris
4. Prepuce of clitoris

Fig. 5.23
Perineal body. Location and size relative to surrounding tissues, with woman sitting.

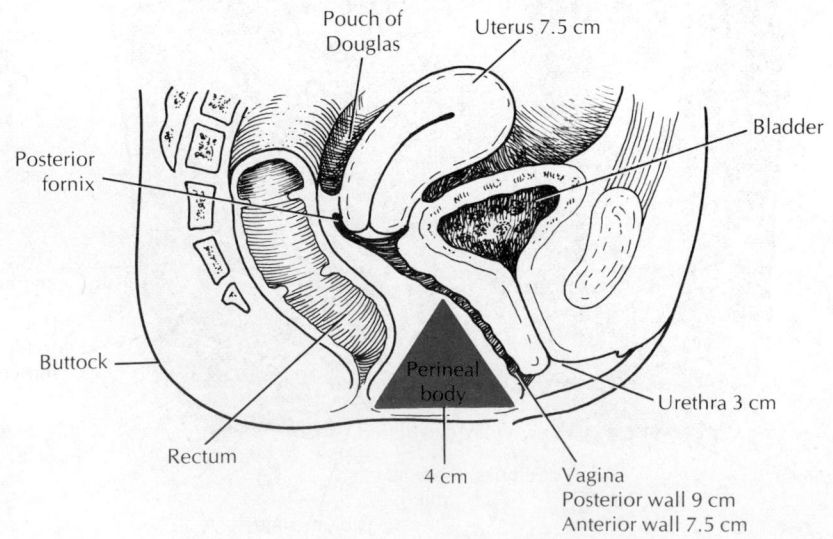

5. Vestibule
   a. Urethral or urinary orifice (meatus)
   b. Lesser vestibular, paraurethral, or Skene's glands
   c. Hymen and vaginal introitus, or orifice
   d. Greater vestibular, vulvovaginal, or Bartholin's glands
6. Fourchet
7. Perineum

The external genitalia are illustrated in Fig. 5.24.

Mons pubis. The mons pubis, or mons veneris, is the rounded, soft fullness of subcutaneous fatty tissue and loose connective tissue over the symphysis pubis. It contains many sebaceous (oil) glands and develops coarse, dark, curly hair at pubarche, about 1 to 2 years before the onset of the menses. Menarche occurs on the average at 13 years of age. In 75% of women the pattern of hair growth (the escutcheon) is a triangle shape with the base along the top of the symphysis pubis, whereas the escutcheon in males is more diamond shaped. In 25% of women, pubic hair extends upward toward the umbilicus along the linea alba. Characteristics of pubic hair vary from sparse and fine among Oriental women to thick, coarse, and curly among black women. The functions of the mons are to play a role in sensuality and to protect the symphysis pubis during coitus.

Labia majora. The labia majora are two rounded lengthwise folds of skin-covered fat and connective tissue that merge with the mons. They extend from the mons downward around the labia minora, ending in the perineum in the midline. The labia majora function as protection for the labia minora, urinary meatus, and vaginal introitus. In the woman who has never experienced vaginal childbirth the labia majora come together in the midline, obscuring the vaginal introitus. Some labial separation and even gaping of the vaginal introitus follow childbirth and perineal or vaginal injury.

On their lateral surfaces the labial skin is thick, usually pigmented darker than the surrounding tissues, and covered with coarse hair (similar to that of the

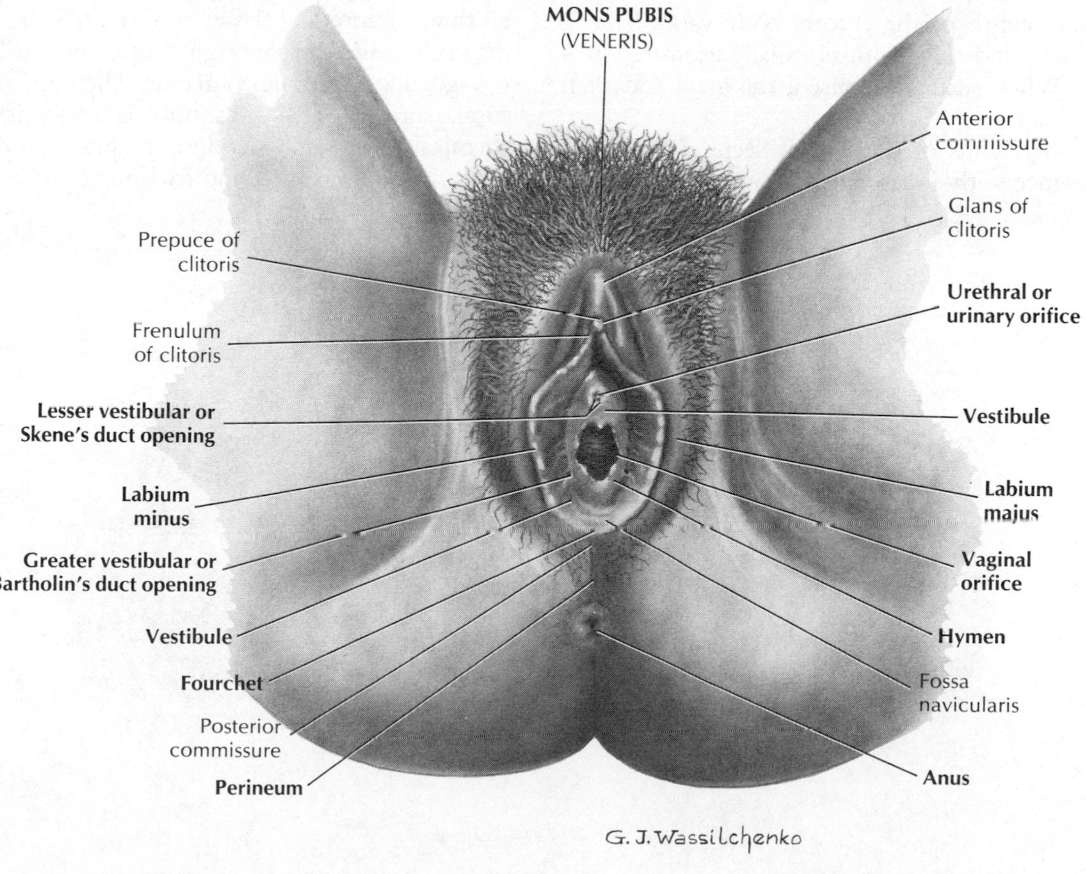

Fig. 5.24
External female genitalia.

G. J. Wassilchenko

mons) that thins out toward the perineum. The medial (inner) surfaces of the labia major are smooth, thick, and without hair. They contain an abundant supply of sebaceous glands and sweat glands and are highly vascular. The extreme sensitivity of the labia majora to touch, pain, and temperature is due to the extensive network of nerves; thus, they function during sensual arousal.

Labia minora. The labia minora, located between the labia majora, are narrow, lengthwise folds of hairless skin extending downward from beneath the clitoris and merging with the fourchet. While the lateral and anterior aspects of the labia are usually pigmented, their medial surfaces are similar to vaginal mucosa: pink and moist. Their rich vascularity gives them a reddish color and permits marked turgescence (swelling) of the labia minora with emotional or physical stimulation. The glands in the labia minora also serve to lubricate the vulva. A rich nerve supply makes them sensitive, enhancing their erotic function. The space between the labia minora is called the vestibule.

Clitoris. The clitoris is a short, cylindric, erectile organ fixed just beneath the arch of the pubis; the visible portion is about 6 × 6 mm or less in the unaroused state. The tip of the clitoral body is called the glans and is more sensitive than its shaft. In healthy women the length of the clitoral body varies from 2 mm to 1 cm, and the width is usually estimated at 4 to 5 mm. When sexually aroused, the glans and shaft increase in size.

Sebaceous glands of the clitoris secrete smegma, a fatty substance with a distinctive odor, which serves as a pheromone (an organic compound that provides communication with other members of the same species to elicit a certain response, which in this case is erotic stimulation of the human male). The term *clitoris* comes from a Greek word meaning "key" because the clitoris was seen as the key to female sexuality.

Its rich vascularity and innervation make the clitoris highly sensitive to temperature, touch, and pressure sensation. The clitoris contains more nerve endings than does its male homologue, the glans penis. Its main function is to stimulate and elevate levels of sexual tension.

Prepuce of clitoris. Near the anterior junction the right and left labia minora separate into medial and lateral portions. The lateral portions unite above the clitoris to form its prepuce, a hoodlike covering; the medial portions unite below the clitoris to form its frenulum. Sometimes the prepuce covers the clitoris. As a result this area has the appearance of an opening that can be mistaken for the urethral meatus if the nurse does not identify vulvar structures carefully. Attempts to insert a catheter into this sensitive area can cause considerable discomfort.

Vestibule. The vestibule is an ovoid or boat-shaped area formed between the labia minora, clitoris, and fourchet. The vestibule contains the openings to the urethra, paraurethral (lesser vestibular, Skene's) glands, the vagina, and the paravaginal (greater vestibular, vulvovaginal, or Bartholin's) glands. The thin, almost mucosal, surface of the vestibule is easily irritated by chemicals (feminine deodorant sprays, bubble bath salts), heat, discharges, and friction (tight jeans).

Fig. 5.25
Hymen and parous introitus.

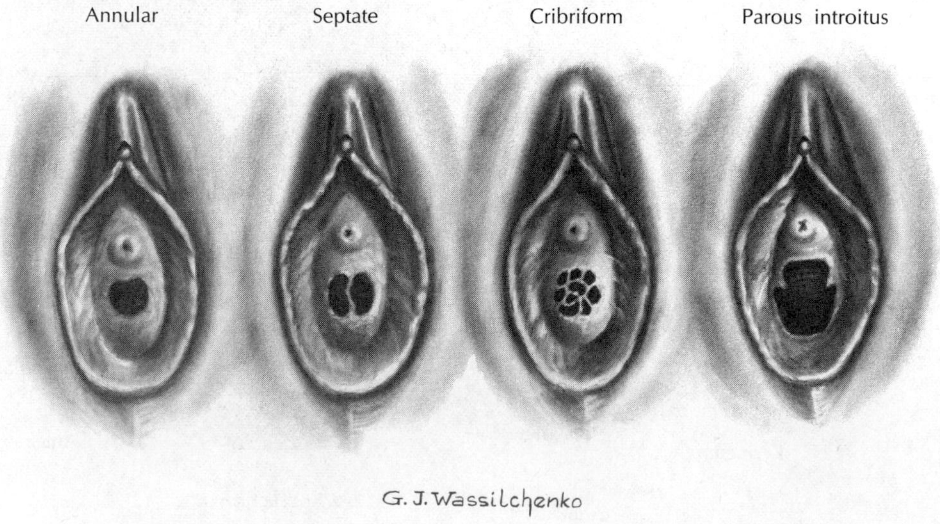

Annular   Septate   Cribriform   Parous introitus

G. J. Wassilchenko

Although not a true part of the reproductive system, the *urinary* (urethral) *meatus* is considered here because of its closeness and relationship to the vulva. The meatus is a pink or reddened opening of varying shapes, often with slightly puckered margins. The meatus marks the terminal, or distal, part of the urethra. It is usually located about 2.5 cm below the clitoris.

The *lesser vestibular* (paraurethral, Skene's) *glands* are short tubular structures situated posterolaterally just inside the urethral meatus, at about the 5 and 7 o'clock positions around the meatus. They produce a small amount of mucus, which functions as lubrication.

The *hymen* (Fig. 5.25) is a partial, rarely complete, elastic but tough mucosa-covered fold around the *vaginal introitus.* In virginal females the hymen may be an impediment to vaginal examination, insertion of internal menstrual tampons, or coitus. The hymen may be elastic and allow distention, or it may be torn easily. Occasionally the hymen covers the orifice completely, resulting in an imperforate hymen that prevents passage of menstrual flow, instrumentation (e.g., with a speculum), or coitus. A hymenotomy may be necessary in some cases. After instrumentation, use of tampons, coitus, or vaginal delivery, residual tags of the hymen (hymenal caruncles or carunculae myrtiformes) may be seen.

One common myth is that one can tell by the condition of the hymen whether a female is a virgin. Sexually active and even parous females may have intact hymens. For other women the hymen may be torn during strenuous physical work or exercise, masturbation, or use of tampons. Some cultural groups cleanse the infant girl so vigorously that the hymen is torn, leaving only vaginal tags in its place. Therefore, the "test for virginity"—evidence of bleeding following sexual intercourse—is an unreliable criterion.

The *greater vestibular* (vulvovaginal, Bartholin's) *glands* are two compound glands at the base of the labia majora, one on either side of the vaginal orifice. Each gland is drained by several ducts, about 1.5 cm long. Each opens into the groove between the hymen and the labia minora. Usually the gland openings are not visible or palpable. The glands secrete a small amount of clear, viscid mucus, especially during coitus. The alkaline pH of the mucus is supportive of sperm.

Fourchet. The fourchet is a thin, flat, transverse fold of tissue formed where the tapering labia majora and minora merge in the midline below the vaginal orifice. A small depression, the fossa navicularis, lies between the fourchet and the hymen.

Perineum. The perineum is the skin-covered muscular area between the vaginal introitus and the anus.

The perineum forms the base of the perineal body. The terms *vulva* and *perineum* occasionally but inaccurately are used interchangeably.

BREASTS

Location and support. The breasts are paired mammary glands located between the second and sixth ribs (Fig. 5.26). About two thirds of the breast overlies the pectoralis major muscle, between the sternum and mid axillary line, with an extension to the axilla referred to as the tail of Spence. The lower one third of the breast overlies the serratus anterior muscle. The breasts are attached to the muscles by connective tissue or fascia.

The breasts of healthy mature women are approximately equal in size and shape but are often not absolutely symmetric. The breasts of women who have never given birth to a child are usually shaped like half cones or hemispheres. The size and shape vary depending on the woman's age, heredity, and nutrition. However, the contour should be smooth with no retractions, dimpling, or masses. If a woman has nursed at some time, her breasts may be pendulous.

Structure. True glandular tissue is called *parenchyma;* supporting tissues, the fat and fibrous connective tissue are called *stroma.* It is the relative amount of stroma that determines the size and consistency of the breast.

Estrogen stimulates growth of the breast by inducing fat deposition in the breasts, development of stromal tissue (i.e., increase in its amount and elasticity), and growth of the extensive ductile system. Estrogen also increases the vascularity of breast tissue.

Once ovulation begins in puberty, progesterone levels increase. The increase in progesterone causes maturation of mammary gland tissue, specifically the lobules and acinar structures. During adolescence fat deposition and growth of fibrous tissue contribute to the increase in the size of the gland. Full development of the breast is not achieved until after the end of the first pregnancy or in the early period of lactation.

Each mammary gland is made up of 15 to 20 lobes, which are divided into lobules. Lobules are clusters of acini (Fig. 5.26). An acinus is a saclike terminal part of a compound gland emptying through a narrow lumen or duct. In discussions of mammary glands the correct anatomic term (acinus) is often used interchangeably with alveolus. The acini are lined with epithelial cells that secrete colostrum and milk. Just below the epithelium is the myoepithelium (myo, muscle), which contracts to expel milk from the acini (Fig. 5.27).

The ducts from the clusters of acini that form the lobules merge to form larger ducts draining the lobes.

Fig. 5.26
Position and structure of mammary gland.

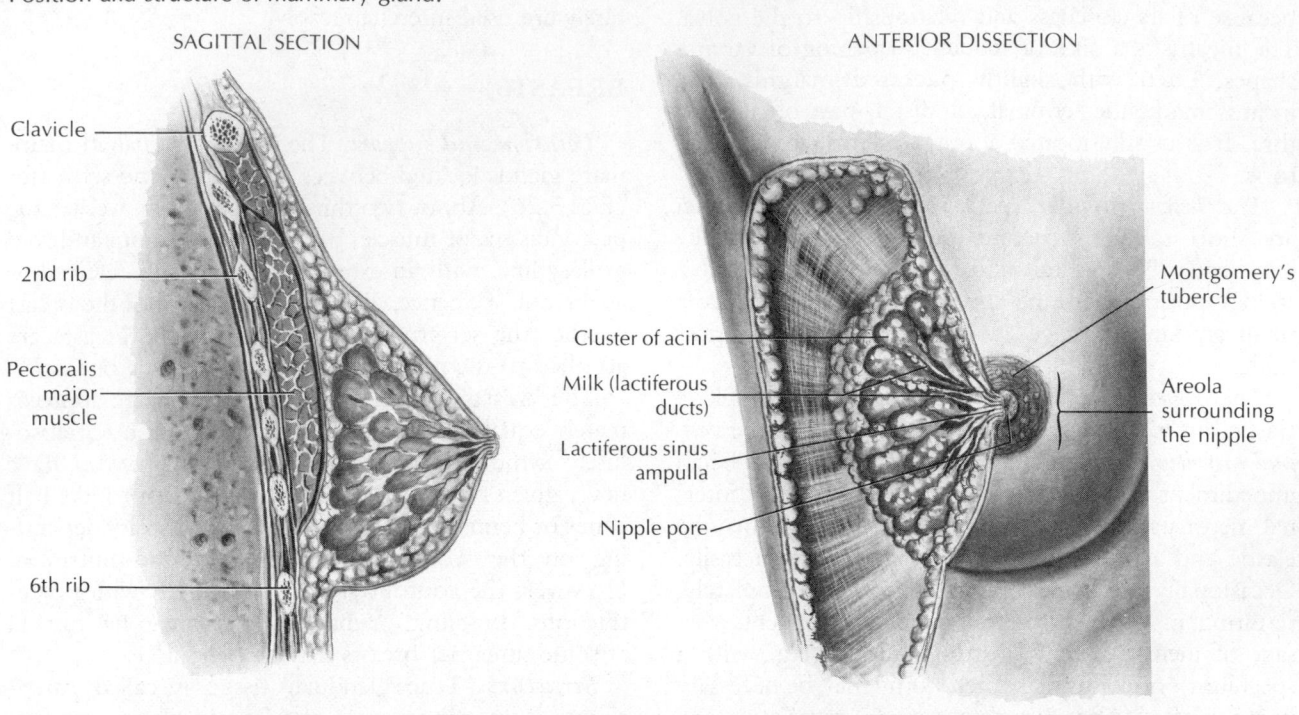

SAGITTAL SECTION

Clavicle

2nd rib

Pectoralis
major
muscle

6th rib

ANTERIOR DISSECTION

Cluster of acini

Milk (lactiferous
ducts)

Lactiferous sinus
ampulla

Nipple pore

Montgomery's
tubercle

Areola
surrounding
the nipple

Ducts from the lobes converge in a single nipple (papilla) surrounded by an areola. Just as the ducts converge, they dilate to form common lactiferous sinuses, which are also called ampullae. The lactiferous sinuses serve as milk reservoirs. Many tiny lactiferous ducts drain the ampullae and exit in the nipple.

The glandular structures and ducts are surrounded by protective fatty tissue and are separated and supported by fibrous suspensory Cooper's ligaments. Cooper's ligaments provide support to the mammary glands while permitting their mobility on the chest wall.

The round nipple is usually slightly elevated above the breast. On each breast the nipple projects slightly upward and laterally. It contains 15 to 20 openings from lactiferous ducts. The nipple (mammary papilla) is surrounded by fibromuscular tissue and covered by wrinkled skin. Except during pregnancy and lactation, there is no discharge from the nipple.

The nipple and surrounding areola are usually more deeply pigmented than the skin of the breast. The rough appearance of the areola is caused by sebaceous glands, the glands of Montgomery (Fig. 5.26) directly beneath the skin. These glands secrete a fatty substance that is thought to lubricate the nipple. Smooth muscle

fibers in the areola contract to stiffen the nipple to make it easier for the nursing child to grasp.

Changes in response to the menstrual cycle. The breasts change in size and nodularity in response to cyclic ovarian changes throughout reproductive life. Increasing levels of both estrogen and progesterone in the 3 to 4 days before menstruation increase vascularity of the breasts, induce growth of the ducts and acini, and promote water retention. The epithelial cells lining the ducts proliferate in number, the ducts dilate, and the lobules distend. The acini become enlarged and secretory, and lipid (fat) is deposited within their epithelial cell lining. As a result, breast swelling, ten-

Fig. 5.27
Acinus in cross section.

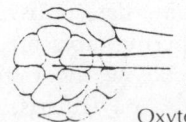

Milk-ejecting myoepithelial cells
Milk-secreting gland cells
Milk-duct opening

Oxytocin from the pituitary gland causes
myoepithelial cells to contract and
eject milk from gland cells into milk ducts

Fig. 5.28
Changes in breast tissue in response to menstrual cycle and their consideration in timing of breast examination.

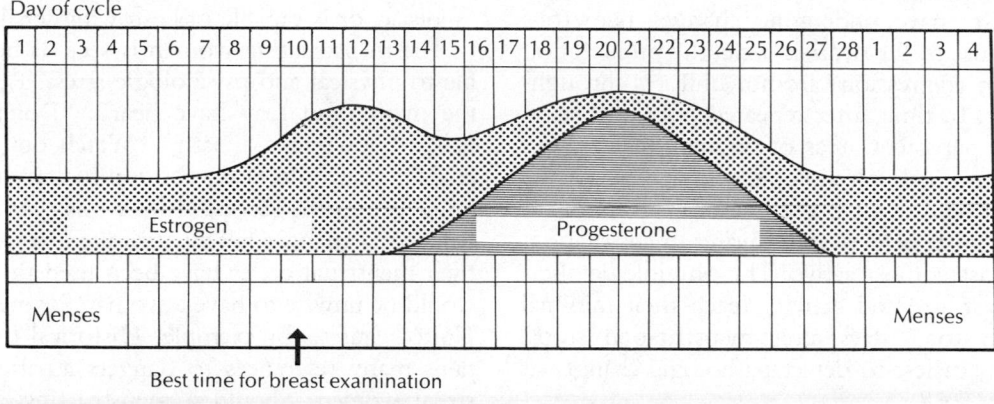

Day of cycle

Best time for breast examination

Fig. 5.29
Mammary gland: lymphatic drainage.

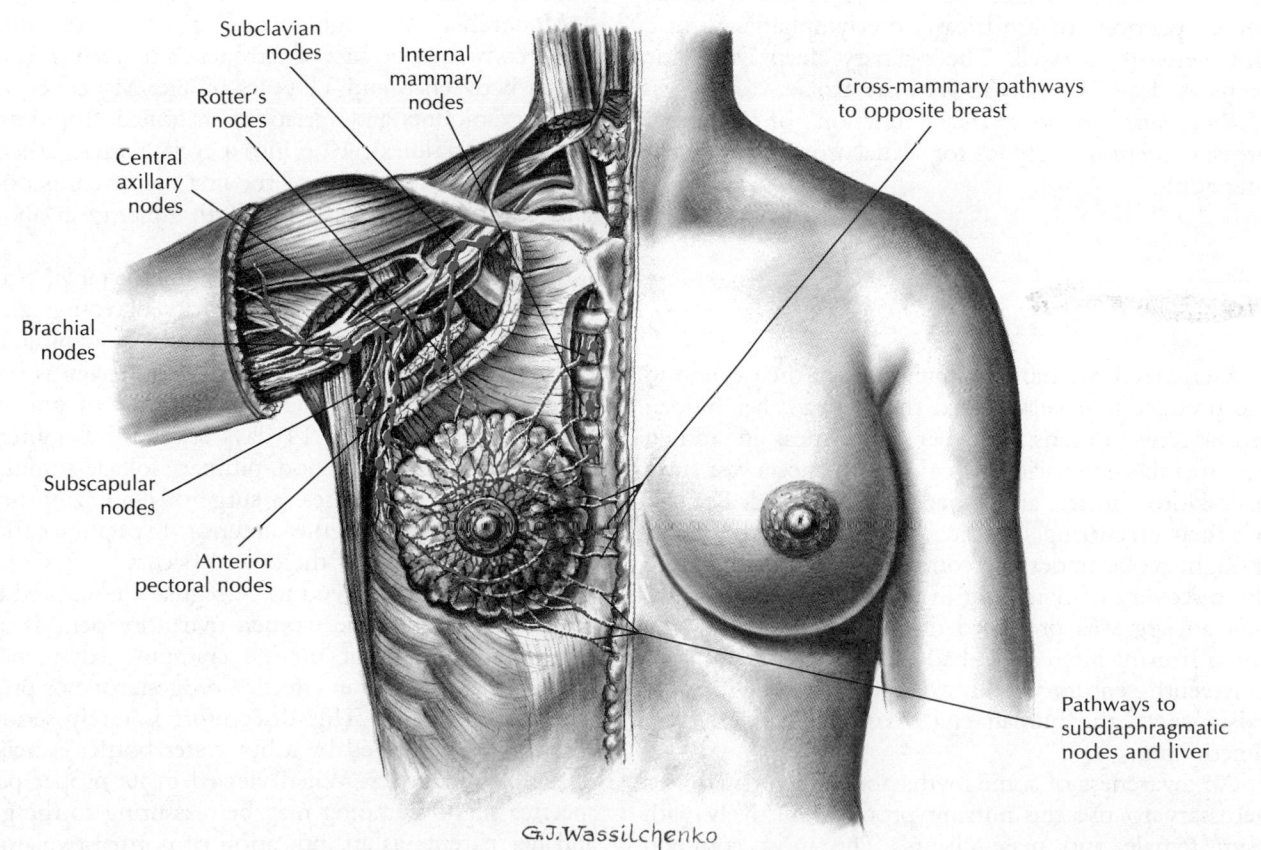

G.J.Wassilchenko

derness, and discomfort are common symptoms just before the onset of menstruation. After menstruation, cellular proliferation begins to regress, acini begin to decrease in size, and retained water is lost.

After breasts have undergone changes numerous times in response to the ovarian cycle, the proliferation and involution (regression) are not uniform throughout the breast. In time, after repeated hormonal stimulation, small persistent areas of nodulations may develop. This normal physiologic change must be remembered when breast tissue is examined. Nodules may develop just before and during menstruation, when the breast is most active. The physiologic alterations in breast size and activity reach their minimal level about 5 to 7 days after menstruation stops. Therefore it is easiest to detect pathologic changes at this time (Fig. 5.28).

Blood vessels and lymphatics. The vascular supply to the mammary gland is abundant. In the nonpregnant state the skin does not have an obvious vascular pattern. The normal skin is smooth without tightness or shininess.

The skin covering the breasts contains an extensive superficial lymphatic network that serves the entire chest wall and is continuous with the superficial lymphatics of the neck and abdomen (Fig. 5.29). In the deeper portions of the breasts the lymphatics form a rich network as well. The primary deep lymphatic pathway drains laterally toward the axillae.

Functions. Besides their function of lactation, breasts function as organs for sexual arousal in the mature adult.

Menstrual Cycle

Menstrual myths. Many myths have their origin in the mystery that surrounded the woman, her hidden reproductive organs, and her uniqueness in adding new members to society. As a consequence a vast store of folklore, fancies, and superstitions evolved. Because of their recurring nature, menstrual cycles were thought to be under the control of the moon. Before the discovery of ovulation in humans, it was thought that an egg was produced during menstruation only when fruitful intercourse had occurred. Not until the nineteenth century was knowledge available about the existence of the human egg, ovulation, and ovarian functioning.

An awareness of some myths about menstruation is necessary to use the nursing process effectively with both female and male clients. The most common myths in existence today include the following:

1. During menstruation the woman is vulnerable and therefore needs to be protected.
2. The menstruating woman can pose a danger.
3. Menstrual blood has healing powers, is an aphrodisiac, or is capable of bestowing fertility.

The menstruating woman is seen as being vulnerable to physical and psychologic stress. Recall some of the myths you may have heard: "Don't wash your hair," "Don't take a bath," "Watch out, you'll catch cold," "That's too heavy for you to carry now."

As late as the second half of this century the many behavioral changes falsely attributed to women during their menstrual cycles have been used to argue why it would be unwise to have a woman for president of the United States, for example. Historical literature contains many references to dangers attributed to menstrual women. Should a menstruating woman walk through a farmer's fields, the crops would not grow and the flowers would wilt; if she tried to bake bread, the dough would not rise. The danger also exists for her husband so that physical contact, especially sexual intercourse, was and in some places still is prohibited. In many cultures the menstruating woman is kept in a separate menstrual hut or in separate quarters. Following a ritualized "cleansing" the woman returns to her place in her family.

Menarche. Although young girls secrete small, rather constant amounts of estrogen, a marked increase occurs between 8 and 11 years of age. Moreover, increasing amounts and variations in gonadotropin and estrogen secretion develop into a cyclic pattern at least a year prior to menarche or the first menstrual period. This occurs in most girls in North America at about 13 years of age.

Initially periods are irregular, unpredictable, painless, and anovulatory in the majority of young girls. After one or more years a hypothalamic-pituitary rhythm develops, and adequate cyclic estrogen is produced by the ovary to mature a number of graafian follicles. Approximately 14 days *before* the beginning of the next menstrual period, pituitary follicle-stimulating hormone (FSH) rises, a surge of luteinizing hormone is released by the anterior hypophysis, and ovulation (extrusion of the ovum) occurs.

Ovulatory periods tend to be regular, monitored by progesterone. In some women ovulatory periods are associated with slight uterine cramping (dysmenorrhea), which may be an effect of progesterone or prostaglandins or both. This discomfort is rarely serious and is readily relieved by a hot water bottle, exercise, or simple analgesics. When viewed in its proper perspective slight cramping may be reassuring to the girl and her parents as an indication of normal ovulatory function.

Although pregnancy may occur in exceptional cases of true (constitutional) precocious puberty, most pregnancies in very young girls occur well after the normally timed menarche. *However, all girls would benefit from knowing that pregnancy can occur at any time after the onset of menses.*

Endometrial cycle

Menstruation. Menstruation is periodic uterine bleeding that begins with the shedding of secretory endometrium approximately 14 days after ovulation. The first day of the menstrual discharge has been designated as *day 1* of the cycle. The average duration of menstrual flow is 5 days (range of 3 to 6 days), and the average blood loss is approximately 50 ml (range of 20 to 80 ml), but there is great variation. During menstruation the average daily loss of iron is 0.5 to 1 mg. If the woman's usual blood loss is over 80 ml, she will most likely need iron supplementation to prevent secondary anemia.

For about 50% of women, menstrual blood does not appear to clot. The menstrual blood clots within the uterus, but the clot is liquefied before it is discharged from the uterus. If the discharge leaves the uterus too rapidly, liquefaction may not be complete so that clots will appear in the vagina. Uterine discharge includes mucus and epithelial cells in addition to blood.

It is generally assumed that the purpose of the menstrual cycle is to prepare the uterus for pregnancy. When pregnancy does not occur, menstruation ensues. The individual's age, physical and emotional status, and environment influence the regularity of her periods.

Phases. The four phases of the menstrual cycle are (1) the menstrual phase, (2) the proliferative phase, (3) the secretory phase, and (4) the ischemic phase (Fig. 5.30). During the *menstrual phase,* shedding of the functional two thirds of the endometrium (the compact and spongy layers) is initiated by periodic va-

Fig. 5.30
Menstrual cycle.

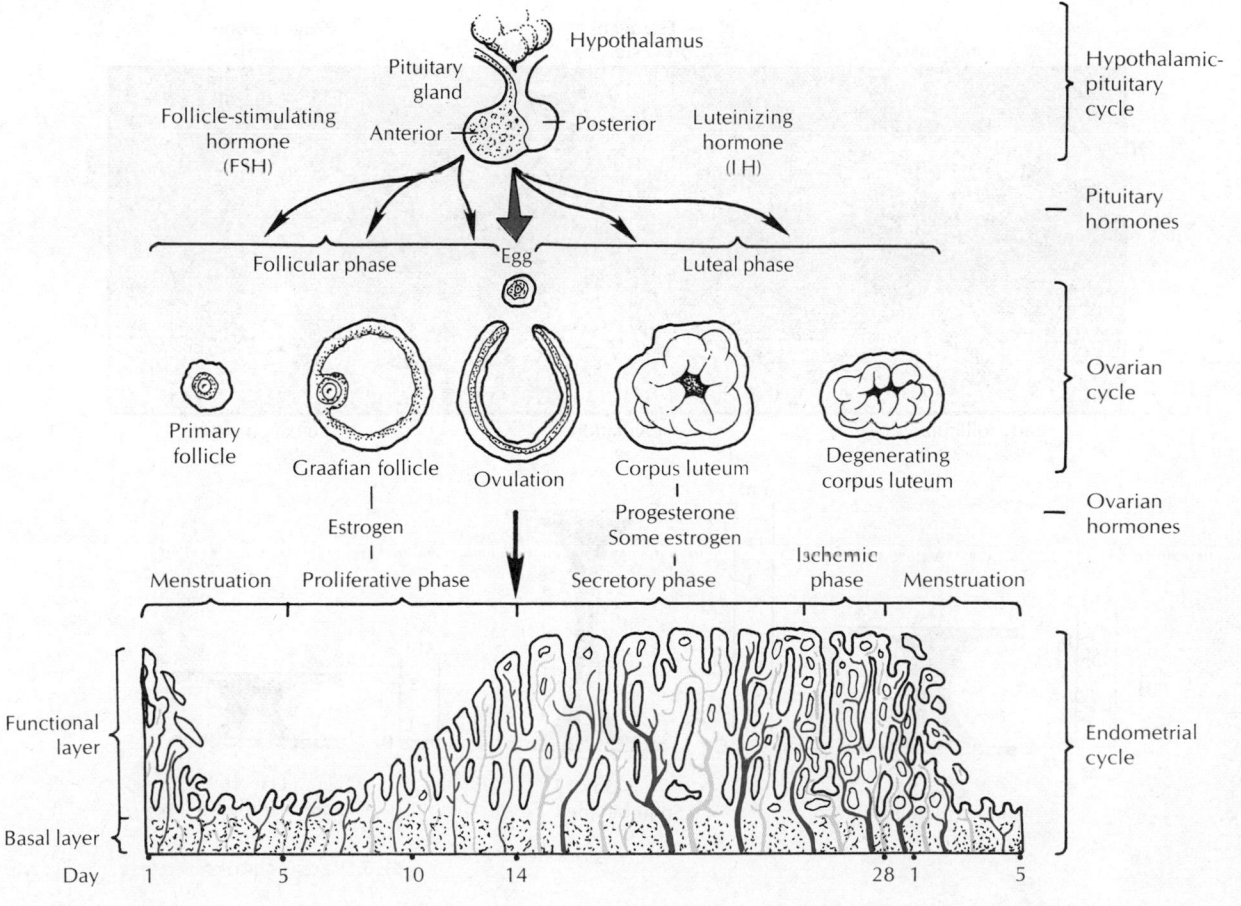

soconstriction of the spiral arterioles most marked in the upper layers of the endometrium. The basal layer is always retained, and regeneration begins near the end of the cycle from cells derived from the remaining glandular remnants or stromal cells in the basalis.

The *proliferative phase* is a period of rapid growth that extends from about the fifth day to the time of ovulation, which would be, for example, day 10 of a 24-day cycle, day 14 of a 28 day cycle, or day 18 of a 32-day cycle. The endometrial surface is completely restored in approximately 4 days or slightly before bleeding ceases. From this point on an eightfold to tenfold thickening occurs, with a leveling off of growth at ovulation. Early in the proliferative phase the functional layer is moderately dense and only slightly vascular. Three of four days before ovulation the glands develop and vascularity is increased. The proliferative phase is dependent on estrogen stimulation derived from ovarian (graafian) follicles.

The *secretory phase* extends from the day of ovulation to about 3 days before the next menstrual period. After ovulation, larger amounts of progesterone are produced. This hormone causes the glands to become tortuous, serrated, and widened. An edematous, vascular, functional endometrium is now apparent. The cells lining the glands secrete a thin, glycogen-containing fluid.

At the end of the secretory phase the fully matured secretory endometrium reaches the thickness of heavy, soft velvet. It becomes luxuriant with blood and glandular secretions, a suitable protective and nutritive bed for a fertilized ovum, should one be available.

Implantation (nidation) of the fertilized ovum generally occurs about 7 to 10 days after ovulation. If fertilization and implantation do not occur, the corpus luteum (yellow body) regresses. With the rapid fall in progesterone and estrogen levels the spiral arteries go into a spasm. During the *ischemic phase* the blood sup-

Fig. 5.31
Changes in cervix and cervical mucus changes during menstrual cycle. **A,** Changes in opening of the cervix and facility for sperm migration. **B,** Characteristic stretchable quality of cervical mucus demonstrated between two glass slides.

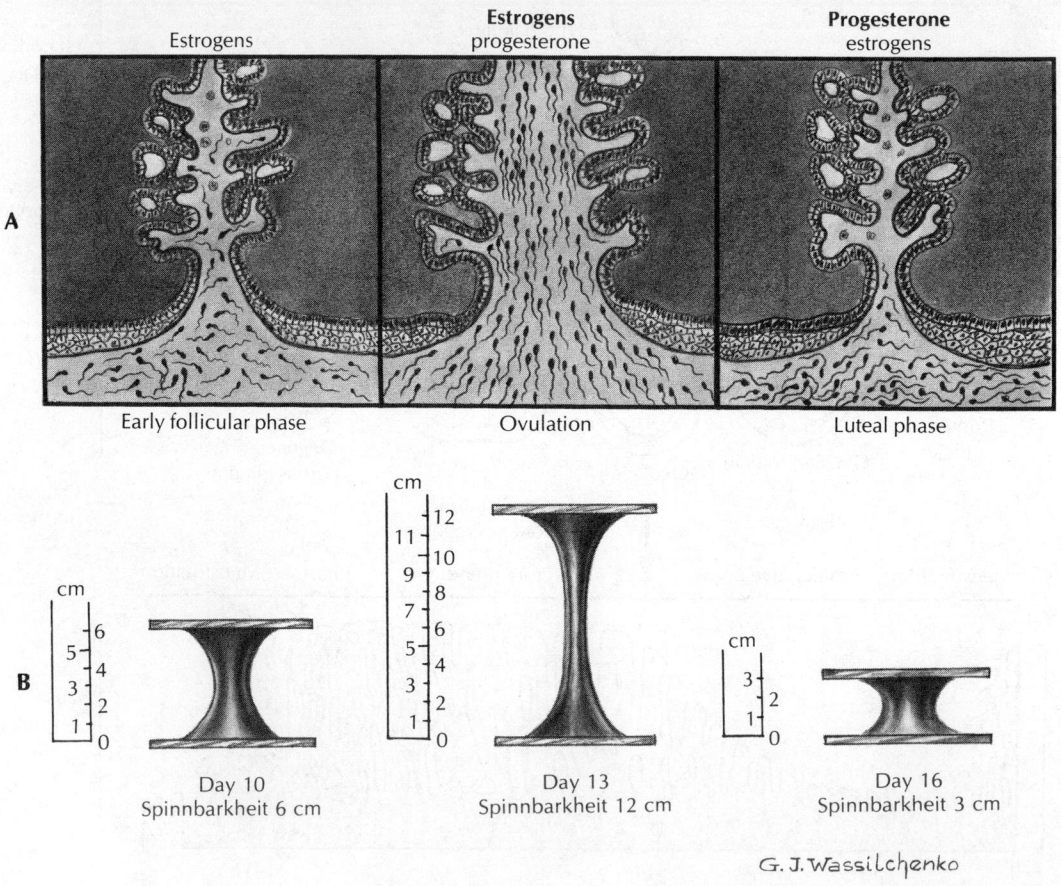

G. J. Wassilchenko

ply to the functional endometrium is blocked and necrosis develops. The functional layer separates from the basal layer, and menstrual bleeding begins, marking day 1 of the next cycle.

Hypothalamic-pituitary cycle. Toward the end of the normal menstrual cycle, blood levels of estrogen and progesterone fall. Low blood levels of these ovarian hormones stimulate the hypothalamus to secrete gonadotropin-releasing hormone (Gn-RH). Gn-RH in turn stimulates anterior pituitary secretion of FSH. FSH stimulates development of ovarian graafian follicles and their production of estrogen. Estrogen levels begin to fall, and hypothalamic Gn-RH triggers the anterior pituitary release of LH. A marked surge of LH and a smaller peak of estrogen precede the expulsion of the ovum from the graafian follicle by about 24 to 36 hours. LH peaks about the twenty-third or twenty-fourth day of a 28-day cycle. If fertilization and implantation (nidation) of the ovum has not occurred by this time, regression of the corpus luteum follows. Therefore the levels of progesterone and estrogen decline, menstruation occurs, and the hypothalamus is once again stimulated to secrete Gn-RH.

Ovarian cycle. The primary graafian follicles contain immature oocytes. Before ovulation, from 1 to 30 follicles begin to mature in each ovary under the influence of FSH and estrogen. The preovulatory surge of LH affects a selected follicle. Within the chosen follicle the oocyte matures, ovulation occurs, and the empty follicle begins its transformation into the corpus luteum. This *follicular phase* (preovulatory phase) of the ovarian menstrual cycle varies in length from woman to woman. Almost all variations in cycle length are the result of variations in the length of the follicular phase. On rare occasions (1 in 100 menstrual cycles), more than one follicle is chosen and more than one oocyte matures and undergoes ovulation (see discussion of twins, Chapter 29).

The *luteal phase* begins immediately after ovulation and ends with the start of menstruation. This postovulatory phase of the ovarian cycle usually *requires 14 days* (range of 13 to 15 days). Eight days after ovulation the corpus luteum reaches its peak of functional activity, secreting both of the steroids, estrogen and progesterone. Coincident with this time of peak luteal functioning the fertilized egg is implanted in the endometrium. If no implantation occurs, the corpus luteum regresses, and steroid levels drop. Two weeks after ovulation, if fertilization and implantation do not occur, uterine endometrium is shed through menstruation.

After ovulation, estrogen levels drop. For 90% of women, only a small amount of *withdrawal bleeding* occurs so that it goes unnoticed. In 10% of women there is sufficient bleeding for it to be visible, resulting in what is known as *midcycle bleeding*.

Other cyclic changes. When the hypothalamic-pituitary-ovarian axis is functioning properly, other tissues undergo predictable responses. Prior to ovulation the woman's basal body temperature (BBT) is lower, often below 98.6° F (37° C); after ovulation, with rising progesterone levels, her BBT rises. Changes in the cervix and cervical mucus follow a generally predictable pattern (Figs. 5.31 and 5.32). At the time of ovulation, cervical mucus is thin and clear. It looks, feels, and stretches like egg white. This stretchable quality is termed *spinnbarkeit* (Fig. 5.31, *B*). Some women experience localized lower abdominal pain called *mittelschmerz* that coincides with ovulation.

These and other cyclic changes enhance fertility awareness and form the basis for the symptothermal

Fig. 5.32

Cervical mucus changes during menstrual cycle. **A,** Fern pattern under estrogen influence. **B,** Mucus receptive to sperm passage under estrogen influence. **C,** Mucus nonreceptive to sperm passage under progesterone influence. (From Fogel, C.I., and Woods, N.F.: Health care of women: a nursing perspective, St. Louis, 1981, The C.V. Mosby Co.)

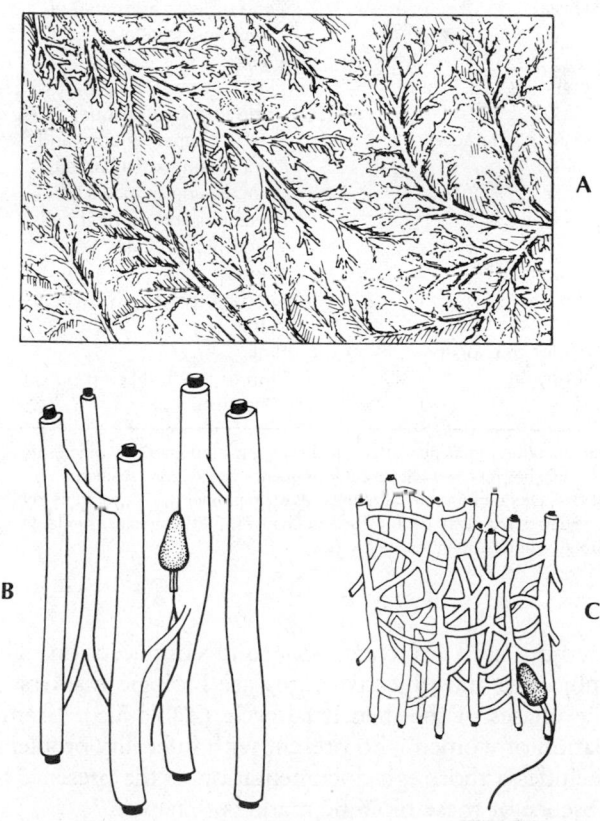

Table 5.3
Markers (Signs and Symptoms) of the Phases of the Menstrual Cycle

Marker	Preovulation	Ovulation	At Least 2 Days After Ovulation up to Menses
Subjective signs			
Physical discomfort			
Breasts	Unreported	Unreported	Heaviness, fullness; enlarged, tender*
Abdomen	Dysmenorrhea: uterine cramping; nausea, vomiting, and diarrhea; dizziness	Intermenstrual pain (mittelschmerz) occurs 1.7 days after peak of cervical mucus and 2.5 days before increase in BBT	Premenstrual syndrome: backaches; feeling of increasing pelvic fullness
General	Increased weight; feeling of heaviness	Unreported	Headache†; acne
Affective changes‡			
Moods	Some depression may persist from premenses	Sense of well-being	Premenstrual syndrome (PMS): increased irritability, passivity, depression
Libido	Unreported	Increases sexual desire	Unreported
Energy levels	Unreported	Unreported	Spurt of energy, followed by fatigue
Objective signs			
BBT	36.2-36.3° C (97.2-97.4°F)	34-36 h before BBT drops 0.2-0.3° F; 24-48 h after, BBT rises 0.7-0.8° F	≥36.7° C (98° F)
Respiration	Unreported	Unreported	Hyperventilation with decrease in alveolar P_{CO_2}
Heart rate	Unreported	Unreported	Increased slightly
Breasts	Time of least hormonal effect and smallest breast size	Increased nipple erectility; increased areolar pigmentation	Increased nodularity; enlarged
Cervix (Figs. 5.31 and 5.32) Mucus characteristics	"Dry" (no mucus) progressing to clear, opaque, watery, slippery mucus and increasing spinnbarkeit; increasing numbers of vaginal and cervical cells and lymphocytes	Abundant, thin, clear (egg white) mucus with spinnbarkeit (4 cm often up to 10 cm]) that dries in a fern pattern (arborization); facilitates sperm transport	Cloudy, sticky, impenetrable to sperm; dries in granular pattern
Mucus pH	About 7.0	7.5	Unreported
Os	Gradual, progressive widening	Open, with mucus seen spilling out	Gradual closing of os
Color of exocervix	Pink	Hyperemic (red)	Gradual return to pink
Body	Firm to touch (like tip of nose)	Soft (like earlobe)	Gradual return to firm

*Sociocultural influences may affect symptoms reported by women. Breast tenderness is rarely reported by Japanese women.
†Headaches reported with greater frequency by Nigerian women.
‡NOTE: Literature usually attributes negative premenstrual symptoms to biology, while good moods and rational behavior are not. When men and women are compared in activity patterns, mood changes, and symptoms, similar variability has been found in *both* men and women even though the changes in women are given more attention by society.

method used for conception and contraception. The subjective and objective signs are biologic markers of the phases of the menstrual cycle (Table 5.3). Examination of women who present with infertility problems includes a thorough documentation of the presence or absence of these biologic markers (Chapter 7).

Prostaglandins. Prostaglandins (PGs) are oxygenated fatty acids now classified as hormones. The different kinds of PGs are distinguished by letters (PGE, PGF), numbers (PGE₂), and letters of the Greek alphabet (PGF₂α).

PGs are produced in most organs of the body but most notably by the prostate and the endometrium. Therefore semen and menstrual blood are potent prostaglandin sources. PGs are metabolized quickly by most tissues and are biologically active in minute amounts in the cardiovascular, gastrointestinal, respiratory, urogenital, and nervous systems. They also exert a marked effect on metabolism, particularly on glycolysis. Prostaglandins play an important role in many physiologic, pathologic, and pharmacologic reactions. $PGF_{2\alpha}$, PGE_1, and PGE_2, are most frequently used in reproductive medicine.

Role in reproductive functions. Prostaglandins affect smooth muscle contractility and modulation of hormonal activity. Indirect evidence supports PGs' effects on the following events:

1. Ovulation
2. Fertility
3. Cervical and cervical mucus changes that affect receptivity to sperm
4. Tubal and uterine motility
5. Sloughing of endometrium (menstruation)
6. Onset of abortion, spontaneous and induced
7. Onset of labor, term and preterm

After exerting their biologic actions, newly synthesized PGs are rapidly metabolized by tissues in such organs as the lungs, kidneys, and liver.

PGs may play a key role in ovulation. If PG levels do not rise along with the surge of LH, the ovum remains trapped within the graafian follicle. Following ovulation, PGs may influence production of estrogen and progesterone by the corpus luteum.

The introduction of PGs into the vagina or into the uterine cavity (from ejaculated semen) increases the motility of uterine musculature, which may assist the transport of sperm through the uterus and into the oviduct. High concentrations of PGs in the semen (about 55 μg/ml) may be necessary for normal fertility in males.

PGs produced by the woman cause regression (return to an earlier state) of the corpus luteum, regression of the endometrium, and sloughing of the endometrium, which results in menstruation. PGs increase myometrial response to oxytocic stimulation, enhance uterine contractions, and cause cervical dilation. They may be one factor in the initiation or maintenance of labor or both. In addition, prostaglandins may be involved in the following pathologic states: male infertility, dysmenorrhea, hypertensive states, preeclampsia-eclampsia, and anaphylactic shock. Further discussion of PGs relevant to abortion may be found in Chapter 27; for a discussion of PGs' role in pregnancy and childbirth, see Chapter 9.

Primary dysmenorrhea. Primary dysmenorrhea (dys, painful; menorrhea, normal menstrual flow) is painful menstruation that occurs in the absence of pelvic pathologic findings. Anovulatory cycles are not accompanied by dysmenorrhea so that it does not occur during the 6 to 12 months following the onset of menarche.

Symptoms of primary dysmenorrhea (premenstrual tension plus uterine cramping and occasionally backache, dizziness, vomiting, and diarrhea) are associated with a functioning corpus luteum. Spasmodic pain starts with the menstrual flow and lasts 1 to 3 days. Intense myometrial contractions lead to uterine ischemia (decreased blood flow) that results in pain. Pregnancy increases vascularity and blood flow to the uterus, so that following pregnancy, intense uterine contractions may no longer lead to ischemia.

PGs have been implicated in primary dysmenorrhea. Significantly elevated $PGF_{2\alpha}$ has been detected in the endometrium and menstrual fluid of women with primary dysmenorrhea. Dysmenorrhea can be produced by administration of $PGF_{2\alpha}$. The symptoms can be relieved by drugs that inhibit production of PGs. Although most of the nonsteroid antiprostaglandin drugs have been recognized for the treatment of primary dysmenorrhea cautious short-term use of mefenamic acid (Ponstel), ibuprofen (Motrin), maproxen (Anaprox), or indomethacin (Indocin) is recommended because of potential adverse side effects. Drug therapy is started with the onset of menstrual flow and continued for 3 days.

Drugs that prevent ovulation, the conventional birth control pills, do not constitute specific therapy for dysmenorrhea, but they are effective for some women. Finally, but of equal importance, the nurse should provide the woman with reassurance and a listening ear. Personal attention, a caring atmosphere, and accurate information help to dispel insecurity and fear, which exaggerate the pain and interfere with therapy.

Male Structures

The male reproductive tract consists of internal organs, located in the pelvic cavity, and external genitalia. The male's reproductive system begins to develop in response to testosterone during early fetal life. Essentially no testosterone is produced during childhood. Resumption of testosterone production at the onset of puberty stimulates growth and maturation of reproductive structures and secondary sex characteristics.

INTERNAL STRUCTURES

Internal structures include the following:

1. Testes: male gonads
2. Ducts of the testes
3. Accessory reproductive tract glands
   a. Seminal vesicles
   b. Prostate glands
   c. Bulbourethral glands
4. Semen

Fig. 5.33
Fascial planes of male lower genitourinary tract. **A,** Transverse section of penis.
B, Relationship of bladder, prostate, seminal vesicles, penis, urethra, and scrotal contents.
(Adapted from Smith, D.R.: General urology, Los Altos, Calif., 1975, Lange Medical
Publications.)

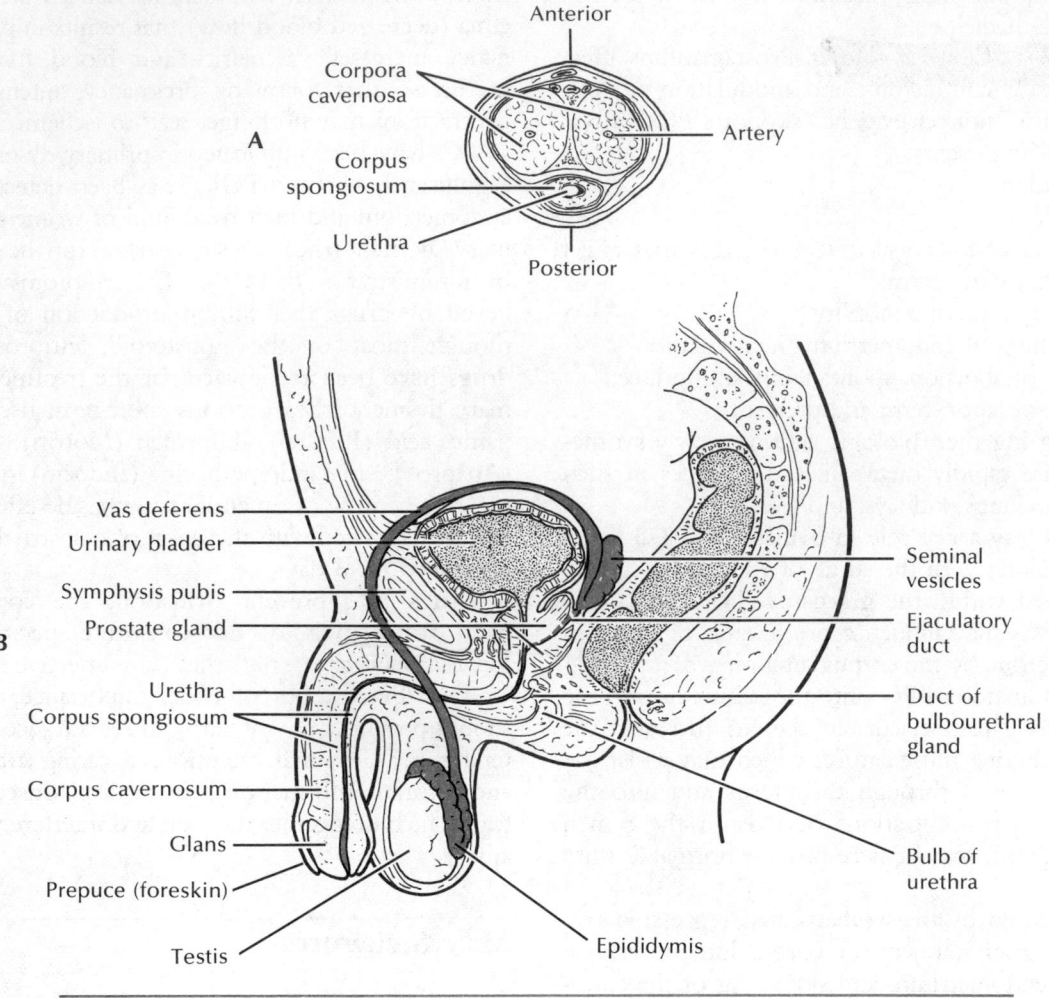

Figs. 5.33 and 5.34 illustrate the male reproductive structures.

Testes: male gonads

Location and support. The testes are two small ovoid glands located within the scrotal sac. Both are suspended by attachment to scrotal tissue and the spermatic cord. Originally located in the abdomen, the testes descend through the inguinal canal by the end of the seventh lunar month of fetal life. At term birth one or both of the testes may still be within the inguinal canals with final descent into the scrotal sac occurring in the early postnatal period. The testes must be within the scrotum for spermatogenesis to occur.

Structure. The testes are similar in origin (homol-ogous) to the ovaries in the female. Each testis is whitish, somewhat flattened from side to side, measures about 4 or 5 cm in length, and weighs 10 to 15 g. White fibrous tissue encases each testis and divides it into several lobules. Within each lobule are one to three long (about 75 cm), narrow, coiled *seminiferous tubules* and clusters of *interstitial cells* (Leydig's cells). Spermatids attach to the germinal epithelium (Sertoli's cells) within the seminiferous tubules and develop into sperm. The interstitial cells are large connective or supportive tissue (stromal) cells responsible for the production of the androgen hormone testosterone.

Functions. The two principal functions of the testes are spermatogenesis and hormone production. Primitive sex cells (spermatogonia) are present in the semi-

Fig. 5.34
Anatomy of urethra and penis.

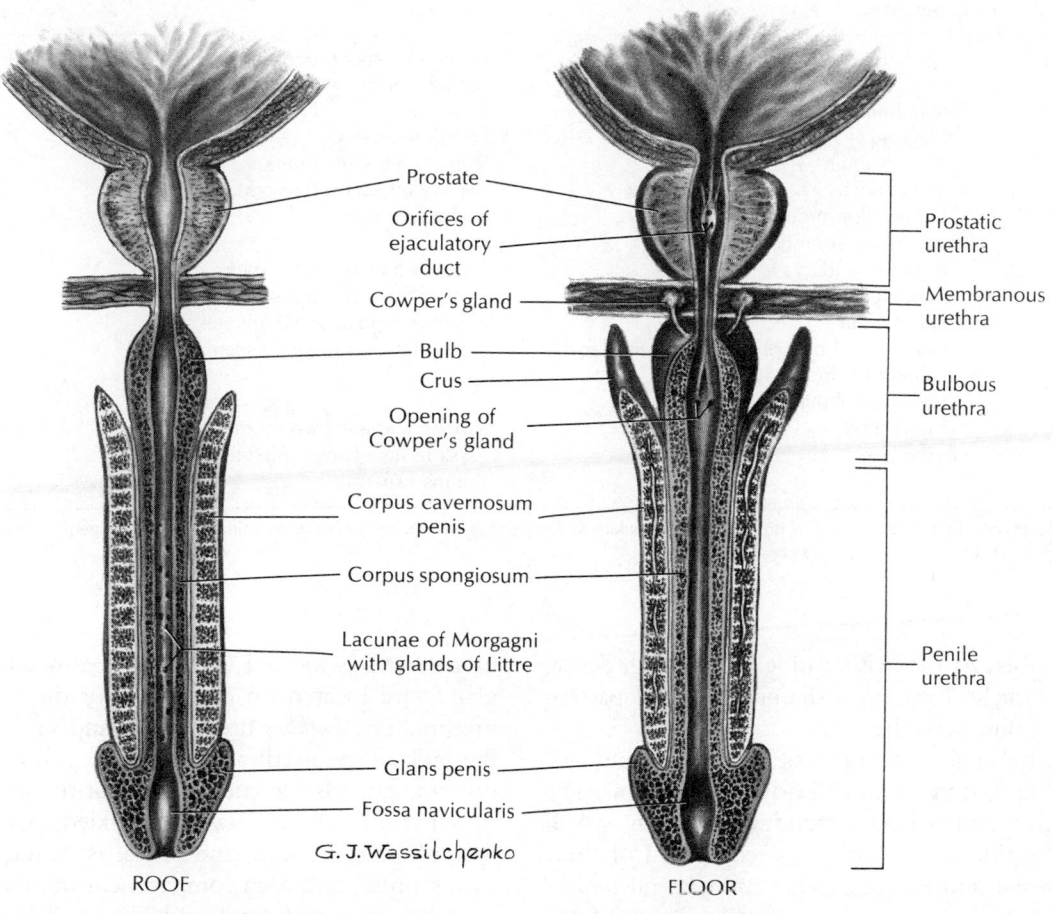

niferous tubules of the male newborn. Spermatogenesis, the maturation process that results in sperm, begins during puberty and normally continues throughout a man's lifetime. The testes secrete the steroid sex hormone testosterone in the amounts that are required for normal male growth, development, and function.

Ducts (canals) of the testes. For sperm to exit the body they must travel the full length of the duct system in succession: seminiferous tubules, epididymides (pl.), vasa deferentia (pl.), ejaculatory ducts, and the urethra. The seminiferous tubules are mentioned above. Each testis has one tightly coiled tube, about 6 m (20 ft) in length. The tube, the *epididymis,* lies along the top and side of each testis. The epididymides are storage sites for maturing sperm and produce a small part of the seminal fluid (semen). Seminiferous tubules are continuous with the epididymides, which in turn connect to the vasa deferentia.

Accessory reproductive tract glands. Accessory re-

productive glands secrete fluids that support the life and function of sperm. These glands include the paired *seminal vesicles,* located along the lower posterior surface of the bladder; the *prostate gland,* which surrounds the prostatic urethra; and the *bulbourethral* (or Cowper's) *glands,* located below the prostate, one at either side of the membranous urethra (Fig. 5.34).

Semen. The components of semen derive from several sources. Each component of semen and its origin, function, and percent of total volume are presented in Table 5.4. At the time of ejaculation, 3 to 5 ml of semen is released.

EXTERNAL STRUCTURES

The structures that make up the external genitalia are presented in the following order:

1. Mons pubis
2. Penis
3. Scrotum

Table 5.4
Composition of Semen

Origin	Component	Functions	Percent of Ejaculate
Testes and epi- didymides	Some fluid Sperm (hundreds of millions)	Vehicle for sperm transport Fertilization of ova to perpetuate species	Under 5%*
Seminal vesicles	Seminal fluid containing:		30%
	Fructose	Energy source	
	Prostaglandins	Increase motility of uterus	
	Thick mucus	Vehicle for sperm transport	
	Coagulation protein	Entrap sperm	
Prostate gland	Prostatic secretion containing:		60%
	Alkaline fluid	Supports and enhances sperm motility	
	Thin mucus	Vehicle for sperm transport	
	Fibrinolysin	Liquefies semen for 10 minutes after ejaculation, to release sperm	
	Citrate, acid phosphatase, spermine, sper- midine, zinc, magnesium		
	Immunoglobulins (IgG and IgA)		
Bulbourethral glands	Alkaline fluid Fibrinolysin	Support and enhance sperm motility Assist in liquefying semen to release en- traped sperm	Under 5%

*Vasectomy affects only the production of this portion of the ejaculate so that there is no noticeable change in volume, even after sperm are no longer available for transport through the remaining canal system.

Mons pubis. At maturity, pubic hair is long, dense, coarse, and curly, forming a diamond-shaped pattern from the umbilicus to the anus.

Penis. The penis, an organ of copulation and urination, consists of the shaft or body and the glans. The shaft of this external male reproductive organ, which enters the vagina during coitus, is composed of three cylindric layers and erectile tissue, two lateral *corpora cavernosa* and a *corpus spongiosum,* which contains the urethra. These corpora terminate distally in the smooth, sensitive *glans penis,* which is the counterpart of the female glans clitoris. Skin and fascia loosely envelop the penis to permit enlargement during erection.

The glans is the enlarged end of the penis that contains many sensitive nerve endings and a urethral meatus at the tip (usually). The *prepuce* (foreskin), an extended fold of skin, covers the glans in uncircumcised males. In the neonate the foreskin is not retractable and may not be retractable for 4 to 6 months or even as long as 13 years. It is easily retractable in the adolescent and the adult. With sexual arousal, neurocirculatory factors cause considerable increase in blood flow to the erectile tissue of the corpora, and enlargement and erection of the penis occur.

The *urethra* is an exiting passageway for both urine and semen (Fig. 5.34). The urethra consists of four anatomic segments: the *prostatic,* or posterior, segment is encircled by the prostate gland and houses the ejaculatory ducts that connect the seminal vesicles with the urethra. The next segment is known as the *membranous*

urethra and is located within the perineum. Cowper's glands are located on either side of the membranous urethra. The *bulbous* urethra is found in the region of the bulb of the urethra. The longest portion, the *penile* urethra, extends the entire length of the male organ.

Scrotum. The *scrotum,* a wrinkled, pouchlike fullness of skin, muscles, and fascia, is divided internally by a septum, and each compartment normally contains one *testis,* one *epididymis,* and one *vas deferens* (seminal duct). The left side of the scrotum hangs somewhat lower (about 1 cm) than the right. Six separate layers of tissue make up the scrotal sac. The skin is abundantly supplied with sebaceous and sweat glands and is sparsely covered with hair. Under the skin is found the *cremaster* fascia and thin smooth muscle layer. Contraction and relaxation of this smooth muscle result in retraction of the testes to protect them from external trauma and cold. During hot external (environmental) or internal (fever) temperature the cremaster muscle relaxes, dropping the testes away from the body. Conversely, cold external temperature stimulates contraction of the cremaster muscle to bring the testes close to the body.

The purpose of this mobility is to maintain the testes within an optimal temperature range for the production and viability of sperm. Hot tubbing, tight underwear (jockey shorts) and pants, and long-term sitting (long-distance truck drivers) present too hot an external environment or prevent testicular mobility so that spermatogenesis and sperm are jeopardized.

Table 5.5
Stages of Sexual Development: Female

Age	Stages	
0-12	I.	Preadolescent. Female pelvic contour evident, breasts flat, labia majora smooth, labia minor poorly developed, hymenal opening small or absent, mucous membranes dry and red, vaginal cells lack glycogen.
8-13	II.	*Breasts:* Elevation of nipple, small mound beneath areola, which is enlarging and begins pigmentation.
		Labia majora become thickened, more prominent and wrinkled, *labia minora* easily identified due to increased size along with clitoris, urethral opening more prominent, mucous membranes moist and pink, some glycogen present in vaginal cells.
		Hair: First appears on mons and then on labia majora about time of menarche, still scanty, soft and straight.
		Skin: Increased activity of sebaceous and merocrine sweat glands and initial function of apocrine glands in axilla and vulva begin.
9-14	III.	Rapid growth peak is passed, menarche most often at this stage and invariably follows peak of growth acceleration.
		Breasts: Areola and nipple further enlarge and pigmentation more evident, continued increase in glandular size.
		Labia minora well developed and vaginal cells have increased glycogen content, mucous membranes increasingly more pale.
		Hair in pubic region, thicker, coarser, often curly (considerable normal variation including a few girls with early stage II at menarche).
		Skin: further increased activity of sebaceous and sweat glands with beginning of acne in some girls; adult body odor.
12-15	IV.	*Breasts:* Projection of areola above breast plane and areolar (Montgomery) glands apparent (this development is absent in about 20% of normal girls). Glands easily palpable.
		Labia: Both majora and minora assume adult structure, glycogen content of vaginal cells begins cyclic characteristics.
		Hair in pubic area more abundant, axillary hair present (rarely present at stage II, often present at stage III).
12-17	V.	*Breasts:* Mature histologic morphology, nipple enlarged and erect, areolar (Montgomery's) glands well developed, globular shape.
		Hair: in pubic area more abundant and may spread to thighs (in about 10% of women it assumes "male" distribution with extension toward umbilicus). Facial hair increased often in form of slight mustache.
		Skin: Increased sebaceous gland activity and increased severity of acne if present before.

Reproduced with permission from Lowrey, G.H.: Growth and development of children, ed. 8, Chicago, 1986, Year Book Medical Publishers.

Table 5.6
Stages of Sexual Development: Male

Age	Stages	
0-14	I.	Preadolescent
10-14	II.	Increasing size of *testes* and *penis* is evident (testis length reaches 2.0 cm or more). Scrotum integument is thinner and assumes an increased pendulous appearance.
		Hair: First appearance of pubic hair in area at base of penis.
		Skin: Increased activity of sebaceous and apocrine sweat glands and apocrine glands on axilla and scrotal area begin.
11-15	III.	*Testes* and *penis:* Further increase in size and pigmentation apparent. Leydig's cells (interstitial) first appear at stage II, are now prominent in testes.
		Hair: In pubic area more abundant and present on scrotum, still scanty and fine textured, axillary hair begins.
		Breasts: Button-type hypertrophy in 70% of boys at stages I and III.
		Larynx: Changes in voice due to laryngeal growth begin.
		Skin: Increasing activity of sebaceous and sweat glands with beginning of *acne*, adult body odor.
12-16	IV.	Rapid growth peak is passed, nocturnal emissions begin.
		Testes: Further increase in size, length 4.0 cm or greater, Increase in size of *penis* greatest at stages III and IV.
		Hair: Pubic hair thicker and coarser and in most ascends toward umbilicus in typical in male pattern, axillary hair increases, facial hair increases over lip and upper cheeks.
		Larynx: Voice deepens.
		Skin: Increasing pigmentation of scrotum and penis, acne often more severe.
		Breasts: Previous hypertrophy decreased or absent.
13-17	V.	*Testes:* Length greater than 4.5 cm.
		Hair: Pubic hair thick, curly, heavily pigmented, extends to thighs and toward umbilicus. Adult distribution and increase in body hair (chest, shoulders, thighs, etc.) continue for more than another 10 years. Baldness, if present may begin.
		Skin: Acne may persist and increase.
		Larynx: Adult character of voice.

Reproduced with permission from Lowrey, G.H.: Growth and development of children, ed. 8, Chicago, 1986, Year Book Medical Publishers.

Fig. 5.35
Hypothalamic-pituitary-gonadal axis: comparison of female and male (RF = releasing factor).

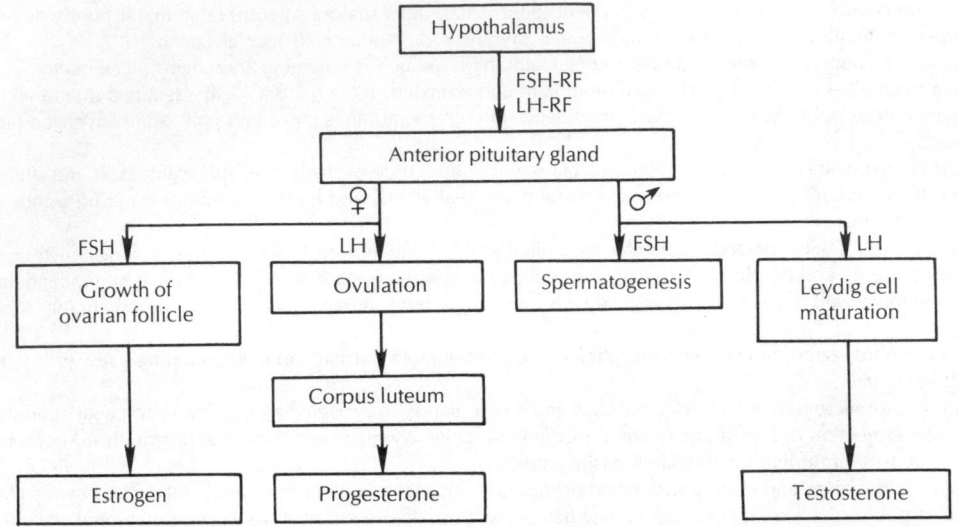

Fig. 5.36
Summary of changes in female reproductive system over life span. (Courtesy Merrill-National Laboratories, Division of Richardson-Merrill, Inc., Cincinnati.)

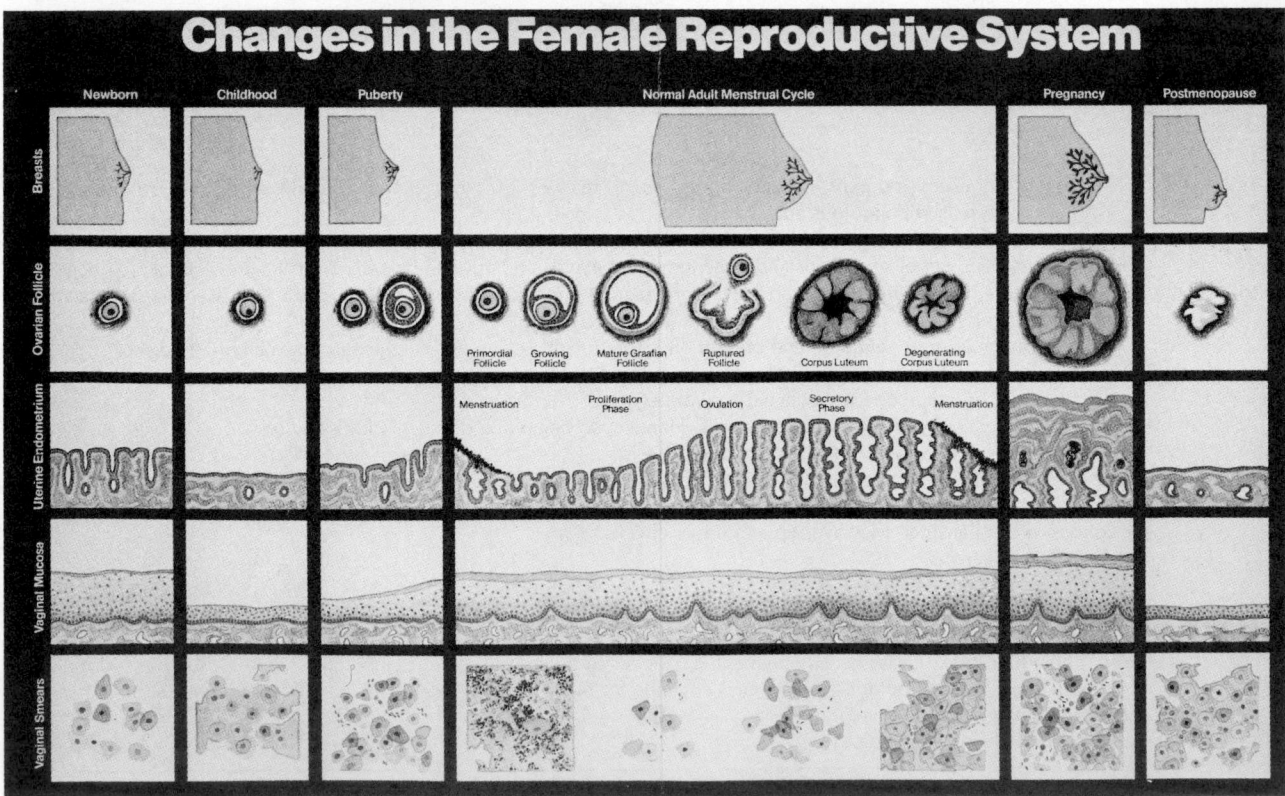

Female and Male Growth and Development Patterns: a Comparison

Female and male growth and development patterns are described and compared in the following tables and figures. A summary of the hypothalamic-pituitary-gonadal axis for the female and the male is presented in Fig. 5.35. Summaries of the stages of sexual development of the female and of the male are presented in Tables 5.5 and 5.6. The changes in the female reproductive system over the life span are illustrated in Fig. 5.36.

Physiologic Response to Sexual Stimulation

Anatomic and reproductive differences notwithstanding, women and men are more alike than different in their physiologic response to sexual excitement and orgasm.* For example, the glans clitoris and the glans penis are homologues with the same number of nerve endings (see Fig. 5.1 and Table 5.1). This explains why the clitoris is so sensitive to sexual stimulation. Not only is there little difference between female and male sexual response, but also it is now accepted that the physical response is essentially the same where the source of stimulation is coitus, fantasy, or mechanical or manual masturbation.

Currently there are two theories to explain the physiologic response to sexual stimulation. The first and most widely used theory is the four-phase response cycle described by Masters and Johnson. The second is Helen Kaplan's biphasic sexual response cycle.

Four-phase response cycle. Physiologically, sexual response, according to Masters and Johnson (1966), can be analyzed in terms of two processes: vasocongestion and myotonia.

1. *Vasocongestion.* Sexual stimulation results in reflex dilation of penile blood vessels (erection) and circumvaginal blood vessels (lubrication), causing engorgement and distention of the genitalia. Venous congestion is localized primarily in the genitalia, but it also occurs to a lesser degree in the breasts and other parts of the body.
2. *Myotonia.* Arousal is characterized by increased muscular tension, resulting in voluntary and involuntary rhythmic contractions. Example of sexually stimulated myotonia are pelvic thrusting, facial gri-

*See Chapter 6 for a discussion of the psychological components of human sexuality.

macing, and spasms of the hands and feet (carpopedal spasms).

The response cycle is arbitrarily divided into four phases: excitement phase, plateau phase, orgasmic phase, and resolution phase. One moves through the four phases progressively, and there is no sharp dividing line between any two phases. However, there are specific bodily changes that take place in sequence. The time, intensity, and duration for cyclic completion also vary for individuals and situations.

The following descriptions and drawings of the female and male genitalia show the major body changes during the four phases of the response cycle.

Excitement phase: women. The first observable reaction to sexual stimulation is vaginal lubrication, which has the biologic function of preparing the vagina for penile penetration. The inner two thirds of the vaginal barrel lengthens and distends. The cervix and fundus are pulled upward.

The external genitalia become congested and darker in color. The clitoris increases in diameter and in tumescence (vascular congestion and swelling) (Fig. 5.37).

Excitement phase: men. The first observable reaction to sexual stimulation is erection of the penis (increase in length and diameter). The scrotal skin be-

---

Fig. 5.37

Female pelvic organs during excitement phase. (From Fogel, C.I., and Woods, N.F.: Health care of women: a nursing perspective, St. Louis, 1981, The C. V. Mosby Co.)

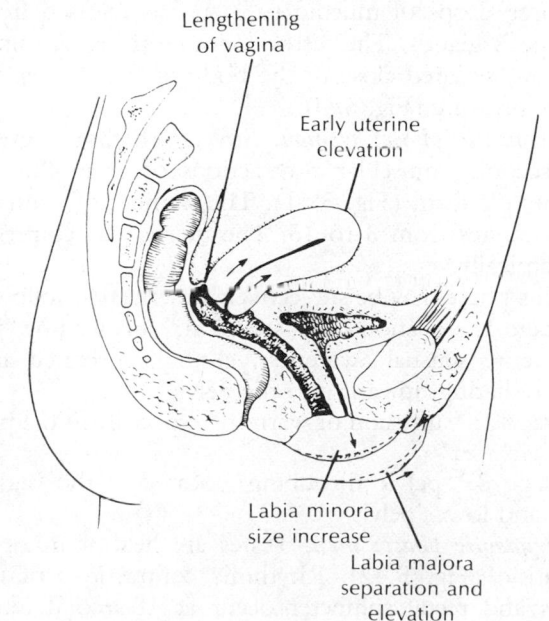

Lengthening of vagina

Early uterine elevation

Labia minora size increase

Labia majora separation and elevation

Fig. 5.38
Male pelvic organs during excitement phase.

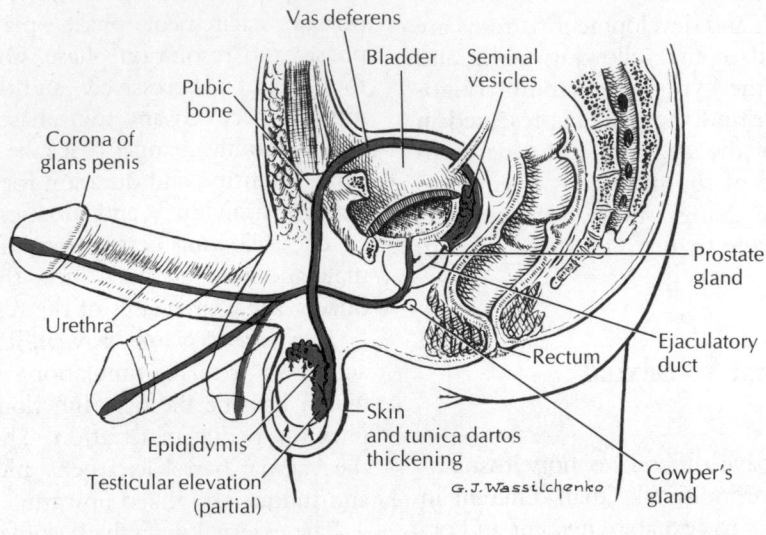

comes congested and thick. The testes elevate because of contraction of the cremasteric musculature (Fig. 5.38).

Plateau phase: women. The wall of the outer one third of the vagina becomes greatly engorged, along with the labia minora, forming the "orgasmic platform." The clitoris retracts under the clitoral hood to protect the clitoris from intense, direct stimulation (Fig. 5.39).

Plateau phase: men. Preorgasmic emission of two or three drops of mucoid substance is released from Cowper's glands. The testes continue to elevate until they are situated close to the body to facilitate ejaculatory pressure (Fig. 5.40).

Orgasmic phase: women. Strong, rhythmic (every 0.8 second), muscular contractions occur in the orgasmic platform (Fig. 5.41). The number of contractions ranges from 3 to 15. The uterus also contracts rhythmically.

This phase may be subjectively described as follows:
Stage 1: sensation of "suspension," followed by "intense sensual awareness, clitorally oriented and radiating upward into the pelvis"
Stage 2: "suffusion of warmth" especially in the pelvic area
Stage 3: "pelvic throbbing" located in the vagina and lower pelvis

Orgasmic phase: men. Testes are held at maximal elevation (Fig. 5.42). Rhythmic contractions of the penis and rectal sphincter occur at 18-second intervals.

This phase may be subjectively described as follows:
Stage 1: point of "inevitability," which occurs just before ejaculation and lasts 2 or 3 seconds; awareness of presence of fluid in the urethra
Stage 2: ejaculation with rhythmic contractions capable of expelling semen up to 60 cm (24 in)

Fig. 5.39
Female pelvic organs during plateau phase. (From Fogel, C.I., and Woods, N.F.: Health care of women: a nursing perspective, St. Louis, 1981, The C. V. Mosby Co.)

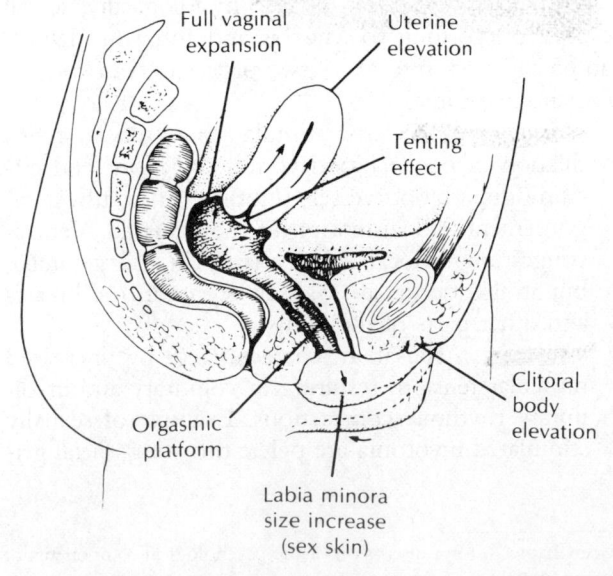

Fig. 5.40
Male pelvic organs during plateau phase.

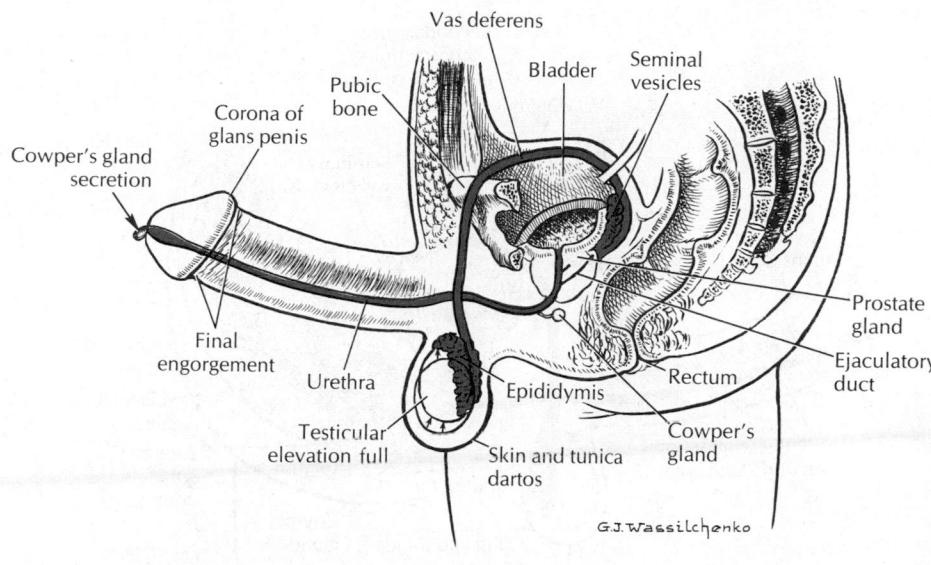

Resolution phase: women. Blood returns from the engorged walls of vagina, and the labia majora and minora rapidly return to their unexcited state. The clitoris rapidly returns from under the hood; however, return to normal size may take longer. Uterus descends, and cervix dips into seminal pool (Fig. 5.43).

Fig. 5.41
Female pelvic organs during orgasmic phase. (From Fogel, C.I., and Woods, N.F.: Health care of women: a nursing perspective, St. Louis, 1981, The C. V. Mosby Co.)

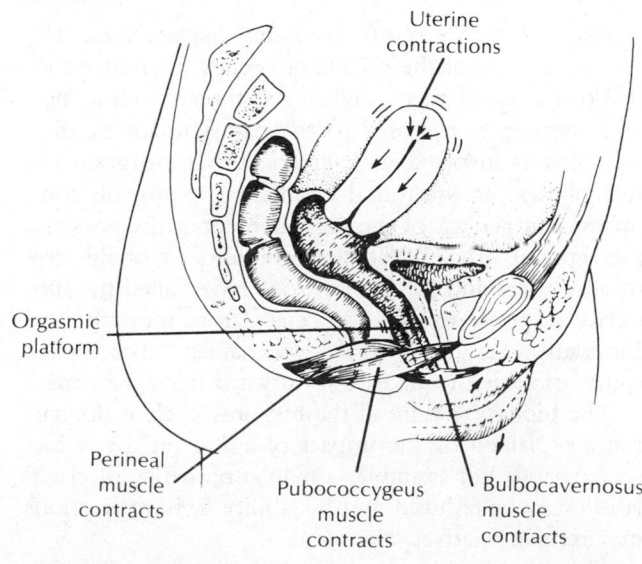

Resolution phase: men. In the first stage of the resolution phase 50% of erection is lost rather rapidly. The second stage can last much longer, depending on the maintenance of physical condition (Fig. 5.44).

The *refractory* period is the time necessary to complete the cycle again. The time varies from a few minutes to a few days, depending on the age and state of physical and emotional health.

Biphasic response. Kaplan (1974) has presented an alternative to the four-phase sexual response of cycle of Masters and Johnson. She believes clinical and physiologic evidence suggests that sexual response is biphasic, with the following two distinct and relatively independent components:

1. Genital vasocongestive reaction—produces vaginal lubrication and swelling in the female and penile erection in the male
2. Reflex clonic muscular contractions—constitute orgasm in both sexes

Phase 1: vasocongestive reaction. Erection in the male is local vasocongestive response. During erection the corpora cavernosa become engorged with blood. Special valves in the penile veins are closed by reflex action, preventing loss of blood. This mechanism is regulated by the parasympathetic division of the autonomic nervous system, which controls the diameter and valves of the penile blood vessels, thus causing erection or loss of erection. Once erection has occurred, excitement can be maintained for some time. Men are physically capable of losing and regaining several erections during love play.

Fig. 5.42
Male pelvic organs during orgasmic phase.

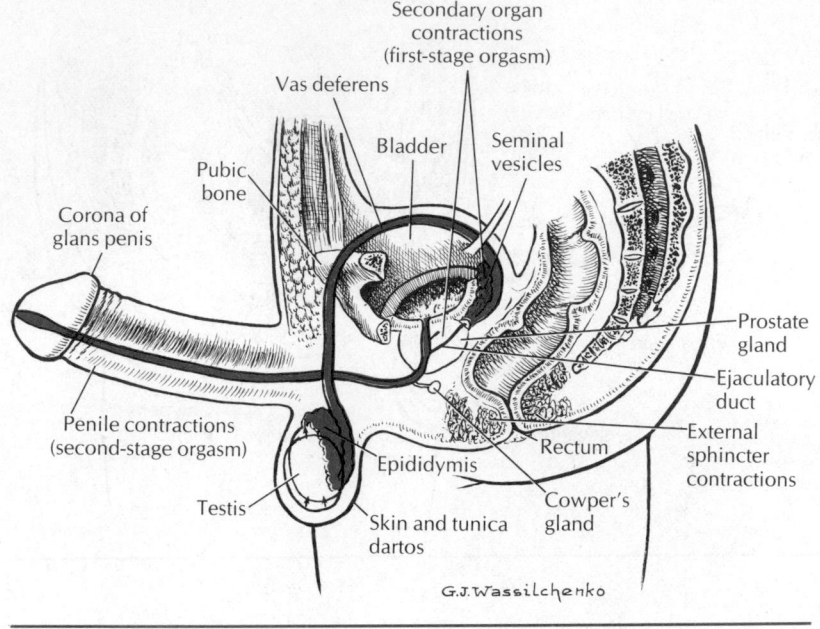

Fig. 5.43
Female pelvic organs during resolution phase. (From Fogel, C.I., and Woods, N.F.: Health care of women: a nursing perspective, St. Louis, 1981, The C. V. Mosby Co.)

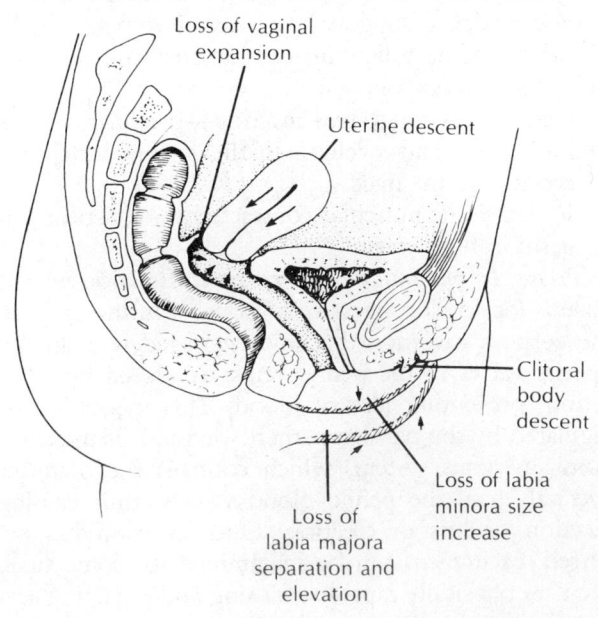

Kaplan calls the vasocongestive reaction in females the "lubrication-swelling" phase. During this phase, dilation of the circumvaginal venous plexus causes a transudate on the walls of the vagina, which results in lubrication. The tissues become the "orgasmic platform" (analogous to erection in the male). In addition the uterus becomes engorged and begins to rise slightly out of the pelvic cavity so that the cervix is placed in a position to increase the likelihood of fertilization.

Phase 2: reflex clonic muscular contractions. The visceral aspects of the ejaculatory reflex are under control of the sympathetic division of the autonomic nervous system, as opposed to the parasympathetic division that is involved with erection. Male orgasm has two phases: emission and ejaculation. Emission comprises contractions of the vasa deferentia, the prostate, the seminal vesicles, and the internal part of the urethra. Masters and Johnson (1966) have called the subjective response to emission "ejaculatory inevitability." Ejaculation is the external mechanism that causes spurts of semen to be forced outward from the penis.

The biphasic nature of the response cycle is dramatically explained by the impact of aging on the refractory period. For example, a man's frequency of ejaculation may be reduced, but his ability to have erections may remain relatively the same.

The woman, like the man, has orgasms consisting

Fig. 5.44
Male pelvic organs during resolution phase.

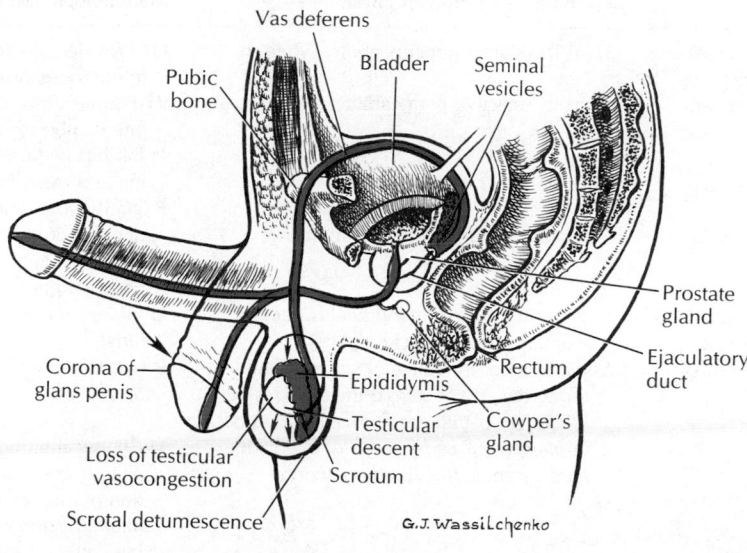

of a series of reflex, involuntary rhythmic contractions of the orgasmic platform.

Clinical significance. There are four important findings from the research of Masters and Johnson that have significance for nurses working with pregnant women and their families. These findings concern (1) multiple orgasm, (2) simultaneous orgasm, (3) clitoral vs. vaginal orgasm, and (4) variations in orgasmic patterns.

Multiple orgasm. Since women never physically have a refractory period, they are capable of having one orgasm after another until exhausted. Multiple orgasms are most frequently reported by women in their late thirties and early forties. Some women have also reported being multiply orgasmic for the first time during the second trimester of pregnancy. The reason is that because of the increased vasocongestion of pregnancy, total completion of the resolution phase never occurs.

Simultaneous orgasm. Many couples have considered simultaneous orgasm the ultimate goal of sexual bliss. The findings of Masters and Johnson and of others show the illogic of such goals, because many couples progress through the response cycle at different rates. The myth of the desirability of simultaneous orgasm has harmed many relationships because of the difficulty of achieving this goal. Although possible, simultaneous orgasm is the exception rather than the rule and is achieved when the woman reaches orgasm easily.

Clitoral vs. vaginal orgasm. Freud taught that women transfer sexual sensation from the clitoris to the vagina when they reach psychosexual maturity. A clitoral orgasm was considered therefore to be an immature orgasm. This belief existed until Masters and Johnson demonstrated that an orgasm is a total body response to sexual stimulation, with the most intense response located in the pelvic area. The response is essentially the same regardless of whether it is experienced through coitus, masturbation, or mechanical stimulation. The clitoris is defined as the "transmitter and conductor" of erotic sensation. Hite (1976) reported that 30% of the women in her sample of 3000 were orgasmic during intercourse without additional clitoral stimulation.

Variations in orgasmic patterns. There are many response patterns for both women and men. These patterns vary in both intensity and duration.

Immunology

Beverly Gaglione

Viewing life as an opportunity to grow and develop through interactions with other systems in the environment enables the nurse to appreciate those factors that monitor and mediate the self-other relationships. A systems theory approach to the concept of immunity is useful in understanding the numerous and complex physiologic factors that serve to maintain the integrity of the body's organization when nonself cells or substances affect the patterns of the body.

Two different types of immunity are addressed in

Table 5.7
Application of Systems Theory to Concept of Immunology

Principles of Systems Theory	Examples from Human Physiology	Immunologic Effect
A system is characterized by degrees of openness—extent to which that system is able to be influenced by another system.	*Skin:* its relative impermeability while intact. *Skin:* its selective permeability. *Skin:* its salty perspiration. *Placenta:* its selective permeability.	U* Provides physical and mechanical barrier to microorganisms and some substances. P† Permits absorption of substances to which one can be sensitive; involves IgE antibody. U Inhibits certain bacterial flora from colonizing and overwhelming system. P IgG humoral antibodies cross placental barrier and provide particularistic (passive natural) immunity, whereas IgM and IgA antibodies do not.
A system exhibits patterns or regularities that permit predictions to be made about behavior and operation of system.	*Vagina:* in a state of good health, fecund woman maintains acidic pH. *Vagina:* under influence of systemic antibiotic therapy or steroid therapy, resident Döderlein bacilli are reduced in number. *Complement cascade:* series of events initiated by antigen-antibody reaction.	U Inhibits growth of certain bacteria and fungi. P *Candida albicans* (fungus) establishes itself on mucosa. U Chemical attraction of leukocytes and phagocytes to site of invasion; degranulation of mast cells (releasing histamine); neutralization of viruses; and lysis of invading cells.
Behavior of whole system is affected by that of its parts and by its interactions with other systems.	*Bone marrow:* treatment with certain antineoplastic drugs suppresses function of marrow. *Exposure* to German measles (rubella), polioviruses, and so on.	U Depression of number and function of phagocytes, monocytes, and B and T lymphocytes, resulting in site of compromised immunocompetency. P Development of IgM humoral antibodies upon first exposure to antigen, to provide protection against invading viruses.
A system is affected by space and time dimensions.	*T cell receptor sites:* only certain places in body have these receptor sites. *Repeated exposure* to an antigen (as through booster injection or second allograft from the same donor) is example of effect of time on immune response	U T cell receptor sites are essential for cell-mediated type of immune response; fact that a woman can be host to embryo formed from mate's sperm cell and surrogate mother's ovum and can continue pregnancy to term‡ is evidence of the female reproductive tract's immune unresponsiveness to foreign protein substances. P Because of existence of memory B and T lymphocyte cells, there is accelerated and stronger antibody or cytotoxic response to substances that body has previously experienced.
Changes occur within system and between systems via communication.	*Histocompatibility complex molecules* permit recognition of self from nonself cells and substances. *Antigens* (antibody generators) are introduced into body via air currents (respiratory tract), pulsating circulating blood, flagellated movements of some cells, and so on.	U Stimulates or inhibits foreign tissue rejection response P Antigens in blood stimulate development of B lymphocyte, humoral antibody, whereas antigens in tissue stimulate T lymphocyte, cell-mediated cytotoxic antibody response.
Nature of systemic change is such that it is progressively more complex and innovative.	Once triggered, *complement cascade,* a complex of 11 proteins, appears to be unidirectional, sustained by enzymes that catalyze subsequent steps. When *blood levels* of appropriate antibiotic drug therapy (according to culture and sensitivity tests) are inadequately maintained, offending microorganism is not effectively brought under control.	U Sum effect of cascade is multifaceted attack on antigenic substance; end result of cascade is lysis of invading cell's wall. P Antigenic bacteria develop resistant strains to antibiotic and may then actually thrive in environment of once effective antibiotic, resulting in overwhelming attack on body system.

*Universalistic or nonspecific effect, a protective immunologic mechanism common to all healthy human beings.
†Particularistic or specific effect, a protective mechanism unique to an individual's system and experience.
‡Bustillo et al., 1984.

Table 5.7: universalistic (or nonspecific) and particularistic (or specific). *Universalistic immunity* consists of those physiologic defense mechanisms common to nearly all humans. It provides general protection against the deleterious effects of nonself cells and substances. *Particularistic immunity* refers to those defense mechanisms unique to an individual because of personal experiences in the environment. This type of immunity not only is peculiar to an individual but also is unique in that it involves resistance to certain specific foreign cells and substances.

Universalistic (nonspecific) immunity. The following immune defense mechanisms are shared by all healthy human beings. Those physiologic defense mechanisms that comprise the body's first line of defense (i.e., those that prevent invasion of the body by foreign cells and substances) include the following:

1. Intact skin, which has a slightly acidic pH and secretes sodium chloride (perspiration) through its sweat glands—both of which discourage many microorganisms but at the same time encourage other bacteria (known as *resident flora*) that function to keep pathogenic bacteria and other nonself matter in check.

2. A ciliated respiratory tract, the operation of which protects the lungs and bronchi from microorganisms, debris, and dirt.

3. A viscous mucous membrane, which lines all the portals (entrances and exits) of the body, including the eye. The character of the mucous membrane inhibits the growth and activity of invading microorganisms. Further, the outward flow of tears, urine, and vaginal secretions hinders the inward movements of microorganisms.

4. The enzyme lysozyme, which is found in tears, saliva, milk, mucus, and other body fluids and is capable of lysing, or breaking down, the cell walls of many different types of bacteria.

5. The very acidic pH of the stomach, which creates a hostile environment for nonself cells and substances, and the resident bacteria of the colon, which discourage the colonization and growth of pathogenic bacteria in the intestines.

6. Eyelids, which can close to protect the eye.

Table 5.8 provides examples of immunologic problems associated with pregnant and parturient women, neonates, and postpartum and perimenopausal women when there is a dysfunction of the first line of defense.

If foreign cells and substances do manage to penetrate through the body's first line of defense, a *second line of defense* is present in all healthy human beings. The various mechanisms of this line of defense include the following:

1. The body has the capability of producing an in-

Table 5.8
Examples of Potential Obstetric, Neonatal, or Gynecologic Immunologic Problems Associated with Dysfunction of Universalistic First Line of Defense Mechanisms

Client Type	First Line of Defense Dysfunction	Immunologic Problem
Obstetric		
Antepartal phase	pH of stomach and mouth altered toward more basic reaction secondary to self-medication with sodium bicarbonate for heartburn (pyrosis).	Prone to invasion of pathologic bacteria in gastrointestinal tract.
Intrapartal phase	Episiotomy, especially a third- or fourth-degree extension of perineal laceration.	Possibility of contamination of suture line (by direct extension) and infection of perineum, vagina, uterus, uterine tubes, and peritoneum with coliform bacteria.
Postpartum phase	If soap or other drying agent is mistakenly applied to "clean" or "disinfect" nipples and areola area of breasts, lubricating glands of Montgomery may cease to function adequately. Also, if breast pads with plastic liners are used, moisture will remain against nipple, predisposing it to maceration and cracking.	Drying may lead to change in secretion of fatty acids and thus to increased susceptibility to tissue breakdown and colonization and invasion of bacteria. With cracking of nipple and subsequent break in integrity of skin comes likelihood of invasion of pathogenic bacteria, leading to mastitis.
Neonatal	If child is born with facial paralysis (Bell's palsy) secondary to birth injury, eye on affected side may remain open (until closed and protected by nurse).	Surface of eye could dry out and be prone to injury and microbial invasion.
Gynecologic	A postmenopausal woman can be expected to have a decrease in vaginal secretions secondary to altered hormonal (estrogenic and progesteronic) influence over mucosal and endometrial secretions.	Prone to vaginitis.

Table 5-9
Role of White Blood Cells in Body's Defense System

Type of White Blood Cell (WBC)	Percentage (%) of Total WBC*	Role Played in Immunity
Granulocytes	51-78	These cells have granules or lysosomes that function to degrade material ingested by WBCs.
Neutrophils ("segs" or polymorphonuclear neutrophils)	50-70	These granulocytes travel in blood to site of invasion; then they adhere to endothelium of blood vessel and proceed to pass through blood vessel to area of invasion and inflammation; here they act by phagocytosis and lysis.
Eosinophils	1-4	Found mostly in tissues of skin, lungs, and gastrointestinal tract, these cells act as phagocytes.
Basophils	0-1	These noncirculating cells are found in connective tissue, where they release heparin and possibly other chemotactic substances that augment and complement inflammatory and allergic response.
Mononuclear (nongranular) leukocytes	22-48	No granules are found in cytoplasm of these cells. They are also known as *agranulocytes*.
Monocytes	2-8	Monocytes travel to site of invasion (like neutrophils) and act as macrophages (very large phagocytes). Some reside in spleen, lymph nodes, connective tissue, and lungs, where they screen out and destroy foreign or damaged self tissues in that environment.
Lymphocytes	20-40	
B type	95%-98% of *circulating* lymphocytes	B lymphocytes travel through body in blood and lymph systems. They proliferate during viral or bacterial infection and form plasma cells (from which *specific* antibodies are made) and memory cells (also *specific* antibodies from which clones are made during subsequent exposure to same antigenic substance). B lymphocytes provide humoral immunity. (See Table 5.11 for more detailed information about role and action of various humoral antibodies.)
T type T "killer" or cytotoxic cells T helper cells T suppressor cells	Approximately 2% of *circulating* antibodies	These lymphocytes act primarily against nucleated cells including body's own cells that may be altered by a foreign substance. When stimulated by an antigen, these lymphocytes also form *specific* monocloned T "killer" (cytotoxic) cells and memory cells. T lymphocytes provide cell-mediated immunity. (See Table 5.11 for more detailed information on role of various subpopulations of T lymphocyte.)

*These percentages are based on the total number of *circulating* white blood cells found in serum; hence it is clear that basophils, eosinophils, and T lymphocytes will be underrepresented in the serum, since they are located in other sites in the body.

flammatory response and "fighting" cells. This response begins with the release of histamine from mast cells, which causes local vasodilatation—distending the capillary beds—resulting in the characteristic warm, reddened inflammatory response. Serous fluid and white blood cells then pass through the distended capillaries and present themselves at the site of invasion, drawn by chemotactic substances released by the invaded cells. Other white blood cells position themselves in strategic places in the body to detect and fight invasive substances. Table 5.9 details the various types of leukocytes (white blood cells) and their roles in the body's defense system.

2. A complementary mechanism of defense acts in a series of steps. The initial step catalyzes subsequent phases, and the overall effect is like a pile of dominoes that have begun to fall against one another. The name of this general mechanism, *complement cascade,* is derived from its function: to complement. The mecha-

nism is comprised of 11 different proteins; the whole effect of their interaction results in chemotaxis (in this instance chemically attracting white blood cells to the site of invasion), triggers the release of histamine from mast cells, neutralizes viruses, and lyses cell membranes of invading cells. Although the complement cascade is said to be a nonspecific defense, it is set into motion by a specific antigen-antibody response. The specific antibody does not have the ability to lyse the invading cell, but the complement cascade results in a multifaceted, combined specific and nonspecific attack on the antigenic substance.

3. *Interferon,* a nonspecific (undifferentiated by viral type) protein, made by any of the body's own cells in response to a viral infection. Interferon is released by cells that have already been invaded by a virus and is used by the noninfected body cells to avert the destructive effects of the viral attack. In the chain of simultaneously occurring body defenses, interferon re-

lease takes place after tissue has been invaded but before the development (in sufficient quantity) of the specific antibodies that will neutralize or otherwise destroy the invading substances. (The time dimension of systems theory is relevant in this context: Once a specific antibody is needed, it takes a certain period of *time* before an effective circulating level, or quantity, of the appropriate antibody is reached. Until that time the white blood cells and the interferon attempt to hold the invading substance in check.)

Interferon continues to be released for the first 24 hours after a cell is invaded by a virus. It is important to realize that the interferon does not arrest a de facto viral infection or invasion that is already established within a cell; it is only of benefit to those cells that have not yet succumbed to the attacking virus. Apparently the half-life of interferon is so short (most sources indicate that it provides protection only for one 24-hour period) that its use artificially (by injection) is expensive. At present its production in laboratories and by genetic engineers entails considerable work and expense.

4. Finally the secondary line of defense mechanisms in the human immune system, present in all healthy adults, also consists of the lymph vessels, lymph nodes, spleen, tonsils, and thymus. The lymph vessels transport interstitial fluid to the lymph nodes and also back to the circulatory system. Lymph fluid contains the agents of trauma, phagocytes, and body tissue that has been damaged from the invasive substances. When these by-products of the invasion reach the lymph nodes (distributed throughout the body, but most frequently checked by palpation in the neck, groin, and axilla), they are trapped there. (Since the lymph nodes adjacent to a cancer site are expected to harbor stray cancer cells, the nodes are usually excised during surgery, for example, during a mastectomy for breast cancer.) Lymphocytes, primarily produced by the bone marrow and the thymus gland, are in abundance in the lymph nodes, along with macrophages (Table 5.9). These two types of cells attack the invading agents lodged in the lymph nodes. Lymphocytes and macrophages are also found in large quantities in the spleen and the tonsils. Because of their location the tonsils function to trap airborne invasive agents, whereas the spleen functions to trap invasive agents borne by the blood. The thymus gland, located behind the sternum, is an organ that plays a vital role in the development of T lymphocytes. (In fact, T lymphocytes take their name from the thymus gland.) The thymus is normally active in fetal life and in early childhood but usually atrophies after puberty. The roles played by the T and B lymphocytes and their specific antibodies are detailed below.

Particularistic (specific) immunity. As defined earlier, particularistic or specific immunity refers to those defense mechanisms developed by an individual in response to environmental stresses or opportunities, the effect of which confers a degree of resistance or nonsusceptibility to specific foreign microorganisms or substances. Table 5.10 depicts four different categories of particularistic immunity, based on distinctions between resistance that is naturally versus artificially acquired and resistance that is obtained actively or acquired passively.

Actively acquired immunity. An actively acquired immunity is obtained by engaging the body in the process of *producing antibodies* specific to the dimensions or characteristics of an antigenic substance. The type of resistance conferred by actively acquired immunity is usually of long duration, sometimes lasting for a lifetime.* The length and strength of the immune response are increased through repeated exposure to small amounts of the antigenic substance. This is the rationale that underlies the sequence of "booster" injections in an immunization series. Repeated or "booster" exposure to small amounts of the antigen or to attenuated (weakened, not so virile) antigen encourages the antibody population to increase. (See Table 5.12 for information regarding the correct interpretation of a titration test.)

Passively acquired immunity. An immunity that is passively acquired provides protection to the body in the event of exposure to specific antigens. The body does not produce its own antibodies in this case; it receives them passively. In general, immunity that is passively acquired is of short duration, since the immune globulin received is of the "fighter" type, not the "memory" type (see Table 5.9 and the discussion that follows); hence its life span is limited.

Naturally acquired immunity. A naturally acquired immunity is developed in response to one's individual experiences throughout life. The body of a person exposed to the viruses that produce diseases such as mumps, German measles, and hepatitis has first-hand experience with the invading agents. Therefore that person's specific immune defenses are stimulated to develop the particular antibodies to fight the invading agents. The passively acquired natural immunity entails a degree of uniqueness because the antibodies received from one's mother (via placenta or colostrum) are dependent upon the antigens to which the mother was exposed and the subsequently devel-

---

*For detailed information about susceptibility and resistance factors (length of immunity following exposure to the antigen) to communicable diseases, refer to the 1981 edition of *Control of Communicable Diseases in Man,* an official report of the American Public Health Association, Washington, D.C.

Table 5.10
Types of Particularistic (Specific) Acquired Immunity

Active	Passive
Naturally acquired	
Body produces an antibody specific to stimulating antigen that has entered body via dysfunction of primary line of defense.	Body receives specific antibodies made by another person and transmitted via a "natural" process (placental transmission or through colostrum).
EXAMPLE: Exposure to measles (rubeola) or German measles (rubella) virus stimulates production of IgM antibodies (see Table 5.11) and memory antibodies that provide protection and resistance to virus on subsequent exposure. Experience with these diseases and their specific antibodies usually confers a permanent type of immunity (long lasting).	EXAMPLE: IgA antibodies are received by infants from their mother's colostrum, and IgG antibodies are received in utero, especially during last several weeks of pregnancy, from mother's circulating humoral antibodies. (Table 5.11 provides more detail regarding different types of immunoglobulins and humoral antibodies.) This type of immunity is transient, lasting only for several months.
Artificially acquired	
Body produces antibody specific to stimulating antigen injected into body. Usually antigen is attenuated (weakened, so as not to produce a full-blown virulent disease).	Body is injected with IgG antibodies produced by another person or animal, to provide protection against antigens to which body has been exposed.
EXAMPLES: Sabin trivalent oral polio virus consists of three types of live but weakened polio virus. When administered, it stimulates production of IgM antibodies and memory cells specific to three types of antigens. When a nonpregnant woman is given rubella vaccine, she is injected with live but attenuated German measles virus. It takes about 3 months for her to develop full immunity to rubella virus subsequent to injection. She must not become pregnant in this 3-month period, since her body is still considered to be "fighting" rubella virus as it develops IgM antibodies against it.	EXAMPLE: When a woman who is Rh negative delivers a baby who is Rh_o (Du) immune positive, or if such a woman has an abortion (miscarriage), she is at risk of being exposed to fetal Rh-positive erythrocytes (secondary to microfracture of placental tissue, with escape of fetal blood cells and their uptake by maternal circulation). If permitted to respond "naturally" to these fetal Rh-positive antigen cells, mother would develop longlasting "fighter" antibody cells against Rh-positive cells. This would pose a problem to subsequent Rh-positive children she would conceive, since her "fighter" antibodies would cross placenta and attack cells of her fetus. Thus woman is given anti-Rh-positive antibodies, so that she will not produce her own antibodies. *Timing* of injection of Rh_o (Du) immune globulin is of utmost importance. If it is given too late after delivery (after 72 hours), mother will have begun process of forming her own long-lasting antibodies against Rh-positive cells. Once a woman has developed long-lasting immunity against Rh-positive cells, she is no longer a candidate for immune globulin, and her Rh-positive offspring are prone to erythroblastosis fetalis (see also Chapter 31).

oped antibodies, the length of pregnancy*; and whether the child was breast fed.

Artificially acquired immunity. An artificially acquired immunity can be said to be iatrogenic, since the antigens (in the case of active artificial immunity) and the antibodies (in the case of passive artificial immunity) introduced into the body are considered to be "legend" drugs, which require a physician's prescriptive order before they can be administered. As pharmacologic categories of drugs, these antigens (e.g., attenuated poliovirus and attenuated rubella virus) and these antibodies (e.g., immune RH_o (D^u) immune globulin and hepatitis B immune globulin) are known as *biologicals,* since they are produced from living cells. In administering these products, it is extremely important to check carefully the expiration dates and lot numbers of the items, since the material can deteriorate or become contaminated.

T lymphocyte response. Two types of lymphocytes are responsible for the development of the antibody-specific immune responses in the body. They are known as T lymphocytes and B lymphocytes. The T lymphocytes, derived from thymus tissue, are activated against eukaryotic (nucleated) cells, and they exert their action at the level of tissues that are invaded by some nonself substance or cells. The type of specific immunity effected by T lymphocytes, then, is known as cell-mediated immunity. Facilitating the body in its job of identifying nonself cells and then attracting cytotoxic (killer) T lymphocytes specific to the offending invading substance are special molecules—known as major histocompatibility complex (MHC) molecules—and T helper (T_H) cells. The MHC molecule is a coded section of a cell that identifies that cell as "self" or "nonself." The MHC code for all your healthy cells is the same. Your best friend's MHC code is different

---

*Prematurely born infants receive less antibody protection than do termbirth neonates because the placental transfer IgG antibodies is greater during the last several weeks of pregnancy (Korones, 1985).

from yours. (In the future with improved technology, nurses may not be identifying neonates by footprinting them but by obtaining a specimen for MHC code discernment.) Hence it is understandable why one person's body tends to reject grafted or transplanted tissue from another person (as an allograft)—unless that person is an identical twin. It is this cell-mediated, T lymphocyte–specific immune reaction that is involved when a body rejects transplanted organs or tissue.

T helper cells. If a virus or another nonself substance invades a person's cells, then the MHC complex becomes somewhat altered, triggering a "nonself" identity and release of some chemotactic substance(s) that attracts the T helper cells. Recently researchers have discovered the existence of T cell receptor sites in the human body (although their sites of distribution have not been discovered to date).* When stimulated by a "nonself" message, these receptor sites would serve to bind the T cells (or perhaps the T helper cells) to the invaded cellular tissue. The T helper cells function to activate cytolytic or cytotoxic (killer) T cells that are specifically made to the dimensions or characteristics of the invading antigenic substance. In addition the T helper cell activates the B lymphocytes in their development of specific circulating antibodies, and so it also indirectly triggers the complement cascade.

Killer T cells: memory cell and fighter cell. It has recently been discovered that killer T cells are of at least two types—a memory cell and a fighter cell—and that the killer T cells are capable of producing monoclones to specific antigens.* The memory cell retains the instructions for producing clones of the specific killer T cell. Because of this conservative strategy the body reacts more quickly (see Table 5.7, space and time dimensions) to a repeated exposure to an antigen. This principle is operational when a person receives a second tissue or organ transplant from the same donor: the graft or tissue rejection response is accelerated and stronger with subsequent exposure to the same antigen. The mechanism for making the specific antibody–killer cell is already in place, and therefore the antigen-antibody is almost immediate.

It is believed that the immune response memory cells (of both the T and B lymphocytes) are stored in lymph nodes and the spleen. It is not unusual for the lymph nodes and the spleen to enlarge during the active acute phase of invasive attack because these areas become productive; they are the focal sites for the replicating monoclones of the requisite T and B specialized lymphocyte cells.

The "fighting" killer T cells act in several different ways: by neutralizing the antigen, by invading it, or by triggering the auxillary macrophages and interferon responses.

T suppressor or T regulator cell. Another type of T cell is the T suppressor or T regulator cell. This cell apparently functions via negative feedback to prevent the killer T cells and even the B lymphocytes from becoming activated or to limit their action.

B lymphocyte response. The B lymphocytes are derived from bone marrow.* They produce antigen-specific antibodies that circulate in the blood, and so the B lymphocytic defense mechanism is known as the effector of the humoral immunity system. Upon stimulation by an antigen the immature (undeveloped or unspecified) B lymphocyte differentiates into plasma cells and memory cells. The antigen-specific antibodies are released by the plasma cells during the first exposure to the antigen. These antibodies function by binding with their antigen and neutralizing, agglutinating, or opsonizing it. The antigen-antibody complex also triggers the complement cascade, which ultimately results in lysis of the cell membrane of the offending invading agent. The memory B lymphocytes continue to circulate (they stay unbound); they travel to the lymph nodes or the spleen or to both to replicate monocloned antibodies in the event of repeated exposure to the specific antigenic substance.

Primary humoral response. Primary humoral response occurs after the initial contact with a specific antigen. It generally takes from 48 to 72 hours before the corresponding B lymphocyte antibody specific to fight that antigen is ready in a quantity sufficient to be effective.

Secondary humoral response. A secondary humoral response entails a short response time to the antigen because of the presence of the memory cells, which reduces the production time. Therefore the response time is generally within 24 to 48 hours, and the strength of the response is greater.

There are five known classes of B lymphocyte antibodies. They are called immunoglobulins (Ig). The gamma globulins of the type IgG are the most widely studied; they are used prophylactically to confer passively acquired immunity status for a short-term period for select clients. (See Table 5.10.) Table 5.11 specifies the role and action of the specific antibodies produced by the B and T lymphocytes.

Assessment of immune responsiveness. If the area of invasion is not quickly resolved by nonspecific and specific defense mechanisms or if it is not confined to

---

*"The T Cell Receptor," 1983.

*The name of the B lymphocyte is taken from the first initial of the bursa of the chicken, from which these cells are derived in that animal.

Table 5.11
Role and Action of Specific Antibodies Produced by T and B Lymphocytes

Antibody Type	Immunity Type	Role and Action
T killer (cytotoxic) lymphocyte	Cell-mediated	Activated against foreign protein (as allografts); intracellular infections (viral, mycobacterial, protozoal, and fungal infections that not only have gained entrance to body but also have lodged within cells in tissue); and self (own) cells that have undergone subtle but significant enough change so as to alter the histocompatibility complex code of cells; converting it to nonself status.
B lymphocyte	Humoral (circulating)	
IgA	Humoral	These antibodies scout, screen, and protect mucosal surfaces of respiratory tract, gastrointestinal tract, and genitourinary tract. They are developed principally in response to viral antigens. They are also found circulating in saliva, colostrum, tears, synovial fluid, and bile, so they are also known as "secretory" immunoglobulins (found in secretions of the body).
IgD	Humoral	Although these antibodies have been identified by researchers, their role and function have not been discerned to date.
IgE	Humoral	These antibodies function during hypersensitivity (allergic) responses. They regulate release of histamine from mast cells when allergens bind with their corresponding IgE antibodies. They are also said to have an antihelminic role (eradicating worms from gastrointestinal tract).
IgG	Humoral	The B lymphocyte antibodies make up greatest number of all five classes of immunoglobulins. Primarily found circulating in serum, they are concerned with secondary humoral response, chiefly to invading viruses and bacteria. This is only type of B lymphocyte antibody that crosses placental barrier and provides natural passively acquired immunity to fetus and neonate. Activates complement cascade when specific antibody binds with antigen.
IgM	Humoral	These large-size antibodies found in serum are manifested during primary humoral response to invading viral and bacterial organisms. They activate complement cascade phenomenon upon binding with antigen.

an area (as by abscess formation), it may spread in either a contiguous fashion or systemically, through the blood or lymph circulation or both. This in turn may be manifested as lymphadenitis (inflammation of the lymph nodes), lymphadenopathy, or septicemia. Symptoms of these processes include swollen and tender lymph nodes (secondary to the accumulation of the agents of trauma, the phagocytes, and the body's own cellular or lymphoid debris resulting from the attack), fever, anorexia, fatigue and lethargy, and leukocytosis (with increased demand there is an increased supply of the necessary white blood cells). In addition to ordering culture and sensitivity tests to determine the causative invading agent (if possible) and the appropriate effective drug therapy to assist the body in combating the infection, a physician frequently orders other types of laboratory tests to determine the body's responsiveness to the invasion. Nurses need to understand the reason(s) why these various tests are performed and the significance of the outcomes of the tests, because the laboratory data provide additional assessment information that guides the nurse and the physician in their approach to the care of the client. Table 5.12 provides information about various laboratory tests of immunologic responsiveness that should be monitored, and the special nursing care implica-

tions that are associated with the tests or their outcomes. Those tests that have specific relevance to maternity, gynecologic, or neonatal clients are italicized in the table.

Factors Affecting Functioning of Immune Defense System

Age: variations across the life span. Although the healthy term neonate is expected to have functioning first-line defense mechanisms, the newborn does not sweat, has no tears, and is not born with resident skin or intestinal flora. For example, the lack of intestinal flora is responsible for the newborn's inability to synthesize vitamin K and thus places the neonate at risk for hemorrhagic disease. Resistance to infection is lowered following hemorrhage for anyone, regardless of age. When the integrity of the skin is broken by an internal fetal scalp electrode, the neonate is predisposed to a blood or tissue invasion by foreign cells or substances. Preterm, small-for-gestational-age, and postterm infants have different qualities of skin that increase their susceptibility to invasive agents. Further, infants whose birth is traumatic or who are born with depleted nutritional stores have even greater susceptibility to infection.

The term infant is expected to have passively ac-

Table 5.12
Using Laboratory Test Data Regarding Activated Immune Defense System to Determine Approach to Health Care

Test Performed	Purpose of Test	Nursing Care Implications
Agglutination and titer levels (blood test)	These two tests permit quantitative and qualitative determination of presence of antibodies to antigen. In quantitative phase, fact of clumping (agglutination) or no clumping is indicative of antibody-antigen reaction (depending on structure of test absence or presence of clumping may be read as positive test for antigen-antibody reaction). *It is a test of this type that is performed as immunologic test for pregnancy (searching for antibody reaction to antigen known as human chorionic gonadotropin, which is formed by fetal tissue).* Qualitative or titration test indicates degree of response aroused in body by antigen. Frequently physician will order two tests of titration separated by a time interval *(as before delivery and after delivery, in case of indirect Coombs test)* to determine if there has been a change—most notably a rise—in titer levels, which would indicate recent experience with antigen in question. *In case of testing for immunity (resistance) to rubella,* titration test is essential to determine if client has adequate number of antibodies to provide protection in event of repeated exposure to rubella virus. Most laboratories consider a titration at level of 1:10 as adequate to ensure a state of immunity against rubella. NOTE: The titration levels conferring immune status differ from disease to disease.	A positive test indicates that exposure has occurred to antigenic substance. *In case of direct Coombs test* (for detection of specific maternal antibodies—IgG—on fetal erythrocytes, antigenic substances): positive test result should alert nurse to fact that neonate is at risk for hyperbilirubinemia, oxygen deficit (secondary to hemolysis of red blood cells), and all sequelae of erythroblastosis fetalis (see Chapter 31). *In case of indirect Coombs test* (for detection of anti-Rh antibodies appearing in mother's serum): if test result is positive and if serial dilutions of serum indicate there is considerable anti-Rh antibody activity in mother's system, mother would not be a candidate for Rh_0 (D^u) immune globulin, since she had already developed the IgM and IgG antibodies against Rh. *If pregnant woman has positive titration test for rubella* at 1:4 dilution (1 part serum to 4 parts diluent) but not positive test at 1:8 dilution, she does not have adequate antibody protection against rubella virus. Woman is then susceptible to acquiring disease if exposed to virus. Compounding risk is fact that rubella that can be demonstrated to have occurred during first trimester of pregnancy (on basis of interval-titration tests) poses a hazard to fetus (see Chapters 8 and 31). Postpartal woman who has demonstrated negative rubella titration test is good candidate to receive rubella vaccine, provided she practices some form of contraception for 3 months following injection of live, attenuated vaccine—until she has developed state of immunity to the disease. Client should also sign informed consent before receiving rubella vaccine to indicate that she is aware of her responsibilities and risks associated with artificially induced active immunity therapy.
Complement (C3, C4) activity (blood test)	Instead of testing for activation of entire complement cascade, usually test is performed for two aspects of cascade sequence, to determine if they have been triggered. In event of immune response, levels of C3 and C4 (2 of 11 proteins involved in cascade) decrease, indicating their having been used.	This is a nonspecific test. It is possible that there may be "normal" test result yet immune response occurring in body. This test is used in combination with other tests (e.g., LE [lupus erythematosus] prep, ANA [antinuclear antibody] and RF [rheumatoid factor] tests) to determine progression of the autoimmune disease processes.
C-reactive protein (blood test)	This is a nonspecific test indicative of inflammatory process. It is sometimes used to rule out viral infection because protein is not present in cases of virally caused inflammation.	Because this test is nonspecific, caution must be used in interpreting results. *It is possible for pregnancy or drug therapy with estrogenic birth control pills to produce false positive test.* Also, test may be positive in other types of inflammatory situations, as during acute myocardial infarction, acute phase of rheumatoid disease, or rheumatoid arthritis.
Culture and sensitivity (C and S)	This test permits identification of type of antigen probably responsible for infectious process. Details about Gram's stain, type of environment (aerobic or anaerobic) that supports growth of antigen, and other characteristics of agent can	Nurse is responsible for collecting correct amount of specimen for culture in appropriate container. It is preferable that specimen be collected before antibiotic therapy is initiated, because this therapy could affect and invalidate test results.

Continued.

Table 5.12, cont'd
Using Laboratory Test Data Regarding Activated Immune Defense System to Determine Approach to Health Care

Test Performed	Purpose of Test	Nursing Care Implications
	be determined. Once a bacteria, virus, or fungus has been identified, test continues to evaluate effectiveness (or sensitivity) of variety of antibiotic drugs in inhibiting growth of agent. Occasionally a C & S test is performed during antibiotic therapy when client has not shown improvement with prescribed medication.	Once results of test are available, it is imperative that client receive medication to which antigenic organisms are sensitive (and not resistant). If client has been receiving a drug to which organism is resistant, nurse must contact physician and report test result immediately.
Immunoelectrophoresis of serum proteins: IgA, IgD, IgE, IgG, IgM (blood test)	Normally this test is used to detect changes in any of immunoglobulins. *In case of a newborn,* this test may be performed to learn if IgM antibodies are present in the cord blood. NOTE: These large IgM antibodies do not cross placental barrier.	*If infant is born with suspicion of intrauterine acquired infection,* nurse should save placenta and cord for laboratory analysis (for IgM antibodies and other tests). A positive IgM cord blood test necessitates contacting physician immediately and initiating protective and supportive care for infected infant (see Chapters 25 and 31).
Immunofluorescence antibody (IFA) tests (blood test)	In direct (searching for antigen), a fluorescent-labeled antibody is mixed with sample of blood. If antigen is present, it binds with antibody and can be detected with ultraviolet light microscope. Indirect test (searching for antibody), known antigen is mixed with blood sample, and then fluorescein antiimmunoglobulin antibodies are mixed in. If a fluorescein-bound antibody-antigen complex is seen, no antibodies were present and so there was no exposure to that antigen (supposedly, unless immune system is compromised or defective).	*Two tests of this type have significance for maternity clients:* fluorescent treponemal antibody (FTA-ABS) test for syphilis exposure and IFA test for toxoplasmosis. (See Chapter 27 regarding care of pregnant women with these infections.) If congenital syphilis of infant is suspected or confirmed, isolation techniques should be instituted for care of infant until such time that she or he is adjudged noncontagious on basis of drug therapy specific to the spirochete.
Sedimentation (erythrocyte) rate (blood test)	During acute systemic inflammatory process, erythrocytes gain in density and therefore fall or settle more rapidly when placed in test tube with anticoagulant. The more quickly cells settle, the more acute and active inflammatory process is said to be.	Change in rate of sedimentation should signal need to reevaluate those limitations placed on client. (This is not a reliable test during pregnancy when sedimentation rate is normally elevated.)
White blood cell (WBC) count and differential	Total count of white blood cells indicates number of leukocytes circulating in serum. An increase is expected during infectious and inflammatory processes. Decreases are associated with certain diseases or certain therapies (antineoplastic drugs or radiation). Differences in the percentages of the various types of leukocytes are associated with activation of or disturbances in the immune responsiveness specific to the role of the type of WBC that is altered (see Table 5.9).	Client with increased levels, indicating active immune response, needs supportive care (adequate rest, fluids, and nutrition) to successfully fight invading organisms. Client with decreased levels or with a number of immature WBCs (on differential assessment) would need protective care, since resistance level (immune responsivity) would be low, and thus client would be prone to overwhelming infection(s). At times, protective or reverse isolation must be practiced, along with blood transfusions and passive artificial immunity therapy. If a client with leukopenia is on drug therapy for any condition, nurse must check to be sure that drug therapy does not coincidentally further deplete number of WBCs (by depressing bone marrow function) as side effect; if it does, conference with physician is indicated for alternate drug therapy or supportive therapy to restore client's immune responsiveness. NOTE: Some elevation of WBCs in pregnancy (up to 16,000/mm^3) and during labor and early postpartal period (up to 25,000/mm^3) is normal. Neonates are expected to have high levels of WBCs (18,000-40,000) during first few weeks of extrauterine life. As in children (up to about age 8), lymphocytes in infants become more prevalent than neutrophils. This is probably because

Continued.

Table 5.12, cont'd
Using Laboratory Test Data Regarding Activated Immune Defense System to Determine Approach to Health Care

Test Performed	Purpose of Test	Nursing Care Implications
		of activity of thymus gland in infancy and early childhood.
		An increase in number of neutrophils is considered a healthy response to invasion, indicating intact and well-functioning immune system.
		If eosinophil content is increased, nurse should assist in assessment of sources of allergy or possible parasitic infestation.
		If lymphocyte count is decreased or if the subpopulations of T helper and T suppressor cells are reversed, client has compromised or deficient immune responsiveness and is in need of protective, supportive care.

quired natural immunity of IgG antibodies via placental transfer that confer resistance to those specific antigens against which the maternal antibodies were developed (Table 5.10). The preterm infant may be deficient in this type of immunity, especially if born before week 36 of gestation. The breast-fed infant who receives colostrum will have additional naturally acquired passive protection of IgA antibodies from the mother.

The neonate is capable of leukocyte activity and will develop IgM antibodies as the initial humoral response to exposure to an antigenic bacteria or virus. The fetus is capable of forming IgM antibodies in response to an intrauterine infection (see Table 5.12, immunoelectrophoresis tests). IgA antibodies produced by the infant (in the process of active natural immune responsiveness) are apparent in mucous membranes, secretions, and tears within a few months after birth.

Theorists have offered immunologic explanations about diseases (e.g., rheumatoid arthritis and adult-onset diabetes mellitus) that generally propose that the body's defense system has been overwhelmed or exhausted after operating efficiently for so many years. This model offers a "compensation, then decompensation," entropic view of physiology rather than the continually compensating, negentropic view* that is characteristic of a systems theory orientation. Some researchers argue that there is a kind of "programming" for dysfunction of the immune system, established and detectable early in life, but more manifest among the elderly. The fact that the thymus gland begins to atrophy after puberty can be used to support this hypothesis.

Negentropy is a systems theory term for negative entropy, which indicates that instead of deteriorating a system increases in complexity over time.

Environment. The environment of each person is significant in determining the challenges posed to one's immune system. The various component factors of one's environment—for example, the quality of air, water, and food, the ventilation, refrigeration, crowding, and cleanliness in the setting—contribute to the risks that a person encounters from nonself microorganisms and substances. With the infectious diseases of tuberculosis and toxoplasmosis, one can readily appreciate the influence of environment in acquisition and transmission. Not every person is exposed to the tubercle bacillus or to the parasite that causes toxoplasmosis. However, if one lives in a setting in which the tubercle bacillus is endemic (e.g., an urban, overcrowded area with poor ventilation), then the risks of exposure are much greater. The cat owner whose pet harbors the toxoplasmosis parasite is at increased risk of acquiring the disease, especially if the person has contact with the cat's feces (i.e., through emptying the litter pan). Although the exact mode of transmission of the parasite from animal to man is not known, it is recognized that the infection can be transmitted from mother to fetus via placental transfer.

The environment of the newborn in a hospital setting is a factor over which a nurse can exert some control to effect fewer challenges to the neonate's immune defense system. Persons who harbor infectious diseases should be barred from the nursery, and the medical aseptic technique employed in the nursery environment should be meticulous (Chapter 20). This is not to suggest that the normal newborn should be provided with a sterile environment but that there is no reason to overtax a relatively meager set of immune defense mechanisms. An overwhelming systemic infection, such as that caused by herpes virus in the neonate, can not only interfere with healthy growth and development of the parent-child relationship because of prolonged separation but also threaten the newborn's life. For this reason the environment into which a fetus will be born must be assessed for its risk potential in posing harm to the newborn. For example, genital herpes infecting a parturient must be identified as quickly as possible so that exposure of the neonate to the virus in the infected birth canal can be avoided by cesarean delivery.

Nutritional status. The notion of environment as a factor in immune responsiveness can also be applied to the internal environment of a person. The adequacy of the diet consumed contributes to the supportive mechanisms of the body that enhance resistance factors to invading organisms and substances. For example, a diet sufficient in protein maintains the correct osmotic fluid pressure in the blood, sustaining the adequate hydration of the body's tissues. Nutritional intake adequate with regard to vitamins, minerals, fluid, and the basic four food groups is supportive of an intact, functionally competent immune defense system. According to various sources of nutritional science the body retains the ability to make immunoglobulins even if the dietary patterns are low in daily consumption of protein and calories, but the synthesis of the proteins that comprise the complement (and are responsible for the complement cascade) are more sensitive to malnourishment and especially protein deficits. It is hypothesized by these sources that nutritional deficiency states also negatively affect the production of interferon and T lymphocytes. Furthermore, the health of lymphoid tissue has been associated with the adequacy of zinc intake.

Although the infant's diet is less varied, frequently consisting of nothing but breast milk for the first several months of life, it is supportive of the body's immune defense system in that breast milk favors the growth of the *Lactobacillus bifidus* in the infant's intestinal tract. This microorganism converts lactose (milk sugar) into lactic acid, which diminishes the growth of pathogenic organisms in the intestine. Also, breast milk provides the necessary amounts of protein, calories, and essential minerals (such as zinc) for healthy functioning of the immune system (Chapter 21).

Life-style. Certain infectious diseases are associated with the patterns of living that people establish for themselves. For instance, the sexually transmitted diseases of syphilis and gonorrhea are more likely to be acquired by those people who have promiscuous sexual contact, and the recently identified problem known as acquired immune deficiency syndrome (AIDS) has been associated primarily with, or has been traced to, people who have had frequent casual homosexual encounters.

Many other aspects comprise the concept of *life-style* besides sexual preference patterns and sexual behavior. These factors include the numerous health behaviors that people practice—such as their patterns of rest, exercise, food and drug intake, relaxation, work performance, selfcare, and use of health care professionals. It is important for the nurse to carefully assess the numerous details about clients' life-styles because these factors affect the clients' susceptibility to invasion by nonself substances. For instance, a pattern of heavy alcohol consumption is associated with certain nutritional deficiencies (notably the B vitamin complex) that decrease the individual's immune responsiveness to vaccines and depress the cell-mediated and humoral lymphocytic activity (Whitney and Cataldo, 1983). Individual's who assume responsibility for their health and who practice health maintenance and preventive strategies (as acquiring artificial active immunity) are more likely to enjoy a competent immune defense system.

Health problems associated with compromised or deficient immune system responsiveness. Four different types of health problems are associated with compromised or deficient immune systems (Table 5.13): (1) acquired immune deficiency syndrome (AIDS), (2) severe combined immunodeficiency disease (SCID), (3) intentionally induced immunosuppression secondary to transplant surgery or treatment, and (4) unintentionally induced immunosuppression secondary to the sequelae accompanying antineoplastic drug or radiation therapy. Table 5.13 distinguishes between those problems that have been contracted directly (actively) or indirectly (passively). All four types create problems of lowered resistance to invasive agents and therefore of increased susceptibility to infections. The types of infection and other problems to which the afflicted clients are prone differ somewhat. These differences are identified in the table.

Other types of diseases that have been associated with immune process, such as rheumatoid arthritis and systemic lupus erythematosus, are not within the scope of this text and so are not discussed at this time. Although some theorists have considered the problem of pregnancy-induced hypertension (PIH) (preeclampsia-eclampsia) to be associated with autoimmunity, there is insufficient evidence to support this theory.

Principles of nursing care for the client with compromised immune responsiveness. When clients have any degree of compromised immune responsiveness, the nurse must take steps to ensure their protection from sources of infection in the hospital and the home environment. Scrupulous attention must be given to practicing medical asepsis by all caregivers who come in contact with the client to prevent superimposed iatrogenic nosocomial infections. In some cases reverse or

Table 5.13
Examples of Four Types of Immunodeficiency Problems

Active (Direct Transmission)	Passive (Indirect Transmission)
Naturally acquired	
EXAMPLE: acquired immune deficiency syndrome (AIDS) via exposure to antigen through direct sexual contact.* *Immunologic symptoms:* there is a normal humoral type of immunity (because this disease characteristically afflicts people after they have had a functionally effective immune system) but reversal of subpopulation of T cells—ratio of T helper to T suppressor cells is reversed. Thus the cell-mediated immune system is not triggered and B lymphocytes and complement cascade are not activated. *Prone* to unusual or rare problems such as Kaposi's sarcoma and opportunistic infections as *Pneumocystis carinii* pneumonia (PCP). it must be remembered that immunity to common microorganisms is developed and that circulating humoral antibodies continue to provide protection from those common invaders. *Treatment:* no therapy has been effective in curing or reversing pathophysiology to date.	EXAMPLE: severe combined immunodeficiency disease (SCID), acquired via heredity either by autosomal-recessive transmission or by sex-linked transmission (X-linked lymphopenic agammaglobulinemia).† *Symptoms:* impaired or absent humoral and cell-mediated immune defense mechanisms. *Prone* to continual bouts of infection with "ordinary" type of microorganisms. SCID manifests itself shortly after birth, when influence of the mother's passively transmitted IgG (via placenta) and IgA (via colostrum) antibodies wear off. *Treatment:* IgG injections, reverse isolation (one child literally existed within a series of sterile "bubble" compartments until 2 weeks before he died at age 12), and bone marrow transplants (frequently not successful; usual problem is graft vs. host rejection).
Artificially acquired (iatrogenic)	
EXAMPLE: intentionally induced immunosuppression that occurs secondary to treatment with certain drugs (e.g., corticosteroids, azathioprine [Imuran], and cyclosporin) to decrease T cell activation and consequent rejection of transplanted foreign protein tissue (allografts). Recently kidneys, hearts, and livers have been transplanted (e.g., cases in which infant is born with biliary atresia). Success of this kind of surgery has been possible only with adjunct therapy of immunosuppression, which prevents rejection of donor cells by recipient cells. *Problems:* client needs protective, supportive nursing care and gradual withdrawal from immunosuppressive agent. Compounding problems experienced by these clients, in addition to pain and fear associated with surgery, are untoward side effects associated with immunosuppressive drug therapy. These include hypersensitivity, anemia, thrombocytopenia, alopecia, steatorrhea, and lesions of the mouth (with azathioprine); and hirsutism, edema, and hyperglycemia (with corticosteroids).	EXAMPLE 1: unintentionally induced immunosuppression that occurs secondary to antineoplastic therapy with radiation or to certain chemotherapeutic drugs that depress bone marrow function. Antineoplastic therapy frequently affects rapidly proliferating bone marrow cells as well as cancer cells for which therapy is given. White blood cells are thereby depressed and unable to engage in phagocytosis. T cell–mediated immunity and, missing cell-mediated type, humoral type are not triggered, nor is complement cascade, CONDITION EXAMPLE: maternity client with treated choriocarcinoma. *Treatment:* supportive and replacement therapy (with blood products), as well as citrovorum (Leucovorin) calcium therapy, a form of folic acid that if given within 1 hour of methotrexate protects bone marrow against destructive effects of chemotherapy. *Problems:* compounding problems experienced by these clients, in addition to dread of cancer therapy (in some cases) and fear of prognosis of cancer diagnosis, are multiple side effects associated with antineoplastic therapy. These may include allergic reactions, depressed clotting factors, abnormal liver function, anemia, nausea and vomiting, alopecia, heart muscle toxicity, and stomatitis. Added to this list are those problems associated with common, rare, and opportunistic infections. EXAMPLE 2: AIDS acquired through acceptance of blood or blood products from an AIDS-afflicted client. Hemophiliacs are especially prone to acquisition of AIDS via this mechanism.

*Since AIDS is transmitted directly through sexual contact as well as indirectly through blood products, the disease is presented here in two different places in the typologic schema
†See Whaley, L.F., and Wong, D.L.: Nursing care of infants and children, ed. 3, St. Louis, 1987, The C.V. Mosby Co.

protective isolation should be instituted to further protect the client.

To devise an individualized plan the nurse assesses for factors that place a person at risk, such as the client's age, overall health status, environment, and life-style. The client requires supportive therapy to maintain good fluid and nutritional status and to

maintain the integrity of this first-line defense mechanism. In some situations the client is further protected with passive immunity support via IgG antibody injections. Those clients who have a poor prognosis (as those with AIDS and SCID) and their families also need supportive psychosocial care and opportunities to discuss and design their future.

Relationship between allergic and immunologic phenomena. An allergen is a foreign substance that induces or generates an allergic reaction in the body. That reaction can be mild (manifested as erythema, local swelling, and pruritis), moderate, or severe (manifested as anaphylaxis, with shock and constricted bronchioles leading to oxygen deficit and even death). The allergic reaction is caused by the histamine released from mast cells by the action of IgE humoral antibodies.

The IgE antibodies, developed from B lymphocytes, are formed as a sensitivity response to certain allergens in the environment. Upon repeated exposure to those allergens, the IgE antibody specific to that foreign substance binds with it and causes the rupture and consequent degranulation of the mast cell. The histamine so released produces peripheral vasodilation, causing local flushing, decrease in blood pressure, and capillary distention (which encourages the movement of intravascular fluid into the interstitial spaces, resulting in edema). It also constricts the smooth muscle of the bronchi, compromising the exchange of oxygen and carbon dioxide in the body.

Although antihistamines have a role to play in the treatment of mild allergic phenomena, they cannot be effective in situations of severe manifestations of allergy (as anaphylaxis). In these cases epinephrine (Adrenalin) is the drug of choice (by injection) to reverse the pathophysiologic condition by dilating the bronchi, by constricting the blood vessels (causing an increase in blood pressure), and by increasing the rate and strength of the heartbeat (and therefore the circulation of oxygen through the body).

The desensitization process—by which minute amounts of the allergen are gradually introduced into the client's system (increasing the exposure, but in amounts that are too small to produce allergic symptoms)—is technically an immunologic treatment aimed at assisting the body to become immune to the allergen by developing IgM antibodies specific to the substance.

Some clients have developed a sensitivity to certain foods, soaps, or drugs as allergens. Although it should be standard procedure for the nurse to assess all clients for sensitivity to foreign foods and substances (including adhesive tape), occasionally the nurse is involved in producing an inadvertent allergic reaction in a client. Such an incident may even occur while the nurse is administering a protective immunization to a client (as the rubella vaccine), since the vaccine is derived from duck egg or human (foreign protein) culture.

It is essential that nurses appreciate the complex operation of the immune system and that they fully understand how to (1) support the healthy defense mechanisms of clients, (2) protect those clients whose immune responsiveness is impaired, and (3) avoid the unintentional stimulation of potentially dangerous (allergic) defense mechanisms.

Summary

Basic knowledge about the female and male reproductive systems is a prerequisite to understanding the process of conception. A systematic investigation of the human reproductive system provides the maternity nurse with a firm foundation for gaining insight into the client's needs and health concerns. The nurse has been provided with information on the similarities and differences of the female and male reproductive organs, growth and development patterns, and human sexual response. Immunology was presented in considerable depth because of its important role in life processes.

References

American Public Health Association: Control of communicable diseases in man: an official report, Washington, D.C., 1981, The Association.

Bustillo, M., and others: Nonsurgical ovum transfer as a treatment of infertile women, J.A.M.A. 251:1171, 1984.

Hite, S.: The Hite report: nationwide study of female sexuality, New York, 1976, Dell Publishing Co.

Kaplan, H.S.: The new sex therapy, New York, 1974, Brunner/Mazel.

Korones, S.F.: High-risk newborn infants: the basis for intensive nursing care, ed. 4, St. Louis, 1985, The C.V. Mosby Co.

Masters, W.H., and Johnson, V.E.: Human sexual response, 1966, Little, Brown & Co.

The T cell receptor: at hand at last, Science 221:444, 1983.

Whaley, L.F., and Wong, D.L.: Nursing care of infants and children, ed. 3, St. Louis, 1987, The C.V. Mosby Co.

Whitney, E.N., and Cataldo, C.B.: Understanding normal and clinical nutrition, New York, 1983, West Publishing Co.

Bibliography

Anthony, C.P., and Thibodeau, G.A.: Textbook of anatomy and physiology, ed. 11, St. Louis, 1983, The C.V. Mosby Co.

Bachmann, G.A.: Menses topics: evaluating menstrual hygiene devices, Contemp. OB/Gyn. 24(5):71, 1984.

Brandeis, V.T., and Bernstein, S.: Menses topics: measuring your patient's menstrual flow, Contemp. OB/Gyn. 25(1):87, 1985.

Brown, M.A., and Woods, N.F.: Correlates of dysmenorrhea: a challenge to past stereotypes, J.O.G.N. Nurs. 13(4):259, 1984.

Can AIDS be a threat to your patient? Contemp. OB/Gyn. 23:163, 1984.

Church, J., and others: IgG subclass deficiencies in children with suspected AIDS, Lancet 1:279, Feb. 4, 1984.

Coyne, C.M., and others: Premenstrual tension syndrome. J.O.G.N. Nurs. 14(6):446, 1985.

Curran, J.W., and others: Acquired immunodeficiency syndrome (AIDS) associated with transfusions, N. Engl. J. Med. 310:69, 1984.

Danforth, D., and others, editors: Obstetrics and gynecology, ed. 4, New York, 1982, Harper & Row, Publishers.

Dawood, M.Y.: Adolescence: an update on dysmenorrhea, Contemp. OB/Gyn. 23(6):73, 1984.

Delaney, J., and others: The curse: a cultural history of menstruation, New York, 1976, New American Library.

Dowdle, W.R.: The epidemiology of AIDS, Public Health Rep. 98:308, 1983.

Fogel, C.I., and Woods, N.F.: Health care of women: a nursing perspective, St. Louis, 1981, The C.V. Mosby Co.

Guyton, A.C.: Textbook of medical physiology, ed. 7, Philadelphia, 1986, W.B. Saunders Co.

Johnson, S.R.: Menses optics: TSS—don't overlook less obvious cases, Contemp. OB/Gyn. 25(6):131, 1985.

Kaiser, H.B.: Allergy and immunology: new discoveries, new treatments, better results, Contemp. OB/Gyn. 21:90 (special issue), May 1983.

Lein, A.: The cycling female: her menstrual rhythm, San Francisco, 1979, W.H. Freeman and Co.

MacVicar, M.G., and others: What do we know about the effects of sports training on the menstrual cycle? M.C.N. 7(1):55, 1982.

Malasanos, L., Barkauskas, V., Moss, M., and Stoltenberg-Ollen, K.: Health assessment, ed. 3, St. Louis, 1985, The C.V. Mosby Co.

Mead, P.B.: Symposium: AIDS in mothers and babies, Contemp. OB/Gyn. 26:126 (special issue), 1985.

Moore, K.L.: The developing human, ed. 2, Philadelphia, 1977, W.B. Saunders Co.

Moore, K.L.: Before we are born: basic embryology and birth defects (revised reprint), Philadelphia, 1977, W.B. Saunders Co.

Office of Public Affairs, U.S. Public Health Service: AIDS information bulletin, Washington, D.C., Jan. 19, 1983, U.S. Government Printing Office.

Orque, M.D., Bloch, B., and Monrroy, L.S.: Ethnic nursing care: a multicultural approach, St. Louis, 1983, The C.V. Mosby Co.

Pritchard, J.A., and others: Williams obstetrics, ed. 17, Norwalk, Conn., 1985, Appleton-Century-Crofts.

Ryan, K.J.: Interpreting the controls of the menstrual cycle, Contemp. OB/Gyn. 26(3):107, 1985.

Scully, D., and Bart, P.: A funny thing happened on the way to the orifice: women in gynecology textbooks, Am. J. Soc. 78:1045, 1973.

Shangold, M.M.: Menses topics: factors affecting menstrual flow, Contemp. OB/Gyn. 25(4):73, 1985.

Shangold, M.M., and Levine, H.S.: The effect of marathon training upon menstrual function, Am. J. Obstet. Gynecol. 143(8):862, 1982.

Whitley, N.: A manual of clinical obstetrics, Philadelphia, 1985, J.B. Lippincott Co.

Willson, J.R., Carrington, E.R., and Ledger, W.J.: Obstetrics and gynecology, ed. 7, St. Louis, 1983, The C.V. Mosby Co.

Woods, N.F.: Relationship of socialization and stress to perimenstrual symptoms, disability, and menstrual attitudes, Nurs. Res. 34(3):145, 1985.

Youngs, D.D., and Works-Lind, M.: Counseling: practical strategies for managing PMS, Contemp. OB/Gyn. 26(4):111, 1985.

Psychosocial Nature of Human Sexuality

A holistic approach to sexual development takes into account the psychosocial nature of human sexuality as well as the biologic nature. These spheres are interdependent and involve processes that progress in an orderly manner to the ultimate physical and psychologic maturity of an individual. The purpose of this chapter is to trace the psychosocial development of sexuality from birth through adulthood. A brief description of cognitive development as proposed by Piaget is included in the presentation. Intellectual response is a critical factor in developing a socially responsible use of sexual potential. As a person's sense of sexual identity is influenced by mastery of psychologic developmental tasks, Erikson's stages of personality development are presented. Social forces that strengthen the concepts of maleness or femaleness are reviewed. The review begins with gender identity in the young child and progresses through the life cycle. Family members are the first significant others in the child's sexual, cognitive, and personality development. As the child matures and ventures into the wider world, peer, educational, and other social groups provide environments that may promote or retard development.

Definitions

Cognition. Cognition is the process by which people recognize, accumulate, and organize the knowledge of their world and use this knowledge to solve problems and change behavior. We will use a young woman for an example. The process begins when she *perceives* or recognizes an event as a problem. She then searches her *memory* to see if the problem is similar to any past experience. Next she *generates ideas* as to a possible solution. Finally she *evaluates* the accuracy of the choice. Obviously the richer the source of ideas, concepts, and past experiences used in successful resolution of problems, the greater the odds for success in resolving current difficulties. Both innate intellectual ability and the quality of the environment are decisive factors in cognitive development.

Personality. Personality is a complex of characteristics that distinguishes a particular individual in his or her relationships with others. It includes emergent tendencies to act and to interact and thereby influence the individual's environment.

Sexuality. Sexual identity begins at conception. At that time, through the chance combination of an ovum and a sperm, a person's biologic sex is determined. Thereafter, intrauterine and extrauterine environmental influences play their part in the realization of each person's sexual potential.

Sexuality pervades the whole of a person's life; it is more than a sum of isolated physical acts. It is a purposeful force in human nature, observable in everyday life in endless variations. It may find expression in the love of parent for child and child for parent, of friend for friend, or a woman for man and man for woman. It can be the source of pleasure or pain, fulfillment or deprivation, and sharing or exploitation. Recognition of the power of such drives has prompted each culture throughout history to develop social codes, religious dogmas, or legal restraints. These help to delineate the sex role models and patterns to be followed in the process of achieving adult sexuality.

Cognitive Development

Piaget (1950), a Swiss scientist, developed theories about how adult thought develops. He contends that two mental activities, *organization* and *adaptation*, continue throughout life. Adaptation derives from two complementary processes: *assimilation,* the absorption of new information interpreted in terms of existing structures, and *accommodation,* the changing of existing

Table 6.1
Summary of Cognitive and Personality Development

Stage	Significant Others	Cognitive Development (Piaget)	Personality Development (Erikson)
Infancy (birth to toddler-hood)	Maternal person	Sensorimotor: reflex → repetition → imitation	Trust vs. mistrust
	+		
Early childhood (2-7 y)	Parental persons and other family members	Preoperational, direct experience (seeing, hearing, feeling) within a well-defined world	Initiative vs. guilt
	+		
Middle childhood (7-12 y)	Neighborhood and school	Concrete thinking (not abstract), humanized (limited inductive reasoning)	Industry vs. inferiority
	+		
Adolescence (12-18 y)	Peer groups and models of leadership	Formal thinking (deductive and abstract reasoning) may be limited up to 15 y	Identity vs. identity confusion
	+		
Early adulthood	Partners in friendship, sex, competition, and cooperation	Formal thinking includes problem solving and separation of fantasy and fact	Intimacy and solidarity vs. isolation
	+		
Young and middle adult-hood	Divided labor and shared household	Formal thinking includes problem solving and separation of fantasy and fact	Generativity vs. self-absorption
	+		
Later adulthood	Humankind, family, and friends	Formal thinking includes problem solving and separation of fantasy and fact	Ego integrity vs.despair

structure to fit new information. According to Piaget, cognitive development progresses in an orderly and sequential manner through four stages. The process is one of gradual evolution, with each stage building on the specific attainments of the previous one. Table 6.1 summarizes cognitive and personality development across the life span.

Sensorimotor stage (birth to 2 years). Reflex activity dominates the beginning of the sensorimotor stage. It gives way to repetitive and finally to imitative behavior. Any problem solving is the result of trial and error, but a sense of "what causes what" begins to emerge. Discovery can be exciting as a child becomes aware of his or her own body as well as other familiar objects. Language begins in a limited fashion, mostly single or double words such as "mine" or "me too." By the end of this period an object can exist without being present (object permanence). As a result, hide-and-seek is no longer frightening but has become a pleasurable game.

Preoperational stage (2 to 7 years). During the preoperational stage children are extremely self-centered or egocentric. As Whaley and Wong (1987) express it, "they are unable to see things from any perspective other than their own; they cannot see

another's point of view, nor can they see any reason to do so." They live in a well-defined world made up of what they see, hear, or otherwise experience. Their thought processes are immature. Characteristically, children are "centered" in that they see one aspect of a situation but are unable to take any other factors into account. They are unaware of the transition process between one static state (the beginning) and another static state (the end). In problem solving adults often retrace their steps to see if their thinking has been logical; they are able to see similarity in apparently dissimilar objects by reversing their properties. By contrast, children see what they see. Gradually their language becomes more complex, and single words progress to phrases and then to sentences. Children grow dramatically through direct experience and an increasing ability to use symbolic communication. Behavior appears to assume *cyclic trends* of equilibrium and disequilibrium.

Concrete operations stage (7 to 12 years). The concrete operations stage is characterized by a gradual increase in problem-solving ability. The method of reasoning used is inductive. Solutions to problems are not based on abstractions but are derived from what has been perceived and categorized. The "social self" appears. Children are no longer exclusively egocentric but can relate to the feelings and thoughts of others.

Formal operations stage (12 to 18 years). Progress through the formal operations stage may be erratic and difficult for the adolescent. By the end of this stage, successful people can consider hypotheses and analyze scientifically. They can deduce conclusions from a set of observations, consider alternatives, and assess risks. In short, they are capable of reasoning logically by using abstractions and of assuming responsibility for the actions taken as solutions to their problems. Piaget notes that formal thinking involves two major dimensions: the use of propositional logic (the ability to think about a problem and thus rearrange aspects of it until it becomes clear) and the ability to separate fantasy from fact.

Personality Development

Erikson (1959) proposed a theory of personality development that defines the process in stages. Each stage focuses on a central conflict and is dependent on the one before it. These problems are envisioned as conflicts between opposites; for example, trust versus mistrust. As each conflict is resolved or mastered to a greater or lesser degree, the individual is ready to move on to the next level. Unresolved conflicts can hamper a person's further development and may persist in residual form throughout life. (See Table 6.1.)

Trust versus mistrust (birth to 1 year). Basic trust develops as a response to being loved and cared for by a giving, and concerned adult. The period from birth to 1 year is a time of "taking in" for the infant, who needs nurturing, security, and a feeling of continuity to develop trust. If such cares makes up the bulk of the infant's experiences, trust takes precedence over mistrust. Successful completion of this stage results in a sense of trust in the child's responses to others throughout life.

Autonomy versus shame and doubt (1 to 3 years). A sense of autonomy develops with the gradual unfolding of the child's control of body, self, and people in the immediate environment. If those who provide care applaud the child's efforts toward self-control and increasing motor skills, autonomy will result. Conversely, feelings of self-doubt and shame can occur if the child experiences frequent failures and frustrations.

Initiative versus guilt (3 to 6 years). The stage of initiative versus guilt ushers in an active exploratory phase in children's development. They learn much from their world by playing games and asking endless questions. They show more evidence of being guided by an inner conscience: the "parent" has been increasingly internalized. This is a time for fears and phobias. Children's developmental tasks revolve around directing their efforts toward purposeful activity and achieving a balance between *daring* and *caution*.

Industry versus inferiority (6 to 12 years). During the period of industry versus inferiority, children develop a sense of being a productive worker. They need opportunities to complete activities and be rewarded for their efforts. Introduction to formal schooling takes place now, and success or failure in this respect can set the stage for later career choice.

Identity versus identity confusion (12 to 18 years). The period of adolescence comes after a period of relative calm. During this time of transition between childhood and adulthood, adolescents have certain tasks to perform: they must establish sexual roles, select an occupation, become independent of the family, and develop a social rather than egocentric response to people and the wider society. The adolescent must accept a new body image that includes the ability to reproduce. Successful mastery of these tasks helps adolescents develop a sense of self and identity that both they and society can accept. With this sense comes the ability for devotion and fidelity. Without it people know not "who they are" or "where they are going," and identity confusion persists.

Intimacy versus isolation (early adulthood). Once people have sense of identity, they can move toward intimate relationships with others. This can be expressed on a personal level as friendship, sexual intimacy, or the intimacy of parent–child relationships. On a social level love of fellow humans is expressed in concern for the welfare of others. Without this sense of freedom to love and be loved, people are isolated and may develop a sense of alienation from family, friends, and society.

Generativity versus self-absorption (young and middle adulthood). During the period of generativity versus self-absorption, people are concerned with creating the next generation and providing the necessary nurturing and caretaking. The tasks in this stage include preparation for assuming the role of parent, participating in the birth of children, and adapting to the reality of parenthood. Some people may become substitute parents in myriad ways: adopting children, being friends to adolescents, teaching, or nursing. Self-absorption, is minimized when involvement of the self with others takes place. Growth of the personality as a person seeks balance between commitment to self and commitment to others leads to a sense of productiveness and fulfillment.

Ego integrity versus despair (late adulthood). Staying productive and involved in the welfare of others increases the satisfaction of elderly people. (In the

United States old age arbitrarily begins at 65 years.) In most cases an elderly person's physical and mental abilities gradually decline, imposing limitations and curtailing his or her sphere of activity. As people confronted the limitations, they must balance acceptance against despair. Wisdom and a sense of satisfaction in their accomplishments come to those who succeed in the search for personal meaning.

Development of Sexuality

We are born into a sexually oriented world, and from birth onward we assume socially defined sexual roles that reflect the basic pattern prescribed by the society. These roles are learned informally through being part of a social group. Development of a concept of sexual roles and sexual identity begins at an early age and continues as a series of developmental tasks throughout a person's life span.

Infancy and childhood. One of the first questions parents ask when their child is born is "Is it a boy or a girl?" The answer sets in motion a series of social influences that will be reflected in the child's concept of "who I am" and "what I can do." The tasks relative to forming a sexual identity include developing core gender identity, acquiring prescribed sex role standards, identifying with the parent of the same sex, and establishing gender preference.

Core gender identity. Core gender identity is the earliest and most stable form of gender identity. By 2 years of age children can differentiate between boys and girls through awareness of dissimilarities in hair and clothing and some awareness of anatomic differences. Core gender identity is developed in normal children by the time they have reached 3 or 4 years of age.

Efforts to determine the importance of biologic versus environmental contributions to a person's gender identity have generated much controversy and research. Some studies indicate certain different biologic responses in male and female newborns and suggest differences in the infants' responses to the environment and readiness for various learning experiences. Other studies reveal the importance of gender labeling on the eventual acceptance of gender identity. Infants whose sex was uncertain at birth accepted the sex role assigned by their parents and identified with that role (Maccoby, 1966).

From the child's perspective, knowing oneself as either a boy or a girl begins before full realization of the implications of sexual identity. The infant establishes his or her gender identity from interactions with the parents. It is largely accomplished by acceptance of parental labeling; for example, "Be a good boy," "That's my girl," and "That is my big boy."

Communication, verbal or nonverbal, provides the child with cues about the sex-appropriateness of his or her behavior. A sense of trust in sexual identity develops through the early reaffirmations of maleness or femaleness.

Sex role standards. The term *sex role standards* refers to the various behaviors, attitudes, and attributes that differentiate the roles. Even 2-year-olds are exposed to this conditioning, because parents choose for them the kinds of clothing, toys, and activities that reflect the parents' expectations of sex role standards.

The child learns by observing the behavior of mothers, fathers, brothers, and sisters. The child formulates a concept of who should perform what tasks, who provides the comforting, who provides the active play, and who is nurturing when there is sickness. The feelings children develop about themselves as people in general and as sexual people in particular are directly related to their experiences with their bodies and the attitudes and values they derive from many sources. One of the most important ways children learn about their bodies is through exploratory sexual behavior (sex play). Sex play is defined by Kinsey and co-workers (1948, 1953) as "actual genital play." Four categories of sex play are listed as follows:

1. Self-exploration and self-manipulation: most common forms of sex play. Fondling of penis and manual stimulation of the clitoris are most common. Infants begin the process of exploring their bodies even by 2 to 3 months of age. As they grow they discover they are able to experience sexual pleasure through self-stimulation. Parents who feel masturbation is harmful will rebuke even young children and forbid them "to play with themselves."

2. Same-sex comparisons: comparison of size and shape. Prepubescent homosexual behaviors do not necessarily lead to adult homosexuality. Children need reassurance that their genitals are similar to others.

3. Coital play: when a boy lies on top of a girl. The activities are largely experimental, imitative, and exploratory. Children become aware of parental sleeping arrangements, bathing, and privacy. They begin differentiating sex role behaviors and will play at being Mommy and Daddy.

4. Exhibitionism: showing and handling genitals in public, especially in the presence of companions. Most children engage in sex play activities only sporadically, especially when these activities are ignored by adults. For example, one out of four boys who had engaged in sex play had done so only during one year, and some had participated in such play only once before puberty (Kinsey and co-workers, 1948). Kinsey and

co-workers (1948, 1953) found that 9 years of age was the peak age for girls, when 14% engaged in some form of sex play. For boys the peak was 12 years of age, when 38% were similarly involved.

During early childhood (2 to 7 years) children are vulnerable to shaming experiences. Parents often use the sense of shame or guilt to encourage children to limit acting out sexually to appropriate places. Children need to be encouraged to develop self-control without loss of self-esteem or the feeling that sexual activity is sinful. During middle childhood the child interacts more freely outside the family. Biologic drives are less pronounced as the child strives for body competence and mastery. Sex role mastery centers on competitiveness, such as "being the fastest runner," or "throwing the ball farther than anyone else."

In Western society the adjectives used to describe a female predominantly express a mothering capacity, that is, "gentle, loving, submissive, patient, warm, and concerned." These qualities suit a person whose central reason for being is assumed to be the care and nurturing of the young and, by extension, anyone who needs such care. Those adjectives used to describe the male, namely, "dominant, aggressive, impatient, objective, and ambitious," portray a person capable of independent, decisive action. These are seen as the qualities needed in the marketplace and the basis for career orientation.

In reality, people of both sexes possess these qualities in common. Some personalities lean more toward the socially defined concept of either male or female; others have no clear demarcation of roles. These latter people, termed *androgynous personalities,* use those qualities most needed at the moment without feeling guilty about usurping another's role. A male nursing student made the following comment during a discussion of mothering:

It is not a case of one or the other, it is what the time calls forth. The most nurturing behavior of "mothering," if you want to call it that, that I've ever seen was in Vietnam when a man was trying to get a wounded friend out of range of fire. He protected him, covering him with his own body, gave him his food and water. No mother could have shown more devotion.

A common way children prepare for a future parenting role is through sibling caretaking. Older children from either the nuclear or extended family care for younger children. Older children are used to provide role flexibility for mothers and for the development of caretaking skills by children. Stereotyped sex roles, so important in many cultures, are maintained when children assume child care responsibilities for younger family members (Weisner and Gallimore, 1977).

Identification with parent of same sex. As a child comes to identify with the parent of the same sex the child internalizes the values, attitudes, and ideals of that parent. The exact method by which the process of identification is accomplished is not yet known. The child does perceive physical and psychologic similarities and is told about similarities by others. Adoption of the same-sex parent's behavior may be motivated by fear of loss of the love of this important person or by awareness of that person's power to control rewards. For a girl to forgo identification with her father, she must love her mother sufficiently to form a positive identification with her. A boy needs to relinquish his early identification with his mother and form a strong commitment to his father.

Gender preference. Gender preference implies not only a knowledge of one's gender and the appropriate sex role but also a liking for it. Development of gender preference involves three main elements: (1) success in the role, (2) liking the same-sex parent, and (3) reinforcement from family, ethnic group, and social institutions as to the value of the role (Newman and Newman, 1975). As with other attitudes, fluctuations in preference can and do occur as people face situations in which one sex role either enhances or hinders personal goals. Deep-seated sex preferences on the part of parents can affect initial parent-child relationships if the child is not of the preferred sex. The parenting lag that results can last a day or a lifetime, depending on whether the parent succeeds or fails in resolving conflicting emotions. Certain ethnic groups have welcoming rituals for one sex and not for the other. These seemingly innocuous societal and personal preferences eventually lead a person to make value judgments about the worthiness of his or her sex. As a result the individual's self-esteem is either increased or diminished.

Implications for nursing. A knowledgeable maternity nurse has many opportunities to help young parents provide a supportive environment for their children's sexual development. *Nurses and parents must be careful not to ascribe adult motives to the sexual behaviors of children.* Katchadourian and Lunde (1972) stated: "It is particularly important not to label the sex play of children as deviant or perverse, no matter what it entails. To do so would be like calling a child who believes in ghosts and fairies delusional or mentally ill." Kolodny and co-workers (1979) caution nurses that contradictory messages about the body (parental encouragement to be aware of the body but to exclude the genitals from awareness) are among the earliest recognizable common determinants of adult sexual problems. For example, parents tell their children to "wash behind their ears" and then remind them to "wash down there." Parents and many health professionals respond to their own insecurities about sex when confronted by the overt but innocent sexuality of children.

Adolescence. Adolescence, the transitional period between childhood and adulthood, begins with puberty. The onset of puberty varies for each person. Biologically the first visible signs of puberty are the development of the secondary sexual characteristics. Shortly thereafter most teenagers experience a rapid increase in linear growth. Concomitantly, emotional changes such as moodiness, tearfulness, or withdrawal are suddenly noticeable in a previously serene youngster. For example, one mother related, "My daughter (aged 12) asked me where I had put her baby teeth. When I replied that I had thrown them away, she burst into tears and cried that I didn't think much of her to throw away something so precious."

Menstruation can be a first indication of puberty, as one woman reported:

The three of us had a routine we followed whenever our mother was away from the house. We trooped into the living room and marched over the tops of the sofa and chairs and piano. Then we rushed outside to walk astraddle the high fence separating us from the neighbors. One Sunday I slipped on the fence and hurt myself. I noticed I was bleeding, but because what I was doing was forbidden, I didn't say anything to my mother but put my panty in the laundry. On Monday night, Mother asked me about it. I told her about falling on the fence. After she examined me for injuries she said, 'You are not hurt, I think you have started to menstruate.' I remember being amazed that I hadn't thought of it. My sister (1 year older) was furious that she hadn't started before I did and wouldn't speak to me for a week. I waited eagerly for the next month and proof. Looking back, it seems such a childish way to start being a woman.

It is not until adolescence that the socially and parentally defined sex role is openly questioned. In recent years changes in the concepts of what constitutes male and female roles have had great impact on teenagers. Conflict can result when the teenager chooses standards consonant with the peer group's attitude rather than with parental expectations.

Developmental tasks. Erikson (1959) has described the adolescent stage of development as the one in which the major task is achieving identity versus identity confusion. A person's identity has many dimensions, including intellectual, interpersonal, and sexual. It is now recognized that the adolescent developmental process proceeds in sequence through three phases. These phases—early, middle, and late adolescence—put a characteristic stamp on the manner of accomplishing the developmental tasks. The developmental tasks of adolescence may be defined as follows (adapted from Havighurst, 1972):

1. *Achieving awareness and acceptance of body image.* The body image is well established by about 15 years of age. Adolescents must cope with normal but rapid changes in physical appearance and concomitant alterations in functional capacity. They must accept their physique and learn to use their bodies effectively. Deviations from the "norm" are a source of stress and may or may not be incorporated into the adolescent's body image.

2. *Achieving emotional independence of parents and other adults.* The movement away from dependence on parents that was begun with the school years is completed in this period of development. Successful accomplishment results in affection and respect for one's parents without a childish dependence on them.

3. *Achieving new and more mature relations with age mates of both sexes.* Adolescents accomplish a satisfactory social adjustment through social activities and experimentation with the peer group. Here they learn to behave as adults as they create, on a small scale, the society of their elders. The influence of the peer group increasingly takes precedence over that of the family.

4. *Achieving a masculine or feminine social role.* Although sex is biologically determined, the masculine and feminine roles are culturally established behavior sets that must be learned.

5. *Establishing a lifestyle that is personally and socially satisfying.* This includes the choice of a career, as well as contemplation of sexual relationships, marriage, family interdependence, and parenthood.

6. *Acquiring a set of values and an ethical system as a guide to socially responsible behavior.* This includes assuming responsibility for his or her own behavior and recognizing the effect that behavior may have on another's welfare.

Early adolescence. Early adolescence begins approximately between 11 and 13 years and merges with midadolescence at 14 or 15 years (Johnson, 1983). It is characterized by an increase in height and the appearance of the secondary sexual characteristics.

In terms of cognitive powers early adolescent thought represents a mixture of two stages, the concrete operational stage and the beginning of the formal operational stage (Piaget, 1950). Although there is a greater capacity for logical reasoning, adolescent thought is still based largely on concrete evidence rather than on abstractions. Some adolescents never reach the final level of cognition (the ability to deal with abstractions), whereas others move smoothly through the intervening period.

Young adolescents tend to see the world around them only in relation to the effect it has on *them.* As their capacity for abstract thought increases, they become intensely interested in themselves, their thoughts, ideas, and fantasies, and what effect they have on others. As a result they are introspective, self-conscious, and easily hurt by real or imagined slights. They feel that everyone is looking at them critically so they demand privacy. The slamming of the bedroom door, the NO ADMITTANCE signs put on retreats, and the long periods of self-enforced isolation from the family are typical of this phase.

The major task of early adolescence is acceptance of a new body image. The rapid changes in appearance cause adolescents to spend much time thinking about their bodies and comparing their physiques with those of others. Girls are interested in their developing breasts and often want to wear brassieres before they are needed. They tend to idealize body structure and feel depressed when their skin, hair, and legs do not compare favorably with the "ideal."

Parents are still in control, and the young adolescent is aware of vulnerability and need for dependence. However, parents and brothers and sisters notice a beginning of the critical appraisal to which they will be increasingly subjected. The adolescent becomes aware of the status of the family in the community and is anxious that his or her family measure up to certain standards.

This is the time of intense relationships with members of the same sex, and these relationships are used primarily for support and mutual understanding. Young adolescents have endless face-to-face and telephone conversations about hypothetical activities; for example, "If Peter speaks to me, I will say . . ." Through these conversations they weigh alternatives, assess risks, evaluate results and in fact practice the problem-solving approach.

Vocational choice is not a source of conflict. The young adolescent's choice is often unrealistic or idealistic. Young adolescents fantasize about what they are able to do, and although their increasing cognitive powers make them accept this as daydreaming, they are defensive about their abilities. They do like to work for money and often take newspaper routes or baby-sit.

Midadolescence. Midadolescence begins around 14 or 15 years and merges with late adolescence at about age 17. Almost all adolescents have reached their growth peak by midadolescence. Many aspects of the body have attained their adult form. For example, in boys the development of the lower jaw alters the contour of the face from the round, childish one to that of the adult. Both boys and girls generally accept their bodies, although this acceptance is tempered by a desire to look otherwise. As a result the interest in their bodies is expressed through efforts to improve themselves. Grooming, makeup, and the right clothes become all important. Stabilizing the body image is very

important in developing a sense of identity. Adolescents of this age can remember that they looked much the same a year ago; body structure has begun to assume permanence.

The midadolescent phase is characterized by increasing competence in abstract thought (Johnson, 1983). The adolescent is capable of perceiving future implications of current acts and decisions. The ability to think in this manner fluctuates. In times of stress the adolescent reverts to concrete operations.

The major task during this phase is emancipation from the family. Adolescents vacillate between acting like responsible adults and acting like dependent children. Their ability to step into the adult role, even if briefly, increases their resentment of being considered children. Role experimentation becomes a central process in the search for identity. Adolescents "try out" many roles in fantasy. They may select movie stars or sports heroes as role models. Vocational choice is related to the midadolescents' concern about obtaining the lifestyle they desire. The settled occupations of their parents and their parents' friends may seem too confining and limiting to their activities. They want to do something new, different, and monetarily rewarding.

There is a definite movement away from the family. Midadolescents are critical of their parents, and the parents' appearance, behavior, dress, and social manners are all subjected to intense scrutiny and disparagement. Brothers and sisters are considered a nuisance, and the adolescent sees himself as being treated unfairly in terms of other members of the family. An adult outside the family group—a nurse, a physician, a coach, or a school counselor, for example—may be taken as a role model. There is increased participation in the adult world. Adolescents become advocates of various ideologies and enjoy debating the merits of current ideas. Many show evidence of leadership potential as they engage in developing their cognitive skills. Rebellion is usually couched in verbal terms rather than physical ones and is more destructive than constructive. Running away is a common phenomenon for adolescents between the ages of 15 and 17 years as an attempt to solve problems and to prove they are not children.

Peer relationships now dominate over family ones. The adolescent looks to the peer group for definitions of the behavioral code. There is a strong need to affirm the newly developed self-image through the affirmation of peers. Most conflicts with parents reflect this change, and communication patterns that were once open may become closed.

There is a change from relationships with members of the same sex to heterosexual relationships. Adolescents test their ability to attract the opposite sex. They continue to define the parameters of femininity and masculinity. They tend to develop plural or rapidly changing serial relationships. As one mother remarked, "I couldn't keep up with the girls' names. I use to just say 'Hello there.' I was afraid I'd call Brenda, Linda or make some other terrible mistake."

Late adolescence. The late adolescent phase extends from age 17 through 21. The upper limit of the phase depends on cultural, economic, and educational factors (Johnson, 1983). The late adolescent is physically mature. Most late adolescents have achieved a stable body image, and the agonizing over this or that real or fancied disability is largely over.

The cognitive development of boys and girls in late adolescence reflects the decentering of thought and production of a life plan, as described by Elkind (1968) and Piaget (1972). They have established abstract thought processes. They are future oriented and capable of perceiving and acting on long-range options.

One of the major tasks confronting the late adolescent is to become a fully *independent* productive citizen. This occurs as the adolescent boy or girl moves from being an idealistic reformer to an achiever. Adolescents finally realize that criticism alone will not bring about changes and that ideals must be linked to a commitment and work. They become self-supporting or begin their professional education. The choice of career pattern is reasonably set. Whatever it may be, it will establish the adult lifestyle. Although young women are now assuming the right to choose careers rather than early marriage, the majority still suspend the final shaping of a career until after commitments to parenthood are fulfilled.

Late adolescents are more tolerant of their families, in part perhaps because they sense the ending of the intense dependence relationship. If, on the whole, parents have permitted growth through role experimentation and have supported the need for increasing independence, the conflicts of parent and child seem to fade. On the other hand, the now self-supporting person may feel totally alienated and break all family ties.

Late adolescents' relationships are still peer-centered, but they realize that with the changes in locale necessitated by job or education these early friendships may end and be replaced by others. The need for approval by the peer group is still strong.

The late adolescent is capable of forming stable relationships. He or she is ready for mutuality and reciprocity in caring for another, in contrast to the former self-centered orientation. Marriage and family become part of present or future plans.

Adolescent sexuality. The adolescent's heightened sexual awareness brings to the surface sexual concerns. These include myths about masturbation and concerns about possible homosexuality, sexual activity and the presence, frequency, and content of sexual fantasies and dreams.

Masturbation. Young adolescents may fear that any deviation from normal, particularly of the genitals, has resulted from masturbation. The adolescent needs to learn that masturbation is a normal, universal behavior that causes neither physical nor mental harm. It is a natural part of learning about human sexuality and can be a useful means of relieving sexual tension (Brookman, 1983).

Homosexuality. Homosexual experience to some degree is part of the psychosexual development of many individuals. The adolescent who is overly affectionate with same-sex peers or adults may cause considerable parental concern. This is a result of society's unresolved position on the meaning or acceptance of homosexuality. Fantasies about sexual encounters with members of the same sex can be very disturbing to the adolescent, especially if the adolescent has not begun dating. Memories of early same-sex explorations compound the adolescent's fear of becoming homosexual.

Sexual activity. Adolescents are surrounded by mixed messages. Parents, religious groups, teachers, health professionals, and others tell them to refrain about sexual contact, to control sexual impulses, and to keep away from temptation. Many of these same adults are asking adolescents to refrain from activities they themselves openly practice. At the same time books, movies, music, and advertisements are laden with sexually stimulating messages.

Questions about whether and when to be sexually active and whether one needs to have sex to be popular become a major part of the lives of adolescents. They express confusion about love and how one expresses love, and concern about sexual adequacy. Pajama parties and locker room discussions are often the only outlet the adolescent has to discuss some of these concerns and to obtain information—and a great deal of misinformation—about sex.

Interest in dating stems from the adolescent's need for companionship and emotional and physical closeness. Intimacy includes hand-holding, kissing, embracing, petting, and sexual intercourse. Approximately two thirds of all teenage males and one half of all teenage females have had intercourse at least once (Brookman, 1983). Many younger adolescents may use intercourse as a means of conforming to peer group expectations, as a challenge to parents, as experimentation, or as a means of relieving loneliness or stress. Some adolescents develop sincere commitments to one another that may persist and lead to marriage. Many have "a series of close committed single-partner relationships, each lasting weeks, months, or longer" (Brookman, 1983). Few adolescents are promiscuous; that is, they do not have multiple partners with little or no commitment.

Adolescents are hesitant to talk to adults, especially parents, because the adult often discounts or invalidates their feelings. Some parents are threatened by their adolescent's budding sexuality. They deal with their own uncertainty about sex by ignoring the reality of adolescent sexuality or by becoming hostile and punitive. At times little attention is given to the teenager who is reluctant to engage in dating at all. The young person who fails to show any interest may need careful evaluation.

Implications for nursing. Health professionals need to be knowledgeable and comfortable with their own sexuality to work effectively with adolescents. Glossing over important issues and making broad generalizations about sexual concerns can be more confusing than helpful. Nurses who counsel young people about specific sexual issues need a) knowledge of sexual anatomy, physiology, and behavior; b) recognition of the importance of local peer influences; and c) understanding of the adolescent's family and ethnocultural background. The approach to adolescents is based on their intellectual and psychosocial maturation. The adolescent usually is willing to express concerns if the discussions are held in a comfortable and nonjudgmental setting.

An increased incidence of adolescent pregnancy and the increased number of adolescents with sexually transmitted diseases make sex education and sex counseling a major task for nurses working with adolescents. Information about their bodies' sexual responses, contraception, pregnancy, and sexually transmitted disease can be made available to them to help them become sexually responsible adults.

It is important for nurses working with adolescents to be aware of adolescents' concern about masturbation and homosexuality. Factual information about masturbation can be given to adolescents, but it is not appropriate for the counselor to advocate masturbation. The decision should be made by each person and rightly includes personal values, such as religious belief.

Brookman (1983) states that reassurance concerning homosexuality may be offered by sharing these points:

1. Strong attraction to same-sex adults is a normal event for most adolescents, representing displacement of such feelings for parents onto others in the separation-individuation process.

2. Strong attraction to same-sex peers is the first step in the shifting of a person's love-object relationship from the parents to age mates. It is also an intermediate early-adolescent stage in the development of the capacity to form intimate interpersonal relationship.

3. Exhibitionism, voyeurism, and mutual masturbation are common experimental experiences, especially among boys age 8 to 13. Group masturbation and ejaculation, often as a contest, are frequent methods of declaring maturity and superiority in the peer group.

4. In many cultures, the expression of affection between same-sex friends and relatives through embracing and kissing is a normal and accepted practice for males as well as females.

5. Few people who have had a homosexual episode in adolescence retain a homosexual preference as adults. There is nothing predictive in such an act alone.

6. Adult sexual identity is not solidified until late adolescence, but as this is most influenced by early childhood factors, ultimate sexual gender preference is well established, albeit nascent, by the advent of adolescence. Homosexual experiences during the early years will not alter a basic heterosexual orientation.

It is important to note that some adult homosexuals report awareness of their homosexuality as early as adolescence. These young people usually begin to be aware of their different feelings by midteens. The nurse counseling these adolescents needs to be accepting and comfortable in communicating with homosexuals. The incidence of sexually transmitted diseases and other infections encountered in homosexuals makes it essential to secure appropriate medical and counseling sources for them. Nurses who are not comfortable with these clients need to refer them to other professionals or agencies who can help them. "Counseling support from within the gay community can be a valuable adjunct to whatever the health professional can provide" (Brookman, 1983).

Adulthood

Adulthood encompasses the period from adolescence to a person's death. Three phases are discernable: early, middle, and late adulthood.

Early adulthood. Early adulthood encompasses that portion of the life cycle devoted to parenting, consolidation of relationships, whether marital or nonmarital, and commitment to a life work. The young adult has attained physical and intellectual maturity. Stature and reproductive growth are virtually complete. The process of aging, beginning in the twenties and continuing in the thirties and forties, causes minimal overt change.

Cognitive powers include the ability to think abstractly, to be future oriented and to act on long-range options (Piaget, 1950). Personality development is related to the task of developing intimacy and solidarity as opposed to existing in isolation (Erikson, 1959). Intimacy involves learning to give and receive love, choosing whether to marry and choosing a sexual partner or partners (Duvall, 1977).

Body image remains a concern for the young adult, particularly in terms of body contour and size (Woods, 1984). Nonacceptance of one's body may inhibit the establishment of sexual relationships.

Family ties are important, but the relationship of parent and child takes on an adult quality. The young adult is expected to be moving toward financial and social independence from the family. He or she is also expected to choose a vocation and obtain the necessary education for it. Establishing a career and advancing in it are major concerns throughout this part of the life cycle.

Social groupings include varying age levels and are often based on similar interests. The need for strong friendships with peers diminishes as individual friendships assume permanence.

Sexuality. Early adulthood has been described as a period of maximum sexual self-consciousness (Offer and Simon, 1976). There is social acceptance and legitimization of sexual experiences. The tasks of sexual development for the young adult include maintaining a long-term commitment to a sexual relationship, practicing responsible reproductive health care, and making rational decisions about childbearing.

1. *Commitment to a relationship* is strengthened by the need to give and receive pleasure. Commitments vary in length and type. For example, some couples remain monogamous throughout their marriage. Others have open marriages, in which the couple agrees that one or both may participate in other sexual encounters. Some couples remain in relationships without formal marriage. Relationships can be terminated by divorce or death. Finally, serial monogamy is practiced by many people in the United States. Serial monogamy is characterized by repeated marriages and divorces. The person is married to only one person at a time but is married a number of times throughout his or her life.

2. *Responsible reproductive health care* includes such actions as women having a Papanicolaou smear at prescribed intervals or both men and women avoiding sexually transmitted diseases.

3. *Rational decisions about childbearing* are important to ensure that every child is a wanted child. The couple

is responsible for using a reliable contraceptive technique when pregnancy is not desired. Unwanted pregnancies and multiple abortions represent a disregard for life and personal well-being. Unwanted children often become targets of abuse and neglect.

There are a variety of sexual orientations and forms of sexual expression open to adults. Heterosexuality, homosexuality, and bisexuality are the three major sexual orientations. The most common forms of sexual expression include vaginal-penile intercourse, anal intercourse, orogenital intercourse, self-stimulation, and mutual masturbation. These are all valid forms of sexual expression and are practiced according to personal preferences.

Myths. In a culture characterized by a rapid increase in knowledge and technology, many people still are misinformed about human sexuality. McCary (1982) has listed 100 of the most common fallacies about human sexuality that plague the United States today. Listed below are common myths about reproduction and birth control:

1. There is an absolutely safe period for sexual intercourse, during which coitus cannot cause impregnation.
2. A couple must have simultaneous climaxes if conception is to take place.
3. A woman can become pregnant only through coitus or artificial insemination.
4. Urination by the woman after coitus or having sexual intercourse in a standing position will prevent pregnancy.
5. Abortion, whether legal or criminal, is always dangerous.
6. Frigid women, prostitutes, and promiscuous women are not as likely to conceive as women whose sexual response or activity is more normal.
7. There must be two acts of sexual intercourse to produce twins, three for triplets, and so on.
8. Sperm from one testis will produce males, and sperm from the other testis will produce females; or the ova from one ovary will produce males, and the ova from the other ovary will produce females.
9. Having only one testis reduces a man's ability to father a child.
10. The woman determines the sex of the child.
11. A woman's diet during pregnancy has a bearing on the sex of the child.

Middle and late adulthood. These phases of the life cycle represent the greatest maximizing of early potential and then a gradual lessening of biopsychosocial attainment through the normal process of aging. Changes in family structure from events such as children leaving home, death of a spouse or role reversal in dealing with aging parents necessitate major changes in life-style. The critical task for these years is maintaining feelings of self-esteem versus despair. The need to love and be loved, to be successful and to feel meaningful prompts involvement in community service and in leisure pursuits.

Cognitive powers continue unabated until physical insults such as Alzheimer's disease or cerebral vascular accident cause a decline. Body image remains an important concern. Western society's accent on health and youth make grooming, weight, nutrition, and exercise a continuous part of adult's daily life.

Sexuality. The sexual developmental tasks of middle and late adulthood focus primarily on adapting to the physical and emotional changes in sexual performance caused by the aging process. The childbearing years are coming to an end. This is a relief for many couples because the threat of pregnancy can be removed from their lovemaking. Others may mourn the loss of the chance for another child.

The fear of growing older in a youth-oriented society can be a source of depression and anxiety. Bodily changes, lower hormone production, and menopause may contribute to anxiety and depression.

The research of Masters and Johnson (1966) has shown that aging does not decrease libido or the capacity to be orgasmic. Men and women are capable of sexual activity well into their old age. Disinterest and abstinence are probably caused by loss of a partner, boredom, ill health, or cultural attitudes about the appropriateness.

Many older people do not understand the impact of aging on their physical response to sexual stimulation. They see these changes as an indication they should terminate sexual activity rather than merely as a need to make minor adaptations. For example, lubrication in women is slower and decreased in amount; in men, erection is slower and erectile firmness decreased. Love play will probably need to be extended, with more direct genital stimulation to produce lubrication and erection. Woman have a shortened orgasmic phase and men's need to ejaculate decreases, resulting in decreased force and volume of ejaculation. These physiologic changes require adaptations in sexual behavior and not cessation of sexual activity.

Mims and Swenson (1980) have stated:

> Sexual fulfillment throughout adulthood and into old age is not only possible but likely. The feeling that older people are not interested in sex (except if they are abnormal—the "dirty old man" syndrome) is largely caused by our inability to imagine our parents or our grandparents as sexually active people. The greatest danger of such attitudes is that they tend to comprise a "self-fulfilling prophecy": if people believe that sexual interest ceases with advancing age, they will find that it does cease. Or, if sexual interest persists, people may believe themselves to be abnormal, sinful, or psychologically sick.

Implications for nursing. The nurse is in a unique position to help adults with health maintenance and detection of problems concerning sexuality. Contacts with adults occur at clinics or hospitals when people seek counseling or care for contraception. Giving nursing care during the pregnancy cycle is an important part of the maternity nurse's role.

The role of sex educator is an important one for nurses working with families during the childbearing and child rearing years. Parents often need help with teaching their children about sex because adults frequently are misinformed about many aspects of reproduction and how their bodies function. Parents therefore need accurate sex information to teach their children to be healthy, responsible sexual beings.

Besides helping with childhood and adult sexuality, the nurse can help prepare clients for the sexual problems and changes occurring with age. Many nurses have not been aware of the importance of sex education for older people because of the myth that the elderly are no longer interested in sex.

Sexual dysfunctional problems often begin after children are born. The mother especially may become so involved with child rearing that her relationship with her husband suffers. At the same time the husband may be actively involved in career establishment, thereby depleting his energies at home. The nurse needs to be aware of how the demands of parenting can adversely affect the marital relationship. Simple counseling provided during these early years may prevent serious marital problems in later years.

The older woman, in particular, who has been able to move gracefully into old age and who continues to recognize herself as a sexual being is probably better able to accept the sexuality of the young. The pregnancy of a daughter then may be accepted as a continuation of her own sexuality rather than as a threat or reminder of her lost youth.

A knowledgeable, nonjudgmental nurse who recognizes personal sexual biases can contribute a great deal to the sexual health of young families. The nurse can recognize potential problems within the marriage and either intervene or refer the couple for further counseling.

Summary

By the time puberty occurs a person has completed most of the developmental tasks of early childhood. Acceptance of childhood sexual identity will have consequences for self-esteem, peer relations, and selection of skills and interest. The concomitant development of moral standards such as honesty and fidelity results in a linkage between sexual identity (role) and moral commitments. Feelings of self-acceptance or guilt can be generated by either upholding or violating standards in these spheres.

By the end of late adolescence the individual is ready to move into the adult world. At this point late adolescents have developed intellectually and socially. Their independence is reflected in their ability to become productive citizens, to establish long-term intimate relationships with others and to emancipate themselves from their families. Their self-image is realistic and they have the capacity to give as well as receive love. They have become socially functioning adults (Handwerker and Hodgman, 1983).

Adulthood represents the longest period in the life cycle. During this time childhood potential is realized and key social roles are assumed. The importance ascribed to the roles of man/woman, husband/wife, and parent/child reflect society's concern with the biopsychosocial nature of adult sexuality.

References

Brookman, R: Adolescent sexuality and related health problems. In Hoffman, A., editor: Adolescent medicine, Menlo Park, Calif., 1983, Addison-Wesley Publishing Co.

Duvall, E.R.: Family development, ed. 5, Philadelphia, 1977, J.B. Lippincott Co.

Elkind, D.: Cognitive development in adolescene. In Adams, J.F., editor: Understanding adolescence, Boston, 1968, Allyn & Bacon.

Erikson, E.: Identity and the life cycle; selected papers. In Psychological issues, New York, 1959, International Universities Press.

Handwerker, L., and Hodgman, C.: Approach to adolescence by Perinatal Staff. In McAnarney, E., editor: Premature adolescent pregnancy and parenthood, New York, 1983, Grune & Stratton.

Havighurst, R.J.: Developmental tasks and education, ed. 3, New York, 1972 David McKay Co.

Johnson, R.: Adolescent growth and development. In Hoffman, A., editor: Adolescent medicine, Menlo Park, Calif., 1983, Addison-Wesley Publishing Co.

Katchadourian, II.A., and Lunde, D.T.: Fundamentals of human sexuality, New York, 1972, Holt, Rinehart and Winston.

Kinsey, A.C., and others: Sexual behavior in human female, Philadelphia, 1953, W.B. Saunders Co.

Kinsey, A.C., and others: Sexual behavior in human male, Philadelphia, 1948, W.B. Saunders Co.

Kolodny, R.C., and others: Textbook of human sexuality for nurses, Boston, 1979, Little, Brown & Co.

Maccoby, E.E., editor: The development of sex differences, Stanford, Calif., 1966, Stanford University Press.

Maccoby, E.E., and Jacklin, C.: The psychology of sex differences, Stanford, Calif., 1974, Stanford University Press.

Masters, W.H., and Johnson, V.E.: Human sexual response, Boston, 1966, Little, Brown & Co.

McCary, J.L.: Human sexuality, ed. 4, New York, 1982, Van Nostrand Reinhold Co.

Mims, F.H., and Swenson, M.: Sexuality, a nursing perspective, New York, 1980, McGraw-Hill Book Co.

Newman, B., and Newman, R.: Development through life: a psychosocial approach, Homewood, Ill., 1975, Dorsey Press.

Offer, D., and Simon, W.: Sexual development. In Sadock, B., Kaplan, H., and Freedman, A., editors: The sexual experience, Baltimore, 1976, The Williams & Wilkins Co.

Piaget, J.: The psychology of intelligence, Boston, 1950, Routledge & Kegan Paul.

Piaget, J.: Intellectual evolution from adolescence to adulthood, Hum. Dev. 15:1012, 1972.

Weisner, T.S., and Gallimore, R.: My brother's keeper: child and sibling caretaking, Curr. Anthropol. 18:169, 1977.

Whaley, L.F., and Wong, D.L.: Nursing care of infants and children, ed. 3, St. Louis, 1987, The C.V. Mosby Co.

Woods, N.F.: Human sexuality in health and illness, ed. 3, St. Louis, 1984, The C.V. Mosby Co.

Bibliography

Catterall, R.D.: Biologic effects of sexual freedom, Lancet 1(8215): 315-319, 1981.

Alan Guttmacher Institute: Teenage pregnancy: the problem that hasn't gone away, New York, 1981, The Institute.

Gordon, S., Scales, P., and Everly, K.: The sexual adolescent: communicating with teenagers about sex, ed. 2, N. Scituate, Mass., 1979, Duxbury Press.

Greydanus, D.E.: Alternatives to adolescent pregnancy: a discussion of the contraceptive literature from 1960 to 1980. Semin. Perinatol. 5(1):53-90, 1981.

Greydanus, D.E., and McAnarney, E.R.: Contraception for the adolescent: current concepts for the pediatrician. Pediatrics 65(1):1-12, 1980.

Masters, W.H., and others: Human sexuality, Boston, 1982, Little, Brown & Co.

Sarrel, L.J., and Sarrel, P.M.: Sexual unfolding: sexual development and sex therapies in late adolescence, Boston, 1979, Little, Brown & Co.

Infertility, Control of Fertility, and Surgical Interruption of Pregnancy

This chapter addresses several fertility-related issues and associated tests, and therapies. A variety of contraceptive methods are discussed in detail. Surgical intervention in elective termination of fertility and some diagnostic and therapeutic techniques for infertility are discussed also. Reproductive issues tend to generate strong emotions in affected people. Because surgical intervention and strong emotional responses are involved in the termination of pregnancy, interruption of pregnancy has been grouped with the reproductive issues of fertility, control of fertility, and termination of fertility.

Infertility

The inability to conceive and bear a child afflicts a surprising number of otherwise healthy adults. It is difficult to be denied the experiences of pregnancy and birth, parenthood, and the expression of love through the care and nurturing of another human being. Disturbance in one's sexual self-concept is often experienced. Couples requesting assistance with infertility problems have already decided that they want a child. They seek acceptance and assistance from the nurse and physician in coping with and possibly resolving these problems.

Infertility is the inability to conceive after at least 1 year of adequate exposure when no contraceptive measures were used. It is also the inability to deliver a live infant after three consecutive conceptions. Generally two thirds of couples who have sexual intercourse without the use of contraceptives achieve pregnancy within 6 months, and 80% within 1 year. For the anxious couple or the older couple (woman over 30 years and man over 40 years) a 6-month effort is sufficient before fertility studies are begun.

Infertility is *primary* if the woman has never been pregnant or the man has never impregnated a woman.

It is *secondary* if the woman has been pregnant at least once but has not been able to conceive again or sustain a pregnancy. Infertility, whether primary or secondary, occurs in one couple in five. For 85% of these couples the underlying cause can be diagnosed; 50% to 70% can be treated successfully. The incidence of infertility seems to be increasing, probably because of (1) the trend to delay pregnancy until later in life when fertility decreases naturally, (2) the increase in pelvic inflammatory disease, and (3) the increase in substance abuse.

Investigation and management of infertility have been aided by the enormous expansion of knowledge in several related fields. Advancements in knowledge have occurred in reproductive physiology, behavioral and environmental influences on sexual functioning, the role of microbiology and immunology, advanced urologic and gynecologic surgical techniques, and in vitro fertilization. Investigation of infertility requires the accumulation of extensive data related to factors essential for or contributing to infertility. A theoretic base is necessary to direct the investigator's assessments to analyze findings and to plan, implement, and evaluate the management of and therapy for infertility.

Some of the data needed are of a sensitive, personal nature. Obtaining these data may be viewed as an invasion of privacy. The tests and examinations are occasionally painful and intrusive and can take the romance out of lovemaking. A high level of motivation is needed to endure the investigation. The attitude, sensitivity, and caring nature of those who are involved in the assessment of infertility lay the foundation for the client's ability to cope with the subsequent therapy and management. All members of the health team must respect the clients' rights to privacy and the confidentiality of client records.

Religious considerations. Civil laws and religious proscriptions about sex must always be kept in mind by the clinician. For example, the Orthodox Jewish husband and wife may face infertility investigaion and management problems because of religious laws that govern marital relations. According to Jewish law the couple may not engage in marital relations during menstruation and through the following 7 "preparatory days." The wife then is immersed in a ritual bath (Mikvah) before relations can resume. The 5 menstrual days and 7 preparatory days collectively are called the "nida state." Any vaginal bleeding of physiologic origin marks the beginning of the nida state. Fertility problems can arise when the woman has a short cycle (i.e., a cycle of 24 days or less, when ovulation would occur on day 10 or earlier). Small doses of estrogen may delay ovulation to allow for the time needed to complete the nida state. Other procedures that induce bleeding may delay intercourse for another 12 days to allow for the nida state. Thus Orthodox Jewish clients as well as observant Catholics may at times question proposed diagnostic and therapeutic procedures because of religious proscriptions. These clients are encouraged to consult their rabbi or priest for a ruling.

Cultural considerations. When the ability to procreate is the norm used to recognize individuals in a culture as whole and complete persons, infertility becomes a tragedy. In Samoa, sterility is serious enough to be a cause for divorce (Clark and Howland, 1978).

Table 7.1
Factors Associated with Fertility and Infertility

Factors Required for Fertility	Conditions Associated with Infertility
Development of reproductive tract is normal	Congenital or developmental factors 　Abnormal external genitals (e.g., enlarged clitoris or fused labia) which may suggest masculinization 　Gynetresia (e.g., absence of vagina or shallow vagina) 　Vaginal anomalies (e.g., double vagina with single or double cervix and single or double uterus or with one vaginal canal ending blindly, the other vaginal canal ending at entrance to a uterus) 　Unusual uterus (e.g., congenitally small, or "infantile," uterus) 　Uterine and tubal defects from exposure to DES as embryo/fetus 　Abnormalities of ovaries (see ovulation)
Ovulation: hypothalamus-pituitary-gonadal axis is normal. An ovum is released from a mature ovarian follicle.	Absence of ovulation 　Malfunctioning of axis with menstrual irregularities 　Abnormal ovaries as seen in Turner's syndrome (see Chapter 28) or Stein-Leventhal syndrome 　Hormonal suppression of hypothalamus-pituitary-gonadal axis with birth control medication 　Emotional problems (e.g., severe psychoneurosis or psychosis or anorexia nervosa, which may be responsible for anovulatory cycles, frequently associated with amenorrhea or oligomenorrhea) 　Menstrual irregularities from vigorous exercise (jogging, sports), especially in thin women
Tubal: ovum enters uterine tube promptly after ovulation. Sperm migrate into uterine tube, where fertilization takes place. Fertilized ovum finds its way down tube into endometrial cavity to implant into hormone-prepared endometrium 7 to 10 days after ovulation.	Uterine tube is blocked or its function is altered 　Blockage of tube by scar tissue formation following infection (pelvic inflammatory disease, ruptured appendix followed by peritonitis) or pelvic surgery 　Blockage of tube by compression or kinking by abnormal growth such as endometriosis and neoplasms 　Alteration in tubal motility by birth control medication or from emotional stress
Uterine: endometrium is adequately prepared to receive fertilized ovum.	Uterus is malformed or endometrium is unreceptive to fertilized ovum (malfunction of hypothalamus-pituitary-gonadal axis; presence of endometrial infection; presence of intrauterine device [IUD])
Vaginal-cervical mucus is receptive and supportive to sperm. Cervix is competent.	Absence of mucous characteristics receptive and supportive to sperm 　Altered vaginal pH from feminine hygiene preparations or douches, infections, antibiotic chemotherapy, disease states (e.g., diabetes mellitus), poor hygiene, or emotional stress 　Presence of spermicidal foams or other preparations used for contraception 　Development of antibodies (an immunologic response) against a specific male's sperm (see discussion of sperm, in assessments of the woman and the man)
Sperm are normal, adequate in number, and ejaculated into female reproductive tract.	Sperm factors discussed later in this chapter
Conceptus develops normally, reaches viability, and is delivered in good condition.	

The person without children in Samoa is pitied. According to Brownlee (1978), in many cultures a woman's inability to conceive may be due to her sins, to evil spirits, or to the fact that she is an inadequate person. The virility of a man in some cultures remains in question until he demonstrates his ability to reproduce by having at least one child.

Determination of a culturally defined cause for sterility is usually accompanied by a culturally proposed solution for the problem. These proposed solutions may or may not be effective. For example, Vietnamese men thought sterility was caused by loss of sperm, or spermatorrhea, during wet dreams at night or through daytime discharge (Coughlin, 1965). Tonics consisting of licorice, aconite, and ginseng might be used to counteract the effect. Certain foods such as cereal were to be eaten, and substances such as alcohol were to be avoided.

In most cultures, infertility is usually blamed on the woman. If infertility is believed to be caused by a misplaced uterus, methods are used to replace it. A Samoan woman may go to a bush doctor who will massage the abdomen over the uterus with oil and attempt to put it back in place (Clark and Howland, 1978).

Assessment of the Woman

History

1. Duration of infertility: length of contraceptive and noncontraceptive exposure
2. Fertility in other marriages of self or spouses
3. Obstetric
   a. Number of pregnancies and abortions
   b. Length of time required to initiate each pregnancy
   c. Complications of any pregnancy
   d. Duration of lactation
4. Gynecologic: detailed menstrual history and leukorrheal history
5. Previous tests and therapy done for infertility
6. Medical: general medical history including chronic and hereditary disease; drug use
7. Surgical: especially abdominal or pelvic surgery
8. Sexual history in detail: libido, orgasm capacity, techniques, frequency of intercourse, and postcoital practices
9. Psychosomatic evaluation
   a. General
   b. As regards infertility problem, particularly her reason for seeking advice at this time

Physical examination

1. General: careful examination of other organs and parts of body; special attention given to habitus, fat and hair distribution, acne
2. Genital tract: state of hymen (full penetration); clitoris; vaginal infection, including trichomoniasis and candidiasis; cervical tears, polyps, infection, patency of os, accessibility to insemination; uterus, including size and position, mobility; adnexae, tumors, evidence of endometriosis

Laboratory data

1. Routine urine, complete blood count, and serologic test for syphilis; additional laboratory studies as indicated
2. Basic endocrine studies in women with irregular menstrual cycles or in amenorrhea, hirsutism, acne, or excessive weight gain

Irregular Menstrual Cycles	Amenorrhea
Protein-bound iodine (PBI) or other thyroid tests	Tomographic x-ray films of skull
17-Ketosteroids	T_4 or other thyroid tests
17-Hydroxycorticoids	17-Ketosteroids
4-Hour glucose tolerance test	17-Hydroxycorticoids
Endometrial biopsy	4-Hour glucose tolerance test
	Endometrial biopsy
	Gonadotropin determination
	Buccal smear and chromosomal studies

Other laboratory tests added as desired for a more complete diagnosis of endocrine problems
3. Rh factor and antibody titer tests—important in abortion and premature delivery problems
4. Sperm antibody agglutination studies. Special laboratory procedure involves obtaining a fresh semen specimen from man and a blood sample from the woman. Sperm are incubated in the blood serum of the woman and checked at intervals for agglutination. The test is negative if no agglutinated sperm are found.

For Mexican-American women and others who subscribe to heat/cold balance and imbalance theories, barrenness is considered to result from having a "cold womb" (Clark, 1970). The cold womb may be heated through external and internal means. Clark (1970) describes two methods used by Mexican-American women. One method requires a barren woman to sit over a washtub of hot water, to which rosemary is added, so that the vapors warm the womb. The other method attempts to build up body heat over a period of 3 days. This is done by avoiding cold foods and water, using a belladonna plaster over the sacral area, and ingesting cathartic pills and hot chocolate.

Factors associated with infertility. Investigation of fertility and identification of the conditions that may be responsible for the infertile state constitute a long and tedious process. Infertility may occur when a single fertility factor is absent. At other times a combination of factors, female and male, is necessary to cause infertility. In Table 7.1 each factor essential to fertility is presented, along with a listing of conditions associated with infertility. Assessment for fertility fac-

Assessment of the Man

History

1. Fertility in other marriages of self or spouses
2. Medical: general medical history, including venereal infections, mumps orchitis, chronic diseases, recent fever, drug use
3. Surgical: herniorraphy, injuries to genitals, or other surgery in genital area
4. Occupational: exposure to chemicals, x-ray equipment, or extreme thermal changes; physical nature of occupation; vacations and work habits
5. Previous tests and therapy done for study of infertility
6. Duration of infertility
7. Sex history in detail, with discussion of actual coital techniques, such as frequency and ability to ejaculate
8. Adequacy of erection

Physical examination

1. General examination: careful examination of other organs and parts of body, with special attention given to habitus, fat and hair distribution
2. Genital tract: penis and urethra; scrotal size; position, size, and consistency of testes; epididymides and vasa deferentia; prostate size and consistency
3. Careful search for varicocele, with man in both supine and upright positions

Laboratory data

1. Routine urine, complete blood count, and serologic test for syphilis
2. Complete semen analysis—essential
   a. Liquefaction: usually complete within 10 to 30 minutes
   b. Semen volume   2-5 ml (range: 1 to 7 ml)
   c. Semen pH   7.2 to 7.8
   d. Sperm density   20 to 200 million/ml
   e. Normal morphology (%) $\geq 60\%$
   f. Motility (important consideration in sperm evaluation); percentage of forward-moving sperm estimated in relationship to abnormally motile and nonmotile sperm. This requires evaluation by a technician with some degree of experience but as the test provides a more accurate diagnosis, it is well worth the time involved; $\geq 50\%$ is normal
   g. Cell count: average normal, 60 million or more per milliliter or a total of 150 to 200 or more million per ejaculate; minimum normal standards: 40 million/ml, with a total count of at least 125 million per ejaculate (average of counts on two or preferably three separate specimens)
   NOTE: These values are not absolute, but only relative to the final evaluation of the couple as a single reproductive unit.
3. Additional laboratory studies as indicated
   a. Basic endocrine studies indicated in men with oligospermia or aspermia:
      (1) Tomographic x-ray films of skull
      (2) T_4 or other thyroid tests
      (3) 17-Ketosteroids
      (4) Gonadotropin determination
      (5) 17-Hydroxycorticoids and pregnanediol
      (6) Buccal smear and chromosomal studies, for example, Klinefelter's syndrome, XXY sex chromosomes
      (7) Test for sperm antibodies; autoimmunization. Autoimmune antibodies (produced by the man against his own sperm) agglutinate or immobilize sperm in less than 5% of men with infertility.
   b. Testicular biopsy, where correct interpretation is available (may give a more accurate diagnosis and prognosis in cases of azoospermia and severe oligospermia), vasography if indicated and available

tors in the woman and in the man are outlined in the boxes on pp. 132 and 133.

INVESTIGATION OF FEMALE INFERTILITY

There are several examinations and tests for female infertility. Each method of assessment is discussed under the following headings: which partner is involved in testing or in collection of the specimen, why the test is done, when the test is scheduled, how and where the test is accomplished, the risks involved, the information that is sought, and specific medical and nursing actions pertinent to the situation.

Self-assessment of basal body temperature (BBT) and cervical mucus involves touching oneself and one's discharges. Therefore self-assessment can be emotionally uncomfortable for some women. The nurse may also be uneasy teaching self-assessment techniques to others. Fertility test findings favorable to fertility are summarized on p. 143.

It is estimated that at least 50% of all female infertility problems can be diagnosed and treated by medical or surgical means. Diagnosis and treatment require considerable physical, emotional, and financial investment over several months or years.

Congenital or developmental factors. If the woman has abnormal external genitals, surgical reconstruction of abnormal tissue and construction of a functional vagina may permit normal intercourse. If internal reproductive tract structures are absent, there is no hope for fertility. Surgical intervention depends entirely on the anatomic development, the surgical feasibility, and the individual's actual gender role.

Vaginal and uterine anomalies and their surgical repair vary from individual to individual. If a functional uterus can be reconstructed, pregnancy may be possi-

ble. After surgical repair of the uterus, cesarean delivery is necessary to prevent uterine rupture during labor. Women with ovarian agenesis or dysgenesis are sterile, and no treatment will improve their fertility.

Ovarian factors

Review of ovarian function. Within healthy ovaries, graafian follicles respond to FSH and LH by the maturation of an ovum and ovulation. The graafian follicle produces estrogen; the empty graafian follicle becomes the corpus luteum and produces estrogen and progesterone.

Impairment of ovarian function. Anovulation may be *primary.* Primary anovulation may be caused by a pituitary or hypothalamic hormone disorder or an adrenal gland disorder such as congenital adrenal hyperplasia. *Secondary* anovulation may be caused by ovarian disease. In amenorrheic states and instances of anovulatory cycles, hormone studies usually reveal the problem.

Treatment and prognosis. In some instances endocrine therapy with so-called fertility drugs such as oral clomiphene citrate (Clomid) or with intramuscular human menopausal gonadotropin (HMG) (Pergonal) may induce ovulation in anovulatory woman (Table 7.2).

Ovarian tumors must be excised; whenever possible, functional ovarian tissue is left intact. Chronic infection, which may cover much or all of the ovary, usually necessitates surgery to free and expose the ovary so that ovulation can occur.

An increasing number of young women are experiencing secondary amenorrhea. Their history reveals a serious interest in jogging and other sports or a considerable weight loss that has been followed by menstrual irregularities. Their dietary history may reveal

Plasma Progesterone Level

Who: Woman
Why: To assess function of corpus luteum
How: A blood sample is drawn
When: Late in menstrual cycle, just before menstruation
Where: Clinic, physician's office, or hospital laboratory
Risk: 1. Low
2. Discomfort from venipuncture

Procedure	Information Sought
■ Woman has blood drawn at the appropriate time.	Findings favorable to fertility: adequate levels of progesterone are found. Progesterone levels correlate well with BBT and cervical mucus characteristics.

meals that consist of lean red meat and calorie-free soda drinks. Examination results frequently reveal amenorrhea or menstrual irregularities and osteoporosis (from loss of calcium). The woman who engages in vigorous exercise with normal menstrual cycles does not need to be concerned about osteoporosis. She may have actually increased her calcium levels in bones and

thereby increased their healthy density. Any woman who has missed two or three periods, however, is urged to consult an endocrinologist or an obstetrician-gynecologist.

Thyroid gland dysfunction may be associated with menstrual abnormalities, infertility, or recurrent fetal waste. Therapy consists of management of the thyroid

Table 7.2
Drug Therapy for Female Infertility

Drug	Indications	Nursing Actions
Ovulatory stimulants		
Clomiphene citrate (Clomid) (O)—a follicular maturing agent	Anovulation caused by hypothalamic suppression (but with an intact hypothalamic-pituitary-ovarian axis)	Counsel regarding oral ingestion of Clomid, maintenance of BBT chart for evidence of ovulation, and potential side effects: ovarian cyst formation, vasomotor effects; visual disturbances, partial alopecia, abdominal disturbances, and multiple pregnancies.
Bromocriptine (Parlodel), a synthetic ergot alkaloid	Anovulation caused by elevated levels of prolactin (inhibits release of prolactin)	Counsel regarding oral ingestion of drug with food to reduce its side effects: nausea, vomiting, lightheadedness, dizziness (tolerance develops within a few weeks; menstruation resumes in 75% of women in 6 to 8 weeks). Should not be taken with drugs that elevate prolactin levels, for example, psychotropic agents. Monitor BBT so that drug is discontinued if pregnancy occurs.
Thyroid stimulating hormone (TSH) (Synthoid)	Anovulation caused by hypothyroidism	Counsel regarding medical regimen: medication and assessment of blood levels of TSH.
Human menopausal gonadotropin (HMG) (Pergonal)	Anovulation caused by hypogonadotropic amenorrhea	Administer or test self-injection of HMG.
Gonadotropin-releasing hormone (GnRH), alone or preceded by clomiphene citrate or HMG	Anovulation caused by hypothalamic-pituitary dysfunction, hypothalamic failure, or failure to ovulate with use of Clomid	Assist with daily injection or teach her self-injection. Overall success rate is 15% to 20%.
Hormone replacement therapy		
Conjugated estrogens and medroxyprogesterone	Hypoestrogenic condition: high stress level, decreased level of body fat caused by eating disorder (e.g., anorexia nervosa) or excessive exercise	Counsel regarding oral ingestion—estrogens on days 1 to 24 and progesterone on days 15 to 24; possible side effects (e.g., fluid retention); stress reduction and so on.
Hydroxyprogesterone supplementation (vaginal suppositories or IM)	Luteal phase defects	Counsel regarding administration: start 3 to 4 days after estimated ovulation and continue to menses (if no menses, a serum pregnancy test is done).
	Endometriosis	Assist with protocol of care.
Other		
Prednisone (O) (a glucocorticoid)	Congenital adrenal hyperplasia	Counsel regarding oral ingestion regimen and associated side effects.
Danazol	Endometriosis	Assist with counseling woman regarding daily dosages and possible side effects: weight gain, hot flushes, night sweats, decrease in breast size, bloody vaginal discharge, atrophic vaginitis.
Mefenamic acid; Naproxen	Dysmenorrhea with pain, nausea, vomiting, headaches, fainting, diarrhea that are induced by danazol therapy for endometriosis	Counsel regarding need to start therapy 48 hours before onset of dysmenorrhea.
Antimicrobial therapy	Infection	Implement usual actions when administering antimicrobial medications.

Hormone Analysis

Who: Woman
Why: To assess endocrine function
How: Blood and urine specimens are obtained
When: At varying times during menstrual cycle
Where: Clinic, physician's office, or hospital laboratory
Risk: 1. Low
2. Discomfort from venipuncture
3. Inconvenience of collecting urine and taking to laboratory (when urine specimens are used)

Procedure	Information Sought
■ Blood sample is drawn.	Findings favorable to fertility:
	1. Levels of progesterone, estrogen, FSH and LH are all appropriate.
■ Urine specimen is obtained.	2. Levels of 17-ketosteroids and 17-hydroxycorticosteroids are within normal limits.

Ultrasound Pelvic Examination

Who: Woman
Why: To visualize pelvic tissues for a variety of reasons (e.g., to identify abnormalities, to verify follicular development and maturity to determine timing for retrieval of ova for preparation of in vitro fertilization or for planning of artificial insemination, to confirm intrauterine [vs. ectopic] pregnancy)
When: Timing depends on the purpose
How: Use of static scanner or a real-time scanner (Chapter 25); it indicated, a bimanual examination
Where: Clinic or office
Risk: Low, diagnostic ultrasound is physically safe; no anesthesia is needed

Procedure	Information Sought
■ Woman's bladder is full to permit visualization of uterus and adnexa.	Findings favorable to fertility:
■ Woman is positioned comfortably and the examination is performed.	1. Size, shape, position of reproductive structures are within normal limits.
■ Findings are discussed with woman.	2. Ovarian changes of follicle development, ovulation, and formation of corpus luteum can be documented and occur within normal limits.
	3. No abnormalities such as ovarian cysts, tubal pathology, masses, or foreign bodies (broken IUDs) are seen.

condition coupled with careful scrutiny of BBT charts for synchrony of sperm deposition with ovulation before fertilization. Continuous monitoring and management of thyroid function during pregnancy is also carried out. The same thyroid aberrations have occasionally been associated with unaltered reproductive ability.

In the presence of severe emotional problems the woman is referred to a mental health therapist. Her condition may require the teamwork of the mental health therapist, the endocrinologist, and an obstetrician-gynecologist.

Diazepam (Valium) ingestion may be responsible for menstrual irregularities or failure to ovulate, changes in libido, and gynecomastia, possibly by raising estrogen levels. These effects can be reversed simply by withdrawing from the drug.

Tubal (peritoneal) factors
Review of tubal function. The fingerlike processes of the fimbriated end of the uterine tube and the tube itself need to be freely movable in order to approach the ovary to "catch" the ovum. The tube must be open, sufficiently long, and capable of ciliary action

Postcoital Test

Who: Both the woman and the man
Why: To test for adequacy of coital technique, cervical mucus, sperm, and degree of sperm penetration
How: Assessment of specimen of cervical mucus following ejaculation of semen into vagina
When: 8 to 24 hours following sexual intercourse that is synchronized with expected time of ovulation (as determined from evaluation of BBT, cervical mucus changes, and usual length of menstrual cycle); performed only in the absence of vaginal infection
Where: Clinic or office
Risk: 1. Low; physically safe; no anesthesia is needed because having this test feels about the same as having a Papanicolaou smear
2. May be difficult to have intercourse with ejaculation "on schedule"; sex "on demand" may strain the couple's interpersonal relationship
3. Expected day of ovulation may occur when facilities or physician is unavailable

Procedure	Information Sought

■ Couple is asked to abstain from intercourse for 48 hours before test commences.
■ Then intercourse with ejaculation into vaginal vault should occur within the 8 hours before the test.
■ Woman may shower but not bathe between time of intercourse and test
■ Within 24 hours after intercourse, but preferably 8 hours, in the office or clinic:
  1. Woman is positioned in lithotomy position and draped; speculum is inserted without lubrication (no lubrication is needed at this time because mucus is abundant and the lubricant may alter the viscosity of the cervical mucus and invalidate the results); cervix is cleansed.
  2. Mucus is removed with a nasal polyp forceps or dressing forceps from the internal and the external cervical os and examined for macroscopic and microscopic characteristics.
	Findings favorable to fertility:
	1. Coital technique is adequate if sperm is found.
	2. Mucus is supportive if many sperm are motile.
	3. If more than 20 motile sperm are found, male most likely produces at least 20 million/ml.*
	4. Mucus is clear and abundant, with good spinnbarkeit.
	5. A drop of each specimen is used for the fern test; with high estrogen at ovulation, fern pattern (arborization) is seen (Fig. 5.32, *A*).

*Postcoital test is *not* a substitute for semen analysis.

and peristalsis to carry the ovum into and down the tube. In most cases fertilization occurs in the ampulla of the tube. Some unknown factor, possibly an enzyme, supplied by the ampulla of the tube seems to be required for the physiologic change or "conditioning" of the sperm called capacitation (see Chapter 8).

Impairment of tubal function. The motility of the tube and its fimbriated end may be reduced or absent as a result of infections, adhesions, or tumors. In rare instances there may be congenital absence of one tube. It is also possible to find one tube relatively shorter than the other. This condition is often associated with an abnormally developed uterus.

Inflammation within the tube or involving the exterior of the tube or the fimbriated ends represents a major cause of infertility. Tubal adhesions resulting from pelvic infections (e.g., ruptured appendix) may cause infertility. Infection with purulent discharge eventually heals by scar formation. In the process the tube may be blocked anywhere along its length. It can

be closed off at the fimbriated end, or it can be distorted and kinked by adhesions. Adhesions may permit the tiny sperm to pass through the tube but may prevent a fertilized egg from completing the journey into the intrauterine cavity. This results in an ectopic pregnancy that may completely destroy the tube (see discussion of ectopic pregnancy).

In other cases, adhesions of the tubes to the ovary or bowel may follow *endometriosis*. Endometriosis is a disease in which endometrial tissue, ordinarily found only within the uterus, is present outside the uterus attached to other organs or tissue in the woman's body. The ectopic endometrial tissue responds to hormonal stimulation in the way that uterine endometrium does. In endometriosis, periodic monthly bleeding from endometrial implants causes dense adhesions, making pregnancy difficult or impossible.

Treatment and prognosis. Treatment must include prevention and early adequate management of infection with appropriate antibiotics. Surgery may be nec-

Rubin's Test

Who: Woman and a driver to take her home
Why: To assess patency of uterine tube or tubes
How: Tubal insufflation with carbon dioxide gas (Fig. 7.1)
When: 2 to 6 days following menses to avoid forcing possible fertilized ovum through tube into peritoneal cavity; in the absence of infection to avoid forcing infectious material through tubes into abdomen
Where: Clinic or physician's office
Risk: 1. Low; no exposure to radiation
2. Discomfort: uterine cramping during procedure; referred shoulder pain after procedure
3. False positive readings

Procedure	Information Sought
■ Woman assumes lithotomy position and is draped. ■ Analgesia may be required. ■ Vaginal speculum is inserted; cannula is inserted into cervical os; carbon dioxide gas is passed through cervix to uterus and tubes with the rate and pressure under careful control	Findings favorable to fertility: 1. Woman experiences referred shoulder pain. 2. Auscultation of abdomen reveals passage of air through tubes. 3. Carbon dioxide pressure is below 150 mm Hg. *False results* (tube is patent, but gas flow is obstructed) may result from poor technique or spasms of the tubes. *Possible therapeutic effects* of test: passage of carbon dioxide may clear out tubes or straighten out kinked tubes.

essary when drainage of a serious focus of infection is required. Hysterosalpingography is useful for identification of tubal obstruction and also for the release of blockage. During laparoscopy, delicate adhesions may be divided and removed and endometrial implants may be destroyed by electrocoagulation. Laparotomy and even microsurgery may be required to do extensive repair of the damaged tube. Prognosis is dependent on the degree to which tube patency and function can be restored.

Uterine factors
Review of uterine functions. The uterus must be of sufficient size and shape to permit maintenance of a pregnancy to term. The endometrium must be prepared by estrogen and progesterone and must be healthy for implantation to occur.

Impairment of uterine function. Congenital abnormalities of the uterus are far more common than might be expected. Minor developmental anomalies of the uterus are fairly common; major anomalies occur rarely. Hysterosalpingography may reveal a double uterus or other anomalous congenital variations that included a T-shaped uterus and a boxlike uterus. These types of uteruses have been described in daughters of women who took diethylstilbestrol (DES) during the early months of pregnancy. Endometrial and myometrial *tumors* (e.g., polyps or myomas) may also be revealed by x-ray studies of infertile women.

Asherman's syndrome, uterine adhesion or scar tissue, is characterized by hypomenorrhea or amenorrhea.

The adhesions, which may partially or totally obliterate the uterine cavity, are sequelae to surgical interventions such as too vigorous curettage (scraping) after an abortion (elective or spontaneous). The hysteroscope is useful in the verification of intrauterine scars as well as for the localization and removal of displaced or broken intrauterine devices (IUDs).

Endometritis (inflammation of the endometrium) may result from any of the causes of infection of the

Fig. 7.1
Carbon dioxide escapes into abdominal cavity through patent left uterine tube.

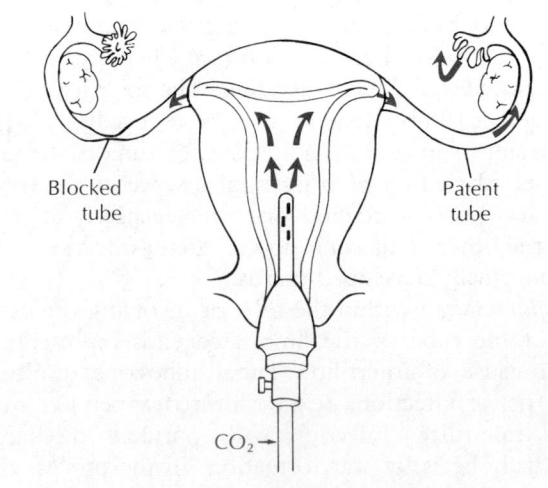

Laparoscopic Examination

Who: Woman and a driver to take her home
Why: To assess visually the organs in the interior of the abdomen; and to perform minor surgical procedures
How: A small telescope is inserted through a small incision in the anterior abdominal wall using cold fiberoptic light sources that allow for superior visualization of the internal pelvis (Fig. 7.2)
When: Laparoscopy is timed depending on the purpose: if tubal patency is to be assessed, it is done 2 to 6 days following cessation of menses; if sites of endometriosis are to be treated, any day of the cycle is appropriate
Where: In a surgical suite with an anesthesiologist present (may be done on an outpatient basis)
Risk: 1. Usually general anesthesia is used
2. A pneumoperitoneum is established by insufflation of carbon dioxide gas via a needle inserted through the abdominal wall.
3. Complications are rare (about 1 in 500): infection; electric burns of intraabdominal tissue
4. Postoperative shoulder (referred) pain or subcostal discomfort may occur for a short time

Procedure	Information Sought
■ Woman signs informed consent and is prepared verbally for the examination.	Findings favorable to fertility:
■ Woman is usually admitted a few hours before surgery having taken nothing by mouth (NPO) for 8 hours.	1. No developmental abnormalities of pelvic structures.
■ Woman voids just before surgery.	2. No lesions, infections, or adhesions.
■ Her pubic area is shaved only if examination is likely to be followed by laparotomy.	3. No complications occur as a result of the examination or procedure.
■ Anesthesia is given: general anesthesia with intubation; occasionally, local.	4. If tubal insufflation is done, the tubes are found to be patent.
■ Woman is placed in a modified lithotomy position, with the legs at 45 degrees.	5. If there is a reparable problem (e.g., adhesions that are kinking the uterine tubes), the problem is repaired through the laparoscope.
■ The vagina, perineum, and abdomen are prepared and draped, and the area from the umbilicus to the vagina is exposed.	
■ An intrauterine probe is inserted except in cases where intrauterine pregnancy may be present.	

■ A needle is inserted and a pneumoperitoneum with carbon dioxide gas is established to elevate the abdominal wall from the organs. The needle may be inserted at lower border of umbilicus.

■ Examination or procedure is performed.

■ After surgery, deflation of most of gas is done by direct expression. Trocar (and needle) sites are closed with a single subcuticular absorbable suture or a skin clip, and an adhesive bandage is applied.

■ Postoperative recovery requires taking of vital signs, assessing level of consciousness, preventing aspiration, monitoring IV fluids, and reassuring client regarding shoulder discomfort. Discharge from hospital usually occurs in 4 to 6 hours.

■ Shoulder or subcostal discomfort (from pneumoperitoneum) usually lasts only 24 hours and is relieved with a mild analgesic.

■ Caution the woman against heavy lifting or strenuous activity for 4 to 7 days, at which time she is usually asymptomatic.

Fig. 7.2

Laparoscopy, in which carbon dioxide lifts abdominal wall off intraabdominal contents, creating an empty space that permits visualization and exploration with laparoscope. Rubin's cannula is used for injections of methylene blue dye to assess for tubal patency.

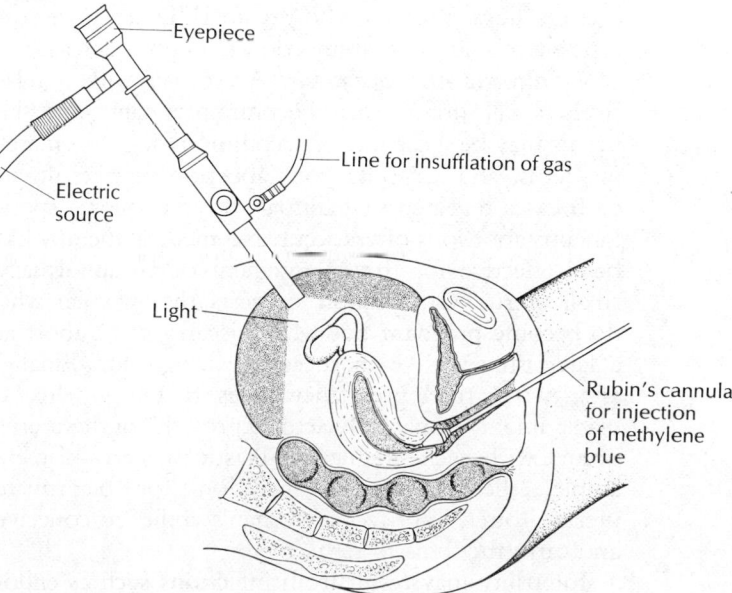

Hysterosalpingography

Who: Woman and a driver to take her home
Why: To assess tubal patency and endometrial cavity to a lesser degree; to assess uterine mobility
How: Fluoroscopic visualization (image intensification fluoroscopy) or spread of radiopaque dye
When: 2 to 6 days after menstruation to avoid flushing a fertilized ovum out through a tube into the peritoneal cavity; if the woman has pelvic inflammatory disease (PID), she is treated with antibiotics first, and the test is rescheduled in 2 to 3 months
Where: Radiology department
Risk:
1. Allergy to radiopaque dye
2. Possible need for premedication
3. Exposure to radiation
4. Discomfort: uterine cramping during procedure; referred shoulder pain after procedure
5. Need for someone to drive her home if medicated or in pain

Procedure	Information Sought

■ Woman may be premedicated.
■ Woman assumes lithotomy position and is draped.
■ Vaginal speculum is inserted.
■ Dye is instilled into uterus with a special cannula inserted into the cervical canal. Dye (Ethiodol*) is injected under controlled pressure.
■ Usually three films are taken:
  1. Before dye instillation
  2. As dye spills out from one or both tubes.
  3. After dye has spread throughout cavity.
■ The shoulder pain:
  1. Subsides with position change.
  2. Disappears usually within 12 to 24 hours.
  3. Is controlled by mild analgesics.
■ Perineal pad is applied to protect clothing from dye.
	Findings favorable to fertility:
	1. Spilling of dye into peritoneum within 10 to 15 minutes.
	2. Spread of dye throughout peritoneal cavity.
	3. Referred shoulder pain. Shoulder pain is indicative of subphrenic irritation from the chemical if the chemical spilled into peritoneal cavity.
	Possible therapeutic effects of test:
	1. Passage of dye may clear tubes of mucous plugs, straighten kinked tubes, or break up adhesions.
	2. Cilia may be stimulated in the lining of the tubes.
	3. It may aid healing as a result of the bacteriostatic effect of dye (iodine).

*Ethiodol, a liquid, oil-based dye, produces a better picture, has a lower incidence of injection pain, and results in better post-hysterosalpingography pregnancy rates than does water-soluble sodium acetrizoate (Salpix). Embolization and possible death are extremely rare but have occurred after hysterosalpingography with either Ethiodol or Salpix. Therefore informed consent should state this fact.

uterine tubes. Women who use an IUD are more susceptible to endometrial infection than are nonusers.

Treatment and prognosis. A woman with a relatively small uterus may become pregnant, but the uterus may be incapable of accommodating the enlarging fetus, and a spontaneous abortion may result. In such cases repeated or habitual (three or more) spontaneous abortions often occur. No medical therapy has been effective for the enlargement of an abnormally small uterus. Observation suggests that women who do become pregnant but who miscarry often abort at a later time with each successive pregnancy. Finally, after two or three pregnancy losses, they may deliver a viable infant. Apparently actual "growth" of the uterus occurs with each pregnancy. Plastic surgery—for example, the unification operation for bicornuate uterus—often improves a woman's ability to conceive and carry the fetus to term.

Infertility may result from infections such as endometrial tuberculosis (from an acid-fast bacillus) or schistosomiasis (from a fluke parasite), which are significant health problems in many parts of the world including the Near East, Puerto Rico, and South America. These disorders often involve the tubes and ovaries. Medical cure of the infection may permit pregnancy despite some scarring of the endometrium.

Surgical removal of tumors involving the endometrium or uterus often improves the woman's chance of conceiving and maintaining the pregnancy to viability. Surgical treatment of uterine tumors or maldevelopment that results in successful pregnancy requires delivery by cesarean surgery near term. The uterus may rupture as a result of weakness of the area of surgical healing.

Vaginal-cervical factors

Review of vaginal-cervical function. Vaginal fluid is acid (pH of 4 or less), whereas cervical mucus is normally alkaline (pH of 7 or more). Ejaculation should place the sperm at or near the cervical os. The alkalin-

Timed Endometrial Biopsy

Who: Woman and a driver to take her home
Why: To assess function of corpus luteum and receptivity of endometrium for implantation; and to check for tuberculosis*
How: Sample of endometrium is removed for histologic study
When: Late in menstrual cycle; 3 to 4 days before expected menses
Where: Clinic or hospital surgical suite
Risk: 1. Analgesia and anesthesia (paracervical block, p. 173) may be needed
2. Discomfort from uterine cramping

Procedure	Information Sought
■ Couple is cautioned to abstain from intercourse during preceding "fertile" period to avoid dislodging a possible pregnancy during procedure. ■ Cervix is dilated with laminaria† 4 to 24 hours before procedure (requires no analgesia). ■ Woman assumes lithotomy position, is draped, and has a speculum inserted. ■ Laminaria are removed. ■ If not previously dilated with laminaria, cervix is dilated now with metal rod dilators. Analgesia/anesthesia is often necessary. ■ Small specimen of endometrium is removed from side wall in fundus to avoid an embryo should conception have occurred.‡	Findings favorable to fertility: 1. Endometrium is negative for tuberculosis, polyps, or inflammatory conditions. 2. Endometrium reflects secretory changes normally seen in presence of adequate luteal (progesterone) phase.

*The incidence of tuberculosis is high today because large numbers of recent refugees have come to the United States with the disease.
†Laminaria are small, thin inserts of packed seaweed, which, when inserted into the cervix, absorb moisture and thus dilate the cervix (Fig. 7.10).
‡When implantation occurs, it is usually high in the fundus, either in the anterior or in the posterior portion.

ity of cervical mucus helps support sperm and permits the ascending transportation of sperm at the time of ovulation.

In addition, endocervical mucus normally obstructs or plugs the cervix, acting as a barrier against infection. The latter is important because, in the woman, ascending infection to the peritoneum is virtually unimpeded with a normally patent genital tract. Alkaline mucus in the cervix not only controls procreation but also is a specific protection to life and health. The amount of cervical mucus and its characteristics are influenced by the hormones estrogen and progesterone (see Table 9.3).

Impairment of vaginal-cervical function. Vaginal-cervical infections (e.g., *Trichomonas* vaginitis) increase the acidity of the vaginal fluid and reduce the alkalinity of the cervical mucus. Thus vaginal infection often destroys or drastically reduces the number of viable, motile sperm before they enter the cervical canal. The amount of mucus and its physical changes are influenced by the presence of blood, pathogenic bacteria, and such irritants as an IUD or a tumor. Severe emotional stress, antibiotic therapy, and diseases such as diabetes mellitus alter the acidity of mucus.

About 20% of infertile women have sperm antibod-ies.* Sperm may be immobilized within the cervical mucus, or they become incapable of migration into the uterus. A greater incidence of sperm agglutination occurs in women with otherwise unexplained infertility. However, the true significance and reliability of tests for sperm immobilization or agglutination are uncertain.

Treatment and prognosis. Therapy for lower genital infection requires the elimination of vaginitis or cervicitis. Appropriate antibiotic or chemotherapeutic drugs generally resolve this problem. In addition to antibiotics, radial chemocautery (destruction of tissue with chemicals) or thermocautery (destruction of tissue with heat, usually electrical) of the cervix, cryosurgery (destruction of tissue by application of extreme cold, usually liquid nitrogen), or conization (excision of a cone-shaped piece of tissue from the endocervix) is effective in eliminating chronic infection. When the cervix has been deeply cauterized or frozen or when extensive conization has been performed, extreme limitation of mucus production by the cervix may result.

*The production of antibodies by one member of a species against something that is commonly found within that species is termed *isoimmunization*.

Therefore sperm migration may be difficult or impossible because of the absence of a mucous "bridge" from the vagina to the uterus. Artificial insemination may be necessary to carry the sperm directly to the *internal os* of the cervix.

If the cervical os is unusually small, it is often called a pinhole os. In such cases, gentle dilatation of the cervix or several shallow radial incisions followed by dilatation are often sufficient to open the lower cervix. In contrast, if the cervix is grossly lacerated after delivery and widely gapping, suturing the cervix (trachelorrhaphy) or cryosurgery may be required to reduce the size of the external os. Prevention of recurrent infection helps to maintain a column of mucus.

Good general hygiene must be practiced to minimize vaginal infections. The woman benefits from good hand washing before and following elimination of urine and stool. To avoid self-contamination, she must wipe from front to back once with each tissue and never wipe back and forth over the perineal area. Feminine deodorants, soaps that are heavily colored and perfumed, bubble-bath salts that cause chemical irritation, and tight clothing that provide a dark damp milieu favorable to microbial growth are avoided. Good nutrition is practiced with the avoidance of large amounts of unrefined sugars which raise the pH of vaginal fluids. To maintain a healthy vaginal-cervical pH during antibiotic therapy, the woman may insert one or two applicators full of cultured yogurt (not pasteurized) once or twice daily. As a general rule, douching is avoided unless by prescription from a physician.

Good mental health helps to prevent some forms of vaginitis that could become secondarily infected. Stress from anxiety, worry, and emotional discomfort increases the vaginal pH so that vaginal infections are more likely to take hold. Concurrent medical conditions such as diabetes mellitus must be controlled to maintain vaginal-cervical pH within normal range.

Treatment is available for women who have immunologic reactions to sperm. Exposure to semen via the orogenital and anal modes is avoided. The use of condoms during genital intercourse for 6 to 12 months will reduce female antibody production in the majority of women who have elevated antisperm antibody titers. After the serum reaction subsides, condoms are used at all times except at the expected time of ovulation. Approximately one third of couples with this problem conceive by following this course of action.

The prognosis for the infertile woman is generally good provided a serious genital or inflammatory disorder is not identified. Most women present numerous so-called minor problems that, although compounded, may be relatively easy to correct (e.g., chronic cervicitis, hypothyroidism). If successful treatment has not been achieved after a year, for example, other alternatives may be considered (e.g., adoption, childlessness, artificial insemination, or in vitro fertilization).

In vitro fertilization. The first successful term delivery of an infant conceived by in vitro fertilization (test-tube pregnancy) in 1978 was the culmination of years of study and experimentation by Robert Edwards and Patrick Steptoe in England. Since then several other "laboratory conceived" and normal-appearing newborns have been delivered.

Many women whose uterine tubes either are obstructed or have been removed are now potential candidates for similar treatment. However, because of the complexity and cost of the procedure, the likelihood is that this approach to infertility must remain limited for the near future. The following steps, ultrasimplified, are necessary for in vitro fertilization.
1. Ovulation is induced by gonadotropin therapy.
2. Mature follicles are identified by laparoscopy, and needle aspiration of ova is carried out.
3. Ova are transferred to tissue culture media, and the sperm are added.
4. After fertilization a second tissue culture transfer allows division to approximately a 12-cell blastocyst (3 to 6 days).
5. Progesterone therapy in the interval induces a late secretory type of endometrium, whereupon the blastocyst is transferred to the uterus, where the implantation (nidation) of the zygote occurs and embryonic development proceeds.

Within an 18-month period, overall success rates for in vitro fertilization worldwide have risen from 1% to 8% to almost 20%. This vast improvement is attributable to increased precision in predicting ovulation and in retrieving the ovum. The conventional methods of predicting ovulation—calendar, BBT, cervical mucus, fertility awareness, and laboratory tests such as vaginal cytology and serum hormone determination—can only approximate the moment of ovulation. The more precise methods are beyond the scope of this text but are mentioned here for interest. These methods are (1) stimulating ovulation with clomiphene citrate (Clomid) or human menopausal gonadotropin (HMG) (Pergonal) given at a precise time during the cycle, (2) monitoring ovulatory function with real-time ultrasound, and (3) performing rapid radioimmunoassay for estrogen level. Through a laparoscope the ovum is retrieved by inserting an aspiration needle into the ripened follicle and removing the ovum. The husband's semen is collected and treated before its use for fertilization of the ovum. The complete procedure is described by Marrs (1982).

Human experimentation and manipulation of this type have been sanctioned by the United States Department of Health and Human Services. The Roman

Table 7.3
Substance Abuse and Male Infertility

Substance	Possible Effects
Alcohol	Causes erectile problems ("impotence").
Marijuana (Cannabis sativa)	Adversely affects spermatogenesis: decreases number and motility, decreases percentages of sperm with the normal oval configuration.
	Potential permanent damage to germ cells (does not seem to affect testosterone production, however).
	Causes gynecomastia, especially if taken in combination with psychoactive and antidepressant drugs.
Monoamine oxidase (MAO) (antidepressant)	Adversely affects spermatogenesis.
Amyl nitrate, butyl nitrate, ethyl chloride, methaqualone (used to prolong orgasm)	Results in changes in spermatogenesis.
Heroin, methadone, barbiturates	Decreases libido.

Catholic Church is strongly opposed to in vitro fertilization. Legal aspects of in vitro fertilization are discussed in Chapter 3.

INVESTIGATION OF MALE INFERTILITY

Factors implicated in male infertility. Male reproductive failure may be caused by many of the difficulties that also affect women, such as nutritional, endocrine, and psychologic disorders. In Table 7.1 each factor essential to fertility is presented, along with a listing of conditions associated with infertility. Assessment for male fertility factors is outlined on p. 133. Substance abuse may have adverse effects on male infertility (Table 7.3).

Semen is analyzed early in the diagnostic process. A sperm analysis is done at least twice to determine whether oligospermia or other abnormalities are likely.

Summary of Fertility Test Findings Favorable to Fertility

1. Follicular development, ovulation, and luteal development are supportive to pregnancy:
   a. BBT(presumptive evidence of ovulatory cycles)
      (1) Is biphasic
      (2) Reveals temperature elevation that persists for 12 to 14 days just before menstruation
   b. Cervical mucus characteristics change appropriately during phases of the menstrual cycle
   c. Findings from endometrial biopsies taken at different times during menstrual cycle are consistent with day of cycle
   d. Laparoscopic visualization of pelvic organs verifies follicular and luteal development
2. The luteal phase is supportive to pregnancy:
   a. Levels of plasma progesterone are adequate
   b. Endometrial biopsy findings indicate a secretory endometrium
3. Cervical factors are receptive to sperm during expected time of ovulation:
   a. Cervical os is open
   b. Cervical mucus is clear, watery, abundant, and slippery and demonstrates good spinnbarkeit and arborization (fern pattern)
   c. Cervical examination is negative for lesions and infections
   d. Postcoital test findings are satisfactory (adequate number of live, motile, normal sperm present in cervical mucus)
   e. No immunity to sperm can be demonstrated
4. The uterus and uterine tubes are supportive to pregnancy:
   a. Uterine and tubal patency is documented by
      (1) Passage of carbon dioxide into peritoneal cavity
      (2) Spillage of dye into peritoneal cavity
      (3) Outlines of uterine and tubal cavities of adequate size and shape with no abnormalities
   b. Laparoscopic examination verifies normal development of internal genitals and absence of adhesions, infections, endometriosis, and other lesions
5. Semen is supportive to pregnancy:
   a. Sperm are adequate in number per milliliter
   b. Majority of sperm show normal morphology
   c. Sperm are motile
   d. No autoimmunity exists
   e. Seminal fluid is normal

Table 7.4
Male Infertility Factors, Tests, and Nursing Actions

Infertility Factor	Tests	Nursing Actions
Physical		
Semen composition	Microscopic analysis: sperm density, motility, structure	Counsel regarding collection of specimen
Absence or decreased number of sperm: ambiguous genitals; disparity of testicular size	Testicular biopsy	Preoperative preparation for general anesthesia Postoperative: ice bag to scrotum, suspensory, mild analgesics
Small gonads, inadequate virilization	Karyotyping for chromosomal abnormality Determination of gonadotropin levels	Assist with protocol of care
Obstructive lesions of vas and epididymis	Vasography often done with testicular biopsy or x-ray examination using contrast medium	Preoperative and postoperative care as above.
Integrity of hypothalamic-pituitary-testicular axis	Clomiphene citrate (Clomid) stimulation of pituitary to release LH and FSH GNRH stimulation* of pituitary to release LH and FSH HCG stimulation of Leydig cell function and increased testosterone production	Counsel regarding oral ingestion for the 5-7 days preceding the test Assist in office or clinic Assist with protocols for test in office or clinic
Infections—viral (mumps) or bacterial (tuberculosis or gonorrhea)	Assessment for current infection	Counsel regarding need to follow directions for antibiotic therapy; use of oral lactinex or lacto-bacillus or cultured yogurt to prevent gastrointestinal upset from antibiotic therapy
Semen volume	Measurement of volume following 2-3 days of abstinence from ejaculation	Counsel regarding protocols for abstention, collection, and transportation to laboratory
Sperm agglutination and *Sperm immobilization antigen-antibody reaction*	Assessment for infection (*E. coli*); Kibrick (agglutination) and Isojima (immobilization) test for circulating and seminal sperm agglutinating autoantibodies	
Sperm antibodies	Serum tests (e.g., Kibrick, Isojima)	Assist with protocols for tests
Retrograde ejaculation†	Measurement of ejaculate volume and assessment for sperm in urine after ejaculation	Assist with protocols for tests
Varicocele	Physical examination	Assist as indicated
Trauma—long-term catheterization, foreign objects in urethra (e.g., hair-pin)	Physical examination	Assist as indicated
Testis torsion	Physical examination; history of sudden onset with intense pain or recurrent, less severe orchidynia (pain)	Assist as indicated; prepare for surgery as above
Psychosocial		
Male sexual dysfunction	Psychiatric and physical work-up	Provide caring, nonjudgmental attitude and an unrushed and confidential milieu; assist the physician to dispel misinformation and reassure client regarding her/his behavior.‡
Religious proscriptions	History	Assist as indicated; counsel regarding approaching clergy/rabbi with problems/concerns.

*Experimental.
†Passage of semen deposited into prostatic urethra during emission back into the bladder through an imcompetent bladder neck.
‡Requires special education and skills.

Table 7.5
Drug Therapy for Male Infertility

Drug	Indications	Nursing Actions
Testosterone enanthate (Delatestryl) and testosterone cypionate (Depotesterone) by injection	Stimulate virilization, especially the adolescent	Teach self-administration or administer every 2 weeks
HCG (Pregnyl), IM (LH activity)	Virilize a hypogonadotropic male to restore Leydig cell function and spermatogenesis	Administer three times a week, perhaps for 18 months.
FSH (human menopausal gonadotropin [HMG], Pergonal)	Aid HCG for completion of spermatogenesis	Administer three times a week
Bromocriptine (ergot derivative and dopamine agonist, Parlodel)	Treat hypogonadotropic hypogonadism-associated prolactin-producing hypothalamic or pituitary tumors; may reduce the tumor	Counsel regarding oral ingestion with food to decrease side effects: dizziness, fainting, hypotension, headache, nausea, vomiting
Adrenal corticoids specific for the condition	Addison's disease Cushing's disease Congenital adrenal hypoplasia	Practice general medical nursing
Clomiphene citrate (Clomid)	Idiopathic subfertility	Counsel regarding oral ingestion every day or every other day in cyclic fashion (25 days followed by 5-day rest period; repeat)
Vitamin C (ascorbic acid, a reducing agent)	Sperm agglutination where there are no autoantibodies	Counsel regarding oral ingestion of 500 mg three times a day indefinitely
Methylprednisolone (Medrol)	Steroid immunosuppression of sperm autoantibodies	Counsel regarding oral ingestion: 96 mg/d for 7 days starting the first regimen on day 21 of the woman's cycle, then every 4 weeks for 3 months
Sputolysin (mucolytic agent)	Increased seminal viscosity; used to wash semen before artificial seminal liquefaction	Counsel regarding use as precoital douching agent
α-Amylase	Delayed seminal liquefaction	Counsel regarding use as precoital douching agent or cocoa-butter vaginal suppository

Before collecting a specimen the man avoids ejaculation for 2 to 3 days. Then he collects a specimen from masturbation in a clean glass jar and takes the sealed jar to the laboratory within 2 hours after emission. Warming or chilling the specimen is not required. The Roman Catholic man may prefer to remove ejaculated sperm from the woman's vagina with a Doyle (vaginal) spoon. A condom should not be used for collection of the semen (unless a special sheath manufactured by the Milex Corporation is used), since any residual rubber solvents and sulfur present would alter the specimen. The semen is examined for gross appearance and other characteristics (p. 133 and Fig. 8.7).

A summary of infertility factors, tests, and nursing actions are presented in Table 7.4. Fertility test findings favorable to fertility are summarized on p. 143.

General therapies. *Medical therapy* for male infertility has been disappointing, especially when pituitary or testicular diseases are discovered. Occasionally it is possible to suppress the production of sperm with injections of testosterone and in that way cause a reduction in the number of autoimmune antibodies present in the man. Following the reduction in sperm autoantibodies, sperm quality improves, and a pregnancy sometimes occurs. Drug therapy for male infertility is discussed in Table 7.5.

The difficulty may be caused by timing and frequency of intercourse. The couple is taught about the menstrual cycle, the peak cervical mucus symptom, and appropriate timing of intercourse.

Penile intromission is often difficult because of chordee and obesity. In these situations the couple is advised to alter positions used for intercourse. Heavy use of alcohol makes penile erection difficult to achieve and maintain until ejaculation. The man is advised to avoid imbibing alcohol during the time of the woman's ovulation.

Infections (e.g., T mycoplasma) are identified and treated promptly. Poor nutritional state is corrected if it exists. Problems with the thyroid or adrenal glands are corrected.

Surgical repair of varicocele* has been relatively

---

*Varicocele refers to varicose veins of the spermatic vein in the groin. The swollen, distended veins press on the testes and impair their function.

successful. A varicocele on the left side is found in a substantial number of subfertile men. Ligation of the varicocele does lead to improvement of the sperm quality and frequently to pregnancy.

Simple changes in life-style may be effective in the treatment of subfertile men. High temperatures in the groin area reduced the number of sperm produced. High temperatures may be caused by the wearing of brief shorts and tight jeans that keep the scrotal sac pressed against the body regardless of environmental temperature changes. The testes are kept at temperatures too high for efficient spermatogenesis. Frequent and prolonged hot tubbing has also been implicated in relative infertility. It must be remembered that these conditions only lead to relative infertility and should not be employed as a means of contraception.

Artificial insemination. The term *homologous insemination* (artificial insemination by husband, or AIH) denotes the use of the husband's semen. The term *heterologous insemination* (artificial insemination by donor, or AID) denotes the use of the semen of a donor other than the husband.

When the husband's sperm has poor quality or mo-

tility, several semen samples are collected from him. The samples consist of split ejaculates, that is, the sperm rich *first portion* only is collected for freezing and later pooling for AIH. Rapid freezing with liquid nitrogen and subsequent thawing do not cause genetic damage even after 10 years' storage using glycerol. Pooling should increase the sperm count and improve the placement of a portion of the total semen specimen at the cervical os.

Assuming normal female fertility, AIH at or about the time of ovulation has resulted in pregnancy in as many as 70% of cases. Numerous inseminations may be necessary to ensure proper timing at ovulation. The basal body temperature (BBT) and cervical mucus record help to determine when to attempt insemination. Approximately 50% of pregnancies with AID will occur within 2 months; almost 90% occur within 6 months.

Insemination directly into the uterine cavity should be avoided because of severe cramping (prostaglandin effect) and possible infection. The recommended procedure is the instillation of about 0.5 ml of the specimen into the cervical canal with the remainder depos-

Table 7.6
Client Behavior Associated with Infertility: Nursing Actions

Behavioral Characteristic	Nursing Actions
Surprise: each person assumes she or he is fertile and that pregnancy is an option	Point out resemblance to grieving process—a normal, expected reaction to loss. Refer to support group.*
	Prepare them for length of time it may take to grieve, types of feelings (psychologic, somatic) to expect.
	Encourage and allow time to talk of past and present feelings of sexuality, self-image, and self-esteem.
Denial: "It can't happen to me!"	Allow time for denial because it gives the body and mind time to adjust a little at a time.
	Do not feed into the client's denial; instead say, "It must be hard to believe such a devastating report."
Anger: toward others (perhaps even at the nurse) or themselves	Explain that the reaction to loss of control and to a feeling of helplessness is often anger, which can easily be projected toward another person. Without release, anger can lead to chronic depression. Anger is a natural feeling.
	Allow time to express anger at losing their sense of control over their bodies and destinies; identify and direct energy directly at the problem. Airing one's anger often eases the intensity of the emotion.
	A helpful approach may be, "It's OK to be angry . . . at those who are pregnant, at people who want abortions, at self, at mate, at care-givers, and so forth."
Bargaining: "If I get pregnant, I'll dedicate the child to God"	Accept bargaining statement without comment.
Depression:	
Isolation: personal	Allow time for both woman and man to talk about how it feels whenever a sight, event, or word serves as a reminder of own infertile state.
	Develop role-playing situations to practice interactions with others under various circumstances to increase the couple's ability to cope and to problem solve (increases their self-confidence).
	The nurse may say, "You must feel so terribly alone sometimes."
Guilt/unworthiness	Allow time to identify feelings that may be based on earlier behaviors (e.g., abortion, premarital sex, contact with sexually transmitted disease [STD]).
	Goal: couple or person comes to the realization that "unworthiness" and infertility are unrelated.
Acceptance (resolution)	Clients need to know that grief feelings are never laid away forever; they may be activated by special reminders (e.g., anniversaries).

*RESOLVE, Inc., P.O. Box 474, Boston, MA 02178.

ited in a cervical cap or a cleanly washed contraceptive diaphragm to be worn by the woman for about an hour.

Insemination with the husband's semen presents no legal problems, but heterologous insemination (insemination with a combination of husband and donor sperm) involves many legal, ethical, and emotional aspects. The couple must know there is no guarantee of pregnancy and that in either instance the spontaneous abortion rate is approximately the same as in a control population. There is no increase in maternal or perinatal complications; that is, the same frequency of anomalies (about 5%) and obstetric complications (between 5 % and 10%) that accompanies normal insemination applies also to AID.

The decision for artificial insemination with donor sperm should be made only after thorough considera-

tion and discussion. The implications for the long-term welfare of the child as well as the parents must be considered.

SUMMARY

The management of infertility is primarily the responsibility of the physician. However, the nurse may assist in a number of ways. Nursing actions vary with the nurse's level of education, position held, and policies of the agency. The nursing actions are planned in collaboration with the physician, with other members of the health team, and with the couple to achieve mutually derived goals. A summary of nursing actions is presented below, and examples of nursing actions for client behavior associated with infertility are provided in Table 7.6.

Summary of Nursing Actions

INFERTILITY

GOALS
1. To identify factors causing infertility.
2. To treat conditions that are treatable.
3. To maintain client's self-esteem and sense of adequacy as a woman or man.
4. To help client maintain control over his or her destiny through active participation in the decision-making process.

PRIORITIES
1. Clients become active partners in the management of their infertility through encouragement, education, and support.
2. Infertility factors are identified and treated, if possible.

ASSESSMENT	EXAMPLES OF POTENTIAL NURSING DIAGNOSTIC CATEGORIES*
Interview	
1. Health history	Disturbance in self-concept: body image, self-esteem, role performance, personal identity
	Powerlessness
	Alteration in family process
	Ineffective individual coping
	Spiritual distress
2. Psychosocial history	Disturbance in self-concept: body image, self-esteem, role performance, personal identity
	Powerlessness
	Alteration in family process
	Ineffective individual coping
	Spiritual distress
3. Review of systems	Disturbance in self-concept: body image, self-esteem, role performance, personal identity
	Anxiety
	Knowledge deficit
Physical examination	Alterations in normal physiologic process
	Knowledge deficit

*Accepted diagnoses from the Seventh National Conference (1986).   *Continued.*

Summary of Nursing Actions

ASSESSMENT	EXAMPLES OF POTENTIAL NURSING DIAGNOSTIC CATEGORIES
Laboratory tests	Knowledge deficit Anxiety Fear Powerlessness Ineffective individual coping Disturbance in self concept: body image, self-esteem, role performance, personal identity

OUTCOME CRITERIA*	PLAN/IMPLEMENTATION
Couple is educated in the anatomy and physiology of the reproductive system. Couple complies with the investigation of infertility. Any abnormalities identified through various tests and examinations are treated (e.g., infections, blocked uterine tubes, sperm allergy, varicocele). Couple receives an estimate of their chances to conceive. Couple resolves guilt feelings and does not need to focus blame. If couple conceives, the couple: a. Accepts their responses to the pregnancy. b. Realigns their goals, aspirations, and identities. c. Is comfortable with their decisions regarding this pregnancy (e.g., abortion, continue with pregnancy and keep the child, give the child up for adoption). If couple does not conceive, the couple: a. Decides on an alternative that is acceptable to both of them (e.g., childlessness, adoption, artificial insemination, or in vitro fertilization). b. Seeks support as necessary (e.g., RESOLVE, National Organization for NonParents). Couple finds acceptable methods for handling pressures they may feel from peers and relatives regarding their childless state. Couple receives list of community agencies that assist with adoptions (OURS†, ARENA) or that provide support (RESOLVE, National Organization for NonParents).	Plan and implement nursing roles of support person, teacher/counselor/advocate, and technician: **Support person** Greet the woman and her family by name. Provide privacy as needed while giving instructions for obtaining specimens and changing clothes and while identifying feelings, myths, misinformation, or "magical thinking" about the cause of infertility. Encourage discussion about the loss of spontaneity and control over the couple's marital relationship and sometimes over one's progress toward career and goals while undergoing the tests. Explore the couple's support systems, their relationship with the couple, their ages, their availability, and available cultural or religious support *If couple conceives,* be prepared for a variety of reactions from anger to joy. Some couples have come to terms with their infertility and have rearranged their lives; pregnancy disrupts the changes. a. Assist couple with identification and expression of their feelings. b. Offer the same type of care offered to other pregnant couples. c. If they choose to continue with the pregnancy, be prepared to offer extra preparation for the realities of pregnancy, labor, and parenthood. *(A history of infertility is considered to be a risk factor for pregnancy.)* d. After delivery, offer information about contraception. *If couple does not conceive,* assist physician in assessing their desire to be referred to help with adoption, artificial insemination or in vitro fertilization, or with choosing childlessness. **Teacher/counselor/advocate** Assists physician in the identification of the client's gaps in knowledge, clarifies information, and reinforces physician's explanations and instructions. Acts as the client's advocate by assisting the client to state a concern or question or to request further explanation. Teaches clients to assess and record BBT and cervical mucus. Helps physician to assess the client's readiness to learn and her or his level of understanding of infertility, diagnostic tests, and therapy.

*Outcome criteria direct the selection of nursing actions (**plan/implementation**) and measure their effectiveness (**evaluation**).
†Lists of such groups throughout the United States can be obtained from OURS, Inc., 20140 Pine Ridge Dr., Anoaka, MN 55303.

Summary of Nursing Actions

OUTCOME CRITERIA	PLAN/IMPLEMENTATION
	Utilizes information in boxes to familiarize clients with tests.
	Provides written and verbal instructions for specific preparation for tests; provides description of sensations client may experience during and after procedures.
	Assists clients to understand and cope with responses/needs commonly associated with infertility (Table 7.6).
	Technician
	Utilizes information in boxes to assemble equipment and to assist physician during testing.
	Assists with pelvic examination, Chapter 11
	Utilizes correct method for obtaining, labeling, and transporting specimens to the laboratory.
	Documents and maintains accurate records.

Evaluation The nurse can be assured that care was effective if the goals have been met.

Control of Fertility: Family Planning and Contraception

The fertile period in humans is relatively short. It is limited to the 24 to 36 hours after ovulation. If 100 normal couples have frequent intercourse, 25% of the couples will conceive the first month, 19% the second, 14% the third, and over the remainder of the year all but four to seven couples will conceive. Therefore if conception is not desired, it is recommended that some method be used to prevent pregnancy.

Contraception is the voluntary prevention of pregnancy having both individual and social implications. It has been established that more than 90% of couples in the United States have used or intend to use some method of birth control (contraception). Family planning is accepted in principle by all religions, but the Roman Catholic Church insists that it be achieved by periodic abstinence alone. The availability of reliable and safe techniques for controlling fertility has meant that parenthood, with its tasks and responsibilities as well as its pleasures, can be willingly assumed by adults who wish to do so. Recent advances in the physiologic safety of prenatal, perinatal, and postnatal existence can now be combined with the psychologic safety of being a wanted child.

Spacing of children is important for promotion of health not only of the mother but also of her children. Quality of the offspring rather than quantity is now emphasized. Moreover, to control excessive world population, voluntary limitation of family size has become important.

Religious considerations. The religion of some groups does not permit the use of contraception. The Catholic Church does not allow contraception. Affonso (1978) studied Filipinos who were predominantly Catholic. In her survey two thirds of the women thought that it would be all right to use contraceptives. Mormons prohibit birth control not as an evil in itself but as an impediment to meeting one's spiritual obligations (Stark, 1982). Samoans represent a variety of religions, but for them contraceptive practices are not highly valued (Clark and Howland, 1978). Rather, priority is placed on demonstration of male and female fertility through childbirth.

Cultural considerations. Cross-cultural information about contraceptive practices is limited. Before modern times, probably the most effective contraception resulted from sexual taboos. Postpartal taboos were generally effective. Kay (1982) points out that the Mexican-Americans she studied continued to place a 40-day restriction on sexual intercourse after childbirth.

In the past, American Indians used herbs as oral contraceptives (Vogel, 1973). Information about these herbs was useful in the development of today's oral contraceptives. Some American Indian groups today favor the use of contraceptives, but others believe that they are against God's will. Although the Japanese were one of the earliest cultural groups to accept the use of birth control and abortion (Okamoto, 1978), Japanese couples are reluctant to use contraception until they have borne one child (Bernstein and Kidd, 1982).

Some subcultural groups in the United States and

Table 7.7
Estimated Annual Deaths Associated with Fertility Control and No Control per 100,000 Fertile Women

Method	Age (years)					
	15-19	20-24	25-29	30-34	35-39	40-44
No method	5.5	5.2	7.1	14.0	19.3	22
Abortion only (legal)	2.3	2.5	2.5	5.2	9.8	6.6
Oral contraceptive only (nonsmoker)	1.3	1.4	1.4	2.2	4.5	3.1
Oral contraceptive only (smoker)	1.5	1.6	1.6	10.8	13.4	59
IUD only	1.1	1.2	1.2	1.4	1.6	1.4
Traditional contraception* only	1.1	1.4	1.9	3.7	4.7	4.0
Traditional contraception with abortion	0.3	0.4	0.4	0.8	1.4	0.8

*Family planning methods, spermicides, and condoms.

in third-world countries believe that the great emphasis placed on family planning is based on the desire of the white middle class to limit minority groups. Darity and Turner (1972) report that a significant group of black Americans is wary of family planning methods.

The ability to control fertility is based on an understanding of the menstrual cycle. According to Scott (1978) a majority of Bahamians, Cubans, Haitians, and Puerto Ricans believe the function of menstruation to be that of ridding the person of unclean waste or unnecessary blood. A large number of Bahamians believe that menstruating means a person is healthy. Less bleeding means that something is wrong. Snow's research (1974) among blacks in parts of western and northern United States also indicates the prevalent belief in impure blood.

If the belief that menstrual flow indicates health or lack of it, anything that would interfere with menstruation would be considered undesirable. The pill, which often reduces the amount of and duration of menstrual-like flow, is considered dangerous to one's health. The intrauterine device (IUD) often affects the cycle and is also considered dangerous.

Family planning and contraception have posed numerous problems for nurses working with persons whose belief systems place a high value on having many children. Nevertheless, many persons with these belief systems are interested in learning about contraception and will listen to explanations if they include respect for another's values. According to Dougherty (1972), health care innovations are accepted or rejected depending on how they fit into the client's cultural pattern.

Methods of control of fertility. There are various contraceptive techniques used in North America. The ideal contraceptive should be safe, easily available, economical, acceptable, simple to use, and promptly reversible. Although no means or method may ever achieve all these objectives, impressive progress has been made recently. Before choosing the "right" con-

traceptive method, several topics need to be discussed: frequency of coitus (once every so often or several times per week); one sexual partner or several; level of involvement each partner wishes to assume; and objections to any methods. The woman or couple must be fully informed of the risks (Tables 7.7 and 7.8), effectiveness, reversibility, and the alternatives (Table 7.9) (see discussion of informed consent, Chapter 3).

Contraception employs one or more of the following methods:

1. Methods available to people without prescription
   a. Natural family planning: biologic periodic abstinence
   b. Chemical barriers: spermicidal creams, gels, or vaginal suppositories and sponges
   c. Mechanical barrier: condoms or sheaths
2. Methods that require periodic medical examination and prescription*
   a. Hormonal therapy: estrogen or progestogen preparations or a combination of these compounds

*Certified nurse-midwives and some certified nurse-practitioners may be educated to provide this service.

Table 7.8
Risk Factors and Degree of Associated Risk by Age for Users of Oral Contraceptives

Risk	Age (years)		
	≤29	30-39	≥40
Heavy smokers (≥15 cigarettes)	2	3	4
Light smokers (≤14 cigarettes)	1	2	3
Nonsmokers with no added risk conditions	1	1,2	2
Nonsmokers with added risk conditions	2	2,3	3,4

1 = Use associated with low risk; 2 = use associated with moderate risk; 3 = use associated with high risk; 4 = use associated with very high risk.

Table 7.9
Contraceptive Methods and Pregnancies per
100 Women

Method of Contraception	Contraceptive Failures (number of pregnancies)*
No method	60-80
Calendar only	14-47
Periodic abstinence	1-47
Jellies/creams	4-36
Condom	3-36
Aerosol foams	2-29
Mucous method	1-25
Diaphragm with spermicide	2-20
BBT only	1-20
BBT with intercourse during postovulatory time	1-7
IUD	1-6
Combination oral contraceptives	1-3

*The fewer the number of pregnancies, the greater the effectiveness.

    b. Mechanical barrier: cervical uterine occlusion by diaphragms or caps
    c. Intrauterine contraceptive devices
3. Methods that require surgical intervention
    a. Female sterilization
    b. Male sterilization

Elective interruption of pregnancy is a surgical procedure that requires sensitivity as well as expert technical skill from health care providers. Methods of elective abortion appropriate for each trimester will be discussed.

METHODS AVAILABLE WITHOUT PRESCRIPTION

Several nonprescription methods for control of fertility are practiced. Prescription and supervision are unnecessary for barrier methods, that is, condom, foam, spermicide, vaginal sponges, and for periodic abstinence. In 1982, among women aged 15 to 44 years practicing contraception, the condom was used by 12.2%, foam by 2.4%, and periodic abstinence by 4% (Bachrach, 1984). Two methods were practiced that are *not* recommended: withdrawal (coitus interruptus). 2% and douching 0.2% (Bachrach, 1984).

Periodic abstinence or "natural" family planning. Periodic abstinence was practiced by 4% of women aged 15 to 44 years practicing contraception in 1982 (Bachrach, 1984). The term *periodic abstinence* is preferred over "natural family planning" for contraceptive methods that rely on avoidance of intercourse during presumed fertile days of the menstrual cycle. Many couples find abstinence for 7 to 18 or more consecutive days of each menstrual cycle to be unnatural (Klaus 1982).

Periodic abstinence methods employ a combination of the following:
1. Rhythm or calendar method
2. BBT method
3. Cervical mucus (Billings, ovulation) method
4. Sympto-thermal method
5. Fertility awareness method
6. Predictor test for ovulation

These methods depend on the continuous observation and recording of events of the menstrual cycle. The woman or couple must be able to assess hormone-induced signs and symptoms that indicate whether she is in the fertile or infertile part of the menstrual cycle. While teaching a woman about fertility awareness, the nurse uses this opportunity for helping the woman or couple learn a great deal about their bodies.

The *mode of action* for these methods of contraception is abstention from intercourse during the fertile period.*

The human ovum can be fertilized no later than 24 to 48 hours after ovulation. Motile sperm have been recovered from the uterus and the oviducts as long as 60 hours after coitus. However, their ability to fertilize the ovum probably lasts no longer than 24 to 48 hours. Pregnancy is unlikely to occur if a couple abstains from intercourse for 4 days before and for 3 or 4 days after ovulation (*fertile period*). Unprotected intercourse on the other days of the cycle (*safe period*) should not result in pregnancy. The principal problems with natural family planning are that the exact time of ovulation cannot be predicted accurately. Couples may also find it difficult to exercise restraint for several days before and after ovulation.

Ovulation usually occurs about 14 days before the onset of menstruation. Therefore variations in the length of menstrual cycles are usually a result of differences in the length of the preovulatory phases. The fertile period can be anticipated by the following:
1. Calculating the time at which ovulation is likely to occur based on the lengths of previous menstrual cycles (*calendar method*)
2. Recording the rise in basal body temperature (BBT), a result of the thermogenic effect of progesterone (*temperature method*)

---

*The World Health Organization (Liskin, 1981) concluded in 1979 that the cervical mucus and sympto-thermal methods "had very limited application, particularly in developing countries, and recommended that the World Health Organization Programme devote no further research to measuring their effectiveness." Similarly, the International Planned Parenthood Federation concluded in 1982 that "couples electing to use periodic abstinence should, however, be clearly informed that the method is not considered an effective method of family planning."

3. Recognizing the changes in cervical mucus at different phases of the menstrual cycle *(ovulation or Billings method)*
4. Using a predictor test for ovulation
5. Utilizing a combination of several methods

Unique developments of monoclonal antibody technology have added a *predictor test* for ovulation. This type of test is a major addition to the natural family planning methods to help women who want to plan the time of their pregnancies and those who are trying to conceive.

Rhythm or calendar method. With the *calendar method* the fertile period is determined after accurately recording the lengths of menstrual cycles for a year. According to the Ogino formula the first unsafe day (beginning of the fertile period) can be determined by subtracting 18 days from the length of the shortest cycle. The last unsafe day (beginning of postovulatory safe period) can be calculated by subtracting 11 days from the length of the longest cycle. If the shortest cycle is 24 days and the longest is 30 days, application of the formula is as follows:

Shortest Cycle	Longest Cycle
24	30
−18	−11
6th day	19th day

To avoid conception the couple would abstain during the "fertile" period, days 6 through 19.

If the woman has very regular cycles of 28 days each, the formula indicates the fertile days to be:

Shortest Cycle	Longest Cycle
28	28
−18	−11
10th day	17th day

To avoid pregnancy, the couple abstains from day 10 through 17 because ovulation occurs on day 14.

Basal body temperature. The BBT during the menses and for approximately 5 to 7 days thereafter usually varies from 36.2° to 36.3° C (97.2° to 97.4° F). If ovulation fails to occur, this pattern of lower body temperature continues throughout the cycle. Infection, fatigue, less than 3 hours of sleep per night, awakening late, and anxiety may cause temperature fluctuations, altering the expected pattern. If a new BBT thermometer is purchased, this fact is noted on the chart because the readings may vary slightly. Jet lag, alcohol taken the evening before, or sleeping in a heated water bed must also be noted on the chart because each will affect the BBT.

About 24 to 36 hours *before* ovulation the temperature may drop 0.2° to 0.3° F and then rise 0.7° to 0.8° F within 24 to 48 hours *after* ovulation. The temperature remains on an elevated plateau until the day before menstruation. Then it drops to the low levels recorded during the previous cycle.

The drop and subsequent rise in temperature are referred to as the *thermal shift*. When the entire month's temperatures are recorded on a graph, the pattern described above is more apparent. It is more difficult to perceive day-to-day variations without the entire picture (Fig. 7.3). To determine if a rise in temperature is indeed the thermal shift, the woman must be aware of other signs approaching ovulation while she continues to assess the BBT. See discussion of sympto-thermal method below for other indicators of ovulation.

Cervical mucus method. The cervical mucus method, also called the *Billings method* or the *ovulation method,* depends on the characteristic changes in the amount and consistency of cervical mucus at the time of ovulation (see Table 5.3 and Figs. 5.31 and 5.32). These changes are easily learned by most couples. The first task is to learn to distinguish changes in the cervical mucus. To ensure accurate assessment of changes, the cervical mucus should be free of semen, contraceptive gels or foams, and blood or discharge from vaginal infections for a least one full cycle. Other factors that create difficulty in identifying mucous changes include douches and vaginal deodorants, being in the sexually aroused state (which thins the mucus), and medications such as antihistamines, which dry up the mucus.

It is difficult to evaluate the mucus in the presence of semen or discharge from vaginal infection. Therefore the woman double checks for fertility by assessing her BBT record and other symptoms of fertility. (NOTE: Each woman has her own unique pattern of mucous changes.)

Whether or not the individual wants to use this method for conception, it is to the woman's benefit to learn to recognize mucus characteristics at ovulation. Assessing changes in cervical mucus can be useful diagnostically for any of the following purposes:

1. To alert the couple to the reestablishment of ovulation while breast-feeding and after discontinuation of oral contraception
2. To note anovulatory cycles at any time and at the commencement of menopause
3. To assist couples in planning a pregnancy

Sympto-thermal method. The sympto-thermal method combines the BBT and cervical mucus methods with awareness of secondary, cycle phase–related symptoms. Both partners take responsibility for assessments, recordings, and evaluation of their findings. Together they determine the days for abstinence. Couples who use the sympto-thermal method frequently report an improvement in their sexual relationship.

The couple gains fertility awareness as they learn

Basal ("Resting") Body Temperature

Who: Woman
Why: To obtain presumptive evidence of ovulation and an adequate luteal (progesterone) phase
How: Obtain and maintain a record of daily rectal temperatures taken each morning after awakening and before *any* physical activity; any physical activity increases the body's metabolic rate; the increased metabolic rate is reflected in a thermal increase, which then may be mistaken for the thermal rise that accompanies ovulation and the secretory phase of the cycle; one suggestion that may help the woman remain at her basal metabolic rate is to ask her to buy a snooze alarm; the first time the snooze alarm goes off, she inserts her thermometer and snoozes; then when the alarm goes off the second time 5 to 10 minutes later, she can take out the thermometer and set it aside to read later when she is awake and can focus
When: Daily throughout several menstrual cycles
Where: At home in privacy of own bedroom
Risk: 1. Low
2. Requires high level of motivation by woman (and cooperation of sexual partner)
3. May be inconvenient to take temperature before any activity (e.g., shaking down the thermometer, going to the bathroom, engaging in lovemaking)
4. Misinterpretation because other factors, when present, elevate the BBT (e.g., tension, infection, headaches, fever, any activity such as coitus before taking BBT, staying up late the previous night, imbibing alcoholic beverages the evening before)
5. Misinterpretation because of inability to use and read the thermometer

Procedure	Information Sought
■ Woman obtains a BBT thermometer that is calibrated in tenths (Fig. 7.3). ■ Woman takes and records her temperature daily before any activity. ■ Woman maintains a record of other events (e.g., fever, tension, cervical mucus characteristics). ■ Woman shakes down the thermometer, washes it in tepid water with a mild soap, and replaces it within easy reach by the bedside. Woman resets the snooze alarm for the next morning.	Factors favorable to fertility: 1. The menstrual cycle is biphasic. 2. The elevated temperature persists for 12 to 14 days before menses. 3. At the time of the slight temperature drop that is followed by a persistent elevation, midcycle bleeding or mittleschmerz may occur; or just prior to the menses, premenstrual syndrome may occur.

Fig. 7.3
A, Special thermometer for recording BBT, marked in tenths to enable person to read more easily. **B,** Basal temperature record shows drop and sharp rise at time of ovulation. Biphasic curve indicates ovulatory cycle.

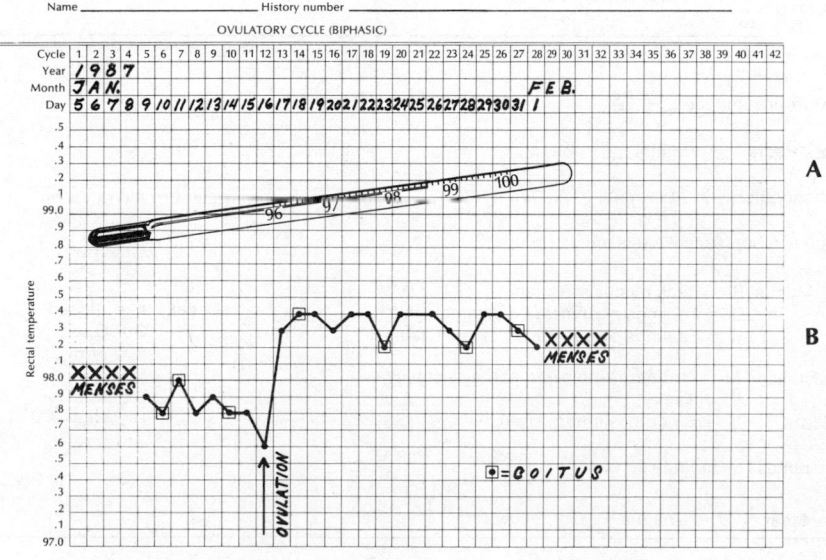

the woman's individual psychologic and physiologic symptoms. These symptoms mark the relatively infertile period (menstrual), fertile period (secretory phase), and infertile period (proliferative phase). Secondary symptoms (see Table 5.3) include increased libido, midcycle spotting, mittelschmerz, pelvic fullness or tenderness, and vulvar fullness. The couple, perhaps using a speculum, looks at the cervix to assess for changes indicating ovulation: that is, the os dilates slightly, the cervix softens and rises in the vagina, and cervical mucus is copious and slippery. To complete their records, the couple notes days on which coitus, changes in routine, illness, and so on have occurred (Fig. 7.4).

Fig. 7.4

Example of completed sympto-thermal method chart. (From Fogel C., and Woods, N.F.: Health care of women, St. Louis, 1981, The C.V. Mosby Co.)

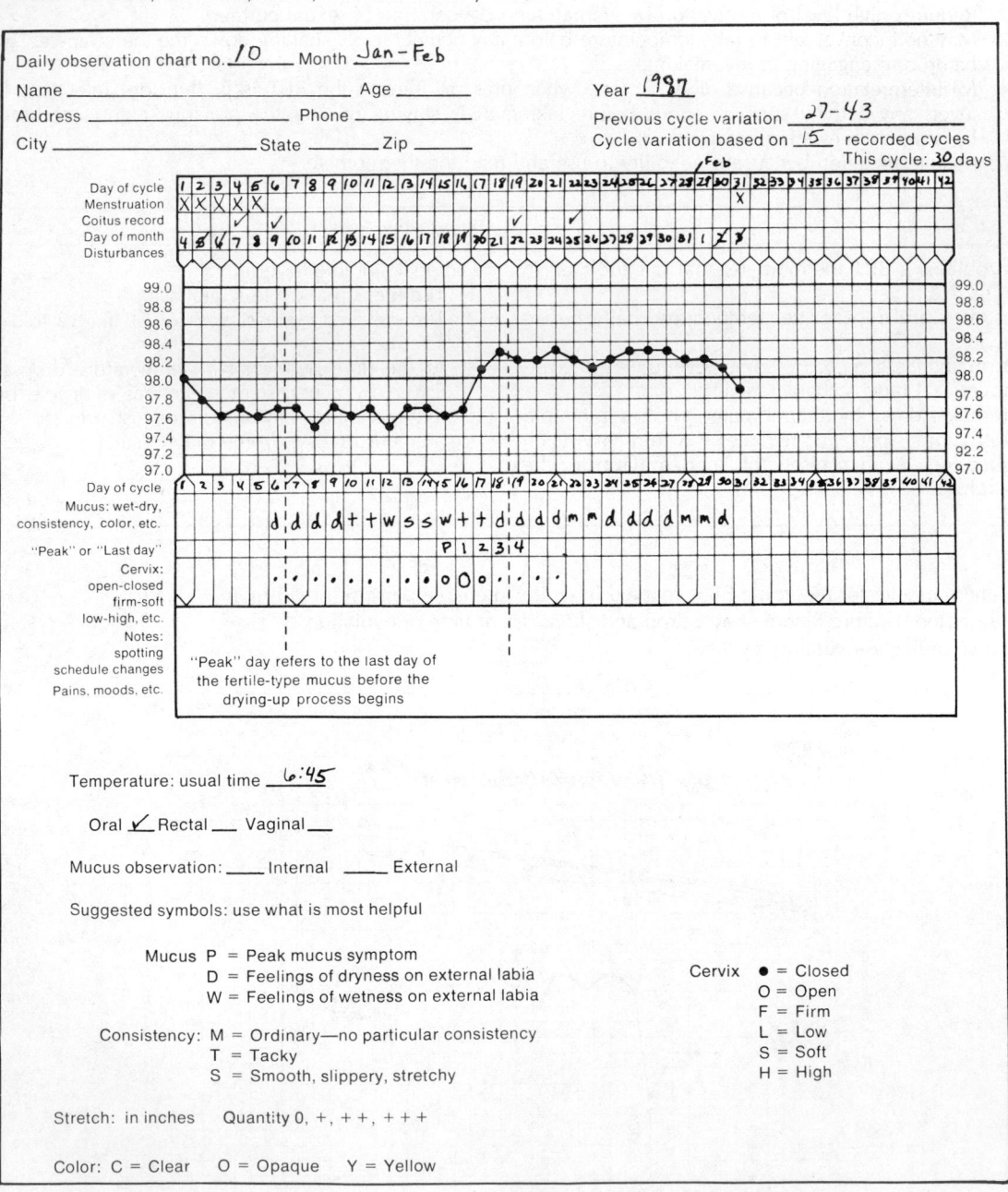

Cervical Mucus Characteristics

Who: Woman (and man)
Why: To obtain presumptive evidence of ovulation and adequacy of estrogen and progesterone phases
How: Obtain and evaluate cervical mucus characteristics through several menstrual cycles (see Figs. 5.31 and 5.32)
When: Daily throughout several menstrual cycles
Where: At home in privacy of own bedroom
Risk: 1. Low
2. Requires high level of motivation by couple. Assessment of mucus characteristics is best learned with mucus that has not been mixed with semen or discharge from infection. The couple is asked to refrain from ejaculation of semen into or near the vagina for a least one full, infection-free cycle. When intercourse is resumed in the following cycle, the difference between cervical mucus and semen will be apparent.
   Good hand washing is imperative to begin and end all self-assessment activities.
3. Evaluation may be difficult in the presence of vaginal discharge from infection, vaginal menstrual bleeding, contraceptive foams, lubricants, and so on.

Procedure	Information Sought
■ Woman learns how to assess for peak mucus sign by practicing with raw egg white. ■ After carefully washing her hands, woman assesses mucus several times per day, perhaps before each time she empties her bladder. Mucus can be obtained from vaginal introitus—no need to reach into vagina to the cervix for mucus. ■ From the last day of the menstrual flow the woman makes daily observations and recordings of changes in her cervical mucus—its quantity, consistency, color, and sensation. ■ Woman records findings on the same record on which her BBT is entered. ■ Woman records any other events or feelings.	For findings favorable to fertility see Table 5.7 and Figs. 5.31 and 5.32. The peak mucus sign appears just before ovulation (e.g., abundant, watery, clear, cloudy or yellowish; spinnbarkeit to 5+ cm; lubricative) and indicates the period of maximal fertility. Sperm deposited in this type of mucus can survive until ovulation occurs. The peak mucus sign may be accompanied by a feeling of fullness around the vagina, mittelschmerz, an increased physical energy, sense of well-being, and libido. Menstruation should follow in 12 to 16 days.

Effectiveness of the sympto-thermal method with abstinence during the fertile period ranges between 73% and 97%.

Fertility awareness method. The fertility awareness method is a combination of the sympto-thermal method and barrier contraception. During the fertile period the couple has the choice of abstinence from genital-genital contact or the use of barrier contraception. After ovulation the couple may enjoy freedom from contraception for the remaining nonfertile days of the menstrual cycle

Predictor test for ovulation. This test detects the sudden surge of LH that occurs approximately 12 to 24 hours prior to ovulation. Unlike BBT, the test is not affected by illness, emotional upset, or physical activity. Available for home use, a test kit contains sufficient material for several days' testing during each cycle. A positive response indicative of an LH surge is noted by color change that is easy to read. Directions for use of this home test kit vary with the manufacturer.

Chemical barriers. A vaginal spermicide is a physical barrier to sperm penetration that also has a chemical action on sperm. Nonoxynol 9 and octoxynol 9 are the most commonly used spermicidal chemicals. Intravaginal spermicides are marketed as aerosol foams, foaming tablets, suppositories, creams, and gels (Fig. 7.5). Preloaded, single-dose applicators small enough to be carried in a small purse are available (Grimes, 1986). This form of contraceptive must be placed deeply in the vagina in contact with the cervix prior to each coitus. Special precautions must be taken. The can of foam must be shaken to distribute the spermicide before use. Tablets and suppositories take from 10 to 30 minutes to dissolve. Maximal spermicidal effectiveness lasts usually no longer than 1 hour. If intercourse is to be repeated, reapplication of additional spermicide must precede it. Douching must be avoided for a least 6 hours after coitus (Grimes, 1986).

Mode of action. Spermicides provide a physical and chemical barrier that prevents viable sperm from entering the cervix. The effect is local, within the vagina.

Advantages. Ease of application, safety, low cost, and ready availability without prescription or previous medical examination characterize this method. The delicate vaginal mucosa is not harmed unless the woman is allergic to a particular preparation. Spermicides aid in lubrication of the vagina. Because their ef-

Fig. 7.5
Vaginal spermicides. **A,** Foam with applicator. **B,** Gel or cream. **C,** Suppository, **D,** Sponge.

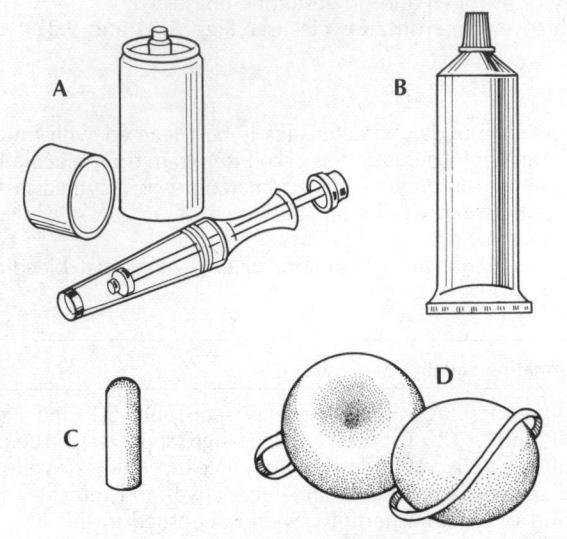

fect is local, spermicides offer an alternative to hormonal contraception, e.g., for the nursing mother (to avoid interfering with lactation), for the premenopausal woman (to prevent masking symptoms of onset of the climacteric), and as a backup for the woman who forgets to take her birth control pill. There is evidence that spermicides provide some protection against sexually transmitted disease through bacteriostatic action. The addition of spermicides increases the effectiveness of the other forms of contraception, e.g., condoms, diaphragms.

Disadvantages and side effects. Users of this method may complain of its "messiness," unpleasant "fizz," stickiness, or unpleasant taste. Allergic response or irritation of vaginal or penile tissue may occur. Some users experience decreased tactile sensation. The need to wait 10 minutes to 30 minutes before coitus initially and to reapply additional spermicide prior to repeated intercourse is not acceptable to all people.

Effectiveness. According to Pritchard, MacDonald, and Gant (1985) the high pregnancy rate seen with this method is probably due to inconsistent use of the spermicide. Correct and regular use could be expected to have a failure rate as low as 5 per 100 woman-years of use (Population Reports,* 1984). Pregnancy rates as low as 2 and as high as 39 per 100 woman-years of use have been reported (Willson, Carrington, and Ledger, 1983).

---

*Population Reports and other references describe effectiveness per 100 woman-years of use.

Nursing actions. The nurse encourages open communication between the sexual partners to discuss intravaginal contraception. Clients are offerred the opportunity to see and handle a variety of samples. To maximize learning, the woman is given the opportunity to insert one application into a medical model or her vagina. The male partner sometimes indicates interest in learning how to insert the spermicide into his female partner. The nurse needs to feel comfortable teaching him as well.

Vaginal sponge. The polyurethane sponge was approved by the FDA in 1983 (Fig. 7.5, *D*). Water is added to activate the spermicide and facilitate insertion. Spermicide is released continuously for 24 hours. A woven loop is used for retrieval from the vagina. It is recommended that at least 6 hours elapse between last intercourse and removal (Grimes, 1986).

Mode of action. The mode of action is the same as that for the spermicides.

The use effectiveness for any contraceptive method can be calculated by determining the number of pregnancies per 100 years of use by Pearl's formula, which permits comparison of methods (Willson, Carrington, Ledger, 1983, p. 177):

Pregnancy rate per 100 years =
$$\frac{\text{Total number of conceptions} \times 1200}{\text{Total months of exposure}}$$

For example, if 100 couples use a method for a total of 3600 months and 12 pregnancies occur, the pregnancy rate is 4:

$$\frac{12 \times 1200}{3600} = \frac{14,400}{3600} = 4/100 \text{ years}$$

Advantages. Like the other spermicides, the sponge is an over-the-counter (OTC) product. It offers spontaneity and is less "messy" than other spermicide delivery systems. Reapplication of spermicide during the 24 hours it is in place is unnecessary.

Disadvantages and side effects. The only reported effects were allergic reactions (2% to 3%) or irritation (2% to 3%) that typically occur with all nonoxynol 9 products. Six percent of users reported difficulty in removing the sponge (Grimes, 1986).

Effectiveness. A relatively high failure rate has been reported during the first year of use, especially in parous women (Grimes, 1986). The failure rate is higher than with the diaphragm, 17/100 vs 13/100 woman-years of use. Effectiveness seems to increase in the second year of use.

Nursing actions. Nursing actions are similar to those for other spermicides. Clients are reminded that each sponge is to be used once, for 24 hours only, and

Fig. 7.6
Mechanical barriers. **A,** Condoms (no prescription required); types of condoms. **B,** Diaphragm. **C,** Cervical cap.

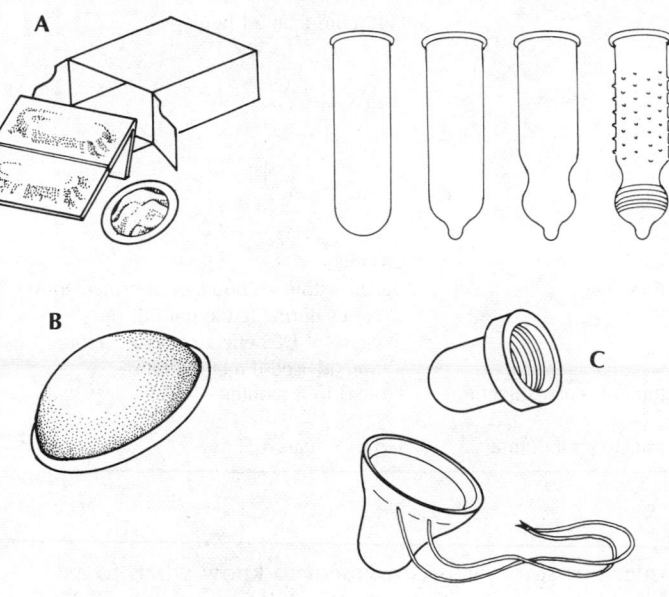

discarded. The woman is coached to "bear down" to facilitate removal of the sponge.

Condom. The condom is a thin, stretchable sheath to cover the penis (Fig. 7.6, *A*). Four basic features differ among condoms marketed in the United States. These features are material, shape, lubricants, and spermicides. Ninety-nine percent are made of rubber. A functional difference in condom shape is the presence or absence of a sperm reservoir tip. To enhance vaginal stimulation, some condoms have lateral ribs. A wet jelly or dry powder lubricates some condoms. Since 1982, spermicide (0.5 g of nonoxynol 9) has been added to the interior or exterior surfaces of some condoms.

The sheath is applied over the erect penis before insertion or loss of preejaculatory drops of semen. Conception is possible even if preejaculatory drops fall around the external vaginal opening because sperm are contained in these drops.

Mode of action. Used correctly, condoms prevent sperm from entering the cervix. Spermicide-coated condoms cause ejaculated sperm to be immobilized rapidly.

Advantages. Condoms are safe, without side effects, and are readily available. Premalignant changes in the cervix can be prevented or ameliorated in women whose partners use condoms (Pritchard, MacDonald,

and Gant, 1985). If the condom is used throughout the act of intercourse and there is no unprotected contact with female genitals, condoms can act as a protective measure against spread of sexually transmitted diseases (STDs). The STDs include gonorrhea, syphilis, herpes, chlamydia, AIDS,* and trichomoniasis (Grimes, 1986; Pritchard, MacDonald, and Gant, 1985; Willson, Carrington, and Ledger, 1983; and *San Francisco Chronicle*, 1/14/86). The unique feature of this method is that the male assumes a major role in contraception (Grimes, 1986).

Disadvantages and side effects. If condoms are used improperly, spillage of sperm can result in pregnancy. Some couples object to interrupting lovemaking to apply the sheath or complain that sensation is blunted. On occasion, condoms have torn during intercourse.

Effectiveness. The pregnancy rate can be as low as three to four pregnancies per 100 woman-years of use, but the general rate is 15 (Willson, Carrington, and Ledger, 1983). The failure rate tends to be higher during the first year of use. Condoms with spermicide are expected to lower the failure rate (Pritchard, MacDonald, and Gant, 1985).

Nursing actions. Both the female and male partner benefit from a discussion of their feelings about this method of contraception. Samples of condoms with different features, a price list, and demonstration of the application and removal of a condom using a medical model offer the clients a focus for discussion and a basis for choice. Clients need to be alerted to the mode of action, advantages, disadvantages, and effectiveness of this method. (See Guidelines for Client Teaching, p. 165.)

METHODS REQUIRING PERIODIC MEDICAL EXAMINATION AND PRESCRIPTION

Several methods for the control of fertility require prescription and supervision. Interview, physical examination, and occasionally laboratory tests are prerequisites for some forms of contraception. These methods of contraception include hormonal therapy, use of diaphragms or caps, and intrauterine devices.

Hormonal contraception. Steroidal contraceptives are available in several preparations. Some are described in Table 7.10.

Oral hormonal contraceptives were used by 28.6% of women aged 15 to 44 years practicing contraception during 1982 (Bachrach, 1984). The minipill ac-

---

*The combination of spermicide and the condom seems to create a synergistic action against a number of sexually transmitted diseases (Grimes, 1986).

Table 7.10
Hormonal Contraception

Composition	Route of Administration	Duration of Effect
Combination of an estrogen and a progestin:	Oral	Not more than 24 hours
Biphasic: constant dose of estrogen and an increase in progestin on day 11		
Triphasic: 3 different products on market—in 2, estrogen is constant and progestin varies; in 1, amounts of both vary. Total hormone dose per cycle is lower than in biphasic combinations		
Sequential: estrogen during first half of cycle, progestin during second half; not sold in United States		
Minipill: progestin (norethindrone, 0.35 mg) only	Oral	24 hours
Morning-after pill: estrogen (diethylstilbestrol [DES]) in very high levels—25 mg	Oral	Taken within 72 hours of unprotected coitus during fertile period; because of DES effect on fetus, abortion advised if method fails
Depo-Provera: progestin only (medroxyprogesterone acetate), 150 mg	Intramuscular injection	From 3 to 6 months
Norplant system: progestin (Levonorgestrel) in silastic containers	Implant, subdermal	Up to 5 years

counts for only 1% of oral contraceptives sold. Because of the wide variety of preparations available the client and nurse need to read the package insert for information about specific products prescribed.

Mode of action. Activation of the hypothalamus and pituitary to release FSH and LH is dependent on fluctuation in the blood concentration of ovarian estrogen and progesterone. The contraceptive action is a combined effect of ovulation inhibition, endometrial changes, and alteration in cervical mucus, and perhaps altered tubal function (Willson, Carrington, Ledger, 1983). The medication suppresses anterior pituitary secretion of the gonadotropins FSH and LH, thereby inhibiting ovulation. It also has a direct effect on the endometrium, so that from 1 to 4 days after the last steroid tablet is taken the endometrium sloughs and bleeds as a result of hormone withdrawal. The *withdrawal bleeding* usually is less profuse than that of normal menstruation and may last only 2 to 3 days. Some women have no bleeding at all.

The cervical mucus remains thick as a result of the effect of the progestin. Cervical mucus under the effect of progesterone does not provide as suitable an environment for sperm penetration as does the thin, viscid mucus at ovulation (Willson, Carrington, and Ledger, 1983).

Advantages. For motivated women it is easy to take an oral contraceptive (OC) at about the same time each day. Taking the pill does not relate directly to the sexual act; this fact increases its acceptability to some women. Frequently, there is an improvement in sexual response once the possibility of pregnancy is not an

issue. For some, it is convenient to know when to expect the next "menstrual" flow. The regular cyclic stimulation of the endometrium may help regulate menstrual cycles and make it possible for conception to occur at a later time. Occasionally, using oral hormone therapy for a period of time may decrease or eliminate premenstrual tension and dysmenorrhea (menstrual cramps).

There has been little publicity about the advantages of hormonal contraceptives. Mishell (1982) and Ory (1982) list the noncontraceptive health benefits of oral contraceptives. The benefits include decreased menstrual blood loss and resultant iron-deficiency anemia, regulation of irregular cycles, protection against endometrial adenocarcinoma, reduced incidence of benign breast disease, protection against the development of functional ovarian cysts, protection against acute salpingitis* and pelvic inflammatory disease (PID), and possible protection against ovarian cancer and rheumatoid arthritis.

Since ovulation is suppressed, the risk for ectopic pregnancy is about one-tenth that of women not using contraceptives. This form of contraception is associated with minimal risk for women aged 15 to 29 years. The mortality rate is 1.2 and 1.4/100,000 for nonsmoking and smoking women, respectively.

Women taking steroidal contraceptives are examined before the medication is prescribed and yearly thereafter. The examination includes medical and fam-

---

*Wolner-Hanssen and others (1985) suggest that this protection may apply to both gonococcal and chlamydial salpingitis.

ily history, weight, blood pressure, general physical and pelvic examination, screening cervical cytologic analysis, and hemoglobin determination. Consistent medical surveillance is valuable in the detection of noncontraception-related disorders as well, so that timely treatment can be initiated.

Disadvantages and side effects

Contraindications. Women must be screened for conditions that present absolute or relative contraindications to oral contraceptive use. *Absolute contraindications* include a history of thromboembolic disorders, cerebrovascular or coronary artery disease, breast cancer, estrogenic-dependent tumors, undiagnosed abnormal genital bleeding, known or suspected pregnancy, liver tumor, sickle cell disease, or migraine headaches (Grimes, 1986; Hatcher and others, 1984; Kols and others, 1982). *Relative contraindications* include age of 40 years or older, diabetes mellitus, hypertension, heavy smoking (more than 15 cigarettes per day), gallbladder disease, gestational cholestasis, history of renal disease, impaired liver function, and hyperlipidemia (Grimes, 1986). The main causes of hospitalization and death are cardiovascular problems, e.g., myocardial infarction (heart attack), cerebrovascular accident (stroke), and thromboembolism (Grimes, 1986).

Estrogen excess/deficiency and progestin excess/deficiency. Certain side effects of anovulatory drugs are attributable to estrogen and progestin or both. Side effects of *estrogen excess* include nausea and vomiting, dizziness, edema, leg cramps, increase in breast size, chloasma (mask of pregnancy), visual changes, hypertension, and vascular headache. Side effects of *estrogen deficiency* include early spotting (days 1 to 14), hypomenorrhea, nervousness, and atrophic vaginitis leading to painful intercourse (dyspareunia). Side effects of *progestin excess* include increased appetite, tiredness, depression, breast tenderness, vaginal yeast infection, oily skin and scalp, hirsutism, and postpill amenorrhea. Side effects of *progestin deficiency* include late spotting and breakthrough bleeding (days 15 to 21), heavy flow with clots, and decreased breast size.

In the presence of side effects, especially those that are bothersome to the woman, a different product, a different drug content, or another method of contraception may be required. The "right" product for a woman contains the lowest dose of sex steroid hormones that prevents ovulation and that has the fewest and least harmful side effects. There is no way to predict the "right" dose* for any particular woman; trial

and error is the main method for prescribing OCs, starting with the lowest possible estrogen dose.

Alteration in metabolism. The *changes in glucose tolerance* that occur in some women taking OCs are similar to those changes that occur during pregnancy. OCs challenge the islets of Langerhans to produce more insulin. If the individual is prediabetic, the use of oral contraception can induce the frank expression of diabetes mellitus.

The OC also affects the woman's *general nutritional needs,* especially for B vitamins. There is considerable evidence that OCs are implicated in deficiencies of vitamin B_6 (pyridoxine) and folic acid in about 20% to 30% of users. Among some OC users, symptoms such as headaches, nausea and vomiting, and emotional disturbances and depression have been alleviated by dietary supplementation of vitamin B_6.

Symptoms of folic acid deficiency are rare, since folate is plentiful in the North American diet. However, if a pregnancy occurs soon after the pill is discontinued, folic acid deficiency is to be expected. Clinical symptoms of folic acid deficiency are those of megaloblastic anemia: increasing fatigue, pallor, moderate depapillation of the tongue, and changes in peripheral blood and bone marrow. Symptoms are rapidly reversed with supplementation of folic acid or if the OC is discontinued.

Although not yet proven, there may be some deficiency of vitamin C and vitamin B_{12} (cobalamin). Vitamins whose metabolism is suspected of being altered by OCs are vitamin A, vitamin B_2, and niacin.

Some women complain of edema, which is associated with administration of estrogens; however, if the dose of estrogen is sufficiently low, fluid retention is not likely to occur or can be compensated for by decreasing the oral intake of sodium compounds.

*Fetal effects after discontinuing the pill.** Women who discontinue oral contraception for a planned pregnancy frequently ask whether they should wait before attempting to conceive. Although data are controversial, there does seem to be some evidence of increased incidence of chromosomal changes in abortuses when pregnancy occurs during the first few (usually one or two) cycles after discontinuation of oral contraception.

Postpill amenorrhea. After discontinuing oral contraception there is usually a delay before ovulation and menstrual cycles recur. However, amenorrhea exceeding 6 months should be investigated.

Neoplastic disease. Some neoplasms of the breast, benign or malignant, may be stimulated by estrogens. If

---

*Warn women, young and old, that using another woman's OCs may not prevent ovulation, if the dose is not correct for them.

*For discussion of effects of the pill on the fetus when the woman continues with oral contraception after conception, see Appendix G.

another hormone-dependent tumor is suspected (e.g., of the endometrium), oral contraception is contraindicated.

There is an association between long-term use of contraceptive pills by women over 30 years of age and the occurrence of a liver tumor known as hepatocellular adenoma (HCA). The risk of developing HCA is higher with increasing use of OCs. The annual incidence of HCA is approximately 3 or 4 per 100,000 long-term users of OCs. In comparison the annual occurrence rate is approximately 1 to 1.3 per 1 million in women aged 16 to 30 years and in women aged 31 to 34 who have never used OCs or have used them for 24 months or less. Of the women who develop HCA, 88% are long-term users of OCs. The development of HCA can be minimized when the lowest possible dose that provides protection against pregnancy is used. Hepatic adenomas are also associated with the use of OCs. Because hepatic adenomas may rupture and cause death through hemorrhage, they should be considered in women with abdominal pain and tenderness, an abdominal mass, or shock.

Hypertension. Infrequently hypertension is first noted after the woman begins oral contraception, especially if she is 30 years of age or older. In some women, higher blood levels of angiotensinogen and plasma renin have been found. It is thought that these factors play a part in the hypertension experienced by some women. After discontinuing oral contraception, hypertension subsides.

Miscellaneous side effects and precautions. Some *laboratory values* may be altered in women taking OCs. These changes are listed, not for memorization, but only for interest and to alert the nurse to the need to ask about contraceptive use when taking a health history. The following laboratory values may be increased: bromsulphalein (BSP), serum glutamic oxaloacetic transaminase (SGOT), serum glutamic pyruvic transaminase (SGPT), alkaline phosphatase, and thyronine-binding protein (a thyroid hormone).

Some conditions are aggravated by fluid retention. Women susceptible to *migraine headaches* may notice an increase in headaches when taking the pill. Since headaches is also a symptom of cerebral thrombosis, there may be confusion with correct diagnosis. Therefore women who experience migraine headaches are counseled to use other forms of contraception. Although many women with *epilepsy* tolerate OCs well, others tend to have an increase in the incidence of seizures.

Some women who wear *contact lenses* experience a change in the curvature of the cornea. Although the reason for this change is unknown, the woman is advised to discontinue use of the contact lenses while taking OCs.

More serious *neuroocular lesions* are associated with use of OCs. Optic neuritis or retinal thrombosis, although rare, has been reported. Symptoms such as sudden or gradual and partial or complete loss of vision and double vision require immediate diagnosis and treatment. **Women must stop taking OCs at the first sign of visual disorders.**

There is an increased risk of *gallbladder disease* after 2 years of use of OCs. The risk doubles after 4 to 5 years of pill use.

Oral contraceptives and drug interactions. The effectiveness of OCs is decreased along with an increased possibility of break-through bleeding if the woman is receiving any of the following drugs:

- Barbiturates (for sedation)
- Phenylbutazone (for arthritis or bursitis; treatment for superficial thrombophlebitis)
- Phenytoin sodium (for seizure disorders)
- Ampicillin (for infections)

Long-term use of OCs slows diazepam (Valium) clearance by the liver; therefore higher blood levels of the drug increase the risk of an overdose of diazepam. Planned Parenthood facilities keep current information about newly identified drug interactions as it becomes available.

Effectiveness. Taken exactly as directed, oral contraceptives prevent ovulation, and pregnancy cannot occur; the overall effectiveness rate is almost 100%. Almost all failures (i.e., pregnancy occurs) are caused by omission of one or more pills during the regimen. The minipill is slightly less effective than the combination pill but can reach 98% reliability if taken exactly as prescribed.

The woman being considered for therapy with the morning-after pill is advised that should pregnancy occur anyway, elective abortion by cervical dilation and curettage (D and C) may be considered. This is because of the adverse effects of DES on the fetus. The effectiveness of the morning-after pill reaches 100% if hormone therapy is followed by D and C.

Nursing actions. There are many different preparations of oral hormone contraceptives. The nurse needs to review the prescribing information in the package insert with the client. Some dosage regimens stipulate that the first pill be taken on day 5 of the menstrual cycle; others start on day 1 or on Sunday. Because of the wide variations, each woman must be clear about the unique dosage regimen for the preparation prescribed for her.

Directions for care after missing one or two tablets also vary. In general, if one or two tablets are missed, another form of contraception needs to be used until the required regimen is reestablished.

Before OCs are prescribed and periodically throughout hormone therapy, the woman is alerted to stop taking the pill and to report any of the following symptoms to the physician immediately. The word *aches* helps in retention of this list:

A—Abdominal pain: may indicate a problem with the liver or gallbladder

C—Chest pain or shortness of breath: may indicate possible clot problem within lungs or heart

H—Headaches (sudden or persistent): may be caused by cardiovascular accident or hypertension

E—Eye problems: may indicate vascular accident or hypertension

S—Severe leg pain: may indicate a thromboembolic process

A general teaching tool for contraceptive methods is presented in Guidelines for Client Teaching on p. 165.

Diaphragm with spermicide. The vaginal diaphragm is a shallow, dome-shaped rubber device with a flexible wire rim that covers the cervix. The diaphragm should feel comfortable. The use of a contraceptive gel or cream with the diaphragm offers both mechanical and chemical barriers to pregnancy.

Mode of action. The diaphragm is a mechanical barrier preventing the meeting of the sperm with the ovum. The diaphragm holds the spermicide in place against the cervix for the 6 hours it takes to destroy the sperm.

Advantages. Except for occasional allergic response to the diaphragm or spermicide, there are no side effects from a well-fitted device. The diaphragm can be inserted several hours before intercourse. The woman who engages in intercourse infrequently may choose this barrier method. The spermicide does offer additional lubrication if it is needed. A decreased incidence of vaginitis and cystitis is noted among women who use contraceptive creams, foams, and gels with the diaphragm.

Disadvantages and side effects. This method is contraindicated for the woman with relaxation of her pelvic support (uterine prolapse) or a large cystocele. It is also not advised for the woman who is "uninformed."

Disadvantages include the reluctance of some women to insert and remove the diaphragm. A cold diaphragm and a cold gel temporarily reduce vaginal response to sexual stimulation if insertion of the diaphragm occurs immediately before intercourse. Some women or couples object to the "messiness" of the spermicide. These annoyances of diaphragm usage, along with failure to insert the device once foreplay has begun, are the most common reasons for failures of this method. Side effects may include irritation of tissues related to contact with spermicides.

Effectiveness. The *effectiveness* of this combined method is approximately 83% to 90%. Highly motivated women may achieve rates of 99%.

Nursing actions. The woman is informed that she needs an annual gynecologic examination and that the device may need to be refitted after the loss or gain of 4.5 kg (10 lb) or more or if she gives birth. Various types of diaphragms are on the market. The nurse uses the package insert for teaching the woman how to use and care for the diaphragm. The directions for one product are given on p. 162.

Cervical cap. Cervical caps come in two types: one is presized in small, medium, and large, and one is custom fitted. The custom cervical cap is a plasticlike cap about 2.5 cm (1 in) in diameter and is fitted to conform to the individual woman's cervix. This cap has several advantages: (1) It can be made in the physician's office in approximately 20 minutes. A mold of the cervix is made with a nontoxic substance used to make contact lenses. A plaster cast is made of the mold, and then the cap is fitted onto the cast. (2) Its design allows menstrual flow out through the cervix and self-cleaning with natural mucous flow, while preventing sperm from entering the cervix. (3) No foreign-matter reaction has been noted in users of this device. (4) It can be left in place indefinitely.

The presized cervical cap, however, cannot be left in place indefinitely (Fig. 7.6, *C*). The custom cervical cap and the presized cervical cap are not yet approved for sale in the United States. They are only available in those clinics involved in studies of this method of contraception.

Intrauterine devices. An intrauterine device (IUD) is a small device inserted into the uterine cavity. Medicated IUDs have taken the place of nonmedicated

Fig. 7.7

Intrauterine devices. **A,** Copper-T 220 and Copper-T 380A are being tested by the Population Council. Both contain copper sleeves. **B,** Multiload devices come in different sizes and are prepared with different loads of copper. Not yet available in the United States, they are widely available outside of the United States.

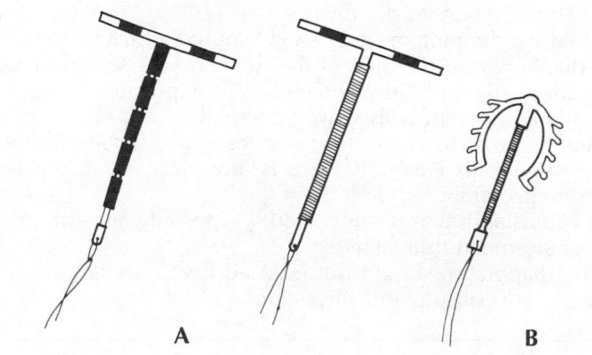

Use and Care of the Diaphragm

Positions for insertion of diaphragm

Squatting

This is the most frequently used position and most women find this position satisfactory.

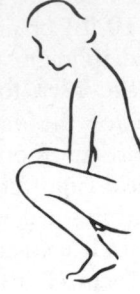

Leg Up Method

A position to suit the convenience of particular women is to raise the left foot (if right hand is used for insertion) on a low stool, and in a bending position the diaphragm is inserted.

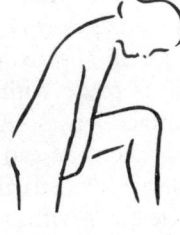

Chair Method

A practical method for diaphragm insertion is for the woman to sit far forward on the edge of a chair.

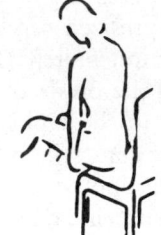

Reclining

In some instances, certain women prefer to insert the diaphragm while in a semi-reclining position in bed.

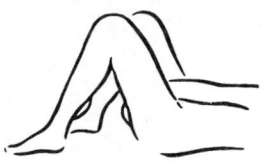

Preparation of diaphragm

Your diaphragm must always be used with a spermicidal lubricant in order to be effective. Pregnancy cannot be prevented effectively by the diaphragm alone.

Always empty your bladder before inserting the diaphragm. Place about 2 teaspoonsful of contraceptive gel, contraceptive jelly, or contraceptive cream on the side of the diaphragm that will rest against the cervix (or whichever way you have been instructed). Spread it around to coat the surface and the rim. This aids in insertion and offers a more complete seal. Many women also spread some gel (jelly) or cream on the other side of the diaphragm. See Fig. A.

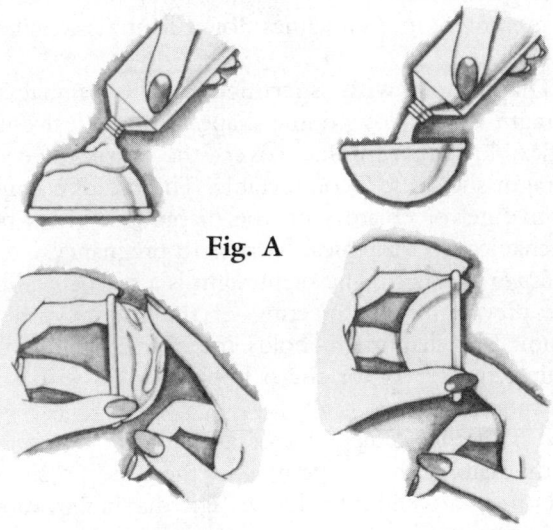

Fig. A

Insertion of diaphragm

The diaphragm can be inserted as much as 6 hours before intercourse. Hold the diaphragm between your thumb and fingers. The dome can either be up or down, as directed by your physician. Place your index finger on the outer rim of the compressed diaphragm. See Fig. B. Use the fingers of the other hand to spread the labia (lips of the vagina). This will assist in guiding the diaphragm into place.

Inspection of diaphragm

Your diaphragm must be inspected carefully before each use. The best way to do this is:

Hold the diaphragm up to a light source. Carefully stretch the diaphragm at the area of the rim, on all sides, to make sure there are no holes. Remember, it is possible to puncture the diaphragm with sharp fingernails.

Another way to check for pinholes is to carefully fill the diaphragm with water. If there is any problem, it will be seen immediately.

If your diaphragm is "puckered," especially near the rim, this could mean thin spots.

The diaphragm should not be used if you see any of the above . . . consult your physician.

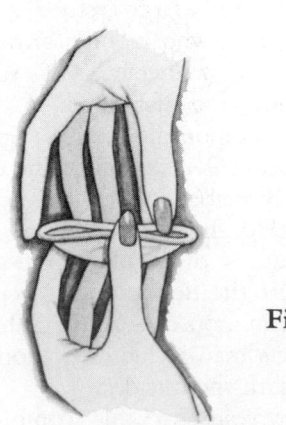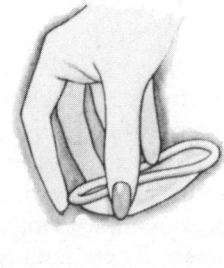

Fig. B

Use and Care of the Diaphragm

Insert the diaphragm into the vagina. Direct it inward and downward as far as it will go to the space behind and below the cervix. See Fig. C.

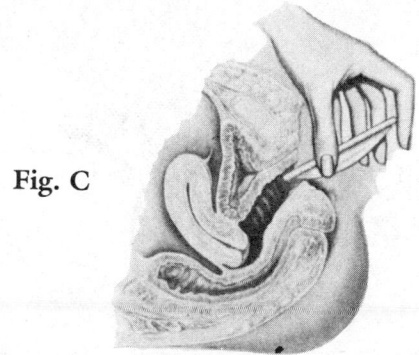

Fig. C

Tuck the front of the rim of the diaphragm behind the pelvic bone so that the rubber hugs the front wall of the vagina. See Fig. D.

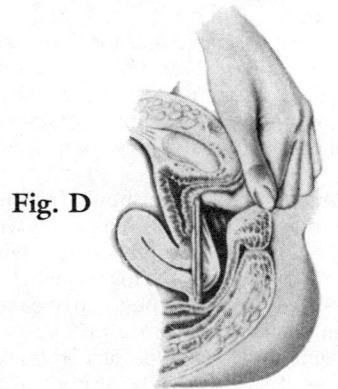

Fig. D

Directions for insertion with diaphragm introducer

Hold the introducer in either hand. Compress the diaphragm, dome up, with the fingers of your other hand. Place one end of the rim in the grooved end of the introducer. See Fig. E.

Fig. E

Fit the other end of the diaphragm over the notch corresponding to the diaphragm size. See Fig. F. Squeeze approximately 1 tablespoonful of gel, jelly, or cream into the folds of the diaphragm. Spread a small amount around the rim.

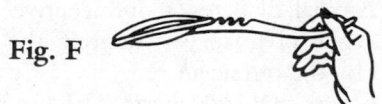

Fig. F

The diaphragm may be inserted while you are lying flat with your legs drawn up. However, any position may be used if more convenient. See positions for insertion of diaphragm.

Insert the diaphragm in a downward direction as far back as it will comfortably go . . . past the cervix. See Fig. G.

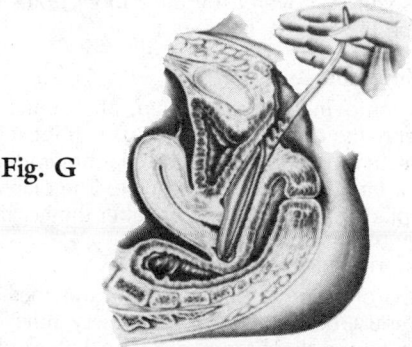

Fig. G

To release the diaphragm, rotate the introducer to the right or left and gently withdraw it. See Fig. H. After the introducer is removed, tuck the front rim of the diaphragm behind the pelvic bone. See Fig. D.

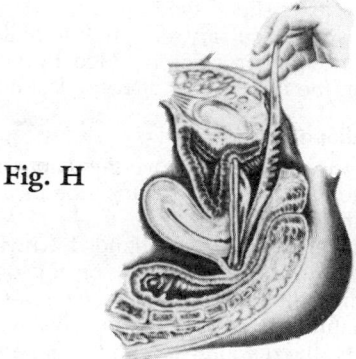

Fig. H

Feel for your cervix through the diaphragm to be certain it is properly placed and securely covered by the rubber dome. See Fig. I.

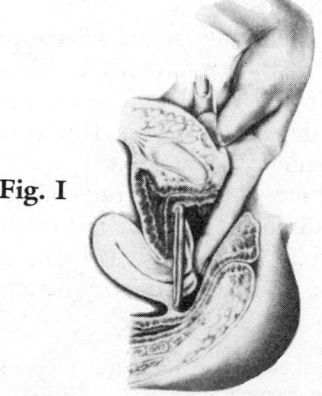

Fig. I

To clean the introducer, wash with mild soap and warm water, rinse and dry thoroughly.

Continued.

Use and Care of the Diaphragm

Final checking

Whether the diaphragm is inserted manually or with the introducer, the finger test must always be made to see that the outer rim of the diaphragm is tucked firmly behind the pelvic bone (see Fig. D). At the same time, you must check to see that the small round knob of the cervix (mouth of the womb) is securely covered by the rubber dome of the diaphragm. See Fig. I.

Repeated intercourse

Without removing the diaphragm, an additional applicatorful of gel (jelly) or cream must be used if intercourse takes place more than 6 hours after the diaphragm has been inserted or for each repeated intercourse. The diaphragm must remain in place for at least 6 hours after the last intercourse.

General information

Regardless of the time of the month, this method of contraception must be used each and every time intercourse takes place. Your diaphragm must be left in place for at least 6 hours after the last intercourse. If you remove your diaphragm before the 6-hour time period, your chance of becoming pregnant could be greatly increased. You should not leave your diaphragm in place for more than 24 hours, to do so may encourage growth of bacteria that could result in infection or toxic shock syndrome.

Douching is not necessary after the use of the diaphragm. However, if desired or recommended by your physician, you must wait the full 6 hours after the last intercourse.

Removal of diaphragm

The only proper way to remove the diaphragm is to insert your forefinger up and over the top side of the diaphragm, and slightly to the side.

Next, turn the palm of your hand downward and backward hooking the forefinger firmly on top of the inside of the upper rim of the diaphragm, *breaking the suction.*

Pull the diaphragm down and out. This avoids the possibility of tearing the diaphragm with the fingernails. The dia-

phragm *should not* be removed by trying to catch the rim from *below* the dome. See Fig. J.

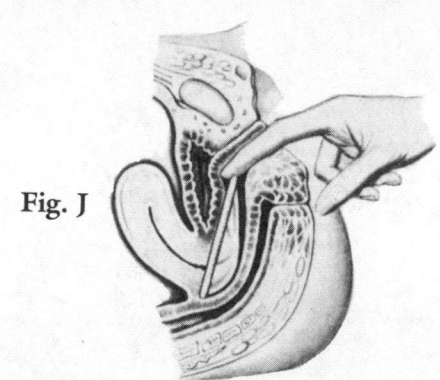

Fig. J

Care of diaphragm

When using a vaginal diaphragm, avoid using products that may contain petroleum such as certain body lubricants, vaginal lubricants, or vaginitis preparations. These products can weaken rubber.

A little care means longer wear for your diaphragm. After each use the diaphragm should be washed in warm water and Ivory soap. Do not use detergent soaps, cold cream soaps, deodorant soaps, and soaps containing petroleum as they can weaken the rubber. *Ivory soap should be the only soap used.*

After washing, the diaphragm should be dried thoroughly. All water and moisture should be removed with your towel. The diaphragm should then be dusted with *cornstarch.* Scented talc, body powder, baby powder, and the like, should not be used because they can weaken the rubber. Remember, only *cornstarch* for dusting.

The diaphragm should then be placed back in the plastic case for storage. It should not be stored near a radiator or heat source, or exposed to light for an extended period of time.

IUDs (Grimes, 1986).* Medicated IUDs are loaded with either copper† (Fig. 7.7) or a progestational agent. These chemically active substances are released continuously to the endometrium, for example, copper-bearing devices for 3 to 4 years (at present) and progesterone devices for 1 year. IUDs are impregnated with barium sulfate for radiopacity.

Mode of action. IUDs alter the endometrium locally and thereby discourage implantation should fertilization occur. Because the effect is local, there is no disruption of the woman's ovulatory pattern.

---

*The last nonmedicated plastic IUD (the Lippes loop) was discontinued by its manufacturer in 1985.

†Searle and Company removed CU-7 and TATUM-7 from the United States market on February 1, 1986.

Advantages. The IUD offers constant contraception without the need to remember to take pills each day or engage in other manipulation prior to or between coital acts. If pregnancy can be excluded, an IUD may be placed at any time during the menstrual cycle. An IUD may be inserted immediately following abortion (Liskin and Fox, 1982).

The absence of interference with hormonal regulation of menstrual cycles makes the IUD more appropriate than hormonal contraception for heavy smokers, women over 35, or those with a history of vascular disease or familial diabetes. Contraceptive effects are reversible. When pregnancy is desired, the IUD may be removed by the physician.

Disadvantages and side effects. The use of an IUD is contraindicated for women with a history of pelvic

Guidelines for Client Teaching
GENERAL CONTRACEPTIVE METHODS

ASSESSMENT

Physical assessment completed in manner appropriate for each method.

Assessment of reason for choice, what she (couple) knows or has heard about method selected, and feelings about touching genital area.

NURSING DIAGNOSES

Potential for infection
Potential for injury
Noncompliance
Alteration in nutrition: less than body requirements (OCs)
Knowledge deficit

GOALS
Short term

Client develops a relationship with care-provider based on trust.

Nurse identifies myths, clarifies misinformation, and fills in knowledge gaps for client.

Client becomes comfortable in the use of the method.

Client learns relevant content, for example, use, action, advantages, disadvantages or side-effects, and effectiveness.

Intermediate

Client confers with care-provider when questions arise regarding use or desire to change to another method.

Client reports complications or suspected pregnancy immediately.

Client returns to care-giver when change in contraceptive use is warranted, for example, pregnancy is desired, age of 35 is reached (hormonal therapy), weight gain or loss exceeds 4.5kg (10 lb) (diaphragm), sterilization is desired.

Client maintains schedule for health supervision.

Long term

Client maintains health, for example, suffers no serious infection (IUD), retains function of hypothalamic-pituitary-ovarian axis (hormonal contraception).

Client achieves desired objective for contraception, that is, no children or desired number of children.

Client indicates satisfaction with care received.

REFERENCES/TEACHING AIDS

Inserts from packages of chosen contraceptive
Hospital/clinic teaching materials
Flip chart showing anatomy of pelvic structures or total body plastic medical models
Hospital or clinic audiovisual teaching materials
Samples of contraceptive device, BBT charts and thermometer, and so on
Fresh egg white (for teaching about cervical mucus)
Mirror
Handouts of printed information

CONTENT/RATIONALE	TEACHING ACTIONS
General discussion about selected method, understanding of its method of action, and reasons for choosing it. Establish basis and direction for cognitive, psychomotor, and affective learning needs.	Encourage general discussion through use of the following: 1. Providing time, privacy, and assurance regarding confidentiality 2. Creating a receptive, nonjudgmental atmosphere. 3. Considering appropriate cultural/ethnic, intellectual/educational, and developmental factors pertinent to the individual woman/couple
Information about action advantages, disadvantages or side effects, and effectiveness.	Using references and equipment listed above, implement the following: ■ Discuss information about the selected method
Illustration or model of method, its placement, locus of action.	■ Indicate on illustration or medical model the placement of device (IUD, diaphragm, cervical cap or sponge, condom), loci of action (hormonal contraceptive vs. diaphragm)
Visualization of use.	■ Demonstrate appliance (diaphragm with spermicide), characteristics of "fertile" cervical mucus (egg white), entering of temperature on BBT chart, calculating fertile times
Hands-on experience in use of method. Testing for mastery of content and experience.	■ Supervise client's return demonstration and practice ■ Assess client's recall of content taught or its availability on printed material supplied
Reaffirmation of health care provider's caring and client's motivation.	■ Ascertain that client has appropriate phone numbers for questions and suggest client call back after implementing method at home

EVALUATION Woman or couple demonstrate degree to which the goals for care are met.

inflammatory disease (PID), known or suspected pregnancy, undiagnosed genital bleeding, suspected genital malignancy, or a distorted intrauterine cavity. IUDs are associated with perforation of the uterus, embedment in endometrium or myometrium, uterine cramping and bleeding, iron-deficiency anemia secondary to blood loss, pelvic infections, pregnancy with IUD in place, and pregnancy following undetected expulsion. Some women allergic to copper develop a rash, necessitating the removal of the copper-bearing IUD.

The incidence of perforation is minimized by delaying insertion until a woman finishes lactation (Liskin and Fox, 1982). Except for the Dalkon Shield, the risk of IUD-associated PID is largely limited to the first few months after insertion (Lee and others, 1983). PID occurs in approximately 1% to 3% of women wearing IUDs of all types (Zatuchni, 1984). PID is linked with involuntary infertility (Dalin, and others, 1985). The risk of PID and primary tubal infection is minimized if a medicated device is used by a woman who has only one sexual partner (Cramer and others, 1985).

The presence of the threads must be checked following menstruation and at the time of ovulation as well as prior to coitus to rule out expulsion of the device. If pregnancy occurs with the IUD in place, it should be removed immediately, if possible (Grimes, 1986). Retention of the IUD increases the risk of septic spontaneous abortion and other obstetric problems (Liskin and Fox, 1982). Because the IUD reduces the absolute number of pregnancies overall, current IUD wearers have only 40% the risk for ectopic pregnancy experienced by women not using contraception (Ory, 1981).

The mean blood loss is increased for the copper IUD but not for the Progestersert. This blood loss may be clinically significant in undernourished populations.

The use of medical diathermy (shortwave and microwave) in a woman with a metal-containing IUD may cause heat injury to surrounding tissue. Therefore medical diathermy to the abdominal and sacral areas should not be used on women using copper-bearing IUDs. Additional amounts of copper available to the body from copper-containing IUDs may precipitate symptoms in women with undiagnosed Wilson's disease. The incidence of Wilson's disease (an inborn error of metabolism) is 1 in 200,000.

Effectiveness. The pregnancy (failure) rates vary from 0.5 to 5 per 100 woman years of use (Population Reports, 1982). Effectiveness and length of effectiveness vary with the type of copper-containing device. The Copper-T 220 and 380 and the multiload Copper 250 (not available in the United States, but probably

the world's largest selling IUD) have lower pregnancy rates then the currently available Copper-T 200 (Zatuchni, 1984). Both the Copper-T 220 and 380 have copper sleeves on the transverse arms of the T as well as copper around the vertical arm (Fig. 7.7). The local effect of copper is extended to the fundal endometrium, where implantation is most likely to occur.

Nursing actions. The nursing actions related to the IUD are presented in the form of teaching tools. A general teaching tool for contraceptive methods is given below.

METHODS REQUIRING SURGICAL INTERVENTION: STERILIZATION

Since 1950, voluntary sterilization has grown rapidly in acceptance and is currently the most prevalent method of contraception in the world. Approximately 100 million couples choose voluntary sterilization, and the demand is expected to grow during this century. In the United States, voluntary sterilization is the most common choice of contraception for couples who are 30 years of age or older.

Motivation for sterilization. Motivation for elective sterilization includes (1) personal preference, (2) obstetric reasons, such as multiparity, (3) medical reasons such as hypertensive, cardiovascular, or renal disease in the woman or recurrent acute epididymitis in the man, and (4) diagnosis of inheritable disease.

Sterilization as a means of contraception may be requested by couples who have almost come to the end of their childbearing years and have the desired number of children. It is also chosen by young adults who have decided not to bear children. Persons in the first group are generally acceptive of the procedure even though there may be some feelings of regret because one of life's phases is over. Persons in the second group need the opportunity to explore the consequences of their choice.

Laws and regulations. All states have strict regulations for informed consent (see Chapter 3). Now many states in the United States permit voluntary sterilization of any mature, rational woman without reference to her marital or pregnancy status. Although the partner's consent is not required, the client is encouraged to discuss the situation with her or his partner.

Sterilization of minors or mentally incompetent females is restricted by most states. The operation often requires the approval of a board of eugenicists or other court-appointed individuals.

If federal funds are used, the person must be at least 21 years of age and mentally competent. Some state and federal regulations govern Medicaid funds for elective sterilization; for example, counseling and a waiting period after the decision is made are mandatory.

Sterilization procedures. Sterilization refers to surgical procedures intended to render the person infertile. Most procedures involve the occlusion of the passageways for the ova and sperm (Fig. 7.8). For the female the oviducts (uterine tubes) are occluded; for the male the sperm ducts (vas deferens) are occluded. Only surgical removal of the ovaries (oophorectomy)

or uterus (hysterectomy) or both will result in absolute sterility for the woman. All other operations have a small but definite failure rate; that is, pregnancy may result.

Female sterilization
Timing of female sterilization. Female sterilization may be done immediately after delivery (within 24 to 48 hours), concomitantly with abortion, or as an interval procedure (during any phase of the menstrual cycle). Most sterilization procedures are performed im-

Fig. 7.8
Sterilization. **A,** Oviduct ligated and severed (tubal ligation). **B,** Sperm duct severed (and ligated) (vasectomy).

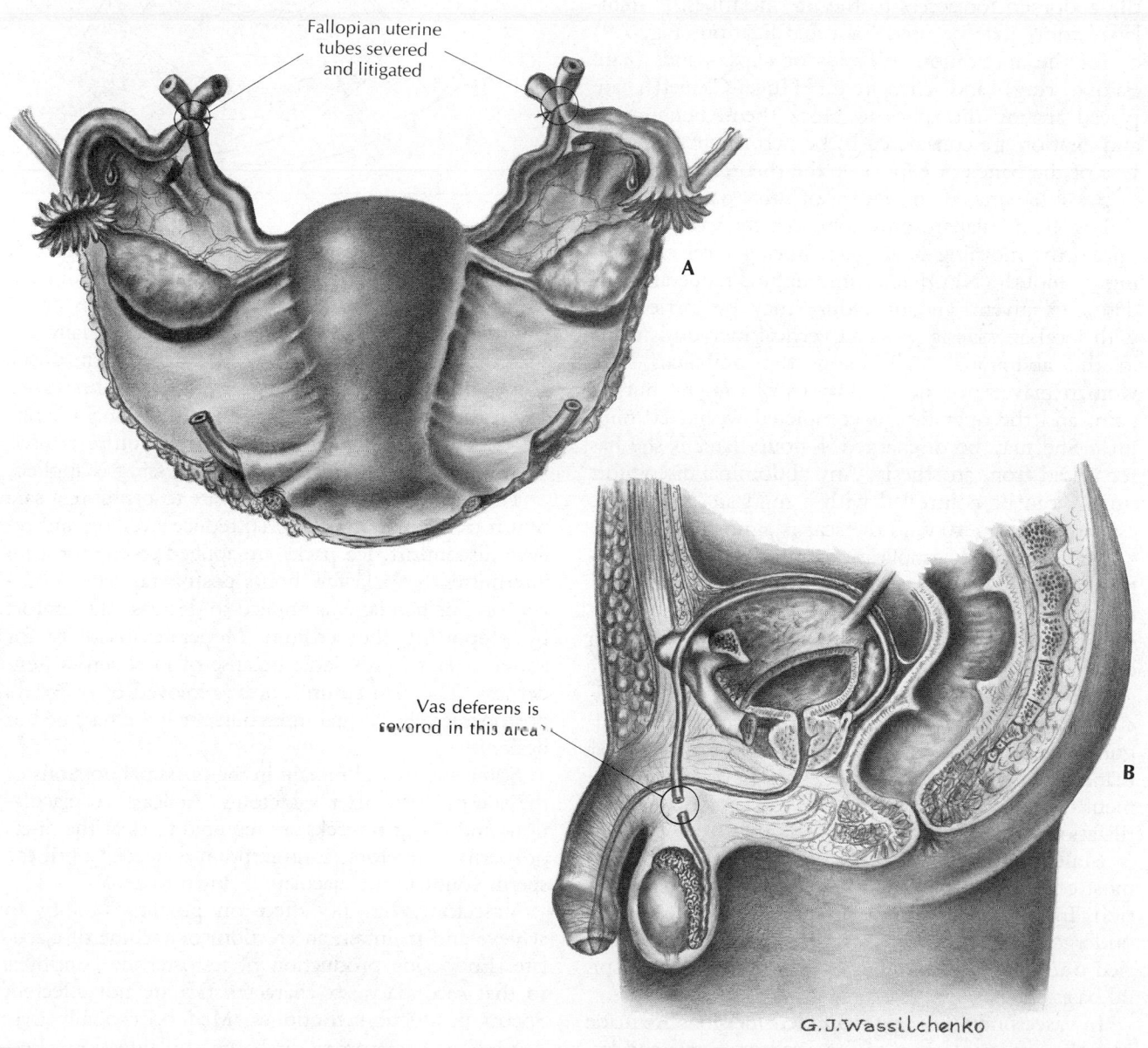

Fallopian uterine tubes severed and litigated

Vas deferens is severed in this area

G.J.Wassilchenko

mediately after a pregnancy, probably because of heightened motivation or increased practicality. Usually the woman is already in the hospital and all preoperative preparations (blood work, physical examination, etc.) have been completed.

However, all sterilization procedures have the lowest morbidity and failure rates when accomplished at a time other than immediately after a pregnancy. Tissue edema continues during the early postpartum period, which may permit the sutures to cut through the tubal wall and leave an opening into the tube.

Tubal occlusion. The operation used frequently is the laparoscopic tubal fulguration (destruction of tissue by means of an electric current). See box (p. 139) for laparoscopy examination, a procedure of entering the abdomen for access to the uterine tubes. A minilaparotomy may be used for tubal ligation (Fig. 7.9) or for the application of bands or clips. Bands (e.g., Falope ring) and clips (e.g., Hulka-Clemens) are placed around the tubes to block them. Fulguration and ligation are considered to be permanent methods. Use of the bands or clips have the theoretic advantage of possible removal and return of tubal patency.

For the minilaparotomy approach the woman is admitted the morning of surgery, having received nothing by mouth (NPO) since midnight. Preoperative sedation is given. The procedure may be carried out with local anesthesia. A small vertical incision is made in the abdominal wall below the umbilicus. The woman may experience sensations of tugging but no pain, and the operation is completed within 20 minutes. She may be discharged 4 hours later if she has recovered from anesthesia. Any abdominal discomfort usually can be controlled with a mild analgesic (e.g., aspirin). Within 10 days the scar is almost invisible.

Major medical complications after elective sterilization are rare. Dysfunctional uterine bleeding or ovarian cyst formation may occur after tubal surgery, presumably because of disturbance of the utero-ovarian circulation.

Tubal reanastomosis. Tubal continuity is not difficult to reestablish except after laparoscopic tubal fulguration. The incidence of successful pregnancy after reanastomosis is only about 15%. The loss of a segment of tube necessary for sperm capacitation and fertilization is the probable cause.

Male sterilization. Vasectomy is the easiest and most commonly employed operation for male sterilization. In the United States since 1975, 1 million men undergo vasectomy each year. Vasectomy can be carried out with local anesthesia and on an out-of-hospital basis.

In vasectomy, short right and left incisions are made into the anterior aspect of the scrotum above and lat-

Fig. 7.9
Use of minilaparotomy to gain access to oviducts for tubal occlusion procedures. Tenaculum is used to lift uterus upward *(arrow)* toward incision.

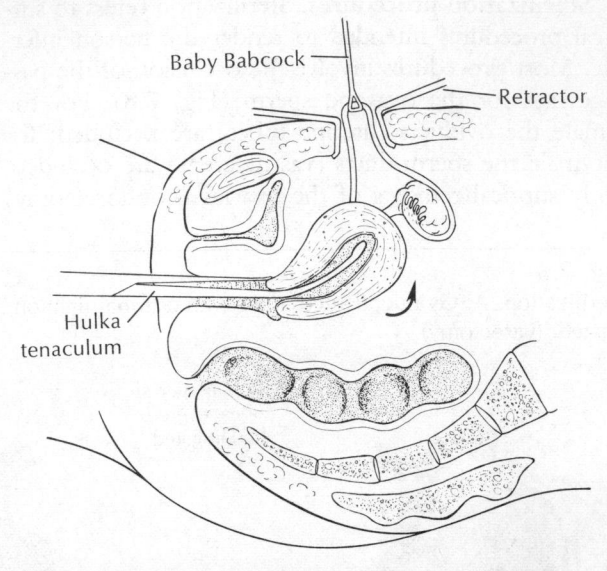

eral to each testis over the spermatic cord (Fig. 7.8, *B*). Each vas deferens is identified and doubly ligated with fine nonabsorbable sutures. Then each vas deferens is incised between the ligatures. Occasionally the surgeon fulgurates the cut stumps of the sperm ducts. Many surgeons bury the cut ends into scrotal fascia to lessen the chance of reunion. Then the skin incisions are closed. Usually one nonabsorbable suture is used for closure of each skin incision. A dressing is applied.

The man is instructed in self-care to promote a safe return to routine activities. To reduce swelling and relieve discomfort, ice packs are applied to the scrotum intermittently for a few hours postoperatively. A suspensory, or bandage, is applied to decrease discomfort by supporting the scrotum. Moderate inactivity for about 2 days is advisable because of local scrotal tenderness. The skin suture can be removed 5 to 7 days postoperatively. Sexual intercourse may be resumed as desired.

Some sperm will remain in the proximal portions of the sperm ducts after vasectomy. At least 10 ejaculations and about 6 weeks are required to clear the ducts of sperm. Therefore, contraception is needed until the sperm count in the ejaculate is down to zero.

Vasectomy has no effect on potency (ability to achieve and maintain an erection) or volume of ejaculate. Endocrine production of testosterone continues so that secondary sex characteristics are not affected. Sperm production continues. Men occasionally may develop a hematoma, discharge, or infection. Less

Table 7.11
Summary of Sterilization Methods: Basis for Counseling

Method and Action	Advantages	Disadvantages and Side Effects	Effectiveness
Woman			
Tubal occlusion: uterine tubes ligated and severed, banded or clipped, or fulgurated, to prevent passage of egg	Abdominal surgery using 2.5 cm (1 in) incision and laparoscopy. Ovaries and endometrium remain intact; menstruation continues	Major surgery with possible complications of anesthesia, infection, hemorrhage, and trauma to other organs Psychologic trauma in some women Sperm may enter peritoneal cavity if tubal ligature slips, and ectopic (abdominal) pregnancy may ensue	100% effective if ligatures, bands, or clips do not slip or cut through
Hysterectomy with salpingo-oophorectomy; no egg produced	No further menstruation	Abrupt loss of ovarian hormones, simulating menopause Possibility of major surgical complications Psychologic trauma if there is a perceived loss of femininity and sexuality	100% effective
Man			
Vasectomy: vas deferens ligated and severed or banded to interrupt passage of sperm	Relatively simple surgical procedure Does not affect endocrine production or function of testosterone Does not alter volume of ejaculate	Possibility of impotence in some men because of psychologic response to procedure Reversible in many cases Even if procedure is reversed, man may remain infertile if he has developed an autoimmune response (antibodies) to his sperm	100% effective after ejaculate is free of sperm that was in vas deferens (about 6 weeks or 10 ejaculations)

common are painful granulomas from accumulation of sperm. Sperm unable to leave the epididymis are lyzed by the immune system.

Complications following bilateral vasectomy are infrequent and usually not serious. They include bleeding (usually external), suture reaction, and reaction to anesthetic agent. Sterilization failures, usually caused by a recanalization, are rare, occurring in about 2 per 1000 men.

Tubal reanastomosis. Microsurgery to reanastomose the sperm ducts can be accomplished successfully in 90% of cases. Yet 30% to 60% of men having the reversal operation remain infertile. The vasectomy may result in permanent changes in the testes that leave men unable to father children. The changes are those ordinarily seen only in the elderly, e.g., interstitial fibrosis (scar tissue between the seminiferous tubules) (Jarow and Marshall, 1985). Some men develop antibodies against their own sperm (autoimmunization). Even if the procedure is successfully reversed, many men remain infertile because of this autoimmune reaction.

Nursing actions

Teaching and counseling. The nurse plays an important role in assisting people with decision making so that all requirements for informed consent are met. People seek information about the various methods of sterilization. Table 7.11 summarizes expected actions,

advantages and side effects, and effectiveness for each method. The table is used as a basis for teaching and counseling. The nurse also provides information about alternatives to sterilization, for examples, contraception.

The nurse acts as a sounding board for people who are exploring the possibility of choosing sterilization and their feelings about and motivation for this choice. The nurse records this information, which may be the basis for referral to a family planning clinic, a psychiatric social worker, or another professional health care provider.

Information about what is entailed in various procedures, how much discomfort or pain can be expected, and what type of care is needed must be given. Many individuals fear sterilization procedures because of the imagined effect on their sexual life. They need reassurance concerning the hormonal and psychologic basis for sexual function and the fact that uterine tube occlusion or vasectomy has no biologic sequelae in terms of sexual adequacy.

Preoperative preparation. Printed instructions are usually available for clients from the physician. The physician performs the preoperative health assessment, which includes a psychologic assessment, physical examination, and laboratory test. The nurse assists with the health assessment, answers questions, and confirms the client's understanding of printed instructions (e.g., NPO after midnight). Ambivalence and extreme fear of the procedure are reported to the physician.

Postoperative care. Postoperative care depends on the procedure performed, for example, laparoscopy,* laparotomy, hysterectomy, or vasectomy. General care includes postanesthesia recovery, vital signs, fluid-electrolyte balance (intake and output, laboratory values), prevention of or early identification and treatment for infection or hemorrhage, control of discomfort, and assessment of emotional response to the procedure and recovery.

Discharge planning. Discharge planning depends on the type of procedure performed. In general, the client is given written instructions about observing for and reporting symptoms and signs of complications, the type of recovery to be expected, and the date and time for a follow-up appointment.

Summary. Personnel who function in infertility and birth control clinics or in hospitals must be carefully selected. Studies indicate that attitudes of personnel significantly affect the client's perception of the quality of care received (World Health Organization, 1971). This consideration is important in planning for the overall delivery of health services. Seeking help for infertility and fertility control is frequently the only contact some people have with the health care system. Positive perceptions of the interest, concern, and technical skill of health workers in this instance may induce wider use of health facilities and care in the future.

Surgical Interruption of Pregnancy

Elective abortion is the purposeful interruption of a previable pregnancy (p. 39). Indications for elective abortion are as follows:

*See p. 139 for discussion of laparoscopy.

1. Preservation of the life or health of the mother (e.g., class III or IV heart disease)
2. Avoidance of the birth of an offspring with a serious developmental or hereditary disorder (e.g., Tay-Sachs disease)
3. Voluntary abortion (e.g., because of inability of the parents to support or care for the child, rape, mental incompetence, or because of severe emotional problems)

The control of birth, dealing as it does with human sexuality and the question of life and death, is one of the most highly emotionalized components of health care. Abortion as one of the surgical alternatives to contraception is regulated in most countries. Regulations exist presumably to protect the mother from the complications of abortion or because of religious constraints. The U.S. Supreme Court set aside previous antiabortion laws in January 1973, holding that first-trimester abortion is permissible in this country inasmuch as the mortality from interruption of early gestation is now less than the mortality after normal term delivery. Second-trimester abortion was left to the discretion of the individual states. Roman Catholic hospitals and some of those maintained by strict fundamentalists forbid abortion (and often sterilization) despite legal challenge.

Before the legalization of abortion, many illegal abortions took place, with little-documented sequelae other than death from infection or hemorrhage or both. Although studies indicate that biologic sequelae do occur after abortion, rates of biologic complications tends to be low, especially if the woman aborts during the first trimester. Studies related to psychologic sequelae reveal that they are short lived. Sequelae are related to circumstances surrounding the abortion, such as rape or the attitudes reflected by friends, family, and health workers. It must be remembered that the

Table 7.12
Interruption of Pregnancy: Basis for Counseling

Methods*	Advantages	Disadvantages and Side Effects	Effectiveness
First-trimester procedures			
Menstrual extraction: forced endometrial extraction through undilated cervix	Performed up to 14 days after missed period No legal proscriptions	Cervical trauma may occur, may lead to incompetence Hemorrhage	100% if implantation site is not missed
Prostaglandin: IV administration or injection into cul-de-sac of Douglas or by vaginal suppository or pessary	Stimulates smooth muscle Causes degeneration of corpus luteum	Requires about 24 hours to take effect May cause vomiting, diarrhea, chills, local tissue reaction Retained placenta necessitates D and C	100%

Adapted from Bobak, I.M.: Nursing during the reproductive years. In Lagerquist, S., editor: Addison-Wesley's graduate nurse review, Menlo Park, Calif., 1982, Addison-Wesley Publishing Co.
*Prophylaxis against Rh isoimmunization, $Rh_0(D)$ immune globulin, is given within 72 hours to every Rh-negative, Du-negative, unsensitized (Coombs' negative) woman.

Table 7.12
Interruption of Pregnancy: Basis for Counseling—cont'd

Methods	Advantages	Disadvantages and Side Effects	Effectiveness
Vacuum (suction) curettage: cannula suction after cervical dilatation, under local anesthesia	Effective with relatively few complications: minimal bleeding, minimal discomfort 5-15 minutes duration Done on out-of-hospital or same-day surgery basis	Pregnancy 12 weeks or less Possibility of cervical trauma (decreased if dilatation accomplished by insertion of laminaria tent 4-24 hours before procedure); endometrial trauma possible Hazards: possible uterine perforation, hemorrhage, or infection	100% if implantation site is not missed and if other reproductive tract anomaly (double uterus) does not exist
Dilatation and curettage (D and C): cervix dilated, endometrium scraped with spoonlike instrument	Duration of 15 minutes Usually few complications	Pregnancy 12 weeks or less Hazards: uterine perforation, infection (25%), effects of general anesthesia, cervical trauma	100% if implantation site is not missed
Second-trimester procedures			
Intraamniotic infusion: between week 14 and 23 or 24 (uterus in abdominal cavity and sufficient amniotic fluid present)	Does not require laparotomy	Increase in complications proportionately with weeks of gestation	Fetal death within 1 hour of injection; abortion completed within 36-40 hours
Transabdominal extraction: amniotic fluid extracted; replaced with equal amount of saline solution (20%) (or 30% urea in 5% D/W)	Ambulation until labor starts (within 24 hours) and during early labor	Reaction to saline solution (hypernatremia): tinnitus, tachycardia, and headache Water intoxication: edema, oliguria ($\leq$200 ml/8 hours), dyspnea, thirst, and restlessness Induced labor, occasionally explosive with an unripe cervix; fetus passes out of posterior vault of vagina and forms fistula Hazards requiring hospitalization (6% readmitted for complications): Hemorrhage and possible D and C May require postabortal D and C or vacuum extraction as well Fever with sepsis	Two thirds of fetuses aborted within 24 hours
Instillation of 40-45 mg PGF$_2\alpha$, E$_2$	Labor usually shorter than with saline solution Avoid complications of water intoxication and hypernatremia	May cause vomiting, diarrhea, nausea Fetus may be born alive D and C may be required to remove placental fragments	100%
Dilatation and evacuation (D and E)	Hospitalization shortened With skilled operator, complication rate lower than with intraamniotic infusion methods	24 hours before procedure, 2 or 3 laminaria tents used to dilate cervix to required 2 cm Fetus possibly born alive	100%
Second- and third-trimester procedures			
Hysterotomy: cesarean incision	Preferred method if woman wishes tubal ligation or hysterectomy to follow	Complications after major surgery—hemorrhage and infection Fetus possibly born alive, opening ethical, moral, religious, and legal problems Mortality risk—combination hysterotomy-hysterectomy 10% greater than with D and C	100%
Hysterectomy: at or before 24 weeks without first emptying uterus	As above	As above	100%

woman facing an abortion is pregnant and will exhibit the emotional responses shared by all pregnant women, including postdelivery depression.

In an attempt to regulate the conflict between professional responsibilities and personal ethics the Nurses' Association of the American College of Obstetricians and Gynecologists (NAACOG) published a position paper on the nurse's role with the abortion client in May 1972, in which the simultaneous rights of each were described (Tyrer, 1973). Women have the right to expect and receive supportive, nonjudgmental care. Nurses have the right to refuse to assist with abortions or sterilizations in keeping with their own moral or religious beliefs, unless the woman's life is in danger.

Compelling medical, surgical, or psychiatric indications for elective abortion are not numerous. The following conditions probably would qualify: class III coronary heart disease; fulminating (pelvic) Hodgkin's disease; stage 1B carcinoma of the cervix; and Marfan's syndrome with early aortic aneurysm. The length of pregnancy and the condition of the woman determine the appropriate type of abortion procedure (Table 7.12).

Early abortion. Methods for performing early therapeutic abortion include the following:

1. Menstrual extraction—early aspiration of the endometrium in women who have not yet missed a period
2. Surgical dilatation and curettage (D and C) when newer aspiration equipment is unavailable
3. Uterine aspiration after one or two missed periods

The insertion of a small laminaria tent retained by a vaginal tampon for 4 to 24 hours usually will facilitate the purposeful interruption of a first-trimester pregnancy by dilating the cervix atraumatically (Fig. 7.10). On removal of the moist, expanded laminaria, the cervix will have dilated two or three times its original (dry) diameter. Rarely will further mechanical dilatation of the cervix be required. The insertion of an adequate-sized aspiration cannula (8.5 to 10.5 mm) is almost always possible. Cervical laceration and bleeding are reduced by the use of laminaria. A disadvantage is the delay necessary and the need for an additional visit to the physician's office or clinic.

The woman comes to the clinic or physician's office the day before the abortion procedure. An antiseptic solution is used to prepare the pelvic area. A vaginal speculum is inserted, and the vaginal canal and cervix are cleansed. Injection of a local anesthetic agent into the cervix may follow (see paracervical block, p. 173). Again the area is cleansed, and the laminaria tent is inserted into the endocervical canal. Prophylactic use of an antibiotic is usually begun. Some women expe-

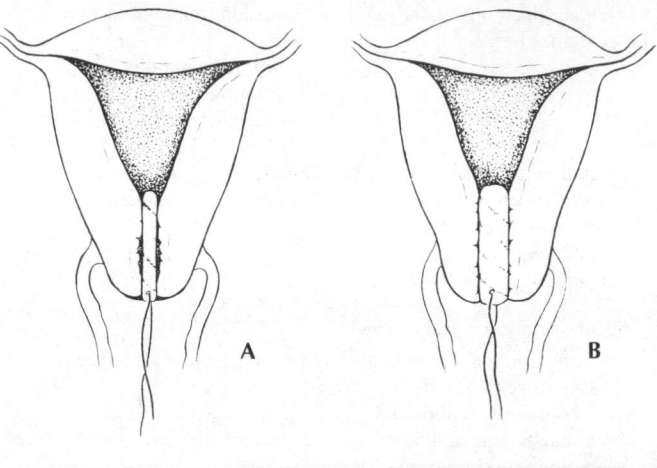

Fig. 7.10
Laminaria tents. **A,** Inserted through narrow cervical canal beyond the internal os. **B,** Cervix dilated 4 to 12 hours later. (From Sanberg, E.C.: Synopsis of obstetrics, ed. 10, St. Louis, 1978, The C.V. Mosby Co.)

rience a mild cramping or have light spotting from the anesthetic injection. Discomfort can usually be controlled with analgesics.

Aspiration abortion may be performed in the physician's office or in the hospital setting. If the woman chooses a hospital setting, she is admitted the day after insertion of the laminaria tent and is given preoperative sedation. The vaginal area is cleansed (shaving is not necessary). The suction procedure for accomplishing an early therapeutic abortion (ideal time is 8 to 10 weeks since last menstrual period) usually requires less than 5 minutes and can easily be effected under paracervical block anesthesia and single sedation. During the procedure the nurse or physician keeps the woman informed as to what to expect next, for example, menstrual-like cramping, sounds of suction machine. The nurse assesses the woman's vital signs and observes her for vagal response (p. 281). The aspirated uterine contents must be carefully inspected to ascertain whether all fetal parts and adequate placental tissue have been evacuated. A single dose of oxytocin is usually sufficient to control bleeding. The woman may remain in the hospital 3 or 4 hours for detection of excessive cramping or excessive bleeding and then is discharged. If the procedure is done in the physician's office, preoperative sedation is usually not given, and the anesthetic of choice is usually paracervical block. After the abortion the woman rests on the table until she is ready to get up. Then she remains in the waiting room until she feels she can travel. She may be discharged in the company of a relative or friend.

Bleeding after the operation normally is about the equivalent of a heavy menstrual period, and cramps are rarely severe. Infection such as endometritis or salpingitis occurs in about 8% of women. Subsequently a D and C procedure for bleeding or sepsis caused by retained placental tissue is necessary in about 2% of women. Serious depression or other psychiatric problems are rare.

Postabortal instructions differ with the institution (e.g., use of tampons may be denied for only 3 days or for up to 6 weeks, and resumption of sexual intercourse may be permitted within 1 week or discouraged for 6 weeks). The woman may bathe or shower daily. Instruction is given to watch for excessive bleeding, cramps, or fever and to avoid douches of any type. The woman may expect her menstrual period to resume 4 to 6 weeks from the day of the procedure. The nurse offers information about the birth control method the woman prefers if this has not been done previously during counseling interview that usually precedes the decision to have an abortion. The woman must be strongly encouraged to return for her follow-up visit so that complications can be avoided and an acceptable contraceptive method prescribed.

Second- and third-trimester abortions. There are four types of techniques used for second- and third-trimester abortions:

1. *Transabdominal intrauterine injection of hypertonic sodium chloride.* The woman is admitted to the hospital for this procedure. Amniocentesis is performed. The physician determines where the needle (an 18-gauge, 7.5 cm [3 in] spinal needle) will be inserted. The area is cleansed, and if desired, a local anesthetic agent is given. Approximately 200 ml of amniotic fluid is withdrawn, and a similar amount of sterile 20% sodium chloride is injected. The woman is instructed to report when uterine contractions begin—generally within 8 to 48 hours. In most cases augmentation with oxytocin is necessary to effect uterine evacuation in a reasonable time. Occasionally reinjection is required. Labor begins, in theory at least, because the hypertonic saline solution releases the placental uterine progesterone blockade that normally prevents the onset of labor. The same careful monitoring of uterine contractions is as necessary as for a term delivery. Instruction in relaxation and breathing techniques is indicated, and analgesia can be administered for discomfort. The assistance of a supportive person at the time of birth of the dead fetus is essential. If the woman wishes to see the fetus, emotional support should be provided before and after the procedure. Many women are relieved to find the fetus normal and frequently inquire as to its sex. After the delivery the standard observations and postpartum care are carried out (see Chapter 24).

Contraceptive counseling is given before discharge. The woman is advised to return should excessive bleeding occur.

Complications of hypertonic saline injection for second-trimester abortion may occur. Complications with the approximate frequency of their occurrence include infection (10%), need for D and C to remove retained tissue (15%), failure to abort (10%), and excessive bleeding, necessitating transfusion (2%). Rarely, disseminated intravascular coagulation (DIC) or expulsion of the fetus through the uterine isthmus occurs.

2. *Injection of urea solution after amniocentesis.* After the removal of about 200 ml of amniotic fluid, 200 ml of 30% solution of urea in 5% dextrose in water is introduced into the uterus by gravity drip. After 1 hour a solution of 5 units of oxytocin in 500 ml of 5% dextrose in water is started intravenously. Fetal death occurs, and delivery ensues in most cases within 12 hours. Complications are less common and are less serious than with hypertonic saline solution.

3. *Transabdominal intrauterine injection of PGF$_{2\alpha}$.* The undesirable side effects of hypertonic saline solution, such as hypernatremia or DIC, do not occur with prostaglandins; therefore it has become the treatment of choice. However, nausea and vomiting are common problems. Abortion usually takes place within 18 to 24 hours after injection. If it does not occur, the procedure is repeated, but only half the dosage is used.

4. *Abdominal or vaginal hysterotomy.* Hysterotomy may be chosen after more than 14 to 16 weeks of pregnancy, after failure of intrauterine injection of saline solution or PGF$_{2\alpha}$, and when sterilization is desired. The vaginal approach is employed when transabdominal surgery should be avoided. The management is comparable to that of cesarean delivery.

Anesthesia for gynecologic procedures: paracervical (uterosacral) block. Paracervical block anesthesia is used for a variety of gynecologic procedures. Tests for infertility such as endometrial biopsy and aspiration abortion are two such procedures.

For paracervical anesthesia (Fig. 16.2) a dilute local anesthetic drug (e.g., 5 ml of 1% procaine) is injected just beneath the mucosa in each fornix posterolateral to the cervix (9- and 3-o'clock positions). The result is excellent pain relief for at least 1 hour. Anesthesia extends from the lower uterine segment and cervix to the upper one third of the vagina; there is no perineal anesthesia. A needle guide (e.g., the "Iowa trumpet") is useful but not indispensable in facilitating the paracervical block. Complications may include vasovagal syncope and intravascular injection.

The procedure is explained to the woman. She is asked to void if her bladder is full. Her vital signs are checked and recorded. The sight of the long needle used to inject the anesthesia may be frightening. The woman can be reassured that only the tip of the needle will be inserted. For this sterile procedure the physician or anesthesiologist will need the nurse's assistance in positioning the woman (dorsal recumbent position with knees flexed), handling supplies, and helping the woman to remain immobile while the injection is made.

Summary of Nursing Actions

INTERRUPTION OF PREGNANCY (ELECTIVE ABORTION)

GOALS

1. To utilize the decision-making process to arrive at a solution acceptable to the woman.
2. To prevent adverse physical or psychologic consequences.

PRIORITIES

1. Providing information and support to assist the woman in decision making.
2. Accurate dating of gestation.
3. Identification of risk factors.
4. Appropriate perioperative management.
5. Follow-up physical and psychologic care.

ASSESSMENT	EXAMPLES OF POTENTIAL NURSING DIAGNOSTIC CATEGORIES*
Interview 1. Health history: risk factors for continuing the pregnancy (health, fetal abnormality, rape, incest), contraceptive failure, last menstrual period. 2. Psychosocial: social problems, financial hardship, inability to give adequate care to a child, interference with educational/vocational goals, no desire to be a parent at this time 3. Review of systems: risk factors for continuing pregnancy (cardiac disease), allergies	Potential for infection Potential for injury Alteration in comfort: pain Knowledge deficit Anxiety Fear Powerlessness Disturbance in self-concept: body image, self-esteem, role performance, personal identity Alteration in family process Anticipatory grieving Alteration in parenting: actual Ineffective individual coping Ineffective family coping Spiritual distress
Physical examination A. Risk factors: concurrent infections, medical disease B. Determination of duration of gestation by manual palpation of uterus, measurement of height of fundus	Potential for infection Potential for injury Alteration in comfort: pain Powerlessness Knowledge deficit Anxiety Fear Disturbance in self-concept: body image, self-esteem, role performance, personal identity
Laboratory tests A. Pregnancy test B. Blood work: HCT, Hgb, Rh, blood type	Potential for isoimmunization† Alteration in nutrition: less than body requirements

*Accepted diagnoses from NANDA's Seventh National Conference (1986).
†Diagnosis not included in NANDA (1986).

Summary of Nursing Actions

OUTCOME CRITERIA*	PLAN/IMPLEMENTATION
Woman arrived at her own decision. The procedure chosen was appropriate for the duration of gestation. Perioperative care was given per accepted protocol. Woman suffers no adverse physical consequences. Woman suffers no adverse psychologic consequences. Woman implements postoperative instructions regarding her care. Woman implements the birth control method suitable/appropriate for her. Woman keeps follow-up appointment.	Plan and implement nursing roles of support person, teacher/counselor/advocate, and technician: **Support person** Encourages verbalization of feelings. Provides information about choices available (having the abortion, carrying the pregnancy to term and then either keeping the child or giving him or her up for adoption; information about the abortion procedure). Involves family members as appropriate for the woman. **Teacher/counselor/advocate** Instructs client regarding what to expect during procedure, for example, sensations, supportive care. Ensures that the woman and significant other know and understand (Tucker, 1984) the following: ■ Importance of reporting bleeding that lasts longer than 7 to 10 days ■ Importance of reporting excessive bright red bleeding with clots ■ Symptoms of infection to report: Nausea or vomiting Severe uterine cramping Temperature about 100° F (37.8° C) Foul odor of vaginal discharge ■ Careful cleaning of perineal area; wipe front to back after each elimination ■ That douching, tampons, and coitus should be avoided for 4 to 6 weeks or as indicated by physician ■ That normal menstrual period should begin in 4 to 6 weeks ■ Importance of follow-up care ■ Contraceptive method of choice, since pregnancy is possible within 2 to 3 weeks **Technician** Assists with interview, physical examination, and laboratory tests. Provides preoperative care: vital signs, blood pressure; abdominal, suprapubic, or perineal cleansing; instruction to empty bladder; sedation per order; intravenous infusion per order. Provides support to the woman and assists physician during procedure. Monitors vital signs, blood pressure, emotional responses. Provides postoperative care: vital signs, blood pressure, recovery from medications, bleeding, postdelivery care, RhoGAM injections as ordered, discharge instructions.

Evaluation The nurse can be assured that care was effective when goals and outcome criteria are achieved.

*Outcome criteria direct the selection of nursing actions (**plan/implementation**) and measure their effectiveness (**evaluation**).

Summary

The roles of the nurse vary in the care of clients requiring treatment for infertility, control of fertility, and termination of fertility (see Summary of Nursing Actions). A solid knowledge base of anatomy and physiology, mastery of nursing skills, and the nurse's self-awareness are all essential factors in meeting client needs. Professional satisfaction is the reward for the nurse who is able to assist clients coping with reproductive issues.

The values, beliefs, and moral convictions of the nurse are involved to the same extent as those of the pregnant woman. The conflicts and doubts of the nurse can be readily communicated to women who are already anxious and overly sensitive. Health professionals need assistance to identify and come to terms with their own feelings. It is not uncommon for confusion to arise as beliefs are challenged by the reality of care. A nursing student reacted to learning experiences associated with in-hospital abortions in the following manner:

I really feel I believe in the rightness of therapeutic abortion, but when I watched the physician insert the needle and then inject the dose of prostaglandin, I felt an unreasoning rage sweep over me. I could have attacked him. Funny, I felt no anger toward the girl at all. I really need to rethink my beliefs.

Responses can also change with life experiences. A nurse who before her marriage had worked as counselor in a municipal clinic established a reputation as a supportive and concerned counselor of young persons with regard to birth control. Four years later she remarked:

I've been trying to get pregnant for the past 3 years. I didn't realize how important it would be to me. You know I can't counsel about abortion any more. I can't be objective. I keep feeling, "Have your baby and please give it to me." I am more concerned about myself now, not them [the pregnant women], and counseling won't work that way.

References

Affonso, D.D.: The Filipino American. In Clark, A., editor: Culture/childbearing/health professionals, Philadelphia, 1978, F. A. Davis Co.

Bachrach, C.A.: Contraceptive practice among American women: 1973-1982, Fam. Plann. Perspect. 16:253, 1984.

Bernstein, J.L., and Kidd, Y.A.: Childbearing in Japan. In Kay, M.A., editor: Anthropology of human birth, Philadelphia, 1982, F.A. Davis Co.

Brownlee, A.T.: Community, culture, and care: a cross-cultural guide for health workers, St. Louis, 1978, The C.V. Mosby Co., p. 202.

Clark, A.L., and Howland, I.H.: The American Samoan. In Clark, A.L., editor: Culture/childbearing/health professionals, Philadelphia, 1978, F.A. Davis Co.

Clark, M.: Health in the Mexican-American culture: a community study, Berkeley, 1970, University of California Press.

Coughlin, R.: Pregnancy and birth in Vietnam. In Hart, D., and others, editors: Southeast Asian birth customs: three studies in human reproduction, New Haven, Conn., 1965, Human Relations Area Files.

Cramer, D.W., and others: Tubal infertility and the intrauterine device, N. Engl. J. Med. 312:941, 1985.

Daling, J.R., and others: Primary tubal infertility in relation to the use of an intrauterine device, N. Engl. J. Med. 312:937, 1985.

Darity, W.A., and Turner, C.B.: Family planning, race consciousness and the fear of genocide, Am. J. Pub. Health 62:1454, 1972.

Dougherty, M.C.: A cultural approach to the nurse's role in health-care planning, Nurs. Forum 11:310, 1972.

Grimes, D.A.: Reversible contraception for the 1980s, JAMA 255(1):69, 1986.

Hatcher, R.A., and others: Contraceptive technology 1984-1985, New York, 1984, Irvington Publishers, Inc.

IPPF International Medical Advisory Panel: Statement on periodic abstinence for family planning, IPPF Med. Bull. 18:2, 1982.

Jarou, J.P., and others: Quantitative pathologic changes in the human testis after vasectomy, N. Engl. J. Med. 313(20): 1252, 1985.

Kay, M.A., editor: Anthropology of human birth, Philadelphia, 1982, F.A. Davis Co.

Klaus, H.: Natural family planning: a review, Obstet. Gynecol. Surv. 37:128, 1982.

Kols, A., and others: Oral contraceptives in the 1980s, Popul. Rep. [A], no. 6, 1982.

Lee, N.C., and others: Type of intrauterine device and the risk of pelvic inflammatory disease, Obstet. Gynecol. 62:1, 1983.

Liskin, L., and Fox, G.: IUDs: an appropriate contraceptive for many women, Popul. Rep. [B], no. 4, 1982.

Liskin, L.S., and Fox, G.: Periodic abstinence: How well do new approaches work? Popul. Rep. [I], no. 3, 1981.

Marrs, R.P.: In vitro fertilization's future looks bright, Contemp. OB/Gyn. 20:135, 1982

Mishell, D.R.: Noncontraceptive health benefits of oral steroidal contraceptives, Am. J. Obstet. Gynecol. 248:184, 1982.

Okamoto, N.J.: The Japanese American. In Clark, A., editor: Culture-childbearing/health professionals, Philadelphia, 1978, F.A. Davis Co.

Ory, H.W.: The Women's Study: ectopic pregnancy and intrauterine contraceptive devices: new perspectives, Obstet. Gynecol. 57:137, 1981.

Ory, H.W.: The noncontraceptive health benefits from oral contraceptive use, Fam. Plann. Perspect. 14:182, 1982.

Population Reports: Barrier Method—new developments in vaginal contraception, series H, no. 7, Jan.-Feb., 1984.

Population Reports: IUDs: an appropriate contraception for many women, series B, no. 4, July 1982.

Pritchard, J.A., MacDonald, P.C., and Gant, N.F.: Williams obstetrics, ed. 17, Norwalk, Conn., 1985, Appleton-Century-Crofts.

San Francisco Chronicle, Jan. 14, 1986, and Feb. 1, 1986.

Scott, C.S.: The theoretical significance of a sense of well-being for the delivery of gynecological health care. In Bauwens, E.E., editor: The anthropology of health, St. Louis, 1978, The C.V. Mosby Co.

Snow, L.: Folk medical beliefs and their implications for care of patients, Ann. Intern. Med, 81:82, 1974.

Stark, S.: Mormon childbearing. In Kay, M.A., editor: Anthropology of human birth, Philadelphia, 1982, F.A. Davis Co.

Tucker, S.M., and others: Patient care standards, ed. 3, St. Louis, 1984, The C.V. Mosby Co.

Tyrer, L.: The new morality, ethics, and nursing, J.O.G.N. Nurs. 2:54, 1973.

Vogel, G.: American Indian medicine, New York, 1973, Ballantine Books, Inc.

Willson, J.R., Carrington, E.R., and Ledger, W.J.: Obstetrics and gynecology, ed. 7, St. Louis, 1983, The C.V. Mosby Co.

Wolner-Hanssen, P., and others: Laparoscopic findings and contraceptive use in women with signs and symptoms suggestive of acute salpingitis, Obstet. Gynecol. 66:233, 1985.

World Health Organization: Induced abortion as public health program: report on working group, Copenhagen, 1971, Regional Office for Europe.

Zatuchni, G.: New devices for intrauterine contraception, Contemp. OB/Gyn. 24 (special issue: technology 1985): 77, Oct. 1985.

Bibliography
Infertility

Asch, R.H., and Smith, C.G.: Effects of marijuana on reproduction, Contemp. Obstet. Gynecol. 22:217, 1983.

Bates, G.: Reproductive failure in women who practice weight control, Fertil. Steril. 37:373, 1982.

Bernstein, J., and Mattox, J.H.: An overview of infertility, J.O.G.N. Nurs. 11:309, 1982.

Bresnick, E.: A holistic approach to the treatment of infertility, J. Marital Fam. Ther. 7:181, 1981.

Clinical News: DES daughters: fighting fear with facts, Am. J. Nurs. 85:639, June 1985.

D'Andrea, K.G.: The role of the nurse practitioner in artificial insemination, J.O.G.N. Nurs. 13:75, March/April 1984.

Darland, N.W.: Infertility associated with luteal phase defect, J.O.G.N. Nurs. 14:212, May/June 1985.

Dugan, K.A.: Diagnostic laparoscopy under local anesthesia for evaluation of infertility, J.O.G.N. Nurs. 14:363, Sept./Oct. 1985.

Edgar, H.S.: The legal implications (in vitro fertilization): are restraints likely? Contemp. OB/Gyn. 20:233, 1982.

Elias, S., and Annas, G.J.: Social policy considerations in noncoital reproduction, JAMA 255:62, 1986.

Estok, P.J. and Rudy, E.B.: Intensity of jogging: relationship with menstrual/reproductive variables, J.O.G.N. Nurs. 13:390, Nov./Dec.1984.

Friedman, B.: Infertility workup, Am. J. Nurs. 81:2041, Dec. 1981.

Garcia, C., and others: Current therapy of infertility, 1984-1985, St. Louis, 1984, The C.V. Mosby Co.

Grimes, E.M.: For infertile couples—a holistic approach, Contemp. OB/Gyn. 23:179, 1984.

Haas, G.G.: Immunologic infertility: which approaches are best? Contemp. OB/Gyn. 22:141, 1983.

McCormick, T.M.: Out of control: one aspect of infertility, J.O.G.N. Nurs. 9:205, July/Aug. 1980.

McCusker, M.P.: The subfertile couple, J.O.G.N. Nurs. 11:157, May/June 1982.

Menning, B.E.: The psychosocial impact of infertility, Nurs. Clin. North Am. 17(1):155, 1982.

Nurses' Association of the American College of Obstetrics and Gynecology: Infertility: an overview. O.G.N. Nursing Practice Resource, no. 7, Nov., 1982.

Ocana R., and McCormick W.: Open laparoscopy: simple and direct, Contemp. OB/Gyn. 23:155, 1984.

Orque, M.D., Bloch, B., and Monrroy, L.S.: Ethnic nursing care: a multicultural approach, St. Louis, 1983, The C.V. Mosby Co.

Problem-patient conference: Habitual aborters. Contemp. OB/Gyn. 27:147, Feb. 1986.

Rosenthal, M.B.: Grappling with the emotional aspects of infertility, Contemp. OB/Gyn. 26:7, July 1985.

Sawatzky, M.: Tasks of infertile couples, J.O.G.N. Nurs. 10:132, 1981.

Shane, J.M., and others: The infertile couple: evaluation and treatment, Clin. Symp. 28:1, 1976.

Shangold, M.M., and Levine, H.S.: The effect of marathon training upon menstrual function, Am. J. Obstet. Gynecol. 143:862, 1982.

Sheinfeld, M.: Helping the infertile orthodox Jewish couple. Contemp. OB/Gyn. 21:137, March 1983.

Smith, C.: Drug effects on male sexual function, Clin. Obstet. Gynecol. 25:525, 1982.

Symposium: Ethical considerations in treating infertility, Contemp. OB/Gyn. 23:226, March 1984.

Tarter, T.H., and Alexander, N.J.: Intricacies of spermatogenesis, Contemp. OB/Gyn. 22:225, 1983.

Valle, R.F.: How endoscopy aids the infertility workup, Contemp. OB/Gyn. 23:191, March 1984.

Wallach, E.E.: Fertility drugs—what effects on the fetus? Contemp. OB/Gyn. 26:171, Aug. 1985.

Wedell, M.A., Billings, T., and Fayez, J.A.: Endometriosis and the infertile patient, J.O.G.N. Nurs. 14:280, July/Aug. 1985.

Control of Fertility

Bartosch, J.C.: Oral contraceptives: selection and management, Nurse Practitioner 8:56, 1983.

Canavan, P.A., and Lewis, C.A.: The cervical cap: an alternative contraceptive, J.O.G.N. Nurs. 10:271, 1981.

Clinical News: The latest in the search for a perfect contraceptive, Am. J. Nurs. 85:126, Feb. 1985.

Connell, E.B.: Oral contraceptives: the current risk-benefit ratio, J. Reprod. Med. 29:513, 1984.

Connell, E.B.: Research on methods of fertility regulation, J.O.G.N. Nurs. 13:50s, 1984.

Cupit, L.G.: Contraception: helping patients choose, J.O.G.N. Nurs. 13:23s, 1984.

Darney, P.D.: Evaluating the pill's long term effects, Contemp. OB/Gyn. 20:57, 1982.

Darney, P.D.: What's new in contraception? Contemp. OB/Gyn. 23:117, June 1984.

DeMoya, D., and DeMoya, A.: Best contraceptive for paraplegic women, RN 48:56, Dec. 1985.

Drug Dispatches: A modified pill, Nurs. 86, 16:76, Jan. 1986.

Hakim-Etahi, E., Contraceptive choice for disabled (handicapped) person. N.Y. State J. Med. 1601, 1982.

Hastings-Tolsma, M.T.: The cervical cap: a barrier contraceptive, M.C.N. 7:382, 1982.

Heartwell, S., and Schlessleman, S.: Risk of uterine perforation among users of intrauterine devices, Obstet. Gynecol. 61:31, 1983.

IPPF International Medical Advisory Panel: Statement on intrauterine devices, IPPF Med. Bull. no. 6, vol. 15, 1981.

Magil, B.: Monoclonals: new frontiers in reproductive medicine, Contemp. OB/Gyn. 26(special issue: technology 1986):75, Oct. 1985.

Mishell, D.R., Jr.: Current status of intrauterine devices, N. Engl. J. Med. 312:984, 1985.

NAACOG OGN nursing practice resource: Natural family planning, no. 9, Dec. 1983.

Norplant researchers await FDA approval: contraceptive sponge, NAACOG newsletter 11:9, 1984.

North, B.B., and Vorhauer, B.W.: Use of the Today contraceptive sponge in the United States, Int. J. Fertil. 30:81, 1985.

Northwestern University Program for Applied Research on Fertility Regulation: Immunologic methods of fertility regulation—report of a workshop, Res. Frontiers Fertil. Reg. 3:1, 1985.

Nurses' Drug Alert: Adverse effects of contraceptive sponges, Am. J. Nurs. 85:171, Feb. 1985.

Nurses' Drug Alert: Vaginal sponge and toxic shock; oral contraceptive failure; spermicides and congenital malformations: no relation, Am. J. Nurs. 85:693, June 1985.

Ollivier, S., and others: Providing infertility care, J.O.G.N. Nurs. 13:85s, 1984.

Orne, B., and Hawkins, J.A.: Reexamining the oral contraceptive issues, J.O.G.N. Nurs. 14:30, Jan./Feb. 1985.

Rosenthal, T.: Voluntary childlessness and the nurse's role, M.C.N. 5:398, 1980.

Roy, S., and others: Long-term reversible contraception with levonorgestrel-releasing Silastic rods, Am. J. Obstet. Gynecol. 148:1006, 1984.

Sasso, S.C.: Biphasic oral contraceptives M.C.N. 9:101, March/April 1984.

Schirm, A.L., and others: Contraceptive failure in the United States: the impact of social, economic and demographic factors, Fam. Plann. Perspect. 14:68, 1982.

Schneider, T.B.: Voluntary termination of pregnancy, J.O.G.N. Nurs. 13:77s, 1984.

Trends: Urine temperature: a key in family planning? Nurs. 85, p. 15, Jan. 1985.

Tyrer, L.B., and Duarte, J.E.: Guiding adolescents' choice of a contraceptive, Contemp. OB/Gyn. 23:172, Jan. 1984.

Washington, A.E., and others: Oral contraceptives, *Chlamydia trachomatis* infection, and pelvic inflammatory disease, J.A.M.A. 253:2246, 1985.

Interruption of Pregnancy and Termination of Fertility

Aby-Nielsen, K.: Physical sensations during stressful hospital procedures: a preliminary study of saline abortion, J.O.G.N. Nurs. 8:105, 1979.

Berger, J.M.: The relationship of age to nurses' attitudes toward abortion, J.O.G.N. Nurs. 8:231, 1979.

Danforth, D. and others, editors: Obstetrics and gynecology, ed. 4, New York, 1982, Harper & Row, Publishers.

DeMoya, D., and DeMoya, A.: Sex Q & A: abortion: no risk to fertility; best contraceptive after rape; when a man won't use a condom, RN 48:77, Feb. 1985.

Executive Board of ACOG: further ethical considerations in induced abortion, J.O.G.N. Nurs. 7:53, 1978.

Mishell, D.R.: State of the art (in vitro fertilization)—what can we offer patients? Contemp. OB/Gyn. 20(5):219, 1982.

Pritchard, J.A., MacDonald, P.C., and Gant, N.F.: Williams obstetrics, ed. 17, Norwalk, Conn., 1985, Appleton-Century-Crofts.

van Lith, D.A., Keith, L.G., and van Hall, E.V., editors: New trends in female sterilization, Chicago, 1983, Year Book Medical Publishers.

Willson, J.R., Carrington, E.R., and Ledger, W.J.: Obstetrics and gynecology, ed. 7, St. Louis, 1983, The C.V. Mosby Co.

Worthington, S.: Genetic screening, J.O.G.N. Nurs. 13:32s, 1984.

UNIT
3

Normal Pregnancy

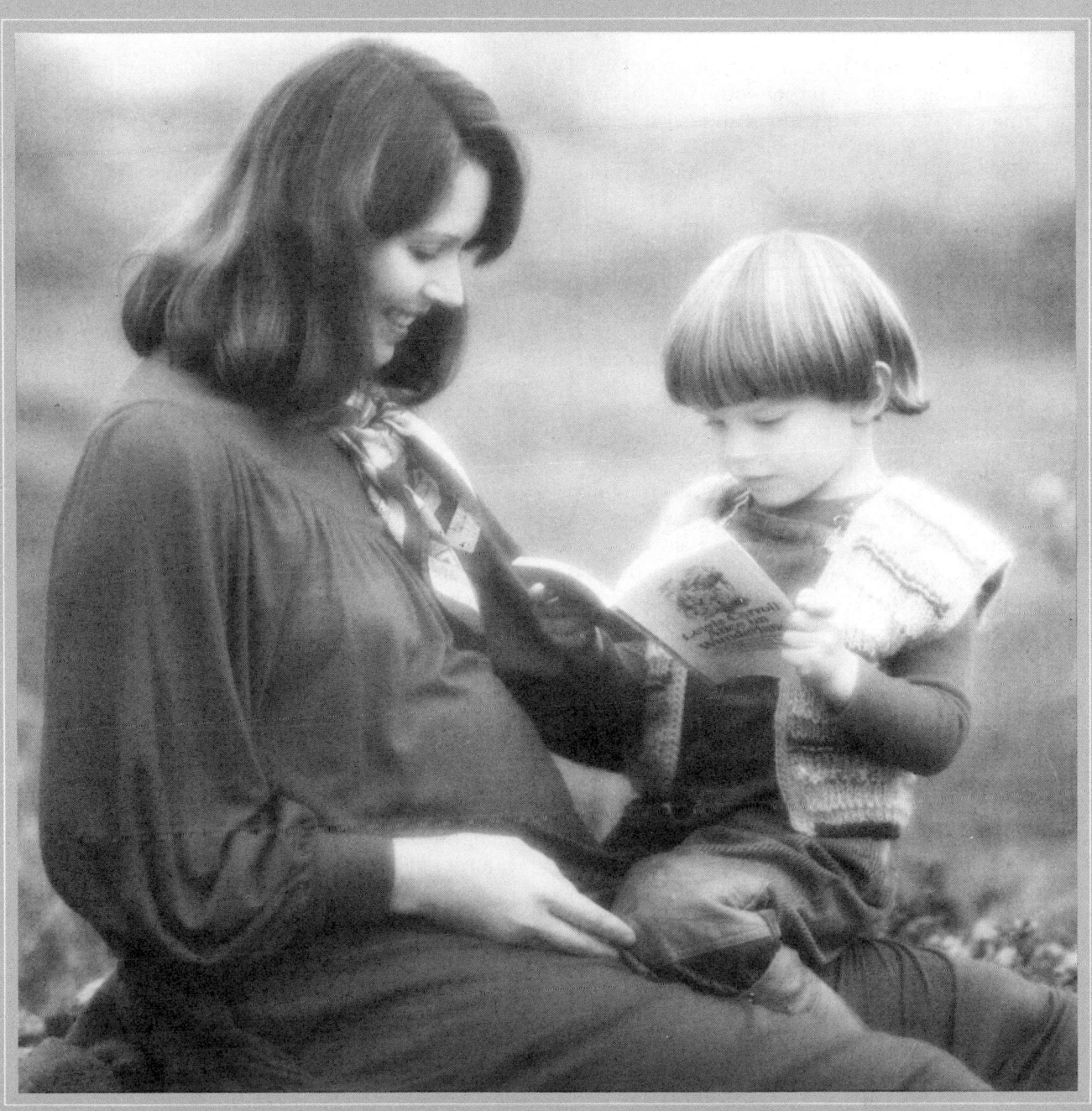

Conception and Fetal Development

The maternity nurse is in the unique position of providing nursing care to the unborn. Gravidas and their families have many questions about fetal development, such as "When is our baby due?" "How big is my baby now?" "My friend had a baby with blue eyes, but both of them have brown eyes. Is that possible?" "My baby jerks every couple of minutes for a short time sometimes. My mother said the baby is hiccuping. Is that so?" "How does the baby breathe in there?" "Everyone smokes in the office where I work. Will it hurt the baby?" "Will having sex (late in pregnancy) put holes in the baby's head or in his heart?" These questions frequently crop up in prenatal classes and private conversations with the woman or her partner. The wide media coverage of substances that affect the unborn can be disturbing to parents. The knowledgeable nurse can advise parents based on understanding of conception and normal fetal development. This chapter is designed to help nurses answer these questions. It gives a brief overview of the genetic basis of inheritance and normal embryonic and fetal development from conception to full-term gestation.

Genetic Basis of Inheritance

Genes and chromosomes. The biologic and behavioral characteristics of each human being are determined by the action of thousands of minute particles of hereditary material contained within the nuclei of all living cells. Each of these particles or *genes,* has a specific function in the control or regulation of cellular activity. Alone or in combination with other genes, they are responsible for all human traits or characteristics, for the orderly pattern and timing of development from conception to death, and for continuity of the species through consistent transmission of these traits from generation to generation.

The genes are composed of tiny segments of *deoxyribonucleic acid (DNA),* which enables them to dupli-cate themselves exactly during cell division. Each body cell contains two sets of genes arranged in a line to form larger structures, the *chromosomes,* within the cell nucleus. Each cell nucleus contains two sets of chromosomes consisting of two matching sets of genes, one set obtained from each parent during the process of fertilization. When a pair of genes are alike and produce the same effect they are called *homozygous;* when they are not alike and produce different effects they are said to be *heterozygous* (Fig. 8.1).

Chromosomes cannot be seen except under a microscope. For analysis they are stained, magnified, and photographed; then each individual chromosome is cut out and arranged in a *karyotype* according to size and shape. They appear as structures with either an X or a Y shape. Fig. 8.2 illustrates the chromosomes in a body cell.

Cell division. Somatic cells divide by the process of *mitosis,* in which the cell components, including the genetic material, divide and are distributed equally to the two newly formed cells (Fig. 8.3). Each new cell contains the same composition and genetic potential as the original cell.

The process of cell division in the reproductive cells is called *gametogenesis.* Gametogenesis takes place by *meiosis,* or *reduction division,* to form *gametes.* It consists of two successive divisions. In the *first* division the pairs of homologous chromosomes randomly separate from each other to form two nonidentical cells containing 23 nonhomologous chromosomes. In the *second* meiotic division the individual chromosomes split to form two identical cells, each with the same genetic complement of 23 chromosomes (Fig. 8.4).

Gametogenesis

Spermatogenesis. Meiosis in the male gonad is a continuous process that begins about the time of puberty and lasts until senescence. A primitive diploid germ cell (spermatogonium) matures to form a *primary spermatocyte,* which divides to form two *secondary*

Fig. 8.1
Genes on a pair of chromosomes illustrating like and unlike gene pairs. (From Whaley, L.F.: Understanding inherited disorders, St. Louis, 1974, The C.V. Mosby Co.)

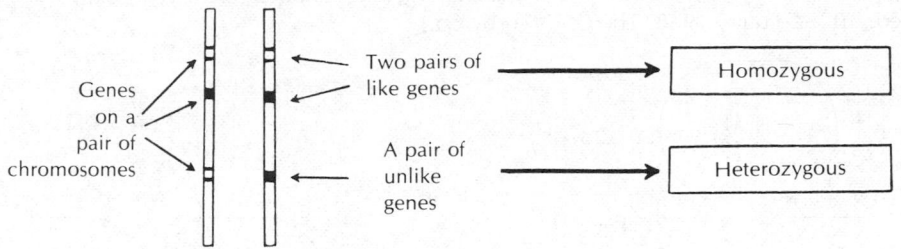

Fig. 8.2
Male chromosomes during cell division. **A,** Example of photomicrograph. **B,** Chromosomes arranged in karyotype. (From Whaley, L.F., and Wong, D.L.: Nursing care of infants and children, ed. 3, St. Louis, 1987, The C.V. Mosby Co.)

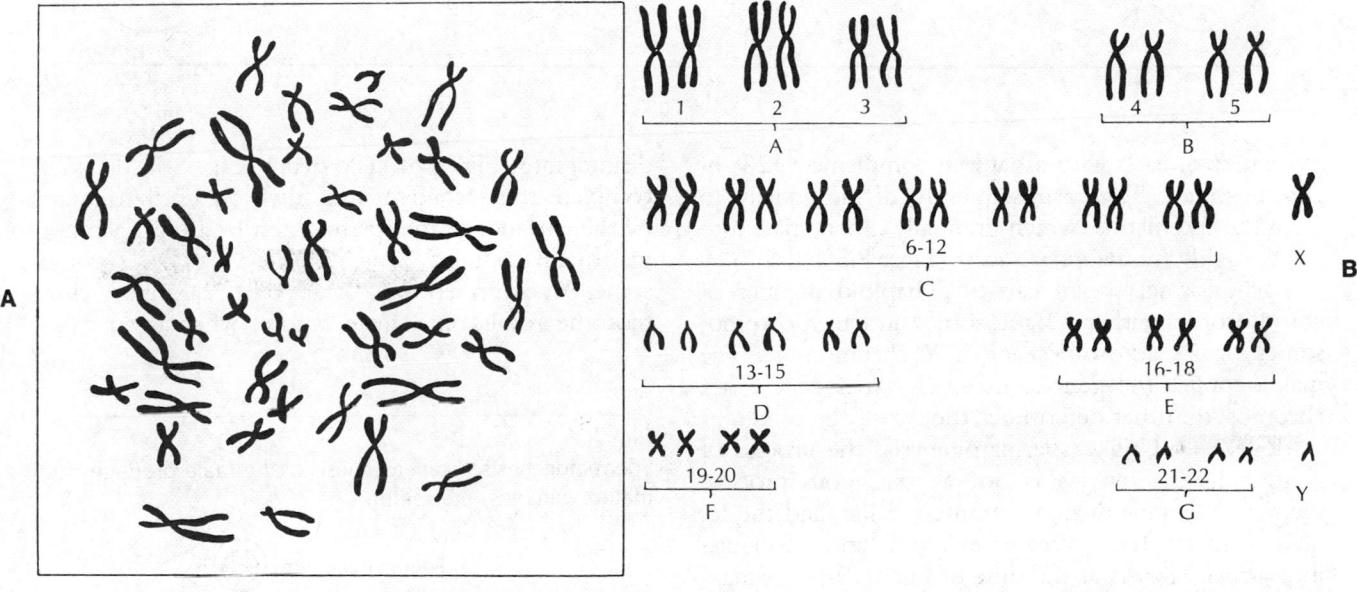

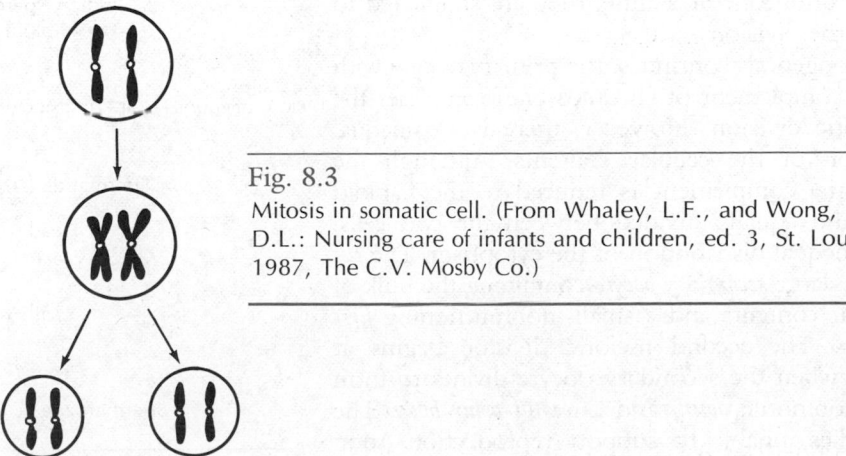

Fig. 8.3
Mitosis in somatic cell. (From Whaley, L.F., and Wong, D.L.: Nursing care of infants and children, ed. 3, St. Louis, 1987, The C.V. Mosby Co.)

Fig. 8.4
Process of meiosis: a premeiotic germ cell with two sets of chromosomes forms four germ cells, each with a single set of chromosomes. Two alternative arrangements of chromosome pairs on first meiotic spindle are diagrammed. (From Sandberg E.C.: Synopsis of obstetrics, ed. 10, St. Louis, 1978, The C.V. Mosby Co.)

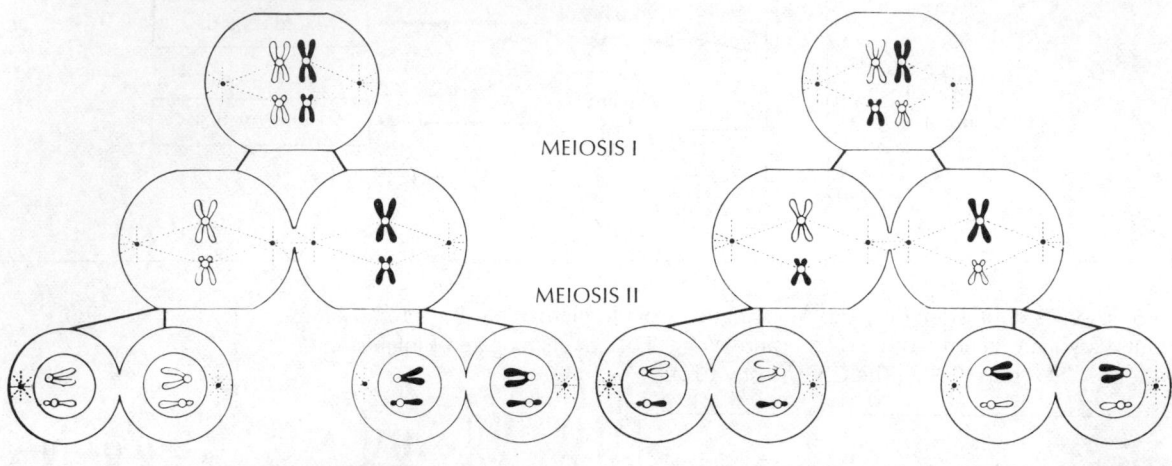

MEIOSIS I

MEIOSIS II

spermatocytes, each with a haploid complement (23) of chromosomes. These subsequently divide equally to form the spermatids, which gradually differentiate into small, highly motile *spermatozoa* (Figs. 8.5 and 8.7).

Each normal sperm carries a haploid number of chromosomes, either 22 autosomes and an X chromosomes or 22 autosomes and a Y chromosome. The male supplies the genetic material (an X or a Y sex chromosome) that determines the sex of the child.

Oogenesis. Unlike spermatogenesis, the process of meiosis in the ovaries is not a continuous process. Oogenesis begins during intrauterine life, and the female gametes have already enlarged and developed into *primary oocytes* at the time of birth. These primary oocytes (approximately 500,000 in number) have begun the first meiotic division but remain suspended at this stage until, one at a time, they are stimulated to complete the division.

When oogenesis continues, the primary oocyte with a diploid complement of chromosomes completes the first meiotic division. However, there is an unequal distribution of the cellular contents. Although the chromosome complement is reduced to the haploid number and equally divided between the two cells, there is unequal distribution of the cytoplasm. The result is one large *secondary oocyte* containing the bulk of the cellular contents and a small, nonfunctioning *first polar body.* The second meiotic division begins at ovulation when the secondary oocyte divides to form a large, nonmotile *ovum* and a *second polar body.* The polar bodies, unable to support reproduction, soon

disintegrate (Fig. 8.6). The ovum (Fig. 8.7) does not complete the second meiotic division until triggered by the entrance of the sperm at fertilization. Each normal ovum contains 22 autosomes and an X chromosome. An ovum fertilized by a sperm bearing a Y chromosome results in a male zygote, whereas an ovum

Fig. 8.5
Spermatogenesis. Gametogenesis of the male produces four mature gametes, the sperm.

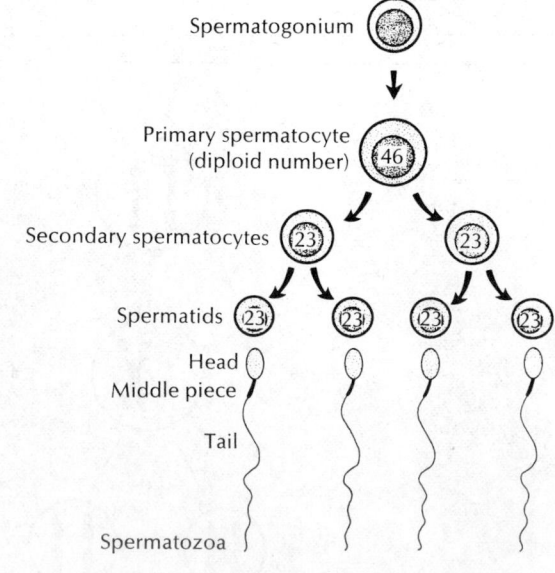

Spermatogonium

Primary spermatocyte
(diploid number)   46

Secondary spermatocytes   23   23

Spermatids   23   23   23   23

Head
Middle piece

Tail

Spermatozoa

Fig. 8.6

Oogenesis. Gametogenesis in the female produces one mature ovum and three polar bodies. Note the relative difference in overall size between the ovum and sperm.

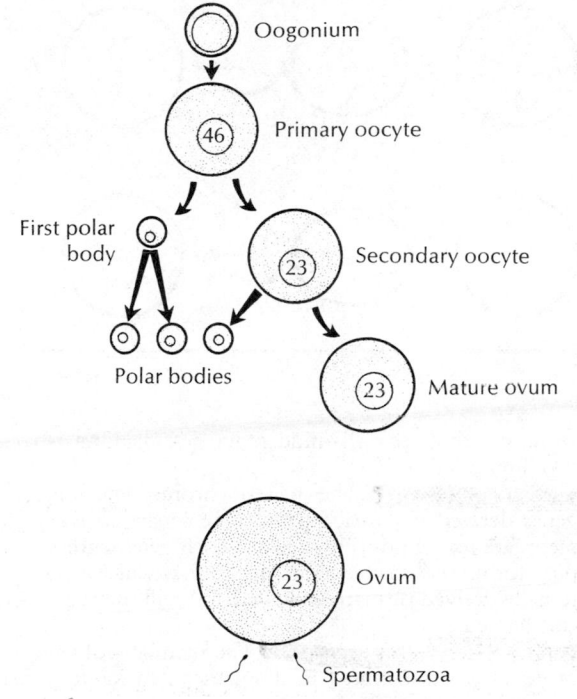

fertilized by an X-bearing sperm results in a female zygote.

Conception (fertilization). During sexual intercourse 2 to 5 ml of semen, usually containing more than 300 million sperm, is ejaculated into the female vagina. By flagellar movement the sperm make their way through the fluids of the cervical mucus (if the mucus is receptive), across the endometrium, and into the uterine tube to meet the descending ovum in the ampulla of the tube (see Chapter 5 for further discussion).

Before fertilization the sperm undergo a physiologic change called *capacitation* and a structural change called *acrosome reaction*. Capacitation refers to the removal of a protective coating from the sperm. Enzymes produced by the lining of the uterine tubes assist in capacitation of the sperm. The acrosome reaction refers to the small perforations that form in the anterior head of the sperm. Enzymes (e.g., hyaluronidase) escape through these perforations and digest a path for the sperm through the corona radiata and zona pellucida of the ovum. Only one sperm is required for actual fertilization, but the presence of many increases the chances for one to penetrate.

Fertilization (conception), the fusion of a *sperm* and an *ovum* (oocyte), is a process that requires about 24 hours. To fertilize an egg the sperm must pass through the *corona radiata* and *zona pellucida* and enter the egg;

Fig. 8.7
Sperm and ovum.

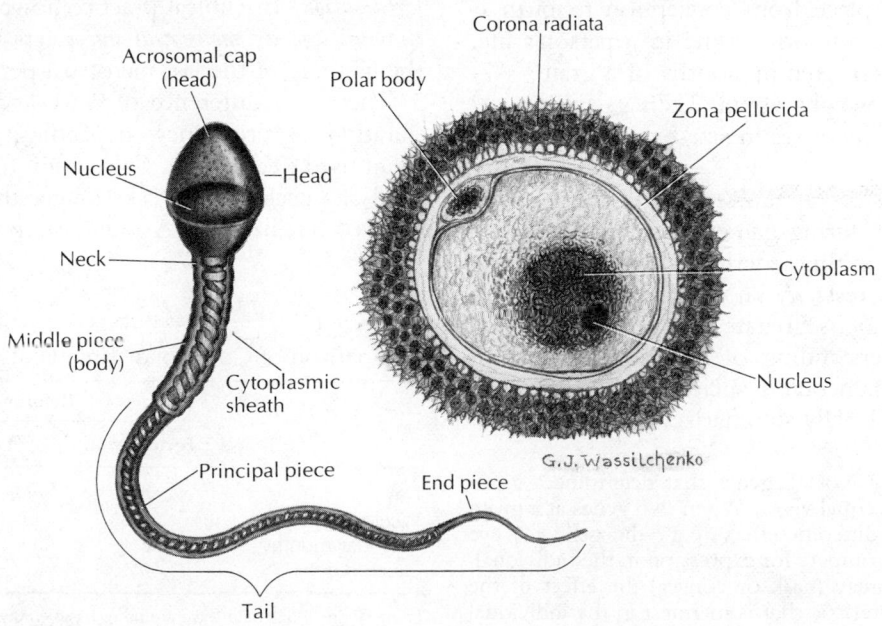

G.J. Wassilchenko

then female and male pronuclei undergo changes that result in a *zygote*.

In general, the process of fertilization takes place as follows: The cells of the corona radiata are dispersed by enzyme action of tubal mucosa and sperm. With the aid of its tail movements, the sperm can pass through this outermost covering of the egg. The acrosomes of several sperm release enzymes that digest a pathway through the zona pellucida. One sperm (usually) attaches to and fuses with the egg's plasma membrane, which then breaks down at the point of contact. At the moment that a sperm makes contact with the egg's plasma membrane, the oocyte reacts in two ways: a "zona reaction" (as yet not understood) occurs, preventing the entry of more sperm, and the oocyte matures (its nucleus is now known as the female pronucleus). The head and tail of the sperm enter the egg, leaving the sperm's plasma membrane (cytoplasmic sheath) attached to that of the oocyte. The tail of the sperm degenerates rapidly; its head enlarges to form the male pronucleus. The female and male pronuclei come together in the center of the oocyte and lose their cell membranes.

When the sperm and the ovum meet and form a *zygote* (fertilized ovum), the diploid number of chromosomes (44 autosomes and 2 sex chromosomes) is restored (Fig. 8.8). At that moment the sex of the new human is determined, and the blueprints for the growth, development, and maturation of a new individual are laid down.

The fertilized ovum begins to divide, differentiate, and grow into a person, a replica of humanity's continuing generations and yet a unique individual. The growth that takes place from conception to birth is more rapid than at any other time in a person's life. The zygote weighs 15 ten-millionths of a gram; a 7-pound term baby weighs about 3175 g. In those 9 months the zygote increases in size by more than 200 billion times.

Gene transmission in families. The genes act in predictable fashion during gamete formation and fertilization, and it is on this orderly performance that the science of genetics rests. A knowledge of the way in which genes combine, segregate, and recombine is essential to an understanding of their distribution in families. The fundamental principles of genetics, or Mendel's laws, are briefly summarized as follows:

principle of dominance Not all genes that determine a given trait operate with equal vigor. When two genes at a given locus produce a different effect (e.g., the gene for eye color), they may compete for expression in the individual. As a result, one may mask or conceal the effect of the other. The characteristic that is manifest in the individual (and the gene that produces the effect) is referred to as

Fig. 8.8

Fertilization. **A,** Ovum fertilized by X-bearing sperm to form female zygote. **B,** Ovum fertilized by Y-bearing sperm to form male zygote.

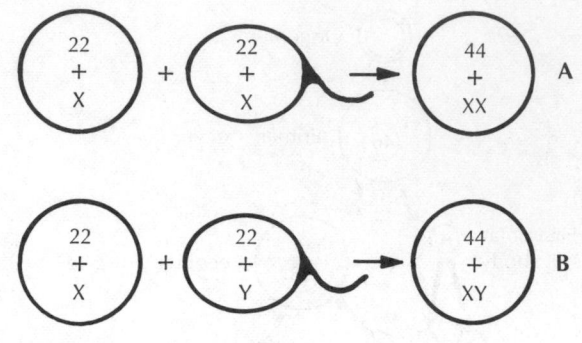

dominant: that which is hidden and not manifest is *recessive* (Fig. 8.9).

principle of segregation The paired chromosomes, bearing genes derived from each parent, are separated when gametes are formed during meiosis. Each gene segregates in pure form, and chance alone determines which gene (paternally derived or maternally derived) will travel to a specific gamete.

principle of independent assortment The members of one pair of genes are distributed in the gametes in random fashion, independent of other pairs.

Gestational time units. The chronology of pregnancy may be referred to in several ways, for example, 10 lunar months (of 4 weeks each), 40 weeks of gestation, or 9 calendar months (3 trimesters of 3 months each). *In this chapter, age in weeks refers to the time since fertilization.* In clinical practice however, the term *gestational age* or *menstrual age* refers to the time since the first day of the last menstrual period (LMP).

There is a difference of 2 weeks in calculating the duration of pregnancy, depending on the reference point used (Table 8.1). Calculation from the LMP (for a 28-day cycle) is 2 weeks longer than that from the time of fertilization. A graphic representation of the

Table 8.1
Comparison of Gestational Time Units

	Reference Point	
	Fertilization	**Last Menstrual Period**
Days	266	280
Weeks	38	40
Calendar months	8¾	9
Lunar months	9½	10

From Moore, K.L.: Before we are born: basic embryology and birth defects, Philadelphia, 1974, W.B. Saunders Co.

Fig. 8.9
Possible offspring in three types of matings. **A,** Homozygous-dominant parent and homozygous-recessive parent. Children all heterozygous, displaying dominant trait. **B,** Heterozygous parent and homozygous-recessive parent. Children 50% heterozygous display dominant trait; 50% homozygous display recessive trait. **C,** Both parents heterozygous. Children 25% homozygous dominant trait; 25% homozygous display recessive trait; 50% heterozygous display dominant trait.

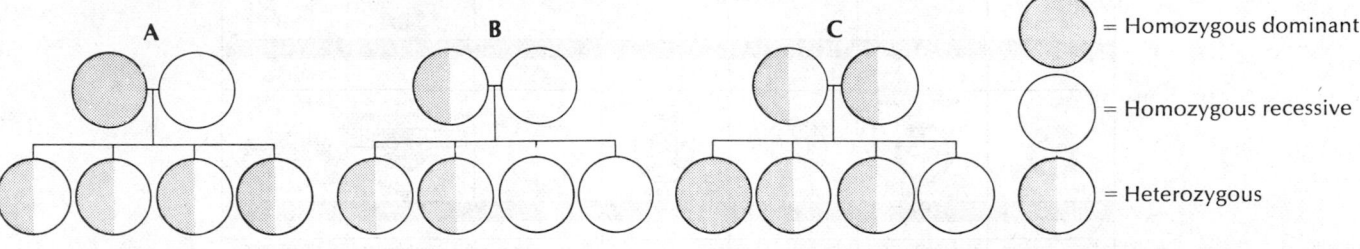

differences is seen in Fig. 8.10. The first square is "day 1 of menses" or day 1 of LMP. Note that 2 weeks pass before fertilization. These 2 weeks are added when discussing *menstrual* age of the pregnancy. The third row of squares identifies the onset of development after fertilization on the first day of the third week of the menstrual cycle.

The date of birth is calculated as about 266 days after fertilization, or 280 days after the onset of the last normal menstrual period. From fertilization to the end of the embryonic period, age is best expressed in days. Thereafter age is commonly given in weeks. Because ovulation and fertilization are usually separated by not more than 12 hours, these events are more or less interchangeable in expressing prenatal age.

Developmental stages. The fusion of the nuclei of the two gametes is called conception, fertilization, fecundation, or impregnation. Fusion initiates the first of the three stages of human prenatal development: ovum, embryo, and fetus.

Ovum. The conceptus is called an ovum during the period from conception until primary villi appear. Villi appear approximately 12 to 14 days after fertilization or about 4 weeks since LMP (see "primary villi" in Fig. 8.10, week 2, day 13). By the end of this period, implantation (nidation) is complete. The conceptus is totally within the endometrium and is covered by surface epithelium.

Embryo. The organism is called an *embryo* during the period from the end of the ovum stage until it measures approximately 3 cm from crown to rump, normally 54 to 56 days (10 weeks since LMP). This period is characterized by rapid cell division and is the most critical time in the development of an individual (Fig. 8.11). All the principle organ systems are being

established and are highly vulnerable to environmental agents (e.g., teratogens such as viruses, drugs, radiation, or infection). Developmental interference during this time can result in major congenital (existing before birth) abnormalities. By the end of this period the beginnings of all the main systems have been established. The embryo attains characteristics that establish it as unquestionably human and is then referred to as a *fetus,* a Latin word meaning *offspring.*

Fetus. The embryo is called a fetus during the period from the end of the embryo stage until the pregnancy is terminated (see Fig. 8.10, week 9, day 57). Changes occurring during the fetal period, although important, are not as dramatic as those in the preceding period. During this period the fetus is less vulnerable to the teratogenic effects of drugs, viruses, or radiation—*malformations.* However, these noxious agents may interrupt normal *functional development* of organs, especially the brain.

Viability

The capability of a fetus to survive outside the uterus at the earliest gestational age is called viability. Until recently it was believed that viability was reached when the fetus weighed more than 1000 g and had reached at least 28 weeks' gestational age. Improvement in maternal and neonatal care now suggests that a new standard of viability must be established (p. 39). On the basis of the limits of available clinical technology, current published literature about fetal lung development, and the age at which the respiratory system is capable of supporting satisfactory gas exchange, fetal viability can be first expected at approximately 22 to 23 weeks'

Fig. 8.10
For legend see opposite page.

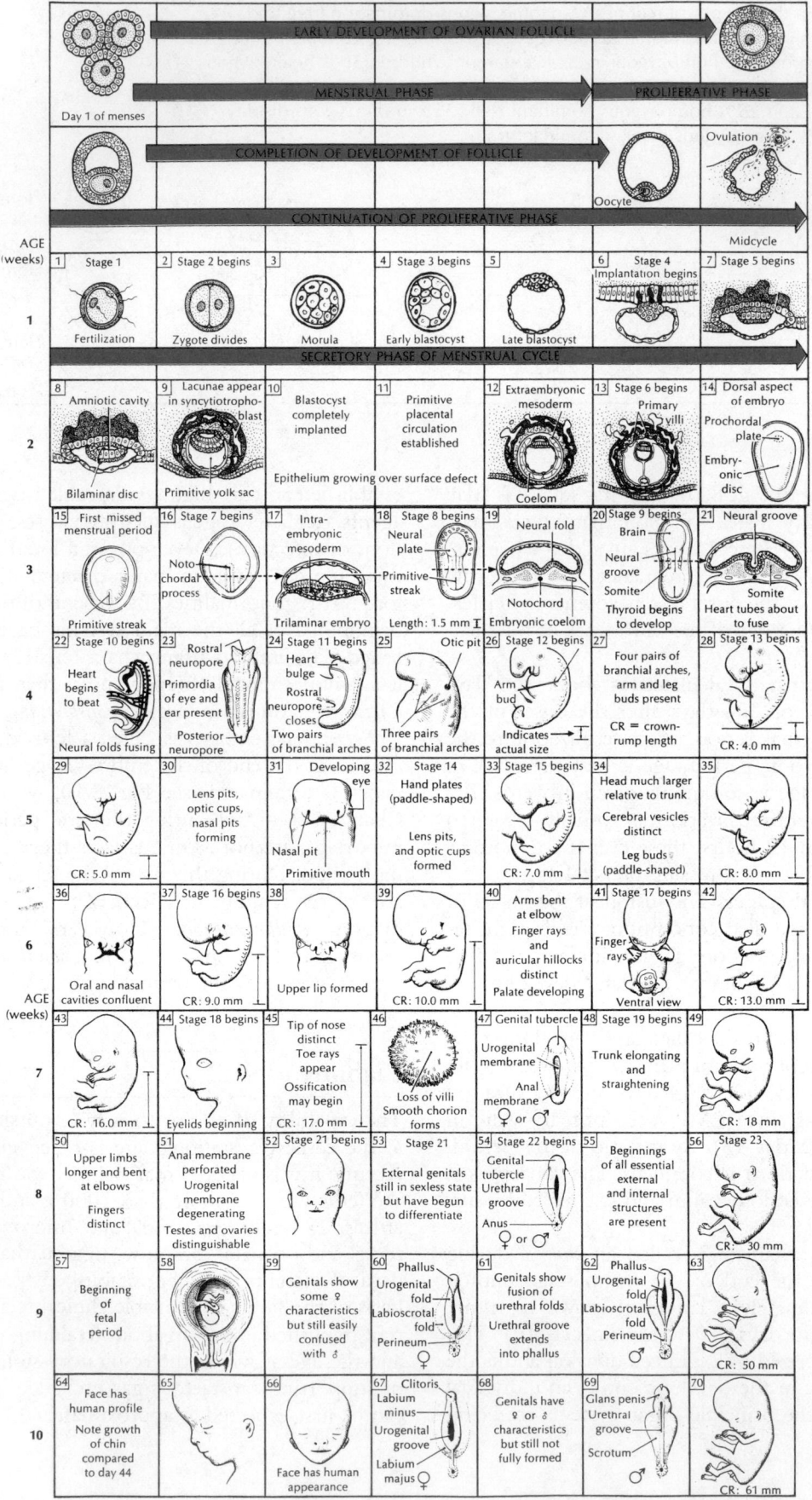

TIMETABLE OF HUMAN PRENATAL DEVELOPMENT
1 to 38 weeks

Fig. 8.10
Timetable of human prenatal development (weeks 1 to 10). (From Moore, K.L.: The developing human: clinically oriented embryology, ed. 2, Philadelphia, 1977, W.B. Saunders Co.)

Fig. 8.11
Sensitive, or critical, periods in human development. Solid red denotes highly sensitive periods; stippled red indicates stages that are less sensitive to teratogens. (From Moore, K.L.: The developing human: clinically oriented embryology, ed. 2, Philadelphia, 1977, W.B. Saunders Co.)

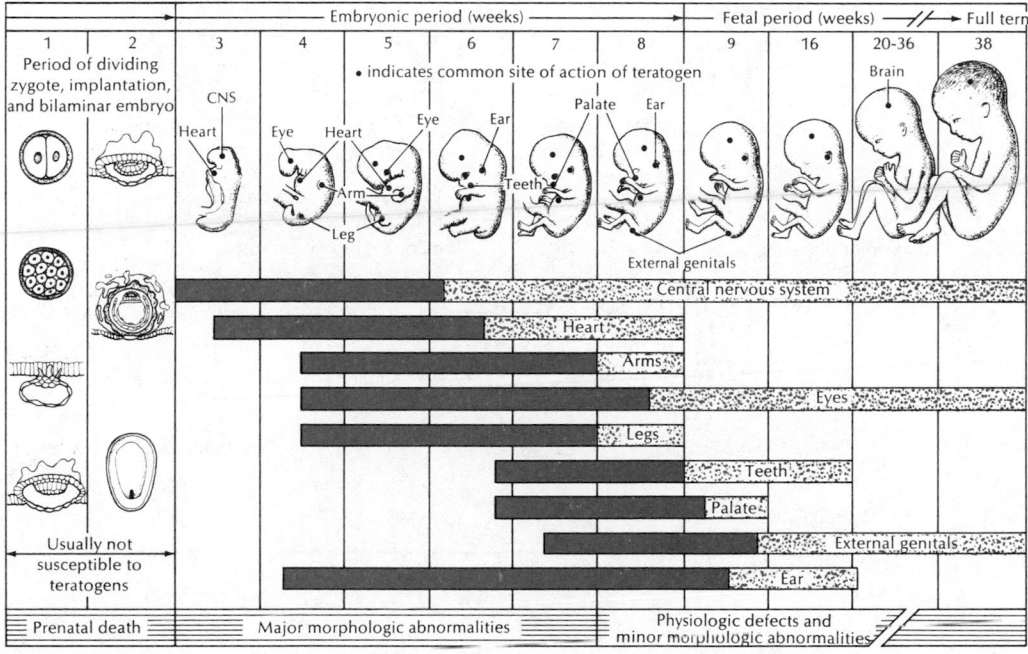

gestation. Since there is a problem with accuracy in estimating gestational age, it is difficult to establish definite criteria.

Survival outside the uterus is dependent on two factors: (1) the maturity of the fetal central nervous system (CNS) for directing rhythmic respirations and controlling body temperature and (2) the maturity of the lungs.

The Decidua

As part of the morphologic changes in the endometrium during the secretory phase (phase of the corpus luteum) of the menstrual cycle, the blood vessels enlarge and the entire lining becomes more succulent and richer in glycogen. After conception the vascularity of the uterine wall increases greatly under the influence of the ovarian hormones, principally progesterone.

After implantation the endometrium is called the *decidua,* which means "to cast off," or "to discard," since this is actually what happens after the infant is born: the prepared lining of the endometrium *is* cast off in a vaginal discharge called lochia (see Chapter 22).

This decidua is divided into three areas (Fig. 8.12):
1. *Decidua vera (parietalis)* is that part of the endometrium not directly associated with the development of the embryo.
2. *Decidua basalis* is the portion of the decidua vera where nidation takes place; that is, the area where chorionic villi (frondosum) invade the maternal blood vessels and develop into the placenta.
3. *Decidua capsularis* is the portion of the decidua vera that covers the blastocyst after nidation occurs, isolating it from the other portions of the uterus. It appears to fuse with the chorion, a fetal membrane, as pregnancy advances.

Implantation (Nidation)

After conception the zygote, propelled by ciliary action and irregular peristaltic contractions, starts to move

Fig. 8.12
Development of fetal membranes. Note gradual obliteration of intrauterine cavity as decidua capsularis and decidua vera meet. Also note thinning of uterine wall. Chorionic and amniotic membranes are in apposition to each other but may be peeled apart.

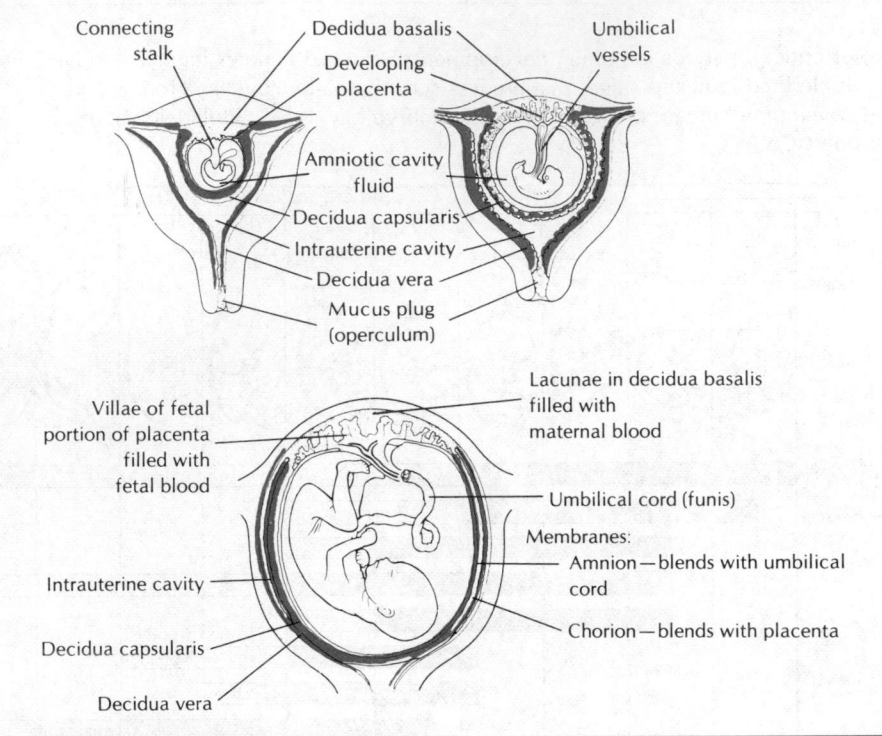

through the uterine tube into the uterine cavity. During the 3- to 4-day period it takes to travel down the uterine tube, the zygote begins a process of rapid cell division called *mitosis,* or *cleavage.* The initial division of the zygote results in two *blastomeres* which subsequently divide into progressively smaller blastomeres. At the end of 3 to 4 days, the developing individual comprises about 16 blastomeres arranged in a ball-like structure called a *morula.* After the morula enters the uterus, a cavity forms within the dividing cells, changing the morula into a *blastocyst.* The blastocyst remains free in the uterus for 1 or 2 days, and then the exposed cells of the *trophoblast* (cellular wall of the blastocyst) implant, generally in the endometrium of the anterior or posterior fundal region.

Cells of the attaching portion of the trophoblast secrete proteolytic (causing breakdown of proteins) and cytolytic (causing breakdown of cells) enzymes to help them burrow their way into the compact layer of the endometrium. This burrowing into the endometrium is called *nidation,* or *implantation.* Slight bleeding, called *implantation bleeding,* occurs in some women. In almost all cases, trophoblastic burrowing stops before it reaches the myometrium. About 7 to 10 days elapse betweeen fertilization and the completion of implantation (Fig. 8.10).

During the first few weeks after nidation, trophoblasts (primary villi) appear over the entire blastodermic vesicle. Trophoblasts are vascular processes that have the power of cytolysis and are able to tap maternal blood vessels as sources of nourishment and oxygen for the embryo. These villi are the first stage of the developing *chorionic villi* (fingerlike projections) that secrete the human chorionic gonadotropic hormone (HCG) and synthesize proteins and glucose for approximately 12 weeks. By 12 weeks, the fetal liver can supply its own glucose and insulin. HCG stimulates continued secretion of progesterone and estrogen by the corpus luteum, thus preventing ovulation and menstruation during pregnancy.

Chorionic villi invasion of the endometrium by enzyme action occasionally opens a maternal vein and artery causing lacunae (small blood lakes) in the decidua basalis. This rich blood supply causes the adjacent villi to multiply rapidly. These villi become the *chorion frondosum,* or fetal portion, of the future placenta.

Placenta

Structure. The maturing placenta (Greek for "flat cake") develops into 15 or 20 subdivisions called *cotyledons*. Each of these is partially separated from other cotyledons by fenestrated septa (windowed partitions); thus in essence each cotyledon is a functioning unit.

Growth of the thickness of the placenta continues until 16 to 20 weeks' gestation. The placental circum-ference continues growing until later pregnancy. The fully developed placenta (afterbirth) is a reddish, discoid organ 15 to 20 cm (6 to 10 in) in diameter and 2.5 to 3 cm (about 1 in) thick (Fig. 8.13). The weight of a term placenta is 400 to 600 g (1 lb to 1 lb, 5 oz) or approximately one sixth the weight of the newborn. About four fifths of the placenta by weight is of fetal origin; the remainder is maternal.

The maternal surface of the placenta, the area orig-

Fig. 8.13

Photographs of full-term placentas. **A,** Maternal (or uterine) surface, showing cotyledons and grooves. **B,** Fetal (or amniotic) surface, showing blood vessels running under amnion and converging to form umbilical vessels at attachment of umbilical cord. **C,** Amnion and smooth chorion are arranged to show that they are (1) fused and (2) continuous with margins of placenta. **D,** Placenta with a marginal attachment of the cord, often called a battledore placenta because of its resemblance to bat used in medieval game of battledore and shuttlecock. (From Moore, K.L.: The developing human: clinically oriented embryology, ed. 2, Philadelphia, 1977, W.B. Saunders Co.)

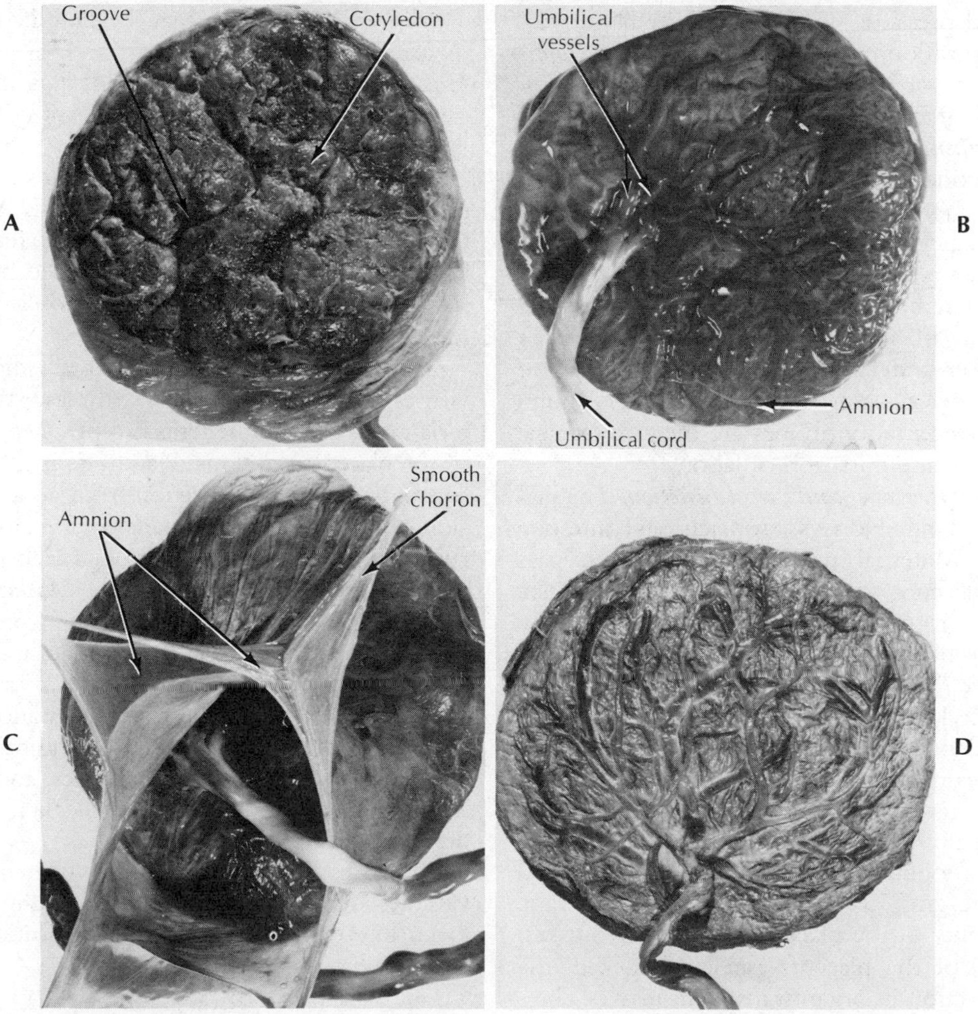

inally adherent to the decidua basalis of the uterus, is rough and beefy red. The cotyledons stand out as segments with shallow clefts between. The fetal surface of the placenta is shiny and slightly grayish. The umbilical vessels that enter the cord can be seen as a branching system just beneath the membranes (Fig. 8.13). The fetal membranes cover the fetal surface of the placenta and extend from the placental margins to envelop the fetus and its amniotic fluid.

In multiple pregnancy, one or more placentas will be present. The number depends on the number of fertilized ova and the manner of ovum segmentation (see discussion of twinning, Chapter 29).

Functions. The placenta has many unique properties. Most of these properties—endocrine, metabolic, and immunologic—are derived from the trophoblasts. Understanding placental functions gives insight into prenatal life and is helpful in providing nursing care to the unborn and the neonate.

Placental function depends almost entirely on maternal circulation. Maternal circulation depends on the woman's blood pressure, condition of her blood vessels, maternal position, and uterine contractions. *Optimal circulation to the placenta and fetus is possible when the woman is lying on her left side* (see Chapter 15).

Endocrine gland. During pregnancy a new group of *protein* hormones of placental origin is seen. One of these, human chorionic gonadotropin (HCG) is the basis for pregnancy tests. At one time it was thought that the placenta was one of the four steroid-producing glands. It may be that the placenta relies for much of the synthesis of steroid hormones on precursors from the mother and fetus (Danforth, 1982). *Steroid* hormones include estrogens and progesterone. Among the actions of placental hormones are the maintenance of pregnancy and the initiation of labor.

Metabolic, respiratory, and renal function. The placenta serves as lung, kidneys, stomach, and intestine for the fetus. Maternal nutrients and oxygen pass through the placenta to the embryo or fetus. Waste materials move from the conceptus to the mother by way of the placenta.

Immunologic function. "The placenta and fetus appear to defy the laws of transplantation immunology" (Pritchard, and others, 1985, p. 110). "The placenta corresponds to a natural homograft in that it is a transplant of living tissue within the same species, yet it does not normally evoke the usual immune response reaction to homografts, resulting in destruction and rejection of the graft" (Willson and others, 1983, p. 132). This quality of the placenta is of major interest. If the "secret" of the placenta can be unlocked, the problem of rejection in organ transplants may be eliminated.

Protective barrier. The placenta serves as a protective barrier against the harmful effects of certain drugs and microorganisms. See discussion of placental transfer.

Transfer. Only two layers of cells separate maternal and fetal circulation for the first 12 weeks of gestation. During the second and third trimesters, only one cell layer separates the two bloodstreams. This so-called *placental barrier* is a partial (semipermeable) barrier; it provides only very limited protection to the fetus.

Passage of materials to and from the fetus is effected by four principal mechanisms:
1. *Diffusion,* such as across a membrane, allows passage of oxygen, carbon dioxide, anesthetic gases, water, electrolytes, and other substances of low molecular weight.
2. *Active,* or *facilitated, transfer,* often by enzyme action, results in the passage of glucose, amino acids, calcium, iron, and other substances of higher molecular weight.
3. *Pinocytosis* is a mechanism by which minute particles, including fats, may be engulfed and carried across the cell.
4. *Leakage* as a result of small defects in the trophoblastic surface *allows slight mixing of maternal and fetal blood cells and plasma.*

Nutrients. The transfer of vitamins to the fetus is only partially understood, but vitamins A, B complex, C, E, and K are transmitted to the fetus. It is not known whether vitamin D is produced by the fetus or supplied by the mother (see discussion of maternal and fetal nutrition, Chapter 12).

Microorganisms. Because of their small size, some viruses traverse the placenta with ease; the larger bacteria rarely involve the fetus except when inflammation of the placenta develops. Placentitis is generally the result of an intranatal infection from an ascending invasion of bacteria from vagina and cervix associated with ruptured membranes and prolonged labor but may occur even if membranes are intact. Maternal, fetal, and neonatal infections are discussed in Chapters 27 and 31.

Drugs. Many drugs cross the placenta readily (e.g., caffeine, alcohol, nicotine, carbon monoxide, pesticides, the over 1000 other toxic substances and gases* inhaled from cigarette smoke, antibiotics, antihistamines, sedatives, analgesics, narcotics, and anesthetics). Most drugs promptly cross the placenta, and many are deleterious to the human fetus.

Examples of these drugs, to which may be added vaccines and excessive amounts of certain vitamins, are given in Appendix G. Because medications may con-

---

*Hydrogen cyanide is present in cigarette smoke. This is the same gas used to execute prisoners in gas chambers.

tain elements harmful to the fetus, all but essential medications should be avoided, particularly during the first trimester of pregnancy.

Oxygen. For a discussion of oxygen transfer, see the discussion of fetal hemoglobin, p. 194.

Fetal Membranes

Two closely applied but separate membranes surround the developing embryo-fetus (Fig. 8.12). Both membranes, the *amnion* (inner membrane) and the *chorion* (outer membrane), arise from the zygote. As the chorion develops, it blends with the fetal portion of the placenta; the amnion blends with the fetal umbilical cord, or *funis*. These deceptively strong, translucent membranes contain not only the fetus but also the amniotic fluid, and they are continuous with the margins of the placenta.

Umbilical Cord

The umbilical cord (funis) is the lifeline that links the embryo and the placenta. It extends from the umbilicus to the fetal portion of the placenta and is attached either centrally or eccentrically. At term this light gray, smooth, vascular attachment is 50 to 55 cm long, slightly longer than the fetus, and is approximately 2 cm in diameter.

The surface of the cord is composed of thin squamous epithelium and is an extension of the skin of the fetus; however, *it contains no pain receptors*. The cord normally contains two umbilical arteries and one umbilican vein (Fig. 17.19). The vein carries oxygenated blood to the fetus, and the arteries return deoxygenated blood to the placenta. Frequently these vessels are longer than the cord and consequently become coiled on themselves, giving the cord a lumpy appearance. They are supported by a loose connective tissue containing a cushioning mucoid material called *Wharton's jelly.* This jelly prevents kinking of the cord in utero and interference with circulation to the fetus.

Approximately 400 ml of blood flows through the cord every minute. The pressure exerted by this rapid flow makes the cord relatively stiff and not flexible as it is after birth. If fetal movements cause the cord to loop, its stiffness prevents the loops from kinking and from knotting tightly. The high water content of Wharton's jelly causes the cord to shrink quickly after birth. In addition, several naturally occurring prostaglandins in Wharton's jelly have a vasoconstrictive effect that inhibits bleeding from the umbilical cord stump when it is cut after birth.

Amniotic Fluid

Origin, composition, and volume. During pregnancy the amniotic fluid volume increases at an average rate of 25 ml per week from 1 to 15 weeks' gestation, and 50 ml per week from 15 to 28 weeks' gestation. The full-term fetus is immersed in about 1000 ml (range of 800 to 1200 ml) of clear, slightly yellowish liquid that has a faint characteristic (not foul) odor. The specific gravity of amniotic fluid is 1.007 to 1.025, and the pH is neutral to slightly alkaline (7.0 to 7.25). It contains albumin, urea, uric acid, creatinine, lecithin, sphingomyelin, bilirubin, fat, fructose, inorganic salts, epithelial cells, a few leukocytes, various enzymes, and lanugo hairs. Amniotic fluid, replaced every 3 hours, is thought to have multiple origins and a composition that changes during pregnancy. Early in pregnancy it probably originates from maternal serum, but as pregnancy proceeds a greater proportion of it is derived from fetal urine.

Functions. Amniotic fluid accomplishes numerous functions for the fetus, including the following:

1. Protects the fetus from direct trauma by distributing and equalizing any impact the mother may receive
2. Separates the fetus from the fetal membranes
3. Allows freedom of fetal movement and permits musculoskeletal development
4. Facilitates symmetric growth and development of the fetus
5. Protects the fetus from loss of heat and maintains a relatively constant fetal body temperature
6. Serves as a source of oral fluid for the fetus
7. Acts as an excretion-collection system

Diagnostic value. There is still much to be learned about amniotic fluid. However, study of its components has provided a great deal of knowledge about the sex, state of health, and maturity of the fetus. Amniocentesis (see p. 734) has made it possible to detect diseases and abnormalities that may suggest the options of therapeutic abortion or intrauterine treatment.

There is great variation within the normal volume; however, more than 2 L (hydramnios) or less than 300 ml (oligohydramnios) is usually associated with fetal disease or abnormality (see Chapter 31).

Embryonic Development and Fetal Maturation

Fetal maturation takes place in an orderly and predictable pattern (Fig. 8.10 and Table 8.2). There is a steady increase in overall growth, and organ systems develop from the three primary germ layers: the ecto-

Table 8.2
Milestones in Human Development Before Birth Since LMP

	4 Weeks	8 Weeks	12 Weeks	16 Weeks
External appearance	Body flexed, C-shaped Arm and leg buds present Head at right angles to body	Body fairly well formed Nose flat, eyes far apart Digits well formed Head elevating Tail almost disappeared Eyes, ears, nose, and mouth recognizable	Nails appearing Resembles a human Head erect but disproportionately large Skin pink, delicate	Head still dominant Face looks human Eye, ear, and nose approach typical appearance on gross examination Arm-leg ratio proportionate Scalp hair appears
Crown-to-rump measurement (CM)	0.4-0.5	2.5-3	6-9	11.5-13.5
Approximate weight (g)	0.4	2	19	100
Musculoskeletal system	All somites present	First indication of ossification—occiput, mandible, and humerus Fetus capable of some movement, definitive muscles of trunk, limbs, and head well represented	Some bones well outlined; ossification spreading Upper cervical to lower sacral arches and bodies ossify Smooth muscle layers indicated in hollow viscera	Most bones distinctly indicated throughout body Joint cavities appear Muscular movements can be detected
Circulatory system	Heart develops; double chambers visible; begins to beat Aortic arches and major veins completed	Main blood vessels assume final plan Enucleated red cells predominate in blood	Blood forming in marrow	Heart muscle well developed Blood formation active in spleen
Gastrointestinal system	Stomach at midline and fusiform Conspicuous liver Esophagus short Intestine a short tube	Intestinal villi developing Small intestines coil within umbilical cord Palatal folds present Liver very large	Bile secreted Palatal fusion complete Intestines have withdrawn from cord and assume characteristic positions	Meconium in bowel Some enzyme secretion Anus open
Respiratory system	Primary lung buds appear	Pleural and pericardial cavities forming Branching bronchioles Nostrils closed by epithelial plugs	Lungs acquire definite shape Vocal cords appear	Elastic fibers appear in lungs Terminal and respiratory bronchioles appear
Renal system	Rudimentary ureteral buds appear	Earliest secretory tubules differentiating Bladder-urethra separates from rectum	Kidney able to secrete urine Bladder expands as a sac	Kidney in position Attains typical shape and plan

Modified from Whaley, L.F., and Wong, D.L.: Nursing care of infants and children, ed. 3, St. Louis, 1987, The C.V. Mosby Co.

20 Weeks	24 Weeks	28 Weeks	32 Weeks	36 Weeks	40 Weeks
Vemix caseosa appears Lanugo appears Legs lengthen considerably Sebaceous glands appear	Body lean but fairly well proportioned Skin red and wrinkled Vernix caseosa present Sweat glands forming	Lean body, less wrinkled and red Nails appear	Subcutaneous fat beginning to collect More rounded appearance Skin pink and smooth Has assumed delivery position	Skin pink, body rounded General lanugo disappearing Body usually plump	Skin smooth and pink; copious vernix caseosa Moderate to profuse hair Lanugo on shoulders and upper body only Nasal and alar cartilage apparent
16-18.5	23	27	31	35	40
300	600	1100	1800-2100	2200-2900	3200+
Sternum ossifies		Astragalus (talus, ankle bone) ossifies	Middle fourth phalanxes ossify Permanent teeth primordia indicated	Distal femoral ossification centers present	
Fetal movements strong enough for mother to feel		Weak, fleeting movements minimum tone	Can turn head to side	Sustained, definite movements; fair tone Can turn and elevate head	Active, sustained movement; good tone May lift head
	Blood formation increases in bone marrow and decreases in liver				
Enamel and dentine depositing Ascending colon recognizable					
Nostrils reopen Primitive respiratory-like movements begin	Alveolar ducts and sacs present Lecithin begins to appear in amniotic fluid (weeks 26-27)	Lecithin forming on alveolar surfaces	L/S ratio = 1.2:1	L/S ratio ≥ 2:1	Pulmonary branching only two thirds complete
				Formation of new nephrons ceases	

Continued.

Table 8.2, cont'd
Milestones in Human Development Before Birth Since LMP

4 Weeks	8 Weeks	12 Weeks	16 Weeks
Nervous system			
Well-marked midbrain flexure No hindbrain or cervical flexures Neural groove closed	Cerebral cortex begins to acquire typical cells Differentiation of cerebral cortex, meninges, ventricular foramens, cerebrospinal fluid circulation Spinal cord extends entire length of spine	Brain structural configuration roughly complete Cord shows cervical and lumbar enlargements Fourth ventricle foramens developed Sucking present	Cerebral lobes delineated Cerebellum assumes some prominence
Sense organs			
Eye and ear appearing as optic vessel and otocyst	Primordial choroid plexuses develop Ventricles large relative to cortex Development progressing Eyes converging rapidly Internal ear developing	Earliest taste buds indicated Characteristic organization of eye attained	General sense organs differentiated
Genital system			
Genital ridge appears (fifth week)	Testes and ovaries distinguishable External genitals sexless but begin to differentiate	Sex recognizable Internal and external sex organs specific	Testes in position for descent into scrotum Vagina open

derm (ecto = outside), the entoderm (ento = inner), and the mesoderm (meso = middle). The *ectodermal* germ layer gives rise to such tissues as the skin and nails, the nervous system, and tooth enamel. The *entodermal* germ layer develops into such tissues as epithelial inner linings of the gastrointestinal and respiratory tracts, endocrine glands, and auditory canal. The *mesodermal* germ layer forms tissues such as the connective tissue, teeth (except for the enamel), muscles, and blood and vascular systems.

Cardiovascular system. The first system to function in the developing human is the cardiovascular system. Blood vessel formation begins early in the third week; it follows the first missed menstrual period of the mother. The cardiovascular system must form early to bring nourishment and oxygen from the mother to the embryo. The cardiovascular system is functional (heart is beating) before the mother's menstrual period is 1 week late. At this time (3 weeks since conception), circulation of blood begins the fetomaternal exchange of oxygen, nutrients, and waste products. This exchange is necessary because the fetal lungs and digestive system are not functional until after birth.

Fetal circulation. The single umbilical vein carries oxygen-enriched blood from the placental (Fig. 19.2).

Upon entering the liver, the vein gives off a number of branches and then enters the ductus venosus. About half the oxygenated blood bypasses the liver through the ductus venosus into the inferior vena cava. There it mixes with deoxygenated blood from the fetal lower extremities, abdomen, and pelvis. Most of this blood then enters the right atrium and is pumped through the foramen ovale into the left atrium, where it mixes with a small amount of deoxygenated blood returning from the lungs through the pulmonary veins. The blood then flows into the left ventricle and exits through the ascending aorta. *As a result, the vessels leading to the heart, head, neck, and upper limbs receive well-oxygenated blood.* This circulatory pattern is the reason for the embryo's cephalocaudal (head-to-tail) development, which persists in subsequent motor development, making it possible for the infant to manipulate his hands long before being able to walk.

A small quantity of oxygenated blood from the inferior vena cava remains in the right atrium and mixes with deoxygenated blood from the superior vena cava and coronary sinus. It then flows into the right ventricle and pulmonary artery, passing through the ductus arteriosus into the aorta; a small amount is diverted to the nonfunctional lungs.

20 Weeks	24 Weeks	28 Weeks	32 Weeks	36 Weeks	40 Weeks
Brain grossly formed Cord myelination begins Spinal cord ends at level S1	Cerebral cortex layered typically Neuronal proliferation in cerebral cortex ends	Appearance of cerebral fissures; convolutions rapidly appearing Indefinite sleep-wake cycle Cry weak or absent Weak suck reflex		End of spinal cord at level (L-3) Definite sleep-wake cycle	Myelination of brain begins Patterned sleep-wake cycle with alert periods Cries when hungry or uncomfortable Strong suck reflex
Nose and ear ossify	Can hear	Eyelids reopen Retinal layers completed; light receptive Pupils capable of reacting to light	Sense of taste present Aware of sounds outside mother's body		
	Testes at inguinal ring in descent to scrotum		Testes descending to scrotum		Testes in scrotum Labia majora well developed

The paired umbilical arteries return most of the mixed blood from the descending aorta to the placenta. There the fetal blood simultaneously gives up carbon dioxide and waste materials and takes up oxygen and nutrients from the maternal blood. The remaining blood circulates through the lower part of the fetal body and ultimately enters the inferior vena cava.

The pattern of blood flow* is as follows:

1. Placenta
   ↓
   Umbilical vein ⟋ Liver, sinusoids, ⟍ Inferior vena
             hepatic veins   cava
            ⟍ Ductus venosus ⟋

2. Inferior vena cava→Right atrium→**Foramen ovale**→Left atrium→Left ventricle→Aorta
3. Inferior vena cava→Right atrium→Right ventricle→Pulmonary artery→Small amount to nonfunctional lungs but most of it through **Ductus arteriosus**→Aorta→Hypogastric arteries→**Umbilical arteries**→Placenta

FHR and fetal hemoglobin. Following are a number of compensatory circulatory factors that benefit the fetus (these values are those of the fetus near term):

1. The fetal heart rate (FHR) is 120 to 160 beats/min, and the fetal cardiac output is approximately 350 to 500 ml/kg/min, or about that of the adult at rest.
2. The hemoglobin of the fetus is primarily fetal hemoglobin (HgF), a type synthesized before birth. HgF is capable of maintaining a high oxygen saturation at a lower pressure (Po_2). It has been estimated that HgF can carry as much as 20% to 30% more oxygen than can maternal hemoglobin.
3. The hemoglobin concentration of the fetus is about 50% higher than that of the mother.

As a result of these compensatory circulatory factors, greater amounts of oxygen can be transported to the fetal tissues.

Hematopoietic system. Hematopoiesis (formation and development of blood cells) begins in the liver about the sixth week of gestation, when vascular channels have been formed. Later, blood formation occurs in the spleen, bone marrow, and lymph nodes.

Platelets are present in the circulation by the eleventh week of gestation. The isoagglutinogens (e.g., the Rh factor) that determine blood grouping are present in the red blood cells soon after the sixth week. Because of the early appearance of red blood cells, the

*The four structures that differentiate fetal circulation from extrauterine circulation are shown in bold type. The foramen ovale and ductus arteriosus allow fetal blood to bypass the fetal lungs.

Rh-negative woman needs to be protected against isoimmunization after each pregnancy that lasts longer than 6 weeks as well as after the birth of each child who is Rh positive (for extensive discussion, see Chapter 3 and Table 5.8).

Respiratory system. As previously mentioned the fetal lungs do not function until after delivery. Simple diffusion (passing from higher to lower concentration across a semipermeable membrane) across the placenta explains the exchange of oxygen and carbon dioxide in the fetus.

Developmental phases. Development of human lungs occurs in four overlapping phases:

1. *Pseudoglandular period* (5 to 17 weeks' gestation): formation of bronchi and terminal bronchi
2. *Canalicular period* (13 to 25 weeks' gestation): enlargement of lumens of bronchi and terminal bronchioles, development of respiratory bronchioles and alveolar ducts, increased vascularity of lung tissue
3. *Terminal sac period* (24 weeks' gestation to birth): growth of primitive alveoli (terminal air sacs) from alveolar ducts; fetuses younger than 24 weeks are not likely to survive if born before the terminal sac period begins
4. *Alveolar period* (late fetal period to approximately 8 years of age): formation of characteristic pulmonary alveoli as the lining of the terminal air sacs thins, with the number of alveoli increasing six to eight times between birth and age 8 years

Pulmonary surfactants. During the terminal sac period *pulmonary surfactants* are produced in increasing amounts by the alveolar cells. Surfactants (surface factors or wetting agents), substances that minimize surface tension, designate a group of surface-active phospholipids. Of this group, *lecithin* (phosphatidylcholine) may be the crucial anti-atelactasis factor responsible for alveolar stability. This biochemical compound is present on the surface of the alveolar cells, creating the minimum surface tension necessary to keep these spaces open on expiration following birth. In extrauterine life, lungs must remain partially expanded at all times.

The effect of decreased surface tension, caused by the presence of lecithin in the lining layer of alveoli, can be compared to powdering rubber gloves so that they do not stick together and to the Teflon coating on cooking utensils. The active ingredient in sprays used to keep foods from sticking to frying pans is lecithin. If insufficient surfactants are present, the lungs cannot be properly inflated and respiratory distress syndrome (RDS) may develop.*

---

*Some diseases in adults result in decreased lecithin production and the development of adult respiratory distress syndrome (ARDS).

Table 8.3
Secretion of Pulmonary Surfactant

Gestation Age (weeks)	L/S Ratio*	Lung Maturity
26-27	Secretion into alveolar space begins	Viability attained
30-32	1.2 to 1	
35	2 to 1	Maturity attained

*Lecithin-sphingomyelin ratio.

Pulmonary surfactants migrate from the lung fluid and mix with amniotic fluid in the upper respiratory tract and then into the amniotic fluid. The presence of surfactants in the amniotic fluid is used as a biochemical marker for determining the degree of fetal lung maturity. Lung maturity is the capacity of lungs to accommodate to normal ventilation after birth. Lecithin builds up in the amniotic fluid from about the twenty-fourth week, and sphingomyelin, another pulmonary phospholipid, remains unchanged. Hence, by determining the amount of lecithin present in relation to sphingomyelin, or the *lecithin-sphingomyelin (L/S) ratio*, an appraisal of fetal lung maturity is possible (Table 8.3).

No consistent relationship exists between fetal weight, age, and pulmonary maturity. Up to 10% of mature fetuses have been reported as having low L/S ratios, whereas normal ratios have been reported in premature infants (Korones, 1986).

Maternal oxygenation. A reduction in the rate and depth of maternal respiration may be reflected in fetal oxygenation. Excessive amounts of barbiturate, narcotic analgesia, or maternal hypoxia during anesthesia may reduce the fetal Po_2. Moreover, heavy maternal sedation by those drugs that readily cross the placenta may depress the fetal CNS respiratory center to further jeopardize the baby at birth. Breathing of pure oxygen (10 to 12 L/min) by the mother before delivery and again before cessation of pulsation in the cord after delivery may aid the infant.

Respiratory movement. *Periodic fetal hiccup* can be seen and palpated, and rhythmic fetal respiratory movements can be demonstrated by ultrasonography in advanced pregnancy. Fetal cellular wastes (squamae) and lanugo fragments are commonly found in the fetal respiratory passages. Hence respirations at birth appear to be an extension of intrauterine respiratory movement.

Renal system. The placenta is the major fetal excretory organ and effectively eliminates waste products from fetal blood. The placenta, in collaboration with maternal lungs and kidneys, maintains fetal water, electrolyte, and acid-base balance. Kidneys are *not* necessary for fetal growth and development. In fact, an infant may be born without kidneys. However, renal excretory and regulatory functions must begin immediately after delivery to maintain life and health.

In preparation for extrauterine existence, the fetal kidneys develop rapidly. The kidneys appear in the fifth week and begin to function during the eighth week. Urine is excreted into and mixes with the amniotic fluid that the fetus swallows.

Neurologic system

Development of the brain. The *neural plate* (a thickened area of embryonic ectoderm), from which the infant's nervous system develops, appears during the third week of gestation. The *neural tube** and *neural crest* evolve from this structure, the first differentiating into the CNS (the brain and cord) and the second into the peripheral nervous system.

The brain, which is formed at the cranial end of the neural tube, consists of the forebrain, midbrain, and hindbrain. The longest part of the neural tube ultimately becomes the spinal cord.

The human brain is only partially developed and functional at birth. It grows in three stages: first, prenatally by hyperplasia (an increase in cell number); second, during the first 6 months of life by a combination of hyperplasia and hypertrophy (an increase in size of existing cells); and third, thereafter until puberty by hypertrophy. An adequate supply of protein and calories is required for this process, particularly during the first and second stages. Prenatal maternal anemia and malnutrition compromise fetal brain development: if the fetus does not receive adequate nutrition early in development, there is a smaller number of cells developed; if the fetus continues to receive inadequate nutrition, the existing cells are smaller in size.

The late fetal and early neonatal phases of maturation are especially critical to later achievement. Disease, trauma, or unfavorable environmental factors may irreparably alter the development of the CNS.

Hypoxia attributable to maternal causes (e.g., premature separation of the placenta), fetal causes (e.g., cord entanglement), or iatrogenic causes (e.g., maternal hypotension after being given spinal anesthesia) may be critical to the infant. Many of the survivors of severe asphyxia develop cerebral palsy, mental retardation, or other neurologic deficits. Newborns of 36 weeks' gestational age or younger are less sensitive to hypoxia but are more sensitive to birth trauma than mature newborns. Fortunately, however, the infant has

remarkable powers of recuperation, and many depressed babies appear to recover satisfactorily. See Chapter 19 for more information on newborn neurologic function.

Neuromuscular behavior. Fundamental to the successive development of behavior patterns is the development of neuromuscular structure and functioning. Behavior advances through five stages: (1) myogenic (originating in the muscle) response, (2) neuromotor (muscle movement stimulated by nerves) response, (3) reflex response, (4) integration of simple reflexes, and (5) integration and control from higher centers. Fetal development of the nervous system parallels fetal behavior.

Response to stimulation. Studies revealed that before the middle of the seventh week of menstrual age, "the human embryo appears incapable of any type of reflex activity" in response to stimulation (Hooker, 1952). During the next 6½ weeks increasing sensitivity was evidenced. By 13½ weeks all areas of the body except the top and back of the head appeared to be sensitive. Stimulation of parts of the body were found to cause a response. For example, lips were pressed together when stroked, the tongue moved when the inside of the mouth was touched, and stimulation of the palm resulted in finger closing and wrist flexion.

Movement. At 9 weeks the whole fetus moves in a jerky, rather convulsive manner, but between 10 and 12 weeks periods of quiet or resting can be noted (Van Dongen and Goudie, 1980); and "instead of the mechanical, stereotyped movement seen earlier, the various activities are graceful and flowing—the fetus is very active" (Hooker, 1952). In one study using ultrasonography the fetus was seen to propel himself around in the amniotic fluid by using paddling movements with the feet, to roll over, turn somersaults, place his hands behind his head and over his ears, suck his thumb, and grasp the umbilical cord (Freud, 1983). Respiratory efforts have been visualized at 18½ weeks, swallowing with tongue movements by 12½ weeks, and sucking by 29 weeks. By 16 weeks fetal muscle movement is strong enough to activate receptors on the maternal abdominal wall; the mother usually interprets this as "the baby moving" and professionals refer to it as "quickening."

Behavioral states. Active and inactive periods noted first between 10 and 12 weeks develop a sequential pattern by 28 weeks. Stainton (1983a) identifies three behavioral states—active, quiet, and sleeping—from data acquired from 23 expectant parents during interviews about their knowledge of their unborn child in the last trimester of pregnancy. Both mothers and fathers described times when the fetus was responsive to their voices or to rubbing of the mother's abdomen by

---

*The nurse may need to explain to parents about neural tube defects, one of several malformations that can be identified in utero through amniocentesis (see test for alpha-fetoprotein).

kicking and moving. Parents noted times when the fetus was quiet but awake and aware. At other times parents said that calling in a loud voice or shaking the abdomen did not result in more than a brief movement. In those pregnancies in which the father's style was expressive (May, 1980), the father's descriptions validated the mother's. Brazelton (1982) notes that most mothers can delineate three behavioral states in the fetus: an active "alert" state, a deep sleep with little or no movement, and an intermediate sleep state with irregular startlelike movement.

Sensory awareness

Touch. Most pregnant women can verify that the fetus touches the uterine wall during pregnancy. In doing so the fetus experiences touch. Fetal response to touch through the uterine wall has not been studied through ultrasonic observation, but parental reports of its effect are consistent. Pregnant women are often seen to be rubbing their abdomens and describe success in assisting their unborn infant to "calm down" or "settle down" when upset (Stainton, 1983b). Prospective fathers also have reported being able to "calm" a restless fetus by patting or rubbing the mother's abdomen (Stainton, 1983a).

Fetal response to painful stimuli can be demonstrated. A fetoscope placed on the mother's abdomen with pressure will usually result in fetal movement away from the site, thus requiring someone to hold the fetus in position to ensure accurate assessment. The insertion of an amniocentesis needle near or touching the fetus will also provoke a moving-away movement (Liley, 1972).

If procedures recognized as painful to a newborn or adult are being considered for the fetus (e.g., intrauterine correction of a defect), fetal anesthesia is warranted. Anesthesia is administered to the mother, and by placental transfer the fetus is anesthetized. Anesthesia is provided during intrauterine transfusions requiring puncture of the fetal abdominal wall and during insertion of catheters to drain urine from the fetus with urinary tract anomalies (Harrison and others, 1981).

Hearing. The fetus is able to hear both internal and external sounds by the fifth month of pregnancy (Liley, 1972). The fetus lives in an environment bombarded with sound. Pulsations of maternal blood flow through the large abdominal vessels supplying the lower body areas, placenta, and uterus and the noise emanating from the mother's digestive tract has been measured to be as high as 85 decibels (Walker and others, 1971; Henshall, 1972). Clements (1977) found that 4- to 5-month-old fetuses discriminated between musical sounds by kicking and moving violently when the music of Beethoven, Brahms, or rock groups was played and quieting with Vivaldi or Mozart.

The sensitive hearing of the fetus has prompted researchers to investigate to what extent the fetus, while in utero, can hear, learn to recognize, and record sounds that contribute to its later social responses, particularly with its mother. Numerous studies (Condon, 1977; Eisenberg, 1979; Simner, 1971) point to a selective listening to the mother's voice sounds and rhythms during intrauterine life that prepares the newborn for recognition and interaction with her or his primary caregiver. Parents have reported feeling gentle movements in response to talking or singing to their fetus (Stainton, 1983a). One mother reported that her baby began "irritable jerky movements" when she changed from vacuuming a carpet to moving the vacuum over a hardwood floor (Stainton, 1983a).

Taste. Taste buds are well developed in the fetus. The fetus has a larger number of taste buds than either a child or an adult and they are more widely distributed (Liley, 1972). Apparently the fetus can distinguish between sweet and sour tastes. In addition, cold solutions can induce hiccups in the fetus.

Sight. Until recently, newborns were thought to be only slightly light sensitive and unable to see. It is now known that light enters the uterus, especially in late pregnancy when the tissues are thin, and that both rods and cones are present at birth (Dobson, 1976). Fetal movement has been elicited through the use of bright light directed on the uterus (Grimwade and others, 1971). Als and co-workers (1979) found that during the last trimester the fetus would startle when a bright light was directed on the mother's abdomen near the head and turned actively but smoothly toward a soft light. These findings were based on reports by mothers and confirmed with ultrasound.

Summary. In summary, the fetus is well equipped with sensory devices to assist in the accumulation of information to promote continued development. The human newborn is not inexperienced at birth—she or he possesses a repertoire of behaviors that meet needs and provide protection. The behavioral state at birth is derived from a gradual development during the fetal period of life. Awareness of fetal response is stimulating research into the concept of prebirth parenting and the effects that mother-father-fetus interactions may have on subsequent parent-child relationships.

Gastrointestinal system. The digestive system forms during the fourth week. The middle portion of the intestine projects out into the umbilical cord during the fifth week of development because there is not enough room in the abdomen (the liver and kidneys are taking up considerable space at this time). The intestines return to the abdomen during the tenth week.

Failure of the intestines to return to the abdomen results in a condition known as omphalocele.

Intrauterine nutrition and elimination occur through the placenta, making it unnecessary for the slowly developing gastrointestinal system to function before birth. During the second trimester the fetus begins to swallow amniotic fluid.

Metabolism. While in utero the fetus exists in a nondemanding physical environment. Constant ambient temperature, minimal physical activity, depressed muscle tone, and effective insulation against heat loss all contribute to a relatively low metabolic rate. The fetus maintains a temperature about 0.4° C above maternal temperature. Oxygen consumption is about one third that of the neonate. Most of the caloric intake is used to accomplish growth and development.

The fetus receives its glucose, its main source of energy, from the mother. *Maternal insulin does not pass to the fetus; the fetus secretes insulin.* The fetus synthesizes glycogen and anabolizes (forms) his own fat rather than receiving these nutrients in these forms from the mother.

Meconium. As term approaches, increasing amounts of meconium (the end product of fetal metabolism) are found in the fetal intestinal tract. Normal meconium is a sterile, dark, greenish brown, semisolid residue of bile and embryonic secretions, plus cellular waste (squamous epithelial cells) and hair swallowed in utero. The presence of meconium in amniotic fluid before delivery usually indicates fetal hypoxia (see Chapter 25).

Hepatic system. Liver function begins at about the fourth week of gestation. Hematopoiesis starts at about the sixth week of intrauterine life; this activity is primarily responsible for the rapid growth and relatively large size of the liver during the second month of gestation.

The fetal liver at term is proportionately much larger than the liver of the 1-year-old infant. It is a metabolic and glycogen storage organ that also secretes bile and acts as a depot for iron. Full liver function is not achieved until well after delivery, however. For example, coagulation factors contributed to or produced by the liver and fibrinogen are low at the time of delivery but adjust in early infancy. The production of fetal liver enzymes is limited, especially in the fetus of less than 36 weeks' gestational age.

Endocrine system. The fetal *adrenal cortex,* or outer part of the gland, produces cortisol. Increasing amounts of cortisol may be important in the initiation of labor.

The *thyroid* gland is the first endocrine gland to develop in the fetus. By the fourth week the thyroid can synthesize thyroxine.

By the twelfth week insulin may be extracted from the beta cells of the fetal *pancreas.* The fetus must supply whatever is needed for its metabolism of glucose. Insulin is the primary hormone regulating the rate of fetal growth.

Reproductive system. Until the end of the ninth week, male and female external genitalia appear somewhat similar (see Fig. 5.1). It is not until the twelfth week that external genitalia are well enough developed to be easily distinguishable.

Female genital development and function. The fetal ovary (see Fig. 5.9) has many primordial (primitive) follicles and produces small but increasing amounts of estrogen. It is the high level of maternal estrogen that stimulates the fetal endometrium; the rapid drop in maternal estrogens in fetal circulation following birth is followed by withdrawal bleeding. Withdrawal bleeding accounts for the brief mucoid vaginal discharge and even slight bloody spotting that may be noted in female neonates.

During childhood a small but continuing secretion of estrogen occurs. Before puberty a much greater production of estrogen accounts for the development of female secondary sex characteristics.

Male genital development and function. Early in embryonic development, the gonads of the genetically male fetus (fetus with a Y chromosome) play a critical role in the formation of the genital tract. As the gonads evolve in the testicular pattern, presumably under the influence of maternal HCG, LH, and fetal adrenal hormones, the testes produce androgenic hormones that result in growth and differentiation of male genitalia.

After delivery a slow increase in the production of androgen and traces of estrogen continue until just before puberty, when much larger amounts of testosterone, in particular, are secreted. This increase causes development of the male secondary sex characteristics (see Table 5.6).

Immune system. See Chapters 5 and 19 for a discussion of the immune system.

Summary

Nurses need to understand basic genetic concepts and the ways hereditary factors interact with the constantly changing environment. This includes knowledge about the genetic basis of inheritance and normal development from conception through full-term gestation. Fig. 8.14 summarizes fetal development, maternal events, common discomforts, remedies, and drug substances to avoid. It was taken from a brochure prepared for coaching parents through pregnancy.

Fig. 8.14

Summary of fetal development, maternal events, common discomforts, remedies, and drug substances to avoid.

	Week 1	Week 2	Week 3	Week 4	Week 5	Week 6	Week 7	Week 8
Baby's Development	The ovum becomes fertilized, divides and burrows into the uterus.	The embryonic disk (ectoderm, entoderm, mesoderm) is formed. These three primitive germ layers will generate every organ and tissue in your baby's body.	The first body segments appear, which will eventually form the primitive spine, brain and spinal cord.	Heart, blood circulation and digestive tract take shape. The embryo is now one-fifth of an inch long, the head one-third of its total length.	The heart starts to pump blood; limb buds appear. Major divisions of the brain can now be discerned.	Eyes begin to take shape; external ears develop from skin folds.	Development is proceeding rapidly. The face is now complete with eyes, nose, lips and tongue — even primitive milk teeth. Tiny bones and muscles appear beneath the thin skin.	The embryo is now a little more than an inch long; its tiny heart beating at about 40-80 times a minutes.

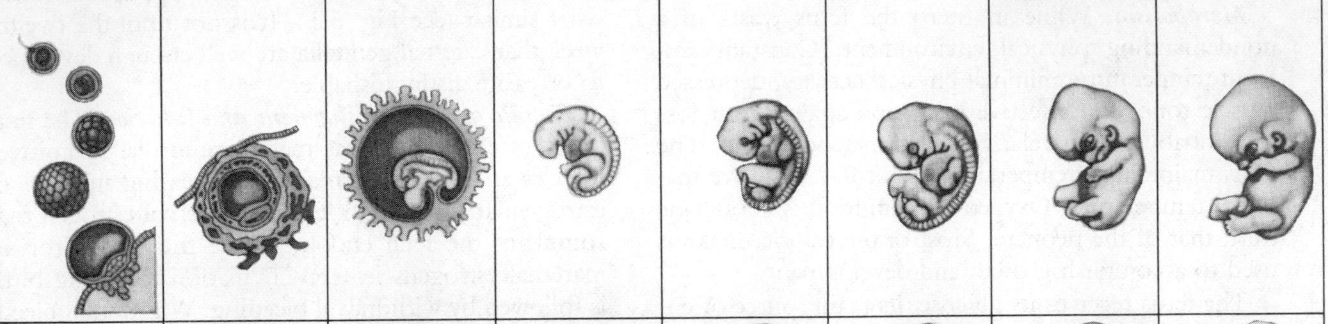

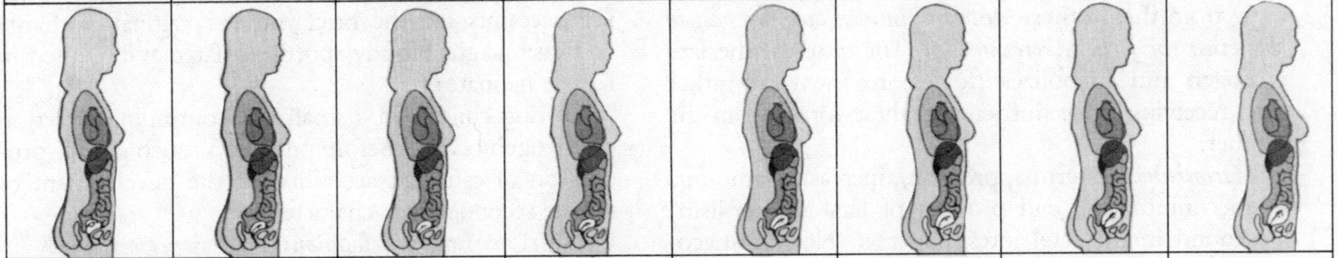

	Week 1	Week 2	Week 3	Week 4	Week 5	Week 6	Week 7	Week 8
Maternal Events	Ovaries increase production of "pregnancy maintaining" hormone, progresterone.	First missed period	Placenta grows to cover one-fifteenth of the uterine interior. Breast may begin to feel tender. No weight gain.			Exchange of fetal and maternal metabolites begin across the placenta, yet the two circulations are completely separate.	No noticeable weight gain.	The placenta now covers about one-third of the uterus lining.
Common Discomforts			**Morning sickness** occurs because increased hormonal activity slows down your digestive system, apprently to enhance the absorption of nutrients for your baby.	**Fatigue** is thought to be caused by a change in ovarian hormone production (progesterone and relaxin), the purpose of which is to relax pelvic ligaments, stimulate breast growth, and soften the cervix.		**Urinary frequency** is caused by the uterus compressing the bladder against the pelvic bones, thus reducing its capacity. Also by hormonal changes which affect the water balance in your body.		
Remedies			Eat a few dry crackers before arising. Frequent, small, low-fat meals during the day should also help. Drink liquids between meals.	Exercise regularly, get plenty of sleep with frequent naps during the day		You can decrease pressure on the bladder at night by sleeping on your side. Also, drink no fluids after 6 p.m.		
Drug Substance to Avoid			**Antiemetics** • cyclizine (Migral® Marezine®) • meclizine (Antivert®, Bonine®) • trimethobenzamide (Tigan®) (Avoid throughout pregnancy)	**Stimulants** • amphetamines • excessive caffine (Avoid throughout pregnancy)				
Acceptable Alternatives	None: Avoid all drugs not prescribed by a physician for a specific condition. Avoid X-rays.							

(From Safe passage: a woman's guide to a healthier pregnancy, McNeil Consumer Products Co., Fort Washington, Pennsylvania.)

	Week 9	Week 10	Week 11	Week 12	Week 13	Week 14	Week 15	Week 16
Baby's Development	Genitalia is now well defined; the baby's sex is determined. Eyelids finish forming and seal shut. The embryo has become a fetus.	The fetus assumes a more human shape as the lower body rapidly develops. Blood and bone cells form. The first movements begin.	Organs begin to function. The pancreas is producing insulin; the kidneys urine.	The lungs have taken shape; primitive breathing motions begin. The swallowing reflex has been mastered as the fetus sucks its thumb while floating weightlessly in the amniotic fluid.		The musculosketetal system has matured. The nervous system begins to exercise some control over the body; blood vessels rapidly develop.	With hands ready to grasp, the fetus — now weighing about 7 ounces — kicks restlessly against the amniotic sac.	All organs and structures have been formed and a period of simple growth begins.

	Week 9	Week 10	Week 11	Week 12	Week 13	Week 14	Week 15	Week 16
Maternal Events	Maternal blood volume has increased 30-40%.	The sensation of these first movements has been described by some women as if something were blowing bubbles through a straw in their stomachs.	2-3 lb weight gain. Possible increase in perspiration.	The placenta has reached complete functional maturity, acting as the baby's lungs, kidneys, liver, digestive and immune systems.		3-4 lb weight gain. Belly beginning to show.		The fetal heartbeart can now be heard with an amplified stethoscope. Placenta begins producing the estrogen hormone.
Common Discomforts		**Sleeplessness** may result from the discomfort or anxieties of pregnancy.				Vaginal secretions are the result of an increased supply of blood and glucose to the vaginal mucosa. Sever itching, irritation and malodor suggest an infection is present.		**Headaches** may occur while your body becomes adjusted to changes in blood volume and vascular tone. Emotional tension may also be a factor.
Remedies		A glass of warm milk before bedtime can work wonders. It's also good for your baby!				If infection is suspected, consult a health professional. Otherwise, cleanse daily with warm water, keeping the area dry to prevent chafing. Apply yogurt for vulvar itch.		Change body positions slowly. Resting with a damp cloth on the forehead helps some women. Drinking milk and/or eatting a small snack also produces relief in some
Drug Substances to Avoid		• tranquilziers • narcotics • antihisamines • alcohol • barbiturates (Avoid throughout pregnancy)				Vaginal Anti-infectives • metronidazole (Flagyl®) (Avoid throughout pregnancy)		**Analgesics** • salicylates (aspirin) • phenacetin/caffeine • propoxyphene (Darvon®) • Idomethacin (Indocin®) **Tranquilizers** (Avoid throughout pregnancy)
Acceptable Alternatives	None: Avoid all drugs not prescribed by a physician for a specific condition. Avoid X-rays.					• AVC™ Cream • Nystatin vaginal tablets (Mycostatin®) • Miconazole vaginal cream (Monistat®)		**TYLENOL®** brand acetaminophen

Continued.

Fig. 8.14, cont'd
Summary of fetal development, maternal events, common discomforts, remedies, and drug substances to avoid.

	Week 17	Week 18	Week 19	Week 20	Week 21	Week 22	Week 23	Week 24
Baby's Development		An oily coating protects the fetus. Fine hair covers the body and keeps the oil on the skin.	Eyebrows, eyelashes and head hair develop.	The fetus is now following a regular schedule of sleeping, turning, sucking and kicking—and has settled upon a favorite position within the uterus.		The skeleton is developing rapidly as the bone-forming cells increase their activity.	Eyelids begin to open and close.	The fetus now weighs about 27 ounces.
Maternal Events		3-4 lb weight gain.	Breasts begin secreting colostrum in preparation for nursing.	The placenta reaches its largest size relative to the fetus, ocering one-half of the uterine lining. There is 400 ml of fluid now present in the amniotic sac.		3-4 lb weight gain.		The placenta becomes thicker rather than wider. Mother can now sense when baby's awake.
Common Discomforts		**Faintness or dizziness** when standing suddenly. This is caused by reduced blood flow to the brain as your body adjusts to new circulatory patterns. Possible shortness of breath.	**Varicose veins** are often the result in rising blood pressure in the lower extremities. This is caused by the enlarged uterus cutting off blood flow back from the legs to the heart.	**Allergies,** such as hay fever, are a common problem for some people.		**Skin changes** such as darkened nipples, stretch marks, splotches on cheeks and forehead, acne, redness on palms of hands and soles of feet are mainly due to increased hormone levels in your blood.		**Nosebleeds** sometime occur because of increased blood volume and nasal congestion.
Remedies		Try to sit with your feet up whenever possible; rise slowly and support yourself.	Whenever sitting, rest legs on footstool with feet elevated; avoid pressure on lower thighs. Many women find support stockings helpful.	Air conditioning (with a clean filter) often helps, and a pollen mask can be worn to screen out allergens.		Be patient. Virtually all of these effects will subside soon after childbirth.		Apply a little petroleum jelly in each nostril; that should stop the bleeding. A humidifier may also help. Do not irritate nasal mucosa.
Drug Substances to Avoid		• tranquilziers • alcohol (Avoid throughout pregnancy)		**Most antihistamines** • hydroxyzine (Atarax®) • trimeprazine (Temaril®) (Avoid throughout pregnancy)		Tetracycline (for acne) (Avoid throughout pregnancy)		
Acceptable Alternatives (occasional use)		• smelling salts • aromotic spirits of ammonia		Chlorpheniramine for congestions; nasal spray for stuffy nose, occasionally. Calamine Lotion for rashes.		If nipples or abdomen itch, a lanolin-based cream or baby oil can provide relief. A mild soap can remove the excessive facial oil produced by acne.		Pseudoephedrine or nasal spray may be used occasionally for stuffy nose, if necessary.

	Week 25	Week 26	Week 27	Week 28	Week 29	Week 30	Week 31	Week 32
Baby's Development		To a certain extent, the baby can now breathe, swallow and regulate its body temperature, but still depends greatly upon maternal support.	A substance called *surfactant* forms in the lungs, preparing them to function independently at birth.	Baby is two-thirds grown.	Fat deposits are building up beneath the skin to insulate the baby against the abrupt change in temperature at birth.	The digestive tract and the lungs are now nearly fully matured and the skin becomes less red and wrinkled.	The baby has grown to about 14 inches.	
Maternal Events		3-4 lb weight gain.	Respiratory movements can be detected by ultrasound. Mother sometimes feels baby's breathing as "hiccups."	The volume of amniotic fluid decreases to make room for growing fetus.		3-5 lb weight gain.		Mother may have trouble sleeping because of baby's activity.
Common Discomforts			**Leg and muscle cramps** may be caused by fatigue, by pressure exerted on the nerves by the uterus, or by too little calcium/too much phosphorus in the diet.	**Heartburn** often occurs as the stomach emptying time is delayed, causing a burning sensation in the throat.		**Swollen ankles.** The pressure of the uterus on the large veins returning blood to the heart may induce water retention.	**Constipation** is another result of the decelerated digestive process. As food moves slowly through your intestines, more water is extracted, leaving the stool drier and harder.	**Hemorrhoids** may also develop.
Remedies			Exercise regularly, walking especially. Elevate legs and flex toes when resting. Increase milk consumption.	Drink milk between small, frequent meals. This problem will disappear soon after your baby's birth.		Elevate legs—once or twice a day for an hour or so—level with your hips. Sleep on your left side.	Eat foods containing roughage, such as raw fruits, vegetables, cereals with bran. Drink liquids and exercise frequently.	Soaking in a warm bath or sitting on soft pillows should soothe the symptoms of hemorrhoids.
Drug Substances to Avoid			• salicylates (aspirin) • tranquilizers (Avoid throughout pregnancy)	**Antacids** • calcium carbonate • magnesium trisillicate (Gaviscon®) • sodium bicarbonate (Baking Soda) • cimetideine (Tagamet®) (Avoid throughout pregnancy)		**Most diuretics** ("water pills") (Avoid throughout pregnancy)	**Laxatives** • mineral oil • castor oil (Avoid throughout pregnancy)	
Acceptable Alternatives (occasional use)			Calcium supplements with little or no phosphorus.	• Maalox® • Mylanta® (also for "gas")			For Constipation: • Metamucil® • Senokot® • teaspoon of milk of magnesia at bedtime	For Hemorrhoids: • Nupercainal® suppositories or cream • Anusol® • Medicone®

Fig. 8.14, cont'd
Summary of fetal development, maternal events, common discomforts, remedies, and drug substances to avoid.

	Week 33		To Term
Baby's Development	Virtually the entire uterus is now occupied by the baby and its activity is restricted.	Maternal antibodies against measles, mumps, rubella, whooping cough and scarlet fever are transferred to the baby, providing protection for about 6 months until the infant's own immune system can take over.	
Maternal Events	The placenta is nearly 4 times as thick as it was 20 weeks ago, and weighs about 20 ounces.	Preparing for birth, the baby descends deeper into the mother's pelvis. 3-5 lb weight gain.	In 9 short months, the miracle is complete: you have transformed a single, microscopic fertilized cell into a six thousand billion celled human being.
Common Discomforts	**Backaches** are often caused by muscles and ligaments relaxing in preparation for the stretching required in delivery. Also by the added off-center weight of the enlarged uterus.	**Urinary frequency** is caused—for the second time in your pregnancy—by the uterus compressing the bladder against the pelvic bones, thus reducing its capacity.	**Uterine contractions** become perceptible as the cervix and lower uterine segment prepare for labor.
Remedies	Back exercises, such as the "pelvic tilt", can help strengthen back and abdominal muscles. Wear low-heeled shoes or flats; avoid heavy lifting.	You can decrease pressure on the bladder at night by sleeping on your side. Urinate frequently.	
Drug Substances to Avoid	**Analgesics** • Salicylates (aspirin) • propoxyphene (Darvon®) • phenacetin/caffeine • indomethacin (Indocin®) • codeine (Avoid throughout pregnancy)		
Acceptable Alternatives (occasional use)	**TYLENOL®** brand acetaminophen		

References

Als, H., and others: Dynamics of the behavioral organization of the premature infant: a theoretical perspective. In Field, T.M. and others, editors: Infants born at risk, New York, 1979, Spectrum Press.

Brazelton, T.B.: Joint regulation of neonate-parent behavior. In Tronick, E.Z.: Social interchange in infancy: affect, cognition, and communication, Baltimore, 1982, University Park Press.

Clements, M.: Observations on certain aspects of neonatal behavior in response to auditory stimuli. Paper presented at the Fifth International Congress of Psychosomatic Obstetrics and Gynecology, Rome, 1977.

Condon, W.S.: A primary phase in the organization of infant responding behavior. In Schaffer, H.R., editor: Studies in mother-infant interaction, New York, 1977, Academic Press.

Danforth, D.N., editor: Obstetrics and gynecology, ed. 4., New York, 1982, Harper & Row, Publishers.

Dobson, V.: Spectral sensitivity of the 2-month infant as measured by visually evoked cortical potential, Vision Res. 16:367, 1976.

Eisenberg, R.B.: Stimulus significance as a determinant of infant responses to sound. In Thoman, E.B., editor: Origins of the infant's social responsiveness, The Johnson & Johnson Baby Products Co., Pediatric Round Table, 2, Skillman, New Jersey, 1979.

Fanaroff, A.A., and Martin, R.J., editors: Behrman's neonatalperinatal medicine: diseases of the fetus and infant, ed. 3, St. Louis, 1983, The C.V. Mosby Co.

Freud, E.: Prenatal attachment and bonding, Paper presented to the First International Congress on Pre- and Peri-natal Psychology, Toronto, July 8, 1983.

Grimwade, J.C., and others: Human fetal heart rate change and movement in response to sound and vibration, Am. J. Obstet. Gynecol. 109:86, 1971.

Harrison, M.R., and others: Management of the fetus with a correctable congenital defect, J.A.M.A. 246:774, 1981.

Henshall, W.R.: Intrauterine sound levels, Am. J. Obstet. Gynecol. 112:576, 1972.

Hooker, D.: The prenatal origin of behavior, Lawrence, 1952, University of Kansas Press.

Korones, S.B.: High-risk newborn infants: the basis for intensive nursing care, ed. 4, St. Louis, 1986, The C.V. Mosby Co.

Liley, A.W.: The foetus as a personality, Aust. N.Z. J. Psychiatry 6:99, 1972.

May, K.A.: A typology of detachment/involvement styles adopted during pregnancy by first-time expectant fathers, West J. Nurs. Res 2:445, 1980.

Moore, K.L.: Before we are born: basic embryology and birth defects, rev. ed., Philadelphia, 1977, W.B. Saunders Co.

Moore, K.L.: The developing human, ed. 2, Philadelphia, 1977, W.B. Saunders Co.

Pritchard, J.A., MacDonald, P.C., and Gant, N.F.: Williams obstetrics, ed. 17, Norwalk, Conn., 1985, Appleton-Century-Crofts.

Simner, M.L.: Newborn's response to the cry of another infant, Dev. Psychol. 5:136, 1971.

Stainton, M.C.: A comparison of pre-natal and post-natal perceptions of their babies by parents, Paper presented to the First International Congress on Pre- and Peri-natal Psychology, Toronto, July 8, 1983a.

Stainton, M.C.: Interview data, 1983b.

Van Dongen, L.G., and Goudie, E.G.: Fetal movement patterns in the first trimester of pregnancy, Br. J. Obstet. Gynaecol. 87:191, 1980.

Walker, D., and others: Intrauterine noise: a component of the fetal environment, Am. J. Obstet. Gynecol. 109:91, 1971.

Willson, J.R., Carrington, E.R., and Ledger, W.J.: Obstetrics and gynecology, ed. 7, St. Louis, 1983, The C.V. Mosby Co.

Bibliography

Athey, P.A., and Hadlock, F.P.: Ultrasound in obstetrics and gynecology, St. Louis, 1981, The C.V. Mosby Co.

Berger, T., and others: Factors affecting human sperm penetration of zona-free hamster ova, Am. J. Obstet. Gynecol. 145:397, 1983.

England, M.A.: Color atlas of life before birth: normal fetal development, 1983. Distributed in North America and Canada by Year Book Medical Publishers, Inc., by arrangement with Wolfe Medical Publications, Ltd.

Kremkau, F.W.: How safe is the obstetric ultrasound? Contemp. Obstet. Gynecol. 20(6):182, 1982.

Lowrey, G.H.: Growth and development of children, ed. 7, Chicago, 1978, Year Book Medical Publishers.

Page, E.W., and others: Human reproduction: essentials of reproductive and perinatal medicine, ed. 3, Philadelphia, 1981, W.B. Saunders Co.

Plauche, W.C., Phosphatidylglycerol and lung maturity, Am. J. Obstet. Gynecol. 144:167, 1982.

Whaley, L.F.: Understanding inherited disorders, St. Louis, 1974, The C.V. Mosby Co.

Whaley, L.F.: Genetic counseling in maternity nursing. In McNall, L.K., and Galeener, J.T., editors: Current practice in obstetric and gynecologic nursing, vol. 1, St. Louis, 1976, The C.V. Mosby Co.

Whaley, L.F.: Genetic counseling. In Curry, J.B., and Peppe, K.K., editors: Mental retardation: nursing approaches to care, St. Louis, 1978, The C.V. Mosby Co.

Williams, S.R.: Nutrition and diet therapy, ed. 5, St. Louis, 1985, The C.V. Mosby Co.

Wilson, M.G.: Genetic counseling, Curr. Probl. Pediatr. 5:1, 1975.

Wohlgemuth, D.J., and Balke, E.M.: Changes in egg and sperm before and during fertilization, Contemp. Obstet. Gynecol. 20(5):196, 1982.

Anatomy and Physiology of Pregnancy

A healthy pregnancy with a physically safe and emotionally satisfying outcome for both mother and infant is the goal of maternity care. Consistent health supervision and surveillance are of utmost importance. Many maternal adaptations are unfamiliar to pregnant women and their families. The knowledgeable maternity nurse can help the pregnant woman recognize the relationship between her physical status and the plan for her care. Sharing in information encourages the pregnant woman to participate in her own care, depending on her interest, need to know, and readiness to learn.

In this and following chapters, terms specific to maternity will be used. Some of the terms are defined below.

Definitions

The following terms refer to the *pregnant woman:*

gravida A woman who is pregnant.
parturient A woman in labor.
parturition or **confinement** The process of labor and delivery.
parity The number of *pregnancies* in which the fetus or fetuses have reached viability, not the number of fetuses delivered. Whether the fetus is born alive or is stillborn after viability is reached does not affect parity.
nulligravida A woman who has never been pregnant.
primigravida A woman who is pregnant for the first time.
multigravida A woman who has had two or more pregnancies.
nullipara A woman who has *not* completed a pregnancy with a fetus or fetuses who have reached the stage of fetal viability (legal definition: 22 to 23 weeks of gestational age).
primipara A woman who has completed one pregnancy with a fetus or fetuses who have reached the stage of fetal viability.
multipara A woman who has completed two or more pregnancies to the stage of fetal viability.

This information is abbreviated as gravidity/parity. For example, "I/0" means that a woman is pregnant for the first time (primigravida) and has not carried a pregnancy to viability (nullipara).

One obstetric abbreviation commonly employed in maternity centers is even more detailed. It consists of five digits with hyphens for separation. The first digit represents the total number of pregnancies, including the present one; the second digit represents the total number of deliveries; the third indicates the number of premature babies; the fourth identifies the number of abortions, and the fifth is the number of children currently living. If a woman pregnant only once with twins delivers at the thirty-fifth week and the babies survive, the abbreviation that represents this information is "1-1-2-0-2." During her next pregnancy the abbreviation is "2-1-2-0-2." Additional examples are given in Table 9.1.

The following terms refer to the *periods of pregnancy:*

prenatal Before birth.
perinatal period Period extending from the twentieth or twenty-eighth week of gestation through the end of the twenty-eighth day after birth.
postnatal After birth.
prepartum Before delivery.
intrapartum Labor and delivery (in reality, delivery of fetus and placenta is part of labor).
postpartum After delivery.

The following terms refer to the *duration of pregnancy:*

term pregnancy A term pregnancy is a gestation of 38 to 42 weeks.
preterm pregnancy A preterm pregnancy is a gestation of less than 38 weeks.
prolonged pregnancy Prolonged or postdate pregnancy, by definition, begins 294 days after the LMP, that is, 14 days after the conventionally accepted normal duration of pregnancy (280 days).

Table 9.1
Gravidity and Parity Using Five-Digit and Two Digit Systems

Condition	Five-digit System					Two-digit System
	A*	B	C	D	E	F
Judith is pregnant for the first time.	1	- 0	- 0	- 0	- 0	i/0
She carries the pregnancy to term and the neonate survives.	1	- 1	- 0	- 0	- 1	i/i
She is pregnant again.	2	- 1	- 0	- 0	- 1	ii/i
Her second pregnancy ends in abortion.	2	- 1	- 0	- 1	- 1	ii/i
During her third pregnancy, she delivers viable twins.	3	- 2	- 0	- 1	- 3	iii/ii

*A, Times uterus has been pregnant; B, number of deliveries, C, number of premature deliveries; D, number of abortions (spontaneous or elective); E, number of living children; F, gravidity/parity; corresponds to A and B of the 5-digit system.

Table 9.2
Comparison of Measurements for Nonpregnant and Pregnant Uterus at 40 Weeks*

Measurement	Nonpregnant	Pregnant (40 Weeks)
Length	6.5 cm (2½ in)	32 cm (12½ in)
Width	4.0 gm (1½ in)	24 cm (9½ in)
Depth	2.5 cm (1 in)	22 cm (8½ in)
Weight	60-70 g (2½ oz)	1100-1200 g (2½ lb)
Volume	1-2 ml	5000 ml

*Note that references vary as to the exact values but all references agree on the magnitude of the growth the uterus undergoes during pregnancy.

Adaptations to Pregnancy

The content in this chapter provides the basis for preventive, curative, and rehabilitative maternity care. Maternal adaptations are thought to be caused by the hormones of pregnancy and by mechanical pressures arising from the enlarging uterus and other tissues. These adaptations serve to protect the woman's normal physiologic functioning, to meet the metabolic demands pregnancy imposes on her body, and to provide for fetal developmental and growth needs. Although pregnancy is a normal phenomenon, problems can occur. The nurse needs an adequate foundation in normal maternal physiology to accomplish the following:

1. Identify potential or actual deviation from normal adaptation in order to initiate remedial care
2. Help the mother understand the anatomic and physiologic changes during pregnancy
3. Allay the mother's (and family's) anxiety, which may result from lack of knowledge
4. Teach the mother (and family) signs and symptoms that must be reported to the physician

Among the expected adjustments to pregnancy are changes that are found in some disease states; for example, low hemoglobin levels, a high erythrocyte sedimentation rate, dyspnea at rest, and alterations in cardiac function and endocrine balance. These changes reflect the body's effort to protect the mother and the fetus. An understanding of these changes is necessary for anyone who participates in the care of the mother and the fetus.

Some of the adaptations are recognized as signs and symptoms of pregnancy. These signs and symptoms appear in **bold print** throughout the chapter. A summary of the signs and symptoms of pregnancy and their order of appearance are presented in Table 11.2.

Reproductive System and Breasts

Hypothalamus-pituitary-ovarian axis. During pregnancy, elevated levels of estrogen and progesterone suppress secretion of FSH and LH. The maturation of a follicle and ovulation of an ovum do not occur. Menstrual cycles cease. The majority of women experience **amenorrhea.** However, at least 20% have some slight, painless spotting during early gestation for unexplained reasons. A great majority of these women continue to term and have normal infants.

Human chorionic gonadotropin (HCG) is produced by the fertilized ovum and by the chorionic villi following implantation. HCG maintains the corpus luteum's production of estrogen and progesterone for the first 8 to 10 weeks of pregnancy until the placenta takes over their production. The production of HCG is the basis for pregnancy tests discussed later in this chapter.

Uterus

Enlargement. The phenomenal uterine growth occurs under the hormonal stimulus of estrogen and progesterone. Enlargement results from (1) increased vascularity and dilation of blood vessels, (2) hyperplasia (production of new muscle fibers and fibroelastic tissue) and hypertrophy (enlargement of preexisting muscle fibers and fibroelastic tissue), and (3) development of the decidua (see Fig. 9.10). By 7 weeks the uterus is the size of a large hen's egg; by 10 weeks, the size of an orange (twice its nonpregnant size); by 12 weeks, the size of a grapefruit. Table 9.2 compares uterine measurements for the nonpregnant and pregnant uterus at 40 weeks' gestation.

As the uterus increases in size, it also changes in

Fig. 9.1
Softening of uterus.

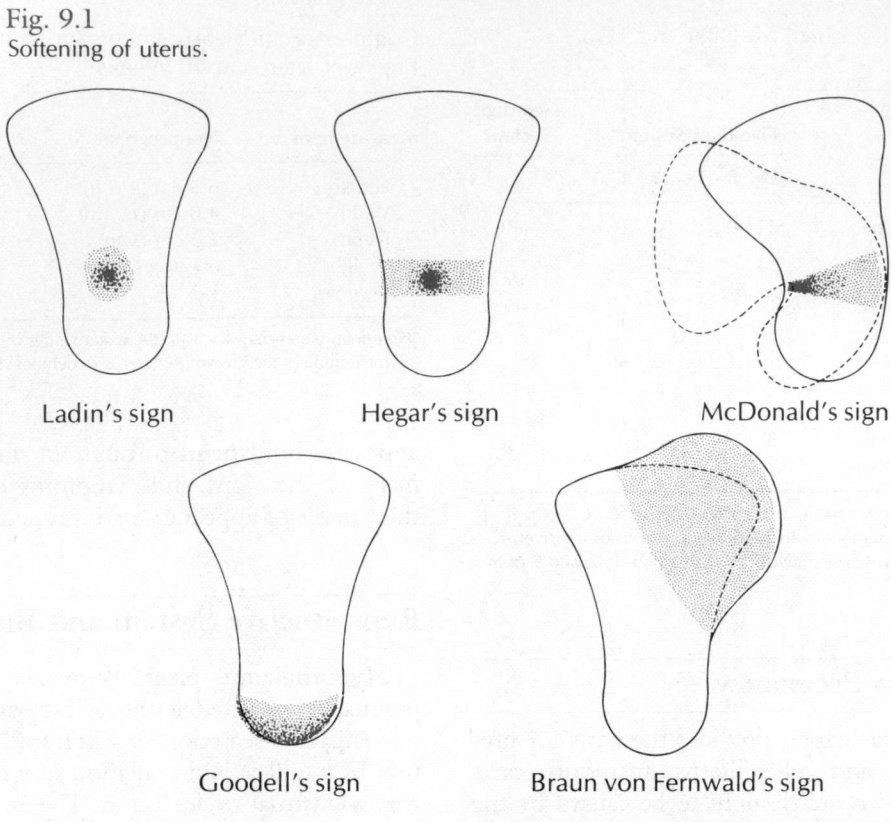

Ladin's sign   Hegar's sign   McDonald's sign

Goodell's sign   Braun von Fernwald's sign

weight, shape, and position. At conception the uterus is shaped like an upside-down pear. During the second trimester it is spheric or globular. Later, as the fetus lengthens, the contour of the uterus becomes more ovoid.

A reasonably accurate correlation of **uterine enlargement** and the duration of amenorrhea in weeks counting from the sixth week to term is possible in most normal pregnant women. Variation in the positions of the fundus or the fetus, variations in the amount of amniotic fluid present, or the presence of more than one fetus reduces the accuracy of this estimation of the duration of pregnancy.

The pregnancy may "show" after the fourteenth week, although this depends to some degree on the woman's height and weight. **Abdominal enlargement** may be less apparent in the primigravida with good abdominal muscle tone (see Fig. 9.7). Posture also influences the type and degree of abdominal enlargement seen.

Consistency. During the early weeks of pregnancy the uterus becomes perceptibly and progressively softer. At about the seventh to eighth week the following

patterns of **uterine softening** are noted: isthmic softening **(Hegar's sign)**, cervical softening **(Goodell's sign)**, easy flexion of the fundus on the cervix (McDonald's sign), softening and slight fullness of the fundus near the area of implantation (Braun von Fernwald's sign), or a soft lateral bulge with cornual implantation (Piskacek's sign) (Figs. 9.1 and 9.2). After the eighth week, general enlargement and softening of the uterine corpus and cervix are likely.

It is believed by some that the nonsteroid ovarian hormone, *relaxin,* may act synergistically along with progesterone. Relaxin contributes to a relaxing effect not only in the uterus but throughout various parts of the body, such as on the joints and walls of blood vessels. Relaxin appears in the blood early in pregnancy and increases in volume gradually to term. The hormone then disappears within 24 hours of delivery.

Position. As the uterus grows it is elevated out of the pelvic area and may be palpated above the symphysis pubis sometime between the twelfth and sixteenth weeks of pregnancy (Fig. 9.3). It rises gradually to the level of the umbilicus at about 22 to 24 weeks and nearly reaches the xiphoid process at term.

Fig. 9.2
Hegar's sign. Bimanual examination for assessing softening of isthmus.

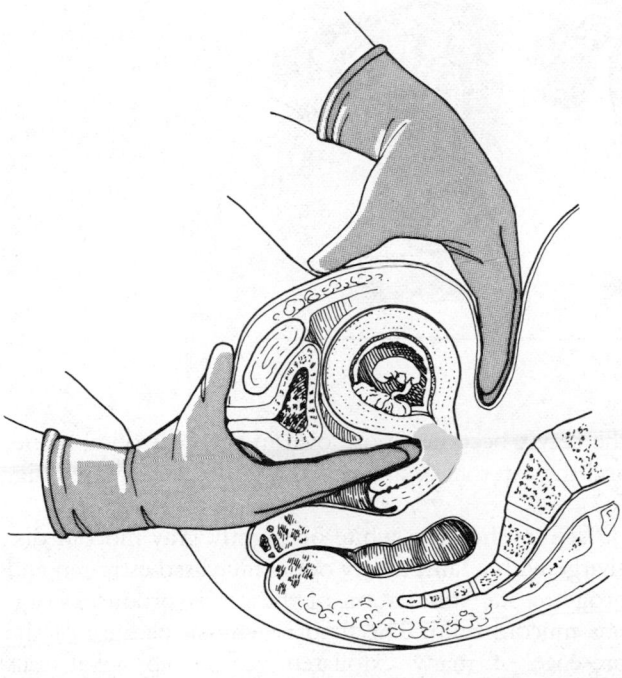

Fig. 9.3
Height of fundus by weeks of normal gestation with a single fetus.

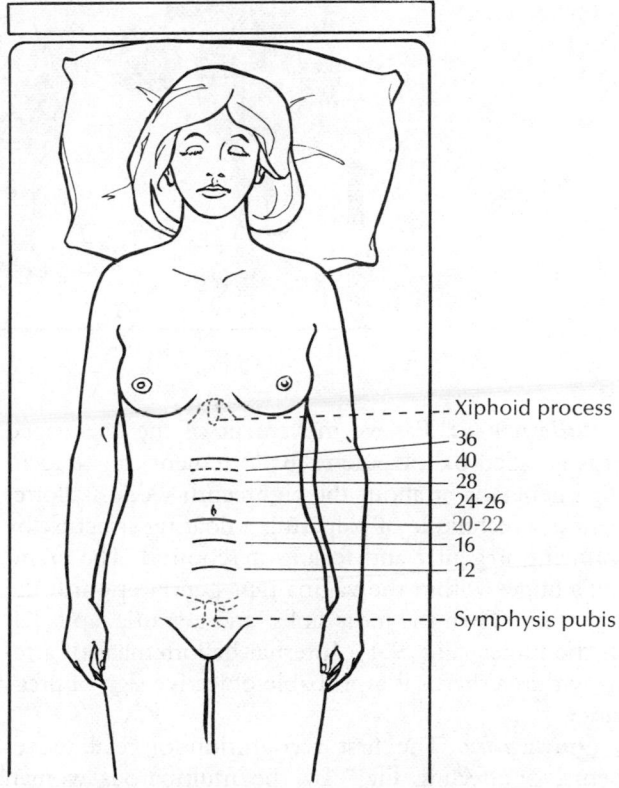

- Xiphoid process
- 36
- 40
- 28
- 24-26
- 20-22
- 16
- 12
- Symphysis pubis

Generally the uterus is rotated to the right as it elevates, probably because of the presence of the rectosigmoid colon on the left side. However, the extensive hypertrophy (enlargement) of the round ligaments keeps the uterus in line. Eventually the growing uterus touches the anterior abdominal wall and displaces the intestines to either side of the abdomen. When a pregnant woman stands, the major part of her uterus rests against the anterior abdominal wall and contributes to altering her center of gravity.

Contractility. Soon after the fourth month of pregnancy, uterine contractions can be felt through the abdominal wall. These contractions are referred to as the **Braxton Hicks sign,** a probable sign of pregnancy. Braxton Hicks contractions are a continuation of the irregular, painless contractions that occur intermittently throughout each menstrual cycle. The contractions are felt as uterine firmness through the abdominal wall or are evident because they raise and push the uterus forward. Contractions facilitate uterine blood flow and thereby oxygenation of the products of conception. Although Braxton Hicks contractions are not ordinarily painful, some women do complain they are annoying. After the twenty-eighth week, contractions become much more definite, especially in slender women. Generally these contractions cease with walking or exercise. Rarely they may be perceived as painful. They may become strong enough during the last few weeks to be confused with the contractions of beginning labor.

Blood flow. In a normal term pregnancy, one sixth of the total maternal blood volume is within the uterine vascular system. The rate of blood flow through the uterus averages 500 ml/min, and oxygen consumption of the gravid uterus averages 25 ml/min. Maternal arterial pressure, contractions of the uterus, and maternal position are three factors known to influence blood flow to this organ throughout pregnancy.

Intrauterine sounds. Using an ultrasound device or a fetal stethoscope, the physician or nurse may hear (1) the **uterine souffle** or bruit, a rushing sound of maternal blood going to the placenta that is synchronous with the maternal pulse, (2) the **funic souffle** caused by fetal blood coursing through the umbilical cord and is synchronous with the fetal heart rate, and (3) the **fetal heart rate (FHR).** For further discussion, see Chapter 16.

Fig. 9.4
Internal ballottement (18 weeks).

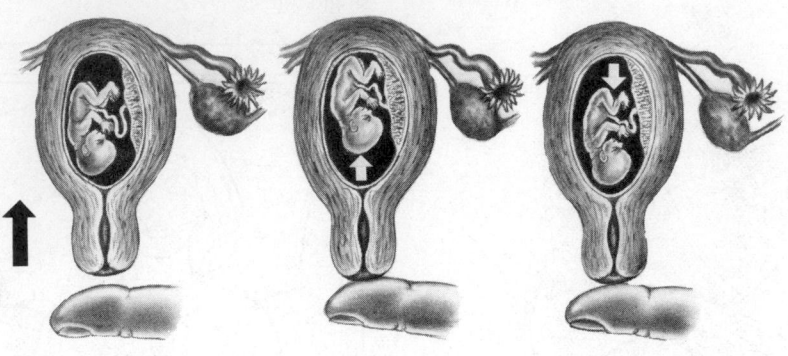

Ballottement. Passive movement of the unengaged fetus is called **ballottement.** Ballottement can be identified generally at about the eighteenth week. Ballottement is a technique of palpating a floating structure by bouncing it gently and feeling it rebound. The examiner's finger within the vagina taps gently upward; the fetus rises. Then the fetus sinks, and a gentle tap is felt on the finger (Fig. 9.4). Internal ballottement of a fetus within a uterus is a probable objective sign of pregnancy.

Quickening. The first recognition of fetal movements, or "feeling life," by the multiparous woman may occur as early as the fourteenth to sixteenth week. The primigravidas may not notice these sensations until the eighteenth week or later. **Quickening** is frequently described as a flutter and is difficult to distinguish from peristalsis. Noting the week in which quickening occurs provides a tentative clue in dating the duration of gestation.

Cervix. A softening of the cervical tip may be observed about the beginning of the sixth week in a normal, unscarred cervix. The softening of the cervix during pregnancy (Goodell's sign, Fig. 9.1) is brought about by increased vascularity, slight hypertrophy, and hyperplasia of the muscle and connective tissue. The connective tissue becomes loose, edematous, highly elastic, and increased in volume. The changes in the cervix, as well as those of the vagina, help to prepare the birth canal for the fetus's passage through it. Friability is increased; that is, the cervix bleeds easily when scraped or touched. Increased friability is the cause of the few drops of blood seen after coitus with deep penetration or vaginal examination. These few drops are usually within normal limits.

The cervix of the nullipara is rounded. Lacerations of the cervix almost always occur during the birth process. With or without lacerations, following childbirth

the cervix becomes more oval in the horizontal plane, and the external os appears as a transverse slit (see Fig. 9.7).

Leukorrhea is a white or slightly gray mucoid discharge with a faint musty odor. Increased estrogen and progesterone stimulation of the cervix produces copious mucoid fluid. The fluid is whitish because of the presence of many exfoliated vaginal epithelial cells caused by normal pregnancy hyperplasia. This vaginal

Fig. 9.5
A, Cervix in nonpregnant woman. **B,** Changes in cervix during pregnancy.

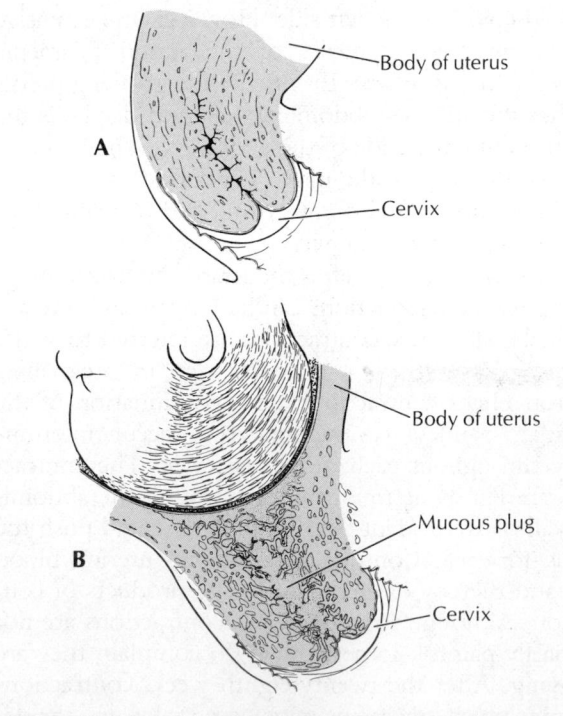

discharge is never pruritic or blood stained. Because of the progesterone effect, *ferning* (see Chapter 5) does *not* occur in the dried cervical mucus smear. The mucus fills the endocervical canal, resulting in the formation of the mucous plug (operculum) (Fig. 9.5). The operculum acts as a barrier against bacterial invasion during pregnancy.

Vagina and vulva

Internal structures. Pregnancy hormones prepare the vagina for distention during labor by producing a thickened vaginal mucosa, loosened connective tissue, hypertrophied smooth muscle, and an increase in the length of the vaginal vault. Increased vascularity results in a violet-bluish color to the vaginal mucosa and cervix. The deepened color, termed **Chadwick's sign** or Jacquemier's sign, may be evident as early as the sixth week, but is easily noted at the eighth week of pregnancy. Desquamation (or exfoliation) of the vaginal, glycogen-rich cells occurs under estrogen stimulation. The cells that are shed contribute to the thick, whitish vaginal discharge, leukorrhea.

During pregnancy the pH of vaginal secretions becomes less acidic. The pH changes from 4 to 5 to about 5.5 to 6.5. The rise in pH makes the pregnant woman more vulnerable to vaginal infections, especially yeast infections. A diet of large quantities of sugars can make the vaginal environment even more suitable for a yeast infection.

The increased vascularity of the vagina and other pelvic viscera results in a marked increase in sensitivity. The increased sensitivity may lead to a high degree of sexual interest and arousal, especially during the second trimester of pregnancy. The increased congestion plus the relaxed walls of the blood vessels and the heavy uterus may result in edema and varicosities of the vulva. The edema and varicosities usually resolve during the postpartal period.

External structures. External structures of the *perineum* are enlarged during pregnancy because of an increase in vasculature, hypertrophy of the perineal body, and deposition of fat (Fig. 9.6). The labia majora of the nullipara approximate and obscure the vaginal introitus; those of the parous woman separate and gape after childbirth and perineal or vaginal injury. Torn residual tags of the hymen remain after the use of tampons, coitus, and vaginal delivery. Fig. 9.7 compares the nullipara and the multipara in relation to several characteristics: pregnant abdomen, vulva, and cervix.

Breasts. Fullness, heightened sensitivity, tingling, and **heaviness** of the breasts begin as early as the sixth week of gestation. Breast sensitivity varies from mild tingling to frank pain (mastodynia). **Nipples** and **areolae** become more **pigmented,** a **secondary pinkish areola** develops, and nipples become more erectile. Hypertrophy of the sebaceous (oil) glands embedded in the primary areola, called **Montgomery's tubercles,** may be seen around the nipples. These sebaceous glands may have a protective role in that they keep the nipples lubricated. Suppleness of the nipples is jeopardized if the protective oils are washed off with soap.

The richer blood supply dilates the vessels beneath the skin. Once barely noticeable, the blood vessels now

Fig. 9.6

A, Pelvic floor in nonpregnant woman. **B,** Pelvic floor at end of pregnancy. Note marked projection (growth of tissue) below line joining tip of coccyx and inferior margin of symphysis. Urethra is elongated, and fat deposits are increased.

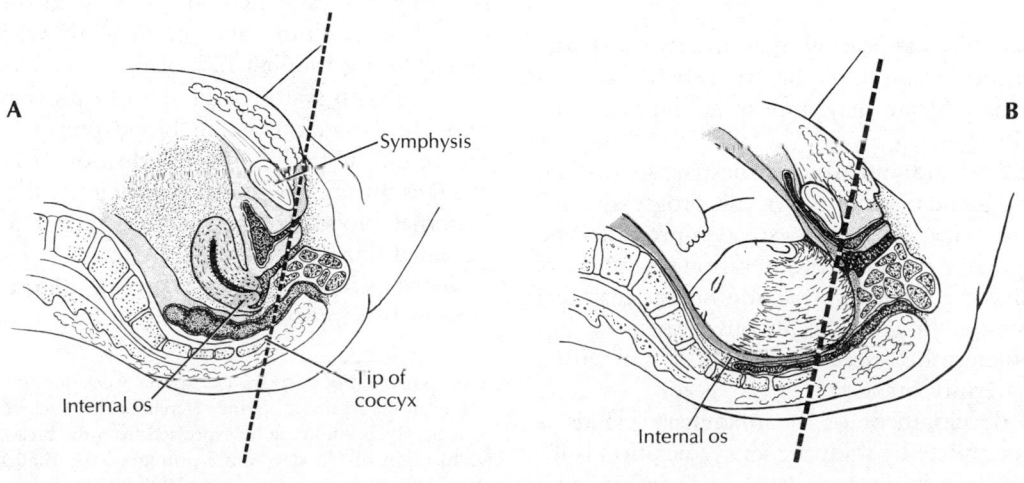

Fig. 9.7
Comparison of abdomen, vulva, and cervix. **A,** Nullipara.
B, Multipara.

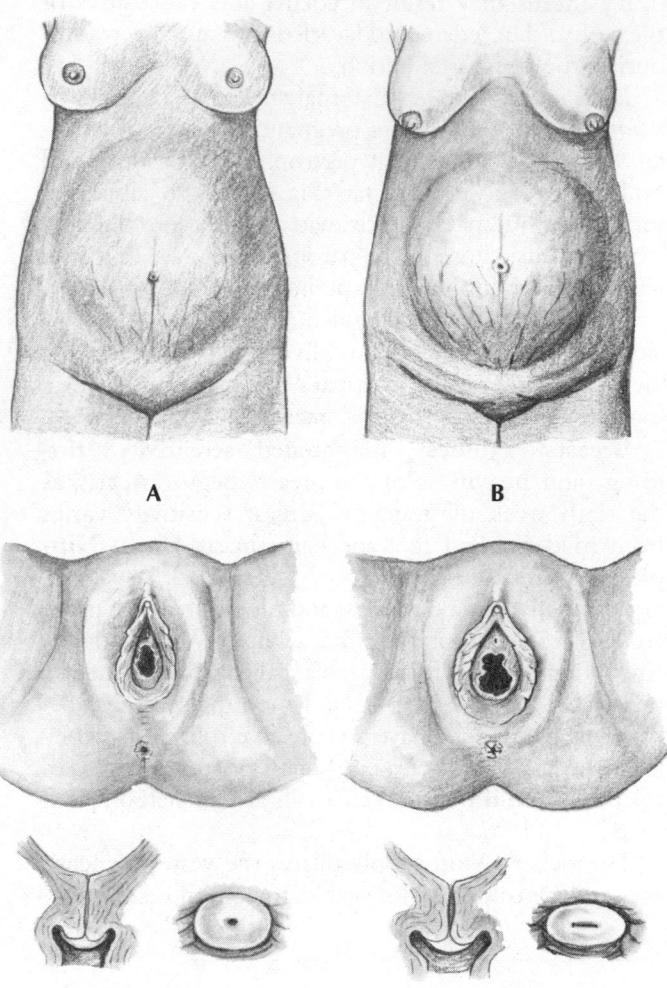

A   B

become visible, often appearing in an intertwining pattern. Venous congestion in the breasts is more obvious in primigravidas. Striae may appear at the outer aspects of the breasts.

During the second and third trimesters, growth of the mammary glands accounts for the progressive increase in breast size. The high estrogen-progesterone levels in pregnancy promote proliferation of the ducts and lobule-alveolar tissue, so that the breasts may feel nodular. Overstretching of the fibrous suspensory ligaments supporting the breasts can be prevented with a well-fitted maternity brassiere.

Although development of the mammary glands is functionally complete by midpregnancy, lactation is inhibited until a drop in estrogen level occurs after deliv-

ery of the fetus and placenta. A thin precolostrum secretion, however, may be expressed from the nipples by the end of the sixteenth week.* This secretion thickens as term approaches and is then known as **colostrum.** Colostrum, the creamy, white to yellowish premilk fluid, may be expressed from the nipples during the third trimester.

General Body Systems

Cardiovascular system. Maternal adjustments to pregnancy involve extensive changes in the cardiovascular system, both anatomic and physiologic. Cardiovascular adaptations serve to protect the woman's normal physiologic functioning, to meet the metabolic demands pregnancy imposes on her body, and to provide for fetal developmental and growth needs.

Anatomic changes: cardiac size and position. Slight cardiac hypertrophy (enlargement) or dilation is probably secondary to increased blood volume and cardiac output. As the diaphragm is displaced upward, the heart is elevated upward and to the left (Fig. 9.8). The apical impulse (PMI) is shifted upward and laterally about 1 to 1.5 cm (½ in). The degree of shift depends on the duration of pregnancy and the size and position of the uterus.

Auscultatory changes. Auscultatory changes accompany the changes in heart size and position. Increases in blood volume and cardiac output also contribute to auscultatory changes common in pregnancy: a third heart sound and an ejection murmur. Between 14 and 20 weeks, *pulse* increases slowly up to 10 to 15 beats per minute, which then persists to term. Palpitations may occur. Bradycardia may occur after delivery and persist for 1 week. *Arterial blood pressure* (brachial artery) varies with age. Blood pressure findings vary with the position of the woman. It is highest when she is sitting, lowest when she is lying in the left lateral recumbent position, and intermediate when she is supine. During the first half of pregnancy, there is a decrease in both systolic and diastolic pressure of 5 to 10 mm Hg. The decrease in blood pressure is probably the result of peripheral vasodilation from hormonal changes during pregnancy. During the third trimester, maternal blood pressure should return to the values obtained during the first trimester.

Blood volume and composition. Blood volume increases by approximately 1500 ml† (normal value:

---

*References differ as to the gestational week during which precolostrum can be expressed. Some references cite week 16 as the earliest time at which fluid may be expressed from the breasts.
†Expansion of blood volume: primigravidas, 1250 ml; multigravidas, 1500 ml; twin pregnancies, 2000 ml.

Fig. 9.8
Changes in position of heart, lungs, and thoracic cage in pregnancy. *Broken line*, Nonpregnant. *Solid line*, Change that occurs in pregnancy.

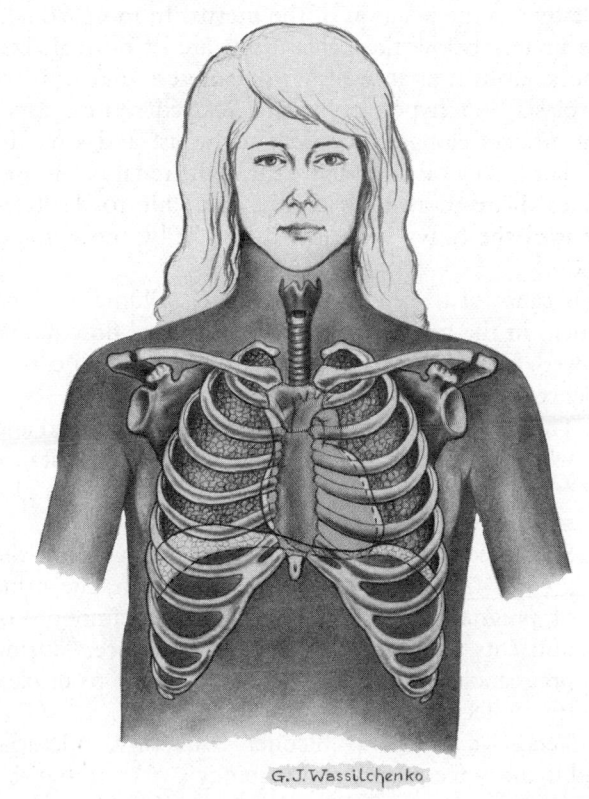

G. J. Wassilchenko

8.5% to 9% of body weight). The increase is made up of 1000 ml *plasma* plus 450 ml red blood cells (RBCs). The increase in volume starts about the twelfth week, peaks at about 25% to 40% at the thirty-second week, then decreases slightly to the fortieth week. The increased volume is a protective mechanism. It is essential for (1) the hypertrophied vascular system of the enlarged uterus, (2) adequate hydration of fetal and maternal tissues when the woman assumes an erect or supine position, and (3) fluid reserve for blood loss during the delivery and puerperium. Peripheral vasodilation maintains a normal blood pressure despite the increased blood volume in pregnancy.

During pregnancy there is an accelerated production of *RBCs* (normal 4 to 5.5 million/mm^3). The percentage of increase depends on the amount of iron available. The RBC mass increases by 30% to 33% by term if an iron supplement is taken. It increases by only 17% in some women if no supplement is taken. For the discussion of iron therapy see Nutrition, Chapter 12, p. 323.

Normal *hemoglobin* values (12 to 16 g/dl blood) and *hematocrit* values (37% to 47%) decrease. The decrease is more noticeable during the second trimester, when rapid expansion of blood volume takes place. If the hemoglobin value drops to 10 g/dl or less, or if the hematocrit drops to 35% or less, the woman is considered anemic.

The total *white cell count* increases during the second trimester and peaks during the third trimester. This increase is primarily in the leukocytes; the lymphocyte count stays about the same throughout pregnancy.

Cardiac output. Cardiac output increases from 30% to 50% by the thirty-second week of pregnancy; it declines to about a 20% increase at 40 weeks. The elevated cardiac output is largely a result of increased stroke volume and in response to increased tissue demands for oxygen (normal value is 5 to 5.5 L/min). The cardiac output decreases with the woman in the supine position (see discussion of supine hypotension, p. 215). Cardiac output increases with any exertion such as labor and delivery.

Circulation and coagulation times. The circulation time decreases slightly by week 32. It returns to near normal near term.

There is a greater *tendency to coagulation* during pregnancy because of increases in various clotting factors. Fibrinolytic activity (the splitting up or the dissolving of a clot) is depressed during pregnancy. During the postpartum period, fibrinolytic activity is depressed, and the woman is again more vulnerable to thrombosis.

Respiratory system. Respiratory adaptations occur during pregnancy to provide for both maternal and fetal needs. Maternal oxygen requirements increase in response to the acceleration in metabolic rate and the need to add to the tissue mass in the uterus and breasts. The conceptus requires oxygen and a way to eliminate carbon dioxide.

Anatomic changes. Increased vascularization in response to elevated levels of estrogen also occurs in the respiratory tract. As the capillaries become engorged, edema and hyperemia develop within the nose, pharynx, larynx, trachea, and bronchi. This congestion within the tissues of the respiratory tract gives rise to several conditions commonly seen during pregnancy. These conditions include nasal and sinus stuffiness, epistaxis (nosebleed), changes in the voice, and marked inflammatory response to even a mild upper respiratory infection. Increased vascularity swells tympanic membranes and eustachian tubes, giving rise to symptoms of impaired hearing, earaches, or a sense of fullness in the ears.

The level of the diaphragm is displaced by as much as 4 cm during pregnancy. With advancing pregnancy, thoracic breathing replaces abdominal breathing and descent of the diaphragm with inspiration becomes less possible.

Pulmonary function. The pregnant woman breathes deeper (increases *tidal volume,* the amount of gases exchanged with each breath) but increases her respiratory rate only slightly (about two breaths per minute). There is a more efficient exchange of lung gases in the alveoli. The oxygen-carrying capacity of the blood is increased accordingly.

During pregnancy, changes in the respiratory center result in a lowered threshold for carbon dioxide. Progesterone and estrogen are presumed to be responsible for the increased sensitivity of the respiratory center. In addition, pregnant women experience increased awareness of the need to breathe; some may complain of dyspnea at rest.

Basal metabolism rate (BMR). The basal metabolism rate usually rises by the fourth month of gestation. It is increased by 15% to 20% by term. The BMR returns to nonpregnant levels by 5 to 6 days postpartum. The elevation in BMR reflects increased oxygen demands of the uterine-placental-fetal unit as well as oxygen consumption from increased maternal cardiac work. Peripheral vasodilation assists in the release of the excess heat production. Gravidas may experience heat intolerance, which is annoying to some women. **Lassitude** and **fatigability** after only slight exertion are described by many women in early pregnancy. These feelings may persist, along with a greater need for sleep. Lassitude and fatigability may be due in part to the increased metabolic activity (see discussion of thyroid gland later in this chapter).

Acid-base balance. By about the tenth week of pregnancy, there is a decrease of about 5 mm Hg in P_{CO_2}. Progesterone may be responsible for increasing the sensitivity of the respiratory center receptors so that tidal volume is increased and P_{CO_2} falls, the base excess (HCO_3, or bicarbonate) falls, and pH rises (becomes more basic). These alterations in acid-base balance indicate that pregnancy is a state of respiratory alkalosis compensated by mild metabolic acidosis.

Renal system. The kidneys are vital excretory organs. Their purpose is to maintain the body's internal environment in the relatively constant homeostatic state necessary for the efficient functioning of the body at the cellular level. The kidneys are responsible for maintenance of electrolyte and acid-base balance, regulation of extracellular fluid volume, excretion of waste products, and the conservation of essential nutrients.

Anatomic changes

Renal pelves and ureters. Changes in renal structure result from hormonal activity (estrogen and progesterone), pressure from an enlarging uterus, and an increase in blood volume. As early as the tenth week of pregnancy, the renal pelves and the ureters dilate. Dilation of the ureters is more pronounced above the pelvic brim, occurring most frequently on the right side due to the position of the uterus. In most women the ureters below the pelvic brim are of normal size. The smooth muscle walls of the ureters undergo hyperplasia and hypertrophy and relaxed muscle tone. The ureters elongate, become tortuous, and kink. In the latter part of pregnancy, the right renal pelvis and ureter dilate more than on the left, due to displacement of the heavy uterus to the right by the sigmoid colon.

Because of these changes, a larger volume of urine is held in the pelves and ureters and urine flow rate is slowed. Urinary stasis or stagnation has several consequences:

1. There is a lag between the time urine is formed and when it reaches the bladder. Therefore clearance test results may reflect substances contained in glomerular filtrate several hours before.
2. Stagnated urine is an excellent medium for the growth of microorganisms. In addition, the urine of pregnant women contains greater amounts of nutrients, including glucose. Therefore, during pregnancy, women are more susceptible to urinary tract infection.

Bladder and urethra. Bladder irritability, nocturia, and **urinary frequency** and **urgency** (without dysuria) frequently is reported in early pregnancy. Near term, bladder symptoms may return.

Urinary frequency results from increased bladder sensitivity and later from compression of the bladder. In the second trimester the bladder is pulled up out of the true pelvis into the abdomen. The urethra lengthens to 7.5 cm (3 in) as the bladder is displaced upward. The pelvic congestion of pregnancy is reflected in hyperemia of the bladder and urethra. This increased vascularity causes the bladder mucosa to be traumatized and bleed easily. There is a decrease in bladder tone, which permits distention of the bladder to approximately 1500 ml. At the same time the bladder is compressed by the enlarging uterus, resulting in the urge to void even if the bladder contains only a small amount of urine.

The causes of dilation of the urine collection and transport system are not fully understood. It has been thought that dilation occurred mainly in response to the high levels of progesterone during pregnancy. There is some evidence that dilation is in response to mechanical pressure as well. Early in pregnancy pressure results from dilated blood vessels, and later, from the enlarging uterus compressing ureters as they pass over the pelvic brim.

Renal function changes. In normal pregnancy, renal function is altered considerably. The woman's kidneys must manage the increased metabolic and circulatory demands of the maternal body and also excretion of fetal waste products. Changes in renal function are caused by pregnancy hormones, an increase in blood volume, the woman's posture, physical activity, and nutritional intake.

Renal function is most efficient when the woman lies in the left lateral recumbent position and least efficient when the woman assumes a supine position. When the pregnant woman is lying supine, the heavy uterus compresses the vena cava and the aorta and cardiac output decreases. The result is a drop in maternal blood pressure and fetal heart rate (vena cava or hypotensive syndrome) and a drop in the volume of blood to the kidneys (see Fig. 15.14). When cardiac output drops, blood flow to the brain and heart is continued at the expense of other organs, including the kidneys and uterus.

Fluid and electrolyte balance

Sodium balance. Selective renal tubular reabsorption maintains sodium and water balance regardless of changes in dietary intake and losses through sweat, vomitus, or diarrhea. From 500 to 900 mEq of sodium is normally retained during pregnancy to meet fetal needs. The need for increased maternal intravascular and extracellular fluid volume requires additional sodium to expand fluid volume and to maintain an isotonic state. To prevent excessive sodium depletion, the maternal kidneys undergo a significant adaptation by increasing tubular reabsorption. As efficient as the renal system is, it can be overstressed by excessive dietary sodium intake or restriction or by use of diuretics. *Severe hypovolemia and reduced placental perfusion are two consequences.*

Water balance. The capacity of the kidneys to excrete water during the early weeks of pregnancy is more efficient than later in pregnancy. Occasionally in early pregnancy the extent of water loss may cause some women to feel thirsty. The pooling of fluid in the legs in the latter part of pregnancy decreases renal blood flow and glomerular filtration rate (GFR). The diuretic response to the water load is triggered when the woman lies down, preferrably on her left side, and the pooled fluid reenters general circulation. This pooling of blood in the lower legs is sometimes referred to as **physiologic edema,** which requires no treatment.

Nutrient, including glucose, excretion. Under normal circumstances, the kidney reabsorbs almost all of the glucose and other nutrients from the plasma filtrate. In pregnant women tubular reabsorption of glucose is efficient so that glucosuria does occur at varying times

and to varying degrees. Normal values are 0 to 20 mg/dl. That is, during any one day, the urine is positive and sometimes it is negative. When it is positive, the amount of glucose varies from $1+$ to $4+$.

In nonpregnant women, blood glucose levels must be at 160 to 180 mg/dl before glucose is "spilled" into the urine (not reabsorbed). During pregnancy, glucosuria occurs when maternal glucose levels are lower than 160 mg/dl. Why glucose, as well as other nutrients such as amino acids, are wasted during pregnancy is not understood nor has the exact mechanism been discovered. Although glucosuria may be found in normal pregnancies (indeed $1+$ levels may be seen with increased anxiety states), the possibility of diabetes mellitus must be kept in mind (see Chapter 28).

Proteinuria. Albumin and globulin are proteins that are not normal constituents of urine at any time. Small (trace) amounts of protein may occasionally be found in very concentrated urine or in first-voided urine following sleep. However, a measurable amount (over 150 mg in 24 hours) of protein in the urine is a significant sign of renal disease at any time.

Integumentary system. Alterations in hormonal balance and mechanical stretching are responsible for several changes in the integumentary system during pregnancy. General changes include increases in skin thickness and subdermal fat, hyperpigmentation, hair and nail growth, accelerated sweat and sebaceous gland activity, and increased circulation and vasomotor activity. There is greater fragility of cutaneous elastic tissues, resulting in striae gravidarum, or stretch marks (Fig. 9.9). Cutaneous allergic responses are enhanced.

Pigmentation is caused by the anterior pituitary hormone melanotropin, which is increased during pregnancy. Facial melasma, also called **chloasma** or **mask of pregnancy,** is a blotchy, brownish hyperpigmentation of the skin over the malar prominences and the forehead, especially in dark-complexioned expectant women. Chloasma appears in 50% to 70% of pregnant women, beginning after the sixteenth week and increasing gradually to delivery. The sun intensifies this pigmentation in susceptible women. Chloasma caused by normal pregnancy usually fades after delivery. Darkening of the nipples, areolae, axillae, and vulva occurs at about the same time.

The **linea nigra** is a pigmented line extending from the symphysis pubis to the top of the fundus in the midline; this line is known as the linea alba before hormone-induced pigmentation. In primigravidas the extension of the linea nigra, beginning in the third month, keeps pace with the rising height of the fundus; in multigravidas the entire line often appears earlier than the third month.

Striae gravidarum, or stretch marks, which appear

Fig. 9.9
Pregnancy with twins at 8 months' gestation. Note striae gravidarum, linea nigra, prominent and deeply pigmented areolae and nipples, fluid retention. Diastasis of abdominal musculature was not noted. Umbilicus is prominent.

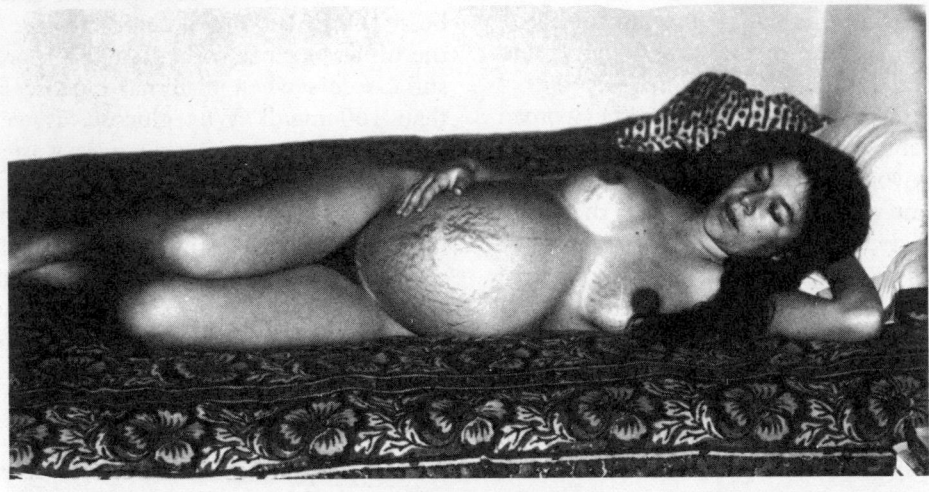

in 90% of gravidas during the second half of pregnancy, may be due to action of adrenocorticosteroids. Striae reflect separation within the underlying connective (collagen) tissue of the skin. These marks tend to occur over areas of maximal stretch (i.e., abdomen, thighs, and breasts). The stretching sometimes causes a sensation that resembles itching. Tendency to the development of striae may be familial. After delivery they usually fade, although they never disappear completely.

Commonly referred to as **vascular spiders,** telangiectasias are tiny, stellate or branched, slightly raised and pulsating end-arterioles. The spiders are usually found on the neck, thorax, face, and arms. They are also described as focal networks of dilated arterioles radiating about a central core. Vascular spiders appear during the second to the fifth month of pregnancy in 65% of white women and 10% of black women. The spiders usually disappear after delivery. Pinkish red, diffuse mottling or well-defined blotches are seen over the palmar surfaces of the hands in about 60% of white women and 35% of black women during pregnancy.

Epulis (gingival granuloma gravidarum) is a red, raised nodule on the gums that bleeds easily. This lesion may develop around the third month and usually continues to enlarge as pregnancy progresses. Treatment by excision is initiated only is it becomes excessive in size, causes pain, or bleeds excessively.

By the sixth week some women notice **thinning and softening of the fingernails and toenails.** Nail polish and nail polish remover may need to be discontinued and the nails kept short to prevent breakage. **Oily skin** and **acne** may occur during pregnancy. For other women the skin clears and looks radiant. **Hirsutism** is reported frequently. An increase in fine hair growth may occur. The fine hair tends to disappear after pregnancy. Growth of coarse or bristly hair does not usually disappear after pregnancy. Some women comment that their hair is thickest and most abundant during pregnancy.

Musculoskeletal system. The gradually changing body and increasing weight of the pregnant woman cause marked alterations in posture and walking. The great abdominal distention, decreased abdominal muscle tone, and increased weight bearing in late pregnancy require a realignment of the spinal curvatures. An increase in the normal lumbosacral curve develops, and a compensatory curvature in the cervicodorsal region (exaggerated anterior flexion of the head) is required to maintain balance. Large breasts and a stoop-shouldered stance will further accentuate the lumbar and dorsal curves. Locomotion is more difficult, and the waddling gait of the gravid woman, termed "the proud walk of pregnancy" by Shakespeare, is well known. The ligamentous and muscular structures of the mid and lower spine may be severely stressed. These and related changes often cause musculoskeletal discomfort.

The young, well-muscled woman may tolerate these

changes without complaint. However, older women or those with a back disorder or a faulty sense of balance may have a considerable amount of back pain during and just after pregnancy.

Slight relaxation and increased mobility of the pelvic joints are normal during pregnancy. This is secondary to exaggerated elasticity of connective and collagen tissue, the result of increased circulating steroid sex hormones and the hormone relaxin. These adaptions permit enlargement of pelvic dimensions. The degree of relaxation varies, but considerable separation of the symphysis pubis and the instability of the sacroiliac joints may cause pain and difficulty in walking. Obesity and multiple pregnancy tend to increase the pelvic disability.

Neurologic system. Little is known regarding specific alterations in function of the neurologic system during pregnancy, aside from hypothalamic-pituitary neurohormonal changes. Specific physiologic alterations resulting from pregnancy may cause the following neurologic or neuromuscular symptomatology:

1. Compression of pelvic nerves or vascular stasis caused by enlargement of the uterus may result in sensory changes in the legs.
2. Dorsolumbar lordosis may cause pain because of traction on nerves or compression of nerve roots.
3. Edema involving the peripheral nerves may result in *carpal tunnel syndrome*. The edema compresses the median nerve beneath the carpal ligament of the wrist. The syndrome is characterized by paresthesia (abnormal sensation such as burning or tingling because of a disorder of the sensory nervous system) and pain in the hand, radiating to the elbow. The dominant hand is usually affected most.
4. Acroesthesia (numbness and tingling of the hands) is caused by the stoop-shouldered stance assumed by some women during pregnancy. The condition is associated with traction on segments of the brachial plexus.
5. Tension headache is common when anxiety or uncertainty complicates gestation. Vision problems such as refractive errors, sinusitis, or migraine may also be responsible for headaches, however.
6. "Lightheadedness," faintness, and even syncope (fainting) are common during early pregnancy. Vasomotor instability, postural hypotension, or hypoglycemia may be responsible.
7. Hypocalcemia may cause neuromuscular problems such as muscle cramps or tetany.

Gastrointestinal system. The functioning of the gastrointestinal tract during pregnancy presents a curiously interesting picture. The appetite increases, and nausea and vomiting may occur. Motility is diminished, and intestinal secretion is reduced. Liver function is altered, and absorption of nutrients is enhanced.

Mouth. The gums are hyperemic, spongy, and swollen, and they tend to bleed easily because the rising level of estrogen causes selective increased vascularity and connective tissue proliferation (a nonspecific gingivitis). There is no increase in secretion of saliva. Women do complain of excessive salivation (ptyalism). This perceived increase is thought to be due to decrease in unconscious swallowing by the woman when nauseated. Epulis and bleeding gums are discussed under Integumentary System.

Teeth. The pregnant woman requires about 1.2 g of calcium and approximately the same amount of phosphorus every day during pregnancy. This is an increase of about 0.4 g of each of these elements over nonpregnant needs. With a well-balanced diet (see Chapter 12), these requirements are satisfied. Serious dietary deficiency, however, may deplete the mother's osseous stores of these elements but does not draw on calcium in her teeth. Demineralization of teeth does not occur during pregnancy. Hence the old adage "for every child a tooth" is untrue. Poor dental hygiene during pregnancy or anytime and gingivitis may contribute to dental caries, which could result in the loss of a tooth.

Esophagus, stomach, and intestine. Herniation of the upper portion of the stomach *(hiatal hernia)* occurs after the seventh or eighth month of pregnancy in about 15% to 20% of gravidas. This condition results from upward displacement of the stomach, which causes a widening of the hiatus of the diaphragm. It occurs more often in multiparas and older or obese women.

Increased estrogen production causes decreased secretion of hydrochloric acid. Therefore peptic ulcer formation or flare-up of existing peptic ulcers is uncommon during pregnancy.

Increased progesterone production causes decreased tone and motility of smooth muscles, so that there is esophageal regurgitation, decreased emptying time of the stomach, and reverse peristalsis. As a result the woman may experience "acid indigestion" or *heartburn* (pyrosis).

In response to increased needs during pregnancy, iron is absorbed more readily in the small intestine. In general, if the individual is deficient in iron, iron absorption is increased.

Increased progesterone (causing loss of muscle tone and decreased peristalsis) results in an increase in water absorption from the colon. **Constipation** may result. In addition, constipation is secondary to hypoperistalsis (sluggishness of the bowel), unusual food choice, lack of fluids, abdominal distention by the pregnant uterus, and displacement of intestines with some

Table 9.3
Hormonal Factors in Pregnancy

Hormone and Source	Principal Effects	Clinical Significance
Fetoplacental unit		
Estrogen: produced by ovary and adrenal cortex as in prepregnant state; however, principal source is placenta. Synthesized from precursors from fetal liver and adrenals. Increase in level of E_3 (estriol) by end of fourth week; by end of pregnancy, 300 × normal. However, low potency of E_3 means estrogenic activity only 30 × normal	Level of circulating estriol rises in pregnancy and so increases in urine and amniotic fluid	Urinary excretion of 30-40 mg/24 h of estriol by end of pregnancy—an indication of fetal well-being (must be repeated, i.e., serial): Significant decrease indicates fetus in jeopardy (or fetal death) Excessive increase may indicate multiple pregnancy, erythroblastosis fetalis

	Enlargement of uterus:
	   Hypertrophy of musculature
	   Proliferation of endometrium
	   Increase in blood supply
		Probable sign of pregnancy
		 Continued growth indicates pregnancy advancing

	Enlargement of breast Growth of glandular tissue ducts, alveoli, nipples Deposition of fat	Breast tenderness

	Enlargement of genitalia
	 Nutrient metabolism altered:
	   Increases elastic properties of connective tissue (relaxation of pubic joints and pelvic ligaments; cervix enlarges, softens, is stretchable [theory])
		Growth of vagina permits passage of infant
		 Softening of connective tissue:
		   Backache, tenderness over pubic area, flank pain
		   Cervical dilation

	Decreased secretion of HCl, pepsin	Digestive upsets, nausea, decreased absorption of fat
	Affects thyroid function: thyroxine production increases, but so does production of thyroxine-binding globulin	No major increase in free thyroxine (BMR rises primarily as result of increased oxygen consumption with growth of uterus, fetus, placenta)
	Interferes with folic acid metabolism Increase in total body proteins	Positive nitrogen balance: protein available for fetal growth
	Sodium and water retention by kidney tubules	Increased plasma volume and interstitial fluid volume →edema, fluid reserve

	Hematologic changes:
	   Hypercoagulability of blood
	   Decrease in fibrinolytic activity
	   Increase in sedimentation rate (SR)
		Safety mechanism vs. hemorrhage
		   Tendency for thrombosis to occur (legs)
		   Affects use in clinical diagnosis using SR tests (no diagnostic value)

	Vascular changes:
	   Telangiectasias (spider nevi)
	   Palmar erythema
		No clinical significance; changes usually disappear after pregnancy

	Stimulation of production of melanin-stimulating hormone	Hyperpigmentation (chloasma, linea nigra, areolar tissue, genitalia)
Progesterone: produced by corpus luteum (Fig. 9.10) for 2 months and by placental trophoblastic cells from about 8-10 days after conception; rises steadily through pregnancy	Promotes development of decidual (secretory) cells in endometrium Decreases contractility of gravid uterus	Glycogen deposits support nutrition of embryo Prevents uterine contractions from causing spontaneous abortion
	Promotes development of secretory portions of lobular-alveolar system	Prepares breasts for lactation

	Nutrient effects:
	   Favors maternal fat deposition
		Nutritional significance:
		   Energy available for maternal and fetal needs

	Reduced gastric motility, sphincters relaxed	Regurgitation (heartburn); small, frequent feedings tolerated
	Increases sodium excretion	Hyponatremia may develop

Table 9.3, cont'd
Hormonal Factors in Pregnancy

Hormone and Source	Principal Effects	Clinical Significance
	Increases sensitivity of respiratory center to CO_2	Respiratory rate increases; decreased alveolar and arterial P_{CO_2} (feeling of breathlessness)
	Reduces tone of smooth muscle	Colonic activity diminishes (constipation)
		Reduced tone of bladder and ureters (distention, urinary stasis, urinary tract infections)
		Vascular tone decreases (venous dilation; stasis in lower limbs with edema, varicosities)
		Decreased tone in gallbladder: reduced motility; incidence of gallbladder disease increases
	Raises body temperature 0.5° C	Feelings of warmth, perspiration increases
Human chorionic gonadotropin (HCG): produced by syncytiotrophoblast. Peak level by day 60-70 of gestation; levels fall after fourth month, disappear 2 weeks after pregnancy ends	Maintenance of corpus luteum in early pregnancy	Corpus luteum not necessary after first few weeks—placenta produces sufficient hormones
	Exerts interstitial-cell-stimulating effect on testes of male fetus	Testosterone levels in male fetus rise
	May have immunologic properties	May inhibit lymphocyte response to foreign protein, the fetal portion of placenta
	May cause allergic response	May be cause of hyperemesis gravidarum
		Diagnostic value:
		Persistence of HCG after spontaneous abortion symptomatic of hydatidiform mole or choriocarcinoma
		Basis for hormone test for pregnancy
		Decreased level in threatened abortion
		Increased level with multiple pregnancies
Human chorionic somatomammotropic hormone (HCS) (also called human placental lactogen [HPL] or chorionic growth hormone [CGH]): produced by syncytiotrophoblast; detectable by week 5 or 6; rises steadily, disappears 2 weeks after delivery	Similar action to pituitary growth hormone: Glucose metabolism:	
	Decreases use of glucose for energy by maternal organism by increasing lipolysis to make fatty acids available for energy (carbohydrate sparer)	Glucose metabolism changes result in: Glucose available for fetal energy needs (only energy source for fetus)
	Glycogen deposition increased, cells saturated (inhibits glyconeogenesis), causing blood glucose levels to rise	Diabetogenic effect in mother (increased blood glucose levels stimulate β cells of islets of Langerhans to produce more insulin)—may "burn out," producing diabetes mellitus
	Carbohydrates and insulin required for hormone activity	Fetal pancreas produces insulin by week 12; maternal insulin does not cross placenta. Fetal pancreas may overproduce if continuous hyperglycemic stimulus is present. At birth infant becomes hypoglycemic and brain growth is endangered
	Protein metabolism: Increases protein synthesis	Protein metabolism: Protein available for fetal and maternal growth needs
	Decreases breakdown and utilization of protein for energy (mobilizes free fatty acids; if excessive, may cause ketosis)	
	Acts synergistically with hydrocortisone and insulin in development of alveoli of breast (lactogenic effect)	Preparation of breasts for lactation
	Amount secreted depends on size of placenta	Research to determine whether level of circulating HCS (HPL, CGH) an indicator of normal pregnancy

Continued.

Table 9.3, cont'd
Hormonal Factors in Pregnancy

Hormone and Source	Principal Effects	Clinical Significance
Origin: multiple organs		
Prostaglandins: widely distributed in human body, including seminal fluid, brain, nerves, most endocrine organs, endometrium, decidua, and amniotic fluid	Reproductive system: play a role in erection, ejaculation, ovulation, formation of corpus luteum, uterine motility, parturition, and milk ejection Cardiovascular system: play a role in platelet aggregation, blood pressure increase	Prostaglandins are used to induce labor in second-trimester abortions; may be used (research in progress) for induction of labor at term
Ovary		
Relaxin	Present in many mammalian species and is thought to: Prevent premature labor Promote relaxation of pelvic joints and cervical softening Stimulate growth of breasts	Same as principal effects
Pituitary		
Pituitary growth hormone: produced by anterior pituitary	Decreases markedly during pregnancy and rises slowly to prepregnancy level 6-8 weeks after delivery	May be reason why insulin requirements decrease after delivery (HCS ↓ with delivery of placenta)
Follicle-stimulating hormone (FSH): produced by anterior pituitary	Decreases markedly during pregnancy; remains low for 10-12 days after delivery Increases then to follicular-phase concentrations during third week after delivery	Ovulation ceases during pregnancy Ovulation recurs 6 weeks after delivery in 10%-15%, 12 weeks in 30% of nonlactating women (first menses usually follows anovulatory cycle)
Prolactin (PRL): produced by anterior pituitary	Lactation: stimulates production of fat, lactose, and casein by mammary glandular cells after placenta is delivered May play role in regulation of fluid exchange across fetal membranes, lung maturation, and pregnancy maintenance	Milk not produced prenatally despite high levels because high levels of estrogen have a local inhibitory effect on mammary gland
Melanocyte-stimulating hormone: produced by anterior pituitary	Causes darkening of integument and nevi: chloasma; linea nigra; darkening of nipples, areolae, and vulva	Pigmentation changes are objective, presumptive signs of pregnancy; usually fade after delivery
Beta-endorphins and encephalins: produced by middle lobe of pituitary	Display analgesic properties	Discomfort is lessened or made more tolerable
Oxytocin: produced by *posterior* pituitary	Causes uterus to contract Action suppressed by action of progesterone until production of oxytocin exceeds that of progesterone Stimulates myoepithelial cells in mammary glands to eject milk	May be used to induce or augment labor Spurt of oxytocin during expulsive phase of labor to ensure efficient muscle contraction during and immediately after birth Sensory receptors in nipple stimulate release of oxytocin via reflex arc. During lactation oxytocin stimulates myoepithelial cells in the mammary gland to eject milk
Thyroid gland		
Thyroxine: produced by thyroid gland with stimulation from anterior pituitary	Gland enlargement with 20% increase in function: BMR increased to 25% near term. BMR returns to nonpregnant level within 1 week after delivery; return to normal size, within 6 weeks	Woman may experience palpitations, tachycardia, emotional lability, heat intolerance, fatigability, and increased perspiration

compression. *Hemorrhoids* (varicose veins of the rectum and anus) may be everted or may bleed during straining at stool. Bowel habits and a characteristic type of stool are established early in life. Variations will be noted with concern and may be perceived as a disease process. A mild ileus (sluggishness, lack of movement) that follows delivery, as well as postdelivery fluid loss and perineal discomfort, contributes to continuing constipation.

Gallbladder and liver. Decreased emptying time of the gallbladder is typical. This feature, together with slight hypercholesterolemia from increased progesterone levels, may account for the frequent development of *gallstones* during pregnancy.

Hepatic function is difficult to appraise during gestation. However, only minor changes in liver function develop during pregnancy. Occasionally, intrahepatic cholestasis (retention and accumulation of bile in the liver, due to factors within the liver) in response to placental steroids, occurs late in pregnancy and may result in *pruritus gravidarum* (severe itching) with or without jaundice. Oatmeal baths and lotions help ease the itching. These distressing symptoms subside promptly after delivery.

Abdominal discomfort. Intraabdominal alterations that can cause discomfort include pelvic heaviness or pressure, round ligament tension, flatulence, distention and bowel cramping, and uterine contractions. In addition to displacement of intestines, pressure from the expanding uterus increases venous pressure in the pelvic organs. Although most abdominal discomfort is a consequence of normal maternal alterations, the physician is constantly alert to the possibility of disorders such as bowel obstruction or an inflammatory process.

Appendicitis (see p. 880) may be difficult to diagnose. The *appendix* is displaced upward and laterally, high and to the right, away from McBurney's point.

Endocrine system. Profound endocrine changes occur that are essential for pregnancy maintenance, normal fetal growth, and postpartal recovery. Each hormone, its source and principal effects, and clinical significance are described in Table 9.3.

Parathyroid gland. Pregnancy induces a slight secondary hyperparathyroidism, a reflection of increased requirements for calcium and vitamin D. When the needs for growth of the fetal skeleton are greatest (during the last half of pregnancy), plasma parathormone levels are elevated; that is, the peak level occurs between 15 and 35 weeks' gestation.

Pancreas. The fetus requires significant amounts of glucose for its growth and development. To meet its need for fuel, the fetus not only depletes the store of maternal glucose but also decreases the mother's ability to synthesize glucose by siphoning off her amino acids. Maternal blood glucose levels fall. Maternal insulin does *not* cross the placenta to the fetus. As a result, in early pregnancy, the pancreas decreases its production of insulin.

However, as pregnancy continues, the placenta grows and produces progressively larger amounts of hormones (i.e., HCS [HPL], estrogen, and progesterone) (Table 9.3). Cortisol production by the adrenals also increases. HCS, estrogen, progesterone, and cortisol collectively decrease the mother's ability to utilize insulin. Cortisol stimulates increased production of insulin but also increases the mother's peripheral resistance to insulin (i.e., the tissues cannot use the insulin). Insulinase is an enzyme produced by the placenta

Fig. 9.10
Changes in endometrium and corpus luteum if pregnancy occurs (in days).

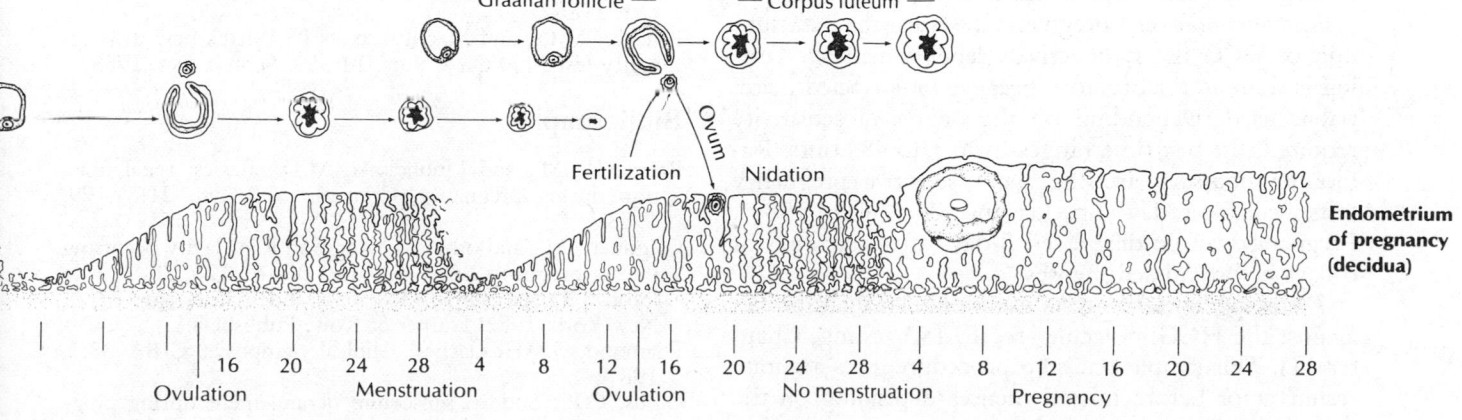

Graafian follicle

Corpus luteum

Fertilization   Ovum   Nidation

Endometrium of pregnancy (decidua)

| | 16 | 20 | 24 | 28 | 4 | 8 | 12 | 16 | 20 | 24 | 28 | 4 | 8 | 12 | 16 | 20 | 24 | 28 |

Ovulation   Menstruation   Ovulation   No menstruation   Pregnancy

to deactivate maternal insulin. Decreasing the mother's ability to utilize her own insulin is a protective mechanism that ensures an ample supply of glucose for the needs of the fetoplacental unit.

The result is an added demand for insulin by the gravida. The normal beta cells of the islets of Langerhans in the pancreas can meet the demand for insulin that continues to increase at a steady rate until term (for a discussion of gestational diabetes mellitus, see Chapter 28).

Pregnancy Tests

Early detection of pregnancy allows early initiation of care. Some tests will diagnose pregnancy as early as 8 days after ovulation or about 22 days since LMP. Other tests are accurate from 4 to 18 days after the missed menstrual period. All tests that are in current use detect levels of HCG. The wide variety of tests precludes discussion of each here; the nurse must read the manufacturer's directions for the test to be used. Several categories of tests are described here.

Latex agglutination inhibition (LAI) tests are easy to do and give results in 2 minutes. They are accurate from 4 to 10 days following missed menses. The first morning urine specimen gives the best results.

Hemagglutination inhibition (HAI) tests are more sensitive than LAI tests but require 1 to 2 hours to obtain results. Except for one test, Neocept, all are accurate about 4 days following missed menses. EPT is an HAI home test. Neocept gives accurate results at or before missed menses. A ring noted at the bottom of the test tube is positve for pregnancy. The first morning specimen is used.

The *radioreceptor assay* is one of the newest categories of pregnancy tests. This 1-hour test requires fairly sophisticated equipment. Radioreceptor assays are usually accurate at time of missed menses (14 days after conception) (Brucker and MacMullen, 1985).

Radioimmunoassay pregnancy tests for the beta subunit of HCG use radioactively labeled markers. Testing is done in a laboratory because radiolabeled material is used. Depending on the degree of sensitivity required, the test time ranges from 1 to 48 hours. Radioimmunoassays are the most sensitive pregnancy tests available today (Brucker and MacMullen, 1985). Pregnancy can be diagnosed 8 days after ovulation or 6 days before missed menses.

Direct agglutination tests use monoclonal antibodies against the HCG molecule (see ELISA testing, Chapter 11). This simple one-step procedure gives accurate results at or before missed menses depending on the test used.

Enzyme immunoassays use complex monoclonal anti-HCG with enzymes.* A visible color change makes the results easy to read. This new test holds promise for the future. Confidot is an immunoenzymatic assay home pregnancy test. The manufacturers of Confidot claim that this self-administered test confirms pregnancy approximately 10 days after fertilization, about 4 days before missed menses.

Interpretation of the results of pregnancy tests requires some judgment. The type of pregnancy test and its degree of sensitivity are interpreted in conjunction with the woman's history. The woman's history includes the date of the last normal menstrual period (LNMP), usual cycle length, and results of previous pregnancy tests. It is important to know if she is a substance abuser. Interactions with other drugs can give false results. Improper collection of the specimen, hormone-producing tumors, and laboratory errors may be responsible for false reports. Where there is any question, serial testing may be the answer (Batzer, 1985). Speed and convenience need to be weighed against accuracy and specificity.

Summary

Adaptation to pregnancy involves all of a woman's body systems. The mother's physical response is assessed in relation to normal expected alterations. Subjective symptoms and objective signs arising from these changes serve as a basis for diagnosis of pregnancy and plan of care during the prenatal period.

---

*Read package inserts for a description of "monoclonal anti-HCG with enzymes."

References

Batzer, F.R.: Guidelines for choosing a pregnancy test, Contemp. OB/Gyn. 26(special issue: technology 1986):37, Oct. 1985.

Brucker, M.C., and MacMullen, N.J.: What's new in pregnancy tests, J.O.G.N. Nurs. 14:353, Sept. 1-Oct. 1985.

Bibliography

Barron, W.M., and Lindheimer, M.D.: Basics: renal function during pregnancy, Contemp. OB/Gyn. 21(5):179, 1983.

Calguneri, M., and others: Changes in joint laxity occurring during pregnancy, Ann. Rheum. Dis. 41:126, 1982.

Danforth, D.N., editor: Obstetrics and gynecology, ed. 4, New York, 1982, Harper & Row, Publishers.

Diamond, S.: Headaches, Clinical Symposia, CIBA 33:2, 1981.

Gibbs, C.E.: Sudden sensorium derangement during pregnancy, Contemp. OB/Gyn. 20:39, 1982.

Goodlin, R.C., and others: Clinical signs of normal plasma volume expansion during pregnancy, Am. J. Obstet. Gynecol. 145:1001, 1983.

Guyton, A.C.: Textbook of medical physiology, ed. 5, Philadelphia, 1976, W.B. Saunders Co.

Hussa, R.O., Rinek, M.L., and Schweitzer, P.G.: Discordant human chorionic gonadotropin and subunit measurements, Obstet. Gynecol. 60:1, 1982.

Malasanos, L., and others: Health assessment, ed. 3, St. Louis, 1985, The C.V. Mosby Co.

Miller, B.K.: How to spot . . . and treat . . . carpal tunnel syndrome . . . early, Nursing '80 10:50, 1980.

National Foundation—March of Dimes: Maternal assessment: urine evaluation, series 2, Prenatal care, module 2, part A, White Plains, New York, 1979.

Ozanne, P., and others: Erythrocyte aggregation during normal pregnancy, Am. J. Obstet. Gynecol. 146:576, 1983.

Patterson, J.A.: Lab tests to establish prenatal profile, Contemp. Obstet. Gynecol. 18:29, 1981 (special issue).

Pritchard, J.A., MacDonald, P.C., and Gant, N.F.: Williams obstetrics, ed. 17, Norwalk, Conn., 1985, Appleton-Century-Crofts.

Resnik, R.: What controls uterine blood flow? Contemp. OB/Gyn. 19:111, 1982.

Rosen, T., and Mills, J.: Tattletale lesions: could this be a "stretchmark"? RN 46(2):49, 1983.

Stauffer, R.A., and others: Gallbladder disease in pregnancy, Am. J. Obstet. Gynecol. 144:661, 1982.

Urban, D.J., and others: Nurse specialization in reproductive endocrinology, J.O.G.N. Nurs. 11(3):167, 1982.

van Geelen, J.M.: The urethral pressure profile in pregnancy and after delivery in healthy nulliparous women. Am. J. Obstet. Gynecol. 144:636, 1982.

Walls, J.L.: Diagnosis and treatment of meralgia paresthetica, Nurse Pract. 9:43, 1984.

Walters, C.A., and others: Human myometrium: a new potential source of prolactin, Am. J. Obstet. Gynecol. 147:639, 1983.

Willson, J.R., Carrington, E.R., and Ledger, W.J.: Obstetrics and gynecology, ed. 7, St. Louis, 1983, The C.V. Mosby Co.

CHAPTER 10

Family Adaptation to Pregnancy

Pregnancy involves all family members. "Conception is the beginning, not only of a growing fetus but also of the family in a new form with an additional member and with changed relationships" (Grossman, 1980). Family members react to pregnancy and interpret its meaning in light of their own needs as well as the needs of the others affected. The process of family adaptation to pregnancy takes place within a cultural environment. "Culture provides the medium through which life experiences are interpreted" (Glass, 1983; Stainton, 1985b).

The role of women has changed in Western societies since women have moved out of the home and participated actively in the economic, social, and political life of their communities. Being successful in life's undertakings is a dominant theme in Western societies. To be successful includes the concepts of maintaining control, being self-reliant, and possessing power (Scott-Palmer and Skevington, 1981; Lederman, 1984; Stainton, 1985b). Maintaining control is applicable in all facets of an individual's life—whether they be emotional, physical, or environmental. Being self-reliant means being capable of making choices, assuming responsibility for one's actions, and showing initiative in solving problems. Possessing power means being able to manipulate the environment to ensure the safety, protection, and support of oneself and significant others. Stainton (1985b) found that parents' interpretation of a successful human being "was one who was self-reliant, social, independent and who could exercise power and control in achieving goals."

The role of mother, while still possessing the qualities of warmth, loving attention, and closeness, now reflects the cultural emphasis on success. Stainton (1985b) found that for mothers representative of upwardly mobile women in a Western society pregnancy was "a project of excellence, the product of which was a perfectly formed and healthy newborn." The changing role of mother has resulted in a corresponding role change for many men. The role of father now includes

more direct participation in preparation for birth, in the birth process, and in caring for the child.

With pregnancy both mother and father are confronted with new tasks. They need to prepare a nurturing and safe environment for the unborn as well as newly born child. During pregnancy, identities change and the possibilities and responsibilities of new roles are explored. The parents assume the major responsibility of integrating the child into an already established family system. In addition, the process of negotiating new roles (parent roles, sibling roles, grandparent roles) for family members will be undertaken by the mother and father. In this chapter the processes of maternal, paternal, sibling, and grandparent adaptation to a pregnancy are reviewed.

Maternal Adaptation

Pregnant women, a varied population, ranging from teenagers to women in their forties, use the 9 months of pregnancy to adapt to the maternal role. The maternal role is a complex, social and cognitive process that is not intuitive but is learned (Rubin, 1967a). In becoming a mother the teenager shifts from being mothered to mothering. The adult moves from "well-established routines to the unpredictable context created by an infant" (Mercer, 1981). Pregnancy for the primigravida is the "period of transition between two lifestyles—two states of being: the woman without child and the woman with child" (Lederman, 1984). For the multigravida the transition is from woman with child to woman with children.

Pregnancy can be described as a developmental change as modifications take place in the woman's self and body in preparation for a new level of caring and responsibility. The dynamic interaction between intrapsychic and biologic processes functions to change the women's self-concept in readiness for parenthood. The woman is involved in a reassessment of her "self-

224

image, beliefs, values, priorities, behavior patterns, relationships with others and problem-solving skills" (Lederman, 1984). As a result of adapting to the maternal role the mother moves from being self-contained and independent to being committed to a life-long concern for another human being. There appears to be a gradual unfolding characterized by a "progressive emphasis in the mother's way of thinking away from the single self and toward the mother-baby unit" (Lederman, 1984). Most women are successful in adapting during the period of pregnancy. They experience stress but not necessarily intense conflict (Grossman, Eichler, and Winickoff, 1980; Leifer, 1980; Wolkind and Zajicek, 1981).

To accomplish the changes in herself the mother undertakes certain developmental tasks. These have been described as accepting the pregnancy, identifying with the role of mother, reordering the relationships between mother and daughter and between husband and wife, establishing a relationship with the unborn child, and preparing for the birth experience (Deutch, 1945; Caplan, 1959; Rubin, 1967a, b; Lederman, 1984; Stainton, 1985b). The mental process accompanying the developmental tasks continue throughout pregnancy. In normal circumstances the mental processes are progressive toward a period of readiness, just before term, in which birth seems to be an essential prerequisite to further development of feelings toward the child. Studies of the interpersonal context of pregnancy have shown a relationship between the accomplishment of these developmental tasks and the extent to which the pregnant woman perceives her social relationships to be supportive of the pregnancy and of her (Ballou, 1978; Entwistle and Doering, 1981; Leifer, 1980; Mercer, 1982).

Acceptance of pregnancy. An initial step in adapting to the maternal role is acceptance of the idea of pregnancy and assimilation of the pregnant state into the woman's way of life (Lederman, 1984). The degree of acceptance is reflected in the woman's readiness for pregnancy and her emotional responses. Her emotional responses include her predominating mood, openness in dealing with others, responses to the discomforts of pregnancy and changes in body image, and ambivalence.

Readiness for pregnancy. For many women the availability of birth control measures permits a pregnancy to be viewed as a joint commitment between responsible partners. Planning for conception is done with consideration for other children, if present, financial stability, and for some, the effect on the woman's career. Planning reflects the cultural emphasis on control as a factor in achieving a pregnancy with the best possible outcome. However, even with a planned pregnancy concerns about changes in life-style can occur. Researchers have found that planning a pregnancy does not necessarily relate to the woman's acceptance of pregnancy (Entwistle and Doering, 1981). For other women pregnancy occurs as a natural outcome of the marital relationship and may or may not be desired, depending on circumstances. For the adolescent, pregnancy can result from sexual experimentation and nonuse of contraception.

The early symptoms of pregnancy can be used to confirm the idea of pregnancy or dismiss it if denial seems necessary, even before the medical diagnosis of pregnancy has been made. Examples of conversational cues to acceptance or denial are given in Table 10.1. Women prepared to accept a pregnancy are prompted by early symptoms to seek medical validation of the pregnancy. Women who have strong feelings of "not me," "not now," and "not sure" may postpone seeking

Table 10.1
Conversational Cues Regarding Possible Pregnancy

Symptom	Acceptance	Denial
Amenorrhea	"I'll wait one more time; the doctor will think I'm crazy if I go in right away."	"This has happened before. My periods are always irregular. When I went away to college I didn't menstruate for nearly a year."
Tingling and tenderness of breasts	"This is always the second symptom I have. Then I'm pretty sure I'm pregnant."	"My breasts always hurt just before I menstruate." "I am gaining weight. I need a new bra." "My breasts are finally developing. I thought they never would."
Nausea and vomiting	"I didn't think I'd be one who gets sick, but you never know."	"I must have the flu—that's what I'll say if old Smith (teacher) says anything. I've had to go out of the room three mornings in a row."
Urinary frequency	"I have to go at the worst times, but now I don't care. I just say, 'Jane take over the class' and go."	"I'm so nervous all the time it makes me want to go to the bathroom constantly. It is so hard to explain to your teacher."
Feeling of fatigue	"When I'm first pregnant I could just sleep all the time."	"Mother asks how come I'm so tired. She doesn't know how hard I work at tennis."

supervision and care (Rubin, 1970). Once pregnancy is confirmed, the first overt reactions to its biologic reality may be manifested. A woman's emotional response to the confirmation of her suspicions may range from great delight to shock, disbelief, and despair, as indicated in the following statements:

"I was just delighted when I heard I was really pregnant. I was so excited I could hardly wait to tell Ron—we talked and talked. I'm still way up there."

"I thought, it can't be; I'm too old! What will he say? We have just finished with the other kids—now to start all over. I can't face it—those 2 AM feedings, diapers, and those terrible 2-year-olds into everything. I feel guilty, but I hate the whole idea."

The reaction of many women to confirmation of their pregnancy is the "someday but not now" response:

There is a real pleasure in finding oneself functionally capable of becoming pregnant. There is pleasure in learning that others are pleased with the promise of having, and being given, a child. But these feelings exist independently of the question of time. Personally and privately she is not ready, not now. (Rubin, 1970)

Caplan (1959) also reports that the majority of his clients were dismayed initially at finding themselves pregnant. However, dismay gave way to an eventual acceptance of pregnancy that paralleled the growing acceptance of the reality of a child. He cautions against equating nonacceptance of the pregnancy with rejection of the child because he believes that women can separate the state of physical pregnancy from the idea of being a parent. Thus a woman may dislike being pregnant but feel love for the child to be born.

Emotional responses

Predominant mood. Women who are happy and pleased about their pregnancies often view pregnancy as biologic fulfillment and part of their life plan. They exhibit high self-esteem. They tend to be confident about outcomes for themselves, their babies, and other family members.

They tactfully asserted initiative in finding solutions to concerns and questions and persevered in defining and attaining goals for themselves. They were relatively self-confident, adjusting to the unexpected and unknown, accepting risk as a reality, and tolerating ambiguity in the future. Their self-confident and inquiring nature enabled them to recover from threat and insult quickly, demonstrating resiliency as opposed to depression. (Lederman, 1984)

Even though a general state of well-being predominates, an emotional lability expressed as rapid mood changes is commonly encountered in pregnant women.

1. *Mood changes.* Disconcerting to the mother-to-be and those around her are the rapid mood changes occasioned by an increased sensitivity to actions and words of persons who are significant to her. Increased irritability, explosions of tears and anger, and feelings of great joy and cheerfulness alternate, apparently with little or no provocation. According to one father-to-be:

"I sometimes think she is crazy—we're going somewhere she wants to go, out to dinner or a concert. She goes upstairs happy as a lark and in 2 minutes is down again in a regular temper, won't go, and shouts at me. I really feel bewildered by it all."

Many reasons, such as sexual concerns or fear of pain during delivery, have been postulated to explain this seemingly erratic behavior. It may be that the profound hormonal changes that are part of the maternal response to pregnancy are also responsible for mood changes, much as they are before menstruation or during menopause.

2. *Openness.* Openness about her feelings toward herself and others becomes a noticeable trait as pregnancy progresses (Caplan, 1959). The layer of reserve that society has hitherto imposed is lifted. The woman exhibits a willingness to talk about matters previously not discussed or discussed only within the family confines. She seems to believe that expression of her thoughts and ideas or description of her symptoms will be of interest to and welcomed by the listener. She appears to enter into a trusting relationship with the outsider she deems protective. This openness, coupled with a readiness for learning, makes working with pregnant women a delight and increases the likelihood of supportive care being therapeutically effective.

Response to discomfort. Not all women suffer from discomforts associated with pregnancy. When the child is wanted, the discomforts experienced tend to be considered as irritations, and the measures taken to relieve them are usually successful. The women derive pleasure from thinking about the unborn child, and this feeling of closeness to the child helps them to adjust to the discomfort.

"I have a terrible time when I'm pregnant; my legs are so swollen and painful and I feel so lumpy and unattractive, but when I am most down, I think of the baby and how much she will mean to us, and I get through another day."

In some instances the woman who frequently complains about physical discomforts may be asking for help with conflicts regarding the mothering role and its responsibilities. Further assessment of coping measures and tolerance is indicated (Lederman, 1984).

Response to body image. The concept we have of our

body (body image) evolves from the perceptions, feelings, and attitudes we have developed during our life. This mental picture has evolved from our earliest experiences. Children incorporate the perceptions and attitudes of parents, adolescents incorporate those of peer groups, and adults incorporate those of intimates. A girl who described herself as very tall noted, "Whenever we have visitors my mother would say, 'Stand up and let them see how tall you are.' Now whenever I feel self-conscious, I feel tall, tall like the Tower of Pisa." A young adult who is now thin remarked, "I see myself as very fat. I wonder if I can get through the doorway. When I was a teenager, I was called 'Fatso'; that image never leaves me."

Body image may be said to encompass two independent dimensions, one relating to an emotional response to the body and another to its physical appearance as it exists in space. The way a woman thinks about her body and her attitude toward pregnancy are related (Rubin, 1968; Lederman, 1984; Strang, 1985). The physiologic changes of pregnancy result in rapid and profound changes in body contour. The woman's and family's responses to this change become more noticeable as pregnancy advances. During the first trimester body shape changes little, but by the second trimester obvious bulging of the abdomen, thickening of the waist, and enlargement of the breasts proclaim the state of pregnancy. The woman develops a feeling of an overall increase in the size of her body and of occupying more space. This feeling intensifies as pregnancy advances (Jessner, 1970). There is a gradual loss of definite "body boundaries" that serve to separate the self from the nonself. These boundaries provide a feeling of safety: "I looked in the mirror and wondered if it were really me. I had a sudden feeling that I was ballooning outward, there was no end, and I did not know how to bring it together and be myself again." Fawcett (1978) describes this feeling as an awareness of the "perceived zone of separation between self and nonself."

These negative feelings may be countered by a "Mother Earth" feeling, one of being a protective shield for the fetus (Deutch, 1945; Colman, 1969; Rubin, 1970). For most women the feeling of liking or not liking their bodies in the pregnant state is temporary and does not cause significant changes in their perception of themselves.

Ambivalence during pregnancy. Ambivalence is defined as simultaneous conflicting feelings, such as love and hate toward a person, thing, or state of being. Ambivalence is a normal response experienced by persons preparing for a new role. Most women have some ambivalent feelings during pregnancy.

Even for women who are pleased to be pregnant,

feelings of hostility toward and a wishing away of the pregnancy or unborn child come and go. Such things as a husband's chance remark about the attractiveness of a slim, nonpregnant woman or hearing about a colleague's promotion when the decision to have a child means relinquishing a job can give rise to ambivalent feelings. Daily events such as body sensations, feelings of dependence, or realization of the responsibilities associated with child care can trigger such feelings.

1. *Body sensations.* Body sensations that come into conscious awareness for the first time can prove unsettling. The concept of pregnancy becomes a set of symptoms—tingling breasts, increased vaginal discharge, frequency and urgency of urination, nausea, vomiting, bizarre food desires, and shortness of breath—all of which under other circumstances would be interpreted as abnormal and in need of treatment. To those who have little knowledge of physiologic responses of the maternal organism to the growing fetus, such symptoms can be alarming as well as uncomfortable. These symptoms can give rise to concern about personal safety or regret about having become pregnant.

2. *Dependence versus independence.* For some women recognition of increasing dependency needs when independence has been attained may give rise to conflict. Independent implies individuation, an ability to stand on one's own. The state has gradually evolved by the process of "emerging from the womb into the arms, from the arms to lap, from lap to yard, to school, and finally to leaving home" (Colman and Colman, 1974). The woman's feelings of being a self-reliant person, someone in control of her own destiny, have become part of her expectations of herself. Pregnancy alters this state: the mother can never be alone. Her baby is always with her as part of her body consciousness. She needs nurturing and support from her husband through birth and child rearing. Adaptation to dependency requires many women to change their self-image as they move from independence to mutual dependency.

3. *Adult responsibilities.* Realization that pregnancy signals the end of girlhood and the beginning of womanhood and that it is accompanied by new tasks and responsibilities can come as a surprise to some people and can be a source of stress to many young women. More than any other happening, pregnancy functions as a rite of passage indicative of reaching maturity in a society that has no other obvious rituals. In many states the pregnant woman is legally an adult regardless of age. She may give personal consent for any type of care for herself or for her newborn. She is entitled to financial and other aid from a government source if needed and, if unwed, is considered the sole legal

guardian of her child. As such she retains the right to care for the child herself, place the child in a foster home, or give the child up for adoption.

Intense feelings of ambivalence that persist through the third trimester may indicate unresolved conflict with the motherhood role (Lederman, 1984). If the birth of a healthy child ensues, memories of these ambivalent feelings are dismissed. If a defective child is born, some women look back at the times of not wanting the child and feel intensely guilty. Even the most enlightened persons tend to give credence in times of stress to the "magical powers of thought." The woman's feelings of ambivalence are seen as instrumental in causing a defect in her child.

Identification with motherhood role. The process of identifying with the motherhood role precedes pregnancy. It begins early in each woman's life, with the memories she has of being mothered as a child. Other experiences also affect each woman's perception of the motherhood role. The emphasis within her social group of what constitutes the feminine role can make the woman lean more to motherhood or a career, to being married or single, to being independent rather than interdependent. Some women have used stepping-stone roles to begin understanding what being a mother entails. They may have played with dolls, baby-sat, or taken care of siblings.

For many women pregnancy and caring for children is regarded as one of the most important goals of their lives. These women have always wanted a baby, liked children, and looked forward to motherhood. They are highly motivated to become parents. Such motivation affects the acceptance of pregnancy and eventual prenatal and parental adaptation (Grossman, 1980; Lederman, 1984). Other women seem not to have considered in any detail what motherhood means to them. During the 9 months of pregnancy, conflicts need to be resolved so that these women can envision themselves as being concerned, loving parents. These conflicts might include not wanting the pregnancy or child or whether to maintain or relinquish a career.

Women use fantasizing and daydreaming to prepare themselves for motherhood. They think of themselves as mothers and what mothering qualities they would like to possess. Expression of desires to be warm, loving, and close to their child are common to expectant parents. They try to anticipate the changes in their lives the child will bring. They wonder how they will react to less freedom, noise, disorder, and caretaking activities. They question their ability to share the love for prior offspring with their unborn child. Rubin (1967a, b) documented that a significant way for women to "try on" and test the motherhood role is for them to take their own mothers or substitute mothers as role models. These persons serve as confidantes or support persons. More importantly the women's own mothers serve as a source of information and experience. Lederman (1984) notes that "the identification of a motherhood role and the renewal and deepening of the mother-daughter relationship are complimentary in pregnancy."

Mother-daughter relationship. The woman's relationship to her mother has proved significant in adapting to pregnancy and motherhood (Deutch, 1945; Caplan, 1959; Rubin, 1967a, b; Ballou, 1978; Leifer, 1980; Mercer, Hackleg, and Bostrom, 1982). Lederman (1984) noted the importance of four components in the gravida's relationship with her mother: the mother's availability, the mother's reactions to the daughter's pregnancy, and the mother's respect for her daughter's autonomy, and the willingness to reminisce.

The availability of the gravida's mother referred to both past and present. During childhood the availability of the mother was perceived as her being there, loving and supportive. Women with such mothers used them as role models for themselves. For other women in the study the mother was perceived as not being available. However, some of these mothers became available during the pregnancy; that is, they showed interest in the daughter and were emotionally supportive as one adult to another. "With the common bond of motherhood and mutual availability, subjects often described a closeness that appeared to facilitate the development and adaptation of both individuals" (Lederman, 1984).

The mother's reaction to the daughter's pregnancy signified her acceptance of the grandchild and of her daughter. If the mother is supportive, the daughter has an opportunity to discuss pregnancy and labor and her feelings of joy or ambivalence with a knowledgeable and accepting woman. Rubin (1975) noted that if the gravida's mother is not pleased with the pregnancy, the daughter begins to have doubts about her self-worth and the eventual acceptance of her child by others.

Mothers who were able to respect their daughters' autonomy prompted feelings of self-confidence in their daughters. These mothers were capable of accepting the daughters as adults, ones who would be self-reliant and in control. The coming child helped the grandmother-to-be move toward a grandmother role. Some grandmothers use the birth of their grandchildren as a second chance at mothering. Grandparents who had helped their children become independent were seen as being willing to help rather than interfere or dominate.

Reminiscing about the gravida's early childhood and sharing the grandmother-to-be's account of her childbirth experience helped the daughter anticipate labor and delivery and prepare for the event (Levy and McGee, 1975). Hearing about themselves as young children gave the gravidas feelings that their parents had loved and wanted them. As a result they drew closer to their parents. They began to feel that in spite of the errors they might make in their own mothering experiences they would continue to be loved by their children.

Wife-husband relationship. The father of her child is probably the most important of the pregnant woman's significant others (Richardson, 1983). There is increasing evidence that the woman who is nurtured by her male partner during pregnancy has fewer emotional and physical symptoms, fewer labor and childbirth complications, and an easier postpartum adjustment (Westbrook, 1978; Lederman, 1979; Grossman, Eichler, and Winickoff, 1980; May, 1982b). Women have expressed two major needs within the wife-husband relationship during pregnancy (Richardson, 1983). The first need relates to the wife's securing indications that she is loved and valued. "The woman repeatedly stressed the importance of feeling that her husband accepted and valued her in her changing roles as wife and mother-to-be. She carefully monitored his attitudes and feelings for indications of acceptance throughout pregnancy" (Richardson, 1983). The second expressed need was related to securing her husband's acceptance of the child. The ever-present reality of being pregnant and the increasing reality of the child impel the woman to prepare for the time when the child will be born. The necessity for feeling secure concerning the father's interest in the child results from the woman's role in assimilating the child into the family. Rubin (1975) states that "as the child-bearer, it devolves on the pregnant woman to ensure the necessary social and physical accommodation within the family and within the household for a new member."

The marital relationship is not a static one but evolves over time. The addition of a child changes forever the nature of the bond between wife and husband. Lederman (1984) reported that wives and husbands grew closer during pregnancy Pregnancy had a maturing affect on the wife-husband relationship as the partners merged into new roles and discovered new aspects of one another. The partners who trusted and supported each other were able to share mutual dependency needs. Women expressed a need for the fathers' active involvement in preparation for birth. To most women the husband was seen as a stabilizing influence, a good listener to expressions of doubts and fears, and a source of physical and emotional reassurance (Grossman, Eichler, and Winickoff, 1980). Most women were aware of the developmental needs of their husbands during pregnancy. They were sympathetic toward the husband's need for reassurance as to his importance to the wife. Wives recognized that the husbands could feel jealous of the closeness of the mother and unborn baby.

Sexuality is a concern for many couples during pregnancy (Zalar, 1976; Ellis, 1980; Swanson, 1980; Lederman, 1984). Sexual expression during pregnancy is affected by physical, emotional, and interactional factors. The couple's relationship is influenced by myths about sex during pregnancy, sexual dysfunction problems, and physical changes in the woman.

Myths about how the body functions and fantasies about the influence of the fetus as a third party in love-making are frequently expressed. Anomalies, mental retardation, and other injuries to the mother and fetus are often attributed to sexual relations at varying points during pregnancy. Many couples have fear that the woman's genitals will be drastically changed by the birth process. Embarrassment and hesitancy because of not wanting to appear foolish often prevent couples from expressing their concerns to the health professional.

Dyspareunia (painful intercourse), differing sexual drives, and impotence are the three major dysfunctional problems experienced by couples during pregnancy. Dyspareunia may be caused by pressure on the woman's abdomen and deep penile thrusting. In addition to pain during coitus, postcoital cramping and backache may occur. Severe breast tenderness has also been reported by multiparous women during the first trimester.

In addition to dyspareunia, differing sexual drives can create problems for expectant parents. The father-to-be may become frustrated by his partner's sporadic lack of interest in sex. The mother-to-be may have difficulty when her partner becomes confused by her libidinal fluctuations. Changes in the man's level of sexual interest may disturb the woman.

As pregnancy progresses, changes in body shape, body image, and levels of discomfort influence the man's and woman's desires for sexual expression. Whether the pregnant body is perceived as beautiful or repulsive has an impact on the couple's comfort and desire for sexual intimacy. During the first trimester the woman is frequently plagued by nausea, fatigue, and sleepiness. However, as she progresses into the second trimester, her combined sense of well-being and increased pelvic congestion profoundly increase her desire for sexual release. In the third trimester, fatigue, fetal demands, and physical bulkiness increase her physical discomfort and lower her libidinal interests.

The woman's expanding abdomen may become an object of ridicule and shame or a source of pride for the couple. A woman who resents losing her shape and wearing waistless maternity clothes may make derogatory comments about her abdomen. Frequently women such as this begin wearing maternity clothes before they actually need to. Men respond in a variety of ways to their wife's changing shape. Some say their wife is most beautiful when pregnant, whereas others make derisive comments about the pregnant contours and are repulsed by them. Both husband and wife need to feel free to discuss their sexual responses during pregnancy. Sensitivity and responsiveness to each other and a willingness to share concerns do much to strengthen their sexual relationship.

Communication between the couple is important during pregnancy. Since pregnancy is a developmental crisis, it is a time of emotional upheaval for both the man and the woman. Partners who do not understand the seemingly rapid physiologic and emotional changes of pregnancy can become confused by the other's behavior. Talking to each other about the changes they are experiencing is of primary importance. Increased communication can lead to the recognition of issues. With increased understanding of the other's point of view, couples are more able to define problems and offer the needed support. The marital bond is strengthened as a result.

Mother-child relationship. Incorporating an infant into an existing family system requires emotional attachment to the child. Researchers have found that attachment to the child begins during the prenatal period (Rubin, 1975; Leifer, 1977; Cranley, 1981a,b; Stainton, 1983, 1985b). Maternal commitment to the unborn child is based on a collegial mother-daughter relationship and a mutually supportive husband-wife relationship.

Development of the relationship. The mother-child relationship progresses through pregnancy as a developmental process (Shereshefsky and Yarrow, 1973; Rubin, 1975; Ballou, 1978; Leifer, 1980). First the mother has to incorporate the idea of a child into her body and self-image, then differentiate the child from herself, and finally, define the nature and characteristics of the child.

Early in pregnancy the mother's thoughts center around herself and the immediate reality of the pregnancy itself. Ballou (1978) found that at this time the child is viewed as "part of one's self." Lumley (1980a,b, 1982a) discovered that the majority of women think of their fetus as "unreal" during the early period of pregnancy. Evidently the pregnancy is experienced as "something happening to *me*."

During the second trimester the egocentric state of the first trimester is balanced by a growing awareness of the child as a separate being. The differentiation of the child from the woman's self permits the beginning of the mother-child relationship. Gilligan (1982) notes that "we experience relationship only insofar as we differentiate other from self."

By the fifth month most women have accomplished the task of identifying the unborn child as a separate person. The mother's sensing of her child as separate from herself encourages not only *caring* but also *responsibility*. With acceptance of the reality of the child (hearing the heartbeat and feeling the child move) and with a subsidence of early symptoms, the woman enters a quiet period. At this time she becomes more introspective, and the fantasy or dream child takes shape. Researchers have noted that women whose pregnancies were planned and who were pleased with their pregnant state felt attachment to the child earlier than other women (Leifer, 1980; Cranley, 1981a,b; Lumley, 1982b). Sometimes a pregnant woman holds her abdomen and gently rocks it as though rocking the child. Conversation reveals the intensity of this intimate mother-baby relationship as women talk freely about their children and their hopes and aspirations for the children's futures. Pet names may be given: "I called all my babies 'Herman' before they were born." Sexual preferences surface: "I just knew I was going to have a boy this time." Some women even begin to plan the child's career: "I saw her as a ballet dancer."

The child becomes precious to the woman, and the feeling that "I am going to have a baby" supersedes all else. The mother seems to withdraw from other relationships and to concentrate her interest on the unborn child. Husbands and other children seem to sense the withdrawal; sometimes husbands comment on feeling "left out," and children become more demanding in their efforts to redirect the mother's attention to themselves.

In the last months of pregnancy the quiet period is superseded by an active period. The active period is more oriented to reality on the part of the mother toward her parental role and toward her child. As discussed in Chapter 8 the unborn child is capable of response to sound, light, and tactile stimulation. Some parents interact a great deal with their child during pregnancy and perceive the child to respond to tactile, verbal, and other environmental stimuli in an individualized, personalized manner (Fig. 10.1). Although the mother is unique in that she alone experiences "the child within," both parents and siblings interact with the child during the later months of pregnancy.

Nature and characteristics of the child. Stainton (1985a) found in her study of 25 couples that al-

Fig. 10.1
Mother talks to her baby: "How are you in there? Are you coming with us to the doctor's?"

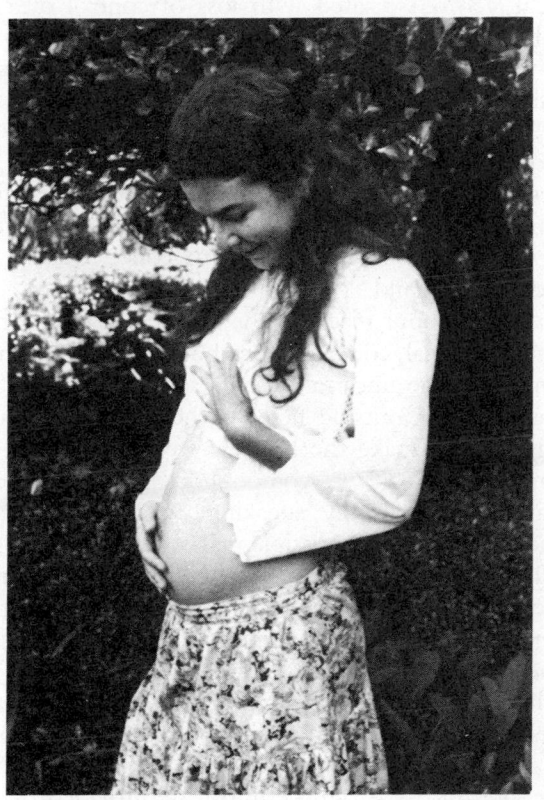

though a couple might disagree on the name or wanted sex of the coming child, they did agree on the nature and characteristics of the child. Sensitivity to the nature and characteristics of the unborn child was expressed in five categories: appearance, communication, gender, sleep-wake cycles, and temperament.

The description of *appearance* of the child included features such as color of hair, size and shape of eyes, and size of the infant. For races other than Caucasian, color of hair and eyes were taken for granted. Both fathers and mothers communicated verbally or nonverbally with the unborn infant. The mothers had more opportunity to talk to their infants when they were alone, either in the bathtub or while dressing. Most parents believe their child listened to them. They felt the child to be responsive to quiet talking, music, or massage by its "settling down." Conversely, the child responded to loud voices or music by moving or kicking excessively.

The *gender* of the child may be known by sono-

graph. If so, the child was usually named and referred to by name. If the sex was not known, the gender was ascribed because of the size of the baby or type of movement. "The movements are graceful and she is gentle" (Stainton, 1985a). Women more than men referred to their unborn infant as "it," but men and women preferred the more concrete reference of a nickname or "baby." Some fathers consistently used "she"; others most commonly used "he," often qualifying this with, "It is not that I want a boy. It's just that it doesn't seem right to say, 'it.' " A few fathers volunteered they used "he" as the nongendered, grammatical pronoun. These data raise the question whether males truly desire male children as often as generally believed or whether they are simply more comfortable using the male pronoun, which readily distinguishes the unborn child from the mother (Stainton, 1985a). Cultural conditioning may color the couple's preference for the sex of the firstborn and subsequent children. Women frequently defer to their husbands' stated preference. Men more than women work at finding an internal fit between the anticipated sex of the child and their own comfort with the imagined future relationship with that child.

The *sleep-wake cycles* of the child are described as three distinct states of alertness: "(1) sleeping, when the unborn child was still and unresponsive to noise, talking or touch; (2) a quiet but calm state in which the child gently rocked or rolled slightly, responding only to loud noises or rubbing on the abdomen; and (3) an upset or alert state in which the child responded readily to touch or noise by kicking, stretching, and until past 30 weeks gestation, rolling over" (Stainton, 1985a).

The temperament of the child was described variously as "calm, cooperative" or "having a temper just like mine." The differing movements of the child were interpreted as indicating pleasure, discomfort, or playfulness.

Concerns. Parental concern for the health of the child seems to vary during the course of pregnancy (Leifer, 1980). The first concern appears in the first trimester and relates to abortion. One woman expressed her feelings as follows: "I spotted [blood] off and on. The doctor said, 'If you are going to hold it, you will; if you abort it, it is probably just as well.' How could he say 'it'? He was talking about my baby." As the child becomes more of a reality, with movement and an audible heartbeat, parental anxiety is focused on possible defects in the mental or physical abilities of the child. Parents talk openly about these anxieties and press for confirmation that the child will be all right. Less identifiable in the later stages of pregnancy is fear about the death of the child; this possibility is evidently remote for parents. Death of the infant comes as a great shock; little or no anticipatory grieving has been done.

Both mothers and fathers expressed eagerness to meet their child. Bringing parental knowledge concerning the unborn child into conscious awareness may assist parents in preparing more realistically to care for their infant. Some parents reported their newborn's activity, responsiveness, and sleep-wake patterns at 2 months of age to be remarkably similar to their description of the unborn child's behavior at 8 months' gestation (Stainton, 1983). Other parents seem to ignore or be less aware of the unborn child's activity. They typically responded with surprise at the similarities in their unborn and newborn infant's characteristics. These expectant parents tended to be well read about pregnancy but demonstrated little knowledge of the social capabilities of the child. More importantly, they did not consider their personal knowledge of the infant acquired during pregnancy important and tended to rely heavily on the theoretical knowledge of others, particularly "experts" (Polanyi, 1958).

Anticipation of labor

Preparation for childbirth. Many women prepare actively for the birth process. They read books, view films, and attend parenting classes. Talking to other women (mothers, sisters, friends, strangers) is a traditional source of information for the gravida. At times the other women tend to recount problems they experienced with deliveries. Such descriptions can frighten primigravidas. The multigravida has her own history of labor and delivery that can either comfort her or make her fearful.

Anxieties. Anxiety can arise from concern about "a safe passage" for herself and her child during the birth process (Rubin, 1975). This may not be expressed overtly, but cues are given as the nurse listens to the plans women make for care of the new baby and other children in case "anything should happen." These feelings persist despite statistical evidence about the safe outcome of pregnancy for the mother. Many women express fear about the pain of delivery. They may fear mutilation because of their ignorance of their body structure and the birth process. Women express concern over what behaviors will be appropriate during the birth process and how the persons who will be caring for them will accept them and their actions. Lederman (1984) found women's fear of loss of control and concommitant loss of self-esteem in labor had physical and emotional dimensions. The women feared a physical loss of control over her body, that is, not being able to work with contractions, failing to relax

or breathe properly. Loss of control was also related to medical decisions regarding physical care made without the women's knowledge (Highley and Mercer, 1978). Associated with loss of control over the body was loss of emotional control. Women worried about crying or becoming hysterical or hostile to their husbands or the staff.

The women's reactions to possible loss of control in labor affected their plans for use of analgesics and anesthesia during labor. These responses varied from complete rejection or acceptance. The use of drugs during labor was also related to concern about the safety of the child.

Anxiety about reaching the hospital in time for the birth, practical concerns for the care of children at home, and the uncertainty of being able to plan specific dates for outside help or the partner's vacation combined to make the last few weeks a time of tension. The tension was compounded by a lack of adequate rest. Generally speaking everyone wishes to function in the best possible manner when confronted with a life event that has great personal implications. The ability to partcipate wholeheartedly in situations that result in growth, joy, and pleasure to the self and others and, conversely, to face pain, separation, disability, or death adequately come in part from the feelings one has about the ability to maintain control, in part from sharing these critical periods with those who care, and in part from the nurturing provided by others in the environment. The best preparation for labor was found to be "a healthy sense of the realistic—an awareness of work, pain, and risk balanced by a sense of excitement and expectation of the final reward" (Lederman, 1984).

Readiness for childbirth. Toward the end of the third trimester a recurrence of symptoms brings the physical nature of pregnancy back to the woman's focus of attention. Breathing is difficult, and movements of the fetus become vigorous enough to disturb the mother's sleep. Backaches, frequency and urgency of urination, constipation, and varicose veins can become troublesome. The bulkiness and consequent awkwardness of her body impede the woman's ability to care for other children, perform routine housekeeping duties, and assume a comfortable position for sleep and rest.

By the ninth lunar month the majority of women become impatient for labor to begin whether the birth is anticipated with joy, dread, or a mixture of both. They have a strong desire to come to the end of the state of pregnancy. "to be over and done with it." Women at this stage are ready to move on to the next stage of pregnancy: childbirth and assuming different aspects of the maternal role.

Paternal Adaptation

Expectant fathers, like the expectant mothers, have been preparing for parenthood throughout their lives. Subconsciously or consciously men give thought to having a wife and children. During courtship and early marriage a couple's discussion of future plans may even include the number, spacing, and names of their children-to-be.

The father's thoughts and feelings during pregnancy are similar to the mother's. His beliefs about the ideal mother and father and his cultural expectations of appropriate behavior during pregnancy will affect his response to his partner's need for him.

The response of the father to pregnancy varies as does the mother's. To one man the pregnant state of his partner may mean freedom to engage in nurturing behavior. To another, it represents a time of loneliness and alienation as the woman becomes physically and emotionally engrossed in the unborn child. He may seek comfort and understanding outside the home or become interested in a new hobby or involved with his work. This is often the time of the husband's first extramarital affair. Some men view pregnancy as a proof of their masculinity and as an outcome of their dominant role. To others, pregnancy as a result of intercourse with a woman has no meaning in terms of responsibility to either mother or child. However, for most women and men pregnancy functions as a time of preparation for the parental role, of fantasy, of great pleasure, and of intense learning.

How fathers adjust to the parental role is the subject of increasing contemporary research. In older societies the man is expected to subject himself to various behaviors and taboos associated with pregnancy and giving birth (Bobak, 1976; May, 1982b). These practices are known as *couvade* (French, "to hatch"). By enacting the couvade through definite patterns of socially prescribed behaviors, the man's new status is recognized and endorsed. In addition, his responses are channeled into acceptable modes of expression. His behavior acknowledges his psychosocial as well as biologic relationship to the mother and child. In Western societies, particularly those of the United States and Canada, participation of fathers in childbirth has risen dramatically over the last 15 years (May, 1982b). The father in the role of labor coach is now well established in United States and Canadian cultures.

The man's responses to becoming a father change during the course of pregnancy, as do those of the mother. Phases of the developmental pattern becomes apparent. Emotional responses, concerns, and informational needs span the entire experience but seem to be more obvious in one phase than another. May (1982c) describes three phases: the announcement phase, the moratorium phase, and the focusing phase.

The early period, the *announcement phase,* may last from a few hours to a few weeks. Men react to the confirmation of pregnancy with joy if the pregnancy is desired or dismay if the pregnancy is unplanned or unwanted. Realization of the reality of the pregnant state seems to come more slowly for the male partner. The woman experiences the early symptoms of pregnancy, but the man sees little physical change in his wife in the first trimester of pregnancy. On seeing a sonograph of his son at 12 weeks, one man remarked, "Until I saw his picture, it was all unreal. I knew intellectually my wife was pregnant, but it didn't mean anything to me. It was amazing—in a few minutes I became a father."

The second phase, the *moratorium phase,* is the period of adjusting to the reality of pregnancy. Men appear to put conscious thought of the pregnancy aside for a time. Fathers seem to become more introspective. They engage in many discussions about their relationships with different family members and friends and about their own philosophy of life, religion, childbearing, and child-rearing practices. Depending on the man's readiness for the pregnancy, this phase may be relatively short or persist until the last few months (May, 1982c).

The third phase, the *focusing phase,* begins in the last trimester and is characterized by the father's active involvement in both the pregnancy and his relationship with his child. In this phase the man concentrates on "his own experience of pregnancy, and in doing so he feels more in tune with his wife. He begins to redefine himself as a father and the world around him in terms of his future fatherhood" (May, 1982c).

Acceptance of pregnancy
Readiness for pregnancy. May (1982c) found in her study that fathers' readiness for pregnancy was reflected in three areas: "(1) a sense of relative financial security, (2) stability in the couple relationship, and (3) a sense of closure to the childless period in their relationship."

Many men express concern for the family's *economic security*. Today the majority of young married women as well as men are employed outside the home. Although pregnant women and mothers with young children may be employed in a work setting, many childbearing and child-rearing women have a phase of unemployment. Length of leave from employment is determined by a combination of factors, such as the couple's economic status, the policies of the employer, and the couple's value system. Some men attempt to compensate for anticipated needs by keeping their current jobs even though they had planned a change. They may put more effort into earning rapid promotions, by working overtime or by taking on extra work. The concern for providing financially may extend beyond the immediate future. Some men acquire new or additional insurance at this time (Bobak, 1976).

Those couples who have a *stable relationship* prior to pregnancy tend to draw closer as a result of their coming parental roles. Pregnancy and parenthood are not remedies for marital problems and conflicts. Those couples who were reasonably conflict free when pregnancy occurs appeared to have agreement on "value systems, areas of responsibility, sex roles, and child care" (Lederman, 1984).

For men their wives' pregnancies bring *to closure the childless period* in their lives. For many men pregnancy is a hoped for and welcome idea. They view having children and being a father as an integral part of their life plan. For some of them the desire to control the time when pregnancy occurs is as culturally relevant as it is to their wives. Couples who plan mutually for pregnancy are more accepting of pregnancy (Lederman, 1984). For some couples pregnancy is unplanned. If the husband had expected to remain childless, a pregnancy can mean alterations in life plans and life-styles. Some men find the change in expectations difficult to accept. They do not necessarily become reconciled to the pregnancy (May, 1982c).

Emotional responses. *Styles of involvement* in pregnancy vary among men. Style refers to the "general patterns of feelings and behaviors that reflect the way men see themselves in relation to pregnancy" (May, 1980). Men's reactions to pregnancy and their involvement in it depend to some extent on their basic personality structure. Their personality structure is reflected in the style in which they project themselves. Three styles characteristic of men studied during their wives' first-time pregnancy have been described by May (1980, 1982a): the observer style, the expressive style, and the instrumental style.

Observer style was defined as a detached approach to involvement in the pregnancy. The fathers in this category fell into two major groupings, those who wanted the pregnancy and those who did not. Those who were happy about the pregnancy were interested in being supportive of their wives and desirous of being good fathers. However, because of cultural values or feelings such as shyness they needed to distance themselves from such activities as prenatal classes, decisions about breast-feeding, or choosing professional care. They appeared to need an "emotional buffer zone." They recognized that by nature they were unemotional and matter-of-fact and that pregnancy had not changed them (May, 1982c).

The other group who were not happy about the pregnancy, reported feelings of ambivalence about pregnancy and the inevitable role of father (May, 1982c). These men believed they needed time to adjust to the idea of pregnancy and fatherhood. They responded to the feelings of ambivalence by becoming involved in careers and resisting their wives' attempt to involve them in preparations for the coming child. "Men established an emotional distance from the pregnancy in relation to the amount of ambivalence they experienced. Women often sensed this distance and attempted to involve their partners more closely. Often the man responded by withdrawing more" (May, 1982c).

Expressive style was defined as a strong emotional response to pregnancy and a desire to be a full partner in the project (Fig. 10.2). These husbands and wives were mutually responsive in their relationships. The husbands showed awareness of their wives' needs for support and were conscious of the times when they were not able to give the wives the support needed. They experienced the same emotional lability that characterizes pregnant women. They were excited and pleased about the baby but also worried about their ability to be a good father. These fathers may experience the discomforts usually associated with women in pregnancy, such as nausea, lassitude, and various aches and pains. *Mitleiden* (suffering along), or psychosomatic symptoms of expectant fathers, has long been

Fig. 10.2
Mother and father walk together. Women respond positively to their spouse's interest and concern. (Courtesy of Marjorie Pyle, RNC, Lifecircle, Costa Mesa, California.)

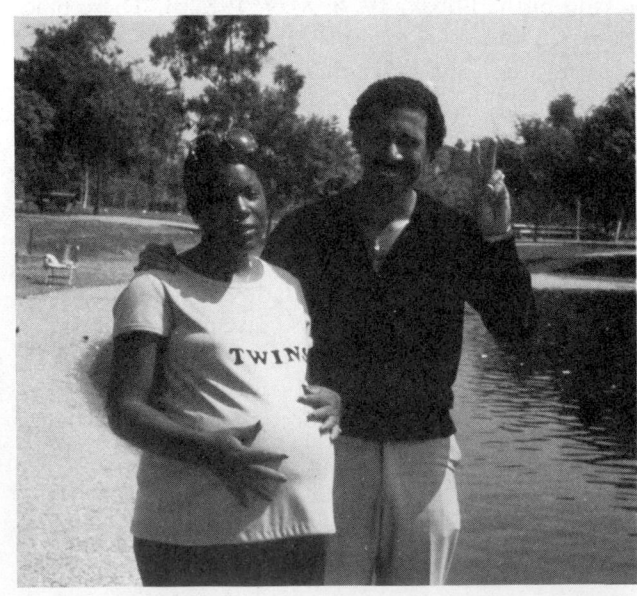

recognized a phenomenon of expectant fatherhood. In 1627 Bacon observed, "That loving and kinde Husbands, have a Sense of their Wives Breeding Childe, by some Accident in their owne Body." And another author in the 1600s commented, "It often falls out, that when the woman is in good health, the husband is sick, yea sometimes being many miles off" (Hunter and Macalpine, 1963). The husband alone may suffer these discomforts. The symptoms can be a positive force that brings the couple closer together and assists the father in becoming more responsive to his wife's and child's needs for love and care.

Instrumental styles were adopted by men who emphasized tasks to be accomplished and who saw themselves as "caretakers or managers of the pregnancy" (May, 1980). They asked questions, became interested in the role of labor coach, and planned for photographs during pregnancy, birth, and the neonatal period. They felt responsible for the outcome of pregnancy and were protective and supportive of their wives.

Description of the three styles of involvement emphasize the differences in the ways men can experience pregnancy. Each needs to feel free to define his role in pregnancy just as the woman does. Freedom to choose a role is particularly applicable in the man's preparation for labor. Not all men are able or willing to attend childbirth classes or act as labor coaches. This can arise from cultural conditioning or personal expression of supportive roles.

Identification with fatherhood role. Every father brings to pregnancy concepts developed over his lifetime that affect his response to his wife's pregnancy, just as her concepts do. Certain experiences have been found to be particularly important in modifying the manner in which the father adjusts to pregnancy and the parental role (Cronenwett and Kunst-Wilson, 1981; Kunst-Wilson and Cronenwett, 1981; Lederman, 1984).

The father's perceptions of the male and father role within his social group will guide his selection of the tasks and responsibilities he will assume. His memories of fathering by his own father and the experiences he has had with child care will affect his response. Some men are highly motivated to nurture and love a child. They may be highly excited and pleased about the anticipated role of father. If men have reasonable self-esteem and control of financial resources and working conditions, they seem more able to incorporate the fatherhood role into their life plans. Lederman (1984) notes that fatherhood identification is a crucial developmental step. "It can temporarily reactivate conflicts with his own parents, intensify feelings of separation, heighten dependency needs, and rekindle feelings of sibling rivalry. The husband who can look at these temporary regressions honestly is more likely to effect attachment and bonding with his newborn."

House (1981) delineated four type of support necessary for the man in the process of preparing for fatherhood:

1. *Emotional support.* During adult life the man's primary source of support is his spouse (Lein, 1979). This support has to be modified to permit nurturing of a third family member and to permit the additional nurturing his wife needs. Therefore the father needs to seek support from family and friends.
2. *Instrumental support.* The father needs to know on whom he can depend for help if necessary, for example, sisters, brothers, parents, or particular friends.
3. *Informational support.* The father needs to know who is available (e.g., professionals or relatives) to provide "tips" on how to solve immediate problems.
4. *Appraisal support.* The father needs to find others to provide comparison information, that is, criteria against which he can measure his performance.

The experience of pregnancy acts as a maturing factor in a man's life. Both husband and wife have to negotiate new role commitments with each other.

Husband-wife relationship. The marital relationship is a reciprocal one. Both partners are required to respect each other's need for support and limitations. Much of what is known about the effect of pregnancy on the husband-wife relationship has resulted from the wife's appraisal of her husband's response. Husbands' responses vary from close involvement with the wife to almost no contact (May, 1980). The responses reflect personal style and cultural concepts.

Ballou (1978) found the husband's role in pregnancy to be one of nurturance and responding to his wife's feelings of vulnerability in both her biologic state and in her relationship with her own mother. The husband's support during pregnancy is thought by his spouse to be an indicator of his involvement in the pregnancy and his preparation for attachment to their child (Caplan, 1959; Grossman, Eichman, and Winickoff, 1980; Leifer, 1980; Lederman, 1984).

In psychoanalytic literature some aspects of the father's behavior are identified as indicators of rivalry. Rivalry between the expectant father and his pregnant wife is not new. In Greek legend, Zeus, angered by his wife's superior wisdom after she conceived, swallowed her and later gave birth to Athena, who emerged full grown from his forehead. In the same instant he both punished and replaced his wife. Direct rivalry with the fetus may be evident, especially during sexual activity. Husbands may protest that fetal movements prevent sexual gratification, making comments such as, "We can't have sex with 'that' kicking around in there" (Bobak, 1976).

The wife's increased introspection may be a source of anxiety to her husband. He may experience a sense of uneasiness as she becomes preoccupied with thoughts of the child and of her mother, with her growing dependence on her male physician, and with her reevaluation of their relationship. He may sense that his wife's support—his key support—is being withdrawn.

Deciding on the infant's feeding method is of concern when the partners' preferences differ or when one partner has intense reactions. Recognized benefits and disadvantages of one method over another appear to be irrelevant. Some expectant mothers are startled by the husband's strong insistance on one method or the other. Some men insist that the wife breast-feed; others are adamantly set against breast-feeding. When the husband refuses to voice an opinion, the wife experiences uneasiness. Inwardly she accuses him of disinterest or feels uncertain about choosing the right way. The wife seems to ask for his support for whatever choice is made.

All these activities speak to the father's involvement and concerns in becoming a father to his own child. Throughout the pregnancy his memories of being fathered as a child emerge. These memories, coupled with his expectations of *himself,* help to define his role as father.

Paternal-child relationship. Research indicates that the father-child attachment can be as strong as the mother-child relationship (Greenberg and Morris, 1974; Jones, 1981; Cronenwett, 1982); fathers can be as competent as mothers in nurturing their infants (Parke and Sawin, 1976). Paternal behavior toward children does not differ significantly from maternal behavior (Field, 1978), with the exception of sociophysical play with their infants.

Men prepare for fatherhood in many of the same ways as women do for motherhood—reading, fantasizing, and daydreaming about the baby. They may adjust working commitments to include new responsibilities. Many fathers plan vacations to coincide with the births of the children, enabling them to spend time with their new families.

Daydreaming is a form of role playing. This form of anticipatory psychologic preparation for the infant is most common in the last weeks before delivery. Rarely do men confide their daydreams unless they are reassured that daydreams are normal and fairly common. Questions such as the following assist the nurse and the parent in identifying concerns and informational needs and allow for reality testing:

1. What do you expect the child to look and act like?
2. What do you think being a father will be like?

3. Have you thought about the baby's crying? Changing diapers? Burping the baby? Being awakened at night? Sharing your wife with the baby?

Occasionally just asking the questions suffices. The father may not wish to share his answers with the nurse at the moment but may need time to think them through or discuss them with his spouse.

If an expectant father can imagine only an older child and has difficulty visualizing or talking about the infant, this area needs to be explored. Information about his unborn child's ability to respond to light, sound, and touch and encouragement to feel and talk to the fetus can be given. Plans for seeing, holding, and examining his newly born child can be made.

As the birth day approaches, questions regarding fetal and newborn behaviors increase: "What do they do in there (in utero)?" "Is he hiccuping?" "Does he suck his thumb?" "How is he breathing?" "What does a newborn baby look like?" Some fathers express shock or amazement about the small size of clothes and furniture for the baby. Other fathers protest, "He'll only be real to me when I can hold him in my arms."

Some fathers become involved with the coming newborn by means of activities such as picking the child's name and anticipating the child's sex. As early as the first month the name of the child may be selected. Family tradition, religious mandate, and continuation of one's own name or names of relatives and friends are important in the selection process. The names chosen are tried on for fit; for example, the father might emphatically state, "I just can't picture myself as being a father to a boy named John." Some strive for originality in the name because "a common name just won't do." Armed with several names, one husband said he would decide on his final choice only after he saw the baby, pointing out that "to be named Eric, he *must* be blue eyed and blond."

At the time of birth most parents are able to accept the sex of the child born to them. Occasionally disappointment is evident and voiced. The parents may experience a grief reaction and a sense of loss at birth as they release the fantasized child and begin to accept the real child.

Anticipation of labor. The days and weeks immediately preceding the expected day of delivery are characterized by anticipation and anxiety. Many husbands (and couples) describe the dimension of time as heavy, slowed down, and distorted. Boredom and restlessness are common. Expectant fathers and their wives focus on the birth process.

During the last 2 months of pregnancy many expectant fathers experience a surge of energy to create and to achieve in the home and on the job. These behaviors could be interpreted as tangible evidence of sharing the wife's childbearing experience while channeling the anxiety or other feelings of the final weeks before birth. Furthermore, these behaviors earn recognition and compliments from friends, relatives, and the wife, and some may even coincide with the wife's nesting activities. Dissatisfaction with present living space increases. The need to alter the environment is acted on wherever possible.

The father's anxieties may be expressed by refusal to think about the coming event, by planning other activities during his wife's labor, or by sleeping and resting to the exclusion of all else. The expectant mother's reactions to the observed behaviors in her mate vary. A prevailing reaction is concern about the possibility of being deserted physically or emotionally when she is feeling most vulnerable.

A major concern of the father is his ability to get the mother to a medical facility in time for the birth. It is a convenient and acceptable focus for his fear and anxiety. Initially some fathers fantasize several ridiculously humorous situations and then move on to plan what they will do. Many rehearse the routes to the hospital, timing each route at different times of the day. Suitcase, car, and essential telephone numbers are readied.

In addition, many fathers want to be able to recognize labor and to determine when it is appropriate to leave for the hospital or call the physician or midwife. The concern here is twofold: getting to the hospital in time and not appearing ignorant.

Many fathers have questions about the labor suite's physical environment and staffing—furniture, nursing staff, location, and availability of physician and anesthesiologist. Other fathers' interests lie in knowing what is expected of them when their wives are in labor.

The father has fears of mutilation and death for his wife and child. While he harbors these fears within, he cannot listen or help his mate with her unspoken or overt apprehensions. Words such as "dropped," "rupture of bag of waters," "bloody show," "tears and stitches," and "labor pains" have violent overtones.

With the exception of parent education classes a father has few opportunities to learn to be involved, active, and needed partner in this rite of passage into parenthood. The unprepared, unsupported father may add to the mother's fears. Tensions and apprehensions are readily transmitted and may increase the mother's difficulties. His own self-doubts and fear of inadequacy may be realized if he is not supported. Self-confidence comes from achieving realistic goals and earning the approval of others.

Sibling Adaptation

The mother with other children faces additional demands when she becomes pregnant. She spends much time and energy reorganizing her relationships with existing children. There is a recognized need to prepare siblings for the birth of the anticipated child and to begin the process of role transition in the family. Parents attempt to include the children in the pregnancy. They are sympathetic to older children's protests against losing their places in the family hierarchy. No child willingly gives up a familiar position (Richardson, 1983).

The response of siblings to pregnancy varies with age and dependency needs. The 1-year-old infant seems largely unaware of the process. However, the 2-year-old child notices the change in mother's appearance and may comment, "Mommy's fat." The 2-year-old child's need for sameness in the environment makes the child aware of any change. Younger children exhibit more "clinging" behavior. Some revert to dependent behaviors in toilet training or eating.

By the third or fourth year of age children like to be told the story of their own beginning (Fig. 10.3) and accept its being compared to the present preg-

Fig. 10.3
Mother-to-be and her 5-year-old son look at his baby pictures.

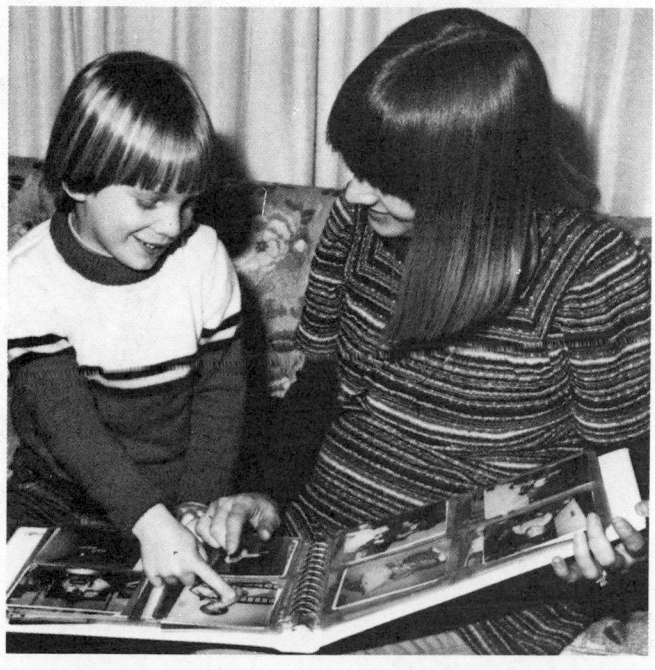

Fig. 10.4
Sharing prenatal care. **A,** Family visits doctor together during prenatal period. **B,** Father holds daughter so she can watch doctor listen to the baby's heart. Note how attentive she is. **C,** Father holds son so he can watch doctor listen to the baby's heart. Note he is reluctant to watch.

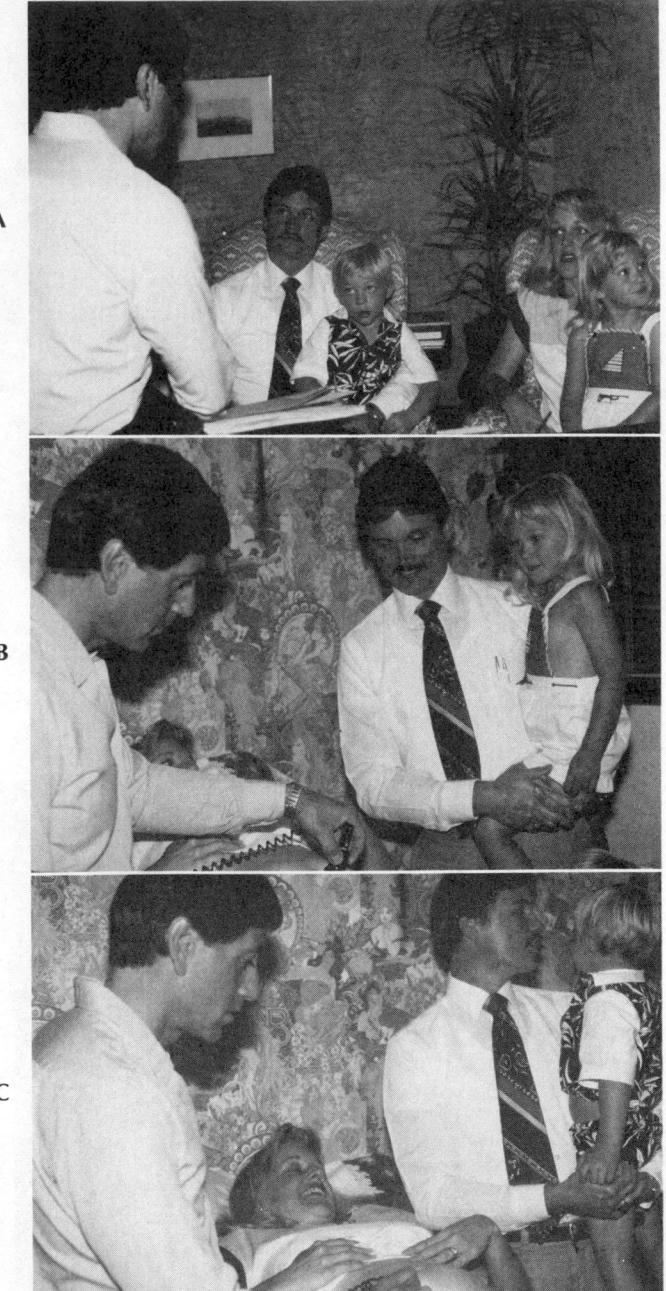

nancy. They like to listen to heartbeats and sometimes worry about how the baby is being fed and what is wears. Parents often take older children with them to antepartal visits, particularly in the last few weeks (Fig. 10.4). Children's responses to feeling the unborn baby moving in utero were often ones of delight. Other mothers reported the child's affectional reactions to the baby in utero. One mother reported, "Near the end [of the pregnancy] he began to kiss my belly. I was surprised by that" (Walz and Rich, 1983). Interference with established routines can cause anger. One 4-year-old boy resented not being able to fit on his mother's lap anymore and was not above shoving at his mother's abdomen; his father resolved the issue by making the child a small ski he could slide down his mother's bosom and over her abdomen ("over the hump"). He could still sit close by, touch her, and accept her abdomen as part of his life. Sharing possessions with the unborn child is often short lived. Mothers have noted that cribs or toys donated to the coming child are mostly reclaimed.

School-age children take a more clinical interest in their mother's pregnancy. They may want to know in more detail, "How did the baby get in there?" and "How will it get out?" Children in this age group notice pregnant women in stores, churches, and schools and sometimes seem shy if they need to approach a pregnant woman directly. On the whole they look forward to the new baby, see themselves as "mothers" or "fathers," and enjoy being included in the preparations of buying baby supplies and readying a place for the baby. Because they still think in concrete terms and base judgments on the here and now, they respond positively to their mother's current good health and do not seem to be anxious about a future injury to her or to the unborn child. They need help to cope with any adverse change in the physical or mental status of the parent or newborn, since they do not anticipate such a change.

For early and middle adolescents preoccupied with the establishment of their own sexual identity, the overwhelming evidence of the sexual activity of their parents may prove very difficult to accept. They reason that if they are "too young" for such activity, certainly their parents are "too old." All the uncertainties about the status of their parents and the appearance of their mothers are compounded by the pregnancy. They seem to take on a critical parental role and may ask, "What will people think?" or "How can you let yourself get so fat?" Many pregnant women with teenage children will confess that their teenagers are the most difficult factor in their current pregnancy.

On the positive side, just as the parents will someday catch a glimpse of the fine person their adolescent will become, so are parents-to-be suddenly confronted by a warm, sensitive person who is able to restore the mother's self-esteem, as illustrated by the following example:

"I came home one day feeling very pregnant, tired, and heavy and dreading the idea of making dinner and being helpful—you know—the mother bit! Mary [age 15 years] was cooking some hamburger, had the table set for dinner, and even had a flower centerpiece. For some reason I just started to cry. She came to me and hugged me and said, 'I think you're doing the loveliest thing in the world, having a baby.' I'll always remember that—she was really *my* mother for the moment."

Late adolescents do not appear to be unduly disturbed. They think that they soon will be gone from home. Parents usually report that offspring in this group are comforting and act more as other adults than as children. One mother delivering her tenth baby remarked, "The only complaint my oldest daughter made was, 'Mother, I'm getting married in August, so don't you dare be too pregnant to come to the wedding.'"

Grandparent Adaptation

Recent research indicates the importance of the grandparent-grandchild relationship. Grandparents act as a potential resource for families. Their support can strengthen family systems by widening the circle of support and nurturance (Barranti, 1985). The parent acts as negotiator in establishing the grandparent-grandchild relationship (Greene and Polivka, 1985). Many women report that their pregnancies bridged the final gap between them and their own mothers. The estrangement that began in adolescence disappeared as the now-pregnant daughter experienced joys, concerns, and anxieties similar to those her mother had felt before her.

Some grandparents-to-be do not welcome the new role for their daughters or sons. It may be seen as notice of their own aging process or as the victory of the exchild in obtaining an equal role with the parent. Some grandparents-to-be not only are nonsupportive but also use subtle means to decrease the self-esteem of the young parents-to-be. Mothers may talk about their terrible pregnancies; fathers may discuss the endless cost of rearing children; and mothers-in-law may describe the neglect of their son as the concern of others is directed toward the pregnant daughter-in-law.

However, most grandparents are delighted with the prospect of a new baby in the family. It reawakens their feelings of their own youth, the excitement of giving birth, and their delight in the behavior of the

parents-to-be when they were infants. They set up a memory store of first smiles, first words, and first steps, which can be used later for "claiming" the newborn as a member of the family. Satisfaction comes with the realization that continuity between past and present is guaranteed.

Summary

Pregnancy represents a developmental crisis in a person's and a family's lives. The concept of crisis implies events that necessitate change in outlook, role responsibilities, and everyday living. The ability to respond to changes with new behaviors and new self-concepts is fostered not only by intrinsic strengths but also by extrinsic strengths, such as the love and support of outsiders. Nurses can act as one source of extrinsic strength. The knowledge they possess of the responses of all family members to a pregnancy enables them to use their responses as the cornerstones of nursing-care plans. The long-term contact nurses have with clients and their families provides unique opportunities for informed supportive nursing that may have a long-term effect on family life.

References

Ballou, J.W.: The psychology of pregnancy, Lexington, Mass., 1978, D.C. Heath & Co.
Barranti, C.: The grandparent/grandchild relationship: family resource in an era of voluntary bonds, Fam. Relat. 34:3, July 1985.
Bobak, I.: Fathers. In Jensen, M.D., Benson, R.C., and Bobak, I.M.: Maternity care, the nurse and the family, St. Louis, 1976, The C.V. Mosby Co.
Caplan, G.: Concepts of mental health and consultation, Washington, D.C., 1959, U.S. Department of Health, Education, and Welfare.
Colman, A.D.: Psychological state during the first pregnancy, Am. J. Orthopsych. 39:778, 1969.
Colman, A.D., and Colman, L.L.: Pregnancy as an altered state of consciousness, Birth Fam. J. 1:7, 1974.
Cranley, M.S.: Development of a tool for the measurement of maternal attachment during pregnancy, Nurs. Res. 30:281, 1981a.
Cranley, M.S.: Roots of attachment: the relationship of parents with their unborn, Birth Defects 17(6):59, 1981b.
Cronenwett, L.R.: Father participation in child care: a critical review, Res. Nurs. Health 5:63, 1982.
Cronenwett, L.R., and Kunst-Wilson, W.: Stress, social support, and the transition of fatherhood, Nurs. Res. 30:196, 1981.
Deutch, H.: The psychology of women, vol. 2, New York, 1945, Bantam Books.
Ellis, D.: Sexual needs and concerns of expectant parents, J.O.G.N. Nurs. vol. 9 Sept.-Oct. 1980.
Entwistle, D.R., and Doering, S.G.: The first birth: a family turning point, Baltimore, 1981, Johns Hopkins University Press.

Fawcett, J.: Body image and the pregnant couple, M.C.N. 3:227, 1978.

Field, T.: The three Rs of infant-adult interactions: rhythms, repertoires, and responsivity, J. Pediatr. Psychol. 3:131, 1978.

Gilligan, C.: In a different voice: psychological theory and women's development, Cambridge, Mass., 1982, Harvard University Press.

Glass, J.: Prebirth attitudes and adjustment to parenthood: when preparing for the worst helps family relations, Fam. Relat. 32:377, 1983.

Greenberg, M., and Morris, N.: Engrossment: the newborn's impact upon the father, Am. J. Orthopsych. 44:520, 1974.

Greene, R., and Polivka, J.: The meaning of grandparent day cards: an analysis of the intergenerational network, Fam. Relat. 34:2, April 1985.

Grossman, F.K., Eichler, L.S., and Winickoff, S.A.: Pregnancy, birth, parenthood, San Francisco, 1980, Jossey-Bass, Inc., Publishers.

Highley, B.L., and Mercer, R.T.: Safeguarding the laboring woman's sense of control, Matern. Child Nurs. J. 3(1):39, 1978.

Hoffman, L.W.: Changes in family roles, socialization and sex differences, Am. J. Psychol. 32:644, 1977.

House, J.S.: Work, stress and social support, Reading, Mass., 1981, Addison-Wesley Publishing Co.

Hunter, R., and Macalpine, I., editors: Three hundred years of psychiatry: 1535-1860, London, 1963, Oxford University Press.

Jessner, L., and others: The development of parental attitudes during pregnancy. In Anthony, E.J., and Benedek, T., editors: Parenthood, Edinburgh, 1970, Churchill Livingstone.

Jones, C.: Father to infant attachment, effects of early contact and characteristics of the infant, Res. Nurs. Health 4:193, 1981.

Kunst-Wilson, W., and Cronenwett, L.: Nursing care for the emerging family: promoting paternal behavior, Res. Nurs. Health 4:201, 1981.

Lederman, R.: Psychosocial adaptation in pregnancy, Englewood Cliffs, N.J., 1984, Prentice-Hall.

Lederman, R., and others: Relationship of psychological factors in pregnancy to progress in labor, Nurs. Res. 28:2, 1979.

Leifer, M.: Psychological effects of motherhood: a study of first pregnancy, New York, 1980, Praeger Publishers.

Leifer, M.: Psychological changes accompanying pregnancy and motherhood, Genet. Psychol. Monogr. 95:57, 1977.

Lein, L.: Male participation in home life: impact of social supports and breadwinner responsibility on the allocation of tasks, Fam. Coord. 28:489, 1979.

Levy, J.M., and McGee, R.K.: Childbirth as a crisis. J. Personal. Soc. Psychol. 31:171, 1975.

Lumley, J.: The development of maternal-fetal bonding in first pregnancy. In Zichella, L., editor: Emotions and reproduction, New York, 1980a, Academic Press.

Lumley, J.: The image of the fetus in the first trimester, Birth Fam. J. 7:5, 1980b.

Lumley, J.: Attitudes to the fetus among primigravidas, Aust. Pediatr. J. 18:106, 1982a.

Lumley, J.: Maternal-fetal bonding. II. Implications for the next three months, unpublished manuscript, Melbourne, 1982b, Monash University.

May, K.A.: A typology of detachment and involvement styles adopted during pregnancy by first-time expectant fathers, Western J. Nurs. Res. 2:445, 1980.

May, K.A.: The father as observer, Matern. Child Nurs. J. 7:319, 1982a.

May, K.A.: Father participation in birth: fact and fiction, J. Calif. Perinat. Assoc. 2:41, fall 1982b.

May, K.A.: Three phases of father involvement in pregnancy, Nurs. Res. 31:337, 1982c.

Mercer, R.T.: A theoretical framework for studying factors that impact on the maternal role, Nurs. Res. 30:2, Mar.-Apr. 1981.

Mercer, R.T.: Patterns of maternal role attainment over the past year, Nurs. Res. 34:119, 1985.

Mercer, R.T., Hackley, K., and Bostrom A.: Factors having an impact on maternal role attainment in the first year of motherhood, San Francisco, 1982, University of California, San Francisco, Department of Family Health Care Nursing.

Parke, R.D., and Sawin, D.B.: The father's role in infancy: a reevaluation, Fam. Coord. 25:365, 1976.

Parke, R.D., and others: The father's role in the family system, Semin. Perinatol. 3(1):25, 1979.

Polanyi, M.: Personal knowledge: towards a post-critical philosophy, Chicago, 1958, University of Chicago Press.

Richardson, P.: Women's perceptions of change in relationships shared with children during pregnancy, Matern. Child Nurs. J. 12:2, summer 1983.

Rubin, R.: Attainment of the maternal role. I. Processes, Nurs. Res. 240:237, 1967a.

Rubin, R.: Attainment of the maternal role. II. Models and referents, Nurs. Res. 16:342, 1967b.

Rubin, R.: Body and image and self-esteem, Nurs. Outlook 16:20, June 1968.

Rubin, R.: Cognitive style in pregnancy, Am. J. Nurs. 70:502, 1970.

Rubin, R.: Maternal tasks in pregnancy, Matern. Child Nurs. J. vol. 4, spring 1975.

Scott-Palmer, J., and Skevington, S.M.: Pain during labor and menstruation: a study of locus of control, J. Psychosom. Res. 25(3), 1981.

Shereshefsky, P.M., and Yarrow, L.J., editors: Psychological aspects of a first pregnancy and early postnatal adaptation, New York, 1973, Raven Press.

Stainton, M.C.: A comparison of prenatal and postnatal perceptions of their babies by parents, paper presented to the First International Congress on Pre- and Peri-natal Psychology, Toronto, July 8, 1983.

Stainton, M.C.: The fetus: a growing member of the family, Fam. Relat. 34:321, 1985a.

Stainton, M.C.: Origins of attachment: culture and cue sensitivity, unpublished doctoral dissertation, University of California, San Francisco, 1985b.

Strang, V.: Body image, attitudes during pregnancy and the postpartum period, J.O.G.N. Nurs. 14:4, July-Aug. 1985.

Swanson, J.: The marital sexual relationship during pregnancy, J.O.G.N. Nurs. vol. 9, Sept.-Oct. 1980.

Walz, B., and Rich, O.: Maternal tasks of taking on a second child in the postpartum period, Matern. Child Nurs. J. 12:3, fall, 1983.

Westbrook, M.T.: The reactions of childbearing and early maternal experience of women with differing marital relationships, Br. J. Med. Psychol. 51:191, 1978.

Wolkind, S., and Zajicek, E.: Pregnancy: a psychological and social study, New York, 1981, Grune & Stratton.

Zalar, M.K.: Sexual counseling for pregnant couples, Matern. Child Nurs. J. 1(3):176, 1976.

Bibliography

Broom, B.: Consensus about the marital relationship during transition to parenthood, Nurs. Res. 33:223 July-Aug. 1984.

Cox, M.: Parent's approach to child rearing is becoming more goal oriented, Wall Street Journal 25, 39, Aug. 9, 1984a.

Cox, M.: Many professional women apply career lessons to job of childbirth, Wall Street Journal 25, 39, Aug. 17, 1984b.

Dubin, B.: Images of the body, Lecture at University of California, Feb. 15, 1985.

Edwards, M.: Communications: dimensions in childbirth education, Pacific Grove, Calif., 1973, M. Edwards.

Griffin, S.: Childbearing and the concept of culture, J.O.G.N. Nurs. 11:181, 1982.

Jordan, B.: Birth in four cultures, Montreal, 1983, Eden Press.

Josselyn, I.M.: Psychology of fatherliness, Smith College Studies Social Work 26:1, Feb. 1956.

Krugen, S., and Maetzold, L.D.: Practices of tradition for pregnancy, Matern. Child Nurs. J. 12:135-139, 1983.

Moore, D.: Prepared childbirth and marital satisfaction during the antepartum and postpartum periods, Nurs. Res. 32:73, Mar.-Apr. 1983.

Phillips, C.R., and Anzalone, J.T.: Fathering, participation in labor and birth, ed. 2, St. Louis, 1982, The C.V. Mosby Co.

Richardson, P.: Women's perceptions of their important dyadic relationships during pregnancy, Matern. Child Nurs. J., vol. 10, fall, 1981.

Rubin, R.: Maternal identity and maternal experience, New York, 1984, Springer Publishing Co.

Stainton, M.C.: Parent infant interactions: putting theory into nursing practice, Calgary, 1981, The University of Calgary.

Standley, K., et al.: Dimensions of prenatal anxiety and their influence on pregnancy outcome, Am. J. Obstet. Gynecol. 135:22, 1979.

Ulrich, S.C.: Psychosocial work of a secundigravida in relation to acceptance of her baby, Matern. Child Nurs. J., vol. 11, spring, 1981.

Weiss, S.J.: The language of touch, Nurs. Res. 28:76, 1979.

Young, I.M.: Pregnant embodiment: subjectivity and alienation, J. Med. Philos., 9:45, 1984.

CHAPTER

11

Nursing Care During Pregnancy

The prenatal period is a preparatory one both physically, in terms of fetal growth and maternal adaptations, and psychologically, in terms of anticipation of parenthood. Becoming a parent represents one of the maturational crises of our lives and as such can represent a time of growth in responsibility and concern for others. It is a time of intense learning for the parents and for those close to them as well as a time for development of family unity.

During a woman's life, pregnancy is unique because only then does the healthy woman seek ongoing health care. Regular prenatal visits, ideally beginning soon after the first missed period, offer opportunities to ensure the health of the expectant mother and her infant. This is done by supervising the course of normal pregnancy. Prenatal health supervision permits diagnosis and treatment of maternal disorders that may have preexisted or may develop during the pregnancy. It is designed to follow the growth and development of the fetus and to identify abnormalities that may interfere with the course of normal labor. The woman and her family can seek support for stress and learn parenting skills.

The professionals who have contact with the gravida and her family will include a cross section of health workers such as nurse, physician, nutritionist, and social worker. It is essential that these persons work as a team to provide holistic care for their clients. The initial visit of the woman to either the physician's office or an obstetric clinic is important in setting the tone for her care. The woman needs to feel welcomed and important. The initial visit may include diagnosing the pregnancy and establishing the data base, depending on the duration of gestation. If pregnancy is too early and cannot be verified, her next appointment is scheduled in 2 weeks. Misdiagnosis may lead to serious emotional and legal consequences; therefore caution is warranted.

The woman's desire for pregnancy is evaluated. If she is pregnant and does not wish to continue the pregnancy, she is referred for abortion counseling (see Chapter 7). If she is not pregnant and does not wish to be, she is referred for family planning, if appropriate (see Chapter 7).

If the woman is pregnant and plans to carry the pregnancy to term, prenatal care is instituted. The nursing care presented in this chapter follows the process of nursing: assessment, formulation of nursing diagnoses, planning, implementation, and evaluation. The descriptions of nursing care are followed by a summary of nursing actions and a case presentation that illustrates the application of nursing knowledge.

Assessment

The process of assessment continues throughout the prenatal period. It begins when a woman makes contact with health professionals because she suspects she is pregnant. Assessment techniques include the interview, the physical examination, and laboratory tests.

TECHNIQUES

Interview. The interview is planned, purposeful communication that focuses on specific content. The initial assessment interview may be the first contact between nurse and client. The interview establishes the therapeutic relationship (see Chapter 4). Two methods are usually used in collecting data: the client's subjective interpretation of health status and the nurse's more objective observations. The client also provides information regarding her reasons for seeking health care, her medical and reproductive history, and her present health care needs.

During the interview the nurse observes the client's

affect, posture, body language, skin color, and other physical and emotional signs. These observations become important data in the assessment.

Often the client will be accompanied by a family member or members. The nurse builds a relationship with these persons as part of the social context of the client. They also are helpful in recalling and validating information related to the client's health problem. With the client's permission, those accompanying her can be included in the initial interview. Wright and Leahey (1984) offer excellent guidance to the nurse in developing skills for interviewing families and assessing the interaction between family members. Observations and information about the client's family are part of the interview. For example, if the client is accompanied by small children, the nurse can inquire about her plans for child care during the forthcoming labor and delivery.

The interview provides information about the client's biopsychosocial status. Although the format for interviewing or recording the client's health history may differ, the information obtained is universal.

Reason for client's request for care. The client's description of the purpose for the request for care is quoted verbatim in the record. For example, "I think I am pregnant," or "My legs get so swollen I can hardly walk." This statement does not constitute a diagnosis, since the client's condition needs to be confirmed by the nurse or physician before any care is instituted. Recording the chief purpose of a visit in the client's own words alerts other personnel to the "priority of need" as seen by the client.

Health history. The present health status of the client is assessed through interview and observation. Any past, chronic, or current health problems are important considerations in planning for care.

The *family history* provides information about the client's immediate family, parents, siblings, spouse, or children. These data help to identify familial, genetic, or environmental disorders or conditions that could affect the present health status of the woman.

The *medical history* describes medical or surgical conditions that may affect the course of pregnancy or be affected by the pregnancy. For example, the pregnant woman who has diabetes or epilepsy will require special care. Because most clients are anxious during the initial interview, reference to cues such as a Medic Alert bracelet will assist the client to explain allergies, chronic diseases, or medications being used (e.g., cortisone, insulin, or anticonvulsants). Often clients who are well adapted to chronic or handicapping conditions forget to mention them because they are so well integrated into their life-style. Special shoes or a limp may indicate a pelvic structural defect, which is an im-

portant consideration in pregnancy. The nurse who observes these special characteristics and can sensitively inquire about them obtains individualized data that will provide the basis for a comprehensive nursing care plan. Observations are vital components of the interview process because they prompt the nurse and the client to focus on the specific needs of the client and her family.

The woman's *sexual and obstetric history* is reviewed. The interviewer will record such information as the woman's menstrual history, sexual activity, and previous pregnancies and their outcomes. The conduct of the *present pregnancy* is predicated on the reports of previous pregnancies.

Psychosocial history. The psychosocial history includes identifying information such as name and place of residence. The nurse elicits the woman's *perceptions* concerning this pregnancy and the expectations the woman and her family have for health care. *Situational factors* such as the family's ethnic and cultural background, socioeconomic status, and availability of health resources are determined. The *patterns of coping* and *interacting* used by the client and her family are noted.

Review of the woman's physical systems. The woman is questioned about physical symptoms she has experienced such as shortness of breath or pain. Pregnancy affects and is affected by all body systems; therefore knowledge of the present status of body systems is important in planning care. In addition to inquiring about health status, the interviewer gains useful information from the woman's physical examination.

Physical examination. The physical examination includes an assessment of all body systems as well as the reproductive system. The initial physical examination provides the baseline for assessing subsequent changes. For example, the pregnant woman's weight and blood pressure are assessed against normative data; but, in addition, the rate of her weight gain and rise or fall in her blood pressure are important notations. A rapid weight gain in excess of the norm for the gestation period may signal the possibility of a multiple pregnancy, developing edema, or both.

The examiner uses a formalized sequence in conducting a physical examination. a cephalocaudal or system-by-system approach will prevent omitting any key information. As the examination proceeds, the client can be questioned about pertinent health concerns or symptoms. The techniques used are observation, palpation, percussion, and auscultation. Each technique is described briefly.

Observation. The general inspection of the client begins with the first meeting and continues through the interview and physical examination. This provides an overall impression of the client's health status. The observations made are noted in the client's record. They include the following: apparent age; sex; race; body type (constitution), stature, and symmetry; weight and nutritional status; posture and motor activity; mental status; speech; general skin condition; apparent state of health; and signs of distress or disorder (Malasanos and others, 1985). These are factors that are not limited to a single system of the body but are instead parameters for the total or whole person—the general appearance from head to toe.

Specific observations are made concerning the various body parts. For example, the os of the cervix changes from a circular opening in the woman who had not delivered an infant to one that has a slitlike appearance in the woman who has delivered one or more infants.

Palpation. By applying light pressure with the fingers over a body surface, the examiner can determine the conditions of parts below the surface. By palpating the uterus the examiner can determine the part of the fetus that will deliver first.

Percussion. The size, density, and position of an internal organ can be determined by tapping a part of the body with short sharp blows of the finger. The sound that is made changes in pitch as the fingers

Table 11.1
Summary of Signs and Symptoms of Pregnancy*

Presumptive	Probable	Positive
Subjective symptoms	**Subjective symptoms**	**Subjective symptoms**
Amenorrhea	Same as presumptive symptoms; when combined with probable signs, strong suspicion of pregnancy	No symptoms positively diagnostic of pregnancy
Nausea, vomiting		
Breast sensitivity		
Urinary symptoms		
Lassitude/fatigue		
Constipation		
Weight gain		
Fingernail changes		
Quickening		
Objective signs	**Objective signs**	**Objective signs†**
Elevation of BBT	Uterine enlargement	FHT
Integumentary changes	Uterine contractions (Braxton Hicks' sign)	Electronic device (8-12 seeks)
Pigmentation		Electrocardiogram (12 weeks)
Chloasma		Auscultation (17-18 weeks)
Nipples, areolae	Ballottement	Palpation of fetal movement
Linea nigra	Uterine souffle	Roentgenographic evidence of fetal skeleton
Striae gravidarum	Laboratory tests (except radioimmunoassay of beta subunit of HCG)	Ultrasonographic (echographic) evidence of pregnancy
Telangiectases (spider nevi)		
Acne		
Hirsutism		
Epulis		
Breast changes		Laboratory tests
Enlargement		Immunologic (6 weeks)
Secondary areolae		Radioimmunoassay (beta subunit of HCG can diagnose pregnancy before missed period)
Montgomery's tubercles		
Colostrum		
Abdominal enlargement		Home pregnancy test (9 days after end of missed period)
Pelvic changes		Clinical test
Vagina (Chadwick's sign; leukorrhea)		Progesterone withdrawal
Cervix (softening; Goodell's sign; dried mucus in granular pattern)		
Uterus (softening; Ladin's sign, Hegar's sign, McDonald's sign, Braun von Fernwald's sign; enlargement)		
Relaxation of bony pelvic joints and ligaments		

*Clinical diagnosis of pregnancy depends on the ability to interpret presumptive, probable, and positive physical signs and symptoms.
†FHT, Fetal heart tones; *HCG*, human chorionic gonadotropin.

move from solid to less solid areas. The size and location of the woman's heart are checked in this way. The nurse uses this technique to assess fullness of the urinary bladder during labor.

Auscultation. Sounds produced within the body can be heard with the unaided ear or by using an instrument. The rate and regularity of the fetal heartbeat is used to monitor fetal health status.

Laboratory tests. The data obtained from laboratory examination of specimens add important information concerning the symptomatology of pregnancy and health status. Both nursing and medical diagnoses stem from such information.

FIRST PRENATAL VISIT

The first phase of prenatal care includes verifying the pregnancy and estimating the date of confinement (EDC). The process of data collection that will act as the basis for care is begun. The examiner responds to the woman's or couple's specific questions and concerns. No opportunity for health teaching is overlooked.

Diagnosis of pregnancy. The clinical diagnosis of pregnancy before the second missed period may be difficult in at least 25% to 30% of women. Physical variability, lack of relaxation, obesity, or tumors, for example, may confound even the experienced obstetrician. Accuracy is most important, however, because social, medical, or legal consequences of an inaccurate diagnosis, either positive or negative, may be extremely serious. A correct date for the last menstrual period (LMP), the date of intercourse, or the basal

body temperature (BBT) record may be of great value in the accurate diagnosis of pregnancy. Reexamination in 2 to 4 weeks may be required for verifying the diagnosis.

Great variability is possible in the subjective and objective symptoms of pregnancy. The diagnosis of pregnancy is classified as follows: presumptive, probable, and positive (Table 11.1). The student is referred to Chapter 9 for an in-depth discussion of the symptoms caused by maternal adaptations to pregnancy. Many of the signs and symptoms of pregnancy are clinically useful in the diagnosis of pregnancy. Table 11.2 presents the signs and symptoms of pregnancy in order of appearance. The presumptive signs and symptoms of pregnancy can be caused by conditions other than gestation. Therefore no one manifestation can be relied on for a final impression, nor are combinations of several manifestations diagnostic. Table 11.3 outlines the differential assessment of signs and symptoms of pregnancy.

The positive signs used to confirm the diagnosis of pregnancy include certain pregnancy tests (see Chapter 9). Enzyme-linked immunosorbent assay (ELISA) testing is currently the most popular testing procedure for pregnancy (Batzer, 1985). It uses a specific monoclonal antibody produced by hybrid cell-line technology. An enzyme rather than a radioactive compound identifies the antigen of the substance to be measured. The enzyme induces a simple color-change reaction. The endpoint of the test can be read with either the eye or a spectrometer.

ELISA testing has many advantages. The antigen enzyme conjugate and test reagents are stable, the

Table 11.2
Summary of Signs and Symptoms of Pregnancy in Order of Appearance

Signs and Symptoms	Approximate Week of Gestation	Signs and Symptoms	Approximate Week of Gestation
Amenorrhea	4	Palpable uterine enlargement—size of an orange	10
"Morning" sickness	4		
Bladder symptoms	6	Palpable uterine enlargement—size of a grapefruit; uterus becomes an abdominal organ	12
Cervical softening	6		
Breasts: increased vascularity and sensation of heaviness	6		
		Internal ballottement	14
Palpable uterine enlargement—size of a large hen's egg	7	Breast: clear fluid (precolostrum) can be expressed	16
Darkening of vaginal mucous membrane and cervix (Chadwick's sign)	8	Quickening ("feeling life")	16-20
Softening of lower uterine segment	8	Palpable uterine contractions (Braxton Hicks' sign)	20
Breast: primary areolae become more pigmented and Montgomery's tubercles also more prominent	8	Palpable fetal movements	20
		External ballottement	24
Ultrasound detection of FHT		Auscultation of fetal heart (fetal stethoscope)	17-18
Vulval varicosities appear	8-12		
	10		

Table 11.3
Differential Assessment of Signs and Symptoms of Pregnancy

Symptoms	Possible Causes of Diagnostic Error
Abdominal enlargement	Obesity, abdominal muscle relaxation, tumors, ascites, ventral abdominal hernia
Amenorrhea	Emotional factors: severe emotional shock, tension, fear of or strong desire for pregnancy
	Endocrine factors: adrenal or ovarian neoplasms, thryoid or pituitary disorders, lactation, menopause
	Metabolic factors: anemia, malnutrition, diabetes mellitus, degenerative disorders
	Systemic disease: acute or chronic infection (tuberculosis, brucellosis) or malignancy
	Local causes (cervical obstruction; jogging)
Braxton Hicks' contractions	Contractions of muscles of abdominal wall
Breast sensitivity (mastalgia; mastodynia)	Infectious processes: mastitis, cystic mastitis, premenstrual tension
	Pseudocyesis (false pregnancy)
	Estrogen excess associated with anovulatory periods or ovarian tumors
Cervical and uterine changes in shape, size, consistency	Tumors, adenomyosis, cervical stenosis with hematometra or pyometra, tubo-ovarian cysts
	Normal-size uterus displaced by a pelvic tumor (fibroid or myoma)
Clinical and laboratory findings	
Elevation of BBT	Poor thermometer, faulty use of thermometer, inaccurate recording
	Corpus luteum cyst
Pregnancy tests	Drug ingestion: progesterone
	False results, incorrect interpretation of results
	Elevation of human chorionic gonadotropin (HCG) levels for a few days after spontaneous abortion
	Elevation of HCG: hydatidiform mole, choriocarcinoma
Lassitude and fatigue	Psychologic: emotional disorders
	Pathologic: anemia, infection, malignant disease
Epulis	Infection, dental calculus, vitamin C deficiency
Hyperpigmentation of skin	Local causes (excessive sunlight, tanning)
	System diseases (Addison's disease)
	Use of oral contraceptives
Leukorrhea	Infections: vaginal, cervical
	Tumors
Nausea or vomiting	Emotional factors: anxiety, pseudocyesis, anorexia nervosa
	Gastrointestinal disorders: hiatal hernia, ulcers, enteritis, appendicitis
	Systemic disease: acute infection—influenza, encephalitis
	Allergies
Nipple discharge (milk-like)	Drug ingestion: oral contraceptives, psychotropic drugs
	Tumors
	Syndromes (also associated with amenorrhea): hypothalamic or anterior pituitary disorders
Pseudocyesis	Emotional factors
	Pituitary tumor
Quickening	Peristalsis; "gas"
Souffle	Heard over vascular tumors or aneurysms or in thin women; may be abdominal aortic pulsation

equipment needs are simple, and there are no nuclear waste products. As an office or home procedure it requires minimal time and offers results in 5 minutes coupled with sensitivities from 25 to 50 mIU/ml of human chorionic gonadotropin (HCG) in the specimen. ELISA technology is the basis for the new over-the-counter tests. The manufacturer provides directions for collection of specimen (serum, plasma, or urine), care of specimen, testing procedure, and reading of results.

Estimated date of confinement. Because the precise date of conception generally must remain conjectural, many formulas or rules of thumb have been sug-

gested to calculate the EDC. No one of these rules of thumb is infallible, but a combination of the results of two or three of the following methods is accurate.

Nägele's rule. Nägele's rule is as follows: add 7 days to the first day of the last menstrual period (LMP), subtract 3 months, and add 1 year. The formula becomes EDC + [(LMP + 7 days) − 3 months] + 1 year; for example, if the first day of the LMP was July 10, 1986, the EDC is April 17, 1987. In simple terms, add 7 days to the LMP and count forward 9 months.

Nägele's rule assumes that the woman has a 28-day cycle and that the pregnancy occurred on the fourteenth day. An adjustment is in order if the cycle is

Fig. 11.1
Measurement of fundal height from symphysis.

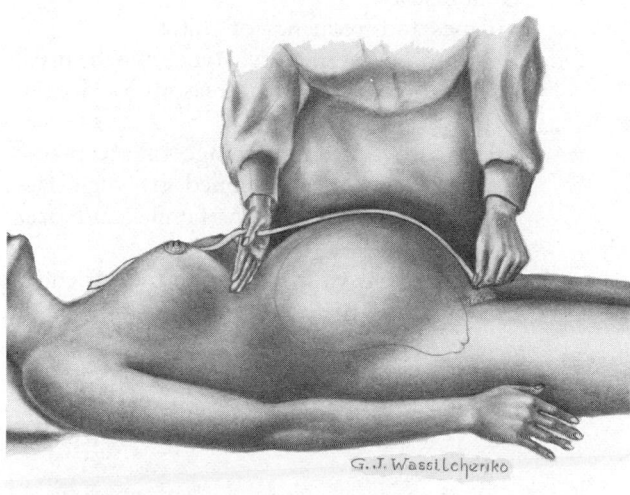

G. J. Wassilcheriko

longer or shorter than 28 days. With the use of Nägele's rule, only about 4% to 10% of gravidas will deliver spontaneously on the EDC. The majority of women will deliver during the period extending from 7 days before to 7 days after the EDC (Appendix D).

Fundal height. During the first and second trimesters of pregnancy the fundal height, as measured on the anterior abdominal wall, provides a gross estimate of the duration of pregnancy. Measurement of fundal height may aid in identification of such high-risk factors as intrauterine growth retardation, multiple gestation, and hydramnios. Among the factors that affect the accuracy of measurement are obesity (subtract 1 cm from the measurement if the gravida weighs 90 kg [200 pounds] or more), the amount of amniotic fluid, multiple gestation, the fetal size and attitude, the tilt of the uterus, and the width of the examiner's finger if fingerbreadths are used.

A pliable (not stretchable) tape measure or a pelvimeter may be used to measure fundal height. The height of the fundus is measured from the notch of the pubic symphysis over the top of the fundus without tipping the corpus back. A metal pelvimeter may be used in place of a pliable tape.

To increase measurement reliability and facilitate management, the same person examines the gravida at each of her prenatal visits, and one protocol is established for use by all examiners providing care to a group of gravidas. The protocol must include the gravida's position on the table and the measuring device and method used. The gravida's position is supine with the knees slightly bent and the head and shoulders slightly elevated. If a pliable measuring tape is used, it should be specified whether the measurement is taken with the tape following the exact contour of the uterus to the fundus or whether the measurement is read with the palm of the hand at the fundus and the tape elevated between the forefinger and middle finger (Fig. 11.1).

Authorities disagree on the exact measurement of fundal height appropriate for each week of gestation. There is no identified protocol for the measuring techniques used to obtain the values listed in Table 11.4. Sandberg (1978) states that during the second trimester the height of the uterine fundus in centimeters above the pubis symphysis generally approximates the menstrual age of the gestation in weeks. *McDonald's rule* adds precision to the measurement of fundal height during the second and third trimesters. It is calculated as follows:

Height of fundus (cm) $\times$ $\frac{2}{7}$ (or + 3.5) =
     Duration of pregnancy in lunar months
Height of fundus (cm) $\times$ $\frac{8}{7}$ =
     Duration of pregnancy in weeks.

Ultrasonography. Ultrasonography may be used to establish the duration of pregnancy if the woman is

Table 11.4
Comparison of Fundal Heights

Week	Height in Fingerbreadths (fb) in Relation to Anatomic Landmarks — McLennan and Sandberg	Height in Centimeters above Pubic Symphysis		
		Spielberg	McDonald	Sandberg
16	3-4 fb above pubis symphysis			
20	2-3 fb below umbilicus		18	20
24	At umbilicus		21	24
28	3 fb above umbilicus	26.7	24.5	28
32	3 fb below xiphoid	29.5-30	28	32
36	2 fb below xiphoid	32	31.5	36
40	2 fb below xiphoid	37.7	35	40

unable to give a precise date for her last menstrual period or if the size of the uterus does not conform to the stated date of the last menstrual period. During the first trimester, ultrasound technique can reveal a gestational sac as early as 6 to 10 weeks. The fetus appears within the sac about 7 or 8 weeks after the last menstrual period. Fetal heart activity can be visualized by 9 or 10 weeks. Fetal breathing movements can be visualized by 11 weeks. For a discussion of the use of ultrasound for estimation of gestational age of the fetus or detection of fetal anomalies, see Chapter 25.

Interview. Through interview techniques and questionaires as much information as possible is obtained concerning subjective symptoms of pregnancy and the woman's general health.

I. Health history
  A. Family history
    1. Health status of woman's parents and her siblings (if deceased, note cause of death)
    2. History of tuberculosis, cancer, diabetes, vascular disease, neuromuscular disease, allergies, other serious illnesses, or complications with pregnancies
  B. Medical history
    1. Age
    2. Racial origin
    3. Ethnic background (e.g., Tay-Sachs disease in Ashkenazic Jews)
    4. Childhood diseases
    5. Other diseases (e.g., sexually transmitted diseases, their treatment, and response to treatment)
    6. Surgery (e.g., abortion may predispose woman to incompetent cervix; uterine surgery or extensive repair of pelvic floor may necessitate cesarean birth; appendectomy rules out appendicitis as cause of right lower quadrant pain; spinal surgery contraindicates spinal or epidural anesthesia)
    7. Injuries, particularly those involving the pelvis
    8. All medications being used (The woman is asked to bring these with her at the next visit.)
    9. Allergies or sensitivities (drugs, foods, previous transfusions)
    10. Immunizations, including rubella
    11. Menstrual history: date of menarche; duration and amount of flow, pain; any other accompanying symptoms
      a. Last menstrual period (LMP)
      b. Previous menstrual period (PMP)
      c. Last normal menstrual period (LNMP)
    12. Date of last Papanicolaou smear for cytology and smear for gonorrhea
  C. Sexual history
    1. Times and frequency of coitus
    2. Contraceptive history: type, when used, any problems, time and reasons for discontinuation.
    3. Attitudes concerning range of acceptable sexual behavior as defined by such factors as culture, religion, family, and peer group
      a. What has your family (partner, friends) told you about sex during pregnancy?
      b. What are your feelings about sex during pregnancy?
      c. Is it all right for married people to masturbate?
      d. How do your ideas and feelings about sex differ from those of your partner?
    4. Sexual self-concept (How one sees oneself sexually influences how one relates to others.)
      a. How do you feel about the changes in your appearance?
      b. How does your partner feel about your body now?
      c. Do maternity clothes make pregnant women attractive?
    5. Level of knowledge, including understanding of how the body functions, sexual anatomy and physiology, and myths and misinformation about sex
    6. Sexual behavior: marital or alternative relationship
    7. Marital relationships
      a. What will it be like to have a baby in the home?
      b. How is your life and that of your partner going to change by having a baby?
      c. What plans do having a baby interrupt?
    8. Physical status (One's state of health affects both sexual interest and ability to perform sexually.)
      a. How is your overall health?
      b. What is your energy level?
      c. When do you feel most alive?
  D. Obstetric history
    1. Gravidity, parity, number of deliveries, premature deliveries, abortions, stillbirths, living children
    2. If woman is a multigravida, description of previous pregnancies: length of gestations;

birth weight; fetal outcome; length of labor; presentation and type of delivery; prenatal, natal, and postdelivery complications

   3. Whether she breast-fed or bottle-fed a previous infant

   4. If woman is Rh negative, whether she received Rho (D) immune globulin (e.g., RhoGAM)

   5. Present pregnancy

     a. Diagnosis of pregnancy

     b. Abnormal symptoms noted

     c. Medications taken, prescription or nonprescription (e.g., aspirin), including alcohol, tobacco, and caffeine

     d. X-ray examinations, if any

II. Psychosocial history (social profile)

  A. Identifying data: birthplace, marital status or history, education, occupation, employment history

  B. Perception of this pregnancy: wanted or not, planned or not, pleased, displeased, accepting, nonaccepting.

   1. Problems engendered by pregnancy: financial, career, and living accommodations

   2. Ideas about childbearing

   3. Expectations of infant's behavior

   4. Outlook on life and female role

   5. What is expected of physician and relationship between woman (couple) and nurse

   6. Perceptions related to age, race, or ethnic background

  C. Support systems

   1. Family support

     a. Meaning of the anticipated baby to the family

     b. Attitude toward health care and particularly care during childbearing

     c. Relationships existing between mother, father, siblings, and in-laws (Is the pregnancy "hers" or "theirs"?)

     d. Primary support available to the mother

     e. Changes needed to promote adequate support for the mother

     f. Preparations being made for the care of the woman and dependent family members during labor and for the care of the infant after birth

   2. Community

     a. Peer group support, friends, relatives

     b. Agency support: financial, educational

  D. Coping mechanisms: knowledge of pregnancy, maternal changes, fetal growth, care of self, and care of newborn, including feeding;

attitudes toward natural or medicated childbirth; knowledge of parent craft classes available; decision-making ability; use of significant others and of community affiliations (church, clubs) as supports; living habits (e.g., exercise, sleep, diet, diversional interests, personal hygiene, clothing)

  E. Parental potential

   1. Mothers psychologic response (Box, p. 251)

   2. Potential disorders in parenting (see Box, p. 257)

III. Review of woman's physical systems (For each symptom presented, obtain the following additional data: body location, quality, quantity, chronology, setting, aggravating or alleviating factors, and associated manifestations [onset, character, course].)

  A. General: energy level, feelings of well-being, recent large gain or loss of weight

  B. Skin, hair, and nails: condition, color, consistency, lesions

  C. Head: injury to, aches, dizziness, syncope

  D. Eyes: vision, prescription glasses or contact lenses, pain, infections, discharges, swelling; last visit to ophthalmologist

  E. Nose and sinuses: pain, bleeding, obstruction, discharge, frequency of colds or sinusitis, sneezing

  F. Oral cavity: hoarseness, toothache, dentures, last visit to a dentist, frequency of dental care, state of lips and gums, problems with chewing or swallowing

  G. Neck: pain, restriction or movement, swelling

  H. Lymph nodes: tenderness, enlargement

  I. Breasts and nipples: pain, lumps, discharge, pigmentation, size, whether woman does breast self-examination

  J. Respiratory system: pain or shortness of breath; frequency and types of infection (bronchitis, pneumonitis, pleurisy); cough, sputum, or wheezing; number of pillows (to elevate head) needed to sleep comfortably; number of cigarettes smoked per day and for how many years

  K. Cardiovascular system: history of congenital heart disease, rheumatic fever, hypertension, hypotension, or anemia; pain; dyspnea; palpitations

  L. Gastrointestinal system: changes in stools; bowel habits, or appetite, including food intolerance; history of disease of gallbladder, liver, or appendix; pain; jaundice; parasites; nausea; vomiting, or diarrhea; drugs taken

M. Genitourinary system: frequency, pain, or discharge; sexual history and contraception history; history of sexually transmitted diseases and treatment

N. Extremities: muscle tone and cramping, vascularity, joint pain or stiffness, gout, bone fragility, flat feet

O. Back: pain, stiffness, movement, sciatica or disc problems, curvature

P. Central nervous system: general, mentation, speech, motor, sensory

Q. Hematopoietic system: blood type, Rh factor, bleeding or coagulation disorders, transfusions, exposure to radiation

R. Endocrine system: history of growth and nutrition, tolerance for heat and cold

S. Immune system

Physical examination

I. Temperature, pulse, respiration, and blood pressure

II. Height and weight

III. General appearance: body type and weight, energy level, grooming, posture

IV. Skin, hair, and nails: condition, color, consistency, lesions

V. Head: face, scalp, hair, and hair pattern distribution, eyes, ears, nose, mouth, breath, teeth, gums, tonsils, salivary glands, lymph nodes

VI. Neck: skin, movement, lymph nodes, pulses (jugular, carotid), trachea, thyroid (tenderness, enlargement, discharge), pain, restriction of movement, swelling

VII. Thorax
A. Anterior: heart, lungs
B. Posterior: heart, lungs, spine, spinal curvature
C. Breasts: masses, skin lesions, and axillary extension, lymph nodes (include axillary), skin, vascularization, pigmentation; nipples assessed for erectility and protraction; changes consistent with pregnancy noted in order of their appearance; woman's ability to complete breast self-examination assessed

VIII. Abdomen
A. Skin: color, turgor, and texture; presence of striae with their number and distribution; rashes, lesions
B. Vascular changes such as dilated veins or spider nevi
C. Pattern and amount of body hair
D. Umbilicus: color, contour, location, condition; hernia
E. Peristalsis: visible, bowel sounds
F. Contour and size of uterus; measurement of fundal height, if appropriate
G. Fetal heart rate, if appropriate
H. Rectus abdominal muscles: diastasis
I. Inguinal hernia, lymph nodes

IX. Reproduction: external structures, speculum, bimanual, and rectovaginal examination of internal structures. If the woman is very tense reexamination may be necessary later in pregnancy. The vagina enlarges and supporting structures are more relaxed as pregnancy advances.
A. External structures
1. Outlet to vagina: may be relaxed (multigravida) or constricted (nulligravida).
2. Skene's and Bartholin's glands inspected and palpated for enlargement, inflammation, or exudate.
3. Size and distribution of varicosities of vulva and vagina.
4. Any skin lesions (e.g., excoriation, ulcerations, growths, leukoplakia).
5. Perineum checked for scars (old lacerations, episiotomies), masses, lesions, or inflammation.
6. Anus examined for prolapse or varices (hemorrhoids).
B. Internal structures
1. Vaginal speculum inserted and vaginal walls examined for lesions or prolapse.
2. Any secretions noted as to clarity, color, odor, and signs of irritation; leukorrhea.
3. Cervix visualized: any bleeding, lesions, or location of cervical lacerations noted.
4. Increased vascularity and deepening color of vestibule and vaginal wall; Chadwick's sign appears at about 6 weeks.
5. Increased softening
   a. Hegar's sign: softening of the lower uterine segment, resulting in its compressibility at about 6 weeks
   b. Goodell's sign: cervical softening occurring about 4 to 5 weeks; infection or fibrosis may mask this presumptive sign
6. Palpate for masses (tumors), although adnexa cannot be readily palpated during pregnancy.
7. Parametria palpated by rectovaginal examination to exclude inflammatory or tumor invasion of broad ligament bases.
8. Pelvic measurements obtained, if possible.

Assessment of Maternal Psychologic Adaptation to Pregnancy and Parenting at 34 to 36 Weeks' Gestation

Score

1. When did you first see a doctor about your pregnancy? Can you tell me why you chose to go at this particular time?

    _____ Saw doctor after third missed menstruation; didn't realize was pregnant; thought lack of menstruation may be due to something else; went to see doctor to have this investigated (1 point)

    _____ Saw doctor after second or third missed menstruation; went to see doctor because husband observed wife's irritability; went to have IUD checked (2 points)

    _____ Vague about when visit to doctor was made; thinks she missed two menstruations; unplanned pregnancy; wanted to validate (3 points)

    _____ Saw doctor about 1 week after second missed menstruation; knew she was already pregnant; planned; wanted to validate (4 points)

    _____ Saw doctor about 1 week after first missed menstruation; wanted to have planned pregnancy validated (5 points)

2. As a child, was there someone in your immediate family that you saw as a loving kind of person? Who was the most loving person in your family? Your mother? Your father? What were your parents like?

    _____ Did not have anyone in family that she saw as a loving person; expresses dislike and negative feelings about early childhood; may have been in numerous foster homes; parents very strict or very lenient (1 point)

    _____ Defines problems in childhood: separations from parents; definite family problems (e.g., alcoholism); parents inconsistent (2 points)

    _____ Vague about family; unable to give definite ideas re "a loving person"; ambivalent feelings expressed; unable to define characteristics (3 points)

    _____ Describes relationship with a parent as being satisfactory, with warmth, but wants relationship with own child to be stronger (4 points)

    _____ Mother or father seen as very positive, very warm person; expresses positive feelings (5 points)

3. What thoughts and ideas have you and your partner had on the changing of life-styles, working hours, or other adjustments pertaining to this pregnancy and new baby?

    _____ Have thought about it but believe no changes or adjustments are necessary; state that they believe this is important, not to change things for the baby (1 point)

    _____ Haven't thought about adjustments and changes; wonder if there will be a need to change; questioning possibility (2 points)

    _____ Have had some thoughts about changes; think they want to wait to see what it will be like once baby arrives; think that it is easier to do after baby comes (3 points)

    _____ Have already made a few changes; think that there will be a need for further changes; have spent time talking about it; have tentative plans (4 points)

    _____ Have made changes to suit wife's needs for increased rest; have spent time thinking about the changes; have plans to help—baby-sister, relatives visiting, etc. (5 points)

4. Do you think you will need help when you get home from the hospital? Have you made any plans for help? If so, what are they?

    _____ No, doesn't want anyone interfering (2 points)

    _____ No, believes can manage well by self (4 points)

    _____ Ambivalent, doesn't know (6 points)

    _____ No help available: has made definite plans on how to try to manage, or plan involves calling someone in case of emergency (8 points)

    _____ Yes, has specific plans for husband or other person to be there for help (10 points)

5. Have you had any thoughts, ideas, or hunches about our baby's appearance and behavior after you bring him home from the hospital?

    _____ Describes very unrealistic behaviors, such as regular sleeping or sleeping through the night; or describes three or four negative aspects (3 points)

    _____ Describes one or two negative aspects along with two or three fears about not knowing what to do; or has no idea, gives it no thought (6 points)

    _____ Unable to describe; can describe only in vague terms; describes fears relating to baby's crying (9 points)

    _____ Can describe a few aspects (one or two) of baby's behavior (12 points)

    _____ Describes realistically baby's sleeping, feeding, and crying behavior; has a few questions to have clarified (15 points)

Key:
 8-20: very high, intervention needed
21-30: questionable, "at risk," further follow-up needed
31-33: low risk
34-40: no risk

Scoring:
Add points from each question:
1. _____
2. _____
3. _____
4. _____
5. _____

TOTAL   _____

Modified from Funke-Farber, J.: Reliability and validity testing of maternal adaptive behavior, Edmonton, 1978, University of Alberta, Faculty of Nursing.

Table 11.5
Summary of Laboratory Tests in Prenatal Period

Laboratory Test	Purpose
Hemoglobin/hematocrit	To detect anemia
Hemoglobin electrophoresis	To identify women with hemoglobinopathies (e.g., sickle cell anemia)
Blood type, Rh, and irregular antibody	To identify those fetuses at risk for developing erythroblastosis fetalis or hyperbilirubinemia in neonatal period
Rubella titer	To determine immunity to rubella
VDRL/FTA-ABS*	To identify women with untreated syphilis
Urinalysis, including microscopic examination of urinary sediment	To identify women with unsuspected diabetes mellitus, renal disease, hypertensive disease of pregnancy
Urine culture	To identify women with asymptomatic bacteriuria
Papanicolaou smear	To screen for cervical intraepithelial neoplasia and herpes simplex, type 2
Gonorrhea culture	To screen high-risk population for asymptomatic infection
Tuberculin skin testing	To screen high-risk population
Renal function tests: BUN,† creatinine, electrolytes, creatinine clearance, total protein excretion	To evaluate level of possible renal compromise in women with a history of diabetes, hypertension, or renal disease
Cardiac evaluation; ECG, chest x-ray film, and echocardiogram	To evaluate cardiac function in women with a history of hypertension or cardiac disease

*FTA-ABS, fluorescent treponemal antibody absorption test.
†BUN, blood urea nitrogen.

X. Extremities: peripheral pulses and capillary filling time, reflexes, muscle mass and tone, varicosities, edema, mobility and condition of joints

Laboratory tests. Collection of specimens is done at this time so that results of their examination will be ready for the next scheduled prenatal visit (Table 11.5).

1. Tine or purified protein derivative of tuberculin (PPD) for exposure to tuberculosis
2. Cervical and vaginal smears for cytology (Papanicolaou smear) and for chlamydia organisms, gonorrhea, and herpes simplex, types 1 and 2
3. Blood: Veneral Disease Research Laboratory (VDRL) test for syphilis, complete blood count (CBC) with hematocrit, hemoglobin, and differential values; blood type and Rh factor; antibody screen (Kell, Duffy, rubella, toxoplasmosis, anti-Rh); sickle cell; level of folacin when indicated
4. Urine: tests for glucose, protein, and acetone; culture and sensitivity tests as necessary

SUBSEQUENT VISITS

The second phase of prenatal care begins with the development of a plan for care suited to the needs of the particular woman. It includes ongoing assessment measures as needed and teaching and counseling the client and her family.

Schedule. The gravida should be seen once each month until the thirty-second week, every 2 weeks until the thirty-sixth week, and each week thereafter until delivery. More frequent visits may be required if there are complications.

Maternal assessment
Interview
1. General well-being, complaints or problems, questions
2. Woman and her family's needs for psychosocial support

Physical examination
1. Temperature, pulse, respirations
2. Blood pressure (right arm, woman sitting)
3. Weight and determination of whether gain (or loss) is compatible with overall plan for weight gain (see Chapter 12).
4. Abdominal palpation
   a. Height of fundus above pubic symphysis (measured with tape); identification of unusual tenderness, masses, herniation, and other important skills (Fig. 11.1).
   b. Auscultation and counting of FHR (FHR may be heard from weeks 8 through 12 using Doppler method) (Fig. 11.2).
   c. Beginning at thirty-second week, identification with aid of Leopold's maneuvers (see Chapter 14) of fetal presentation, position, and station (engagement); assessment of uterine measurements and size (weight) of fetus as compared with supposed duration of pregnancy. Although

Fig. 11.2
Detecting fetal heartbeat. **A,** Fetoscope. **B,** Stethoscope with rubber band. **C,** Doppler principle.

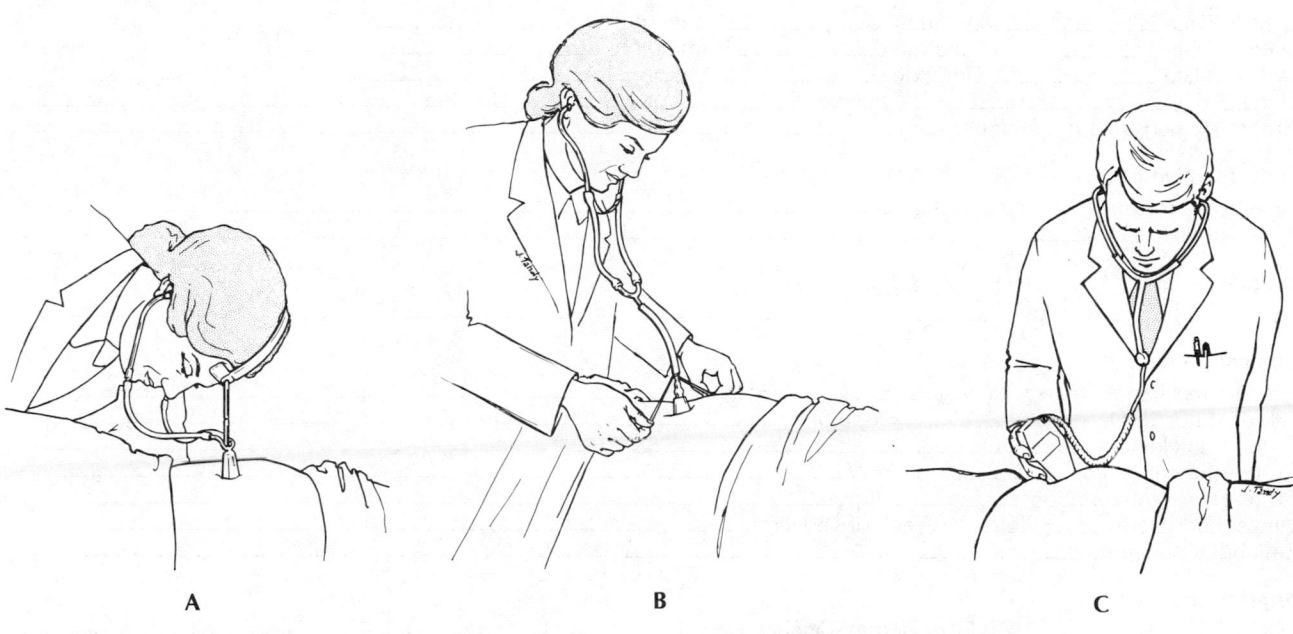

A   B   C

some clinicians can estimate fetal weight with unbelievable accuracy, estimations are generally inconsistent and unreliable. Accuracy in estimating fetal weight improves with ultrasound determination of biparietal diameter. Possible growth retardation of fetus, multiple pregnancy, or inaccuracy of the EDC may be disclosed by ultrasound (see Chapter 31).

5. Vaginal or rectal examination at any time (unless gravida is bleeding) to investigate leukorrhea, confirm presenting part, corroborate station, and determine cervical dilation and effacement; may be especially important if labor is impending or induction is anticipated

Laboratory tests (see Table 11.5)
1. Cervical and vaginal smears (repeat at 32 weeks or as necessary): chlamydia organisms, gonorrhea, and herpes simplex, types 1 and 2
2. Blood (repeat at 32 weeks or as necessary): VDRL test for syphilis: complete blood count (CBC) with hematocrit, hemoglobin, and differential values; blood type and Rh factor; antibody screen (Kell, Duff, rubella, toxoplasmosis, anti-Rh); sickle cell; level of folacin when indicated; packed cell volume (PCV) may be done at each visit in some offices
3. Urine: tests for glucose, protein, and acetone; culture and sensitivity as necessary

Fetal assessment
Fetal gestational age. In a normal pregnancy, fetal gestational age is estimated by determining the duration of pregnancy and the date of delivery. In some centers ultrasonography is used with all pregnancies, and a more exact estimation of gestational age can be made (Box, p. 254). However, ultrasonography is not a universally recommended procedure (see Chapter 25).

Fetal health status. Assessment of fetal health status includes consideration of fetal movement, FHR, and abnormal maternal or fetal symptoms.

Fetal movement. The mother is instructed to note the extent and timing of fetal movements and to report immediately if the pattern changes or if movement ceases. Regular movement has been found to be a reliable determinant of fetal health (Cohen, 1985).

Fetal heart rate. The FHR is checked on routine visits once it has been heard (see Fig. 11.2 and Chapter 9). Normal rate and rhythm is another good indicator of fetal health. Absence of FHR, once heard, requires immediate investigation.

Abnormal maternal or fetal symptoms. Intensive investigation of fetal health status is initiated if any maternal or fetal complications arise (e.g., maternal hypertension, premature rupture of membranes, or irregular or absent fetal heart rate). (For a discussion of electronic fetal monitoring, see Chapter 16; for other monitoring techniques of the fetus at risk, see Chapter 25.)

Correlation of Data in Determining Fetal Gestational Age*

Menstrual history

LNMP: Date _____ Duration _____ Amount _____
LMP: Date _____ Duration _____ Amount _____
PMP: Date _____ Duration _____ Amount _____
Menarche _____ Interval _____ Duration _____
History of menstrual irregularity _____

Contraceptive history

Type of contraceptive _____
When stopped _____

Pregnancy test

Date _____ Type _____ Result _____

Clinical evaluation

First uterine size estimate: Date _____ Size _____
FHT first heard: Date _____ Dopptone _____ Fetoscope _____
Date of quickening _____
Current fundal height _____ EFW _____
Current week of gestation _____
Ultrasound: Date _____ Week of gestation _____ BPD _____
Reliability of dates _____

Impression

EDC _____ Estimated gestational age _____
Estimation based on _____
Comments _____
Signature _____ Date _____

LNMP, Last normal menstrual period; PMP, previous menstrual period (before LMP); EFW, estimated fetal weight; BPD, biparietal diameter.

Nursing Diagnoses

Each client and family will have a unique set of responses to pregnancy. To attend to these responses the nurse begins by formulating appropriate nursing diagnoses. Following are examples of nursing diagnoses arising during the course of the prenatal period (see Summary of Nursing Actions, pp. 284 and 285).

1. From the family history: Potential injury to mother or fetus related to knowledge deficit of relevant symptomatology of previous pregnancy
2. From the present pregnancy: Potential alteration in fetal development related to substance abuse (tobacco)*
3. From the psychosocial history: Potential alteration in health maintenance related to cultural beliefs
4. From the laboratory examinations: Potential injury to mother or fetus related to poor nutrition as evidenced by low maternal hematocrit

---

*Diagnosis not included in those of the North American Nursing Diagnosis Association (NANDA), 1986.

Planning

Planning care for clients during the prenatal period is based on the biopsychosocial assessment of the client and her family. For each client a plan is developed that relates specifically to her clinical and nursing problems. The information in this chapter is general in nature; that is, not all women will experience all problems discussed nor require all facets of the care described. The nurse selects those aspects of care revelant to the client and the client's family.

GOALS

Goals directed to the maternity population as a whole include the following:

1. To develop health services that are available to all pregnant women and their fetuses or newborns and families (Appendix C).
2. To develop standards of maternity care applicable to all women and their families (Tucker and others, 1984; NAACOGs, 1985; Appendix B).

3. To develop nursing strategies with sound scientific bases.

Goals directed toward women and their families include both physiologic and psychosocial goals.

Physiologic care. The following goals relate to physiologic care:

1. To alert clients to the symptoms that indicate deviations from normal progress and the protocols for reporting them.
2. To detect deviations from the normal progress of pregnancy and to initiate prompt remedial therapy.
3. To provide clients with pertinent knowledge of the adaptation of the maternal body to a developing fetus as a basis for understanding the rationale and necessity for modalities of care.
4. To provide clients with information and counseling, including those relating to nutritional needs, sexual needs, activities of daily living, and discomforts of pregnancy.

Psychosocial care. The following goals relate to psychosocial care:

1. To encourage participation by clients and their families in their care during pregnancy.
2. To provide support for clients and their families as they experience stress during pregnancy.
3. To establish an environment that promotes an emotionally satisfying pregnancy.

Implementation

Nurses assume many caretaking roles during the prenatal period. The nurse acts as support person, teacher/counselor/advocate, and technician.

SUPPORT PERSON

The nurse-client relationship is critical in setting the tone for further interactions (see Chapter 4). The techniques of listening with an attentive expression, touching, and using eye contact have their place, as does recognition of the client's feelings and her right to express them. The intervention may occur in various formal or informal settings. For certain persons, involvement in goal-directed health groups is neither feasible nor acceptable. Encounters in hallways or clinic examining rooms, home visits, or telephone conversations provide the only opportunities for contact and can be used effectively. One nurse described her intervention with a gravid woman as follows:

I tried to teach her about relaxation and breathing techniques during childbirth, but she was not interested. When she phoned to tell me she was at the hospital in labor, she said, "What was all that stuff you were saying about breathing?" In between the next few contractions I repeated the salient points.

Sometimes women seek information about a particular problem repeatedly, not so much for the advice given, but to direct the nurse's attention toward themselves. The nurse can help these women by asking for a client-generated solution and a report of its effectiveness. The need for additional attention is recognized and provided in other ways.

In supporting a client it must be remembered that both the nurse and the client are contributing to the relationship. The nurse has to accept the client's responses as a factor in trying to be of help. An example of one nurse-client relationship follows:

Mrs. _____ had been very forthright in saying that this pregnancy was unplanned but had countered this statement with comments such as "All things happen for the best," "We always wanted the boys to have a family to turn to," and "Children bring their own love." Over a period of time, as our relationship developed to one of *mutual* trust, she complained increasingly of her fear of pain, her hating to wear maternity clothes, and her having to give up helping the family. Finally I ventured to say, "Sometimes when a pregnancy is unplanned, women resent it very much and are angry about it." Her relief was evident, She said, "Oh, you don't know how angry I've been." As a result the whole tenor of support being offered changed, and the plan was adjusted to meet her real needs.

The nurse also needs to accept the fact that the woman must be a willing partner in a relationship that is a purely voluntary one. As such, the relationship can be refused or terminated at any time by the pregnant woman or her family.

Supportive care involves developing, augmenting, or changing the mechanisms used by women and families in coping with stress. An effort is made to promote active participation by the individuals in the process of solving their own problems. Clients are helped to gather pertinent information, explore alternative actions, make decisions as to choice of action, and assume responsibility for the outcomes. These outcomes may be any or all of the following:

1. Living with a problem as it is
2. Mitigating effects of a problem so that it can be accepted more readily
3. Eliminating the problem through effecting change

Expectations of success in the area of emotional supportive care must of necessity be flexible. It is not within the province of any outsider to assure another person a rewarding, satisfying experience. The mother and persons significant to her are crucial elements in this process. Many of their problems are beyond the scope or capabilities of any professional worker. In describing her work with young and poor persons, Edwards (1973) notes: "They did not usually change their living situation and I was not instrumental in modifying home or drug problems." However, this did not deter her from encouraging clients to use the decision-making process as a means of coping with problems rather than merely complaining about injustice.

At other times a successful outcome can be readily documented. A woman who early in her pregnancy had predicted a severe depressive state in the postdelivery period was elated when such a state did not materialize. She remarked to the nurse who had provided support during the pregnancy and birth, "You're the best nerve medicine I've ever had!"

TEACHER/COUNSELOR/ADVOCATE

Health maintenance is an important aspect of prenatal care. Client participation in the care ensures prompt reporting of untoward responses to pregnancy. Client assumption of responsibility for health maintenance is prompted by understanding of maternal adaptations to the growth of the unborn child. Nurses in their roles of teacher/counselor/advocate provide clients with the knowledge necessary for compliance with health care measures.

Instruction regarding danger signals. One of the first responsibilities of persons involved in the care of the pregnant woman is to alert her to signs and symptoms that indicate a potential complication of pregnancy. The client needs to know how to report such danger signals (Boxes above and on p. 257). When one is stressed by a disturbing symptom, it is difficult to remember specifics. Therefore the gravida and her family are reassured if they receive a printed form listing the signs and symptoms that warrant an investigation and the phone numbers to call in an emergency.

Nutrition counseling. Nutritional intake is an important factor in the maintenance of maternal health during pregnancy and in the provision of adequate nutrients for fetal development. Assessing nutritional status and providing nutritional information are part of the nurse's responsibilities in prenatal care. For detailed information concerning maternal and fetal nutritional needs, see Chapter 12.

Childbirth and parenthood education. Formal classes in childbirth and parenthood education have proved successful for some women and families. The various methods (e.g., Lamaze, Bradley) have certain premises in common:

Physical Danger Signals

1. Visual disturbances—blurring, double vision, or spots
2. Swelling of face, fingers, or sacrum
3. Severe, frequent, or continuous headaches
4. Muscular irritability or convulsions
5. Epigastric pain
6. Persistent vomiting beyond first trimester or severe vomiting at any time
7. Fluid discharge from vagina—bleeding or amniotic fluid (anything other than leukorrhea)
8. Signs of infections: chills, fever, burning on urination, diarrhea
9. Severe or unusual pain in abdomen
10. Absence of fetal movements after quickening (Physicians want women to report any unusual change in pattern or amount of fetal movements.)

1. The partners wish to share the birth of their child as part of their concept of family unity.
2. The mother gains the support of a partner who is trained to provide it.
3. Opportunity is provided to develop mechanisms for coping with pain or discomfort during labor and delivery (relaxation, diversion, or disassociation). These mechanisms assist in maintaining self-controlling behaviors and control of the environment.
4. Parent craft activities are discussed and practiced.

For a complete discussion of childbirth and parenthood education, see Chapter 13. If the woman (or couple) does not ask about prenatal classes in preparation for childbirth, the nurse provides the information and encourages participation.

Common questions. Women and their families have many questions concerning the pregnancy and the physical and emotional changes they experience in themselves as well as those they perceive in others. Questions about activities of daily living are common.

Clothing. Comfortable, loose clothing is best. Washable fabrics (e.g., absorbent cottons) are often preferred. Since maternity clothes are expensive and rarely wear out, hand-me-downs or used clothes from garage sales can suffice. Tight brassieres and belts, stretch pants, garters, tight-top knee socks, panty girdles, and other constrictive clothing should be avoided. Tight clothing over the perineum encourages vaginitis and miliaria (heat rash). Impaired circulation in the lower extremities favors varices.

A well-fitted maternity girdle, frequently readjusted, may be used for backache by obese women or those

Potential Parenting Disorders

Parents	Child or Pregnancy
1. Mother is extremely depressed over pregnancy.	1. Mother seems overly concerned with baby's sex.
2. Mother is frightened and alone, especially in anticipation of delivery. Careful explanations do not seem to dissipate fears.	2. Mother exhibits denial of pregnancy (not willing to gain weight, no plans for baby, refusal to talk about situation).
3. Mother not supported by husband or family.	3. This child could be "one too many."
4. Mother or father previously wanted an abortion or seriously considered relinquishment and have changed their minds.	4. Ambivalence concerning child or pregnancy intensifies to term.
5. Parents come from an abusive or neglectful background.	5. Crying of infants noted as stressful.
6. Parents' living situation is overcrowded, isolated, unstable, or intolerable to them.	6. Rigid expectations of infant's behavior.
7. Parents do not have a telephone.	
8. Parents have no supportive relatives or friends.	

Adapted from Gray, J.D., Christy, A.C., Dean, G.D., and Kempe, C.H.: Prediction and prevention of child abuse, Semin. Perinatol. **3:**86, Jan. 1979.

with a multiple pregnancy. The woman should be cautioned to begin fastening the girdle from the pubic symphysis upward to support the uterus from below. An old, even very large, girdle meant for the nonpregnant woman is unsuitable during pregnancy because it pushes the abdomen (uterus) inward. A nonmaternity girdle may also aggravate backache and leg ache.

Maternity brassieres are constructed to accommodate the increased breast weight, chest circumference, and size of breast tail tissue (under the arm). These brassieres have drop flaps over the nipples to facilitate actual nursing. A good brassiere can help prevent neck ache and backache.

Elastic hose or leotards may give considerable comfort to women with large varicose veins or swelling of the legs. Comfortable shoes that provide firm support and promote good posture and balance are advisable. Very high heels and platform shoes are not recommended because of the woman's changed center of gravity. She has a tendency to lose her balance. In the third trimester her pelvis tilts forward and her back arches. Leg aches and leg cramps are aggravated by nonsupportive shoes.

Bathing and swimming. Tub bathing is permitted even in late pregnancy, because water does not enter the vagina unless under pressure. However, tub bathing is contraindicated after rupture of the membranes. Baths can be therapeutic because they relax tense tired muscles, help counter insomnia, and make the pregnant woman feel fresh. Physical maneuverability presents a problem (increased chance of falling) late in pregnancy. Swimming is also permitted during normal pregnancy, although diving is discouraged because of possible traumatic injury.

Employment. Many women continue to work during pregnancy. A recent American study found an employment rate of 60% among pregnant women (Marbury and others, 1984). Pregnant women, particularly those with young children, who have regular jobs in addition to home responsibilities are carrying one of the heaviest loads of all workers (Bryant, 1985).

Whether the expectant mother can or should work and for how long depends on the physical activity involved, industrial hazards, medical or obstetric complications, and employment regulations of the company. A prime consideration is the avoidance of a fetotoxic environment (e.g., chemical dust particles or gases such as inhalation anesthesia). Operating room personnel who are pregnant need to be aware of the dangers of their working environment to the fetus. The latest Occupational Safety and Health Administration New Hazard Communication Standard (labeled the federal right-to-know law), November, 1985, requires chemical manufacturers to assess exposure health hazards and inform employees of those hazards (NAACOG, 1985). Nurses who are pregnant are not to be assigned to the care of infants or others with infectious diseases that can be dangerous to the fetus (e.g., measles or cytomegalovirus [CMV]).

The Pregnancy Discrimination Act of 1978 designates the conditions under which a woman can obtain maternity leave.

Women affected by pregnancy, childbirth, or related medical conditions shall be treated the same for all employment related purposes, including receipt of benefits under fringe benefits programs, as other persons not so affected but similar in their ability or inability to work.*

Part of the anticipatory guidance given during pregnancy should include discussion of maternity leave and discussion of plans to return to work (Leap and others, 1980). The following questions need to be reviewed with the client (Brucker and Reedy, 1983):

1. Does the client's employer cover her health care? If so, pregnancy is included if the prescribed waiting period of employment has been completed.
2. What policies for leave are granted by the employer?
3. What provisions are made for coverge of the infant's health care (coverage for infants is not addressed in the Pregnancy Discrimination Act)?
4. What should be done if the company policy is at variance with the Pregnancy Discrimination Act? (One answer is that the U.S. Department of Labor investigates and handles complaints regarding Pregnancy Discrimination Act violations or suspected violations.)

Activities that depend on a good sense of balance should be discouraged, especially during the last half of pregnancy. Frequently, excessive fatigue is the deciding factor in the termination of employment. Women in sedentary jobs need to walk around at intervals and should neither sit nor stand in one position for long periods. Activity is necessary to counter the usual sluggish, dependent circulation that potentiates development of varices and thrombophlebitis. The pregnant woman's chair should provide adequate back support. A footstool can prevent pressure on veins, relieve strain on varices, and minimize swelling of feet. Work breaks are best spent resting in the left lateral side-lying position (employers are required to have an area where women can lie down).

The nurse can encourage each woman to consider the effects of working postnatally on herself and her newborn. Flexible scheduling of working hours, if possible, can allow for breast feeding. Also, women who plan to return to work after giving birth may appreciate information about daycare centers. Continued assessment during the prenatal period is necessary to determine if working is causing undue fatigue or stress. It may be possible for the woman to change the type of work being done with a recommendation from her physician (Bryant, 1985). Some women may lose interest in work as they become more introverted during pregnancy. This response may be difficult to accept for

---

*Public Law 95-555; 92 Stat. 2076; Oct. 31, 1978, and the 1979 amendment to Title VII, the Pregnancy Discrimination Act.

Fig. 11.3
Proper use of safety belt. Both shoulder and lap belts should be used. The lap belt should be worn low across the hip bones and as snug as is comfortable. The shoulder belt should be worn above the gravid uterus and below the neck to avoid chafing. The pregnant woman should sit upright. The headrest should be used to avoid a whiplash injury.

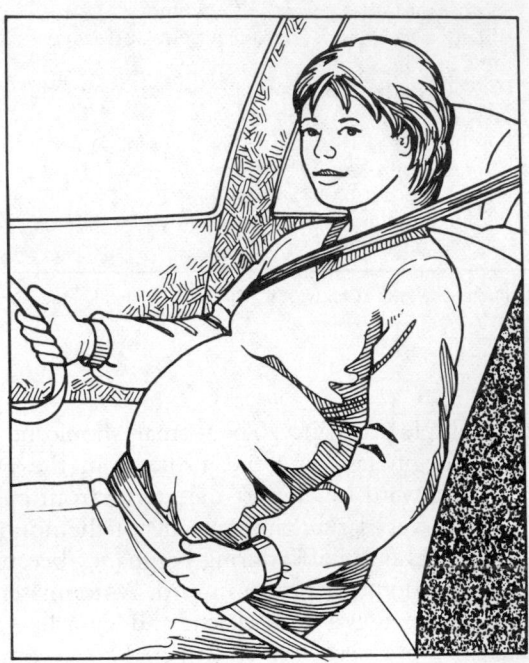

the woman who has always been competent and independent before pregnancy.

Travel. Although travel in itself is not a cause of either abortion or premature labor, certain precautions are recommended. A woman who does not wear automobile restraints risks injury to herself and her fetus (Krozy and others, 1985). Maternal death as a result of injury is the most frequent cause of fetal death (Crosby, 1983). The next most frequent cause is placental separation. Body contours change in reaction to the force of a collision. The uterus as a muscular organ can adapt its shape to that of the body. The placenta lacks the resiliency to change, and placental separation can occur (Crosby, 1983). A combination lap belt and shoulder harness is the most effective automobile restraint (Fig. 11.3) (Chang, 1985).

In high-altitude regions, lowered oxygen levels may cause fetal hypoxia. Women who travel widely expose themselves to the risk of serious accident and may find themselves far removed from good maternity care. In addition, fatigue or tension, as well as altered regular personal habits and diet during arduous travel, may be

Exercise Tips for Pregnant Women

Consult your health-care provider when you know or suspect you are pregnant. Discuss your medical and obstetric history, your current regimen, and the exercises you would like to continue throughout pregnancy.

Seek help in determining an exercise routine that is well within your limit of tolerance, especially if you have not been exercising regularly. Don't push too hard.

Consider decreasing weight-bearing exercises (jogging, running) and concentration on non-weight-bearing activities such as swimming, cycling, or stretching. The latter cut down on bouncing motions, decrease the workload, and may be better tolerated by the fetus. If you are a runner, you may wish to walk instead, starting in your seventh month.

Because strenuous exercise during the last few weeks of pregnancy increases the risk of low birthweight, stillbirth, and infant death, reduce exercise sharply 4 weeks before your due date.[19,25]

Avoid risky activities such as surfing, mountain-climbing, sky-diving, and racquetball. As your pregnancy progresses, your increasing weight, a shift of your center of gravity, and the softening and mobility of your joints and ligaments may alter coordination.[26] Activities requiring precise balance and coordination may be dangerous.

Exercise regularly at least three times a week, as long as you are healthy, to improve muscle tone and increase or maintain your stamina. Sporadic exercises may put undue strain on your muscles.

Limit activity to shorter intervals. Exercise for 10 to 15 minutes, rest for 2 to 3 minutes, then exercise for another 10 to 15 minutes. During exercise, blood flow is redistributed from the internal organs to the skeletal muscle system. The decreased blood flow to the uterus may be risky for the fetus if it continues too long. This decrease reverses rapidly, when exercise stops.

Decrease your exercise level as your pregnancy progresses. The normal alterations of advancing pregnancy, such as decreased cardiac reserve and increased respiratory effort, may produce physiologic stress if you exercise strenuously for a long time.[27,28] Your greater body weight calls for a larger energy output, so you will feel more fatigue. If you are a runner, switch to walking during the last 4 weeks before delivery.

Take your pulse every 10 to 15 minutes while you are exercising. If it's more than 140 beats per minute, slow down until it returns to a maximum of 90.

Avoid becoming overheated for extended periods. It's best not to exercise for more than 35 minutes, especially in hot, humid weather. As your body temperature rises, the heat is transmitted to your fetus. Prolonged or repeated fetal temperature elevation may result in birth defects, especially if done during the first 3 months.[29,30]

Limit the time you spend in hot tubs, saunas, or hot baths. Here are some guidelines:

- Hot tub: water temperature 39.0° C (102.2° F) for less than 15 minutes or 41.0° C (105.8° F) for less than 10 minutes
- Sauna: room temperature 81.4° C (178.5° F) for less than 5 minutes.
- Hot bath: water temperature 39.0° C (102.2° F) for less than 15 minutes.

Ask your health club about the temperature of its hot tubs and saunas, and measure your water temperature at home.

Warmup and stretching exercises prepare your joints for more strenuous exercise and lessen the likelihood of strain or injury to your joints.

A cool-down period of mild activity after exercising will help bring your respiration, heart, and metabolic rates back to normal and avoid pooling of blood in the exercised muscles.

Rest for 10 minutes after exercising, lying on your left side. As the uterus grows, it puts pressure on your inferior vena cava, a major vein carrying blood to your heart, on the right side of your abdomen. Lying on your left side takes the pressure off the vena cava and promotes return circulation from your extremities and muscles to your heart, increasing blood flow to your placenta and fetus.

Drink two or three 8-ounce glasses of water after you exercise, to replace the body fluids you lost through perspiration. While exercising, drink water whenever you feel the need.

Increase your caloric intake to replace the calories burned during exercise. Eat enough to satisfy your hunger and support a weight gain of 1 pound a week, beginning in your fourth month. Choose such high-protein foods as fish, cheese, eggs, or meat.

Take your time. This is not the time to be competitive or train for activities requiring long endurance.

Wear a supportive bra. Your increased breast weight may cause changes in posture and put pressure on the ulnar nerve.

Wear supportive shoes. As your uterus grows, your center of gravity shifts and you compensate by arching your back. In addition, your pelvic muscles and ligaments soften and become more mobile.[26] These natural changes may make you feel off balance and more likely to fall.

Stop exercising immediately if you experience shortness of breath, dizziness, numbness, tingling, abdominal pain, or vaginal bleeding, and consult your health-care provider.

From Paglone, A., and Worthington, S.: Cautions and advice on exercise during pregnancy, Contemp. OB/Gyn. **25** (special issue):160, May 1985.

detrimental. If long-distance travel is necessary, the trip should be made by air. Perhaps fortuitously, flight regulations do not permit pregnant women aboard during the last month without a statement from an obstetrician.

Many women experience a sense of uneasiness when traveling by any vehicle. They describe feelings of fear for the safety of their unborn baby.

Physical activity. Physical activity promotes a feeling of well-being in the pregnant woman. It improves circulation, assists relaxation and rest, and counteracts boredom as it does in the nonpregnant state.

Exercise. A number of researchers have recommended moderate exercise (Bullard, 1981; Dean, 1981; Hutchinson and others, 1981; Jopke, 1983). However, activities continued to the point of exhaustion or fatigue compromise uterine perfusion and fetoplacental oxygenation (Dale and others, 1982). If the woman is accustomed to jogging, she may continue; however, she should not reach the point of fatigue. Heat stress may also endanger the fetus. Furthermore, as gestation advances the woman's center of gravity changes, her bony pelvic support loosens, her coordination usually decreases, and she notices a sensation of awkwardness. Awkwardness may cause her to lose balance and fall injuring herself (Box, p. 259).

Exercises such as those depicted in Fig. 11.4 are taught either at prenatal classes or by the nurse in the clinic or the physician's office. The exercises promote comfort and assist in preparing the woman for labor. Posture and how to lift and move objects safely also

are discussed and demonstrated to counteract the awkwardness experienced toward the end of pregnancy (Fig. 11.5).

Kegel's exercises. Kegel's exercises can strengthen the muscles around the reproductive organs and improve muscle tone. If practiced on a regular basis at least three times a day, the exercises also help to prevent stress incontinence.

Women can be taught to do Kegel's exercises easily and in any position. To locate the correct muscle, women are asked to imagine that they are urinating. Then they are asked to imagine that they are stopping the flow of urine. The muscles that stop the flow are the pubococcygeal muscles. Doing Kegel's exercises during urination helps the woman to know whether she is doing them correctly. If she can stop the stream of urine, her tone is good.

After a woman has located the correct muscles, Kegel's exercises can be done in the following ways:
1. *Slow:* Tighten the muscle, hold it for the count of three, and relax it.

Fig. 11.4
Exercises. **A-C,** Pelvic rocking relieves low backache (excellent for relief of menstrual cramps as well). **D,** Abdominal breathing aids relaxation and lifts abdominal wall off uterus.

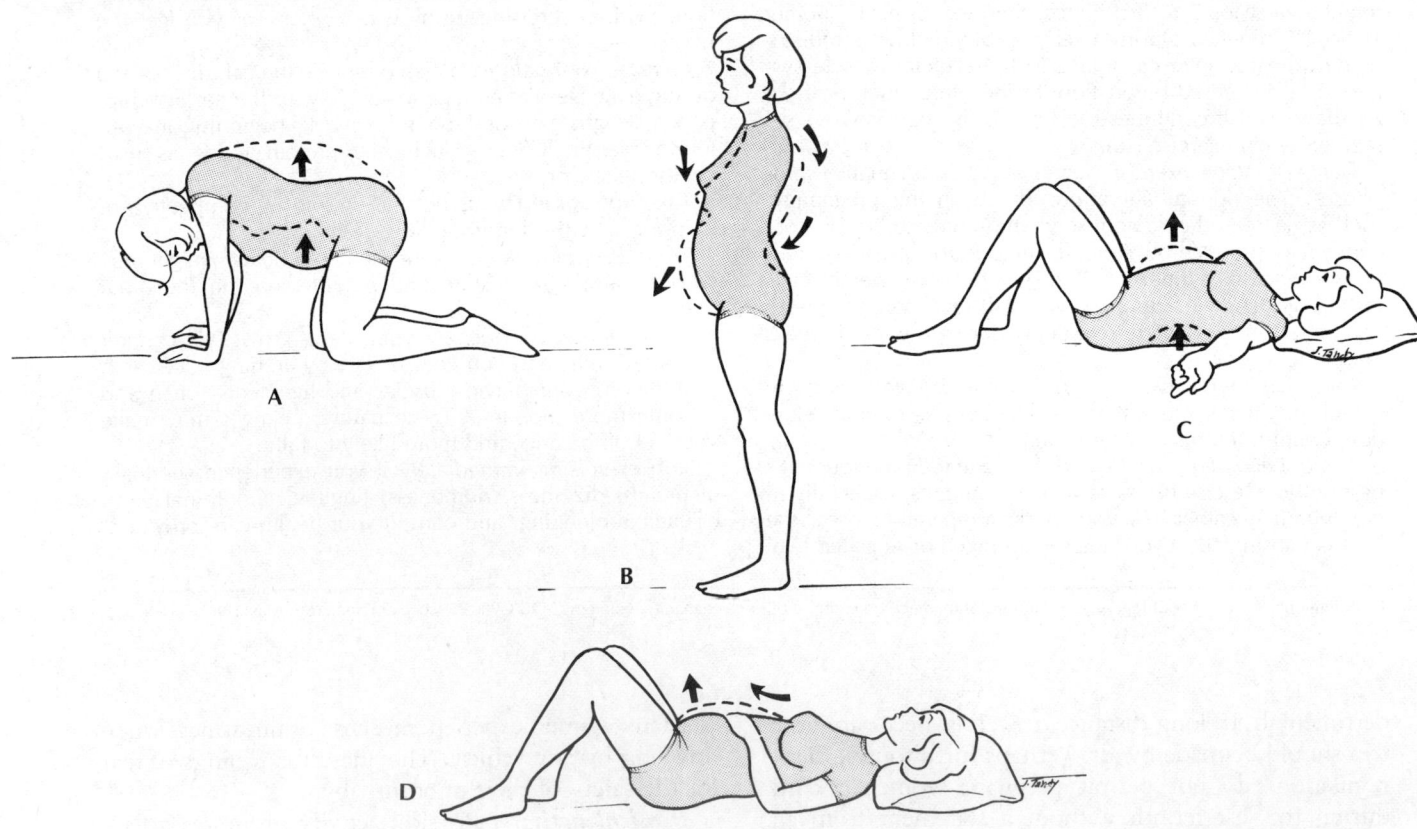

2. *Quick:* Tighten the muscle, and relax it as rapidly as possible.
3. *Push out-pull in:* Pull up the entire pelvic floor as though trying to suck up water into the vagina. Then bear down as if trying to push the imaginary water out. This uses abdominal muscles also.

Rest and relaxation. The pregnant woman is encouraged to plan regular rest periods particularly as pregnancy advances (Fig. 11.6). The side-lying position is recommended to promote uterine perfusion and fetoplacental oxygenation by eliminating pressure on the ascending vena cava (supine hypotension). During shorter rest periods, the woman can assume the position in Fig. 11.7 to promote venous drainage from the legs and relieve edema and varicose veins. The mother is shown how to rise slowly to minimize the hypotension secondary to changes in position common in the latter part of pregnancy (Fig. 11.8).

Dental health. Dental care during pregnancy is especially important. Nausea during pregnancy may lead to poor oral hygiene, and dental caries may develop.

No physiologic alteration during gestation can cause dental caries. Calcium and phosphorus in the teeth are fixed in enamel. Therefore the old adage "for every child a tooth" need not be true.

There is no scientific evidence that filling teeth or even dental extraction with the use of local or nitrous oxide-oxygen anesthesia causes abortion or premature labor. Antibacterial therapy should be considered for sepsis, however, especially in gravidas who have had rheumatic heart disease or nephritis. Extensive dental surgery is postponed until after delivery for the woman's comfort, if possible (Martin and Reeb, 1982, 1983).

Immunization. There has been some concern over the safety of various immunization techniques during pregnancy. The recommendations of the American College of Obstetricians and Gynecologists (1982) with appropriate updating for specific immunizations during pregnancy are summarized in Table 11.6 (Pritchard and others, 1985):

Fig. 11.5
Posture. **A,** Standing. **B,** Stooping. **C,** Lifting.

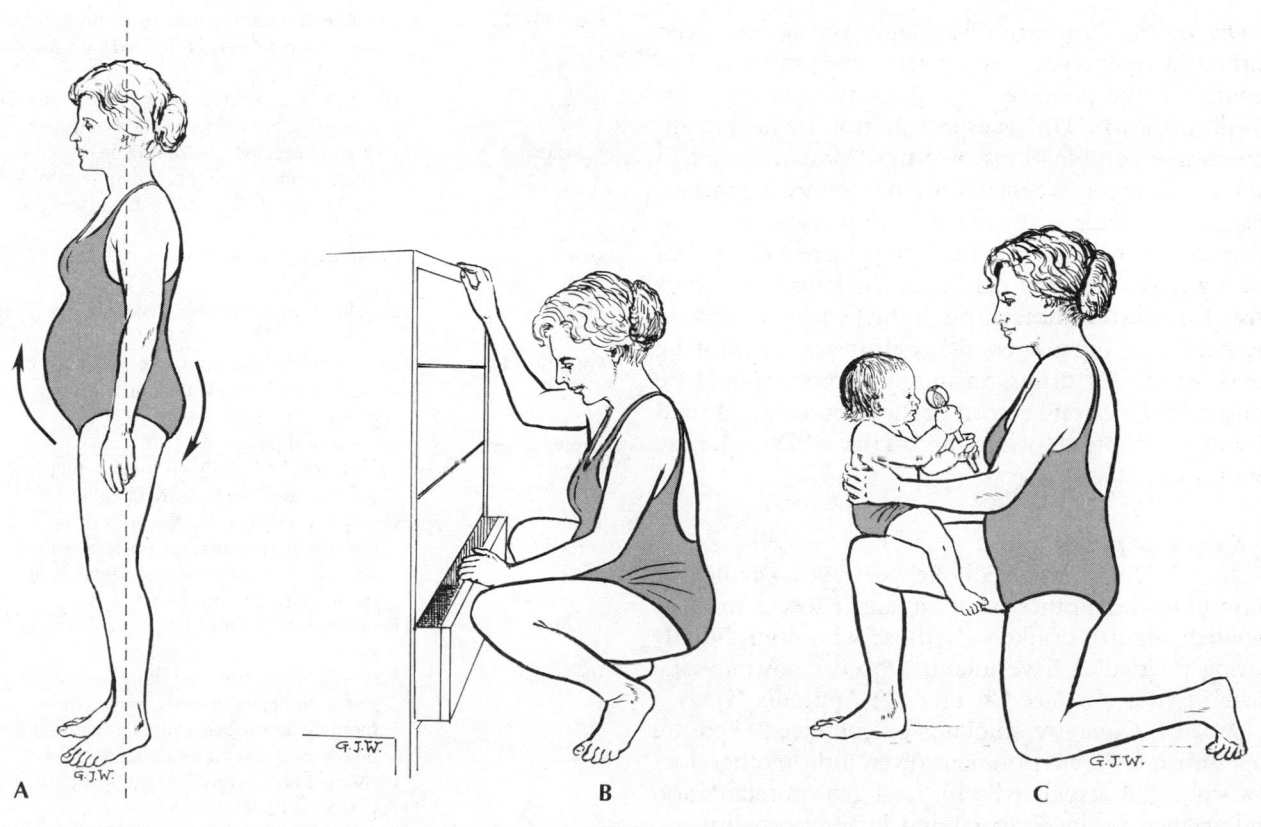

A   B   C

Fig. 11.6
Positions for rest and relaxation. **A,** Side-lying position. Some women prefer to support upper leg with pillows. **B,** Tailor sitting position aids in relaxing muscles of pelvic floor. **C,** Squatting helps to relax the pelvic floor. **D,** Position for pushing. All these positions can be assumed during labor.

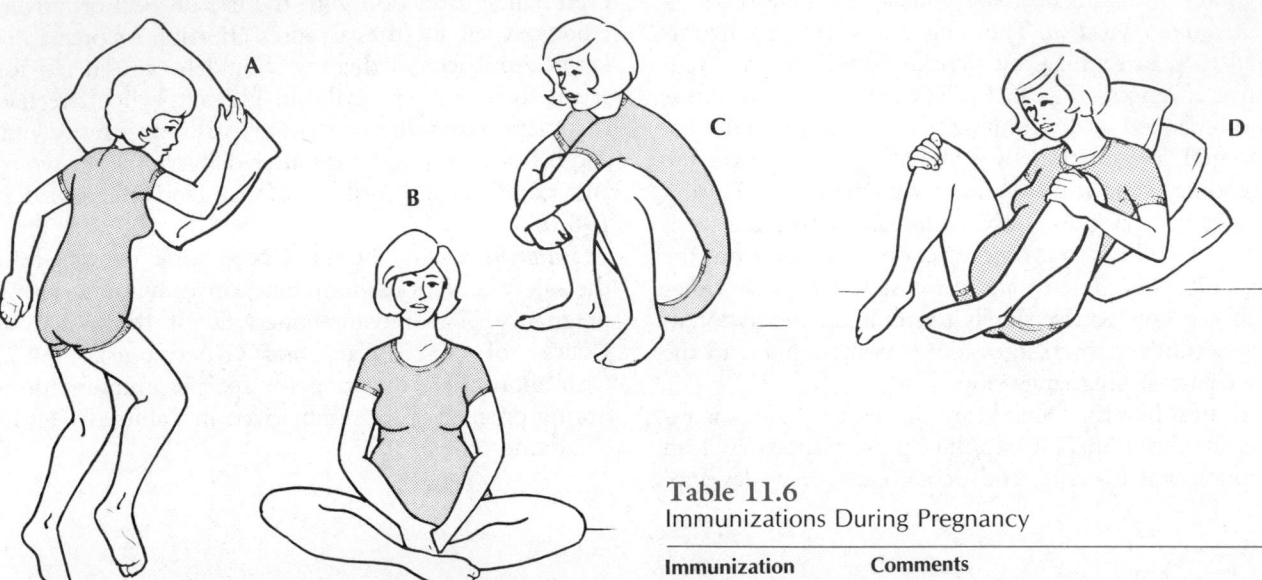

Drugs (medication). Although much has been learned in recent years about fetal drug toxicity (Appendix G), the possible teratogenicity of many drugs is still unknown. This is especially true for new medications and combinations of drugs. Moreover, certain subclinical errors or deficiencies in intermediate metabolism in the fetus may convert an otherwise harmless drug into a hazardous one. The greatest danger of causing developmental defects in the fetus from drugs exists from fertilization through the first trimester (i.e., the period of organogenesis). Self-treatment must be discouraged. All drugs, including aspirin, should be limited, and a careful record of therapeutic agents used should be kept (Howard and Hill, 1979; McKay, 1980; Luke, 1982).

Substance abuse

Alcohol. Occasional alcoholic beverages *may* not be harmful to the mother or her infant. Excesses must be avoided; regular drinkers or those who drink heavily during pregnancy have infants who demonstrate fetal alcohol syndrome (see Chapter 27; Appendix G).

Smoking. Cigarette smoking or continued exposure to a smoke-filled environment (even if the mother does not smoke) is associated with fetal growth retardation and an increase in perinatal and infant morbidity and

Table 11.6
Immunizations During Pregnancy

Immunization	Comments
Cholera	Only meet international travel requirements
Hepatitis A	After exposure; newborns of mothers who are incubating or ill should receive 1 dose after birth
Hepatitis B	Hepatitis B hyperimmune globulin to infant soon after delivery, followed by vaccination
Influenza	Evaluate pregnant woman for immunization according to criteria applied to others
Measles	Live virus vaccine contraindicated on theoretic grounds during pregnancy; pooled immune globulins for postexposure prophylaxis
Mumps	Contraindicated on theoretic grounds during pregnancy
Plague	Should be used only if substantial risk of infection
Poliomyelitis	Not recommended routinely for adults but mandatory in epidemics or when traveling to endemic area
Rabies	Same as nonpregnant
Rubella	Contraindicated although teratogenicity of vaccine appears to be negligible
Tetanus-diphtheria	Give toxoid if no primary series or no booster in 10 years; for postexposure prophylaxis with unvaccinated tetanus immune globulin and toxoid
Typhoid	Recommended if traveling in endemic region
Varicella	Varicella-zoster immune globulin may be given; indicated for newborns whose mothers developed varicella within 4 days before or 2 days after delivery
	Immunize before travel to high-risk area but postpone travel if possible

Fig. 11.7
Position for resting legs and reducing swelling, edema, and varicosities. Encourage women
with vulvar varicosities to add pillow under her hips.

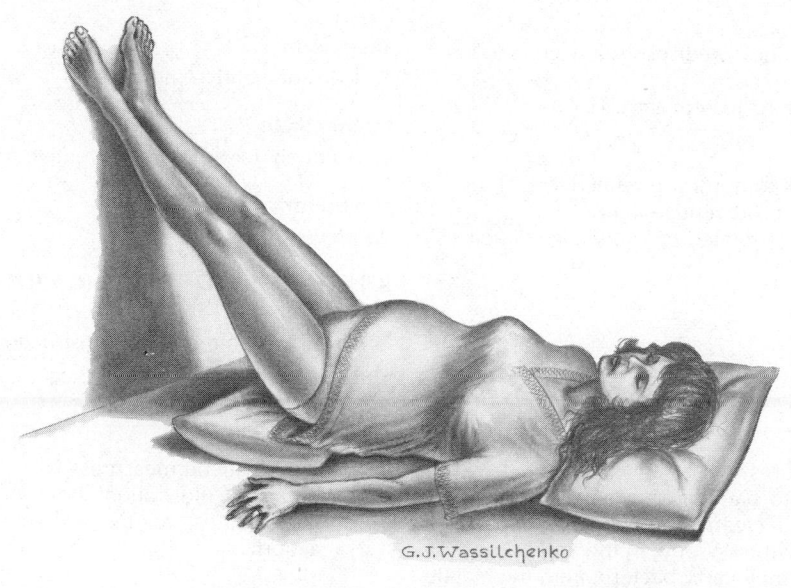

Fig. 11.8
Student in nursing laboratory practices helping mother rise slowly: turn on side, lower legs
over side of bed, come to sitting position, and wait a minute before standing. Rising by
this method also minimizes pull on round ligament.

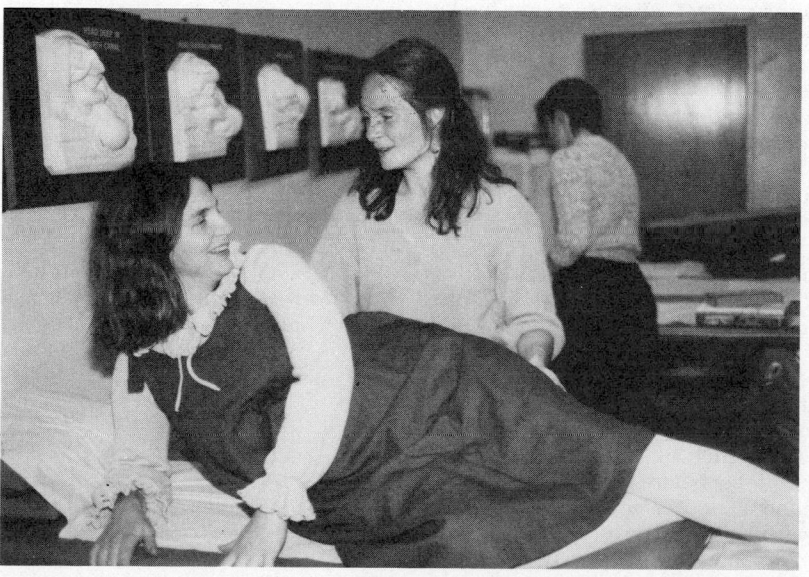

Guidelines for Client Teaching

PREVENTION OF URINARY TRACT INFECTION

ASSESSMENT
Woman is pregnant (pregnancy predisposes a woman to urinary tract infection [UTI]).
Woman is unaware of actions to prevent UTI.

NURSING DIAGNOSES
Potential for maternal/fetal compromise related to UTI.*
Knowledge deficit related to preventive actions.
Potential for noncompliance related to knowledge deficit.

GOALS
Short-term
To learn preventive methods.

Intermediate
To routinely incorporate preventive methods.

Long-term
To prevent UTI.

REFERENCES AND TEACHING AIDS
Texts
Hospital or Clinic prepared instructions, illustrations

CONTENT/RATIONALE

1. General hygiene measures
   a. Always wipe front to back after urinating or moving your bowels. Use a clean piece of toilet paper for each front to back wipe. Wiping in the opposite way, from back to front, may carry bacteria from the rectal area (anus) to the urethral opening and increase the risk of infection. Use soft, absorbent toilet paper, preferably white. Harsh, scented, or printed toilet paper may cause irritation.
   b. Change tampons, sanitary napkins, or panty shields often. Bacteria can multiply in menstrual blood or soiled panty shields.
   c. Wear underpants and panty hose with a cotton crotch. Avoid wearing tight fitting slacks for long periods. A build up of heat and moisture in the genital area may contribute to the growth of bacteria.
2. Fluid and food intake
   a. Drink 2 to 3 quarts of liquid a day. You may include 8 to 10 ounces of cranberry juice a day. Cranberry juice is more acidic than other fluids and can lower the pH of the urinary tract. A more acidic urinary tract is a less hospitable medium to developing bacteria.
   b. Include lactobacilli in the diet. Yogurt that contains the live culture and acidophilus milk may help prevent urinary tract infection as well as vaginal infections. Lactobacilli, which are normally found in the vagina and the urinary tract, maintain the normal pH balance.
3. Urination
   a. Urinate frequently. Maintain fluid intake to ensure urination; do not limit fluids to reduce frequency of urination. Do not ignore signals that indicate the need to use the bathroom. Holding your urine increases the time bacteria are in the bladder and allows them to multiply. Plan ahead when you are in situations where you will not be able to urinate for a long period of time, such as a car ride; urinate in advance. Always urinate before going to bed at night.
   b. Urinate before and after intercourse. Then drink a large glass of water so that you urinate again. This helps eliminate a medium for bacteria that are introduced during intercourse.

TEACHING ACTIONS

1. General hygiene measures
   a. Using an illustration show woman locations of urinary meatus, vagina, and anus. Provide rationale for action.

   b. Encourage discussion about perineal hygiene, for example, feelings regarding odors, vaginal discharges, touching oneself.

2. Fluid and food intake
   a. Elicit feelings or ideas reflecting cultural, ethnic, religious, or other factors affecting food and fluid intake. Provide rationale.

3. Urination
   a. Elicit information about daily schedule, for example, if working, can she get to bathroom often. Provide rationale.

*Diagnosis not included by NANDA, 1986.

mortality. Laboratory studies indicate a lowered Po_2 level in both mother and fetus during exposure to cigarette smoke. Smoking is deleterious to women with asthma, chronic respiratory infections, and allergy to pollen, dust, or dander. Smoking may result in a lessened supply of milk during lactation, and harmful substances may be transferred to the fetus in the milk.

Mind-altering drugs. The use of the drugs marijuana, heroin, and cocaine is most reported. These drugs have a deleterious effect on the fetus and should not be used (see Chapter 27, Appendix G).

Radiation. For a discussion of the dangers of radiation during pregnancy, see Chapter 9 and Appendix G.

Prevention of urinary tract infection. Pregnancy predisposes women to urinary tract infections. Women may develop a type of asymptomatic bacteriuria. They do not have cramping, pain, or burning on voiding. Most urinary tract infections are limited to the urethra and the bladder. Occasionally a urinary tract infection involves the kidney, a serious complication. Signs of serious infection include fever, chills, vomiting, and pain in the back over the kidneys (costovertebral angle tenderness) (see Chapter 29). An example of a teaching tool for the prevention of urinary tract infection, is given on p. 264.

Preparation for feeding the newborn. Pregnant women are usually eager to discuss their plans for feeding the newborn. Breast milk is the food of choice, and breast feeding is associated with a decreased incidence in perinatal morbidity and mortality. However, immaturity of the infant, deep-seated aversion to breast feeding by mother or father, and certain medical complications, such as pulmonary tuberculosis, are contraindications to breast feeding. The woman and her partner are encouraged to decide which method of feeding is suitable for them.

The decision to breast feed or bottle feed the baby is most often made for psychologcial rather than physical reasons (Dawson et al., 1979). Nicholson (1985) notes that fears mothers may have about breast-feeding, such as inadequate milk supply, may influence their choice. A mother who is the sole supporting parent may find it impossible to breast feed. In most traditional societies no alternative to breast feeding is perceived or practiced. Mothers from these societies require little or no encouragement to breast feed. Nurses need only to support their decisions.

Anticipatory guidance during pregnancy contributes to later success in breast feeding (Nicholson, 1985). The topic of infant feeding can be introduced early in pregnancy and brought up again later. Most

Fig. 11.9

A and **B,** When stimulated, normal nipples evert (protract). **C,** Unstimulated, normal, and inverted nipples look the same. **D,** and **E,** When stimulated, inverted nipples retract.

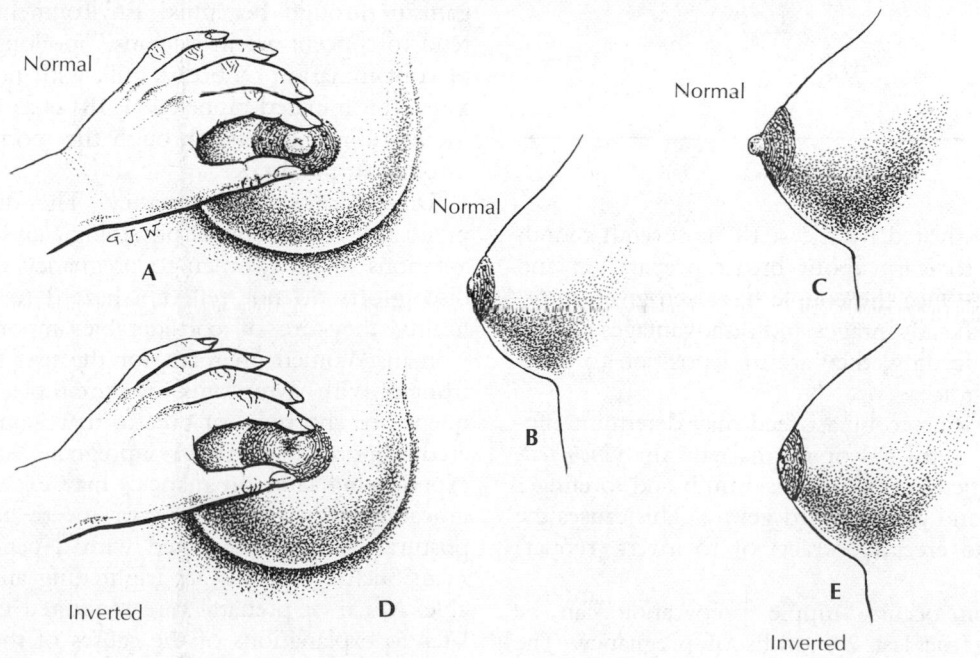

Fig. 11.10
A, and **B**, Nipple stretching. **C**, Nipple rolling. **D**, Nipple cup.

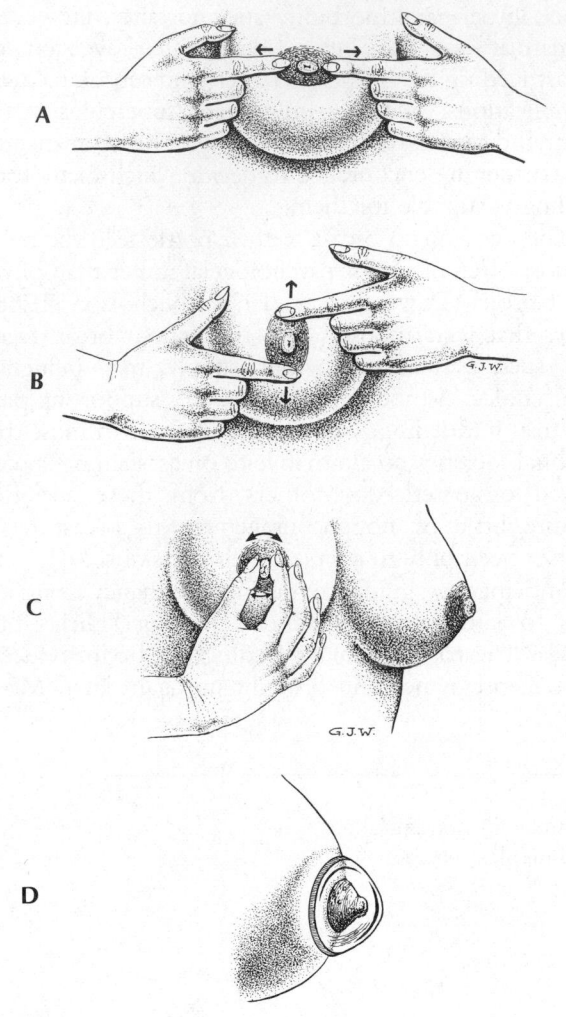

vent blocking with dried colostrum and are dried with a rough towel. The breasts are milked to remove colostrum and keep the milk ducts clear. To ensure correct usage, the nurse needs to supervise the woman's use of the following measures (Fig. 11.10).

1. *Nipple stretching.* The thumbs are placed close to the inverted nipple, pressing firmly into the breast tissue, and gradually pushing away from the areola. The massage is done vertically and horizontally and is repeated five times (Fig. 11.10, *A* and *B*).
2. *Nipple rolling.* The nipple is stimulated by gently rolling it between the fingers (Fig. 11.10, *C*).
3. *Nipple cups.* Plastic doughnut-shaped cups are available for correcting inversions or retractions (Fig. 11.10, *D*). A continuous, gentle pressure exerted around the areola pushes the nipple through a central opening in the inner shield. Nipple cups should be worn during the last two trimesters of pregnancy for 1 to 2 hours daily. The time for wearing them should be increased gradually. Brand names for these cups include Woolwich, Netsy, La Leche League Cups, Nurse-Dri, Free and Dry, and Hobbit Shields. They can also be worn after childbirth. However, because body warmth can foster rapid bacterial growth and contamination, milk that collects in the cup should be discarded and not fed to the infant (Riordan, 1983).

The possibility of contaminants in breast milk concerns many women, both consumers and professionals (Doucette, 1978). Breast milk can be potentially hazardous as illustrated in the following examples. The mother harboring *Salmonella kottbus* transmits this organism through her milk. Environmental pollutants tend to concentrate in humans. The long-term effects of contamination of breast milk with pollutants such as polybrominated biphenyl (PBB) is as yet unknown. Medications that pass through the mother's milk are listed in Appendix K.

Discomforts of pregnancy. The discomforts of pregnancy are a result of physiologic and anatomic adaptations of the woman to pregnancy. Although the discomforts do not reflect a hazard to the woman's health, they are of considerable importance to the woman. Women pregnant for the first time are confronted with symptoms, for example, urinary frequency or shortness of breath, that would be considered abnormal in the nonpregnant state. Women experiencing later pregnancies may experience an aggravation of varicose veins or severe backache from postural changes associated with a pendulous abdomen. Such symptoms are frightening and uncomfortable. Much of prenatal care requested by women relates to explanations of the causes of the discomforts and what measures can be taken to relieve them. The

women are motivated by the sixth or seventh month of pregnancy to learn about breast preparation and breast feeding. Once the couple has been given information about the advantages and disadvantages of bottle and breast feeding, they are in a position to make an informed choice.

Women desiring to breast feed may determine nipple formation (retracted or normal) by the *pinch test*. They are instructed to place the thumb and forefinger on the areola and press inward gently. This causes the nipple to stand erect (protract) or to invert (retract) (Fig. 11.9).

If retraction occurs, nipple preparation can be started during the last 2 months of pregnancy. The nipples are cleansed with mild soap and water to pre-

discomforts are fairly specific to each trimester of pregnancy:

First trimester
Pain and tingling in the breasts
Urgency and frequency of urination
Languor and malaise
Nausea and vomiting
Second trimester
Constipation
Heartburn
Increased pigmentation
Leg cramps
Pica
Third trimester
Hemorrhoids
Varicosities
Leg cramps

Hypermobility of joints
Backache
Urinary frequency

Nurses can anticipate the appearance of these symptoms and provide anticipatory guidance for women. Table 11.7 contains information about the physiology, prevention, and treatment of the discomforts. Women who have a knowledge of the physical basis for the discomforts of pregnancy are less apt to become overly anxious concerning their health. An understanding of the rationale for treatment promotes their participation in their own care. Nurses need to use terminology the woman (or couple) can understand. To help a woman cope with the discomforts of pregnancy, they can advocate use of the conscious relaxation guide and flying exercise.

Text continued on p. 272.

Table 11.7
Discomforts Related to Maternal Adaptations to Pregnancy

Discomfort	Physiology	Prevention	Treatment
Gastrointestinal (GI) tract			
"Morning" sickness—occurs in 50% to 75% of pregnant women; starts between first and second missed periods and lasts until about fourth missed period; may occur any time during day; if mother does not have symptoms, expectant father may; may be accompanied by "bad taste" in mouth	Cause unknown (may result from hormonal changes, possibly human chorionic gonadotropin [HCG]; may be partly emotional, reflecting pride in, ambivalence about, or rejection of pregnant state)	Avoid empty or overloaded stomach, offending odors, or foods hard to digest; maintain good posture—give stomach ample room; stop or decrease smoking	Eat dry carbohydrate on awakening; remain in bed until feeling subsides, *or* alternate dry carbohydrate one hour with fluids such as hot tea, milk, or clear coffee the next hour until feeling subsides; eat 5 to 6 small meals per day; avoid fried, odorous, spicy, greasy, or gas-forming foods; consult physician if intractable vomiting (hyperemesis gravidarum, food poisoning, infectious disease) occurs; reassurance
Food cravings	Cause unknown; cravings determined by culture or geographic area	Not preventable	Satisfy craving unless it interferes with well-balanced diet; report unusual cravings (eg., pica: laundry starch, clay, dirt) to physician
Ptyalism (excessive salivation)—may occur starting 2 to 3 weeks after first missed period	Elevated estrogen levels (?)	Not preventable	Astringent mouth wash; chewing gum
Gingivitis and epulis (hyperemia, hypertrophy, bleeding, tenderness)	Increased vascularity and proliferation of connective tissue from estrogen stimulation	Well-balanced diet with adequate protein and fresh fruits and vegetables; avoid trauma; good dental hygiene	Gentle brushing and good dental hygiene; avoid infection; reassurance that condition will disappear spontaneously 1 to 2 months after delivery
Heartburn, pyrosis, or acid indigestion: burning sensation in lower chest or upper abdomen, occasionally with	Progesterone slows GI tract motility and digestion, reverses peristalsis, relaxes cardiac sphincter, and de-	Limit or avoid gas-producing or fatty foods and large meals; maintain good posture to give GI tract ample	Sips of milk for temporary relief; hot tea, chewing gum; physician may prescribe antacid (aluminum hydrox-

Continued.

Table 11.7, cont'd
Discomforts Related to Maternal Adaptations to Pregnancy

Discomfort	Physiology	Prevention	Treatment
Gastrointestinal (GI) tract—cont'd			
burping and raising of a little sour-tasting fluid	lays emptying time of stomach; stomach displaced upward and compressed by enlarging uterus; may be associated with tension, nausea, and vomiting in early pregnancy	space; keep torso upright to reach below the waist (bend down at knees)	ide, magnesium trisilicate, or magnesium hydroxide [Amphojel, Gelusil, Maalox, milk of magnesia]) between meals (NOTE: *Do not* use baking soda or Alka-Seltzer [both have high salt content] or patent medicines); flying exercise; refer to physician for persistent symptoms to rule out hiatal hernia or peptic ulcer
Constipation	GI tract motility slowed because of progesterone, resulting in increased resorption of water and drying of stool; intestines compressed by enlarging uterus; predisposition to constipation (some women respond with diarrhea) because of oral iron supplementation	Six glasses of water per day; roughage in diet: bran, course ground cereals, fresh fruits and vegetables; moderate exercise; sit on toilet seat with feet supported on footstool and maintain regular schedule for bowel movements; use relaxation techniques and deep breathing	Treatment same as prevention; *do not* take stool softener, laxatives, other drugs, or enemas without first consulting physician; *never* ingest mineral oil, since this inhibits absorption of fat-soluble vitamins
Hemorrhoids—see Cardiovascular system			
Flatulence with bloating and belching	Reduced GI motility because of hormones, allowing time for bacterial action that produces gas; swallowing air	Chew solid foods slowly and thoroughly; avoid gas-producing foods, fatty foods, large meals	Treatment same as prevention; exercise; regular bowel habits
Cardiovascular system (CVS)			
Faintness and, rarely, syncope (orthostatic hypotension)	Vasomotor lability or postural hypotension from hormones; in late pregnancy may be caused by venous stasis in lower extremities	Moderate exercise, deep breathing, vigorous leg movement; avoid sudden changes in position* and warm crowded areas; move slowly and deliberately; keep environment cool; avoid hypoglycemia by eating 5 to 6 small meals per day	Treatment same as prevention; elastic hose; sit down as necessary; rise slowly so CVS has time to adjust to upright position (Fig. 11.8); if symptoms are serious, refer to physician for possible neurologic disorder or hypoglycemia
Supine hypotension (vena cava syndrome)	Posture induced by pressure of gravid uterus on ascending vena cava when woman is supine; reduces uterine-placental and renal perfusion	Side-lying position or semi-sitting posture, with knees slightly flexed	Treatment same as prevention
Palpitations	Unknown; should not be accompanied by persistent cardiac irregularity	Not preventable	Reassaurance; refer to physician if accompanied by symptoms of cardiac decompensation
Ankle edema (nonpitting) to lower extremities	Posture aggravated by prolonged standing, sitting, or hot weather	Good posture; avoidance of prolonged standing or sitting; moderate exercise; avoidance of constrictive clothing (e.g., *garters*); ample fluid intake for "natural" diuretic effect	Treatment same as prevention; put on support stockings before arising; rest periodically with legs and hips elevated; refer to physician if generalized edema develops even if other symptoms of preeclampsia are not found; diuretics *contraindicated*

*Caution woman to rise slowly and sit on edge of bed or to assume hands-and-knees posture before rising, and to get up slowly after sitting or squatting.

Table 11.7, cont'd
Discomforts Related to Maternal Adaptations to Pregnancy

Discomfort	Physiology	Prevention	Treatment
Varicose veins (large distended, tortuous, superficial veins—may be associated with aching legs and tenderness; may be present in legs, vulva, and perianal area (hemorrhoids, piles)	Hereditary predisposition; relaxation of smooth muscle walls of veins because of hormones, causing pelvic vasocongestion; condition aggravated by enlarging uterus, gravity, and bearing down for bowel movements or during second stage of labor; thrombi from leg varices rare but may be produced by hemorrhoids	Avoidance of obesity, lengthy standing or sitting, constrictive clothing, and constipation and bearing down with bowel movements; moderate exercises	Treatment same as prevention; rest with legs and hips elevated (Fig. 11.7); support stockings applied before rising—may need assistance with this as abdominal size increases; thrombosed hemorrhoid may be evacuated; outlet forceps delivery may prevent enlargement of hemorrhoids; relieve swelling and pain with hot sitz baths, local application of astringent compresses (witch hazel)
Spider nevi (telangiectases)—appear during trimesters 2 or 3 over neck, thorax, face, and arms (in that order) in two thirds of women	Focal networks of dilated arterioles (end-arteries) from increased concentration of estrogens	Not preventable	Reassurance that they fade slowly during late puerperium; rarely disappear completely
Palmar erythema occurs in 50% of pregnant women; may accompany spider nevi	Diffuse reddish mottling over palms and suffused skin over thenar eminences and fingertips may be caused by genetic predisposition or hyperestrogenism	Not preventable	Reassurance that condition will fade within 1 wk after giving birth
Respiratory system			
Shortness of breath and dyspnea—occur in 60% of pregnant women	Expansion of diaphragm limited by enlarging uterus (compensated for in part by other maternal adaptations); may be caused by increased sensitivity to or compensation for slight acidosis ("breathing for two")	Not preventable; avoid anemia	Good posture; flying exercise; sleep with extra pillows; avoid overloading stomach; stop smoking; refer to physician if symptoms worsen to rule out anemia, emphysema, and asthma
Nasal stuffiness	Increased vascularization because of hormones	Not preventable	Reassurance that condition will return to normal during puerperium
Musculoskeletal system			
Leg cramps (gastrocnemius spasm)—especially when reclining	Compression of nerves supplying lower extremities because of enlarging uterus; reduced level of diffusible serum calcium or elevation of serum phosphorus; aggravating factors: fatigue, poor peripheral circulation	Avoid pointing toes when stretching legs and lead with heel of foot when walking; avoid drinking more than 1 L (1 qt) of milk per day (may need to limit to 0.5 L [1 pt]); avoid fatigue and cold legs; diet with adequate calcium	Rule out blood clot by checking for Homans' sign; if Homans' sign negative, use massage and heat over affected muscle; stretch affected muscle by standing up and leaning forward on affected leg or by having another person extend knee and dorsiflex foot of affected leg until spasm relaxes (Fig. 11.11); stand on cold surface; treatment same as prevention; oral supplementation with calcium carbonate or calcium lactate tablets, 0.6 g, three times a day before meals; aluminum hydroxide gel, 1 oz, with each meal removes phosphorus by absorbing it

Continued.

Table 11.7, cont'd
Discomforts Related to Maternal Adaptations to Pregnancy

Discomfort	Physiology	Prevention	Treatment
Musculoskeletal system—cont'd			
Joint pain, backache, and pelvic pressure; hypermobility of joints	Relaxation of symphyseal and sacroiliac joints because of hormones, resulting in unstable pelvis; exaggerated lumbar and cervicothoracic curves caused by change in center of gravity from enlarging abdomen	Maternity girdle; good posture and body mechanics; tuck pelvis under baby; bend at knees; avoid fatigue; wear shoes with 5 cm (2 in) heels; conscious relaxation; exercises to strengthen back muscles; firm mattress	Treatment same as prevention; local heat and back rubs; pelvic rock exercise; rest; reassure that condition will go away 6-8 wk after delivery
Renal system			
Urinary frequency and urgency	Vascular engorgement and altered bladder function caused by hormones; bladder capacity reduced by enlarging uterus and fetal presenting part	Not preventable; Kegel exercises to strengthen pubococcygeal muscle; limit fluid intake before bedtime to ensure rest	Treatment same as prevention; reassurance; wear perineal pad; refer to physician for pain or burning sensation
Integumentary system			
Spider nevi—see Cardiovascular system			
Pruritus (noninflammatory)	Unknown cause; various types as follows:	Keep fingernails short and clean	Refer to physician for diagnosis of cause
	Nonpapular	Not preventable	Symptomatic: Keri baths; mild sedation
	Closely aggregated pruritic papules	Not preventable	As for nonpapular type
	Increased excretory function of skin and stretching of skin possible factors	Distraction; tepid (not hot) baths with sodium bicarbonate or oatmeal added to water	Treatment same as prevention; lotions and oils; change of soaps or reduction in use of soap; loose clothing
Deepened pigmentation (striae gravidarum, chloasma, linea nigra, fingernails, hair) acne, oily skin			Usually resolved during puerperium; reassurance given to women and their families about these manifestations of pregnant state
Rashes	Various causes; infection, reaction to drugs, allergies	Dependent on underlying condition	Refer to physician for diagnosis: drug reactions; allergies; herpes gestationis
Breast changes, new sensations	Hypertrophy of mammary glandular tissue and increased vascularization, pigmentation, and size and prominence of nipples and areolas caused by hormone stimulation	Not preventable; supportive maternity brassiere with pads to absorb discharge may be worn at night; wash with warm water and keep dry	Treatment same as prevention; see Maternal physiology and sexual counseling
Neurologic system			
Feelings during pregnancy (Chapter 10): mood swings, mixed feelings	Hormonal and metabolic adaptations; plus feelings about female role, sexuality, timing of pregnancy, and resultant changes in one's life and life-style	Not preventable; reassurance and support; supportive significant other who can reassure woman about her attractiveness, etc.; improved communication with her partner, family, and others	Treatment same as prevention; both partners need support; refer to social worker, if needed, or supportive services (financial assistance, food stamps)

Table 11.7, cont'd
Discomforts Related to Maternal Adaptations to Pregnancy

Discomfort	Physiology	Prevention	Treatment
Faintness and syncope—see Cardiovascular system			
Headaches	Emotional tension (more common than vascular migraine headache); eye strain (refractory errors); vascular engorgement and congestion of sinuses from hormone stimulation	Emotional support; prenatal teaching timed to need; conscious relaxation	Treatment same as prevention; refer to physician for constant "splitting" headache, either frontal, sincipital, occipital, or bilateral after assessing for pregnancy induced hypertension (PIH)
Carpal tunnel syndrome (involves thumb, second and third fingers, lateral side of little finger)	Compression of median nerve from changes in surrounding tissues: pain, numbness, tingling, burning; loss of skilled movements (typing); dropping of objects	Not preventable	Elevation of affected arms; splinting of affected hand may help; surgery is curative
Periodic numbness, tingling of fingers (acrodysesthesia)—occurs in 5% of pregnant women	Brachial plexus traction syndrome from drooping of shoulders during pregnancy (occurs especially at night and early morning)	Maintain good posture; wear good supportive maternity brassiere	Treatment same as prevention; reassurance that condition will disappear if lifting and carrying baby does not aggravate it
Miscellaneous conditions			
Fatigue (early pregnancy, usually)	Unexplained; may be due to increasing levels of estrogen, progesterone, and HCG or to elevated basal body temperature (BBT)	Not preventable; avoid anemia	Reassurance; rest prn; well-balanced diet to prevent anemia
Insomnia (later weeks of pregnancy)	Fetal movements, muscular cramping, urinary frequency, shortness of breath, or other discomforts	Not preventable; conscious relaxation	Reassurance; conscious relaxation; back massage; support of body parts with pillows; warm milk or warm shower before retiring
Abdominal discomfort			
Pressure	Pressure from enlarging uterus, especially when standing or walking; multiple gestation	Not preventable	Rest, conscious relaxation and good posture; maternity girdle; refer to physician for assessment and treatment if pain is present (appendicitis, urinary tract infection, abruptio placentae, gallbladder disease, torsion of adnexa); if near term, rule out labor
Braxton Hicks' contractions	Intensification of uterine contractions in preparation for work of labor	Necessary uterine function	Reassurance; rest; change of position; practice breathing techniques when contractions are bothersome
Round ligament pain (tenderness)	Stretching of ligament caused by enlarging uterus	Not preventable; avoid further stretching (e.g., to get out of bed, roll on side first, then push self to sitting position with hands)	Reassurance, rest, good body mechanics to avoid overstretching ligament; relieve cramping by squatting or bringing knees to chest
GI discomforts—see Gastrointestinal tract			
Leukorrhea	Hormonally stimulated cervix becomes hypertrophic and hyperactive, producing abundant amount of mucus	Not preventable; do not douche	Hygiene; perineal pads; reassurance; refer to physician if accompanied by pruritis, foul odor, or change in character of color

Fig. 11.11

Relief for muscle spasm (leg cramps). Have another person extend woman's knee and dorsiflex foot until spasm relaxes. (From Lerch, C.: Maternity nursing, St. Louis, 1970, The C.V. Mosby Co.)

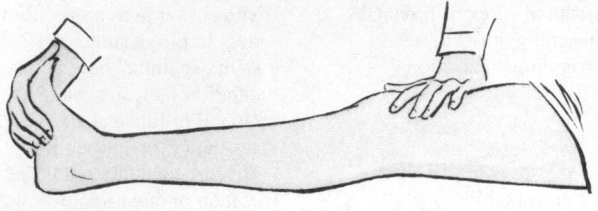

Conscious relaxation guide

Definition and rationale. Relaxation is the release of the mind and body from tension through conscious effort and practice. The ability to relax consciously and intentionally can be beneficial for the following reasons:

1. Relief of normal discomforts related to pregnancy
2. Reduction of stress and therefore diminished pain perception during the childbearing cycle
3. Heightened self-awareness and trust in own ability to control one's responses and functions
4. Coping with stress in everyday life situations, pregnant or not

The techniques for conscious relaxation are numerous and varied. The following guidelines can be used by anyone:

1. Preparation: Loosen clothing, assume a comfortable sitting or side-lying position with all parts of body well-supported.
2. Beginning: Allow self to feel warm and comfortable. Inhale and exhale slowly, and imagine peaceful relaxation coming over each part of the body starting with the neck and working down to the toes. Often persons who learn conscious relaxation speak of feeling relaxed even if some discomfort is present.
3. Maintenance: Imagine (fantasize or daydream) to maintain the state of relaxation. With active imagery the person imagines herself as moving or doing some activity and experiencing its sensations. With passive imagery, one imagines watching a scene, such as a lovely sunset.
4. Awakening: The return to the wakeful state is gradual. The person begins slowly to take in the stimuli from the surrounding environment.
5. Further retention and development of the skill: Regular practice for regular periods of time each day, for example, at the same hour for 10 to 15

minutes each day, is refreshing, revitalizing, and invigorating.

Flying exercise (Fig. 11.12)

1. Sit tailor or Indian fashion. *Keep back straight throughout exercise.*
2. Raise arms over head. Elbows are straight and palms are held toward each other.
3. With palms facing upward, lower arms out to sides.
4. Reach behind back and try to bring backs of hands together briskly; repeat five times.
5. With hands in lap, shrug shoulders (upward toward ears) while breathing in through the nose.
6. Passively and slowly let out breath while letting go of shoulders.

Sexual counseling during pregnancy. Counseling couples concerning sexual adjustment during pregnancy demands self-assessment by the nurse as well as a knowledge of the physical, social, and emotional responses to sex during pregnancy (Zalar, 1976). Pregnant women or couples continue to be sexual beings. The expectant woman or couple needs information about sexual activities and possible changes that may be encountered in feelings and behaviors. Not all maternity nurses are comfortable dealing with the sexual concerns of their clients. The nurse who is aware of her personal stengths and limitations in dealing with sexual content is in a better position to make referrals when necessary.

The role of the maternity nurse in sexual counseling is defined by the origin and severity of the sexual problem encountered. There are a significant number of clients who merely need *permission* to be sexual during pregnancy. Many other clients need *information* about the physiologic changes that occur during pregnancy and an opportunity to debunk myths associated with sex during pregnancy. Giving permission and providing information are within the purview of the maternity nurse and should be an integral component of providing health care.

A smaller number of couples must be referred for either *sex therapy* or *family therapy.* Couples with sexual dysfunction problems of long standing that may be intensified by pregnancy should be referred for sex therapy. When a sexual problem is a symptom of a more serious interactional problem, the couple would benefit from family therapy.

Obtaining a history. The history provides a baseline for sexual counseling. History taking is an ongoing process. Receptivity to changes in attitudes, body image, marital relationships, and physical status is relevant throughout pregnancy. When changes occur, unexpected problems may develop that require intervention. The history reveals the client's knowledge

Fig. 11.12
Flying exercise.

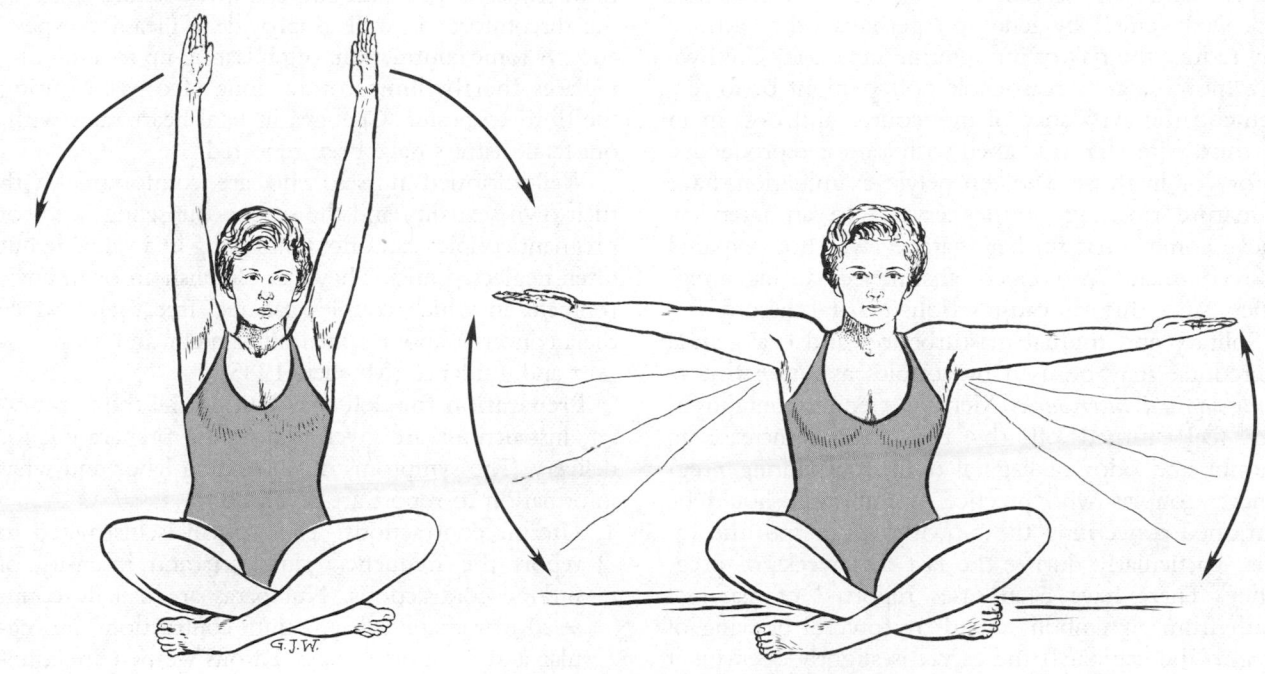

of female anatomy and physiology, attitudes about sex during pregnancy, as well as perceptions of the pregnancy, the health status of the couple, and the quality of their marital relationship. Identification of the couple's subjective experience provides the direction and focus of sexual counseling. Sexual counseling includes countering misinformation, providing reassurance of normalcy, and suggesting alternative behaviors. The uniqueness of each couple is considered within a biopsychosocial framework.

Countering misinformation. Many myths and much of the misinformation related to sex and pregnancy are masked behind seemingly unrelated issues. For example, a question about the baby's ability to hear and see in utero may be related to the baby's role as a third person in lovemaking. The counselor must be extremely sensitive to questions behind the question when counseling in this highly charged emotional area.

Fetal heart rate decreases during orgasm; however, fetal distress has not been noted. Although it has been suggested that premature delivery may be induced by the effect of oxytocin released during maternal response, by orgasmic contractions, or by prostaglandins in the male ejaculate, researchers have not validated these hypotheses. When possible the couple is counseled together. Expectant parent education classes can

also be an effective way to explore these kinds of concerns because of the support and sharing offered by the group.

Providing reassurance of normalcy. Couples are relieved to learn that their fears and concerns do not make them "weird" or "crazy." A breast-feeding mother may welcome the knowledge that her erotic response to suckling is normal. At the same time the father may be relieved to know that many fathers are jealous of their suckling infants.

It is important for the counselor to view sexuality in its broadest sense. Kissing, hugging, massaging, petting, and increased gentleness and sensitivity are valid forms of sexual expression and signs of affection. Each of these behaviors is pleasurable in itself and is not always a preliminary behavior leading to intercourse. When a couple cannot have, or chooses not to have, penile-vaginal intercourse, the need for closeness and intimacy can be expressed in many other ways.

Suggesting alternative behaviors. To date research has not proved conclusively that coitus and orgasm are contraindicated at any time during pregnancy for the obstetrically and medically healthy woman (Mill and others, 1981; Naeye, 1981; Flood and Naeye, 1984). However, a history of more than one spontaneous abortion or a threatened abortion in the first trimester, impending miscarriage in the second trimester, or premature rupture of membranes, bleeding, or abdominal pain during the third trimester warrant precaution against coitus and orgasm. Naeye (1979) suggests that improved genital hygiene and perhaps other actions may reduce the risk of intrauterine infection. Until we have more data, "a reasonable policy might be to recommend the avoidance of intercourse and orgasm in the third trimester in women with a poor reproductive history or in those who, on pelvic examination, have premature ripening of the cervix." In an interview Naeye commented further that he "was not prepared to recommend prolonged abstinence during pregnancy, since this can cause serious marital discord."

Solitary and mutual masturbation and oral-genital intercourse may be used by couples as *alternatives to penile-vaginal intercourse*. Men who enjoy cunnilingus may feel "turned off" by the normal increase in amount and odor of vaginal discharges during pregnancy. Couples who practice cunnilingus should be cautioned concerning the blowing of air into the vagina, particularly during the last few weeks of pregnancy. There have been cases reported of maternal death from air emboli caused by forceful blowing of air into the vagina. If the cervix is slightly open (as it may be near term), there is the possibility that air will be forced between the membranes and the uterine wall. Some air may enter the maternal placental lakes, thus gaining entrance into the maternal vascular bed.

The woman or couple should also be cautioned against masturbatory activities when orgasmic contractions are contraindicated. Studies have shown that orgasm is often more intense when induced by masturbation. After being cautioned against orgasm, some women require reassurance if they experience erotic dreams.

Pictures of possible variations of *coital position* are often helpful. The female-superior, side-by-side, and rear-entry positions are possible alternative positions to the traditional male-superior position. The woman astride (superior position) allows her to control the angle and depth of penile penetration as well as to protect her abdomen. The side-by-side position is the one of choice, especially during the third trimester, since it requires reduced energy and pressure on the pregnant abdomen. For other positions, the reader is referred to Bing and Colman (1977) and McCary (1982).

Multiparous women have reported severe *breast tenderness* in the first trimester. A coital position that avoids direct pressure on the woman's breasts and decreased breast fondling during love play can be recommended. The woman should also be reassured that this condition is normal and temporary. *Lactating mothers* lose milk in uncontrolled spurts in response to sexual stimulation. The couple that is forewarned can be prepared for this eventuality.

Some women complain of lower abdominal cramping and backache after orgasm during the first and third trimesters. A back rub can often relieve some of the discomfort, as well as provide a pleasant experience. A tonic contraction, often lasting up to a minute, replaces the rhythmic contractions of orgasm during the third trimester. Changes in fetal heart rates without fetal distress have been reported.

Well-informed nurses who are comfortable with their own sexuality and the sexual counseling needs of pregnant couples can offer counseling in a valuable but often neglected area. They can establish an open environment in which couples can feel free to introduce their concerns about sexual adjustment and seek support and guidance (Mueller, 1985).

Preparation for delivery. During the third trimester, instructions are given concerning preparation for delivery. The symptoms of impending labor and what information to report are reviewed:

1. Uterine contractions: The woman is instructed to report the frequency, duration, and intensity of uterine contractions. Nulliparas are usually counseled to remain at home until contractions are regular and 5 minutes apart. Parous women are counseled to remain at home until contractions are regular and 10 minutes apart. If the woman lives more than 20 minutes from the hospital or has a history of rapid labors, these instructions are modified accordingly.
2. Rupture of the membranes (see Chapter 16).
3. Bloody "show": The "show" is scant, pink in color, and sticky (contains mucus).

If the woman or couple is not attending classes in preparation for parenthood, the clinic or office nurse assumes responsibility for instruction. The instruction includes information about the following:

1. Process of labor
2. Methods to control pain (e.g., analgesia and anesthesia, breathing-relaxing techniques)
3. Responsibilities of the spouse, family member, or friend who will be accompanying the woman through labor and delivery
4. Care of the newborn (i.e., clothing, feeding, daily hygienic care)

If a hospital delivery is planned, the woman is required to register at the hospital of choice. Most hospitals now provide pamphlets containing information such as where to report when labor begins and policies pertaining to visitors and visiting hours. Many facilities also conduct tours.

Counseling is provided to relieve emotional tensions. These tensions often relate directly to the childbirth experience (e.g., anxiety about pain or possible delivery of the child before reaching the hospital). Nursing strategies include providing an opportunity for discussing the woman's specific fears or anxieties, helping her make definite plans concerning what she will do when labor starts, repeating instructions willingly, and having "sharing sessions" with mothers who have recently delivered. If possible, involve significant others in preparation for the birth. Arrange to have them participate in a supportive way during labor and delivery. These techniques may be effective in allaying or diffusing anxiety.

Most men whose wives are approaching labor may have their anxieties decreased through intervention before the event. Fantasies can be replaced by knowledge gained through activities such as the following:

1. A hospital tour to enable visualization of the labor room and waiting areas (This will allow him to envision the environment, familiarize himself with the delivery room and determine what his role will be.)
2. A demonstration of helping and supportive measures to comfort his wife during labor
3. A brief review of what to expect from his wife during the labor process if she has medication or anesthesia or if she delivers without medication or anesthesia (e.g., irritability, breathing, grunting)
4. A description of what to expect of the staff during his wife's labor

A realistic discussion of all known factors helps the father problem-solve more rationally and plan for the event. Such discussions are ego strengthening because they help focus the father's energies toward more appropriate coping strategies by helping alleviate anxieties about the unknown. Today many men elect to participate actively during labor and the delivery of their child. However, some men through personal or cultural concepts of the father role neither wish to nor intend to participate. *The important concept is that the partners agree on the other's roles.* For nurses to advocate any changes in these roles may cause confusion or feelings of guilt.

TECHNICIAN

The technical aspects of prenatal care center around assessment techniques designed for health maintenance and detection of disability. These techniques also can be used for teaching purposes. Careful and concise recording of client responses or laboratory results contribute to the continuous supervision vital to the mother and fetus.

Pelvic examination. The pelvic examination is essential to provide baseline data for care during pregnancy. Some women have experienced the pelvic examination as part of their gynecologic care. For others the pelvic examination early in pregnancy is their first experience. Every effort needs to be made to put them at ease. The examination causes less discomfort in the

relaxed woman and more information can be obtained. The woman is instructed to refrain from douching or using vaginal medications for 24 hours before the examination. Douching and medications cloud diagnosis, which is based on secretions, cells, and odor. In addition, douching removes vaginal secretions and makes insertion of the vaginal speculum more difficult. Some women have a hard time complying with this request; they cannot go to a doctor feeling unclean in the genital region. Procedure 11.1 outlines the care of a woman undergoing this examination.

Collection of specimens. Collection of specimens for examination is an important part of prenatal care. Once the diagnoses have been made, treatment for protection of mother and fetus can be instituted. **Carcinogenic conditions,** potential or actual, can be determined by examination of cells from the cervix collected during the pelvic examination (Procedure 11.2).

Infection also can be diagnosed through examination of specimens collected during the pelvic examination. These infections include gonorrhea, *Chlamydia trachomatis,* and herpes simplex 1 and 2.

Gonorrheal culture. A culture for gonorrhea is done to screen women for gonorrheal infection that could compromise the woman, her fetus, and her partner. The woman is told the reason for the test (e.g., test for vaginal infection) and that the test is done routinely at the first prenatal visit and repeated toward the end of pregnancy (thirty-sixth week).

The specimen is obtained at the same time as the Papanicolaou smear, and the same precautions regarding use of digital examinations and lubricant are followed. A specimen is obtained from the endocervical canal using a sterile cotton-tipped applicator (Fig. 11.13). The applicator is rolled on a culture plate with a special medium (Thayer-Martin). The plate is then incubated.

Chlamydia trachomatis examination. Smears of urethral or cervical secretions are collected during the initial pelvic examination, following the same precautions used for the Papanicolaou smear (News, 1985). Slides containing the smears are incubated for 30 minutes with fluorescein-labeled antibodies. The physician than examines the slides using a fluorescent microscope.

Research indicates that certain prenatal infections can be diagnosed by use of the monoclonal tests. Tissue cultures are still sometimes used, although they are more expensive and it takes longer to obtain results with them than with the monoclonal tests.

*Herpes simplex, types 1 and 2 culture.** If an open lesion is present at the time of the initial pelvic examination, a viral culture is obtained from the lesion and

---

*See also Chapter 29.

Procedure 11.1

PELVIC EXAMINATION

PURPOSE

1. To provide a data base for medical diagnoses, medical therapy, nursing diagnoses, and nursing care plans
2. To promote a trust relationship with the client
3. To involve the client as an active participant in her own health supervision, maintenance, and care

EQUIPMENT

1. Lithotomy table and drapes
2. Supplies and equipment (see Fig. 11.13)

NURSING ACTIONS	RATIONALE
Ask client to empty her bladder before examination.	A full bladder makes the pelvic examination uncomfortable for the client and difficult for the examiner.
Instruct woman to remove her clothing and don a cover gown. Assist woman into the lithotomy position (the woman's hips and knees are flexed with the buttocks at the edge of the table and her feet supported by heel or knee stirrups).	The lithotomy position is the position of choice; however, other positions can be used (Figs. 11.14 and 11.15).
Assess for and treat imminent **untoward responses** (Boxes, p. 281).	
Support client. Explain the procedure as it is performed: inspection of external genitals, insertion of speculum for examination of vagina and cervix (Fig. 11.16), bimanual examination of internal organs (Fig. 11.17).	Health teaching can be carried out while performing care. Knowledge reduces tension.
Refrain from questioning the client extensively. Hold questions until she is sitting up and at eye level with the examiner.	Questioning during the procedure, especially if she cannot see the questioner's eyes, may make the woman tense.
Assist with relaxation techniques. Have the woman place her hands on her chest at about the level of the diaphragm, breathe deeply and slowly (in through her mouth and out through her O-shaped mouth), concentrate on the rhythm of breathing, and relax all body muscles with each exhalation (Malasanos and others, 1985).	Many women express feelings of vulnerability and strangeness when in the lithotomy position. Women express fears of being hurt during the examination. This breathing technique is particularly helpful for the adolescent or the woman whose introitus may be especially tight. Others for whom the experience may be new or tension provoking can also benefit from using the relaxation technique.
Encourage the woman to become involved with the examination; for example, a mirror can be placed so that the area being examined can be seen by the client.	This type of participation helps with health teaching as well.
Distract the woman's attention by placing interesting pictures or mobiles on the ceiling over the head of the table.	Distraction is an effective method of reducing tension.
Remind the woman not to squeeze her eyes closed, clench her fists, or squeeze the nurse's hand.	Tightening these muscles encourages tightening of the perineal muscles.
Instruct client to bear down when speculum is being inserted (Fig. 11.16).	Bearing down helps open vaginal introitus and relax perineal muscles so insertion of speculum is easier.
Assist examiner with collection of cytology specimens such as Papanicolaou smear (see Procedure 11.2).	Reduces possibility of contamination of specimens if performed prior to bimanual examination.
Explain purpose and how procedure is accomplished. Describe sensations to expect.	Reduces anxiety related to knowledge deficit.
Lubricate examiner's fingers with water prior to bimanual examination (Fig. 11.17).	Reduces friction and thereby discomfort. Other types of lubricant distort findings.
Assist woman at completion of examination into a sitting position and then standing position.	Most women, particularly toward the end of pregnancy, find it difficult to attain a sitting position without help. Rising slowly helps to overcome transient hypotension.
Provide tissues to wipe lubricant from perineum.	Provides comfort and cleanliness.
Provide privacy for client to dress.	Recognition of client's needs promotes feelings of security.
Inform her as to the next step in the assessment protocol.	Knowledge reduces tension.
Record findings on the appropriate form.	Fosters continuity of care.

Fig. 11.13

Equipment used for pelvic examination. **A,** Thayer-Martin medium for isolation of Neisseria gonorrhoeae. Cylindrical container *(arrow)* is for pellet that releases carbon dioxide; medium and specimen are refrigerated until transport to laboratory. **B,** Vaginal speculum. **C,** Culturette, modified Stuart's bacterial transport medium with self-contained sterile swab. **D,** Vaginal pipette with rubber bulb. **E,** Plastic spatula for Papanicolaou smear and cytology. **F,** Slides for cytology specimens (Pap smear) or for wet mounts for diagnosing cause of vaginitis. **G,** Spray can of fixative for slide specimens. When dry, slides are packaged in cardboard for transport to laboratory. **H,** Normal saline and 10% potassium hydroxide (KOH) for wet mounts of vaginal fluids. **I,** Cotton pledget stick. **J,** Tenaculum. **K,** Ring (sponge or stick) forceps. **L,** Tissue forceps. **M,** Uterine sound (slightly curved for insertion). **N,** Sterile lubricant; may be antiseptic. **O,** Glove for vaginal and rectal examinations (sterile for vaginal, clean for rectal).

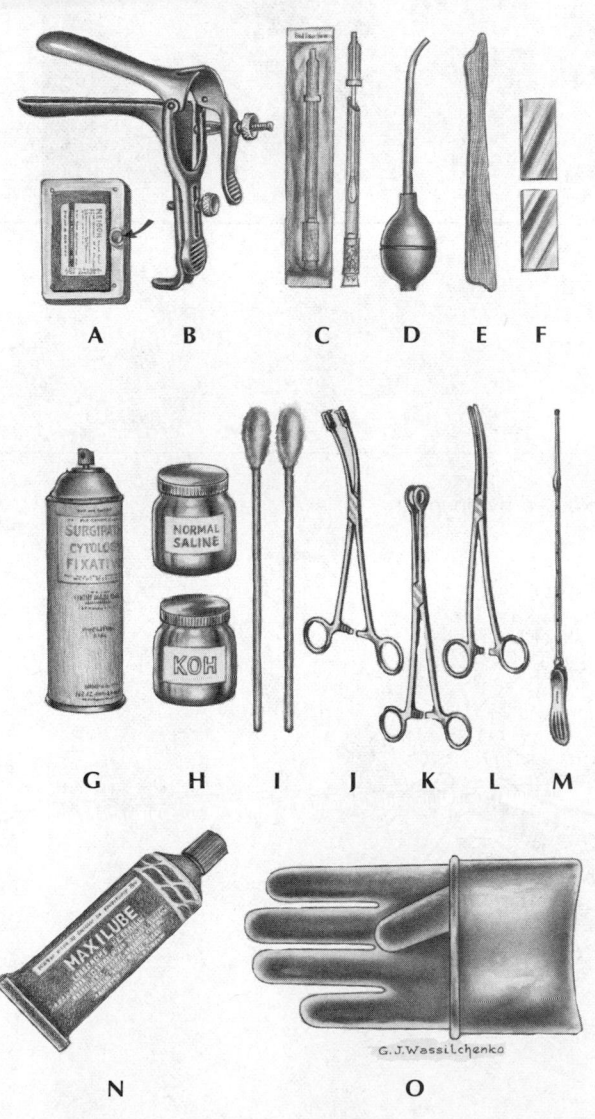

Fig. 11.14

Lithotomy position for pelvic examination. Note draping that acknowledges need for modesty but still allows for eye contact with examiner. Foot rests are padded for added comfort. (Courtesy Nanci Newell.)

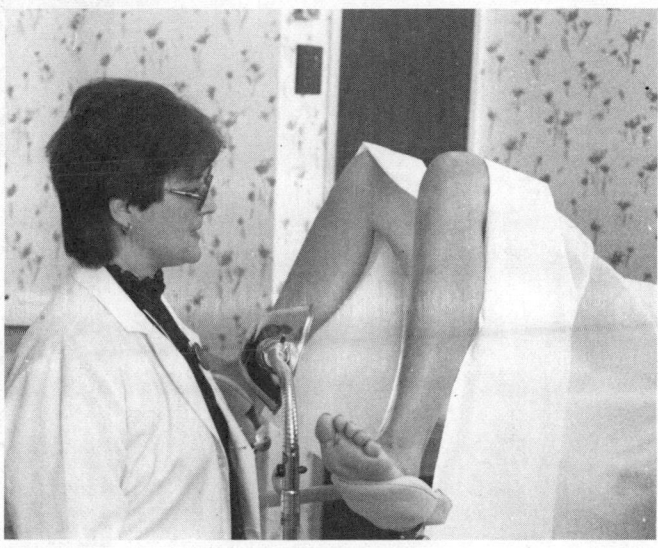

is repeated at intervals. A positive Papanicolaou smear may be caused by the presence of herpes simplex, type 2.

Urinalysis. Urinalysis provides data relating to urinary infections or medical complications of pregnancy such as pregnancy-induced hypertension (Procedure 11.3).

Hazards during the pelvic examination. The nurse needs to remain alert to the woman's clues that indicate imminent untoward response such as supine hypotension, vasovagal syncope, and possible cardiac arrest.

Supine hypotension. When a woman is lying in the lithotomy position, the weight of the abdominal contents may compress the vena cava and aorta, resulting in a drop in blood pressure. Pallor, breathlessness, and clammy skin are other objective signs. Nursing actions are presented on p. 281.

Vasovagal syncope. Vasovagal syndrome is a poorly defined but very real emergency. It occurs without warning, is of brief duration but without predictable effects, and *can be fatal.* Those who have an attack should be managed by basic principles of cardiopulmonary resuscitation (Queenan, 1982).

The syndrome occurs when two conditions are operative: (1) There is actual or threatened physical harm. Often the experience the woman is facing is either a new one or one that was hard for her to face on

Fig. 11.15
Alternate positions for examination of genitals. **A,** Left lateral position. **B,** Semi-Fowler's
position. (**A** from Malasanos, L., Barkauskas, V., Moss, M., and Stoltenberg-Allen, K.:
Health assessment, ed. 3, St. Louis, 1985, The C.V. Mosby Co. **B,** photograph by Irene M.
Bobak.)

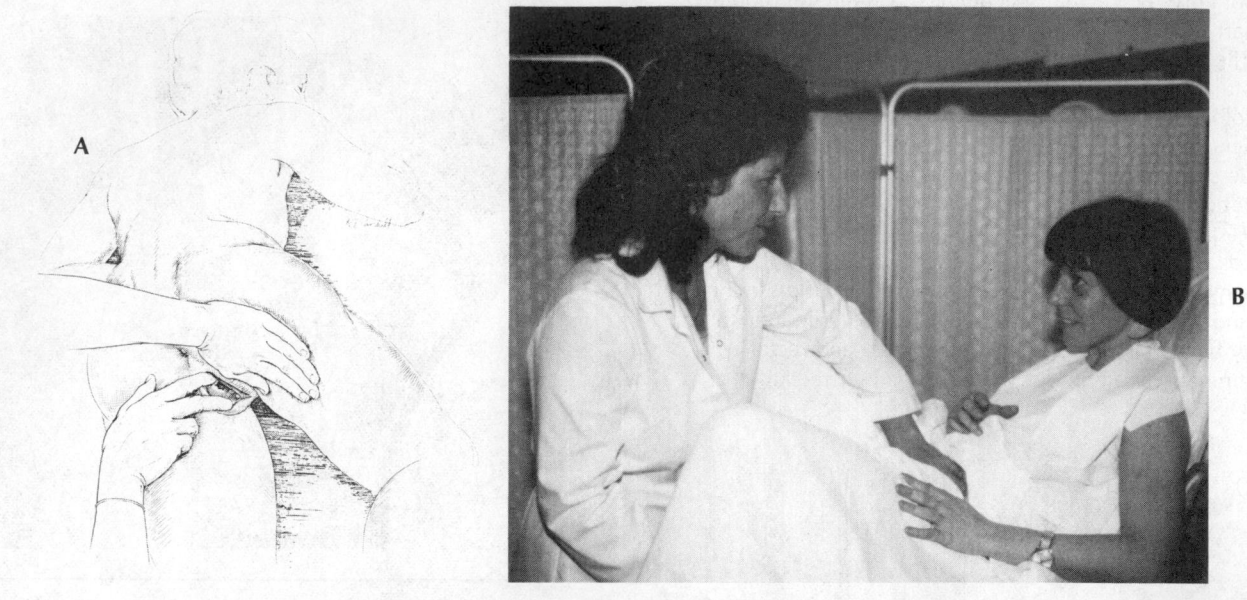

Fig. 11.16
Bivalve speculum examination. Cervix and vaginal mucosa are exposed by opening
blades.

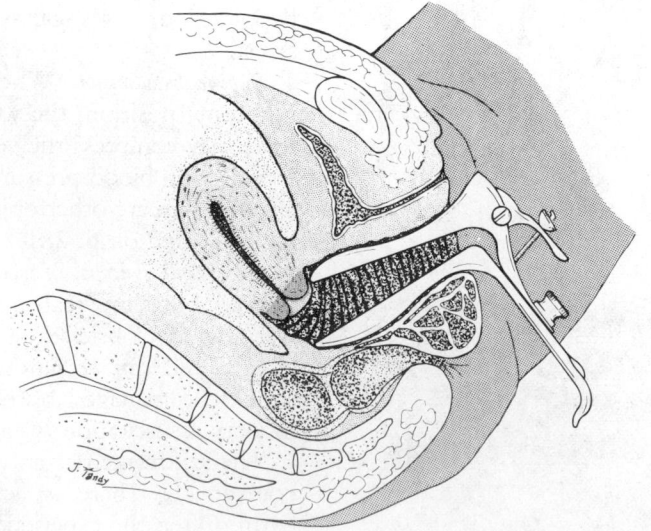

Fig. 11.17
Bimanual (abdominovaginal) palpation of uterus, **A,** and adnexa, **B.** (From Malasanos, L., Borkauskas, V., Moss, M., and Stoltenberg-Allen, K.: Health assessment, ed. 3, St. Louis, 1985, The C.V. Mosby Co.)

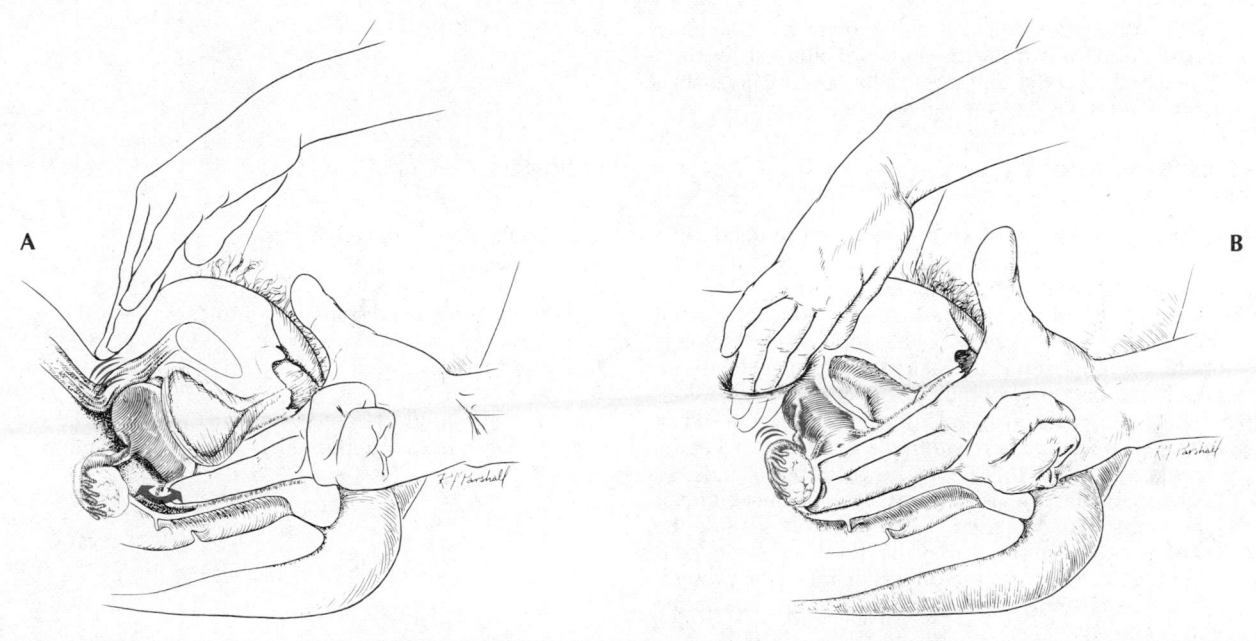

Fig. 11.18
A, Cervical smear. **B,** Endocervical smear. (From Malasanos, L., Borkauskas, V., Moss, M., and Stoltenberg-Allen, K.: Health assessment, ed. 3, St. Louis, 1985, The C.V. Mosby Co.)

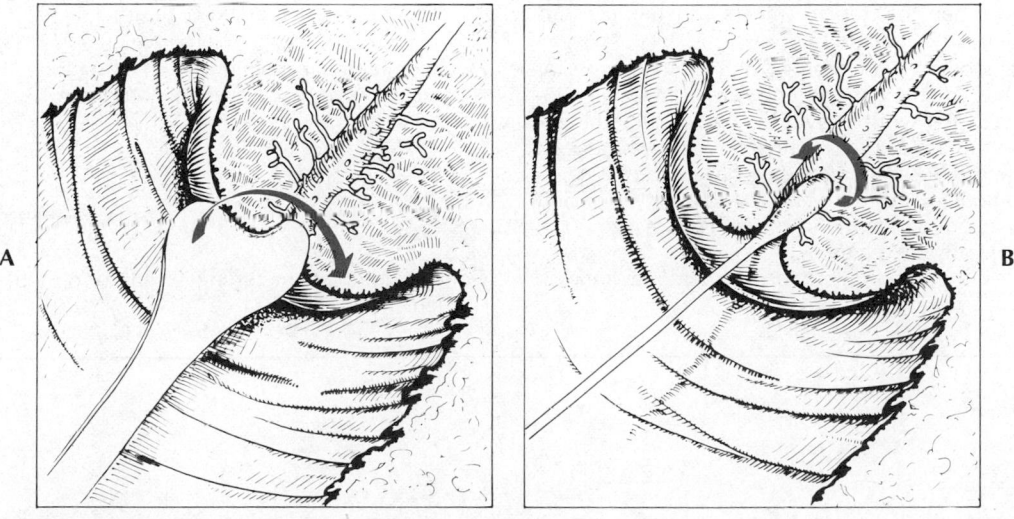

Procedure 11.2

PAPANICOLAOU SMEAR

PURPOSE

To detect abnormalities of cell growth by examining secretions and cells from the squamocolumnar junction (Fig. 5.19), the cervix, and the vagina. During pregnancy it is done at the time of the pelvic examination.

EQUIPMENT

See Fig. 11.13.

NURSING ACTIONS	RATIONALE
Explain to the woman the purpose of the test and what sensations she will feel as the specimen is obtained (i.e., pressure but not pain).	Knowledge helps reduce tension.
Assist examiner with test. The cytologic specimen is obtained before any digital examination of the vagina is made, or endocervical bacteriologic specimens are taken with cotton swabbing of the cervix.	The findings may be distorted by lubricant.
The specimen is taken by placing the S-shaped end of the cervical spatula just *within the cervical canal at the external os* (Fig. 11.18, *A*). The blade is rotated 360 degrees so that the surface at the squamocolumnar junction is firmly scraped. If the junction is inside the cervical canal, a swab may be used to obtain cells (Fig. 11.18, *B*). If gross exudate or mucus is present, the excess is gently pushed away from the os with the end of the spatula.	The mucus around the cervix contains more carcinoma cells than mucus found in other parts of the vagina.
The mucus is spread on a slide without drying or rubbing, sprayed lightly with fixative, and allowed to dry.	The first slide will contain mainly cells from the endocervix and ectocervix in the area where cervical cancer is most often found.
Some mucus is obtained from the *posterior fornix* (vaginal pool) with the rounded end of the spatula, spread on another slide, sprayed, and dried.	The second slide may reveal cells from the endometrium, endocervix, ectocervix, and vagina.
Label the slides with woman's name and site. Include on the form to accompany the slides the woman's name, age, parity, and chief complaint or reason for taking the cytologic specimens.	Minimizes chance of loss or mismatching of specimens.
Send specimens to the pathology laboratory promptly for staining, evaluation, and a written report, with special reference to abnormal elements, including cancer cells.	Delay may cause change in specimen and false report.
Advise the woman that repeat smears may be necessary if specimen is not adequate.	To reduce anxiety if asked to return.
Instruct the woman concerning routine check-ups for cervical and vaginal cancer. The American Cancer Society advises that women over the age of 20 and those under 20 who are sexually active have the test at least every 3 years, *but only after they have had two negative Papanicolaou tests a year apart.* A pelvic examination is recommended every 3 years from age 20 to 40 and annually thereafter.	Health maintenance information is included as part of procedures to reach as many people as possible.
Record the examination date and untoward reactions on the woman's prenatal record.	Concise complete recording is vital for providing care for clients.

Supine Hypotension

Signs and Symptoms
Blood pressure drops
Pallor
Breathlessness
Clammy skin

Nursing Actions	Rationale
1. Remove her from lithotomy position.	1. When a woman is lying in the lithotomy position, the weight of abdominal contents may compress the vena cava and aorta.
2. Position her on her side until signs and symptoms abate (Fig. 11.16).	2. Reduce pressure on vena cava and aorta.
3. Provide frank explanation.	3. Knowledge reduces fear of the unknown.

a previous occasion. (2) The injury or potential harm is one that the woman is expected to face with ease, for example, venipuncture or gynecologic examination.

The vasovagal response is biphasic: (1) the *sympathetic nervous system* (fight or flight) discharges, and pulse rate, blood pressure (especially systolic), cardiac output, and vascular resistance increase. The woman appears apprehensive and pale but says she is fine. Then, if the woman perceives the threat as overwhelming and just cannot face it, the *parasympathetic nervous system* (conservation and withdrawal) discharges. All physical changes reverse suddenly. Pulse, blood pressure, cardiac output, and vascular resistance decrease. The woman is diaphoretic and feels weak, muscle tone relaxes, and she complains of lightheadedness and vertigo and loses consciousness. Vomiting, bowel movement, and seizures may occur. Nursing actions are presented below.

Vasovagal Syncope

Signs and Symptoms

Shock	State of Consciousness	Cardiopulmonary Arrest
Apprehension	Vomiting	Absence of breathing
Pallor	Seizures	Absence of heart beat
Diaphoresis	Incontinence, bowel or bladder	
Generalized weakness	Loss of consciousness	
Lightheadedness		
Vertigo		

Nursing Actions	Rationale
1. Alert physician.	1. Immediate care essential.
2. Assess pulse and blood pressure.	2. To determine extent of shock response.
3. Assess level of consciousness.	3. To determine state of consciousness.
4. Ensure adequate airway. 　a. Extend head or use jaw thrust maneuver. 　b. Suction as required.	4. To permit oxygenation.
5. Provide oxygen when airway is clear.	5. To prevent cellular death.
6. Begin seizure precautions.	6. To protect from injury.
7. Assist with cardiopulmonary resuscitation (CPR). 　a. Airway 　b. Breathing: mouth-to-mouth or artificial intermittant pressure breathing with oxygen (1:5 compression) 　c. Circulation: external cardiac compression 60-80/min	7. To prevent death.
8. Assist with drugs: atropine, 0.5-1 mg. intravenously, and epinephrine, 0.5 mg intravenously (Queenan, 1982).	
9. Assist with direct current defibrillation, 200-400 J (Queenan, 1982).	

Procedure 11.3

CLEAN-CATCH URINE SPECIMEN

PURPOSE

A specimen of urine is needed at the initial visit for routine urinalysis and at subsequent visits for evaluation for glucose and protein.

EQUIPMENT AND SUPPLIES

1. A clean container with lid
2. Identifying label
3. Tissue wipes

NURSING ACTIONS	RATIONALE
Instruct woman to: Wash hands. Spread labia and wipe from front to back, using moistened toilet paper or wipes. Begin voiding and then obtain specimen during midstream in a clean container; 30-60 ml (1-2 oz) of urine is sufficient.	Minimize contamination of specimen.
Wash hands. Label container and fill in data for laboratory: name, to be tested for glucose, protein, and acetone; microscopic assessment for pus, red blood cells, and casts; culture and sensitivity as necessary.	Health teaching. To assess for potential complications such as pregnancy-induced hypertension.
Instruct woman to bring a specimen each time she comes for prenatal follow up. Ideally the specimen is obtained immediately after rising in the morning. A clean container must be used. It does not have to be kept cool.	Urinalysis profiles important information regarding health status, e.g., excess protein may indicate pregnancy-induced hypertension.
Record findings on the appropriate form.	Fosters continuity of care.

RECORDER

Recording complete and concise records during the prenatal period is essential for the documentation of maternal and fetal progress. Many standard printed record forms are available. The best records incorporate medical, laboratory, nursing, and dietary data assessments and plans in an easily readable arrangement from the first through subsequent office or clinic visits.

CULTURAL VARIATION IN PRENATAL CARE

Prenatal care as we know it is a phenomenon of Western medicine. The Western biomedical model of care encourages women to seek prenatal care as early as possible in their pregnancy by visiting a physician or clinic. Visits are usually routine and follow a systematic sequence, with the initial visit followed by a monthly and then weekly visits. Monitoring weight and blood pressure; testing blood and urine; teaching specific information about diet, rest, and activity; and preparing for childbirth are common components of prenatal care.

The preceding model not only is unfamiliar but frequently seems strange to many groups (Artschwager, 1982). Even when the prenatal care described is familiar, some practices may conflict with a subcultural group's beliefs and practices. Because of these and other factors, such as lack of money, lack of transportation, and poor communication on the part of health care providers, many groups do not participate in the prenatal care system. Their behavior may be misinterpreted by nurses as uncaring, lazy, or ignorant. For example, Muecke (1976) points out that the Northern Thai do not focus on the prenatal period at all. They only focus on the childbirth and postpartum periods. According to their beliefs, they personally perceive themselves as having little influence on pregnancy until the time of birth. For them spiritual influences, apart from human beings, control what occurs before birth. Western prenatal care, which does not deal with the spiritual influences, appears irrelevant.

Horn's research (1982) with a group of Northwest Coast Indians elicited the strongly held belief that visible preparation for the coming infant was frequently associated with the infant's death. Women could identify many instances when preparation such as buying infant clothes or preparing a crib was followed by the death of the infant. A high infant mortality supported this belief. Another group not favoring preparation by the mother before birth is the Arab-American population. Meleis and Sorrell (1981) stress that Egyptian and Arab mothers do not have a layette or room set aside for newborns at the time of birth. They believe that planning ahead has the potential of defying God's will. Also planning ahead only to have those plans not materialize can be disappointing. Women on the Caribbean island of St. Kitt prefer not discussing the coming infant, mentioning its name, or referring to it directly until it is christened (Gussler, 1982). Until the time of christening, spirits of the dead would come and make the infant ill or kill it. This same concern for the dead spirit's influence was expressed by the Muckleshoot, who kept a candle burning to keep the spirits from coming to get the baby. Kendall (1979) tells of a pregnant Iranian woman's grandmother who prepared a complete set of clothing for her expected grandchild during the sixth or seventh month of pregnancy. She placed among the clothing a triangular scarf with beads, amulets, and shells to ward off the evil eye and thus protect the newborn infant.

A concern for modesty is also a deterrent for prenatal care for many persons. Exposing one's body parts, especially to a man, is a major violation of modesty. Puerto Ricans (Parken, 1978), Mexicans (Kay, 1982), and Japanese (Bernstein and Kidd, 1982) express great concern over body exposure. Arab women also value modesty (Meleis and Sorrell, 1981). Besides being fully clothed, the Arab woman is expected to manifest modesty through diffidence, shyness, and bashfulness when interacting with men and strangers. For many women invasive procedures such as vaginal examination may be so threatening that they cannot be discussed, even with one's own husband. Thus many Arab women prefer a midwife over a male physician. Recent immigrants such as Southeast Asians also prefer a midwife (Gallo and others, 1980; Hollingsworth and others, 1980).

For numerous cultural groups a physician is deemed appropriate only in times of illness. A physician is considered inappropriate when pregnancy is considered a normal process and the woman is in a state of health. Even when problems with pregnancy develop according to beliefs of Western medicine, they may not be perceived as problems but may be considered normal. Muecke (1976) notes that Thai women do not perceive weakness, fainting spells, palpitations, tremors, and diarrhea as abnormal. Many Muckleshoot women view puffiness of hands, eyes, and feet and frequent headaches as normal (Horn, 1982).

Although pregnancy is considered normal by many, certain practices are expected of women of all cultures to ensure a good outcome. Prescriptions tell women what to do, and proscriptions establish taboos. The purposes of these practices are to (1) prevent maternal illness from a pregnancy-induced imbalanced state, (2) protect the vulnerable infant, and (3) protect other persons from illness caused by a woman in state of imbalance. Prescriptions and proscriptions discussed in the chapter are related to emotional response, clothing, activity and rest, sexual activity, and dietary practices.

Emotional response. Virtually all cultures emphasize the importance of a socially harmonious and agreeable environment. Absence of stressful relationships is important for a successful outcome for mother and baby. Harmony with other persons must be fostered. Visits from extended family members may be required to demonstrate continued pleasant and noncontroversial relationships. If dissonance exists in any relationship with others, it is usually dealt with in culturally prescribed ways. For example, a pregnant woman on the Muckleshoot reservation described how she became ill after eating chili, a food to avoid during pregnancy because of its spiciness. The pregnant woman's mother had specifically warned her about eating chili. Thus the woman had created disharmony in two areas, physiologic and social, by eating a proscribed food and by not following the mother's admonitions. To remedy the situation and to reestablish harmony, the pregnant woman attended a Shaker prayer service. She prayed for herself and was "brushed off"; that is, a church member symbolically brushed the problem away by touching her shoulder lightly. She believed she had now regained a state of physiologic and social harmony.

Imitative magic functions in other proscriptions in addition to food. Mexicans advise against pregnant women witnessing an eclipse of the moon because they believe it may cause a cleft palate in the infant. Exposures to an earthquake may result in premature delivery or miscarriage. A breech may occur if the earthquake was exceptionally strong (Clark, 1970). Snow (1974) notes that among blacks a pregnant woman must not ridicule someone with an affliction for fear her child might be born with the same handicap. A mother should not hate a person lest her child resemble that person, and dental work should not be done during pregnancy because it may cause a baby to have a harelip. Carrington (1978) describes a widely held folk belief in many cultures that includes refraining from raising one's arm above one's head and refraining from tying knots, so that the umbilical cord does not wrap around the baby's neck and become knotted.

Clothing. Although most cultural groups do not prescribe specific clothing for pregnancy, modesty is an expectation for many (Clark, 1970; Meleis and Sorrell, 1981). Spanish-speaking people of the Southwest wear a cord beneath the breast and knotted over the umbilicus. This cord, called a *muneco,* is thought to prevent morning sickness and ensure a safe delivery (Brown, 1976). Amulets, medals, and beads may be worn to ward off evil spirits.

Activity and rest. Norms that regulate physical activity of mothers during pregnancy vary tremendously. Many groups (Carrington, 1978; Horn, 1982; Stringfellow, 1978) encourage women to be active, to walk, and to engage in normal although not strenuous activities to ensure that the baby is healthy and not too large. On the other hand, the Filipino woman is cautioned that any activity is dangerous, and others willingly take over work (Affonso, 1978; Stern, 1981). The belief among Filipinos is that inactivity constitutes a protection for mother and child. The mother is encouraged to simply produce the succeeding generation. Health care providers could misinterpret this behavior as laziness or noncompliance with the health regimen desired in prenatal care. Again it is important for the nurse to find out the meaning of activity and rest for each culture.

Sexual activity. In most cultures sexual activity is not prohibited until the end of pregnancy. Among blacks sexual relations are viewed as natural because pregnancy is a state of health (Carrington, 1978). Mexican-Americans view sexual activity as necessary to keep the birth canal lubricated (Kay, 1982). On the other hand, Vietnamese have definite proscriptions about sexual intercourse, requiring abstinence as early as the sixth month (Hollingsworth and others, 1980; Stringfellow, 1978). Sexual taboos are more common after delivery.

Diet. Nutritional information given by Western health care providers may be a source of conflict for many cultural groups. The conflict is frequently not known by the health care providers unless they have an understanding of dietary beliefs and practices of the persons for whom they are caring (see Chapter 12).

Evaluation

Evaluation is a continuous process. To be effective, evaluation needs to be based on measurable criteria. The criteria reflect the parameters used to measure the goals for care. The maternal and fetal areas consistently assessed as indicators of maternal and fetal well-being and the clinical findings that represent normal response are presented as outcome criteria in the Summary of Nursing Actions. These criteria are used as a basis for selecting appropriate nursing actions and evaluating their effectiveness.

Summary

The prenatal period is one of growth and change in the woman's personal and social context. Achieving a goal of a safe and satisfying pregnancy for a woman and her family requires a mutual effort on the part of the woman and the professionals involved. Practitioner and client need a clear understanding of their objectives, roles, and capabilities. Nursing care provided during this period can act as a stimulus for the continued use of the health care system by the woman and her family. Nursing actions reflect the changes experienced by the woman as she progresses through the three trimesters of pregnancy. For further details see the Summary of Nursing Actions and Application of Nursing Process.

Summary of Nursing Actions

NURSING CARE DURING PREGNANCY

GOALS
1. For the mother: to have a physically safe and emotionally satisfying pregnancy.
2. For the unborn child: to have an uncomplicated intrauterine existence.
3. For the family: to have an experience that promotes loving and concerned parenting for the child and enhances the personal growth of all individuals involved.

PRIORITIES
1. Establish plan of care related to woman's EDC and family circumstances.
2. Monitor woman, fetus, and family for normal adaptations to pregnancy.
3. Initiate remedial therapy for abnormal adaptations to pregnancy.
4. Promote client recognition of normal and abnormal adaptations to pregnancy.
5. Promote client and family participation in care.
6. Provide supportive care to client and family.

Summary of Nursing Actions—cont'd

ASSESSMENT	EXAMPLES OF POTENTIAL NURSING DIAGNOSTIC CATEGORIES

FIRST VISIT*
Interview
A. Health history
    1. Family history
    2. Medical history
    3. Sexual history
    4. Obstetric history
    5. Present pregnancy
	Potential for maternal or fetal compromise†

B. Psychosocial history
    1. Identifying data
    2. Perception
    3. Support systems
       a. Family
       b. Community
    4. Coping mechanisms
    5. Parenting potential
	Anxiety
	Impaired verbal communication
	Ineffective individual (or family) coping
	Knowledge deficit
	Potential alteration in family process
	Potential disturbance in self-concept: body image, self-esteem, role performance, personal identity
	Potential spiritual distress
	Powerlessness

C. Review of woman's physical systems	Potential for maternal or fetal compromise†
Physical examination A. Vital signs, blood pressure, weight B. Head C. Neck D. Thorax E. Abdomen F. Extremities G. Pelvic examination	Potential for maternal compromise† Alteration in normal physiologic process†
Laboratory tests A. Tine or PPD (purified protein derivative [of tuberculin]) for exposure to tuberculosis. B. Cervical and vaginal smears for cytology (Papanicolaou) and for chlamydia, gonorrhea, and herpes simplex, types 1 and 2. C. Blood (repeat at 32 weeks as necessary): VDRL test for syphilis, complete blood count (CBC) with hematocrit, hemoglobin, and differential values; blood type and Rh; antibody screen (Kell, Duffy, rubella, toxoplasmosis, anti-Rh); sickle cell; level of folacin when indicated; packed cell volume (PCV)—may be done at each visit in some offices. D. Urine: tests for glucose, protein, and acetone; culture and sensitivity as necessary. E. Pregnancy tests if indicated (Tables 11.1 to 11.3).	Potential for maternal or fetal compromise† Potential alteration in health maintenance Anxiety related to uncertainty of diagnosis of pregnancy

*The protocol for the first visit is the same regardless of whether it occurs early in the first trimester or later during pregnancy.
†Diagnosis not included by NANDA, 1986.

Continued.

Summary of Nursing Actions—cont'd

OUTCOME CRITERIA*	PLAN/IMPLEMENTATION

Emotional support

A. Nurse and client
  1. Client and family respond positively to personnel.
  2. Anxiety appears lessened. Client able to question nurse regarding learning needs.
  3. Client able to work with nurse to plan care appropriate to her needs.

B. Maternal emotional health
  Client able to express feelings openly (i.e., pleasure, dismay, anger, anxiety, fear).

C. Client and family
  Client expresses feelings of support from family and friends.

Knowledge and skills

A. Client able to describe plan of care.

B. Client verbalizes understanding of danger signals and to whom to report problems.

C. Client asks questions freely about anticipated problems.

D. Client verbalizes understanding of physiologic basis, prevention, and treatment of common discomforts.

Support Person

A. Client
  1. Establish caring relationship with woman (or couple).
  2. Orient to initial visit.
     a. Interview
     b. Physical examination
     c. Laboratory tests
  3. Encourage woman to express her likes and dislikes.
B. Maternal emotional health
  Listen to description of emotional responses to pregnancy (i.e., words, tone of voice, affect). Observe body language (i.e., tension, eyes averted).
C. Client and family
  Encourage spouse to accompany wife on prenatal visits. Include him in discussion of maternal and fetal well-being.

Teacher/counselor/advocate

A. Establish a plan of care based on EDC.
  1. Develop a plan of care for continuing assessment of maternal and fetal well-being and of significant others.
  2. Schedule regular office or clinic visits every 4 weeks for 32 weeks, every 2 weeks until week 36, and then weekly until term or until labor begins.
  3. Review plan of care with woman and family.
     a. Schedule: check for convenience of timing, problems in transportation, and care of other children; provide written copy of schedule.
     b. Need for continuity of care: check for woman's understanding of reasons for periodic reassessment.
     c. Physical examinations: describe routine physical examinations, including instructions for obtaining clean-catch urine specimens for routine analysis.
B. Provide written list of danger signals and written directions for obtaining medical care if abnormal symptoms occur.
C. Instruct woman on general health care:
  1. Personal hygiene
  2. Diet
  3. Rest and exercise
  4. Dental care
  5. Use of medications
  6. Sexual counseling
D. Instruct woman to avoid supine position. Provide information concerning physiologic basis, prevention, and treatment of physical symptoms woman may be experiencing (e.g., urgency and frequency of urination, languor and malaise, and nausea and vomiting).

---

*Outcome criteria direct the selection of nursing actions (**plan/implementation**) and measure their effectiveness (**evaluation**).

Summary of Nursing Actions —cont'd

OUTCOME CRITERIA	PLAN/IMPLEMENTATION
Physical care A. Maternal 　1. Client is in general good health. Age and physical condition are within low-risk category. 　2. Appearance is healthy, grooming adequate, energy level normal. B. Fetal 　Findings related to fetal well-being are appropriate for gestational age.	**Technician** A. Maternal 　1. Inquire as to general health of client. 　2. Note appearance, grooming, energy level. 　3. Assist with examinations. B. Fetal 　Check FHR and other systems if appropriate to gestational age.

ASSESSMENT	EXAMPLES OF POTENTIAL NURSING DIAGNOSTIC CATEGORIES
FIRST AND SECOND TRIMESTER **Interview** A. Health history 　1. Current family happenings and their effect on woman 　2. Problems she may be experiencing 　3. Knowledge and understanding of danger signals and to whom to report 　4. Knowledge of diet 　5. Amount of participation woman (or couple) desires in childbirth and whether classes are appropriate 　6. Woman's knowledge of infant care, including methods of feeding B. Psychosocial history 　1. Reactions to pregnancy 　2. Understanding of sexual responses 　3. Self-image 　4. Understanding of plan of care 　5. Awareness of fetal movements C. Review of woman's physical systems	Ineffective individual or family coping Maternal or fetal compromise† Alteration in normal physiologic processes† Alteration in health maintenance Knowledge deficit Alteration in nutrition: less or more than body requirements Disturbance in self-concept: body image, self-esteem, role performance, personal identity Alteration in family process Powerlessness Noncompliance Alteration in tissue perfusion: cerebral, cardiopulmonary, renal, gastrointestinal, peripheral Alteration in bowel elimination: constipation or diarrhea Alteration in pattern of urinary elimination Alteration in fluid volume: excess (i.e., edema)
Physical examination A. Temperature, pulse, respiration (TPR), blood pressure: (BP), and weight B. Fundal height and gestational age C. Fetal heart rate and fetal activity D. Edema E. Skin F. Pelvic examination (as necessary) 　1. Vagina 　2. Cervix 　3. Uterus G. Breasts (as necessary)	Alteration in normal physiologic process† Potential maternal or fetal compromise related to complications† Impairment of skin integrity
Laboratory tests (as necessary) A. Blood B. Urine C. Other (e.g., for infection)	Alteration in normal physiologic process† Potential maternal or fetal compromise related to complications†

Continued.

Summary of Nursing Actions—cont'd

OUTCOME CRITERIA	PLAN/IMPLEMENTATION

Emotional support
A. Nurse and client
  1. Client family participation in interview
	Support person
	A. Nurse and client
	  1. Use appropriate interview techniques
	    a. Greet by name in unhurried manner.
	    b. Provide a relaxed and trusting atmosphere.
	    c. Provide privacy.
	    d. Validate normalcy of their responses (if they fall within normal limits).
	    e. Provide information as needed.
	    f. Respect cultural, ethnic, religious, or other responses.
	    g. Ensure confidentiality.

2. Client verbalizes understanding of schedule, need for continuity of care, physical examination to be done, reporting of abnormal symptoms.
  3. Client complies with plan of care.
    Client follows diet plan, takes only prescribed medications, refrains from smoking and drinking alcohol beverages, and exercises.
	2. a. Review protocol for schedule and care.
	    b. Set next appointment time.
	  3. a. Inquire as to convenience of appointments.
	    b. Discuss problems, work mutually toward solutions.
	    c. Review problems associated with noncompliance.

B. Maternal emotional health
  Reactions indicative of positive psychologic response to pregnancy, including birth process and parenthood.
  1. During second trimester, woman usually is reasonably free of symptoms; she is more tranquil and at ease; reality of child is now recognized, and most women come to accept their pregnant state; however, feelings of ambivalence come and go.
	B. Maternal emotional health
	  1. Provide support related to emotional responses or problems.
	    a. Mood changes
	    b. Relationship between mother and pregnant daughter
	    Acceptance
	    Use of gravida's mother as role model
	    c. Relationship between mother and unborn child
	    Consciousness of fetal movement
	    Feelings of closeness to child
	    Concern for self enlarges to include concern for unborn child.

2. Negative feelings about self-image are recognized as temporary; expresses pride or pleasure about being pregnant.	2. Initiate discussions related to the woman's self-concept
	    a. Body image
	    b. Self-esteem
	    c. Ambivalence
	    d. Happiness or depression
	    e. Anxiety, fear, or anger

C. Client and family
  1. Partner's expression of commitment to pregnancy accepted (e.g., observer, style, ethnic expression).
	C. Client and family
	  1. a. Welcome partner participation in routine visits, preparation for parenthood classes.
	    b. Accept partner's definition of amount of support to be given.
	    c. Assist mother to broaden her network of support people.

2. Verbalizes understanding of sexual responses and reports that sexual relationships are mutually accepted and serve as a means of communication.
  3. Sibling acceptance of idea of new brother or sister is beginning.
	2. a. Listen to client's comments of satisfaction or problems with husband-wife relationships.
	    b. Discuss alternatives in sexual expression.
	  3. a. Encourage mother to include siblings in routine visits for care.
	    b. Begin discussion of sibling participation in preparation classes.

4. Grandparents act as an important part of support network.	4. Encourage discussion of client's relationships with her parents.

Summary of Nursing Actions—cont'd

OUTCOME CRTIERIA	PLAN/IMPLEMENTATION
Knowledge and skills A. Woman or couple verbalize understanding of physiologic basis, need for immediate treatment, and how to obtain necessary care for complications of pregnancy.	**Teacher/counselor/advocate** A. Review danger signals of complications of pregnancy 1. Vaginal bleeding 2. Burning or pain on urination 3. Chills or elevated temperature 4. Exposure to communicable disease (e.g., rubella) 5. Nausea and vomiting beyond week 12 or persistent or severe vomiting anytime 6. Abdominal pain or cramping 7. Reduction in or absence of fetal movement (after quickening) 8. Woman reports abnormal symptoms promptly

B. Women or couple verbalize understanding of physiologic basis, prevention, and treatment of problems common to first and second trimester.	B. Review changes common to first and second trimesters, physiologic basis, prevention, and treatment
	1. *First trimester*
	  a. Pain and tingling in the breasts
	  b. Urgency and frequency of urination
	  c. Languor and malaise (fatigue)
	  d. Nausea and vomiting (morning sickness)
	2. *Second trimester*
	  a. Constipation
	  b. Heartburn
	  c. Increased pigmentation
	  d. Leg cramps
	  e. Pica
	  f. Food cravings and food avoidances
	  g. Leukorrhea
	  h. Round ligament pain

C. Woman and family verbalize understanding of rationale for answers to common questions	C. Provide answers to common questions relating to:
	1. Clothing
	2. Bathing and swimming
	3. Employment
	4. Travel
	5. Physical activity
	6. Dental problems
	7. Immunization
	8. Drugs
	9. Substance abuse
	10. Radiation
	11. Resources available
	  a. Education
	  b. Dental evaluation
	  c. Medical service
	  d. Social service
	  e. Emergency room

D. Woman and family verbalize 1. Understanding of fetal development, FHR, and fetal movement, adaptation, and status. 2. Understanding of fetal and maternal needs during pregnancy.	D. 1. Instruct woman and family concerning fetal development, maternal adaptations, maternal and fetal symptomatology and significance. (This is a gradual process and may take weeks to complete). 2. Instruct woman and family concerning maternal and fetal needs (e.g., care during travel, continuity of care).

E. 1. Woman and family verbalize understanding of maternal and fetal nutritional needs.
2. Physical response indicates compliance with nutritional counsel.
	E. 1. Provide nutritional guidance (see also Chapter 12).
	  a. Weight gain
	  b. Balanced diet
	  c. Special nutritional needs: iron supplements
	2. Comment on appearance and energy level.

Continued.

Summary of Nursing Actions—cont'd

OUTCOME CRITERIA	PLAN/IMPLEMENTATION
Knowledge and skills—cont'd	**Teacher/counselor/advocate—cont'd**
3. Woman verbalizes understanding of choices regarding infant feeding.	3. Instruct regarding choices in infant feeding.
F. Woman verbalizes understanding of choices and availability of prenatal education classes.	F. Instruct regarding choices in prenatal education classes.
G. Woman seeks assistance for problems such as infections (cold), allergies, or substance abuse (smoking and drinking).	G. 1. Instruct regarding effect for woman or unborn child related to such problems. 2. Suggest or institute remedial care.
Physical care	**Technician**
A. Maternal	1. Implement appropriate techniques for physical assessment and analyze findings. Share findings with woman or couple as appropriate.
1. Findings from physical assessment are within normal limits.	
2. Appearance is healthy, grooming is adequate, energy level is normal.	2. Comment in positive manner about her appearance Inquire about energy level. Review exercise and relaxation techniques.

3. Temperature, pulse, respiration, blood pressure, and weight
a. Temperature, normal range
b. Pulse, normal range
c. Respiration, 18-20/min
d. Blood pressure, normal range of less than +30 systolic and +15 diastolic over baseline; may decrease slightly in midpregnancy
e. Weight gain
  (1) Weeks 1-13: about 3-4 lb (1.4 to 1.8 kg)
  (2) Weeks 12-26: about 12-14 lb (5.6-6.3 kg)
  (3) Weeks 27-40: approximately 0.5 lb (0.23 kg) per week.
	3. Share findings prn.

4. Edema, dependent edema not yet apparent.	4. Instruct woman regarding significance of findings. Review resting positions.
5. Abdomen, gradual enlargement, see height of fundus	5. Review significance of findings.

6. Uterus
a. Progressive enlargement to accommodate growing products of conception.
b. Fundal height:
  (1) 12-13 weeks: felt just above pubic symphysis;
  (2) 16 weeks: felt 3-4 cm above pubic symphysis;
  (3) 20 weeks: felt 2-3 cm below umbilicus
  (4) 24 weeks: felt at umbilicus
	6. Review significance of findings.

7. Skin, changes not noticeable.	7. Review anticipated changes.
B. Fetal	
1. FHR heard by Doppler principle (Dopptone) at 8-12 weeks, by fetoscope at 17-18 weeks	1. Let woman and family listen to FHR. Review significance of findings.
2. Fetal movements felt at 17-19 weeks (quickening)	2. Review significance of findings. Review procedure for reporting changes in fetal movements.
3. Fetal breathing movements detected by sonography by 18½ weeks	3. Review significance of findings if appropriate (in normal pregnancy, sonography may not be utilized).

Summary of Nursing Actions—cont'd

ASSESSMENT	EXAMPLES OF POTENTIAL NURSING DIAGNOSTIC CATEGORIES

THIRD TRIMESTER
Interview
A. Health history
   1. Current family happenings and their effect on woman
   2. Problems she may be experiencing
   3. Knowledge and understanding of danger signals
   4. Preparation for emergency arrangements
   5. Knowledge and understanding of labor process and of symptoms of beginning labor
   6. Understanding of responsibilities related to preparing for hospital or home delivery
	Anxiety
	Alteration in bowel elimination: constipation or diarrhea
	Alteration in health maintenance
	Knowledge deficit
	Noncompliance
	Alteration in normal physiologic processes†
	Alteration in nutrition: less or more than body requirements
	Potential maternal or fetal compromise†
	Alteration in respiratory functions†
	Sleep pattern disturbance
	Alteration in tissue perfusion: cerebral, cardiopulmonary, renal, gastrointestinal, peripheral
	Alteration in patterns of urinary elimination

B. Psychosocial history
   1. Emotional status (e.g., anxiety about labor and control of pain).
   2. Client and family responses to unborn child
   3. Sibling and grandparent response to coming birth of child
   4. Preparation for care of family at home during woman's absence
   5. Plans for postdelivery care of infant and understanding of infant's needs
   6. Anticipatory worry concerning new parenting responsibilities, sibling rivalry, recuperation from pregnancy and birth, and family planning
   7. Knowledge of diet
   8. Knowledge of fetal movements
   9. Knowledge of positions for rest and relaxation
	Alteration in family process
	Potential alteration in parenting
	Disturbance in self-concept: body image, self-esteem, role performance, personal identity
	Ineffective family coping: compromised or disabling
	Powerlessness
	Sexual dysfunction

C. Review of woman's physical systems	Potential for maternal or fetal compromise†

Physical examination
A. TPR, BP, weight
B. Fundal height and gestational age
   1. FHR and fetal activity
   2. Additional measures other than palpation may be employed to determine presentation, position, and size of infant (e.g., ultrasonography and area of maximum density of fetal heartbeat).
   3. Precise calculations of fetal age may be made with use of various techniques.
D. Edema
E. Skin
F. Pelvic examination is made on weekly visits from week 38 to term to permit evaluation of amount of cervical softening, effacement, and dilatation, and station of presenting part
G. Breasts
	Changes in breasts†
	Alteration in normal physiologic process†
	Potential for maternal or fetal compromise†

Laboratory tests A. Blood B. Urine C. Cervical and vaginal smears for gonorrhea (repeated at 36 weeks).	Alteration in normal physiologic process† Potential for maternal or fetal compromise related to complications†

Continued.

Summary of Nursing Actions—cont'd

OUTCOME CRITERIA	PLAN/IMPLEMENTATION

Emotional support
A. Nurse and client
  1. Client and family participate in interview.
	Support person
	A. Nurse and client
	  1. Use appropriate interview techniques.
	    a. Greet by name in unhurried manner.
	    b. Provide a relaxed and trusting atmosphere.
	    c. Provide privacy.
	    d. Validate normalcy of their responses (if they fall within normal limits).
	    e. Provide information as needed.
	    f. Respect cultural, ethnic, religious, or other responses.
	    g. Ensure confidentiality.

2. Client verbalizes understanding of schedule, need for continuity of care, physical examination to be done, reporting of abnormal symptoms.	2. a. Review protocol for schedule and care. b. Set next appointment time. Medical and nursing care is increased to permit detection of any abnormal maternal or fetal response: woman is examined every 2 weeks between 32 and 36 weeks every week between 36 and 40 weeks; if indicated, plan of care is modified.

3. Client complies with plan of care: client follows diet plan, takes only prescribed medications, refrains from smoking, drinking alcoholic beverages, and exercises.	3. a. Inquire as to convenience of appointment.
	    b. Discuss problems: work mutually toward solutions.
	    c. Review problems associated with noncompliance.

B. Maternal emotional health
  1. Client verbalizes acceptance of pregnancy and unborn child. Ambivalent feelings lessen. Mother expresses feelings of closeness to her unborn child and assigns personal characteristics.
  2. Client expresses satisfaction with herself, her relationships, her feelings of competence.
  3. Client expresses feelings of closeness to her own mother or accepts feelings of distance.
  4. Client verbalizes feeling of tension arising from fears or anxieties pertaining to labor, parental responsibilities, safety of mother and child, and relationships with significant others.
	B. Maternal emotional health
	  1. Discuss parental awareness of unborn child's response to stimuli, such as light, sound, maternal posture or tension, and patterns of sleeping and waking.
	  2. Discuss woman's feeling relating to her self-concept (i.e., self-image self-esteem, sense of power and being in control).
	  3. Discuss mother and daughter relationships: acceptance and use of mother as role model.
	  4. Provide opportunities for discussion of probable emotional tensions related to:
	    a. Childbirth experience such as fear of pain, loss of control, and possible delivery of child before reaching hospital.
	    b. Responsibilities and tasks of parenthood
	    c. Mutual parental concerns arising from anxiety for safety of mother and unborn child.
	    d. Mutual parental concerns related to siblings and their acceptance of new baby.
	    e. Mutual parental concerns about social and economic responsibilities.
	    f. Mutual parental concerns for cognitive dissonance arising from conflicts in cultural, religious, or personal value systems.

5. Mother expresses confidence in her knowledge of her own body.	5. Provide opportunities for discussion of mother's awareness of her body's responses such as "this pregnancy feels O.K." or "something is wrong" and provide acknowledgment of mother's ability.

Summary of Nursing Actions—cont'd

OUTCOME CRITERIA	PLAN/IMPLEMENTATION

Emotional support—cont'd
C. Client and family
  1. Husband and wife express feelings of acceptance of husband and wife's choice of role in pregnancy and in labor.
  2. Mother, father, and siblings talk about unborn child as part of the family.
  3. Woman and partner verbalize understanding of various modes of sexual expression (which are safe, which to avoid) and of medical acceptance of sexual intercourse with penile penetration until rupture of membrane; feelings of frustration and resentment over abstinence expressed early in third trimester and acceptance expressed toward end of third trimester.
	Support person—cont'd
	C. Client and family
	  1. Discuss husband and wife's relationships; partner's commitment to pregnancy, and coping with ambivalence and mood changes.
	  2. Discuss the growing relationship between mother and unborn child and other family members.
	  3. Discuss sexual relationships if partners wish to do so. Instruct as to techniques for sexual expression.

Knowledge and skills
A. Woman or couple verbalizes understanding of physiologic basis, need for immediate treatment, and how to obtain necessary care for complications of pregnancy.
	Teacher/counselor/advocate
	A. Review prenatal danger signals and instruct woman to report the following signs and symptoms immediately:
	  1. Vaginal bleeding: Rule out brownish spotting occurring 48 h after vaginal examination. Rule out "show" of pinkish mucus. Woman is to come to hospital's emergency area immediately for diagnosis and treatment if bleeding is other than one of preceding types.
	  2. Symptoms of preeclampsia-eclampsia.
	  3. Cessation, noticeable diminution, or acceleration in amount of fetal movement: woman is to come to clinic or physician's office for evaluation.
	  4. Rupture of membranes: woman is to come to clinic or physician's office for evaluation.
	  5. Burning or pain on urination: woman is to come to clinic or physician's office for evaluation and to bring urine sample for analysis.
	  6. Chills or elevated temperature.
	  7. Abdominal pain.
	  8. Persistent nausea and vomiting.
	  9. Signs and symptoms of premature labor: woman is to come to labor unit for evaluation.
	  10. Modify original plan of care if maternal or fetal complications are detected. Institute specific remedial interventions.

B. Woman or couple verbalizes understanding of physiologic basis, prevention, and treatment of problems common to third trimester.	B. Discuss physiologic basis, prevention, and treatment for changes common in the third trimester (discomforts):
	  1. Hemorrhoids, vulvar varicosities
	  2. Varicosities
	  3. Leg cramps, ache or edema
	  4. Hypermobility of joints
	  5. Backache
	  6. Return of urinary frequency
	  7. Shortness of breath
	  8. Round ligament pain
	  9. Discomfort from Braxton Hicks' contractions and differentiation from "false labor"
	  10. Emotional changes
	  11. Sexual needs and changes; intercourse

Continued.

Summary of Nursing Actions —cont'd

OUTCOME CRITERIA	PLAN/IMPLEMENTATION
Knowledge and skills—cont'd C. Woman and family verbalize understanding of rationale for answers to common questions	**Teacher/counselor/advocate—cont'd** C. Provide answers to common questions relating to: 　1. Clothing 　2. Bathing and swimming 　3. Employment 　4. Travel 　5. Physical activity 　6. Dental problems 　7. Immunization 　8. Drugs 　9. Substance abuse 　10. Radiation 　11. Resources available 　　a. Education 　　b. Dental evaluation 　　c. Medical service 　　d. Social service 　　e. Emergency room
D. Woman and family verbalize 　1. Understanding of fetal development, fetal heart rate, and fetal movements, and maternal adaptation and status. 　2. Understanding of fetal and maternal needs during pregnancy.	D. 1. Instruct woman and family concerning fetal development, maternal adaptations, maternal and fetal symptomatology and significance. (This is a gradual process. It may take weeks to complete). 　2. Instruct woman and family concerning maternal and fetal needs (e.g., care during travel, continuity of care).
E. 1. Woman and family verbalize understanding of maternal and fetal nutritional needs. 　2. Physical response indicates compliance with nutritional counsel. 　3. Verbalizes understanding of choices regarding infant feeding.	E. 1. Provide nuritional guidance (see also Chapter 12). 　　a. Weight gain 　　b. Balanced diet 　　c. Special nutritional needs 　　d. Supplements 　2. Comment on appearance, energy level. 　3. Instruct regarding choices in infant feeding.
F. Verbalizes understanding of choices and availability of prenatal education classes.	F. Instruct regarding choices in prenatal education classes.
G. Woman seeks assistance for problems such as infections, colds, allergies, and substance abuse (smoking or drinking).	G. 1. Instruct regarding effects on woman or unborn child or such problems. 　2. Suggest or institute remedial care.
H. Verbalizes readiness for labor. 　1. Expresses eagerness to be done with pregnancy; complaints about awkwardness, annoyance about symptoms (shortness of breath and backache) expressed; questions asked about how soon appearance will be back to "normal." 　2. Interest centered around preparing for labor and delivery. 　3. Anxiety may be expressed over pain in labor, behavior during labor, care of other children.	H. Encourage client and family to discuss feelings.
I. Verbalizes understanding of preparation for delivery; symptoms of impending labor (i.e., uterine contractions, rupture of membranes, bloody "show"), what to report, and where to go for delivery.	I. Discuss preparation for labor. 　1. Symptoms of impending labor and what information to report. 　2. Breathing and relaxation techniques. 　3. Involvement of husband or significant other. 　4. Provision for needs of other children. 　5. Plans to get to hospital.

Summary of Nursing Actions —cont'd

OUTCOME CRITERIA	PLAN/IMPLEMENTATION
Knowledge and skills—cont'd	**Teacher/counselor/advocate—cont'd**
J. Verbalizes understanding of delivery process.	J. Review plans of labor, terminology, and what care to expect.
K. Requests information relative to caring for new baby: a. Plans for care of newborn; help at home; preparation of siblings.	K. Discuss preparation for baby.
Physical care	**Technician**
A. Maternal	A. Maternal
1. Appearance is healthy, grooming adequate, energy level normal.	1. Comments in positive manner about her appearance. Inquire about energy level. Review rest and relaxation techniques.
2. TPR, BP, weight	2. Shares findings prn.
a. Temperature, normal range	
b. Pulse, gradual rise of $+8$ to $+10$ by thirty-fifth week	
c. Respirations, 18-20/min; occasional shortness of breath and sighing breaths may be troublesome at times.	
d. Blood pressure, systolic no greater than $+30$ and diastolic no greater than $+15$ over baseline, which is normally higher ($+6$ to $+10$) as term approaches.	
e. Weight gain, week 27 to term: no more than 1 lb. (0.45 kg) per week; approximately 27 ± 4 lb (11 kg) gain over prepregnancy weight (less than 20 lb [9 kg] puts fetus at risk).	
f. Edema, dependent edema of lower legs, ankles, and feet.	3. Instruct woman regarding significance of findings. Review resting position.
4. Abdomen, enlargement continues: see fundal height. Toward end of pregnancy striae gravidarum may occur; in multipara glistening silvery lines of striae from earlier pregnancies may be seen. Linea nigra at midline of abdomen.	4. Review significance of findings.
5. Uterus, continued progressive enlargement of uterus.	5. Review significance of findings.
a. Fundal height at 36 weeks: almost to xiphoid process; 40 weeks; 2 cm below caused by "lightening."	
b. Readiness for labor: Braxton Hicks' contractions may be felt.	
6. Fetus, fetal heart rate and rhythm are normal (120-160 beats/min) and regular; will be less if fetus is asleep and greater with fetal movement.	6. Let woman and family listen to FHR. Review significance of findings.
a. Fetal movements increase with maternal movements, may lessen during fetal sleep, same pattern of movements every 24 hours.	
b. Fundal heights, abdominal growth, and estimation of weight within normal limits for the estimated gestational age; presentation, size of infant and maternal pelvic configuration permit vaginal delivery.	
c. Engagement occurs about 2 weeks before term in nullipara; may not occur until labor is well established in parous woman.	
7. Skin, may develop chloasma (mask of pregnancy), vascular spiders, palmar erythema (red palms).	7. Review physiologic basis for skin changes, varicosities.
8. Varicose veins may appear in lower legs and vulva.	8. Instruct regarding posture and resting.

Continued.

Summary of Nursing Actions—cont'd

OUTCOME CRITERIA	PLAN/IMPLEMENTATION
Physical care—cont'd	**Technician—cont'd**
9. Pelvic examination, findings are within normal limits.	9. Review significance of findings.
a. Vagina, highly distensible. Leukorrhea persists.	
b. Cervix, readiness for labor: Cervix becomes more softened as term approaches. In parous women, external os of cervix may be about 3 cm dilated by week 35.	
c. Pelvis, pelvic measurements adequate in relation to size of fetus (reexamined near term).	
10. Breasts, striations may appear if increase in size of breasts is extensive.	10. Review significance of findings.
a. Areola become larger and more deeply pigmented and glands of Montgomery's appear.	Begin preparation of breasts for breast feedings.
b. Lactogenesis begins with secretion of colostrum; may be expressed by gentle massage.	
c. Preparation of breasts for breast feeding begins.	
Laboratory tests	Review significance of findings.
A. Blood tests, RBC, at sea level for week 27 to term: Hgb, 10 g/dl; hematocrit, 33%; RBC repeated at 32-34 weeks; sexually transmitted disease (VDRL), negative.	Review necessity for repetition of tests as necessary. Review prevention and treatment of anemia.
B. Urinalysis, negative for protein and acetone, no greater than 1+ for glucose; lactose is present as hormone prolactin increases.	
C. Tests for infection are negative.	

Application of the Nursing Process

PRENATAL PERIOD

Carol (age 29) and Si (age 30) are expecting their second child. A review of Carol's prenatal record reveals the following information:

First pregnancy 1983, normal pregnancy, delivered 8 lb 4 oz. (3742 g) boy.

Second pregnancy 1985, ended in abortion at 10 weeks.

Present pregnancy EDC September 15, 1987.

Carol works as a computer programmer. Si is an electrical engineer. Both come from large families and want another child. Peter (age 4) attends nursery school five mornings a week. Carol is in her 36th week of pregnancy and has maternity leave for 3 months.

At her regular checkup, Carol reports the following:

1. She finds it increasingly difficult to sleep at night. She gets short of breath and leg cramps in the middle of the night.
2. Peter's behavior has changed. He cries when she leaves him at school. He took back all the toys he had put in the baby's room. He is clinging, wants to be picked up and held. He makes her impatient.
3. Carol describes her feelings of love for the unborn baby. "We don't even know her, yet we love her."

Application of the Nursing Process—cont'd

FUNCTIONAL PATTERN: ASSESSMENT	NURSING DIAGNOSIS	RATIONALE: PLAN/ IMPLEMENTATION	EVALUATION
SLEEP-REST ■ Sleep difficult ■ Shortness of breath ■ Leg cramps	Sleep pattern disturbance related to a. Shortness of breath	*To faciliatate sleep and rest:* 1. Review physiologic basis. a. Shortness of breath: expansion of diaphragm limited by enlarging uterus (compensated for in part by other maternal adaptations); may be caused by increased sensitivy to or compensation for slight acidosis ("breathing for two").	Carol reports relief of symptoms and that measures were successful.
	b. Leg cramps	b. Leg cramps: compression of nerves supplying lower extremities because of enlarging uterus; reduced level of diffusible serum calcium or elevation of serum phosphorus; aggravating factors: fatigue, poor peripheral circulation.	

		2. Demonstrate.
		  a. Relieve shortness of breath.
		    (1) Sleep with extra pillows.
		    (2) Do flying exercises.
			Carol demonstrates use of pillow, flying exercises.

		b. Prevention and treatment of leg cramps. (1) Avoid pointing toes when stretching legs and lead with heel of foot when walking; avoid drinking more than 1 L (1 qt) of milk per day (may need to limit to 0.5 (1 pt); avoid fatigue and cold legs; take diet with adequate calcium.	Carol demonstrates techniques.

Continued.

Application of the Nursing Process—cont'd

FUNCTIONAL PATTERN: ASSESSMENT	NURSING DIAGNOSIS	RATIONALE: PLAN/ IMPLEMENTATION	EVALUATION
SLEEP-REST—cont'd		(2) Oral supplementation with calcium carbonate or calcium lactate tablets, 0.6 g three times a day before meals; aluminum hydroxide gel, 1 oz (30 ml) with each meal, removes phosphorus by absorbing it. (3) Use massage and heat over affected muscle; stretch affected muscle by standing up and leaning forward on affected leg or by having another person extend knee and dorsiflex foot of affected leg until spasm relaxes (Fig 11.12); stand on cold surface; treatment same as prevention.	
ROLE-RELATIONSHIP ■ Peter's behavior.	Alteration in family processes related to 4 year old's response to mother's pregnancy (i.e., fear of being deserted; anger toward unborn; need to focus mother's attention on himself; need for mother's interest and body contact).	*To enhance role relationships:* 1. Encourage Carol to tell what she is doing to cope. Praise her successes. 2. Review 4-year-old child's concepts (cognitive); concrete here-and-now world, little understanding of future, need to keep mother's attention, regressive behavior is coping mechanism. 3. Discuss ways of: a. Paying attention to Peter and resting at same time (i.e., reading to him; playing table games).	At next visit have Carol describe what she has done and what has helped.

Application of the Nursing Process—cont'd

FUNCTIONAL PATTERN: ASSESSMENT	NURSING DIAGNOSIS	RATIONALE: PLAN/ IMPLEMENTATION	EVALUATION
ROLE-RELATIONSHIP —cont'd	Keeping Peter close by (i.e., bring Peter on clinic visits, have him listen to baby's heart beats; take him on daily walk; let him help with house-work).		
		4. Suggest she talk with other mothers as this behavior is a common oc-curence.	Ask what other moth-er's are doing.
		5. Review good body me-chanics for lifting and carrying Peter (i.e., bend knees, keep back straight, lift by straight-ening legs) (Fig. 11.5).	Ask about back stretch and if body mechan-ics helped.
SELF-PERCEPTION–SELF-CONCEPT	Disturbance in self-con-cept related to her feel-ing:	*To enhance self-concept:*	Inquire at next visit how she and her son are managing.
■ Peter's behavior is changed.	1. That her mother-son relationship is chang-ing.	1. Raise her conscious awareness of feelings.	
■ He makes her impa-tient.	2. That she is depriving her son by having an-other child.	2. Note normalcy of such feelings shared by other mothers.	
	3. That she will not be able to love two chil-dren as much as one.	3. Encourage her to talk about her feelings.	
		4. Encourage her to talk about her feelings to-ward her own siblings.	
COGNITIVE-PERCEPTUAL	Knowledge deficit related to lack of awareness of how much mother and father know about un-born baby.	*To increase knowledge base:*	At next visit, question Carol as to growing knowledge of unborn child.
■ We don't know her (the unborn baby).		1. Review knowledge re-lating to unborn (i.e., vision, hearing; re-sponse to heat, cold, touch; sleep and wake patterns).	
		2. Assist Carol to identify what she knows of this baby.	
		3. Question Carol as to why sex has been as-signed (no ultrasono-graph has been done).	
		4. Compare with what other parents have ex-pressed (i.e., girl is smaller, gentler move-ments).	
		5. Anticipate possible disappointment, "not always correct."	

Continued.

Application of the Nursing Process

FUNCTIONAL PATTERN: ASSESSMENT	NURSING DIAGNOSIS	RATIONALE: PLAN/ IMPLEMENTATION	EVALUATION
ROLE-RELATIONSHIP ■ We love her.	Alteration in parenting relating to growth of love to include two children.	*To enhance role relationships:* 1. Comment on how family structure has already changed; unborn child is a real child to them. 2. Note how parents have begun process of integrating child into family.	Comment on Carol and Si's positive statements about newborn.

References

Affonso, D.D.: The Filipino American. In Clark A., editor: Culture/childbearing/health professionals, Philadelphia, 1978, F.A. Davis Co.

American Cancer Society, 535 Race St., San Jose, CA, 1986.

Artschwager, M.: Anthropology of human birth, Philadelphia, 1982, F.A. Davis Co.

Batzer, F.R.: Guidelines for choosing a pregnancy test, Contemp. OB/Gyn. 26:37(special issue), Oct. 1985.

Bernstein, J.L., and Kidd, Y.A.: Childbearing in Japan. In Kay, M.A., editor: Anthropology of human birth, Philadelphia, 1982, F.A. Davis Co.

Bing, E., and Colman, L.: Making love during pregnancy, New York, 1977, Bantam Books.

Bracken, M.B., and Holford, T.R.: Exposure to prescribed drugs in pregnancy and association with congenital malformations, Obstet. Gynecol. 58:336, 1981.

Brown, M.S.: A cross-cultural look at pregnancy, labor, and delivery, Obstet. Gynecol. Nurs. 5:35, 1976.

Brucker, M.C., and Reedy, N.J.: Maternity leaves and the Pregnancy Discrimination Act, J.O.G.N. Nurs. 12:341, 1983.

Bryant, H.: Antenatal counseling for women working outside the homes, Birth 12:4, Winter 1985.

Bullard, J.A.: Exercise and pregnancy, Can. Fam. Physician 27:977, 1981.

Carrington, B.W.: The Afro-American. In Clark, A.L., editor: Culture/childbearing/health professionals, Philadelphia, 1978, F.A. Davis Co.

Chang, A.: Auto safety in pregnancy, a neglected area, Contemp. OB/Gyn. 254:117, 1985.

Chung, H.J.: Understanding the Oriental maternity patient, Nurs. Clin. North Am. 12:67, Mar. 1977.

Clark, M.: Health in the Mexican-American culture: a community study, Berkeley, 1970, University of California Press.

Cohen, A.: Movement as a yardstick for fetal well-being, Contemp. OB/Gyn. 26:61, Aug. 1985.

Crosby, W.M.: Traumatic injuries during pregnancy, Clin. Obset. Gynecol. 26(4):902, 1983.

Dale, E., and others: Exercise during pregnancy: effects on the fetus, Can. J. Appl. Sport Sci. 7:98, June 1982.

Dameron, G.W.: Helping couples cope with sexual changes pregnancy brings, Contemp. Obstet. Gynecol. 21:23, Feb. 1983.

Dawson, K.P., and others: Keeping abreast of the times: the Tauranga infant feeding survey, N.Z. Med. J. 89:75, 1979.

Dean, J.: Pregnancy and exercise: how much and what kind? On this the experts agree: more research is needed, Sportwest 1:30, Dec. 1981.

Doucette, J.S.: Is breast-feeding still safe for babies? M.C.N. 3:354, 1978.

Dressendorfer, R.H., and Goodlin, R.C.: Fetal heart rate response to maternal exercise testing, Phys. Sportsmed. 8:90, Nov. 1980.

Edwards, M.: Communications: dimensions in childbirth education, Pacific Grove, Calif., 1973, M. Edwards.

Flood, B., and Naeye, R.: Factors that predispose to premature rupture of fetal membranes, J.O.G.N. Nurs. 13:4, Mar.-Apr. 1984.

Gallo, A.M., and others: Little refugees with big needs, R.N. 43:45, 1980.

Gussler, J.: Poor mothers and modern medicine in St. Kitts. In Kay, M.A., editor: Anthropology of human birth, Philadelphia, 1982, F.A. Davis Co.

Hollingsworth, A.O., and others: The refugees and childbearing: what to expect, R.N. 43:45, 1980.

Horn, B.M.: Northwest coast Indians: the Muckleshoot. In Kay, M.A., editor: Anthropology of human birth, Philadelphia, 1982, F.A. Davis Co.

Howard, F.M., and Hill, J.M.: Drugs in pregnancy, Obstet. Gynecol. Surv. 34:643, 1979.

Hutchinson, P.L., and others: Metabolic and circulatory responses to running during pregnancy, Phys. Sportsmed. 9:55, Aug. 1981.

Jopke, T.: Pregnancy: a time to exercise judgement, Phys. Sportsmed. 11:139, July 1983.

Kay, M.A., editor: Anthropology of human birth, Philadelphia, 1982, F.A. Davis Co.

Kendall, K.: Maternal and child care in an Iranian village. In Leininger, M., editor: Transcultural nursing '79, New York, 1979, Masson Publishing U.S.A.

Krozy, R.E., and others: Auto safety, pregnancy and the newborn, J.O.G.N. Nurs. 14:1, Jan.-Feb. 1985.

Leap, T.L., and others: Equal employment opportunity and its implications for personnel practices in the 1980s, Labor Law J. 31:669, 1980.

Luke, B.: Does caffeine influence reproduction? M.C.N. 7:240, July-Aug. 1982.

Malasanos, L., Barkauskas, V., Moss, M., and Stoltenberg-Allen, K.: Health assessment, ed. 3, St. Louis, 1985, The C.V. Mosby Co.

Marbury, M.C., and others: Work and pregnancy, Occup. Med. vol. 26, 1984.

Martin, B.J., and Reeb, R.M.: Oral health during pregnancy: a neglected nursing area, M.C.N. 7:350, 1982.

Martin, B.J., and Reeb, R.M.: The nurse as the first line of defense against periodontal disease, J.O.G.N. Nurs. 12:333, 1983.

McCary, J.L.: Human sexuality: physiological factors, ed. 4, New York, 1982, Van Nostrand Reinhold Co.

McKay, S.: Smoking during the childbearing years, M.C.N. 5:46, Jan.-Feb. 1980.

Meleis, A.I., and Sorrell, L.: Bridging cultures: Arab American women and their birth experiences, M.C.N. 6:171, 1981.

Mill, J., and others: Should coitus late in pregnancy be discouraged: Lancet 1:136, 1981.

Muecke, M.A.: Health care systems as socializing agents: childbearing the North Thai and Western ways, Soc. Sci. Med. 10:377, 1976.

Mueller, L.: Pregnancy and sexuality, J.O.G.N. Nurs. 14:4, July-Aug. 1985.

NAACOG: Reproductive health hazards: women in the workplace, vol. 11, Feb. 1985, NAACOG, 600 Maryland Ave., S.W. Suite 2000, Wash. DC 20024.

Naeye, R.L.: Coitus and associated amniotic-fluid infections, N. Engl. J. Med. 301:1198, 1979.

Naeye, R.L.: Coitus and antepartum hemorrhage, Br. J. Obstet. Gynecol. 88:765, 1981.

News: Monoclonals: new frontiers in reproductive medicine in Technology 1986. Contemp. OB/Gyn. 26:75, Oct. 1985.

Nicholson, W.: Midwives, mothers, and breastfeeding, Nursing Mothers Association of Australia, 5 Glendale St., Nunawading, Victoria 3131, 1985.

Parken, M.: Culture and preventive health care, J.O.G.N. Nurs. 7:40, 1978.

Pritchard, J., and others: Williams/Obstetrics, ed. 17, Norwalk, Conn., 1985, Appleton-Century-Crofts.

Queenan, J.T., editor: Managing ob/gyn emergencies: a contemporary ob/gyn book, Oradell, N.J., 1982, Medical Economics Co.

Riordan, J.M.: Breastfeeding: a guide for nurses, St. Louis, 1983, The C.V. Mosby Co.

Sandberg, E.C.: Synopsis of obstetrics, ed. 10, St. Louis, 1978, The C.V. Mosby Co.

Snow, L.: Folk medical beliefs and their implications for care of patients, Ann. Intern. Med. 81:82, 1974.

Stern, P.M.: Solving problems of cross-cultural health teaching: the Filipino childbearing family, Image 13:47, 1981.

Stringfellow, L.: The Vietnamese. In Clark, A., editor: Culture/childbearing/health professionals, Philadelphia, 1978, F.A. Davis Co.

Tucker, S.M., and others: Patient care standards, ed. 3, St. Louis, 1984, The C.V. Mosby Co.

Wright, L.M., and Leahey, M.: Nurses and families: a guide to family assessment and interaction, Philadelphia, 1984, F.A. Davis Co.

Zalar, M.K.: Sexual counseling for pregnant couples, M.C.N. 1:176, May-June 1976.

Ziskin, D.E., and Neese, G.J.: Pregnancy gingivitis: history, classification, etiology, Am. J. Orthod. 32:390, 1980.

Bibliography

Afaf Ibraheim Meltas, L.: Arab American women and their birth experiences, M.C.N. 6:171, May-June 1981.

Bash, D.: Jewish religious practices related to childbearing, J. Nurse Midwife 25(5):39, 1980.

Benson, F.C., editor: Current obstetric and gynecologic diagnosis and treatment, ed. 4, Los Altos, Calif., 1982, Lange Medical Publications.

Bentz, J.M.: Missed meanings in nurse/patient communication, M.C.N. 5:55, Jan.-Feb. 1980.

Gray, J.D., and others: Prediction and prevention of child abuse, Semin. Perinatol. 3:86, Jan. 1979.

Gross, C., and others: The Vietnamese American family—and grandma makes three, M.C.N. 6:177, May-June 1981.

Shanghold, M.: Keeping fit during pregnancy, Fit 6:68, June 1982.

Wheeler, L.A.: Sexuality during pregnancy and the puerperium, Perinatal Press 3:131, Oct. 1979.

Maternal and Fetal Nutrition

A woman can select foods and dietary patterns associated with a healthy pregnancy and a healthy outcome. Considerable resources and information are available to assist her. To promote successful reproduction, however, the dissemination of nutrition information must be directed to persons in all stages of the life cycle, not only to expectant parents, whose motivation to change may temporarily be great. Nutrition education can be effective throughout the life cycle.

The Policy Statement on Nutrition and Pregnancy issued by the American College of Obstetricians and Gynecologists (ACOG) contains the following statements:

a woman's nutritional status before, during and after pregnancy contributes to a significant degree to the well-being of both herself and her infant. Therefore, what a woman consumes before she conceives and while she carries the fetus is of vital importance to the health of succeeding generations.

This chapter presents information on nutrition applicable to the nursing process that the nurse can use in working with families.

Physiologic Adjustments and the Basis for Nutrition Needs in Pregnancy

Many physiologic changes occurring during pregnancy influence the need for nutrients and the efficiency with which the body uses them. Several of these changes are apparent early in the first trimester, an indication that they are an integral part of the maternal-fetal system. Physiologic adjustments create the favorable environment and growth, and prepare the mother for labor, childbirth, and lactation.

Functional alterations
Alimentary. A decrease in gastric motility and intestinal tonus is common in pregnancy. Slowing the passage of food through the gastrointestinal tract may enhance absorption of nutrients. On the other hand, it may be a factor in nausea of pregnancy and may lead to considerable discomfort when it results in constipation.

Respiratory and cardiovascular systems. In addition to serving as a lifeline for nutrients, the placenta functions in the exchange of respiratory gases between the mother and fetus. In the presence of normal concentrations of hemoglobin, maternal blood can deliver up to 16 ml/dl of oxygen. If maternal hemoglobin levels are depressed, the quantity of oxygen per deciliter of blood is reduced. Since the fetus can tolerate little variation in the rate at which oxygen is supplied, the mother must compensate by increasing her cardiac output, which increases her basal metabolic rate (BMR).

Renal system. Renal blood flow and glomerular filtration rate (GFR) are increased somewhat during pregnancy. These accelerations facilitate the clearance of creatinine, urea, and other waste products of fetal and maternal metabolism. Normally most of the glucose, amino acids, and water-soluble vitamins that are filtered by the glomerulus are reabsorbed in the tubules, but in pregnancy substantial quantities of these nutrients appear in the urine. One explanation is that the high GFR offers the tubules greater quantities of nutrients than they can feasibly resorb.

Pregnancy is accompanied by a considerable increase in total body water. Except for women with generalized edema, all the water gained until about 30 weeks' gestation can be accounted for in the products of conception and increases in maternal blood volume and reproductive organs.

At term there is a surplus of about 1 or 2 L. All or most of the gain is lost through perspiration and urine within 6 to 8 weeks after delivery. These calculations have important implications for monitoring and interpreting body weight gained during pregnancy.

Table 12.1
Comparison of Distribution of Weight Gain During Pregnancy Assuming a Minimum Gain of 11 kg.*

Maternal components	A		B†	
Uterus	1,100 g (2.5 lb)		Uterus and breasts	1,600 g (3.5 lb)
Breasts	1,400 g (3 lb)		Blood volume	2,000 g (4.5 lb)
Blood volume	1,800 g (4 lb)		Fluid	1,600 g (3.5 lb)
Maternal stores	1,800-3,600 g (4-8 lb)		Other (fat)	800 g (1.75 lb)
Fetal components	**A**		**B†**	
Fetus	3,400 g (7.5 lb)		Fetus	3,400 g (7.5 lb)
Placenta	450 g (1 lb)		Placenta	600 g (1.5 lb)
Amniotic fluid	900 g (2 lb)		Amniotic fluid	1,000 g (2.25 lb)
TOTAL	11 to 13 kg (24-28 lb)		TOTAL	11 kg (24.5 lb)

*A from Williams, S.R.: Nutrition and diet therapy, ed. 5, St. Louis, 1985, The C.V. Mosby Co.; **B** from Schneider, H.A., and others: Nutritional support of medical practice, New York, 1977, Harper & Row, Publishers.
†Compare B with Fig. 12.1.

Endocrine system. Progesterone causes the deposit of fat in subcutaneous tissues over the abdomen, back, and upper thighs. The fat serves as a caloric reserve for both pregnancy and lactation.

Increases in several hormones affect nutrition, including increased secretion of the following:

1. Aldosterone, which conserves salt, by the adrenal gland
2. Thyroxin, which regulates metabolism, by the thyroid gland
3. Parathyroid hormone, which controls calcium and magnesium metabolism, by the parathyroid gland
4. Human chorionic somatomammotropin (HCS), which also acts as a growth hormone, by the placenta
5. Human chorionic gonadotropin (HCG), which induces nausea and vomiting in some women in early pregnancy, by the placenta

Weight gain during pregnancy. The weight gained in a normal pregnancy will vary among individual women. The acceptable weight gain for most healthy women of normal weight for height carrying a single fetus is 12 kg (27 lb) (Naeye, 1979) with a range of 10 to 14.5 kg (22 to 32 lb).

Along with growth of the developing fetus itself, a concurrent increase in supporting maternal tissue occurs (Table 12.1). The components of maternal weight gain shown in Fig. 12.1 indicate that normal pregnancy calls for considerable weight gain over and above that represented by the size of the fetus. The weight gain ascribed to each component of the maternal weight gain varies by author (Table 12.1). All authors support a *minimum* weight gain of 11 kg.

Pattern of weight gain. A pattern of desirable prenatal gain in weight is shown in Fig. 12.1. To monitor the desirable weight gain as compared to deviations in weight gain, a grid may be used for plotting the pregnant woman's weight throughout pregnancy.

There is general agreement that the normal curve of weight gain should show little gain during the first trimester, a rapid increase during the second, and some slowing in the rate of increase during the third. During the first trimester, growth takes place almost entirely in maternal tissue, gain is primarily in maternal tissue during the second trimester and in fetal tissue in the third trimester.

Deviations in weight and weight gain. Deviations from usual values for either prepregnant weight or weight gain during pregnancy are relatively common. The following are considered to be deviations from the norm:

1. Underweight: prepregnant weight less than 85% of standard weight for age and height* (Appendix F).
2. Overweight: prepregnant weight more than 120% of standard weight for age and height (Appendix F).
3. Inadequate gain: gain of 1 kg (2.2 lb) or less per month in the second or third trimester. Weight loss or failure to gain during pregnancy is a sign of nutritional difficulties.
4. Excessive gain: gain of 3 kg (6.6 lb) or more per month is likely to have been caused by tissue fluid retention rather than by excessive caloric intake. A total weight gain of over 14.5 kg (32 lb) is associated with higher rates of perinatal mortality.

Hazards of restricting adequate weight gain. There are potential hazards for both mother and infant from restricting weight gain during pregnancy. The mother's weight gain and prepregnancy weight are the two strongest influences (except gestational age) on birth weight. Infant birth weights, in turn, have been stud-

---

*The female suffering from anorexia nervosa, the ultimate in malnourishment, is usually amenorrheic and therefore would not be capable of conceiving.

Fig. 12.1

Pattern and components of weight gain throughout course of pregnancy, assuming an 11 kg (24.5 lb) weight gain. (From Schneider, H.A., et al.: Nurtritional support of medical practice, New York, 1977, Harper & Row, Publishers.)

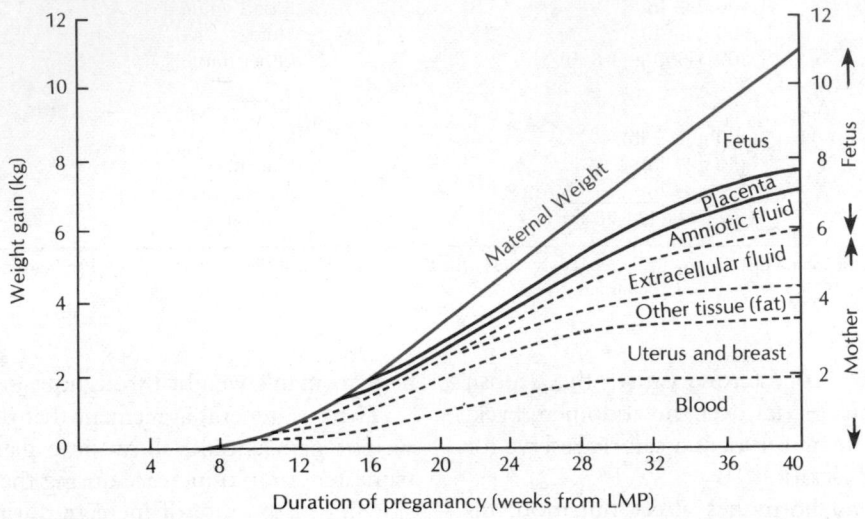

ied intensively with respect to infant mortality and morbidity, brain development, and learning disabilities in later life. Birth weights serve as practical indicators of the health and nutrition of a population.

The obese woman entering pregnancy faces an increased risk of severe complications, notably hyperten-sive disorders and diabetes mellitus, which have adverse effects on pregnancy outcome. Obesity should not be equated with overall good nutrition; excessive caloric ingestion may mask other nutritional problems (e.g., anemia, inadequate protein intake). Some persons have advocated restriction of weight gain in such

Table 12.2

Recommended Daily Dietary Allowances (RDAs) Designed for the Maintenance of Good Nutrition of Practically All Healthy People in the United States*

		Weight		Height				Fat-soluble vitamins		
	Age (years)	kg	lb	cm	in	Energy (kcal)	Protein (g)	Vitamin A (µg RE)†	Vitamin D (µg)‡	Vitamin E (mg α TE)§
Females	11-14	46	101	157	62	2500	46	800	10	8
	15-18	55	120	163	64	2400	46	800	10	8
	19-22	55	120	163	64	2400	44	800	7.5	8
	23-50	55	120	163	64	2300	44	800	5	8
	51+	55	120	163	64	2300	44	800	5	8
Pregnant						+300	+30	+200	+5	+2
Lactating						+200	+20	+400	+5	+3

From Food and Nutrition Board, National Academy of Sciences—National Research Council, Washington, D.C., 1980.
*The allowances are intended to provide for individual variations among most normal persons as they live in the United States under usual environmental stresses. Diets should be based on a variety of common foods in order to provide other nutrients for which human requirements have been less well defined.
†Retinol equivalents. 1 Retinol equivalent = 1 µg retinol or 6 µg 8 carotene.
‡As cholecalciferol. 10 µg cholecalciferol = 400 IU vitamin D.
§α tocopherol equivalents. 1 mg d-α-tocopherol = 1 α TE.

women so that they conclude pregnancy with a net loss. However, the advisability of such a course seems questionable on several grounds. First, dietary restrictions to limit calories may also result in displacement of other nutrients from the diet. Second, optimal protein utilization in pregnancy apparently requires a minimum of approximately 30 kcal/kg/24 hours. This weight gain may be excessive, however, if calculated on obese weight. Third, dietary restriction results in catabolism of fat stores, which in turn produces ketonemia. Ketonemia jeopardizes the development of the fetus.

Nutrient Needs

The nutrients the mother must consume to supply the fetus and her own changing body are given in the Recommended Daily Dietary Allowances (RDAs) for pregnancy (Table 12.2). The RDAs may be used as a guide for evaluation of the gravida's diet. Nutrient needs of pregnancy, reasons for increased nutrient need in pregnancy, and food sources are summarized in Table 12.3.

Energy (kilocalories): RDA nonpregnant, 2400; pregnant, 2700. To support good energy status during pregnancy, sufficient energy is required for the following:
1. Growth of new tissue
2. Deposition of nutrients
3. Increased metabolic expenditure of energy to maintain the tissue and nutrient deposition

4. Increased activity level associated with the movement of a heavier body as pregnancy progresses and with other activities such as work and play

Tissue growth
Uterine-placental-fetal unit. Placentas of poorly nourished mothers often contain fewer and smaller cells. Poorly developed placentas have a reduced ability to synthesize substances needed by the fetus, to facilitate flow of needed nutrients, and to inhibit passage of potentially harmful substances. Therefore it is understandable that the infant of a poorly nourished mother would be poorly nourished and would be small for gestational age (SGA) (see Chapter 30). Maternal uterine adaptations are discussed in Chapter 9.

Maternal blood volume and constituents. Total blood volume is known to increase about 33% above normal levels. Plasma volume increased 50% in nulliparas and higher in multiparas. Red blood cell (RBC) production is stimulated during pregnancy. The number of RBCs increase gradually; the expansion of plasma volume proceeds more rapidly. This relatively more rapid increase in plasma volume over RBC mass results in hemodilution referred to as physiologic (pseudo) anemia of pregnancy. At the same time, a deficiency of iron or of folic acid may contribute to the development of true anemia.

Blood levels of many nutrients decrease during pregnancy secondary to hemodilution, for example, total protein. Most plasma lipid fractions rise during pregnancy. For example, cholesterol increased from under 200 mg/dl to between 250 and 300 mg/dl.

Water-soluble Vitamins							Minerals					
Vitamin C (mg)	Thiamin (mg)	Riboflavin (mg)	Niacin (mg NE)‖	Vitamin B$_6$ (mg)	Folacin¶ (µg)	Vitamin B$_{12}$# (µg)	Calcium (mg)	Phosphorus (mg)	Magnesium (mg)	Iron (mg)	Zinc (mg)	Iodine (µg)
50	1.1	1.3	15	1.8	400	3.0	1200	1200	300	18	15	150
60	1.1	1.3	14	2.0	400	3.0	1200	1200	300	18	15	150
60	1.1	1.3	14	2.0	400	3.0	800	800	300	10	15	150
60	1.0	1.2	13	2.0	400	3.0	800	800	300	18	15	150
60	1.0	1.2	13	2.0	400	3.0	800	800	300	10	15	150
+20	+0.4	+0.3	+2	+0.6	+400	+1.0	+400	+400	+150	**	+5	+25
+40	+0.5	+0.5	+5	+0.5	+100	+1.0	+400	+400	+150	**	+10	+50

‖1 NE (niacin equivalent) is equal to 1 mg of niacin or 60 mg of dietary tryptophan.

¶The folacin allowances refer to dietary sources as determined by *Lactobaccilus casei* assay after treatment with enzymes ("conjugates") to make polyglutamyl forms of the vitamin available for the test organism.

#The RDA for vitamin B$_{12}$ in infants based on average concentration of the vitamin in human milk. The allowances after weaning are based on energy intake (as recommended by the American Academy of Pediatrics) and consideration of other factors such as intestinal absorption.

**The increased requirement during pregnancy cannot be met by the iron content of habitual American diets nor by the existing iron stores of many women; therefore the use of 30-60 mg of supplemental iron is recommended. Iron needs during lactation are not substantially different from those of nonpregnant women, but continued supplementation of the mother for 2 to 3 months after parturition is advisable in order to replenish stores depleted by pregnancy.

Table 12.3
Nutrient Needs of Pregnancy

Nutrient	Amount (NRC) Nonpregnant Adult Need (19-22 yr)	Amount (NRC) Pregnancy Need	Reasons for Increased Nutrient Need in Pregnancy	Food Sources

Protein	44 g	74 g	Rapid fetal tissue growth
			Amniotic fluid
			Placental growth and development
			Maternal tissue growth: uterus, breasts
			Increased maternal circulating blood volume:
			  Hemoglobin increase
			  Plasma protein increase
			Maternal storage reserves for labor, delivery, and lactation
				Milk
				Cheese
				Egg
				Meat
				Grains
				Legumes
				Nuts

Calories	2400	2700	Increased BMR, energy needs Protein sparing	Carbohydrates Fats Proteins
Minerals				
Calcium	800 mg	1200 mg	Fetal skeleton formation Fetal tooth bud formation Increased maternal calcium metabolism	Milk Cheese Whole grains Leafy vegetables Egg yolk Milk
Phosphorus	800 mg	1200 mg	Fetal skeletal formation Fetal tooth bud formation Increased maternal phosphorus metabolism	Milk Cheese Lean meats
Iron	18 mg	18+ mg (+30-60 mg supplement)	Increased maternal circulating blood volume, increased hemoglobin Fetal liver iron storage (primarily in third trimester) High iron cost of pregnancy	Liver Meats Egg Whole or enriched grain Leafy vegetables Nuts Legumes Dried fruits
Iodine	150 µg	175 µg	Increased BMR—increased thyroxine production	Iodized salt
Magnesium	300 mg	450 mg	Coenzyme in energy and protein metabolism Enzyme activator Tissue growth, cell metabolism Muscle action	Nuts Soybeans Cocoa Seafood Whole grains Dried beans and peas
Vitamins				
A	800 RE* (4000 IU)	1000 RE* (5000 IU)	Essential for cell development, hence tissue growth Tooth bud formation (development of enamel-forming cells in gum tissue) Bone growth	Butter Cream Fortified margarine Green and yellow vegetables
D	5 µg† (200 IU)	10 µg† (400 IU)	Absorption of calcium and phosphorus, mineralization of bone tissue, tooth buds	Fortified milk Fortified margarine

Adapted and revised from Williams, S.: Handbook of maternal and infant nutrition, Berkeley, Calif., 1976, SRW Productions, Inc.
*Retinol equivalents (RE) replace international units (IU).
†400 IU (international units) = 10 µg of pure crystalline vitamin D_3 (cholecalciferol).
‡Total vitamin E activity, estimated to be 80% as alpha-tocopherol and 20% as other tocopherols.

Table 12.3, cont'd
Nutrient Needs of Pregnancy

Nutrient	Amount (NRC)		Reasons for Increased Nutrient Need in Pregnancy	Food Sources
	Nonpregnant Adult Need (19-22 yr)	Pregnancy Need		
E	8 mg alpha-TE‡	10 mg alpha-TE‡	Tissue growth, cell wall integrity Red blood cell integrity	Vegetable oils Leafy vegetables Cereals Meat Egg Milk
C	60 mg	80 mg	Tissue formation and integrity Cement substance in connective and vascular tissues Increases iron absorption	Citrus fruits Berries Melons Tomatoes Chili peppers Green peppers Green leafy vegetables Broccoli Potatoes
Folic acid (Folacin)	400 µg	800 µg (+200-400 µg supplement)	Increased metabolic demand in pregnancy Prevention of megaloblastic anemia in high-risk women Increased heme production for hemoglobin Production of cell nucleus material Coenzyme in energy metabolism Coenyzme in protein metabolism	Meat Peanuts Beans and Peas Enriched grains
Riboflavin	1.2 mg	1.5 mg	Coenzyme in energy metabolism and protein metabolism	Milk Liver Enriched grains
Thiamin	1.1 mg	1.5 mg	Coenzyme for energy metabolism	Pork, beef Liver Whole or enriched grains Legumes
B_6 (pyridoxine)	2.0 mg	2.6 mg	Coenzyme in protein metabolism Increased fetal growth requirement	Wheat, corn Liver Meat
B_{12}	3.0 µg	4.0 µg	Coenzyme in protein metabolism, especially vital cell proteins such as nucleic acid Formation of red blood cells	Milk Egg Meat Liver Cheese

Maternal mammary changes. Preparation of mammary glands for lactation is presented in Chapter 21.

Deposition of nutrients. Both fat and protein are deposited during pregnancy. By term about 3.8 kg of fat, representing about 36,000 kcal, has been deposited. Protein stores total about 925 g at term, and deposition of protein represents about 5200 kcal. Thus total fat and protein deposits require about 41,000 kcal.

Metabolic needs. Basal metabolic rates (BMR), when expressed as kilocalories per minute, are about 20% higher in pregnant women than in nonpregnant women. This increase includes the energy cost for tissue synthesis. The increased basal energy need over the entire pregnancy period plus the energy needed for new tissue brings the total energy cost for pregnancy to about 80,000 kcal, or about 300 kcal/in 24 hours.

Activity level. Energy required for activity essential for ordinary living as well as for planned physical exercise is probably the most variable contributor to energy expenditure. The additional energy required for activity per kilogram of body weight is the same in pregnant and nonpregnant women.

If the woman participates regularly in weight-bearing activities, her energy needs will be greater than that recommended. Since the energy needs for activity vary from one woman to another, it is best to advise women to eat enough to satisfy their physiologic hunger and to support a weight gain of about 0.4 kg (13 to 14 oz) per week during the last 30 weeks of pregnancy.

Water fluid needs. Water as an essential nutrient is frequently overlooked during assessment. Among its many functions, water assists digestion by dissolving food and aiding its transport. Essential during the exchange of nutrients and wastes across cell membranes, water is the main substance of cells, blood, lymph, and other vital body fluids. It also aids in maintaining body temperature.

Six to eight glasses (1500 to 2000 ml) of water and juices every 24 hours are recommended. Other types of fluids contain ingredients that are best used sparingly or omitted during pregnancy. For instance, fluids containing high levels of sodium, artificial sweeteners, and other additives are discouraged.

Protein: RDA nonpregnant, 44 g; pregnant, 74 g. The efficiency of protein utilization depends on the protein's digestibility and amino acid composition. Proteins that do not contain all eight essential amino acids in amounts proportional to human requirements are utilized less efficiently. The utilization of even high-quality protein is only about 70%.

Protein utilization also depends on caloric intake. This means that calories from nonprotein sources (i.e., carbohydrate, fat) have a sparing effect on protein. If these calories are inadequate, protein requirements would increase.

Recommended protein intake is adjusted to the body size of individuals. The following guidelines are suggested:
1. Mature women: 1.3 g protein per kilogram of pregnant weight
2. Adolescent girls (15 to 18 years of age): 1.5 g protein per kilogram of pregnant weight
3. Younger girls: 1.7 g protein per kilogram of pregnant weight

A greater amount is recommended for adolescents and younger girls to support possible continued maturation. If a multiple birth (e.g., twins) is expected, the need for protein and other nutrients in the mother's diet is increased.

Major minerals

Iron: RDA nonpregnant, 18 mg; pregnant, 18+ mg (+30-60 mg supplement). The changes in maternal red blood volume and cell mass accompanying pregnancy represent a fundamental physiologic adjustment.

Since full-term average-for-gestational-age (AGA) infants are born with high hemoglobin levels of 18 to 22 g/dl and with a supply of iron stored in the liver to last 3 to 6 months, the maternal organism must transfer about 300 mg of iron to the fetus during gestation.

If dietary iron is not available to meet the needs of the maternal-placental-fetal unit, iron stores will be depleted and there will be a reduction in expansion of the maternal red cell mass rather than impairment of fetal iron reserves. If the mother has no iron reserves, which occurs frequently in young women, especially teenagers, maternal hemoglobin levels will drop more than usual and iron deficiency anemia may be superimposed on the physiologic anemia of pregnancy. Iron supplementation is usually started during the second trimester to maintain maternal reserves and to meet fetal requirements during pregnancy.

Calcium: RDA nonpregnant, 800 mg; pregnant, 1200 mg. Almost all the additional calcium required during pregnancy is utilized by the fetus. Because it is virtually impossible to meet these requirements with foods other than dairy products, milk is considered by many to be particularly essential during pregnancy. One liter of milk contains 1200 mg of calcium, precisely the amount suggested in the RDAs. Individuals who do not consume milk or milk products—for example, persons with lactose intolerance or reduced intake of dairy foods—will require calcium supplementation.

Calcium and phosphorus are found in the same foods. If calcium needs are met, adequate phosphorus will be assured.

Sodium: RDA not given. During pregnancy there is a slight increase in the need for most nutrients, including sodium. Routine restriction of sodium is unphysiologic and unfounded. Diets low in calories and sodium place the normal mother and her fetus at unneccesary risk (Worthington-Roberts, Vermeersch and Williams, 1985; Williams, 1981). When sodium is restricted, the maternal organism undergoes a series of hormonal and biochemical changes in an effort to conserve sodium.

Sources of excessive sodium are discouraged, however. Excessive sodium is found in many canned and processed foods. Products devoid of nutritive value and excessively high in sodium include pretzels, potato chips, soft drinks, and bouillion cubes. Hidden sources of sodium occur in medications such as bicarbonate of soda. Some people are unaware that table salt contains sodium.

The use of diuretics during pregnancy should be discouraged because their use leads not only to loss of sodium but also to electrolyte imbalance, thereby placing the pregnant woman and her unborn child in double jeopardy. Diuretics and sodium restriction are of no value in the prevention or treatment of pregnancy-induced hypertension (PIH) (see Chapter 29). The problem in PIH is not with the sodium ion but with the role of plasma proteins in hypovolemia (Williams, 1985).

Fat-soluble vitamins

Vitamin A: RDA nonpregnant, 800 RE (4000 IU); pregnant, 1000 RE (5000 IU). The added allowance for pregnancy relates to fetal storage of the vitamin. The RDA can readily be provided by dietary sources. There appears to be no need for routine supplementation. Certain food faddists advocate massive amounts of vitamin A. Pregnant women should be cautioned against this practice. Toxicity related to *hypervitaminosis A* represents a potential danger to both the pregnant woman (liver damage) and to her unborn child (congenital malformations).

Vitamin D: RDA nonpregnant, 5 μg (200 IU); pregnant, 10 μg (400 IU). Vitamin D plays an important role in promoting positive calcium balance in pregnancy. It is present naturally in only a few animal foods such as fatty fish, eggs, butter, and liver. It is also produced in the skin by the action of ultraviolet light on dehydrocholesterol. Excessive amounts in the mother may cause *hypervitaminosis D* expressed as hypercalcemia in infants. Since most milk in the United States is fortified with vitamin D at a level of 10 μg per quart, the daily consumption of a quart of milk provides the full allowance of vitamin D and of calcium as well for most gravidas.

Water-soluble vitamins. The water-soluble vitamins, in contrast to those soluble in fat, are readily excreted in urine. The daily diet must supply the RDA because storage is limited. Toxicity with overdosage is less likely than with fat-soluble vitamins.

Folic acid: RDA nonpregnant, 400 μg; pregnant, 800 μg (+200-400 μg supplement). The augmented maternal erythropoiesis of pregnancy requires substantially increased amounts of folic acid (folacin). Moreover, because folic acid is intimately involved in DNA synthesis, requirements are particularly high in rapidly growing cells such as fetal and placental tissues. In view of the evidence indicating increased folic acid needs during pregnancy and dietary survey data suggesting that the usual American diet is marginal in folic acid content, some authorities have advised routine folic acid supplementation for pregnant women.

B vitamins. An important function of thiamin (vitamin B_1), riboflavin (B_2), pyridoxine (B_6), and cobalamin (vitamin B_{12}) is that of coenzyme in metabolism. Suggested increased RDAs during pregnancy can usually be provided by the diet. Low maternal levels of

vitamin B_{12} are associated with prematurity and occur more often in smokers than in nonsmokers.

Ascorbic acid (vitamin C): RDA nonpregnant, 60 mg; pregnant, 80 mg. The entire requirement of vitamin C may be readily provided by dietary sources. Some people do not think of vitamins as medications. Pregnant women should be cautioned against unprescribed use of any vitamin preparation, including vitamin C. The possibility of beneficial effects of extremely large ascorbic acid supplements for prevention of the common cold has created considerable interest. Aside from the controversial aspect of this type of pharmacologic treatment, its use in pregnancy is open to serious question.

Trace minerals

Zinc: RDA nonpregnant, 15 mg; pregnant, 20 mg. The metal zinc is a constituent of numerous enzymes involved in major metabolic pathways. It may be noteworthy that maternal zinc deficiency is highly teratogenic in rats. The incidence of malformations of the central nervous system (CNS) in humans appears to be increased in geographic areas where zinc deficiency is prevalent.

Flourine: RDA not given. Flourine in small amounts (1 part per million in drinking water) is associated with dental health. Excessive flourine acts on teeth in their budding stage of formation so that by the time they erupt, the enamel is mottled, pitted, and discolored.

Vitamin and mineral supplements: their role in pregnancy. Nutrition counselors (nurses, nutritionists) must assess whether the woman has sufficient knowledge, motivation, and income to follow the nutrition guidance given. If needs can be met through diet, vitamin and mineral supplementation may not be necessary. However, in some instances a careful selection of vitamin and mineral supplements is of some value if problems are anticipated in a particular person. It must be noted that supplementation cannot compensate for poor food habits. In some instances the prescriptions of supplements may give both the woman and the health care professional a false sense of security.

Nutrition Risk Factors in Pregnancy

To assess effectively the nutritional status of the pregnant or lactating woman, the nutrition counselor needs to understand the major risk factors and their implications for nutrition. Nutrition risk factors include those present at the onset of pregnancy and those that may occur during the course of pregnancy.

Risk factors at the onset of pregnancy

Adolescence. See Chapter 30 for a discussion of the nutrition risk factors for pregnant adolescents.

Frequent pregnancies. The woman who has had three or more pregnancies within 2 years, as well as the multiparous woman who has progressed from one pregnancy directly to another, is considered to be at increased risk. These women are prone to depleted nutrient stores. This situation can potentially compromise maternal and fetal health and well-being.

Poor reproductive history. Special attention should be paid to the woman's obstetric history. Poor weight gain in pregnancy, PIH, a previous stillbirth or delivery of a low-birth-weight infant, premature delivery, and perinatal infection are all common in women who are or have been poorly nourished in the past. As a result the woman with a poor reproductive history may need more than usual nutrition guidance.

Economic deprivation. For economically deprived women there are several programs that help with the purchase of food or that offer supplements, for example, the federal food stamp program and the supplemental food program for women, infants, and children, sometimes known as the WIC program.

Bizarre food patterns. A woman may enter pregnancy either having been or continuing to be on a faddish or otherwise nutritionally inadequate diet. The woman who practices pica may not consume adequate levels of nutrients. Pica is defined as regular and excessive ingestion of nonfood items (Argo starch or red clay) or of foods with limited nutritional value. The practice often relates to cultural or geographic factors or both (pp. 311 and 319 to 321).

Recently megavitamin supplementation has become popular. Persons on a megavitamin regimen ingest massive amounts of vitamins far above the RDA levels. There is no documentation that these large amounts of vitamins are beneficial (Luke, 1985; Mirkin, 1985).

Vegetarian diets. There are various types of vegetarian diets (see pp. 321 to 323). The lactoovovegetarian eats no meat, fish, or poultry but will use either eggs (ovo) or dairy products (lacto) or both. Of particular concern is the strict vegetarian (vegan), who eliminates all products of animal origin, including meat, poultry, fish, cheese, eggs, and milk. The pregnant woman who practices strict vegetarianism may not receive adequate quantities of complementary and complete proteins and may not obtain enough vitamin B_{12}. Thoughtful nutrition counseling will be required to work out a diet pattern for a strict vegetarian during the prenatal period.

Smoking, drug addiction, and alcoholism. The person who is a heavy smoker (more than 6 cigarettes per day), drug addict, or alcoholic (chronically using more than 150 ml [5 oz] of whiskey per day or its equivalent of beer or wine) is likely to have major physiologic problems. The effects of smoking during pregnancy include reduction in gestation length (with onset of premature labor) and infants who are small for gestational age (SGA). In addition, there is always the possibility that women who indulge excessively in the use of cigarettes, drugs, or alcohol may not consume sufficient quantities of nutritious food. (For detailed discussion, see Chapter 28 and Appendix G.)

Medical problems. Medical problems such as anemia, thyroid dysfunction, and chronic medical or surgical gastrointestinal disorders may be associated with interference with the ingestion, absorption, or utilization of nutrients. Drugs utilized in treatment of these conditions may also affect nutrition by similar interference. Nutrition counseling should combine general nutrition guidelines for prenatal care *and* diet therapy recommended for a particular woman's medical condition.

Women who were born with the genetic inborn error of metabolism *phenylketonuria (PKU)* usually conceive genetically normal offspring. These women must follow a rigorously restricted low phenylalanine diet during pregnancy to prevent mental retardation in the child (Worthington-Roberts, 1985; Barnico and Cullinane, 1985; Lipson, 1984; Lenke, 1980). Concern has even been expressed about the potential hazard of aspartame use to all pregnant women. Aspartame is the popular new sugar substitute composed of a dipeptide containing phenylalanine and aspartic acid. While no data confirm that aspartame use by normal pregnant women elevates circulating phenylalanine to levels of concern, several United States researchers have urged the federal government to monitor aspartame use carefully (Worthington-Roberts, 1985).

Risk factors in pregnancy

Anemia. The iron needs during pregnancy are obtained from maternal iron stores, diet, and supplementation. True anemia occurring during pregnancy is most often caused by iron deficiency. Many healthy American women do not have iron stores large enough to meet the demands of pregnancy. Iron supplementation will aid greatly in maintaining the hemoglobin at normal levels.

Pregnancy-induced hypertension. The cause of PIH is not known. It is characterized by an elevation in blood pressure, proteinuria, and rapid weight gain caused by edema. There is considerable controversy over the influence of nutrition (particularly sodium and protein) on the development of PIH (Worthington-Roberts, 1985; Zlatnik, 1983).

Inadequate weight gain. Normal pregnancy is a

time of progressive maternal weight gain. The following are presumptive signs of maternal and fetal malnutrition: (1) failure to gain weight (less than 0.9 kg [2 lb] per month during the second and third trimesters), (2) actual weight loss, (3) significant nausea and vomiting during early pregnancy, and (4) poor or delayed uterine-fetal growth.

Inadequate maternal weight gain has been associated with lowered birth weight and evidence of intrauterine growth retardation (IUGR). It is therefore important to document the pattern of weight gain in pregnancy as well as the total amount gained.

Excessive weight gain. Total maternal weight gain during the 40 weeks of pregnancy averages 11.5 kg (25 lb). This amounts to about 1.4 to 1.8 kg (3 to 4 lb) per month. Rapid accumulation of weight in a singleton pregnancy—that is, 0.9 to 2.3 kg (2 to 5 lb) per week results only from tissue fluid retention and may be associated with PIH. The woman must be carefully assessed for development of this condition.

Excessive weight gain associated with accumulation of fat is less dramatic and is best assessed by evaluating the woman's eating habits and by measuring subcutaneous fat stores by means of skinfold calipers (Chapter 20). Sources of calorically rich but nutritionally poor food should be identified and eliminated. Weight reduction in pregnancy or lactation by dietary manipulation or drug administration or both is contraindicated because of the potentially adverse and possibly toxic effects on fetal nutrition, growth, and development.

Demands of lactation. Increased nutritional demands of lactation can also be a risk factor. Storage of 2 or 3 kg of fat during pregnancy provides the gravida with a reservoir of some 14,000 to 24,000 kcal for lactation needs. Ordinarily, fat stores will be gradually utilized for the first 4 to 6 months of lactation.

Without the demands of nursing, fat stores may remain a permanent addition to the maternal frame and increase the potential for obesity with advancing age and parity. A modest reduction in caloric intake after delivery is appropriate for the woman who does not nurse her infant. This is particularly true if she uses an oral contraceptive agent. For discussion of nutrition and oral hormone contraception refer to p. 159.

Nursing Process

Adequate nutrition is vital throughout the life span. During pregnancy, nutrition plays a key role in achieving an optimal outcome for the mother and her unborn baby. Motivation to learn about nutrition is usually higher during pregnancy, as parents strive to "do what's right for the baby." Optimal nutrition cannot eliminate all problems that may arise in pregnancy, but it establishes a good foundation for supporting the needs of the mother and her unborn child.

Assessment. An individual assessment of nutritional status must be made at the beginning of prenatal care and supported by continuing evaluation throughout the pregnancy (Brennan, 1979). The following methods of assessment provide the data necessary to determine need:
1. Interview (individual and family history, dietary assessment)
2. Physical examination, including assessment for skinfold thickness
3. Laboratory tests

Interview
Health history. Data from the pregnant woman's history are among the most important elements in nutrition assessment. These data must include basic information carefully taken from the medical, obstetric, nutrition, family, and social portions of the history, all of which have a bearing on nutritional status (Chapter 11). From the obstetric history it is important to note the woman's age, number of pregnancies and their outcomes, and the interval between pregnancies. Several medical problems have a nutritional base. These problems include diabetes mellitus, cystic fibrosis, PKU, anemia, and lactose intolerance (White and Owsley, 1983).

Background data. Food habits and attitudes cannot be viewed in isolation: life situations and values as well as physical and emotional factors must also be considered. Thus, if nutrition counseling is to be valid, it must be based on an individual plan of care.

A woman's living situation will have an influence on her eating behavior. Therefore the data on the home setting, housing, life-style, family members, occupation, general socioeconomic status, food assistance needs, and family roles and attitudes concerning foods are important. What is her activity level? Is she a housewife, office worker, or farm laborer? Are there other "special" circumstances, for example, is she a model or dancer? How many people eat together for each meal? How many meals are taken per day?

Nutrition-related folklore and myths need to be identified. Some beliefs may prevent the gravida from complying with sound nutritional guidelines. A number of old wives' tales are given here: eating for two; a tooth for every pregnancy; if you eat green peppers, your baby will be hairy; eating prunes may cause the infant's face to be wrinkled; eating pickles could give the baby a sour disposition; eating carrots gives the baby red hair; eating a lot of eggs or chicken makes the baby an early riser; eating cheese causes the womb to rot. Cultural-ethnic food and religious practices need to be explored.

It is important to determine special diet practices such as faddish or unusual patterns. Strict vegetarian diets or various forms of pica may be nutritionally unsound. The use of *all* medications and vitamin and mineral supplements should be discussed with the woman.

Food allergies and milk or lactose intolerance need to be explored (White and Owsley, 1983). Lactose intolerance is a problem for certain ethnic groups and individuals. The nurse's help is often needed for the family to plan for protein and calcium intake from sources other than milk. One food, tofu (soybean cake), contains considerable calcium but no lactose. Of the cheeses, Swiss cheese contains the least amount of lactose.

Dietary assessment. A *nutrition questionnaire* covering the background information is a useful tool in dietary assessment. The California Department of Health Services (1975) developed an excellent instrument to be used specifically by the physician, nurse, dietitian, or nutritionist with the pregnant woman. The nutrition questionnaire below groups questions into 11 sections that identify factors that may influence prenatal nutrition.

Additional information is gathered with the follow-

Nutrition Questionnaire

Name: _____ Date: _____

Please answer the following by checking the appropriate box or filling in the blank. Answer only those questions that apply to you. All information is confidential.

1. a. Before this pregnancy, what was your usual weight? _____ kg (_____ lb)
       ☐ Don't know
    b. During your last pregnancy, how much weight did you gain? _____ kg (_____ lb)
       ☐ Don't know
    c. How much weight do you expect to gain during this pregnancy? _____ kg (_____ lb)
       ☐ Don't know
    d. Have you ever had any problems with your weight?
       ☐ Yes ☐ No If yes, what? ☐ Underweight ☐ Overweight ☐ Other _____

2. a. How would you describe your appetite?
       ☐ Hearty ☐ Moderate ☐ Poor
    b. With this pregnancy, have you experienced either of the following? ☐ Nausea ☐ Vomiting

3. How would you describe your regular eating habits?
       ☐ Regular ☐ Irregular

4. a. Indicate the person who does the following in your household:
       Plans the meals _____
       Buys the food _____
       Prepares the food _____
    b. How much is spent on food each week for your household? _____ ☐ Don't know
       How many people does this feed? _____
    c. Indicate the type of kitchen equipment you have in your home:
       ☐ Refrigerator ☐ Hot plate ☐ Stove

5. a. Are you *now* taking any vitamin or mineral supplement? ☐ Yes ☐ No
    b. Do you take any pills to control your weight?
       ☐ Yes ☐ No
    c. Do you take diuretic (water) pills?
       ☐ Yes ☐ No

6. a. Are you now on a diet to lose weight?
       ☐ Yes ☐ No
    b. Are you *now* on a special diet (low salt, diabetic, gallbladder, etc.)?
       ☐ Yes ☐ No
       If yes, what kind of diet? _____
    c. If you have been on a special diet in the past, indicate what kind and when._____
       _____
       _____

7. a. Is there any food you *cannot* eat?
       ☐ Yes ☐ No
       If yes, what food(s)? _____
       _____
       What happens when you eat this food? _____
       _____
    b. Do you have any cravings for things such as
       ☐ Cornstarch ☐ Plaster ☐ Dirt or clay
       ☐ Other _____

8. Do you have either of the following problems?
       ☐ Constipation ☐ Diarrhea

9. a. Do you smoke? ☐ Yes ☐ No
    b. Do you drink any alcoholic beverages (liquor, wine, beer)? ☐ Yes ☐ No

10. Are you receiving either of the following?
       ☐ Food stamps ☐ WIC vouchers

11. How do you want to feed your baby? ☐ Breast milk
       ☐ Evaporated milk formula ☐ Commercial formula ☐ Undecided

Adapted from Nutrition during pregnancy and lactation, Sacramento, Calif., 1975, Maternal and Child Health Branch, California Department of Health Services.

ing questions. How many meals and snacks are served per day and how are these spaced? What is a typical menu? What quantities are served? How are foods selected and cooked? What is the woman's level of understanding of good nutrition? What does she consider to be "good nutrition"?

Psychosocial history. Since pregnancy is a time in the life cycle when nutrition is of special importance, it is essential to learn who the mother is, what her needs are, and how these needs can best be met. What does she perceive as nutritional problems and solutions? Only in this context can realistic guidance be provided.

Review of woman's physical systems. Several functional gastrointestinal problems are common during pregnancy. Nausea and vomiting, constipation and hemorrhoids, heartburn, or a full feeling may interfere with optimum nutrition. These complaints are highly individual in character. Their existence is usually uncovered during the review of the physical systems (see Chapter 11).

Physical examination. Two problems bear on the validity of the physical examination. First, the lack of standard definitions and the nonspecificity of most clinical manifestations of malnutrition result in considerable variation in interpretation of physical signs. Second, pregnancy may complicate specific interpretation of physical signs. Despite these shortcomings the physical assessment of nutritional status can be useful if it is utilized in conjunction with the biochemical analyses and dietary assessment (Table 12.4).

General screening for *dental health status* provides helpful information on nutritional status. The most common clinical nutrition-related disorders that are likely to be encountered during the reproductive years are caries and periodontitis. These conditions cause mechanical and mastication difficulties that interfere with the ingestion of certain types of food.

Anthropometry, the study of human body measurements, provides both short- and long-term indications of the level of nutrition and is therefore a valuable component of the nutrition assessment profile. Assessment of height, weight, and skinfold thickness is performed. Care must be taken to ensure that proper equipment and techniques are used for anthropometric assessment; for example, the scale is calibrated to zero before a weight is taken.

Measurements of weight-for-age and weight-for-height are used in assessing obesity, but they do fail to distinguish muscular and skeletal tissue mass from fat. On the other hand, serial weight measurements give a reasonable indication of excessive weight gain and likely obesity.

Lean body mass can be estimated from the triceps fat-fold thickness and upper arm circumference. Mea-

surement of skinfold thickness is the most convenient method of objectively assessing relative fatness. In general, two fat-fold measurements, one on a limb (left triceps) and one on the trunk (left subscapular), are advised to account for differing distributions of fat.

Erroneous information regarding specific indexes such as height and weight measurements can lead to inappropriate conclusions. An incomplete or inaccurate data base can result in poor decisions and client care management.

Laboratory tests. Laboratory data provide vital baseline information for nutrition assessment at the beginning of pregnancy as well as a means of monitoring nutritional status throughout gestation. In general, laboratory tests provide a more objective and precise determination of nutritional status than do other assessment indexes.

Blood-forming nutrients. Measures of the blood-forming nutrients—iron, folacin, and vitamins B_6 and B_{12}—are important guides for use in preventing and treating anemias often associated with pregnancy (see Chapter 27). The following can be measured in routine tests:

1. Hemoglobin levels
2. Hematocrit levels
3. Mean corpuscular volume (MCV)
4. Mean corpuscular hemoglobin concentration (MCHC)
5. Serum iron levels and percentage of concentration in saturation
6. Transferrin levels

Other tests include those for folic acid deficiency:

1. MCV
2. Hypersegmented polymorphonuclear leukocytes
3. Serum folic acid
4. RBC folic acid
5. Serum protein

Some of these tests are expensive. Care must be taken to order those that benefit the client most, at the least expense.

Serum albumin. An adequate level of serum albumin is important during pregnancy. Serum albumin helps to maintain normal flow of tissue fluids from the circulating blood through the tissue for nourishment of cells and back into circulation by means of capillary fluid shift mechanisms. A protein deficit would contribute to a lowered plasma albumin level and in turn to an imbalance in the fluid shift mechanism, resulting in edema. An acceptable level of serum albumin during pregnancy is 3.5 g/dl or above.

Other minerals and vitamins. Depending on individual situations, tests for other vitamin and mineral levels may be performed, including determinations of the water-soluble vitamins (thiamin, riboflavin, niacin, and

Table 12.4
Physical Assessment of Nutritional Status

Body Area	Signs of Good Nutrition	Signs of Poor Nutrition
General appearance	Alert, responsive	Listless, apathetic, cachectic
Weight	Normal for height, age, body build	Overweight or underweight (special concern for underweight)
Posture	Erect, arms and legs straight	Sagging shoulders, sunken chest, humped back
Muscles	Well developed, firm, good tone, some fat under skin	Flaccid, poor tone, undeveloped, tender, "wasted" appearance, cannot walk properly
Nervous control	Good attention span, not irritable or restless, normal reflexes, psychologic stability	Inattentive, irritable, confused, burning and tingling of hands and feet (parasthesia), loss of position and vibratory sense, weakness and tenderness of muscles (may result in inability to walk), decrease or loss of ankle and knee reflexes
Gastrointestinal function	Good appetite and digestion, normal regular elimination, no palpable organs or masses	Anorexia, indigestion, constipation or diarrhea, liver or spleen enlargement
Cardiovascular function	Normal heart rate and rhythm, no murmurs, normal blood pressure for age	Rapid heart rate (above 100 beats/min: tachycardia), enlarged heart, abnormal rhythm, elevated blood pressure
General vitality	Endurance, energetic, sleeps well, vigorous	Easily fatigued, no energy, falls asleep easily, looks tired, apathetic
Hair	Shiny, lustrous, firm, not easily plucked, healthy scalp	Stringy, dull, brittle, dry, thin and sparse, depigmented, can be easily plucked
Skin (general)	Smooth, slightly moist, good color	Rough, dry, scaly, pale, pigmented, irritated, easily bruised, petechiae
Face and neck	Skin color uniform, smooth, pink, healthy appearance, not swollen	Greasy, discolored, scaly, swollen, skin dark over cheeks and under eyes, lumpiness or flakiness of skin around nose and mouth
Lips	Smooth, good color, moist, not chapped or swollen	Dry, scaly, swollen, redness, angular lesions at corners of mouth, fissured, scarred (cheilosis, stomatitis)
Mouth, oral membranes	Reddish pink mucous membranes in oral cavity	Swollen, boggy oral mucous membranes
Gums	Reddish pink, healthy, no swelling or bleeding	Spongy, bleed easily, marginal redness, inflamed, gums receding
Tongue	Healthy pink or deep reddish in appearance, not swollen or smooth, surface papillae present, no lesions	Swollen, scarlet and raw, magenta color, beefy (glossitis), hyperemic and hypertrophic papillae, atrophic papillae
Teeth	No cavities, no pain, bright, straight, no crowding, well-shaped jaw, clean, no discoloration	Unfilled caries, absent teeth, worn surfaces, mottled (fluorosis), malpositioned
Eyes	Bright, clear, shiny, no sores at corners of eyelids, membranes moist and healthy pink color, no prominent blood vessels or mound of tissue on sclera, no fatigue circles beneath	Eye membranes pale (pale conjunctiva), redness of membrane (conjunctival injection), dryness, signs of infection, Bitot's spots, redness and fissuring of eyelid corners (angular palpebritis), dryness of eye membrane (conjunctival xerosis), dull appearance of cornea (corneal xerosis), soft cornea (keratomalacia)
Neck (glands)	No enlargement	Thyroid enlarged
Nails	Firm, pink	Spoon shaped (koilonychia), brittle, ridged
Legs, feet	No tenderness, weakness, or swelling; good color	Edema, tender calf, tingling, weakness
Skeleton	No malformations	Bowlegs, knock-knees, chest deformity at diaphragm, beaded ribs, prominent scapulas

From Williams, S.R.: Nutritional guidance in prenatal care. In Worthington, B.S., Vermeersch, J., and Williams, S.R.: Nutrition in pregnancy and lactation, St. Louis, 1977, The C.V. Mosby Co.

vitamin C), the fat-soluble vitamins (A, D, E, and K), and trace minerals.

Blood lipids, glucose, and enzymes. Routine testing for urine sugar and ketone bodies is often done to screen for latent diabetes mellitus or gestational glycosuria. However, more definitive tests are necessary for accurate assessment for endocrine disturbances such as diabetes mellitus (Chapter 28). Other tests may be performed if there is a complicating chronic disease, particularly cardiovascular or renal disease.

Nursing diagnosis. Each gravida and her family will present the nurse with a unique set of nutritional needs. The nurse formulates appropriate nursing diagnoses based on the identified needs from the assessment data. Following are examples of nutrition-related nursing diagnoses arising from the course of the prenatal period (see Summary of Nursing Actions).

From the health history: Alteration in nutrition: less than body requirements related to imbalance of intake vs activity expenditures.

From the psychosocial history: Alteration in nutrition: less than body requirements related to inability to procure food.

From the physical examination: Alteration in nutrition: less than body requirements related to chewing difficulties secondary to poor dental hygiene.

From the laboratory tests: Potential alteration in normal physiologic processes of pregnancy* related to knowledge deficit of RDAs.

Planning. The information in this chapter is general in nature. A plan is developed for each gravida utilizing content that relates specifically to her and her family's nutritional needs. Collaboration between the nurse and the client is basic to the following step in the nursing process: setting the goals in client-centered terms, prioritizing the goals, and selecting nursing actions that will assist the client to meet the goals.

Goals. General goals directed to the maternity population as a whole include the following:

1. To provide nutrition-related services for all pregnant women and their fetuses or newborns and families
2. To ensure optimum nutrition for women of childbearing age
3. To ensure optimum nutrition for the gravida and her fetus
4. To involve the woman as a participant in her own care

Implementation. Nurses assume many caretaking roles during the prenatal period: support person, teacher/counselor/advocate, and technician.

Support person. The nurse-client relationship is important in setting the tone for further interactions (Chapter 4). The techniques of listening with an attentive expression, touching, and using eye contact have their place, as does recognition of the client's feelings and her right to express them. One common complaint of gravidas is the weighing-in at the start of a prenatal visit. Weighing-in should be ego-building and psychologically unthreatening. Many women state that they "shake in their boots" while waiting to hear remarks of disgust and condemnation for gaining too much. To avoid this disapproval, some starve themselves the evening before the visit or take diuretics ("water pills"). Both alternatives are detrimental to the health of the mother and her unborn child.

Nutrition counseling provides the nurse with the opportunity to commend the gravida for her knowledge and use of good nutrition practices. The nurse can assist the woman to set her own goals and make her own decisions.

Teacher/counselor/advocate. There are several tools that are useful in providing nutrition information to the pregnant woman. The tools include a daily food guide and a list of food groups, a sample meal pattern and sample menus, and information on ethnic preferences and vegetarian diets.

Daily food guide and list of food groups. A diet consisting of a variety of foods can supply needed nutrients (Table 12.5). The increased quantities of essential nutrients needed during pregnancy may be met by skillful planning around a daily food guide based on the RDAs.

The list of food groups on pp. 316 and 317 presents six categories according to the nutrients they contribute. Comparable amounts of specific nutrients are provided in each group, although portion sizes differ for various foods. Because of the comparable amounts of specific nutrients, it is possible to substitute, or "exchange," foods within each group. The six food groups are described in some detail, and the list includes nutrients found in significant amounts and foods that can be exchanged.

Sample meal pattern and sample menus. It is necessary to show the woman how the daily food guide and list of food groups can be used. Table 12.6 provides a sample daily meal pattern and sample menus. A mutually developed plan is more likely to be followed by the client. Gravidas find a collaboratively written shopping list helpful in implementing the planned menus.

Ethnic cultural influences on dietary practices. Consideration of a woman's cultural food preferences enhances the communication between her and her counselor, thus providing a greater opportunity to obtain compliance with a prescribed diet. However, within one

---

*Diagnosis not included in those of NANDA, 1986.

Food Groups

Protein foods include both animal and vegetable foods. Animal protein foods supply protein, iron, riboflavin, niacin, vitamins B_6 and B_{12}, phosphorus, zinc, and iodine. Vegetable protein foods supply protein, iron, thiamin, folacin, vitamins B_6 and E, phosphorus, magnesium, and zinc.

Animal protein foods*: a serving is a 60-90 g (2-3 oz) cooked (boneless) of the following unless otherwise noted.
Bacon, 6 slices
Beef: ground, cube, roast, chop
Canned tuna, salmon, crab, etc., ½ C
Cheese (see milk list)
Chitterlings (tripe)
Clams, 4 large or 9 small
Crab
Duck
Eggs, 2
Fish: fillet, steak
Fish sticks, breaded, 4
Frankfurters, 2
Hog maws
Lamb: ground, cube, roast, chop
Lobster
Luncheon meat, 3 slices
Organ meats: liver, kidney, sweetbreads, heart, tongue
Oysters, 10-15 medium
Pigs' feet, ears, snouts
Pork, ham: ground, roast, chop
Poultry: ground, roast
Rabbit
Sausage links, 4
Shrimp, scallops, 5-6 large
Spareribs, 6 medium ribs
Veal: ground, cube, roast, chop

Vegetable protein foods: a serving is 1 C cooked unless otherwise stated.
Canned garbanzo, lima, kidney beans
Canned pork and beans
Dried beans and peas
Lentils
Nut butters, ¼ C
Nuts, ½ C
Sunflower seeds, ½ C
Tofu (soybean curd)

Milk and milk products constitute an exchange group of foods containing calcium, phosphorus, vitamin D, and riboflavin. In addition, these foods supply protein, vitamins A, E, B_6, and B_{12}, magnesium, and zinc. For some people, milk and milk products serve as primary sources of protein in the diet.

A serving is 240 ml (8 oz. or 1 C) unless otherwise noted.
Cheese: hard and semisoft (except blue, Camembert, and cream), 42 g (1½ oz)
Cheese spread, 56 g (2 oz)
Cottage cheese, creamed, 1 ⅓ C
Cow's milk: whole, nonfat, low fat, nonfat dry reconstituted, buttermilk, chocolate milk, cocoa made with milk
Cream soups made with milk, 360 ml (12 oz)
Evaporated milk, 90 ml (3 oz)
Goat's milk (low B_{12} content)
Ice cream, 1½ C
Ice milk
Instant breakfast made with milk, 120 ml (4 oz)
Liquid diet beverage, 150 ml (5 oz)
Milkshake, commercial, 240 ml (8 oz)
Puddings, custard (flan)
Soybean milk (low B_{12} content)
Yogurt
NOTE: Tofu is also a source of calcium; 1 C tofu may be exchanged for one serving of the above foods.

Grain products supply thiamin, riboflavin, iron, phosphorus, and zinc. This exchange group is divided into two parts: whole grain items and enriched products. The enriched breads, cereals, and pastas provide significantly lower amounts of magnesium and zinc. For this reason, people should be urged to choose whole grain products.

Whole grain items
Brown rice, ½ C
Cereals, hot: oatmeal (rolled oats), rolled wheat, cracked wheat, wheat with malted barley, ½ C cooked
Cereals, ready-to-eat: puffed oats, shredded wheat, wheat flakes, granola, ¾ C
Wheat germ, 1 tbsp

Enriched breads, cereals, and pastas
NOTE: California law requires that bread and bakery products be made with enriched flours. The following should comply with this requirement.
Bread, 1 slice (all other forms)
Cereals, hot: cream of wheat, cream of rice, farina, cornmeal, grits, ½ C cooked
Cereals, ready to eat, ¾ C
Cornbread, 1 piece (5 cm [2 in] square)
Crackers, 4 (all kinds)
Macaroni, noodles, spaghetti, ½ C cooked
Muffin, biscuit, dumpling, 1
Pancake, 1 medium
Rice, cooked, ½ C
Roll, bagel, 1
Tortilla, corn, 2
Tortilla, flour, 1 large
Waffle, 1 large

Vitamin C–rich fruits and vegetables supply ascorbic acid. Fresh, frozen, or canned forms may be used, although vitamin C content of canned products is lower.

Juices
Orange, grapefruit, 120 ml (4 oz)
Tomato, pineapple, 360 ml (12 oz)
Fruit juices and drinks enriched with vitamin C, 180 ml (6 oz)

Adapted from Nutrition during pregnancy and lactation, Sacramento, Calif., 1975, Maternal and Child Health Branch, California Department of Health Services.
*An alternate protein food is a combination of animal (70%) and vegetable (30%) protein foods. Most commonly used is a mixture of meat and textured vegetable protein (TVP). Such foods have the advantage of being more economical than 100% animal protein foods.

Food Groups—cont'd

Fruits
- Cantaloupe, ½
- Grapefruit, ½
- Guava, ¼ medium
- Mango, 1 medium
- Orange, 1 medium
- Papaya, ⅓ medium
- Strawberries, ¾ C
- Tangerine, 2 small

Vegetables
- Bok choy, ¾ C
- Broccoli, 1 stalk
- Brussels sprouts, 3-4
- Cabbage, cooked, 1⅓ C
- Cabbage, raw ¾ C
- Cauliflower, raw or cooked, 1 C
- Greens: collard, kale, mustard, Swiss chard, turnip greens, ¾ C
- Peppers, chili, ¾ C
- Peppers: green, red, ½ medium
- Tomatoes, 2 medium
- Watercress, ¾ C

Leafy green vegetables are an exchange group containing folacin. In addition, these foods supply vitamins A, E, and B₆, riboflavin, iron, and magnesium.
A serving is 1 C raw, or ¾ C cooked.
- Asparagus
- Bok choy
- Broccoli
- Brussel sprouts
- Cabbage
- Dark, leafy lettuce: chicory, endive, escarole, red leaf, romaine
- Greens: beet, collard kale, mustard spinach, Swiss chard, turnip
- Scallions
- Watercress

Other fruits and vegetables include yellow fruits and vegetables that supply significant amounts of vitamin A. Vitamin A is also found in outstanding amounts in the leafy green vegetable group. Other fruits and vegetables also contribute varying amounts of B-complex vitamins, vitamin E, magnesium, zinc, and phosphorus.
A serving is ½ C (fresh, frozen, or canned) unless otherwise indicated.

Vegetables
- Artichoke
- Bamboo shoots
- Bean sprouts: alfalfa, mung
- Beet
- Burdock root
- Carrot
- Cauliflower
- Celery
- Corn
- Cucumber
- Eggplant
- Beans: green, wax
- Hominy
- Lettuce: head, Boston, bib
- Mushrooms
- Nori seaweed
- Onion
- Parsnip
- Peas
- Pea pods
- Potato
- Radishes
- Summer squash
- Sweet potato
- Winter squash
- Yam
- Zucchini

Fruits
- Apricot, fresh, 1 large
- Nectarine, 2 medium
- Peach, fresh, 1 medium
- Persimmon, 1 small
- Prunes, 4 (also significant iron source)
- Pumpkin, ¼ C
- Apple, 1 medium
- Banana, 1 small
- Berries
- Cherries
- Dates, 5
- Figs, 2 large
- Fruit cocktail
- Grapes
- Kumquats, 3
- Pear, 1 medium
- Pineapple
- Plums, 2 medium
- Raisins (also significant iron source)
- Watermelon

cultural group there may occur several variations. Women in most cultures are encouraged to eat a normal diet. The nurse needs to know what constitutes a normal diet for each ethnic group. Thus careful exploration of individual preferences is needed (Table 12.7).

Among Chinese-Americans, herbal teas, such as ginseng, may be used as a tonic in early pregnancy, and to strengthen the womb during the seventh and eighth month (Campbell and Chang, 1973; Dunn, 1978). Chung (1977) refers to the use of ginseng tea as a dietary supplement by Chinese mothers, but these same women refuse iron supplements supplied by Western medicine because they believe their bones will harden and they will have a difficult delivery.

Table 12.5
Daily Food Plan for Pregnancy and Lactation

Food	Nonpregnant Woman	Pregnant Woman	Lactating Woman
Milk, cheese, ice cream, skimmed milk or buttermilk (food made with milk can supply part of requirement)	2 C	3-4 C	4-5 C
Meat (lean meat, fish, poultry, cheese, occasional dried beans or peas)	1 serving (3-4 oz)	2 servings (6-8 oz); include liver frequently	2½ servings (8 oz)
Eggs	1	1-2	1-2
Vegetable* (dark green or deep yellow)	1 serving	1 serving	1-2 servings
Vitamin C–rich food* Good source—citrus fruit, berries, cantaloupe Fair source—tomatoes, cabbage, greens, potatoes in skin	1 good source or 2 fair sources	1 good source and 1 fair source or 2 good sources	1 good source and 1 fair source or 2 good sources
Other vegetables and fruits	1 serving	2 servings	2 servings
Bread† and cereals (enriched or whole grain)	3 servings	4-5 servings	5 servings
Butter or fortified margarine	As desired or needed for calories	As desired or needed for calories	As desired or needed for calories

From Williams, S.R.: Nutrition and diet therapy, ed. 5, St. Louis, 1985, The C.V. Mosby Co.
*Use some raw daily.
†One slice of bread equals 1 serving.

Table 12.6
Sample Menus

	Nonpregnant Woman	Pregnant Woman	Lactating Woman
Breakfast	120 ml (4 oz) orange juice ½ C oatmeal 240 ml (8 oz) milk Coffee or tea*	120 ml (4 oz) orange juice ½ C oatmeal 240 ml (8 oz) milk Coffee or tea*	120 ml (4 oz) orange juice ½ C oatmeal 240 ml (8 oz) milk Coffee or tea*
Morning snack		Fruit and/or cheese†	Fruit and/or cheese†
Lunch	1 tuna fish sandwich made with: 2 slices whole wheat bread ½ C tuna fish Diced celery and onion to taste, mayonnaise,* lettuce* 1 medium apple 240 ml (8 oz) milk	1 tuna fish sandwich made with: 2 slices whole wheat bread ½ C tuna fish, 1 hard-boiled egg Diced celery and onion to taste,* mayonnaise,* lettuce* 1 medium apple 240 ml (8 oz) milk	1 tuna fish sandwich made with: 2 slices whole wheat bread ½ C tuna fish, 1 hard-boiled egg Diced celery and onion to taste,* mayonnaise,* lettuce* 1 medium apple 240 ml (8 oz) milk
Afternoon snack		½ C salted peanuts 120 ml (4 oz) milk	½ C salted peanuts 240 ml (8 oz) milk
Dinner	3 oz roast beef ½ C egg noodles* with sautéed poppy seeds* ¾ C cut asparagus Salad made with: 1 C torn spinach Sliced mushrooms and radishes to taste* Oil and vinegar* Coffee or tea†	6 oz roast beef ½ C egg noodles* with sautéed poppy seeds,* 1 pat butter ¾ C cut asparagus Salad made with: 1 C torn spinach Sliced mushrooms and radishes to taste,* tomato Oil and vinegar* 240 ml (8 oz) milk Coffee or tea	6-9 oz roast beef ½ C egg noodles* with sautéed poppy seeds,* 1 pat butter ¾ C cut asparagus Salad made with: 1 C torn spinach Sliced mushrooms and radishes to taste,* tomato Oil and vinegar* 240 ml (8 oz) milk Coffee or tea
Evening snack		1-2 oatmeal raisin cookies* 120 ml (4 oz) milk	2 oatmeal raisin cookies* 240 ml (8 oz) milk

Adapted from nutrition during pregnancy and lactation, Sacramento, 1975, Maternal and Child Health Branch, California Department of Health Services
*This food is optional and is added to the basic diet.
†Serving size determined by caloric or dietary need.

Table 12.7
Characteristics of Some Cultural Food Patterns

Ethnic Group	Milk Group	Meat Group	Fruits and Vegetables	Breads and Cereals	Possible Dietary Problems
American Indian (many tribal variations; many "Americanized")	Fresh milk Evaporated milk for cooking Ice cream Cream pies	Pork, beef, lamb, rabbit Fowl, fish, eggs Legumes Sunflower seeds Nuts: walnut, acorn, pine, peanut butter Game meat	Green peas, beans Beets, turnips Leafy green and other vegetables Grapes, bananas, peaches, other fresh fruits Roots	Refined bread Whole wheat Cornmeal Rice Dry cereals "Fry" bread Tortillas	In California, major problems: obesity, diabetes, alcoholism, nutritional deficiencies expressed in dental problems and iron deficiency anemia Inadequate amounts of all nutrients Excessive use of sugar
Middle Eastern (Armenian, Greek, Syrian, Turkish)	Yogurt Little butter	Lamb Nuts Dried peas, beans, lentils	Peppers Tomatoes Cabbage Grape leaves Cucumbers Squash Dried apricots, raisins	Cracked wheat and dark bread	Fry many meats and vegetables Lack of fresh fruits Insufficient foods from milk group (use olive oil* in place of butter) Like sweetenings, lamb fat, and olive oil
Black	Milk Ice Cream Puddings Cheese: longhorn, American	Pork: all cuts, plus organs, chitterlings Beef, lamb Chicken, giblets Eggs Nuts Legumes Fish, game	Leafy vegetables Green and yellow vegetables Potato: white, sweet Stewed fruit Bananas, and other fresh fruit	Cornmeal and hominy grits Rice Biscuits, pancakes, white breads Puddings: bread rice Molasses†	Extensive use of frying, "smothering," or simmering Fats: salt pork, bacon drippings, lard, and gravies Like sweets Insufficient citrus and enriched breads Vegetables often boiled for long periods Limited amounts from milk group
Chinese (Cantonese most prevalent)	Cheese Milk: water buffalo	Pork sausage‡ Eggs and pigeon eggs Fish Lamb, beef, goat Fowl: chicken, duck Nuts Legumes	Many vegetables Radish leaves Bean, bamboo sprouts Soybean curd (tofu)§	Rice/rice flour products Cereals, noodles Wheat, corn, millet seed	Tendency of northern China (Mandarin), coastal China (Shanghai), and inland China (Szechwan) immigrants to use more grease in cooking Limited use of milk and milk products Often low in protein, calories, or both May wash rice before cooking Soy sauce, ginger
Filipino (Spanish-Chinese influence)	Flavored milk Milk in coffee Cheese: gouda, cheddar	Pork, beef, goat, deer, rabbit Chicken Fish Eggs Nuts Legumes	Many vegetables and fruits	Rice, cooked cereals Noodles: rice, wheat	Limited use of milk and milk products Tend to prewash rice May have only small portions of protein foods
Italian	Cheese Some ice cream	Meat Eggs Dried beans	Leafy vegetables Potatoes Eggplant Spinach Fruits	Macaroni White breads, some whole wheat Farina Cereals	Prefer expensive imported cheeses; reluctant to substitute less expensive domestic varieties Tendency to overcook vegetables Limited use of whole grains Enjoys sweets Extensive use of olive oil Insufficient servings from milk group

Continued.

Table 12.7, cont'd
Characteristics of Some Cultural Food Patterns

Ethnic Group	Milk Group	Meat Group	Fruits and Vegetables	Breads and Cereals	Possible Dietary Problems
Japanese (Isei, more Japanese influence; Nisei, more westernized)	Increasing amounts being used by younger generations	Pork, beef, chicken Fish Eggs Legumes: soya, red, lima beans Nuts	Many vegetables and fruits Seaweed Tofu	Rice, rice cakes Wheat noodles Refined bread, noodles	Excessive salt: pickles, salty crisp seaweed Insufficient servings from milk group May use refined or pre-washed rice
Mexican-Spanish, Mexican-American	Milk Cheese Flan Ice Cream	Beef, pork, lamb, chicken, tripe, hot sausage, beef intestines Fish Eggs Nuts Dry beans: pinto, chick-peas (often eaten more than once daily)	Spinach, wild greens, tomatoes, chilies, corn, cactus leaves, cabbage, avocado, potatoes Pumpkin, zapote, peaches, guava, papaya, citrus	Rice, oats, cornmeal Sweet bread Tortilla: corn, flour Biscuits Vermicelli (fideo)	Limited meats primarily due to economics Limited use of milk and milk products Some tendency toward increasing use of flour tortillas over more nutritious corn tortillas Large amounts of lard (manteca) Abundant use of sugar Tendency to boil vegetables for long periods
Polish	Milk Sour cream Cheese Butter	Pork (preferred) Chicken	Vegetables Cabbage Roots Fruits	Dark rye	Like sweets Tendency to over-cook vegetables Limited fruits (especially citrus), raw vegetables, and meats
Puerto Rican	Limited use of milk products Coffee with milk (café con leche)	Pork Poultry Eggs (Fridays) Dried codfish Beans (habichuelas)	Avacado, okra Eggplant Sweet yams Starchy vegetables and fruits (viandas)	Rice Cornmeal	Use small amounts of pork and poultry Use fat, lard, salt pork, and olive oil extensively Lack of butter and other milk products
Scandinavian: Danish, Finnish, Norwegian, Swedish	Cream Butter	Wild game Reindeer Fish Eggs	Fruit berries Dried fruit Vegetables: cole slaw, roots, avocado	Whole wheat, rye, barley, sweets (molasses for flavoring)	Insufficient fresh fruits and vegetables Like sweets, pickled salted meats, and fish
Southeast Asian: Vietnamese, Cambodian	Generally not taken Coffee with condensed cow's milk Plain yogurt Ice cream (rare) Soybean milk	Fish (daily): fresh, dried, salted Poultry/eggs: duck, chicken Pork Beef (seldom) Dry beans Bean curd	Seasonal variety: fresh or preserved Green, leafy Yams Corn Bean noodles	Rice: grains, flour, noodles, "cellophane" French bread	Fresh milk products generally not consumed Poultry/eggs: dependent on family wealth Meat considered "unclean" is avoided Pregnant women prefer a diet high in salt and pepper as well as rice and pork High intake of monosodium glutamate (MSG) and soy sauce
Jewish: orthodox	Milk Cheese	Meat (bloodless; Kosher prepared): beef, lamb, goat, deer, poultry (all types) Fish with fins and scales only No crustaceans	Wide variety	Wide variety	Milk and milk products not eaten with meat; milk may be taken before the meal or 6 hours following meal; different sets of dishes and silverware are used to serve milk and meat products

*Olive oil is all fat, with no other nutrient value.

†Light molasses (first extraction): 1 tbsp = 50 calories, 33 mg of calcium, 0.9 mg of iron, 0.01 mg each of vitamins B_1 and B_2; dark molasses (third extraction): 1 tbsp = 45 calories, 137 mg of calcium, 3.2 mg of iron, 0.02 mg of vitamin B_1, 0.04 mg of vitamin B_2, 0.4 mg of niacin.

‡Lower in fat content than Western sausage.

§Good source of protein.

Food taboos are more common than food prescriptions. Vietnamese women are to avoid "unclean" foods such as beef, dog, rat, and snake meat (Hollingsworth et al., 1980). Japanese women are cautioned against hot, spicey, and salty food, as are Filipino women. Filipino women are to avoid sweet foods because they may cause a big baby and a difficult delivery (Affonso, 1978), whereas Japanese women are encouraged to gain as much weight as they are comfortable with, believing that a large weight gain is good for the baby (Bernstein and Kidd, 1982). Blacks in the southern United States, Guatemalans, Mexicans, and Mexican-Americans should not eat acid foods or fresh fruits and vegetables (Kay, 1982). According to Snow (1974), red meat should be avoided by blacks because it is too strong and virile a food.

Food taboos often follow the principles of imitative magic, in which physical characteristics of food eaten by the mother may be transmitted to the child. Filipinos avoid eating prunes (Affonso, 1978) and Chinese avoid eating soy sauce (Campbell and Chang, 1973), in both instances to prevent a dark-skinned infant. Birthmarks and their pigmentation are often associated with the shape and color of the food eaten, such as the strawberry mark (Carrington, 1978). Campbell and Chang (1973) report that some Chinese mothers shun shellfish during the first trimester, believing it is responsible for allergies in the latter life of the child. Filipino mothers have said that they are not to eat squid during pregnancy for fear that the mother's insides will become tangled and the baby's cord will tie around its neck (Affonso, 1978).

Food cravings during pregnancy are considered normal by many cultures, but the specific kinds of cravings may be culturally specific (Carrington, 1978; Obeyesekere, 1963). In most cultures women crave acceptable foods, such as chicken, fish, and greens among blacks (Carrington, 1978) or fruits, nuts, bird meat, and taro among the Gadsup (Leininger, 1979). Satisfaction of food cravings is considered vital for culturally specific reasons. For example, Obeyesekere (1963) describes the foods craved by Sinhalese women as being extremely difficult to obtain. Sinhalese women have very low status in their society and are unable to express their anger about it or ever to demand anything for themselves. Their demand for foods difficult to obtain is interpreted as the only time hostility toward their role as women is acceptable. Sinhalese men are required to obtain the food even at great cost to themselves. Affonso (1978) notes that the Filipinos believe cravings should be satisfied to prevent the premature arrival of the infant.

Women in some cultures desire nonnutritive substances such as laundry starch, clay, and dirt. Eating of these substances is called *pica*. Kay (1982) describes Mexican-American women eating clay. All of these nonnutritive substances are used by black women (Carrington, 1978). A longitudinal study indicated that 40% of pregnant women in Mississippi eat clay (Vermeer and Frate, 1975). One Canadian Ojibwa woman who had had five children stated that with each pregnancy she craved and ate large quantities of "clean" dirt.

Certain ethnic groups have been identified as having a greater incidence of pica than others. Lackey (1978) studied groups of black women and white women and found that women in both groups ate substances such as clay and starch, although the percentage of black women was higher. Causes of pica have been attributed to a variety of reasons and may be engaged in by children as well as pregnant women. Pica may be a psychologic response of someone needing attention, a truly cultural phenomenon, a response to hunger, or the body's response to needed nutrients. Scientific controversy exists about whether the iron deficiency observed in persons with pica is the cause or the effect of the anemia. Whatever the reason, according to Leiderman and co-workers (1977), a documented sequela is increased iron deficiency anemia because of interference with absorption of necessary nutrients when clay is eaten.

Stern (1981) found that Filipino-Americans rarely attempt to explain their dietary beliefs to maternity nurses and obstetricians. They concur politely with dietary instructions and then return home to follow their traditional diet. However, nurses need to remember that dietary patterns, although ingrained, actually change rapidly, sometimes within one generation, and

Table 12.8
Modified Food Guide for Vegetarian Diets

	Recommended Number of Servings			
	Lactovegetarian		Lactoovovegetarian	
Food group	Adult	Pregnant Adult	Adult	Pregnant Adult
Milk	4	5	4	5
Protein				
Eggs (2 = 1 serving)	0	0	½	1
Legumes	2	3	2	3
Nuts	1	1	1	1
Fruits and vegetables				
Vitamin C	3	3	3	3
Vitamin A	1½	2	1½	2
Other	3	4	3	3
Whole grain products	6	7	5	6
Others	0	1	0	1

an individual food history is an important adjunct to knowledge of cultural food habits.

Vegetarian diet practices. Vegetarianism has gained popularity in recent years. Foods basic to almost all vegetarian diets are vegetables, fruits, legumes, nuts, and grains. Vegetarian diets may not satisfy all nutrient requirements for the pregnant and lactating woman. The use of eggs and of milk and milk products varies. There are four basic types of vegetarians:

1. *Lactoovovegetarian.* The vegetable diet is supplemented with milk, eggs, and cheese. There is no problem in securing adequate protein with this diet.

2. *Lactovegetarian.* The vegetable diet is supplemented

Table 12.9
Vegetarian Food Guide*

General guidelines†

1. Follow nutrition guide for regular food plan during pregnancy.
2. Eat a wide variety of foods, including milk and milk products and eggs.
3. If no milk is allowed, use a supplement of 4 µg of vitamin B_{12} daily. If goat and soy milk are used, partial supplementation may be needed.
4. If no milk is taken, also use supplements of 12 mg of calcium and 400 IU of vitamin D daily. Partial supplementation will be necessary if less than 4 servings of milk and milk products are consumed.
5. Select a variety of plant foods (especially grains, legumes, nuts, and seeds) to obtain "complete" proteins by complementary combinations, as indicated in the list below.
6. Use iodized salt.
7. Increase intake of legumes, dried seeds, and nuts for protein and iron.
8. Increase intake of dairy foods for calcium, protein, and vitamin B_{12}.
9. Cut "empty" calories (sugars, concentrated sweets, and visible fats) at least by half.
10. Increase intake of whole grain breads and cereals for B vitamins, protein, and iron.
11. Increase intake of fruits and vegetables for vitamins A and C and for minerals.

Complementary plant protein combinations‡

Careful planning is necessary to complement incomplete plant proteins with each other and with dairy foods.

Food	Amino acids deficient	Complementary protein food combinations
Grains	Isoleucine Lysine	Rice + legumes Corn + legumes Wheat + legumes Wheat + peanut + milk Wheat + sesame + soybean Rice + brewer's yeast
Legumes	Tryptophan Methionine	Legumes + rice Beans + wheat Beans + corn Soybeans + rice + wheat Soybeans + corn + milk Soybeans + wheat + sesame Soybeans + peanuts + sesame Soybeans + peanuts + wheat + rice Soybeans + sesame + wheat
Nuts and seeds	Isoleucine Lysine	Peanuts + sesame + soybeans Sesame + beans Sesame + soybeans + wheat Peanuts + sunflower seeds
Vegetables	Isoleucine Methionine	Lima beans Green beans Brussels sprouts } + Sesame seeds or Cauliflower Brazil nuts or Broccoli mushrooms Greens = millet or rice

*Adapted from Williams, S.R.: Nutritional guidance in prenatal care. In Worthington, B.S., Vermeersch, J., and Williams, S.R.: Nutrition in pregnancy and lactation, ed. 3, St. Louis, 1985, The C.V. Mosby Co.
†Nutritional considerations when meat, poultry, and fish are omitted from the diet.
‡Adapted from Lappe, F.M.: Diet for a small planet, New York, 1971, Friends of the Earth/Ballantine.

with milk and cheese. Milk products add complete protein to this diet.

3. *Pure vegetarian, or vegan.* The all-vegetable diet includes vegetables, fruits, legumes, nuts, and grains but is not supplemented with any animal foods, dairy products, or eggs. More careful planning is required to achieve combinations providing the necessary amounts of the essential amino acids. Vitamin B_{12} deficiency is a potential problem.

4. *Fruitarian.* The fruitarian diet consists of raw or dried fruits, nuts, honey, and olive oil. Potential inadequacy is greater in this diet than in other diets.

In general, protein is not a problem for the vegetarian when caloric intake is adequate and a wide variety of plant proteins are selected. It is necessary to eat certain combinations of plant foods to obtain complete proteins. These complete proteins contain the eight essential amino acids in amounts necessary for growth

Guidelines for Client Teaching
IRON SUPPLEMENTATION

ASSESSMENT

Gravida is in her second trimester. She states she "eats beets each day to keep her blood strong . . . I hate to take pills so I always wash them down with milk . . ." Laboratory values: hemoglobin 10.5 g/dl; hematocrit, 35%.

NURSING DIAGNOSIS

Alteration in nutrition: less than body requirements related to knowledge deficit of needed nutrients.

GOALS
Short-term

Gravida takes iron supplement, as prescribed, immediately.
Gravida's laboratory data for hemoglobin and hematocrit indicate beginning improvement with the next test.

Intermediate

Gravida continues to take iron supplement as long as prescribed.
Gravida understands anemia and its potential effects on her and her baby.

Long-term

Woman and her baby do not suffer adverse effects of anemia.

REFERENCES/TEACHING AIDS

Printed instructions for using iron supplements
Hospital-supplied pamphlets on nutrition, including information on food groups and supplements
Laboratory slips showing her blood values

CONTENT/RATIONALE	TEACHING ACTIONS

1. Laboratory report: to facilitate understanding of her condition.
   a. Definitions and values of hemoglobin, hematocrit, red blood cells, anemia.
   b. Gravida's values and normal parameters.
	1. Laboratory report.
	
	   a. Review; assess her level of understanding.
	
	   b. Discuss clinical significance of differences.

2. Building blood through diet: to increase her knowledge of nutrition.
   a. Types and amounts of bloodforming nutrients.
   b. Food sources of nutrients.
	2. Building blood through diet.
	
	   a. Review; help her identify food sources of nutrients in her current diet; praise her.
	   b. Assist her to make choices she can add to her diet.
	   c. Inform her that beets, some calcium, and some vitamin A and C are good additions.

3. Building blood through iron supplementation (30-60 mg of elemental iron [150-300 mg of ferrous sulfate]); to increase her knowledge of medical therapy for anemia.
   a. Daily dose is divided into 3 doses and is taken with a source of vitamin C to aid absorption and utilization of iron.
   b. Taken after meal or with food to minimize gastrointestinal irritation.
	3. Building blood through iron supplementation.
	
	   a. Discuss need to take iron with a vitamin C source. Emphasize value of milk in diet, but that it keeps iron from being absorbed.
	   b. Discuss timing of medication to fit her family's meal time and her convenience.

4. Side effects: to encourage compliance and to relieve anxiety.
   a. Constipation or diarrhea and black colored stools.
	4. Side effects
	
	   a. Discuss side effects.
	   b. Review dietary treatment of constipation and need to report diarrhea to physician.
	   c. Review directions for taking medication.

and maintenance. Unlike animal foods, most plant foods do not contain all the essential amino acids in these appropriate amounts. If one essential amino acid is missing, the protein is incomplete and cannot be utilized to build body tissues. The appropriate combination of two or more plant foods eaten at the same meal can make a "complete" protein. Tables 12.8 and 12.9 illustrate combinations of plant foods that are complementary, that is, that constitute complete proteins.

Iron supplementation and nutrition counseling. An important responsibility of the nurse is to teach women about meeting nutritional needs for themselves and

Table 12.10
Examples for Nutrition Counseling During Pregnancy

Client Knowledge Needs	Goals	Nursing Actions	Outcome Criteria
Why are nutrient needs increased during pregnancy?	Woman will know reason for increased nutrient and energy needs during pregnancy.	Explain that pregnancy is like building a house (the baby). You need materials (nutrients) and labor (energy). If you do not have enough materials or labor, the house will not be big or strong. This is also true for the baby.	Woman will explain why she needs more nutrients and energy while she is pregnant.
What are extra nutrients needed during pregnancy? How can they be obtained?	Woman will know additional nutrients needed during pregnancy and how to fulfill this need. Woman will meet her nutrient needs.	Explain that although all nutrient needs are increased during pregnancy, *seven* nutrients are particularly essential: *calories, protein, calcium, iron supplements, vitamin A, vitamin C,* and *folic acid.* Use 24-hr recall to point out areas of concern. Discuss daily food guide (see Table 12.5).	Woman will identify which nutrients should be increased, including calories, protein, calcium, iron, vitamin A, vitamin C, and folic acid. Woman will suggest how she might fulfill these needs.
What is normal pattern of weight gain during pregnancy? What are components of normal weight gain in pregnancy?	Woman will know normal weight gain pattern and components of total weight gain during pregnancy.	Explain that normal weight gain pattern is about 1.4 kg (3 lb) in first trimester, 4.5 kg (10 lb) in second, and 4.5 kg (10 lb) in third. Discuss components of total weight gain as follows: 27%, fetus 12%, placenta and fluid in uterus 50%, increased maternal organs (uterus, fat, breasts) 10%, increased blood volume	Woman will explain what normal weight gain pattern is and will list following components that make up total weight gain: 27%, fetus 12%, placenta and fluid in uterus 50%, increase in maternal organs 10%, increased body volume
What is relationship between good nutrition and normal weight gain in pregnancy?	Woman will know that good nutrition leads to normal weight gain in pregnancy.	Explain that monitoring weight is a way to measure whether fetus is receiving adequate supply of nutrients.	Woman will state that adequate supply of nutrients promotes normal development of infant and normal weight gain.
What is my weight gain?	Woman will achieve normal weight gain.	Explain that normal weight gain indicates that fetus is receiving adequae nutrients.	Woman will state how much she has gained.
How does it compare to average weight gain?	Woman will know how her weight gain compares to average weight gain.	Using pregnancy gain-in-weight grid, record weight gain at each visit. Discuss weight gain pattern.	Complete each time throughout second and third trimesters. Woman will state how her weight gain compares to average.
What are dangers of poor nutrition during pregnancy?	Woman will know that poor nutrition can lead to anemia, preeclampsia-eclampsia, obesity, or prematurity.	Explain that poor nutrition during pregnancy may lead to several problem conditions. Poor supply of iron, folic acid, protein, or vitamin C may lead to *anemia.* Generally poor nutrition may lead to *prematurity.* Poor selection of food may lead to *obesity.*	Woman will identify following problems that may result from poor nutrition in pregnancy: anemia, preeclampsia-eclampsia, obesity, and prematurity.

Adapted from Pregnancy protocol for nutrition counseling, Phoenix, 1978, Nutrition Services, Arizona Department of Health; and Detroit, 1979, Nutrition Division, City of Detroit Department of Health.

their unborn babies. Guidelines for client teaching about iron supplementation are given on p. 323. Table 12.10 is another format that can be used for nutrition counseling during pregnancy.

Referral for additional services. A problem of sufficient income to purchase foods may cause an individual to have a nutritionally inadequate diet. Nutrients such as protein and iron are among those more likely to be deficient in diets of low-income groups. To help improve the nutritional quality of the diet, the person with limited income should be encouraged to participate in federal food programs such as the supplemental feeding program for women, infants, and children (WIC) and the food stamp program. Nutrition education and counseling are important to ensure the benefits of such programs.

The referral system has two functions. First, a comprehensive network of services can offer solutions to problems that a particular program may not have the resources to solve. Second, the referral system informs women about a program by making them aware of their needs for benefits from that service. Food assistance programs such as the WIC program are a particularly good example of resources that can be tapped for pregnant women.

Technician. The technical aspects of nutrition counseling center around assessment and teaching techniques. Careful and concise recording of client responses or laboratory results contribute to the continuous supervision vital to the care of the mother and unborn baby.

Evaluation. Evaluation is a continuous process that begins during assessment. To be effective, evaluation is based on measurable outcome criteria. Nurses are accountable for measuring and documenting client outcomes. The nurse can be assured that nursing interventions relevant to nutrition have been effective when outcome criteria have been met (Table 12.10 and Summary of Nursing Actions).

Summary

Nutrition is an important component of care during the prenatal period. Scientific research has identified the nutrient needs for optimal body function, growth, development, maintenance and repair of body tissues, and prevention of disease. The nurse is in a strategic position to assist clients meet their nutrition needs. Among the nurse's tools are a sound knowledge of maternal physiologic adjustments to pregnancy and nutritional needs and the nursing process.

Summary of Nursing Actions

NURSING CARE RELATED TO MATERNAL AND FETAL NUTRITION

GOALS
1. For the mother: To consume adequate amounts of required nutrients each day.
2. For the unborn baby: To have adequate nutrients and a healthy maternal-placental unit.
3. For the family: To increase the family's knowledge of adequate nutrition within their cultural-ethnic context.

PRIORITIES
1. Pregnancy reaches term with both mother and newborn in optimum nutritional state.
2. Mother's and family's knowledge needs regarding nutrition are met.
3. Family is able to purchase, store, and prepare needed foods.

ASSESSMENT	EXAMPLES OF POTENTIAL NURSING DIAGNOSTIC CATEGORIES*
Interview A. Health history B. Psychosocial history: background data and dietary assessment	Potential for maternal or fetal compromise† Alteration in nutrition: less or more than body requirements Impaired verbal communication Ineffective coping by individual or family Alteration in health maintenance Potential for injury Noncompliance Spiritual distress Potential for maternal or fetal compromise† Knowledge deficit

*All diagnoses except those indicated by a dagger were approved by the Seventh National Conference (1986) of the North American Nursing Diagnosis Association (NANDA).
†Diagnoses not included by NANDA, 1986.

Continued.

Summary of Nursing Actions—cont'd

ASSESSMENT	EXAMPLES OF POTENTIAL NURSING DIAGNOSTIC CATEGORIES
Interview—cont'd C. Review of woman's physical systems	Potential for maternal or fetal compromise† Alteration in bowel elimination: constipation or diarrhea Potential for injury Alteration in nutrition: less or more than body requirements Knowledge deficit
Physical examination	Alteration in nutrition: less or more than body requirements Alteration in oral mucous membrane Alteration in health maintenance Alteration in nutrition: less than body requirements
Laboratory tests	Potential for maternal or fetal compromise† Knowledge deficit

OUTCOME CRITERIA‡	PLAN/IMPLEMENTATION

OUTCOME CRITERIA‡

Maintain adequate nutrition throughout pregnancy

By the end of the second prenatal visit:
1. The gravida is assessed for nutritional status.
2. Nutrition risk factors are identified.
3. Nutrition care plan is developed and initiated (e.g., education, mineral/vitamin supplementation).

Throughout pregnancy:
1. Gravida's dietary intake is maintained at appropriate levels for calories and all needed nutrients.
2. Gravida's pattern of weight gain is within normal limits; gravida gains approximately 454 g (1 lb) per month during the first trimester, and 425 g (15 oz) per week during the last two trimesters.
3. Gravida's hemoglobin and hematocrit remain at or above minimal values (sea level):

	HGB	HCT
First trimester	11 g/dl	37%
Second trimester	10.5 g/dl	35%
Third trimester	10 g/dl	33%

4. Intrauterine fetal growth remains appropriate for gestational age.
5. Gravida's urine remains negative for glucose and ketones.
6. Referrals are made to community agencies as necessary for assistance with acquisition of necessary food, food preparation, and food storage.

By end of pregnancy
1. Gravida has attained appropriate weight gain.
2. Gravida is knowledgeable regarding nutrition: calories, needed nutrients, food preparation.
3. Gravida is knowledgeable regarding effects of drugs, alcohol, and tobacco on nutrition; pica; weight below and above normal limits; special needs for the adolescent (if appropriate); nutrition-related conditions (PKU, diabetes, if appropriate).
4. Gravida has had opportunity to explore the choices for feeding the newborn (breast, bottle).

PLAN/IMPLEMENTATION

Plan and implement nursing roles of support person, teacher/counselor/advocate, and technician

Support person
1. Greet woman and her family by name.
2. Provide privacy as needed.
3. Obtain translator, as necessary.
4. Acknowledge effort woman makes in altering or maintaining diet. Praise when appropriate.
5. Refer woman (and family) to appropriate community agencies for additional assistance as needed (school, welfare, public health nurse).

Teacher/counselor/advocate
1. Make the woman a participant in her own care.
2. Refer woman to physician and registered dietitian for special dietary and pharmaceutic prescriptions for unique circumstances (e.g., PKU, cystic fibrosis, diabetes, anemia). Confer with physician and registered dietitian§ or refer to flow sheet regarding those therapies to ensure team approach to care.
3. After analyzing woman's understanding of nutrition and food preparation, briefly discuss physiologic demands (maternal and fetal) on body stores and daily intake.
4. Share with woman laboratory results, weight gain, and blood pressure. Discuss how these reflect her nutritional status. Point out areas where her laboratory values reflect her efforts to improve her nutrition.
5. Discuss nutrition-related folklore and myths with woman.
   a. Utilizing openings gained from identifying myths, explore realities and clarify or correct misinformation.
   b. If some beliefs are firmly held, discuss alternative food sources for nutrients needed.
6. Check to see how woman is managing her iron, vitamin, and mineral supplements. Initiate teaching tool for iron supplementation, as necessary.
7. Discuss discomforts of pregnancy that can be managed by means of foods and fluids, for example, nausea and vomiting, constipation, leg cramps, and fatigue.

---

‡Outcome criteria direct the selection of nursing actions (**plan/implementation**) and measure their effectiveness (**evaluation**).

§In some rural and other areas, registered dietitians may not be readily available. Contact the local hospital for a registered dietitian or the local health department WIC program. It may become the nurse's and physician's responsibility to be thoroughly informed as to particular food habits in that community, that is, nutritive values, usual means of preparation, and other characteristics.

Summary of Nursing Actions—cont'd

OUTCOME CRITERIA	PLAN/IMPLEMENTATION
Pregnancy outcome 1. Pregnancy reaches term. 2. Mother suffers no adverse sequelae. 3. Newborn's weight and condition are within normal limits.	**Technician** 1. Obtain weight. 2. Obtain blood pressure. 3. Test urine specimens for glucose, protein, acetone (ketones). 5. Obtain blood specimen to send to laboratory (in some hospitals, nurses have this responsibility). 6. Record all data.

Application of the Nursing Process

MATERNAL/FETAL NUTRITION

Laura is a 22-year-old married woman who is 10 weeks' pregnant with her second child. John, her first child, now a healthy 18 months of age, was born at term weighing 3500 g (7 lb, 12 oz). Laura expressed concern that she would not have enough calcium because she "just had a baby 18 months ago and never could stand drinking milk." During the dietary assessment she reveals that she cannot drink orange juice. During her last pregnancy she drank castor oil in orange juice for "chronic constipation." History, physical examination, and laboratory results are not remarkable.

FUNCTIONAL HEALTH PATTERN: ASSESSMENT	NURSING DIAGNOSIS	RATIONALE: PLAN/ IMPLEMENTATION	EVALUATION
NUTRITIONAL-METABOLIC ▪ 10 weeks' pregnant; first baby 18 months old. ▪ Does not drink milk. ▪ Cannot drink orange juice.	Alteration in nutrition: less than body requirement related to inability to drink milk or orange juice.	*To ensure adequate intake of nutrients present in milk and orange juice:* ▪ Explore alternate food sources. ▪ Encourage her to choose sources she likes and can afford.	Laura is able to choose alternate sources of nutrients. Laura ingests sufficient quantities of nutrients to meet RDAs and her own needs. Laura will not experience constipation.
ELIMINATION ▪ Experienced chronic constipation during first pregnancy.	Alterations in bowel elimination: constipation related to pregnancy.	*To prevent constipation during this pregnancy or to treat constipation with nonpharmaceutic means:* ▪ Review her usual bowel habits and explore changes during her pregnancy. ▪ Review maternal adaptations to pregnancy that alter alimentary function. ▪ Review methods of prevention and treatment (Chapter 11).	Laura will not experience constipation or will be able to control it with nonpharmaceutic means.

Continued.

Application of the Nursing Process—cont'd

FUNCTIONAL HEALTH PATTERN: ASSESSMENT	NURSING DIAGNOSIS	RATIONALE: PLAN/ IMPLEMENTATION	EVALUATION
SELF-PERCEPTION—SELF-CONCEPT ■ Concerned that she is unable to use the usual food sources of nutrients.	Disturbance in self-concept related to perceived lack of self-control in meeting nutritional needs.	*To increase her perceived control of what happens to her and to enhance her self-concept:* *Nutrients* ■ Compliment her on her expressed concern and her knowledge of needed nutrients. ■ Introduce her to the four food groups and distribution of nutrients. ■ Compliment her on choosing equivalent alternatives. ■ Write out shopping list and sample menus.	Laura participates in her own care. Laura practices problem solving by exploring alternatives and making choices to meet changing needs.
■ Experienced chronic constipation during first pregnancy.	Alteration in bowel elimination: constipation related to knowledge deficit of self-help methods of prevention and treatment.	*Constipation* ■ Help her incorporate knowledge into menu plan as necessary and set schedule for water intake, bowel elimination, exercise, and so on. ■ Commend her on her participation in problem solving.	Laura learns methods of preventing or treating constipation. Laura expresses pleasure with her ability to master these two situations.

References

Affonso, D.D.: The Filipino American. In Clark, A.L., editor: Culture/childbearing/health professionals, Philadelphia, 1978, F.A. Davis Co.

Barnico, L.M., and Cullinane, M.M.: Maternal phenylketonuria: an unexpected challenge, M.C.N. 10:108, Mar./Apr. 1985.

Bernstein, J.L., and Kidd, Y.A.: Childbearing in Japan, In Kay, M.A., editor: Anthropology of human birth, Philadelphia, 1982, F.A. Davis Co.

Brennan, R.E., Caldwell, M., and Rickard, K.A.: Assessment of maternal nutrition, J. Am. Diet. Assoc. 75:152, Aug. 1979.

Campbell, T., and Chang, B.: Health care of the Chinese in America, Nurs. Outlook 21:245, 1973.

Carrington, B.W.: The Afro-American. In Clark, A.L., editor: Culture/childbearing/health professionals, Philadelphia, 1978, F.A. Davis Co.

Chung, J.J.: Understanding the Oriental maternity patient, Nurs. Clin. North Am. 12:67, 1977.

Committee on Nutrition: Nutrition in maternal health care, Chicago, 1974, The American College of Obstetricians and Gynecologists.

Dunn, F.L.: Medical care in the Chinese communities of peninsular Malaysia. In Kleinman, A., et al., editors: Culture and healing in Asian societies, Cambridge, Mass., 1978, Schenkman Publishing Co.

Food and Nutrition Board: Recommended dietary allowances, rev. ed., Washington, D.C., 1980, National Academy of Sciences—National Research Council.

Hollingsworth, A.O., et al.: The refugees and childbearing: what to expect, R.N. 43:45, 1980.

Kay, M.A., editor: Anthropology of human birth, Philadelphia, 1982, F.A. Davis Co.

Lackey, C.J.: Pica—a nutritional anthropology concern. In Bauwens, E.E.: The anthropology of health, St. Louis, 1978, The C.V. Mosby Co.

Leiderman, P.H., et al.: Culture and infancy, New York, 1977, Academic Press, Inc.

Leininger, M.: The Gadsup of New Guinea and early child-caring behaviors with nursing implications. In Leininger,

M., editor: Transcultural nursing '79, New York, 1979, Masson Publishing U.A.S., Inc.

Lenke, R.R., and Levy, H.L.: Maternal phenylketonuria and hyperphenylalaninemia, N. Engl. J. Med. 303:1202, 1980.

Lipson, A., et al.: Maternal hyperphenylalaninemia and fetal effects, J. Pediatr. 104:216, 1984.

Luke, B.: Megavitamins and pregnancy: a dangerous combination, M.C.N. 10:18, Jan./Feb., 1985.

Mirkin, G.: Assailing vitamin abuse: facts about mega- and pseudo-vitamins, Contemp. OB/Gyn. 25:86 (special issue), May 1985.

Naeye, R.L.: Effects of maternal nutrition on fetal and neonatal survival, Birth 10:109, Summer 1983.

Naeye, R.L.: Weight gain and the outcome of pregnancy, Am. J. Obstet. Gynecol. 135:3, 1979.

Nutrition during pregnancy and lactation, Sacramento, Calif., 1975, Maternal and Child Health Branch, California Department of Health Services.

Obeyesekere, G.: Pregnancy cravings (dola-duka) in relation to social structure and personality in a Sinhalese village, Am. Anthropol. 65:323, 1963.

Schneider, H.A., and others: Nutritional support of medical practice, New York, 1977, Harper & Row, Publishers.

Smith, N.: Personal communication, San Francisco State University, Department of Nursing, 1986.

Snow, L.: Folk medical beliefs and their implications for care of patients, Ann. Intern. Med. 81:82, 1974.

Stern, P.N.: Solving problems of cross-cultural health teaching: the Filipino childbearing family, Image 13:47, 1981.

Truong, T.: Personal communication, San Francisco State University, Department of Nursing, 1986.

Vermeer, D.E., and Frate, D.A.: Geophagy in a Mississippi county, Ann. Assoc. Am. Geographers 65:414, 1975.

White, J.E., and Owsley, V.B.: Helping families cope with milk, wheat, and soy allergies, M.C.N. 8:423, Nov./Dec. 1983.

Williams, S.R.: Nutrition and diet therapy, ed. 5, St. Louis, 1985, The C.V. Mosby Co.

Worthington-Roberts, B.: Nutrition deficiencies and excesses: impact on pregnancy, part 1, J. Perinat. 5:9, Summer 1985.

Worthington-Roberts, B.S., Vermeersch, J., and Williams, S.R.: Nutrition in pregnancy and lactation, ed. 3, St. Louis, 1985, The C.V. Mosby Co.

Zlatnik, F.J., and Burmeister, L.F.: Dietary protein and preeclampsia, Am. J. Obstet. Gynecol. 147:345, 1983.

Bibliography

Edwards, L.E., et al.: Pregnancy in the massively obese: course, outcome and obesity prognosis of the infant, Am. J. Obstet. Gynecol. 131:479, 1978.

Edwards, L.E., et al.: Pregnancy in the underweight woman: course, outcome and growth patterns of the infant, Am. J. Obstet. Gynecol. 135:297, 1979.

Frank, D.W., et al.: Nutrition in adolescent pregnancy, J. Calif. Perinatal Assoc. 1:21, 1983.

Grosso, C., et al.: The Vietnamese American family . . . and grandma makes three, M.C.N. 6:177, 1981.

Hattner, J.: Personal communication, Dietetics Department, Stanford University Hospital, Stanford, Calif.

Haworth, J.C., et al.: Fetal growth retardation in cigarette-smoking mothers is not due to decreased maternal food intake, Am. J. Obstet. Gynecol. 137:719, 1980.

Hurley, L.S.: Developmental nutrition, Englewood Cliffs, N.J., 1980, Prentice-Hall.

Jacobson, H.N.: Diet therapy and the improvement of pregnancy outcomes, Birth 10:29, Spring, 1983.

Jensen, M.D., and Bobak, I.M.: Handbook of maternity care: a guide for nursing practice, St. Louis, 1980, The C.V. Mosby Co.

Jensen, M.D., and Bobak, I.M.: Maternity and gynecologic care: the nurse and the family, ed. 3, St. Louis, 1985, The C.V. Mosby Co.

Laboratory indices of nutritional status in pregnancy, pub. no. F-427, Washington, D.C., Sept. 1977, National Academy of Sciences–National Research Council.

Leonard, L.G.: Pregnancy and the underweight woman, M.C.N. 9(5):331, Sept./Oct. 1984.

Naeye, R.L.: Teenaged and pre-teenaged pregnancies: consequences of the fetal-maternal competition for nutrients, Pediatrics 67:146, 1981.

Orque, M.S., Bloch, B., and Ahumada-Monrroy, L.S.: Ethnic nursing care: a multicultural approach, St. Louis, 1983, The C.V. Mosby Co.

Pritchard, J.A., MacDonald, P.C., and Gant, N.F.: Williams obstetrics, ed. 17, Norwalk, Conn., 1985, Appleton-Century-Crofts.

Willson, J.R., Carrington, E.R., and Ledger, W.J.: Obstetrics and gynecology, ed. 7, St. Louis, 1983, The C.V. Mosby Co.

Worthington-Roberts, B.: Nutrition deficiencies and excesses: impact on pregnancy, part 2, J. Perinat. 5:12, Fall 1985.

Zuspan, F., and Quilligan, E.J., editors: Practical manual of obstetrical care: a pocket reference for those who treat the pregnant patient, St. Louis, 1982, The C.V. Mosby Co.

Family Preparation for Birth of a Child

In its publication *Guidelines for Childbirth Education* (1981) the Nurses' Association of the American College of Obstetricians and Gynecologists (NAACOG) defines *childbirth education* as follows:

The process designed to assist parents in making the transition from the role of expectant parents to the role and responsibilities of parents of a new baby which includes the period from the time of conception to approximately three months after birth.

This statement implies that childbirth education is more than preparation for a labor and birth experience. It is also *preparation for parenting*.

Comprehensive parent education programs are needed to meet the numerous and varied learning needs of expectant and new parents. Classes in preparation for the birth itself are only one part of preparation-for-parenthood programs. Such programs recognize that pregnancy is not a disease state but a state of wellness. During pregnancy people move from the role of expectant parents to the role and responsibilities of parents of a new baby. Pregnancy can be a meaningful growth experience.

Traditionally, teaching has occurred within a formalized structure in the United States and Canada. However, it also has been recognized that all of life educates and that teaching occurs in many ways. Too often, education for birth and parenting has been limited to a classroom. Formal classes may be effective for people socialized into structured education, but structured education can be ineffective for people who have not found the classroom atmosphere stimulating.

Nurses have limitless opportunities to teach parents in formal classes, in small group sessions, in office and clinic waiting rooms, and at home. Education for childbirth and for parenting is an integral part of the nursing process.

Nursing Process in Prebirth Education

Since the days of Florence Nightingale, nurses have attempted to state the essence of nursing. Through these efforts, rationales have been developed for classification systems, rules of categorization, and implications of systems for nursing practice, education, and research. In her work published in 1859, Florence Nightingale identified the elements that constitute good nursing. She emphasized the necessity of careful observation, systematic preparation, and ongoing management.

Authors of contemporary nursing literature seem to agree that nursing is a decision-making process. In its simplest form the process of nursing consists of five problem-solving steps: (1) assessment, (2) formulation of nursing diagnoses, (3) planning, (4) implementation, and (5) evaluation.

Teaching is a process involving interactions between a teacher and a learner. Assessment, formulation of educational diagnoses, planning, implementation, and evaluation are also stages in the teaching process. **Teaching** can be defined as a deliberate intentional action taken to help another person learn to do what that person cannot presently do. **Learning** involves measurable behavior change resulting from practice and experience.

The nursing process and the teaching process can be seen as parallel. Both provide the basis for childbirth education as an integral part of the teaching component of nursing.

Nursing process in parent education assessment involves data collection for the purpose of identifying client needs (Fig. 13.1). Pertinent data include the ages of the learners, their culture or ethnicity, and their readiness to learn. This data gathering is a continuous collection of information from a variety of valid and reli-

Fig. 13.1
The nursing process in parent education. Arrows indicate direction of communication.

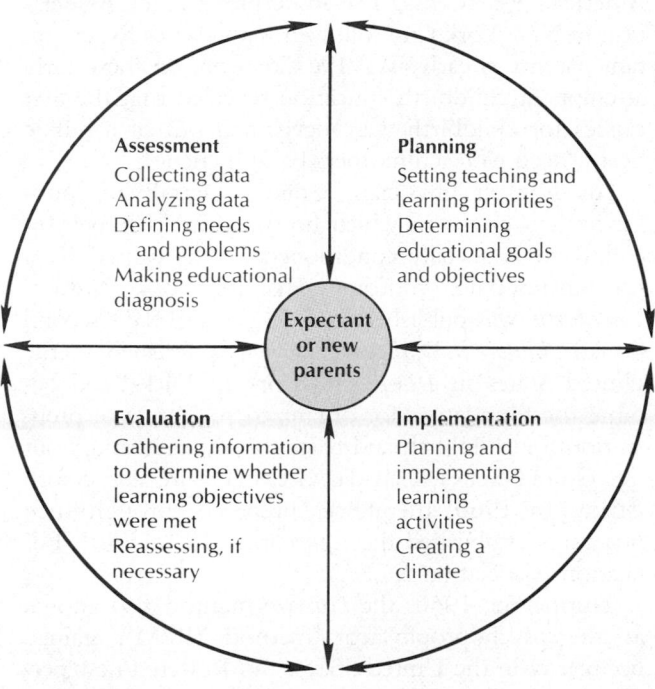

Assessment
Collecting data
Analyzing data
Defining needs
   and problems
Making educational
   diagnosis

Planning
Setting teaching and
learning priorities
Determining
educational goals
and objectives

Expectant
or new
parents

Evaluation
Gathering information
to determine whether
learning objectives
were met
Reassessing, if
necessary

Implementation
Planning and
implementing
learning
activities
Creating a
climate

The physical and emotional needs of the learner are given priority. An atmosphere conducive to learning is created in a climate of friendliness and acceptance.

Evaluation determines teaching effectiveness in relation to the stated objectives. Constructive evaluation promotes individual growth. Methods commonly used by nurses to evaluate client learning are (1) direct observation, (2) client records, (3) reports, (4) tests, (5) interviews and questionnaires with clients and their families, (6) interviews and questionnaires with staff, and (7) research using statistical comparisons. Effective evaluation occurs as a result of careful planning.

The goal of teaching in preparation for birth and parenting is to enable the nurse and clients to enter each other's worlds, recognize mutual values, and learn more about each other and themselves. Concerns are shared, and mutual learning goals are accepted. We indoctrinate when we teach a "set of beliefs" and teach them in such a way that their validity seems beyond question. To avoid indoctrination, it is important to consider all sides of the issues. Learning is a lifelong search for truth.

able sources. Examples of sources are group discussion, observation, and a formal pen-and-pencil assessment of learning needs, personal interviews, client health records, other health-care team members, family members, and review of pertinent literature. An **educational diagnosis** can be formulated after the collected data have been analyzed and learning needs and problems defined. An **educational diagnosis** identifies the client's learning needs and suggests a plan of action.

Planning involves specifics. The nurse establishes teaching and learning priorities for the identified needs using his or her personal philosophy of childbirth and parent education as a guide. Educational goals are then identified as the nurse works with the family. Next, educational objectives are established. These are statements related to the goal. They are specific, measurable, attainable, and agreed on by the family and the nurse.

Implementation involves carrying out the learning activities designed to meet the learning objectives. The emphasis is on principles, content, level, and scope of learning. Implementation encompasses selecting instructional methods. These methods include (1) discussion, (2) role playing, (3) repetition, (4) testing, (5) rewards, and (6) the use of audiovisual materials.

Prebirth Education for the Family

Preparation for parenthood. A typical preparation-for-parenthood program recognizes the expectant parents and their families have different interests and information needs as the pregnancy progresses. Consequently, the program is designed to meet the information needs of parents at the three major stages of pregnancy and after birth.

Early pregnancy classes. Early pregnancy ("early bird") classes provide fundamental information. Classes are developed around the following areas: (1) early fetal development, (2) physiologic and emotional changes of pregnancy, (3) human sexuality, and (4) the nutritional needs of the mother and fetus. Environmental and workplace hazards have become important concerns in recent years. Even though pregnancy is considered a normal process, danger signs, drugs, and self-medication are topics of interest and concern.

Midpregnancy classes. Midpregnancy classes emphasize the woman's participation in self-care. Classes provide information on (1) preparation for breast and bottle feeding, (2) basic hygiene, (3) health maintenance (rest, exercise, and nutrition), (4) common complaints and simple, safe remedies, (5) infant health, and (6) parenting.

Late pregnancy classes. Late pregnancy classes are designed to meet the needs of the entire family: (1) couple discussion groups, (2) expectant father discussion groups, (3) sibling classes, (4) grandparents'

Fig. 13.2
Teenage expectant mothers learn about maternal adaptations to pregnancy. (Courtesy Marjorie Pyle RNC, Lifecircle, Costa Mesa, California.)

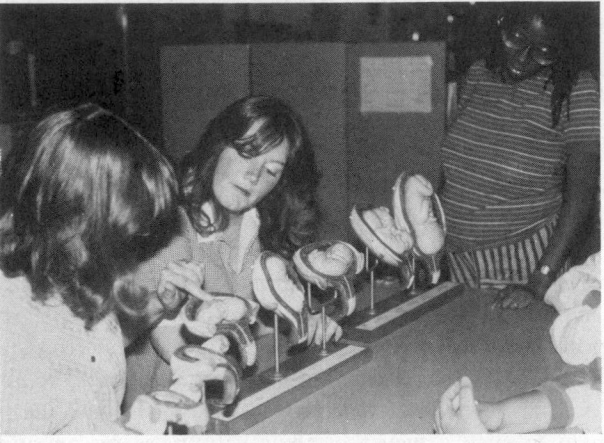

classes, and (5) newborn care classes. Special classes are developed for teenage parents (Fig. 13.2), for parents expecting a cesarean delivery (Hart, 1980), and for parents of twins. Refresher courses for those who feel they are prepared through previous childbirth experience but would like to review a few things are also available (Mercer, 1979).

Throughout the series of classes there is discussion of support systems that people can use during pregnancy and after birth; such support systems help parents function independently and effectively. During all the classes the open expression of feelings and concerns about any aspect of pregnancy, birth, and parenting is welcomed.

After-birth classes. After-birth classes help parents meet the tasks and responsibilities of their new roles. Topics for discussion can include (1) coping mechanisms for the reality of parenting, (2) use of support systems, and (3) infant care and growth and development. Birth control methods and adapting to new roles (wife-lover ⇌ mother and husband-lover ⇌ father) are explored.

Parent preparation for childbirth

Historical overview. Since colonial times in America, women shared their information on childbirth with other women. Births occurred in the family's home with a midwife in attendance. However, in the nineteenth century, male physicians gradually came to be recognized as experts to whom women went for information about birth. By 1900 physicians had usurped the age-old skills of women concerning child-

birth and became for many the sole authorities.

In the United States the first formal classes in childbirth education were offered nationally in 1913 by the American Red Cross. The Maternity Center Association in New York City followed with classes for expectant parents as early as 1919. Literature on these early attempts at childbirth education revealed that the first classes for childbirth were developed out of a public health need to teach mothers basic hygiene.

An English physician, Grantly Dick-Read, published two books in which he theorized that pain in childbirth is socially conditioned and is caused by a fear-tension-pain syndrome. His first book, *Natural Childbirth,* was published in 1933. Dick-Read's second book, *Childbirth Without Fear,* was published in the United States in 1944. The work of Dick-Read became the foundation for organized programs of preparation for childbirth and teacher training throughout the United States, Canada, Great Britain, and South Africa. In 1960, the nurses prepared through such programs established the International Childbirth Education Association (ICEA).

During the 1960s the Lamaze method also known as the psychoprophylactic method (PPM), gained popularity in the United States. PPM offered new perspectives on preparation for childbirth by emphasizing mind control. Marjorie Karmel introduced PPM to the United States in her book, *Thank You, Dr. Lamaze,* which was published in the United States in 1959. Others have written extensively on PPM. This system grew out of Pavlov's work on the higher nervous activity of humans and animals in which he proposed that every vital activity of an organism is a complex reflex process capable of conditioning.

In 1960 the American Society for Psychoprophylaxis in Obstetrics (ASPO) was formed in New York as a national organization to promote use of the Lamaze method and to prepare teachers of the method. The National Association of Childbirth Education, Inc. (NACE) (formerly the Childbirth Without Pain Education League, Inc. [CWPL]), was formed in 1970 to teach the Lamaze method and prepare teachers. The Council of Childbirth Education Specialists, Inc. (CCES) was founded in New York City in 1971 and offered teacher training seminars throughout the United States.

A Denver obstetrician, Robert Bradley, published *Husband-Coached Childbirth* in 1965. In the book he advocates what he calls true natural childbirth, without any form of anesthesia or analgesia and with a husband-coach and breathing techniques for labor. The American Academy of Husband-Coached Childbirth (AAHCC) was founded to make the Bradley method available and to prepare teachers.

Of the other techniques developed, the most widely known include the work of Kitzinger and Wright, developed in England. Wright's work is based on PPM and is described as "levels of breathing." Kitzinger's work is designed around a psychosexual approach, which proposes that birth is a sexual experience. As such, birth is perceived as a normal physiologic process in which the woman works in harmony with her body.

Hypnosis as a method of relieving pain in childbirth has been used since the 1800s. Through hypnosis the woman reaches a trancelike state, remaining awake but responsive to the hypnotist (Johnson, 1980). Hypnosis requires an extensive time commitment by the hypnotist. It is impractical for use with large numbers of women.

Components of childbirth methods. All preparation techniques have three components, which are (1) psychophysical, (2) psychologic, and (3) intellectual. The psychologic principles involved are suggestion and distraction. The confidence and assurance derived from participation in the classes help women (couples) to cope with labor and delivery (Myles, 1981). Women benefit from learning the techniques for coping with pain and loss of control (Lederman, 1984).

Psychophysical component. Various studies have been undertaken to determine the physiologic effectiveness of prepared childbirth methods. These studies analyze data in terms of the amount of pain experienced during labor and birth, maternal and fetal complications, and the length of labor. Chertok (1967) and Velvovsky and co-workers (1960) reviewed many studies in which investigators demonstrated the effectiveness of preparation-for-birth approaches to pain relief during childbirth. Huttel and co-workers (1972) reported observations of less "complaint" and "tension" behaviors among women who were prepared for birth when compared with women who did not attend preparation classes. Huttel suggested that preparation for birth enables the mother to experience a shorter labor.

Psychologic component. Although physiologic benefits of prepared childbirth are important, additional benefits have been claimed. A review of the literature by Buxton in 1962 concluded by emphasizing the critical importance of the psychologic benefits of preparation for birth. Unlike some of the contradictory material found on physiologic effects, research on psychologic effects continues to be overwhelmingly in agreement. Tanzer (1967) found the prepared women had a more positive subjective experience during delivery. It is particularly notable in this research how many of the women stressed the importance of having either their husband or another support person present during labor. Tanzer's results indicate that women experience a positive and highly desirable effect when their mates

are present during birth. Other studies report that support and participation in labor and birth by the infant's father contribute to positive perceptions of the birth experience.

Intellectual component. The intellectual components of preparation for childbirth are closely tied to the psychologic components. Research has indicated that the more knowledge a woman gains concerning pregnancy, labor, and birth as a result of childbirth preparation classes, the more favorable will be her attitude toward the pregnancy and the labor and delivery experience. A woman's perception of maintaining control is closely associated with satisfaction, according to studies by Willmuth (1975), Felton and Segelman (1978), Cronenwett (1980), and Cronenwett and Brickman (1983). Although the mechanisms by which preparation-for-childbirth classes affect the birth experience are not yet fully understood, it is clear that these classes affect the subjective experience in a positive manner.

• • •

Major methods taught in the United States are (1) the Dick-Read method, (2) the Lamaze method (PPM), and (3) the Bradley method. Each will be discussed, outlining the three components of prepared childbirth.

Dick-Read method: Childbirth without fear
Psychophysical component. Dick-Read basically recommended three techniques: deep breathing both in abdominal respirations and thoracic respirations; shallow breathing; and breath holding for the second stage of labor.* The Dick-Read method also incoporates physical exercise to prepare the body for labor.

For most of labor the pattern of breathing is basically abdominal breathing. The woman is taught to force her abdominal muscles to rise during a contraction. In this way she lifts the abdominal muscles off the uterus as it rises forward during a contraction. Teachers of the Dick-Read method contend that the weight of the abdominal musculature on the contracting uterus increases pain.

Relaxation is an important part of the Dick-Read method. Women are taught to use conscious relaxation methods that involve progressive relaxation of the muscle groups in the entire body. Consequently, during labor the woman is able to relax completely between contractions. Using conscious relaxation techniques, some women are actually able to sleep between contractions.

---
*Breath holding is no longer advised.

Psychologic component. According to Dick-Read (1959):

Fear, tension and pain are three veils opposed to the natural design which have been concerned with preparation for and attendance at childbirth. If fear, tension, and pain go hand in hand, then it must be necessary to relieve tension and to overcome fear in order to eliminate pain. The implementation of my theory demonstrates the methods by which fear can be overcome, tension may be eliminated and replaced by physical and mental relaxation.

Intellectual component. Dick-Read's program educated women to exchange understanding and confidence for fear of the unknown. Adequate prenatal education included information on nutrition and basic hygiene as well as information on labor and birth.

In the Dick-Read method, support for the woman in labor was originally to be provided by nursing and medical attendants. However, in the adaptations of the Dick-Read method in use today, labor support is provided by the father or a support person chosen by the mother.

Lamaze method: psychoprophylaxis method (PPM)

Psychophysical component. Controlled muscular relaxation and breathing techniques are combined in the Lamaze method. Active relaxation is an integral part of the Lamaze method (Lamaze, 1970). The woman is taught to relax uninvolved muscle groups (neuromuscular control) while she contracts a specific muscle group (Fig. 13.3). By this process the woman can relax the uninvolved muscles in her body while her uterine musculature contracts. Women who attended Lamaze-type childbirth preparation classes maintained a significantly higher level of neuromuscular control during the first stage of labor than women who were self-prepared (Bernardini and others, 1983, p. 111).

The breathing techniques use the chest muscles. Lamaze teachers believe that chest breathing lifts the diaphragm off the contracting uterus, thus giving it more room to expand. These chest breathing patterns vary according to the intensity of the contractions and the progress of labor.

Psychologic component. According to the Lamaze method, pain in labor is a conditioned response and women can be conditioned not to experience pain in labor. Instead of crying out and losing control during uterine contractions, women are taught to respond with conditioned relaxation and breathing patterns. The psychologic experience of maintaining control appears to be intimately related to the physiologic experience of maintaining control (Bernardini and others, 1983, p. 106).

Fig. 13.3
Teaching relaxation. Women are exhaling slowly and performing effleurage. Coaches are watching a clock and counting off the seconds of this "contraction." (Courtesy Lisa Livingston, R.N., B.S.N., director, Maternal Child Health Education, Community Birth Center, Community Hospital, Santa Cruz, California.)

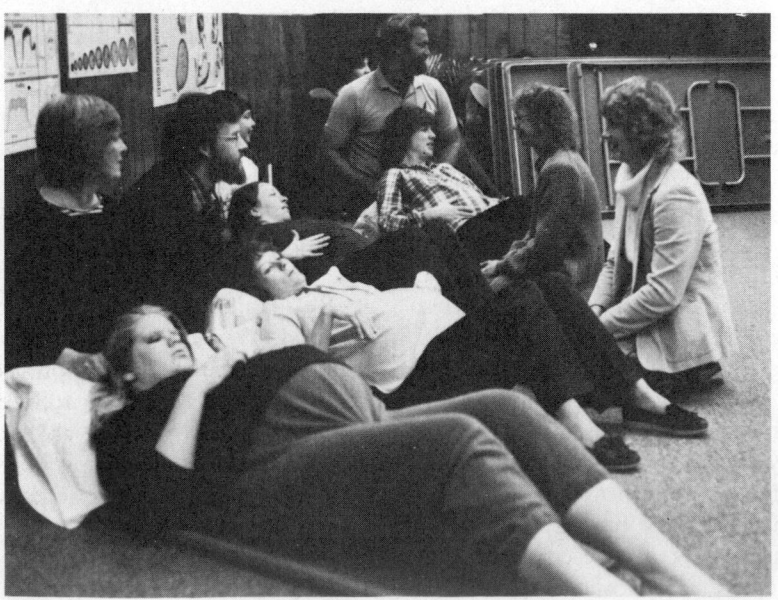

Intellectual component. The Lamaze method emphasizes understanding the body and how it works. It offers a flexible but structured program to remove fear by education, thus eliminating distressing associations. This method finds its rationale in the neurophysiology of pain.

In the Lamaze method, support for the woman in labor is provided by her husband or other support person. Specially trained labor attendants termed *monitrices* sometimes provide support for the laboring mother using the Lamaze method.

Bradley method

Psychophysical component. Breath control, abdominal breathing, and general body relaxation are used in the Bradley method. Working in harmony with the body is emphasized (Bradley, 1965). Bradley based his method on observations of animal behavior during birth. His technique focuses on environmental variables such as darkness, solitude, and quiet to make childbirth a more natural experience. Women using the Bradley method often appear to be sleeping during labor. However, they are not asleep but simply in a state of deep mental relaxation.

Psychologic component. The importance of the husband's support is foremost in this method. In fact, the method is also referred to as "husband-coached childbirth."

Intellectual component. Preparation-for-birth teaching concentrates on minimizing the need for analgesics or anesthetics for birth. There is also an emphasis on nutrition, omitting foods containing preservatives and added salt and sugar.

■ ■ ■

Each of the three methods just discussed emphasizes intellectual and physical components. However, the Dick-Read and Bradley methods emphasize the naturalness of childbirth, whereas Lamaze emphasizes active mental and physical conditioning. These methods have mutually influenced each other so that it is unusual to find classes in a pure "method" anymore. Different teachers develop their own methods, which may change with each group of expectant couples. Education in preparation for birth is continually evolving. The teachers themselves are being taught by the experiences of each expectant couple. Books, journal articles, magazine articles, and audiovisual aids in childbirth education are proliferating. A list of some of the organizations involved in parent education can be found at the end of this chapter.

Recent trends. Childbirth education in the 1980s is at a crossroads. Once a small consumer movement, childbirth education gained momentum in the 1970s, paralleling the growth of the women's movement. Childbirth education has evolved into large professional organizations with significant influence on maternity care in the United States. Responding to this movement, health care professionals and hospitals are offering childbirth education programs in rapidly growing numbers. At the same time these hospital-sponsored programs are proliferating, there is a widening gap between the "medical" model of childbirth and the "physiologic" model. If the new programs are truly education and not indoctrination, they will present all known options for the birth experience and discuss both risks and benefits of obstetric procedures. Childbirth education must offer choice and not just hospital policy.

There also seems to be a gap forming *within* the original consumer-based childbirth education movement. Critics of methods to prepare for birth are presenting physiologic evidence that specific breathing techniques (such as breath holding while pushing) may be harmful to the fetus and have no influence on the progress of the second stage (see Chapter 17). Fresh approaches to old techniques are being proposed. These emphasize tuning into the laboring woman's body cues and encouraging her to do what feels natural. In this holistic approach to childbirth education the emphasis is on how the mind, body, and spirit are related and affect one another.

Women are encouraged to incorporate their natural responses into coping with the pain of labor and birth. Valuable tools to incorporate include vocalization or "sounding" to relieve tension in pregnancy and labor, massage with a light touch to encourage relaxation, visualization to guide women into positive spaces ("seeing" the vagina open up around the baby), hot compresses to the perineum, perineal massage, relaxing music and subdued lighting, and the use of warm water for showers or bathing during labor. In response to the critics, organizations also are adapting their teaching methods to changing times.

There are times when the woman or couple will choose not to cope with labor and request analgesia or anesthesia (total or partial). Each person has a right to labor and give birth in whatever way she chooses, provided the way is safe for both mother and baby.

Grandparent preparation. The definition of "grand" is extensive and includes descriptions such as impressive or imposing; stately, majestic, dignified; highest, or very high, in rank or official dignity; of great importance or distinction; first-rate, very good, splendid; princely, regal, royal, and exalted. A grandparent is an ancestor, one generation more remote—a founder or originator of a family. Grandparents are a vital link between generations (Horn and Manion, 1985).

Every pregnancy affects all family relationships. In particular, a first pregnancy is undeniable evidence that one is now old enough to have a child who is soon to bear a grandchild. Many think of a "grandparent" as old, white-haired, and becoming feeble of mind and body. Being "old" carries a stigma for some in predominantly youth-oriented societies. Some people face grandparenthood when still in their 30s and 40s. A mother-to-be announcing her pregnancy to her mother may be greeted by, "How *dare* you do that to me! *I* am not ready to be a grandmother!" Both daughter and mother may be startled and hurt by the outburst.

The proliferation of literature, visual aids, and classes for expectant and new parents projects these as *the* sources for information. Rapid advances in technology, increased mobility of families, and establishment of nuclear families sometimes thousands of miles distant have added to the reliance of these sources for information and guidance (Newell, 1984). Under these conditions opportunities to become "grand" become minimal or unavailable.

Fortunately, childbirth educators are becoming more aware of the unique role of the grandparent and are forming classes for grandparents (Hassid, 1984; McKay and Phillips, 1984; Horn and Manion, 1985). An outline for such classes, developed by childbirth educators at The Woman's Hospital of Texas (Houston), is presented on p. 337. The various grandparental roles are acknowledged (Kornhaber and Woodward, 1981): (1) historian who transmits the history of the family and provides continuity with the present, (2) resource person who shares knowledge gleaned from experience, (3) role model, and (4) support person.

Grandparents' anxieties and concerns and their relationships with expectant parents and with grandchildren should be opened to discussion during courses for expectant parents as well (see Fig. 13.4 and Guidelines for Client Teaching: Grandparent Preparation). The expectant parents may use this opportunity to begin to resolve conflicts and perceived differences with their parents, a task that can enhance their ability to relate to their own children. In addition, another potential problem can be averted. Consider the difficulty a child faces when a beloved grandparent is belittled by a beloved parent; the child is caught in the middle (Satir, 1972) thus negatively influencing the relationship with the parent and that with the grandparent. To be truly *family-oriented,* maternity care must consider the grandparent when implementing the nursing process with childbearing families. (See also Chapters 10 and 23.)

Sibling preparation. Sibling preparation has a definite place in family-centered maternity care (Johnsen and Gaspard, 1985). Many expectant parents are concerned about an older child's response to the birth of a new brother or sister. Parents want to provide as much support as possible for the older child or children (see also Chapters 10, 15, 17, 18, and 23). Professional groups of clinics and hospitals are developing classes to prepare children for the birth of a new brother or sister (Fig. 13.5). A general teaching plan used for young children is found on p. 339. The general plan can be modified to fit needs of children of different ages and the needs of children who will be present during the birth.

Parent preparation for cesarean birth. Concerned professional and lay groups in the community have established councils for cesarean birth in an attempt to meet the needs of women and their families. Such groups advocate including preparation for cesarean birth in all parenthood preparation classes. This is encouraged even if parents-to-be "tune out" such discussions and feel later that they have been betrayed by not having been made aware of this eventuality. No woman can be guaranteed a vaginal delivery, even if she is in good health and there is no indication of danger to the fetus before the onset of labor. Every woman needs to be aware of and prepared for this eventuality. The unknown and unexpected is ego weakening. Each woman or couple needs accurate data to build new coping abilities or to strengthen old ones. "Walking through," role playing, or worry work before a crisis situation increases one's sense of control in

Fig. 13.4
Grandparents learn about fetal monitoring procedures in labor room. (Courtesy Jane Rohan, Educational Department, The Women's Hospital, Houston.)

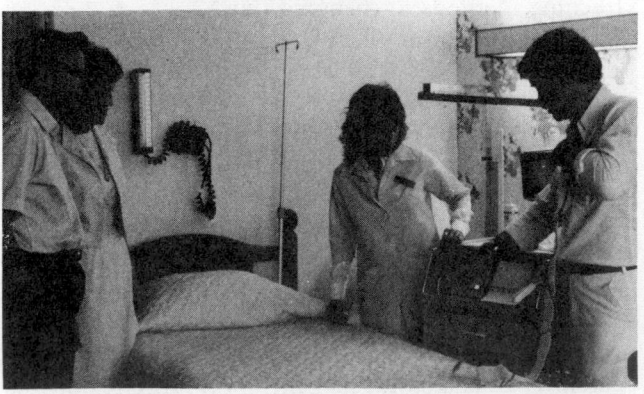

Grandparents' Tour and Class

Objectives

Participants will be able to:
1. State policies and procedures of labor and delivery, nursery, and family-centered unit.
2. Explain purpose and reason for Bililites and infant warmers.
3. Describe circumcision and cord care.
4. Summarize total care of family unit at hospital.

Outline

I. Meet in administrative office and move to classroom
   A. Slides on family-centered care
   B. Discussion of options available to couple of today
     1. LeBoyer
     2. Birthing room
     3. Lamaze
   C. Changing role of father in family unit
     1. Education
     2. Participation
   D. Changing role of grandparent
     1. Mobility
     2. Transient society
     3. Retirement
II. Tour through labor and delivery area
   A. Science and technology and birth process
     1. Why fetal monitoring (Fig. 13.4)
     2. Why IVs
   B. Complications in labor
   C. Anesthesia of today

   D. Gown and mask for delivery room
     1. Position of father
     2. Explanation of warmer
III. Nursery
   A. Transitional care nursery (use check sheet to explain care)
   B. General nursery: Bililites
   C. Intensive care nursery and family-centered care
IV. Skylight room: visiting anytime at mother's choice
V. Family-centered care
   A. Visit to empty room on family unit
   B. Explanation of channel 5 (in-hospital)
VI. Return to classroom for demonstrations and explanations (coffee and doughnuts)
   A. Cord care (demonstrate with doll)
   B. Circumcision care
   C. Temperature regulation of newborn
   D. Bonding
   E. Breast-feeding
   F. Normal newborn skin conditions (use pictures)
VII. Questions and answers

Courtesy Jane Rohan, Education Department, The Woman's Hospital of Texas, 7600 Fannin St., Houston, Texas, 77054.

Fig. 13.5
Sibling preparation class for preschool children, Community Birth Center, Community Hospital, Santa Cruz, California. (Courtesy Marjorie Pyle, RNC, Lifecircle, Costa Mesa, California.)

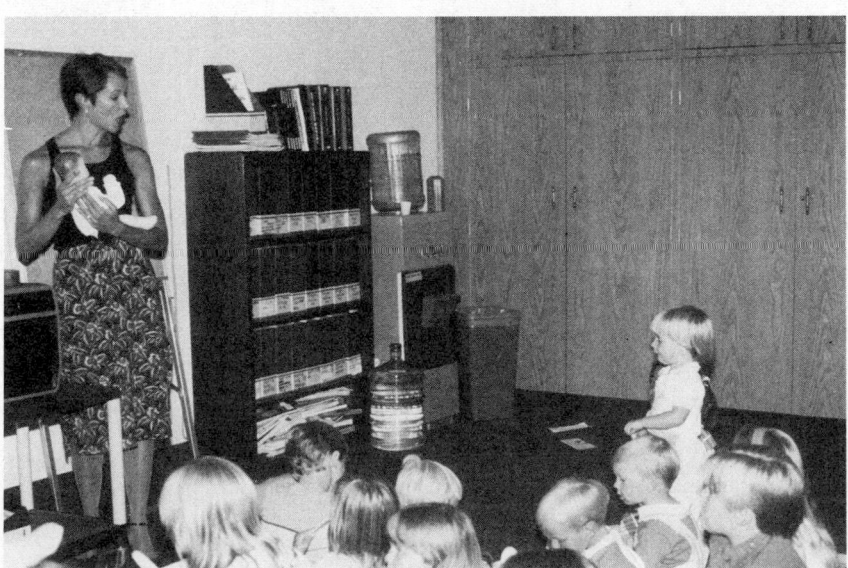

Guidelines for Client Teaching

GRANDPARENT PREPARATION

ASSESSMENT

Expectant parents voice concerns about role of grandparents and request assistance (readiness to learn).

Expectant grandparents request information about hospital policies and procedures, childbirth today, new parents' needs, and their own roles.

NURSING DIAGNOSES

Alterations in health maintenance
Knowledge deficit
Powerlessness
Disturbance in self-concept
Alteration in family processes
Alteration in parenting
Social isolation
Ineffective individual coping
Ineffective family coping
Spiritual distress

GOALS

Short-term

Grandparents are oriented to hospital routines and policies to be experienced by daughter or son and newborn.

Grandparents are oriented to childbirth experience expected by the daughter or son.

Grandparents learn current techniques of child care.

Intermediate

Grandparents prepare for role transition from parent to grandparent.

Grandparents begin to define mutually acceptable role-relationship with daugher or son.

Grandparents come to terms with own childbirth experiences.

Long-term

Grandparents develop a mutually satisfying role-relationship with daughter or son.

Grandparents develop a mutually satisfying role-relationship with grandchild.

Grandparents become effective and creative grandparents.

REFERENCES AND TEACHING AIDES

Values clarification or attitude awareness exercise (Horn and Manion, 1985)

Audiovisual materials: films, slides, charts

List of references available for the lay public

Tour of maternity unit, gowns, shoe covers, caps

CONTENT/RATIONALE	TEACHING ACTIONS
To explore values and attitudes: Values-clarification, attitude-awareness exercise: ■ When I think about myself as a grandparent, I feel* ____ ■ Children bring a couple* ____ ■ Breast feeding is* ____ ■ Pacifiers are* ____ ■ Labor is ____ ■ During their child's labor and delivery, grandparents should ____ ■ The happiest (most satisfying) memory of my (my wife's) labor and childbirth was ____ ■ The unhappiest (least satisfying) memory of my (my wife's) labor and childbirth was ____	Develop and administer values and attitudes exercise. Use exercise as basis for facilitating small-group discussion. Encourage members of group to compare and contrast own experiences, values, and attitudes
To explore knowledge base of science and technology and the birth process: See Grandparents tour and class, p. 337.	Encourage questions regarding topics they wish to discuss. Write topics on chalkboard. Ask group to prioritize list of topics. Begin lecture or discussion with the prioritized list. During lecture or discussion, use appropriate audiovisual materials: charts, film, slides.
To expand learning and orient to environment to maternity area, provide: ■ Tour of unit ■ Hands-on experience with equipment and supplies ■ Introduction of personnel ■ Description of personnel's services and responsibilities.	Offer or conduct a tour of the maternity area, including restrooms, waiting area. Inform them of location of cafeteria. Encourage hands-on experience with selected supplies (gowns, shoe covers) and equipment (fetoscope). Introduce to available personnel. Review roles of personnel.

---

*Horn, M., and Manion, J.: Creative grandparenting: bonding the generations, J.O.G.N. N. 14:233, May/June 1985.

Guidelines for Client Teaching —cont'd

CONTENT/RATIONALE	TEACHING ACTIONS
To bring closure to class: Questions	Return group to classroom. Provide refreshments. Encourage questions. Encourage them to compare and contrast their experiences with this class content. Provide printed materials. Summarize the experience. Thank the group for their interest.

EVALUATION: The nurse can be assured that the class was effective if the goals have been achieved.

Guidelines for Client Teaching
SIBLING PREPARATION

ASSESSMENT

Parents express desire for preparation of older siblings.
Age-related developmental needs of children determine to a great extent readiness to learn and experiential readiness to learn.

NURSING DIAGNOSES

Noncompliance
Potential for injury
Knowledge deficit
Anxiety
Disturbance in self-concept
Impaired verbal communication (child's developmental level)
Alteration in family process
Alteration in parenting
Ineffective individual coping

GOALS
Short-term

Child and parent feel less anxious about the mother's impending hospitalization.
Child begins to develop realistic expectations of newborn.
Parent begins to develop strategies to prepare the older child for the mother's hospitalization and newborn sibling.

Intermediate

Child begins to prepare for role transition to big sister or big brother.
Parent begins to develop strategies for caring for older sibling and new child.
Parent begins to prepare for role transition necessitated by addition of new member of the family.

Long-term

Child develops realistic expectations of newborn.
Child learns how to participate with family to cope with changes.
Child and parent learn new coping skills.
Parent successfully makes role transition necessitated by addition of new member to the family.

REFERENCES AND TEACHING AIDES

Audiovisual materials: film, slides, doll, cassette recordings, materials with which to draw pictures, finger puppets
See Bibliography for list of references available to parents and small children.

CONTENT/RATIONALE	TEACHING ACTIONS
To allay anxiety related to an unknown environment: Concrete experiences (Johnsen and Gaspard, 1985): ■ Visit hospital classroom. ■ Dress up in hospital clothing. ■ Prior to tour, children learn hospital "rules": walk slowly, speak quietly. ■ Tour maternity area: birthing room, postpartum room; see and touch telephone that they can use to talk to their mothers. ■ See naked newborn.	In the hospital (clinic) prepare a room to convey warmth and friendliness. Dressed in uniform, greet children as they arrive with parents. Explain hospital clothing. Change to scrub outfit worn by nurses and fathers. Help children try on hospital gowns, caps, masks. During tour, answer questions and expect children to abide by hospital "rules."

Continued.

Guidelines for Client Teaching—cont'd

CONTENT/RATIONALE	TEACHING ACTIONS
To help child form realistic expectations of newborn: Practice in new role: ■ By listening to stories about what newborns can do and how older children react to the newborn. ■ By holding a doll with care to support the head. ■ By exploring what they can do when the baby cries. Hear sound of newborn cries and cooing as they vary with hunger, contentment, desire for company, and complaining about a dirty or wet diaper. *To help child substitute acceptable behavior for unacceptable behavior with the newborn:* Practice through role-playing: ■ When newborn gets a present and older child does not. ■ When parent spends time with newborn. ■ When the child gets angry with the newborn. *To help child recognize their feelings:* ■ Watch a film depicting jealousy, anger, and being left out (Johnsen and Gaspard, 1985). ■ Participate in discussion of film and how to ask for help when needed. ■ Participate in drawing a picture to show how they feel and what they understand of their mother's pregnancy and the coming baby. ■ Discuss puppet play; identify and discuss individual puppet characters. *To help parents with older child's preparation for the birth and with coping with an additional family member, see Chapters 10 and 23.*	Read stories and employ role-playing. Ask children leading questions (Johnsen and Gaspard, 1985): "Do you dress yourself? Can the new baby do that?" Help children with holding the doll. Demonstrate ways to console a crying baby, such as singing, talking. Caution children against picking up baby. Play cassette of baby sounds and encourage questions and discussions. Role-play situation demonstrating positive responses to newborn in selected situations. Involve older child in problem solving in selected situations. Show film and encourage discussion. Lead discussion: encourage each child to comment. Provide equipment, space, and directions for drawing, such as "draw a picture of your family." Ask children to tell a story about their pictures. Put on a play with finger puppets.

EVALUATION: The nurse can be assured that the class was effective if the goals have been met.

---

that situation and serves to minimize the sense of loss experienced.

Childbirth educators stress the importance of emphasizing the similarities as well as differences between cesarean and vaginal births. Also, in support of the philosophy of family-centered birth, many hospitals have changed policies to permit fathers to share in cesarean births as they have vaginal ones (see Chapter 29). Women undergoing cesarean birth stress that the continued presence and support of their partners have helped them to experience a positive response to the whole process:

Knowing that he would be there and that he would be among the first to hold and nurture our baby made a tremendous difference to me. Even though "I" as the woman couldn't participate as directly as I had anticipated, "we" as the family could. I felt a sense of control, not a sense of being a passive . . . well . . . organ.

In many hospitals today care of parents experiencing a cesarean birth is family centered rather than surgery centered. As education on cesarean birth is being incorporated into prenatal classes, couples are becoming aware of options available to them if a cesarean delivery is necessary. Some of the alternatives available to women and their families who experience cesarean birth include the following:

1. Cesarean delivery that is performed in the labor and delivery area, rather than in the general surgery area
2. The choice of regional instead of general anesthesia, whenever possible
3. The option of having a support person (preferably father) present during the birth
4. The opportunity for skin-to-skin contact with baby and parents immediately after birth
5. Initiation of early rooming-in with help from staff until mother is able to assume responsibility for baby care
6. Encouragement of breast feeding
7. Extended and unlimited visiting privileges for the immediate family members

Cesarean delivery is a birth experience and must be incorporated as such. The goal is a positive birth experience brought about by cooperation between parents, physicians, and hospital personnel.

Organizations involved in parent education. The following organizations can provide information on parent education:

American Academy of Husband-Coached Childbirth (AAHCC)
P.O. Box 5224
Sherman Oaks, Calif. 91413

American Society for Psychoprophylaxis in Obstetrics (ASPO)
1411 K Street N.W., Suite 200
Washington, D.C. 20005

Childbirth Without Pain Education Association
20134 Snowden
Detroit, Mich. 48235

Council of Childbirth Education Specialists, Inc. (CCES)
168 West 86th Street
New York, N.Y. 10024

International Childbirth Education Association (ICEA)
P.O. Box 20048
Minneapolis, Minn. 55420

Maternity Center Association
48 East 92nd St
New York, N.Y. 10028

National Association of Childbirth Education, Inc. (NACE)
3940 11th Street
Riverside, Calif. 92501

Nurses' Association of the American College of Obstetricians and Gynecologists (NAACOG)
600 Maryland Avenue S.W. #300
Washington, D.C. 20024

Read Natural Childbirth Foundation, Inc.
1300 S. Eliseo Drive, Suite 102
Greenbrae, Calif. 94904

Education for Choice

Birth is a life event that has significant impact on human behavior. Childbirth requires sensitive management and attention to the psychosocial health of the family.

In June 1978 the American College of Obstetricians and Gynecologists (ACOG) published a joint statement, "The Development of Family-Centered Maternity/Newborn Care in Hospitals." The statement was prepared by the Interprofessional Task Force on Health Care of Women and Children, which included representatives from the American Academy of Pediatrics (AAP), the American College of Nurse-Midwives (ACNM), the American Nurses' Association (ANA), ACOG, and the Nurses' Association of the American College of Obstetricians and Gynecologists (NAACOG). These five organizations endorsed the concept of family-centered childbirth and supported efforts to develop alternative childbirth centers along the lines described in the statement. The American Hospital Association added its support. The definition of family-centered care in the joint statement follows:

Family-centered maternity/newborn care can be defined as the delivery of safe, quality health care while recognizing, focusing on, and adapting to both the physical and psychological needs of the client-patient, the family, and the newly born. The emphasis is on the provision of maternity/newborn health care which fosters family unity while maintaining physical safety.

The statement recommends significant changes in hospital maternity care, including the following:
1. The option of a homelike birthing room
2. Flexible rooming-in with maximal mother-child contact during the first 24 hours
3. Breast feeding and handling of the baby immediately after delivery
4. Allowing the father or other support persons to be present throughout the labor, delivery, and recovery periods
5. Allowing siblings to visit in a special family room
6. Optional early discharge from the hospital with careful follow-up after discharge
7. Childbirth preparation classes offered by the hospital

The alternative birth movement is the practical application of the family-centered concept of maternity-newborn care. However, family-centered care requires more than just a proper physical environment. The attitude of the health care providers is the most important aspect of family-centered care. Family-centered care recognizes birth as a vital life event and not a surgical procedure. The philosophic approach to family-centered care and alternative childbirth programs is that which gives people the right to make informed choices regarding their childbirth experiences.

Organizations such as ICEA and ASPO and the National Association of Parents and Professionals for Safe Alternatives in Childbirth (NAPSAC) have increased the public's knowledge of prepared childbirth techniques and their impact on birth outcomes. The prepared childbirth movement has fostered greater acceptance of birth as a normal, rather than a pathologic, event and has encouraged expectant parents to become more knowledgeable about and accountable for their participation. As women began to experience childbirth awake and aware, they began to feel greater self-esteem and control over their lives. Also, the social significance of the birth experience became very clear to many women and their mates.

Consumer response has been varied, demonstrating the intensely personal quality of every birth experience and the need for safe, sensible choices in care during this important life event. Some couples wish to exercise maximal control over the birth of their child, with minimal technology and intervention by the health care team. Other couples choose a more traditional approach. The key element in optimal care of the childbearing family is *informed choice* about the place of birth, the plan of care, and the people present. In fact, the ICEA has always subscribed to the motto, "Freedom of choice based on knowledge of alternatives."

Choice and the nurse. Since choices for childbirth vary widely from one community to the next, nurses should be aware of all alternatives available in their community. Nurses should evaluate their own values and beliefs about childbearing and attempt to understand why they feel as they do. During their educational and socialization process, nurses have been socialized into a provider culture. The "provider" emphasis in professional socialization tends to view health care from an illness perspective or medical-model viewpoint. This unique preparation of nurses can create values and beliefs that often do not sanction any methods of health care other than those that are "scientifically proved." As a result, there is often incongruity of beliefs and value systems between nurses and consumers. Such incongruity can lead to conflict between the family's choices for childbirth and what the nurse sees as the best choice.

Understanding why families choose alternatives to traditional hospital birth is imperative. Cohen (1982) compared women who chose two different childbirth alternatives: a hospital or a freestanding alternative birth center (ABC). He found that women choosing the birth center planned to emphasize autonomy and independence rather than intimacy in their child rearing. Also, their closest relationship were much more supportive and involved in the birth than those women choosing hospital births. Women delivering at the Childbearing Childrearing Center (CCC) at the University of Minnesota, Minneapolis (Rising and Lindell, 1982) reported the three major reasons they chose the center were (1) to have control over their experience, (2) to have family-centered care, and (3) to have no routine procedures administered. Kieffer (1980) compared the attitudes of 109 women before

and after experiencing birth using the birthing room concept. The four highest ranking reasons for choice of the birth room were (1) philosophy, (2) no separation of mother and baby, (3) personal involvement in the birth, and (4) freedom to make choices regarding labor and birth. These studies seem to indicate that attitudes toward issues of choice in the childbirth experience are related to the degree of control that families expect to exert over the birth event (Fullerton, 1982).

Most people who choose home birth are very sincere and concerned about their own safety and the health and safety of their unborn child (Searles, 1981). In fact, there are probably as many sincere and well-considered reasons for choosing home birth as there are home births. For many individuals experiencing home birth, birth is a very special, intensely personal event to be shared only with family and friends, and not with assorted hospital personnel who are strangers. For many others, birth is an intensely spiritual experience for which a hospital setting is totally inappropriate. Still others do not relish giving up responsibility for their births to hospital personnel; instead, these people want to control their own experience. Most people choosing home birth understand fully the risk involved but also understand that there are risks in hospital birth.

The nurse's concern is to encourage expectant couples to explore the birth alternatives available to them so they can make a responsible, informed decision. It is the nurse's responsibility to become actively involved in ensuring that a variety of options for safe childbirth are available in communities.

Birth-setting choices. The concept of family-centered maternity care is implemented in birth rooms or alternative birth centers (ABCs) in the hospital. Hospital ABCs as well as freestanding birth centers are originally designed to offer families an alternative to home birth. The ABCs were designed to be a compromise between hospital and home. More and more, consumers and professionals are accepting and using birth rooms and ABCs. These birth-setting choices have been shown to be safe alternatives to birth in a traditional delivery setting (Mann, 1981; Marieskind, 1980).

Birth rooms. In Manchester, Connecticut, an obstetrician, Philip Sumner, and his colleagues have had over 12 years of experience with labor and birth in hospital birthing rooms. Unlike ABCs in hospitals, there is very little admission or risk criteria for the use of these rooms. The program at Manchester Memorial Hospital incorporates labor support by highly trained nurses, or *monitrices.* Prenatal education is stressed, and client feedback is overwhelmingly positive.

Fig. 13.6
The Borning Bed.

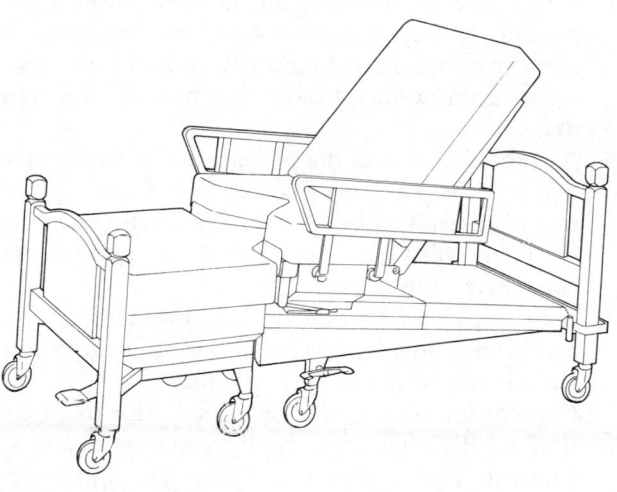

Women labor, give birth, and spend the first bonding time with their families in birthing rooms. Transfer to a postpartum room is usually the only room change they have to make.

Birth rooms offer families a comfortable, private space for childbirth (Sumner and Phillips, 1981; Rosen, 1980). Fig. 13.6 shows the *Borning Bed,* which provides safe options for positioning of the mother in the event of labor or birth complications. The borning bed has the ability to "break," so the woman can quickly be put into stirrups. Generally, this option is not used unless an episiotomy is performed or laceration occurs. Even in the unbroken mode a simple push of a button will cause the upper half of the bed to raise approximately 25 cm (10 in) and allow the easy management of an unsuspected shoulder dystocia.

Giving birth in a birth room rather than moving from a labor room to a delivery room has the advantage of not interfering or disrupting the progress of labor. The woman is able to concentrate on pushing her baby out without expending energy moving to a stretcher and then moving again to the delivery table. Her vital signs may be taken continuously if necessary, and the fetal monitor may remain in place until the baby is born. The father is able to provide continuous support and does not have to be redirected to the new location. If rapid delivery is necessary, the woman's legs may be placed in the leg supports and the baby born quickly without time being wasted in transport to a delivery room. Other advantages of a birth room include the following:

1. The nursing staff no longer has to make decisions on when to move the mother to the delivery room.
2. There is no second room to be set up, so the nurses have ample time to prepare for an in situ delivery.
3. It may be possible to reduce costs, since fewer rooms are used, less laundry and equipment are involved, and there is better use of hospital space.

The concept underlying hospital birthing rooms is that of humanizing the birth experience, minimizing intervention, and affording continuity of care. Since these facilities are not a response to the home birth movement, they do not employ rigid screening criteria. Instead, they offer a two-tiered model of care (low risk and high risk) and emphasize individualizing the birth experience. When deemed necessary by the physician, nurse, or mother, local anesthesia, forceps, fetal monitoring, and so on are used to facilitate a safe but still joyous birth.

Alternative birth centers. Alternative birth centers usually are in hospital suites away from the traditional obstetric department. They are located close to the delivery and operating rooms and medical or neonatal intensive care facilities for use when serious problems arise.

ABCs have homelike accommodations, including a double bed for the couple and a crib for the newborn. Emergency equipment and drugs are discreetly stored within cupboards, out of view, but easily accessible. Private bathroom facilities are incorporated into each birth center. There may be an early labor lounge or living room and small kitchen. There is careful screening of each applicant so that the ABC can rule out women with risk factors (see Chapter 25). Only low-risk and prepared women or couples are accepted.

The family is admitted to the ABC, labors there, and gives birth there. They may remain there until discharge if the time interval and requirements for room use permit. If the family has to remain in the hospital for more than 24 hours postpartum, the demand for use of the ABC by more prospective families may require transfer of the new family to a regular postpartum room.

Ideally the ABC becomes the private space for one childbearing family throughout their birth experience and until they are ready to go home. It is a warm, private, friendly space within a complex, fully equipped medical constellation. While emphasizing normalcy, self-help, and family participation, ABCs are fully supported by the presence of an obstetric nurse or nurse-midwife and by the availability of obstetric and pediatric house staff at all times, with attending staff backup.

If a situation that could threaten the safety of the mother or baby should arise at any time in labor, the mother would be moved to the regular labor and delivery area. In such a situation the ABC nurse and the father of the baby would go with her.

Families who choose birth in the ABC may experience a warm, positive, family-centered, highly personalized, highly emotional birth within a structure offering safe and preventive perinatal care. Immediately outside the door of their alternative birth space, this family has available to them the sophistication of technical resources for management of complicated obstetric situations—truly the best of two worlds!

By agreement, medication and instrumentation (forceps, monitoring) are limited. Delivery can be accomplished in the woman's bed with skin-to-skin contact on the mother's abdomen after (usually) spontaneous birth. During labor and delivery, family, including older siblings, and friends of the mother's choosing may remain. Early discharge from the center, often during the day of delivery, must meet medical criteria. Many centers arrange for the mother and infant to be seen within 24 hours of discharge by a nurse-midwife or neonatal nursing specialist.

Ideally, an ABC should also offer childbearing couples alternative prices, in contrast to the high cost of obstetric care. Since alternative birth requires that the family occupy fewer spaces, less hospital time, and fewer supplies, linen, and staff, it is usually possible to reduce the overall cost of birth to the hospital and consumer.

The establishment of an ABC requires the hospital maternity personnel, childbirth educators, physicians, and parents to come together to develop a common philosophy from which can be elicited specific goals and objectives. The next step is to develop specific policies and procedures to provide uniform standards that will achieve the designated goals. An example of criteria relative to a couple's admission to an ABC follows*:

1. The program is designed for healthy pregnant women who expect a normal labor, birth, and postpartum course.
2. The expectant mother should discuss with her physician or midwife her desire to give birth in the alternative birth center as early as possible in pregnancy.
3. When an agreement has been reached that the alternative birth center will be used, the woman and her partner or support person should register for the alternative birth center orientation classes. All

*Hillcrest Medical Center, Tulsa, Oklahoma. From McKay, S., and Phillips, C.R.: Family-centered maternity care: implementation strategies, Rockville, Md., 1984. Reprinted with permission of Aspen Systems Corp.

those who will be present during labor and birth are asked to attend the class series.
4. Attendance at childbirth preparation classes is important. If the expectant mother and her primary support person have attended classes during a previous pregnancy, a refresher class may be chosen by them.
5. A prenatal visit with the pediatrician or family physician of the parents' choice should be arranged so that plans can be made for the specific follow-up of the infant after birth and after discharge from the alternative birth center.
6. A specific plan for family participation during labor and birth should be developed during pregnancy in consultation with the birth attendant.
7. Consent forms that must be signed prior to admission to the alternative birth center are Patient's Consent Form, Physician/Midwife's Agreement, Verification of Infant Care, and Consent for Sibling Participation.

Freestanding birth centers. Although most ABCs or birthing rooms are located in hospitals, there is a growing number of freestanding birth centers. These units are outside the hospital but are often close to a major hospital so that quick transfer to that institution is possible if necessary.

Most freestanding birth centers are staffed by physicians who have privileges at the local hospital, and certified nurse-midwives. Both groups are equipped to attend low-risk gravidas through the puerperium. Ambulance service and emergency procedures are readily available. Fees vary with the services provided and the ability of the family to pay (reduced-fee sliding scale). Several insurance companies, as well as Medicaid, recognize and reimburse these clinics.

Services provided by the freestanding birth centers include those necessary for safe management during the childbearing cycle. There are some significant additions, however:
1. Attendance at childbirth and parenting classes is required of all clients. Prenatal supervision of the woman in good nutritional and health status must begin in the first trimester. All clients must be familiar with situations requiring transfer to a hospital.
2. Each expectant family identifies their "birth plan" (Arms, 1978). This is an explanation of practices and procedures they would like to include in or exclude from their childbirth experience. Although the family is given a wide range of choices, they are asked to "assume that there will be no overriding medical or legal necessity for or against any of them in (their) individual case." A sampling of choices follows:

a. *Preparation:* enema, "miniprep," hospital gown instead of own clothing?

b. *Labor:* electronic monitor or fetoscope, freedom to choose positions and activity in labor (walking, squatting), analgesia, presence of siblings, translator?

c. *Birth:* presence of mate or chosen person, presence of siblings, draping, mirror, dimmed lights, Leboyer bath?

d. *Recovery:* recovery with or without baby or mate or chosen person?

e. *After recovery:* rooming-in, sibling visitation, vitamin K for baby, circumcision, demand feeding—breast or bottle?

Birth centers usually have available a lending library, reference files on related topics, recycled maternity clothes and baby clothes and equipment, supplies and reference materials for childbirth educators, and referral files for community resources that offer services relating to childbirth and early parenting, including support groups (such as single parents, postdelivery support group, parents of twins), genetic counseling, women's issues, and consumer action.

Home birth. Home birth has always been popular in certain advanced countries, such as Great Britain, Sweden, and the Netherlands. In developing countries, hospitals or adequate lying-in facilities often are unavailable to most pregnant women, and home birth is a necessity. In the United States and Canada home birth is rapidly gaining popularity.

National groups supporting home birth are HOME (Home Oriented Maternity Experience) and NAPSAC (National Association of Parents for Safe Alternatives in Childbirth). These groups support changes toward more humane childbearing practices at all levels, integrating the alternatives for childbirth to meet the needs of the total population.

The literature on childbirth contains excellent statistics on medically directed home birth services with skilled nurse-midwives and medical backup. Two examples of such services are the Chicago Maternity Center with 12,000 home births from 1950 to 1960 without a single maternal death and the home delivery statistics of the Frontier Nursing Service in Appalachia with 23 years without a single maternal death. In the United States there are reports of very low risk home delivery populations who have very low levels of difficulty and consequently have excellent statistics. However, there is danger in taking these data on very select populations and applying them to the total population. It must be recognized that even though labor and delivery are normal physiologic events, they do present potential hazards to the mother and fetus both before and after birth. These hazards require provisions for emergency intervention and medical backups that are available only in hospitals and some birthing homes or in independent birth centers.

Selective home birth in uncomplicated pregnancies is feasible, provided those women at high risk can be identified during the prenatal period and referred for hospital delivery and assuming that a transport system is available for transfer of women with suddenly complicated labors to a nearby adequate medical facility. Another acceptable plan provides for specialist care to be brought to the home by means of a so-called flying squad service, which is utilized in Great Britain, for example.

Collaboration with and supervision of midwives are the obstetrician's duty in many countries. Moreover, obstetric nursing practitioners or nurse-midwives have proved to be invaluable components of the health care team. Thus nurse specialists, general practitioners, and obstetric specialist consultants have become incorporated into home delivery units. A midwife or general practitioner can call on or refer women or infants to numerous essential backup services for study or specialty care during pregnancy and the early puerperium. When a woman is to be assisted by a midwife, it is the practice in most areas for the general practitioner to supervise her; meanwhile, both are under the direction of the obstetric specialist.

Although some physicians and nurses are proponents of home births that use good medical and emergency backup systems, many health care professionals regard this practice as exposing the mother and the fetus to unnecessary danger.

Advantages. One advantage of home birth is that delivery may be more natural or physiologic in familiar surroundings. The mother may be more relaxed and less tense than she might be in the impersonal, sterile environment of a hospital. The family can assist in and be a part of the happy event, and mother-father-infant (and sibling-infant) contact is sustained and immediate. In addition, home birth may be less expensive than a hospital confinement. Serious infection may be less likely, assuming strict aseptic principles are followed. People generally are relatively immune to their own home bacteria.

Disadvantages. Because home births are not generally accepted by the medical community, a family may have difficulty finding a qualified health care professional to give prenatal care and to attend the delivery. Also, backup emergency care by a physician in a hospital may be difficult to arrange in advance. And, emergency transfer to a hospital could be life threatening if the hospital were more than a 10-minute distance from the home or if emergency care were not available during the transfer from home to hospital.

Contraindications. Hospital, not home, birth is indicated for the following:

1. High-risk women (fetal or maternal jeopardy) (see Chapter 25)
2. Women who cannot be transferred easily to a hospital should the need arise unexpectedly
3. Women who are opposed to home birth
4. Women with inadequate home facilities

Family's preparation for home birth. If a home birth is planned, it will usually be possible to obtain and store the necessary articles in advance. In contrast, if birth in the home or elsewhere is an emergency or is determined by circumstances beyond control, considerable improvisation may be necessary.

Facilities and supplies can approximate those available in hospitals. The family will work closely with the physician, nurse, or midwife to complete preparations well in advance of delivery. Attendance by both parents-to-be at childbirth classes (prenatal classes for vaginal and abdominal birth; instructions about the actual delivery of the child if this should occur before the midwife, physician, or other attendant arrives) adds to the competence and also to the pleasure of the parents and other family members. Classes for siblings and grandparents are recommended.

Detailed descriptions for preparation are required and may be obtained from either the physician's office or from local health agencies. The agencies may provide some of the equipment and supplies.

A visit to the home by the community health nurse is recommended well before the expected date of birth. At that time the process of birth can be discussed, so that all are aware of the characteristics of normal labor and birth and of the newborn, deviations from normal, and the plan of care for each stage.

Home birth is a selected alternative to hospital birth for some women and couples and a necessity for many. A physically and emotionally safe outcome can be anticipated for most women and couples and their infants, especially if they are prepared and have adequate health care support.

Summary

The nurse encourages the childbearing family to participate in prenatal classes. Attendance at such classes permits sharing of experiences with other couples and families. The couple is reassured by knowing that their thoughts, feelings, and concerns are common to others. Classes can increase confidence and self-assurance and help parents develop new coping skills.

Consumers learn about birth-setting choices from a variety of sources. Classes offered by community agencies, the media, newspapers, and advertisements alert consumers to available services. The knowledgeable nurse serves as a valuable resource for couples who want to individualize their childbirth experience.

References

American College of Obstetricians and Gynecologists: The development of family-centered maternity/newborn care in hospitals, Washington, D.C., 1978, The College.

Arms, S.: Five women, five births, film, 1978, Davidson Films, Inc.

Bernardini, J.Y., Maloni, J.A., and Stegman, C.E.: Neuromuscular control of childbirth-prepared women during the first stage of labor, J.O.G.N. Nurs. 2:105, Mar./Apr. 1983.

Bradley, R.: Husband-coached childbirth, New York, 1965, Harper & Row, Publishers.

Buxton, C.L.: A study of psychological methods for relief of pain in childbirth, Philadelphia, 1962, W.B. Saunders Co.

Chertok, L.: Psychosomatic methods of preparation for birth, Am. J. Obstet. Gynecol. 98(5):698, 1967.

Cohen, R.L.: A comparative study of women choosing two different birth alternatives, Birth 9:1, Spring 1982.

Cronenwett, L.R.: Elements and outcomes of a postpartum support group program, Res. Nurs. Health 3(3):33, 1980.

Cronenwett, L.R., and Brickman, P.: Models of helping and coping in childbirth, Nurs. Res. 32:84, Mar./Apr. 1983.

Dick-Read, G.: Childbirth without fear, ed. 2, New York, 1959, Harper & Row, Publishers.

Felton, G.S., and Segelman, F.B.: Lamaze childbirth training and changes in belief about personal control, Birth Fam. J. 5:141, Fall 1978.

Fullerton, J.D.T.: The choice of in-hospital or alternative birth environment as related to the concept of control, J. Nurse Midwife, 27:2, Mar./Apr. 1982.

Hart, G.: Maternal attitudes in prepared and unprepared cesarean deliveries, J.O.G.N. Nurs. 9:243, 1980.

Hassid, P.: Textbook for childbirth educators, ed. 3, New York, 1984, J.B. Lippincott Co.

Horn, M., and Manion, J.: Creative grandparenting: bonding the generations. J.O.G.N.N. 14:233, May/June 1985.

Huttel, F.A., and others: A quantitative evaluation of psychoprophylaxis in childbirth, J. Psychosom. Res. 16:81, 1972.

Johnsen, N.M., and Gaspard, M.E.: Theoretical foundations of a prepared sibling class, J.O.G.N. Nurs. 14:237, May/June 1985.

Johnson, J.M.: Teaching self-hypnosis in pregnancy, labor, and delivery, M.C.N. 5:98, 1980.

Kieffer, M.J.: The birthing room concept at Phoenix Memorial Hospital. II. Consumer satisfaction during one year, J.O.G.N. Nurs. 9:158, May/June 1980.

Kornhaber, A., and Woodward, K.L.: Grandparents/grandchildren: the vital connection, Garden City, N.Y., 1981, Anchor Press/Doubleday.

Lamaze, F.: Painless childbirth: the Lamaze method, Chicago, 1970, Henry Regnery Co.

Lederman, R.P.: Psychosocial adaptation in pregnancy: assessment of seven dimensions of maternal development, Englewood Cliffs, N.J., 1984, Prentice-Hall.

Mann, R.J.: San Francisco General Hospital Nurse-midwifery practice: the first thousand births, Am. J. Obstet. Gynecol. 140:6, July 1981.

Marieskind, H.I.: Women in the health system: patients, providers, and programs, St. Louis, 1980, The C.V. Mosby Co.

McKay, S., and Phillips, C.R.: Family-centered maternity care: implementation strategies, Rockville, Md., 1984, Aspen Systems Corp.

Mercer, R.T.: "She's a multip . . . she knows the ropes," M.C.N. 4:301, Sept./Oct. 1979.

Myles, M.F.: Textbook for midwives, with modern concepts of obstetric neonatal care, ed. 9, New York, 1981, Churchill Livingstone.

Newell, N.J.: Grandparents: the overlooked support system for new parents during the fourth trimester, NAACOG Update Series, 1:lesson 21, 1984.

Nurses' Association of the American College of Obstetricians and Gynecologists: Guidelines for childbirth education, Washington, D.C., 1981, The Association.

Rising, S.S., and Lindell, S.G.: The Childbearing Childrearing Center: a nursing model, Nurs. Clin. North Am. 17:1, March 1982.

Rosen, E.L.: The birth room: implementation of an alternative, Can. Nurse, p. 30, March 1980.

Satir, V.: Peoplemaking, Palo Alto, Calif., 1972, Science and Behavior Books.

Searles, C.: The impetus toward home birth, J. Nurse Midwife 26:3, May/June 1981.

Sumner, P., and Phillips, C.: Birthing rooms: concept and reality, St. Louis, 1981, The C.V. Mosby Co.

Tanzer, S.: The psychology of pregnancy and childbirth: an investigation of natural childbirth, unpublished doctoral dissertation, Waltham, Mass, 1967, Brandeis University.

Velvovsky, I., and others: Painless childbirth through psychoprophylaxis, Moscow, 1960, Foreign Languages Publishing House.

Willmuth, L.R.: Prepared childbirth and the concept of control, J.O.G.N. Nurs. 4(5):38, 1975.

Bibliography

Anderson, S.V.: Siblings at birth: a survey and study. Birth Fam. J. 6:80, 1979.

Anderson, S.V., and Simken, P.: Birth through children's eyes. Seattle, 1981, The Penny Press.

Bookmarks. ICEA Bookcenter, P.O. Box 20048, Minneapolis, MN 33420, Jan. 1984. (A source of books on pregnancy and related topics.)

Gates, S.: Children's literature: it can help children cope with sibling rivalry, M.C.N. 5:351, 1980.

Holt, J.R.: Best laid plans: pre- and postpartum comparison of self and spouse in primiparous Lamaze couples who share delivery and those who do not, Nurs. Res. 29:20, Jan./Feb. 1980.

Humenick, S.S.: Pregnant adult learners. NAACOG Update Series 1: lesson 24, 1984.

Imprints. Birth and Life Bookstore, P.O. Box 70625, Seattle, WA 98107, Sept., 1983. (A source of books on birth and life.)

Karmel, M.: Thank you, Dr. Lamaze, New York, 1965, Doubleday & Co.

Keuscher, M.B., and Oliver, M.: An overview of childbirth education, J. Calif. Perinatal Assoc. 2(1):79, 1982.

Kitzinger, S.: The experience of childbirth, Middlesex, England, 1970, Pelican Publishing Co.

Knowles, M.: The modern practice of adult education (from pedagogy to androgogy), Chicago, 1980, Follett Publishing.

Libresco, M.: Creative teaching: beyond lecture and demonstration, In Humenick, S.S., editor: Expanding horizons in childbirth education, Washington, D.C., 1983, ASPO/Lamaze (P.O. Box 33429 Farragut Station, Wash. DC 20033).

Lumley, J.: Preschool siblings at birth: short-term effects, Birth 10:11, Spring 1983.

Milstein, J.M.: Alternative birthing sites: interference versus intervention, J. Calif. Perinatal Assoc. 2(1), 1982.

Nicholas and the baby (16 mm film or ¾ inch videocassette), Centre Productions, Inc., Suite A, 1312 Pine St., Boulder, Colo. 80302. (Film available for preparing older preschool and school-age children for participation in the birth experience.)

Oehler, J.: The frog family books: color the pictures "sad" or "glad," M.C.N. 6:281, 1981.

Olson, M.L.: Fitting grandparents into new families, M.C.N. 6(6):419, 1981.

Rankin, S.H., and Duffy, K.L.: Patient education issues, principles, and guidelines, Philadelphia, 1983, J.B. Lippincott Co.

Redman, B.K.: The process of patient education, ed. 5, St. Louis, 1984, The C.V. Mosby Co.

Stephany, T.: Supporting the mother of a patient in labor, J.O.G.N. Nurs. 12(5):345, 1983.

Sweet, P.T.: Prenatal classes especially for children, M.C.N. 4:82, March/April 1979.

Waller, M.M.: Siblings in the childbearing experience, NAACOG Update Series 1: lesson 17, 1984.

Normal Childbirth

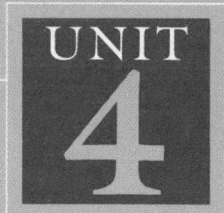

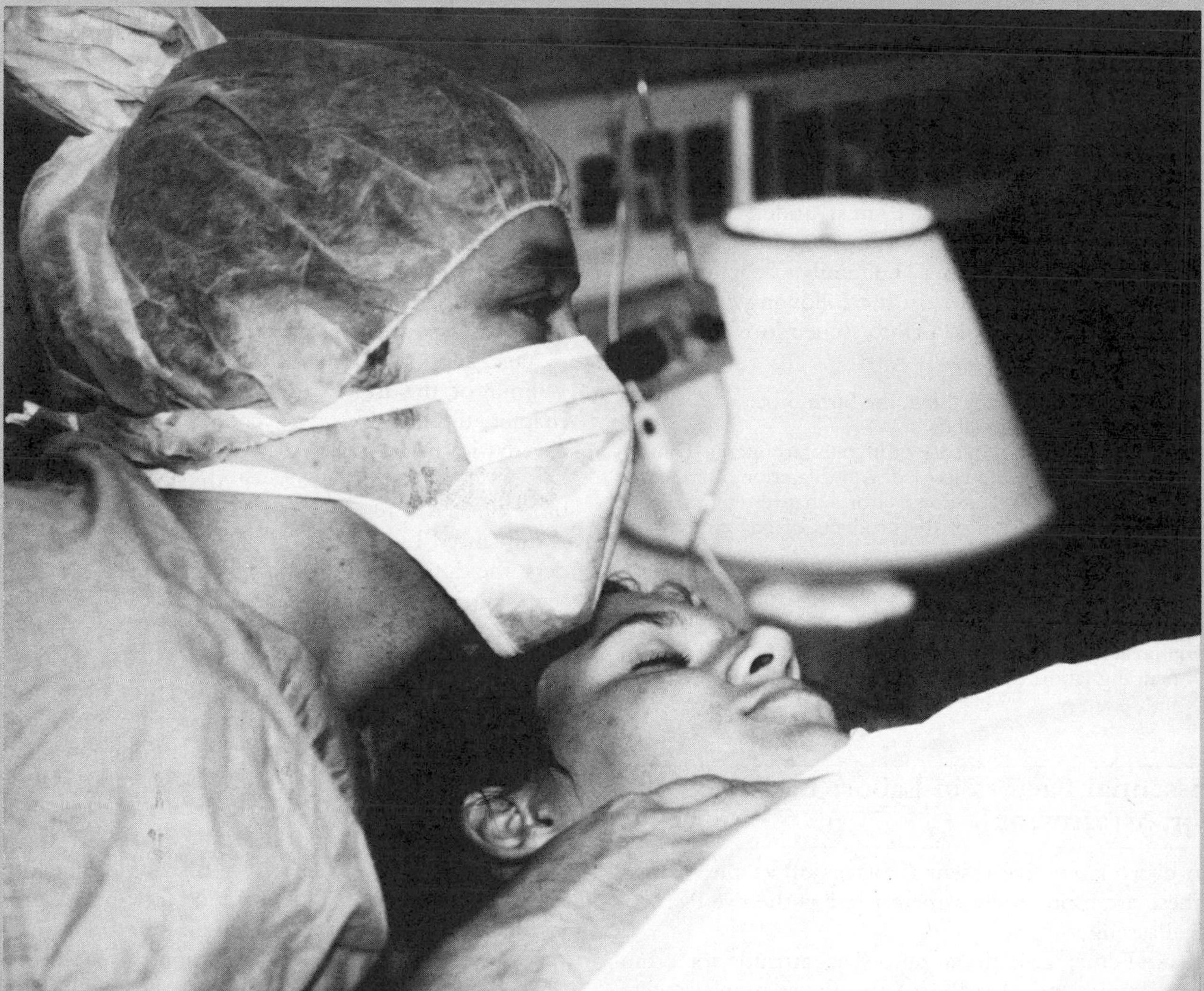

CHAPTER 14

Labor: Essential Factors and Processes and Maternal and Fetal Adaptations

During pregnancy the mother's anatomic and physiologic adaptations have prepared her for childbirth. The fetal-placental unit has grown and developed in preparation for life outside the uterus. Labor is an intense period during which the fetus and placenta are expelled from the uterus and the vagina. To implement the nursing process, a nurse must understand the essential factors and processes of labor, and maternal and fetal adaptations to labor. The family's adaptations are discussed in Chapter 15. In the following chapter, essential terms are in **bold print.** Some terms are defined below:

parturition Childbirth, birthing, the birth process.
parturient A woman in labor.
labor A coordinated sequence of involuntary uterine contractions that result in effacement and dilatation of the cervix and voluntary bearing-down efforts that result in delivery; the actual expulsion of the products of conception—the fetus and placenta.
toko- and toco- (Greek) Combining forms meaning childbirth or labor.
eutocia Normal labor.
prodromal labor Early or premonitory manifestations of impending labor; events before the onset of true labor.

Essential Factors in Labor: Basis for Assessment

In every labor five essential factors affect the process. These are more easily remembered as the five P's:
1. Passenger
   a. Fetus: gestational age, size, attitude, presentation, and position of the fetus; number of fetuses
   b. Placenta: type, sufficiency of and site of insertion
2. Passageway
   a. Configuration and diameters of the maternal pelvis

   b. Distensibility of the lower uterine segment, cervical dilatation, and capacity for distension of vaginal canal and introitus
3. Powers
   a. Primary powers: intensity, duration, and frequency of uterine contractions
   b. Secondary powers: bearing-down efforts
4. Position of the mother: standing, walking, side-lying, squatting, hands and knees
5. Psychologic response: previous experiences, emotional readiness, preparation, cultural-ethnic heritage, support systems, and environment

Four of the five factors will be discussed in this chapter; the fifth factor, psychologic response, will be covered in the next chapter.

Passenger. The passage of the fetus through the birth canal is a result of several interacting factors. It is influenced by the size of the fetal head and shoulders, the dimensions of the pelvic girdle, and fetal presentation and position.

Fetal head. Because of its size and relative rigidity, the fetal head has a major effect on the birth process. The external cranial vault is composed of two parietal bones, two temporal bones, the frontal bone, and the occipital bone (Fig. 14.1, A). These bones are united by membranous sutures: the sagittal, lambdoidal, and coronal. At the points of intersection, these sutures become enlarged to form the fontanels ("soft spots") (Fig. 14.1, B and C). The two most important fontanels are the anterior and posterior fontanels. During labor, vaginal palpation of fontanels and sutures reveals fetal presentation and position. Assessment of their size reveals information about the age and well-being of the newborn.

The larger of the two, the anterior fontanel or bregma is diamond-shaped and closes at about 18 months of age. The posterior fontanel is at the junction of the sutures of the two parietal bones and one occipital bone and is therefore triangular in shape. It

Fig. 14.1
Fetal head at term. **A,** Bones. **B** and **C,** Sutures and fontanels.

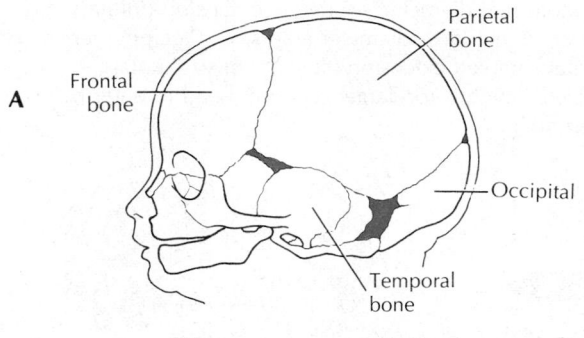

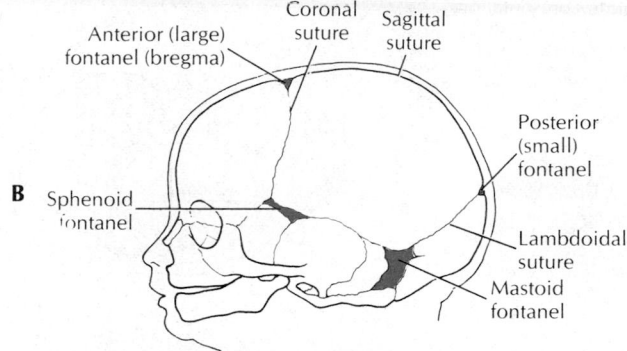

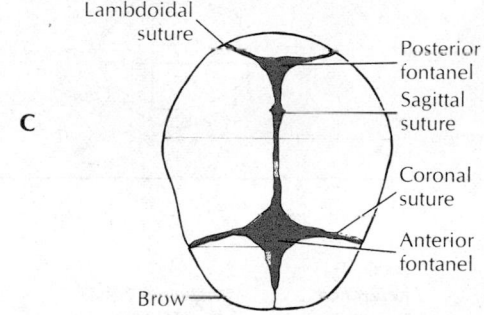

Fig. 14.2
Cephalic landmarks. **A,** Cephalic presentations: occiput, vertex, and sinciput; and cephalic diameters: suboccipitobregmatic, occipitofrontal, and occipitomental. **B,** Cephalic presentations and biparietal diameter.

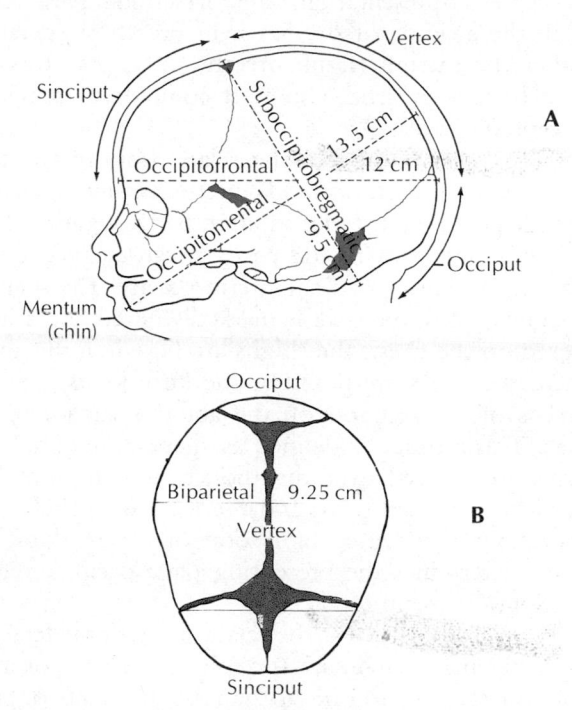

is smaller than the anterior fontanel and closes by about the twelfth week of life. The sutures and fontanels allow the brain to continue growing.

The bones of the cranial vault are not firmly united, and slight overlapping of the bones, or **molding** of the shape of the head, occurs during labor. This capacity of the bones to slide over one another permits adaptation to the various diameters of the maternal pelvis. Molding can be extensive, but with most neonates the head assumes its normal shape within about 3 days after birth.

Principal measurements of the fetal skull are in centimeters (Fig. 14.2). The **biparietal diameter** is the largest transverse diameter. Of the anteroposterior diameters shown in Fig. 14.2, it can be seen that the attitudes of flexion or extension allow diameters of different sizes to enter the maternal pelvis. With the head in complete flexion, the smallest diameter, **suboccipitobregmatic,** presents and enters the true pelvis easily (Fig. 14.3).

Shoulders and pelvic girdle. Because of their mobility, the position of the shoulders (the shoulder girdle) can be altered during labor, so that one shoulder may occupy a lower level than the other. This permits a small shoulder diameter to negotiate the passage. The circumference of the hips, or pelvic girdle, is usually small enough not to create problems.

Fetal lie. Lie is the relationship of the long axis (spine) of the fetus to the long axis (spine) of the mother. There are two lies: longitudinal or vertical in which the long axis of the fetus is parallel with the long axis of the mother, and transverse or horizontal in which the long axis of the fetus is at right angles to that of the mother (Figs. 14.4 and 14.5). Longitudinal lies are either cephalic (head) or sacral (breech) presentations, depending on the fetal structure that first enters the mother's pelvis.

Presentation. **Presentation** refers to that portion of the fetus that enters the pelvis first and covers the internal os of the cervix, such as cephalic (head), breech, or shoulder (Figs. 14.4 and 14.5). Presentation may also be more precisely described as a presenting part; in cephalic presentation, the presenting part varies with the attitude of the fetus; in breech presentation either the sacrum (frank breech) or a foot (footling breech) may present. The most common presentation is **cephalic** (96%).

Attitude. **Attitude** is the relationship of the fetal body parts to each other. The fetus assumes a characteristic posture (attitude) in utero partly because of the mode of fetal growth and partly because of accommodation to the shape of the uterine cavity. The shape is roughly ovoid, the back is markedly flexed, the head is flexed on the chest, the thighs are flexed on the abdomen, the knees are flexed at the knee joints, and the arches of the feet rest on the anterior surface of the legs. This attitude is defined as "general flexion." The arms are crossed over the thorax, and the umbilical cord lies between them and the legs. In cephalic presentations the degree of flexion of the head on the chest determines the presenting part: occiput, vertex, sinciput, or mentum.

Position. **Position** is the relationship of the fetal reference point or landmark (occiput, brow, chin or mentum, or sacrum) to one of the four quadrants or sides of the mother's pelvis. In other words the most prominent and dependent portion of the presenting part is related to one of the four quadrants of the mother's pelvis.

Fig. 14.3
Head entering pelvis. Biparietal diameter is indicated in black. **A,** Suboccipitobregmatic diameter: complete flexion of head on chest so that smallest diameter enters. **B,** Occipitofrontal diameter: moderate extension (military attitude) so that large diameter enters. **C,** Occipitomental diameter: marked extension (deflection) so that largest diameter, which is too large to permit head to enter pelvis, is presenting.

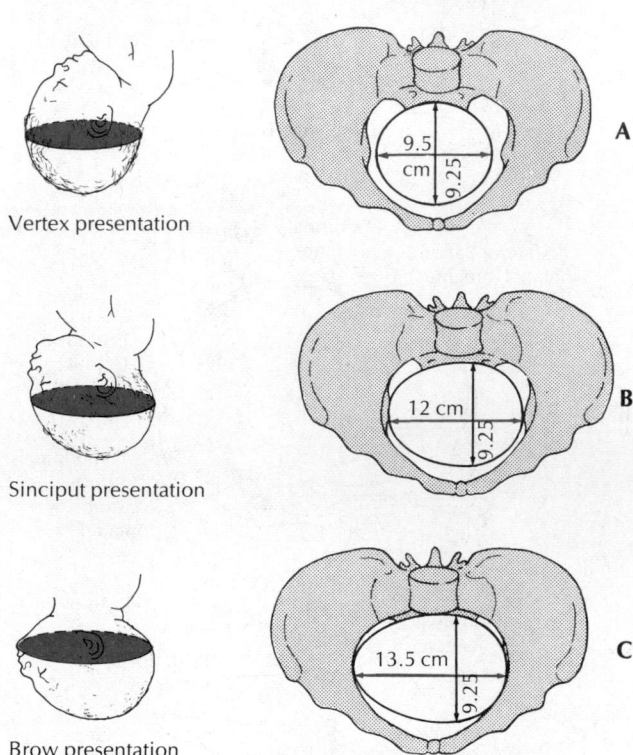

Vertex presentation

Sinciput presentation

Brow presentation

Table 14.1
Fetal Lie, Presentation, and Position

	Presenting Part	Example of Position
Longitudinal lie		
Cephalic		
Vertex	Occiput	*Left occiput transverse* (LOT)
Brow	Brow	*Left brow anterior* (LBA)
Face (chin) (rare)	Mentum	*Right mentum posterior* (RMP)
Pelvic		
Breech	Sacrum	*Right sacrum anterior* (RSA)
Transverse lie		
Shoulder	Scapula	*Right scapula anterior* (RScA)

Maternal Pelvis Side	Fetal Reference Point	Maternal Pelvis Quadrant
L—Left	O—Occiput	A—Anterior (front)
R—Right	M—Mentum	T—Transverse (side)
	B—Brow	P—Posterior (back)
	S—Sacrum	
	Sc—Scapula	

These quadrants formed by drawing an imaginary line from the mother's sacral promontory to the upper edge of the symphysis pubis and bisecting it transversely with a line from one side to the other, are termed the *right posterior* and *anterior quadrants* and the *left posterior* and *anterior quadrants* (Fig. 14.4). In a vertex presentation, if the occiput (fetal reference point) is the most prominent portion of the presenting part and is located in the right anterior quadrant, the position is noted as right occiput anterior (ROA). Ex-

Fig. 14.4
Examples of fetal vertex (occiput) presentations in relation to quadrant or side of maternal pelvis. Modified from Iorio, J.: Childbirth: family-centered nursing, ed. 3, St. Louis, 1973, The C.V. Mosby Co.

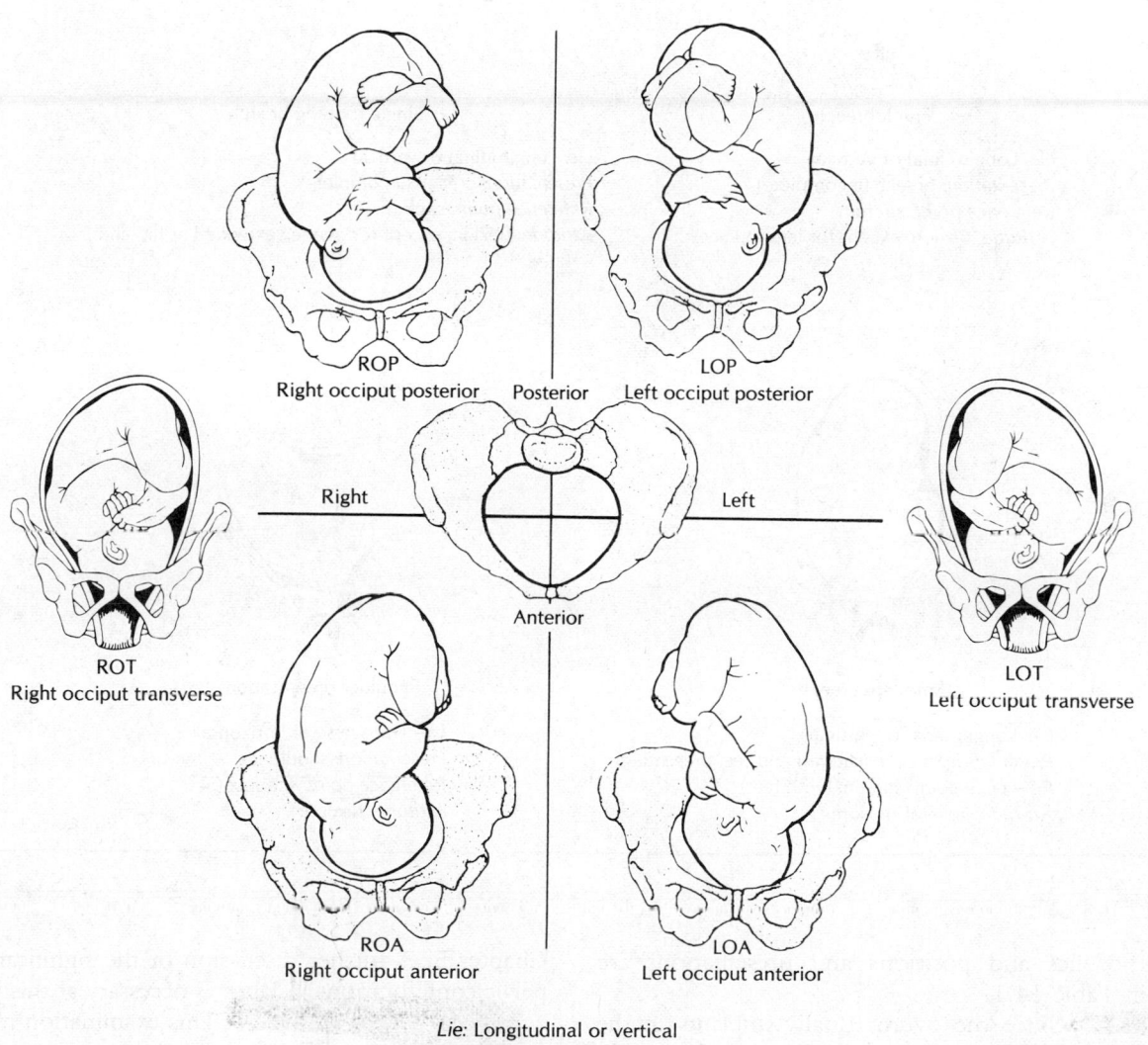

ROP
Right occiput posterior

Posterior

LOP
Left occiput posterior

Right

Left

ROT
Right occiput transverse

LOT
Left occiput transverse

Anterior

ROA
Right occiput anterior

LOA
Left occiput anterior

Lie: Longitudinal or vertical
Presentation: vertex
Reference point: occiput
Attitude: complete flexion

Fig. 14.5
Fetal presentations. **A** to **C**, Breech (sacral) presentation. **D,** Shoulder presentation.

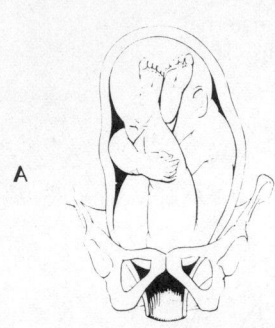

Frank breech

Lie: Longitudinal or vertical
Presentation: breech (incomplete)
Reference point: sacrum
Attitude: flexion, except for legs at knees

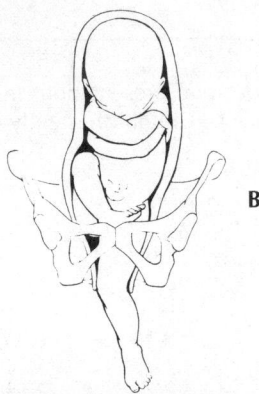

Single footling breech

Lie: Longitudinal or vertical
Presentation: breech (incomplete)
Reference point: sacrum
Attitude: flexion, except for one leg extended at hip and
    knee

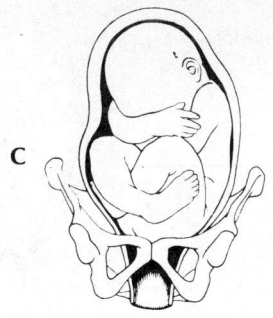

Complete breech

Lie: Longitudinal or vertical
Presentation: breech (sacrum and feet presenting)
Reference point: sacrum (with feet)
Attitude: general flexion

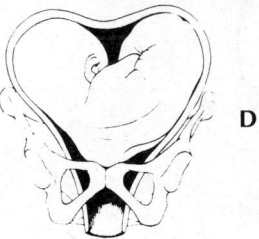

Shoulder presentation.

Lie: Transverse or horizontal
Presentation: shoulder
Reference point: scapula (Sc)
Attitude: flexion

amples of lies and positions and presentations are given in Table 14.1.

Placenta. Since the ovum usually implants in the fundal portion of the uterus, the developed placenta rarely acts as an impediment to labor. Placenta-related problems are included with content on dystocia (complications of pregnancy and childbirth).

Passageway. The passageway, or birth canal, is composed of the rigid bony pelvis and the soft tissues of the cervix, vagina, and introitus.

Pelvis. The anatomy of the pelvis was reviewed in Chapter 5. A further discussion of the significance of pelvic configurations in labor is necessary at this point.

Assessment of the bony pelvis. This examination may be performed during the first prenatal evaluation and need not be repeated if the pelvis is of adequate size. In the third trimester of pregnancy, the examination may be more thorough and the results more accurate because there is a relaxation of pelvic joints and ligaments. The four pelvic joints are the symphysis pubis, the right and left sacroiliac joints, and the sacrococcygeal joint (Fig. 14.6). The hormones of pregnancy, es-

Fig. 14.6
Female pelvis. **A,** Pelvic brim (inlet, linea terminalis, or iliopectineal line) from above. **B,** Pelvic outlet from below.

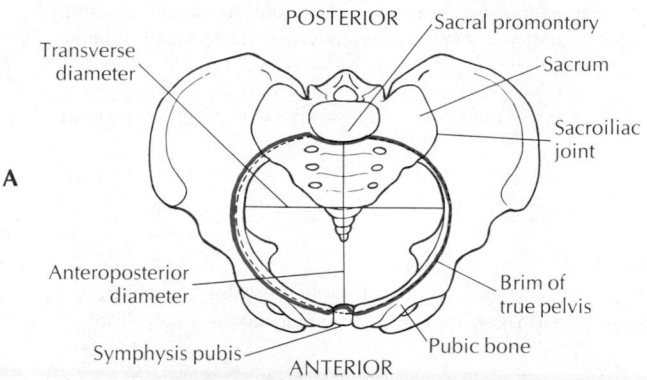

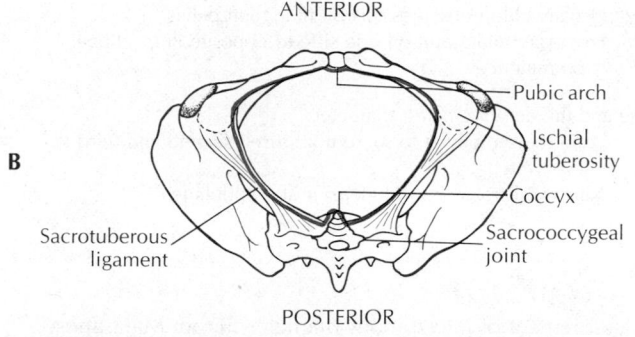

Fig. 14.7
Pelvic cavity. **A,** Inlet and midplane. Outlet not shown. **B,** Cavity of true pelvis. **C,** Note curve of sacrum and axis of birth canal.

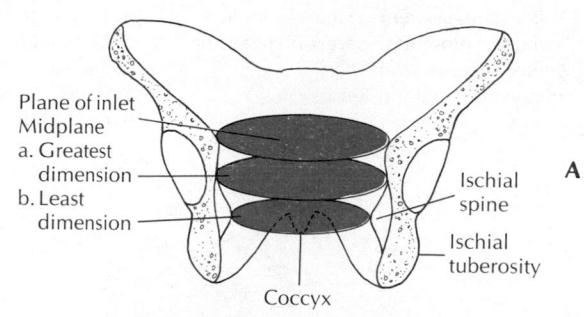

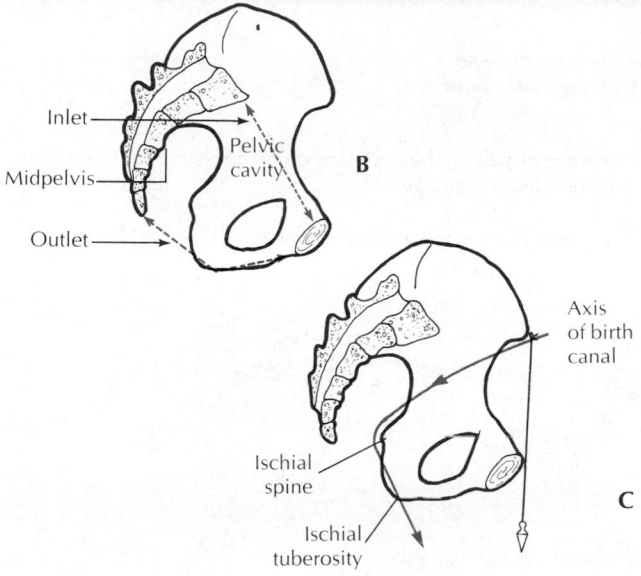

pecially the ovarian hormone progesterone, cause considerable mobility to develop. Widening of the symphyseal joint and instability may cause pain in any or all of the joints.

Because the examiner does not have direct access to the bony structures and because the bones are covered with variable amounts of soft tissue, estimates are approximate. Precise bony pelvis measurements can be determined using computed tomography and ultrasound, or x-ray films. However, x-ray examination is not indicated for the vast majority of gravidas.

The bony pelvis is separated by the brim or inlet into two parts: the **false pelvis** and the **true pelvis** (see Fig. 5.4). The false pelvis is that part above the brim and is of no obstetric interest.

The *true pelvis* is divided into three planes: the inlet or brim, the midpelvis or cavity, and outlet:

1. The **pelvic inlet** or brim of the pelvis, is formed anteriorly by the upper margins of the pubic bone, laterally by the iliopectineal lines along the innominate bones, and posteriorly by the anterior, upper margin of the sacrum, the sacral promontory (Figs. 5.4 and 14.6, *A*).

Fig. 14.8
Estimation of angle of subpubic arch. Using both thumbs, examiner externally traces descending rami down to tuberosities. (From Malasanos, L., Barkauskas, V., Moss, M., and Stoltenberg-Allen, K.: Health assessment, ed. 3, St. Louis, 1986, The C.V. Mosby Co.)

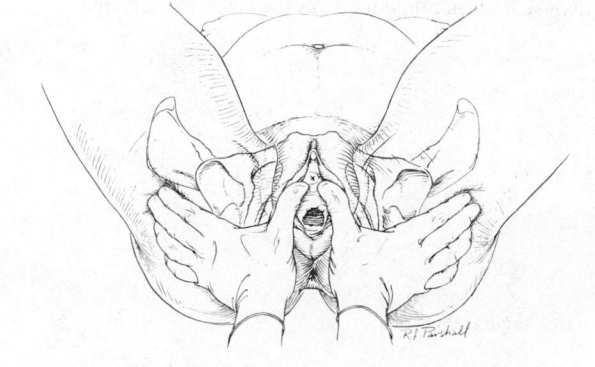

Table 14.2
Obstetric Measurements

Plane of inlet (superior strait). The principal pelvic diameters of the plane of the inlet are as follows:

Conjugates

Diagonal	12.5-13 cm	From *inferior border* of symphysis pubis to sacral promontory
Obstetric: measurement that determines whether presenting part can engage or enter superior strait	1.5-2 cm greater than diagonal (radiographic)	From *posterior surface* of symphysis pubis to sacral promontory
True (vera) (anteroposterior)	≥11 cm (12.5) (radiographic)	From *upper margin* of symphysis pubis to sacral promontory

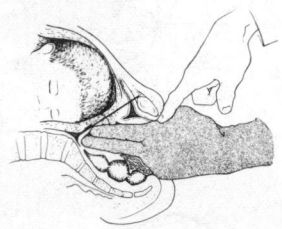

Fig. 14.9
Length of diagonal conjugate (solid red line), obstetric conjugate (broken red line), true conjugate (black line).

Transverse diameter	≥13 cm	Usually colon obscures this by filling left pelvis
Oblique diameter (R or L)	≥12.75 cm	From sacroiliac joint on one side to opposite iliopectineal prominence

Midplane of pelvis. The midplane of the pelvis normally is its largest plane and the one of greatest diameter.

Anteroposterior diameter	≥11.5 cm	From midsymphysis to sacrum (at fused second and third sacral vertebras)
Transverse diameter (interspinous diameter)	10.5 cm	Narrowest transverse diameter in the midplane

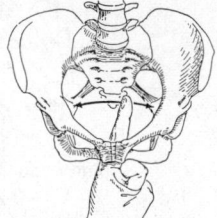

Fig. 14.10
Measurement of interspinous diameter. (From Malasanos, L., Barkauskas, V., Moss, M., and Stoltenberg-Allen, K.: Health assessment, ed. 3, St. Louis, 1986, The C.V. Mosby Co.)

Posterior sagittal diameter	4.5 cm	Segment of anteroposterior diameter dorsal to line between ischial spines; although midplane is comparatively large, critical shortening of interspinous or posterior sagittal diameter of midplane may cause pelvic dystocia

Plane of pelvic outlet. The outlet presents the smallest plane of the pelvic canal. It encompasses an area including the lower portion of the symphysis pubis, the ischial tuberosities, and the tip of the sacrum. The significant diameters are as follows:

Anteroposterior diameter	11.9 cm	From lower border of symphysis pubis to tip of sacrum; coccyx may be displaced posteriorly during labor and is not considered to be a fixed bone
Transverse diameter (intertuberous diameter)	≥8 cm	From inner border of one ischial tuberosity to other

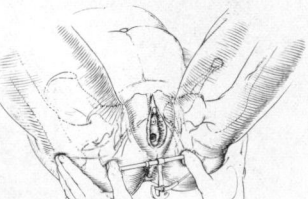

Fig. 14.11
Use of Thom's pelvimeter to measure intertuberous diameter. (From Malasanos, L., Barkauskas, V., Moss, M., and Stoltenberg-Allen, K.: Health assessment, ed. 3, St. Louis, 1986, The C.V. Mosby Co.)

Posterior sagittal diameter	9 cm	Projected from tip of sacrum to a point in space where intertuberous diameter transects anteroposterior projection

2. The **pelvic cavity** or midpelvis, is a curved passage having a short anterior wall and a much deeper concave posterior wall. It is bounded by the posterior aspect of the symphysis pubis, the ischium, a portion of the ilium, and the sacrum and coccyx (see Fig. 5.5).

3. The **pelvic outlet** when viewed from below is ovoid, somewhat diamond shaped, bounded by the pubic arch anteriorly, the ischial tuberosities laterally, and the tip of the coccyx posteriorly (Fig. 14.6, *B*). In the latter part of pregnancy the coccyx is movable (unless it had been broken in a fall while skiing or skating, for example, and had fused to the sacrum during healing).

The pelvic canal varies in size and shape at various levels. The diameters at the plane of the pelvic inlet, midpelvis, and outlet plus the axis of the birth canal (Fig. 14.7) determine whether vaginal delivery is possible and the manner by which the fetus may pass down the birth canal (mechanism of labor).

The **subpubic angle,** which indicates the type of pubic arch, together with the length of the pubic rami and the intertuberous diameter, is of great importance. Because the presenting part must pass beneath the pubic arch, a narrow subpubic angle will be less favorable than a rounded, wide arch. Measurement of the subpubic arch is shown in Fig. 14.8. A summary of obstetric measurements is given in Table 14.2. The most important measurements are depicted in Figs. 14.8 through 14.11.

Classification of pelves. The four basic types of pelves are as follows:

1. Gynecoid (the classic female type)

Fig. 14.12

Pelves. **A,** Gynecoid, female. **B,** Android, male. Compare shape of brim and angle of subpubic arch.

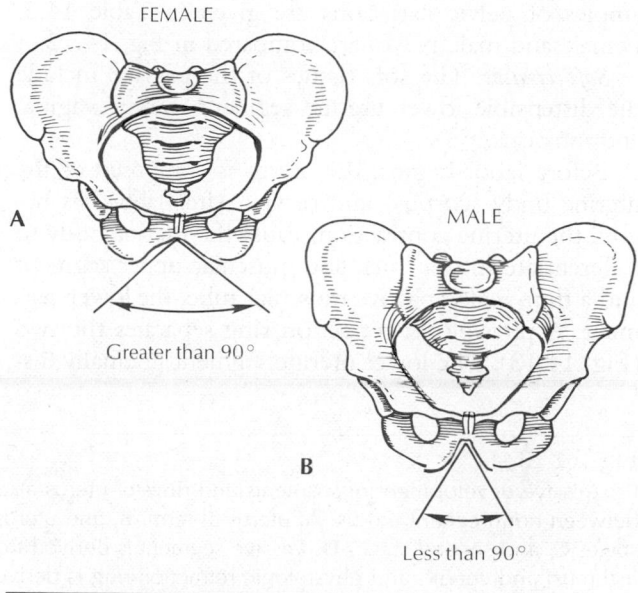

2. Android (resembling the male pelvis)
3. Anthropoid (resembling the pelvis of anthropoid apes)
4. Platypelloid (the flat pelvis)

Major gynecoid pelvic features can be expected in about half of all pregnant women; significant anthro-

Table 14.3
Comparison of Pelvic Types

	Gynecoid (About 50% of Women)	Android (About 20% of Women)	Anthropoid	Platypelloid
Brim	Slightly ovoid or transversely rounded	Heart shaped, angulated	Oval, wider anteroposteriorly	Flattened anteroposteriorly, wide transversely
	◯ Round	♡ Heart	◯ Oval	▢ Flat
Depth	Moderate	Deep	Deep	Shallow
Side walls	Straight	Convergent	Straight	Straight
Ischial spines	Blunt, somewhat widely separated	Prominent, narrow interspinous diameter	Prominent, often with narrow interspinous diameter	Blunted, widely separated
Sacrum	Deep, curved	Slightly curved, terminal portion often beaked	Slightly curved	Slightly curved
Subpubic arch	Wide	Narrow	Narrow	Wide
Usual mode of delivery	Vaginal Spontaneous OA position	Cesarean Vaginal Difficult with forceps	Vaginal Forceps/spontaneous OP or OA position	Vaginal Spontaneous

poid features will be present in slightly less than one fourth of gravidas; android configuration will affect almost one fifth of pregnant women; and the small remainder of gravidas will have a platypelloid pelvis. Examples of pelvic variations are given in Table 14.3. Female and male pelves are compared in Fig. 14.12.

Soft tissues. The soft tissues of the passage include the distensible lower uterine segment, cervix, vagina, and introitus.

Before labor begins, the uterus is composed of the uterine body (corpus) and cervix. After labor has begun, the uterine contractions cause the uterine body to differentiate into a thick and muscular upper segment and a thin-walled passive muscular tube, the lower segment. A physiologic retraction ring separates the two (Fig. 14.13). The lower uterine segment gradually distends to accommodate the intrauterine contents as the walls of the upper segment become thicker and its content is reduced.

The downward pressure caused by contraction of the fundus is transmitted to the cervix. The cervix then effaces (thins) (Fig. 14.13, *B* and *C*) and dilates (opens) (Fig. 14.13, *C* and *D*) sufficiently to allow descent of the presenting part into the vagina. Actually, the cervix is drawn upward and over the presenting part as the vertex or breech descends.

The vagina in turn distends to permit passage of the fetus into the external world. As noted earlier, the soft tissues of the vagina develop throughout pregnancy until at term the vagina can dilate to accommodate the fetus.

Fig. 14.13
Progressive development of segments and rings of uterus at term. Note comparison between nonpregnant uterus, **A,** uterus at term, **B,** and uterus in normal labor in early first stage, **C,** and second stage, **D.** Passive segment is derived from lower uterine segment (isthmus) and cervix, and physiologic retraction ring is derived from anatomic internal os. (Modified from Willson, J.R., Carrington, E.R., and Ledger, W.J.: Obstetrics and gynecology, ed. 7, St. Louis, 1983, The C.V. Mosby Co.)

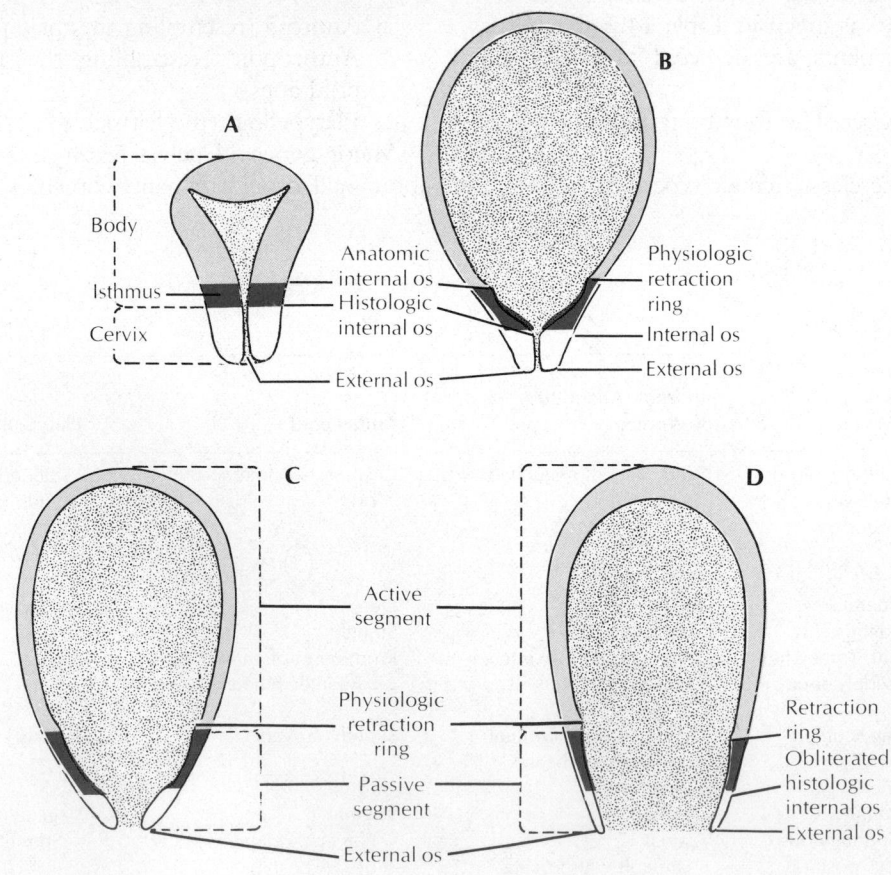

Powers. The forces acting to expel the fetus and placenta are derived from the **primary powers,** the involuntary uterine contractions. Following the first stage of labor, **secondary powers,** voluntary bearing-down efforts, augment the force of the involuntary contractions.

Primary powers: involuntary uterine contractions. Contractions originate at pacemaker points in the myometrium near the uterotubal junction. From the pacemaker points, contractions move over the uterus like a wave. Successive downward waves of contractions are separated by short rest periods.

Description of primary forces. The following is a description of the primary forces from Willson, Carrington, and Ledger (1983, p. 386).

The ultimate effect of a normal labor contraction . . . is a gradient of force directed from the fundus to the least active and weakest area of the uterus, the cervix. This is called *fundal dominance.* The force generated by each contraction is applied to the amniotic fluid and directly against the pole of the infant that occupies the upper segment. Therefore each time the muscle contracts, the uterine cavity becomes smaller, and the presenting part of the infant or the forebag of waters lying ahead of it is pushed downward into the cervix. This tends to force it open, or *dilate* it.

A more potent factor in cervical dilatation, however, is the *retraction of the upper segment.* As this area of the uterus becomes shorter and thicker, it pulls the lower segment and the dilating cervix upward around the presenting part at the same time the uterus contracting directly against the infant tends to push it through the cervical opening (Fig. 14.14). The cervix opens or is dilated by a combination of these two factors. Retraction is probably more important than the pressure of the presenting part, since dilatation will occur even though the presenting part does not descend into it. A *completely dilated cervix* that will permit a term infant to pass through it has a diameter of about 10 cm. . . . Less work is required to dilate the multiparous cervix because the uterus works more effectively; the time required to dilate the cervix completely is less for multiparas than it is for nulliparas.

Function of uterine contractions. The primary powers are responsible for the effacement and dilatation of the cervix and descent of the fetus. **Effacement** of the cervix means the shortening and thinning of the cervix during the first stage of labor. The cervix, normally 2 to 3 cm in length and about 1 cm thick, is obliterated or "taken up" by a shortening of the uterine muscle bundles during the thinning of the lower uterine segment in advancing labor. Eventually only a thin edge of the cervix can be palpated when effacement is complete. Effacement generally is advanced in nulliparas at term before more than slight dilatation occurs. In multiparas, effacement and dilatation of the cervix tend to progress together. Degree of effacement is expressed in percentages (for example, a cervix that is 50% effaced) (Fig. 14.15).

Dilatation of the cervix is the enlargement or widening of the cervical os and the cervical canal during the first stage of labor. The diameter increases from perhaps less than 1 cm to approximately 10 cm to allow delivery of a term fetus. When the cervix is fully dilated (and completely retracted), it can no longer be palpated (Fig. 14.15 and back cover of book).

Dilatation of the cervix occurs by the drawing upward of the musculofibrous components of the cervix with strong uterine contractions. Pressure exerted by the amniotic fluid while the membranes are intact or force applied by the presenting part also encourages cervical dilatation. Scarring of the cervix as a result of infection or surgery may retard cervical dilatation.

Secondary powers: voluntary bearing-down efforts. As soon as the presenting part reaches the pelvic floor, the woman experiences an urge to push, a voluntary bearing-down effort (secondary power). The bearing-down effort is similar to that used in the process of defecation. However, a different set of muscles is used; the parturient contracts her diaphragm and abdominal muscles and pushes out the contents of the birth canal. Bearing down results in increased intraabdominal pressure. The pressure compresses the uterus on all sides

---

Fig. 14.14

Lower uterine segment and cervix are pulled up (retracted) as the fetus and amniotic sac are pushed downward. **A,** Cervix is effaced and partially dilated. It has not yet retracted around the presenting part. **B,** Cervical dilatation is complete. Cervix is being pulled upward as presenting part descends. Intrauterine space is decreasing. (From Willson, J.R., Carrington, E.R., and Ledger, W.J.: Obstetrics and gynecology, ed. 7, St. Louis, 1983, The C.V. Mosby Co.)

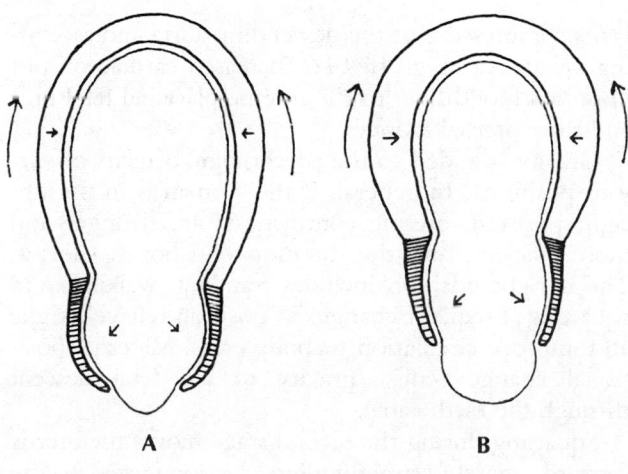

A   B

Fig. 14.15
Cervical effacement and dilatation. Note how cervix is drawn up around presenting part (internal os). Membranes are intact, and head is not well applied to cervix. **A,** Before labor. **B,** Early effacement. **C,** Complete effacement (100%). Head is well applied to cervix. **D,** Complete dilatation (10 cm). Some overlapping of cranial bones. Membranes still intact.

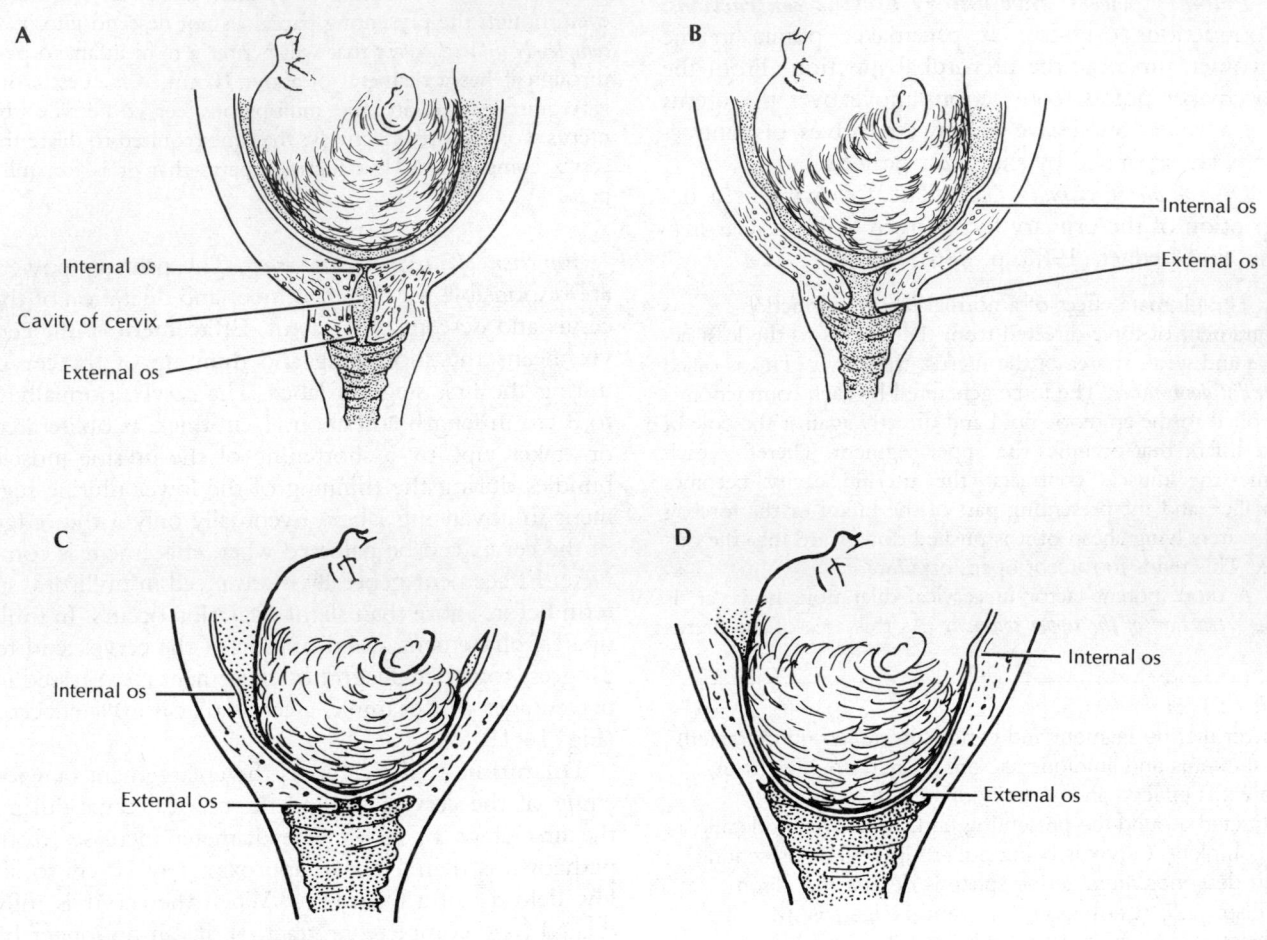

and adds to the power of the expulsive forces. The secondary forces have no effect on cervical dilatation, but they are of considerable importance in aiding the expulsion of the infant from the uterus and vagina after the cervix is fully dilated (10 cm).

Any voluntary bearing-down efforts by the woman earlier in labor are counterproductive to cervical dilatation. Straining will exhaust the woman and cause cervical trauma (pp. 398 and 399).

Position of the mother. The mother's position affects her anatomic and physiologic adaptations to labor. Her cardiac output normally increases during labor as uterine contractions return blood into the maternal vascular bed (Table 14.4). The increase in cardiac output is possible if the maternal position prevents compression of the descending aorta and ascending vena cava (Fig. 15.14). Increased cardiac output improves blood flow to the uterine-placental-fetal unit and the maternal kidneys.

Gravity is added to the psychologic benefits of various positions. In general, if the woman is in the upright position, uterine contractions are stronger and more efficient, and the duration of labor is shorter. The upright position includes standing, walking, and squatting. Frequent changes in position relieve fatigue and improve circulation to body parts. Maternal positional changes enlist gravity to aid fetal descent through the birth canal.

Squatting during the second stage moves the uterus forward, thereby straightening the long axis of the birth canal (McKay, 1984). As the fetus descends in the birth canal, the pressure of the presenting part on stretch receptors of the pelvic floor stimulates the woman's bearing-down reflex. Stimulation of the stretch receptors in turn stimulates the release of oxytocin from the posterior pituitary (Ferguson's reflex). Oxytocin increases the intensity of the uterine contractions. In a sitting position, such as squatting, abdominal muscles work in greater synchrony with uterine contractions during bearing-down efforts.

Process of Labor

The phenomena of normal labor consist of the mechanism and stages of labor. The cardinal movements of the **mechanism of labor** are **descent, flexion, internal rotation, extension, external rotation,** and **expulsion** of the baby. There are three stages of labor. The **first stage** is the stage of dilatation of the *cervix* from 0 to 10 cm or full dilatation. The **second stage,** expulsion, begins with complete cervical dilatation and ends with the *birth of the baby.* The **third stage** begins with the delivery of the baby and ends with the *delivery of the placenta.* The first 1 to 2 hours after delivery constitute the period of recovery. This *recovery period* is referred to as the **fourth stage** of labor. Prodromal signs and symptoms are among the first indicators that the reproductive system is preparing for the childbirth.

Reproductive system changes
Prodromes to labor. In nulliparas the uterus gradually sinks downward and forward about 2 weeks before term, when the fetus's presenting part (usually the fetal head) descends into the true pelvis. This settling is called lightening or "dropping" and usually happens gradually (Fig. 14.16). After lightening, women feel less congested and breathe more easily. However, there is usually more bladder pressure as a result of this shift and consequently a return of urinary frequency. In multiparas, lightening may not take place until after uterine contractions are established and true labor is in progress.

Persistent low backache and sacroiliac distress due to relaxation of the pelvic joints may be described. Occasionally strong, frequent, but irregular uterine (Braxton Hicks) contractions may be identified by the gravida.

Before the onset of labor the vaginal mucus becomes more profuse in response to the extreme congestion of the vaginal mucous membranes. Brownish or blood-tinged cervical mucus may be passed (bloody show). The cervix becomes soft (ripens) and partially effaced and may begin to dilate. The membranes may rupture spontaneously.

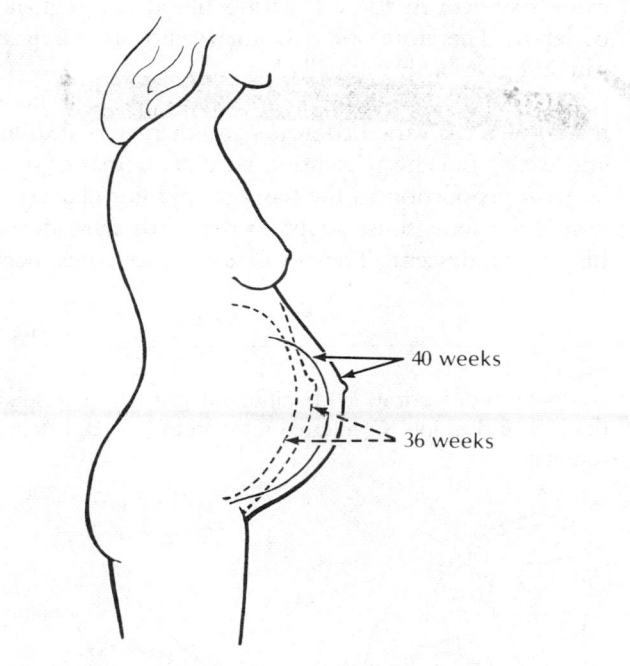

Fig. 14.16
Lightening.

40 weeks

36 weeks

Two other phenomena are common in the days preceding labor: (1) loss of 0.5 to 1.5 kg (1 to 3 lb) in weight, caused by water loss resulting from electrolyte shifts that in turn are produced by changes in estrogen and progesterone levels, and (2) a burst of energy. Women speak of a burst of energy that they often use to clean the house and put everything in order. This activity has been described as the "nesting instinct."

Onset of labor. The onset of labor cannot be ascribed to a single cause. Many factors, including changes in the maternal uterus, cervix, and pituitary gland are involved. Hormones produced by the normal fetal hypothalamus, pituitary, and adrenal cortex probably contribute to the **initiation of labor.** Progressive uterine distension, increasing intrauterine pressure, and aging of the placenta seem to be associated with increasing myometrial irritability. This is a result of increasing concentrations of estrogen and prostaglandins, and decreasing progesterone levels. In actuality, many factors may be responsible for initiating labor. The mutually coordinated effects of these factors result in strong, regular, rhythmic uterine contractions. Normally, these factors working in concert terminate in the birth of the fetus and the delivery of the placenta. It is still not completely understood how certain alterations trigger others and how proper checks and balances are maintained.

Afferent and efferent nerve impulses to and from

the uterus alter its contractility. Although nerve impulses to the uterus will stimulate contractions, the denervated uterus still contracts well during labor because oxytocin in the circulating blood is a regulator of labor. Therefore some women who are paralyzed can still give birth vaginally.

Mechanism of labor: vertex presentation. The female pelvis has varied contours and diameters at different levels, and the presenting part of the passenger is large in proportion to the passageway. For delivery to occur, the fetus must adapt to the birth canal during his or her descent. The turns and other adjustments necessary in the human birth process are termed the **mechanism of labor** (Fig. 14.17).

The phases of the mechanism of labor in vertex presentation are called (1) engagement, (2) descent, (3) flexion, (4) internal rotation, (5) extension, and (6) external rotation. Restitution is a phase of external rotation. The fetus is born by expulsion. Although these phases will be discussed separately, a combination of movements is occurring simultaneously; for example, engagement involves both descent and flexion.

Engagement. When the biparietal diameter of the head passes the pelvic inlet, the head is said to be en-

Fig. 14.17

Mechanism of labor in left occiput anterior (LOA) presentation. **A,** Engagement and descent. **B,** Flexion. **C,** Internal rotation to OA. **D,** Extension. **E,** Restitution. **F,** External rotation.

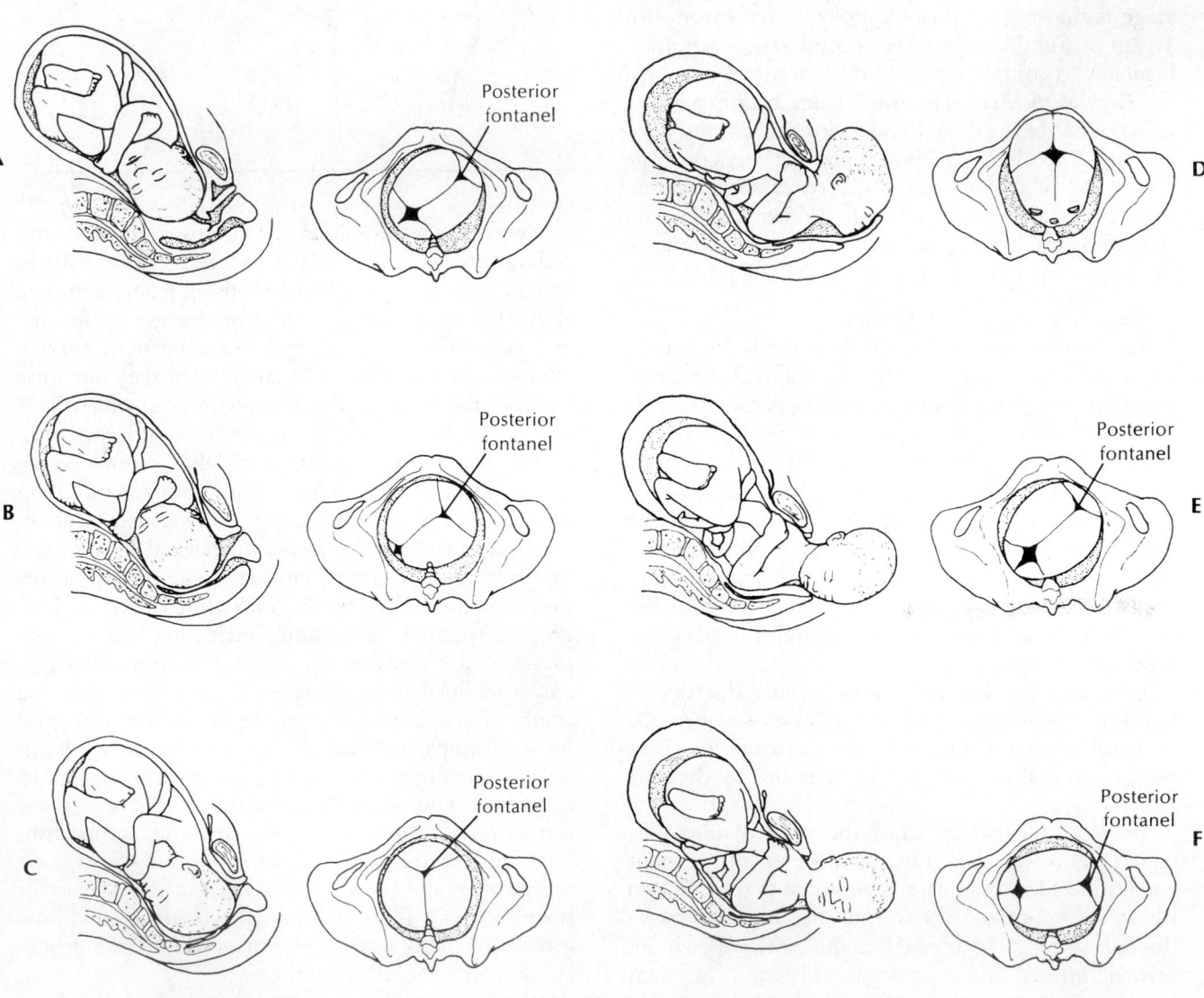

gaged, or fixed, in the pelvic. In most nulliparous women this occurs prior to the onset of active labor because the firmer abdominal muscles direct the presenting part into the pelvis. In multiparous women with more relaxed musculature the head often remains freely movable above the pelvic brim ("floating") until labor is established. In the majority of cases the head of a normal-sized fetus enters the pelvis with the sagittal suture transverse to the pelvic inlet (Fig. 14.4, *B*).

Descent. **Descent** refers to the progress of the presenting part through the pelvis. As **partograms** (labor curves) (Figs. 15.9 and 15.10) indicate, there is little progress in descent during the latent phase of the first stage of labor. Descent becomes more rapid in the latter part of the active phase when the cervix has dilated to 5 to 7 cm. It is apparent especially when the membranes have ruptured.

Descent depends on three forces: (1) pressure of the amniotic fluid, (2) direct pressure of the contracting fundus on the fetus, and (3) contraction of the maternal diaphragm and abdominal muscles in the second stage. The effects of these forces are modified by the size and shape of the maternal pelvic planes and the size and capacity of the fetal head to mold.

The degree of descent is gauged by the station of the presenting part. **Station** is expressed in centimeters above (minus) and below (plus) the level of the ischial spines (Fig. 14.18). If the lowest point of the present-

ing part is at the level of the spines, it is at station 0; if 1 cm above the spines, at station minus 1; if 2 cm above the spines, at station minus 2; and so on. If the lowest level of the presenting part is above the plane of the pelvic inlet, it is said to be floating. If the presenting part is 1 cm below the plane of the spines, it is at station +1, and so on. When the presenting part reaches station +3, it usually has just reached the pelvic floor. The speed of descent increases in the second stage of labor. In nulliparas this descent is slow but steady; in multiparas the descent may be rapid. Progress in the descent of the presenting part is determined by vaginal examination until the presenting part can be seen at the introitus.

Flexion. As soon as the descending head meets resistance from the cervix, pelvic wall, or pelvic floor, **flexion** normally occurs, and the chin is brought into more intimate contact with the fetal chest (Fig. 14.17, *B*). Flexion permits the smaller suboccipitobregmatic diameter (9.5 cm) rather than the larger diameters to present to the outlet.

Internal rotation. The maternal pelvic inlet is widest in the transverse diameter. Therefore the fetal head passes the inlet into the true pelvis in the occiput transverse position (Fig. 14.4, *B*). The outlet is widest in the anteroposterior diameter, however. To exit, the fetal head must rotate. **Internal rotation** begins at the level of the ischial spines but is not completed until the presenting part reaches the lower pelvis. As the oc-

Fig. 14.18
Stations of presenting part, or degree of descent. Silhouette shows head of infant approaching station +1. (Courtesy Ross Laboratories, Columbus, Ohio.)

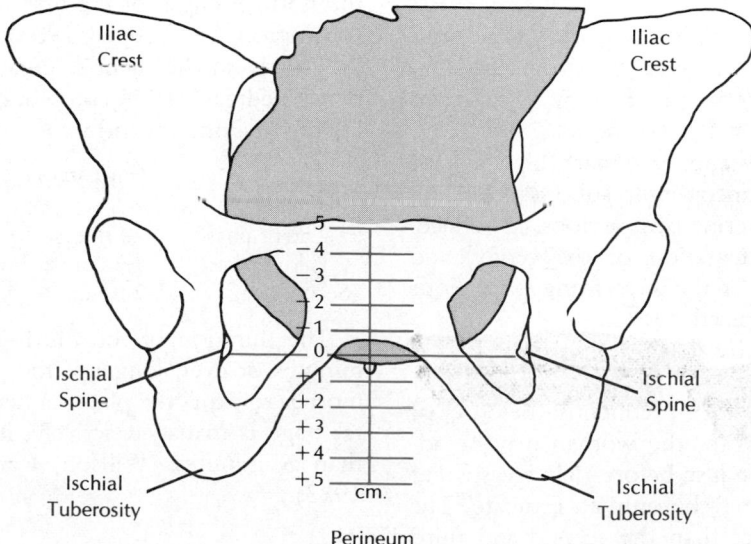

ciput rotates anteriorly, the face rotates posteriorly. With each contraction the fetal head is guided by the bony pelvis and levator ani muscle sling, eventually to lie in the midline beneath the pubic arch. The head is almost always rotated by the time it reaches the pelvic floor (Fig. 14.17, *C*). Both the levators and the bony pelvis are important for anterior rotation. Previous childbirth injury or regional anesthesia compromises the function of the levator sling.

Extension. When the fetal head reaches the perineum to be born, it is deflected anteriorly by the perineum. The occiput acts as the fulcrum as it passes under the lower border of the symphysis pubis. As a result the **head is born by extension:** first the occiput, then the face, and finally the chin (Fig. 14.17, *D*).

Restitution and external rotation. After delivery of the head, it rotates briefly to the position it occupied when it was engaged in the inlet. This movement is referred to as **restitution** (Fig. 14.17, *E*). The 45-degree turn realigns the infant's head with his or her back and shoulders. The head can then be seen to rotate further. **External rotation** occurs as the shoulders engage and descend in maneuvers similar to those of the head. As noted earlier the anterior shoulder presents first. When it reaches the outlet, it remains impinged beneath the pubic arch. The posterior shoulder is forced up over the perineum until it is free of the introitus (Fig. 14.17, *F*). The head then falls toward the maternal anus, and the anterior shoulder is delivered.

Expulsion. After delivery of the shoulders the rest of the infant's body is born quickly. No particular mechanism is involved in this cardinal movement of labor **expulsion.** When the *entire infant* has emerged from the mother, birth is said to be complete. *This is the time noted on the records.*

Stages of labor. Normal labor (eutocia) is recorded when the woman is at or near term, without complications, when a single fetus presents by vertex, and when labor is completed within 24 hours.

The course of normal labor is remarkably constant and consists of three concomitant subprocesses: (1) regular progression of uterine contractions, (2) effacement and progressive dilatation of the cervix, and (3) progress in descent of the presenting part. Four stages of labor are recognized.

First stage of labor. The first stage of labor is considered to last from the onset of regular contractions to full dilatation of the cervix. Frequently the onset of labor is difficult to establish; the woman may be admitted to the labor floor just before delivery so that the beginning of labor may be only an estimate. The first stage is much longer than the second and third combined. Great variability is the rule, however, depending on the essential factors discussed earlier. Some

multiparas may become fully dilated in less than an hour, or, infrequently, a nullipara may not be completely dilated even in 24 hours.

The first stage of labor has been divided into two phases: a *latent phase* and an *active phase.** During the latent phase there is more progress in effacement of the cervix and little increase in descent. During the active phase there is more rapid dilatation of the cervix and descent of the presenting part. If the degree of dilatation and descent is plotted in a graph, it forms an S curve. This curve can be used as a basis for assessment of progress in labor (Figs. 15.9 and 15.10).

Second stage of labor. The second stage of labor lasts from full dilatation of the cervix to delivery of the fetus. Labor of up to 2 hours is considered within the normal range for the second stage.

Third stage of labor. The third stage of labor lasts from delivery of the fetus to delivery of the placenta. The placenta normally separates with the third or fourth strong uterine contraction after the infant has been delivered. Then it should be delivered with the next uterine contraction after placental separation. Placental separation usually begins with the contraction that delivers the baby's trunk and is normally completed with the first contraction after the birth of the baby. However, delivery of the placenta within 45 to 60 minutes is generally considered within normal limits.

Fourth stage of labor. The fourth stage of labor arbitrarily lasts about 2 hours after delivery of the placenta. It is the period of immediate recovery, when homeostasis is reestablished. It serves as an important period of observation for complications, such as abnormal bleeding.

Duration of labor. There are no absolute values for the normal length of the first stage of labor (Willson, Carrington, and Ledger, 1983). Variations may reflect differences in the client population or in clinical practice. Friedman (1978) provides statistical upper limits for the first and second stage:

	Nulliparous	Multiparous
First stage		
Latent phase	20 hours	14 hours
Active phase	1.2 cm per hour	1.5 cm per hour
Second stage	2 hours	1.5 hours

The duration of the third stage will be 15 to 30 minutes or even longer if the physician waits for the mother to expel the placenta herself. When the placental stage is managed actively, its duration can be less than 5 minutes (Willson, Carrington, and Ledger, 1983).

---

*Transition is a part of the active phase of the first stage of labor (see Chapters 15 and 29).

A description of the labor experience of a significant number of parturients is given in Figs. 15.9 and 15.10. Friedman and Sachtleben (1965) used the information to predict the duration of normal labor for the first and second stages.

Anatomic and Physiologic Adaptations

The mother and fetus must adapt anatomically and physiologically during the birth process. Accurate assessment of the parturient and fetus requires a knowledge of expected adaptations. Maternal and fetal responses are addressed in the content that follows.

MATERNAL ADAPTATIONS

Body systems. A thorough understanding of maternal adaptations to pregnancy (see Chapter 9) is fundamental to anticipating and meeting the parturient's needs. Table 14.4 summarizes normal adaptations by body systems, including objective and subjective symptomatology.

Discomfort during labor

Origins. The discomfort experienced during labor has two origins. During the *first stage* of labor, uterine contractions cause (1) cervical dilatation and effacement and (2) uterine ischemia (decreased blood flow and therefore local oxygen deficit) from contraction of the arteries to the myometrium.

The discomfort from cervical changes and uterine ischemia is *visceral.* The discomfort is located over the lower abdomen and radiates to the lumbar area of the back and down the thighs. Usually the woman experiences discomfort only during contractions and is free of pain between contractions.

During the *second stage* of labor, the stage of expulsion of the baby, the woman experiences perineal or *somatic* pain. Perineal discomfort results from traction on the peritoneum and uterocervical supports during contractions. It can also be produced by expulsive forces or from pressure by the presenting part on the bladder, bowel, or other sensitive pelvic structures.

Pain may be *local,* with cramplike pain and a tearing or bursting sensation because of distension and laceration of the cervix, vagina, or perineal tissues. It may also be *referred,* with the discomfort felt in the back, flanks, or thighs. Emotional tension from anxiety and fear may increase pain and perception of pain during labor.

Pain impulses during the first stage of labor are transmitted through the spinal nerve segment of T11-12 and accessory lower thoracic and upper lumbar sympathetic nerves. Pain impulses during the second stage of labor are carried through S1-4 and the para-

sympathetic system. Pain experienced during the third stage, as well as so-called afterpains, is uterine, similar to that experienced early in the first stage of labor. Areas of discomfort during labor are illustrated in Fig. 14.19.

Symptomatology. Pain results in both psychic responses and reflex physical reactions. The quality of physical pain has been described as pricking, burning, aching, throbbing, sharp, nauseating, or cramping. Pain in childbirth gives rise to symptoms that are identifiable. It may cause increased activity of the sympathetic nervous system. As a result there are changes in blood pressure, pulse, respirations, and skin color. Bouts of nausea and vomiting and excessive perspiration are also commonplace. Certain affective expressions of suffering are familiar to all. Affective changes include increasing anxiety with lessened perceptual field, writhing, crying, groaning, gesturing (hand clenching and wringing), and excessive muscular excitability throughout the body. Childbirth pain is of a limited duration (at most 2 to 3 days).

Perception of pain

Pain threshold. Although the pain threshold is remarkably similar in all people regardless of sexual, social, ethnic, or cultural differences, these differences play a definite role in the individual's perception of the pain experience. The reasons for the effects of such factors as culture, use of counterstimuli, or distraction in coping with pain are not fully understood. The meaning of pain and the verbal and nonverbal expressions given to pain are apparently learned from interactions within the primary social group. It is personalized for each individual. As pain is experienced, people develop various coping mechanisms to deal with it. Pain or the possibility of pain that has unknown qualities can induce fear in which anxiety borders on panic. Fatigue and sleep deprivation magnify pain.

Gate control theory. At times, pain stimuli that are particularly intense can be ignored. It may be that certain nerve cell groupings within the spinal cord, brain stem, and cerebral cortex have the ability to modulate the pain impulse through a blocking mechanism. This gate control theory is helpful in understanding the approaches used in education-for-childbirth programs or the use of hypnosis in labor. According to this theory, local physical stimulation such as massage or stroking of the woman in labor can balance the pain stimuli. It is thought to work by closing down a hypothetical "gate" in the spinal cord, thus blocking pain signals from reaching the brain. Also, when the laboring woman performs neuromuscular and motor skills, activity within the spinal cord itself further modifies the transmission of pain. Cognitive activities of concentration on breathing and relaxation skills require selective

Table 14.4
Maternal Anatomic and Physiologic Adaptation to Labor

Body System	Normal Adaptation to Labor	Observable Findings
Cardiovascular		
Cardiac output	Increases; during each contraction 400 ml blood is emptied from uterus into maternal vascular system	Pulse slows BP increases No alteration in FHR
WBC	Mechanism unknown; possible WBC level changes secondary to physical/emotional stress	$\geqslant$25,000/mm^3
Peripheral vascular system	Response to cervical dilatation; compression of vessels by fetus passing through birth canal	Malar flush Hot or cold feet Hemorrhoids
Respiratory		
Rate	Increased physical activity with increased oxygen consumption	Rate increases
Acid/base balance	Hyperventilation may be cause of increased pH early in labor; pH returns to normal by end of first stage	None if hyperventilation is controlled
Renal		
Fluids/electrolytes	Diaphoresis Increased insensible water loss through respirations Occasionally NPO	Possible temperature elevation Thirst
Bladder	Becomes an abdominal organ starting with the second trimester	When filling, palpable above symphysis pubis
	Deterrents to spontaneous voiding: tissue edema secondary to pressure from presenting part, discomfort, sedation, embarrassment	Possible inability to void spontaneously
Urine constituents	Breakdown of muscle tissue from the physical work of labor	1+ proteinuria
Integument	Great distensibility in area of vaginal introitus; degree of distensibility varies with the individual	Minute tears in skin around vagina
Musculoskeletal	Marked increase in muscle activity (in addition to uterine activity)	Diaphoresis Fatigue 1+ proteinuria ? Increased temperature
	Backache and joint ache (unrelated to fetal position) secondary to increased joint laxity at term	Verbal/nonverbal cues indicating back discomfort
	Leg cramps secondary to labor process and pointing of toes	Verbal/nonverbal cues
Neurologic	Sensorium alterations change as woman moves through phases of first stage of labor and as she moves from one stage to the next	Euphoria to increased seriousness to amnesia between contractions to elation or fatigue after delivery
	Discomfort (see discussion on pain during childbirth) Endogenous endorphins and encephalins and physiologic anesthesia of perineal tissues with decreased perception of discomfort	Verbal/nonverbal cues absent or minimal
Gastrointestinal	Mouth breathing, dehydration, emotional response to labor	Verbal/nonverbal cues indicating dry mouth
	Decreased motility and absorption; delayed stomach emptying time	Nausea/vomiting of undigested foods eaten after onset of labor
	Nausea as a reflex response to full cervical dilatation	Nausea/vomiting Belching
	History of diarrhea concurrent with onset of labor or	Verbal cue
	Presence of hard or impacted stool in rectum	Palpable on vaginal examination Fecal material extruded during delivery
Endocrine	Level of estrogen decreases; levels of progesterone, prostaglandins, and oxytocin increase	Labor is initiated and maintained
	Metabolism increases	Blood glucose may decrease

Fig. 14.19
Discomfort during labor. **A,** Distribution of labor pain during first stage. **B,** Distribution of
labor pain during later phase of first stage and early phase of second stage. **C,** Distribution
of labor pain during later phase of second stage and actual birth.

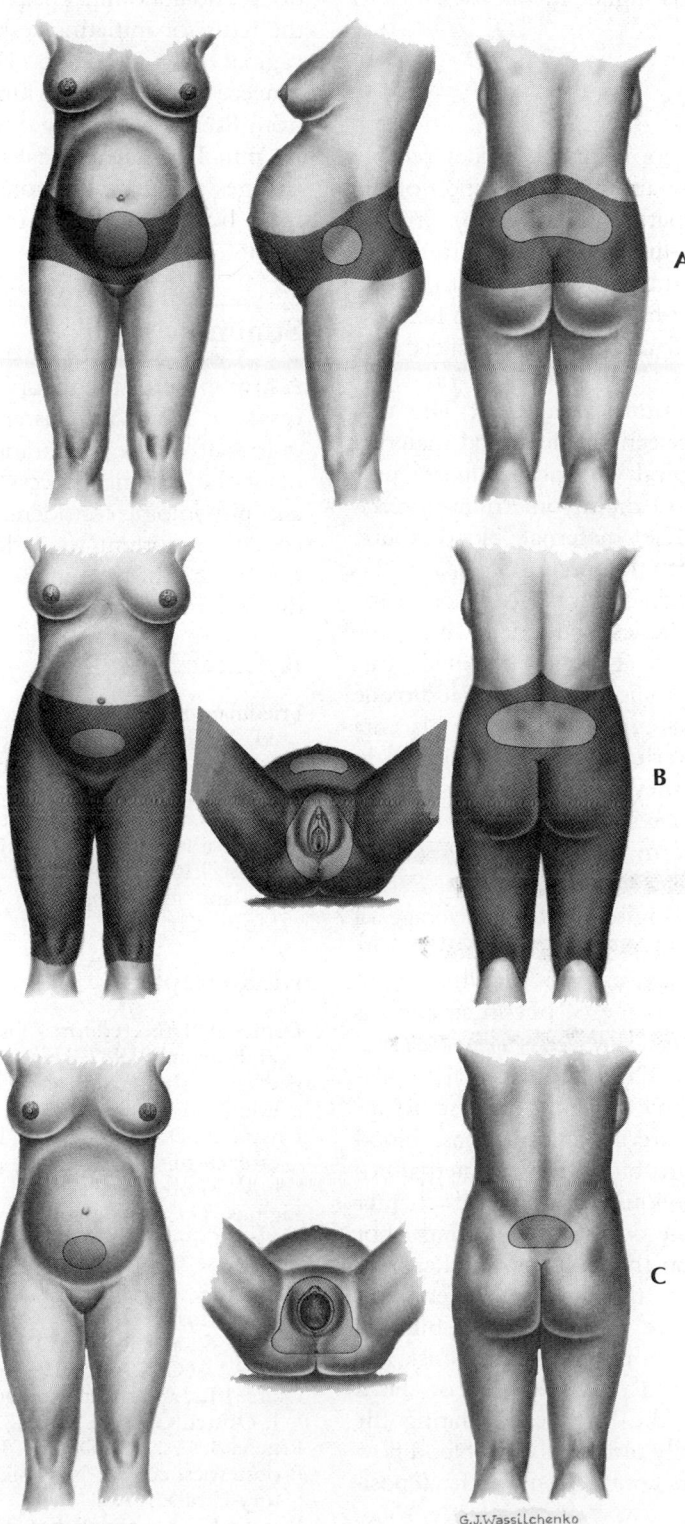

G.J.Wassilchenko

and directed cortical activity, which activates and closes the gating mechanism as well. The gate control theory emphasizes the need for a supportive setting for birth. In such an environment the laboring woman can relax and allow the various higher mental activities to be implemented.

FETAL ADAPTATIONS

Fetal heart rate (FHR) monitoring provides reliable and predictive information about the condition of the fetus as it relates to oxygenation (Chapter 16). Stresses to the uterofetoplacental unit result in characteristic FHR patterns. It is important for the nurse to have a basic understanding of the factors involved in fetal oxygenation and of the fetal responses that reflect adequate fetal oxygenation.

Review of uteroplacental circulation. The placenta serves as a link between the fetal and maternal circulations. Uterine spiral arterioles must pass through the full thickness of the myometrium to reach the intervillous space. The maternal blood spurts through these arterioles into the intervillous space. Oxygen, nutrients, and inherent warmth are absorbed by the thin-walled fetal capillaries contained within the chorionic villi of the placenta. These are eventually carried to the fetus by the umbilical vein. Carbon dioxide and fetal waste products circulate back to the placenta through the umbilical arteries and fetal capillaries in the chorionic villi. Here they cross back through the intervillous space to the maternal circulation.

The average FHR at term is 140 beats per minute (bpm); the normal range is 120 to 160 bpm. Earlier in gestation the FHR is higher, with an average of approximately 160 bpm at 20 weeks' gestation. The rate decreases progressively as the maturing fetus reaches term. The normal range of pH in an adult is 7.35 to 7.45. The average fetal range is 7.30 to 7.35.

Origins of fetal stress. Uterofetoplacental circulation can be affected by many factors. These factors include maternal position, uterine contractions, blood pressure, and umbilical cord blood flow. Maternal position is discussed in a previous section of this chapter and in Chapter 16. Uterine contractions during labor tend to decrease circulation through the spiral arteries and subsequent perfusion through the intervillous space. This stress seems to be well within the ability of the fetus to compensate for in most gestations. The fetus is exposed to increased pressure as he or she is moved passively through the birth canal during the mechanism of labor. Usually umbilical cord blood flow is undisturbed by uterine contractions or fetal position.

Normal adaptations to stress of labor. A healthy fetus with an adequate uterofetoplacental circulation will respond in fairly predictable ways to stresses. Transitory accelerations and slight decelerations can be expected in response to spontaneous fetal movement, vaginal examination, fundal pressure, uterine contractions, and abdominal palpation. These changes prepare the fetus for initiating respirations after birth. During vaginal delivery, 7 to 42 ml of amniotic fluid is squeezed from the fetal lungs. Normally, fetal Po_2 falls from 80 to 15 mm Hg, arterial Pco_2 rises from 40 to 70 mm Hg, and arterial pH falls below 7.35. These changes stimulate chemoreceptors in the aorta and carotid bodies to initiate respirations immediately after birth.

Summary

A firm grasp of the theory of essential factors and processes in labor and maternal and fetal adaptations is only half of the preparation a nurse needs to implement the nursing process with parturients. Anatomic and physiologic considerations are important, but it is equally important to understand the family's adaptation to childbirth. Family responses and adaptation are discussed in Chapter 15.

References

Friedman, E.A.: Labor: clinical evaluation and management, ed. 2, New York, 1978, Appleton-Century-Crofts.

Friedman, E.A., and Sachtleben, M.R.: Station of the fetal presenting part, Am. J. Obstet. Gynecol. 93:522, 1965.

McKay, S.: Squatting: an alternate position for the second stage of labor. M.C.N. 9:181, May/June 1984.

Willson, J.R., Carrington, E.R., and Ledger, W.J.: Obstetrics and gynecology, ed. 7, St. Louis, 1983, The C.V. Mosby Co.

Bibliography

Danforth, D.N., editor: Obstetrics and gynecology, ed. 4, Philadelphia, 1982, Harper & Row, Publishers.

Feetham S.L.: Acute and chronic pain in maternal-child health, M.C.N. 9:249, July/Aug. 1984.

Jensen, M.D., and Bobak, I.M.: Handbook of maternity care: a guide for nursing practice, St. Louis, 1980, The C.V. Mosby Co.

Liggins, G.C.: New concepts of what triggers labor, Contemp OB/Gyn. 19(5):131, 1982.

Malasanos, L., Barkauskas, V., Moss, M., and Stoltenberg-Allen, K.: Health assessment, ed. 3, St. Louis, 1986, The C.V. Mosby Co.

McKay, S., and Roberts, J.: Second stage labor: what is normal? J.O.G.N.N. 14:101, Mar./Apr. 1985.

Okita, J.R., and others: Initiation of human parturition, Am. J. Obstet. Gynecol. 142:432, 1982.

Pritchard, J.A., MacDonald, P.C., and Gant, N.R.: Williams obstetrics, ed. 17, Norwalk, Conn., 1985, Appleton-Century-Crofts.

Romond, J.L., and Baker, I.T.: Squatting in childbirth: a new look at an old tradition, J.O.G.N.N. 14:406, Sept./Oct. 1985.

CHAPTER 15

Nursing Care During the First Stage of Labor

The first stage of labor begins with the onset of regular contractions and is complete when the cervix is fully dilated. The symptoms the expectant mother has been prepared to recognize herald the beginning of labor. The waiting period of pregnancy is at an end. The time has come for the child to be born. The mother or couple are about to undergo one of the most meaningful events of their lives.

Care of the woman in labor begins with the woman's report of the following:

1. Onset of progressive, strong, frequent, sustained uterine contractions
2. Rupture of the membranes
3. Bloody vaginal discharge (bloody show)

If a hospital delivery has been elected, the woman is admitted to the labor unit (Fig. 15.1). If a home or birthing center delivery has been planned, the family follows the instructions previously agreed upon.

When the woman arrives on the unit, greet her warmly, using her name. Extend a welcome to her and her family. Welcoming the family will be discussed in greater detail under implementation of the nursing process with the family in labor. Assessment is the first priority.

Initial Assessment

The admission form can be used to guide the nurse's assessment of the woman being admitted to a labor unit. The data for the admission record is obtained from several sources (Fig. 15.2):

1. The prenatal record
2. Interview
3. Physical examination
4. Laboratory tests

Although childbirth is essentially a normal process, some complications may develop during the clinical course of labor (see Unit 7). Knowledge of the pregnancy, careful initial assessment, and follow-up of progress are necessary during any labor.

Prenatal record. Before the nurse's first meeting with the woman who is in labor, a review of her prenatal record is made. Significant items are noted. If the woman has not had any prenatal care, the needed information must be obtained on admission. It is best to complete her data base before active labor begins.

General information. **Age** is important. The needs of a 12-year-old girl and those of a 42-year-old woman vary in some respects. **Height** and **weight** also are significant. A woman who stands 4 ft 10 in (145 cm) and weighs 170 lb (77 kg) may require interventions different from those needed by the woman who also weighs 170 lb but is 5 ft 11 in (177.5 cm) tall. **General health,** any **medical conditions,** and history of **surgical interventions** are carefully noted.

Past obstetric history. **Parity** and **gravidity** are recorded (Chapter 9). Previous obstetric experience is reviewed for the following:

1. Problems: spontaneous abortions, preterm labors, stillbirths, premature rupture of membranes, bleeding, hypertension, anemia, gestational diabetes
2. Type of labors: duration of labors, anesthesia used
3. Type of deliveries: normal spontaneous vaginal delivery (NSVD), forceps assisted, cesarean
4. Condition of babies at birth: weight, Apgar scores, singleton (one baby) or multiple (twins, triplets) births

History of this pregnancy. Pertinent information includes the date of the last normal menstrual period, date of quickening, growth of height of the fundus, and estimated weight of the fetus. These data are used to confirm the **EDC** or "expected date of confinement." The woman's vital signs, blood pressure, weight and pattern of weight gain, and results of urinalysis help confirm the normalcy of this pregnancy.

Fig. 15.1
Couple arrives on labor/birth unit accompanied by maternal grandmother. (Courtesy Marjorie Pyle, RNC, Lifecircle, Costa Mesa, California.)

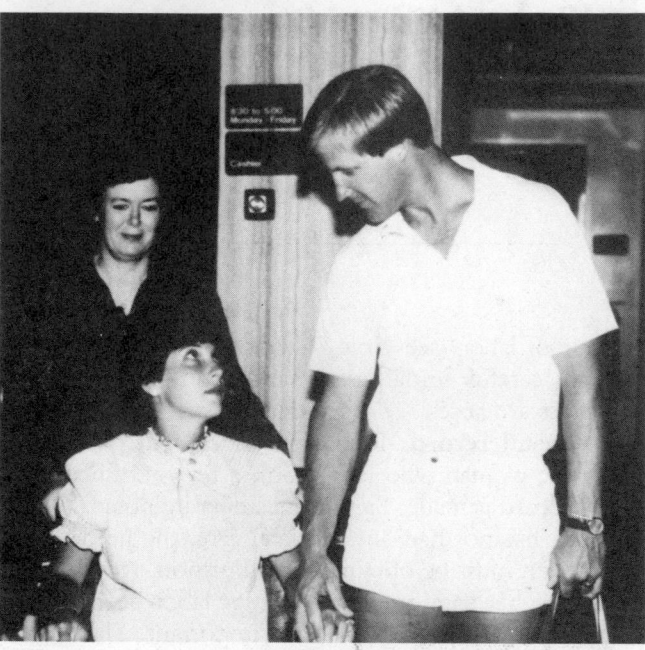

Table 15.1
Comparison of True and False Labors

True Labor	False Labor
Show: usually present; pinkish mucus; may contain mucous plug from cervix	Show: usually none or brownish-stained mucus (inquire whether she had vaginal examination within last 48 hr)
Contractions: occur regularly; interval between has shortened; intensity has gradually increased; located in lower back (may feel like gastrointestinal upset with some diarrhea); intensified by walking	Contractions: occur irregularly; intervals remain long; intensity unchanged; located in abdomen; relief with walking or no effect (Braxton Hicks contractions)
Cervix: becomes effaced and dilates progressively	Cervix: no change
Descent: progressive	Descent: no change
Fetal movement: no significant change	Fetal movement: intensifies (for a short period) or remains the same

The FHR and its location provide a baseline against which the nurse can compare findings of initial assessment.

Data noted include the gestational week of initial visit, diagnostic studies done, and problems encountered. The medications used during this pregnancy are carefully documented. Frequently, prenatal records indicate the woman's preferences for anesthesia, feeding her newborn, and the name of her pediatrician.

Laboratory tests performed during this pregnancy and the findings are recorded. These tests include the initial blood test for blood group and Rh factor, hemoglobin and hematocrit, and sickle cell trait, if indicated. Antibody titers are determined. As necessary, throughout the pregnancy, tests are repeated for hematocrit and hemoglobin and antibody titers. Urinalysis is usually recorded for each visit. Urine is assessed for protein, acetone, and glucose.

To complete the admission form, the nurse uses the assessment techniques of interviewing, physical examination, and laboratory tests. Each of these techniques will be discussed individually.

Interview. Any information not found in the prenatal record is requested on admission. Pertinent data include choice of infant feeding method, anesthesia,

and pediatrician. A client profile is obtained; this profile indicates the woman's preparation for childbirth, supportive persons desired and available, and ethnic or cultural expectations or needs.

The woman's chief complaint or reason for coming to the hospital is determined. The chief complaint may be rupture of membranes with or without contractions. In this case she is in for an **obstetric check.** The obstetric check is reserved for women who are unsure about onset of labor. This designation allows time on the unit for diagnosis of labor without official admission, and cost to the client is minimized or avoided.

False labor may be experienced from the thirty-eighth week onward. It is frustrating for the woman to find that the contractions she was experiencing were not true labor and that she must return home until more definitive symptoms are present. For those who experience false labor two or three times, the onset of true labor comes as an anticlimax. Only attentive care eradicates the feelings of disappointment and even anger. (For a comparison of false and true labors, see Table 15.1.)

The woman may have been scheduled for induction of labor. (Induction of labor and the nursing care involved are discussed in Chapter 29.) Induction of labor and other complications of labor, such as premature rupture of membranes, do require special alterations in the nursing care plan. However, even in those instances some nursing care remains the same.

The onset of labor may be difficult to determine even for the experienced gravida. The woman is asked to recall the events of the previous days. She is assessed

Fig. 15.2
Obstetric labor admission record. (Courtesy Stanford University Medical Center, Stanford, California.)

STANFORD UNIVERSITY HOSPITAL
Stanford University Medical Center
Stanford, California 94305

OBSTETRICAL LABOR ADMISSION RECORD

_____ addressograph stamp _____

Admission Date _____ Time _____ M.D. Notified _____ Time _____
Patient's Age _____ EDC _____ Parity _____ Patient's Blood Type _____ Father's Blood Type _____
□ In Labor: Began On _____ 19 _____ Time _____ Membranes _____
□ Not in Labor: Admitted for   □ Induction   □ Suspected Labor   □ Other _____
Anesthesia Preferred _____ Feeding: □ Breast   □ Bottle
Time of Last Meal _____ Type of Food _____ Pediatrician _____
Room Type _____ Rooming In _____

COMPLICATIONS AND MEDICATIONS DURING PREGNANCY

Initial Visit:
□ 1st trimester
□ 2nd trimester
□ 3rd trimester

Diagnostic Studies Done:
□ None
□ Estriols
□ NST & CST
□ NST only
□ CST only
□ Ultrasound
□ Amniocentesis: □ L/S
            □ Shake
            □ Other _____

Cardiovascular:
□ None
□ Mild pre-eclampsia
□ Severe pre-eclampsia
□ Eclampsia
□ Chronic hypertension
□ Heart Disease

Bleeding ($\geq$ 20 wks GA):
□ None
□ Placenta previa
□ Abruptio placenta
□ Vasa previa
□ Other bleeding

Diabetes:
□ None
□ Non-insulin
□ Insulin dependent
□ With vascular disease
□ Suspected macrosomia

Pre-term Labor
($\geq$ 20 wks and < 37 wks GA):
□ None
□ Spontaneous w/o underlying cause
□ PROM
□ Pre-eclampsia
□ Eclampsia
□ Bleeding
□ Multiple births
□ Hydramnios
□ Infection
□ Incompetent cervix
□ Other uterine anomalies
□ Other known etiology _____

Other Problems:
□ None
□ Anemia
□ Renal disease
□ Urinary tract infection
□ Rh incompatibility
□ Other _____

Medications Used:
□ None
□ Antibiotics
□ Antihistamines
□ Aspirin
□ Barbiturates
□ Decongestants
□ Diuretics
□ Iron/Vitamins
□ Tranquilizers
□ Insulin
□ Tocolytic _____
□ Steroids _____
□ Other _____

ADMISSION PREPARATION AND EXAMINATIONS

Admission Preparations: □ Half Prep.   □ Abdominal Prep.   □ Enema   □ No Prep.
Temp. _____ R. _____ P. _____ BP. _____ Ht. _____ Wt. _____
Head: □ Normal   □ Other _____   Neck: □ Normal   □ Other _____
Heart: □ Normal   □ Other _____   Lungs: □ Normal   □ Other _____
Abdomen: □ Normal   □ Other _____
          Fetal presentation _____   Estimated Fetal Wt. _____
          Fetal Heart Rate _____   Uterine Contractions _____
Vagina: Dilation _____ Effacement _____   Consistency _____ Position _____
         Fetal Position _____   Station ___ _____
Other Significant Findings: _____

_____ M.D. _____ R.N.

□ Taken to Delivery Room without further examinations.

15-108 Rev. 6-82   WHITE - Mother's Medical Record   CANARY - Nursery   PINK - Perinatal Outreach

for the prodromes of labor (Chapter 14) and for the onset of regular contractions. She is asked to describe the following:

1. Frequency and duration of contractions.
2. Location and character of discomfort from contractions.
3. Persistence of contractions despite changes in maternal position, when walking or lying down.
4. Presence and character of vaginal discharge or show.
5. Status of amniotic membranes, such as gush or seepage of fluid. If there is a discharge that may be amniotic fluid, she is asked the date and time the fluid was first noted. This information is recorded and followed by physical examination to confirm rupture of membranes.

In case general anesthesia may be required at a moment's notice, it is important to know about the woman's respiratory status. The nurse asks if the gravida has a "cold" or related symptoms, "stuffy" nose, sore throat, or cough. Allergies are rechecked. Some allergic responses cause swelling of mucous membranes of the respiratory system. Because vomiting and subsequent aspiration into the respiratory tree can complicate an otherwise normal labor, the nurse records the type and time of the woman's last meal.

Procedure 15.1

MEASUREMENT OF VITAL SIGNS AND BLOOD PRESSURE

PURPOSE

1. To establish baseline data against which future readings can be compared
2. To identify any abnormalities that could interfere with normal progress of labor and with maternal or fetal health

EQUIPMENT (varies with facility)

1. Thermometer: glass reusable, electronic with probe and probe covers, or chemical disposable
2. Watch with second hand
3. Mercury or aneroid sphygmomanometer and stethoscope for indirect measurement of systemic blood pressure
4. Appropriate size blood pressure cuff
   a. Cuff that is 20% wider than diameter of the extremity around which it is wrapped: about 12-14 cm (about 6 in) for average-size individuals and 18-20 cm (about 8 in) for obese individuals
   b. Too small a cuff → False high BP
   c. Too large a cuff → False low BP

NURSING ACTION	RATIONALE
Use the protocols of care for the unit regarding vital signs and blood pressure.	Meets the hospital's standard of care.
	Checks equipment, for example, looks for breaks in thermometer, appropriate size cuff.
Obtain temperature.	Establishes baseline value.
	Identifies deviations from normal findings, such as fever.
Count pulses and assess quality of pulse.	Establishes a baseline value.
	Identifies deviations from normal findings, such as tachycardia.
Count respirations and assess respiratory effort.	Establishes a baseline value.
	Identifies deviations from normal findings, such as signs of a "cold."
Measure blood pressure (Fig. 15.3)	Establishes a baseline value.
	Identifies deviations from normal findings, such as elevation in blood pressure often seen if woman is anxious.
Remeasure blood pressure after woman has had a chance to relax.	Helps in identifying cause of elevation.
Measure blood pressure between contractions.	Rules out elevations related to normal blood pressure response to uterine contractions.
Charting: Chart findings using the established protocol for the facility.	Provides data base against which to compare prenatal values.
	Provides data base for implementation of the next steps in the nursing process.
	Promotes collaboration with other members of the health team.

Physical examination. The initial examinations serve to confirm the onset of true labor. The findings serve as a baseline for assessing the woman's progress from that point in time. Physical examinations performed include the following:

1. Vital signs and blood pressure
2. Brief physical assessment: heart, lungs; presence of edema of the legs, face, hands, or sacrum (see Chapter 11)
3. Abdominal palpation: Leopold's maneuvers
4. Fetal heart rate (FHR), rhythm, area of maximal intensity (MI)
5. Vaginal examination
6. Assessment of vaginal discharge
7. Assessment for rupture of membranes
8. Uterine contractions

The assessment procedures that follow can be used as a basis for teaching clients and their families. The purpose, equipment needed, and nursing actions and rationale of each procedure can be shared with the woman. All procedures are preceded by excellent handwashing. The procedure and findings are explained to the woman whenever possible. Findings and the time the procedure is performed are carefully noted and initialed in the chart. Handwashing is also important after the examinations. Accurate charting is done as soon after interaction with a client as possible.

Vital signs and blood pressure. Vital signs and blood pressure are assessed on admission to the hospital of any client. Findings are assessed for normalcy and are used for comparison with future values. Assessment for vital signs and blood pressure is found in Procedure 15.1.

Abdominal palpation: Leopold's maneuvers. The four maneuvers of Leopold provide a systematic examination. Proficiency in determining presentation and position by abdominal palpation requires considerable practice, so every opportunity to learn must be used to perfect the technique. Gross maternal obesity, excessive amniotic fluid (hydramnios), or tumors may make it difficult to feel the fetal contours.

Auscultation of FHR. The area of maximal intensity (MI) of the FHR is the location of the maternal abdomen where the FHR is heard the loudest. The MI is an aid in determining the fetal position (Fig. 15.5). In vertex and breech presentations, with the head well flexed on the fetal chest, the FHR is heard loudest through the fetal back. In vertex presentations the FHRs commonly are heard below the mother's umbilicus in a lower quadrant of the abdomen (Fig. 15.4, *A*). In breech presentations the FHRs are usually heard loudest above the level of the umbilicus (Fig.

Fig. 15.3
Assessment of blood pressure (Courtesy Marjorie Pyle RNC, Lifecircle, Costa Mesa, California.)

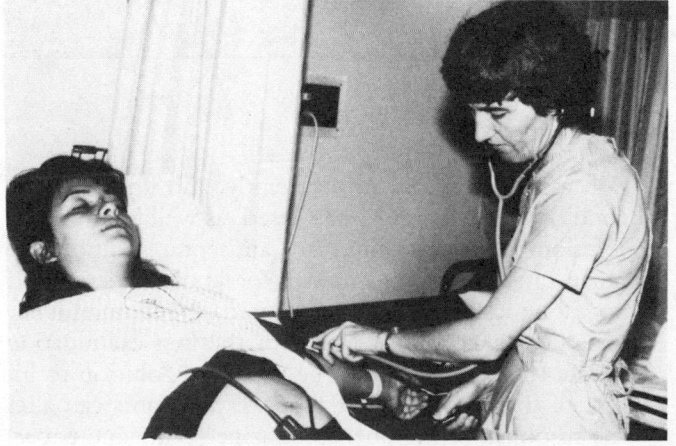

Fig. 15.4
The area of the FHR. **A,** With fetus in ROA position. **B,** Changes in area of MI as fetus undergoes internal rotation from ROA to OA for delivery. **C,** With fetus in LSP (left sacral posterior) position. (**A** and **C** courtesy Ross Laboratories, Columbus, Ohio.)

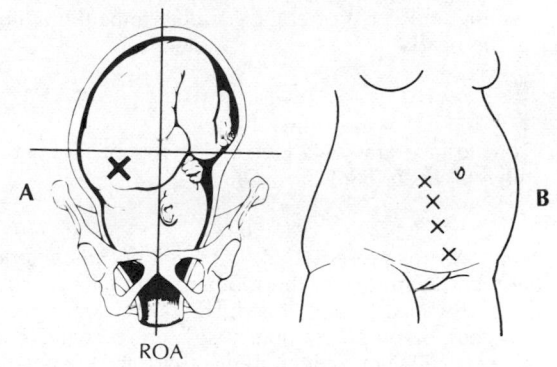

ROA

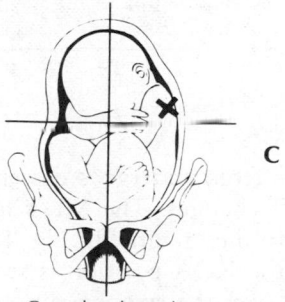

C

Complete breech

Lie: vertical
Presentation: breech (sacrum and feet presenting)
Reference point: sacrum (with feet)
Attitude: general flexion

Procedure 15.2

ABDOMINAL PALPATION: THE FOUR MANEUVERS OF LEOPOLD

PURPOSE
1. To identify number of fetuses
2. To identify fetal presentation, lie, presenting part, degree of descent, attitude

EQUIPMENT
None needed

NURSING ACTION	RATIONALE
Ask woman to empty her bladder.	Prevents maternal discomfort during examination. Facilitates accurate measurement.
Position woman supine with one pillow under her head and her knees slightly flexed.	Ensures comfort. Relieves tension of abdominal musculature.
Place small rolled towel under her right hip.	Displaces uterus to left, off of major blood vessels.
If right-handed, stand at woman's left, facing her.	Facilitates examination by using dominant hand.
1. Identify the fetal part that occupies the fundus. The head feels round, firm, freely movable, and palpable by ballottement; the breech feels less regular and softer (Fig. 15.5, *A*).	Identifies fetal lie (vertical or horizontal) and presentation (vertex or breech).
2. Using palmar surface of one hand, locate and palpate the smooth convex contour of the fetal back and the irregularities that identify the small parts (feet, hands, elbows) (Fig. 15.5, *B*).	Assists in identifying fetal presentation.
3. With the right hand, determine which fetal part is presenting over the inlet to the true pelvis. Gently grasp the lower pole of the uterus between the thumb and fingers, pressing in slightly. If the head is presenting and it is not engaged, determine the attitude of the head.	Confirms presenting part. Helps in identifying degree of descent. If the presenting part is not engaged, it can be rocked from side to side; if engaged, it cannot be rocked. If the cephalic prominence is found on the same side as the small parts, the head must be flexed, and the vertex is presenting (Fig. 15.5, *C*). If the cephalic prominence is on the same side as the back, the presenting head is extended (Fig. 14.3, *C*).
4. Turn to face gravida's feet. Using two hands, outline the fetal head (Fig. 15.5, *D*).	When presenting part has descended deeply, only a small portion of it may be outlined. Palpation of cephalic prominence assists in identifying attitude of head.
Charting: Vertex presentation, LOA (left occiput anterior: the fetal occiput is in the mother's left anterior quadrant). The head is well flexed; station is "floating" (not engaged). Some practitioners use a line drawing to depict results. When written in the chart, this information reads, "Vtx, LOA, floating."	Provides data base against which to compare future findings. Provides data base for implementation of the next steps in the nursing process. Promotes collaboration with other members of the health team.

15.4, *C*). As the fetus undergoes descent and internal rotation, the MI changes. The MI is found to move downward and to the midline. In Fig. 15.4, *B*, the MI of the fetus in the ROA position is seen to move to the midline just over the symphysis pubis. Just before delivery the fetal position is OA and the fetal back is directly above the symphysis pubis.

Vaginal examination. The condition, effacement, and dilatation of the cervix and the descent of the fetus are determined by vaginal examination. The examina-

tion must be done carefully, gently, and under aseptic conditions. Sterile gloves are used, as well as antiseptic solution. Prior to using any antiseptic solution the nurse must assess the mother for known allergies. If povidone-iodine (Betadine) is used, the woman is assessed for allergy to iodine. For the first examination in labor, sterile water can be used as a solution to lubricate the fingers. Other types of lubricants can alter the response of the phenaphthazine (Nitrazine paper) if it is to be used to diagnose rupture of membranes.

Fig. 15.5
Leopold's maneuvers.

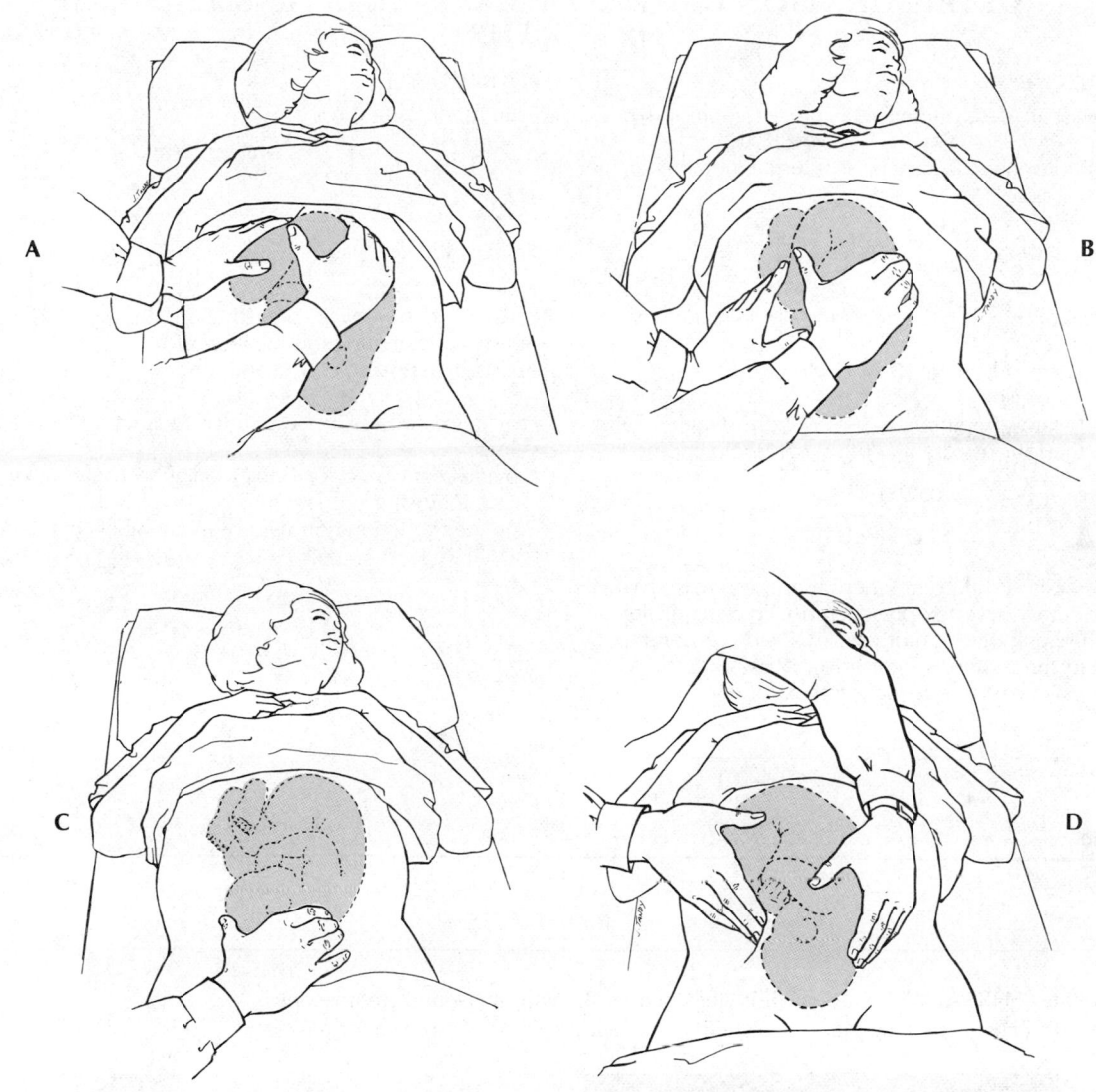

Vaginal examinations must never be performed by a nurse if bleeding (as distinguished from bloody show) is present. Until the source of the bleeding is diagnosed, no vaginal or rectal examinations should be done nor should any enemas be given (see discussion of placenta previa in Chapter 27).

Assessment of vaginal discharge. Effacement and dilatation of the cervix loosens the membranes from the area of the internal os, resulting in slight bleeding. These cervical changes set free the mucous plug or operculum. This bloody mucus discharge is the "show." The appearance of show is not an invariable prelude to labor; it may occur after labor begins.

Assessment for rupture of membranes. Labor is initiated by spontaneous rupture of the membranes (SRM) in almost 25% of gravidas. The lag period, rarely exceeding 24 hours, precedes the onset of labor. Loss of urine by the incontinent woman or leukorrhea must be differentiated from amniotic fluid for appropriate management. Three simple procedures are useful in the diagnosis of ruptured membranes. Usually only the Nitrazine paper test is performed by the nurse. Two other tests are discussed that are performed by physicians in most facilities.

Uterine contractions. The primary powers, the uterine contractions, and their function are described in

Procedure 15.3

DETERMINATION OF AREA OF MAXIMAL INTENSITY (MI) OF THE FHR

PURPOSE

1. To assist in determining fetal presentation and position
2. To monitor the descent and internal rotation of the fetus

EQUIPMENT

Fetal monitoring device

NURSING ACTION	RATIONALE
Perform abdominal palpation: the four maneuvers of Leopold.	Locates the fetal back, presentation, and position.
Auscultate the FHR (Fig. 15.6).	Assists in estimating the location of MI.
Apply monitor prn	Assists in assessing fetal well-being.
Charting: Many practitioners use a two-line figure to indicate the four quadrants of the maternal abdomen:	Provides data base against which to compare future findings.

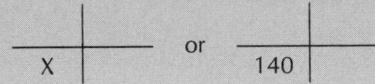

RUQ	LUQ
RLQ	LLQ

The umbilicus is the point where the lines cross. The MI for the fetus in vertex presentation, in general flexion with the back on the mother's right side, is commonly found in the mother's right lower quadrant. The MI of this fetus's heart rate is recorded as follows:

X | or   140 |

Provides data base for implementation of the next steps in the nursing process.
Promotes collaboration with other members of the health team.

Fig. 15.6
Nurse auscultates FHR. **A,** With DeLee-Hillis stethoscope. **B,** With ultrasound stethoscope. Mother listens to FHR. (Courtesy Marjorie Pyle RNC, Lifecircle, Costa Mesa, California.)

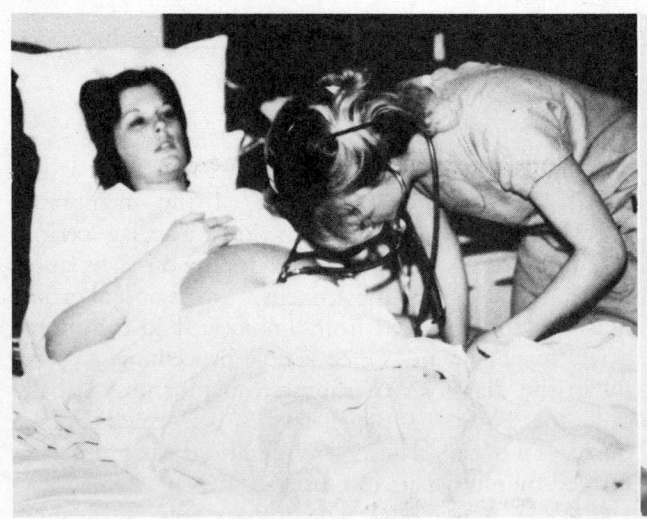
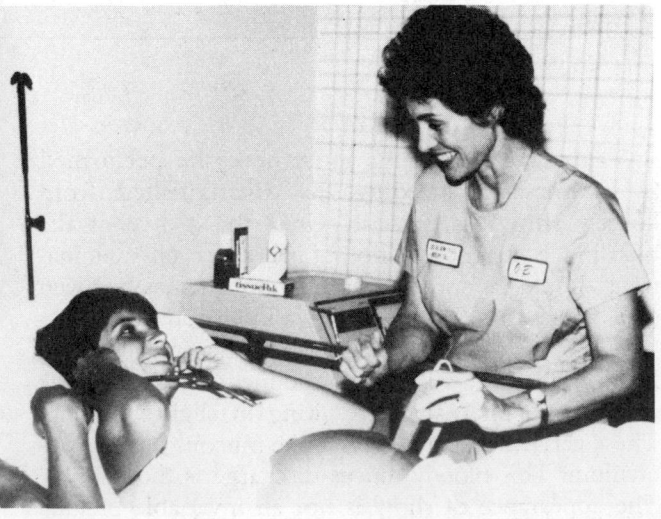

PERFORMING OR ASSISTING WITH A VAGINAL EXAMINATION

PURPOSE

1. To assess the cervix: degree of softness (readiness for labor), effacement and dilatation
2. To assess presentation and position of the fetus
3. To assess degree of descent or station
4. To assess degree of molding of the fetal head, if presenting
5. To assess the membranes: intact, bulging, or ruptured
6. To assess how well the presenting part is applied to the cervix
7. To assess the presence and amount of stool in the rectum

EQUIPMENT

1. Sterile gloves
2. Antiseptic solution or sterile water
3. Drapes
4. Light source
5. Nitrazine paper

NURSING ACTION	RATIONALE
Prior to the Examination	
Assess for vaginal bleeding.	Vaginal bleeding is contraindication to vaginal examination, as trauma from examination could cause life-threatening hemorrhage if placenta previa exists.
If No Bleeding is Present	
Ask woman to empty bladder.	Prevents maternal discomfort. Facilitates accurate assessment.
Drape appropriately.	Respects modesty, protects privacy.
Position the light.	Permits visualization of vulva.
Assist the woman into the supine position with one pillow under her head and her knees flexed and separated.	Reduces tension of abdominal musculature. Facilitates examination.
Place a small rolled towel under her right hip.	Displaces uterus to left, off of major blood vessels. Prevents supine hypotension (pp. 393, 395, and 396).
Apply gloves (assist examiner to don gloves).	Maintains asepsis for the mother and the examiner.
Lubricate examining fingers with sterile water or antiseptic solution (see assessment for rupture of membranes).	Facilitates examination; maintains asepsis; prevents interference with Nitrazine paper when water is used.
Separate labia with one gloved hand, introduce the middle and index finger of examining hand into vagina with palmer surface downward. Maintain downward pressure toward less sensitive posterior vaginal wall.	Prevents rolling of labia into vagina as fingers of examining hand enter vagina; aids in preventing infection. Lessens discomfort by directing pressure toward less sensitive posterior vaginal wall.
Curl last two fingers (Fig. 15.7).	Lessens chance of contamination or infection from anal area.
Place other hand on fundus and exert a gentle downward pressure.	Facilitates assessment by steadying the fetus and applying the presenting part to the cervix.
Rotate fingers as necessary to complete assessment of fetus, station, cervix, status of amniotic membranes, and rectal fullness.	Performs assessment. Assesses need for enema.
During Examination	
Coach woman with breathing and focusing.	Assists in keeping perineum relaxed. Assists woman to "stay in control."
Remind woman to keep her eyes open and her hands relaxed.	Facilitates examination and decreases woman's discomfort by helping her relax her perineum.
If she shows signs of supine hypotension or the vagal nerve reflex (see p. 281) (for example, she becomes pale, breathless, and faint, and her skin becomes clammy), turn her onto her left side.	Relieves the signs and symptoms (see boxes, p. 281).

Continued.

Procedure 15.4 —cont'd

After the Examination

Clean the parturient's vulva; place a clean pad on bed under her; reposition bed covers according to her preference.

Answer questions regarding findings.

Aids comfort, both physical and emotional.
Maintains cleanliness to decrease possibility of infection.
Respects woman's dignity.
Helps decrease anxiety and increase woman's (couple's) sense of control over situation.

Charting

The nurse enters initial findings on the admission form (see Fig. 15.2):

Cervix	
Dilation	0 to 100%
Effacement	0 to 10 cm
Consistency	Thick/firm to soft ("ripe")
Position	Anterior, posterior
Fetal position	Vtx, LOA
Station	Floating to 0 to +4

Provides data base against which to compare future findings.
Provides data base for implementation of the next steps in the nursing process.
Promotes collaboration with other members of the health team.

Fig. 15.7

Vaginal examination. **A,** Undilated, uneffaced cervix. Membranes intact. **B,** Palpation of sagittal suture line. Cervix effaced and partially dilated.

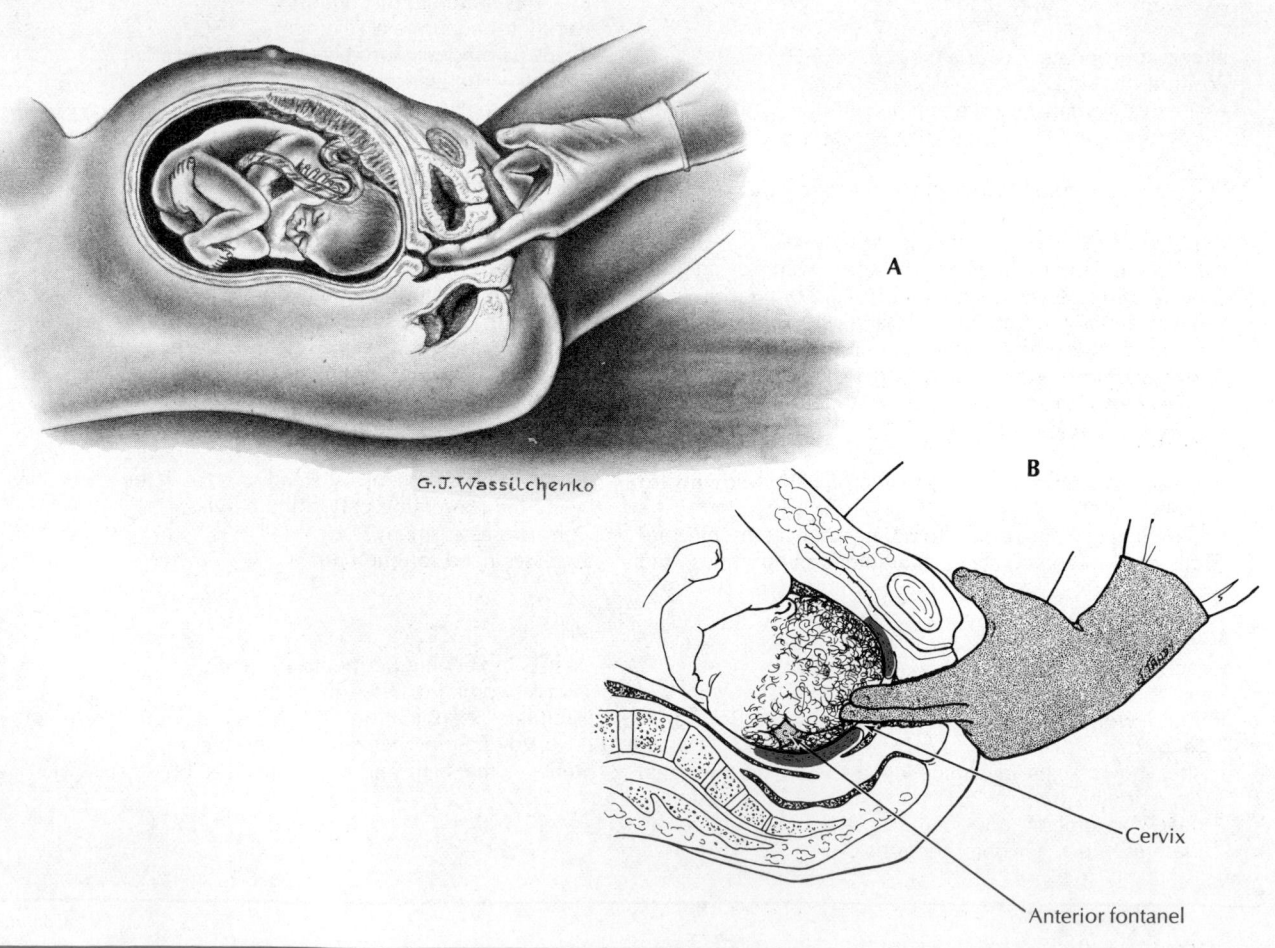

G.J. Wassilchenko

A

B

Cervix

Anterior fontanel

Procedure 15.5

ASSESSMENT OF VAGINAL DISCHARGE

PURPOSE

1. To confirm onset of labor if discharge is bloody show
2. To differentiate between bloody show (mucous plug) and bleeding due to a complication

EQUIPMENT

None needed

NURSING ACTION	RATIONALE
Observe and assess nature of the vaginal discharge. Note its amount, color, and character.	Distinguishes bloody show from bleeding that may indicate a serious complication.
Look for show that is pink in color and feels sticky from the mucus it contains.	Characterizes bloody show seen at onset of labor.
Charting: Pink-streaked, mucuslike discharge noted on panties on admission.	Provide data base against which to compare future findings.
	Provides data base for implementation of the next steps in the nursing process.
	Promotes collaboration with other members of the health team.

detail in Chapter 14. There are three methods of assessing contractions: by the subjective description given by the woman, by palpation and timing by a nurse or physician, and by electronic monitoring devices.

Describing uterine contractions. Each contraction exhibits a wavelike pattern; it begins with a slower increment, gradually reaches an acme, and then diminishes rather rapidly (decrement). Next there is an interval of rest (intrauterine pressure is 8 to 15 mm Hg), which is broken when the next contraction begins.

In describing a uterine contraction (Fig. 15.8), reference is made to the following characteristics:

1. **Frequency.** Contractions occur intermittently throughout labor. They begin at about 20 to 30 minutes apart and become closer together until, at the height of the expulsive efforts, they are as frequent as every 2 to 3 minutes.
2. **Regularity.** Contractions occur more and more regularly as labor becomes well established.
3. **Duration.** The length of time a contraction lasts increases from 30 seconds to between 60 and 90 seconds near full dilatation of the cervix. Then the duration becomes about 60 seconds until delivery of the fetus is accomplished.
4. **Intensity.** The strength of the contraction also increases as labor progresses, from weak contractions noted early in labor to strong expulsive contractions (intrauterine pressure measured at 50 to 75 mm Hg) evidenced near the time of delivery.

Uterine contractions are measured in **Montevideo units** in some parts of the United States; the intensity of the contractions is measured in total millimeters of mercury per 10 minutes. Until the thirtieth week of pregnancy, contractions are fewer than 20 Montevideo units. Contractions increase thereafter from 30 to 80 Montevideo units as pregnancy approaches term. During early labor, uterine activity averages 80 to 120 Montevideo units. Near the end of labor (five contractions per 10 minutes) the average of 250 Montevideo units is reached.

Palpation of uterine contractions is less precise. Practice is required to discern between mild, moderate, and strong contractions. The definitions of these descriptive terms are as follows:

mild contractions: Slightly tense fundus that is easy to indent with fingertips

moderate contractions: Firm fundus that is difficult to indent with fingertips

strong contractions: Rigid, boardlike fundus that is almost impossible to indent

Laboratory tests. If there is time and the membranes are not ruptured, a urine specimen is obtained. The urine is tested for routine analysis and the presence of protein, glucose, and acetone. The urine is tested on admission and usually with each voiding while the woman is in labor.

The woman who has had no prenatal care needs blood drawn for blood grouping, determination of Rh factor, hematocrit, hemoglobin, antibody titer, and

Procedure 15.6

TESTS FOR RUPTURE OF MEMBRANES

PURPOSE
To determine if the membranes have ruptured.

EQUIPMENT
1. Nitrazine paper
2. Sterile glove, water, swab
3. Microscope, clean glass slide
4. Nile blue stain

NURSING ACTION	RATIONALE
Nitrazine Test for pH	
Use Nitrazine paper, a dye 1-1 impregnated test paper for pH.	Differentiates amniotic fluid, which is slightly alkaline, from urine and pus, which are acidic.
Wearing a sterile glove lubricated with water, place a piece of test paper at the cervical os.	Maintains asepsis.
	Does not affect pH.
	Ensures testing for amniotic fluid.
OR	
Use a sterile, cotton-tipped applicator to dip deep into vagina to pick up fluid; touch applicator to test paper.	Maintains asepsis.
	Ensures testing for amniotic fluid.
Read results:	Completes the test.
Membranes probably intact:	Vaginal and most body fluids are acidic.
Yellow pH 5.0	
Olive yellow pH 5.5	
Olive green pH 6.0	
Membranes probably ruptured:	Amniotic fluid is alkaline.
Blue-green pH 6.5	
Blue-gray pH 7.0	
Deep blue pH 7.5	
Realize that false readings are possible.	False readings can occur because of presence of bloody show or insufficient amniotic fluid.
Test for Fern Pattern	
Spread a drop of fluid on a clean glass slide with a sterile, cotton-tipped applicator.	Obtains specimen.
Allow fluid to dry.	Maintains asepsis.
	Dried amniotic fluid will show a frondlike crystalline pattern when viewed under a microscope.
Reads a positive fern test if ferning occurs,* indicative of ruptured membranes.	Urine, vaginal discharge, or blood will not show a crystalline pattern.
Test for Lanugo Hairs or Fetal Squamous Cells	
Aspirate fluid from posterior vaginal vault with sterile aspiration syringe.	Obtains specimen.
Place on clean glass slide.	Maintains asepsis.
Study under microscope.	Prepares specimen for examination.
Stain with Nile blue stain.	Fetal lanugo hairs or fetal squamous cells may be noted.
	Some squamous cells contain lipids that stain yellow after Nile blue is added; other squamous cells and hairs stain blue.
Assess findings.	
Charting: Membranes	
Nitrazine positive.	Provides data base against which to compare future findings.
Positive fern test.	Provides data base for implementation of the next steps in the nursing process.
Nile blue stain shows some yellow squamous cells and some blue squamous cells and hair.	Promotes collaboration with other members of the health team.

*It should not be confused with the cervical mucus test. That test also shows a fernlike formation for high levels of estrogen.

Fig. 15.8
Assessment of uterine contractions. **A,** Changes in abdominal contour before and during uterine contraction. **B,** Assessing contractions.

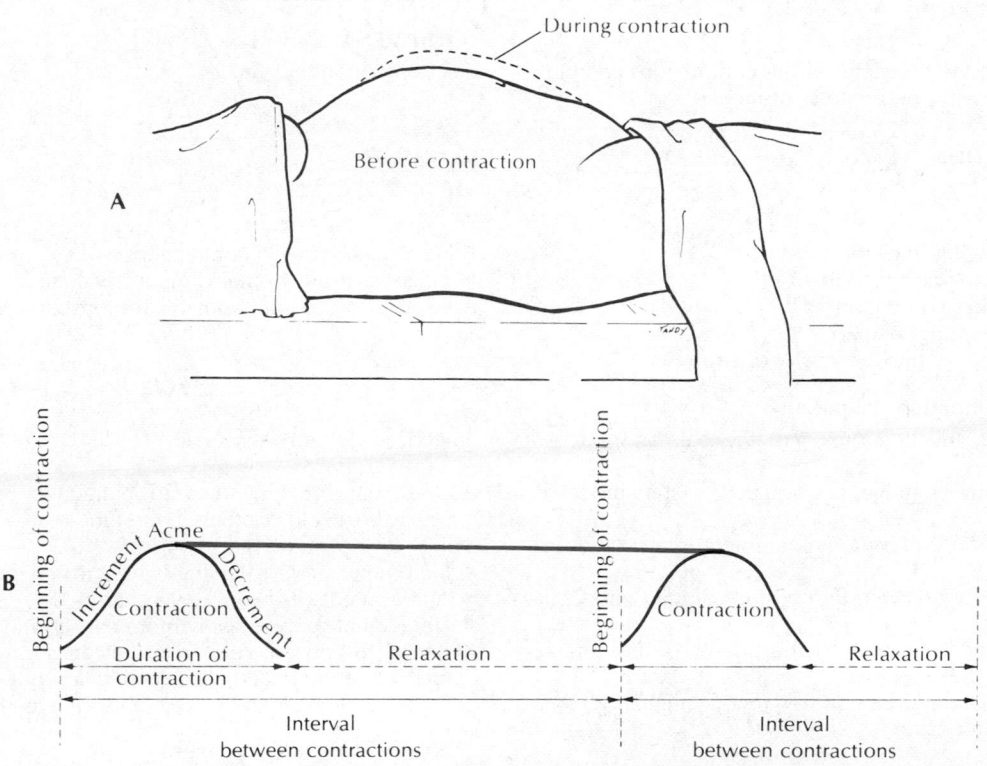

screening for sexually transmitted diseases (Chapter 11). Until the results of these tests are back, precautions for infection control are instituted. If there is no time for test results prior to the birth of the child, cord blood is obtained for evaluation.

Assessment of the gravida's psychologic response. The woman's general appearance and behavior (and that of her partner) provide valuable clues as to the type of supportive care she will need. The nurse notes the following:

1. *Verbal interaction.* Is she talkative or mute? Does she talk to staff members freely or only in response to questions? How does she talk to her support person? Does that person do all the talking?

2. *Body posture and set.* Is she relaxed or tense? What is her anxiety level? Does she lie rigidly on her back or sit up tailor fashion? Where does her partner sit?

3. *Perceptual acuity.* Does she have any helpful or harmful background knowledge? Does her anxiety level require repeated explanations? Does she understand what the nurse says? Can she repeat what has been said or demonstrate that she understands (for example, use the call bell correctly)?

4. *Energy level.* Does she look tired? How much rest has she had in the previous few days? Does excitement mask a depleted energy reserve?

5. *Discomfort or pain.* How much does the woman relate what she is experiencing? How does she react to a contraction?

6. *Cultural background.* How does the woman's cultural background influence her perception of pain? Does she want male or female support while in labor?

Subsequent Assessment of Progress During Labor

Findings from initial assessments serve as a basis for comparison to expected symptomatology of labor (Tables 15.1 and 15.3). Assessment is continuous throughout labor. The routine for assessment of progress and of the continued well-being of the mother and fetus is usually set on a minimal level by hospital policy (Table 15.2). Any unusual findings would prompt an increase in the timing of assessment procedures.

The symptomatology of progress in labor is well de-

Procedure 15.7

ASSESSMENT OF UTERINE CONTRACTIONS

PURPOSE
To determine the character of the contractions and compare them with the progress of labor

EQUIPMENT
Electronic monitor

NURSING ACTION	RATIONALE
Interview Ask the following questions: ■ When did the contractions start? ■ How often are they coming? ■ Are they coming regularly? ■ Would you say they are weak or strong?	Adds to data base on contractions. Indicates that the woman's input is valued. Adds to data base on woman's response to contractions.
Physical Examination: Palpation Palpate using the fingertips, not the palmer surface of hand. Keep fingers moving over uterus as contraction proceeds. Assess contraction during its increment, acme, and decrement. Compare sensations with descriptions of mild, moderate, and strong. Assess mother's response to the phases of the contraction. Assess the contractions for frequency, regularity, duration, and intensity.	Fingertips are more sensitive. Adds to data on total uterine contraction pattern. The uterus begins to contract in the fundal area. Ability to indent the uterus varies: ■ Increment: progressively less easy to indent. ■ Acme: uterus feels firm, even hard. ■ Decrement: progressively more easy to indent. Maternal response is related to the sensation of discomfort. Therefore maternal subjective description may not be as accurate as the nurse's objective assessment.
Electronic Monitoring Device See Fetal Monitoring, Chapter 16	
Charting 1. Gravida's description: write gravida's subjective description on admission record. On admission record also write in time and date when contractions began. 2. Palpation of uterine contractions: intensity, frequency, regularity, and duration are entered in abbreviated form as follows: Contr mild to moderate, q5-10 min, 30-45 s. 3. Electronic monitoring device: see Fetal Monitoring, Chapter 16.	Provides data base against which to compare future findings. Provides data base for implementation of the next steps in the nursing process. Promotes collaboration with other members of the health team.

fined (Table 15.3). The character of the woman's uterine contractions and her behavior and appearance correlate with the phase of labor she is experiencing.

The woman's response to labor may also be reflected in vital signs and blood pressure. Fear, anxiety, and fatigue can cause alterations in the baseline findings. Continued fetal well-being is monitored through assessment of the FHR and of the character of the amniotic fluid discharge.

Careful assessment provides the cues for selection and implementation of nursing actions. *The nurse assumes much of the responsibility for making the assessment of progress. It is the nurse's responsibility to keep the physician informed about progress and any deviations from normal findings.*

Uterine contractions, cervical dilatation, and descent. A general characteristic of effective labor is regular uterine activity. Uterine activity is not directly related to labor progress. Minimal activity may cause rapid progress in some women. For other women a large amount of uterine activity may produce slow progress or no progress. Several methods available for evaluation of uterine contractions are presented in Procedure 15.7.

Table 15.2
Minimal assessment of Progress of First Stage of Labor

	Cervical Dilatation		
	0-5 cm	**6-7 cm**	**8-10 cm**
Vital signs*	Every 4 h	Every 4 h	Every 4 h
Blood pressure	Every 60 min	Every 30 min	Every 30 min
Contractions	Every 30 min to 1 h	Every 15 min	Every 5-10 min
FHR	Every 15 min†	Every 15 min†	Every 5 min†
Show	Every 60 min	Every 30 min	Every 10-15 min
Behavior, appearance, energy level	Every 30 min	Every 15 min	Every 5 min
Vaginal examination‡	To be done only for following reasons: 1. To confirm diagnosis when symptoms indicate change (e.g., strength, duration, or frequency of contractions; increase in amount of bloody show; membranes rupture; or woman feels pressure on her rectum) 2. To determine whether dilatation and descent are sufficient for administration of anesthetic 3. To reassess progress if labor takes longer than expected 4. To determine station of presenting part		

*If membranes have ruptured, check temperature every 2 hours.
†For a period of 30 seconds immediately after a uterine contraction (Zuspan and others, 1982).
‡In presence of vaginal bleeding, physician performs vaginal examination, usually under double setup.

Table 15.3
Maternal Progress in First Stage of Labor Within Normal Limits

Criterion	Phases Marked by Cervical Dilatation*		
	0-3 cm	**4-7 cm**	**8-10 cm Transition**
Duration	About 8-10 h	About 3 h	About 1-2 h
Contractions			
Magnitude (strength)	Mild	Moderate	Strong to expulsive
Rhythm	Irregular	More regular	Regular
Frequency	5-30 min apart	3-5 min apart	2-3 min apart
Duration	10-30 s	30-45 s	45-60 (few to 90) s
Descent			
Station of presenting part	Nulliparous: 0 Multiparous: 0 to −2 cm	About +1 to +2 cm About +1 to +2 cm	+2 to +3 cm +2 to +3 cm
Show			
Color	Brownish discharge, mucus plug or pale, pink mucus	Pink to bloody mucus	Bloody mucus
Amount	Scant	Scant to moderate	Copious
Behavior and appearance	Excited; thoughts center on self, labor, and baby; may be talkative or mute, calm or tense; some apprehension; pain controlled fairly well; alert, follows directions readily; open to instructions	Becoming more serious, doubtful of control of pain, more apprehensive; desires companionship and encouragement; attention more inner directed; fatigue evidenced; malar flush; has some difficulty following directions	Pain described as severe; backache common; feelings of frustration, fear of loss of control, and irritability surface; vague in communications; amnesia between contractions; writhing with contractions; nausea and vomiting, especially if hyperventilating; hyperesthesia; circumoral pallor, perspiration on forehead and upper lips; shaking tremor of thighs; feeling of need to defecate, pressure on anus

*The pace of progress in cervical dilatation (according to Friedman and Sachtleben, 1965) varies as follows: from 0 to 2 cm (**latent phase**), progress is slow; from 2 to 4 cm (**phase of acceleration**), pace quickens; from 4 to 9 cm (**phase of maximal acceleration**), pace is most rapid; and from 9 to 10 cm (**phase of deceleration**), pace slows again (Figs. 15.9 and 15.10).
In the nullipara, effacement is often complete before dilatation begins; in the multipara, it occurs simultaneously with dilatation.

Fig. 15.9
Partogram showing relationship between dilatation and descent of presenting part. **A,**
Nulliparous labor. **B,** Multiparous labor. (**B** adapted from Friedman, E.A., and Sachtleben,
M.R.: Am. J. Obstet. Gynecol. 93:522, 1965.)

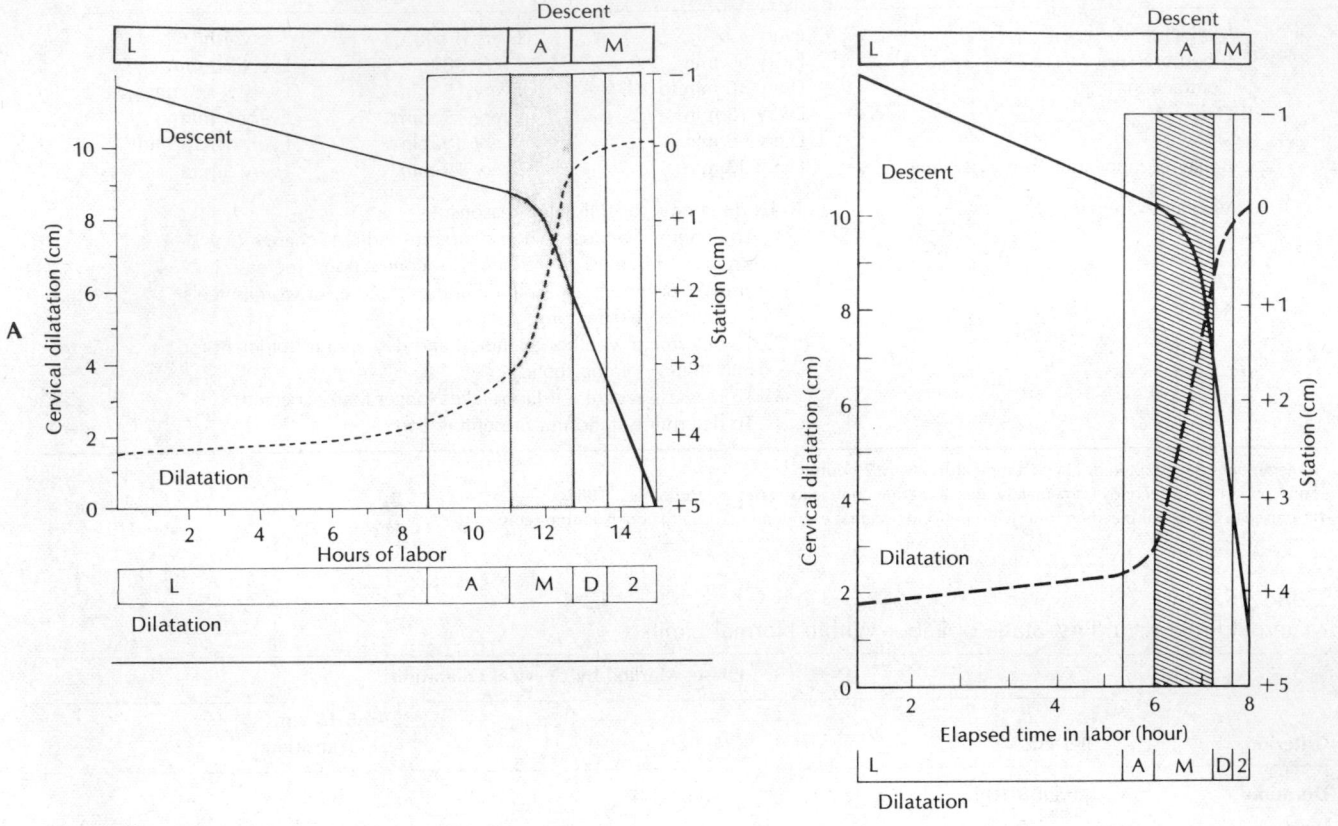

Any time uterine activity is discussed it must be related to (1) its effect on progress in cervical effacement and dilatation and descent of the presenting part and (2) its effect on the fetus (see Fetal Monitoring). Graphing labor progress with both cervical dilatation and station (descent) of the presenting part validates the normalcy of labor progress. It also facilitates early identification of deviations from normal patterns. The normal pattern of cervical dilatation and descent in a nulliparous labor is shown in Fig. 15.9, *A*. The pattern in a parous labor is shown in Fig. 15.9, *B*.

Each time an assessment is made, the findings are plotted on the **partogram** (a graphic chart) and a pattern emerges (Fig. 15.10). Nurses are expected to record findings on a partogram. In addition, nurses are responsible for notifying the physician should an abnormal pattern begin to emerge. Therefore an understanding of the partogram is necessary. As a result of the clinical research of Friedman and Sachtleben (1965) a standardized graph was developed. The early

recognition of normal and abnormal labor patterns has been facilitated.

Cervical effacement. Effacement precedes cervical dilatation in the nullipara. It often accompanies dilatation in the multipara. The process of effacement plays a role in dilatation. As the cervix is retracted upward, it becomes a part of the lower uterine segment. The "taking up" of the cervix reduces the length of the cervix from about 2 cm to a few millimeters when it is 100% effaced. This upward pull on fibers of the lower uterus and downward push on the fetus presses the presenting part onto the cervix. As uterine contraction and retraction continue, the cervical os dilates (opens) progressively. Effacement does not appear on the partogram.

Cervical dilatation. On the partogram the phases of cervical dilatation are identified by the letters L, A, M, and D. The "2" refers to the second stage of labor. The **latent phase** (L) of the first stage of labor is that time between the onset of labor and onset of accelera-

Fig. 15.10

Partogram for assessment of patterns of cervical dilatation and descent. Individual woman's labor patterns (*red*) superimposed on prepared graph (*black*) for comparison. **A,** Nulliparous labor. **B,** Multiparous labor.

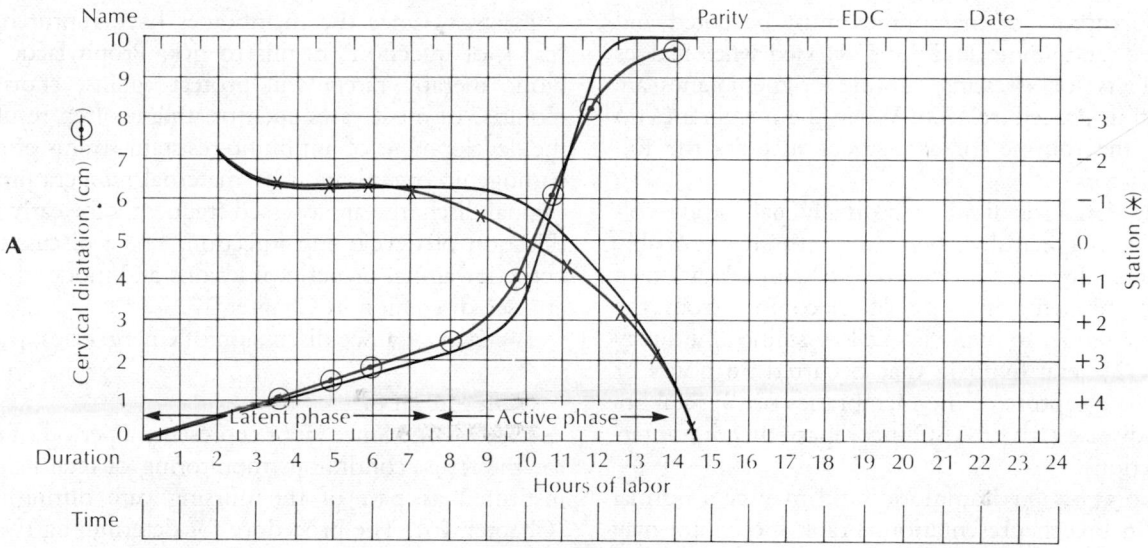

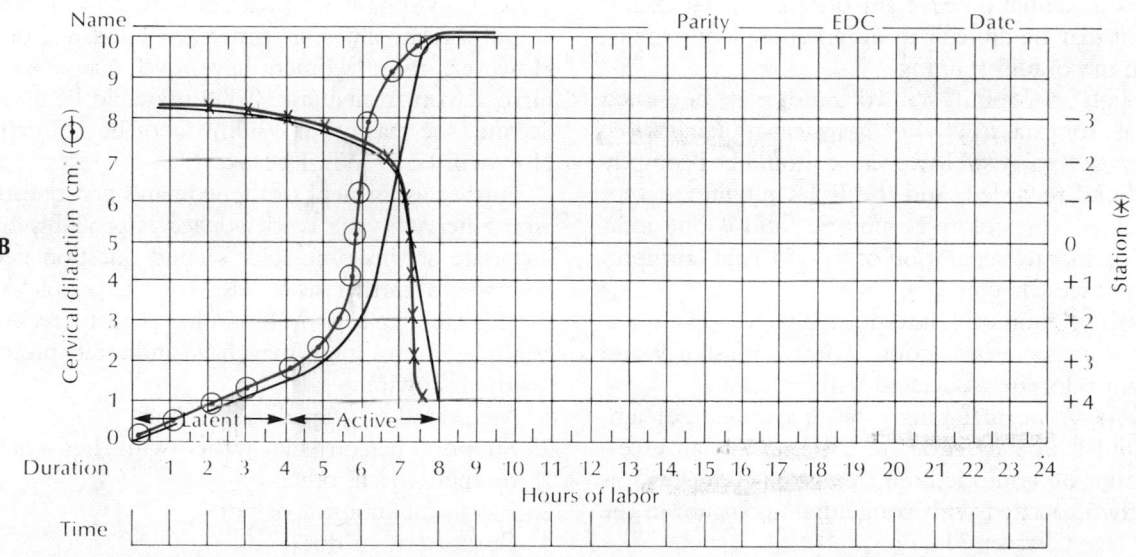

tion. The **active phase** spans the time between the upswing of the dilatation curve and complete cervical dilatation. The active phase is subdivided into three parts: (1) *acceleration* (A), (2) *linear phase of maximum slope* (M), and (3) *deceleration* (D). The dotted line in Fig. 15.9 denotes cervical dilatation. In Fig. 15.10 the rate of dilatation is indicated by the symbol Ø. A line drawn through the symbols reveals the slope of the curve.

Descent. Located over the graph are the letters L, A, and M. The L refers to the latent phase of minimal descent. **Active descent** (A) generally begins when the cervical dilatation curve reaches its phase of maximum slope. The rate of descent reaches its maximum at the beginning of the deceleration phase of cervical dilatation. **Maximum descent** (M) continues in a linear manner until the perineum is reached (Zuspan and Quilligan, 1982). In Fig. 15.9 the solid line shows the rate of descent. In Fig. 15.10, station is indicated with an x. A line drawn through the xs reveals the pattern of descent.

Rupture of membranes and amniotic fluid. Rupture of membranes may occur at any time during labor. The rupture of membranes must be noted and confirmed, and amniotic fluid is assessed when it does occur. Tests for assessing rupture of membranes are discussed in Procedure 15.6. When the membranes do rupture, the routine for assessment includes the following factors.

Color. Amniotic fluid is normally pale straw colored. If it is greenish brown, the fetus has probably undergone a hypoxic episode resulting in relaxation of the anal sphincter. Passage of meconium from the bowel is a sequel to hypoxia. Yellow-stained fluid may indicate (1) fetal hypoxia that occurred 36 hours or more before rupture of the membranes or (2) fetal hemolytic disease (Rh or ABO incompatibility, intrauterine infection).

Meconium-stained amniotic fluid may be a normal finding in breech presentation. Frank meconium may often be seen exuding into the birth canal. However, even in the case of a breech presentation the passage of meconium may indicate fetal distress and not just pressure on the fetal rectum. If an iodine preparation is used as a vaginal disinfectant during vaginal examinations, it may be difficult to differentiate iodine staining from meconium staining.

Although meconium-stained fluid may be noted with fetal asphyxia, *its presence is not always diagnostic of prospective fetal distress.* However, it should be promptly reported and recorded, and the FHR monitored very closely. Port wine-colored amniotic fluid is one indicator of premature separation of the placenta (abruptio placentae) (see Chapter 27).

Character. Amniotic fluid normally looks like water and has a characteristic odor. Thick consistency and unpleasant odor are associated with infection.

Amount. A normal range for the amount of amniotic fluid is 500 to 1200 ml. *Hydramnios,* an excessive amount of amniotic fluid (more than 2000 ml), is frequently associated with congenital anomalies in the neonate (see Chapter 31).

Oligohydramnios, an abnormally small amount or virtual absence of amniotic fluid (less than 500 ml) may be accompanied by such abnormalities as agenesis or malformation of the ears. In the presence of oligohydramnios, genitourinary tract anomalies, particularly renal agenesis may be seen (see Chapter 31).

The nurse should not be too quick to diagnose oligohydramnios or hydramnios on the basis of the amount that trickles or gushes out when the membranes rupture or are ruptured artificially. The engaged vertex may prevent the escape of amniotic fluid.

Complications. Complications associated with ruptured membranes may include infection and prolapsed cord.

Infection. Once the membranes have ruptured, the "clock of infection" begins to tick. Prophylactic antibiotic therapy rarely will protect against chorioamnionitis. In most cases such treatment often results in the development of antibiotic-resistant strains of many pathogenic organisms. The maternal temperature and vaginal discharge are assessed frequently for early identification of developing infection. For a discussion of herpetic vaginal or perineal lesions and mode of delivery, see discussion in Chapter 27.

Prolapsed cord. See discussion of emergencies, p. 389.

Stress in labor

Fetal stress. Since labor represents a period of stress for the fetus, continuous monitoring of fetal health is instituted as part of the nursing care during labor (Chapter 16). The procedure for determining the area of maximal intensity (MI) of the FHR is given in Procedure 15.3.

Maternal stress. Women and their families approach labor with a feeling of satisfaction that the preparatory phase of pregnancy is now at an end; within a relatively short time their child will be born. However, most women have two major concerns: First, a woman may ask, "Will my child be all right?" Second, she may ask, "Will my labor be as I expected? How will I act? Will I be okay?"

Further assessment of the woman's first question by asking her why she is so worried is probably not appropriate at this time. Her second question needs to be assessed further now. Her (or the couple's) goals for this labor may be noted in her prenatal record. For example, she or they may have indicated preferences for the following:

1. Medicated or unmedicated labor
2. Support person she wants with her—husband, mother, coach, other
3. Electronic monitor or not
4. Episiotomy or not

Some women and couples want an active role in decision making; others want to leave it all in the hands of the physicians and nurses. Each individual has her or his own self-expectations and expectations of others. Regardless of the actual labor and delivery experience, the woman's or couple's *perception of the birth experience* is most positive if she or they evaluate the events and performance as meeting expectations.

Women from various cultures are taught from

childhood the "right" way to behave during labor. They are taught that they should moan, scream, remain silent, or be totally anesthetized, depending on the culture. If a woman can follow through with the social expectations of her culture, she perceives herself as having mastery, as having had control over her labor. Her self-esteem receives a boost.

The woman's level of anxiety may rise when she does not understand what is being said. Observe the facial expression and body language of the woman who has just been examined vaginally when the physician, within the parturient's hearing, tells the nurse, "She's a primigravida, EDC 2 weeks from now. She's 50% effaced but I can barely get a fingertip in there. She has bloody show but she'll have to drop the head some yet. If her membranes don't break by themselves, I'll pop them myself. The contractions are weak now; they'll have to get a lot harder to get the job done." To the nurse, the physician may say, "Do a mini-prep on her." Understandably, the woman who is unfamiliar with these terms could panic. Many of the terms—bloody show, drop the head, membranes break—sound violent and could conjure up thoughts of injury or pain. If she had thought that her "weak" contractions were uncomfortable, she may become tense anticipating the more intense uterine contractions that are needed "to get the job done."

The woman's or couple's body language, facial expressions, and verbal cues (such as "Huh?" "What's wrong?") are all noted by the observant nurse. Symptoms and signs of discomfort are described and discussed in Chapter 14 (pp. 365 and 367).

Paternal stress. The father's behavior is also assessed. Is he hesitant to go into the labor room? Does he appear confident? Does he appear aggressive or hostile as he strides into the labor room? (He may be asserting his felt need to be with his wife or just covering up his anxieties.) Is he hungry? (He could faint from low blood sugar.) Is he sleepy, red eyed, or glassy eyed from fatigue? Does he look worried? Does he pull back and say that he is "just an onlooker" (observer)?

The nurse assesses the father's and mother's perception and preference as to the type and amount of participation he is to have. Is he prepared through classes? Which kind? How does the couple interpret information given them in classes (for example, does natural childbirth mean the woman is not to receive medication?) Does he want to provide comfort measures? Which comfort measures does he need to learn? Is he considering accompanying her at the birth?

Has the father been on a hospital tour? Does he want a tour? Is he oriented to the unit? To this hospital? Which questions does he have regarding the mother's room, delivery area, nursery, and postdelivery care?

Nursing Diagnoses

Nursing diagnoses lend direction to types of nursing actions needed to implement a plan of care. Before establishing nursing diagnoses, the nurse analyzes the significance of findings collected during assessment.
1. Initial assessment
   a. *Prenatal record:* Impaired verbal communication related to foreign language barrier
   b. *Interview:* Knowledge deficit related to lack of previous experience or preparation-for-parenthood classes
   c. *Physical examination:* Anxiety related to knowledge deficit regarding physical examination procedures
   d. *Laboratory tests:* Potential for injury related to lack of prenatal testing of blood and urine
2. Subsequent assessments
   a. Alteration in comfort-pain related to bedrest
   b. Fluid volume deficit related to decreased fluid intake
   c. Impaired gas exchange related to hyperventilation
   d. Impaired physical mobility related to station of fetal presenting part, status of fetal membranes, or fetal monitoring
   e. Alteration in pattern of urinary elimination related to bed rest, lack of privacy, analgesia, or anesthesia
3. Assessment of stress during labor
   a. Impaired gas exchange, fetal, related to maternal position
   b. Spiritual distress, maternal, related to inability to meet expectations of self
   c. Ineffective family coping related to knowledge deficit of comfort measures that can be used for parturient

Planning

During this important step, goals are set in client-centered terms, and the goals are prioritized. Nursing actions are selected, with the client where appropriate, to meet the goals. The speed and accuracy with which planning is accomplished depends on the nurse's level of competence (Chapter 2).

Goals

1. To confirm labor
2. To identify any abnormalities that would interfere with normal progress and fetal and maternal health and to intervene appropriately
3. To support the woman's and her family's degree of involvement and participation in this momentous event in their lives

Implementation

Procedures

General nursing actions. Standards of care guide the nurse in preparing for and implementing procedures with the maternity client (Chapter 3). The reasonably prudent nurse is expected to know and follow hospital policies and protocols. The nursing student gains competency by reviewing general nursing techniques, practicing manual skills in simulated laboratory settings, reading hospital protocols, and requesting supervision as needed. Protocols for care include guidelines such as the following:

1. Check the physician's orders.
2. Assess the physician's orders for appropriateness and accuracy; for example, see When Not to Give an Enema.
3. Read labels on any solutions, ointments, or other material used in the procedure.
4. If sterilized packs of supplies are needed, check for sterility by noting appropriate indicator for sterility (such as disks or crystals that change color or diagonal black stripes over the tape) and the expiration date.
5. Examine prepackaged supplies, such as intravenous fluid bags and bottles. Check for defects (cracks in bottle) and possible contamination (floating particles).
6. Check the woman's identification band and hospital number.
7. Use a nurturing approach to the woman:
   a. Explain procedure and purpose.
   b. Use a calm manner and gentleness in carrying out necessary procedures.
   c. Accept the woman's definition of discomfort or pain.

Procedure 15.8

PREPARATION OF THE VULVA AND THE MINI-PREP

PURPOSE

1. To cleanse the vulva
2. To shave or cut pubic and perineal hair to facilitate repair and curtail infection

EQUIPMENT

1. Soap
2. Water
3. Bedpan prn
4. Razor (sterile, disposable) or scissors

NURSING ACTION	RATIONALE
Cleanse vulvar area with soap solution or nonirritating detergent preparation: ■ On admission ■ After elimination ■ After vaginal examination ■ For vaginal discharge	Maintains cleanliness. Curtails infection. Promotes comfort.
If voided urine specimen is indicated, obtain after cleansing vulva. Check the physician's orders. A mini-prep varies with the hospital and physician. It is either a clipping of vulvar hair with scissors or a shaving of a very small area between the vagina and the anus, the site for episiotomies.	Minimizes potential for contamination with vaginal discharge. Shaving is undesirable because even in expert hands the razor leaves nicks and scrapes that serve as portals of entry for infection. There may be small warts or moles that could be cut inadvertently. The procedure is uncomfortable, especially if the woman is trying to work with her contractions.
If a shave is ordered: ■ Use extreme care in shaving. ■ Explain to the woman that she may experience itching as the hair grows back.	Regrowth of the hair is accompanied by itching.

d. Repeat instructions as needed.
e. Modify the time taken to carry out procedures as needed.
f. Make woman comfortable before leaving the bedside. Put call bell close at hand, and clean up area.
g. Wash hands.
8. Complete follow-up work; for example, label specimens, chart procedure completion and maternal response, and initial the chart entry.

The procedures as presented can be used for teaching clients and their families. For each procedure, the purpose, equipment needed, nursing actions and rationales can be shared with the woman. The procedures that follow can be categorized under protective nursing interventions (Chapter 4). The procedures include preparation of the vulva and the mini-prep (Procedure 15.8), enema (Procedure 15.9), and intravenous therapy (Procedure 15.10).

Times Not to Give an Enema

1. Vaginal bleeding
2. Premature labor
3. Presenting part not engaged or abnormal (e.g., breech, transverse lie)

Emergency interventions

Prolapsed cord. Prolapse of the umbilical cord is displacement of the cord downward, often below the presenting part (Fig. 15.11). Occasionally, the cord may even slip through the cervix into the vagina or beyond. A long, loose cord and an unengaged presenting part or breech presentation, frequently associated with rupture of membranes, may allow prolapse of the cord. When membranes rupture, the cord may be carried downward with a sudden gush of fluid. The gravida

Procedure 15.9

GIVING AN ENEMA

PURPOSE
1. To add to the space available for stretching of the birth canal by emptying the bowel
2. To prevent bowel movements later in labor
3. To stimulate uterine contractions*

EQUIPMENT
1. Gloves, nonsterile
2. Extra lubricant
3. Toilet tissue
4. Enema kit
5. Bedpan

NURSING ACTION	RATIONALE
Assess for: ■ Vaginal bleeding	Enemas may stimulate uterine contractions. If vaginal bleeding is caused by a placenta previa (Chapter 27), contractions could result in cervical dilatation, separation of the placenta, and life threatening complications to the fetus especially hemorrhage.
■ Premature labor ■ Fetal station and lie	Labor could be stimulated. If the presenting part is not yet engaged, uterine contractions could cause rupture of membranes and possible prolapsed uterine cord.
Assess for diarrhea prior to admission. If it occurred, alert the physician.	If the onset of labor was preceded by diarrhea, there is no need for the enema. Enemas do add to the discomfort and unpleasantness of labor.
During vaginal examination, note distension of rectum with stool. Record and report findings. When an enema is necessary because of a full rectum, follow hospital protocol for enema solution. A physiologic solution is preferable.	A full rectum could impede the progress of the fetus through the vaginal canal. Use of soapsuds enemas is controversial. Soapsuds enemas have been implicated in soapsuds emboli and damage to intestinal mucosa (Mitchell, 1981).
Several prepared formulas in individual dose bottles are available commercially. Give enema according to directions on the label. Give fluid slowly *between* contractions.	Minimizes discomfort.

*Enemas are *not* used to stimulate labor. The infamous "3H" enema ("high, hot, and hell of a lot") has no place in obstetrics (Pritchard and others, 1985).

Procedure 15.10

INTRAVENOUS THERAPY

PURPOSE

1. To provide fluids and calories if the woman is unable to take anything by mouth for a period of time
2. To prevent dehydration that can result in fatigue, increased temperature, and generalized discomfort
3. To provide a ready "life line" if complications occur and the woman requires fluids for the treatment of hypovolemic shock, or if she needs medications
4. To ensure adequate hydration in the event she requires anesthesia

EQUIPMENT

Equipment and infusate as required by hospital protocol and manufacturer's specifications

NURSING ACTION	RATIONALE
Assess woman's status: ■ Desire for nonmedicated labor ■ Physical condition ■ Ability to take oral fluids	Each woman should be evaluated as an individual. Intravenous fluids are not necessary for every woman in labor. The woman whose labor is progressing normally, who is able to take oral clear fluids with sugar, and who is planning to receive no analgesics or anesthesia is not usually in need of intravenous fluids.
Check physician's orders. If parturient has an intravenous line in place, the nurse follows hospital's protocols for its care.	Maintains standard of care.
The protocols may include the following: ■ Recheck physician's order with label on solution container. Monitor flow rate accurately and record level of solution every hour. Check for possible contamination of solution (cloudy or discolored fluid). ■ On the tape at the venipuncture site, write the type of needle that is in place, the date and time it was placed, and initial it. ■ Check security and comfort of tape. ■ Inform woman of purpose and importance of fluid therapy. Caution her to avoid touching or lying on the tubing. ■ Check patency of all tubing and position of extremity. ■ Check venipuncture site for pain, warmth, redness, swelling, leakage of fluid or oozing of blood; assess for elevated temperature, tachycardia, and hypotension. ■ Assess for headache, tachycardia, neck vein distension, elevated blood pressure, respiratory distress, shortness of breath, shock, and pulmonary edema.	Assures accuracy of type of fluid and drip rate. Prevents adverse response to contaminant, such as infection, allergy, disseminated intravascular coagulation (DIC). Alerts staff so proper technique is employed when needle is removed. Promotes comfort and protects venipuncture site. Meets knowledge needs. Respects gravida's right to know. Enlists woman's participation in her care. Assures infusion of fluid. Alerts staff to possible complications, such as **infection, thrombosis,** and **infiltration.** These are **symptoms of fluid overload,** which requires prompt medical attention.

may feel the cord slither into the vagina when the membranes rupture. More often, vaginal examination by an alert nurse or physician immediately after a sudden gush of fluid may lead to the diagnosis of prolapsed cord. Prompt recognition of prolapse of the cord, which occurs in 1 of every 400 late pregnancies and more often in immature gestations (under 37 weeks), is important. The cord may become compressed between the presenting part and the bony pelvis. Fetal hypoxia from prolonged cord compression (more than 5 minutes) usually causes central nervous system (CNS) damage or death of the fetus.

Both Trendelenburg's position and the vaginal support of the presenting part to keep the presenting part away from the prolapsed cord are continuously maintained until delivery is accomplished (see box p. 392 and Fig. 15.12). Immediate cesarean birth is indicated unless the cervix is fully dilated. If the cervix is dilated sufficiently, rapid forceps delivery of a vertex or extraction of a breech presentation may be feasible. Prompt

Fig. 15.11

Prolapse of umbilical cord. Note pressure of presenting part on umbilical cord, which endangers fetal circulation. **A,** Occult (hidden) prolapse of cord. **B,** Complete prolapse of cord. Note membranes are intact. **C,** Cord presenting in front of fetal head and may be seen within vagina. **D,** Frank breech presentation with prolapsed cord.

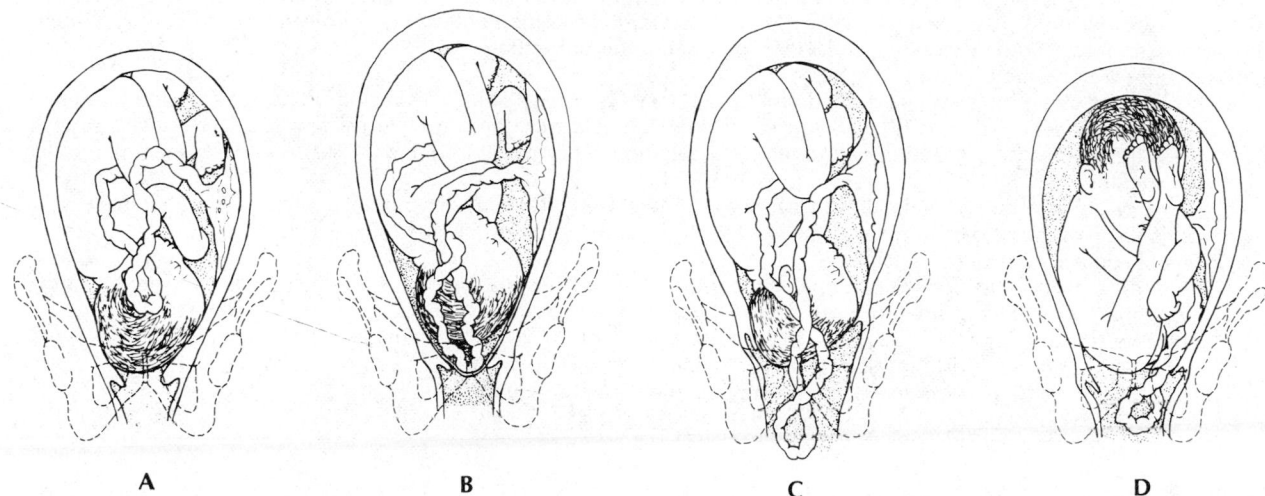

A   B   C   D

Fig. 15.12

Arrow indicates direction of pressure of examiner's fingers against presenting part to relieve compression of prolapsed umbilical cord in vertex presentation, **A,** and in breech position, **B.** Modified Sims' position helps relieve pressure of presenting part on prolapsed umbilical cord. NOTE: hips are elevated as high as possible with pillows, **C.**

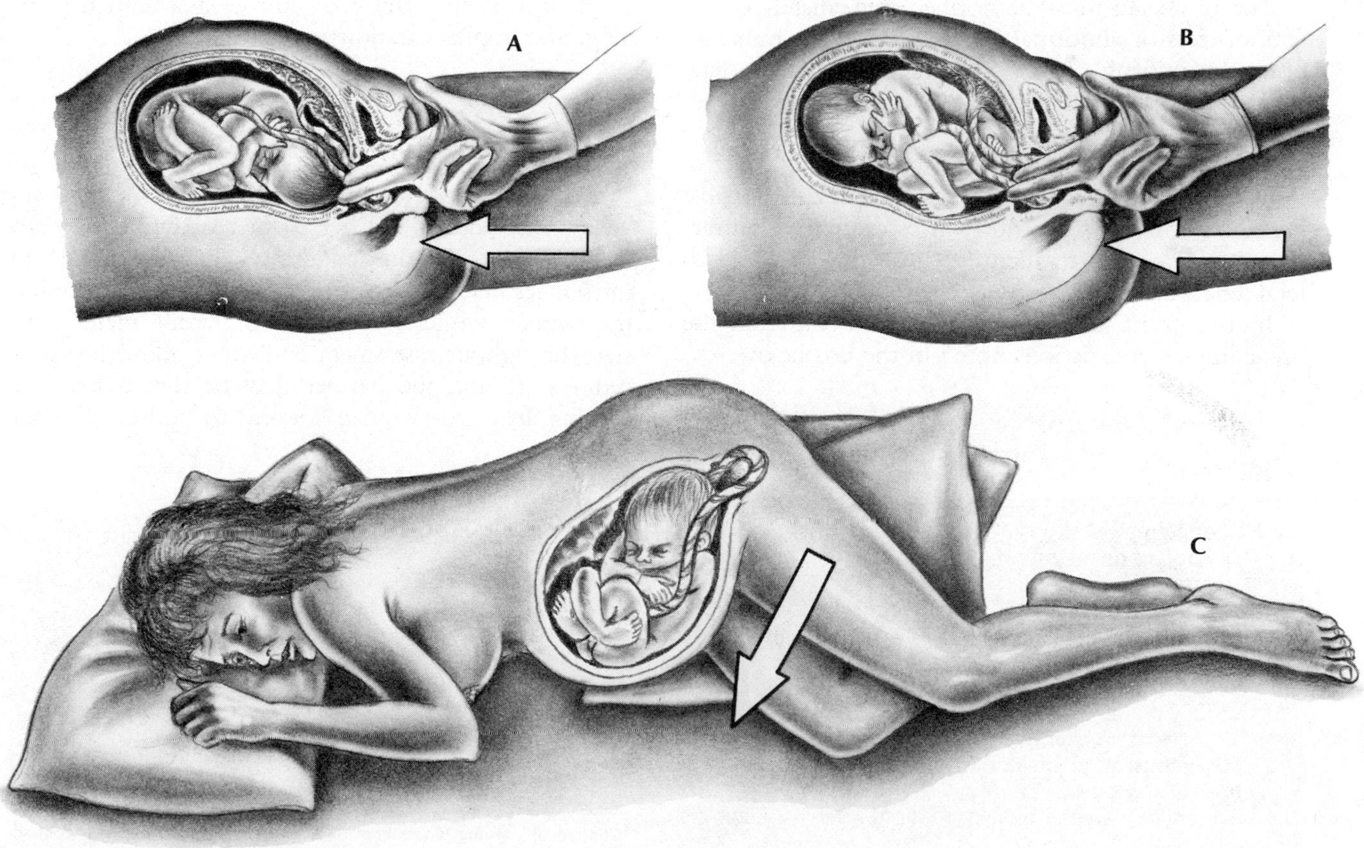

Rupture of Membranes and Prolapse of Cord

1. Auscultate FHR immediatedly after rupture of the membranes and perform a vaginal examination. If no prolapse is evident at that time, reassess FHR within 10 minutes; strong uterine contractions stimulated by rupturing of membranes can force the cord down to, beside, or in front of the presenting part.
2. If prolapse is suspected, immediately:
   a. If possible, glove the examining hand rapidly and insert two fingers into the vagina to the cervix. With one finger on either side of the cord or both fingers to one side—do not compress the cord with fingers—exert upward pressure against the presenting part to relieve the compression of the cord (Fig. 15.12, A and B), keeping a rolled towel under her right hip.
   b. Assist or direct others to assist the woman into extreme Trendelenburg's or modified Sims' position so that gravity pulls the presenting part down and thus relieves the compression of the cord (Fig. 15.12, C).
   c. Direct someone to notify physician.
3. If the cord is protruding from the vagina, direct others to wrap it loosely in a sterile towel wet with sterile normal saline while you maintain upward pressure against presenting part.
4. Direct others to apply a face mask for oxygen. Give oxygen at 10 to 12 L/min until delivery is accomplished.
5. Direct others to increase drip rate of maintenance intravenous fluid.
6. Direct others to prepare for delivery, including possible cesarean delivery.

delivery in the manner least harmful to mother and infant is imperative.

Fetal distress or abnormal FHR pattern. Fetal distress may occur in the absence of prolapsed cord. If distress is noted, the nurse implements the measures given in the box below.

The physician must be notified immediately of the fetal distress or abnormal FHR pattern. The nurse reports the nursing actions implemented, and the fetal response to the interventions recorded. For further discussion, see Chapter 16.

Inadequate uterine relaxation. Uterine contractions can be stressful to the fetus. To prevent possible damage to the fetus, the nurse assesses uterine contractions continuously to identify those that can lead to fetal jeopardy.

In the event of inadequate uterine relaxation the nurse implements actions noted in the box below.

Fetal Distress or Abnormal FHR Patterns

1. Change maternal position:
   a. For late deceleration, place mother in the left lateral position.
   b. For prolapsed cord, place mother in Trendelenburg's, modified Sims', or any other position that corrects the problem.
2. Correct maternal hypotension:
   a. Elevate her legs.
   b. Increase rate of maintenance IV.
3. Stop stimulation of uterine contractions by discontinuing oxytocin infusion.
4. Administer oxygen by face mask at 10 to 12 L/min.

Evaluation

Evaluation of outcomes is an ongoing activity. During each encounter with the parturient and her family the nurse evaluates the degree to which goals for care are being met. If the evaluation shows that results fall short of achieving any goal, further assessment, planning, and implementation are warranted.

Motherhood with Dignity

Admission to the labor unit. First impressions are vivid. The woman and her partner or family need to feel welcome. The nurse addresses them by name and introduces herself. The nurse then determines whether the woman wishes her partner or family member to stay throughout assessment and other admission procedures. If not, the partner may be directed to the waiting area. The woman is asked to undress and get

Inadequate Uterine Relaxation*

1. Change maternal position.
2. Stop stimulation of uterine contractions by discontinuing oxytocin infusion.
3. Notify physician.
4. Administer oxygen by face mask at 10 to 12 L/min until physician arrives and permits oxygen to be discontinued.

*Contractions lasting longer than 90 seconds; relaxation between contractions inadequate or less than 30 seconds.

into bed. Her personal belongings are put away safely. For legal reasons, most hospitals have a check list or other method of recording her belongings that becomes part of her permanent record. If the woman prefers to wear some items of her own (such as knee socks), these are noted on her chart.

Her understanding of the use of the call bell (or light) is checked. She is told the reasons that bathroom privileges are permitted or not. If the membranes have ruptured, have her remain in bed until assessment for potential prolapse of the umbilical cord is completed. The routine of care is reviewed, that is, which techniques will be used to assess progress, the reasons for using them, and how the woman or couple may assist in reporting her progress. For the minimal schedule for assessment of progress during the first stage of labor, see Table 15.2.

If the woman has not already done so, she signs the necessary papers giving permission for care for herself and her newborn. Her identification bracelet is secured. Legally a permit for care must be signed before the woman receives any medication for discomfort or any procedures are done to her.

If parking is a problem at that facility, the nurse inquires if she came by car and where the car is parked. The nurse may need to advise a family member to repark the car, or, as in a recent case where the woman drove in herself and therefore could not repark the car, the nurse must inform the hospital's security forces. Some women, especially those who arrive in labor unexpectedly (for example, directly from the physician's office), welcome the offer of a telephone to notify their families. In some instances the nurse may have to make the calls to the family.

Do not increase the woman's anxiety by quizzing her about her understanding of terms commonly used during labor. As the nurse reviews the woman's prenatal record, the nurse can add short definitions or explanations for technical terms and abbreviations. The woman's interest and response serve to guide the nurse in choosing the depth and breadth of the explanations. The nurse's openness and willingness to explain can be reassurance in itself—it indicates to the woman and her family that there need be no "secrets."

Fluid intake, voiding, bowel elimination, and general hygiene. Intake, elimination, and general hygiene are basic human needs. The parturient has the same needs. However, nursing care of the parturient is modified somewhat. A summary of nursing actions and rationales is presented in Table 15.4.

Maternal position during labor. The position women assume during labor and birth has not been dictated as much by physiology as by culturally patterned behavior. Women may walk, stand, squat, sit, or kneel (Fig. 15.13, A). There is no "right" position; each has a positive and a negative effect. For example, the squatting position in the second stage of labor enlarges the pelvic outlet and makes use of the forces of gravity; however, if assumed before engagement, it impedes descent. Research has shown that women in the upright position during labor (Fig. 15.13, B) and birth have stronger and more efficient contractions. This results in shorter labor duration, and increased comfort.

The dorsal recumbent or semirecumbent position came into use in the nineteenth century with the advent of the obstetric forceps. It is still advocated in most developed countries because it is more conve-

Table 15.4
Fluid Intake, Voiding, Bowel Elimination, and General Hygiene: Nursing Actions and Rationales

Need	Nursing Actions	Rationale
Oral	Per physician's orders: Offer clear fluids, which are fluids you can see through, tea with honey and lemon, homemade broth (not salt-loaded bouillon), apple juice, and lollipops are examples of clear fluids.	Meets standard of care Provides hydration Provides calories Warm teas are used by many cultural groups to counteract the effects of heat loss during labor and delivery. Absorb quickly and are less likely to be vomited. Provides positive emotional experience.
	Offer small amounts of ice chips, if ordered.	Deters vomiting and its potential sequelae, aspiration and tracheal irritation.
IV	Establish and maintain IV, which is often 5% dextrose in Ringer's lactated solution.	See Procedure 15.10, IV therapy.
NPO	Inform family of NPO and rationale.	A precautionary measure if anesthesia is a possibility. Deters vomiting and its possible sequelae.
	Provide mouth care.	Promotes comfort.

Continued.

Table 15.4, cont'd

Fluid Intake, Voiding, Bowel Elimination, and General Hygiene: Nursing Actions and Rationales

Need	Nursing Actions	Rationale
Voiding	Encourage voiding at least every 2 hours.	A full bladder may impede descent of presenting part. Overdistension may cause bladder atony and injury and difficulty in voiding postnatally.
Ambulatory	Ambulate to bathroom per physician's orders, *if*	Reinforces normal process of labor.
	■ The presenting part is engaged, or	Precautionary measure against prolapse of umbilical cord.
	■ The membranes are not ruptured, and	
	■ The woman is not medicated.	Precautionary measure against injury.
Bedrest	Offer bedpan.	Prevents hazards of bladder distension and ambulation.
	Turn on the tap water to run; pour warm water over the vulva; and give positive suggestion.	Encourages voiding.
	Provide privacy.	Shows respect for gravida.
	Put up side rails on bed.	Prevents injury from fall because of narrow bed or medication effects.
	Place call bell within reach.	
	Offer washcloth for hands	Maintains cleanliness and comfort.
	Wash vulvar area.	Maintains standard of care.
Catheterization	Catheterize per physician's order using hospital protocols.	Prevents hazards of bladder distension.
	Insert catheter between contractions.	Minimizes discomfort.
	Avoid force if obstacle to insertion is noted.	"Obstacle" may be due to compression of urethra by presenting part.
	If presenting part is low, introduce 2 fingers of free hand into introitus to apply upward pressure on presenting part while other hand inserts the catheter.	Minimizes potential for injury and subsequent infection to urethra.
Bowel elimination	After careful assessment an *experienced* nurse ambulates woman to bathroom or offers and retrieves bedpan.	Women often misinterpret rectal pressure from the presenting part as the need to defecate.
General hygiene		Improves woman's morale and comfort. Maintains cleanliness.
Showers/bed baths	Assess for progress in labor.	Determines appropriateness for the activity.
	Supervise showers closely if gravida is in true labor	Prevents injury from fall.
		Labor may accelerate.
	Suggest allowing warm water to strike lower back.	Aids relaxation.
		Increases comfort.
Vulva	See Procedure 15.8.	
Oral hygiene	Offer every hour. Offer toothbrush, mouthwash, or wash the teeth with an ice-cold wet washcloth.	Refreshes mouth.
		Improves morale.
		Helps counteract the dry, thirsty feeling, a complaint of many women.
Hair	Comb, braid per gravida's wishes	Improves morale.
		Helps maintain a "nonsick" attitude.
Hand-washing	Offer washcloths before and after voiding and prn.	Maintains cleanliness.
		Improves morale and comfort.
Gowns/linens	Change prn; fluff pillows.	Improves morale and comfort, probably through the **Hawthorn effect.**
		The Hawthorn effect is the "phenomenon that occurs when a person in pain begins to feel more comfortable as the nurse talks soothingly, fluffs a pillow, and promises to stay nearby. Positive support, especially by one in authority, enhances the ability to cope with stress" (Jimenez, 1983).

Fig. 15.13
Maternal positions for labor. **A,** Squatting. **B,** Walking with husband.
(Courtesy Marjorie Pyle, RNC, Lifecircle, Costa Mesa, California.)

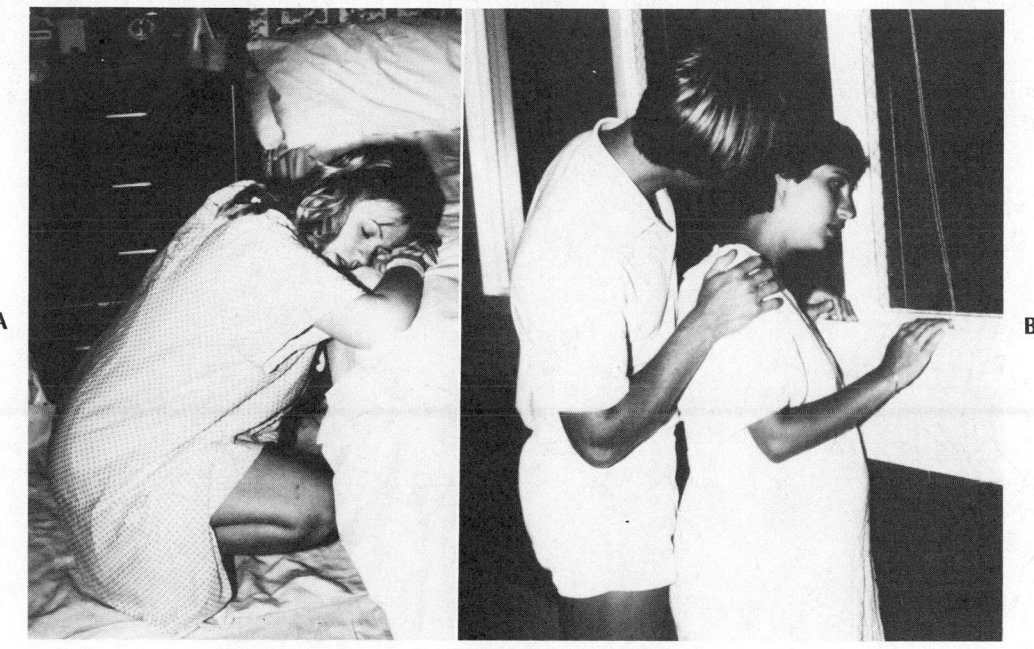

nient for auscultation of the fetal heart, administration of anesthetics, application of forceps, and management of postdelivery hemorrhage. However, this position* results in the development of supine hypotension (Fig. 15.14). The weight of the gravid uterus compresses the ascending vena cava, impeding blood return to the right atrium with a resultant drop in cardiac output and maternal hypotension. To maintain placental perfusion the systolic pressure (brachial artery) must remain above 100 mm Hg. To minimize this danger, any woman who desires or is required to remain in bed during labor should assume a left lateral position. If she prefers to lie supine, she should have a wedge placed under the right hip to maintain a tilt to the left. She is encouraged to assume a sitting position (45-degree angle) as much as possible.

Many authorities are now suggesting that women in labor walk and assume any position that feels comfortable. Delivery occurs with the woman supported in a semisitting or semireclining position, her feet resting on the bed and her legs supported with pillows. Beds and chairs are now designed to function both for labor

and for birth (Fig. 13.9). The traditional delivery table is still widely used, however.

Much research is presently being directed toward a better understanding of the physiologic and psychic effects of maternal position in labor. It is important to appreciate that clinical entities such as fetal presentations or mechanisms of labor may be helped or hindered by maternal posture.

Support measures. Important components of the nursing care of the woman in labor relate to (1) helping the parturient participate to the extent she wishes in the delivery of her infant, (2) meeting her goals for herself, (3) helping her conserve her energy, and (4) helping to control her discomfort.

An understanding, competent nurse acts as an advocate for the woman and her family. Couples who have attended childbirth education programs using the psychoprophylactic approach will know something about the labor process, coaching techniques, and comfort measures (see Chapter 13). However, the staff's role is to be supportive and keep them informed of progress. Even if the couple has not attended such classes, the various techniques may be taught to a degree during the early phase of labor. The nurse will be expected to do more of the coaching and give suppor-

---

*For other factors that impede circulation to the maternal-fetal-placental unit, see discussion of fetal monitoring, Chapter 16.

Fig. 15.14
Supine hypotension—Vena cava syndrome. Note relationship of gravid uterus to ascending vena cava in standing posture, **A,** and in supine posture. Note how enlarged uterus compresses vena cava, especially during contraction, **B,** reducing return of blood to heart. Reduced cardiac output causes maternal hypotension and reduced flow of blood to placenta, with consequent fetal distress. **C,** Compression of aorta and inferior vena cava with woman in supine position. **D,** Use of a wedge pillow placed under woman's right side to shift weight of fetus off woman's aorta and inferior vena cava.

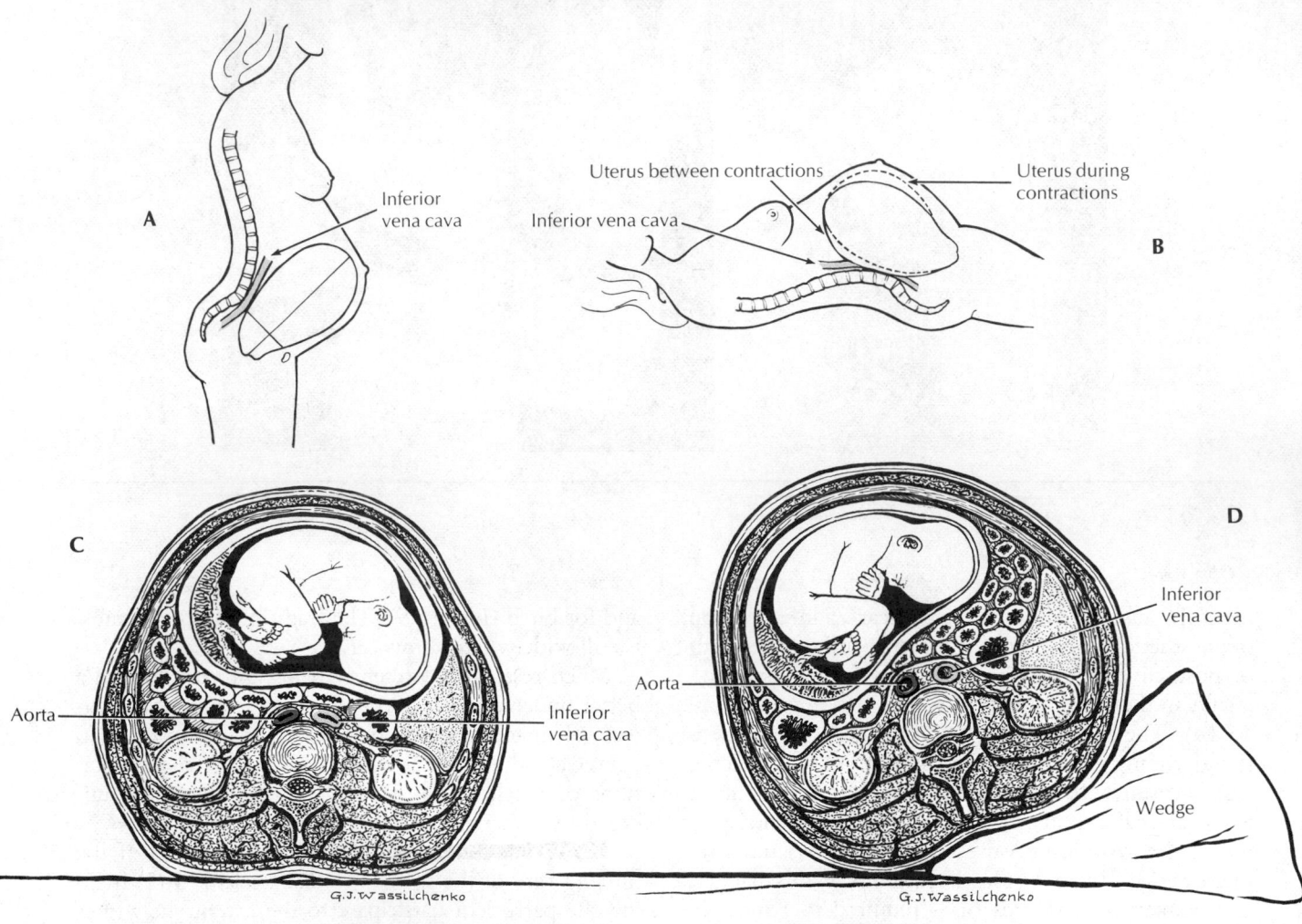

tive care. If the women is alone, the nursing staff acts as the substitute family. Staff members coach and support her. They help her use her energy constructively in relaxing and working with the contractions.

Comfort measures vary with the situation (Fig. 15.15). The nurse can draw on the couple's repertoire of comfort measures learned during the pregnancy. The comfort measures to be discussed below include maintaining a comfortable, supportive atmosphere in the labor and delivery area; using touch therapeutically; nonpharmacologic management of discomfort; and administering analgesics when necessary; but, most of all, just *being there*.

Atmosphere of the labor and delivery area. Labor rooms need to be light and airy. However, the bright overhead lights are turned off when not needed. The area should be large enough to accommodate the woman's partner in a comfortable chair, as well as the monitoring equipment and hospital personnel. In some hospitals, couples are urged to bring extra pil-

Fig. 15.15
Father providing comfort by supplying warmth with an extra blanket, **A,** and with a cool cloth to forehead, **B.**

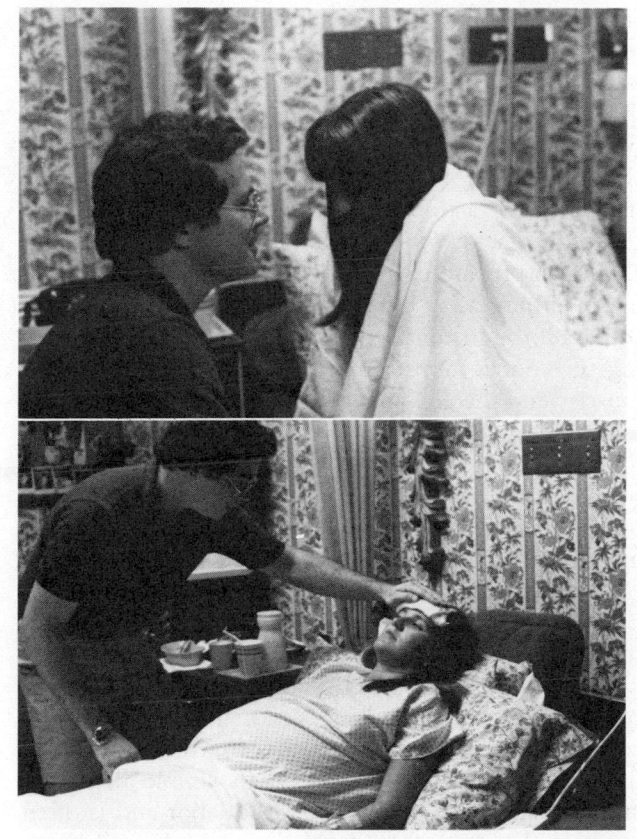

lows to help make the hospital surrounding more homelike. Labor areas *should be constructed with windows* that can be hung with colorful curtains. When people stay in any area for a period of time and do not have access to a view of the outside world, it is easy to become disoriented to time and to focus unnaturally on whatever is happening to them.

The room temperature is kept at a comfortable level—between 20° and 22.2° C (68° and 72° F). Although most women feel very warm during labor, a number complain of feeling cold. A warm blanket placed over the woman and one wrapped around her feet are comforting. Many women wish to wear socks. For those who feel too warm, a cool moist cloth placed on the forehead can be soothing, as can ice chips given for sucking (where permissible) (Fig. 15.15).

Touch. Most women respond positively to touch in labor. They appreciate gentle handling by the staff. Effleurage (pp. 401-402) may be effective in helping them relax between contractions. Counterpressure against the sacrum during a contraction results in relief from discomfort (Fig. 15.16). Back rubs, including over the sacral area and the buttocks (especially for women who have been in labor a long time), every hour or two and as necessary between contractions help to ease tension. If possible, warm foot baths followed by foot massage can result in general body relaxation.

The woman's awareness of the soothing qualities of touch changes as labor progresses. Many women develop hyperesthesia (increased sensitivity, especially in the skin) as labor progresses. They may tell their coach

Fig. 15.16
Father applies sacral pressure with a tennis ball while nurse provides verbal encouragement. (Courtesy Marjorie Pyle RNC, Lifecircle, Costa Mesa, California.)

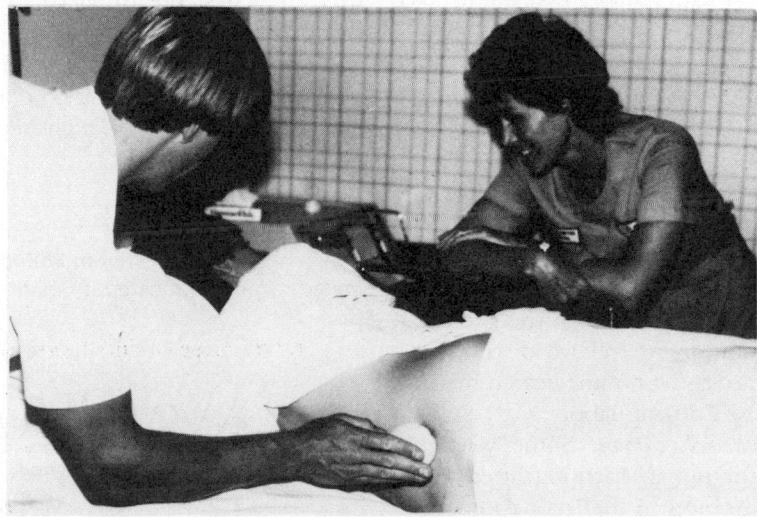

to "leave me alone," or they may say, "Don't touch me." The partner who is unprepared for this normal response may feel rejected and may react by withdrawing active support. The nurse can point out that this response on the part of the woman is a positive indication that the first stage is ending and that the transitional stage is approaching. The woman's aggressive behavior is accepted; negative comments toward the woman are unwarranted and inappropriate.

Sound is the touching of sound waves against the tympanic membrane of the ear. The nurse can use soft tones in speaking to the woman. Even firm commands to breathe a certain way or to pant-breathe to avoid pushing at the wrong time can be done without resorting to harsh, vibrant speech.

The manner in which a woman is touched during her labor is often reflected in the manner in which she touches others. This may influence her response toward her infant after birth. She must be mothered in order to mother.

Nonpharmacologic management of discomfort. The alleviation of pain is important. Frequently it is not the amount of pain the woman experiences, but *whether or not she meets her goals for herself in coping with the pain* that influences her perception of the birth experience as "good" or "bad." The observant nurse looks for cues to identify the woman's desired level of control in the management of pain and its relief.

The origins of discomfort during labor, the symptomatology of pain, pain threshold, and the gate control theory of pain are discussed in Chapter 14. Pharmacologic control of discomfort is discussed in Chapter 16. The pain associated with parturition was accepted as a necessary part of childbirth until the discovery of the first anesthetics, nitrous oxide and ethyl ether. Since that time much research has gone into the development of methods of pain control that can bring effective relief for the mother without harm to the child. The perfect solution is yet to be found; therefore at times the safety of the child must take precedence over the comfort of the mother.

Nonmedicated methods of relief of discomfort are taught in many different types of prenatal preparation classes. In Chapter 13, three methods are described: Dick-Read, Lamaze, and Bradley. Whether or not a woman or couple has attended these classes or read from the various books and magazines on the subject, the nurse can teach techniques to relieve discomfort during labor. Following are some nonmedicated methods of managing discomfort during labor.

Focusing and feedback relaxation. Some women bring a favorite device for use in focusing attention. Others choose some fixed object in the labor room. As the contraction begins, they may focus on this object to reduce their perception of pain. This technique, coupled with feedback relaxation, helps the woman work with her contractions rather than against them. The coach monitors this process, giving the woman cues as to when to begin the breathing techniques. After the degree of relaxation has been assessed, she can be reminded to use relaxation techniques practiced in the prenatal period. The coach also keeps her from being disturbed by routine examination for progress or checking of FHR. These procedures are postponed until the contraction is completed.

Breathing techniques. Different approaches to childbirth preparation stress varying techniques for using breathing as a "tool" to help the woman maintain control through contractions. In the first stage, breathing techniques can promote relaxation of abdominal muscles and thereby increase the size of the abdominal cavity. This lessens friction and discomfort between the uterus and the abdominal wall. Since the muscles of the genital area also become more relaxed, they do not interfere with descent. In the second stage, breathing is used to increase abdominal pressure and thereby assist in expelling the fetus. It is also used to relax the pudendal muscles to prevent precipitate expulsion of the head.

For those couples who have prepared for labor by practicing such techniques, occasional reminders to the couple may be all that is necessary. For those who have had no preparation, instruction in simple breathing and relaxation can be given early in labor and is often surprisingly successful. Motivation is high, and learning readiness is enhanced by the reality of labor.

Cervical dilatation to 3 cm. As the woman feels the onset of a contraction, she takes a deep, cleansing breath in through the nose and out through pursed lips. Then she is encouraged to concentrate on slow, rhythmic chest breathing (6 to 9 breaths per minute) through the contraction (Fig. 15.17). When the contraction is over, she takes a final deep breath in and then "blows the contraction away" through pursed lips. She may focus on a chosen fixed point or simply close her eyes.

Fig. 15.17

Slow chest breathing. (From Phillips, C.R.: Family-centered maternity/newborn care, St. Louis, 1980, The C.V. Mosby Co.)

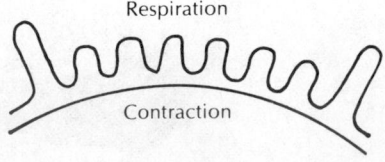

Respiration

Contraction

Cervical dilatation of 4 to 7 cm. Breathing during this phase is similar to that advocated in the early phase. When cervical dilatation reaches 5 cm, some women begin to concentrate seriously on the strength of the contractions and the discomfort accompanying them. At this time a change to shallower, lighter breathing can be suggested (no more than 16 breaths per minute to prevent hyperventilation). Other women can be helped by changing to slow abdominal breathing. Another technique that is often successful is to have the woman slowly raise her abdomen as she breathes in, following the support person's hand "up the ceiling" (if she is supine) or "out to the side of the bed" (if she is in side-lying position). This focusing mechanism results in the lifting of the abdominal wall away from the contracting uterus.

Cervical dilatation of 8 to 10 cm: transition. The most difficult time to maintain control during contractions comes when cervical dilatation reaches 8 to 10 cm. This period is also called the **transition period.** Even for the woman who has prepared for labor, concentration on breathing techniques is difficult to maintain. The type used may be the 4:1 pattern: breath, breath, breath, breath, puff (as though blowing out a candle). This ratio may increase to 6:1 or 8:1. These patterns begin with the routine cleansing breath and end with a deep breath exhaled to "blow the contraction away." An undesirable side effect of this type of breathing may be **hyperventilation.** The woman must be aware of the accompanying symptoms of the resultant **respiratory alkalosis:** lightheadedness, dizziness, tingling of fingers, or circumoral numbness. Alkalosis may be overcome by having the women breathe into a paper bag that is tightly held around the mouth and nose. This enables her to rebreathe carbon dioxide and replace the bicarbonate ion. She can breathe into her cupped hands if no bag is available.

As the fetal head reaches the pelvic floor, the woman will experience the urge to push and will automatically begin to exert downward pressure by contracting her abdominal muscles. Descent cannot continue until the cervix is fully dilated and the presenting part is free to move down the birth canal. *Pushing before full dilatation* is reached compresses the cervix between the fetal head and the pubic bone. This compression *may result in fetal distress or in cervical edema.* It may even slow the dilatation process. The women can control the urge to push by taking panting breaths or by slowly exhaling through pursed lips. This is good practice for the type of breathing to be used as the fetal head is slowly delivered.

Transcutaneous electrical nerve stimulation (TENS). The application of pressure to or rubbing of a part of the body that is sore is an age-old remedy to relieve discomfort. Effleurage and sacral pressure or massage are two methods that have brought relief to many women during the first stage of labor. The gate control theory may supply the reason for the effectiveness of these measures (Chapter 14). TENS may operate on the same principle. TENS may also be effective because of the "placebo effect"; that is, confidence in TENS may stimulate the release of endogenous opiates (enkephalins) in the woman's body and thus alleviate the discomfort.

Two pairs of electrodes are taped on either side of the thoracic and sacral spine. Continuous mild electrical currents are applied from a battery-operated device. During a contraction the woman increases the stimulation by turning control knobs on the device. Women describe the sensation as a tingling or buzzing and pain relief as good or very good. The use of TENS poses no risk to the mother or fetus. TENS is credited with reducing or eliminating the need for analgesia and with increasing the woman's perception of control over experience.

The nurse assists the mother who is using TENS by explaining the device and its use, by carefully placing and securing the electrodes, and by closely evaluating its effectiveness.

Sociocultural aspects of coping and helping. The quality of the nurse-client relationship is a factor in the woman's ability to cope with the discomfort of the labor process. A competent nurse who is aware of sociocultural aspects of helping and coping acts as a protective agent for the woman. The responsibility for initiating and maintaining such a therapeutic relationship rests with the nurse.

An area in which the nurse and the pregnant woman from different cultures could misunderstand each other is pain (Table 15.5).

A study of nurses from the United States, Japan, Puerto Rico, Korea, Thailand, and Taiwan revealed that nurses from diverse cultures make different inferences about physical pain and psychologic distress (Davitz and others, 1977). Reviewing these nurses' responses to a questionnaire composed of vignettes describing different client situations, it was found that Korean and Japanese nurses in this sample made the highest inferences of physical pain. Taiwanese nurses inferred a moderate degree of physical pain with the smallest variability in ratings. Regarding psychologic distress, Korean and Puerto Rican nurses inferred the greatest degree of psychologic discomfort. Nurses sampled from the United States were midway between the other national groups and showed the smallest variability. Taiwanese nurses inferred the least suffering of all the groups.

An important implication of these findings is that

Table 15.5
Sociocultural Basis of Pain Experience

	Woman in Labor	Nurse
Perception of meaning	Origin: Cultural concept of and personal experience with pain; for example: Pain in childbirth is inevitable, something to be borne Pain in childbirth can be avoided completely Pain in childbirth is punishment for sin Pain in childbirth can be controlled	Origin: Cultural concept of and personal experience with pain; in addition, nurse becomes accustomed to working with certain "expected" pain trajectories. For example, in obstetrics, pain is expected to increase as labor progresses, be intermittent in character, and have end point; relief can be derived from drugs once labor is well established and fetus or newborn can cope with amount and elimination of drug; relief can also come from woman's knowledge and attitude and support from family or friends
Coping mechanisms	Woman may do the following: Be traditionally vocal or nonvocal; crying out or groaning or both may be part of ritual of her response to pain Use counterstimulation to minimize pain; for example, rubbing, applying heat, or counterpressure Have learned to use relaxation, distraction, autosuggestion as pain-countering techniques Resist any use of "needles" as modes of administering pain relief	Nurse may do the following: Have learned to use self effectively; for example, tone of voice, closeness in space, touch, as media for message of interest and caring Use avoidance, belittling, or other distancing actions as protective devise for self Use pharmacologic resources at hand judiciously Be skilled in use of comfort measures Assume accountability for control and management of pain
Expectations of others	Nurse may be seen as someone who will accept woman's statement of pain and act as her advocate Medical personnel may be expected to relieve woman of all pain sensations Nurse may be expected to be interested, gentle, kindly, and accepting of behavior exhibited	Nurse may accept only certain verbal or nonverbal behaviors as responses to pain Nurse may expect couple who are prepared for childbirth to refuse medication and to wish to "do everything on their own" Nurse may find it difficult to accept woman's definition of pain; that is, woman may wish to experience and participate in controlling pain or may not be able to accept any pain as reasonable

Oriental national groups differ among themselves in terms of response to pain, just as one would expect groups from various Western societies to differ. A Puerto Rican nurse interestingly interpreted these findings to indicate that the amount of physical pain cannot always be judged by the woman's behavior. This nurse stated that pregnant Puerto Rican women might be very emotional despite the absence of unusual labor pains (Davitz and others, 1977).

Indochinese women walk around during labor and do not ask for medications. These women and others exert great self-control, to the point that the nurse may not recognize an impending delivery (Hollingsworth, 1980). Black women frequently find comfort in having another woman such as a mother or sister pray with them during the discomfort of labor. Based on these data, the nurse need not label clients from the same cultural group as alike in their responses to pain. Not all Orientals are stoic, nor do all Western people respond to pain in the same manner. Mormons have a special rule not to behave badly and not to cry out

during labor and delivery. The Mormon woman must remember that she is of pioneer stock and should behave as a strong woman (Stark, 1982). Zborowski (1952) found that people of Irish, Jewish, Italian, and "old American" descent respond to pain differently. Although Irish clients may admit that they are suffering to relatives and friends, when in pain, these clients tended to prefer to suffer in physical isolation. Old Americans of Anglo-Saxon origin, usually of Protestant faith, and whose ancestors came to the United States more than three generations ago, did not express their pain. They tended to be precise in describing their pain. However, when their pain became severe, they withdrew from people and cried only when alone.

Zborowski reported that Italian and Jewish people had a low tolerance for pain and were emotional in expressing pain. People from these two groups demanded instant relief and gave an impression of having extraordinary sensitivity. Apparently, Jewish clients' intense reactions to pain were intended to mobilize others (doctors, family members) to give them the best possible care. This purpose did not seem to be a major concern to Italian clients, who were reluctant to complain for fear that this would drive family members and friends away. When compared to Jewish clients, Italians were more concerned with the immediate amelioration of pain and its effects rather than with any future-oriented reason.

General nursing actions. Even if the laboring woman and her partner (or family or support persons) are well prepared, the nurse remains an important member of the childbirth team. Labor is a crisis time, and all people, no matter how well prepared, enter labor with some level of anxiety. The following are some helpful actions that the nurse as a support person can use to offer both verbal and practical support during labor:

1. Remember that labor is stressful, even if the couple is prepared. Continually encourage relaxation. They need you. Do not leave them totally alone. Provide support when they need it—and privacy when they need it.

2. Minimize adverse environmental stimuli. Control glaring lights. Decrease traffic flow and noise in the birth setting.

3. Remind the mother that she is to select the *position* in which she feels most comfortable during labor and to change her position whenever she wishes. Encourage walking in early labor.

4. Provide privacy and a space with adequate room temperature and ventilation.

5. Talk of contractions, not pains. Remember, the woman is having "contractions!"

6. Relax and get as near to the woman's level as possible. Sit by the bedside. Do not tower over her. Touch!

7. Adjust the labor bed to provide a comfortable position (usually elevating the top of the bed to 45 degrees). She should never be flat on her back because the weight of the uterine contents puts too much pressure on major blood vessels, thus reducing the blood flow back to the brain. Use pillows to support all dependent body parts.

8. Use comfort measures such as cold cloths, backrubs, and ice chips. Showers or tub baths may be taken depending on the progress of labor. Allowing warm water to strike the lower part of the back may be very relaxing.

9. Try **effleurage** (a light rhythmic stroking over the woman's abdomen in rhythm with breathing during contractions). Effleurage is best done by the woman herself, although it may be done for her.

10. Carry on a conversation only between contractions if necessary.

11. Talk with the father or other support **person.** Give reassurance and remember that the **father** has needs for nourishment, rest, and elimination as well as the mother. Let him know where the bathroom is and where he may purchase food. Also, reassure him that you will stay with the laboring woman if he needs to leave for a while to tend to his own needs.

12. Do not ask irrelevant questions. Keep talk to a minimum. It uses energy needed to cope. Be aware of attitudinal changes as labor progresses.

13. Keep your voice well modulated at all times.

14. Remind the mother to urinate frequently. A full bladder can slow down the descent of the baby.

15. Encourage rest between contractions.

16. Keep the couple informed of what is happening: how many centimeters dilated, station, effacement, and fetal position.

17. Assure the mother she is doing well, offer encouragement, agree with her if she says it hurts but offer positive comments, too.

18. Do not distract her during contractions. Wait until a contraction is over to do a nursing procedure.

19. Remember that transition (8 to 10 cm) may be the most intense time during labor. Because the woman may fall asleep between contractions, they may get ahead of her. She may become very irritable.

20. During the actual birth stage, trust her and work with her body. This is not an athletic contest; the goal is pelvic floor release and relaxation. Encourage a series of quick breaths, holding one for 5 seconds while pushing and then taking another breath. Give verbal support such as, "Beautiful! Go with it! Let it flow! Open up below! Soft and loose! Open the door!" You might even give the woman a mirror so that she can watch her own progress as she pushes the baby out.

21. If the couple is giving birth in the delivery room, give the father or other support person the clothes to wear in the delivery room well in advance so that there is no last-minute rush.

22. As you encourage relaxation, encourage *release* toward your touching hand on her body. This will help the woman to increase her body awareness.

23. Always encourage the breathing that *feels* right for each woman. She may have practiced one type of breathing before labor only to find that it is not helpful during a certain part of labor. If this happens, be flexible. Encourage her to find what is working for her and stick with it.

24. There is no failure! Some people who have prepared faithfully for a "natural" childbirth will not be able to achieve that goal because of circumstances beyond their control. They may need analgesia, anesthesia, or a cesarean birth. If they are disappointed,

Table 15.6
Summary of Woman's Expected Responses and Support Person's Actions by Phase of Cervical Dilatation

	Woman	Support Person
Dilatation of cervix 0-3 cm		

Contractions 10-30 s long, 5-30 min apart, mild to moderate
Mood: alert, happy, excited, mild anxiety
	Settles into labor room; selects focal point
	Rests or sleeps if possible
	Uses breathing techniques
	  Begin contraction with deep breath in through nose and out through pursed lips
	  Slow chest breathing, 6-9/min through contraction
	  End contraction with deep breath in and out
	Uses effleurage (gentle stroking of abdomen, using both hands, begin at pubes and stroke upward and outward); focusing and relaxation techniques
		Provides encouragement, feedback for relaxation, companionship
		Assists with contractions
		  Alerts woman to the following:
		    Beginning of contraction
		    Time called out at 15 sec, 30, etc.
		    Ending of contraction
		  Uses focusing techniques
		    Concentration on fixed point in room
		    "Listen to me and follow my breathing"
		    "Watch my face"
		  Concentration on breathing technique
		Uses comfort measures
		  Position most comfortable for woman
		  Keeps woman aware of progress, explains procedures and routines
		  Gives praise
		  Offers ataractics as ordered (Chapter 16)

Dilatation of cervix 4-7 cm		

Contractions 30-40 s long, 3-5 min apart, moderate to strong
Mood: seriously labor oriented, concentration and energy needed for contractions, alert, more demanding
	Continues relaxation, focusing techniques
	Uses breathing techniques
	Begin contraction with deep breath in and out, then slow chest breathing until contraction intensifies, then shallow, effortless breathing, moderate pace, high in chest through peaking of contraction; slow chest breathing as contraction subsides
	or
	Use abdominal breathing to raise abdominal wall away from uterus; end contraction with deep breathing in and out
		Acts as buffer, limits assessment techniques to between contractions
		Assists with contractions
		  May need to encourage woman to help her to maintain breathing techniques
		  Uses same instructions
		  Uses same focusing devices as in early phase
		Uses comfort measures
		  Positions woman on side to minimize pressure of uterus on vena cava and aorta
		  Encourages voluntary relaxation of muscles of back, buttocks, thighs, and perineum; effleurage
		  Uses counterpressure to sacrococcygeal area
		  Encourages and praises
		  Keeps woman aware of progress
		  Offers analgesics and anesthetics as ordered
		  Checks bladder, encourages to void
		  Gives mouth care, ice chips

Dilatation of cervix 8-10 cm (transition)		

Contractions 45-60-90 s long, 2-3 min apart, strong
Mood: irritable, intense concentration, symptoms of transition
	Continues relaxation, needs greater concentration to do this
	Breathing techniques
	Uses 4:1 pattern if possible
	Uses panting to overcome response to urge to push
		Stays with woman, provides constant support
		Assists with contractions
		  Probably will need to remind, reassure, and encourage to reestablish breathing pattern and concentration
		  If sedated or drowsy, woman needs warning to begin breathing pattern before contraction becomes too intense
		  If woman begins to push, institutes panting respirations
		Uses comfort measures
		  Accepts woman's inability to comply with instructions
		  Accepts irritable response to helping, such as counterpressure
		  Supports woman who has nausea and vomiting, gives mouth care as needed, gives reassurance regarding symptomatology of end point of first stage
		  Uses countertension techniques (effleurage and voluntary relaxation)
		  Keeps woman aware of progress, tells woman when time to push

encourage them to talk about their disappointment and then help them to work through it by emphasizing that there is no failure. When they have achieved a meaningful and safe birth experience, they have achieved their goal.

25. Throughout the entire labor process be constantly and consistently aware of the needs of the fetus. When the couple has prepared diligently for labor and are extremely intent on what they are doing, it is often easy for the support person to get caught up in that intensity and feel reluctant to do any procedure that might "spoil" their experience. Continually think of yourself as a fetal advocate and use your knowledge and skills to make sound judgments that will lead to a meaningful and safe birth experience for all family members.

26. Share in the couple's joy (or in their grief).

The helpful actions for labor support given in this unit are very useful for all laboring women (Table 15.6). However, if there is no family or friend to support the laboring woman, then the nurse's role becomes even more crucial. A woman should never have to labor alone! If the realities of staffing shortages prevent constant attendance to women laboring alone, seek labor support persons from community volunteer groups. A few days spent in teaching and preparation of these volunteers could provide countless hours of labor support for women alone at this crisis time in their lives. Until labor support groups can be formed, you can communicate openly and honestly with women laboring alone. Inform them of the constraints on your time. Let them know where you will be when you leave their side, how they can communicate with you, and when you will be back.

Women alone or couples who have not attended preparation-for-birth classes can learn relaxation and slow chest breathing techniques with your help during labor. Inform them that there are ways to cope with labor and that you can help them to learn these techniques right then and there. A motivated learner is the best learner, and most laboring women are highly motivated for relief of discomfort.

Fatherhood with Dignity

Miller (1966) remarked, "There is joy in having a baby, and joy is an experience worth sharing." Conception is a psychologic as well as a physiologic experience of a man and woman creating a new life; birth can be no less. Conception is the experience of two people; birth, the experience of three (or more) people.

Involving the father in the birth of his child dispels

feelings of alienation, isolation, impotence, helpless inaction, and insignificance. *Ethnic definition and role expectations govern the type and degree of the individual's involvement.*

Individual preference for the kind of involvement spans a full spectrum of possibilities. One family, recent arrivals from Italy, is a case in point. The father absented himself to the waiting room while the female relatives took turns attending his wife and reporting her progress to him at intervals. After delivery, wife and son were wheeled back to the labor area. The father entered proudly as the female relatives stepped aside. He made what sounded like endearing comments to wife and son and kissed them both; then all the relatives left. The new mother beamed. The students present expressed negative reactions about this father, whose participation in this event was perceived as tangential and unsupportive. One student was assigned to this mother's postdelivery care and to make a home visit. Her report and discussion of her experience with the group clarified the situation as "right" for this family.

Other men seek a different type of involvement. What are their hopes and expectations for this experience for themselves and their wives? What is the nurse's role in relation to their decisions? These questions will be discussed in the following sections.

Birth process as seen through father's eyes. The nurse should recall her feelings the first time she witnessed a woman in active labor. The father's experience can be no less intense. In addition, the woman in labor is not a client to him; she is birthing their baby.

During the delivery he may see the following:

1. Her facial and physical expression of pain; grimace and effort written on her face while pushing
2. Blood, mucus, and watery drainage from her vagina
3. Fecal discharge
4. Bulging perineum just before birth
5. Episiotomy, if done, and repair
6. Delivery by forceps, if used
7. Her postures for vaginal examinations, for observations of the perineum, and for delivery
8. Dry heaves or vomiting

He may hear the following:

1. Her moans and grunts (especially while pushing)
2. Dry heaves or efforts at vomiting
3. Hospital noises (such as call lights, page systems, clanging, sterilizer buzzers, fetal monitoring devices)
4. Protests about fathers who "belong in a waiting room" and who "should leave this to us"
5. Extraneous, irrelevant social or business chatter among staff

He may smell the following:
1. Vaginal drainage
2. Fecal drainage
3. Vomitus (occasionally)
4. Cleaning solutions or anesthetics

With the emergence of the infant, the father will see and hear the following:
1. Small patch of scalp and hair at the introitus
2. Prolonged (usually) emergence of the molded fetal head (one father commented, "and then when all that kept coming out was head and more head and no eyes or ears, I wondered when they would come")
3. Blue-purple coloration of the fetal scalp and body along with blood, amniotic fluid, vernix, and occasionally meconium
4. Cord being loosened around the child's neck and or being eased over his head or shoulders
5. Mucus draining from nose and mouth and the physician or nurse suctioning the infant
6. Sounds of suctioning
7. Cutting the cord
8. Verbal communications between physician and nurse regarding position, cord, placement of episiotomy, and similar medical matters in terms often unfamiliar to him

Father in labor suite. "He'll just be underfoot." "He'll add confusion and increase the chance of infections and the number of lawsuits." These typical statements for years kept the father apart from his wife and child. These fears proved largely unfounded when fathers were reunited with their laboring wives. Fathers proved helpful, comforting, and reassuring to their wives. There was no change in the incidence of infection or lawsuits. Furthermore, it was found that it was easier for the physician and parents to cope with the birth of a child with a defect when both parents were active participants on an adult-to-adult level with the physician.

The father may be an adjunct to the nurse-physician team in several ways. For example, he may assist with comfort measures such as pillows, ice chips, washcloths to forehead, and back rubs. He may provide almost constant companionship to offset the aloneness of labor and the anxiety it can foster. Should something occur when the nurse or physician is out of the room, the father can call for help. In addition, he is usually better equipped to interpret the mother's wishes and needs to the staff.

Participation in the birth is ego building. The father *can* be of assistance; his presence *is* important. It is frequently observed that a caring person can be his or her weight in Demerol (meperidine). Recently a 16-year-old unwed mother in labor with her first child thrashed about, moaning and screaming with each contraction. A nurse remained at her bedside, coaching and comforting to no avail. The unwed adolescent father arrived and was immediately escorted into her room. The young woman continued her labor calmly and unmedicated through delivery.

When the father is active and supportive, the mother turns to him. The physician remains the medical-surgical expert, without his taking on the father-or husband-surrogate role as well. The couple's future relationship and their relationship to their child may be positively influenced. Mutuality is fostered when the mother can turn to the father and say, "I could never have done it without you. You were my pillar of strength."

Supporting the father during labor. Supporting the father* as well as the mother in labor elevates the nurse's role. It is another step forward from merely providing custodial care to enacting a therapeutic role. Supporting the father reflects the nurse's orientation and commitment to the person, the family, and the community. Therapeutic nursing actions convey to the father several important concepts.

First, he is of value as a person. He is not a comic strip character, inept and bungling or idle, nervous, and inconsequential. Second, he can learn to be a partner in the mother's care. Finally, childbearing is a partnership.

Even if the father enters the labor unit without any parent education classes, he can be taught "on the job," and his choices can be supported. The nurse can support the father in the following ways:
1. Regardless of the degree of involvement desired, orient him to the maternity unit, including wife's labor room and what he can do there (sleep, telephone, smoke or not), restroom, cafeteria, Dads' Room, nursery, visiting hours, and names and functions of personnel present.
2. Respect his or their decisions as to his degree of involvement, whether the decision is active participation in the delivery room or just being kept informed. When appropriate, provide data on which he or they can base decisions; offer freedom of choice as opposed to coercion one way or another. This is *their* experience and *their* baby.
3. Indicate to him when his presence has been helpful.
4. Offer to teach him comfort measures to the degree he wants to know them. Reassure him that he is not assuming the responsibility for observation and management of his wife's labor. Supportive behav-

---

*These measures recognize parents' need for the nurse to be psychologically as well as physically present. They may be accomplished by the physician or nurse as the situation warrants.

ior can be classified into three categories:
a. Physical care
b. Nonverbal care (such as holding her hand, smiling, kissing)
c. Verbal care (coaching breathing and relaxation techniques, complimenting)
5. Communicate with him frequently regarding her progress and his needs. Keep father or couple informed of procedures to be done, what to expect from procedures, and what is expected of him.
6. Prepare him for changes in her behavior and physical appearance.
7. Remind him to eat; offer snacks and fluids if possible.
8. Relieve him as necessary; offer blankets if he is to sleep in a chair by the bedside. Acknowledge the stress of the situation on each partner and identify normal responses. The nonjudgmental attitude of staff helps the father and mother accept their own and the other parent's behavior.
9. Attempt to modify or eliminate unsettling stimuli (such as extra noise, extra light, chatter); keep the woman clean and dry.

A well-informed father can make a significant contribution to the health and well-being of the mother and child, their family interrelationship, and his self-esteem. It has been found that a significantly lower percentage of women suffered postdelivery emotional upsets when their partners received support and assistance from prenatal classes, physicians, and nurses throughout the childbearing cycle. This is continued by the care from community health nurses in the home.

Culture and father participation. Many hospitals encourage the father's presence during labor and delivery. If he is not able to be there, another significant person may be present. In several cultures the father may be available, but his presence with the mother may not be appropriate and he may resist involvement at this time. His behavior could be misconstrued by the nursing staff as lack of concern, caring, or interest. Griffith (1982) identifies the importance of the affectional bond between a Mexican woman and her mother and sisters or other female relatives in regard to home-related activities such as childbearing. This is also true for many other groups, and the presence of another woman or women is highly desired. If childbearing occurs in the hospital, at least one woman must be present for assistance. Southeast Asians (Hollingsworth and others, 1980), blacks (Carrington, 1978; Johnson and Snow, 1978), and American Indians (Farris, 1978; Horn, 1982) are some of the major cultural groups indicating a preference for a woman's assistance during childbearing.

According to Pillsbury (1978), the Chinese husband is not allowed in the delivery room, lest he becomes polluted by the woman's blood. A nurse from a different culture might think it odd that a Chinese husband did not seem to have given any emotional support to his wife during labor and delivery. There are various reasons for the husband's behavior: (1) Oriental men are usually embarrassed to show their emotions in public, (2) Oriental men consider childbirth as solely the woman's work, and (3) Oriental women feel embarrassed and uncomfortable about their husbands' involvement with a function that they consider their prerogative (Chung, 1977). Nevertheless, Oriental men have as much emotion as Western men. However, Oriental women have significant others who can provide emotional support—mothers, inlaws, cousins, other members of the extended family, or close friends. In the absence of these significant others the husband provides the wife with as much emotional support as possible (such as interpreting for a wife who doesn't speak English).

In India all attendants at birth are women; men are totally excluded (Flin, 1982). On the other hand, in Guatemala, a husband may assist his wife and the midwife during delivery (Cosminsky, 1982). During the labor process of the Navajo in the Southwestern United States, people passing by the hogan are encouraged to enter and provide support for the mother (Newton, 1972). Because of the wide variation in who comprises the preferred person or persons, it is critical for the nurse to determine from the woman and her family what persons are wanted during labor and delivery.

Grandparenthood with Dignity

Support of grandparents is similar to that provided the father as discussed in the preceding pages. The nurse acts as a role model for parents. By treating grandparents with dignity and respect, by acknowledging the value of their contributions to parental support, and by recognizing the difficulty parents have in witnessing their child's discomfort or crisis, regardless of the child's age.

Of particular value is the availability of another person or persons to relieve the father or coach. This may be necessary to assist the parturient with walking, especially if IV poles are to be pushed; and to help the parturient when she needs two tasks performed simultaneously.

Whenever possible the nurse offers the grandparent emotional support. This can be done by providing liquid refreshment even if unsolicited and by initiating discussion with open-ended questions or statements, such as "It is sometimes hard to watch a daughter in labor. . . ."

These nursing actions are therapeutic for the entire family unit. According to Barnard (1978), "Rather than compete with family members, we can use them, provide support to them, and teach them. The family's influence will far outlast our contact with the client. If we can improve this social unit's ability to care, we will have a powerful health care system indeed." Support for the mother of a laboring woman—mothering *her* mother—is an important place to begin (Stephany, 1983).

Siblings During Labor

Preparation for acceptance of the new child helps with the attachment process. Parents, brothers and sisters, and other extended family members benefit from *cognitive rehearsal* for the new addition to the family. Preparation for and participation during pregnancy and labor may help the older children accept this change. The older child or children become *active* participants who are important to the family (Bliss, 1980). Rehearsal for the event before labor is essential. Preparation for the entire family includes the additional support person who is to be responsible for the older children during the entire childbirth process.

The age and developmental level of the children influence their responses. The child under 2 years of age shows little interest in pregnancy and labor; for the older child the experience may reduce fears and misconceptions. Preparation is adjusted to the age and developmental level of the child. Most parents have a "feel" for the maturational level and ability to cope of their children. Preparation includes description of anticipated sights and sounds. The children must learn that their mother will be working hard. She will not be able to talk to them during contractions. She may groan and pant at times. Labor is uncomfortable, but their mother's body is made for the job. The sights, sounds, smells, and behavior of participants will be similar to those for which fathers are prepared (pp. 403 to 405). The film *Nicholas and the baby* is available for preparing older preschool and school-age children for participation in the birth experience.

Leonard and associates (1979) observed the behavior of children present during labor, delivery, and the postpartum period. In general the preschool-age children tended to interact eagerly with their parents during early labor. They were seen to withdraw from the happenings as labor progressed. None of the children seemed to become acutely distressed during the expe-

rience. Other researchers (Anderson, 1979) report similar findings.

Preparation for Giving Birth in the Delivery Room

If any parturient, nullipara or multipara, states, **"The baby is coming!"** it is too late for the transfer. The baby is coming *now*—prepare to assist her if the physician is not yet present. See When the Nurse Must Assist the Woman to Give Birth, pp. 465 to 471.

The delivery room attendant is responsible for seeing that the facility is properly prepared and that all supplies and equipment are in working order at all times. The role of the woman's partner is reviewed and suitable operating room clothing provided. It is essential that the woman's record be up-to-date, because her condition can change quickly.

All nursing care and the woman's or couple's responses must be recorded to (1) ensure continuity of care, (2) ensure appropriate assessment of the woman's progress, and (3) document the nursing and other care given. Courts of law insist that the nursing and medical care that is not documented on the client's record has not been given.

The following are suggestions for preparation for delivery. These items may vary among different facilities so that the protocols from each facility's procedure manual should be consulted.

1. Scrubbing facilities, scrub brushes, cuticle sticks, cleaning agent, and masks are available.
2. The following have been done:
   a. Sterile gowns and gloves for physician or nurse-midwife, sterile drapes and towels for draping the woman, and sterile instruments and other supplies (such as bulb syringe, sutures, and anesthetic solutions) are arranged for convenience in use on sterile table.
   b. Sterile basin and water for hand washing during delivery process are readied for use.
   c. Supplies for cleansing vulva are available (sterile basin, sterile water, and cleaning solution).
   d. Delivery area is warmed and free of drafts.
   e. Infant receiving blankets and heated crib are

Transfer to the Delivery Room

Nulliparas	When the presenting part begins to distend the perineum
Multiparas	When they are 8 to 9 cm dilated

readied. Material for prophylactic care of infant's eyes is available (see p. 469).

3. Equipment is in working order: delivery table (bed or chair), overhead lights, and mirror.
4. Emergency equipment, anesthesia, cardioscope, and supplies are available and in working order if needed for emergency situations such as control of maternal hemorrhage or fetal respiratory distress.
5. Additional supplies (anesthetics, oxytocics for injection, and obstetric forceps) are available.
6. Woman's record is up-to-date and ready for use in delivery area. In areas such as labor unit, recordings are made concomitantly as symptoms are noted, assessments are made, and care is given. Since woman's condition can change quickly, it is imperative to have recordings complete at all times.

Summary

The childbearing family has special needs and concerns during the first stage of labor. These needs can only be met by a skillful, knowledgeable, caring provider. The nurse who uses the nursing process as a systematic approach can provide comprehensive nursing care. Consideration of clients' cultural diversity allows the nurse to personalize the approach to the childbearing family. All members of the family unit are given an opportunity to participate in this meaningful event if the woman desires. The first stage of labor sets the stage for the actual birth of the infant.

Summary of Nursing Actions

NURSING CARE DURING THE FIRST STAGE OF LABOR

GOALS
1. For the mother: A safe and satisfying first stage of labor.
2. For the unborn: An uncompromised adjustment to the labor process.
3. For the family: An experience that fulfills their expectations for the first stage of labor.

PRIORITIES
1. Validate onset of true labor.
2. Determine maternal and fetal status.
3. Identify and initiate immediate therapy for deviations from normal labor processes.
4. Facilitate family's achievement of personal goals.

ASSESSMENT	EXAMPLES OF POTENTIAL NURSING DIAGNOSTIC CATEGORIES*
PRIOR TO ADMISSION TO UNIT Review prenatal record if possible.	
Interview A. Health history: family history, medical history, sexual history, obstetric history, present pregnancy. B. Psychosocial history: identifying data such as age. C. Review of systems.	Potential for maternal or fetal compromise† Alteration in health maintenance Ineffective individual or family coping Alteration in family process Impaired verbal communication Spiritual distress Potential alteration in normal physiologic processes† Knowledge deficit
Physical examination Findings during this pregnancy, such as pattern and amount of weight gain, blood pressure, symptomatology experienced, height, nutritional status.	Potential alteration in normal physiologic processes Alteration in health maintenance Alteration in nutrition: less than or more than body requirements
Laboratory tests Hemoglobin, hematocrit, blood type, Rh, CBC, antibody titers; urinalysis; amniocentesis and ultrasound, if done; other.	Potential alteration in normal physiologic processes† Potential for injury Alteration in nutrition: less than or more than body requirements Potential for maternal or fetal compromise† Health maintenance

*Accepted diagnoses from Seventh National Conference (1986) of NANDA, except for those diagnoses carrying a dagger.
†Diagnosis not included by NANDA, 1986.

Continued.

Summary of Nursing Actions—cont'd

ASSESSMENT	EXAMPLES OF POTENTIAL NURSING DIAGNOSTIC CATEGORIES
Following admission to unit	
A. Assess general appearance and behavior.	Anxiety Alterations in comfort: pain Impaired verbal communication Ineffective individual or family coping Alteration in nutrition: less than or more than body requirements
B. Check vital signs and blood pressure (if elevated, repeat 30 minutes after woman has relaxed to obtain true reading).	Anxiety Potential for maternal or fetal compromise†

C. Assess for fetal health status:
  1. FHR: regularity and area of maximum intensity.
  2. Leopold's maneuvers: fetal presentation, lie, position, engagement.
  3. Fetal activity level.
	Potential for fetal compromise†

D. Assess for onset of true labor.	Powerlessness Disturbance in self-concept: body image, self-esteem, role performances, personal identity Knowledge deficit Alteration in comfort: pain Alteration in normal physiologic processes†

E. Assess progression of labor:
  1. Contractions: time begun, intensity, frequency, regularity.
  2. Vaginal discharge, bloody show.
  3. Effacement and dilatation of cervix.
  4. Station of presenting part.
  5. Degree of molding of fetal head (if head is presenting).	

F. Assess status of amniotic membranes:
  1. Bulging.
  2. If ruptured—time; color, character, amount, odor; pH response to Nitrazine paper; ferning present or absent on drying.
	Potential for fetal compromise†

G. Assess bladder distension and presence and amount of stool in rectum.	Potential for maternal compromise† Alteration in normal physiologic processes†

H. Assess for complications:
  1. Inquire regarding symptoms of infection.
  2. Recheck for allergies.
  3. Check for edema.
  4. Obtain specimen of urine for routine analysis and presence of albumin, glucose, and acetone.
  5. Check woman's dietary intake for last 4 hours.
	Potential for maternal or fetal compromise†
	
	Potential for ineffective airway clearance

I. Assess psychologic status and support:
  1. Preparation for childbirth.
  2. Expectations of woman and family.
  3. Response to first stage.
	Knowledge deficit
	Powerlessness
	Disturbance in self-concept: body image, self-esteem, role performance, personal identity
	Ineffective individual or family coping
	Anxiety
	Fear
	Ineffective breathing pattern
	Ineffective relaxation pattern†
	Sensory-perceptual alteration: visual, auditory, kinesthetic, gustatory, tactile, olfactory
	Sleep pattern disturbance

Summary of Nursing Actions—cont'd

OUTCOME CRITERIA*	PLAN/IMPLEMENTATION
Admission routines are completed.	Admit to unit per hospital protocol; ascertain that necessary permits are signed and identification bracelet is accurate and secure.
Woman, family, and personnel establish a therapeutic relationship.	Welcome and greet by name, orient to personnel and unit, and to procedures, as necessary.
Parturient	
A. Vital signs and blood pressure remain within normal limits. 1. Pulse: same as during antepartum period. 2. Respirations: change with use of breathing techniques and discomfort. 3. Blood pressure: may be elevated during a contraction or with excitement. 4. Temperature: does not increase beyond 37.2° C (99° F) as a result of dehydration and labor	Measure vital signs and blood pressure, record findings, and report any deviations from normal limits per hospital protocol and physician directives.
B. Abdominal palpation (Leopold's maneuvers) is performed to determine fetal presentation, position, lie, attitude, and descent.	1. Complete the examination. 2. Include gravida (family) in palpating fetal parts, if appropriate. 3. Share with gravida (family) findings and their significance, as appropriate. 4. Record findings and report as necessary.

C. Maternal progress in labor within normal limits.
1. Baseline data is obtained and recorded.
2. Contractions:
  a. Magnitude: from mild to moderate to strong to expulsive.
  b. Rhythm: from irregular to regular.
  c. Frequency: from one every 30 minutes to one every 2 to 3 minutes.
  d. Duration: from 10 to 60 seconds (few at 90 seconds).
3. Show: from scant, brownish pink mucus to copious bloody mucus.
4. Cervix: 1 to 10 cm dilation; 0-100% effacement.
5. Descent (station): from floating to +2 or +3 cm.
	1. Assist physician or midwife with general and obstetric examinations to determine:
	  a. General health of body systems.
	  b. Diagnosis of true labor.
	  c. Progress of labor.
	  d. Maternal and fetal health status.
	2. Follow medical directives for preparation of vulva, administration of enema.
	3. Monitor contractions by uterine palpation or by electronic monitor; record findings; report deviations from normal limits.
	4. Share findings and their significance with gravida and family, if appropriate.
	5. Record findings and report deviations from normal limits.
	6. Complete vaginal examination using aseptic technique.

D. Membranes: rupture of membranes may occur at any time; amniotic fluid is pale and straw colored; FHR remains stable; cord does not prolapse.	1. Advise gravida that ambulation and bedrest are directed by fetal station and status of amniotic membranes. 2. Following rupture of membranes, institute appropriate assessments, reporting and recording; if cord prolapses, institute emergency care.
E. Duration of labor within normal limits for nullipara and multipara.	Record on partogram; assess and report deviations from expected pattern for nullipara or multipara.
F. Fluid and nutrient needs are met.	Limit dietary intake to clear fluids (ice chips) as ordered by physician. Monitor intravenous fluids (may be ordered to counteract dehydration and to meet energy needs). If permitted, offer ice chips, tea with lemon and sugar, and hard sour candy suckers.
G. Elimination: woman voids every 2 hours or more often if bladder is palpable over pubic symphysis; bladder is emptied before anesthesia is initiated.	Encourage woman to void frequently; catheterize as necessary.

*Outcome criteria direct the selection of nursing actions (**plan/implementation**) and measure their effectiveness (**evaluation**).

Summary of Nursing Actions—cont'd

OUTCOME CRITERIA	PLAN/IMPLEMENTATION
Stress in labor	Provide comfort measures to control stress:
A. Maternal and paternal stress is minimized.	1. Maintain supportive attitude: calm manner, gentleness in carrying out necessary procedures, and acceptance of gravida's definition of pain and desires for alleviation of discomfort; willingly repeat instructions and stay with gravida having unavoidable pain; orient partner to unit and inform where fluids or meals may be obtained.
B. Support person(s) participates in supporting relaxation and in providing comfort measures; partner meets self and parturient's expectations.	
	2. Work through a number of contractions with gravida and husband, noting effectiveness of their method of relaxation, breathing, and other supportive techniques. If none are used, introduce techniques and coach husband in their use (for example, counterpressure against sacrum during contractions, effleurage, assuming position of comfort, breathing techniques).
C. Parturient and family express satisfaction with labor experience.	3. Provide for general hygiene: showers or bed baths, if allowed; frequent washing of vulva; mouthwash and mouth care.
	4. Although most women feel very warm as result of labor, a number complain of feeling cold—promote comfort by placing warm blanket over her and wrapping another around her feet; if available, apply bedsocks.
	5. Maintain comfortable, quiet environment and control temperature, light, and ventilation in room.
	6. Administer analgesia as ordered.
	7. Assist with anesthesia as necessary.
D. Grandparental stress is minimized or eliminated.	1. Orient to unit.
	2. Provide information as requested and if appropriate
	3. Treat with respect (refer to them by name, offer coffee).
	4. Support them if husband needs a break and if they and couple wish.
E. Sibling stress is minimized or eliminated.	1. Involve siblings per hospital protocol.
	2. Orient the babysitter to place where siblings can wait if not involved in the labor or birth or when distraction is needed.
F. Maternal behavior follows the expected course: from excited (usually) and alert to introspective (concentrating on self and and what is happening inside her); to perhaps irritable, vague in communication, amnesic between contractions; to appearance of circumoral pallor, perspiration on forehead and upper lip, shaking, belching, and feeling need to defecate.	1. Provide acceptance of behaviors.
	2. Explain behavior to family.
	3. Provide continual support, comfort measures, and explanations.
	4. Help partner with or provide coaching.
Fetus	
A. Perfusion of uterus is maintained as evidenced by FHR.	1. Position woman on her side.
B. Fetal response throughout first stage indicates continued well-being, as follows:	2. Monitor FHR per hospital protocol.
1. Rate: between 120-160 beats per minute	3. Recheck consent forms.
2. Normal baseline variability	4. Prepare woman and family for delivery.
3. No abnormal variability	5. Prepare equipment and supplies needed for delivery.
4. No periodic changes	6. Complete the labor records.
C. Preparation for delivery is completed.	
D. Records are completed concurrently with care given; all care given is documented thoroughly.	

*Outcome criteria direct the selection of nursing actions (**plan/implementation**) and measure their effectiveness (**evaluation**).

References

Anderson, S.V.: Siblings at birth. A survey and study, Birth Fam. J. 6:80, 1979.

Barnard, R.: The family and you, M.C.N. 3:83, 1978.

Bliss, J.: New baby in the family, Can. Nurs 76:42, 1980.

Carrington, B.W.: The Afro-American. In Clark, A.L., editor: Culture/childbearing/health professionals, Philadelphia, 1978, F.A. Davis Co.

Chung, J.J.: Understanding the Oriental maternity patient, Nurs. Clin. North Am. 12:67, 1977.

Cosminsky, S.: Knowledge and body concepts of Guatemalan midwives. In Kay, M.A., editor: Anthropology of human birth, Philadelphia, 1982, F.A. Davis Co.

Davitz, L.L., Davitz, J.R., and Higuchi, Y.: Cross-cultural inferences of physical pain and psychological distress, Nurs. Times 73:556, 1977.

Farris, L.: The American Indian. In Clark, A.L., editor: Culture/childbearing/health professionals, Philadelphia, 1978, F.A. Davis Co.

Flint, M.: Lockmi: an Indian midwife. In Kay, M.A., editor: Anthropology of human birth, Philadelphia, 1982, F.A. Davis Co.

Friedman, E.A., and Sachtleben, M.R.: Station of the presenting part, Am. J. Obstet. Gynecol. 93:522, 1965.

Griffith, S.: Childbearing and the concept of culture, J.O.G.N. Nurs. 11:181, 1982.

Hollingsworth, A.O., and others: The refugees and childbearing: what to expect, RN 43:45, 1980.

Horn, B.M.: Northwest coast Indians: the Muckleshoot. In Kay, M.A., editor: Anthropology of human birth, Philadelphia, 1982, F.A. Davis Co.

Jimenez, S.L.: Application of the body's natural pain relief mechanisms to reduce discomfort in labor and delivery, NAACOG Update Series, lesson 1, vol. 1, 1983.

Johnson, S.M., and Snow, L.F.: The profile of some unplanned pregnancies. In Bauwens, E.E., editor: The anthropology of health, St. Louis, 1978, The C.V. Mosby Co.

Leonard, C.H., Irvin, N., Ballard, R.A., and others: Preliminary observations on the behavior of children present at the birth of a sibling, Pediatrics 64:949, 1979.

Miller, J.S.: Return the joy of home delivery with fathers in the delivery room, Hosp. Top. 44:105, Jan. 1966.

Mitchell, P.H., and Loustan, A.: Concepts basic to nursing, New York, 1981, McGraw-Hill Book Co.

Newton, N.: Childbearing in broad perspective: pregnancy, birth and the newborn baby, Boston, 1972, Delacorte Press.

Nicholas and the baby (16 mm film or ¾ inch videocassette), Centre Productions, Inc., 1312 Pine St., Suite A, Boulder Colo. 80302.

Pillsbury, B.L.K.: "Doing the month": confinement and convalescence of Chinese women after childbirth, Soc. Sci. Med. 12:11, 1978.

Pritchard, J.A., MacDonald, P.C., and Gant, N.F.: Williams obstetrics, ed. 17, Norwalk, Conn., 1985, Appleton-Century-Crofts.

Stark, S.: Mormon childbearing. In Kay, M.A., editor: Anthropology of human birth, Philadelphia, 1982, F.A. Davis Co.

Stephany, T.: Supporting the mother of a patient in labor, J.O.G.N. Nurs. 12(5):345, 1983.

Zborowski, M.: Cultural components in responses to pain, J. Soc. Issues 3:16-30, 1952.

Zuspan, F.F., and Quilligan, E.J., editors: Practical manual of obstetric care, St. Louis, 1982, The C.V. Mosby Co.

Bibliography

Andrews, C.M., and Andrews, E.C.: Nursing, maternal postures, and fetal position, Nurs. Res. 32:336, Nov./Dec. 1983.

Bates, B., and Turner, A.N.: Imagery and symbolism in the birth practices of traditional cultures, Birth 12:29, Spring 1985.

Bauwens, E., and Anderson, S.: Home births: a reaction to hospital environmental stressors. In Bauwens, E.E., editor: The anthropology of health, St. Louis, 1978, The C.V. Mosby Co.

Benner, P.: From novice to expert—excellence and power in clinical practice, Menlo Park, Calif., 1984, Addison-Wesley Publishing Co.

Bentz, J.M.: Missed meanings in nurse/patient communications, M.C.N. 5(1):55, 1980.

Bjorkman La Du, E.: Childbirth care for Hmong families, M.C.N. 10(6):382, 1985.

Bloom, K.C.: Assisting the unprepared woman during labor, J.O.G.N. Nurs. 13:303, Sept./Oct. 1984.

Campbell, A., and Worthington, E.L.: Teaching expectant fathers how to be better childbirth coaches, M.C.N. 7(1):28, 1982.

Chute, G.E.: Expectation and experience in alternative and convential birth, J.O.G.N. Nurs. 14:61, Jan./Feb. 1985.

Craig, J.: Birth of a grandchild brings time of reflection, Menninger Perspect. 23, 1980.

Danforth, D.N., editor: Obstetrics and gynecology, ed. 4, Philadelphia, 1982, Harper & Row, Publishers.

Erikson, E.H.: Childhood and society, New York, 1964, W.W. Norton & Co.

Fullerton, J.D.: The choice of in-hospital or alternative birth environment as related to the concept of control, J. Nurse Midwife 27(2):17, 1982.

Grosso, C., and others: The Vietnamese American Family . . . and grandma makes three, M.C.N. 6:177, 1981.

Hassid, P.: Textbook for childbirth educators, ed. 2, Philadelphia, 1984, J.B. Lippincott Co.

Haun, N.: Nursing care during labor, Can. Nurs 80:26, Oct. 1984.

Horn, M., and Manion, J.: Creative grandparenting: bonding the generations, J.O.G.N. N. 14:233, May/June 1985.

Howe, C.L.: Physiologic and psychosocial assessment in labor, Nurs. Clin. North Am. 17(1):49, 1982.

Howley, C.: The older primipara: implications for nurses, J.O.G.N. Nurs. 10(3):182, 1981.

Investigators: A look at endorphins in reproductive medicine, Contemp. OB/Gyn. 20(3):117, 1982.

Jensen, M.D., and Bobak, I.M.: Handbook of maternity care: a guide for nursing practice, St. Louis, 1980, The C.V. Mosby Co.

Jensen, M.D., and Bobak, I.M.: Maternity and gynecologic care: the nurse and the family, ed. 3, St. Louis, 1985, The C.V. Mosby Co.

Jimenez, S.L.: The pregnant woman's comfort guide, Englewood Cliffs, N.J., 1983, Prentice-Hall.

Johnsen, N.M., and Gaspard, M.E.: Theoretical foundations of a prepared sibling class, J.O.G.N. N. 14:237, May/June 1985.

Kay, M.A., editor: Anthropology of human birth, Philadelphia, 1982, F.A. Davis Co.

Kitzinger, S.: The experience of childbirth, Baltimore, 1972, Pelican Books.

Kowba, M.D., and Schwirian, P.M.: Direct sibling contact and bacterial colonization of newborns, J.O.G.N. N. 14:412, Sept./Oct. 1985.

Lang, R.: The birth book, Ben Lomond, Calif., 1972, Genesis Press.

Leininger, M.: Transcultural nursing: an essential knowledge and practice field for today, Can. Nurs 80:41, Dec. 1984.

MacDonald, J.: Birth attendants: another choice, Can. Nurse 80:22, Oct. 1984.

Malinowski, J.S., and others: Nursing care of the labor patient, ed. 2, Philadelphia, 1983, F.A. Davis Co.

Maloney, R.: Childbirth education classes: expectant parents' expectations, J.O.G.N. N. 14:245, May/June 1985.

Marecki, M., and others: Early sibling attachment, J.O.G.N. N. 14:418, Sept./Oct. 1985.

May, K.A.: The father as observer, M.C.N. 7(5):319, 1982.

McKay, S., and Phillips, C.R.: Family-centered maternity care: implementation strategies, Rockville, Md., 1984, Aspen Systems Corp.

Mead, M.: Culture and commitment: a study of the generation gap, Garden City, N.Y., 1979, Doubleday & Co.

Miller, F.C., and others: Effects of position change during labor on intrauterine resting pressure, J. Calif. Perinatal Assoc. 2(2):50, 1982.

Namikoshi, T.: The complete book of shiatsu therapy, Tokyo, 1981, Japan Publications.

Olson, M.L.: Fitting grandparents into new families, M.C.N. 6(6):419, 1981.

Orque, M.S., and others: Ethnic nursing care: a multicultural approach, St. Louis, 1983, The C.V. Mosby Co.

Perez, P.: Nurturing children who attend the birth of a sibling, Am. J.M.C.N. 4(4):215, 1979.

Phillips, C.R., and Anzalone, J.T.: Fathering: participation in labor and birth, ed. 2, St. Louis, 1982, The C.V. Mosby Co.

Poole, C.: Educating new labor and delivery room nurses, J.O.G.N. N. 14:459, Nov./Dec. 1985.

Powers, B.A.: The use of orthodox and Black-American folk medicine, Adv. Nurs. Sci. 4:35, 1982.

Roberts, J.: Alternative positions for childbirth: first stage, J. Nurse Midwife 25:11, 1980.

Robertson, J.F.: Grandmotherhood: a study of role conception, J. Marriage Fam. 39:165, 1977.

Romond, J.L., and Baker, I.T.: Squatting in childbirth: a new look at an old tradition, J.O.G.N. Nurs. 14:406, Sept./Oct. 1985.

SantoPietro, M.C.: How to get through to a refugee patient, RN 44:43, 1981.

Satir, V.: Peoplemaking. Palo Alto, Calif., 1972, Science & Behavior Books.

Siegel, D.: The gate-control theory, Am. J. Nurs. 74:498, 1974.

Stanton, M.E.: The myth of "natural" childbirth: the practices of people in traditional cultures, J. Nurs. Midwife 24(2):25, 1979.

Sweet, P.T.: Prenatal classes especially for children, M.C.N. 4:82, 1979.

Trause, M.A., and Irvin, N.A.: Care of the sibling. In Klaus, M.H., and Kennell, J.H., editors: Parent-infant bonding, St. Louis, 1982, The C.V. Mosby Co.

Waller, M.M.: Siblings in the childbearing experience, NAACOG Update Series, Lesson 17, vol. 1, 1984.

Whaley, L.F., and Wong, D.L.: Nursing care of infants and children, ed. 3, St. Louis, 1987, The C.V. Mosby Co.

Willson, J.R., Carrington, E.R., and Ledger, W.J.: Obstetrics and gynecology, ed. 7, St. Louis, 1983, The C.V. Mosby Co.

Zepeda, M.: Selected maternal infant care practices of Spanish-speaking women, J.O.G.N. Nurs. 11:371, 1982.

Pharmacologic Control of Discomfort and Fetal Monitoring

Nursing care of the parturient may include pharmacologic control of discomfort and fetal monitoring. These two topics are discussed separately in this unit for four reasons. (1) The flow of the content on the normal processes of labor is disrupted by interjecting two such large content areas. (2) Fetal monitoring may be used in both the first and second stages of labor. (3) Medications for discomfort are used for all stages of labor. (4) Content can be found more quickly when not buried within a broader content area.

Analgesia and Anesthesia

Nursing management of obstetric analgesia and anesthesia combines the nurse's expertise in maternity care with knowledge and understanding of techniques and medications and their potential desired effects and complications. A general knowledge of analgesia and anesthesia is basic to implementation of the nursing process in relation to use of medications during labor. Analgesia and anesthesia are defined:

analgesia Alleviation of pain; the raising of one's threshold for pain perception.
anesthesia Abolition of pain perception by interrupting the nerve impulses going to the brain.

Four general categories of analgesia and anesthesia. Table 16.1 defines the four general categories of analgesia and anesthesia. In Table 16.2 the four categories are discussed under the following headings: category and desired effects, assessment and comments, and planning and implementation. Figs. 16.1 and 16.2 illustrate the spinal cord and nerve pathways.

Table 16.1

Four General Categories of Pharmacologic Analgesia and Anesthesia

Category	Definition	Examples
Systemic medication	Medication that is ingested or injected with a syringe; affects central and peripheral nervous systems, but total unconsciousness does not result.	Sedatives Narcotic analgesics Analgesic-potentiating drugs (ataractics, tranquilizers)
Inhalation analgesia	Inhalation of drugs in subanesthesia concentrations; some may be self-administered.	Methoxyflurane Nitrous oxide
General anesthesia	Medication that is administered intravenously or by inhalation, resulting in unconsciousness.	Intravenously Thiopental (Pentothal) sodium Inhalants

Regional (conduction) anesthesia	Local anesthetics injected to block primary sensory (pain) neuropathways that pass from uterus to spinal cord by accompanying sympathetic nerves.	Peripheral nerve block
		  Pudendal
		  Local infiltration
		  Paracervical*
		Regional block
		  Peridural block
		  Caudal
		  Subarachnoid (low spinal, saddle block)

*Paracervical (uterosacral) block is *not* recommended during labor because of its effects on the fetus, but it is well suited for gynecologic procedures. It is discussed in Chapter 7.

Fig. 16.1
Membranes and spaces of spinal cord.

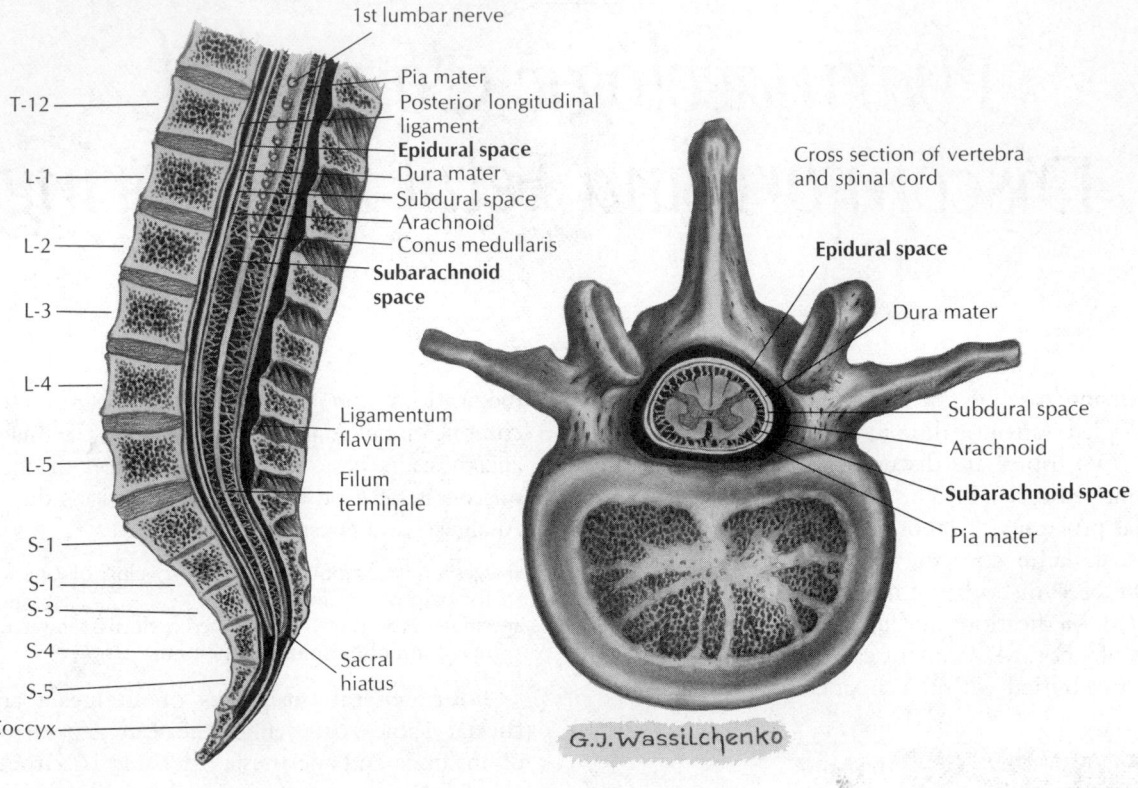

1st lumbar nerve
Pia mater
Posterior longitudinal
ligament
Epidural space
Dura mater
Subdural space
Arachnoid
Conus medullaris
Subarachnoid space

T-12
L-1
L-2
L-3
L-4
L-5
S-1
S-1
S-3
S-4
S-5
Coccyx

Ligamentum flavum
Filum terminale
Sacral hiatus

Cross section of vertebra and spinal cord

Epidural space
Dura mater
Subdural space
Arachnoid
Subarachnoid space
Pia mater

G.J.Wassilchenko

Fig. 16.2
Pain pathways and sites of pharmacologic interruption. **A,** Pudendal block; suitable during
second and third stage of labor and for repair of episiotomy. **B,** Paracervical (uterosacral)
block: suitable during first stage of labor. **C,** Lumbar sympathetic block: given as shown,
suitable during first stage of labor (not usually method of choice; caudal is preferable).
D, Lumbar epidural block: suitable during all stages of labor and for repair of episiotomy.

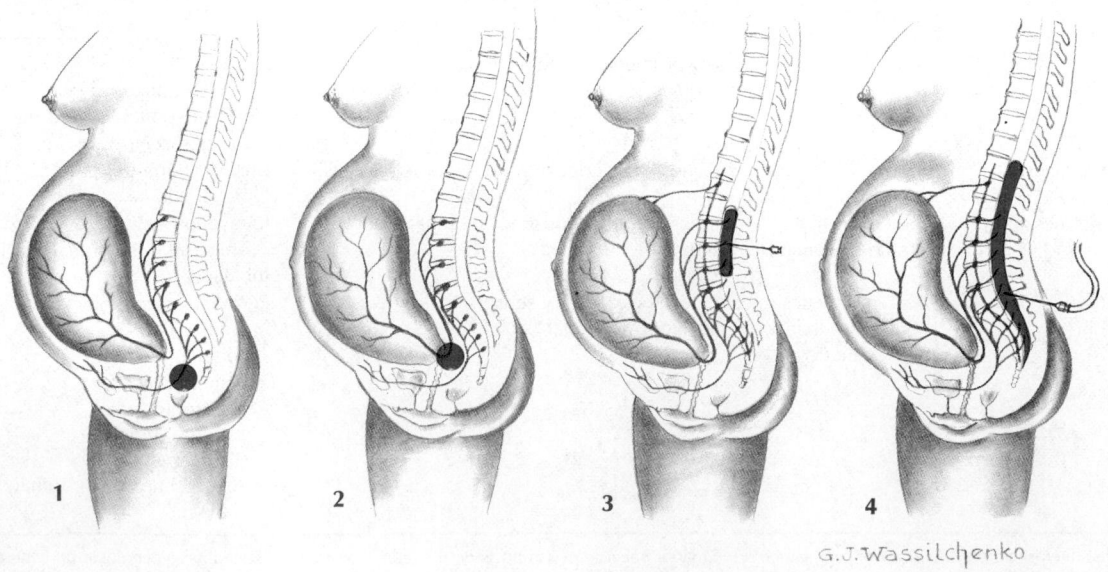

1   2   3   4

G.J.Wassilchenko

Routes of administration of analgesic medications

Intravenous route. The preferred route of administration is through intravenous tubing. The medication is given slowly in small doses at the *beginning* of three to five consecutive contractions. Since uterine blood vessels are constricted during contractions, the medication stays within the maternal vascular system for several seconds before the uterine blood vessels reopen. Through this method of injection, the amount of drug crossing the placenta to the fetus is minimized. With decreased placental transfer, the mother's degree of pain relief is maximized. The intravenous route has the following results:

1. Pain relief is obtained with small doses of the drug.
2. Onset of pain relief is more predictable.
3. Duration of effect is more predictable.

Intramuscular route. Intramuscular injections of analgesics, although still used, are no longer the preferred route of administration to the laboring woman. Identified disadvantages of the intramuscular route include the following:

1. Onset of pain relief is delayed for several minutes.
2. Higher doses of medication are required.
3. Medication is released from the muscle tissue at an unpredictable rate and is available for transfer across the placenta to the fetus.

Intramuscular injections are given in the upper arm if regional anesthesia is planned later in the labor. This is because the autonomic blockade from the regional (e.g., epidural) anesthesia increases blood flow to the gluteal region and accelerates absorption of the drug. The maternal plasma level of the drug necessary to bring pain relief usually is reached 45 minutes after intramuscular injection, followed by a decline in plasma levels. The maternal drug levels (after intramuscular injections) are unequal because of uneven distribution (maternal uptake) and metabolism. The advantage of using the intramuscular route is quick administration.

Subcutaneous route. Another quick method of administering medications that generally does not involve changing the woman's position is the subcutaneous injection. Subcutaneous administration does have the same disadvantages as the intramuscular route. When using the subcutaneous route, small amounts of highly soluble, nonirritating drugs in solution are given by means of a hypodermic syringe and needle. This is usually accomplished with a fine 25-gauge needle. Alphaprodine hydrochloride (Nisentil), a synthetic narcotic analgesic chemically related to meperidine, is usually administered subcutaneously on the outer surface of the upper arm.

Timing for administration of analgesia. Many medication orders are written to be given on the nurse's judgment. These prn orders require clinical knowledge and expertise. To assist the nurse in decision making, a quick reference is provided in Table 16.2. Table 16.3 compares different modalities for relief of discomfort and gives usual parenteral dose, time of administration, advantages for the parturient, disadvantages for the neonate, and nursing concerns.

Text continued on p. 423.

Table 16.2
Pharmacologic Control of Discomfort During Childbirth and Nursing Process

Category and Desired Effect	Assessment and Comments	Planning and Implementation
Systemic medication		

Examples: *sedatives*
   Short duration (1 h): secobarbital (Seconal)
   Intermediate (2 h): pentobarbital (Nembutal)
   Long duration (3 h): phenobarbital (Luminal sodium)
Desired effect: relieve anxiety and induce sleep only in prodromal or early latent labor
Route: oral or intramuscular
	Before administration of medication note:
	   Prenatal history of allergies or medical disorders
	   Prodromal labor
	   Degree of apprehension
	      Woman states she is anxious
	      Woman is clenching fists, restless, seems tense
	   Absence of pain
	After administration of medication note:
	   Strength and frequency of uterine contractions should not decrease appreciably
	   Little change in maternal vital signs; with decreased anxiety, pulse, respirations, and blood pressure do decrease but should not fall below woman's normal baseline in her prenatal record
	   Assess woman's response to medication
	   Assess FHR
	   Assess for pain
		Alert physician if chart reveals history of drug allergy, other disorders
		Administer if
		   Woman is apprehensive, tense
		   Woman is in early latent phase of first stage of labor
		Do not give without an analgesic if woman has pain
		Continue with comfort measures and general hygiene given to any woman in labor
		If changes occur in contractions or in maternal or fetal vital signs, record and notify physician
		If woman becomes uncomfortable, confer with physician regarding need for analgesic relief

Continued.

Table 16.2, cont'd

Pharmacologic Control of Discomfort During Childbirth and Nursing Process

Category and Desired Effect	Assessment and Comments	Planning and Implementation
Systemic medication—cont'd		
Examples: *narcotic analgesics*	Before administration of medication note:	Do not administer if birth is expected within 2 h
Morphine	Prenatal information regarding	Explain expected effect
Meperidine hydrochloride (Demerol)	Drug allergies	
Pentazocine (Talwin)	Liver and kidney damage	
Fentanyl	Substance (drug) abuse	
Desired effect: relief of severe, persistent, or recurrent pain, without nausea and vomiting or respiratory depression of mother or fetus	History of asthma	
	Stage of labor; progress in labor	
	Nullipara: before full dilatation	
	Multipara: before 7 cm dilatation	
Route: intramuscular or intravenous	Degree of discomfort	
	Mother states she is having pain; cries out with pain; clenches teeth, fists	
	Maternal and fetal vital signs	
	After administration of medication note:	
	Time between administration of narcotic and time of baby's birth	If baby is born when drug reaches maximum effect, baby may be depressed and require resuscitation; prepare Narcan (0.01/kg) to be given intramuscularly into baby's thigh
	Maximum effect (IM) in 15 min, duration of 2 h	
	Drug may slow labor, or it may accelerate labor as woman relaxes	
	Adverse side effects assessed every 5-30 min	
	Respiratory depression	
	FHR deceleration and loss of short-term variability noted by electronic fetal monitor	
	Nausea, vomiting, dizziness, sweating, dysphoria	
	Bronchospasm in women who suffer from asthma	
Examples: *narcotic antagonists*	Note which drug was given, time, amount, route; respiratory depression from any drug other than a narcotic cannot be reversed with these drugs	Do not give Narcan to mother addicted to narcotics because this causes instant withdrawal symptoms; Narcan given to mother reverses pain relief instantly, so that she must be prepared for return of pain or a second form of pain relief is given (e.g., epidural)
Naloxone hydrochloride (Narcan)*		
Levallorphan tartrate (Lorfan)		
Nalorphine (Nalline)		
Desired effect: Reversal of narcotic depression of mother and/or baby		
Route: intravenous		
Examples: *analgesic-potentiating drugs (ataractics, tranquilizers)*	Same as for narcotic analgesics	Same as for narcotic analgesics
Promethazine hydrochloride (Phenergan)		
Propiomazine hydrochloride (Largon)		
Hydroxyzine pamoate (Vistaril)		
Promazine hydrochloride (Sparine)		
Route: intravenous, intramuscular		
Desired effects: increase desirable effects of analgesics without increasing dose of analgesics (i.e., ataractic potentiates effects of analgesic that is given with it and acts as antiemetic)		

*Preferred drug because it does not intensify depressive effects if depression is caused by drugs other than narcotics.

Table 16.2, cont'd
Pharmacologic Control of Discomfort During Childbirth and Nursing Process

Category and Desired Effect	Assessment and Comments	Planning and Implementation
Inhalation analgesia		
Mother breathes subanesthetic concentrations of inhalation anesthetic; if given properly, woman remains conscious but has profound pain relief		
Example: *methoxyflurane (Penthrane)*	Monitor vital signs closely (be alert for cardiac arrhythmias) every 30 min and FHR every 15 min	Stay with woman; never administer drug for woman because overdose is a risk
Route: self-administered (usually) from a capsule and mask strapped to wrist; physician sets desired concentration; mother inhales drug during contractions.	Assess mother's level of consciousness (LOC) and responsiveness. Mother should remain conscious and not become delirious or excited	Alert physician and remove from mother's hand if:
Desired effect: profound analgesia while remaining conscious; some amnesia for painful events		Mother has cardiac arrhythmia Mother loses consciousness; FHR abnormalities occur
Example: *nitrous oxide (N₂O₂)*	Monitor maternal-fetal vital signs every 15 min	Trained personnel must remain with woman
Route: administered by trained personnel, during contractions, or continuously via face mask		
Desired effect: analgesia		
General anesthesia		
Rarely indicated for uncomplicated vaginal delivery; woman is not awake; danger of aspiration and respiratory depression; safer than regional anesthesia for hypovolemic clients; does not depress neonate unless mother is anesthetized deeply	Anesthetist assesses woman continuously (intubation is necessary) Monitor fetal response continuously Provide postanesthesia recovery care: assess every 15 min until vital signs are stable and woman is alert and reactive.	If general anesthesia is being considered, keep woman NPO and see that an intravenous infusion is established; premedicate with cimetidine to neutralize acid contents of stomach Assist with **cricoid pressure** before intubation (p. 423)
Examples: *Thiopental (Pentothal) sodium IV* produces rapid induction of anesthesia; depresses neonate; useful in controlling convulsions	If woman delivered by cesarean birth, do routine postsurgery assessment—wound assessment, intake and output, etc.	Recovery room care Maintain open airway Maintain cardiopulmonary functions Prevent postpartal hemorrhage
Halothane (fluothane) (inhalation)—relaxes uterus quickly, facilitates intrauterine manipulation, version, and extraction	Routine postpartum assessment Assess readiness to see baby Assess her response to anesthesia and event that necessitated general anesthesia delivery (e.g., giving birth by cesarean delivery when vaginal delivery was anticipated)	Routine postpartum care Facilitate parent-child attachment as soon as possible Answer mother's questions
Desired effect: produces general loss of sensitivity to touch, pain, and other stimulations		
Regional (conduction) anesthesia		
Local anesthetics injected to block primary neuropathways that result in temporary interruption of conduction of nerve impulses, notably pain; mother remains awake		
Examples: common agents in 0.5% to 1.0% solution		
Lidocaine (Xylocaine) hydrochloride		
Bupivacaine (Marcaine) hydrochloride		

Continued.

Table 16.2, cont'd
Pharmacologic Control of Discomfort During Childbirth and Nursing Process

Category and Desired Effect	Assessment and Comments	Planning and Implementation
Regional (conduction) anesthesia—cont'd		
Chloroprocaine*		
Tetracaine (Pontocaine) hydrochloride		
Mepivacaine hydrochloride (Carbocaine)		
Types of nerve blocks		
Peripheral nerve block	Monitor fetal response continuously.	See general nursing actions below.
Pudendal (5-10 ml on each side) (Fig. 16.3): anesthetizes lower two thirds of vagina and perineum; of short duration (30 min)—given for delivery and repair; local anesthesia, may be done by physician or anesthetist; simple and safe, does not depress neonate; may inhibit bearing-down reflex	Assist physician or anesthetist as necessary.	
Local infiltration: useful for perineal repairs (Fig. 16.4)	Assist physician or anesthetist as necessary.	See general nursing actions below. Nurse informs physician of medication in syringe.

*Based on assessment using the Apgar score, blood gas analysis, drug concentration, and the assessment of newborn neurobehavioral response, it was found that bupivacaine and chloroprocaine offered some advantages over the other drugs: the newborns scored higher when these anesthetics were used than when the other agents were used (Lundberg, 1983).

Fig. 16.3
Use of needle guide ("Iowa trumpet") in pudendal anesthetic block. A Luer-Lòk syringe is used. (Modified from Benson, R.C.: Handbook of obstetrics and gynecology, ed. 5, Los Altos, Calif, 1974, Lange Medical Publications.)

Fig. 16.4
Tray for local infiltration anesthesia. Note Luer-Lòk syringe, a glass syringe with a mechanism to attach the needle securely, and with finger holds on barrel, and with a thumb rest on plunger (also shown in Fig. 16.3). (Courtesy Stanford University Hospital, Stanford, California.)

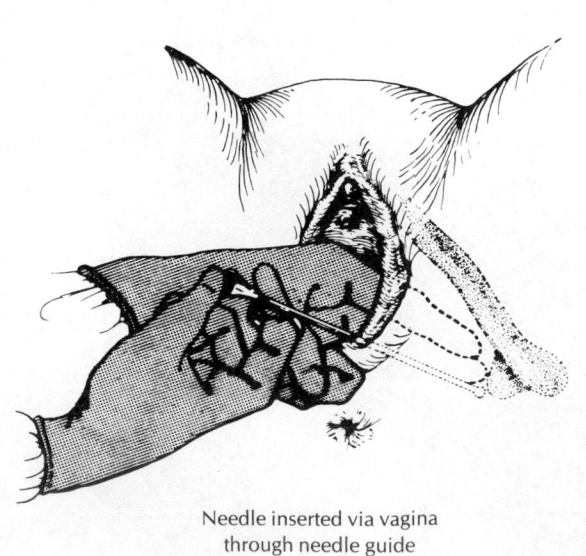
Needle inserted via vagina
through needle guide

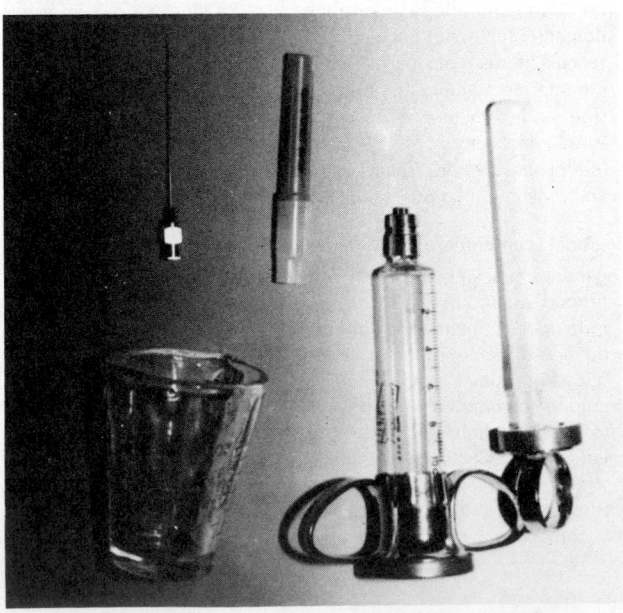

Table 16.2, cont'd
Pharmacologic Control of Discomfort During Childbirth and Nursing Process

Category and Desired Effect	Assessment and Comments	Planning and Implementation

Regional block (Figs. 16.5 and 16.6): requires trained anesthesiologist; with proper administration, relieves pain completely, may prolong labor if given too early; hypotension from vasodilation (below anesthesia level) is likely; fetal bradycardia may occur as a result of maternal hypotension; bearing-down reflex partially or completely eliminated,	General assessment for all nerve blocks: note degree of hydration, history of allergy, skin infection over back, previous neural or spinal injury or disease, and attitude toward anesthesia
	Predelivery monitor
	  Maternal vital signs and FHR
	  Assess for return of pain
	  Monitor labor if anesthesia is established during late first stage
	  Rate of IV fluid infusion
		General nursing actions for all nerve blocks
		  Hydrate by intravenous infusion
		  Explain to woman expected feelings as anesthesia begins (warm toes) and as it wears off (tingling); help position her, offering reassurance and support; it is very frightening not to be able to see the procedure and to deal with only sensations and sounds; do not make promises of complete pain relief; each woman may have a differing perception of pain, or block may not provide complete relief

Continued.

Fig. 16.5
A, Regional block anesthesia in obstetrics. **B,** Level of anesthesia necessary for cesarean delivery and for vaginal delivery. (Courtesy Ross Laboratories, Columbus, Ohio.)

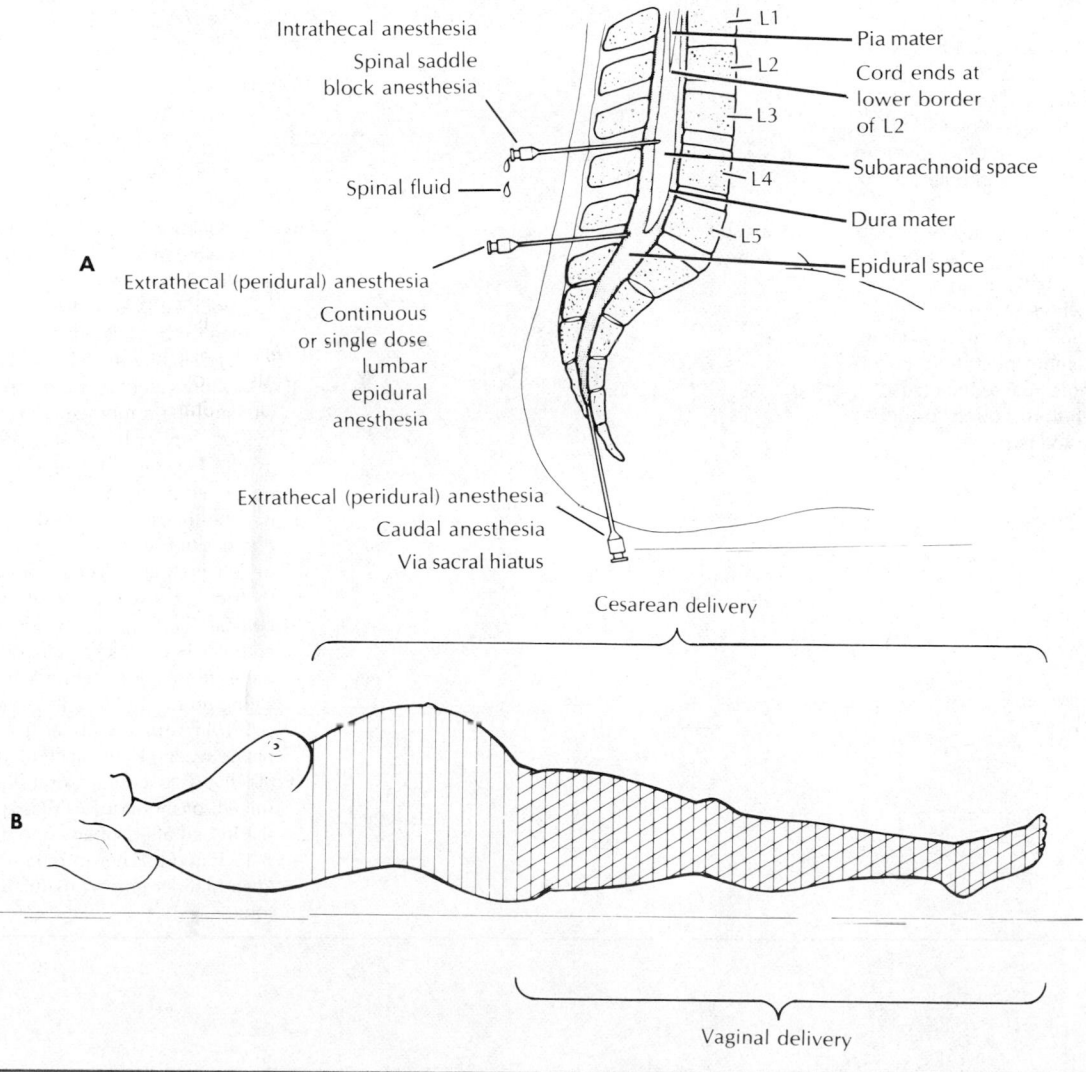

Table 16.2, cont'd
Pharmacologic Control of Discomfort During Childbirth and Nursing Process

Category and Desired Effect	Assessment and Comments	Planning and Implementation
Types of nerve blocks—cont'd		
necessitating outlet forceps at delivery: mother remains awake throughout delivery; absence of pain may facilitate maternal-child attachment; can be used for women with metabolic, lung, and heart diseases.	Perineum to see if delivery is imminent (or monitor progress by vaginal examination)	Treat hypotension: maintain lateral position or elevate legs; administer humidified oxygen by mask at 10-12 L/min; increase rate of IV maintenance fluids
Epidural (Figs. 16.5 and 16.6): useful during first and second stages; can be given as "one shot" or over a period of time; given on top of (or over) dura through third, fourth, or fifth lumbar interspace; risk of dural puncture During labor, analgesic doses are given For delivery, anesthetic dose is given	Postdelivery, monitor Uterine tone Bladder tone Return of sensation	If contractions become less frequent, of less intensity, or of shorter duration, report to physician immediately; physician may need to augment labor; assist as necessary Add forceps to delivery table Provide assistance to move from delivery table to bed; maintain good uterine tone; prevent bladder distention; prevent injury by keeping side rails up and assisting her when she ambulates
Caudal (through sacral hiatus) (Figs. 16.1 and 16.5): useful during first and second stages; can be given as "one shot" or over a period of time; given in peridural space through sacral hiatus		Assist with positioning woman
Subarachnoid (low spinal, saddle nerve block [Figs. 16.1 and 16.5]); usually given as "one shot" when fetal head is on perineum; medication is mixed with cerebrospinal fluid in subarachnoid space; injected through third, fourth, or fifth lumbar interspace	After subarachnoid block, observe for headache	For introduction of epidural anesthesia, position woman as for subarachnoid block or in modified Sims' position (Fig. 16.6). For modified lateral Sims' position, place woman on her left side, shoulders parallel, legs slightly flexed, and back arched. If indwelling catheter is threaded and woman feels a momentary twinge down her leg, hip, or back, anesthetist or nurse assures her it is not a sign of injury. An alternate position may be preferred by the anesthetist: position woman in a sitting position with her buttocks near edge of delivery table, feet supported on a footstool; ask woman to place her arms between her knees, flex her head, and arch her back "like a rainbow." After medication is injected, ask her to remain sitting up for 20-30 s; then place her supine with a pillow under her head and a pelvic wedge to displace uterus to left. Postdelivery: encourage oral fluids (if permitted) or monitor IV fluids; position her flat in bed after subarachnoid block for 8-12 h and ask her to report headache; keep bladder empty; maintain uterine tone.

Fig. 16.6
A, Lateral decubitus position for epidural and subarachnoid block and anatomic landmarks to locate needle insertion site. **B,** Epidural anesthesia. Skin has been prepared with antiseptic solution (Betadine). Anesthesiologist is explaining procedure step by step. Area is draped with sterile towels. Nurse continues to support woman. Test dose is administered. **C,** Catheter is taped to woman's back; port segment is taped near her shoulder. (**B** and **C** courtesy Stanford University Hospital, Stanford, California.)

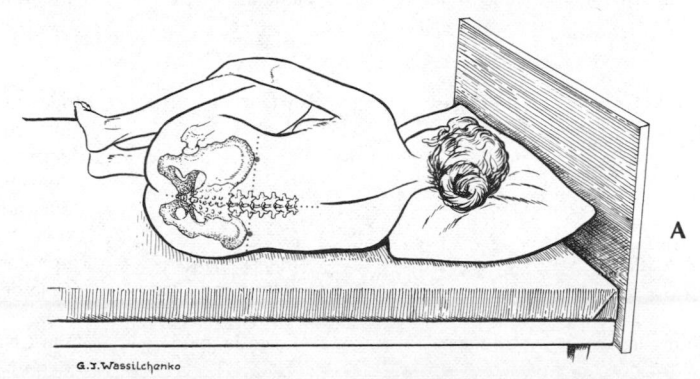

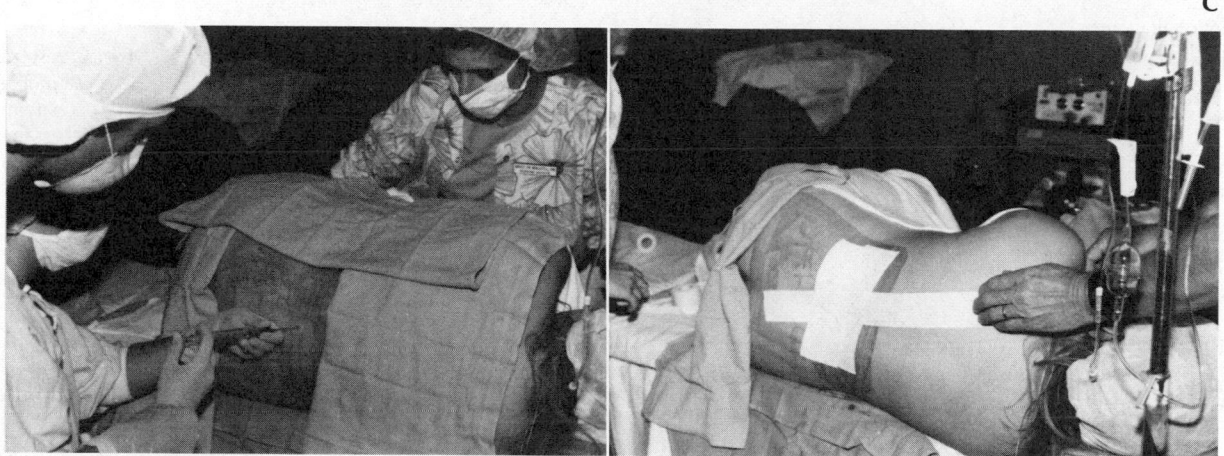

Table 16.3
Comparison of Modalities for Obstetric Analgesia

Therapeutic Modality Drug	Usual Parenteral Dose	Time of Administration	Advantages for Parturient	Disadvantages for Neonate	Nursing Concerns
Psychoprophylaxis		Late pregnancy Labor stages 1-3	No drugs Training in self-reliance	None	Pain controlled but not eliminated
Hypnosis		Late pregnancy Labor stages 1-3	No drugs In rare women, pain free	None	Suggestion reinforcement essential
Medications *Sedatives-hypnotics*					
Secobarbital sodium (Seconal)	50-100 mg IM	Early stage 1, mid-stage 1, or postdelivery	Disinhibition or somnolence (no pain relief in usual doses)	Hypoactive "sleepy" neonate	Either subdued or excited; may become dehydrated

Continued.

Table 16.3, cont'd
Comparison of Modalities for Obstetric Analgesia

Therapeutic Modality Drug	Usual Parenteral Dose	Time of Administration	Advantages for Parturient	Disadvantages for Neonate	Nursing Concerns
Medications—cont'd					
Sedatives-hypnotics—cont'd					
Pentobarbital sodium (Nembutal)	50-100 mg IM	Same as above	Same as above	Same as above	Same as above
Narcotic analgesics					
Morphine	8-15 mg IM or IV	Mid-stage I	Analgesia excellent	Moderate to marked CNS depression if delivery <2 h after administration	Emesis common
Alphaprodine (Nisentil)	40-60 mg SC or IV	Late stage 1	Amnesia partial plus good analgesia	Respiratory and CNS depression	Routine care
Meperidine	50-100 mg IM or IV	Mid-stage 1	Analgesia good	Slight CNS depression	Routine care
Narcotic antagonists					
Nalorphine (Nalline)	Adult—5 mg IM or IV Neonate—0.5 mg IM or IV	Stage 2 or to neonate	Prompt termination of narcotic effect but ineffective against depression caused by barbiturates or anesthetics	Overdose may be toxic	Physical resuscitation of mother or neonate may be necessary despite narcotic antagonist
Levallorphan tartrate (Lorfan)	Adult—1.0 mg IM or IV Neonate—0.05-0.1 mg IM or IV	Same as above	Same as above	Same as above	Same as above
Naloxone hydrochloride (Narcan)	Adult—0.4 mg IM or IV Neonate—0.01 mg/kg body weight, IV or SC	Same as above	Same as above	Same as above	Abrupt reversal of narcotic reaction (nausea, vomiting, tachycardia, hypertension, tremors in narcotics addicts)
Analgesic-potentiating drugs (ataractics, tranquilizers)					
Promethazine (Phenergan)	25-50 mg IM	Early stage 1, mid-stage 1, and postdelivery	Apprehension, anxiety, depression relieved; narcotic effects potentiated; antiemetic	Drug enchances narcotic effect (CNS depression)	Closer supervision may be necessary because of mild pseudohypnotic state
Promazine (Sparine)	50 mg IM	Early stage 1, mid-stage 1, or postdelivery	Apprehension, anxiety, depression relieved; narcotic effects potentiated; antiemetic	Drug enhances narcotic effect (CNS) depression	Closer supervision may be necessary because of mild pseudohypnotic state
Hydroxyzine pamoate (Vistaril)	25-50 mg IM or SC	Same as above	Same as above	Same as above	Same as above
Diazepam (Valium)	5 mg IM or IV	Same as above	Same as above	Same as above	Same as above

Effects of analgesia and anesthesia on mother and newborn. All the drugs and procedures used to alleviate the discomforts of giving birth have some advantage or desirable characteristic, but none is perfect. Widespread reappraisal of medications and methods used to relieve pain in obstetrics is important because at least 10% of maternal deaths are now due to problems with anesthesia. The two biggest problems are aspiration of vomitus and complications of high spinal anesthesia. Perinatal morbidity and mortality are greatly dependent on the analgesia and anesthesia employed.

There is an ongoing debate concerning the effects of epidural anesthesia on the neonate's neurobehavioral responses. Studies of associations between neurobehavioral outcome and epidural anesthesia are far from consistent (Avard and Nimrod, 1985). One author found a beneficial effect (Hodgkinson and others, 1977). Some authors found that neonates did not score as well (Rosenblatt and others, 1981). Others found no difference (Marx, 1984; Abboud and others, 1982). However, the findings suggest a mild transient effect on newborn behavior.

Combination anesthesia for cesarean birth. *Light general anesthesia*, considered by many to be ideal for cesarean delivery, is achieved with a combination of *thiopental, nitrous oxide–oxygen, and succinylcholine.* The woman is given oxygen for 3 minutes, followed by almost simultaneous rapid administration of thiopental and succinylcholine. During intubation, cricoid pressure is maintained to prevent aspiration of vomitus (Fig. 16.7). Cricoid pressure is often maintained by the nurse. When the woman is somnolent, a nitrous oxide–oxygen mixture is given. Excellent tolerance of the anesthetic is widely reported. Rapid resuscitation of the mother and even small-for-gestational-age and growth-retarded infants can be achieved.

Epidural narcotic method. Epidural narcotic usage in obstetrics is being reported in the literature. There is a high concentration of receptors in the spinal column that are open to the action of the opiates to block pain. These receptors are reached by a catheter placed in the epidural space. When used in labor, 1.5 mg morphine sulfate is administered through the epidural catheter. The women feel contractions, but no pain is noted by them or observers. Since the pushing reflex is not lost, the mother can cooperate during delivery. Maternal vital signs are normal during labor, and no motor or sympathetic block is noted. Women may experience itching of the face, mouth, and eyes. These symptoms are treated with promethazine or metoclopramide.

Women who deliver by the abdominal route are given epidural morphine 1 hour after surgery through the epidural catheter. The catheter is then removed, and the women are pain free for 24 hours. Ability to be up with ease and to care for the baby are two of the advantages to epidural morphine. The women cannot believe the effects of the morphine on pain. To women who have had a previous cesarean delivery

---

Fig. 16.7

Technique of applying pressure on cricoid cartilage to occlude esophagus prevents pulmonary aspiration of gastric contents during anesthesia induction.

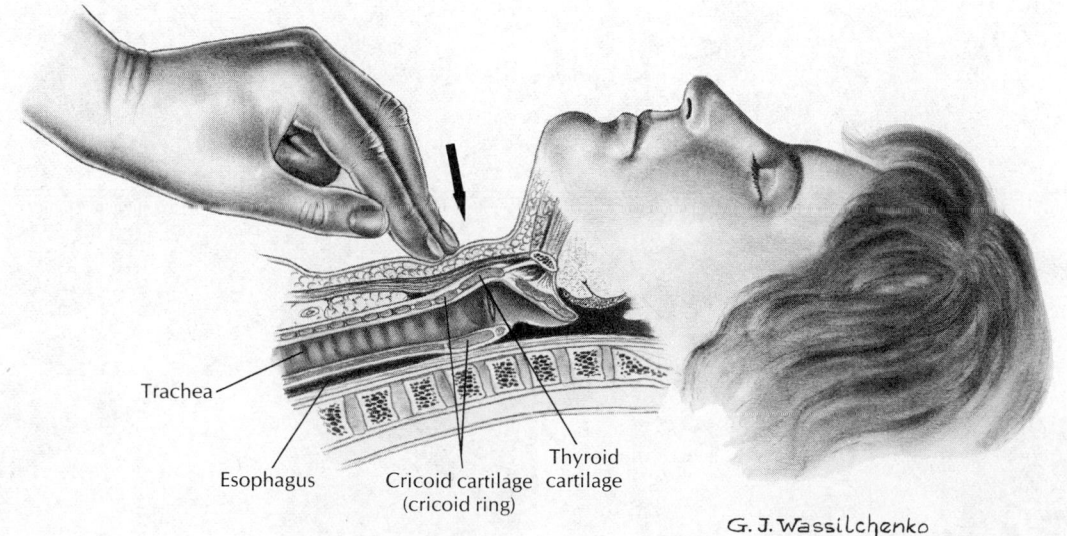

Trachea

Esophagus   Cricoid cartilage   Thyroid
             (cricoid ring)   cartilage

G. J. Wassilchenko

with the usual postoperative pain, the effects of the epidural morphine seem miraculous. The nurse caring for the woman who has been given epidural morphine generally is amazed at the mother's ease in ambulation and relative freedom from pain.

The side effects of epidural morphine are nausea, vomiting, pruritus (itching), urinary retention, or delayed respiratory depression. Antiemetics, antipruritics, and naloxone hydrochloride (Narcan) are used to relieve the nausea, vomiting, and pruritus.

The reversal drug for morphine is naloxone, 0.4 mg. Morphine is believed to have no effect on the course of labor. The pain relief continues up to 11 hours after injection.

Early ambulation and freedom from pain facilitate bladder emptying. The serious concern is for delayed respiratory depression. The woman is observed frequently and is placed on an apnea monitor for 24 hours (Fig. 16.8). Delayed respiratory depression is caused by absorption of morphine from the spinal fluid by the respiratory centers in the brain.

Summary. The physiologic requirements of the woman (e.g., adequate hydration, preventing hypotension) receiving pharmacologic control of discomfort have been presented. Effects on the unborn and newborn baby (e.g., uterine blood flow, oxygenation, and glucose) have been discussed. The key is to provide the childbearing family with a choice in pain relief. It is then the duty of caring professionals to provide the safety in that choice by using their knowledge of drugs and techniques (Petree, 1983).

Fig. 16.8

A, Epidural morphine. After epidural anesthesia for cesarean delivery, dose of morphine is injected into indwelling catheter. Anesthetist is applying apnea monitor on woman. Her respirations will be monitored for 24 hours. **B,** Husband supports wife as nurse begins routine postpartum assessments following cesarean birth.

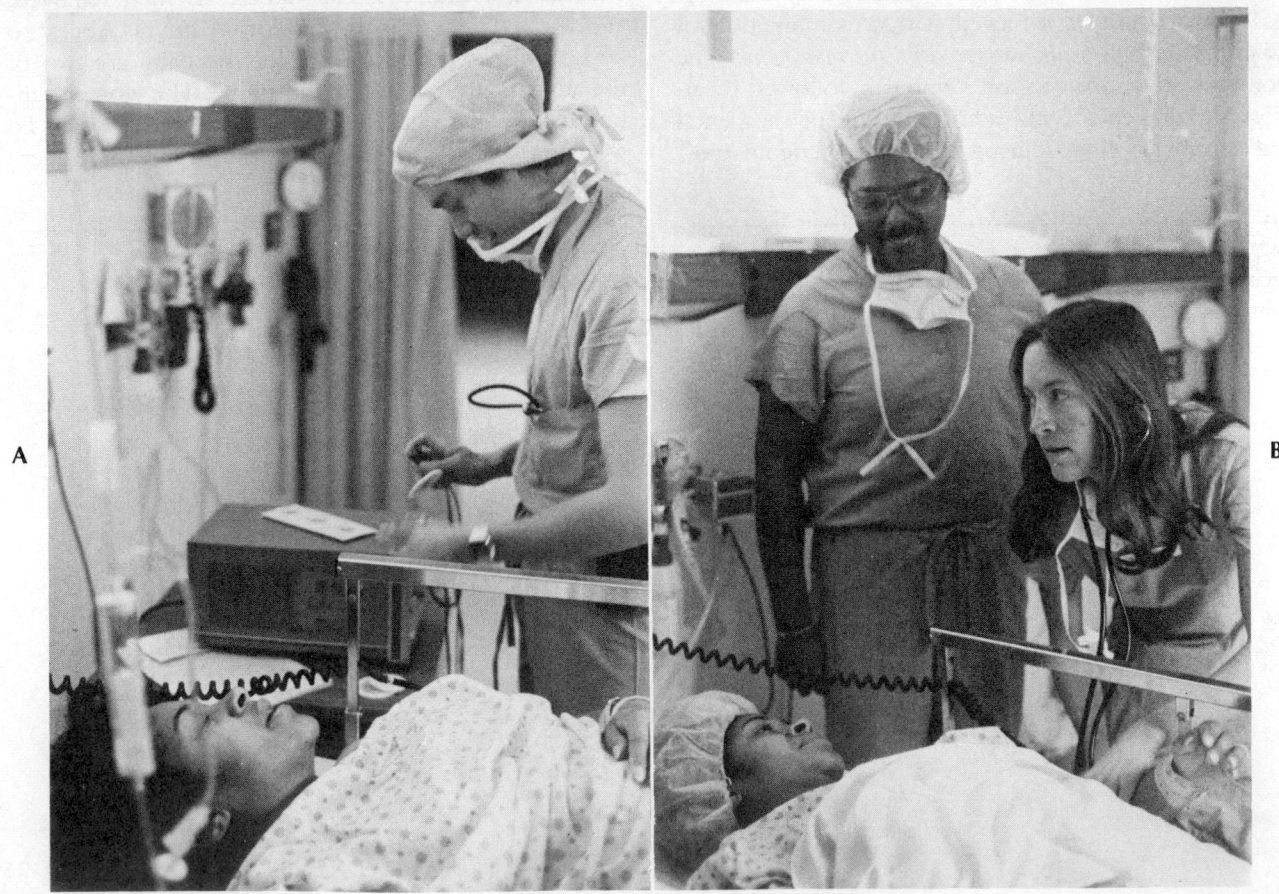

Summary of Nursing Actions

PHARMACOLOGIC CONTROL OF DISCOMFORT

GOALS

1. For the mother: To achieve adequate pain relief without adding to maternal risk.
2. For the unborn and newborn: To maintain well-being and adjustment to extra-uterine life.
3. For the family: To know of their needs and rights in relation to use of analgesia or anesthesia.

PRIORITIES

1. Differentiate between the woman's need for pharmacologic control and her need for physiologic control of discomfort.
2. Select the most effective techniques for each woman.
3. Prepare the medication and administer it correctly.
4. Monitor the effects of pharmacologic control on maternal, and fetal, and newborn well-being and maternal pain relief.

ASSESSMENT	EXAMPLES OF POTENTIAL NURSING DIAGNOSTIC CATEGORIES*
Interview A. Health history: allergies or unusual reactions to medications B. Psychosocial: level of understanding of analgesia or anesthesia; preferences; assessed need for pharmacologic relief; fatigue C. Review of systems: present respiratory problem (cold); amount, type, time of last food taken	Alteration in respiratory function† Alteration in maternal or fetal well-being† Potential for injury Anxiety Fear Knowledge deficit Powerlessness Disturbance in self-concept, body image, self-esteem, role performance, personal identity Ineffective individual coping Alteration in comfort: pain
Physical examination Vital signs, blood pressure, FHR; uterine contractions, station, effacement and dilatation; degree of hydration	Alteration in maternal or fetal well-being† Alteration in tissue perfusion (fetal): cerebral, cardiopulmonary, renal, gastrointestinal, peripheral Potential for injury Alteration in comfort: pain Fluid volume deficit
Laboratory tests None specific	None specific to laboratory tests
Informed consent	Spiritual distress Powerlessness Knowledge deficit
Physician's orders	Potential for injury Knowledge deficit
Before administration of analgesia/anesthesia A. Labor: contractions, cervical effacement and dilatation, station; FHR; maternal response and desire for medication B. Degree of hydration: input and output; moisture of mucous membranes, skin turgor, temperature C. Bladder distension D. Client understanding of the analgesia or anesthesia to be administered	Alteration in maternal or fetal well-being† Potential for maternal or fetal compromise† Alteration in normal physiologic response† Fluid volume deficit Potential for injury Anxiety Fear Powerlessness Spiritual distress Knowledge deficit
During administration of analgesia/anesthesia Maternal or fetal response	Alteration in normal physiologic response† Potential for injury (during administration)

*Diagnoses approved by the Seventh National Conference (1986) of NANDA except for those indicated by a dagger.
†Diagnosis not included by NANDA, 1986.

Summary of Nursing Actions—cont'd

ASSESSMENT	EXAMPLES OF POTENTIAL NURSING DIAGNOSTIC CATEGORIES
Following administration of analgesia/anesthesia A. Safety precautions: side rails; use of restraints on stirrups B. Labor: maternal or fetal response (as given above) C. Bladder distension	Alteration in normal physiologic response† Potential for injury (sensory deficits resulting from medication) Sensory-perceptual alteration: visual, auditory, kinesthetic, gustatory, tactile, olfactory Knowledge deficit Alteration in patterns of urinary elimination Impaired physical mobility

OUTCOME CRITERIA*	PLAN/IMPLEMENTATION

Before administration of analgesia/anesthesia
A. Woman decides on the type of medication she wants.
B. Woman states she understands the medication selected.
C. Woman signs the Informed Consent form
 	
During administration of analgesia/anesthesia
A. Injury does not occur from needle if woman moves during injection.
B. Woman receives the correct medication and dose by the appropriate method.
C. Aseptic technique is used.
 	
After administration of analgesia/anesthesia
A. Injury does not occur from falls or from prolonged pressure on anesthetized tissues.
B. Physician is informed when
  1. Pain sensation returns.
  2. Maternal vital signs change.
  3. Uterine contractions change—decrease in intensity, frequency, duration.
  4. FHR pattern changes.
C. Hydration is maintained with solutions such as lactated Ringer's.
D. Nurse maintains records.
  1. Evidence of need for medication.
  2. Medication: type, amount, dose, time, route of administration.
  3. Effects of woman ("discomfort lessened") or effects on fetus ("FHR 140").
	Implements roles as support person, teacher/counselor/advocate, and technician.
	
	Support person
	Provides explanation of procedure and what will be asked of the woman (e.g., maintain flexed position during insertion of epidural).
	Coaches woman regarding sensations she can expect.
	
	Teacher/counselor/advocate
	Reviews or validates woman's choices for relief from discomfort.
	Clarifies mother's information, as necessary
	Describes how medication is to be given, degree of discomfort to expect from administration of medication, skin preparation, time requirement for administration, interval before medication "takes hold"
	Explains need for keeping bladder empty
	
	Technician
	  1. Monitors labor: contractions, cervical effacement and dilatation, descent, status of membranes.
	  2. Monitors maternal and fetal response to labor: vital signs, blood pressure, FHR.
	  3. Monitors maternal perception of, response to, and coping with discomfort.
	  4. Assists mother to keep bladder empty.
	  5. Assists mother with position changes, hygiene needs, fluids and calories, as needed.
	  6. Initiates and maintains intravenous infusions.
	  7. Administers medications as needed.
	  8. During administration of anesthesia
	    a. *Ensures safety* by selecting wrapped supplies that are sterile and are not outdated; prepares mother's skin (nurse [and physician] practices *good handwashing techniques*).
	    b. Aids woman in assuming proper position and assists her in maintaining appropriate position.
	    c. Assists physician, as appropriate, if needed; opens sterile trays and packages; adds medications.

*Outcome criteria direct the selection of nursing actions (**plan/implementation**) and measure their effectiveness (**evaluation**).

OUTCOME CRITERIA	PLAN/IMPLEMENTATION
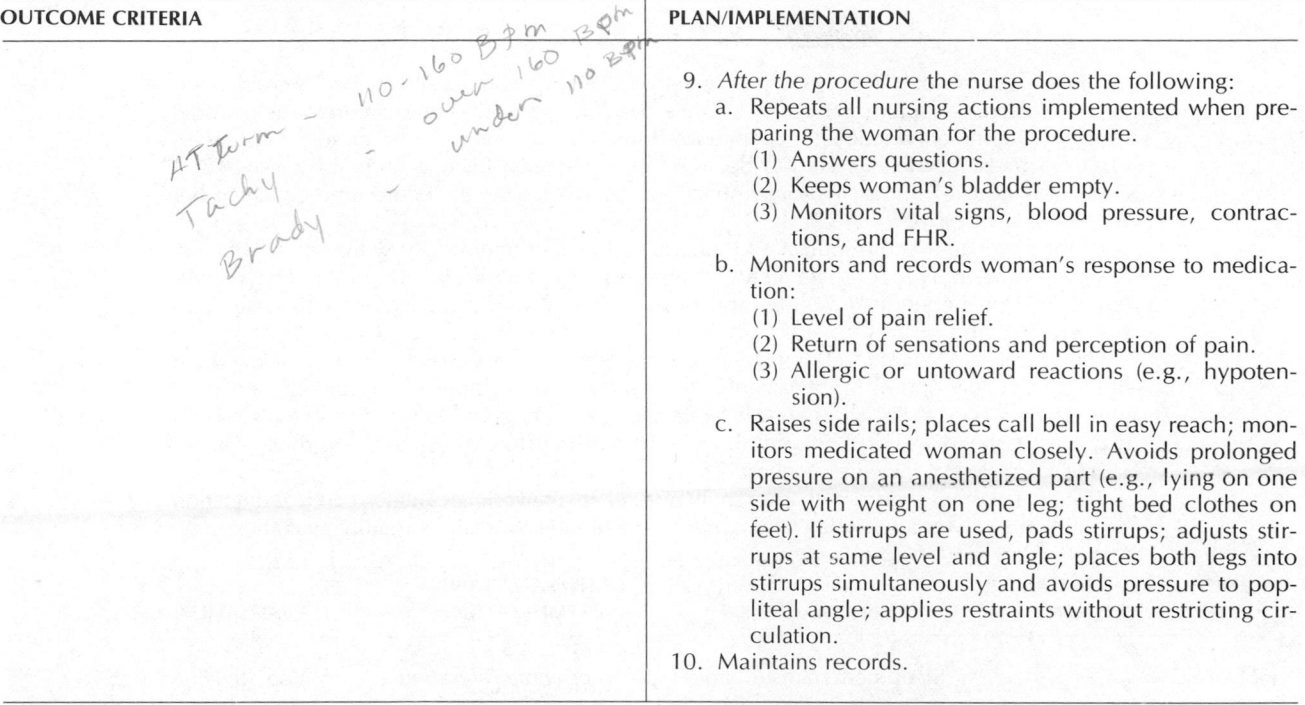	9. *After the procedure* the nurse does the following: a. Repeats all nursing actions implemented when preparing the woman for the procedure. (1) Answers questions. (2) Keeps woman's bladder empty. (3) Monitors vital signs, blood pressure, contractions, and FHR. b. Monitors and records woman's response to medication: (1) Level of pain relief. (2) Return of sensations and perception of pain. (3) Allergic or untoward reactions (e.g., hypotension). c. Raises side rails; places call bell in easy reach; monitors medicated woman closely. Avoids prolonged pressure on an anesthetized part (e.g., lying on one side with weight on one leg; tight bed clothes on feet). If stirrups are used, pads stirrups; adjusts stirrups at same level and angle; places both legs into stirrups simultaneously and avoids pressure to popliteal angle; applies restraints without restricting circulation. 10. Maintains records.

EVALUATION The nurse is assured that care was effective when the goals and outcome criteria have been met.

Fetal Monitoring

Fetal stress. Since labor represents a period of stress for the fetus, continuous monitoring of fetal health is instituted as part of the nursing care during labor. The fetal oxygen supply must be maintained during labor to prevent severe debilitating conditions after birth. Fetal stress can result in death in utero or shortly after birth. The fetal oxygen supply can be reduced in a number of ways:

1. Reduction of blood flow through the maternal vessels as a result of maternal hypertension or hypotension (Systolic blood pressure of 100 mm Hg in brachial artery is necessary for placental perfusion.)
2. Reduction of the oxygen content of the maternal blood as a result of hemorrhage or severe anemia
3. Alterations in fetal circulation, occurring with compression of the cord, placental separation, or head compression (Head compression causes increased intracranial pressure and vagal nerve stimulation with slowing of the heart rate.)

Before discussing the various techniques available to detect fetal responses to such stresses, current knowledge concerning baseline FHR and FHR responses to uterine contractions will be reviewed.

Baseline fetal heart rate. The fetal autonomic nervous system exerts primary control over the FHR. An increase in sympathetic response results in acceleration of the FHR. An augmentation in parasympathetic response produces a slowing of the FHR. Usually there is a balanced increase of sympathetic and parasympathetic response during contractions, with no observable change in the FHR.

Baseline FHR is the average rate between contractions. At term this average is about 135 beats/min, a decrease from 155 beats/min early in pregnancy. The normal range at term is 120 to 160 beats/min. Tachycardia refers to rates above 160 beats/min, and bradycardia refers to rates below 120. (Bradycardia should be distinguished from prolonged deceleration patterns, which are *periodic changes* that are described later in this chapter.)

Tachycardia may result from maternal or fetal infection and maternal hyperthyroidism. It may also be an early response to fetal hypoxemia and can be produced by use of parasympathetic blocking drugs (e.g., atropine). **Bradycardia** is a later response to fetal hypoxemia and may occur for a brief period just before fetal demise. It may also result from placental transfer of drugs such as local anesthetics.

Application of the Nursing Process

ANALGESIA DURING LABOR

Lynne, 24-years-old, married, G_2P_1, is in active labor: membranes intact, 5 to 6 cm dilated, 100% effaced, 0 station; FHR 140, average baseline variability, and no ominous periodic changes; uterine contractions: moderate to strong intensity, every 3 to 4 minutes, lasting 45 to 60 seconds. Lynne's cervix has been 5 to 6 cm dilated for one hour. Labor started at 7 AM; it is now 11:30 AM. Husband-coach has been with her the entire time coaching her with each contraction.

Lynne's prenatal record indicates no allergies. All other findings are within normal limits. A signed Consent Form is in her chart for analgesia and anesthesia. Her physician has written orders for meperidine, 75 mg, and hydroxyzine (Vistaril), 25 mg, intramuscularly, as needed for pain.

Lynne states, "I didn't get any sleep last night because my 2-year-old was sick. I'm so tired! I can't stay on top of these contractions. I really want something to take the edge off these contractions!" She does appear tense and is not able to follow her husband's coaching. Her husband leaves the room about once per hour to call to check on their ill older child's condition at his wife's request.

The nurse knows that sometimes a small dose of an analgesic facilitates cervical dilatation by helping the woman to relax. Naloxone hydrochloride (Narcan) is readily available.

FUNCTIONAL HEALTH PATTERN: ASSESSMENT	NURSING DIAGNOSIS	RATIONALE PLAN/ IMPLEMENTATION	EVALUATION
SLEEP-REST ■ Labor following loss of night's sleep; worry over ill child at home. **COGNITIVE-PERCEPTUAL** ■ Labor pain and fatigue ■ Concern for older child ■ Separation from ill older child ■ No progress in labor for 1 hour **HEALTH PERCEPTION–HEALTH MANAGEMENT** ■ Medication alters pain perception	Sleep-pattern disturbance related to sleep deprivation, fatigue, and labor. Alteration in comfort: pain related to labor. Powerlessness related to concern for older ill child and unavoidable separation. Powerlessness related to lack of progress in labor. Potential for injury related to sensory-perceptual alteration.	*To promote relaxation and labor progress and to enhance her sense of control:* ■ Implement nursing actions outlined in Summary of Nursing Actions: Pharmacologic Control of Discomfort. ■ Implement Summary of Nursing Actions: First Stage of Labor. *To prevent injury and to ensure her safety:* ■ Implement Summary of Nursing Actions: Pharmacologic Control of Discomfort.	Body tension eases. Dozes between contractions. Able to work with her husband-coach. One hour later: 8-9 cm dilated, station +1. States she is eager to push. Three hours after medication: baby is born, alert and in good condition with Apgar scores of 9-9. Mother recovers quickly and is ready for discharge home 6 hours after delivery. Mother (couple) state their satisfaction with relief from discomfort with medication. Mother sustains no injury.

Fig. 16.9

Fetal heart rate variability. Short- and long-term variability tend to increase and decrease together. (From Tucker, S.M.: Fetal monitoring and fetal assessment in high-risk pregnancy, St. Louis, 1978, The C.V. Mosby Co.)

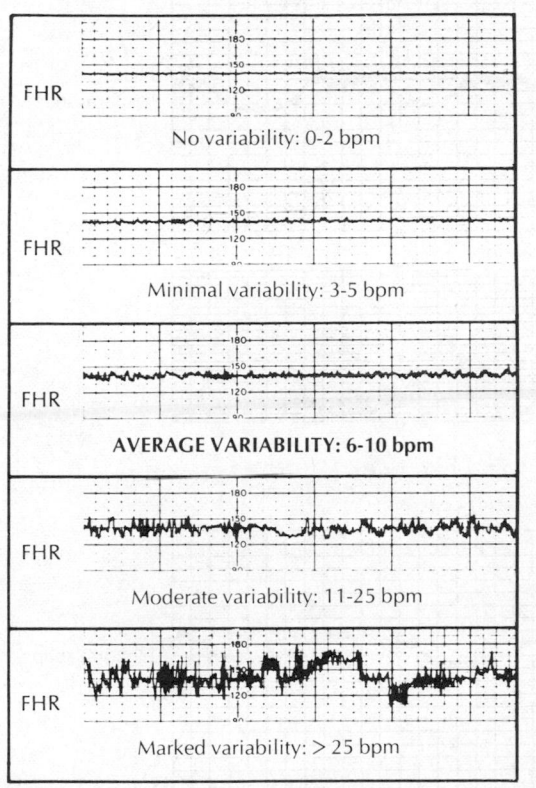

No variability: 0-2 bpm

Minimal variability: 3-5 bpm

AVERAGE VARIABILITY: 6-10 bpm

Moderate variability: 11-25 bpm

Marked variability: > 25 bpm

Another important aspect of the baseline FHR is the degree of **baseline variability** (beat-to-beat variations) (Fig. 16.9). Two types of variability have been described: long-term changes of 3 to 5 cycles/min and short-term changes of 120 to 180 cycles/min. These fluctuations correlate well with normal acid-base status and fetal health. Variability increases with gestation. Variability decreases with fetal sleep and the administration of certain drugs such as atropine, diazepam (Valium), promethazine hydrochloride, magnesium sulfate, and most sedatives and narcotic agents. Minimal baseline variability (3 to 5 beats/min) indicates central nervous system depression and is associated with fetal hypoxemia. No variability (0 to 2 beats/min) is described as a **smooth or flat baseline** and is considered to be an important warning sign of possible fetal jeopardy.

Response to uterine contractions. Fetal well-being during labor is measured by the response of the FHR to uterine contractions. In general, normal, active labor is characterized by:

1. A FHR between 120 and 160 beats/min with normal baseline variability and no ominous periodic changes.
2. Uterine contractions with the following characteristics (Tucker, 1978):
   a. Frequency of every 3 to 5 minutes.
   b. Duration of 30 to 60 seconds.
   c. Intensity resulting in a rise in intrauterine pressure to 50 to 70 mm Hg at the peak of a contraction.
   d. An average resting intrauterine pressure of between 8 and 15 mm Hg.

Fig. 16.10

A, Acceleration of fetal heart rate with uterine contractions. **B,** Acceleration of fetal heart rate with fetal movement. (From Tucker, S.M.: Fetal monitoring and fetal assessment in high-risk pregnancy, St. Louis, 1978, The C.V. Mosby Co.)

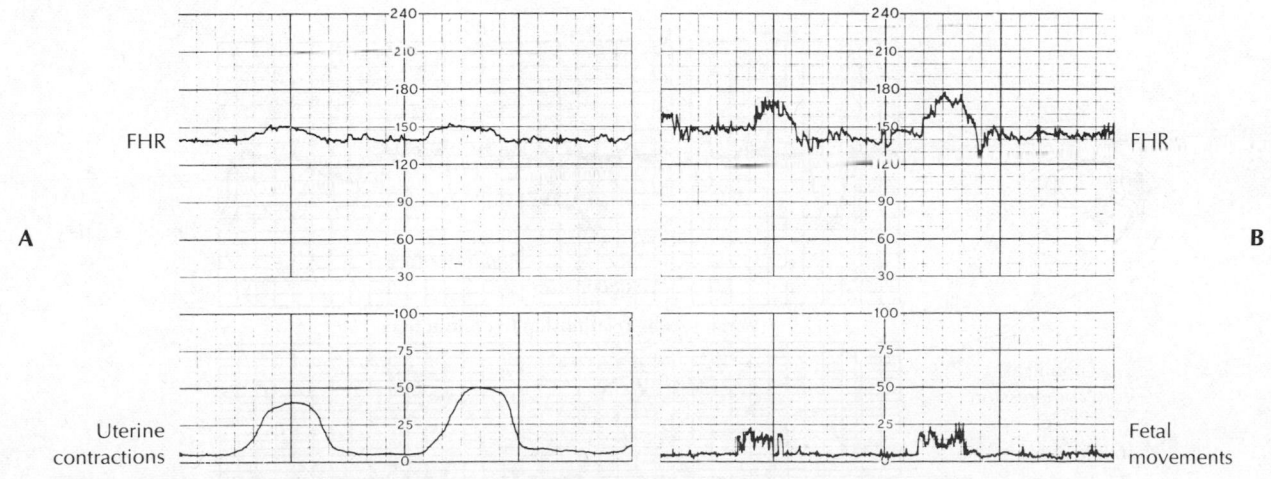

Fig. 16.11
A, Early decelerations caused by head compression. **B,** Late deceleration caused by uteroplacental insufficiency. **C,** Variable deceleration caused by cord compression.

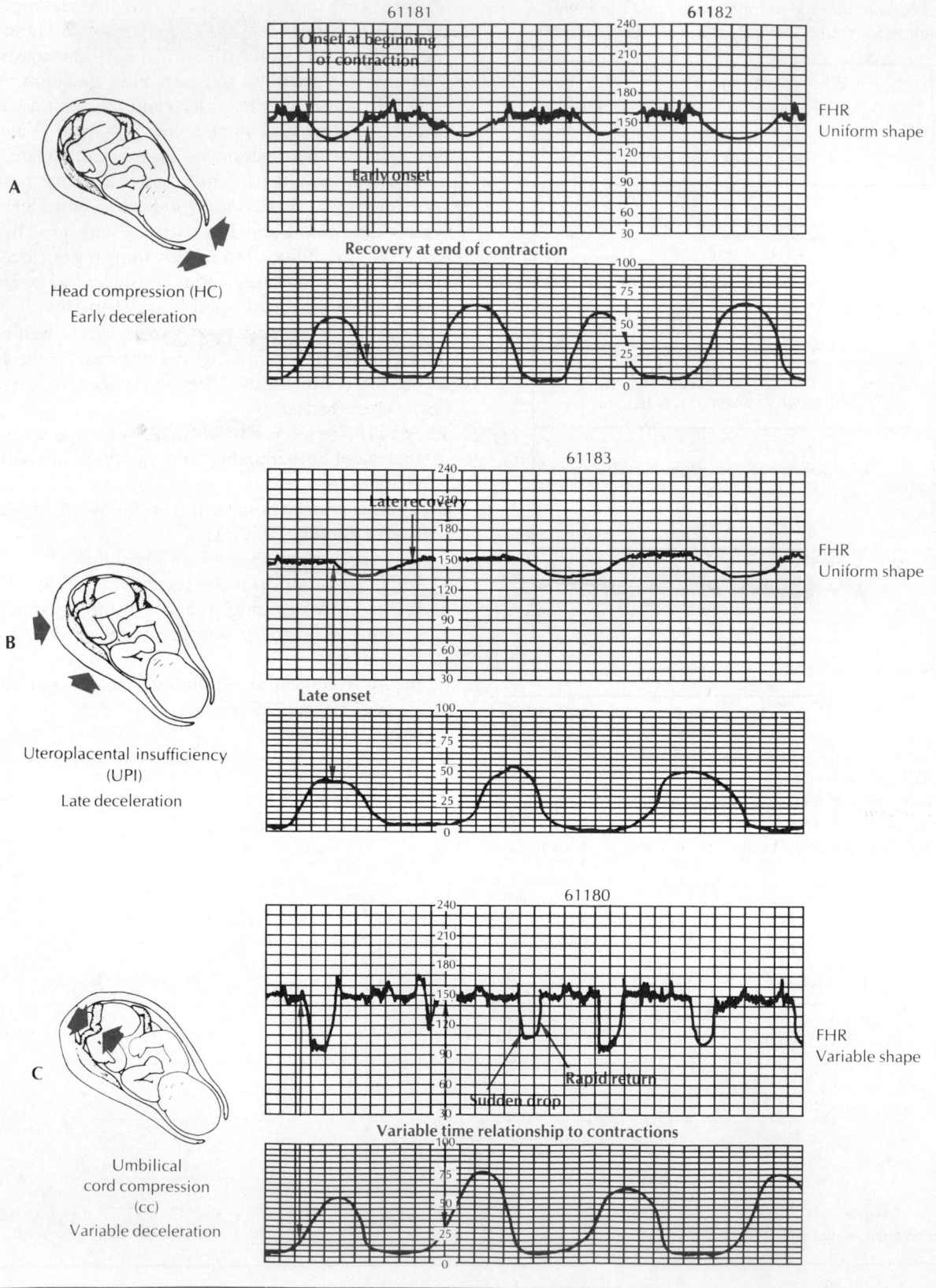

Head compression (HC)
Early deceleration

Uteroplacental insufficiency
(UPI)
Late deceleration

Umbilical
cord compression
(cc)
Variable deceleration

Periodic changes in the FHR are referred to as accelerations or decelerations, and the latter are described as early, late, or variable depending on their characteristics of timing, shape, and repetitiveness in relation to uterine contractions. **Periodic accelerations** (caused by dominance of the sympathetic response) are usually encountered with breech presentations (Fig. 16.10). Pressure applied to the infant's buttocks results in accelerations, whereas pressure applied to the head results in decelerations. Accelerations may occur, however, during the second stage of labor in cephalic presentations. **Nonperiodic accelerations** (Fig. 16.10) of the FHR occurring during fetal movement are indications of fetal well-being (nonstress test, p. 25).

Periodic decelerations (caused by dominance of parasympathetic response) may be benign or ominous. The three types of decelerations that are encountered during labor are early, late, and variable. Fetal decelerations are described by their relation to the onset and end of a contraction and by their shape. **Early** and **late** decelerations are described as uniform and bell shaped. **Variable** decelerations are U or V-shaped. Nursing actions for each type are described later in this chapter.

Early deceleration (slowing of heart rate) in response to compression of the fetal head is normal and usually does not indicate fetal distress (Fig. 16.11, *A*). Tracing is characterized by a uniform shape and an early onset corresponding to the rise in intrauterine pressure as the uterus contracts. It is not a common occurrence but when present usually occurs during the first stage of labor when the cervix is dilated 4 to 8 cm. Early deceleration is sometimes seen during the second stage when the parturient is pushing.

Late deceleration is also a smooth, curvilinear, uniform heart rate pattern that mirrors the pattern of intrauterine pressure during a contraction. However, the deceleration necessarily begins *after* the contraction has been established and consistently *persists into the interval after the contraction* (Fig. 16.11, *B*). **Late deceleration** when persistent or recurrent usually indicates fetal hypoxia because of deficient placental perfusion. Any drop in the FHR of more than 30 beats/min is sufficient for the diagnosis of late deceleration. It is usually associated with maternal hypotension or excessive uterine activity (e.g., during induction of labor). However, it may result from any maternal, placental, umbilical cord, or fetal factors that limit effective oxygenation of the fetus. If associated with minimum baseline variability, it is increasingly significant as an indicator of fetal distress.

Variable deceleration indicates a transient drop in the FHR before, during, or after a uterine contraction (Fig. 16.11, *C*). There is no uniformity to the FHR pattern. Variable deceleration may be related to partial, brief compression of the cord. If encountered in the first stage of labor, it can usually be eliminated by changing the mother's position, such as from one side to the other. It is most frequently encountered during the second stage of labor as a result of cord compression during fetal descent. Variable deceleration is associated with neonatal depression only when cord compression is severe or prolonged (e.g., tight nuchal cord). Variable and late deceleration patterns then occur simultaneously or are replaced by persistent bradycardia.

Bradycardia that is persistent is an ominous sign, especially when it follows a uterine contraction. Bradycardia during several contractions may indicate cord compression or separation of the placenta. **Tachycardia,** when continued for an hour or more and accompanied by late deceleration, is an indication of fetal distress.

Monitoring techniques. Following are methods of determining the degree of fetal distress throughout labor:

- Fetal heart rate monitoring
- Fetal blood sampling (pH and concentrations of oxygen and carbon dioxide [Po_2 and Pco_2])
- Noting the presence of meconium-stained amniotic fluid

Fetal heart rate monitoring

Periodic auscultation. Periodic auscultation of the fetal heart may reveal tachycardia, bradycardia, or arrhythmia that may occur during the brief examination (Fig. 16.12).

In the low-risk woman auscultation of the FHR may be done every 15 minutes in the first stage of labor and every 5 minutes during the second stage of labor. In both instances, auscultation is done for a period of 30 seconds immediately after a uterine contraction. However, ominous FHR patterns of a fetus in severe jeopardy may not occur during the periods of auscultation and may pass unrecognized by the examiner. Only marked degrees of fetal distress can be identified by listening to the FHR periodically (Pritchard and Mac Donald, 1985, p. 290).

An improved method that is more likely to aid in diagnosing fetal compromise in the high-risk pregnancy is the counting of FHR during sequential contractions and for a full 3 minutes thereafter. Persistent, postcontraction bradycardia (e.g., FHR of 100 beats/min, or a persistent drop of 30 beats/min or more below baseline) or gross irregularity indicates fetal distress.

Fig. 16.12
A, Leffscope. **B,** DeLee-Hillis scope. **C,** Ultrasound fetoscope; amplifies sound to those in immediate area. **D,** Ultrasound stethoscope; amplifies mechanical movement of fetal heart to listener by means of ear pieces. (From Ingalls, A.J., and Salerno, M.C.: Maternal and child health nursing, ed. 5, St. Louis, 1983, The C.V. Mosby Co.)

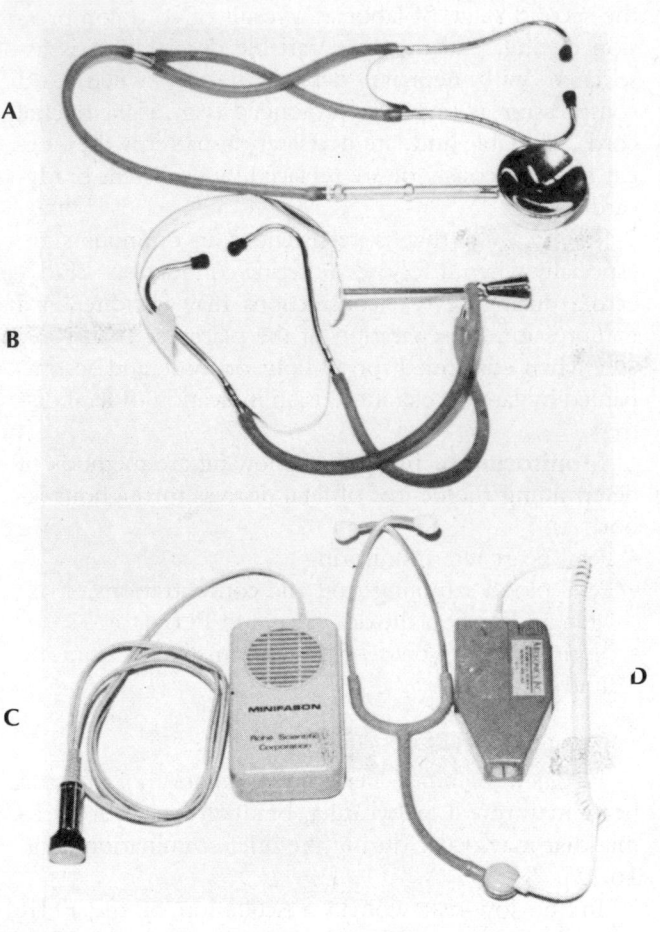

placed on the maternal abdomen to assess heart rate and uterine activity. The internal mode uses a spiral electrode applied to the fetal presenting part to assess the fetal electrocardiogram and the intrauterine catheter to assess uterine activity and pressure. A brief description contrasting the external and internal modes of monitoring is provided in Table 16.4.

External electronic monitoring. Separate transducers monitor the FHR and uterine contractions (Fig. 16.13). The *ultrasound transducer* acts through the reflection of high-frequency sound waves from a moving interface, in this case the fetal heart and valves. Therefore short-term variability and beat-to-beat changes in the FHR cannot be assessed by this method. It is also difficult to reproduce a continuous and precise record of the FHR because of artifacts introduced by fetal and maternal movement. The fetal heart rate is transcribed to a strip chart, and a consistent waveform is observed on the oscilloscope. Once the *area of maximum intensity of FHR* has been located, conductive gel is applied to the crystals on the ultrasound transducer, and the transducer is then positioned below the umbilicus (Fig. 16.13, *B*).

The *tocotransducer* (tocodynamometer) measures uterine activity transabdominally. A pressure-sensitive button on the side next to the abdomen is depressed by uterine contractions or fetal movement. The device is placed over the fundus above the umbilicus (Fig. 16.13, *B*). The tocotransducer can measure and record the frequency, regularity, and duration of uterine contractions but not their intensity. This method is especially valuable during the first stage of labor in women with intact membranes or for use in the nonstress test (NST) or oxytocin challenge test (OCT).

The equipment is easily applied by the nurse but must be repositioned as the mother or fetus changes position. The woman is asked to assume a semisitting position or left-lateral position (Fig. 16.13, *B*). It is removed periodically to permit washing of the applicator sites and giving of back rubs. This type of monitoring confines the woman to bed. Portable monitors allow observation of the FHR and uterine contraction patterns by means of centrally located electronic display units. These portable units permit ambulation during electronic monitoring (Fig. 16.14).

Internal electronic monitoring. The technique of continuous internal monitoring provides an accurate appraisal of fetal well-being during labor (Fig. 16.15). For this type of monitoring the membranes must be ruptured and the presenting part must be low enough for placement of the electrode. A small electrode attached to the presenting part yields a continuous rate on a graph and a visual report of the fetal cardiograph

The woman becomes anxious if the examiner cannot count the FHR. For the inexperienced listener it often takes time to locate the heartbeat and find the area of maximum intensity. The mother can be told that the nurse is "finding the spot where the sounds are loudest." If it has taken considerable time to locate them, offer the mother an opportunity to hear them too, to reassure her. If the examiner cannot locate the FHR, an experienced nurse should be asked for assistance.

There are two modes of electronic monitoring. The external mode employs the use of external transducers

Table 16.4
External and Internal Modes of Monitoring

	External Mode	**Internal Mode**
Fetal heart rate	*Ultrasound transducer:* High-frequency sound waves reflect mechanical action of the fetal heart. Used during the antepartum and intrapartum period. *Phonotransducer:* Microphone amplifies sound, reflects excessive noise when woman is in labor. Used infrequently for antepartum monitoring. *Abdominal electrodes:* Fetal ECG is obtained when electrodes are properly positioned. Used infrequently for antepartum monitoring because of ease and reliability of ultrasound transducer.	*Spiral electrode:* Electrode converts fetal ECG as obtained from the presenting part to FHR via a cardiotachometer. This method can only be used when membranes are ruptured and cervix sufficiently dilated during the intrapartum period. Electrode penetrates fetal presenting part 1.5 mm and must be on securely to ensure a good signal.
Uterine activity	*Tocotransducer:* This instrument monitors frequency and duration of contractions by means of pressure-sensing device applied to the maternal abdomen. Used during both the antepartum and intrapartum periods.	*Intrauterine catheter:* This instrument monitors frequency, duration, and *intensity of contractions.* Catheter filled with sterile water is compressed during contractions, placing pressure on a strain gauge converting the pressure into millimeters of mercury on the uterine activity panel of the strip chart. It can be used when membranes are ruptured and cervix sufficiently dilated during the intrapartum period.

Fig. 16.13

Diagrammatic representation of external noninvasive fetal monitoring with tocotransducer and ultrasound transducer, **A,** with ultrasound transducer placed below umbilicus and tocotransducer placed on uterine fundus, **B.** Note that client is lying in left lateral position. (**B** from Tucker, S.M.: Fetal monitoring and fetal assessment in high-risk pregnancy, St. Louis, 1978, The C.V. Mosby Co.)

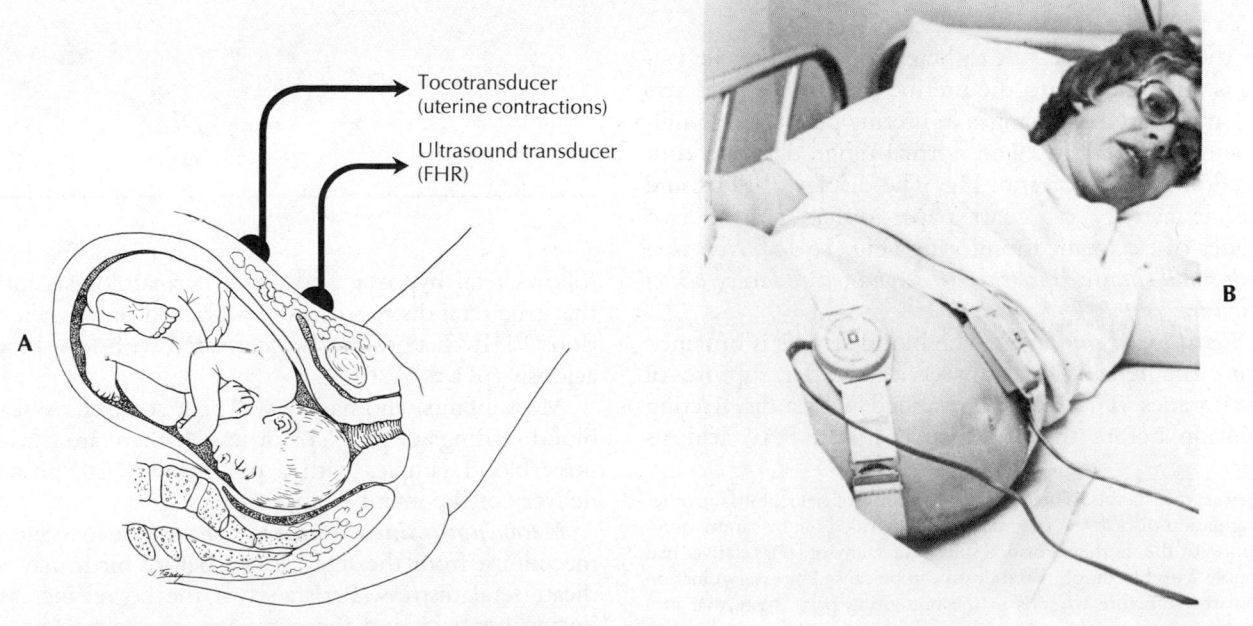

Tocotransducer
(uterine contractions)

Ultrasound transducer
(FHR)

A

B

Fig. 16.14

Woman wearing portable fetal monitor while working. (Courtesy Colleen Stainton.)

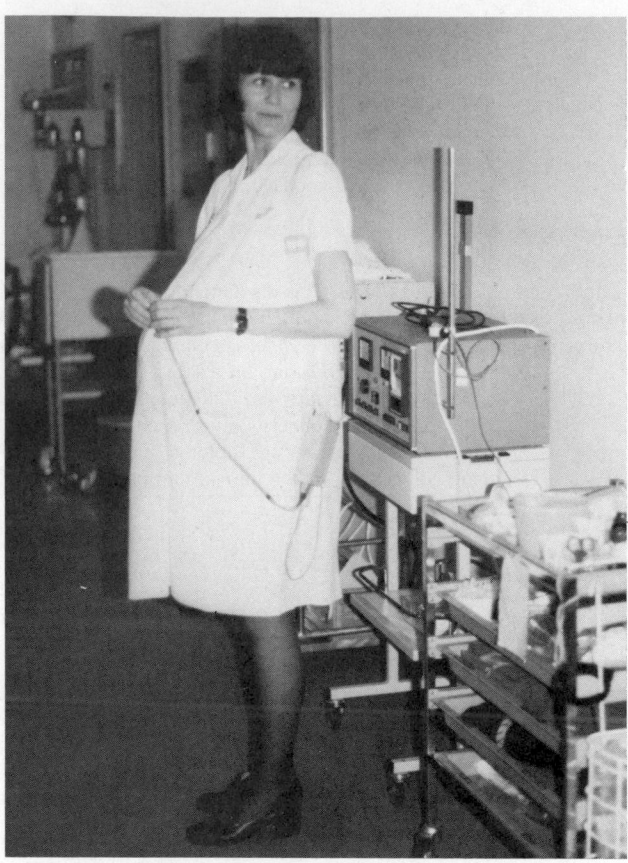

Fig. 16.15

Diagrammatic representation of internal invasive fetal monitoring with intrauterine catheter and spiral electrode in place, **A** (membranes ruptured and cervix dilated), and secured to woman's thigh, **B.** (From Tucker, S.M.: Fetal monitoring and fetal assessment in high-risk pregnancy, St. Louis, 1978, The C.V. Mosby Co.)

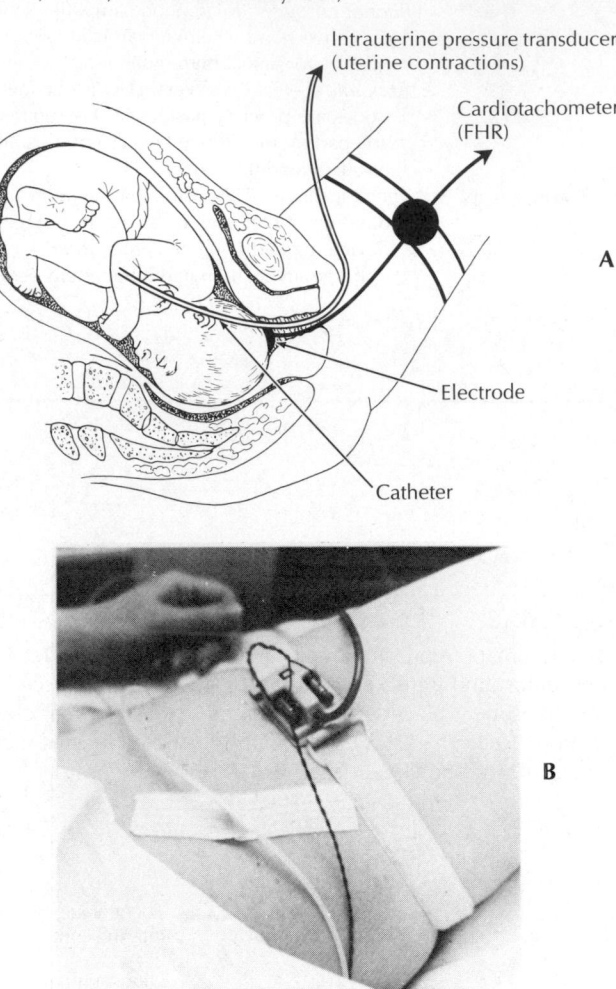

Intrauterine pressure transducer (uterine contractions)

Cardiotachometer (FHR)

A

Electrode

Catheter

B

on the oscilloscope.* A catheter filled with sterile water is introduced into the uterine cavity. The fluid acts as a transmitter of changes in uterine pressure into millimeters of mercury. The normal range during a contraction is 50 to 75 mm Hg. The display of FHR and uterine activity on chart paper differs for the two modes of electronic monitoring (Fig. 16.16). *Note that each small square represents 10 seconds; each larger box of 6 squares equals 1 minute.*

Fetal blood sampling. The blood sample is obtained from the fetal scalp transcervically after rupture of membranes. The scalp is swabbed with a disinfecting solution before the puncture is made. Fetal acidosis

*Before this method is used, the possibility of hemophilia or other coagulation disorder in the infant must be ruled out by careful questioning of the mother. For example, "Have any of your relatives had trouble with bleeding?" Fetal death can be caused by exsanguination from the puncture wounds in the presenting part. (Note that in a vertex presentation, the electrode is placed over a bone—*not* over a suture or fontanel.)

follows fetal hypoxia, and some perinatologists insist that true fetal distress can be diagnosed only when serious FHR changes can be correlated with fetal blood acidosis (pH $\leq$ 7.20).

Most infants who have low Apgar scores have scalp blood readings of pH 7.15 or less. If there are consecutive blood samples with a pH below 7.20, prompt delivery of the infant is imperative.

Meconium-stained amniotic fluid. The passage of meconium from the fetal bowel before birth may indicate fetal distress. Peristalsis of the bowel increases during hypoxia, and the contents are likely to be expelled. Although the presence of meconium-stained

Fig. 16.16
Display of FHR and uterine activity on chart paper. **A,** External mode with ultrasound and tocotransducer as signal source. **B,** Internal mode with spiral electrode and intrauterine catheter as signal source. (From Tucker, S.M.: Fetal monitoring and fetal assessment in high-risk pregnancy, St. Louis, 1978, The C.V. Mosby Co.)

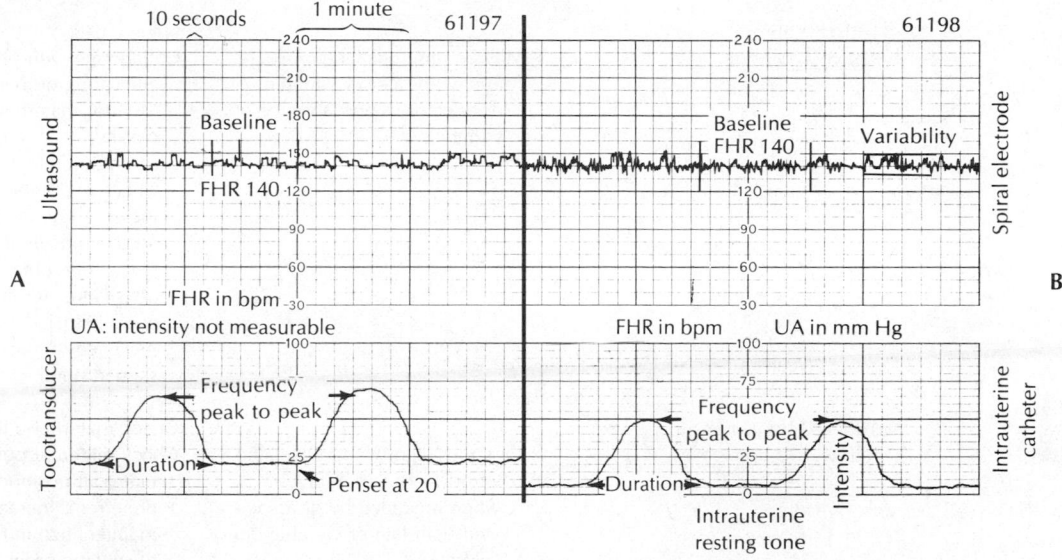

amniotic fluid is not always an indication of fetal difficulty, its presence requires immediate notification of the physician (see Chapter 15).

Pattern recognition and nursing standards: electronic fetal monitoring. Many factors must be evaluated to determine if an FHR pattern is reassuring or nonreassuring. This includes an assessment and evaluation of baseline rate, variability, accelerations, and decelerations, as well as consideration of the frequency and strength of uterine contractions. These factors must be evaluated based on other obstetric information, including parity, maternal and obstetric complications, progress in labor, and analgesia or anesthesia. The estimate of anticipated delivery time must also be considered. Intervention and interruption of labor are therefore based on medical judgment of a complex, integrated process.

It is the responsibility of the labor and delivery room nurse to assess FHR patterns, perform independent nursing interventions, and report nonreassuring patterns to the physician.

Nurses planning to work with electronic monitors require additional education and training in their use. Review Chapter 3, Legal Issues and Risk Management, for a clearer understanding of the legal responsibilities involved.

Table 16.5 presents nursing standards for electronic fetal monitoring (Blank, 1985). Fetal heart rate patterns and characteristics are described, clinical significance is indicated, and related nursing interventions are addressed in this reference table. Following Table 16.5 is the statement on electronic fetal monitoring. The statement is jointly prepared by the American College of Obstetricians and Gynecologists and the NAACOG, the organization for obstetric, gynecologic, and neonatal nurses.

Electronic Fetal Monitoring: Joint ACOG/NAACOG Statement

The primary goal of obstetric and neonatal care is to ensure optimal maternal and fetal outcome. An important tool in attaining this goal is electronic monitoring of the fetal heart. Nurses and physicians who perform fetal monitoring are responsible for their actions and will be held to the established standard of care as defined by their professional organization, the standards of practice in their hospitals, and the laws governing practice in their respective states. Hospitals should have a policy for the use of electronic fetal monitoring (EFM) in their obstetric patients. It is recommended that high-risk patients be monitored with continuous EFM.

Recognition and documentation. Physicians and nurses who use EFM must be able to recognize fetal heart rate patterns, beat-to-beat variability, and uterine activity. Fetal monitoring patterns have been given descriptive names (e.g.,

Table 16.5
Nursing Standards: Electronic Fetal Monitoring*

Fetal Heart Rate Patterns	Characteristics	Clinical Significance	Nursing Interventions
Baseline changes	Normal 120-160 bpm†		
1. Tachycardia			
a. Moderate	160-180 bpm		None
b. Marked	Above 180 bpm	May be ominous when associated with later or variable decelerations and absence of variability.	Collaborate with physician in alleviating primary cause. Monitor maternal vital signs closely, change maternal position (left lateral preferred). Check hydration status and increase rate of maintenance intravenous until specific order can be obtained from physician. Administer oxygen at 5 L/min.‡ Observe for presence of meconium-stained fluid.
2. Bradycardia			
a. Moderate	100-120 bpm, transitory		Check maternal pulse.
b. Marked	Below 100 bpm	Ominous sign when associated with loss of variability or when preceded by or associated with late or variable decelerations.	Check maternal pulse. Change maternal position (left lateral preferred). Increase rate of maintenance intravenous until specific order can be obtained from physician. Discontinue Pitocin drip, if infusing. Administer oxygen at 5 L/min. Observe for presence of meconium-stained fluid. Notify physician.
3. Variability	Normal fluctuations of fetal baseline. Refers to the intervals between beats.		
a. Marked			None
b. Average			None
c. Minimal		May be ominous if associated with changing baseline or decelerations.	Observe closely for signs of decelerations and absence of variability. Optimize fetal blood flow by changing maternal position. Notify physician.

Table 16.5, cont'd
Nursing Standards: Electronic Fetal Monitoring*

Fetal Heart Rate Patterns	Characteristics	Clinical Significance	Nursing Interventions
d. Absent		Ominous sign of fetal distress when preceded by a period of acute insult.	Change maternal position (left lateral preferred). Increase rate of maintenance intravenous until specific order can be obtained from physician. Administer oxygen at 5 L/min. Observe for presence of meconium-stained fluid. Notify physician.
4. Sinusoidal	Predominant pattern of rhythmic long-term variability with absence of beat-to-beat changes	When persistent, this pattern may be ominous.	Collaborate with physician in determining the significance and treatment of this pattern.
Decelerations§			
1. Early	Uniform shape, onset, and recovery correspond with contraction. Repetitive. Degree of deceleration usually does not exceed 110 bpm.		None
2. Late	Uniform shape with late onset (usually 20 s after beginning of contraction). Depth of deceleration proportional to amplitude of contraction. Repetitive.	May be ominous sign, especially when associated with change in baseline and absence of variability.	Change maternal position, (left lateral preferred). Increase rate of maintenance intravenous until specific order can be obtained from physician. Discontinue Pitocin if infusing. Administer oxygen at 5 L/min. Observe for presence of meconium-stained fluid. Notify physician. Anticipate fetal scalp sampling.
3. Variable deceleration a. Mild	Variable shape with sudden drop not to go below 00, lasting less than 30 s. Onset can be anytime. Recovery occurs rapidly. Baseline rate and variability remain unchanged.		Try alternate positions to minimize effects of cord compression. Notify physician.

From Blank, J.J.: Electronic fetal monitoring: nursing management defined, J. O. G. N. Nurs. **14:**463, Nov./Dec., 1985.
*As part of fetal assessment and in keeping with NAACOG standards, the intrapartum nurse has the responsibility of observing, assessing, evaluating information received from the fetal monitor, and intervening appropriately. The ability to recognize and interpret fetal heart rate patterns and uterine activity is inherent in the nurse's role in electronic fetal monitoring (EFM).
†Beats per minute.
‡Some hospital protocols specify 10-12 L/min.
§See Fig. 16.11.

Continued.

Table 16.5, cont'd
Nursing Standards: Electronic Fetal Monitoring

Fetal Heart Rate Patterns	Characteristics	Clinical Significance	Nursing Interventions
b. Deep	Variable shape with sudden drop below 80 lasting longer than 30 s. Onset can be any time. Recovery slow, may be accompanied by overshoot of baseline. Associated with rising or falling baseline or decrease in variability.	May be ominous pattern when associated with changing baseline and loss of variability.	Try alternate position to minimize effects of cord compression. Increase rate of maintenance intravenous until order can be obtained from physician. Discontinue Pitocin if infusing. Administer oxygen at 5 L/min. Notify physician.
4. Prolonged deceleration	Drop in fetal heart rate at least 30 bpm, lasting 2½ min or more. Not necessarily in relation to contraction pattern.		Collaborate with physician in eliminating primary cause such as hyperstimulation. Alternate maternal position (left lateral preferred). Increase rate of maintenance intravenous until order can be obtained from physician. Discontinue Pitocin if infusing. Check maternal BP and pulse. Administer oxygen at 5 L/min. Observe for presence of meconium-stained fluid. Notify physician.

accelerations and early, late, or variable decelerations). It is appropriate for physicians and nurses to use these terms in written chart documentation and verbal communication. It is especially important that when a change in fetal heart rate patterns is noted that a subsequent return to normal patterns be documented as well.

The medical record should include observations and assessments of fetal heart rate and characteristics of uterine activity as well as specific actions taken when changes in fetal heart rate patterns are observed. The monitor tracing is a legal part of the medical record and should include identifying information about the patient as well as times and events related to the patient's ongoing care.

Nonreassuring patterns. After the identification of a nonreassuring pattern, the nurse is responsible for initiating appropriate nursing interventions, as indicated by the pattern identified, and for notifying a physician. Once the physician is notified of a nonreassuring pattern, the nurse can expect the physician to respond. There should be established hospital policy for the nurse to follow in the event the physician is unable to respond in a timely fashion.

Staffing. To implement adequate intrapartum care of the patient in labor, staffing should be adequate in the labor and delivery area. Appropriate recommendations can be found in AAP/ACOG *Guidelines for Perinatal Care.*

Education. Electronic fetal heart rate monitoring requires the presence of skilled individuals to recognize heart rate pattern changes and the availability of physicians capable of proper diagnosis. It is the responsibility of the hospital to verify the knowledge base of health professionals in the clinical application of electronic fetal monitoring and to encourage the continuous updating of their skills.

Monitoring in the delivery room. When continuous electronic fetal heart rate monitoring had been used during labor, the guidelines as recommended in *Standards for Obstetric-Gynecologic Services (Sixth Edition, page 36) should be followed.*

References

American Academy of Pediatrics/American College of Obstetricians and Gynecologists: Guidelines for Perinatal Care, Elk Grove Village, IL, AAP/ACOG, 1983.
American College of Obstetricians and Gynecologists: Standard for Obstetric-Gynecologic Services, 6 ed. Washington, DC, ACOG, 1985.

Summary. Normal FHR patterns correlate with high Apgar scores and low neonatal morbidity. An abnormal pattern is equated with fetal hypoxia, low Apgar scores, and high neonatal morbidity in many but by no means in all cases. Because FHR patterns suggesting hypoxia may occur in the absence of fetal distress, intermittent and continuous FHR assessments are screening rather than diagnostic devices. More investigation and clarification of the factors and findings involved will be necessary to perfect the interpretation of fetal monitoring.

Summary of Nursing Actions

FETAL HEART MONITORING

GOAL
To maintain fetal well-being during labor and delivery.

PRIORITIES
1. To maintain adequate fetal oxygenation.
2. To identify and treat fetal distress.

ASSESSMENT

The interview, physical examination, and laboratory tests reveal normal findings.

EXAMPLES OF POTENTIAL NURSING DIAGNOSTIC CATEGORIES*

Alteration in normal physiologic processes†
Knowledge deficit

OUTCOME CRITERIA‡

A. FHR and pH remain within normal limits; no meconium-stained amniotic fluid is seen.
B. Gravida receives nursing care specific to the mode of monitoring used.
C. Gravida and family understand functions of the monitor.
D. Gravida is able to use learning derived from prepared childbirth classes.
E. The monitor functions accurately.

PLAN/IMPLEMENTATION

In the nursing care of gravidas and fetuses electronically monitored during labor the roles assumed by the nurse are support person, teacher/advocate/counselor, and technician.

Support person
A. To allay anxiety the nurse:
   1. Explains the basic functions of the monitor.
   2. Describes briefly the type of information printed on the upper and lower panels of the chart paper.
   3. Explains that the information regarding fetal status can be assessed continuously, even during contractions.
   4. Explains that although the digital display cannot print out every heart beat, it provides a sampling of FHR.
   5. Explains that the fluctuations and variability in the heart rate result in numbers such as 88 and 156 when the baseline rate is actually 120 beats/min.
B. To reassure and encourage some women, set the volume to an audible beep.

Teacher/advocate/counselor
A. To help gravida and family to adapt learning from prepared childbirth classes:
   1. Teaches them to effleurage upper thighs instead of abdomen.
   2. Teaches them to look at monitor to identify onset of the contraction to coach her to start the desired breathing sequence before she senses the contraction. The coach can note the peak of the contraction and relay this information to the woman so that she knows the contraction is half over and that the intensity will diminish.
B. To assist couples who are adamantly opposed to the fetal monitor:
   1. Notes that the physician has obtained a signed informed consent.
   2. Answers questions as necessary.
   3. Monitors FHR intermittently per hospital protocol.

*Diagnoses approved by the Seventh National Conference (1986) of NANDA except for those indicated by a dagger.
†Diagnosis not included by NANDA, 1986.
‡Outcome criteria direct the selection of nursing actions (**plan/implementation**) and measure their effectiveness (**evaluation**).

OUTCOME CRITERIA	PLAN/IMPLEMENTATION

	Technician
	A. To ensure the woman's comfort and proper functioning of the monitor:
	1. Cleans the ultrasound transducer and reapplies transmission gel every 2 hours as needed.
	2. Repositions the belts and tocotransducer every 1 to 2 hours; massages any reddened areas; provides a light dusting of powder under the belts often.
	3. Repositions the leg plate strap when ECG paste is reapplied.
	4. Uses a checklist to trouble-shoot the monitor (pp. 440 and 441).
	  a. Avoids dropping the transducers.
	  b. Avoids tight rolling of the cords (damages the wires and leads to an unsatisfactory signal).
	B. If an abnormal tracing appears, to ensure fetal well-being, the nurse immediately effects the following measures:
	1. Changes the woman's position from supine to side or from one side to another.
	2. Administers oxygen by mask (10 to 12 L/min).
	3. Stops oxytocin administration; changes to bottle of Ringer's lactate solution or 5% dextrose in water and increases drip rate to deliver 80 to 125 ml/h or more.
	4. Notifies the physician of the tracing and the effect of repositioning and oxygen administration.
	5. Completes preparation for cesarean delivery if the pattern persists.

Checklist for Fetal Monitoring Equipment

Name: ——————————————————— Evaluator: ———————————————

Date: ———————————————————

Items to be Checked	Yes	No	Remarks
Preparation of monitor 1. Is the paper inserted correctly? 2. Are transducer cables plugged into the appropriate outlet of the monitor?			
Ultrasound transducer 1. Has ultrasound transmission gel been applied to the crystals? 2. Was the FHR tested and noted on the chart paper? 3. Does a consistent wave form appear on the oscilloscope? 4. Is the strap secure and snug?			
Tocotransducer 1. Is the tocotransducer firmly strapped where the least maternal tissue is in evidence? 2. Has it been applied without gel or paste?			

From Tucker, S.M.: Fetal monitoring and fetal assessment in high-risk pregnancy, St. Louis, 1978, The C.V. Mosby Co.

*Uterine activity.

Checklist for Fetal Monitoring Equipment—cont'd

Items to be Checked	Yes	No	Remarks
3. Are there any accumulations of gel around the pressure button?			
4. Was the pen-set knob adjusted between 20 and 25 mm marks and noted on chart paper?			
5. Was this setting done between contractions?			
6. Is the strap secure and snug?			
Spiral electrode			
1. Are the wires attached firmly to the posts on the leg plate?			
2. Is the spiral electrode attached to the presenting part of the fetus?			
3. Is the inner surface of the leg plate covered with electrode paste?			
4. Is the leg plate properly secured to the woman's thigh?			
Internal catheter/strain gauge			
1. Is the strain gauge located about half the height of the uterus (approximately at maternal xiphoid)?			
2. Is the catheter filled with sterile water?			
3. Is the black line on the catheter visible at the introitus?			
4. Is it noted on the chart paper that the stopcock was opened to room air (reading 0 on paper)?			
5. Was the uterine activity (UA) tested at 50 for 10 seconds?			
6. Is the stopcock turned off to the syringe during monitoring?			
Charting			
1. Are testings of FHR and UA* written on chart paper at least every 4 hours?			
2. Is the chart paper properly labeled with the following:			
a. Woman's name			
b. Identification number			
c. Date			
d. Time monitor attached and mode			
e. High-risk conditions (pregnancy-induced hypertension, diabetes, etc.)			
f. Membranes intact or ruptured			
g. Gestational age			
h. Dilatation and station			
3. Are the following noted?			
a. Maternal position and repositioning in bed			
b. Vaginal examinations			
c. Paracervical block			
d. Medication given			
e. BP and TPR			
f. Voidings			
g. O$_2$ given			
h. Emesis			
i. Pushing			
j. Fetal movement			
k. Notations of baseline or periodic changes			
l. Any change in mode of monitoring			
m. Adjustments of equipment, i.e.:			
(1) Relocation of transducers			
(2) Flushing catheter			
(3) Replacement of electrode			
(4) Replacement of catheter			

Comments:

Application of the Nursing Process

INTERMITTENT FETAL MONITORING

Denise is an unmarried, 18-year-old primigravida whose EDC is 2 days from now. She has arrived on the labor unit to determine if true labor has begun. The prenatal record reveals that this pregnancy is progressing normally. She shares an apartment with another woman. While the nurse is listening to the FHR, Denise states, "I feel OK, but I have never been in a hospital before." She asks, "Why do you listen to the baby all the time? Do you have to do that when I'm in labor too? I don't want to sound dumb, but I've been dying to ask someone. Did my girlfriend call? She's going to be my coach if she can get off work."

FUNCTIONAL HEALTH PATTERN: ASSESSMENT	NURSING DIAGNOSIS	RATIONALE: PLAN/ IMPLEMENTATION	EVALUATION
COGNITIVE-PERCEPTUAL ■ Stated an interest in learning about need for fetal monitoring	Knowledge deficit related to inexperience	*To facilitate learning:* ■ Explain need for FHR; offer her opportunity to listen to it.	States she understands need for fetal monitoring. Continues to pose questions about pregnancy-related concerns without prefacing them with "I don't want to sound dumb." States she knows she won't feel as strange when she does return in labor.
SELF PERCEPTION–SELF CONCEPT ■ Age 18 years ■ First stay in hospital ■ First pregnancy	Potential for improved self-concept related to increase in knowledge base Powerlessness related to knowledge deficit and inexperience	*To enhance self-concept and perception of control:* ■ Encourage and answer all questions. ■ Review signs of true labor and any concerns she may have. ■ Introduce her to staff. ■ Orient her to facilities and routines of care.	
HEALTH PERCEPTION–HEALTH MANAGEMENT ■ Age 18 years ■ First hospitalization	Noncompliance related to knowledge deficit and inexperience	*To increase compliance:* ■ Demonstrate interest in her. ■ Explain. ■ Teach. ■ Introduce her to staff.	States she is pleased to learn about self-care.
ROLE RELATIONSHIP ■ Only support seems to be a woman with whom she shares an apartment. ■ First experience in a hospital.	Social isolation related to lack of assurance of presence of her coach.	*To decrease the sense of isolation:* ■ Reassure her that a nurse will be available to assist her coach or substitute for her coach.	States she is happy to know a nurse will be available to assist or substitute for her coach.

References

Abboud, T.K., and others: Maternal, fetal and neonatal responses after epidural anesthesia with bupivacaine, 2-chloroprocaine or lidocaine, Anesthesth. Analges. 61:638, 1982.

Avard, D.M., and Nimrod, C.M.: Risks and benefits of obstetric epidural analgesia: a review, Birth 12:215, Winter 1985.

Blank, J.J.: Electronic fetal monitoring, J.O.G.N. Nurs. 14:463, Nov./Dec. 1985.

Hodgkinson, R., and others: Neonatal neurobehavioral tests following vaginal delivery under ketamine, thiopental, and extradural anesthesia, Anesthesth. Analges. 56:548, 1977.

Jensen, M.D., and Bobak, I.M.: Maternity and gynecologic care: the nurse and the family, ed. 3, St. Louis, 1985, The C.V. Mosby Co.

Marx, G.F.: Pain relief during labor—more than comfort, J. Calif. Perinat. Assn. 4:36, Winter 1984.

Nurses Association of the American College of Obstetricians and Gynecologists: Statement: electronic fetal monitoring, joint ACOG-NAACOG statement, Washington, DC, 1986, The Association.

Petree, B.: A nursing perspective of obstetrical analgesia/anesthesia, NAACOG update series, 1:lesson 12, 1983.

Pritchard, J.A., MacDonald, P.C., and Gant, N.F., editors:

Williams' obstetrics, ed. 17, Norwalk, Conn. 1985, Appleton-Century-Crofts.

Rosenblatt, D.B., and others: The influence of maternal analgesia on neonatal behavior. II. Epidural bupivacaine. Br. J. Obstet. Gynaecol. **88**:407, 1981.

Tucker, S.M.: Fetal monitoring and fetal assessment in high-risk pregnancy, St. Louis, 1978, The C.V. Mosby Co.

Bibliography

Albright, G.A.: Neurobehavioral assessment—a prospective, J. Calif. Perinatal Assoc. 1:60, 1981.

Amiel-Tison, C., and others: A new neurologic and adaptive capacity scoring system for evaluating obstetric medications in full-term newborns, Anesthesiology 56:340, 1982.

Bonica, J.J.: Obstetric analgesia and anesthesia, ed. 2, Amsterdam, 1980, World Federation of Societies of Anaesthesiologists.

Bradley, R.: Husband-coached childbirth, New York, 1965, Harper & Row, Publishers.

Bromage, P.R., and others: Epidural narcotics for postoperative analgesia, Anesthesth, Analges. 59:473, 1980.

Cavanaugh, D., and others: ICF: obstetrical emergencies, ed. 2, New York, 1978, Harper & Row, Publishers.

Clark, P.E., and Clark, M.J.: Therapeutic touch: is there a scientific basis for the practice? Nurs. Res. 33:37, Jan.-Feb., 1984.

Clark, R.B.: Conduction anesthesia, Clin. Obstet. Gynecol. 24:601, 1981.

Dailey, P., et al.: Neurobehavioral testing of the newborn infant, Clin. Perinatal. 9:1, Feb. 1982.

Danforth, D.N., editor: Obstetrics and gynecology, ed. 4, New York, 1982, Harper & Row, Publishers

Datta, S., and others: Neonatal effect of prolonged anesthetic induction for cesarean section, Am. J. Obstet. Gynecol. 58:331, 1981.

Dilts, P.V.: Selection of analgesia and anesthesia, Clin. Obstet. Gynecol. 24:521, 1981.

Fishburne, J.I.: Systemic analgesia during labor, Clin. Perinatol. 9:29, 1982.

Freeman, R.K., and Garite, T.J.: Fetal heart rate monitoring, Baltimore, 1982, Williams & Wilkins.

Gibbs, R.F., editor: Legal perspectives on anesthesia, vol. 4, Jan-Feb. 1984. (Entire issue; McMahon Publishing Co., Georgetown, Conn. 06829.)

Hughes, S.C.: Intraspinal narcotics in obstetrics, Clin. Perinatol. 9:167, 1982.

James, F.M., and Wheeler, A.S.: Obstetric anesthesia: the complicated patient, Philadelphia, 1982, F.A. Davis Co.

Lundberg, G.D., editor: Anesthetics and neonatal response, J.A.M.A. 250:2133, 1983.

Nursing photobook. Using monitors. Nursing '81 books, Horsham, Pa., Intermed Communications, Inc.

Redick, L.F.: Epidural anesthesia, Clin. Perinatol. 9:63, 1982.

Roberts, W.E., and others: Pros and cons of meperidine for intrapartum analgesia. Contemp. OB/Gyn. 23:69, April 1984.

Schwarz, T.: Prolong regional analgesia with morphine—epidurally, R.N. 45(5):32, 1982.

Shnider, S.M.: Choice of anesthesia for labor and delivery, Am. J. Obstet. Gynecol. 58(5):24, 1981.

Smith, C.M.: Epidural anesthesia in labor: various agents employed, J.O.G.N. Nurs. 13(1):17, 1984.

Yurth, D.A.: Placental transfer of local anesthetics, Clin. Perinatol. 9:13, 1982.

Zuspan, F.P., and Quilligan, E.J., editors: Practical manual of obstetric care: a pocket reference for those who treat the pregnant patient, St. Louis, 1982, The C.V. Mosby Co.

CHAPTER 17

Nursing Care During the Second and Third Stages of Labor

In this chapter the physiologic and psychosocial processes of the second and third stages of labor are presented. Nursing care of the woman who experiences the rhythmic nature of the second stage of labor and birth will be discussed. Nursing responsibilities for the woman who delivers in a traditional setting are addressed. Nursing care of the newborn during the mother's third stage of labor is covered. While the third stage is primarily the focus of the physician or nurse-midwife, most responsibility for the normal newborn rests with the nurse. Terminology during the two stages are defined.

Definitions

second stage of labor Stage of expulsion of the fetus; from full cervical dilatation (10 cm) through birth of the baby. The three phases of the second stage are **latency/resting, descent,** and **final/transitional.**

Ferguson's reflex Pressure of presenting part on stretch receptors of pelvic floor stimulates release of oxytocin from posterior pituitary, resulting in more intense uterine contractions.

caul Hood of intact amniotic membranes covering head during birth. In Scotland a child born with a caul is thought to be gifted with "second sight." In the past, pieces of the caul were sold to sailors as a good luck token against being drowned at sea.

bearing down Tensing of abdominal muscles to push out or deliver the fetus; an involuntary reflex response to the pressure of the presenting part on stretch receptors of pelvic musculature. A strong expiratory grunt may accompany the push.

bulging of perineum Phase of descent when fetal presenting part is distending the perineum but is not yet visible at the introitus.

crowning Phase of descent when the crown, the largest diameter of the baby's head, is encircled by the vaginal introitus.

episiotomy Surgical incision of the perineum to enlarge the vaginal opening for delivery; perineotomy.

Ritgen maneuver Procedure used by the physician or nurse-midwife to control the birth of the head to protect the musculature of the perineum.

Valsalva maneuver Straining and breath holding with a closed glottis, often associated with adverse effects on fetus and mother; silent pushing.

ring of fire Burning sensation of acute pain as vagina stretches and fetal head crowns (Carr, 1983).

third stage of labor The stage of separation and expulsion of the placenta.

placenta The "afterbirth"; flat cake; specialized fetal vascular disc-shaped organ for maternal and fetal gas and nutrient exchange.

Apgar scoring system Standardized system permitting rapid assessment of the infant's physical condition for identification of infants requiring immediate intervention.

accoucheur One who delivers a child.

Second Stage of Labor

There is a rhythmic nature to the second stage of labor (Carr, 1983). The rhythm and movement emerge for the woman encouraged to listen to her body as she progresses through this stage. She responds by changing positions, pushing *with* the urge to push, and vocalizing as she bears down. This natural rhythm is lost if the woman labors recumbent in bed and must push on command. The rhythm is disturbed if she is then transferred to another room and onto the delivery table to deliver in the lithotomy position. In most non-Western societies, labor and delivery occur in one room. Women use a variety of positions for labor such as kneeling, sitting, standing, or squatting.

"In the majority of cases, labor and delivery are physiologic processes, and do not, in the true sense, require 'management'" (Danforth, 1982, p. 643). In response to the question of whether the accoucheur should interfere with the process of labor during the second stage, Warrington (1842) replied, "He should

Table 17.1
Maternal Progress in Second Stage of Labor

Criterion	Latent/Resting (10-20 min)	Descent	Final/Transition
Contractions 　Magnitude (intensity) 　Frequency 　Duration	Period of physiologic lull for all criteria Period of peace and rest (Carr, 1983; Mahan and McKay, 1984)	Significant increase 2½ min 90 s	Overwhelmingly strong Expulsive 2½ min 90 s
Descent		Increases and Ferguson's reflex activated	Rapid
Show: color and amount		Significant increase in dark red bloody show	Fetal head visible at introitus; bloody show accompanies birth of head
Spontaneous bearing-down efforts	Slight to absent except with peaks of strongest contractions (Carr, 1983)	Increased urgency to bear down	Greatly increased
Vocalization		Grunting sounds or expiratory vocalization (Carr, 1983; Mahan and McKay, 1984)	Grunting sounds and expiratory vocalizations continue
Maternal behavior (Carr, 1983)	Experiences sense of relief that transition to second stage is finished Feels fatigued and sleepy Feels a sense of accomplishment and optimism, since the "worst is over" Feels in control	Senses increased urgency Alters respiratory pattern: has short 4 to 5 s breath-holds with regular breaths in between, 5-7 times per contraction Makes grunting sounds or expiratory vocalizations	Expresses sense of extreme pain Expresses feelings of powerlessness Shows decreased ability to listen or concentrate on anything but giving birth Describes the "ring of fire" Often shows excitement immediately following delivery of head

let it alone if he has ascertained that the position is correct" (p. 228).

Assessment

Identification of second stage. The only positive objective sign that the second stage has begun is obtained by vaginal examination. The cervix is fully dilated and cannot be felt on vaginal examination (Myles, 1981). Other signs that suggest the onset of the second stage include the following:

1. Sudden appearance of sweat on the upper lip
2. An episode of vomiting
3. An increase in bloody show

These signs are thought to appear at the time the cervix reaches full dilatation (Danforth, 1982; Myles, 1981). Other indicators for each of the phases of the second stage are listed in Table 17.1.

Schedule of assessments. Assessment is continuous during the second stage of labor. The specific type and timing of assessments are determined by hospital protocol. These may include the following types of assessments (see Chapter 15 for assessment procedures). During the second stage *each* contraction is monitored for frequency, strength, duration, intensity, and fetal response. Descent of the presenting part is confirmed

by vaginal examination until the presenting part can be seen at the introitus. The degree of bladder filling is assessed.

If the FHR is monitored intermittently with a fetoscope, it is checked after every contraction or every 5 minutes. If continuous FHR monitoring is used (Chapter 16), the nurse checks the tracings on the monitor with each contraction. Mild, brief bradycardia and decelerations can occur in 90% or more of women during the second stage of labor (Mahan and McKay, 1984). If recovery of the FHR from the deceleration is prompt after the contraction and expulsive forces cease, the labor is permitted to continue (Pritchard, MacDonald, and Gant, 1985).

Maternal vital signs and blood pressure are checked every 30 minutes. The blood pressure is obtained between contractions (see Procedure 15.1). The presence of amnesia between contractions is noted. The partner's or father's response is assessed.

All protocols include assessment of show and amniotic fluid. Show is checked for evidence of excessive bleeding. The amniotic fluid is checked for meconium staining and amount. Vaginal examinations are avoided or the number restricted whenever possible. Characteristics given in Table 17.1 can be used to plot

Table 17.2
Duration of Second Stage

Parity	Range (min)	Average (min)
Nulliparas	25-75	57
Multiparas	13-17	14.4

Table 17.3
Duration of Second Stage by Bearing-down Technique

Number	Technique	Duration (min)
5	Traditional (coached)	74.2
5	Spontaneous	67.4

progress for a labor that is within normal limits.

Duration of second stage. Controversy continues over the precise duration of this stage within normal limits. Friedman's curve (Figs. 15.9 and 15.10) is one tool by which to assess the progress of the second stage. Application of Friedman's curve is "often erroneously misinterpreted as meaning that all labors must be completed within a prescribed time" (Mahan and McKay, 1984, p. 37). Mahan and McKay (1984) compared duration findings from 16 researchers, which are noted in Table 17.2.

In a pilot study, Yeates and Roberts (1984) compared spontaneous and traditional bearing-down techniques of 10 nulliparas to duration of second stage. The findings appear in Table 17.3.

Danger signs. Early identification and prompt intervention are required if the normal processes are disrupted. A second-stage duration of more than 2 hours for a nullipara and more than 1 hour for a multipara must be reported to the physician. Signs that alert to potential problems are listed below (Mahan and McKay, 1984).

Timing for transfer to the delivery room. If birth is expected to occur in the delivery room, it is best to transfer the woman early enough to avoid a last-min-

ute rush. Criteria for transfer to the delivery room are repeated from Chapter 15. See also Table 17.4, Nurse/Support Person's actions during the descent phase of the second stage of labor.

If any parturient, nullipara or multipara, states, "The baby is coming!" the baby *is* coming, and it is too late for the transfer. The baby is coming *now*—prepare to assist her if the physician is not yet present. See When the Nurse Assists the Mother to Give Birth, pp. 465 to 471.

Nursing diagnosis. Nursing diagnoses lend direction to types of nursing actions needed to implement a plan of care. Before establishing nursing diagnoses, the nurse analyzes the significance of findings collected during assessment.

1. Potential for injury to mother and fetus related to persistent use of Valsalva maneuver
2. Disturbance in self-concept, related to knowledge deficit of normal, beneficial effect of vocalizations during bearing-down efforts
3. Ineffective individual coping, related to coaching that contradicts her physiologic urge to push
4. Ineffective individual (sibling) coping, related to absence of appropriate care-giver
5. Alteration in comfort, pain, related to knowledge deficit of underlying reasons for perineal sensations

Planning. During this important step, goals are set in client-centered terms and prioritized. Nursing actions are selected, with the client where appropriate, to meet the goals. The speed and accuracy with which planning is accomplished depends on the nurse's level of competence (Chapter 2).

Goals
1. A second stage that is physically safe and emotionally satisfying
2. A cheerful, comfortable, and supportive environment
3. Participation of woman in the process of labor
4. Inclusion of family members of her choice

Implementation. A variety of support measures can be used for the woman during the second stage. The woman is encouraged to indicate other support measures she would like. Some options are not univer-

---

Danger Signs During Second Stage

Duration Over 2 hours for nullipara; over 1 hour for multipara
FHR pattern Abnormal; loss of variability
Descent Arrest in progress of descent and rotation
Uterine contractions Poor quality
Fetal blood pH Under 7.20

Transfer to Delivery Room

Parity	Stage	Characteristic
Nulliparas	Second	When the presenting part begins to distend the perineum
Multiparas	First	When the cervix is dilated to 8 to 9 cm

Table 17.4
Summary of Woman's Expected Responses and Support Person's Actions by Phase of Second Stage of Labor

Phase	Woman	Nurse/Support Person
Latent/resting	Experiences a short period (10-20 min) of peace and rest	Encourages woman to listen to her body (Carr, 1983) Continues support measures (Chapter 15, Implementation) If descent phase does not begin after 20 min, suggests upright position to encourage progression of descent
Descent	Senses increased urgency to bear down as Ferguson's reflex is elicted Notes increase in intensity of uterine contractions Demonstrates change in respiratory pattern, e.g., 5-second breath-holds, 5 to 7 per contraction Makes grunting sounds or expiratory vocalizations	Endorses respiratory pattern (short breath-holds with glottis closed) Stresses normalcy and benefits of grunting sounds and expiratory vocalizations Encourages pushing *with* urge to push Encourages/suggests maternal movement and position changes (upright, if descent is not occurring) If descent is occurring, encourages woman to listen to her body regarding movement and position change Discourages long breath holding If transfer to a delivery room cannot be avoided, nurse transfers her early to avoid rushing or offers her option of walking to DR if permitted If descent is too fast, places her in lateral recumbent position to slow descent (Carr, 1983)
Final/transitional	Behaves in manner similar to transition during first stage (8-10 cm) Experiences a sense of severe pain and powerlessness (Carr, 1983) Shows decreased ability to listen Concentrates on delivery of baby until head is born Experiences contractions as overwhelming in intensity Reports "ring of fire" as head crowns Maintains respiratory pattern of 3 to 5, 5-second breath-holds per contraction followed by forced expiration Eases head out with short expirations Responds with excitement and relief after head is born	Encourages slow, gentle pushing (Carr, 1983) Explains that "blowing away the contraction" facilitates a slower birth of the head Provides mirror or guides woman to see/touch emerging fetal head (best to extend over 2 to 3 contractions) to help her understand the perineal sensations Coaches relaxation of mouth, throat, and neck to relax pelvic floor Applies warm compresses to perineum to aid relaxation

sally available, for example, the warm tub at Pithiviers, France, or a warm shower. A summary of the woman's expected responses and some suggested actions by the support person are found in Table 17.4.

Maternal position. The woman may want to assume positions such as squatting. For this position a firm surface (not the mattress on a bed) is required, and the woman will need side support. Another position is the side-lying position with the upper leg held by the nurse or coach or placed on a pillow. Some women prefer Fowler's position, which can be attained with the support of a wedged pillow or with the father supporting the woman. Others prefer the hands and knees or standing position when bearing down.

Bearing-down efforts. As the fetal head reaches the pelvic floor, most women experience the urge to push. Automatically the woman will begin to exert downward pressure by contracting her abdominal muscles while relaxing her pelvic floor. When helping women to push, the nurse encourages them to push as *they* feel like pushing. The nurse monitors the woman's breath-

ing so that the woman does not hold her breath more than 5 seconds at a time. If breath is held more than 5 seconds, the Valsalva maneuver may be triggered. This results in the woman's closing the glottis, thereby increasing intrathoracic and cardiovascular pressure. In addition, holding her breath for more than 5 seconds diminishes the perfusion of oxygen across the placenta and results in fetal hypoxia. The nurse reminds the woman to take deep breaths to refill her lungs.

To ensure slow delivery of the fetal head, the nurse encourages the woman to control the urge to push. The urge to push is controlled by coaching the woman to take panting breaths or to exhale slowly through pursed lips as the baby's head crowns. The woman needs simple, clear directions from *one* coach.

Birth beds and chairs. There is no single position for childbirth. Labor is a dynamic, interactive process between the mother's uterus, pelvis, and voluntary muscles. Angles between the baby and the mother's pelvis constantly change as the infant turns and flexes down the birth canal. If able to, a mother will con-

Fig. 17.1

Delivery room. **A,** Starting at left top of picture and proceeding to right and bottom: door to warmer; roller; x-ray viewing box, fetal heart monitor; Apgar scoring chart; suction; socket for stirrup. Nurse is responsible for seeing that the room is kept clean and ready for use at a moment's notice. Behind delivery table on left is anesthesia machine, intravenous pole with fluid, table of supplies and emergency cart, second clock and regular clock with second hand. Fetal heart monitor with its extension arm that swings over mother is out of the way. Wedge pillow elevates head of bed. **B,** Note foot pedal to raise and lower entire table; crank to raise or lower head or foot; lever to loosen or tighten stirrup; and hand grip for woman to use as she wishes. Nurse needs to know how to operate this table. One foot pedal is not shown—the pedal that stabilizes (brakes) the table. **C,** Infant Kreisselmann resuscitator with overhead heat panel. Emergency equipment and supplies and drug tray are positioned next to the resuscitator under infant-sized stethoscope. Nurse is responsible for seeing that resuscitator is plugged in and functional at all times in event of an emergency.

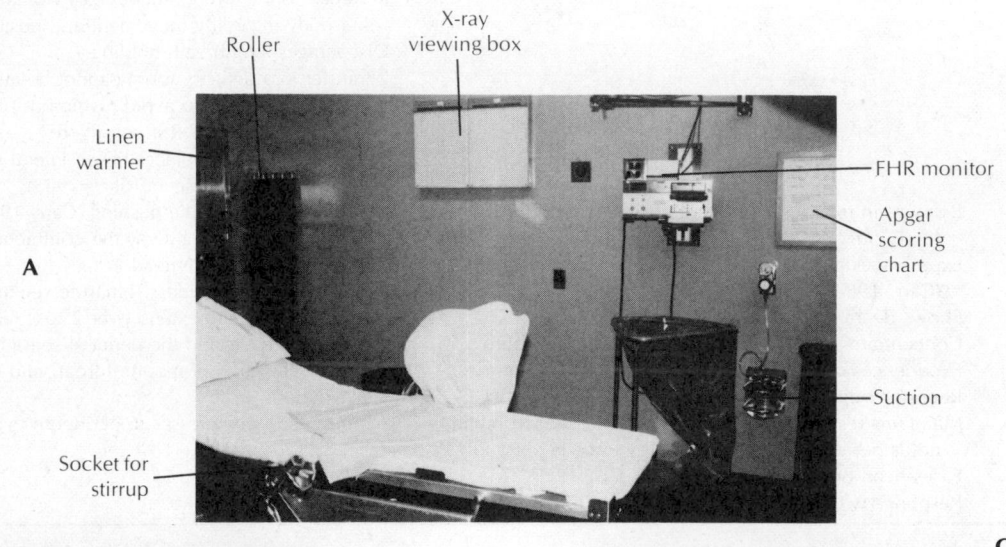

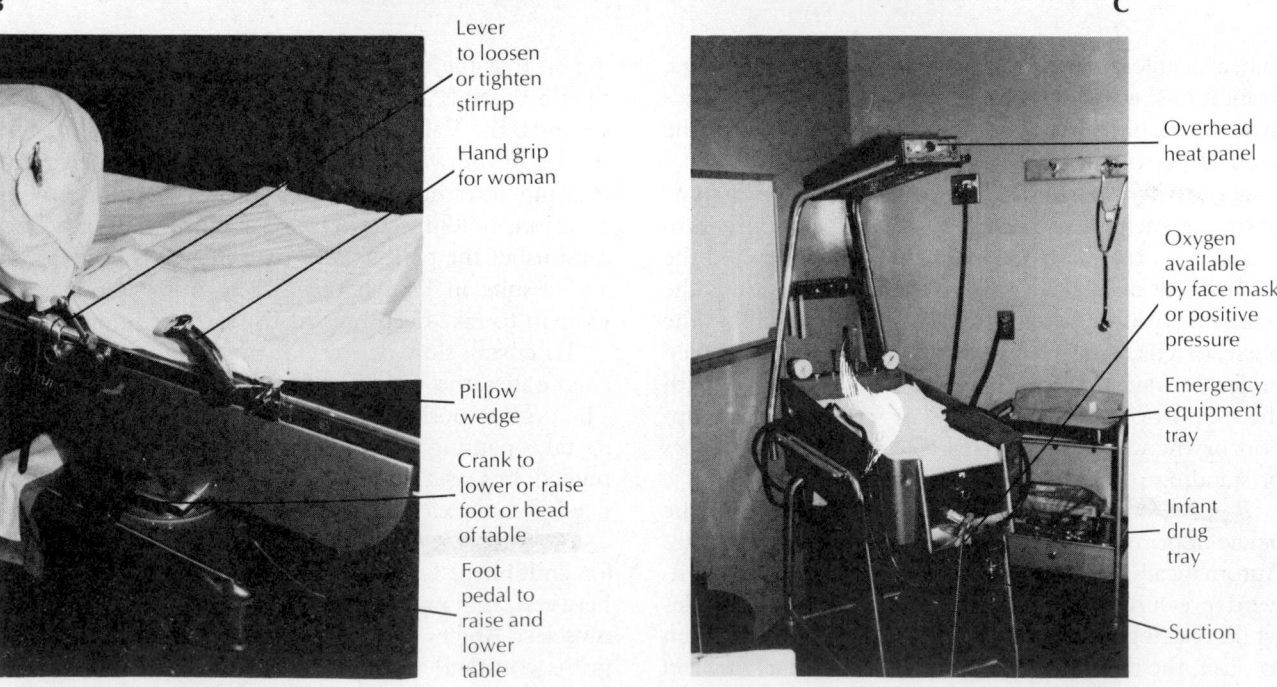

stantly change position in labor. The Borning Bed (see Fig. 13.9) changes shape according to the mother's needs. She can squat, kneel, recline, or sit, whatever is most comfortable. At the same time, there is excellent exposure for examination, electrode placement, fetal scalp sampling, and delivery. The mother has full control of both seat and back functions. She can adjust her position for maximal comfort. The mother and father can maintain close personal contact and a new degree of involvement in the birth if they desire. The bed can be positioned for administering anesthesia, the V-shaped perineal cut-out is adaptable to both forceps and spontaneous birth, and the bed can be used for transport to surgery in the event of a cesarean birth.

Birth chairs provide some women with a better physiologic position during childbirth, although some women feel restricted by the chair. There is a psychologic advantage to the upright position. The chair is designed so that, in the event of emergency, it can be adjusted to the horizontal or Trendelenburg's position.

Fetal heart rate. If the FHR begins to drop, or if there is a loss of variability, prompt therapy is initiated (Table 16.5). The woman can be turned on her side, oxygen can be administered by face mask at 10 to 12 L/min. If a maintenance intravenous line is in, the drip rate can be increased. This is often all that is required

to restore the normal FHR. If a normal FHR does not resume immediately, quickly notify the physician. Medical intervention to hasten the birth may be indicated (see box, p. 446).

Coach. During the second stage the woman needs continuous support and coaching. The coaching process can be emotionally tiring for the father. The nurse can offer him nourishment, fluids, and short breaks. If the father is to attend the delivery in the delivery room, he is given instructions as to donning cover gown, mask, hat, and shoes.

Preparation for birth in a delivery room. If the woman is to be transferred to a delivery area for completion of the birth process, the nurse uses the guidelines stated earlier in box on p. 446.

The delivery room birth table. Delivery rooms are specifically designed to facilitate care during delivery (Fig. 17.1) The delivery table is designed with many features: the entire table can be raised or lowered, and the head or foot may be raised or lowered. A wedge pillow or bolster can be inserted under the top of the mattress to raise it slightly, or the head of the table can be raised to prevent supine hypotension and to facilitate pushing. The table is equipped with stirrups for supporting the legs and handle grips to aid in bearing down. If stirrups are used, the bed can be "broken";

Fig. 17.2

Instrument table (all equipment sterile). *Top, left to right:* receiving blanket, perineal pad, vaginal roll, medicine glasses (for anesthetic agent), hand cover for spotlight, urine specimen bottle, towels, and placenta bowl and paper towel for covering scales. *Bottom, left to right:* syringe (anesthetic) needle guard, episiotomy scissors, bulb syringe (covered with gauze for aspirating newborn), two artery forceps, scissors, cord clamp, ring forceps, needle holder, thumb forceps (for repair of episiotomy), extra instruments (ring forceps, small artery forceps, toothed forceps, Allis clamps and sharp hook forceps for holding drapes in place), and kidney basin.

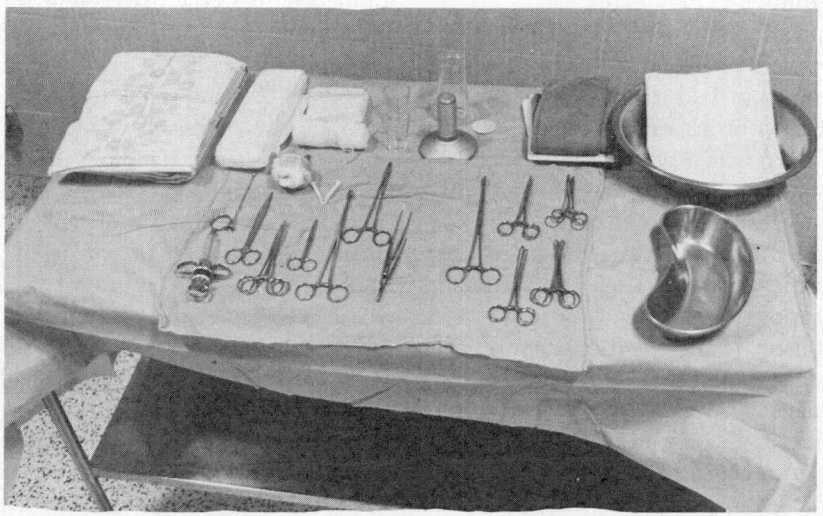

Fig. 17.3
Sterile delivery pack with a strip of nonsterilized heat-sensitive tape to illustrate difference between a pack that has been sterilized and one that has not. Lower pack illustrates proper labeling and dating of packs. Nurse is responsible for ensuring that all supplies used are sterile. (Courtesy Stanford University Medical Center, Stanford, California.)

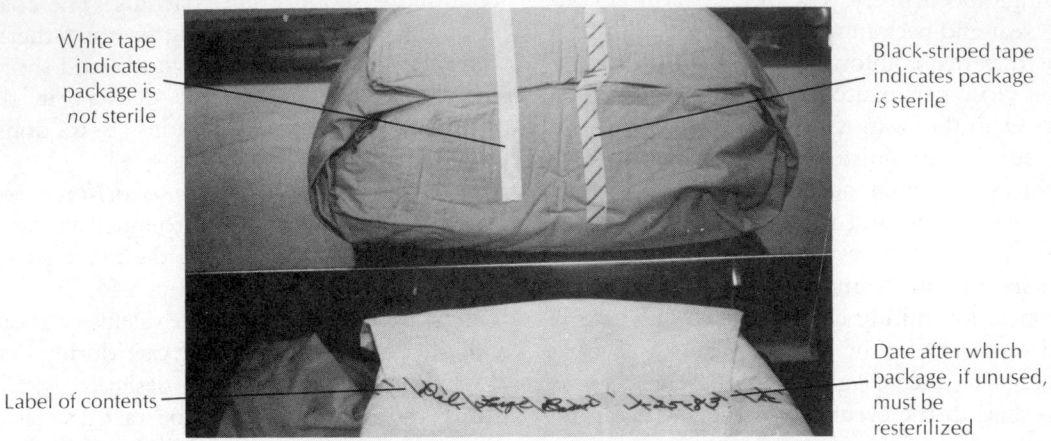

that is, the lower half of the bed can be lowered and rolled back to fit under the top half.

Supplies, instruments, and equipment. The delivery table is prepared. Fig. 17.2 illustrates one way to arrange the instrument table. Procedures for several delivery-related activities include the following:

1. Identifying a sterile pack (Fig. 17.3)
2. Opening sterile packages (Fig. 17.4)
3. Adding sterile supplies to the instrument table (Fig. 17.5)
4. Gloving (Fig. 17.6)
5. Perineal cleansing (Fig. 17.7)
6. Unwrapping and handing sterile forceps to physician or nurse-midwife (Fig. 17.8)

The crib and equipment are readied for the infant.

Birth in a delivery room. The woman will need assistance to move from the labor bed to the delivery table. If this is done between contractions, the mother can help, but because of her awkwardness, she cannot be rushed.

The position assumed for delivery may be (1) modified Sims' position (if this is the case, the attendant will need to support the upper leg), (2) dorsal position, or (3) lithotomy position.

The lithotomy position is the position most commonly used for delivery in Western cultures. The lithotomy position makes it more convenient for the physician to deal with any complications that arise. For this position the buttocks are brought to the edge of the table, and the legs are placed in stirrups. Care must be taken to pad the stirrups, raise and place both legs simultaneously, and adjust the shank of the stirrups so that the calf of the leg is supported. There should be no pressure on the popliteal space. If the stirrups are uneven in height, the woman can develop strained ligaments in her back as she bears down. This strain causes considerable discomfort in the postdelivery period. The lower portion of the table may be dropped down and rolled back under the table.

Once the woman is positioned for delivery, the vulva is washed thoroughly with soap and water or a surgical disinfectant (Fig. 17.7). The physician or midwife dons cap and mask, scrubs hands, and puts on the sterile gown and gloves. The woman may then be draped with sterile towels and sheets. The husband or coach helps the mother to remember not to touch the sterile drapes.

The circulating nurse will continue to coach and encourage the parturient. Once the woman's legs are in the stirrups, the handle grips can be used to pull against. The nurse will check FHR after every contraction and notify the physician as to the rate and regularity. The equipment for taking the blood pressure should be readied for instant use if signs of shock develop. However, the readings are distorted (increased) by the increase in thoracic and abdominal pressures as the woman pushes. A reading will be taken after delivery before transferring the woman to the recovery room. An oxytocic medication such as Syntocinon may be prepared for administration after delivery. Observations and procedures are recorded on the chart.

Fathers are encouraged to be present at the birth of

Fig. 17.4

Opening sterile packages. *1,* Remove heat-sensitive tape closing package and check tape for color change indicating sterility. Start unwrapping package with point of wrapper facing you. In this way the part of the package next to you will remain covered and protected for the longest period possible. *2,* Pull back point and let it drop down after assuring that outside of dangling wrapper will not contaminate any nearby sterile surface. *3,* Pull back two side folds by little turnback flaps. Uncover end on side, supporting under hand first, then side next to active hand. If you are preparing inner package for a drop onto a sterile surface, stabilizing pack by bringing your thumb over top of wrapper before completely exposing inner pack is sometimes helpful. *4,* Pull back last fold covering inner wrap to expose sterile surface. Inner pack can now be picked up by a gloved associate or it can be "scooted" onto a sterile table while ends of outer wrapper are held back to prevent contamination. *5,* If hand thumb grip is used, pack can be dropped in manner pictured. Care must be taken not to get too close to a sterile table or field while adding supplies. (From Ingalls, A.J., and Salerno, M.C.: Maternal and child health nursing, ed. 5, St. Louis, 1983, The C.V. Mosby Co.)

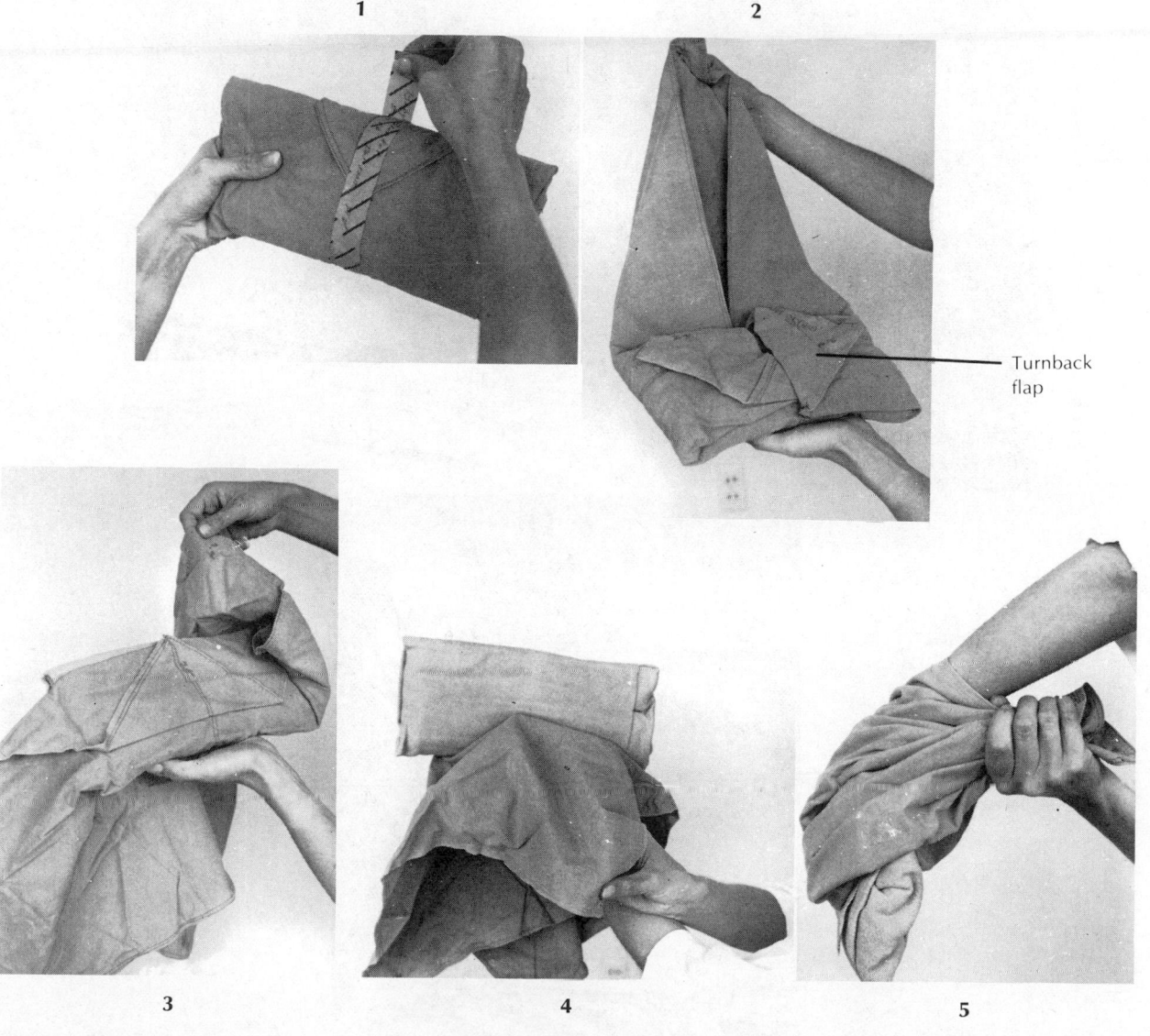

Turnback flap

Fig. 17.5

Adding sterile supplies to the instrument table. *1,* Extracting a sterile catheter with ring forceps from a commercially prepared peel-back package. *2,* Dropping sterile suture from a commercially prepared peel-back package. *3,* Lifting sterile instruments using ring forceps (uterine forceps or sponge sticks). For beginners this is a good grip. Curved Kelly forcep is balanced and is far from surface of table. Note sharp hooked instruments used for clipping drapes together in lower right corner of photograph. (From Ingalls, A.J., and Salerno, M.C.: Maternal and child health nursing, ed. 5, St. Louis, 1983, The C.V. Mosby Co.)

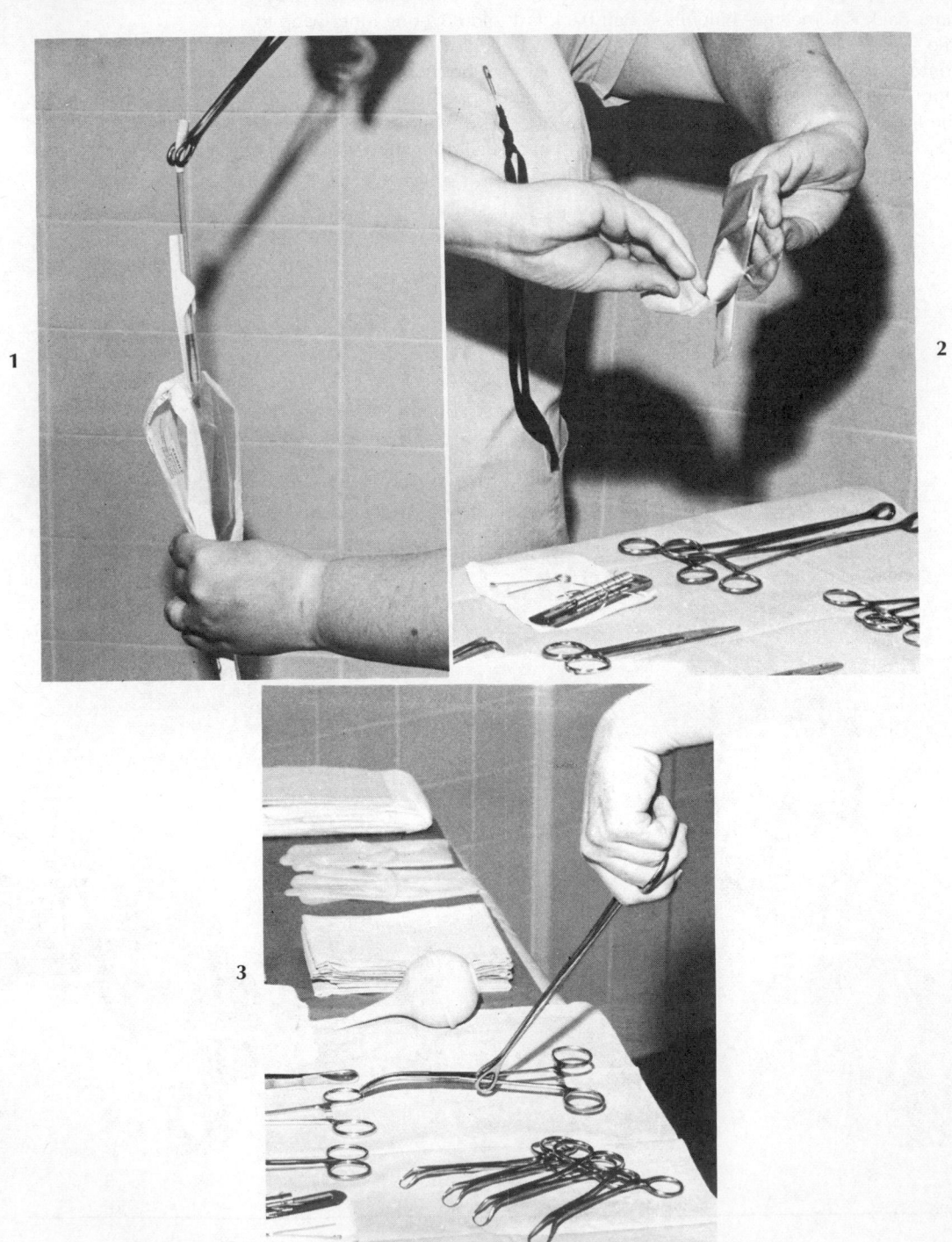

Fig. 17.6
Gloving procedure. *1,* Sterile gloves usually lie side by side with thumbs on top at outside edges, left glove on left and right glove on right. Pick up glove by pinching cuff folded down over palm of glove. If right-handed, slide on right-hand glove first. Your bare fingers may touch any area of the glove that represents the inside of tne glove. *2,* Slide your hand in with a rotating motion while pulling on turned-down cuff. *3,* Pick up second glove with your gloved hand by sliding your sterile fingers *under* turned-down cuff. *4,* Place your other hand into glove, sliding and rotating your hand as you pull out and up against inside of cuff with your gloved fingers. Keep your thumb back out of the way. Remember, your arm and top of cuff are contaminated and must not be touched with your fingers. When only gloves are worn, it is permissible to retain narrow cuffs at tops of gloves; but they, of course, are not sterile and should not be treated as such. *5,* After you are gloved, you may adjust the fingers. Learning to glove takes time, patience, and usually more than one pair of gloves. (From Ingalls, A.J., and Salerno, M.C.: Maternal and child health nursing, ed. 5, St. Louis, 1983, The C.V. Mosby Co.)

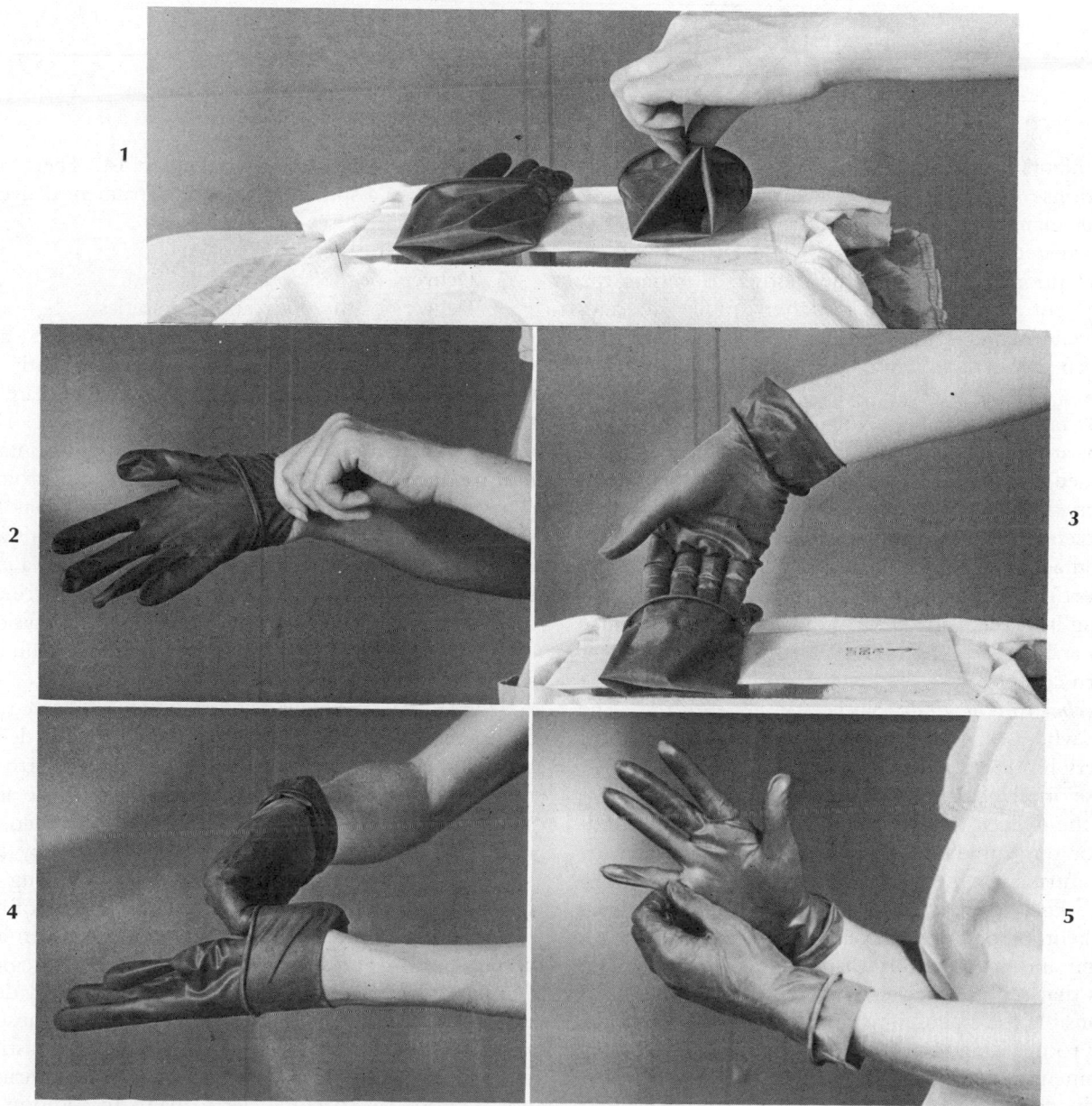

Fig. 17.7
Perineal cleansing. Use cotton swabs or gauze squares well moistened with disinfectant
solution. Discard swab after each step. Finish cleansing with wash of sterile water.

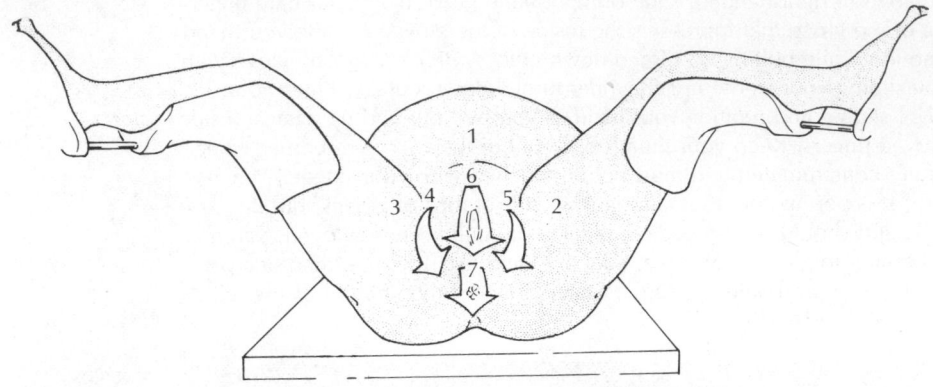

their infants if this is in keeping with their cultural expectations. The psychologic closeness of the family unit is maintained, and the father can continue the supportive care given in labor. The father needs as much opportunity as does the mother to initiate the attachment process with the baby. Studies indicate, however, that it is the continuous long-term contact between father and child that acts to cement the bonds.

The father is usually gowned in a clean scrub outfit and wears a cap and a mask. These supplies need to be provided in ample time for him to don them before the delivery. If the couple has decided that the father is not to be present, their decision should be respected.

Contact with parents is maintained by touch, verbal comforting instructions as to reasons for care, and sharing in parents' joy at birth of their child. The nurse notes and records the time of birth (i.e., when infant is born completely).

Mechanism of delivery: vertex presentation. The nurse who is knowledgeable about the mechanism of delivery has increased skills as support person, teacher/counselor/advocate, and technician. While most of the time the delivery remains in the hands of the obstetrician or nurse-midwife, there may be a time when the nurse must assist the woman to give birth (p. 465). The nurse's knowledge of the birth process provides a basis for client preparation before and during pregnancy. During and after delivery many new parents need answers that require specialized knowledge. The nurse is responsible for maintaining an adequately supplied delivery room. This responsibility requires knowledge of equipment needed and maintenance of asepsis.

Prior to reading this section, review Mechanisms of

Labor: Vertex Presentation, Chapter 14. There are three phases to a spontaneous, noninstrument delivery of the fetus in a vertex presentation:

1. Delivery of the head
2. Delivery of the shoulders
3. Delivery of the body and extremities

The presenting part, in this instance the vertex, advances with each contraction and recedes slightly as the contraction wanes; descent is constant, and late in the second stage the head reaches the pelvic floor. The occiput generally rotates anteriorly, and with voluntary bearing-down efforts the head distends the introitus (Fig. 17.9). Although more and more caput may be seen with each push, the head "crowns" when its widest part (the biparietal diameter) distends the vulva just before birth. Immediately before delivery, the perineal musculature becomes greatly distended. If an episiotomy is necessary, it is done at this time to minimize soft tissue damage.

Delivery of head. The vertex first appears, followed by the forehead, face, chin, and neck. The speed of delivery of the head must be controlled, or sudden birth of the head may cause severe lacerations through the anal sphincter or even into the rectum. The physician or nurse-midwife controls the birth of the head by (1) applying pressure against the rectum, drawing it downward to aid in flexing the head as the back of the neck catches under the symphysis pubis; (2) then applying upward pressure from the coccygeal region (modified Ritgen maneuver) to extend the head during the actual delivery, thereby protecting the musculature of the perineum (Fig. 17.10); and (3) assisting the mother with voluntary control of the bearing-down efforts by coaching her to pant. In addition to

Fig. 17.8

Unwrapping and handing sterile forceps to physician or midwife. *1,* Grasp one end of package, remove outer tape, and unwind outer wrapper. *2,* Pull back inner turnback at top of package and continue to uncover inner wrap (rather like peeling a banana!). *3,* Grasp carefully all dangling ends of outer wrap and pull them out of the way toward your wrist. Do not touch inner wrap! (From Ingalls, A.J., and Salerno, M.C.: Maternal and child health nursing, ed. 5, St. Louis, 1983, The C.V. Mosby Co.)

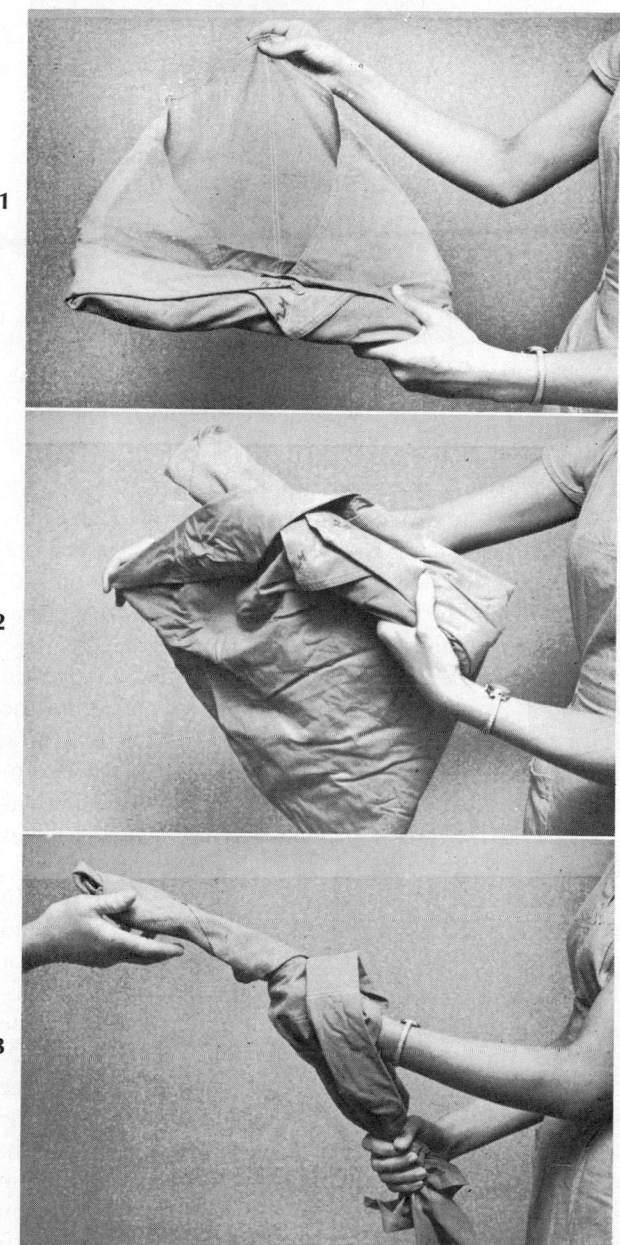

Fig. 17.9

Perineal bulging. (Courtesy Marjorie Pyle, RNC, Lifecircle, Costa Mesa, California.)

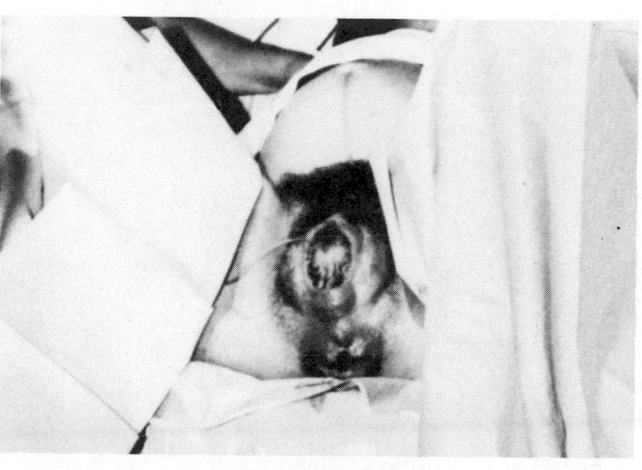

Fig. 17.10

Delivery of head by modified Ritgen maneuver. Note control to prevent rapid delivery of head.

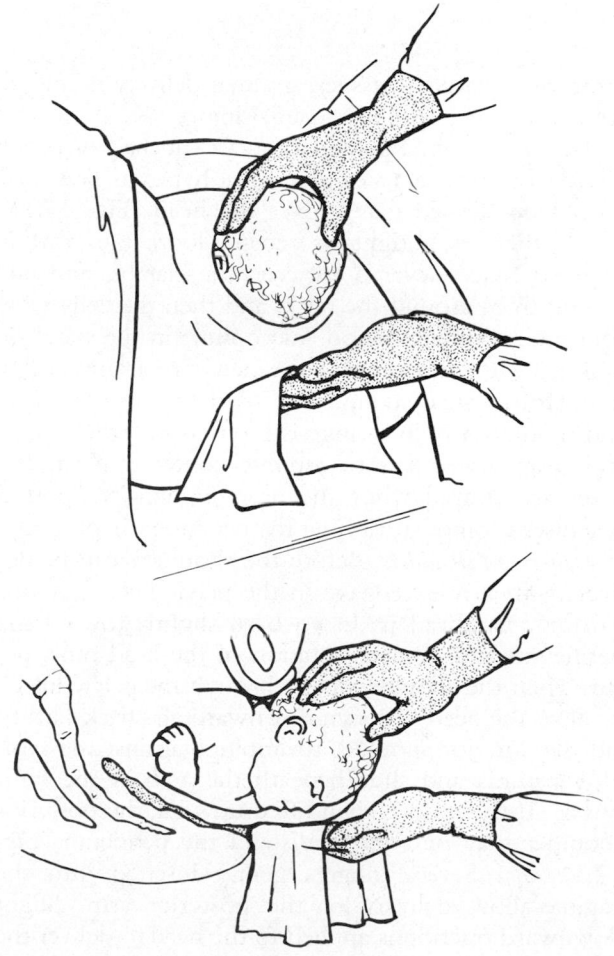

Fig. 17.11
A, Loosening nuchal cord. **B,** Birth of posterior shoulder. (Courtesy of Marjorie Pyle, R.N.C., Lifecircle, Costa, Mesa, Calif.)

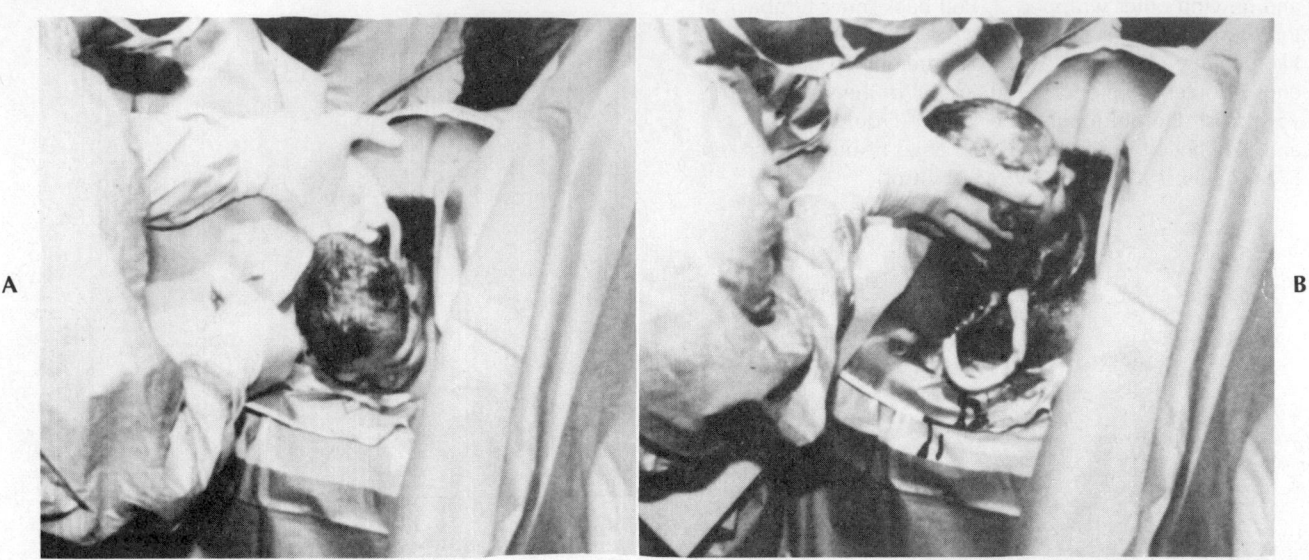

protecting maternal tissues, gradual delivery is imperative to prevent fetal intracranial injury.

The cord often encircles the neck (nuchal cord) but rarely so tightly as to cause critical hypoxia. The cord should be slipped gently over the head (Fig. 17.11, *A*). If there is a tight or second loop, the cord is clamped twice, severed between the clamps, and unwound from around the neck, and then the delivery is continued. Mucus, blood, meconium in the nasal or oral passages may prevent the newborn from breathing. Moist gauze sponges are used to wipe the nose and mouth. A bulb syringe is inserted into the mouth and oropharynx first to aspirate contents. Next, the nares are cleared while the head is being supported (see discussion of suctioning the neonate, Chapter 20).

Delivery of shoulders. Before the shoulders can be delivered, they must engage in the pelvic inlet. For this to occur the head is drawn back slightly toward the perineum, and external rotation of the head must occur. Then the shoulders pass through the pelvic inlet.

Now the head is drawn downward and backward to aid the anterior shoulder to impinge against the symphysis pubis and slide beneath the arch of the symphysis. If the head is then lifted upward, the posterior shoulder may be seen to distend the perineum (Fig. 17.11, *B*). Several fingers gently inserted into the vagina allow delivery of the posterior arm. Slight downward traction is applied to the head to deliver the anterior shoulder and arm. On occasion, it may be eas-

ier to deliver the anterior shoulder first.

Occasionally a hand may present with or after the head. If this occurs, the hand and arm are swept out gently before delivery of the shoulder. Traction and pressure must be limited to avoid damage to the brachial plexus or the neck vessels (see Chapter 29).

Delivery of body and extremities. Easy, gradual traction should now deliver the baby. Slight rotation to the right or left may facilitate the birth. The "time to be born" has come. The infant, with all his or her potential, is now part of this world. The **time of birth** is considered the precise time when the whole baby is out of the mother.

Preparation for birth in a birth room or ABC. In some hospitals, parents have the option to labor and give birth in one room, without changing rooms or beds (Fig. 13.9). Expectant parents and siblings usually attend classes to prepare for the experience. One couple's birth experience is recorded in Fig. 17.12. The mother had marked her progress by feeling the baby's head distend the perineum. She had chosen the side-lying position for bearing down and giving birth.

Local anesthesia with episiotomy is an option in many birth rooms (Fig. 17.13). External restitution (Fig. 17.14, *A*) rotation (Fig. 17.14, *B*), and expulsion (Fig. 17.14, *C*) occur slowly in this gentle birth. The physician had wiped the baby's face with sterile gauze squares and used the bulb syringe while awaiting rotation.

Fig. 17.12
Side-lying position. **A,** Perineal bulging. **B,** Slow expulsion of fetus/newborn. (Courtesy of Marjorie Pyle, R.N.C., Lifecircle, Costa Mesa, Calif.)

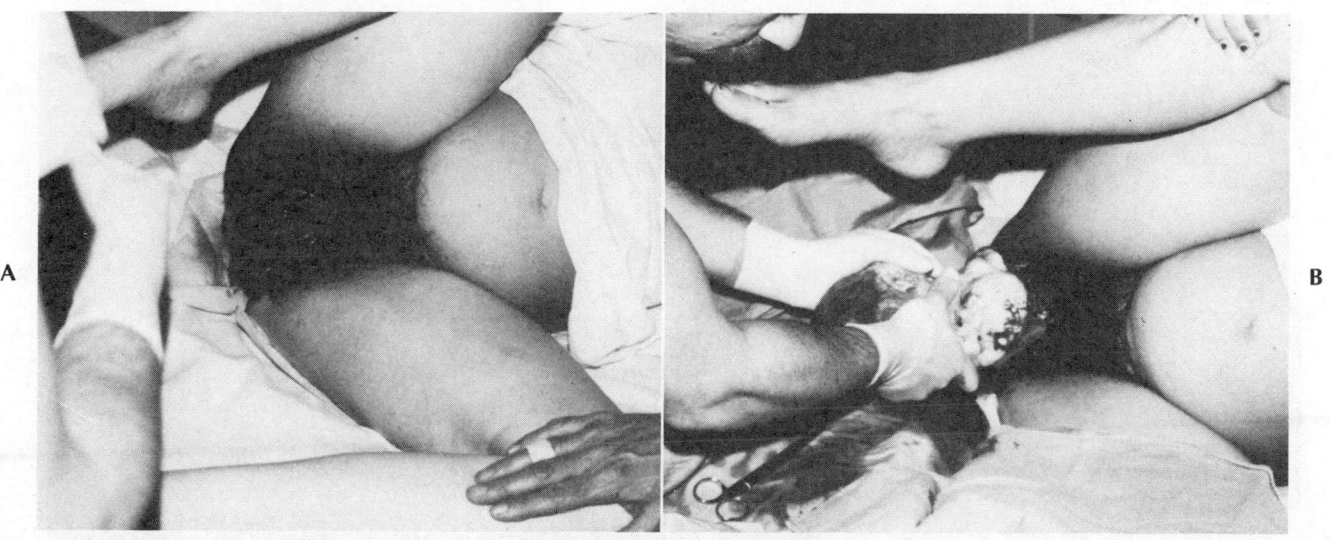

Siblings during the second stage. A young child may become frightened by the intensity of the second stage. Sights such as the rupture of the membranes and sounds such as their mother's moans, screams, and grunts can be unsettling (Quinlan, 1983). The child needs someone to be close, to be held by, and to give explanations simply and calmly. Long-term effects on young children witnessing birth are not yet known.

Evaluation. Evaluation of outcomes is an ongoing activity. During each encounter with the woman and her family during the second stage of labor the nurse evaluates the degree to which goals for care are being met. If the evaluation shows that results fall short of achieving any goal, further assessment, planning, and implementation are warranted.

Fig. 17.13
Birth room. **A,** Local infiltration anesthesia. **B,** Episiotomy. (Courtesy of Marjorie Pyle, R.N.C., Lifecircle, Costa Mesa, Calif.)

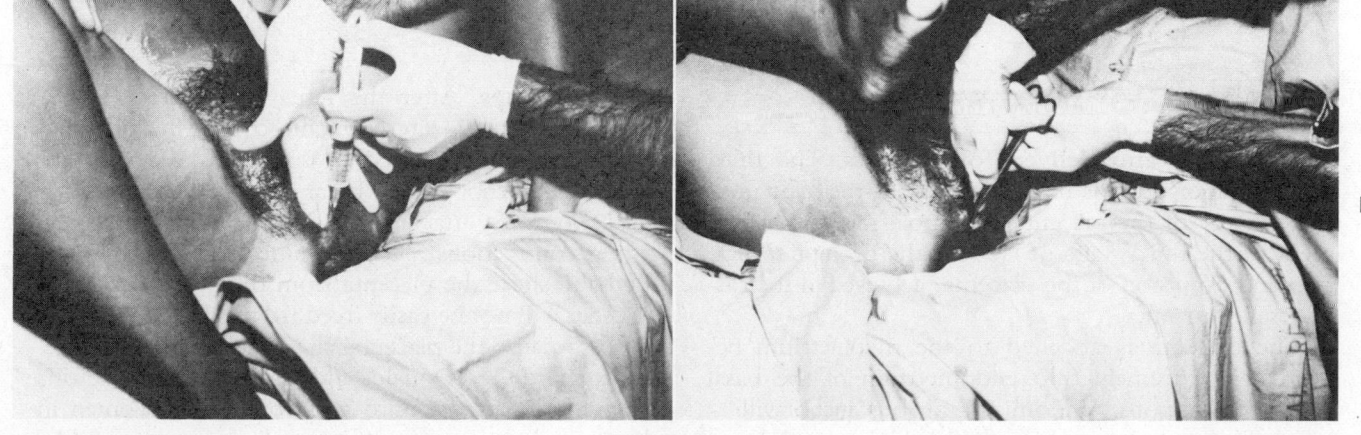

Fig. 17.14
Mechanism of labor. **A,** Restitution. **B,** External rotation. **C,** Slow expulsion of fetus/
newborn. (Courtesy of Marjorie Pyle, R.N.C., Lifecircle, Costa Mesa, Calif.)

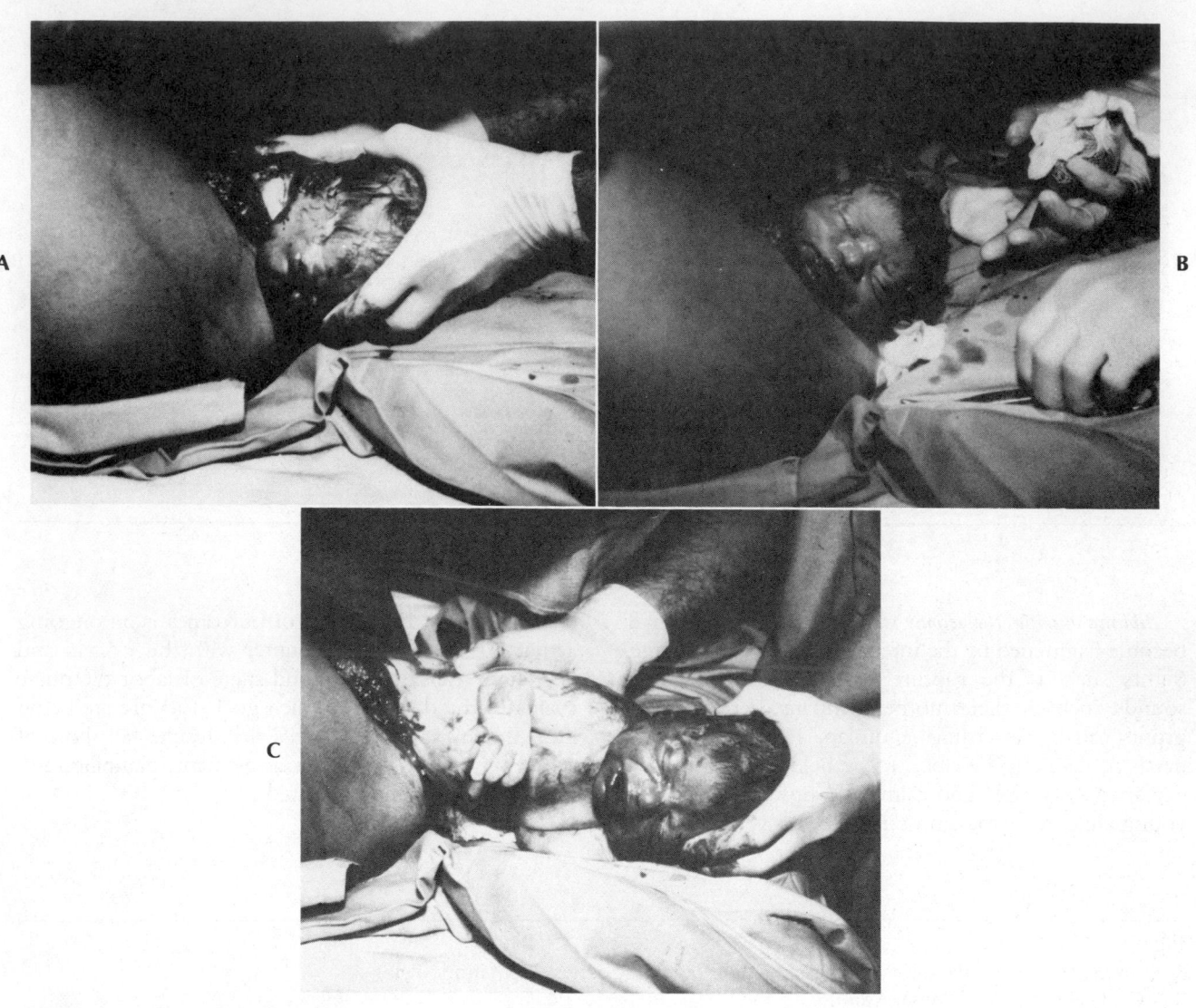

Third Stage of Labor: the Mother

Separation and delivery of placenta. The third stage of labor extends from the birth of the baby until the delivery of the placenta. The goal in the management of the third stage of labor is the prompt separation and expulsion of the placenta, achieved in the easiest, safest manner.

The placenta is attached to the myometrium beneath the extremely thin endometrium of the basal plate by numerous, randomized, fibrous anchor villi—much like a postage stamp is attached to a sheet of postage stamps. After the fetus is delivered, in the presence of strong uterine contractions, the placental site is markedly reduced in size. This reduced size causes the anchor villi to break and the placenta separates from its attachments. Normally the first few strong contractions 5 to 7 minutes after the birth of the baby shear the placenta from the myometrium. A placenta will not be easily freed from a flaccid (relaxed) uterus because the placental site is not reduced in size.

Pritchard, MacDonald, and Gant (1985) make this comment about the third stage of labor: "Women in the recumbent position frequently cannot expel the

Fig. 17.15
Third stage of labor. **A,** Placenta begins by separating in central portion with retroplacental bleeding. Uterus changes from discoid to globular shape. **B,** Placenta completes separation and enters lower uterine segment. Uterus is globular in shape. **C,** Placenta enters vagina, cord is seen to lengthen, and there may be increase in bleeding. **D,** Expression (birth) of placenta and completion of third stage.

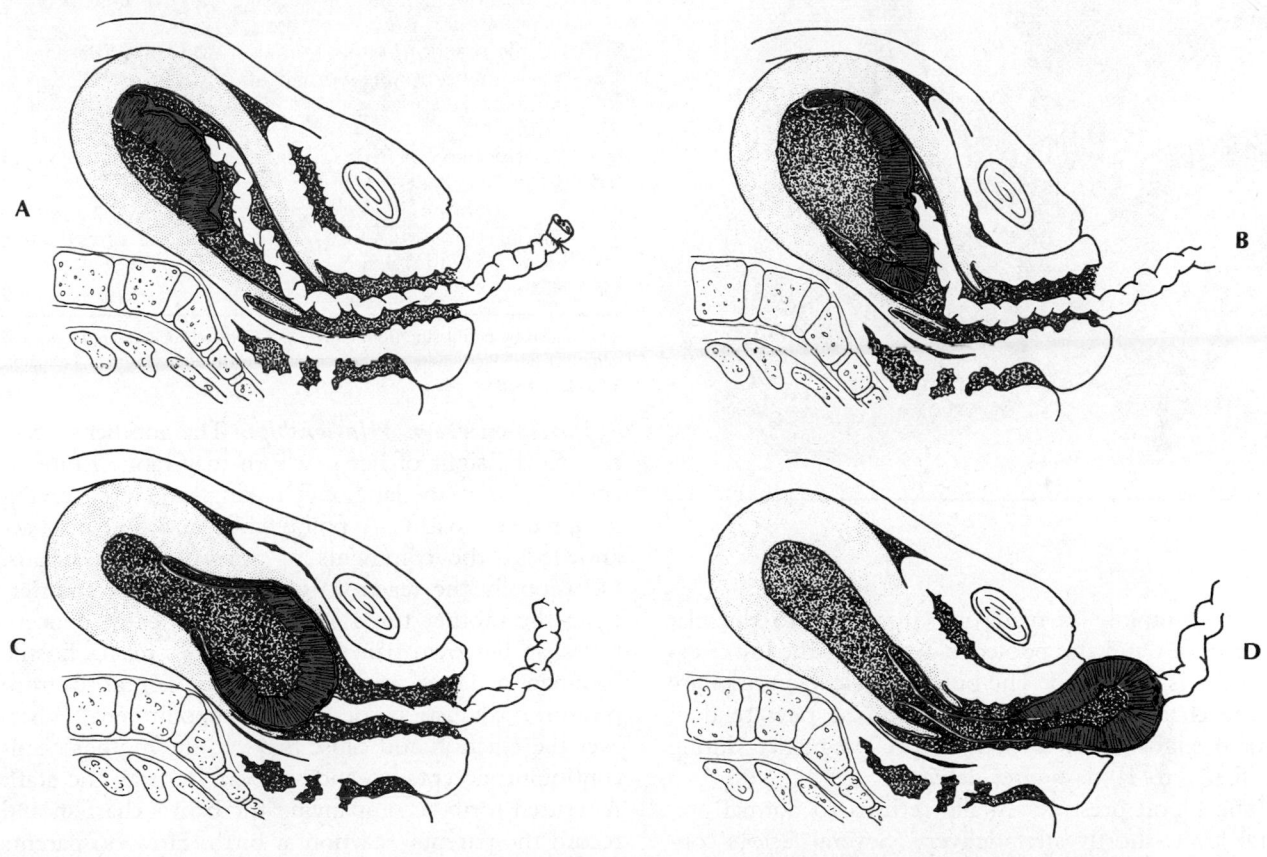

placenta spontaneously. Therefore, an artificial means of completing the third stage generally is required. The usual method employed is *alternate compression and elevation of the fundus,* while *minimal* traction is exerted on the umbilical cord."

Assessment
Identification of the third stage. Placental separation is indicated by the following, in sequence (Fig. 17.15).
1. A firmly contracting fundus
2. A change in the uterus from a discoid to a globular shape
3. A visible and palpable rounded bulge above the symphysis (the bladder must be empty to avoid confusing a full bladder with a change in the uterus)
4. A sudden gush of dark blood from the introitus
5. Apparent lengthening of the umbilical cord as the placenta gets closer to the introitus
6. A vaginal fullness (the placenta) noted on vaginal or rectal examination, or fetal membranes seen at the introitus.

Whether the placenta presents by the shiny fetal surface (Schultze mechanism) or whether it turns to show first its dark roughened maternal surface (Duncan mechanism) is of no clinical importance. At one time it was believed that the Duncan mechanism was associated with a significantly greater blood loss, but this has been disproved. After the placenta with its membranes is born, it is examined for intactness to be certain that no portion of it remains in the uterine cavity (that is, no retained placental fragments of the placenta or membranes) (Fig. 17.16).

Maternal physical status. Physiologic changes following delivery are profound. The cardiac output is

Fig. 17.16
Examination of the placenta. (Courtesy of Marjorie Pyle, R.N.C., Lifecircle, Costa Mesa, Califor.)

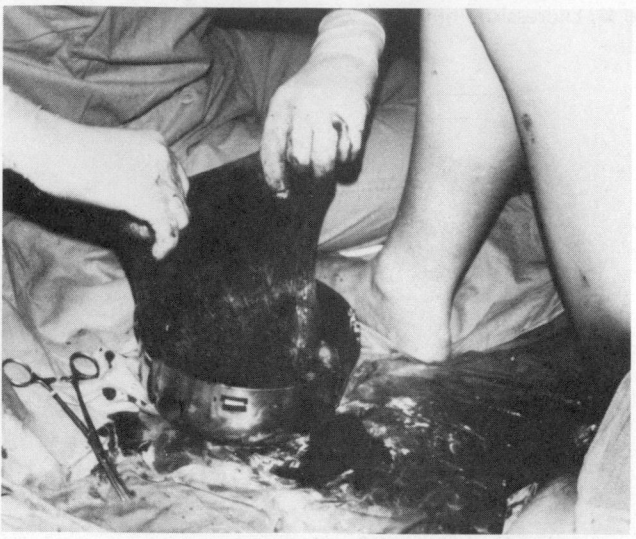

Warning Signs: Parent-Newborn Relationships Immediately Following Delivery

1. Passive reaction, either verbal or nonverbal (Parents do not touch, hold, or examine baby or talk in affectionate terms or tones about baby.)
2. Hostile reaction, either verbal or nonverbal (Parents make inappropriate verbalization, glances, or disparaging remarks about physical characteristics of child.)
3. Disappointment over sex of baby
4. No eye contact
5. Nonsupportive interaction between parents (If interaction seems dubious, talk to nurse and physician involved with delivery for further information.)

Reproduced by permission from Gray, J.D., Christy, A.C., Dean, G.D., and Kempe, C.H.: Prediction and prevention of child abuse, Semin. Perinatol. 3:85, Jan. 1979.

increased rapidly as maternal circulation to the placenta ceases and the pooled blood from the lower extremities is mobilized. The pulse rate slows in response to the change in cardiac output. Pulse rates tend to remain slightly slower than before pregnancy during the first 7 to 10 days after delivery.

The blood pressure usually returns to normal prenatal levels shortly after delivery. Several factors contribute to an elevated blood pressure: the excitement of the second stage, certain medications, and the time of day (blood pressure is highest during the late afternoon). Analgesics and anesthetics may lead to hypotension in the hour following birth.

Even as the physician or nurse-midwife is completing the third stage of labor, the nurse observes the mother for signs of an altered level of consciousness (LOC) or alteration in respirations. Because of the rapid cardiovascular changes (e.g., the increased intracranial pressure during pushing and the rapid increase in cardiac output), this period presents the risk of rupture of a preexisting cerebral aneurysm and of pulmonary emboli. The risk of pulmonary amniotic fluid emboli arises from another source as well. As the placenta separates, there is a possibility of amniotic fluid entering the maternal circulation if the uterine musculature does not contract rapidly and well. The incidence of these possible complications is small; however, the alert nurse can contribute to their immediate recognition and the prompt initiation of therapy.

Parent-newborn relationships. The mother's reaction to the sight of her newborn may range from excited outbursts of laughing, talking, and even crying to apparent apathy. A polite smile and nod may acknowledge the comments of nurses and physicians. Occasionally the reaction is one of anger or indifference; the mother turns away from the baby, concentrates on her own pain, and sometimes makes hostile comments. These varying reactions can arise from pleasure, exhaustion, or deep disappointment. Whatever the reaction and cause may be, the mother needs continuing acceptance and support from all the staff. A written form accompanying the baby's chart should record the parents' reaction at birth. How do parents *look?* What do they *say?* What do they *do?*

Some warning signs in parent-child relationships apparent immediately following delivery are listed above.

Nursing diagnoses. Before establishing nursing diagnoses, the nurse correlates the events of the third stage and the mother's physical and emotional responses to the third stage of labor. The following is an example of a nursing diagnosis: Ineffective individual (mother) coping related to knowledge deficit of sensations to expect during the third stage of labor.

Planning. During this important step, goals are set in client-centered terms. The goals are prioritized. Nursing actions are selected, with the client where appropriate, to meet the goals. The speed and accuracy with which planning is accomplished depends on the nurse's level of competence (Chapter 2).

Goals
1. A third stage that is physically safe for the mother and newborn

2. A cheerful, comfortable, and supportive environment

3. The inclusion of family members of her choice

Implementation

In the delivery area. To assist in the delivery of the placenta, the nurse or coach instructs the mother to push as contractions are felt. If an oxytocin medication is ordered, the nurse administers the medication in the dosage and by the route indicated by the physician or nurse-midwife. When the delivery of the placenta is complete and the episiotomy is sutured, the vulva is gently cleansed with sterile water by the physician or nurse-midwife. The circulating nurse (sometimes assisted by the physician) then performs the following:

1. Applies a sterile perineal pad
2. Removes the drapes
3. Repositions the delivery table or bed
4. Lowers the mother's legs simultaneously from the stirrups
5. Assists the woman onto her bed if she is to be transferred from the delivery area to the recovery area (The nurse will need assistance to move the woman from a delivery table onto a bed if the woman has had anesthesia and does not have full use of her lower extremities.)
6. Dresses the woman in a clean gown and covers her with a warmed blanket
7. Raises the side rails of the bed during the transfer (In some hospitals, the mother is given the baby to hold during transfer; in some hospitals, the father carries the baby; in other hospitals, the nurse carries the baby either to the nursery or to the recovery area for the duration of the mother's recovery period.)

NOTE: The nurse is to observe excellent body mechanics to avoid injury to own back or other body structure.

If the woman labors, gives birth, and recovers in the same bed and room, she is refreshed as described above. After the woman is discharged, the delivery area is cleaned as necessary.

The family during the third stage. Most parents enjoy being able to handle, hold, and examine the baby right after birth. The newborn is placed on the mother's abdomen, which has been draped with a warm receiving blanket. Both parents can assist with the thorough drying of the infant.

The mother may cut the cord or the cord may be left long enough so that the father can clamp it and cut off the extra portion. The mother can hold the infant next to her skin to maintain the baby's body heat and provide skin contact; care must be taken to keep the head warm as well. It is the nurse's responsibility

Fig. 17.17
Nurse assists big brother to become acquainted with sibling.

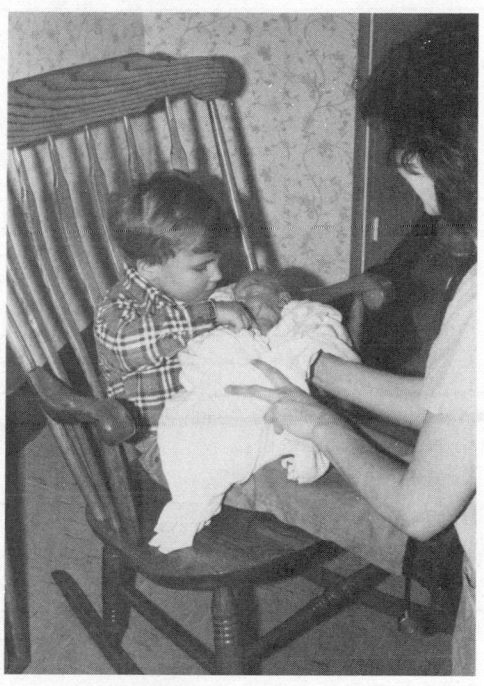

to make sure the baby is kept warm and is in no danger of slipping from the parents' grasp.

Many women wish to begin to breast feed their infants at this time to take advantage of the infant's alert state and to stimulate the production of oxytocin that promotes contraction of the uterus. Others wish to wait until the infant, mother, father, and older siblings are together in the recovery room.

While the physician carries out the postdelivery vaginal examination and, if necessary, repairs the episiotomy, the mother usually feels discomfort. Therefore, while the process is being completed, the infant can be weighed and measured, wrapped in warm blankets, and given to the father to hold.

Big brother, who had appeared only remotely interested in the final phases of the second stage, experiences renewed interest and excitement as he holds the new family member (Fig. 17.17).

Parents are responsive to praise of their newborn. Many require reassurance that the blue appearance of the baby after delivery is normal until respirations are well established. The reason for the molding of the baby's head must be reviewed with parents. Information about hospital routine as to future parent-child contacts can be repeated. The hospital staff, by their interest and concern, can do much to make this a satisfying experience for both parents.

Fig. 17.18
Physical assessment of the newborn. (Modified from form used by Kaiser-Permanente Hospital, Santa Clara, California.)

Addressograph

Mother's room number _____

Date _____

Antepartum
(1) G ____ _____
(2) EDC ____ _____
(3) ABO ____ _____
(4) Titre ____ _____
(5) VDRL _____
(6) Br ____ Bottle _____

(7) RI* ____ NRI _____
(8) PPTL† _____
(9) Adoption _____
Comments _____
_____
_____

Complications
(1) Family history of
bleeding _____
(2) Preeclamptic _____
(3) Gestational diabetic _____
(4) Prenatal meds _____
(5) Pertinent history _____

Intrapartum
(1) Induction or augmentation
(2) Amniotic fluid
(A) PROM ____ hr.
(B) Hydramnios _____
Heavy _____
(C) Mec. stained ____ Light _____
Terminal _____

(3) Monitored‡ _____ ED ____ V ____ LD ____ Baseline ____
(4) Fetal blood sample X _____ Reason _____
(5) Maternal problems _____
(6) Pertinent meds & time _____
_____
(7) Comments _____

Postnatal
(1) Sex: M _____ F _____
(2) Del. date _____
(3) Time _____ AM _____
(4) Weight _____ g
_____ lb _____ oz
(5) Length _____ cm _____ in
(6) ID band # _____
(7) Void _____ Stool _____
(8) Eye prophylaxis: AgNO₃ _____ Other _____
(9) Cord around neck X
  1   2   3
(10) # vessels   2   3
(11) Method of delivery
(A) Spontaneous
Mid _____ Low _____
(B) Forceps
(C) Breech _____
(D) C/B _____
(why)

(12) Placenta
(A) Normal _____
(B) Small _____
(C) Abruptio _____ Previa _____
(D) Other _____

Apgar score

Apgar score		0	1	2	1 min	5 min
	Heart rate	Absent	Less than 100	Over 100		
	Resp. effort	Absent	Slow irreg.	Good cry		
	Muscle tone	Limp	Some flexion	Active motion		
	Reflex irritability	No response	Grimace	Cry		
	Color	Pale	Body pink, ext. blue	All pink		

(13) Comments _____
_____
_____
_____
_____
Signature _____

* RI, rooming in; NRI, not rooming in.
†PPTL, postpartum tubal ligation (or occlusion).
‡Monitored (electronic): ED, early deceleration;
 V, variable deceleration; LD, late deceleration.

Fig. 17.18, cont'd
Physical assessment of the newborn.

Postnatal resuscitation

(1) Pediatrician: Notified_____ AM _____ PM _____
          In attendance_____
(2) O₂ _____ Mask _____ Bag _____
(3) Oral suction _____ Mec _____ Mucus _____
(4) Delees suction _____
(5) Intubation: Successful _____ Unsuccessful _____
     (A) Suctioned: Clear_____
                    Thick _____
                    Mec. _____ Thin _____
     (B) Lavaged_____
(6) Cardiac massage_____
(7) Med and route_____
(8) Comments_____
     _____
     _____
     _____
     _____
     _____

Nursery

(1) Admit to nsy _____ @ _____ (AM/PM or
                                      military time)
(2) Admit to ICN _____ @ _____ AM _____ PM
     (or transferred via _____
     to regional center) _____
(3) MD notified, i.e. problem/client _____
                        _____ AM _____
                        _____ PM _____
(4) Admission v.s.: T_____ P_____ R_____
(5) Est. gest. age_____wk
(6) Color _____
(7) Cry _____
(8) O₂ _____
(9) Suctioned _____
(10) Head_____Chest_____
(11) Comments_____
     _____
     _____

                    Signature

Item	Findings	Clinical significance
Posture		
Measurements Weight		
Length		
Head circumterence		
Chest circumterence		
Vital signs Blood pressure		

Evaluation. Evaluation of outcomes is an ongoing activity. During each encounter with the new mother during the third stage of labor, the nurse evaluates the degree to which goals for care are being met. If the evaluation shows that results fall short of achieving any goal, further assessment, planning, and implementation are warranted.

Third Stage of Labor: the Newborn

Assessment. Before birth, the nurse evaluates the maternal history, including labor, to identify potential problems for the neonate. Although an extensive examination will be performed later, a minimal examination of the neonate is completed immediately following birth. The physician or nurse performs the following assessments and records findings (Fig. 17.18):

1. Assesses respirations and neonate's ability to keep airway clear
2. Estimates infant's health status using Apgar rating at 1 and 5 minutes of age
3. Examines the cord for anomalies and verifies the presence of two arteries and one vein (Fig. 17.19)
4. Collects cord blood from placenta for analysis (Rh factor, blood grouping, and hematocrit)
5. Assesses weight, length, and gestational age
6. Notes passage of meconium or urine
7. Performs minimal physical examination and assessment of neonate such as the following (see Chapter 20 for more in-depth discussion and techniques):
   a. *External:* notes skin color, staining, peeling, or wasting (dysmaturity); considers length of nails and development of creases on soles of feet; checks for presence or absence of breast tissue; assesses nasal patency by closing one nostril at a time while observing the infant's respirations and color; notes meconium staining of cord, skin, fingernails, or amniotic fluid (may indicate fetal hypoxia; offensive odor may indicate intrauterine infection)
   b. *Chest:* palpates for site of maximal cardiac impulse and auscultates for rate and quality of heart tones, compares and notes character of respirations and presence of rales or rhonchi by holding stethoscope in each axilla
   c. *Abdomen:* verifies presence of a domed abdomen and absence of anomalies (Chapter 31)
   d. *Neurologic:* checks muscle tone and reflex reaction and appraises Moro's reflex (at 1 and 5 minutes); palpates large fontanel for fullness or bulge; notes by palpation the presence and sizes of the sutures and fontanels

Fig. 17.19
Cross section of umbilical cord. Note collapsed appearance of thin-walled umbilical vein and contour of thicker, muscular-walled arteries.

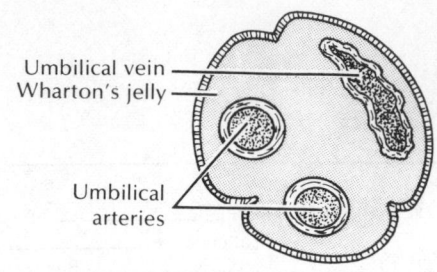

Umbilical vein
Wharton's jelly
Umbilical arteries

   e. *Other observations:* notes gross structural malformations obvious at birth (described in general terms and recorded on delivery record)
8. Assesses parents' response to newborn and to each other. Assessment of the parent-child relationship is discussed under the nursing care of the mother during the fourth stage of labor.

Nursing diagnoses. Nursing diagnoses lend direction to the type of nursing actions needed to implement a plan of care. Before establishing nursing diagnoses, the nurse analyzes the significance of findings collected during assessment. Following are some examples of nursing diagnoses.

1. Ineffective airway clearance related to airway obstruction with mucus and amniotic fluid
2. Alteration in thermal regulation related to environmental factors
3. Alteration in health maintenance related to congenital disorders

Planning. During this important step, goals are set in client-centered terms. The goals are prioritized. Nursing actions are selected to meet the goals. The speed and accuracy with which planning is accomplished depend on the nurse's level of competence (Chapter 2).

Goals. The nurse provides continuous care during the neonate's initial adjustment to extrauterine life by selecting nursing actions that accomplish the following:

1. Maintenance of a clear airway to facilitate respirations
2. Prevention of heat loss (cold stress) to conserve neonate's energy and prevent respiratory distress
3. Maintenance of a safe environment (e.g., to prevent infection)
4. Identification of any potential or actual problem that may require immediate medical or surgical intervention
5. Completion of accurate records

Abnormal Neonatal Breathing

If the infant fails to breathe normally after delivery, immediate resuscitative measures (e.g., aspiration of the trachea through an infant laryngoscope, administration of oxygen by mask) are initiated. Obtain immediate pediatric assistance if needed. Transfer the critical or seriously compromised infant to the pediatric neonatal intensive care unit as soon as possible. Parents should be informed that additional care in an intensive care nursery is required.

Implementation. Events move rapidly during this time period. Assessment must be followed quickly by appropriate implementation. The physician/midwife may be concentrating on the progress of the third stage for the mother. The nurse assumes responsibility and accountability for accurate assessment of and timely intervention for the newborn.

Abnormal neonatal breathing. Initiation and maintenance of respiration is the top priority. Abnormal breathing must be recognized and treated (see box).

General nursing actions. Nursing actions that usually apply to this period include a variety of activities. Among them are actions relevant to the care of the **airway, cord clamping, attachment and warmth, Apgar score, eye prophylaxis, measurement of weight and length,** and **identification.** A summary of these nursing actions and the rationale for each are given in Table 17.5.

Eye prophylaxis. Instillation of a prophylactic agent in the eyes of all newborns is required by law. The agent used is specified in hospital protocols. The method of instillation of the medication in the conjunctival sacs is important (see Box, p. 468).

Evaluation. Evaluation of outcomes is an ongoing activity. During each encounter with the newborn during the third stage of labor the nurse evaluates the degree to which goals for care are being met. If the evaluation shows that results fall short of achieving any goal, further assessment, planning, and implementation are warranted.

Emergency Childbirth: When the Nurse Assists the Mother to Give Birth

Even under the best of circumstances there will probably come a time when the maternity nurse will be required to deliver an infant without medical assistance. Consider the precipitous multipara who arrives at the community hospital fully dilated in the middle of the night. As it is impossible to prevent an impending delivery, the maternity nurse needs to be able to function independently and to be skilled in safely delivering a vertex fetus.

Emergency birth of fetus in vertex presentation. The following measures are necessary for the emergency birth of a fetus in the vertex position:

1. The woman will usually assume the position most suitable for her. If she is in a bed and there is time, elevate the head of the bed about 45 degrees. This position, in addition to facilitating perfusion of the uterus, allows you to maintain eye-to-eye contact with the woman. Occasionally the woman will assume the crawling position, on hands and knees. Some women will stand and lean over a bed or their support person's shoulder. Others will assume a side-lying position.

2. Reassure her verbally with eye-to-eye contact and a calm, relaxed manner. If there is someone else available (e.g., the father), that person could help support her in position, assist with coaching, and compliment her on her efforts.

3. Wash your hands with soap and water or wash-and-dry pledgets if possible.

4. Place under her buttocks whatever clean material or clean newspapers are available.

5. Avoid touching the vaginal area to decrease the possibility of infection. (If there is time, scrub your hands and fingernails for 5 minutes before touching the parturient.) If hands can be clean or sterile gloves are available, massage or support perineum as needed.

6. The perineum thins and distends. As the head begins to crown, the birth attendant should do the following:

   a. Tear the amniotic membrane (caul) if it is still intact.

   b. Instruct woman to pant or pant-blow, thus avoiding the urge to push.

   c. Place the flat of the hand on the exposed fetal head and apply *gentle* pressure toward the vagina to prevent the head from "popping out" (see Fig. 17.10). The mother may participate by placing her hand under yours on the emerging head.

   NOTE: Rapid delivery of the fetal head must be prevented because (1) it is followed by a rapid change of pressure within the molded fetal skull, which may result in dural or subdural tears, and (2) it may cause vaginal or perineal lacerations.

7. Instruct the mother to pant or pant-blow as you check for an umbilical cord. If the cord is around

Text continued on p. 468.

Table 17.5
Nursing Care of the Neonate: Implementation and Rationales

Implementation	Rationale
Airway	
Hold baby with head lowered (10 to 15 degrees).	Uses gravity to help remove fluids.
Suction oral pharynx with a small bulb syringe as soon as head is born.	Expedites drainage and prevents aspiration of amniotic fluid, mucus, and blood (maternal).
Suction nares next.	Prevents inspiration following stimulation of nares before mouth is clear.
Avoid deep suctioning with a catheter, if possible.	May cause bradycardia or laryngospasm or both.
Avoid suspending neonate by the ankles.	Results in hyperextension of baby whose entire development occurred in the flexed position (may be detrimental or painful).
Cord clamping	
Immediately following birth, neonate is kept at about the same level as the uterus, until cord clamp is applied or until cord has stopped pulsating. Cord pulsations usually cease within seconds after respiration is initiated.	If neonate is held above level of uterus, allows gravity to drain blood to the placenta. If neonate is held below level of uterus, allows gravity to drain blood from placenta to neonate.
Without "stripping" ("milking") it, the cord is clamped close to the umbilicus approximately 30 seconds after birth if neonate appears normal and mature (Figs. 17.20 to 17.22).	Some parents want the baby to receive an extra supply of blood and advocate "stripping" the cord toward the baby. Ordinarily it is unwise to strip the cord before clamping and cutting because postdelivery red blood cell destruction, which normally occurs neonatally, will be increased and hyperbilirubinemia (see Chapter 31) may ensue. In addition, polycythemia (increased number of red blood cells) increases blood viscosity, leading to cardiopulmonary problems in the neonate.
The cord is clamped 8 to 10 cm from the umbilicus if there is a possibility for exchange transfusion (see erythroblastosis, Chapter 31).	Permits access to umbilical vessels.
Assess cord for two arteries and one vein.	Alerts physician for need of further assessment if there is only one artery (Chapter 31)
Attachment and warmth	
If neonate is full term, of adequate weight for gestational age, and in good condition, dry quickly and place her or him on mother's abdomen and cover both of them with a warm blanket. Or wrap neonate in warm blanket first.	Facilitates attachment, especially if there is skin-to-skin contact. Assures and relaxes mother. Prevents cold stress to neonate.
Caution parents to keep neonate's head covered.	Prevents cold stress to neonate (Chapter 20).
Apgar score	
Appraise neonate at 1 minute and again at 5 minutes. Use the Apgar scoring method (Fig. 17.23).	Permits a rapid and semiquantitative assessment based on five signs indicative of the physiologic state of the neonate (Fig. 17.23): heart rate, based on auscultation with stethoscope; respiration, based on observed movement of chest wall; muscle tone, based on degree of flexion and movement of the extremities; reflex ability, based on response to gentle slaps on the soles of the feet; and color (pallid, cyanotic, or pink). The 5-minute score correlates with neonatal mortality and morbidity.
Eye prophylaxis	
Instill medication in conjunctival sacs (Figs. 17.24 and 17.25). OR	Meets the legal requirement for all newborns to have treatment to prevent conjunctival infections: gonococcal, pneumococcal, or chlamydial. Such infections, known as ophthalmia neonatorum, can lead to varying degrees of blindness. Recommendations of the National Society to Prevent Blindness, Committee on Ophthalmia Neonatorum, June 15, 1981, are given on p. 468.
If family objects to eye prophylaxis, physician requests parent(s) to sign an informed consent. Note parents' refusal in neonate's record.	
May delay instillation safely until the fourth stage (about 2 hours after birth).	
Newborn weight and length	
Weigh and measure the neonate. This may be delayed until the fourth stage.	Pleases parents who are anxious to know and who want to spread the word to relatives and friends.
Identification	
Identify the neonate by one of a number of techniques *before mother or baby leaves the delivery area.*	Although rare, an occasional mix-up in the identity of newborns occurs. Identification and care to check both mother's and baby's ID numbers prevent unnecessary anxiety and legal complications.

Fig. 17.20
Hollister cord clamp. **A,** Position clamp close to umbilicus.
B, Secure cord. **C,** Cut cord. **D,** Remove clamp, using
scissors, after cord dries (about 24 hours).

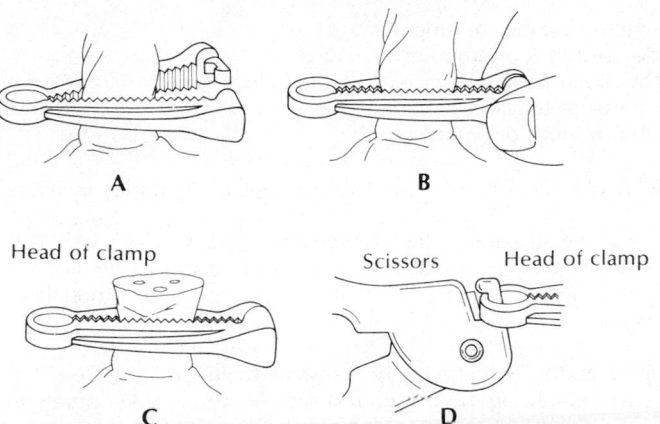

Fig. 17.21
Hesseltine cord clamp.

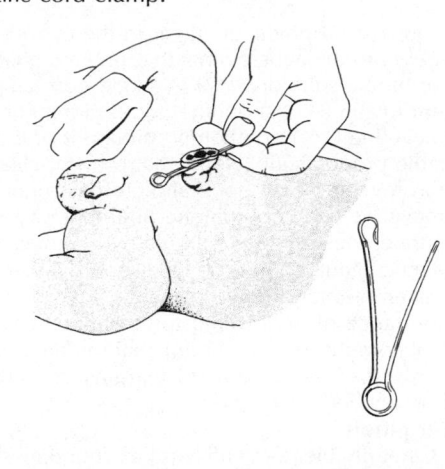

Fig. 17.22
Technique of tying off umbilical cord using, **A,** soft flat
tape to prevent cutting through cord as it is drawn tight
and, **B,** square knot to prevent slippage.

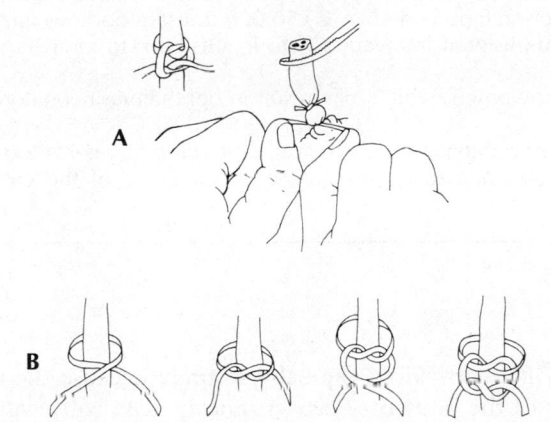

Fig. 17.23
Apgar scoring chart.

Sign	0	1	2
Heart rate	Absent	Slow (below 100)	Over 100
Respiratory effort	Absent	Slow, irregular	Good, crying
Muscle tone	Flaccid	Some flexion of extremities	Active motion
Reflex irritability	No response	Grimace	Cry
Color	Blue, pale	Body pink, extremities blue	Completely pink

Recommendations for Neonatal Treatment of Conjunctiva

1. Instillation of a prophylactic agent in the eyes of all newborn infants.
2. Acceptable prophylactic agents that prevent **gonococcal ophthalmia neonatorum** include the following:
   a. Silver nitrate solution (1%) in single-dose ampules
   b. Erythromycin (0.5%) ophthalmic ointment or drops in single-use tubes or ampules
   c. Tetracycline (1%) ophthalmic ointment or drops in single-use tubes or ampules
3. Acceptable prophylactic agents that prevent **chlamydial ophthalmia neonatorum** include the following:
   a. Erythromycin (0.5%) ophthalmic ointment or drops in single-use tubes or ampules
   b. Tetracycline (1%) ophthalmic ointment or drops in single-use tubes or ampules
   Silver nitrate does not prevent chlamydial infections.
4. Prophylactic agents should be given shortly after birth. A delay of up to 1 hour* is probably acceptable and may facilitate initial maternal-infant bonding.
5. The importance of performing the instillation so the agent reaches all parts of the conjunctival surface is stressed. This can be accomplished by careful manipulation of the lids with fingers to ensure spreading of the agent. If medication strikes only the eyelids and lid margins but fails to reach the cornea, the instillation should be repeated. Prophylaxis should be applied as follows:
   a. **Silver nitrate**
      (1) Carefully clean eyelids and surrounding skin with sterile cotton, which may be moistened with sterile water.
      (2) Gently open baby's eyelids and instill two drops of silver nitrate on the conjuntival sac. Allow the silver nitrate to run across the whole conjunctival sac. Carefully manipulate lids to ensure spread of the drops. Repeat in the other eye. Use two ampules, one for each eye.
      (3) After 1 minute, gently wipe excess silver nitrate from eyelids and surrounding skin with sterile water. *Do not irrigate eyes.*
   b. **Ophthalmic ointment (erythromycin or tetracycline)**
      (1) Carefully clean eyelids and surrounding skin with sterile cotton, which may be moistened with sterile water.
      (2) Gently open baby's eyelids and place a thin line of ointment, at least 1 to 2 cm (½ in), along the junction of the bulbar and palpebral conjunctiva of the lower lid. Try to cover the whole lower conjunctival area. Carefully manipulate lids to ensure spread of the ointment. *Be careful not to touch the eyelid or eyeball with the tip of the tube.* Repeat in other eye. Use one tube per baby.
      (3) After 1 minute, gently wipe excess ointment from eyelids and surrounding skin with sterile water. *Do not irrigate eyes.*
   c. **Ophthalmic drops (erythromycin or tetracycline)**
      (1) Apply as for silver nitrate.
6. The eye should not be irrigated after instillation of a prophylactic agent. Irrigation may reduce the efficacy of prophylaxis and probably does not decrease the incidence of chemical conjunctivitis.
7. Infants born to mothers infected with agents that cause ophthalmia neonatorum may require special attention and systemic therapy as well as prophylaxis. A single dose of aqueous crystalline penicillin G, 50,000 units/kg body weight for term and 20,000 units for low-birth-weight infants should be administered intravenously to infants born to mothers with gonorrhea.
8. The detection and appropriate treatment of infections in pregnant women, which may result in ophthalmia neonatorum, are encouraged.
9. All physicians and hospitals should be required to report cases of ophthalmia neonatorum and etiologic agents to state and local health departments so that incidence data may be obtained to determine the effectiveness of the control measures.

From National Society to Prevent Blindness, NSPB Committee on Ophthalmia Neonatorum, June 15, 1981.
*Center for Disease Control, Atlanta, specifies up to 2 hours' delay is safe.

the neck, try to slip it up over the baby's head or pull *gently* to get some slack so that it can slip down over the shoulders.

8. Support fetal head as restitution (external rotation) occurs. After restitution, with one hand on each side of the baby's head, exert *gentle* pressure downward so that the anterior shoulder emerges under the symphysis pubis and acts as a fulcrum; then as *gentle* pressure is exerted in the opposite direction, the posterior shoulder, which has passed over the sacrum and coccyx, is delivered.

9. Be alert! Hold the baby securely because the rest of the body may deliver quickly. The baby will be slippery!

10. Cradle the baby's head and back in one hand and the buttocks in the other, keeping the head down to drain away the mucus. Use a bulb syringe to remove mucus if one is available.
NOTE: Do not hold the baby upside down by the ankles because to do so (1) hyperextends the spine, which has been flexed since conception, (2)

Text continued on p. 470.

Fig. 17.24
Silver nitrate for prophylactic eye care of newborn. **A,** Silver nitrate, 1%, in wax
containers.**B,** Puncture wax containers with needle. **C,** Squeeze to release drops.
Administer by placing 1 or 2 drops in lower conjunctival sac of lower lid and close eye to
spread medication. **D,** New-style sterile container with twist-off top for silver nitrate in a
see-through package. **E,** Silver nitrate for prophylactic eye care of newborn. (**E,** from
Ingalls, A.J., and Salerno, M.C.: Maternal and child health nursing, ed. 5, St. Louis, 1983,
The C.V. Mosby Co.)

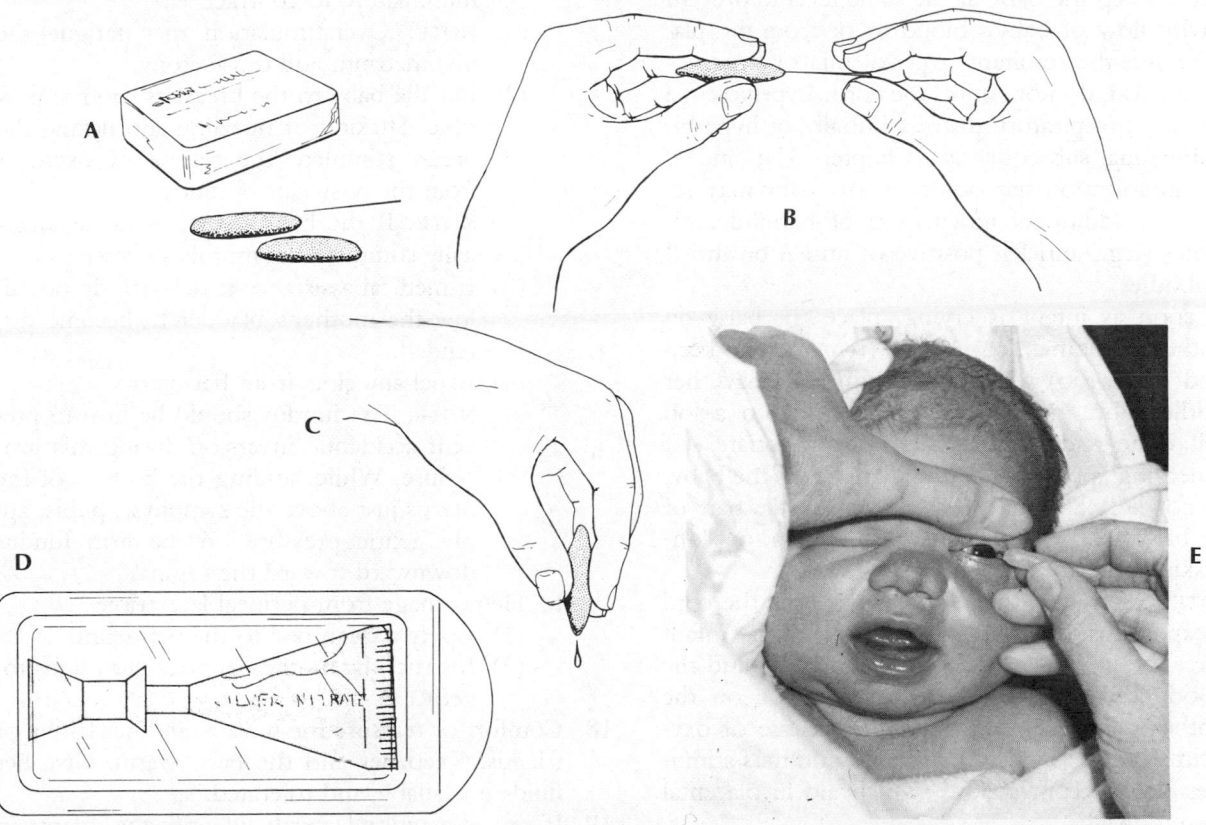

Fig. 17.25
Instillation of ophthalmic erythromycin drops using
needleless syringe. Drops are instilled into conjunctival
sac. (Photograph by I.M. Bobak.)

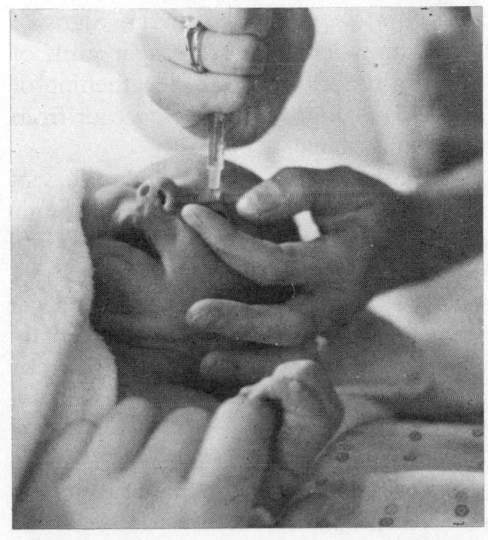

increases intracranial pressure and the danger of capillary rupture, (3) may cause direct tissue trauma to the ankles, and (4) increases the possibility of dropping a wet, slippery baby.

11. Dry the baby rapidly (to prevent rapid heat loss), keeping the baby at the same level as the mother's uterus.

    NOTE: Keep the baby at the same level to prevent gravity flow of baby's blood to or from the placenta and the resultant hypovolemia or hypervolemia. Also, do not "milk" the cord: hypervolemia can cause respiratory distress initially or hyperbilirubinemia subsequently (Chapter 31); and if isoimmunization has occurred, the baby may receive an additional inoculation of harmful antibodies (e.g., anti-Rh positive or anti-A or anti-B antibodies).

12. As soon as infant is crying, place the baby on mother's abdomen, cover baby (remember to keep head warm too) with her clothing, and have her cuddle baby. Compliment her (them) on a job well done and on the baby if appropriate. (If something appears to be the matter with the baby, do not lie!) She may wish to expose the part of the baby that will be touching her skin for skin-to-skin contact.

    NOTE: Soon after the Wharton's jelly in the cord is exposed to cool air and shrinks and the infant cries, the umbilical vessels stop pulsating and the blood flow ceases. The baby's presence on the mother's abdomen stimulates the release of oxytocin from the posterior pituitary and thus stimulates uterine contractions, which aid in placental separation.)

13. *Wait* for the placenta to separate; *do not* tug on the cord.

    NOTE: Injudicious traction may tear the cord, separate the placenta, or invert the uterus. Signs of placental separation include (1) a slight gush of dark blood from the introitus, (2) lengthening of the cord, and (3) change in uterine contour from discoid to globular shape.

14. Instruct the mother to push to deliver the separated placenta. Gently ease out the placental membranes, using an up-and-down motion until membranes are removed. To minimize complications do not cut the cord without proper clamps or ties and a sterile cutting tool and inspect the placenta for intactness. Place the baby on the placenta and wrap the two together for additional warmth.

    NOTE: There is no hurry to cut the cord. The infant will not lose blood through the placenta because the cord circulation ceases (clots) within minutes of birth.

15. Check the firmness of the uterus. Gently massage the uterus and demonstrate to the mother how she can massage her own uterus properly.

16. Clean the area under the mother's buttocks.

17. Prevent or minimize hemorrhage.
    a. Hemorrhage from uterine atony.
       (1) *Gently* massage fundus to stimulate uterine musculature to contract.
           NOTE: Overstimulation may fatigue the myometrium and cause atony.
       (2) Put the baby to the breast as soon as possible. Sucking or nuzzling and licking the breast stimulate the release of oxytocin from the posterior pituitary.
           NOTE: If the baby does not nurse, manually stimulate the mother's breasts.
       (3) If medical assistance is delayed, do not allow the mother's bladder to become distended.
       (4) Expel any clots from her uterus.
           NOTE: The fundus should be firm to prevent accidental inversion during this procedure. While holding the bottom of the uterus just above the symphysis pubis, apply gentle pressure on the firm fundus downward toward the vagina.
    b. Hemorrhage from perineal lacerations.
       (1) Apply a clean pad to the perineum.
       (2) Instruct the mother to press her thighs together.

18. Comfort or reassure the mother and her family or friends. Keep her and the baby warm. Give her fluids if available and tolerated.

19. If this is a multiple birth, identify the infants in order of birth.

20. Make notations on the birth.
    a. Fetal presentation and position
    b. Presence of cord around neck or other parts and number of times cord encircles part
    c. Color, character, and amount of amniotic fluid
    d. Time of delivery
    e. Estimate time of Apgar score, resuscitation, and ultimate condition of baby
    f. Sex of baby
    g. Approximate time of placental expulsion, its appearance, and completeness
    h. Maternal condition: affect, amount of bleeding, and status of uterine contractions
    i. Any unusual occurrences during the delivery

Lateral Sims' position for delivery. A lateral Sims' posture may be the position of choice for delivery when (1) the delivery is progressing rapidly and there is insufficient time for slow distention of the perineum; (2) the fetal head seems too large to pass through the introitus without laceration, and episiotomy is not possible; or (3) the apparent size of the fetus is consistent with possible shoulder dystocia.

In the lateral Sims' position, less stress is placed on the perineum and better visualization of the perineum is possible. In the event of shoulder dystocia, lateral Sims' posture increases the space needed for delivery.

Birth and management of preterm infant. The actual process of birthing the preterm infant does not vary from that of the term infant. However, the care of the infant after birth requires some modification as follows:

1. Warmth is essential.
2. Minimize handling, maintain a clear airway, and feed and change the infant.
3. Nutrition may be a problem if a medical facility is not available. Although the infant may be unable to nurse at the breast, slow feeding is important, using a medicine dropper, for example.
4. Urge the preterm infant to breathe by stimulating him *gently* when he "forgets."

5. Transport the infant to a medical facility equipped to handle preterm infants as early as possible (see Chapter 25).

Summary

Nursing care during the second and third stages of labor considers all members of the childbearing family. The new mother has now completed what in most instances is an exhilarating and rewarding experience. The maternity nurse is in an ideal position to encourage and promote early family participation and attachment and to focus on the individual health care needs of each member of the childbearing family. The nurse's expertise takes into consideration the management of a challenging emergency vertex childbirth in a calm, supportive, and professional manner. The maternity nurse uses specialized skills to provide safe, quality nursing care during the second and third stages of labor.

Summary of Nursing Actions

Nursing Care During the Second and Third Stages of Labor

GOALS

1. For the mother: a safe and satisfying second and third stage of labor
2. For the unborn child: a continuing state of well-being
3. For the newborn: a satisfactory adjustment to extrauterine existence
4. For the family: a satisfying experience in the second stage of labor and in the first meeting with the newborn

PRIORITIES

1. Early identification and immediate therapy for any deviations from normal processes
2. Cheerful, comfortable, and supportive environment
3. Encouragement to facilitate the natural rhythm of the second stage
4. Safe transition into extrauterine life for the neonate
5. Environment to facilitate individual and family coping and growth

ASSESSMENT	EXAMPLES OF POTENTIAL NURSING DIAGNOSTIC CATEGORIES*
Second stage	
A. Monitor the following continuously:	
1. FHR	Alteration in normal physiologic processes†
2. Contractions	Alteration in normal physiologic processes†
3. Show, excessive bleeding	Potential for maternal or fetal compromise†
4. Amniotic fluid	Potential for fetal or maternal compromise†
5. Maternal response to labor: energy level, ability to relax between contractions, ability to push	Ineffective relaxation patterns†
	Alteration in comfort: pain
	Powerlessness
	Disturbance in self-concept: body image, self-esteem, role performance, personal identity
	Ineffective individual or family coping

*Approved diagnoses from NANDA's Seventh National Conference (1986).
†Diagnosis not included by NANDA, 1986.

Continued.

Summary of Nursing Actions—cont'd

ASSESSMENT	EXAMPLES OF POTENTIAL NURSING DIAGNOSTIC CATEGORIES
Second stage—cont'd	
B. Monitor per hospital protocol:	
1. Descent of presenting part and readiness for delivery	Potential for fetal compromise†
2. Respirations and blood pressure (between contractions)	Potential for maternal compromise†
C. Assess family's response	Knowledge deficit
	Powerlessness
	Ineffective family coping
D. Assess physician's or midwife's need for equipment and supplies	Potential for injury
E. Assess woman for comfort and safety needs	Potential for injury
	Alteration in comfort: pain
Third stage: mother and family	
A. Assess mother's level of anxiety, excitement, or restlessness	Potential for alteration in parenting
B. Assess for signs of placental separation and note time of delivery of placenta	Potential for maternal compromise†
	Alteration in normal physiologic processes†
C. Observe physician or midwife in case other supplies or equipment is needed while:	Potential for injury
	Alteration in normal physiologic processes†
1. Cervix, vagina, perineum, placenta, and membranes are checked	
2. Uterine fundus is checked for degree of firmness and position	
3. Episiotomy or laceration is repaired	
D. After physician or midwife completes care, assess:	Potential for injury
1. Uterine fundus	Alteration in normal physiologic processes†
2. Lochia	
3. Perineum	
4. Comfort level	Alteration in comfort: pain
5. Maternal response to baby and family	Ineffective individual or family coping
6. Family's response to baby (taking into consideration the family's culture and ethnicity)	Spiritual distress
7. Mother's mobility of lower limbs (postanesthesia effects)	Impaired physical mobility
	Potential for injury
8. Check labor and delivery records	
Third stage: newborn	
A. Assess respirations	Potential for ineffective airway clearance
B. Estimate infant's health status using Apgar rating at 1 and 5 minutes of age	Potential for impaired gas exchange
	Potential for impairment of thermal regulation
C. Examine cord and count vessels	Potential for alterations in thermal regulation
D. Complete the physical examination	Potential for injury
E. Confirm time of birth, sex, and presentation and position (e.g., LOA) for medical records	Potential alteration in cardiac output: decreased
F. Collect cord blood for analysis (Rh factor, blood group, and hematocrit)	
G. Assess for safety and comfort	

OUTCOME CRITERIA*	PLAN/IMPLEMENTATION
Second stage: parturient-mother	
A. Vital signs and blood pressure: remain within normal limits	Monitor respirations, blood pressure, and maternal progress in labor per hospital protocol; record findings; and report deviations from normal limits.
1. Pulse: assessed when indicated	

*Outcome criteria direct the selection of nursing actions (**plan/implementation**) and measure their effectiveness (**evaluation**).

Summary of Nursing Actions—cont'd

OUTCOME CRITERIA	PLAN/IMPLEMENTATION
2. Respirations: altered by pushing, hyperventilation prevented 3. Blood pressure: altered by pushing or anesthesia; hypertension or hypotension prevented 4. Temperature: assessed when indicated	

B. Maternal progress through second stage: within normal limits
  1. Cervix: completely effaced and dilated; lacerations do not occur during birth
  2. Show: copius amounts of mixed blood and mucus with no evidence of excessive bleeding
	Assist woman to use her expulsive powers to expedite descent and birth of infant.
	  ■ Encourage woman to push with urge to bear down until vertex crowns.
	  ■ When presenting part crowns, instruct woman to control urge to push by panting to permit slow delivery of head and eventually of entire infant.
	  ■ Give woman simple, clear directions.

3. Contractions: magnitude is expulsively powerful (50-75 mm Hg); frequency, 2-3 min; duration, 60 s; rhythm, regular
  4. Descent: constant
    a. *For nulliparas,* it takes ½-1 h for descent from station +1 to station +4 cm; from station +4 cm to birth of infant, approximately 20 contractions needed
    b. *For multiparas,* it takes 10-30 min for descent from station 0 to station +4 cm; from station +4 cm to birth of infant, approximately 10 contractions needed
  5. Duration of labor: within normal limits for nullipara or multipara
	If necessary, transfer woman to delivery area at appropriate time for nullipara and rate of progress of labor.
	If stirrups are used, use care to pad stirrups and to position and restrain woman's legs properly.

C. Birth: no lacerations of vagina or perineum	Provide care for delivery. Record time of birth, sex, and other items required on the delivery record. Report any findings that deviate from normal limits.
D. Fluids/nutrients: intravenous flow rate maintained	Monitor flow rate. Adjust arm position and protect IV site during woman's movements or transfer from bed to table. Moisten lips and teeth with cold, wet washcloths, but usually prohibit oral fluids.
E. Elimination: bladder and urethra not traumatized by labor or delivery	Encourage voiding, or catheterize bladder if fullness is seen as interfering with descent or if bladder is in danger of trauma.
F. Maternal behavior and appearance: pain sensations decrease in early phases of second stage; urge to push controlled by panting; woman eager to cooperate and give birth to infant and fretful and irritable if progress is not deemed fast enough; needs coaching to work with contractions and will experience amnesia between contractions; fatigue becomes apparent, especially in nulliparas; woman can follow simple, clear directions; will often comment with surprise at sensation of birth	Monitor maternal behavior. Coach as necessary; use simple, clear instructions. NOTE: only one person should coach at a time; all other conversation is avoided.

Second stage: fetus
Well-being continues
  1. Fetal heart rate: within normal pattern
  2. No evidence of meconium staining of amniotic fluid (in vertex presentations)
	Monitor FHR continuously electronically or manually after each contraction; report any deviations immediately; implement emergency action for ominous FHR decelerations immediately; when appropriate, record event, therapy given, and results.

Third stage: parturient/mother A. Maternal progress through third stage of labor: within normal limits 1. Placenta: delivered intact, with membranes, within 30 min (usually 3-5 min)	Assist physician or midwife as needed.

Summary of Nursing Actions—cont'd

OUTCOME CRITERIA	PLAN/IMPLEMENTATION
Third stage: parturient/mother—cont'd 2. Uterine muscles: contract sufficiently to limit loss of blood from placental site 3. Bleeding from cervical tears: within normal limits or controlled by ligation of torn vessels 4. After delivery, uterus remains firm, positioned in midline 5. At birth: 2 cm below or at the umbilicus B. Vital signs and blood pressure: remain within her normal range C. Immediate maternal response to infant within normal limits (e.g., open expression of concern for infant's health, joy or disappointment tempered by her physical state and amount of pain or fatigue experienced); reactions vary from euphoria to sleepy exhaustion, with lack of awareness of surroundings D. Opportunity for parent(s) to begin attachment to (or acquaintance with) newborn	Administer oxytocin as ordered. Check respirations and blood pressure before transferring from delivery area. Provide opportunities for parents to verbalize reactions to newborn and to the experience. Share in excitement and joy over birth. Facilitate mother-father-sibling-newborn attachment. Accept any expressions of disappointment from parents and reassure them that such feelings are expected. Reassure mother that her behavior during labor was acceptable if she appears worried about this. Assist with breast feeding if desired. Remove legs from stirrups; put perineal pad in place. Cover with warm blanket and change gown. Help woman to move from delivery table to bed or stretcher (if epidural or spinal anesthetic has been used, with help, lift or roll her into position on her bed). Transfer woman to recovery area.
Third stage: newborn A. Infant is in good health: Apgar rating of 7-10 (at birth); respirations present; color dusky to pink; muscle tone good; if neonate is crying, crying is strong; reflexes present; no obvious malformations B. Apgar score: 7-10 at 5 min C. Respirations: established within 30-60 s D. Cord clamped and cut after pulsations cease and respirations are established; no obvious malformations noted E. Gestational age characteristics are appropriate for estimated date of confinement F. Infant identified G. Findings from minimal physical examination are within normal limits H. Cold stress is avoided	Ensure clear airway. Ensure warm environment; prevent cold stress. Protect from injury and infection. Report findings that deviate from normal limits. Complete and record Apgar score at 1 and 5 min. Initiate resuscitation as necessary. Identify the newborn per hospital protocol (bands, footprints). Assist with breast feeding if mother wishes.

EVALUATION The nurse can be assured that care was effective if goals and outcome criteria are achieved.

References

Carr, K.C.: Management of the second stage of labor, NAA-COG Update Series, Lesson 9, vol. 1, 1983.

Danforth, D.: Obstetrics and gynecology, ed. 4, Philadelphia, 1982, Harper & Row, Publishers.

Mahan, C.S., and McKay, S.: Are we overmanaging second-stage labor? Contemp. OB/Gyn. 24:37, Dec. 1984.

Myles, M.F.: Textbook for midwives, with modern concepts of obstetric and neonatal care, ed. 9, New York, 1981, Churchill Livingstone.

Pritchard, J.A., MacDonald, P.C., and Gant, N.F.: Williams obstetrics, ed. 17, Norwalk, Conn., 1985, Appleton-Century-Crofts.

Quinlan, P.: Genevieve's birth at Pithiviers, Birth 10:187, Fall 1983.

Warrington, J.: The obstetric catechism, Philadelphia, 1842, Crolius & Clading, p. 228.

Yeates, D., and Roberts, J.: A comparison of 2 bearing-down techniques during the second stage of labor, J. Nurs. Midw. 29:3, 1984.

Bibliography

Andrews, C.M., and Andrews, E.C.: Nursing, maternal postures, and fetal position, Nurs. Res. 32:336, Nov./Dec. 1983.

Bates, B., and Turner, A.N.: Imagery and symbolism in the birth practices of traditional cultures, Birth 12:29, Spring 1985.

Bjorkman La Du, E.: Childbirth care for Hmong families, MCN 10:382, Nov./Dec. 1985.

Caldeyro-Barcia, R.: Report given at ICEA International Convention, Kansas City, Mo., June 1978.

Childbirth sitting up, Newsweek, p. 79, March 2, 1981.

Chute, G.E.: Expectation and experience in alternative and conventional birth, J. O. G. N. Nurs. 14:61, Jan./Feb. 1985.

Haun, N.: Nursing care during labor, Canadian Nurse 80:26, Oct. 1984.

Horn, M., and Manion, J.: Creative grandparenting: bonding the generations, J. O. G. N. Nurs. 14:233, May/June 1985.

ICEA Review: Maternal position during labor and birth, Milwaukee, 1978, International Childbirth Education Association, Inc.

ICEA Review: Second stage labor: labor, Milwaukee, 1978, International Childbirth Education Association, Inc.

Jensen, M.D., and Bobak, I.M.: Maternity and gynecologic care: the nurse and the family, ed. 3, St. Louis, 1985, The C.V. Mosby Co.

Johnsen, N.M., and Gaspard, M.E.: Theoretical foundations of a prepared sibling class, J. O. G. N. Nurs. 14:237, May/June 1985.

Kowba, M.D., and Schwirian, P.M.: Direct sibling contact and bacterial colonization in newborns, J. O. G. N. Nurs. 14:412, Sept./Oct. 1985.

Leininger, M.: Transcultural nursing: an essential knowledge and practice field for today, Canadian Nurse 80:41, Dec. 1984.

Macdonald, J.: Birth attendants: another choice, Canadian Nurse 80:22, Oct. 1984.

Malinowski, J.S., and others: Nursing care of the labor patient, ed. 2, Philadelphia, 1983, F.A. Davis Co.

Maloney, R.: Childbirth education classes: expectant parents' expectations, J. O. G. N. Nurs. 14:245, May/June 1985.

Maloni, J.: The birthing room: some insights into parents, M.C.N. 5(5):314, 1980.

Marecki, M., and others: Early sibling attachment, J. O. G. N. Nurs. 14:418, Sept./Oct. 1985.

McKay, S.: Squatting: an alternate position for the second stage of labor, M.C.N. 9:181, May/June 1984.

McKay, S., and Roberts, J.: Second stage labor: what is normal: J. O. G. N. Nurs. 14:101, March/April 1985.

National Society to Prevent Blindness, NSPB Committee on Ophthalmia Neonatorum, June 15, 1981.

Poole, C.: Educating new labor and delivery room nurses, J. O. G. N. Nurs. 14:459, Nov./Dec. 1985.

Roberts, J.: Alternative positions for childbirth. First stage, J. Nurs. Midw. 25:11, July/Aug. 1980.

Roberts, J.: Alternative positions for childbirth. II. Second stage of labor, J. Nurs. Midw. 25:13, Sept./Oct. 1980.

Romond, J.L., and Baker, I.T.: Squatting in childbirth: a new look at an old tradition, J. O. G. N. Nurs. 14:406, Sept./Oct. 1985.

Shannon-Babitz, M.: Addressing the needs of fathers during labor and delivery, M.C.N. 4(6):378, 1979.

Simkin, P.: Preparing parents for second stage, Birth Fam. J. 9:229, Winter 1982.

Sumner, P.E., and Phillips, C.R.: Birthing rooms: concept and reality, St. Louis, 1981, The C.V. Mosby Co.

Nursing Care During
the Fourth Stage of Labor

The fourth stage of labor, the stage of recovery, is a critical period for the mother and neonate. While both the mother and neonate are recovering from the physical process of birth, they are also initiating new relationships.

During the next 2 hours, the maternal organism makes its initial readjustment to the nonpregnant state, and body systems begin to stabilize. The neonate's anatomy and physiology continue with the transition from intrauterine to extrauterine existence. Many parents are opting for early discharge from the hospital. Parents and the health care team must be reasonably assured that there is no potential for disruption in the normal processes for the mother or newborn. The nurse's skills as a technician, teacher/advocate/counselor, and support person can make a critical difference during the fourth stage. The focus of this chapter is the application of the nursing process with the mother.

Definitions

puerperium Variable period, usually 6 to 8 weeks, that begins with the delivery of the placenta and ends either with the resumption of ovulatory menstrual periods or when involutionary changes that result in the nonparous state are complete (e.g., after postdelivery hysterectomy); the postpartum period; the postnatal period; the postdelivery period.
   p. immediate The 24 hours after delivery.
involution Process that results in the healing of the birth canal and the return of the uterus and all systems to or almost to the prepregnant state. Generally, changes reflect reversals of the anatomic and physiologic adaptation to pregnancy.
lochia Uterine discharge after delivery.

Assessment

If the nurse is unfamiliar with the new mother, assessment begins with a review of the prenatal and labor record. Of primary importance are conditions that could predispose the mother to hemorrhage. Hemorrhage is a potential danger during the fourth stage for any woman.

The fourth stage is a busy one for the nurse. The recovery of the mother depends on frequent assessments and timely interventions. To assist the nurse to provide comprehensive care, a worksheet is suggested (p. 477). On a busy unit even experienced nurses appreciate a checklist.

During the first hour in the recovery room, physical assessment of the mother is frequent. All factors except temperature are assessed every 15 minutes for 1 hour (Table 18.1). After the fourth 15-minute assessment, if values are stabilized within the woman's normal range, assessment is repeated twice more, 30 minutes apart.

The procedure for the physical assessment of the mother during the fourth stage of labor is given in Procedure 18.1. The area of examination and purpose, the method of assessment, and findings within normal limits are discussed briefly.

Nursing Diagnoses

Nursing diagnoses lend direction to types of nursing actions needed to implement a plan of care. Before establishing nursing diagnoses, the nurse analyzes the significance of findings collected during assessment.

1. Potential for hemorrhage related to uterine atony.*
2. Potential for injury related to ambulating the first time without assistance.
3. Alteration in comfort: pain related to childbirth trauma.
4. Potential for alteration in parenting, related to postpartum pain or fatigue.

*Diagnosis not included by NANDA, 1986.

476

Worksheet: Fourth Stage of Labor

G _____ P _____ AB _____   Analgesia/anesthesia _____

Type of delivery _____ Sex _____ Apgar _____ Episiotomy _____ Lac _____

Time	Admit	15 min	30 min	45 min	1 h	1 h 15 min	1 h 30 min	1 h 45 min	2 h
Fundus									
Lochia: color and amount									
Blood pressure									
Temperature, pulse and respirations									
Perineum									
Pain: type and location									
Intake and output									
Parent-child interactions									
Medications									
Comments:									

Table 18.1
Physical Assessment of the Mother During Fourth Stage of Labor

Factors	Minimal Assessment	Findings and Comments
Blood pressure	Every 15 min for 1 h or until stable, then every 30 min times two	Slightly elevated from excitement and effort of delivery; returns to normal within 1 h
Pulse	Every 15 min for 1 h or until stable; then every 30 min times two	Normal rate for individual within 1 h; slight bradycardia may occur (50-70 beats/min)
Temperature	Once, at 1 h; then as per hospital protocol	May be elevated if dehydrated or fatigued.
Fundus	Every 15 min for 1 h or until stable; then every 30 min times two.	Firm: midline, 2 cm below or at umbilicus Soft: massage until firm and express clots until contracted to midlevel Right of midline: check bladder for distension
Bladder	Every time fundus is assessed.	Fills quickly because of postdelivery diuresis and intravenous fluids.
Lochia	Every 15 min (in conjunction with assessment of fundus)	Moderate flow: normal; if flow comes in spurts, suspect cervical tear Heavy flow: recheck in 3-5 min and report
Perineum	Check in conjunction with assessment of lochia.	Condition of episiotomy and perineum: clean, edematous, discolored, stitches intact

METHOD OF ASSESSMENT AND FINDINGS WITHIN NORMAL LIMITS DURING THE FOURTH STAGE OF LABOR

AREA OF EXAMINATION AND PURPOSE	METHOD OF ASSESSMENT	FINDINGS WITHIN NORMAL LIMITS
Blood pressure To obtain baseline data (Fig. 18.1).	Measure BP according to assessment schedule (Table 18.1)	Stabilizes at prelabor values during first hour
Pulse To obtain baseline data.	Count pulse, assess rate, amplitude (indicating volume), rhythm and symmetry, regularity	Stabilizes at prelabor levels during first hour; bradycardia, 50-70 beats/min
Temperature To obtain baseline data.	Determine temperature	Stabilizes within woman's normal range during first hour, or Slight elevation to 38° C (100.4° F) related to dehydration.
Fundus (Fig. 18.2) To prepare woman. To locate fundus. To stimulate contraction of a tonic (boggy) uterus to stimulate the "living ligature" To expel clots while uterus is firm (contracted) to allow uterus to remain contracted. To measure degree of involution with uterus in midline and bladder empty.	Ask her to empty bladder. Position her with knees flexed. Just below umbilicus, cup hand, press firmly into abdomen. Place hands appropriately, massage gently only until firm. Overstimulation causes muscle fatigue. Keep hands placed as in Fig. 18.2. With upper hand firmly apply pressure downward toward vagina. Observe perineum. Lay fingers flat on abdomen under umbilicus; measure how many fingerbreadths fit between umbilicus and top of fundus.	Bladder is empty. Tension on the abdomen is relieved. Entire fundus feels firm like tip of nose (i.e., has good tone). Uterus is supported during assessment, massage, and expulsion of clots. Slightly boggy uterus begins to contract immediately. Clots are expelled. Uterus retains tone. Most authors identify a level below the umbilicus.*
Bladder To assess distension. To assess return of bladder function.	Note fundal height and tone. Gently massage boggy uterus to restore tone and return uterus to midline. Observe and palpate area cephalad to symphysis pubis. Measure amount of urine voided. Assess tone and level of fundus and repalpate bladder.	If bladder is distended, it is seen as a suprapubic rounded bulge that is dull to percussion and fluctuates like a water-filled balloon. When the bladder is distended, the uterus may be boggy, well above umbilicus, and usually to her right side. Amount varies. Fundus firm, in midline; bladder nonpalpable.
Lochia (Fig. 18.3) To assess for normal color and amount. To assess odor. To rule out non-lochia bleeding.	Observe lochia on perineal pads and on linen under mother's buttocks. Note odor. Observe perineum for source of bleeding (e.g., episiotomy, lacerations) (see Chapter 27).	Lochia rubra is moderate and may contain some small clots. Odor of normal menstrual flow. Lochia does not come out in a continuous trickle or in spurts.
Perineum To assess delivery trauma. To assess repair of episiotomy or lacerations.	Ask or assist woman to turn on her side and flex upper leg on hip. Lift upper buttock. Observe perineum in good lighting.	Vaginal birth: mild edema or labial swelling; slight bruising. Episiotomy or laceration repair is intact, dry, mildly edematous but not inflamed.

*Level of contracted fundus immediately after expulsion of placenta:

Midway between umbilicus and symphysis, or slightly higher (Pritchard, MacDonald, and Gant, 1985, p. 367).

At a level below umbilicus, size of 15- to 16-week gestation (Danforth, 1982, p. 787).

Superior surface can be felt below the umbilicus (Willson, Carrington, and Ledger, 1983, p. 584).

At 2 cm above level of umbilicus descending by 1 cm in 12 hours (Quistad, 1984, p. 40).

Midway between symphysis and umbilicus. Rises to level of umbilicus within a few hours. Remains at level of umbilicus or 1 fingerbreadth below for a day or two (Varney, 1980, p. 348).

Fig. 18.1
Nurse prepares to assess for blood pressure, pulse, and respirations. As she interacts with new mother, nurse also assesses for maternal alertness, signs of discomfort, and cues to reaction to her birth experience and newborn. (Photograph by I.M. Bobak.)

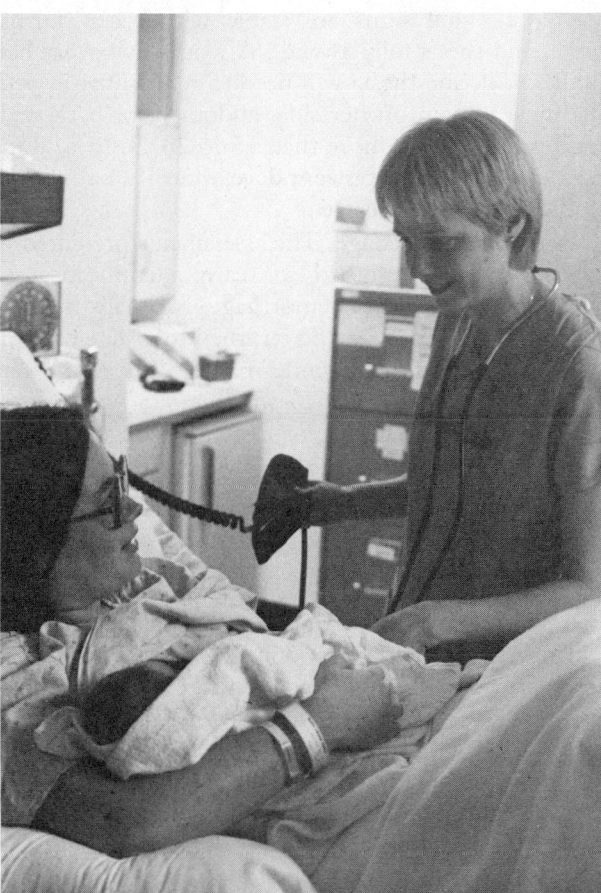

Fig. 18.2
Palpating fundus of uterus during first hour after delivery. Note that upper hand is cupped over fundus; lower hand dips in above symphysis pubis and supports uterus while it is massaged gently.

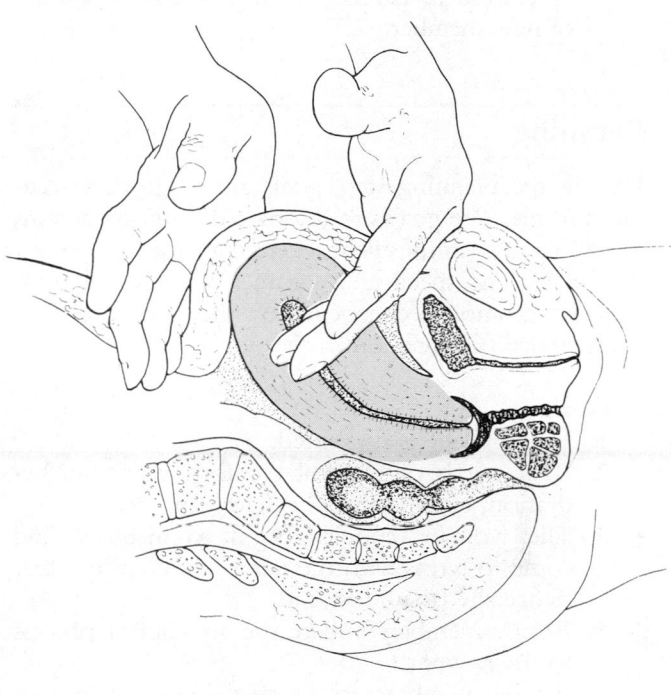

Fig. 18.3
Peripad-saturation volumes. (Reprinted with permission from Jacobsen, H.: A standard for assessing lochia volume, M.C.N. 10:175, May/June 1985. Copyright © 1985 American Journal of Nursing Co.)

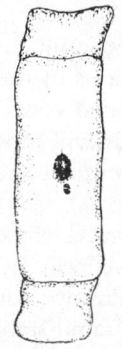 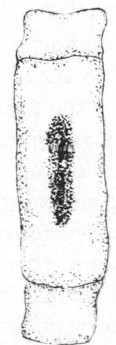 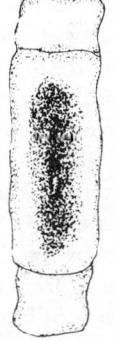 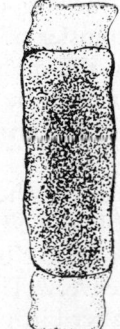

Scant amount
Blood only on tissue when wiped or less than 1-inch stain on peripad

Light amount
Less than 4-inch stain on peripad

Moderate amount
Less than 6-inch stain on peripad

Heavy amount
Saturated peripad within 1 hour

5. Potential for alteration in parenting, related to breast-feeding difficulties.
6. Alteration in family process related to addition of new member.

Planning

During the planning step, goals are set in client-centered terms. The goals are prioritized. Nursing actions are selected, with the client where appropriate, to meet the goals. The speed and accuracy with which planning is accomplished depends on the nurse's level of competence (Chapter 2).

Goals
1. Hemorrhage is prevented.
2. Basic needs of physical comfort, nutrition, hydration, elimination, and safety are met.
3. The woman (couple) begin to integrate and come to terms with the labor and delivery experience she (they) just had.
4. Family members initiate the attachment process to the newborn.
5. Family members are satisfied by the degree of involvement each had during the fourth stage.

Implementation

During the fourth stage, the nurse must organize care to meet the demands of accepted protocol while not appearing rushed. The nurse is concerned about several matters. These concerns include the following: the maternal position in bed, the prevention of hemorrhage, the prevention of urinary bladder distention, the maintenance of cleanliness, the maintenance of comfort, the maintenance of fluid balance and nutrition, and the support of parental emotional needs before the transfer of the family to the postdelivery unit. Following the discussion of each of these items is an outline of care. In Table 18.2 goals, assessment findings, nursing actions, teaching, and evaluation are addressed.

Position mother. The nurse settles the woman comfortably in bed. A new mother needs to remain in bed for at least 2 hours even if she has had an unmedicated delivery. The rapid decrease in intraabdominal pressure after birth results in a dilation of blood vessels supplying the intestines (known as splanchnic engorgement). **Splanchnic engorgement** pools blood in the viscera. Therefore when the woman stands up, she may feel faint (orthostatic hypotension). Women and their families need to be forewarned so that they know

to call for assistance, especially the first time or two that the woman gets out of bed.

The woman who has received analgesics needs to be watched until she is fully recovered from the medications (i.e., vital signs are stable within her normal range, and she is fully awake). A woman who has had saddle block anesthesia will need to remain flat in bed. She must remain on her side, abdomen, or back with her head raised not more than 15 to 20 cm (6 to 8 in) for 8 to 12 hours to prevent development of a "spinal" headache (see Chapter 16).

Prevent hemorrhage. The assessments presented in Table 18.1 are designed for early identification of events that may lead to hemorrhage. Normally the fundus remains firm or may be returned to a state of firmness with intermittent gentle massage. As noted earlier, *atony (relaxation) of the uterine musculature* may occur. As the relaxed uterus distends with blood and clots, blood vessels in the placental site are not clamped off by the "living ligature," and bleeding results. It is necessary to express gently the accumulated blood and clots before the uterus can again contract. If atony is not controlled by such treatment, medical intervention must be instituted (see Chapter 28).

The nurse notes the amount of *lochia*. Lochia may be described as scant, light, moderate, or heavy (profuse). As the effect of the oxytocic medication administered after delivery wears off, the amount of lochia will increase because the myometrium relaxes somewhat. The nurse always checks under the mother's buttocks as well as on the perineal pad. Bleeding may flow between the buttocks onto the linens under the mother while the amount on the perineal pad is slight. A perineal pad that is soaked through from tail to tail contains approximately 100 ml of blood. If a pad is found to be soaked through in 15 minutes, or if blood is seen pooled under the buttocks, continuous observation of blood loss, vital signs, and maternal color and behavior is indicated (see Box, p. 481).

If bleeding is in the form of a continuous trickle or is seen to come in spurts, lacerations of the vagina or cervix or the presence of an unligated vessel in the episiotomy is suspected. The woman will most likely be returned to the delivery area to permit visualization of the site and surgical correction.

Danger signs: hypovolemic shock. Hemorrhage and early hemorrhagic shock may occur in an otherwise normal fourth stage of labor. Prompt identification and intervention usually result in rapid stabilization of the woman's pulse, blood pressure, and other signs. The box on p. 481 is a quick reference for signs and symptoms, goals, and interventions.

Prevent bladder distension. Palpation to determine the amount of *bladder distension* accompanies the

Danger Signs: Hypovolemic Shock

Signs and symptoms

Marked bleeding persists: a second perineal pad is soaked in 15 min, *whether or not bleeding is accompanied by a change in vital signs or maternal color or behavior.*

Mother states she feels light-headed, "funny," "sick to [her] stomach," or "sees stars."

Mother begins to act anxious, her color turns ashen or grayish, her skin feels cool and clammy (wet), or she exhibits air hunger.

Pulse rate is increasing, and blood pressure is falling.

Goals	Interventions
Bring help *to you. Do not* leave woman.	Call for help fast—push emergency button; yell, if necessary.
Increase circulating blood volume; prevent supine hypotension.	Tilt woman onto her side.
	Increase flow of intravenous drip.
	Raise woman's legs *high.*
Prevent further loss of blood, by stimulating uterine contractions.	If uterus is atonic, massage gently and expel clots to allow uterus to contract; compress uterus manually, as needed, using two hands.
	Add oxytocic to intravenous drip, per standing order.
Facilitate oxygenation. ■ Stimulate respirations. ■ Increase available oxygen.	Break ampule of aromatic ammonia, a respiratory stimulant*; give oxygen by face mask at 8-10 L/min.

*Reflex stimulation of the vasomotor center results in a rise in blood pressure; therefore observe caution for woman with cardiovascular disorders.

palpation of the fundus. The full bladder forces the uterus upward and to the right of the midline. Such a position interferes with the contractility of the uterine muscle, and hemorrhage results. The nurse encourages the woman to void. If necessary, the nurse obtains an order for catheterization. In addition to the possibility of causing uterine relaxation, distension of the urinary bladder can result in atony of the bladder wall. Atony leads to urinary retention. Retention provides a favorable environment for infection. The nurse encourages the woman to void naturally. The nurse may employ one or more of the following: the nurse places a bedpan under the mother, gives her water to drink if the physician has ordered oral fluids, turns on the water faucet, helps her to walk (if ordered), and provides privacy. If the woman cannot void, most physicians write an order for catheterization. If the woman is catheterized, a urine specimen is saved for laboratory studies as necessary (e.g., culture and sensitivity).

Spirits of peppermint are sometimes used to aid the woman to void naturally. "Spirits" are concentrated alcohol solutions of volatile substances; they are also known as essences. Spirits of peppermint give off vapors. These vapors have an external, local relaxing effect on the sphincter muscle of the urinary meatus. Use of *peppermint spirits* may make it unnecessary to catheterize. The nurse places a bedpan under the woman and pours a few drops of peppermint spirits *into the bedpan.* The vapors rise to flow over the vulvar area, the urinary meatus relaxes, and urine is released. Nothing touches the woman except the vapors; the woman feels no sensation, only notices the aroma of peppermint. We know of no hospital that requires a physician's order for this technique.

Maintain cleanliness. The nurse changes perineal pads as necessary and cleanses the vulvar areas with each pad change. While demonstrating good hand-washing technique before touching the mother's perineal area, the nurse verbally emphasizes the action. The nurse reminds the woman to cleanse the vulvar area using a separate tissue for one swipe from front to back, applying the pad from front to back and then rewashing the hands. Some hospitals routinely offer a bed bath during this period.

Maintain comfort. The nurse refreshes the mother, her bed, and the area around the bed as necessary. *Cleanliness* is one measure that increases the mother's comfort. The nurse's attention to the mother's needs demonstrates a sense of caring. The woman feels more comfortable even if the same amount of discomfort is still present. The increase in perception of comfort is known as the Hawthorne effect.

Uterine contractions may result in discomfort known as *afterpains*. The volume within the uterus is decreased after delivery. The force of the myometrial contractions is considerable; the intrauterine pressure is much greater than that during labor, reaching 150 mm Hg or more.

During the first 2 hours after delivery, uterine contractions are regular and strong, especially in multiparas. The nurse adds to the woman's comfort by the following measures:

1. Explaining the normal physiology of afterpains
2. Helping the mother keep her urinary bladder empty
3. Providing a warmed blanket to the mother's abdomen
4. Administering analgesics ordered by the physician
5. Encouraging relaxation and breathing exercises

A filling bladder pressing up against the uterus causes it to relax. The uterus attempts to stay firm by increasing the force of contractions, thereby increasing the discomfort of afterpains.

Gentle massage of the fundus increases uterine contractions, thereby intensifying afterpains. To help the new mother cope with the discomforts of assessment measures, the nurse explains what is being done and why.

The *episiotomy area* or *hemorrhoids* may contribute to the new mother's discomfort. Ice packs wrapped in gauze or other protective cloth are placed against the area of the episiotomy. Cold therapy is used to numb the area and to minimize the amount of edema that occurs, thus reducing discomfort. The ice pack is most effective in minimizing edema if it is used for the first hour or two after delivery. The physician may order any one of several antiseptic or anesthetic ointments or sprays in order to ease discomfort in the perineal area. A side-lying position relieves direct pressure on the area.

If the woman had had a saddle block or other regional anesthetic, the nurse's description of sensations to expect as the anesthetic wears off can be very reassuring. Women describe the sensation as tingling or prickly. The sensation is much like that experienced by people after they have been sitting cross-legged for a long time and the legs have "gone to sleep."

Some women experience intense *tremors* after delivery that resemble the shivering of a chill. This chilling may be related to the sudden release of pressure on pelvic nerves. According to another theory, chilling may be symptomatic of a fetus-to-mother transfusion that sometimes occurs during placental separation. The feeling of a "chill" may be a reaction to epinephrine (adrenaline) production during delivery. The nurse can help the woman to relax or to feel comforted by providing her with warm blankets and an explanation that the tremors are commonly seen after delivery and are not related to infection.

If the nurse administers analgesics, the sedating effect of these analgesics necessitates such protective care as raising side rails, placing call bell within reach, and cautioning about remaining in bed. The woman must be warned about the "head-spinning" effect of the medications.

Maintain fluid balance and meet nutritional needs. Because of the restrictions on fluid intake and the loss of fluids (blood, perspiration, or emesis) during labor, many women are thirsty and request fluids soon after giving birth. If fluids are ordered, the nurse may offer any clear fluids in moderate amounts and should instruct the mother to drink slowly. Excessive fluids or drinking too quickly often precipitates bouts of nausea and vomiting. After the first hour, the nurse may offer the mother a light diet if ordered by the physician. The nurse records the type of fluids and foods taken, the time, the amount, and the mother's tolerance of the fluids or foods ingested. The physician may order continued parenteral fluids at a "keep open" rate in the event of hemorrhage or need for intravenous medications.

Support parental emotional needs. It is acceptable for the nurse openly to share in the excitement and joy of birth. The nurse assists the parents by accepting any expressions of disappointment (about the child's sex or appearance) and reassures them that these feelings are within normal limits. The nurse may reassure the mother that her behavior during labor was acceptable if the mother appears worried about this.

Psychic states of new mothers range from euphoria, a feeling of well-being, to a sleepy state marked by an unawareness of surroundings. As noted earlier, first reactions of new mothers and fathers to their newborns vary widely. These reactions give the obstetric team cues to use in individualizing plans of care. Women who have experienced long, difficult labors or who are in pain are frequently too exhausted to extend interest to the child. The nurse can offer to take the baby to the nursery until the mother is rested. After sufficient rest their attitudes can be surprisingly different. The child unwanted for diverse reasons may continue to be rejected or given only mild interest. The attitude of the husband is often reflected in the mother. His pleasure arouses a responsive pleasure, or his disappointment arouses corresponding disappointment.

Ethnic or cultural origins dictate behaviors that are deemed appropriate for special occasions. Some parents may not be able to express their delight openly; others wish to welcome the newcomer noisily.

The single mother may think she is not expected to express joy or pleasure in her baby. The nurse can encourage the woman to express her feelings of pleasure. If the single mother does not wish to see or touch the child, the nurse, verbally or nonverbally, can indicate to the mother that her decision is acceptable.

Some mothers, particularly with their firstborn, are surprised and disturbed by the passivity or disinterest they experience on seeing their long-awaited infant. The nurse can reassure the mother of the normalcy of these feelings. The idealized mother love does not necessarily come into being right after delivery. The gradual growth of such love comes to some as they assume the care and responsibility for their child.

The nurse can facilitate parent-child attachment or acquaintance by providing a warm, quiet, darkened environment. An infant responds by opening the eyes. Parents are encouraged to hold the infant *en face*. In the *en face* position, parents and newborns gaze into each other's eyes. Newborns focus best at about 20.3 cm (8 in) distance. Body odor can be noticed (mothers have remarked that each child smells different), and the infant can be put to breast.

During the fourth stage of labor, the nurse uses every opportunity to teach the new mother. Regardless of parity, new mothers can benefit from explanations for the various nursing actions during the immediate puerperium (Mercer, 1979). Examples of teaching are correlated with goals, assessment findings, nursing actions, and evaluation in Table 18.2.

Transfer of the mother and neonate to postdelivery area. At the end of the second hour after delivery the nurse assesses the new mother thoroughly. If her

physical state has stabilized, the mother has completed the fourth stage of labor. The mother is ready for transfer to the postdelivery area. The nurse checks the mother's record for completeness and prepares the record for transfer to the postdelivery area. In the postpartum area the delivery nurse assists the mother into bed and introduces her to the nurse on the postpartum unit and to other women who may be sharing her room. The delivery nurse gives a report to the postpartum nurse (Table 18.3).

The neonate is transferred to either the postpartum unit to room-in with the mother or to the newborn nursery. The recovery nurse gives a report on the newborn to the appropriate nurse. An example of pertinent information to relay is given in Table 18.4.

Table 18.2
Teaching the New Mother During the Fourth Stage of Labor

Goal and Assessment Findings	Nursing Actions	Teaching	Evaluation
Prevent hemorrhage			
Uterus			
Firm	None needed	Rationale: living ligature. Identify location and size.	Retains tone.
Boggy	Gentle massage and expel clots as needed. Medication Intravenous drip	Self-message Meaning of term *involution*.	Mother locates and massages uterus.
Lochia		Rationale for assessing.	
Scant	None needed	Meaning of terms.	Lochia is moderate or less
Light	None needed		with no clots or just a few
Moderate	None needed; observe	Expected regression (color and amount) during involution.	small clots.
Heavy	Reassess source of bleeding, uterine tone, degree of bladder distension. Intervene as needed. Continue to observe.	Atony and subsequent hemorrhage can be the result of distended bladder. Or bleeding can be from another source (e.g., unrepaired laceration).	
Clots	Expel. Note size and amount. Observe.	Clots prevent living ligature from working.	
Bladder		Rationale for keeping empty: prevent uterine atony and trauma to bladder.	
Voids	Measure, record amount Reassess uterine tone, position, and degree of bladder filling.	Postdelivery, diuresis and intravenous fluids result in rapid bladder filling.	Voids completely so that uterus is firm, in midline, and below umbilicus.
Unable to void	Provide privacy, sound of running water, fluids to drink. Catheterize.	Same as above. Direct trauma to tissues, edema, analgesia/anesthesia, impair normal urination pattern.	Voids completely. Bladder is emptied without additional trauma and by using strict aseptic technique.
Interested in *breast feeding* and newborn and is healthy and ready to nurse.	Assist her with breast feeding (Chapter 21).	Nipple stimulation results in release of oxytocin, which causes the uterus to contract and assists involution.	Uterus retains tone. Mother understands cause of possible sensation of afterpains during breast feeding.

Continued.

Table 18.2, cont'd
Teaching the New Mother During the Fourth Stage of Labor

Goal and Assessment Findings	Nursing Actions	Teaching	Evaluation
Comfort			
Woman presents nonverbal cues, indicating discomfort.	Determine that discomfort is "normal" and take appropriate actions:	Validate that this discomfort is expected.	Woman's nonverbal and verbal responses validate that she is comfortable.
Woman states she is uncomfortable and specifies location and characteristics of discomfort	■ *Episiotomy:* Position Icepacks Medication	Explain expected results of chosen intervention.	Woman is able to rest comfortably.
Discomfort is located at site of repair of episiotomy or laceration and is due to hemorrhoids, or "afterpains"	■ *Afterpains* Warm blanket Empty the bladder Medications Refer abnormal or suspicious findings to physician (e.g., headache).		
Hydration			
Woman complains of fatigue	Provide oral fluids as ordered.	Explain relationship of fluid deficit to temperature rise and fatigue.	Woman is well hydrated (elevated temperature and fatigue take time to resolve).
Woman's temperature is elevated	Caution her against drinking rapidly or drinking large amounts at one time.		
Woman has just completed labor and given birth within previous two hours	Maintain intravenous fluid infusion at rate specified.	Explain need to drink small amounts slowly to prevent nausea and vomiting.	Woman takes oral fluids without difficulty.
Woman's fluid intake (oral and intravenous) were limited			
Nutrition			
Prenatal record shows time and amount of food intake before admission	Provide foods as ordered.	Begin postpartum nutrition counseling by simple statements such as, "the vitamin C in this juice will. . . ."	Woman's hunger is satisfied. Woman takes food without incident.
Labor record shows calorie intake (intravenous/oral)		Explain relationship of food deficit and fatigue.	
Woman states she is hungry			
Woman complains of fatigue			
Elimination: bladder			
Woman has just given birth and diuresis begins	Encourage woman to void.	Explain reason for need to prevent bladder distension.	Bladder distension is prevented.
Labor record shows amount of intake and output	Catheterize as needed, per physician's orders.		
Bladder filling is observed and palpated			
Uterine fundus may be rising			
Safety			
Woman delivered within the previous 2 hours	Request that woman ask for assistance to ambulate.	Explain possible hypotension and fainting due to natural causes during this time.	Woman requests assistance. Woman ambulates without difficulty.
Woman had analgesia or anesthesia	Promote safety as appropriate: ■ Put side rails up. ■ Prevent ambulation until anesthesia wears off. ■ Help woman maintain flat position for specified time after spinal anesthesia.	Explain reasons for specific nursing actions to woman and her family.	Woman incurs no injury.
Woman just gave birth	Promote good hygiene.	Explain rationale to promote comfort and healing and to prevent infection.	Woman understands rationale.

Table 18.2, cont'd
Teaching the New Mother During the Fourth Stage of Labor

Goal and Assessment Findings	Nursing Actions	Teaching	Evaluation
Integration of experience			
Woman has completed labor and given birth within previous 2 hours Woman gives verbal cues such as, "I was such a baby." "I'm sorry for screaming." "What did the doctor say?" "This [labor and delivery] was not like the last time."	Implement communication techniques (Chapter 4). Listen to mother's replay of her experience.	Phrases questions and answers in manner that indicates that her responses during all stages of labor were within expected range.	Woman indicates by nonverbal cues (relaxed) and nonverbal responses that she is is beginning to accept her behavior and the experience.
Attachment process			
Woman indicates desire to hold newborn; other family members indicate desire to hold newborn Woman indicates desire to breast feed	Assess newborn's condition to be within normal limits. Wrap baby warmly. Position baby in person's arms for maximum safety. Ensure woman's comfort. Point out newborn's individual characteristics. Accept parents' decisions.	Attachment to newborn is a continuous process. Fatigue of either mother or baby may delay but will not adversely influence attachment response.	Mother (family) begins attachment process; or if sedated or fatigued, mother indicates she can accept the delay.
Individual and family satisfaction Woman and family talk about their expectations before experience and how they perceive whether their goals have or have not been met. Woman and family express reactions to the newborn.	Meet family's ethnic and cultural expectations for care: ■ Accept degree of involvement of individuals regarding overt expression of joy or love. ■ Accept family's desires regarding neonate (e.g., some may want newborn to be cared for in nursery).	Each ethnic and cultural group has developed workable ways for family interactions. There is no one "right" way.	Family indicates satisfaction with the experience.

Table 18.3
Recovery Nurse's Report to Postpartum Nurse

Item	Example
Type of labor and delivery; unusual observations, if any, of the placenta	Spontaneous or assisted (forceps) vaginal delivery; vertex presentation
Gravidity and parity, age	G I, P I, 22 years old.
Anesthesia and analgesia used	None; epidural, low spinal, local
Condition of perineum	Episiotomy; repair of lacerations
Events since delivery	Vital signs, blood pressure, fundus, lochia, intake and output, medications (dosage, time of administration, and results), response to newborn, observation of family interactions, including siblings, if present
Condition and sex of newborn; other information	Apgar at 1 and 5 min; time of birth; eye prophylaxis given; weight; whether breast or bottle feeding; if breast feeding, whether newborn was at breast; name of pediatrician
Relevant information from prenatal record	Need for rubella vaccination
Miscellaneous information	
■ Intravenous drip	If intravenous drip is infusing, rate of infusion, medications added (e.g., Pitocin), whether to keep open or discontinue after completion of bag that is hung
■ Social factors	If woman is giving baby up for adoption, whether she wants to see baby, breast feed, allow visitors, or other preferences she may have

Table 18.4
Recovery Nurse's Report to Newborn's Nurse

Item	Example
Type of labor and delivery; unusual events (e.g., cord around neck)	Spontaneous or assisted (forceps, vacuum extractor) vaginal birth in vertex presentation
Gravidity and parity, age of mother	G I, P I, 22 years old
Analgesia and anestheisa	None; epidural, low spinal, or local
Condition at birth	Apgar scores at 1 and 5 min
Sex and weight	Male; 3400 g (7 lb, 8 oz)
Events since birth*	Nursed at breast; took nipple well Voided ×I; meconium ×I Eye prophylaxis Vitamin K injection Held by siblings who are happy (or have other response) to newborn
Relevant information from prenatal record	Unremarkable pregnancy

*Neonatal adjustment to extrauterine existence and recovery of the neonate are discussed in detail in Chapter 17 and Unit 5.

Evaluation

Ongoing evaluation and moment-to-moment adjustment of the nursing care plan are common during the fourth stage of labor. The nurse uses the goals of care as guides to nursing actions. Care is evaluated as effective if the goals have been achieved.

Summary

During the fourth stage of labor the new mother's recovery from childbirth is monitored closely. Her basic needs for comfort, fluids, nutrients, elimination, cleanliness, and safety are met. She and her family begin to integrate the experience and the newborn into their lives. A data base is prepared for use in continuing care on the postpartum unit or after return to the home.

Summary of Nursing Actions

Nursing Care During the Fourth Stage of Labor

GOALS
1. For the mother: an uncomplicated immediate recovery from the birth process and an adequate beginning for integration of the birth experience.
2. For the newborn: a continuation of a healthy extrauterine existence.
3. For the family: a continuation of a positive process of attachment to the newborn and an adequate beginning for integration of the birth experience.

PRIORITIES
1. Identification of the potential risks for hemorrhage and initiation of preventive measures if needed.
2. Implementation of immediate interventions if hemorrhage does occur.
3. Promotion of recovery through the use of supportive and comfort measures (e.g., nourishment, fluids, safety precautions, and medications).
4. Promotion of attachment of family members to newborn.
5. Promotion of opportunities for family to begin to integrate the experience.

ASSESSMENT	EXAMPLES OF POTENTIAL NURSING DIAGNOSTIC CATEGORIES*
Mother Obtain information from delivery room personnel (or check record) regarding significant findings from prenatal and intrapartum periods.	Potential for maternal compromise† Potential fluid volume deficit Alteration in normal physiologic processes† Ineffective individual family coping Knowledge deficit Potential fluid volume deficit (blood loss) Alteration in comfort: pain
Complete assessment for physical findings every 15 min: ▪ Fundus ▪ Lochia ▪ Perineum ▪ Blood pressure ▪ Pulse ▪ Bladder distension	Alteration in patterns of urinary elimination

*Accepted diagnoses from the Seventh National Conference (1986).
†Diagnosis not included by NANDA, 1986.

Summary of Nursing Actions—cont'd

ASSESSMENT	EXAMPLES OF POTENTIAL NURSING DIAGNOSTIC CATEGORIES
Assess temperature before transfer to postpartum unit.	Potential fluid volume deficit (decreased fluid intake)
	Potential for infection
Assess comfort level and character and location of discomfort.	Alteration in comfort: pain
	Potential for maternal compromise†
Assess energy level.	Sleep pattern disturbance
	Energy depletion (exhaustion)†
Assess recovery from analgesia or anesthesia.	Impaired physical mobility
	Potential for injury
Assess emotional response to birth, to the newborn, taking into consideration cultural and ethnic variations.	Ineffective individual or family coping
	Alteration in parenting
	Alteration in family process
	Potential disturbance in self-concept: body image, self-esteem, role performance, personal identity
Assess need for fluids and nutrients.	Fluid volume deficit
	Alteration in nutrition: less than body requirements
Assess mother's (family's) educational needs:	Knowledge deficit
■ Postpartum care and recovery	Disturbance in self-concept: body image, self-esteem, role performance, personal identity
■ Breast or bottle feeding	Alteration in parenting
■ Newborn characteristics	Ineffective individual or family coping
■ Newborn care	Potential for injury (nipples etc.)
Assess and summarize findings before transfer to postpartum area.	Any or all of the categories given above
Newborn	
Evaluate maternal history, including labor, to identify potential problems for newborn.	Potential for ineffective airway clearance
Assess respirations and newborn's ability to keep airway clear.	Potential for impaired gas exchange
	Potential for impairment of thermal regulation
Assess for meconium staining of fingernails, vernix, or cord.	Potential for ineffective thermoregulation
Assess temperature and color.	Potential for injury
Assess weight, length (may be delayed until temperature is stabilized).	
Reassess for gestational age and possible complications, including structural malformations.	
Note passage of meconium or urine.	

OUTCOME CRITERIA*	PLAN/IMPLEMENTATION
Mother	
Physical findings are assessed every 15 min × 4 (at least) until stable within normal limits:	Settle the mother comfortably in bed; explain routine care.
■ Uterus remains firm, in midline, at or slightly above umbilicus for first 2 hours.	Massage gently as necessary to maintain firmness; expel clots if present.
■ Lochia is moderate.	Teach mother how and why this is done.
	Change perineal pads as necessary; wash vulva with soap and water as needed.
	Teach mother about lochia—amount and color to expect and time periods for change in character and amount.
■ Perineum is intact; or repair of episiotomy or laceration is intact; perineal edema is minimal.	Apply ice pack to perineum per physician's order.
■ Blood pressure remains within her normal limits.	If blood pressure is too low: turn her on her side, give oxygen by face mask if she is breathless, give intravenous fluids; massage uterus until firm; place in trendelenburg position; call physician if blood pressure does not return to normal quickly.

*Outcome criteria direct the selection of nursing actions (**plan/implementation**) and measure their effectiveness (**evaluation**).

Continued.

Summary of Nursing Actions—cont'd

OUTCOME CRITERIA	PLAN/IMPLEMENTATION
Mother—cont'd	
	If elevated: assess deep tendon reflexes (DTR) and for other signs of pregnancy-induced hypertension (PIH); record and report to physician.
■ Pulse may be slow, often between 50 and 70 beats/min. ■ Bladder distension is prevented.	Encourage to void completely. If distension occurs and woman is unable to void, catheterize and record amount, character, and type. Send specimen to laboratory if indicated.
Temperature is within normal limits.	Provide fluids, oral or intravenous, per hospital and physician protocol. If infection is diagnosed, treat per physician order.
Woman states she feels comfortable and rested. Desire to rest not hampered because of discomfort from pain, thirst, hunger, or emotional upset.	Teach regarding "afterpains," lochia, reasons for checking fundus and expressing clots, return of sensation to legs after regional anesthesia, and need to keep bladder empty. Give medications for pain if other comfort measures do not work, if woman desires medication, and if appropriate. Provide general hygiene. Help her into positions of comfort. Make environment conducive to rest (e.g., temperature, ventilation, quiet). Provide emotional support as needed (e.g., answer questions).
Mother's fluid and nutrient needs are met.	Provide fluids and nourishment per hospital and physician's protocol. Record amounts and types.
Mother takes fluids and food without nausea or vomiting.	Caution her to drink fluids slowly and in small amounts to prevent nausea or vomiting.
Mother is recovered from analgesics or anesthetics.	Explain return of sensation to legs after spinal or epidural anesthestics. Monitor vital signs and blood pressure. Assist to ambulate for the first time to prevent injury in case of fall secondary to splanchnic engorgement. Keep side rails up and call bell within easy reach until woman is fully recovered.
Mother's and family's questions are answered.	Provide assurance by answering questions simply and directly; encourage questions regarding labor and recovery experience. Share in excitement and joy over birth.
Initial mother-family-child interactions are enough to satisfy the need to touch, hold, and examine the newborn; to reassure as to the normalcy of the newborn's appearance and behavior; to provide eye contact with the newborn (if possible); and to initiate breast feeding of the newborn (if desired). Maternal behavior and appearance are within normal limits. Initial excitement replaced with drowsy satisfaction.	Facilitate mother-family-child attachment: provide a warm, quiet, darkened environment (newborn is more apt to open eyes), encouraging parents to hold newborn en face within 2.5 to 20 cm (1 to 8 in, the distance at which most newborns can focus). Accept any expressions of disappointment from parents and reassure them that such feelings are common. Reassure mother and family that her behavior during labor was acceptable if she or they appear worried about it. Assist with breastfeeding as necessary.
Mother and family indicate that care given is within their religious, cultural, and ethnic prescriptions and proscriptions.	Inquire of mother and family what they expect in terms of care during the recovery from childbirth. Accommodate them as much as possible. Use services of interpretor if indicated.
Transfer to postdelivery area is accomplished when mother's condition is stabilized within normal limits, fundus is remaining contracted, bladder is empty, and record is complete.	Check record for completeness and prepare record for transfer to postdelivery area. Collect woman's possessions; raise side rails on bed; check intravenous bottle, lines, and pole to ensure safe transfer.

Summary of Nursing Actions—cont'd

OUTCOME CRITERIA	PLAN/IMPLEMENTATION
Mother—cont'd	
	Give report to admitting nurse (Table 18.3).
	Assist nurse to help woman into bed.
	Introduce her to postpartum nurse and to other women sharing her room.
If woman does not want to breast feed, administer antilactogenic medications. If antilactogenic hormones are used, in some hospitals the woman is asked to sign an informed consent (before delivery) before receiving these hormones.	Check record to see that consent form has been signed.
	Administer the medication per physician's order.
	If woman is to receive bromocriptine mesylate (Parlodel), delay administration until the vital signs have been stabilized and administer no sooner than 4 hours after delivery.
Newborn	
Physical health is satisfactory as measured by the following:	Ensure clear airway.
■ Temperature: 37° C (98.6° F)	Maintain warmth by mother's body heat, warm blankets, a stockinette cap for head, overhead heating panel, or a warmed bassinet, following hospital protocol.
■ Heart rate, rhythm, regularity are within normal limits.	
■ Color and respiration are within normal limits.	
Data base established through physical examination and assessment for gestational age; by end of 2 hours after birth, newborn is weighed, length and suboccipital bregmatic diameter are measured, and eye prophylaxis is completed.	Share data with parents, if appropriate.
	Meet parents' needs for knowledge regarding eye prophylaxis; provide eye prophylaxis.
Newborn is alert with eyes open during first 30-60 min, followed by sleep; during alert period when sucking reflex is present, newborn is put to the breast.	Facilitate mother-father-child attachment.
	Suggest breast feeding and assist with process if mother indicated she planned to breast feed.
Transfer of newborn is accomplished per parent's choice and hospital protocol, e.g., to transitional nursery where constant surveillance, external heat sources, and emergency care are available until newborn is stabilized; then to normal newborn unit or rooming-in unit; or, from delivery area directly to rooming-in unit where nursing personnel, mother, or family member share responsibility for continuous surveillance and care needed by newborn.	Keep newborn with parents during recovery phase if newborn remains in good condition. Check record for transfer to postdelivery area.
	Accomplish transfer per hospital protocol, e.g., father may carry newborn to nursery and place in heated crib; mother may carry baby in bed with her; nurse may carry newborn.
	Give report to admitting nurse (Table 18.4).
	Give postpartum nurse information regarding mother's (family's) knowledge as well as noting this on her record.

Nursing Care During the Four Stages of Labor

Mrs. G. (G I P O) was admitted to the labor room at 8:30 AM today. Her labor began at home at 2:30 AM with contractions every 20 minutes, lasting 50 to 20 seconds. Her membranes are intact. The couple has attended childbirth classes. Fetal heart rate is 144. At 10:00 AM the assessment shows the following:

Effacement: 100%
Dilation: 6 cm
Presentation, station: vertex, −1
Membranes: intact
Show: scant bloody mucus
Behavior: serious, apprehensive; does not want to be alone
Contractions: every 7 minutes; of moderate intensity; lasting approximately 40 seconds

It is now 10:40 AM. As you begin your assessment, the membranes rupture spontaneously.

At 12 noon, Mrs. G. complains of nausea, perspiration is seen on her upper lip, and vaginal examination confirms full cervical dilatation. At 12:10 PM, Mrs. G. begins to bear down spontaneously with contractions. At 1:00 PM the fetal head is distending the perineum. Mrs. G. indicates she desires to assume the squatting position. The bed is adjusted to support her in the squatting position. Fifteen minutes later a girl is born. Her Apgar scores at 1 and 5 minutes are 9 and 10 respectively. The newborn girl is assessed, wrapped in warm blankets, and given to the father while the placenta is expelled. Within 20 minutes the newborn girl is placed at her mother's breast while Mr. G. completes taking pictures. Mrs. G.'s bladder is noted to be filling. One hour after giving birth, Mrs. G. voids spontaneously.

FUNCTIONAL HEALTH PATTERN: ASSESSMENT	NURSING DIAGNOSIS	RATIONALE: PLAN/ IMPLEMENTATION	EVALUATION
FIRST STAGE			
Activity-Exercise	Potential for impairment of gas exchange in fetus related to prolapse of umbilical cord.	*To ensure gas exchange:*	Cord does not prolapse. FHR stays within normal limits, indicating adequate gas exchange.
■ Spontaneous rupture of membranes.		■ Assess FHR stat; repeat in 10 min.	
		■ If FHR stays within normal limits, note time on record, and return to usual protocol for care.	
Coping–stress tolerance	Ineffective individual coping, related to first stage of labor, active phase.	*To meet need for support person:*	After delivery, woman perceives the experience in a positive manner regarding care she received, husband's role, and her performance.
■ Behavior: serious, apprehensive; does not want to be alone.		■ Stay with her.	
		■ Assist husband to participate in implementing comfort measures as appropriate.	
		■ Keep couple informed regarding progress in labor.	
		■ Reassure couple that responses are understandable and acceptable	
SECOND STAGE			
Cognitive-perceptual	Sensory-perceptual alteration related to knowledge deficit of normal processes.	*To counter knowledge deficit and remedy sensory-perceptual alteration during last phase of the second stage:*	Mother responds in positive manner to care received:
■ As fetal head is distending the perineum, Mrs. G. screams that something is wrong because she feels herself tearing apart.		■ Assist woman or engage husband to assist her into position so she can see and place her hand over emerging head.	1. By signs of reduced anxiety or increased interest in seeing or feeling fetal head 2. By verbal expression after delivery.

Application of the Nursing Process—cont'd

FUNCTIONAL HEALTH PATTERN: ASSESSMENT	NURSING DIAGNOSIS	RATIONALE: PLAN/ IMPLEMENTATION	EVALUATION
		■ Remind her of sensations common to this time in labor. ■ Focus her on closeness to giving birth. ■ Reassure couple that responses are understandable and acceptable.	
THIRD STAGE **Coping–stress tolerance** ■ Mrs. G. cries out, "It's a girl." "Look honey how beautiful she is!" "She looks like you!"	Family coping: potential for growth related to pleasure in newborn.	*To promote parent-child attachment:* ■ Compliment them on the baby, as appropriate. ■ When appropriate, support parents' desire to hold baby, put her to breast, and soon.	Parent's verbal and nonverbal responses indicate pleasure with newborn and each other.
FOURTH STAGE **Elimination** ■ Bladder distension is noted by observation, palpation, and height of uterine fundus.	Alteration in patterns of urinary elimination related to post childbirth decrease in sensation or perception of sensation to void.	*To facilitate complete voiding:* ■ Implement measures that facilitate voiding (e.g., privacy, sound of running water, suggestion).	Woman voids spontaneously. Bladder cannot be palpated. Fundus remains firm, in midline, and below umbilicus.

References

Danforth, D.: Obstetrics and gynecology, ed. 4, Philadelphia, 1982, Harper & Row, Publishers.

Jacobsen, H.: A standard for assessing lochia volume, M.C.N. 10:174, May/June 1985.

Mercer, R.T.: "She's a multip . . . she knows the ropes," 4:301, Sept./Oct. 1979.

Pritchard, J.A., MacDonald, P.C., and Gant, N.F.: Williams obstetrics, ed. 17, Norwalk, Conn., 1985, Appleton-Century-Crofts.

Quistad, C.: How to smooth mom's postpartum path, R.N. 47:40, April 1984.

Varney, H.: Nurse-Midwifery, Boston, 1980, Blackwell Scientific Publications.

Willson, J.R., Carrington, E.R., and Ledger, W.J.: Obstetrics and gynecology, ed. 7, St. Louis, 1983, The C.V. Mosby Co.

Bibliography

Bentz, J.M.: Missed meanings in nurse/patient communications, M.C.N. 5(1):55, 1980.

Chute, G.E.: Expectation and experience in alternative and conventional birth, J.O.G.N. Nurs. 14(1):61, Jan./Feb. 1985.

Ellison, S.L., et al.: Sucking in the newborn infant during the first hour of life, J. Nurse Midwife. 24:6, 1979.

Gorrie, T.M.: Postpartal nursing diagnosis, J.O.G.N. Nurs. 15(1):52, Jan./Feb. 1986.

Hans, A.: Postpartum assessment: the psychological component, J.O.G.N. Nurs. 15(1):49, Jan./Feb. 1986.

Haun, N.: Nursing care during labor, Can. Nurse, 80(9):26, Oct. 1984.

Honig, J.C.: Preparing preschool-aged children to be siblings, M.C.N. 11(1):37, Jan./Feb. 1986.

Horn, M., and Manion, J.: Creative grandparenting: bonding the generations, J.O.G.N. Nurs. 14(3):233, May/June 1985.

Jensen, M.D., and Bobak, I.M.: Maternity and gynecologic care: the nurse and the family, ed. 3, St. Louis, 1985, The C.V. Mosby Co.

Johnsen, N.M., and Gaspard, M.E.: Theoretical foundations of a prepared sibling class, J.O.G.N. Nurs. 14(3)237, May/June 1985.

Kowba, M.D., and Schwirian, P.M.: Direct sibling contact and bacterial colonization in newborns, J.O.G.N. Nurs. 14:412, Sept./Oct. 1985.

Leininger, M.: Transcultural nursing: an essential knowledge and practice field for today, Canadian Nurse 80:41, Dec. 1984.

Macdonald, J.: Birth attendants: another choice, Canadian Nurse 80:22, Oct. 1984.

Maloney, R.: Childbirth education classes: expectant parent's expectations, J.O.G.N. Nurs. 14:245, May/June 1985.

Maloni, J.: The birthing room: some insights into parents, M.C.N. 5(5):314, 1980.

Marecki, M. and others: Early sibling attachment, J.O.G.N. Nurs. 14:418, Sept./Oct. 1985.

McKay, S., and Mahan, C.S.: Ways to upgrade postpartal care, Contemp. OB/Gyn. 27:63, Nov. 1985.

Myles, M.F.: Textbook for midwives with modern concepts of obstetric and neonatal care, ed. 9, New York, 1981, Churchill Livingstone.

Phillips, C.R., and Anzalone, J.T.: Fathering: participation in labor and birth, ed. 2, St. Louis, 1982, The C.V. Mosby Co.

Stolte, K.M.: Nursing diagnosis and the childbearing woman, M.C.N. 11:13, Jan./Feb. 1986.

Taubenheim, A.M.: Paternal-infant bonding in the first-time father, J.O.G.N. Nurs.10:261, 1981.

Wieser, M.A., and Castiglia, P.T.: Assessing early father-infant attachment. M.C.N. 9:104, Mar./Apr. 1984.

Wiggins, J.D.: Childbearing: physiology, experiences, needs, St. Louis, 1979, The C.V. Mosby Co.

Zuspan, F.P., and Quilligan, E.J., editors: Practical manual of obstetric care, St. Louis, 1982, The C.V. Mosby Co.

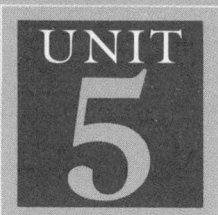

UNIT
5

The Normal Newborn

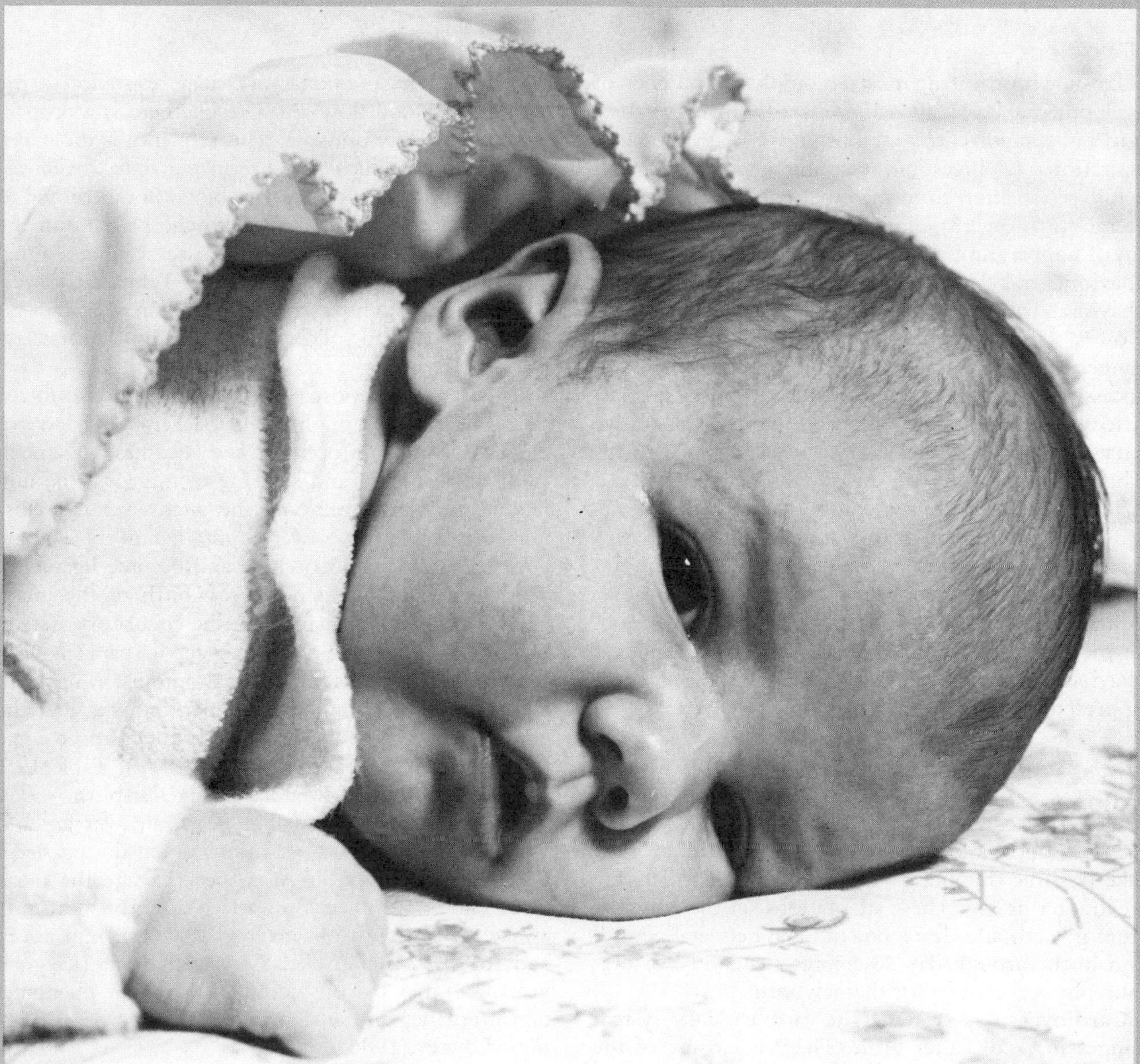

CHAPTER 19

Biologic and Behavioral Characteristics of the Newborn

The newborn infant must accomplish a number of developmental tasks to achieve autonomy. The biologic tasks involve (1) establishing and maintaining respirations, (2) ingesting, retaining, and digesting nutrients, a transition from maternal parenteral to infant enteral nutrition, (3) elimination of waste, (4) regulation of temperature, and (5) regulation of weight. The behavioral tasks include (1) establishing a regulated behavioral tempo independent of the mother, which involves self-regulation of arousal, self-monitoring of changes in his or her state, and patterning of sleep, (2) processing, storing, and organizing the multiple stimuli to which he or she is exposed, which is cognitive in nature, and (3) establishing a relationship with his or her caretakers and with the environment (Lewis and Zarin-Ackerman, 1977) (see also Chapter 20).

By term the infant's various anatomic and physiologic systems have reached a level of development and functioning that permits a physical existence apart from the mother and a readiness for social interaction. For the purpose of clarity a separation of biologic and behavioral characteristics has been made in the following presentation.

Biologic Characteristics

The profound biologic adaptations that occur at birth make possible the infant's transition from intrauterine to extrauterine life. These adaptations set the stage for future growth and development. The neonatal period, from birth through day 28, represents a time of dramatic physical change for the newborn.

Cardiovascular system. The cardiovascular system changes markedly after birth. There is closure of the foramen ovale, ductus arteriosus, and ductus venosus. The umbilical arteries and vein and the hepatic arteries become ligaments (Fig. 19.1).

The infant's first breath inflates the lungs and

thereby reduces pulmonary vascular resistance to the pulmonary blood flow. As a result there is a drop in pulmonary artery pressure. This sequence is the major mechanism by which pressure in the *right atrium declines*. The increased pulmonary blood flow returned to the left side of the heart *increases* the pressure in the *left atrium*. This change in pressures causes a functional closure of the foramen ovale. Temporary reversal of flow through the foramen ovale may occur with crying and lead to mild cyanosis during the first few days of life.

The ductus arteriosus constricts in response to the establishment of a high oxygen level in the arterial blood. Eventually it occludes and becomes a ligament. With the clamping and severing of the cord, the umbilical arteries and vein and the ductus venosus close immediately and are converted into ligaments. The hypogastric arteries also occlude and become ligaments. The changes in blood flow with birth of the infant have the effect of transforming the circulatory system. Before birth the two ventricles act in parallel, with shunts adjusting possible unequal outputs. After birth the two pumps act in series, which requires that the outputs of the right and left sides of the heart be equal (Vaughan, McKay, and Behrman, 1979). Table 19.1 summarizes the cardiovascular changes at birth.

Heart rate and sound. The heart rate averages 140 beats/min at birth with variations noted during sleeping and waking states. At 1 week of age the mean heart rate is 128 beats/min asleep and 163 beats/min awake; at 1 month of age it is 138 beats/min asleep and 167 beats/min awake. Sinus arrhythmia (irregular heart rate) may be considered a physiologic phenomenon in infancy and an indication of good heart function (Lowrey, 1986).

Heart sounds after birth reflect the series action of the heart pump. They are described as the familiar "lub, dub, lub, dub" sound. The "lub" is associated with closure of the mitral and tricuspid valves at the

494

Fig. 19.1

Fetal circulation. *Before birth*. Arterialized blood from the placenta flows into the fetus through the umbilical vein and passes rapidly through the liver into the inferior vena cava; from there if flows through the foramen ovale into the left atrium, soon to appear in the aorta and arteries of the head. A portion bypasses the liver through the ductus venosus. Venous blood from the lower extremities and head passes predominantly into the right atrium, the right ventricle, and then into the descending pulmonary artery and ductus arteriosus. Thus the foramen ovale and the ductus arteriosus act as bypass channels, allowing a large part of the combined cardiac output to return to the placenta without flowing through the lungs. Approximately 55% of the combined ventricular output flows to the placenta; 35% perfuses body tissues; and the remaining 10% flows through the lungs (Fanaroff, 1983). *After birth*. The foramen ovale closes; the ductus arteriosus closes and becomes a ligament; the ductus venosus closes and becomes a ligament; and the umbilical vein and arteries close and become ligaments. (Courtesy Ross Laboratories, Columbus, Ohio.)

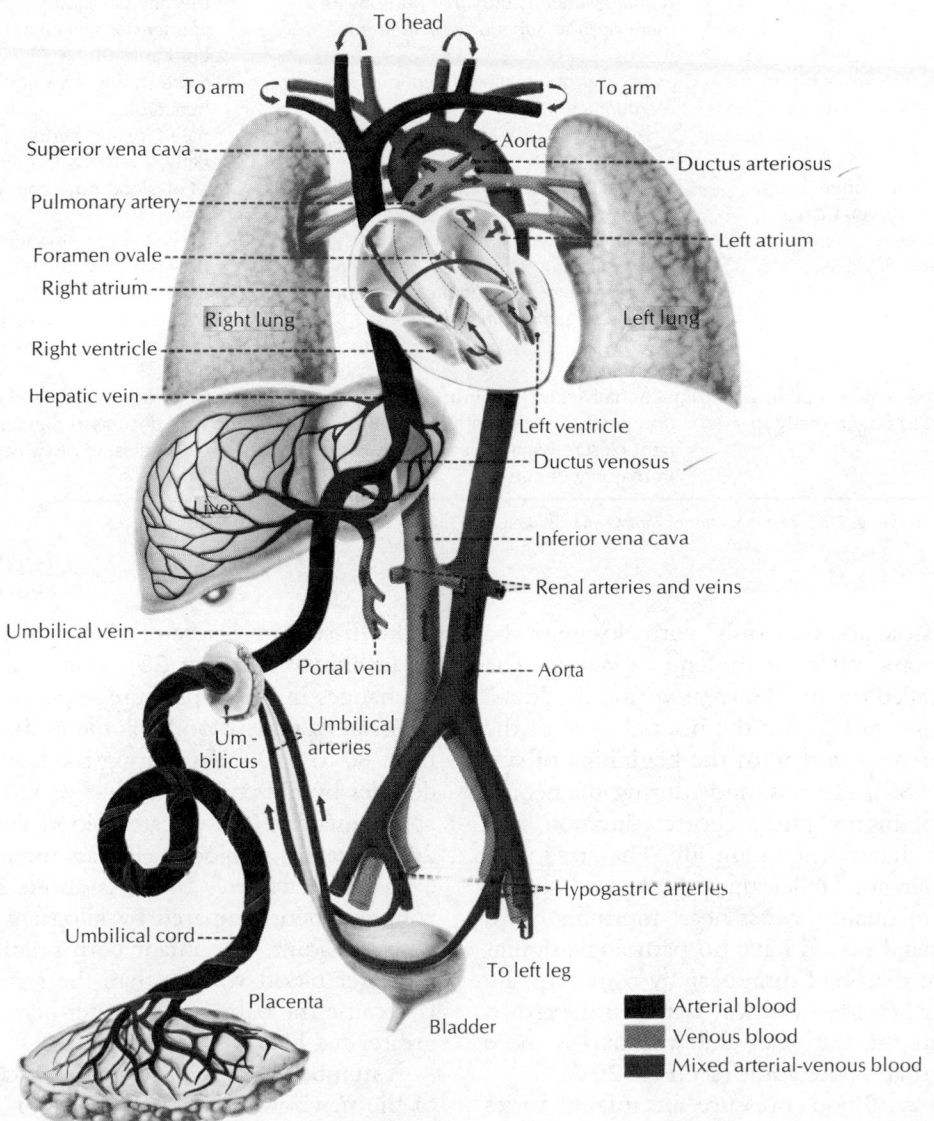

Table 19.1
Cardiovascular Changes at Birth

Prenatal Status	Postdelivery Status	Associated Factors
Primary changes		
Pulmonary circulation: high pulmonary vascular resistance; increased pressure in right ventricle and pulmonary arteries	Low pulmonary vascular resistance; decreased pressure in right atrium, ventricle, and pulmonary arteries	Expansion of collapsed fetal lung with air
Systemic circulation: low pressures in left atrium, ventricle, and aorta	High systemic vascular resistance; increased pressure in left atrium, ventricle, and aorta	Loss of placental blood flow
Secondary changes		
Umbilical arteries: patent; carry blood from hypogastric arteries to placenta	Functionally closed at birth, obliteration by fibrous proliferation may take 2-3 months; distal portions become *lateral vesicoumbilical ligaments;* proximal portions remain open as *superior vesicle arteries*	Closure precedes that of umbilical vein; probably accomplished by smooth muscle contraction in response to thermal and mechanical stimuli and alteration in oxygen tension; mechanically severed with cord at birth
Umbilical vein: patent; carries blood from placenta to ductus venosus and liver	Closed; after obliteration it becomes *ligamentum teres hepatis*	Closure shortly after umbilical arteries; hence blood from placenta may enter neonate for short period after birth; mechanically severed with cord at birth
Ductus venosus: patent; connects umbilical vein to inferior vena cava	Closed, after obliteration it becomes *ligamentum venosus*	Loss of blood flow from umbilical vein
Ductus arteriosus: patent; shunts blood from pulmonary artery to descending aorta	Functionally closed almost immediately after birth; anatomic obliteration of lumen by fibrous proliferation requires 1-3 months; becomes *ligamentum arteriosum*	High systemic resistance increases aortic pressure; low pulmonary resistance reduces pulmonary arterial pressure
		Increased oxygen content of blood in ductus arteriosus creates vasospasm of its muscular wall
Foramen ovale: forms a valve opening that allows blood to flow directly to left atrium	Functionally closes at birth; constant apposition gradually leads to fusion and permanent closure within a few months or years in majority of persons	Increased pressures in left atrium together with decreased pressure in right atrium cause closure of valve over foramen

From Whaley, L.F., and Wong, D.L.: Nursing care of infants and children, ed. 3, St. Louis, 1987, The C.V. Mosby Co.

beginning of systole and the "dub" with closure of the aortic and pulmonic valves at the end of systole. The "lub" sound is called the *first heart sound* and the "dub" the *second heart sound* because the normal cycle of the heart is considered to start with the beginning of systole (Guyton, 1985). Heart sounds during the neonatal period are of higher pitch, shorter duration, and greater intensity than during adult life. The first sound is typically louder and duller than the second sound, which is sharp in quality. Most heart murmurs heard during the neonatal period have no pathologic significance, and more than half disappear by 6 months. By term the infant's heart lies midway between the crown of the head and the buttocks, and the axis is more transverse than that of the adult (see Fig. 20.3).

Blood pressure. Blood pressure in infants varies from day to day. A drop in systolic blood pressure (about 15 mm Hg) the first hour after birth is common. Values from several hours after delivery through the neonatal period average a systolic pressure of 78

and a diastolic pressure of 42 (see discussion of Doppler technique, Chapter 25). Crying and moving result in changes in blood pressure, especially systolic.

Blood volume. Blood volume in the newborn ranges from 80 to 110 ml/kg during the first several days and doubles by the end of the first year. The newborn has approximately 10% greater blood volume and nearly 20% greater red blood cell mass than the adult. However, the newborn's blood is about 20% less plasma volume when compared by kilogram of body weight with the adult. The infant born prematurely will have a greater blood volume than the term newborn. This is because the baby has a greater plasma volume, not a greater red blood cell mass.

A number of differences in the circulatory dynamics of the newborn result from early or late clamping of the cord. Late clamping results in an expansion of blood volume from the so-called placental transfusion, an increase of close to 60%. This in turn causes an increase in heart size, higher systolic blood pressure, and an increased respiratory rate. Pulmonary rates and transient cyanosis are also encountered more frequently. To date the value of early or late clamping of the cord has not been determined (Pritchard and others, 1985).

Hematopoietic system. The hematopoietic system of the newborn exhibits certain variations from that of the adult. There are differences in red blood cells and leukocytes and relatively few differences in platelets.

Red blood cells and hemoglobin. At birth the average values of red blood cells and hemoglobin are higher than those values in the adult. These fall and reach the average levels of 11 to 17 g/dl and 4.2 to 5.2/mm,³ respectively, by the end of the first month. The blood values may be affected by delayed clamping of the cord, which results in a rise in hemoglobin, red blood cells, and hematocrit. The source of the sample is another significant factor, since capillary blood will give higher values than venous blood. Also, the time after birth when the blood sample was obtained is significant, since the slight rise in red blood cells after birth is followed by a substantial drop. At birth the infant's blood contains about 80% fetal hemoglobin, but because of the shorter life span of the cells containing fetal hemoglobin, the percentage falls to 55% by 5 weeks and 5% by 20 weeks. Fortunately iron stores generally are sufficient to sustain normal red blood cell production for 6 months, and thus the slight brief anemia is not serious.

Leukocytes. Leukocytosis, with the white blood cell count approximately 18,000/mm,³ is normal at birth. The number, largely polymorphs, increases to about 23,000 to 24,000/mm³ during the first day after birth. A resting level of 11,500/mm³ normally is maintained during the neonatal period. Serious infection is not well tolerated by the newborn, and a marked increase in the white blood cell count is unlikely even in critical sepsis. In most instances sepsis is accompanied by a decline in white cells, particularly in neutrophils. The activity of the marrow is accurately reflected by the number of circulating cells—both erythrocytes and leukocytes. The early high white blood cell count of the newborn decreases rapidly. A relative leukopenia found in black children and adults is apparent by 1 year of age and is primarily caused by a decreased number of neutrophils. By 6 years of age the peripheral blood picture is approximately the same as that of an adult (see Appendixes E and I).

Platelets. Platelet count and aggregation are essentially the same in neonates as in adults. One exception is the infant of a mother who has taken acetylsalicylic acid (aspirin) or chlorpromazine, both of which interfere with the release of adenosine diphosphate (ADP). Otherwise bleeding tendencies in the newborn are rare, and unless there has been a marked vitamin K deficiency, clotting is sufficient to prevent hemorrhage.

Blood groups. The infant's group is established early in fetal life. However, during the neonatal period there is a gradual increase in the strength of the agglutinogens present in the RBC membrane.

Respiratory system. At birth, air must be substituted for fluid that has filled the respiratory tract to the alveoli. During the course of normal vaginal delivery, between 7 and 24 ml of amniotic fluid is squeezed or drained from the newborn's lungs (Aladjem and others, 1979). After delivery the major portion of the fetal lung fluid is absorbed across the alveolar membrane into the blood capillaries. This is largely a result of the pressure gradient from alveoli to interstitial tissue to blood capillary. Reduced vascular resistance also accommodates this flow of lung fluid; however, it is the diminished intravascular pressure that is ultimately responsible.

Initial breathing. Abnormal respiration and failure to completely expand the lungs retard the egress of fetal lung fluid from alveoli and interstices into the pulmonary circulation. Retention of fluid in turn alters pulmonary function.

Initial breathing is probably the result of a reflex triggered by pressure changes, chilling, noise, light, and other sensations related to the birth process. In addition the chemoreceptors in the aorta and carotid bodies initiate neurologic reflexes when the arterial Po_2 falls from 80 to 15 mm Hg, arterial Pco_2 rises from 40 to 70 mm Hg, and arterial pH falls below 7.35. (When these changes are extreme, however, depression ensues.) In most cases an exaggerated respiratory reaction follows within 1 minute of birth, and the infant takes a first gasping breath and cries.

With the first breath the infant develops a considerable negative intrathoracic pressure. Air is drawn in, and about half of this remains as residual pulmonary volume. Normally only a few breaths are required to expand the lungs well; subsequently the pressure will be lower than at the onset of respiration.

Respirations. After respirations are established, they are shallow and irregular, ranging from 30 to 60 breaths per minute, with short periods of apnea (less than 15 seconds). Apnea (periodic breathing) is characteristic of the newborn. It occurs most often during the active (rapid eye movement [REM]) sleep cycle and decreases in frequency and duration with age. However, any apneic period should be evaluated.

Infants are obligatory nose breathers. The reflex response to nasal obstruction is opening the mouth to maintain an airway. This response is not present in most babies until 3 weeks after birth but may occur earlier in certain races (Freedman, 1979). Therefore

Fig. 19.2
Normal respiration. Chest and abdomen rise with inspiration. (Courtesy Mead Johnson & Co., Evansville, Indiana.)

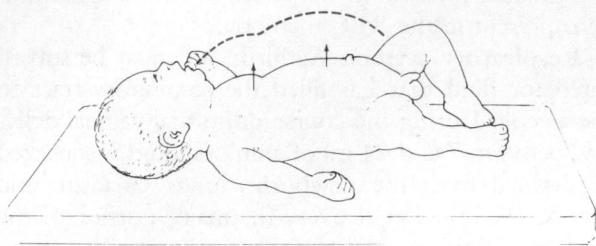

Fig. 19.3
Seesaw respiration. Chest wall retracts and abdomen rises with inspiration. (Courtesy Mead Johnson & Co., Evansville, Indiana.)

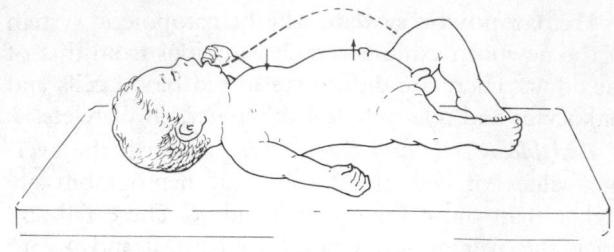

cyanosis or asphyxia may occur with nasal blockage.

The chest circumference is approximately 30 to 33 cm (12 to 13 in) at birth. The ribs of the infant articulate with the spine at a horizontal rather than a downward slope; consequently the rib cage cannot expand as readily as does the adult's with inspiration. Neonatal respiratory function is largely a matter of diaphragmatic contraction. The negative intrathoracic pressure is created by the descent of the diaphragm, much like negative pressure is created in the barrel of a syringe when medication is drawn up by retracting the plunger. The infant's chest and abdomen rise simultaneously with inspiration (Fig. 19.2). *Seesaw respirations are not normal* (Fig. 19.3).

Auscultation of the chest of an infant reveals loud, clear breath sounds that seem very near, because little chest tissue intervenes. Several significant differences exist between the respiratory system of the infant and the adult:

1. Infants are obligate nose breathers.
2. The infant's tongue is relatively large (macroglossia), whereas the glottis and trachea are small.
3. All lumens of the infant are narrower and more easily collapsed.
4. Respiratory tract secretions of the infant are more abundant than those of the adult.
5. The mucous membranes of the infant are more delicate and therefore more susceptible to trauma. The ciliated columnar epithelium just below the vocal cords is especially prone to edema.
6. The alveoli of the infant are more sensitive to changes in pressures.
7. The capillary network of the infant is less well developed. Capillaries are more friable and have less well developed vasoconstrictive and dilatative ability.
8. The infant's bony rib cage and respiratory muscles are not as well developed.

Renal system. At term the kidneys occupy a large portion of the posterior abdominal wall. The bladder lies close to the anterior abdominal wall and is partially an abdominal, as well as a pelvic, organ. In the newborn almost all palpable masses in the abdomen are renal in origin.

Maturation of kidney function to that comparable to the adult's is well advanced only after the first year of life. The neonate has a minimal range of chemical balance and safety. Diarrhea, infection, or improper feeding can lead rapidly to acidosis and fluid imbalances—dehydration or edema. Renal immaturity also limits the neonate's ability to excrete drugs.

Small amounts of urine are usually present in the bladder at birth; however, the newborn may not void for 12 to 24 hours. Voiding after this period is frequent. Six to ten voidings of pale, straw-colored urine are indicative of adequate fluid intake. The usual urinary output by 10 days is 50 to 300 ml/24 hours.

Fluid and electrolyte balance. Differences from adult physiologic response include the following:

1. The distribution of extracellular and intracellular fluid differs from that of the adult. About 40% of the body weight of the newborn is extracellular fluid, whereas in the adult it is 20%.
2. The rate of exchange of extracellular fluid is different. The newborn daily takes in and excretes 600 to 700 ml of water, which is 20% of the total body fluid, or 50% of the extracellular fluid. In contrast, the adult exchanges 2000 ml of water, which is 5% of the total body fluid and 14% of the extracellular fluid.
3. The composition of body fluids shows variations. There is a higher concentration of sodium, phosphates, chloride, and organic acids and a lower concentration of bicarbonate ions. These findings mean that the newborn is in a compensated acidotic state and in a state of potential manifest edema.
4. The glomerular filtration rate is about 30% to

50% of that of the adult. This results in a decreased ability to remove nitrogenous and other waste products from the blood. However, the newborn's ingested protein is almost totally metabolized for growth.

5. The decreased ability to excrete excessive sodium results in hypotonic urine compared to plasma.

6. The sodium reabsorption is decreased as a result of a lowered sodium-potassium-activated adenosine triphosphatase (ATPase) activity.

7. The newborn can dilute urine down to 50 milliosmols (mOsm). An osmol is a measure of total number of particles. One gram molecular weight (mole) of nondiffusible and nonionizable substance is equal to 1 osmole. Capacity to dilute urine exceeds capacity to concentrate it. There is some limitation in the ability to increase urinary volume.

8. The newborn can concentrate urine to 600 to 700 mOsm compared to the adult's capacity of 1400 mOsm. The inability to concentrate urine is not absolute, but in terms of adult function, it is somewhat limited.

9. The infant has a higher renal threshold for glucose.

Neuromuscular system. Until the late 1950s the human newborn was considered to be immature, disorganized, and able to function only at a brainstem level. Neurobehavioral assessment of the neonate was therefore based mainly on evaluation of muscle tone and primitive reflexes. Recent studies have recognized the term newborn to be a vital, responsive, and reactive being. The newborn shows remarkable sensory development and an amazing ability for self-organization and social interaction (Fanaroff, 1983).

Postdelivery growth of the brain follows a predictable pattern: rapid during infancy and early childhood, more gradual during the remainder of the first decade, and minimal during adolescence. The cerebellum ends its growth spurt, which began at about 30 gestational weeks, by the end of the first year. This is perhaps why it is vulnerable to nutritional or other trauma in early infancy (see discussion of newborn nutrition, Chapter 21, and kernicterus, Chapter 31).

The brain requires glucose as a source of energy and a relatively large supply of oxygen for adequate metabolism. Oxygen requirements range from 5 to 8 ml/100 g. Such requirements signal a need for careful assessment of the infant's ability to maintain an open airway and of respiratory conditions requiring oxygen therapy. The necessity for glucose requires an awareness of those neonates who may have hypoglycemic episodes.

Spontaneous motor activity may be seen in transient tremors of mouth and chin, especially when crying, and of extremities, notably the arms and hands. Persistent tremors or tremors involving the total body may be indicative of pathologic conditions. Marked tonicity, clonicity, and twitching of facial muscles are signs of convulsions. There is a need for the physician to differentiate among normal tremors, tremors of hypoglycemia, and CNS disorders so that corrective care can be instituted, as necessary.

Neuromuscular control in the newborn, although still very limited, can be noted. If newborns are placed facedown on a firm surface, they will turn their heads to the side to maintain an airway. They attempt to hold their heads in line with their bodies if they are raised by their arms. Various reflexes serve to promote their safety and an adequate food intake. This is described further in this chapter under behavioral characteristics of the newborn.

Gastrointestinal system. In the adequately hydrated infant the mucous membrane of the mouth is moist and pink. Pallor and cyanosis of the mucous membrane are normally not present. Drooling of mucus is common in the first few hours after birth. There are no clefts in the palate. Retention cysts, small whitish areas, may be found on the gum margins and at the juncture of the hard and soft palate. The cheeks are full because of well-developed sucking pads. These, like the labial tubercles (sucking calluses) on the upper lip, disappear when the sucking period is over.

A special mechanism present in the normal newborns weighing more than 1500 g coordinates the breathing, sucking, and swallowing reflexes necessary for oral feeding. Sucking in the newborn takes place in small bursts of three or four sucks at a time. In the term newborn, longer and more efficient sucking attempts occur in only a few hours. The infant is unable to move food from the lips to the pharynx; therefore it is necessary to place the nipple (breast or bottle) well inside the baby's mouth. Peristaltic activity in the esophagus is uncoordinated in the first few days of life. It quickly becomes a coordinated pattern in normal infants, and they swallow easily.

Bacteria are not present in the infant's gastrointestinal tract at birth. Soon after birth, oral and anal orifices permit entrance of bacteria and air. Bowel sounds can be heard 1 hour after birth. Generally the highest bacterial concentration is found in the lower portion of the intestine, particularly in the large intestine. The normal intestinal flora help synthesize vitamin K, folic acid, and biotin.

The capacity of the stomach varies from 30 to 90 ml depending on the size of the infant. Emptying time for the stomach is highly variable. Several factors, such as time and volume of feedings, type and temperature of food, and psychic stress, may affect the emptying time. This can range from 1 to 24 hours. Regurgitation may be noted in the neonatal period. The cardiac sphincter and nervous control of the stomach are still immature.

Digestion. Two principal types of cells make up the lining of the stomach. The first type, chief cells, synthesizes and secretes pepsinogen, which aids protein digestion. The second type, parietal cells, secrete hydrochloric acid, which forms the gastric acidity. The enzyme pepsin and gastric acidity are necessary for preliminary digestion of milk before its entrance into the small intestine. The infant's gastric acidity at birth normally equals the adult level but is reduced within a week and may remain reduced for 2 to 3 months. The reduction in gastric acidity may lead to "colic." Infants with colic usually remain awake, crying in apparent distress between 2 feedings, often the same ones every day. Nothing seems to appease them. They appear to "grow out" of this behavior by age 3 months.

Further digestion and absorption of nutrients occur in the small intestine. This complex process is made possible by pancreatic secretions, secretions from the liver through the common bile duct, and secretions from the duodenal portion of the small intestine.

The infant's ability to digest carbohydrates, fats, and proteins is regulated by the presence of certain enzymes. Most of these are functional at birth. One exception is *amylase,* produced by the salivary glands after about 3 months and by the pancreas at about 6 months of age. This enzyme is necessary to convert starch into maltose. The other exception is *lipase,* also secreted by the pancreas; it is necessary for the digestion of fat. Thus the normal newborn is capable of digesting simple carbohydrates and proteins but has a limited ability to digest fats (see Chapter 21 for more detail).

Stools. At birth the lower intestine is filled with meconium. Meconium is formed during fetal life from the amniotic fluid and its constituents, intestinal secretions and shed mucosal cells. Meconium is greenish black and viscous and contains occult blood. The first meconium passed is sterile, but within hours all meconium passed contains bacteria. The first passage of meconium occurs within 24 hours in 90% of normal infants. Most of the rest do so within 36 hours (Pritchard, 1985).

The number of stools varies considerably during the first week, being most numerous between the third and sixth days. Transitional stools (thin, slimy, and brown to green because of the continued presence of meconium) are passed from the third to sixth day. Therefore the stools of breast-fed babies and bottle-fed babies differ. The stools of the breast-fed baby are loose, golden yellow in color, and nonirritating to the infant's skin. It is normal for the baby to have a bowel movement with each feeding or a bowel movement

every 3 to 4 days. Even if the latter is the case, the stools remain loose and unformed. The stools of the bottle-fed baby are formed but soft, are pale yellow, and have a typical stool odor. They tend to be irritating to the infant's skin. The number of stools decreases in the first 2 weeks from five or six each day (after every feeding) to one to two per day.

Distension of the stomach muscles causes a corresponding relaxation and contraction of the muscles of the colon. As a result, infants often have bowel movements during or just after a feeding. (Breast-fed babies are more likely to stool during a feeding than bottle-fed babies.) Stooling at these times has been attributed to the gastrocolic reflex.

The infant develops an elimination pattern by the second week of life. With the addition of solid food the baby's stool gradually assumes the characteristics of an adult's stool.

Feeding behaviors. Variations occur among infants regarding interest in food, symptoms of hunger, and amount ingested at any one time. The amount that the infant takes at any one bottle feeding depends, of course, on the size of the infant; but other factors seem to play a part: if put to breast, some infants nurse immediately, whereas others require a learning period of up to 48 hours before nursing can be said to be effective. Random hand-to-mouth movement and sucking of fingers have been seen in utero. These actions are well developed at birth and are intensified with hunger.

Hepatic system. The liver performs a number of functions, one of which is to control the amount of circulating unbound bilirubin. The pigment bilirubin is derived from the hemoglobin released with the breakdown of red blood cells (90% to 95%). The remaining pigment is derived from the myoglobin in muscle cells. The hemoglobin is phagocytized by the reticuloendothelial cells, converted to bilirubin, and released in an unconjugated form. Unconjugated bilirubin, termed *indirect bilirubin,* is relatively insoluble and is almost entirely bound to circulating albumin, a plasma protein. The unbound bilirubin can leave the vascular system and permeate other extravascular tissues (e.g., the skin, sclera, oral mucous membranes). The resultant yellow coloring is termed *jaundice.*

In the liver the unbound bilirubin is conjugated with glucuronide in the presence of the enzyme glucuronyl transferase. The conjugated form of bilirubin is excreted from liver cells as a constituent of bile. It is termed *direct bilirubin* and is soluble. Along with other components of bile, direct bilirubin is excreted into the biliary tract system that carries the bile into the duodenum. Bilirubin is converted to urobilinogen and stercobilin within the duodenum through the action of

Fig. 19.4
Formation and excretion of bilirubin. (From Whaley, L., and Wong, D.: Nursing care of infants and children, St. Louis, 1987, The C.V. Mosby Co.)

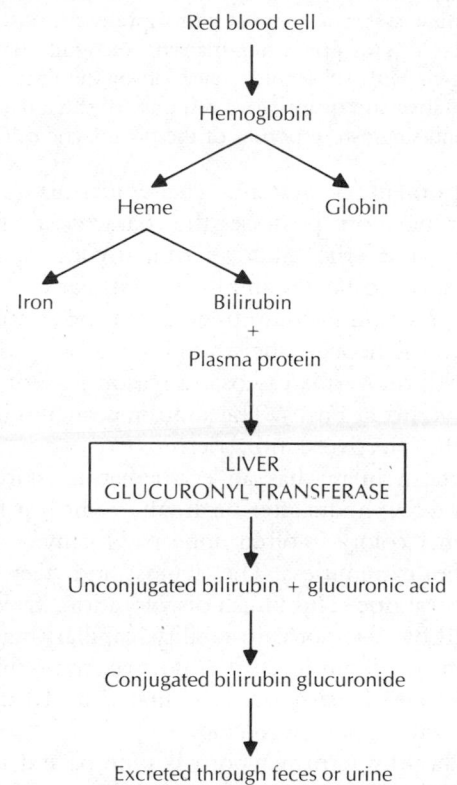

1. The newborn has a higher rate of bilirubin production. The number of fetal red blood cells per kilogram of weight is greater than the adult. The fetal red blood cells have a shorter survival time, 40-90 days compared to 120 days in the adult.
2. There is considerable reabsorption of bilirubin from the neonatal small intestine.

Although physiologic jaundice is considered benign, bilirubin may accumulate to hazardous levels and become pathologic (Chapter 31). Physiologic jaundice fulfills the following specific criteria (Korones and Lancaster, 1986):

(1) the infant is otherwise well; (2) in term infants, jaundice first appears after 24 hours and disappears by the end of the seventh day; (3) in premature infants, jaundice is first evident after 48 hours and disappears by the ninth or tenth day; (4) serum unconjugated bilirubin concentration does not exceed 12 mg/100 ml, either in term or preterm infants; (5) hyperbilirubinemia is almost exclusively of the unconjugated variety, and conjugated (direct) bilirubin should not exceed 1 to 1.5 mg/100 ml; (6) daily increments of bilirubin concentration should not surpass 5 mg/100 ml. Bilirubin levels in excess of 12 mg/100 ml may indicate either an exaggeration of the physiologic handicap or the presence of disease. *At any serum bilirubin level, the appearance of jaundice during the first day of life or persistence beyond the ages previously delineated usually indicates a pathologic process.*

Jaundice is noticeable first in the head and then progresses gradually toward the abdomen and extremities because of the neonate's circulatory pattern (cephalocaudal developmental progression). The appearance of jaundice in the various body locations gives a rough estimate of the circulating levels of unbound bilirubin. For example, when jaundice appears over the nose, the circulating level of unbound bilirubin is approximately 3 mg; levels at which other body areas appear jaundiced are as follows:

Approximate Level of Hyperbilirubinemia by Cephalocaudal Distribution

Nose: 3 mg/dl	Abdomen: 10 mg/dl
Face: 5 mg/dl	Legs: 12 mg/dl
Chest: 7 mg/dl	Palms: 20 mg/dl

Several nursery practices may influence the appearance and degree of physiologic hyperbilirubinemia. *Early feeding* tends to keep the serum bilirubin level low by stimulating intestinal activity and the passage of meconium and stool. Removal of intestinal contents prevents the reabsorption (and recycling) of bilirubin from the gut, a residual mechanism left over from fetal life (Rosta, 1970; De Carvalho, 1982; and Ostler, 1979).

Chilling of the neonate may result in acidosis and raise the level of free fatty acids. In the presence of

the bacterial flora. Urobilinogen is excreted in urine and feces; stercobilin is excreted in the feces (Fig. 19.4). Total serum bilirubin is the sum of conjugated (direct) and unconjugated (indirect) bilirubin.

The full-term newborn's liver is usually sufficiently mature and the production of glucuronyl transferase great enough to conjugate the circulating unconjugated bilirubin. Adequate serum albumin–binding sites are also available unless the infant experiences asphyxia neonatorum, cold stress, or hypoglycemia. Maternal prebirth ingestion of drugs such as sulfa drugs and aspirin can reduce the amount of serum albumin–binding sites in the newly born. Although the neonate has the functional capacity to convert bilirubin, physiologic hyperbilirubinemia occurs in most infants.

Physiologic hyperbilirubinemia. Physiologic hyperbilirubinemia or neonatal jaundice is a normal occurrence in 50% of full-term and 80% of preterm newborns. Korones and Lancaster (1986) note that neonatal jaundice occurs because:

acidosis, albumin binding of bilirubin is *weakened* and biluribin is freed. Bilirubin is *displaced* from its serum albumin–binding sites by the free fatty acids and as unbound bilirubin can be deposited in body tissues. Kernicterus, the most serious *complication* of neonatal hyperbilirubinemia, is caused by the precipitation of bilirubin in neuronal cells, resulting in their destruction (see Chapter 31). Cerebral palsy, epilepsy, and mental retardation are expected in survivors.

There is an increase in the number of mothers and infants being discharged from the hospital between 2 and 48 hours after birth and others who have elected birth at home. As a result the professional attendant may not be available to assess pathologic rises in circulating unbound bilirubin. *Therefore all parents need instruction in how to assess jaundice and to whom to report the findings* (see Chapter 21).

Breast milk jaundice. Breast milk jaundice (BMJ) has been defined as progressive indirect hyperbilirubinemia beyond the first week of life. Jaundice from ingestion of breast milk occurs in 0.5% to 2% of full-term neonates (Saul and Warburton, 1984). It is thought that an enzyme present in the milk of some women inhibits the enzyme glucuronyl transferase, which is necessary for the conjugation of bilirubin. Although breast milk jaundice is a form of physiologic jaundice, it occurs after the mature milk has come in and persists longer—up to 6 weeks. Unconjugated bilirubin rises beyond physiologic limits (15 to 20 mg/dl) by the seventh day. The levels subside by 5 to 10 mg if nursing is discontinued for 12 to 24 hours. Then usually 3 to 5 days pass before the previous high level is again reached. Guthrie (1978) believes that it is not necessary to completely discontinue breast feeding. It is unfortunate that many breast-feeding women have been made to feel their milk is pathogenic for their offspring.

Immune system. All newborns and especially preterm newborns are at high risk for infection during the first several months of life. During this period, infection represents one of the leading causes of morbidity and mortality. The newborn is unable to limit the invading pathogen to the portal of entry because of a generalized hypofunction of the inflammatory and immune mechanisms (Medici, 1983).

Resistance to infection (immunity) includes both nonspecific and specific protective mechanisms (see Chapter 8). Medici (1983, pp. 25-26) summarizes the newborn's defense mechanisms as follows:

The term and preterm neonate has an increased incidence of infection for the first four to six weeks of life. This reflects the immaturity of a number of protective systems which significantly increases the risk of infection in this patient population. Natural barriers such as the acidity of the stomach or the production of pepsin and trypsin which maintain sterility of the small intestine are not fully developed until three to four weeks. The membrane protective IgA is missing from the respiratory and urinary tracts, and unless the newborn is breast fed, it is absent from the gastrointestinal tract as well. The immune system is in great part suppressed; possibly this is a mechanism for preventing maternal recognition of paternal antigens with subsequent rejection of the fetus. Finally, the qualitative and quantitative response of the inflammatory factors and sluggish responses of the phagocytic cells.

Integumentary system. The epidermis (skin) of the term newborn possesses the characteristic five layers (strata) of the adult: germinativum, spinosum, granulosum, corneum, and on the palmar and plantar surfaces, stratum lucidum underneath the stratum corneum. In the neonate the stratum corneum is thin and fused with the vernix caseosa (a reason for not removing the vernix at birth). The stratum corneum later becomes the effective skin barrier.

The term infant has an erythematous skin (beefy red) for a few hours after birth, after which it fades to its normal color. It often appears blotchy, especially over the extremities. The hands and feet appear slightly cyanotic. This bluish discoloration, *acrocyanosis*, is caused by vasomotor instability, capillary stasis, and a high hemoglobin level; it is normal, transient in occurrence, and persists over the first 7 to 10 days, especially with exposure to cold.

The healthy term newborn is plump, and the skin may be slightly tight, suggesting fluid retention. Fine *lanugo hair* may be noted over the face, shoulders, and back. Actual edema of the face and *ecchymosis* (bruising) may be noted as a result of face presentation or forceps delivery.

Caput succedaneum. Caput succedaneum is a localized, easily identifiable edematous area of the scalp (Fig. 19.5, *A*). The sustained pressure of the presenting vertex against the cervix results in compression of local vessels, thus slowing venous return. The slower venous return causes an increase in tissue fluids within the skin of the scalp, and an edematous swelling develops. This boggy edematous swelling present at birth extends across suture lines of the fetal skull and disappears spontaneously within 3 to 4 days. Excessive pressure to the presenting vertex as it passes over the bony maternal pelvis may cause a cephalhematoma to develop.

Cephalhematoma. Cephalhematoma is a collection of blood between a skull bone and its periosteum. Therefore a cephalhematoma never crosses a cranial suture line (Fig. 19.5, *B*). Cephalhematoma is caused by pressure during delivery. Bleeding may occur with spontaneous delivery from pressure against the maternal bony pelvis. Low forceps delivery, as well as diffi-

Fig. 19.5

Differences between caput succedaneum and cephalhematoma. **A,** Caput succedaneum: edema of scalp noted at birth; crosses suture line. **B,** Cephalhematoma: bleeding between periosteum and skull bone appearing within first 2 days; does not cross suture lines.

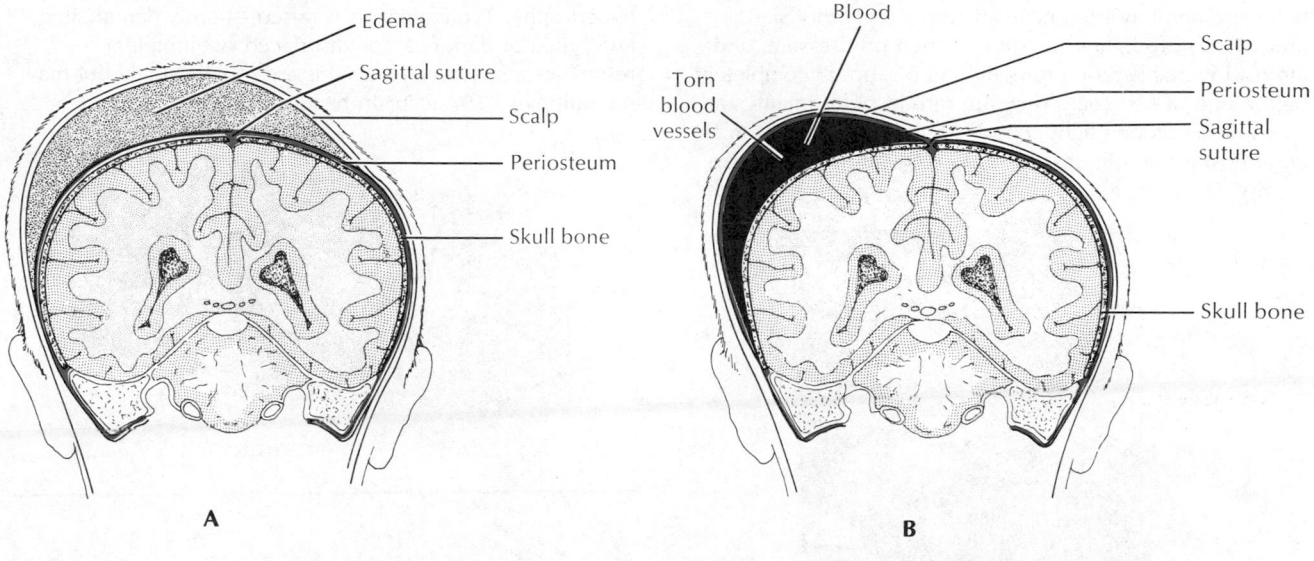

cult forceps rotation and extraction, may also cause bleeding. This soft, fluctuating, irreducible fullness does not pulsate or bulge when the infant cries. It appears several hours after birth or the day after delivery or becomes apparent following absorption of a caput succedaneum (Fig. 19.5, *A*). It is usually largest on the second or third day, by which time the bleeding stops. The fullness of cephalhematoma spontaneously resolves in 3 to 6 weeks. It is not aspirated because infection may develop if the skin is punctured.

As the hematoma resolves, the hemolysis of RBCs occurs. Hyperbilirubinemia (jaundice) may result after the newborn is home. Therefore the parents are instructed to observe the newborn for jaundice and may be asked to bring the infant in to be rechecked before the usual 4-week visit.

Desquamation. Desquamation of the skin of the term infant does not occur until a few days after birth. Its presence at birth is an indication of postmaturity. *Subcutaneous fat* accumulated during the last trimester acts to insulate the newborn. The preterm infant has difficulty maintaining an even body temperature because of the lack of this fat.

Sweat glands. Sweat glands are present at birth but do not function effectively (i.e., do not respond to increases in ambient or body temperature), perhaps because the neurogenic stimuli are still immature. There is some fetal *sebaceous gland* hyperplasia and secretion of sebum as a result of the hormonal influences of pregnancy. Vernix caseosa, a cheeselike substance, is a product of the sebaceous glands. Distended sebaceous glands, noticeable in the newborn, particularly on the cheeks and nose, are known as *milia.* Although sebaceous glands are well developed at birth, they are only minimally active during childhood. They become more active as androgen production increases before puberty.

Mongolian spots. Mongolian spots, bluish-black areas of pigmentation, may appear over any part of the extensor surface of the body, including the extremities. They are more commonly noted on the back and buttocks. The occurrence of Mongolian spots is not primarily related to race. Thus these pigmented areas are noted in babies whose origins are from the shores of the Mediterranean, Latin America, Asia, or a number of other areas in the world. They are more common in dark-skinned individuals regardless of race. They fade gradually over a period of months or years.

Telangiectatic nevi. Known as "stork bites," telangiectatic nevi are pink and easily blanched (Fig. 19.6). They appear on the upper eyelids, nose, upper lip, lower occiput bone, and nape of the neck. They have no clinical significance and fade between the first and second years. Other birthmarks include nevus vasculosus (strawberry mark) (Fig. 19.7) and nevus flammeus (port-wine stain) (Fig. 19.8).

Erythema toxicum. An evanescent rash, erythema toxicum is also called *erythema neonatorum,* or "flea-

Fig. 19.6
Telangiectatic nevi (stork bite). Pale pink or mauve spots seen frequently on eyelids, glabella, and occipital areas of newborn infants are considered by some to be a type of nevus flammeus, or true vascular nevus. Certainly they behave differently from nevus flammeus in other skin areas. They are lighter in color, blanch on pressure, and almost invariably fade promptly and disappear completely before end of first year. They are rare in older infants and so common among light-complexioned newborns as to be an almost routine finding. (Courtesy Mead Johnson & Co., Evansville, Indiana.)

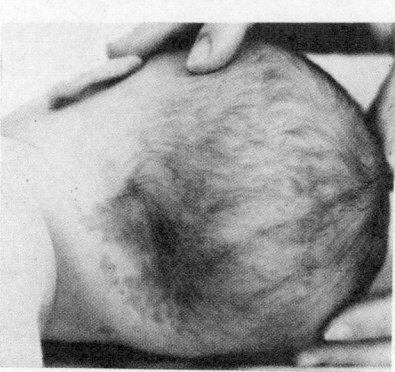

Fig. 19.7
Nevus vasculosus, or strawberry mark, is second most common type of capillary hemangioma. It consists of dilated, newly formed capillaries occupying entire dermal and subdermal layers with associated connective tissue hypertrophy. Typical lesion is raised, sharply demarcated, and bright or dark red, roughsurfaced swelling that resembles a strawberry. Lesions are usually single but may be multiple; 75% occur in head region.

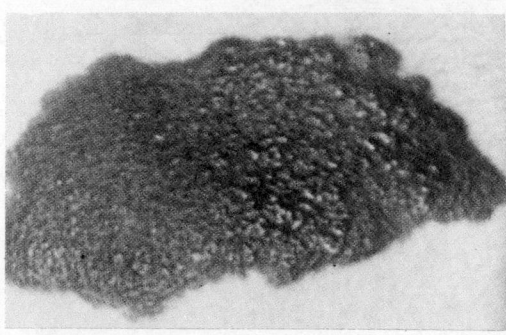

bite" dermatitis. It has lesions in different stages, erythematous macules, papules, or small vesicles, and may appear suddenly anywhere on the body. The rash is thought to be an inflammatory response. Eosinophils, which help decrease inflammation, are found in the vesicles. The rash is found only in term neonates (36 or more weeks gestational age) during the first 3 weeks of age (Medici, 1983). Although the appearance is alarming, it has no clinical significance and requires no treatment.

The intact skin of the infant acts as an effective barrier to infection; however, the fragility of the skin makes it more vulnerable to disruption of the surface when traumatized by too vigorous handling, rubbing, or excoriation.

Reproductive system

Female. At birth the ovaries contain thousands of primitive germ cells. These represent the full complement of potential ova, since no oogoniums form after delivery in term infants. The ovarian cortex, which is made up primarily of primordial follicles, forms a thicker portion of the ovary in the newborn than in the adult. The number of ova decreases from birth to maturity by approximately 90%.

Hyperestrogenism followed by a drop after delivery results in a mucoid vaginal discharge and even some slight blood spotting. The infant's uterus also responds by undergoing involution in the first weeks of life and decreasing in size and weight. Vaginal tags are common findings and have no clinical significance.

Male. The testes have descended into the scrotum in 90% of newborn boys. Although this percentage drops with premature birth, by 1 year of age the incidence of undescended testes in all boys is less than 1%. Spermatogenesis does not occur until puberty (see Chapter 5).

Adhesions of the foreskin (prepuce) are almost universally present in newborn boys. During prenatal development the tissue of the prepuce is continuous with the epidermis that covers the glans. Gradually the preputial space between the prepuce and glans forms. The complete separation of the two tissue areas is generally not complete at birth. For this reason the prepuce of the newborn is usually not retractable.

Swelling of breast tissue. Swelling of the breast tissue in infants of both sexes is caused by the hyperestrogenism of pregnancy. In a few infants a thin discharge (witch's milk) can be seen. The finding has no clinical significance, requires no treatment, and will subside as the maternal hormones are eliminated from the infant's body.

Thermogenetic system. Thermogenesis means the production of heat (thermo = heat, genesis = origin). Effective neonatal care is based on the maintenance of an optimal thermal environment. In homoiothermic individuals the narrow limits of normal body temperature are maintained by producing heat in response to

Fig. 19.8
Port-wine stain, or nevus flammeus, is usually observed at birth and is composed of plexus of newly formed capillaries in papillary layer of corium. It is red to purple, variable in size, shape, and location, and not elevated. True port-wine stains do not blanch on pressure and do not disappear spontaneously. (Courtesy Mead Johnson & Co., Evansville, Indiana.)

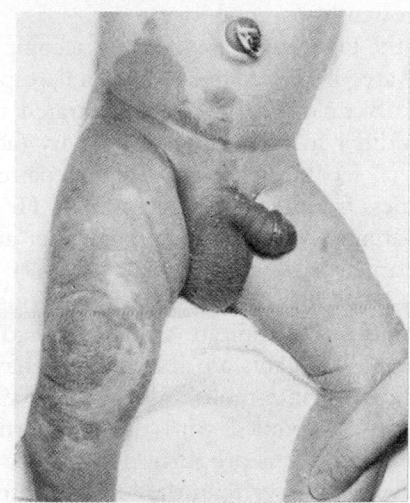

its dissipation. Hypothermia from excessive heat loss is a prevalent and dangerous problem in neonates. The newborn infant's ability to produce heat often approaches the capacity of the adult. However, the tendency toward rapid heat loss in a suboptimal thermal environment is increased in the newborn and is often hazardous to well-being.

Heat production. The shivering mechanism of heat production is rarely operable in the newborn. Nonshivering thermogenesis is accomplished primarily by brown fat and secondarily by increased metabolic activity in the brain, heart, and liver. Brown fat is unique to the newborn (Davis, 1980). It is located in superficial deposits in the interscapular region and axillas, as well as in deep deposits at the thoracic inlet, along the vertebral column, and around the kidneys. Brown fat has a richer vascular and nerve supply than does ordinary fat. Heat produced by intense lipid metabolic activity in brown fat can warm the neonate by increasing heat production as much as 100%. Reserves of brown fat, usually present for several weeks after birth, are rapidly depleted with cold stress. The less mature the infant, the less reserve of this essential fat is available at birth.

Heat loss. Heat loss occurs in four ways:

1. *Convection:* the flow of heat from the body surface to cooler ambient air. For this reason nursery ambient temperatures are kept at 24° C (75° F), and newborns are wrapped to protect them from the cold.

2. *Radiation:* the loss of heat from the body surface to cooler solid surfaces not in direct contact but in relative proximity to each other. Nursery cribs and examining tables are placed away from outside windows.

3. *Evaporation:* the loss of heat that occurs when a liquid is converted to a vapor. In the newborn, heat loss by evaporation occurs as a result of vaporization of moisture from the skin. This process is invisible and is known as insensible water loss (IWL). This heat loss can be intensified by not drying the newborn directly after birth or by bathing and drying the infant too slowly.

4. *Conduction:* the loss of heat from the body surface to cooler surfaces in direct contact. The newborn when admitted to the nursery is placed in a warmed cot to minimize heat loss. Loss of heat must be controlled to protect the infant. As noted above, control of such modes of heat loss is the basis for care-taking policies and techniques.

Temperature regulation. Anatomic and physiologic differences among the newborn, child, and adult are notable:

1. The newborn's thermal insulation is less than an adult's. Blood vessels are closer to the surface of the skin. Changes in environmental temperature alter that of blood, thereby influencing temperature-regulating centers in the hypothalamus.

2. The newborn has a larger body surface to body weight (mass) ratio. The flexed position that the newborn assumes is a safeguard against heat loss because it substantially diminishes the amount of body surface exposed to the hostile thermal environment.

3. The neonate's vasomotor control is less well developed. However, the ability to constrict subcutaneous and skin vessels is as efficient in premature infants as it is in adults.

4. The newborn produces heat primarily by nonshivering thermogenesis.

5. The neonate's sweat glands have little homoiothermic function until the fourth week or later of extrauterine life.

In response to the discomfort of lower environmental temperature, the normal term infant may try to increase body temperature by crying or by increased motor activity. Crying increases the work load, and the cost of energy (calories) may be expensive, particularly in a compromised infant.

Cold stress. Cold stress imposes metabolic and physiologic problems on all infants, regardless of gestational age and condition. The respiratory rate is increased as a response to the increased need for oxygen when the oxygen consumption increases significantly in cold stress. Oxygen consumption and energy in the cold-stressed infant are diverted from maintaining normal brain cell and cardiac function and growth to thermogenesis for survival.

If the infant cannot maintain an adequate oxygen tension, vasoconstriction follows and jeopardizes pulmonary perfusion. As a consequence, arterial blood gas levels of Po_2 are decreased, and the blood pH drops. These changes aggravate existing respiratory distress syndrome (RDS), also known as hyaline membrane disease (HMD). Moreover, decreased pulmonary perfusion and oxygen tension may maintain or reopen the right-to-left shunt across the patent ductus arteriosus.

The basal metabolic rate will be increased with cold stress. If cold stress is protracted, anaerobic glycolysis occurs, resulting in increased production of acids. Metabolic acidosis develops, and if there is a defect in respiratory function, respiratory acidosis also develops. Excessive fatty acids displace the bilirubin from the albumin-binding sites. The increased level of circulating unbound bilirubin that results increases the risk of kernicterus even at serum bilirubin levels of 10 mg/dl or less.

Behavioral Characteristics

The healthy infant must achieve both biologic and behavioral tasks in order to develop normally. Behavioral characteristics form the basis of the social capabilities of the infant. Through the first half of this century the focus of developmental research was on how the infant was affected by the environment. Infants were considered to have been born with neither personality nor ability to interact.

Today it is recognized that newborns are well equipped to begin social interactions with their parents. The behavioral characteristics of the newborn represent a second phase in human development. The first phase, fetal phase, of development was discussed in Chapter 8. Research now indicates that the individual personalities and behavioral characteristics of infants play a major role in the ultimate relationship between infants and their parents.

Brazelton (1973) and others have brought the behavioral states of the newborn into prominence. It is their contention that the behavioral responses of infants are indicative of cortical control, responsiveness, and eventual management of the infant's environment.

They emphasize the importance of infant-parent interaction. By their responses infants act to either consolidate relationships or alienate the persons in their immediate environment. By their actions they encourage or discourage attachment and care-taking activities. The development of parent-child love does not occur without feedback. The absence of feedback because of separation or incorrectly interpreted feedback can impair the growth of parental love.

One of the first tasks parents must accomplish is to become aware of the unique behavioral responses of their child. Brazelton (1969) demonstrated that normal babies differ in such things as activity (active, average, quiet), feeding patterns, sleeping patterns, and responsiveness from the moment of birth. He suggests that the parents' reaction to their infants are determined in part by these differences.

Sensory behaviors. From birth, infants possess sensory capabilities that indicate a state of readiness for social interaction. Infants are able to use behavioral responses effectively in establishing their first dialogues. These responses, coupled with the newborns' "baby appearance" (the face is proportioned so that the forehead and eyes are larger than the lower portion of the face) and their smallness and helplessness, rouse feelings of wanting to hold, protect, and interact with them.

Vision. The infant's eyes drift off target because muscle control and coordination are immature. This glancing away permits the image being viewed to fall on the fovea (retinal area of clearest vision) more directly. The clearest visual distance is 17 to 20 cm (7 to 8 in), which is about the distance the infant's face is from the mother's face as she breast feeds or cuddles. Infants are sensitive to light. They will frown if a bright light is flashed in their eyes and will turn toward a soft red light. If the room is darkened, they will open their eyes widely and look about. This is noticeable when the delivery area is darkened after birth. By 2 months of age they can detect color, but under 5 days of age they seem more attracted by black-and-white patterns (Frantz, 1966).

Response to movement is noticeable. If a bright object is shown to newborns (even at 15 minutes of age), they will visually follow it, and some will even turn their heads to do so. Because human eyes are bright, shiny objects, newborns will track their parents' eyes. Parents will comment on how exciting this behavior is.

Visual acuity is surprising; even at 2 weeks of age infants can distinguish patterns with stripes 3 mm (1/8 in) apart. By 6 months their vision is as acute as that of an adult (Frantz and Miranda, 1975). They prefer to look at patterns rather than plain surfaces, even if the latter are brightly colored. They also prefer more complex patterns to simple ones. They prefer novelty (changes in pattern) by 2 months of age. This is significant knowledge, since it means the infant of a few weeks of age is capable of responding actively to an enriched environment.

From birth onward, infants are able to fix their eyes and gaze intently at objects. They gaze at their parents' faces and respond to changes in them with apparent imitative effect. This ability permits parents and children to gaze into each other's eyes, and a subtle communication pattern is thereby set up. Some researchers have indicated that there may be an ethnic component to this pattern. Freedman (1979) reported a study comparing Navaho and Anglo mothers in their efforts to get their babies' attention. The Anglo mothers became animated, smiled, and used gestures and high-pitched vocal sounds. The Navaho mothers gazed quietly at their babies until their eyes met and the infant gazed quietly back. It is conjectured that such responses may persist over time and influence behavior, as indicated by the following example:

■ A 7-month-old Indian infant admitted for treatment of an ear infection seemed lonely and depressed. He would stare solemnly at me with his big brown eyes. I tried to cheer him by talking and shaking toys at him, but he would lie stiffly in my arms and gave no indication of noticing me. One evening when giving him his bottle I did not respond to his look by talking (I don't know why) but just looked back at him. After a bit he seemed to give a sigh, I could feel his little body relax against mine, and he reached up and patted the bottle.

Whether such conjectures are true or not, the need to have eye contact is a compelling one (Robson, 1967). Children of blind parents and parents who have blind children must circumvent this obstacle for the formation of a relationship (see Chapter 23).

Hearing. It has been demonstrated that newborns, at 1 minute of age, can correctly look toward sound presented alternately to them on the right and the left side. They were especially good at detecting sound directly in front of them. The newborns were also able to discriminate frequencies of sound in the range of the human voice (500 to 900 decibels) (Wertheimer, 1961; Clifton and others, 1981).

Even more discrete differentiation of sound can be demonstrated by a newborn's consistent, preferential turning toward the sound of his mother's voice immediately after birth (Brazelton, 1977). This occurs even when another female voice has previously captured the neonate's attention. The phenomenon can be demonstrated to mothers with consistent success. The origins of this behavior have been discovered by Truby, a linguist, who with a Swedish pediatrician and an American dentist developed highly sophisticated measuring devices to record and analyze the cry of newborns. They discovered that cry imprints produced for each newborn had, like footprints and fingerprints, an individual uniqueness (Truby and Lind, 1965). When a newborn's cry print was compared with the mother's speech patterns, unmistakable similarities were present. Later studies of the cries of very young premature babies, as small as 900 g (2 lb), corresponded to the mother's speech patterns (Truby, 1975). Infants of mute mothers did not cry or cried strangely. It was hypothesized that the fetus receives and stores speech features from the mother through hearing and listening while in utero.

All these studies indicate a selective listening to the maternal voice sounds and rhythms during intrauterine life that prepare newborns for recognition and interaction with their primary caregivers—their mothers. One of us (M.J.) remembers a mother in the transitional stage of labor who gave a sudden loud scream when a contraction began. The nurse was listening to the fetal heart rate at the time and noted that both she and the fetus jumped with surprise. Newborns are accustomed in the uterus to hearing the regular rhythm of the mother's heartbeat. As a result they respond by relaxing and ceasing to fuss and cry if a regular heartbeat simulator is placed in their cribs.

The acute sensitivity to the human voice has been experimentally tested. In observations of the responses of quiet, alert newborns to computer-simulated cries and the cries of human newborns, more restlessness and crying occurred in response to the genuine cry. Newborns less than 35 hours old typically began to cry when submitted to the cry of other newborns but quieted at the sound of their own cry (Martin, 1981).

Condon and Sander (1974) describe normal patterns of response to speech sounds. In these patterns the listener's body motions are synchronous with those of the speaker. The researcher termed these patterns *interactional synchrony.* Condon and Sander found that alert, moving newborns coordinated their movements to the sounds of adult speech patterns and continued to do so when tested again the following day. Movement of head, shoulders, elbows, hips, and feet occurred without eye contact with the speaker (an adult male voice). Some newborns received recorded voices and other direct voice contact. The results were the same—sustained, coordinated movement. No change in the findings occurred when the language was changed to Chinese nor when infant posture was changed from being held to being supine in their cribs.

However, when disconnected vowel and tapping sounds were made, the degree of correspondence of body movement with the sound disappeared. The human infant appears to be particularly *tuned in* to the rhythms of human speech in preference to all other sounds.

Touch. Sensory pathways for kinesthetic (movement) and tactile (touch) activities are the first to complete myelinization in the infant (Kolb, 1959; Purpura, 1975). The newborn's responses to touch suggest this sensory system is well prepared to receive and process tactile messages. Many of the reflexes of the newborn demonstrated a response to tactile stimulation (see Chapter 20).

The new mother uses touch as one of the first interaction behaviors: fingertip touch, soft stroking of the face, and gentle massage of the back. Since touch between strangers is avoided in some cultures, it would seem that this automatic maternal touching behavior evidences an already intimate relationship. Birth trauma or stress and depressant drugs taken by the mother decrease the infant's sensitivity to touch or painful stimuli.

Taste. Newborns have repeatedly demonstrated a preference for sweet fluids over sour or bitter ones. Facial expressions indicating newborn response to taste have been recorded in a series of studies. The facial expressions of a selected variety of people were photographed as various tastes were presented (Steiner, 1973, 1979). Premature and normal newborns; anencephalic newborns; mentally retarded, facially deformed, or congenitally blind adolescents; and normal adults showed the same responses. Sour fluids precipitated puckering of the lips; bitter fluids caused retching or spitting, and sweet tastes resulted in relaxed expressions interpreted as enjoyment and satisfaction. These studies demonstrate not only the newborn's response to various tastes but also the strength of the taste response and its independence from cortical levels of the nervous system.

It is generally accepted that young infants are particularly oriented toward the use of their mouths both for meeting their nutritional needs for rapid growth and for releasing tension through sucking. The early development of circumoral sensation and muscle activity as well as taste would seem to be preparation for survival in the extrauterine environment.

Smell. Several studies have tested newborn response to odors. The findings demonstrate not only a preference for smells deemed pleasant by adults but also that newborns have the ability to learn and remember.

Steiner (1979) experimented with newborns responses to smell. Using photographic recordings of facial expressions, Steiner found that newborns, some of whom were only hours old and inexperienced with food odors, showed a preference for the odors of banana, vanilla, and strawberry. The newborns rejected smells of fish or rotten eggs. These odors were presented to the newborns on cotton swabs held under their noses.

One of the most well-known studies of infant learning through the olfactory tract was done by Macfarlane (1975). Newborns were tested for recognition of their mother's breast pads. By age 2 to 7 days, infants turned more often toward their mother's used breast pad than an unused one when both were placed above them. Within another few days these infants turned preferentially toward their own mother's used breast pad than that of another nursing mother.

The significance of smell in maternal identification of offspring and vice versa in the animal world is well documented. Maternal identification of the human newborn by smell has not been studied extensively. Stainton (1985) noted that mothers reported their infants smell differently from birth onward.

Response to environmental stimuli. Each newborn has a predisposed capacity to handle the multitudinous stimuli in the external world (Brazelton, 1961). Individual variations in the primary reaction pattern of newborns have been described and termed *temperament* (Thomas, 1961, 1970). The style of behavioral response to stimuli is guided by the temperament that affects the newborn's sensory threshold, ability to habituate, and response to maternal behaviors.

Habituation. The newborn is able to control the type and amount of incoming stimuli processed with the ability to *habituate*. Habituation is a psychologic and physiologic phenomenon whereby the response to a constant or repetitive stimuli is decreased (Bridger, 1975; Ornstein, 1972). In the term newborn this can be demonstrated in several ways. Shining a bright light into a newborn's eyes will cause a startle or squinting the first two to three times and possibly a hand or arm will be brought up over the eyes. The third or fourth flash will elicit a diminished response and by the fifth or sixth flash, the infant ceases to respond (Brazelton, 1973, 1977). The same response pattern holds true for the sounds of a rattle, a bell, or a pinprick to a heel. A newborn presented with new stimuli will become wide-eyed and alert, gaze for a time, but eventually show a diminished interest.

As well as shutting out repetitive stimuli, the ability to habituate enables the newborn to select stimuli that potentiate continued learning about the social world, avoiding overload. The intrauterine experiences seem to have programmed the newborn to be especially responsive to human voices, soft lights, soft sounds, sweet tastes, and perhaps patting and rubbing.

Habituation is an early form of learning (Stone, 1973). The newborn quickly learns the constant sounds in a newborn nursery and in the home environment and is able to sleep in their midst. The selective responses of the newborn indicate cerebral organization capable of remembering and making choices. The ability to habituate is dependent on state of consciousness, hunger, fatigue, and temperament. These factors also affect consolability, cuddliness, irritability, and crying.

Consolability. Korner (1971) reports on studies conducted over several years that describe variations in the ability of newborns to console themselves or to be consoled. In the crying state, most newborns will initiate one of several ways to reduce their distress and move to a lower state. Hand-to-mouth movements are common with or without sucking, as well as alerting to voices, noises, or visual stimuli in the environment.

Cuddliness. The degree to which a newborn will mold into the contours of the person holding them varies. Korner and Thoman (1970) tested the effect of body contact and vestibular stimulation in both soothing babies and creating alertness. The vestibular stimulation of being picked up and moved had the greater effect. Schaffer and Emerson (1964) classified newborns into "cuddlers," "noncuddlers," and an "intermediate group."

Irritability. Some newborns cry longer and harder than others. For some the sensory threshold seems low. They are readily upset by unusual noises, hunger, wetness, or new experiences and respond intensively. Others with a high sensory threshold require a great deal more stimulation and variation to reach the active, alert state (Korner, 1971).

Crying. Crying in an infant may signal hunger, pain, desire for attention, or fussiness. As mother and infant become more adept at interpreting each other's behavior, some mothers state that they are able to distinguish the reasons for crying.

■ I can tell when she's hungry. Crying starts in a plaintive way and then becomes more and more demanding. When she is hurt, she lets out a startled yell as though she couldn't believe it was happening to her. Sometimes when she is put down to sleep, she starts a kind of talking cry, jerky and demanding; it gets louder, and if nothing happens, fades away in little spurts. The fussy cry is the hardest to take—nothing seems to work; like a complaining sound it goes on and on.

A report such as this means that the mother and baby are communicating effectively.

Temperament. The behavioral styles of infants and children "show distinct individuality in temperament in the first weeks of life, independently of their parents' handling or personality style"; "the original characteristics of temperament tend to persist in most children over the years" (Chess, 1969; Chess and Thomas, 1977).

Chess (1969) developed nine categories of primary reactivity to evaluate behavioral style:

1. Activity level: the diurnal proportion of diurnal active to inactive periods.
2. Rhythmicity: the regularity and predictability of bodily functions and sleep-wake cycle.
3. Approach or withdrawal: the response to a new stimulus.
4. Adaptability: the speed and ease with which current behavior is modified in response to environmental changes.
5. Intensity of reaction: the energy in a response regardless of its quality or direction.
6. Threshold of responsiveness: the intensity of stimuli required to evoke a response.
7. Quality of mood: the proportion of happy behavior to unhappy behavior.
8. Distractibility: the efficacy of external stimuli in changing the direction of ongoing behavior.
9. Attention span and persistence: the length of time one activity is pursued and the effect of distraction.

These nine categories were then grouped into three major patterns of behavioral style or temperament:

1. The easy child who demonstrates regularity in bodily functions, readily adapts to change, has a predominantly positive mood, a moderate sensory threshold, and approaches new situations or objects with a response of moderate intensity.
2. The slow-to-warm-up child who has a low activity level, withdraws on first exposure to new stimuli, is slow to adapt, low in intensity of response, and is somewhat negative in mood.
3. The difficult child who is irregular in bodily functions, intense in reactions, generally negative in mood, resistant to change or new stimuli, and often cries loudly for long periods.

The human newborn possesses sensory receptors capable of responding selectively to various stimuli present in the internal and external environment. The infant also possesses individual characteristics that define him or her as a unique personality.

Sleep-wake cycles. Infant variations in *state of consciousness* are called the sleep-wake cycles (Brazelton, 1973). They form a continuum with deep sleep, narcosis, or lethargy at one end and extreme irritability at the other end. There are two sleep states, deep sleep and light sleep, and four wake states, drowsiness, quiet alert, active alert, and crying. Brazelton (1973) has

Fig. 19.9
Summary of sleep-wake states of newborn. States of consciousness: deep sleep, light sleep, drowsy, quiet alert, active alert, crying. (Courtesy March of Dimes.)

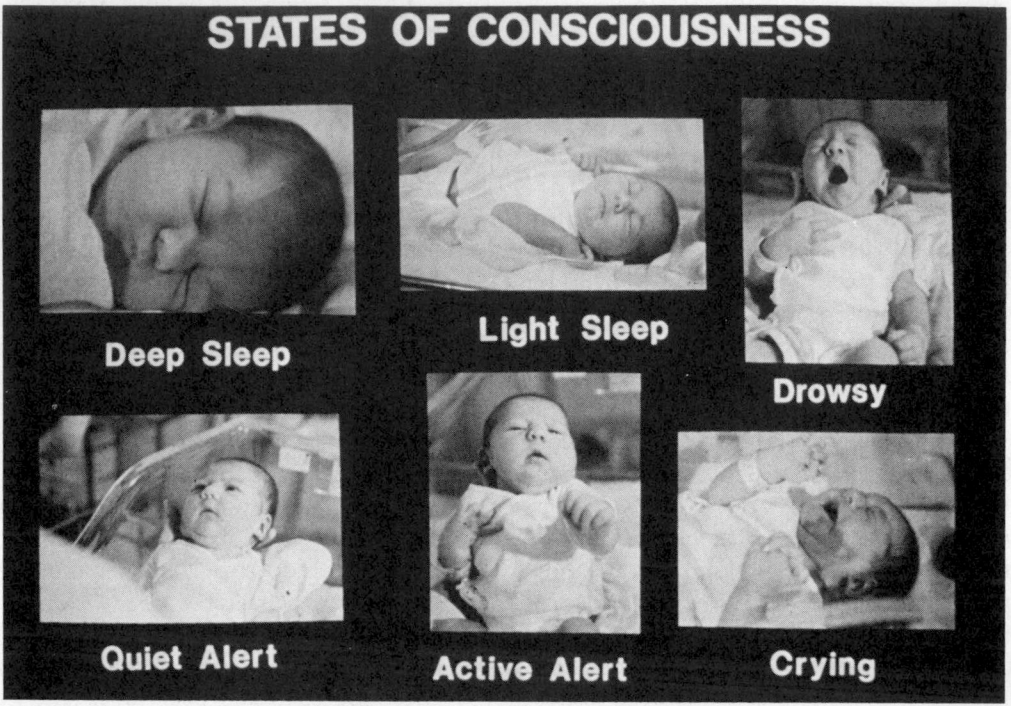

noted that the infant's state of consciousness is the most important element in assessing the baby's reactions to stimulation. This state is affected by a number of variables: hunger, dehydration, exhaustion.

As shown in Table 19.2 and Fig. 19.9, each state has its distinguishing characteristics. The quiet alert state is also termed the optimal state of arousal. This state "allows sustained attention to external stimuli, purposeful hand-eye coordinated movements and active manipulation of the outside world" (Lewis and Zarin-Ackerman, 1977). During this state infants may be observed smiling, vocalizing, or moving in synchrony. Even during the first day of life, smiling is evident in a surprising number of infants (Wolff, 1969). They seem to watch their parents' faces carefully and respond to other persons talking to them. They move their bodies in coordination with the parent's voice and the simultaneous movement of the parent's body (Condon and Sander, 1974). Brazelton (1969) notes that this "dancing in tune" gives feedback to the speaker and encourages more interaction. Infants have been shown to imitate parents' actions by 2 weeks of age (Meltzoff and Moore, 1977). Many infants begin a type of vocalizing by the time they are 2 weeks of age,

making cooing, small, throaty noises while feeding.

The infant employs purposeful behavior to maintain the optimum arousal state: (1) active withdrawal by increasing physical distance, (2) a rejecting motion of pushing away with hands and feet, (3) decreasing sensitivity by falling asleep or breaking eye contact by turning the head, or (4) use of signaling behavior, fussing, or crying (Brazelton, 1973). Use of such behaviors permits infants to quiet themselves and reinstate readiness to interact again.

Transition period. Desmond and associates (1966) noted that infants pass through phases of instability in the first 6 to 8 hours after birth; these phases collectively are termed the *transition period* between intrauterine and extrauterine existence (Fig. 19.10). The first phase lasts up to 30 minutes after birth and is called the *first period of reactivity.* The *second period of reactivity* occurs at about the fourth to eighth hour after birth. This sequence occurs in all newborns, regardless of gestational age or type of delivery (vaginal or cesarean). There will be variations, however, in the length of time the periods last, depending on amount and kind of stress experienced by the fetus. Following are clinical findings in the first period:

Table 19.2

Behavioral States and State Behavior

State	Body Activity	Eye Movements	Facial Movements	Breathing Pattern	Level of Response
			Characteristics of State		
Sleep states					
Deep sleep	Nearly still, except for occasional startle or twitch	None	Without facial movements, except for occasional sucking movement at regular intervals	Smooth and regular	Threshold to stimuli is very high so that only very intense and disturbing stimuli will arouse infants.
Light sleep	Some body movements	Rapid eye movements (REM), fluttering of eyes beneath closed eyelids	May smile and make brief fussy or crying sounds	Irregular	More responsive to internal and external stimuli. When these stimuli occur, infants may remain in light sleep, return to deep sleep, or arouse to drowsy.
Awake states					
Drowsy	Activity level variable, with mild startles interspersed from time to time. Movements usually smooth	Eyes open and close occasionally, are heavy-lidded with dull, glazed appearance	May have some facial movements; often there are none, and face appears still	Irregular	Infants react to sensory stimuli although responses are delayed. State change after stimulation frequently noted.
Quiet alert	Minimal	Brightening and widening of eyes	Faces have bright, shining, sparkling looks	Regular	Infants attend most to environment, focusing attention on any stimuli that are present. Optimal state of arousal.
Active alert	Much body activity, may have periods of fussiness	Eyes open with less brightening	Much facial movement; faces not as bright as quiet alert state	Irregular	Increasingly sensitive to disturbing stimuli (hunger, fatigue, noise, excessive handling).
Crying	Increased motor activity, with color changes	Eyes may be tightly closed or open	Grimaces	More irregular	Extreme response to unpleasant external or internal stimuli.

From Barnard, K.E., and others: Behavioral states and state behaviors. In Early parent-infant relationships, copyright 1978 by the March of Dimes Birth Defects Foundation, White Plains, NY. Reprinted by permission.

1. Infant is awake, alert, and active; eyes are open; the infant looks around and may appear hungry; there is a good sucking reflex.
2. Respirations are rapid and irregular; there may be some grunting and barreling of chest.
3. Heart rate is rapid (tachycardia) with some irregularity.
4. Body temperature falls.

The infant's activity gradually diminishes, alertness fades, and sleep comes. Air enters the gastrointestinal tract, and by about the end of the first hour bowel sounds can be heard.

In the second period the infant again wakens and is alert. There is usually a gagging episode with regurgitation of mucus and maternal blood from the birth canal. The meconium stool is usually passed, and the infant again appears hungry and ready to suck.

Neonatal period. The first 6 weeks of life involve a steady decrease in the proportion of active REM sleep to total sleep. A steady increase in the proportion of quiet sleep to total sleep time also occurs. There is a 25% increase in wakefulness over the first 3 or 4 weeks. For the first few weeks the wakeful periods seem dictated by hunger, but soon thereafter a need

Fig. 19.10
Some physiologic changes occurring in newborn in adjustment to extrauterine life. (From
Pierog, S., and Ferrara, A.: Medical care of the sick newborn, ed. 2, St. Louis, 1976, The
C.V. Mosby Co. Adapted from Desmond, M.M., and others: Pediatr. Clin. North Am.
13:651, 1966.)

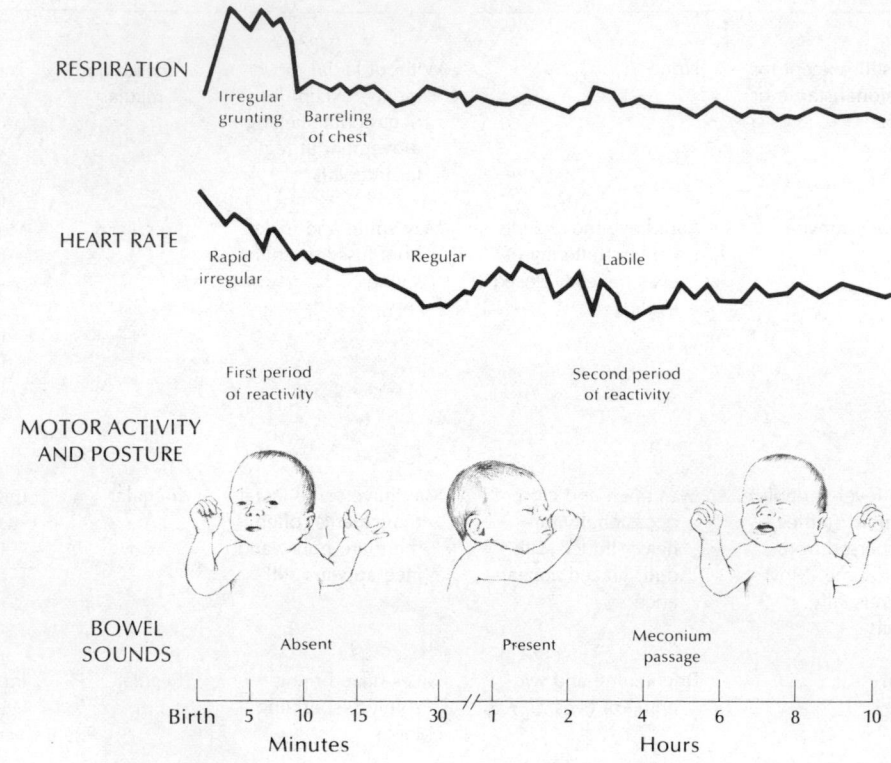

for socializing appears to function as well. The newborn sleeps a total of about 17 hours a day, with the periods of wakefulness gradually increasing. By the fourth week of life, some infants are staying awake from one feeding session to the next. It is not until 4 or 5 years of age that children achieve the adult pattern of sleeping.

Summary

During the period of infancy the infant within the "protective envelope of nurturing adults" (Brazelton, 1982) can learn complex coping mechanisms and control systems. These in turn help the infant to be alert, to pay attention, and to master rules of communication. The newborn and adult learn about each other and about themselves—a feeling of mutuality, of identification with the "other" is accomplished.

The nurse uses knowledge of the biologic and behavioral characteristics of the newborn as a basis for the care of the infant and the teaching and counseling of the parents. Chapter 20 presents the assessment strategies and tools that provide information for devising nursing diagnoses in order to plan and implement nursing actions for the care of the child. The criteria used to evaluate progress toward the goal of a healthy, happy infant are presented to complete the phases of the nursing process.

References

Aladjem, S.A., and others: Clinical perinatology, ed. 2, St. Louis, 1979, The C.V. Mosby Co.

Brazelton, T.B.: Psychophysiologic reactions in the neonate. I. The value of observation of the neonate, J. Pediatr. 58:508, 1961.

Brazelton, T.B.: Infants and mothers, ed. 1, New York, 1969, Dell Publishing Co.

Brazelton, T.B.: Effect of maternal expectations on early infant behavior, Early Child Dev. Care 2:259, 1973.

Brazelton, T.B.: The remarkable talents of the newborn, Paper presented at Parent to Infant Attachment Conference, Cleveland, November 6, 1977.

Brazelton, T.B.: Joint regulation of neonate-parent behavior. In Tronick, E.Z., editor: Social interchange in infancy: affect, cognition, and communication, Baltimore, 1982, University Park Press.

Bridger, W.H.: Sensory discrimination and autonomic function in the newborn, Am. Acad. Child Psychiatry 15:257, 1975.

Chess, S.: Individuality and baby care, Dev. Med. Child. Neurol. 11:749, 1969.

Chess, S., and Thomas, A.: Temperament and the parent-child interaction, Pediatr. Ann. 6(9):26, 1977.

Clifton, R.K., and others: Newborns' orientation toward sound: possible implications for cortical development, Child Dev. 52:833, 1981.

Condon, W.S., and Sander, L.W.: Neonate movement is synchronized with adult speech: interactional participation and language acquisition, Science 183:99, 1974.

Danforth, D.: Obstetrics and gynecology, Philadelphia, 1982, Harper and Row, Publishers.

Davis, V.: The structure and function of brown adipose tissue in the neonate, J.O.G.N. Nurs. 9(6):368, 1980.

De Carvalho, M., and others: Frequency of breast-feeding and serum bilirubin concentration, J. Dis. Child. 136:737, 1982.

Desmond, M.M., and others: The transitional care nursery, Pediatr. Clin. North Am. 13:651, 1966.

Fanaroff, A., and Martin, R.: Behrman's neonatal-prenatal medicine, St. Louis, 1983, The C.V. Mosby Co.

Frantz, R.L.: Pattern discrimination and selective attention as determinants of perceptual development from birth. In Kidd, A.J., and Rivaire, J.L., editors: Perceptual development in children, New York, 1966, International University Press.

Frantz, R.L., and Miranda, S.B.: Newborn infant attention to form and contour, Child Dev. 46:224, 1975.

Freedman, D.G.: Ethnic differences in babies, Hum. Nature, p. 4, Jan. 1979.

Guthrie, R.A.: Breast milk and jaundice: keep abreast, J. Hum. Nutr. 3:47, 1978.

Guyton, A.: Textbook of medical physiology, Philadelphia, 1985, W.B. Saunders Co.

Kolb, L.: Disturbances of the body image. In Arieti, S., editor: American handbook of psychiatry, vol. 1, New York, 1959, Basic Books, Inc., Publishers.

Korner, A.F.: Individual differences at birth: implications for early experiences and later development, Am. J. Orthopsychiatry 41:608, 1971.

Korner, A.F., and Thoman, E.B.: Visual alertness in neonates as evoked by maternal care, J. Exp. Child Psychol. 10:67, 1970.

Korones, S.B., and Lancaster, J.: High-risk newborn infants: the basis for intensive nursing care, ed, 4, St. Louis, 1986, The C.V. Mosby Co.

Lewis, M., and Zarin-Ackerman, J.: Early infant development. In Behrman, R.E., and others, editors: Neonatal-perinatal medicine: diseases of the fetus and infant, ed. 2, St. Louis, 1977, The C.V. Mosby Co.

Lowrey, G.: Growth and development of children, ed. 8, Chicago, 1986, Year Book Medical Publishers.

Macfarlane, A.: Olfaction in the development of social preferences in the human neonate. In Parent-infant interaction: CIBA Symposium, 1975.

Martin, C.: Newborns pacified by tapes of their own crying, Brain/Mind Bulletin 10:2, 1981.

Medici, M: The fight against infection: the neonates' defense mechanisms, J. Calif. Perinat. Assoc. 3(2):25, 1983.

Meltzoff, A., and Moore, M.: Imitation of facial and manual gestures by human neonates, Science 198:75, 1977.

Minegeot, R., and Herbert, M.: The functional status of the newborn infant: a story of 5,370 consecutive infants, Am. J. Obstet. Gynecol. 115:1138, 1973.

Ornstein, R.E.: The psychology of consciousness, San Francisco, 1972, W.H. Freeman & Co.

Ostler, C.W.: Initial feeding time of newborn infants: effect upon first meconium passage and serum indirect bilirubin levels, Health Care Wom. 1:1, 1979.

Pritchard, J., McDonald, P., and Gant, N.: Williams' obstetrics, ed, 17, East Norwalk, Conn., 1985, Appleton-Century-Crofts.

Purpura, D.: Dendrite differentiation in human cerebral cortex: normal and aberrant developmental patterns, Adv. Neurol. 12:91, 1975.

Robson, K.S.: The role of eye-to-eye contact in maternal-infant attachment, J. Child Psychol. Psychiatry 8:13, 1967.

Rosta, J., and others: Delayed meconium passage and jaundice in newborn infants, Pediatr. Acad. Sci. Hungar. 11:295, 1970.

Saul, K., and Warburton, D.: Increased incidence of early-onset hyperbilirubinemia in breast-fed versus bottle-fed infants, J. Perinatol. 4(3):36, 1984.

Schaffer, H., and Emerson, P.: Patterns of response to physical contact in early human development, J. Child Psychol. Psychiatry 5:1, 1964.

Stainton, C.: Origins of attachment, culture and cue sensitivity. Unpublished doctoral dissertation, University of California, San Francisco, 1985.

Steiner, J.E.: The gustofacial response: observation on normal and anencephalic newborn infants. In Bosma, J.F., editor: Fourth symposium on oral sensation and perception: development in the fetus and infant, Bethesda, Md., 1973, U.S. Dept. of Health, Education and Welfare.

Steiner, J.E.: Human facial expressions in response to taste and smell stimulation, Adv. Child Dev. Behav. 13:257, 1979.

Stone, L.J., and others: The competent infant: research and commentary, New York, 1973, Basic Books, Inc., Publishers.

Thomas, A., and others: Individuality in responses of children to similar environmental situations, Am. J. Psychiatry 117:798, 1961.

Thomas, A., and others: The origin of personality, Sci. Am. 223:102, 1970.

Truby, H.M.: Prenatal and neonatal speech, prespeech and an infantile speech lexicon. In Child language—1975, Word 27 (special issue).1, 1975.

Truby, H., and Lind, J.: Cry sounds of the newborn infant. In Lind, J., editor: Newborn infant cry, Acta Pediatr. Scand. 163(suppl.):7, 1965.

Vaughan, V.C., McKay, R., and Behrman, R.: Nelson's textbook of pediatrics, Philadelphia, 1979, W.B. Saunders Co.

Wertheimer, M.: Psychomotor coordination of auditory and visual space at birth, Science 134:1962, 1961.

Whaley, L.F., and Wong, D.L.: Nursing care of infants and children, ed. 3, St. Louis, 1987, The C.V. Mosby Co.

Wolff, P.H.: Observations on newborn infants, Psychosom. Med. 21:110, 1969.

Bibliography

Ainsworth, M.D.S.: The development of mother-infant attachment, Rev. Child Dev. Res. 3:1, 1973.

Apostolakis, E.: Visual preferences of preterm and term infants, J. Calif. Perinat. Assoc. 11:61, Spring 1982.

Brazelton, T.: Infants and mothers, ed. 2, New York, 1983, Dell Publishing Co.

Bushnell, I.W.R.: Discrimination of faces by young infants, J. Exp. Child Psychol. 33:298, 1982.

Clark, D.A.: Times of first void and first stool in 500 newborns, Pediatrics 60:457, 1977.

Dayton, G.O., Jr., and Jones, M.H.: Analysis of characteristics of fixation reflex in infants by use of direct current electroculography, Neurology 14:1152, Dec. 1964.

Fleming, J.: Common dermatologic conditions in children, M.C.N. 6:346, 1981.

Foss, B.M., editor: Determinants of human behavior, New York, 1963, John Wiley & Sons.

Guyton, A.: Textbook of medical physiology, Philadelphia, 1980, W.B. Saunders Co.

Kohn, C.L., and others: Gravidas' responses to realtime ultrasound fetal image, J.O.G.N. Nurs. 9:177, March-April 1980.

Krantz, D.H., Human color vision, Contemp. Psychol. 27:88, 1982.

Lang, R.: Birth book, Ben Lomond, Calif., 1972, Genesis Press.

Leifer, A.D., and others: Effects of mother-infant separation on maternal attachment behavior, Child Dev. 43:1203, 1972.

Ludington-Hoe, S.: What can newborns really see? Am. J. Nurs. 83:1286, 1983.

Schachter, J., and others: Heart rate and blood pressure in black newborns and white newborns, Pediatrics 58:283, 1976.

Seil, E., and Carrigan, J.: Platelet counts, fibrinogen concentrations, and factor V and factor VII levels in healthy infants according to gestational age, J. Pediatr. 82:1028, 1973.

Slater, A.M., and Findley, J.M.: Binocular fixation in the newborn baby, J. Exp. Child Psychol. 20:248, 1975.

Winick, M.: Malnutrition and brain development, J. Pediatr. 74:667, 1969.

Wolff, P.H.: The natural history of crying and other vocalization in early infancy. In Foss, B.M., editor: Determinants of infant behavior, vol. 4, New York, 1969, Barnes & Noble Books.

Wolff, P.H.: Observations on the early development of smiling. In Stone, L.J., and others, editors: The competent infant, research and commentary, New York, 1973, Basic Books, Inc., Publishers.

Nursing Care of the Normal Newborn

During the neonatal period the prenatal and post-delivery characteristics of the infant merge. Gradually the former disappear as the infant grows and matures outside the womb. Although most infants make the necessary biopsychosocial adjustment to extrauterine existence without undue difficulty, their well-being depends on the care they receive from others. The nursing care described in this chapter is based on careful assessment of biologic and behavioral responses and formulation of nursing diagnoses. It includes planning and implementing appropriate nursing actions and evaluating their effectiveness. The chapter concludes with the Summary of Nursing Actions: Nursing Care of the Newborn Infant and Application of the Nursing Process.

Assessment

Assessment is a continuous process; the newborn changes rapidly, both physically and psychologically, during the neonatal period. The nurse includes in the assessment pertinent information from:

1. The mother's prenatal record
2. The record of events during the mother's labor, during the newborn's birth, and during the newborn's first hours and days of life

Physical assessment. The first *physical assessment* of the infant is done at birth, using the Apgar scoring technique and a brief physical assessment (see Chapter 18). The assessment for gestational age, if considered necessary, is done within the first 2 hours after birth (see Chapter 29).

A second more thorough physical examination is done within 24 hours after delivery. The *goal* is to compile a complete record of the newborn that will act as a data base for subsequent assessment and care. Having the parents present during the examination permits prompt discussion of parental concerns. It involves the parents actively in the health care of their child from birth. At the same time, *parental interactions with the child* can be observed; this aids in early diagnosis of problems in parent-child relationships.

The area used for the examination should be well lit, warm, and free of drafts. The child is undressed as needed and placed on a firm, flat surface. The infant may need to be picked up and cuddled at times for reassurance. The examination is carried out in a systematic manner. It begins with a general evaluation of such characteristics as appearance, maturity, nutritional status, activity, and state of well-being. This general evaluation is followed by more specific observations (Table 20.1).

Text continued on p. 532.

Table 20.1
Physical Assessment of Newborn

Area Assessed and Appraisal Procedure	Normal Findings		Deviations from Normal Range (Possible Problems)
	Average Findings	Normal Variations	
Posture			
Inspect newborn before disturbing for assessment	Vertex: arms, legs in moderate flexion; fists are clenched (Fig. 20.1)	Frank breech: more straight and stiff, so that newborn will assume intrauterine position in repose for a few days	Lack of muscle tone, relaxed posture while awake: prematurity or hypoxia in utero
Refer to maternal chart for fetal presentation, position, and type of birth (vaginal, surgical), since newborn readily assumes prenatal position	Newborn resists having extremities extended for examination or measurement and will cry when this is attempted	Prenatal pressure of limb or shoulder may cause temporary facial asymmetry (Fig. 20.2) or resistance to extension of extremities	Hypertonia: drug dependence, CNS disorder
	Crying ceases when allowed to reassume curled-up fetal position		Opisthotonos: CNS disturbance
	Normal spontaneous movement is bilaterally asynchronous (legs move in bicycle fashion) but equally extensive in all extremities		Limitation of motion in any of extremities: see Extremities, below
Vital signs			
Blood pressure (BP)	75/42 (approximately)	Varies with change in activity level: awake, crying, sleeping	Difference between upper and lower extremity pressures may provide early clue to coarctation of aorta
Electronic monitor	At birth		
BP cuff: BP cuff width affects readings; use cuff 2.5 cm (1 in) wide and palpate radial pulse (see Chapter 25)	Systolic: 60-80 mm Hg Diastolic: 40-50 mm Hg At 10 days Systolic: 95-100 mm Hg Diastolic: slight increase		Hypotension Hypertension: coarctation of aorta
Heart rate and pulses	Pulsations visible in left midclavicular line; fifth intercostal space	100 (sleeping) to 160 (crying); may be irregular for brief periods, especially after crying	Tachycardia (persistent; ≥170): RDS
Thorax	Apical pulse; fourth intercostal space 120-140/min (Fig. 20.3)	Murmurs, especially over base or at left sternal border in interspace 3 or 4 (foramen ovale anatomically closes at about 1 year)	Bradycardia (persistent; ≤120): congenital heart block
Inspection			
Palpation			Murmurs: may be functional
Auscultation	Quality: *first sound* (closure of mitral valves) and *second sound* (closure of aortic and pulmonic valves) should be sharp and clear	Average pulses (slightly faster for girls)	Arrhythmias: irregular rate
Apex: mitral valve			Sounds
Second interspace, left of sternum: pulmonic valve		2 year: 105	Distant: pneumomediastinum
Second interspace, right of sternum: aortic valve		6 year: 100	Poor quality
Junction of xiphoid process and sternum: tricuspid valve		8-12 year: 85-90 16 year: 80 18 year: 70	Extra Heard on right side of chest: dextrocardia (often accompanied by reversal of intestines)
Femoral pulse palpation: flex thighs on hips; place fingers along inguinal ligament about midway between symphysis pubis and iliac crest; feel bilaterally at same time (Fig. 20.4)	Femoral pulses should be equal and strong		Weak or absent femoral pulses Hip dysplasia Coarctation of aorta Thrombophlebitis

Continued.

Fig. 20.1
A newly born baby. Note the relaxed posture with arms and legs in flexion. (Courtesy Marjorie Pyle, RNC, Lifecircle, Costa Mesa, California.)

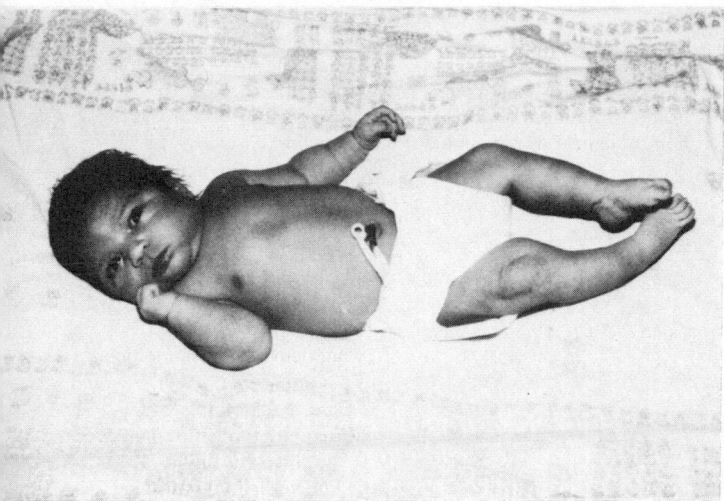

Fig. 20.2
A, Facial asymmetry. Asymmetric appearance is caused by displacement of mandible and presence of more or less pronounced fossa, or excavation, in neck, representing former position of shoulder. Some malocclusion is apparent. Confirmatory evidence may be provided by observing position of comfort newborn often assumes. **B,** Lopsided appearance disappears spontaneously in few weeks or months, depending on its severity. (Courtesy Mead Johnson & Co., Evansville, Indiana.)

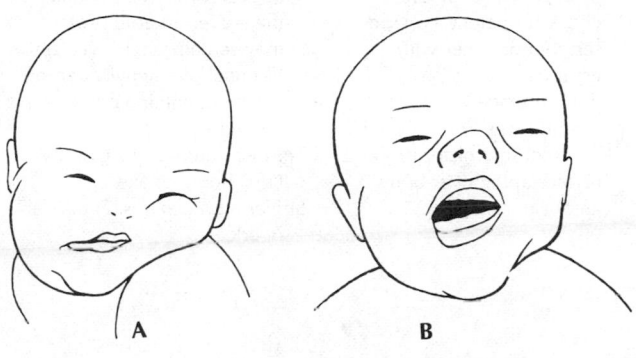

Fig. 20.3
Note differences in location of apical pulse in newborn from that of adult. **A,** Apical impulse (PMI) in the neonate is at the fourth intercostal space and to the left of the midclavicular line. The PMI is often visible. **B,** Apical impulse (PMI) in the adult is at the fifth intercostal space at or just medial to (to the right of) the midclavicular line. (From Whaley, L.F., and Wong., D.L.: Nursing care of infants and children, ed. 3, St. Louis, 1987, The C.V. Mosby Co.)

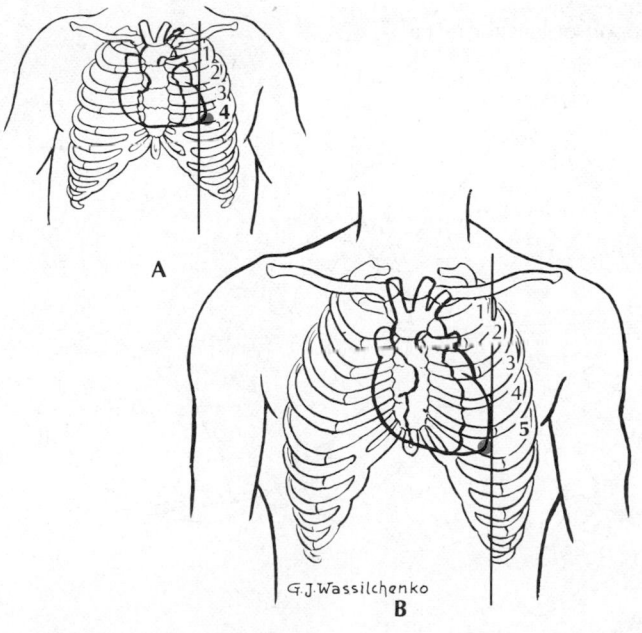

Fig. 20.4
Pulses are palpated simultaneously with tips of fingers along inguinal ligament about midway between iliac crest and pubic symphysis. (From Whaley, L.F., and Wong, D.L.: Nursing care of infants and children, ed. 3, St. Louis, 1987, The C.V. Mosby Co.)

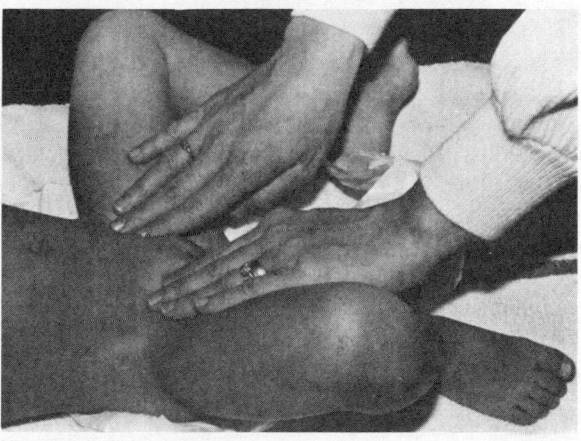

Table 20.1, cont'd
Physical Assessment of Newborn

Area Assessed and Appraisal Procedure	Normal Findings		Deviations from Normal Range (Possible Problems)
	Average Findings	Normal Variations	
Temperature	Axillary: 36.5°-37° C (97.6°-98.6° F)	35.7°-37.2° C (96°-99° F) Heat loss: 200 kcal/kg/min from evaporation, conduction, convection, radiation	Subnormal—may reflect the following:
Axillary (Fig. 20.5, *A*): method of choice until 6 years of age			Prematurity
Rectal (Fig. 20.5, *B*): before passage of meconium, check for patent anus; insert thermometer with great caution, gently; hold in place for 90 s, keeping legs immobilized	Rectal: 35.5°-37.5° C (96°-99.5° F): may be misleading—even in cold stress may remain unchanged until metabolic activity can no longer maintain core temperature		Infection Low environmental temperature Inadequate clothing Dehydration Increased (pyrexia)—may reflect the following: Infection
Electronic: thermistor probe (avoid taping over bony area) (see Chapter 25)	Temperature stabilization by 8-10 hours of age Shivering mechanism undeveloped		High environmental temperature Excessive clothing Proximity to heating unit or in direct sunshine Drug addiction (following increased activity level of infant) Diarrhea and dehydration Temperature not stabilized by 10 hours after birth If mother received magnesium sulfate, newborn is less able to conserve heat by vasoconstriction; maternal analgesics may reduce thermal stability in newborn

Fig. 20.5
A, Taking axillary temperature. **B,** Taking rectal temperature. Support of legs for rectal temperature. Attendant maintains support during entire procedure.

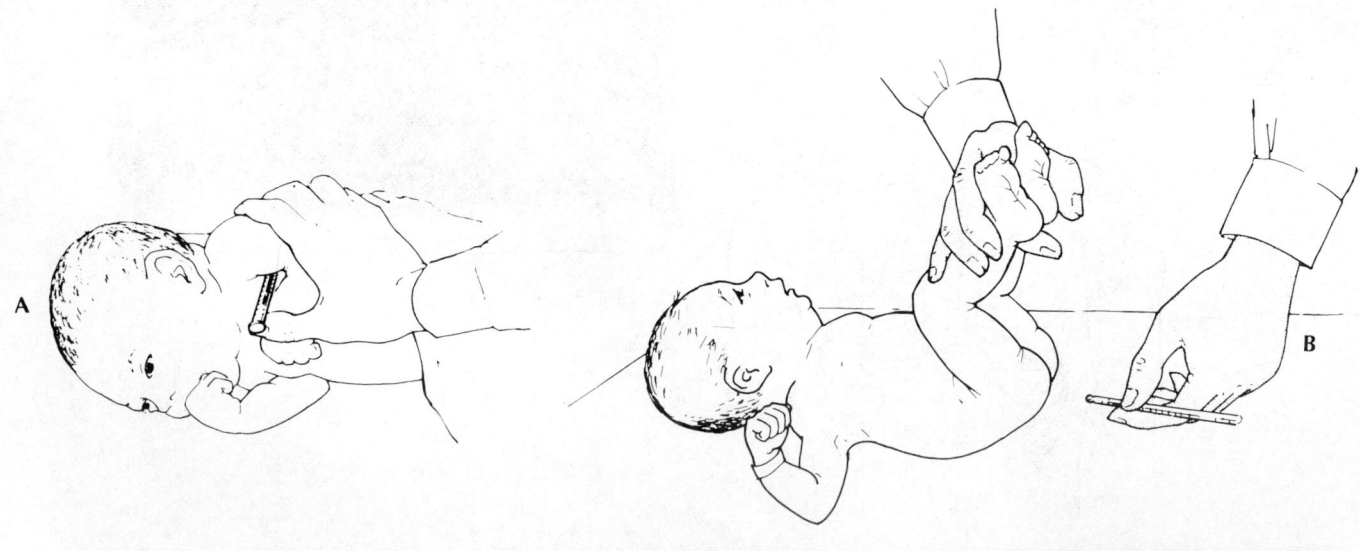

Table 20.1, cont'd
Physical Assessment of Newborn

| Area Assessed and Appraisal Procedure | Normal Findings | | Deviations from Normal Range (Possible Problems) |
	Average Findings	Normal Variations	

Respiratory rate and effort
  Observe respirations when infant is at rest
  Count respirations for full minute
  Apnea monitor
  Listen for sounds audible without stethoscope
  Observe respiratory effort (see Chapter 19)
	40/min
	Tend to be shallow, and when infant is awake, irregular in rate, rhythm, and depth
	No sounds should be audible on inspiration or expiration
	Breath sounds: bronchial; loud, clear, near (see Chapter 19)
		30-60/min
		May appear to be Cheyne-Stokes with short periods of apnea and with no evidence of respiratory distress
		
		First period (reactivity): 50-60/min
		Second period: 50-70/min
		Stabilization (1-2 days): 30-40/min
			Apneic episodes: ≥15/s
			  Preterm or premature infant: "periodic breathing"
			  Rapid warming or cooling of infant
			
			Bradypnea: ≤25/min
			  Maternal narcosis from analgesics or anesthetics
			  Birth trauma
			Tachypnea: ≥60/min
			  RDS
			  Aspiration syndrome
			  Diaphragmatic hernia
			Sounds
			  Rales, rhonchi, wheezes
			  Expiratory grunt
			Distress
			  Nasal flaring
			  Retractions
			  Chin tug
			  Labored breathing

Weight*
Put protective liner cloth or paper in place and adjust scale to 0 (Fig. 20.6)
Take weight at same time each day
Protect newborn from heat loss
	3400 g (7 lb 8 oz)
	Regains birth weight within first 2 weeks
		2500-4000 g (5 lb 8 oz to 8 lb 13 oz) (Fig. 20.7)
		Acceptable weight loss: 10% or less (to estimate percent of weight loss, see Chapter 25)
			Weight ≤2500 g
			  Prematurity
			  Small for gestational age
			  Rubella syndrome
			Weight ≥4000 g
			  Large for gestational age (LGA): maternal diabetes
			Hereditary: normal for these parents
			Weight loss over 10%: dehydration?

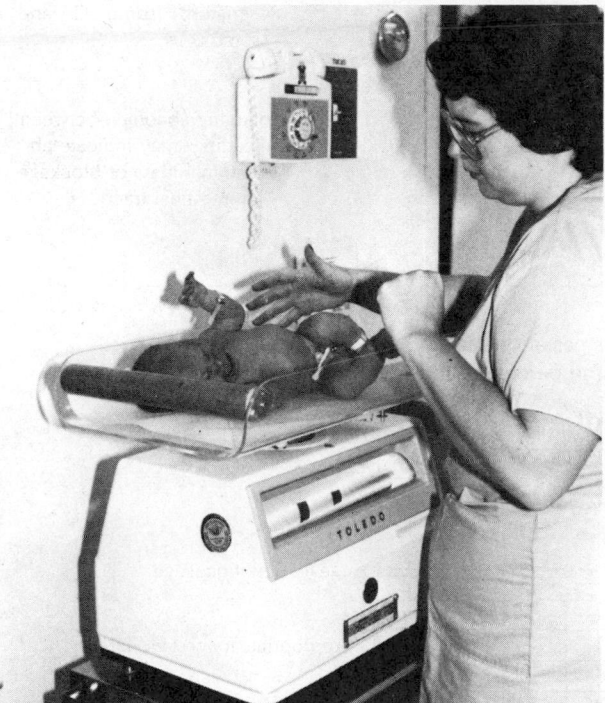

Fig. 20.6
Weighing infant. Note hand is held over infant as safety measure. Scale is covered to provide warmth and protection against cross infection. Scale is adjusted to zero reading after cover is in place. Note newborn's flexed extremities. (Photograph by I.M. Bobak.)

*NOTE: Weight, length, and head circumference should all be close to same percentile for any child.   *Continued.*

Table 20.1, cont'd

Physical Assessment of Newborn

Area Assessed and Appraisal Procedure	Normal Findings		Deviations from Normal Range (Possible Problems)
	Average Findings	Normal Variations	
Head circumference			
Measure head at greatest diameter: occipitofrontal circumference (Fig. 20.8, *A*) May need to remeasure on second or third day after resolution of molding and caput succedaneum	33-35.5 cm (13-14 in) Circumferences of head and chest may be about the same for first 1 or 2 days after birth	32-36.8 cm (12½-14½ in)	Microcephaly (under 32 cm) Rubella Toxoplasmosis Cytomegalic inclusion disease (CMV) Hydrocephaly (≥4 cm more than chest) Increased intracranial pressure Hemorrhage Space-occupying lesion
Chest circumference			
Measure at nipple line (Fig. 20.8, *B*)	2 cm (¾ in) less than head circumference; averages between 30-33 cm (12-13 in)		Prematurity: ≤30 cm Postmaturity: some SGA and some LGA
Abdominal circumference			
Measure below umbilicus (Fig. 20.8, *C*)	Abdomen enlarges after feeding because of lax abdominal muscles		Enlarging abdomen between feedings may indicate abdominal mass or blockage in intestinal tract

Fig. 20.7

Intrauterine growth status as determined by birth weight at various gestational ages. Note: Weight, length, and head circumference should all be close to same percentile for any child.

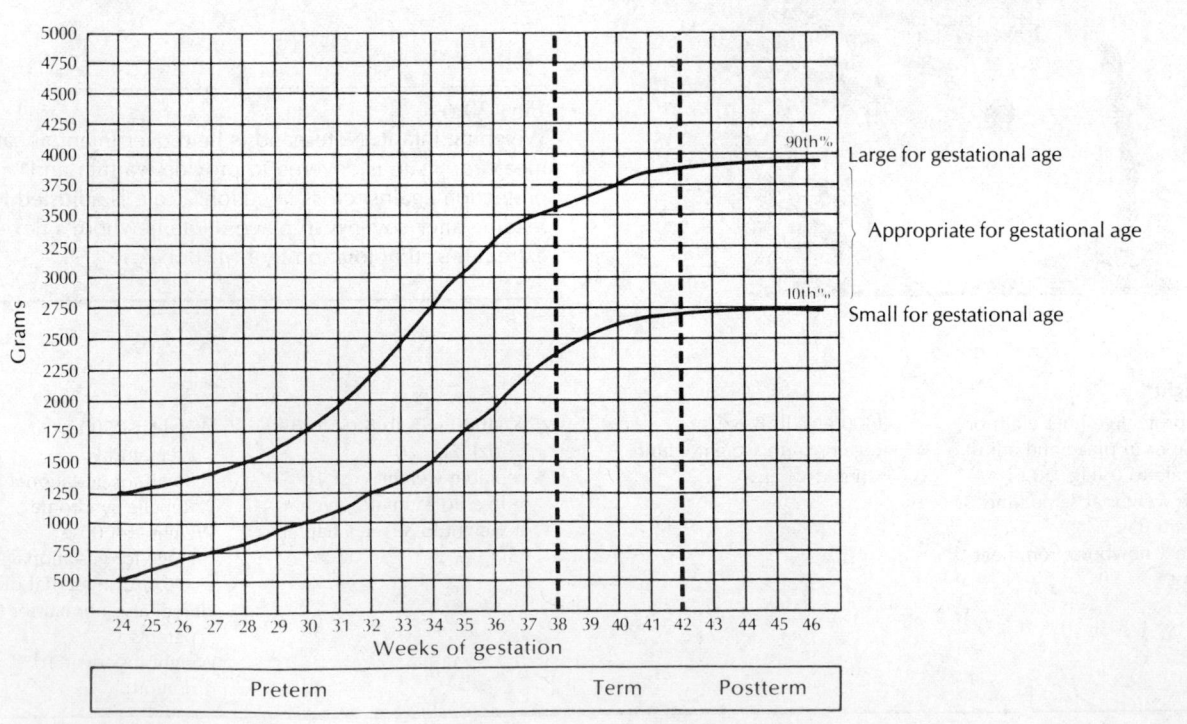

Table 20.1, cont'd
Physical Assessment of Newborn

Area Assessed and Appraisal Procedure	Normal Findings		Deviations from Normal Range (Possible Problems)
	Average Findings	Normal Variations	
Length			
Measure recumbent length from top of head to heel; difficult to measure in full-term infant because of presence of molding, incomplete extension of knees (Fig.20.8, D)	50 cm (20 in)	45-55 cm (18-22 in)	Chromosomal aberration Heredity: normal for these parents
Integument			
Color			
Inspection and palpation Inspect naked newborn in well-lit, warm area without drafts; natural daylight provides best lighting Inspect newborn when quiet and when active	Varies with ethnic origin; skin pigmentation begins to deepen right after birth in basal layer of epidermis Generally pink Acrocyanosis, especially if chilled	Mottling Harlequin sign Plethora Telangiectases ("stork bites" or capillary hemangiomas) Erythema toxicum neonatorum ("newborn rash")	Dark red: prematurity Pallor Cardiovascular problem CNS damage Blood dyscrasia; blood loss; twin transfusion Nosocomial problem (e.g., infection)

Fig. 20.8
Measurements. **A,** Measuring circumference of head. **B,** Measuring circumference of chest.
C, Measuring infant's length, crown to rump. To determine total length, length of legs is
included. **D,** Measuring abdominal circumference.

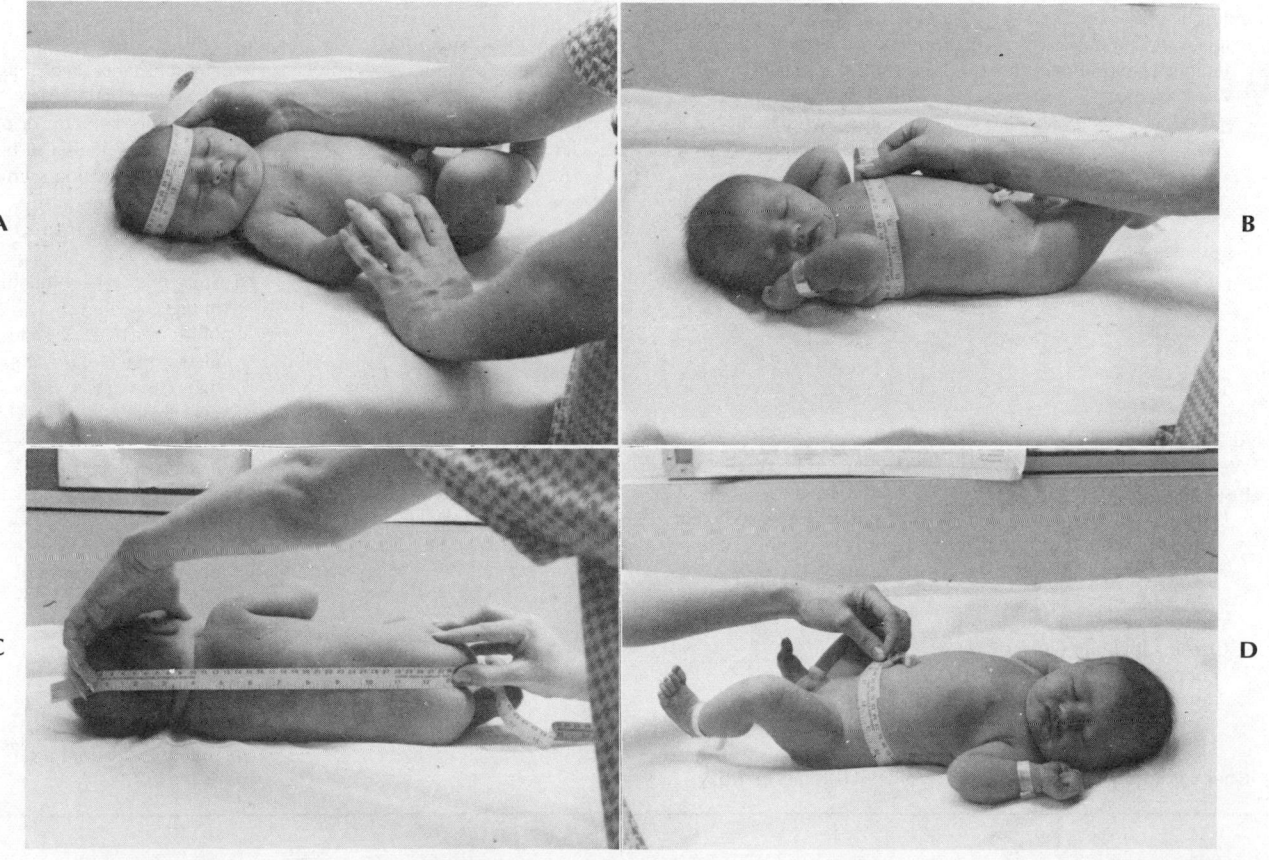

Continued.

Table 20.1, cont'd
Physical Assessment of Newborn

Area Assessed and Appraisal Procedure	Normal Findings		Deviations from Normal Range (Possible Problems)
	Average Findings	Normal Variations	

			Cyanosis
			  Hypothermia
			  Infection
			  Hypoglycemia
			  Cardiopulmonary diseases
			  Malformations: cardiac, neurologic, or respiratory

Check for jaundice (see Chapter 19)			Jaundice Gray: hypotension, poor perfusion

		Petechiae over presenting part	Petechiae over any other area may be caused by the following:
			  Clotting factor deficiency
			  Infection

		Ecchymoses from forceps in vertex births or over buttocks and legs in breech births	Ecchymoses in any other area: hemorrhagic disease

Birthmarks
  Inspect and palpate for location, size, distribution, characteristics, color (see Chapter 19)
	Transient hyperpigmentation
	  Areolae
	  Genitals
	  Linea nigra
		Mongolian spotting
		  Infants of black, Oriental, and American Indian origin; 70%
		  Infants of white origin: 9%
			Hemangiomas (vascular tumors)
			  Nevus flammeus (port-wine stain)
			  Strawberry mark
			  Cavernous hemangiomas

Condition
  Inspect and palpate for intactness, smoothness, texture, edema
	No skin edema
	Texture: thick; superficial or deep cracking
	Opacity: few large blood vessels seen indistinctly over abdomen
		Slightly thick; superficial cracking, peeling, especially of hands, feet
		No blood vessels seen; a few large vessels clearly seen over abdomen
		Some fingernail scratches
			Prematurity
			  Edema on hands, feet; pitting over tibia
			  Texture thin, smooth, or of medium thickness; rash or superficial peeling seen
			  Numerous vessels easily seen over abdomen
			Postmaturity
			  Texture thick, parchmentlike
			  Skin tags; webbing
			  Papules, pustules, vesicles, ulcers, maceration: impetigo, candidiasis, herpes
			  Diaper rash

Hydration and consistency
  Weigh infant routinely
  Inspection and palpation
    Gently pinch skin between thumb and forefinger over abdomen and inner thigh to check for turgor
    Check subcutaneous fat deposits (adipose pads) over cheeks, buttocks
	Dehydration: best indicator is loss of weight
	After pinch is released, skin returns to original state immediately
		Normal weight loss after birth is up to 10% of birth weight
		May feel puffy
		Amount of subcutaneous fat varies
			Loose, wrinkled skin
			  Prematurity
			  Postmaturity
			  Dehydration: fold of skin persists after release of pinch
			Tense, tight, shiny skin: edema, extreme cold, shock, infection
			Lack of subcutaneous fat (e.g., clavicle or ribs prominent): prematurity, malnutrition

Check voiding	Voids 6-10 times per day		

Table 20.1, cont'd
Physical Assessment of Newborn

Area Assessed and Appraisal Procedure	Normal Findings		Deviations from Normal Range (Possible Problems)
	Average Findings	Normal Variations	
Vernix caseosa			
Observe amount		Amount varies; usually more is found in creases, folds	Absent or minimal: postmaturity
			Excessive: prematurity
Observe its color and odor before bath or wiping	Whitish, cheesy, odorless		Yellow color
If not readily apparent over total body, check in folds of axilla and groin			Possible fetal anoxia 36 hours or more before birth
			Rh or ABO incompatibility (see Chapter 31)
			Green color: possible inutero release of meconium because of fetal anoxia less than 36 hr before birth or presence of bilirubin
			Odor; possible intrauterine infection (e.g., amnionitis)
Lanugo			
Inspect for this fine, downy hair: amount, distribution	Over shoulders, pinnas of ears, forehead	Amount varies	Absent: postmaturity
			Excessive: prematurity, especially if lanugo is abundant and long and thick over back
Head			
Palpate skin	See Integument, p. 521	Caput succedaneum; may show some ecchymosis	Cephalhematoma (appears after third day)
Palpate, inspect, measure fontanels	Anterior fontanel 5 cm diamond; increases as molding resolves	Fontanel size varies with degree of molding	Fontanels
		Fontanels may be difficult to feel because of molding	Full, bulging: possible intracranial lesion (e.g., tumor, hemorrhage, infection)
	Posterior fontanel triangle; smaller than anterior		Large, flat, soft: malnutrition, hydrocephaly, retarded bone age (hypothyroidism)
			Depressed: dehydration
			Large mastoid and sphenoid fontanels: hydrocephaly
Palpate sutures	Sutures palpable and not joined	Sutures may overlap with molding (Fig. 20.9)	Sutures
			Widely spaced: hydrocephaly
			Premature synostosis (closure)
Inspect pattern, distribution, amount of hair; feel texture	Silky, single strands, lies flat; growth pattern is toward face and neck	Amount varies	Fine, wooly: prematurity
			Unusual swirls, patterns, hairline or coarse, brittle: endocrine or genetic disorder
Inspect shape and size	Makes up one fourth of body length	Slight asymmetry from intrauterine position	Molding (Fig. 20.9)
	Molding		Severe molding may result from birth trauma
			Lack of molding: prematurity, breech presentation, cesarean birth
			Circumference ≥4 cm larger than chest circumference: hydrocephaly; ≤32 cm: prematurity, microcephaly

Continued.

Fig. 20.9
Molding.

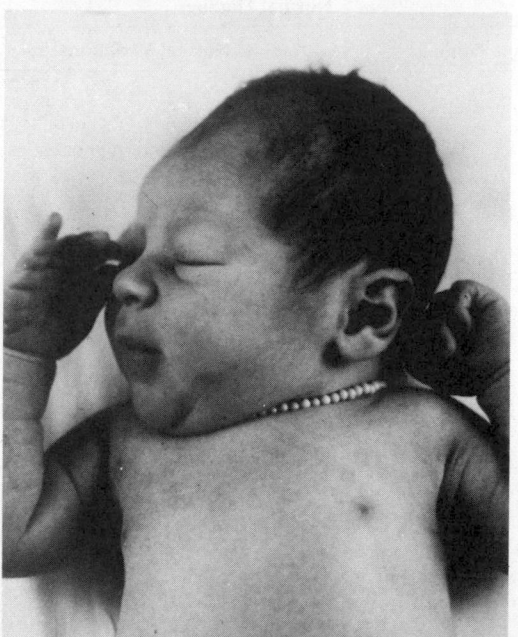

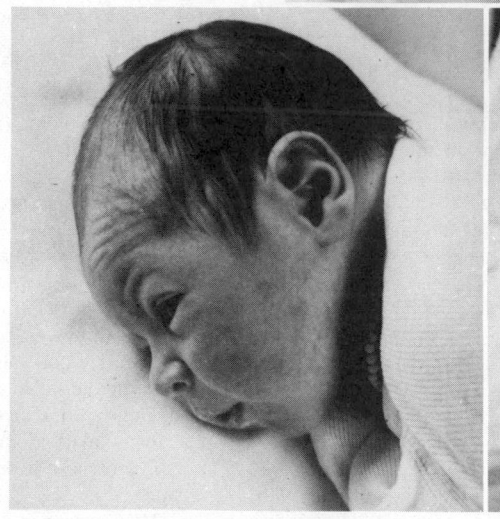
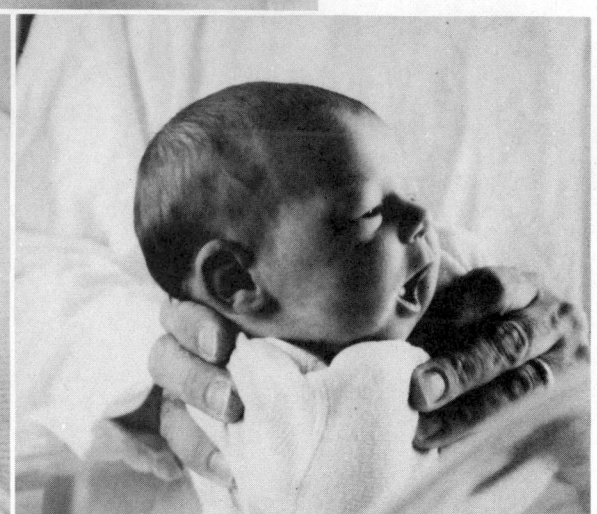

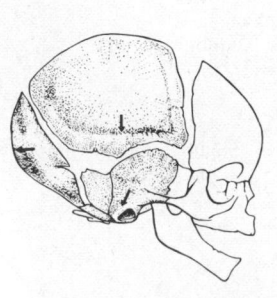
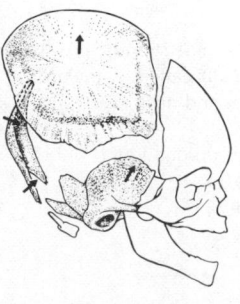

Table 20.1, cont'd
Physical Assessment of Newborn

Area Assessed and Appraisal Procedure	Normal Findings		Deviations from Normal Range (Possible Problems)
	Average Findings	Normal Variations	
Eyes (Fig. 20.10) Placement on face Symmetry in size, shape Eyelids: size, movement, blink	Symmetric in size, shape Blink reflex Epicanthal folds: normal racial characteristic	Edema from instilling silver nitrate	Epicanthal folds when present with other signs, may be caused by chromosomal disorders (e.g., Down's syndrome, cri du chat syndrome)
Discharge	None	Some discharge from silver nitrate	
Eyeballs: presence, size, shape	No tears Both present and of equal size; both round, firm	Occasionally has some tears Subconjunctival hemorrhage	Agenesis or absence of one or both eyeballs Small eyeball size: rubella syndrome Lens opacity or absence of red reflex: congenital cataracts, possibly from rubella Lesions: coloboma (absence of part of iris) Pink color of iris: albinism Jaundiced sclera Discharge: purulent Pupils: unequal, constricted, dilated, fixed

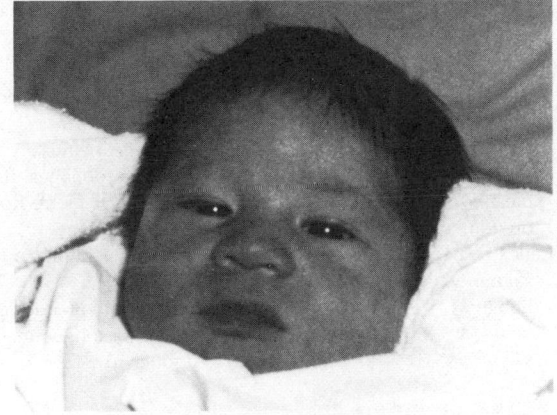

Fig. 20.10
Eyes. Pseudostrabismus. Inner epicanthal folds cause eyes to appear malaligned; however, corneal light reflexes fall perfectly symmetric. Eyes are symmetric in size and shape and well placed. Note the *folds of cheeks* are present and symmetric, indicating an absence of facial palsy. *Hair* on head consists of individual strands and is growing toward face. *Eyebrows* are well shaped and do not converge in midline. *Mouth* is of appropriate size and has a distinct vermilion border.

Eyeball movement	Random, jerky, uneven, can focus momentarily, can follow to midline	Transient strabismus or nystagmus until third or fourth month	Persistent strabismus
Eyebrows: amount, pattern	Distinct		
Nose			
Observe shape, placement, patency, configuration of bridge of nose	Midline Apparent lack of bridge, flat, broad Some mucus but no drainage Obligatory nose breathers Sneezes to clear nose	Slight deformity from passage through birth canal	Copious drainage, with or without regular periods of cyanosis at rest and return of pink color with crying: choanal atresia, congenital syphilis Malformed: congenital syphilis, chromosomal disorder Flaring of nares

Continued.

Table 20.1, cont'd
Physical Assessment of Newborn

Area Assessed and Appraisal Procedure	Normal Findings		Deviations from Normal Range (Possible Problems)
	Average Findings	Normal Variations	
Ears			
Observe size, placement on head, amount of cartilage, open auditory canal Hearing	Correct placement: line drawn through inner and outer canthi of eye should come to top notch of ear (at junction with scalp) Well-formed, firm cartilage	Size: small, large, floppy Darwin's tubercle (nodule on posterior helix)	Agenesis Lack of cartilage: possible prematurity Low placement: possible chromosomal disorder, mental retardation, kidney disorder Preauricular tags Size: may have overly prominent or protruding ears
Facies			
Observe overall appearance of face	Infant looks "normal"; features are well placed, proportionate to face	"Positional" deformities (Fig. 20.2)	Infant looks "odd" or "funny" Usually accompanied by other features, such as low-set ears and other structural disorders
Mouth			

Inspection and palpation
Placement on face
Lips: color, configuration, movement, rooting reflex, sucking
Gums
Tongue: attachment, mobility, movement, size
Cheeks
Palate (soft, hard)
  Arch
  Ulva
Saliva: amount, character
Chin
Reflexes
	Pink gums
	Symmetry of lip movement
	Tongue does not protrude, is freely movable; symmetric in shape, movement
	
	Sucking pads inside cheeks
	
	Soft and hard palates intact
	Ulvula in midline
	Reflexes present
		Transient circumoral cyanosis
		Short frenulum
		
		Anatomic groove in palate to accommodate nipple; disappears by 3-4 years of age
		Epsteins pearls (Bohn's nodules): whitish, hard nodules on gums
		Reflex response dependent on state of wakefulness and hunger
			Gross anomalies
			  Placement, size, shape
			  Cleft lip and/or palate, gums
			Cyanosis; circumoral pallor
			Asymmetry in movement of lips: seventh cranial nerve paralysis
			Macroglossia
			  Prematurity
			  Chromosomal disorder
			Excessive saliva
			  Esophageal atresia
			  Tracheoesophageal fistula
			Micrognathia: Pierre Robin or other syndrome
			Teeth: predeciduous or deciduous
			Thrush: white plaques on cheeks or tongue that bleed if touched

Neck			

Inspection and palpation
  Length
  Movement of head
  Sternocleidomastoid muscles; position of head
  Trachea: position; thyroid gland
 	
Reflex response (Table 20.2)
	Short, thick, surrounded by skinfolds; no webbing
	Head held in midline, i.e., sternocleidomastoid muscles are equal; no masses
	Freedom of movement from side to side and flexion and extension; cannot move chin past shoulder
	Thyroid not palpable
		Transient positional deformity apparent when neonate is at rest: head can be moved passively	Webbing
			Restricted movement; head held at angle; possible torticollis (wryneck), opisthotonos
			Masses: enlarged thyroid
			Distended veins: cardiopulmonary disorder
			
			Skin tags
			Positive owl's sign: prematurity
			Absence of head control: prematurity; Down's syndrome

Table 20.1, cont'd
Physical Assessment of Newborn

Area Assessed and Appraisal Procedure	Normal Findings		Deviations from Normal Range (Possible Problems)
	Average Findings	Normal Variations	
Chest			

Inspection and palpation
  Shape
  Clavicles
  Ribs
  Nipples: size, placement, number
  Breast tissue
  Respiratory movements
  Amount of cartilage in rib cage
Auscultation
  Heart tones and rate and breath sounds (see Vital signs, above)
	Almost circular; barrel shaped
	Symmetric chest movements; chest and abdominal movements synchronized during respirations
	Breast nodule: approximately 6 mm
	Nipples prominent, well formed; symmetrically placed
		Occasional retractions, especially when crying
		
		Breast nodule: 3-10 mm
		Secretion of witch's milk
			Bulging of chest
			  Pneumothorax
			  Pneumomediastinum
			Malformation: funnel chest (pectus excavatum)
			Fracture of clavicle
			Nipples
			  Supernumerary, along nipple line
			  Malpositioned or widely spaced
			Lack of breast tissue: possible prematurity
			Poor development of rib cage and musculature: possible prematurity
			Sounds: bowel sounds (see Abdomen, below)
			Retractions with or without respiratory distress

Abdomen			
Inspect, palpate, and smell umbilical cord	Two arteries, one vein (AVA) Whitish gray Definite demarcation between cord and skin; no intestinal structures within cord Dry around base; drying Odorless	Reducible umbilical herniation	One artery: internal anomalies Bleeding or oozing around cord: hemorrhagic disease Redness or drainage around cord: infection, possible persistence of urachus Hernia: herniation of abdominal contents into area of cord (e.g., omphalocele); defect covered with thin, friable membrane, may be extensive Gastroschisis: congenital fissure of abdominal cavity Meconium stained: intrauterine distress

Inspect size of abdomen and palpate contour (Fig. 20.8, C)
Auscultate for bowel sounds
	Rounded, prominent, dome shaped because abdominal musculature is not fully developed
	No distension
	Bowel sounds heard 1 hour after birth
		Some diastasis of abdominal musculature	Distension
			  At birth
			    Ruptured viscus
			    Genitourinary masses or malformations: hydronephrosis; teratomas
			    Abdominal tumors
			  Mild
			    Aerophagia
			    Overfeeding
			    High gastrointestinal tract obstruction
			  Marked
			    Lower gastrointestinal tract obstruction
			    Imperforate anus
			  Intermittent or transient
			    Aerophagia
			    Overfeeding

Continued.

Table 20.1, cont'd
Physical Assessment of Newborn

Area Assessed and Appraisal Procedure	Normal Findings		Deviations from Normal Range (Possible Problems)
	Average Findings	Normal Variations	
			Partial intestinal obstruction from stenosis of bowel
			Annular pancreas
			Malrotation of bowel or adhesions
			Sepsis
Auscultate bowel sounds and note number, amount, and character of stools, and behavior—crying, fussiness— before or during elimination	Sounds present within 1-2 hours after birth		Scaphoid, with bowel sounds in chest and respiratory distress: diaphragmatic hernia
	Meconium stool passes within 24-48 hours after birth		
Color		Linea nigra may be apparent; possibly caused by hormone influence during pregnancy	
Movement with respiration	Respirations primarily diaphragmatic; abdominal and chest movements synchronous		Decreased abdominal breathing
			Intrathoracic disease
			Diaphragmatic hernia
Genitals (Fig. 20.11)			
Girl			
Inspection and palpation			
General appearance	Female genitals	Increased pigmentation caused by pregnancy hormones	Ambiguous genitals—enlarged clitoris with urinary meatus on tip; fused labia: chromosomal disorder; maternal drug ingestions
Clitoris	Usually edematous		
Labia majora	Usually edematous; cover labia minora in term neonates	Edema and ecchymosis following breech birth	
Labia minora	May protrude over labia majora	Vaginal tag	Stenosed meatus
Discharge	Smegma	Blood-tinged discharge from pseudomenstruation caused by pregnancy hormones	Labia majora widely separated and labia minora prominent: prematurity
Vagina	Orifice open		Absence of vaginal orifice or imperforate hymen
	Mucoid discharge	Some vernix caseosa may be between labia	Fecal discharge: fistula
Urinary meatus	Beneath clitoris; hard to see— watch for voiding	Rust-stained urine (uric acid crystals) (To determine whether rust color is caused by uric acid or blood, wash under running warm tap water. Uric acid washes out, blood does not.)	
Boy			
Inspection and palpation			
General appearance	Male genitals	Increased size and pigmentation caused by pregnancy hormones	Ambiguous genitals
Penis	Meatus at tip of penis		Urinary meatus not on tip of glans penis
Urinary meatus seen as slit			
Prepuce	Prepuce (foreskin) covers glans penis and is not easily retractable	Prepuce removed at circumsion	Hypospadias / Epispadias } may be associated with other anomalies
		Size of genitals varies widely	
Scrotum	Large, edematous, pendulous; covered with rugae	Scrotal edema and ecchymosis if breech birth	Adherent or tight prepuce: phimosis
Rugae (wrinkles)		Hydrocele, small, noncommunicating	Scrotum smooth and testes undescended: prematurity, cryptorchidism
			Hydrocele

Table 20.1, cont'd
Physical Assessment of Newborn

Area Assessed and Appraisal Procedure	Normal Findings		Deviations from Normal Range (Possible Problems)
	Average Findings	Normal Variations	
Testes	Palpable on each side	Bulge palpable in inguinal canal	Inguinal hernia Round meatal opening If not palpable may be in abdomen
Urination	Voiding before 24-48 hours, stream adequate, amount adequate	Rust-stained urine (uric acid crystals)	
Reflexes			
Erection	Erection may occur when genitals are touched		
Cremasteric	Testes are retracted, especially when neonate is chilled		

Fig. 20.11
A, Genitals in female term infant. Note mucoid vaginal discharge. **B,** Genitals in male infant. Uncircumcised penis. Rugae cover scrotum, indicating term gestation. Cord has been swabbed with ethylene blue to prevent infection. (Photographs by I.M. Bobak.)

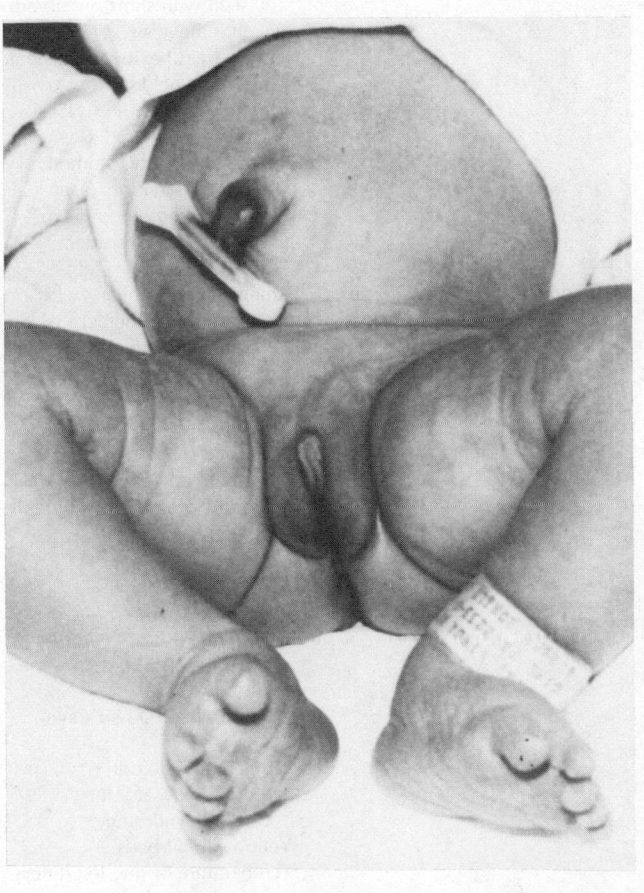

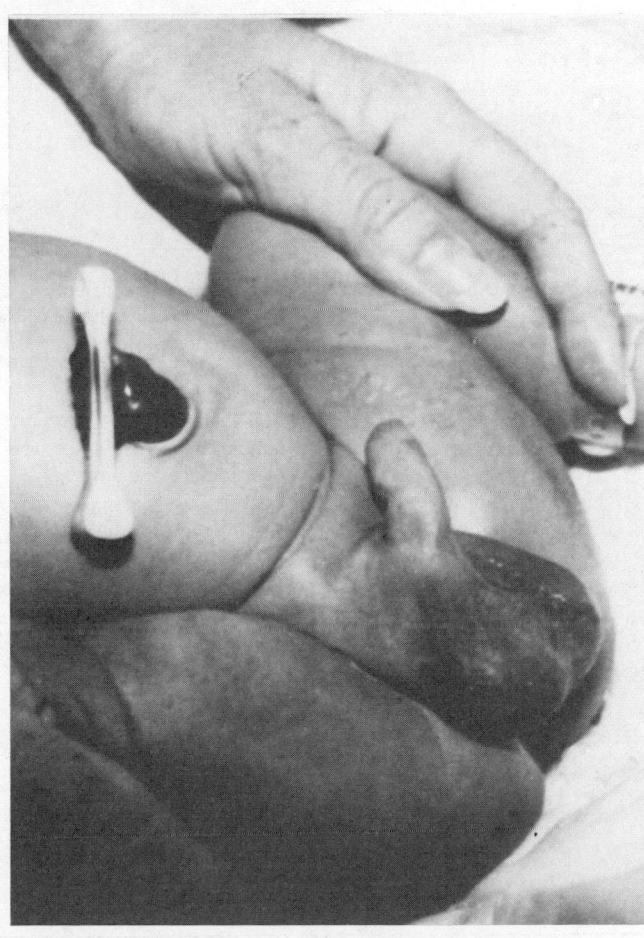

Continued.

Table 20.1, cont'd
Physical Assessment of Newborn

Area Assessed and Appraisal Procedure	Normal Findings		Deviations from Normal Range (Possible Problems)
	Average Findings	**Normal Variations**	

Extremities

General

Inspection and palpation	Assumes position maintained in utero	Transient (positional) deformities	Limited motion: malformations
Degree of flexion	Attitude of general flexion		Poor muscle tone
Range of motion	Full range of motion, spontaneous movements		Positive scarf design (see Chapter 29)
Symmetry of motion			
Muscle tone			

Arms

Inspection and palpation	Longer than legs in newborn period	Slight tremors may be seen at times	Assymetry of movement
Color	Contours and movement are symmetric	Some acrocyanosis, especially when chilled	Fracture
Intactness	Should be intact		Brachial nerve trauma
Appropriate placement	Fist often clenched with thumb under fingers		Malformations
Number of fingers	Full range of motion; symmetric contour		Asymmetry of contour
Palpate humerus			Malformations
Joints			Fracture
Shoulder			Amelia or phocomelia
Elbow			Webbing of fingers: syndactyly
Wrist			Absence or excess of fingers
Fingers			Palmar creases
Reflex: grasp (Table 20.2)			Simian line (commonly seen in Down's syndrome) seen with short, incurved little fingers
			Strong, rigid flexion; persistent fists; fists held in front of mouth constantly: CNS disorder
			Increased tonicity, clonicity, prolonged tremors (especially if whole body is involved): CNS disorder

Legs

Inspection and palpation	Appear bowed since lateral muscles more developed than medial muscles	Feet appear to turn in but can be easily rotated externally, also positional defects tend to correct while infant is crying	Amelia, phocomelia
Intactness	Major gluteal folds even		Chromosomal defect
Length—in relation to arms and body and to each other	Femur should be intact	Acrocyanosis	Teratogenic effect
Major gluteal folds	No click should be heard; femoral head should not override acetabulum (Fig. 20.12)		Webbing, syndactyly: chromosomal defect
Number of toes	Feet flat; soles well lined (or wrinkled) over two-thirds		Absence or excess of digits
Femur	Plantar fat pad gives flat-footed effect (Fig. 20.13)		Chromosomal defect
Head of femur as legs are flexed on hips and abducted; placement in acetabulum; femoral pulses	Inspection and palpation		Familial trait
Color	Joints		Femoral fracture: after difficult breech delivery
	Hip		Congenital hip dysplasia
	Knee		Absent femoral pulses
	Ankle		Soles of feet
	Toes		Poorly lined: prematurity
	Reflexes (Table 20.2)		Covered with lines: postmaturity
			Simian line: Down's syndrome
			Congenital clubfoot
			Hypermobility of joints: Down's syndrome
			Yellowed nail beds
			Temperature of one leg differs from that of the other

Continued.

Fig. 20.12
Method of assessing for hip dysplasia using Ortolani's maneuver. **A,** Examiner's middle fingers are placed over greater trochanter and thumbs over inner thigh opposite lesser trochanter. **B,** Gentle pressure is exerted to further flex thigh on hip, and thighs are rotated outward. If hip dysplasia is present head of femur can be felt to slip forward in acetabulum and slip back when pressure is released and legs returned to their original position. A click is sometimes heard (Ortolani's sign).

A 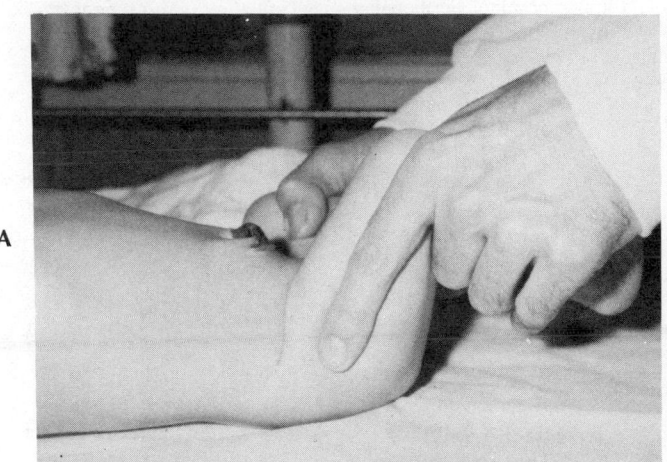 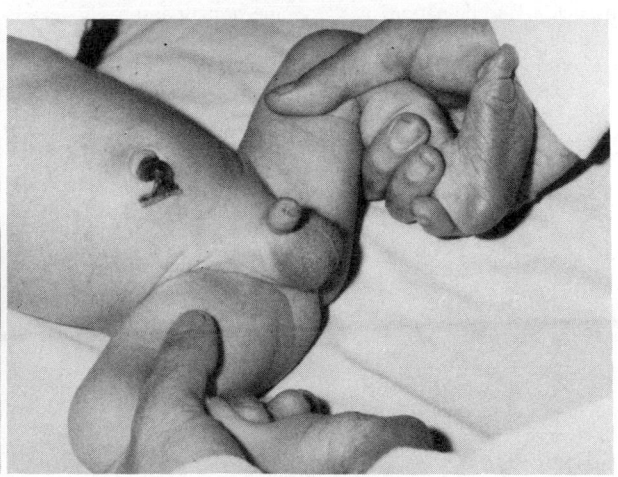 B

Fig. 20.13
Normal absence of arch in newborn.

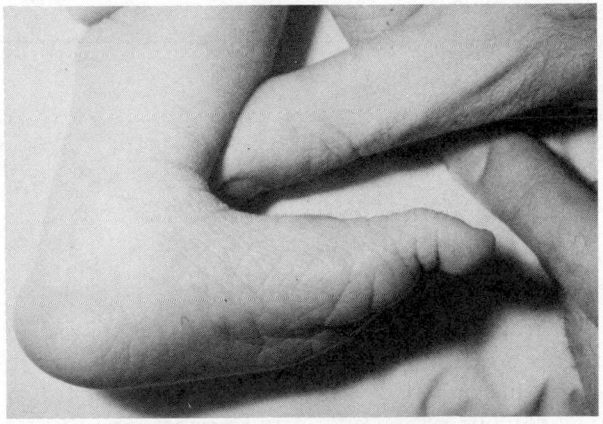

Fig. 20.14
Examining back. Infant's back should be slighty flexed, freely movable, and free of defects. Infant should kick both legs.

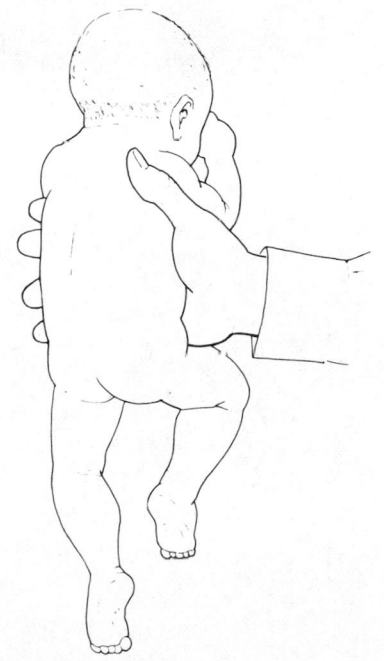

Table 20.1, cont'd
Physical Assessment of Newborn

Area Assessed and Appraisal Procedure	Normal Findings		Deviations from Normal Range (Possible Problems)
	Average Findings	Normal Variations	
Back			
Anatomy (Fig. 20.14)			
Inspection and palpation	Spine straight and easily flexed	Temporary minor positional deformities, which can be corrected with passive manipulation	Limitation of movement: fusion of deformity of vertebras
Spine	Infant can raise and support head momentarily when prone		Pigmented nevus with tuft of hair when located anywhere along the spine is often associated with spina bifida occulta
Shoulders			
Scapulae	Shoulders, scapulae, and iliac crests should line up in same plane		
Iliac crests			
Base of spine—pilonidal area			Spina bifida cystica
			Meningocele
			Myelomeningocele
Reflexes (spinal related)			
Test reflexes (Table 20.2)			
Anus			
Inspection and palpation	One anus with good sphincter tone	Passage of meconium within 48 hours after birth	Low obstruction: anal membrane (thermometer cannot be inserted)
Placement			
Number	Passage of meconium within 24 hours after birth		High obstruction: anal or rectal atresia (thermometer may be inserted, but there is no passage of meconium)
Patency			
Test for patency and sphincter response (active "wink" reflex)	Good "wink" reflex of anal sphincter		
Observe for following:			Drainage of fecal material from vagina in female or urinary meatus in male: possible rectal fistula
Abdominal distention			
Passage of meconium			
Passage of fecal drainage from surrounding orifices			
Stools	See Chapter 19		

Neurologic assessment. The physical assessment includes a neurologic assessment of the newborn's reflexes. This provides useful information about the infant's nervous system and state of neurologic maturation. Many of the reflex behaviors are important for survival, for example, sucking and rooting. Others act as safety mechanisms, for instance, gagging, coughing, and sneezing. The assessment needs to be carried out as early as possible because abnormal signs present in the early neonatal period may disappear. They may reappear months or years later as abnormal functions. Table 20.2 gives the techniques for eliciting significant reflexes and characteristic responses.

Text continued on p. 540.

Table 20.2
Assessment of Newborn's Reflexes

Reflex	Eliciting the Reflex	Characteristic Response	Comments
Sucking and rooting (Figs. 20.15 and 20.16)	Touch infant's lip, cheek, or corner of mouth with nipple	Infant turns head toward stimulus, opens mouth, takes hold, and sucks	Difficult if not impossible to elicit after infant has been fed; if weak or absent, consider prematurity or neurologic defect Parental guidance Avoid trying to turn head toward breast or nipple; allow infant to root. Disappears after 3-4 months but may persist up to 1 year
Swallowing	Swallowing usually follows sucking and obtaining fluids, suck and swallow are often uncoordinated in early-born infant and may also occur during first few hours of term (normal) infant's life	Swallowing is usually coordinated with sucking and usually occurs without gagging, coughing, or vomiting	If weak or absent, may indicate prematurity or neurologic defect
Extrusion Glabellar (Myerson's)	Touch or depress tongue Tap over forehead, bridge of nose, or maxilla of neonate whose eyes are open	Newborn forces tongue outward Newborn blinks for first 4 or 5 taps	Disappears at about fourth mo Continued blinking with repeated taps is consistent with extrapyramidal disorder

Fig. 20.15
Sucking. Also note hand-to-mouth facility with prolonged sucking. (Courtesy Joan Edelstein and Ralph Levy, San Jose, California.)

Fig. 20.16
Rooting reflex is apparent when corner of newborn's mouth is touched. Bottom lip lowers on same side; tongue moves toward stimulation. (Courtesy Joan Edelstein and Ralph Levy, San Jose, California.)

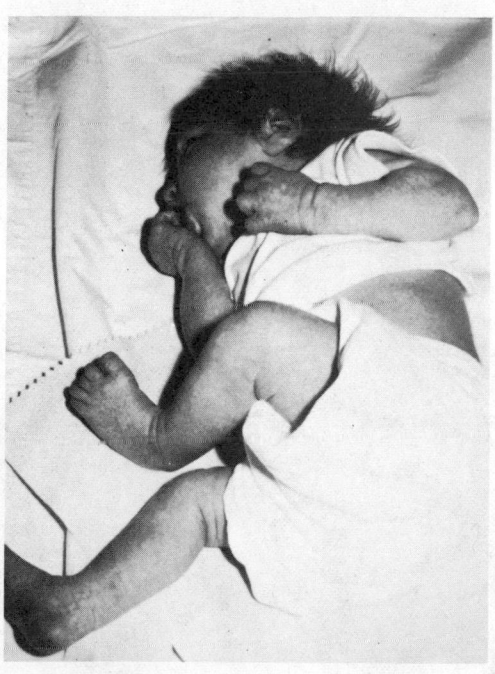

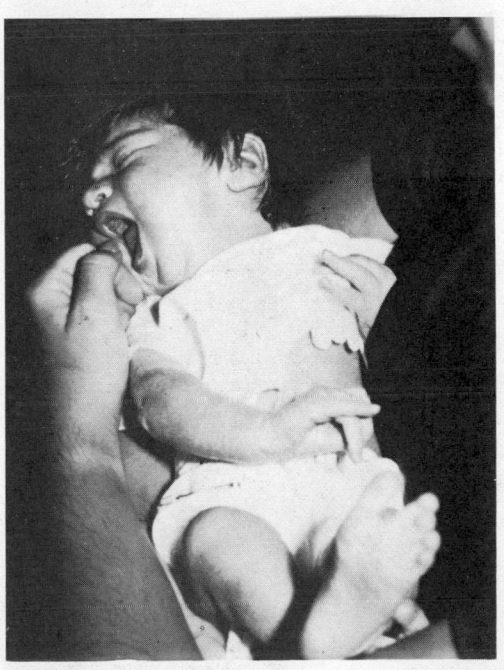

Continued.

Fig. 20.17
Classic pose in spontaneous tonic neck reflex finds infant on his back with head turned to one side and arm and leg on same side extended. If baby's head is passively rotated in opposite direction, reversal of position of extremities may occur. (Courtesy Mead Johnson & Co., Evansville, Indiana.)

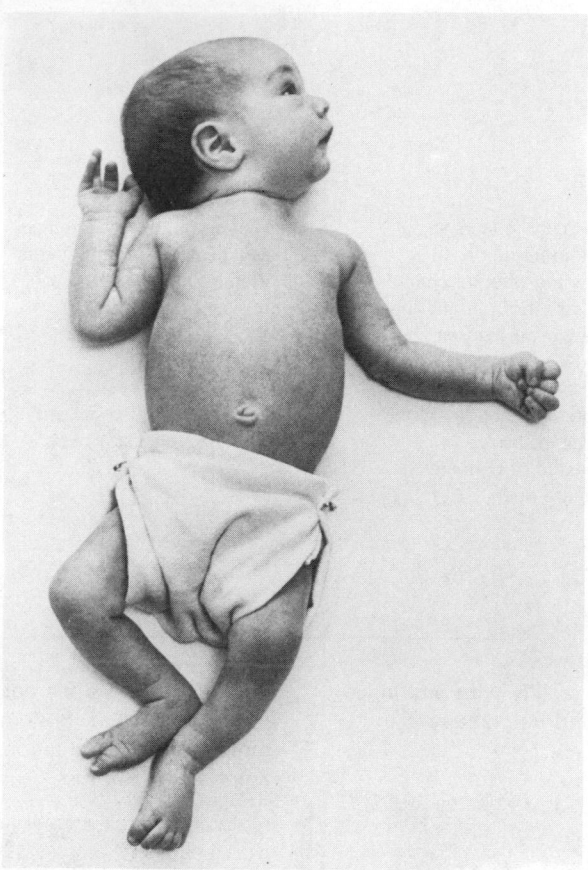

Fig. 20.18
A, Palmer (hand) grasp. **B,** Plantar grasp. (Courtesy Joan Edelstein and Ralph Levy, San Jose, California.)

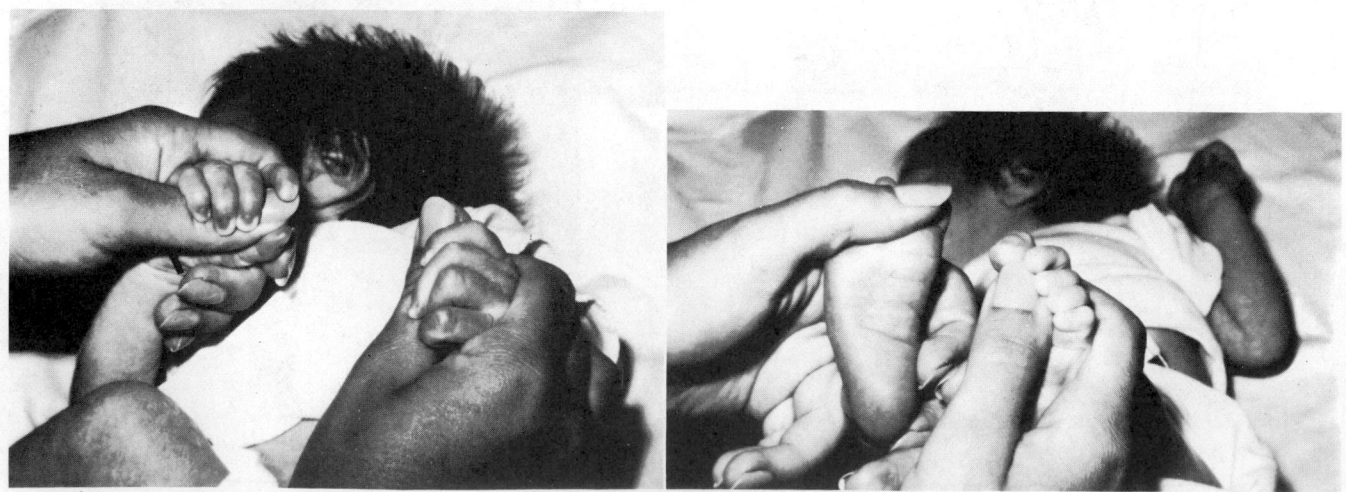

Table 20.2, cont'd
Assessment of Newborn's Reflexes

Reflex	Eliciting the Reflex	Characteristic Response	Comments
Tonic neck or "fencing" (Fig. 20.17)	With infant falling asleep or sleeping, turn head quickly to one side	With infant facing left side, arm and leg on that side extend; opposite arm and leg flex (turn head to right, and extremities assume opposite postures)	Responses in legs are more consistent Complete response disappears by 3-4 months; incomplete response may be seen until third or fourth year After 6 weeks persistent response is sign of possible cerebral palsy
Grasp (Fig. 20.18) Palmar Plantar	 Place finger in palm of hand Place finger at base of toes	Infant's fingers curl around examiner's fingers; toes curl downward	Palmar response lessens by 3-4 months; parents enjoy this contact with infant; plantar response lessens by 8 months
Moro (Fig. 20.19)	Hold infant in semisitting position; allow head and trunk to fall backward to an angle of at least 30 degrees Place infant on flat surface; strike surface to startle infant	Symmetric abduction and extension of arms; fingers fan out and form a **C** with thumb and forefinger; slight tremor may be noted; arms are adducted in embracing motion and return to relaxed flexion and movement	Present at birth; complete response may be seen until 8 weeks* of age; body jerk only, between 8-18 weeks; absent by 6 months if neurologic maturation is not delayed; may be incomplete if infant is deeply

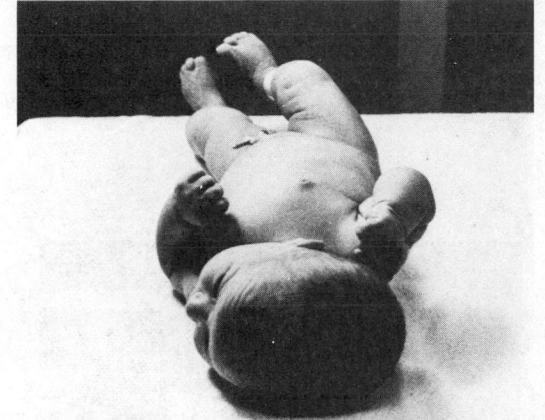

A

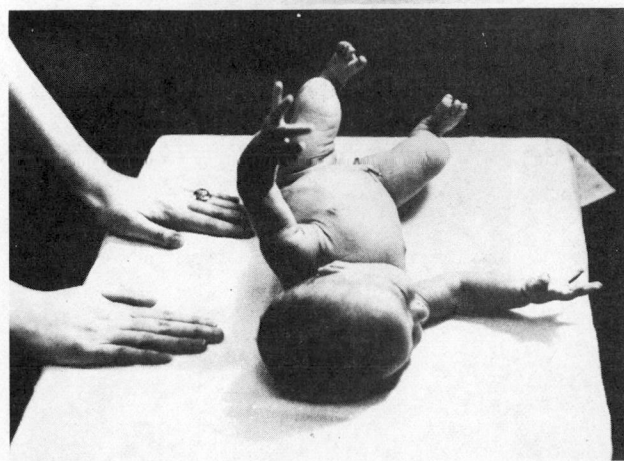

B

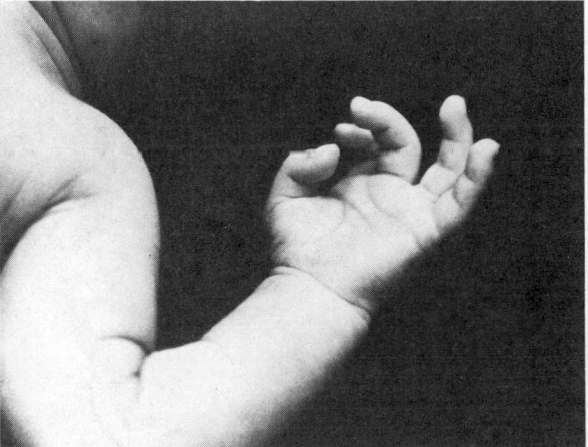

C

Fig. 20.19
A, Position of rest. **B,** Moro's reflex consists predominantly of abduction and extension of arms. **C,** Interesting subtlety of Moro's response in newborn infants is C position of fingers: digits extend, except finger and thumb, which are often semiflexed, forming shape of C. (Courtesy Mead Johnson & Co., Evansville, Indiana.)

*All durations for persistance of reflexes are based on time elapsed since 40 weeks' gestation, that is, if this newborn was born at 36 weeks' gestation, add 1 month to all time limits given.

Continued.

Table 20.2, cont'd
Assessment of Newborn's Reflexes

Reflex	Eliciting the Reflex	Characteristic Response	Comments
		Legs may follow similar pattern of response	asleep; give parental guidance about normal response
		Premature infant does not complete "embrace," instead, arms fall backward because of weakness	Asymmetric response; possible injury to brachial plexus, clavicle, or humerus
			Persistent response after 6 months: possible brain damage
Startle	Loud noise of sharp hand clap elicits response; best elicited if newborn is 24-36 hours old or older	Arms abduct with flexion of elbows; hands stay clenched	Should disappear by 4 months Elicited more readily in premature newborn (inform parents of this characteristic)
Pull-to-sit (traction) (Fig. 20.20)	Pull infant up by wrists from prone position	Head will lag until infant is in upright position; then head will be held in same plane with chest and shoulder momentarily before falling forward; head will right itself spontaneously for a few moments	Depends on general muscle tone and maturity and condition of infant

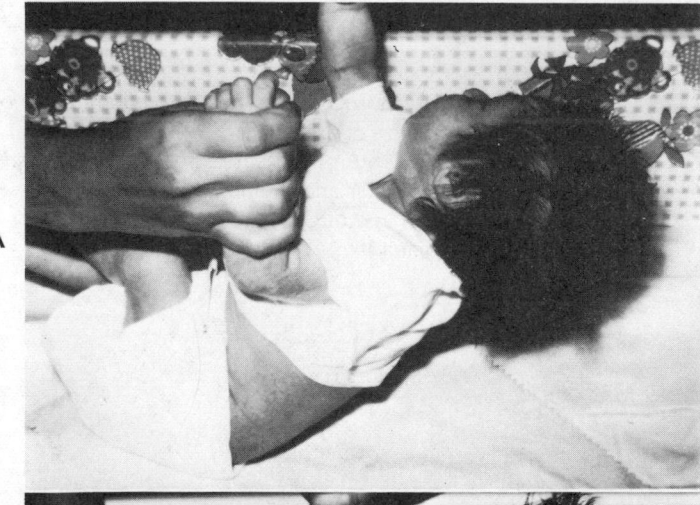
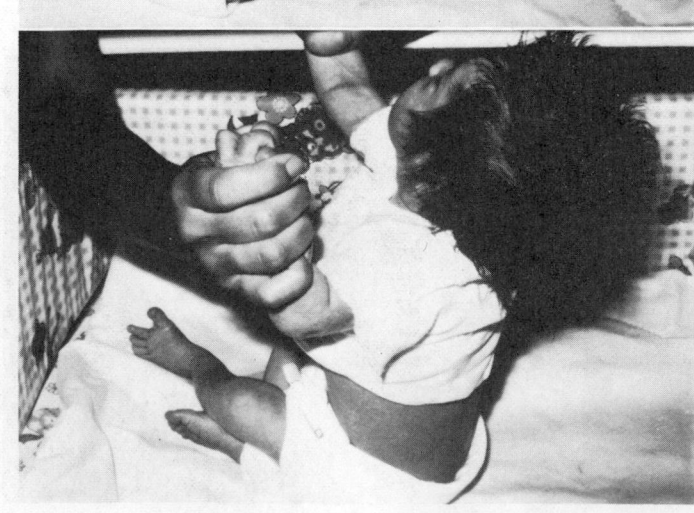
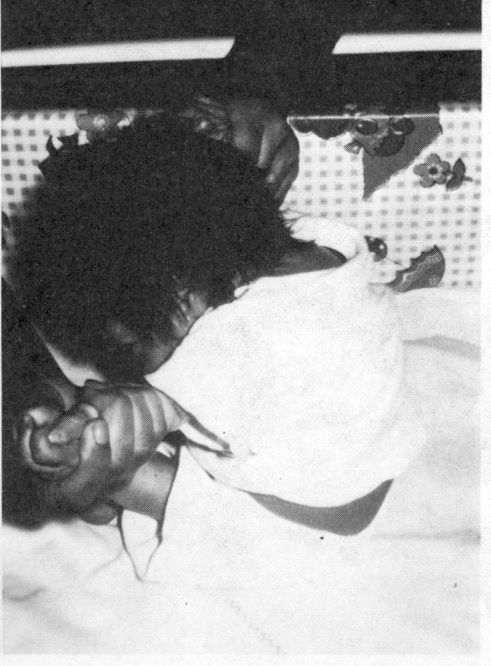

Fig. 20.20
Pull-to-sit (or traction reflex). **A,** Head falls backward. **B,** Infant attempts to right head. **C,** Infant unable to maintain head up. (Courtesy Joan Edelstein and Ralph Levy, San Jose, California.)

Table 20.2, cont'd
Assessment of Newborn's Reflexes

Reflex	Eliciting the Reflex	Characteristic Response	Comments
Trunk incurvation (Galant) (Fig. 20.21)	Infant should be prone on flat surface; run finger down back about 4-5 cm (1½-2 in) lateral to spine, first on one side, and then down other	Trunk is flexed and pelvis is swung toward stimulated side	Response disappears by fourth week
Magnet (Fig. 20.22)	Infant should be supine; partially flex both lower extremities and apply pressure to soles of feet	Both lower limbs should extend against examiner's pressure	
Crossed extension (Fig. 20.23)	Infant should be supine; extend one leg, press knee downward, stimulate bottom of foot; observe opposite leg	Opposite leg flexes, adducts, and then extends	
Babinski's sign (plantar) (Fig. 20.24)	On sole of foot, beginning at heel, stroke upward along lateral aspect of sole, then move finger across ball of foot	All toes hyperextend, with dorsiflexion of big toe	Absence requires neurologic evaluation; should disappear after 1 year of age
Stepping or "walking" (Fig. 20.25)	Hold infant vertically, allowing one foot to touch table surface	Infant will simulate walking, alternating flexion and extension of feet; term infants walk on soles of their feet, and premature infants walk on their toes	Normally present for 3-4 weeks
Neck righting	Place newborn in supine position and turn head to one side	Shoulder and trunk and then pelvis will turn to be in alignment with head	Disappears at 10 months of age; absence: implications same as for absent tonic neck reflex
Otolith righting	Hold newborn erect and tilt body	Head returns to erect, upright position	Absence: implications same as for absent tonic neck reflex
Crawling (Fig. 20.26)	Place newborn on abdomen	Newborn makes crawling movements with arms and legs	Should disappear about 6 weeks of age

Fig. 20.21
Trunk incurvation reflex. In prone position, infant responds to linear skin stimulus (pin or finger) along paravertebral area by flexing trunk and swinging pelvis toward stimulus. With transverse lesions of cord, there will be no response below that level. Complete absence of response suggests general depression or nervous system abnormality. Response may vary but should be obtainable in all infants, including premature ones. If not seen in the first few days, it is usually apparent by 5 to 6 days. (Courtesy Mead Johnson & Co., Evansville, Indiana.)

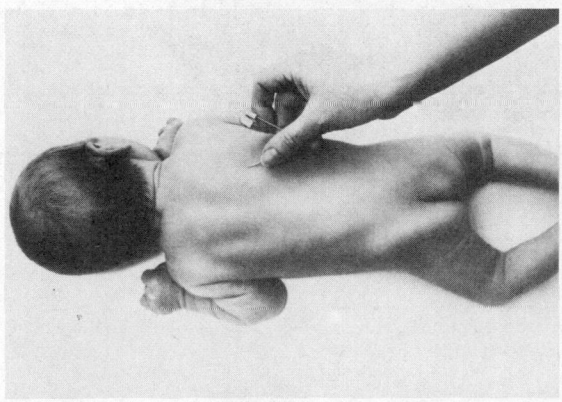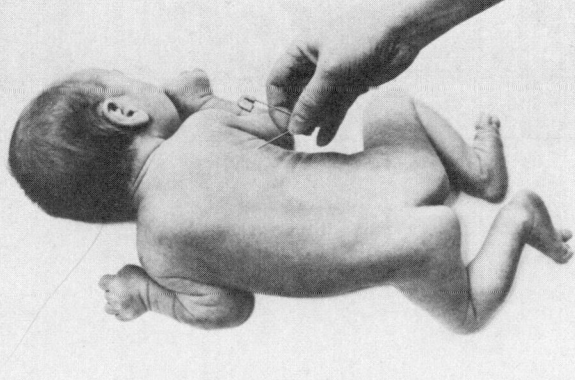

Continued.

Fig. 20.22
Magnet reflex. With child in supine position and lower limbs semiflexed, light pressure is applied with fingers to both feet. Normally, while examiner's fingers maintain contact with soles of feet, lower limbs extend. Absence of this reflex suggests damage to spinal cord or malformation. Weak reflex may be seen following breech presentation *without* extended legs or may indicate sciatic nerve stretch syndrome. Breech presentation *with* extended legs may evoke an exaggerated response. (Courtesy Mead Johnson & Co., Evansville, Indiana.)

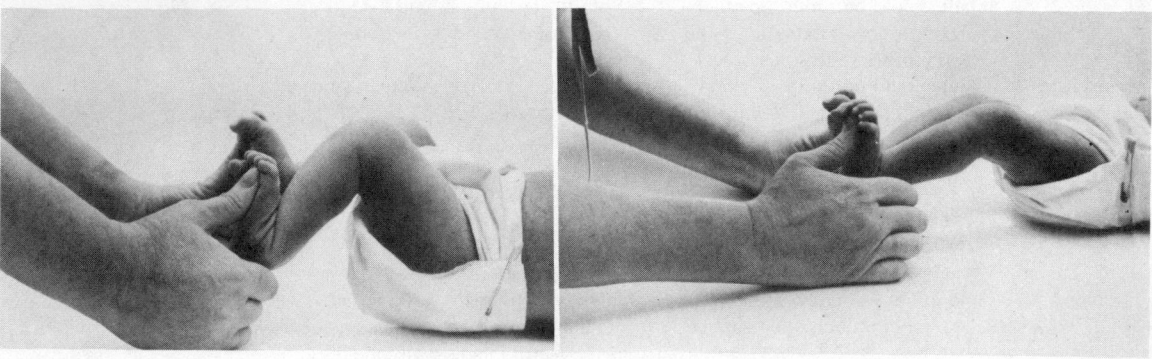

Fig. 20.23
Crossed extension reflex. With child in supine position, examiner extends one of infant's legs and presses knee down. Stimulation of sole of foot of fixated limb should cause *free* leg to flex, adduct, and extend as if attempting to push away stimulating agent. This reflex should be present during newborn period. Absence of response suggests a spinal cord lesion; weak response suggests peripheral nerve damage. (Courtesy Mead Johnson & Co., Evansville, Indiana.)

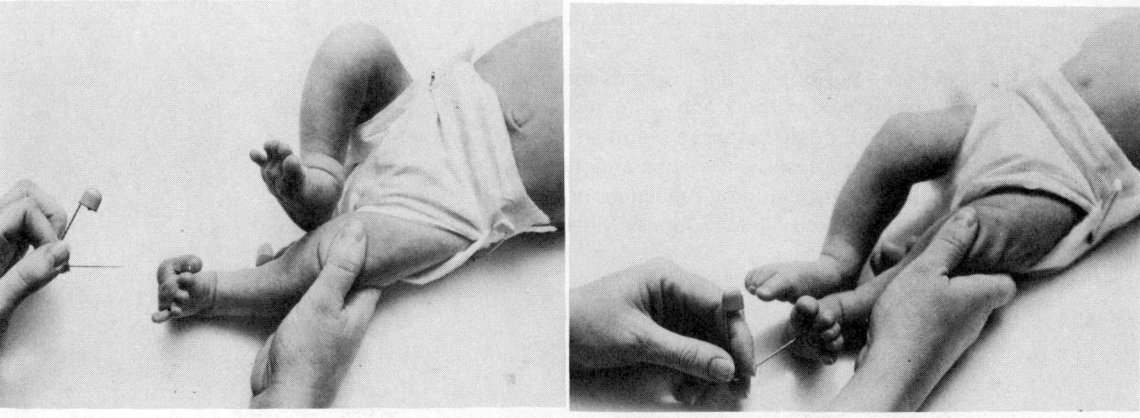

Fig. 20.24
Babinski's reflex (line drawing). **A,** Direction of stroke. **B,** Dorsiflexion of big toe.
C, Fanning of toes. **D,** Babinski's reflex (newborn). (From Whaley, L.F., and Wong, D.L.:
Essentials of pediatric nursing, ed. 3, St. Louis, 1987, The C.V. Mosby Co.)

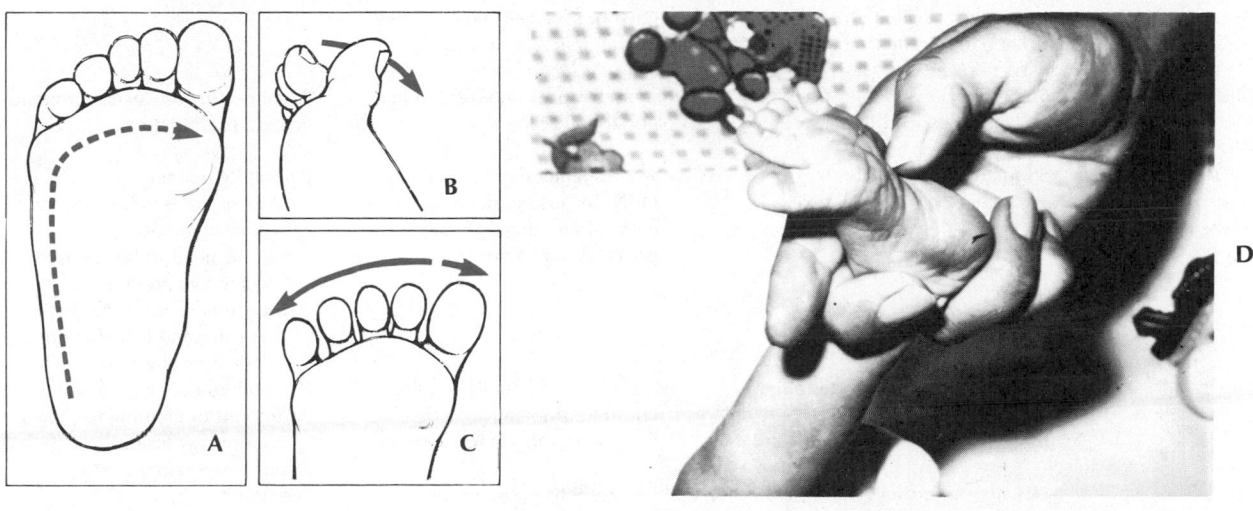

Fig. 20.25
A, Standing. **B,** Placing. **C,** Automatic walking reflex is phase of neuromuscular maturity
from which infant normally graduates after 3 to 5 weeks. If infant is held so that sole of his
foot touches table, reciprocal flexion and extension of leg occur, simulating walking.
(Courtesy Joan Edelstein and Ralph Levy, San Jose, California.)

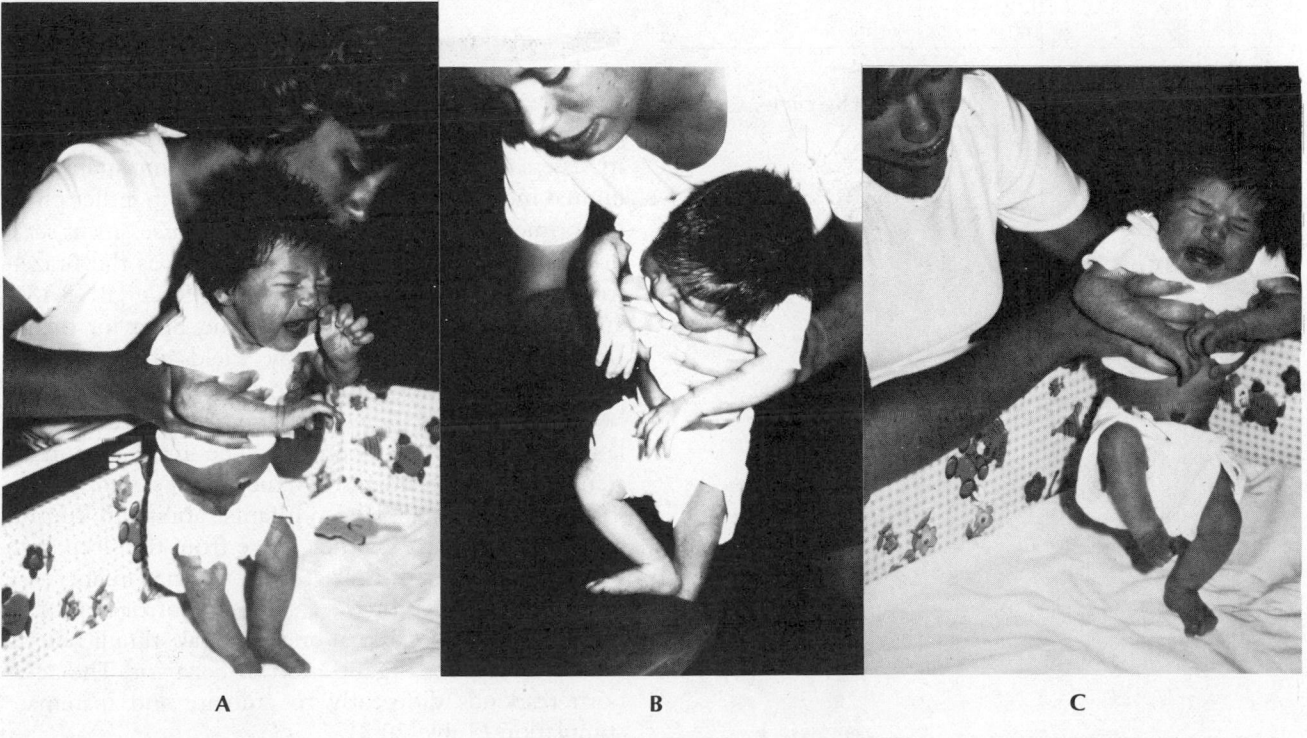

Table 20.2, cont'd
Assessment of Newborn's Reflexes

Reflex	Eliciting the Reflex	Characteristic Response	Comments
Deep tendon	Use finger instead of percussion hammer to elicit patellar, or knee jerk, reflex; newborn must be relaxed	Reflex jerk is present; even with newborn relaxed, nonselective overall reaction may occur	
Landau	Over a crib or a table, using two hands, suspend infant in prone position	Infant attempts to hold spine in horizontal plane	Absence suggests need for neurologic examination
Yawn, stretch, burp, hiccup, sneeze	Spontaneous behaviors	May be slightly depressed temporarily because of maternal analgesia of anesthesia, fetal hypoxia, or infection	Parental guidance Most of these behaviors are pleasurable to parents Parents need to be assurred that behaviors are normal Sneeze is response to lint, etc., in nose and (usually) not an indicator of a cold
Sweat	Usually not present in term newborn	Sweat response usually not present in term infant; may be seen in infants with cardiac response	Parental guidance Amount of clothing for infant: indoors, outside Room temperature
Shiver	Usually not present in term newborn	Shiver response usually not present in term infant; if seen, check infant for postmaturity	See above
Kernig's sign	Flex thigh on hip and extend leg at knee	Procedure should be accomplished easily and without inflicting pain	Pain and resistance to extension of knee suggest meningeal irritability
Brudzinki's sign	Place infant in supine position; flex neck and observe knees	Infant does not move legs when neck is flexed	Spontaneous flexion of knees suggest meningeal irritability
Paradoxic irritability	Ascertain that infant is not hungry; hold and cuddle infant	Infant usually responds by quieting down	Infant cries when touched and held; response suggests meningeal irritability

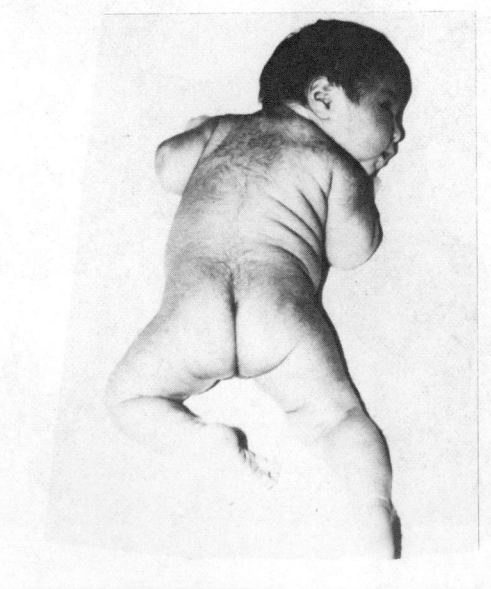

Fig. 20.26
Crawling. (Courtesy Marjorie Pyle, RNC, Life circle, Costa Mesa, California.)

Behavioral assessment. The behavioral assessment of the newborn is receiving increasing attention. For some years the only tool used routinely was the neurologic and reflex activity assessment. The reflex activity assessment (Table 20.2), although important, is a limited indicator of the child's potential in either physical or mental capacity. The behavioral assessment scale developed by Brazelton (1978) (known as the Brazelton Neonatal Behavioral Assessment Scale [BNBAS]) and the Mother's Assessment of the Behavior of her Infant (MABI) developed by Field and associates (1978) provide a psychologic assessment of a newborn's capabilities. These capabilities are relevant to later personality development. The most important element in the evaluation is the infant's *state of consciousness* (see Table 19.2). Infants' ability to control their response varies as they move from the sleep state to the waking state. Brazelton notes that infants' use of a particular sleep or wake state to control or modify their reactions to external and internal stimuli reflects their potential for organization of behavior. The newborn responds differently to animate and inanimate stimulation (Table 20.3).

Table 20.3
Infant State-Related Behavior Chart

Behavior	Description of Behavior	Infant State Consideration	Implications for Caregiving
Alerting	Widening and brightening of the eyes. Infants focus attention on stimuli, whether visual, auditory, or objects to be sucked.	From drowsy or active alert to quiet alert.	Infant state and timing are important. When trying to alert infants, one may try to: 1. unwrap infants (arms out at least) 2. place infants in upright position 3. talk to infants, putting variation in your pitch and tempo 4. show your face to infants 5. elicit the rooting, sucking, or grasp reflexes. Being able to alert infants is important for caregivers, as alert infants offer increased feedback to adults.
Visual response	Newborns have pupillary responses to differences in brightness. Infants can focus on objects or faces about 7-8 inches away. Newborns have preferences for more complex patterns, human faces, and moving objects.	Quiet alert.	Newborn's visual alertness provides opportunities for eye-to-eye contact with caregivers, an important source of beginning caregiver-infant interaction.
Auditory response	Reaction to a variety of sounds, especially in the human voice range. Infants can hear sounds and locate the general direction of the sound, if the source is constant and remains coming from the same direction.	Drowsy, quiet alert, active alert.	Enhances communication between infants and caregivers. The fact that crying infants can often be consoled by voice demonstrates the value this stimulus has to infants.
Irritability	How easily infants are upset by loud noises, handling by caregivers, temperature changes, removal of blankets or clothes, etc.	From deep sleep, light sleep, drowsy, quiet alert, or active alert to fussing or crying.	Irritable infants need more frequent consoling and more subdued external environments. Parents can be helped to cope with more irritable infants through the items listed under "Consoling by caregivers."
Readability	The cues infants give through motor behavior and activity, looking, listening, and behavior patterns.	All states.	Parents need to learn that newborns' behaviors are part of their individual temperaments and not reflections on their parenting abilities or because their infants do not like them. By observing and understanding an infant's characteristic pattern, parents can respond more appropriately to their infant as an individual.
Smile	Ranging from a faint grimace to a full-fledged smile. Reflexive.	Drowsy, active alert, quiet alert, light sleep.	Initial smile in the neonatal period is the forerunner of the social smile at 3-4 weeks of age. Important for caregivers to respond to it.
Habituation	The ability to lessen one's response to repeated stimuli. For instance, this is seen where the Moro response is repeatedly elicited. If a noise is continually repeated, infants will no longer response to it in most cases.	Deep sleep, light sleep, also seen in drowsy.	Because of this ability families can carry out their normal activities without disturbing infants. Infants are not victims of their environments. Infants can shut out most stimuli, similar to adults not hearing a dripping faucet after a period of time. Infants who have more difficulty with this will probably not sleep well in active environments.

From Barnard, K.E., and others: Infant state-related behavior chart. In Early parent-infant relationships, copyright 1978 by the March of Dimes Birth Defects Foundation, White Plains, N.Y. Reprinted by permission.   *Continued.*

Table 20.3, cont'd
Infant State-Related Behavior Chart

Behavior	Description of Behavior	Infant State Consideration	Implications for Caregiving
Cuddliness	Infant's response to being held. Infants nestle and work themselves into the contours of caregivers' bodies versus resist being held.	Primarily in awake states.	Cuddliness is usually rewarding behavior for the caregivers. It seems to convey a message of affection. If infants do not nestle and mold, it would be wise to discuss this tendency and show the caregivers how to position infants to maximize this response.
Consolability	Measured when infants have been crying for at least 15 seconds. The ability of infants to bring themselves or to be brought by others to a lower state.	From crying to active alert, quiet alert, drowsy, or sleep states.	Crying is the infant behavior that presents the greatest challenge to caregivers. Parents' success or failure in consoling their infants has a significant impact on their feelings of competence as parents.
Self-consoling	Maneuvers used by infants to console themselves and move to a lower state: 1. hand-to-mouth movement 2. sucking on fingers, fist, or tongue 3. paying attention to voices or faces around them 4. changes in position	From crying to active alert, quiet alert, drowsy, or sleep states.	If caregivers are aware of these behaviors, they may allow infants the opportunity to gain control of themselves instead of immediately responding to their cues. This does not imply that newborns should be left to cry. Once newborns are crying and do not initiate self-consoling activities, they may need attention from caregivers.
Consoling by caregivers	After crying for longer than 15 seconds, the caregivers may try to: 1. show face to infant 2. talk to infant in a steady, soft voice 3. hold both infant's arms close to body 4. swaddle infant 5. pick up infant 6. rock infant 7. give a pacifier or feed	From crying to active alert, quiet alert, drowsy, or sleep states.	Often parental initial reaction is to pick up infants or feed them when they cry. Parents could be taught to try other soothing maneuvers.
Motor behavior and activity	Spontaneous movements of extremities and body when stimulated versus when left alone. Smooth, rhythmical movements versus jerky ones.	Quiet alert, active alert.	Smooth, nonjerky movements with periods of inactivity seem most natural. Some parents see jerky movements and startles as negative response to their caregiving and are frightened.

Factors influencing the behavior of the newborn
Gestational age. The gestational age of the infant and level of CNS maturity will affect observed behavior. An infant with an immature CNS will have an entire body response to a pinprick of the foot. The mature infant will withdraw the foot. CNS immaturity will also be reflected in reflex development and sleep-wake cycles.

Time. Length of time to recuperate from labor and delivery will affect the behavior of infants as they attempt to become initially organized. Time since the last feeding and time of day may influence infants' responses.

Stimuli. Environmental events and stimuli will have an effect on the behavioral responses of infants. Nurses in intensive care nurseries observe that infants respond to loud noises, bright lights, monitor alarms, and tension in the unit. It has been well documented that infants are affected by nonverbal behavior in the environment. Infants of mothers who are tense have more muscle activity and their heart rates change parallel to their mothers during feeding.

Medication. There is controversy concerning the effects of maternal medication (analgesia, anesthesia) during labor on infant behavior. Some researchers have noted that infants of mothers who were given medications may continue to demonstrate poor state organization beyond the fifth day (Murray, 1981). Others maintain that the effect can be beneficial or that there is no effect (Chapter 16).

Culture. Some of the most interesting research findings have been the differences in infant behavior across

Table 20.4
Infant Behavioral Patterns and Sensory Capabilities

Item	Parameters of Normal	Deviations From Normal/Probable Conditions
Behavioral patterns	Cortical control and responsiveness	CNS disorders
Feeding	Variations in interest, hunger; usually feeds well within 24 hours of birth	Lethargic, tires easily or may perspire while attempting to feed; poor suck, poor coordination with swallow, cyanosis, choking
Social	Cry is lusty, strong; soon indicative of hunger, pain, attention seeking	Weak or absent; high pitched
	Smiling, focusing evident within first week	Absence; no focusing on person holding him; unconsolable
	Responds by quietness and increased alertness to cuddling, voice	
Sleep-wakefulness (Fig. 27.9)	Transitional period with 2 periods of reactivity: at birth and 6-8 hours later	Lethargy; drowsiness
	Stabilization with wakeful periods about every 3-4 hours	Disorganized pattern
Elimination	Develops own pattern within first 2 weeks:	See "Elimination behaviors"
	Stooling: see "Elimination behaviors"	
	Urination:	Diminished number: dehydration
	First few days: 3-4 times daily	
	End of first week: 5-6 times daily	
	Later: 6-10 times daily with adequate hydration	
Reflex response	Brainstem development and musculoskeletal intactness	Present in anencephalic neonates also
	See "Reflexes"	Absence; hyperreactive; incomplete; asynchronous
Sensory capabilities		
Vision	Limited accommodation with clearest vision within 18-20 cm (7-8 in)	Absence of these responses may be caused by absence of or diminished acuity or by sensory deprivation
	Detects color by 2 months but attracted by black-white pattern at 5 days or less	
	Focuses and follows by 15 min of age	
	Prefers patterns to plain surfaces	
	Prefers changes in patterns by 2 months	
	At birth, can gaze intently	
Hearing	By 2 min of age, moves eyes in direction of sound	Absence of response: deafness
	Responds to high pitch by "freezing," followed by agitation; to low pitch (crooning) by relaxation	
	Can hear beginning in last trimester of fetal life	
Touch	Sensitivity to pain may be diminished (because of β-endorphins present prenatally)	
	Soothed by massaging, warmth, weightlessness (as in warm water bath)	Unable to be comforted; possible drug dependence
Smell	By days 2 to 7 can distinguish between own mother's used breast pads and those of another woman	
Taste	By 3 days of age, can distinguish between sucrose and glucose and grimaces in response to drop of lemon juice on tongue	
Motor	Coordinates body movement to parent's voice and body movement; imitates parent's actions by 2 weeks of age	Absence

cultures (Freedman, 1979). Freedman and Freedman (1969) found that Chinese-American infants had more self-quieting activities, fewer state changes, and more rapid responses to consoling activities than white infants. The Zinacanteco Indians in southern Mexico demonstrated greater motor maturity and increased ability to maintain quiet alert states for longer times than U.S. infants (Brazelton, 1969).

Coll and co-workers (1981) determined that Puerto Rican infants had lower scores on habituation and higher scores on both orientation and maintaining organization than black and white infants. Interestingly, studies done on infants delivered by the Leboyer method have not revealed any differences in behavior from those infants delivered by conventional methods (Nelson, 1980; Saisal, 1981). The range of the infant's responses may impress the examiner with the newborn's formidable neurologic capacity. The newborn's innate ability is truly amazing (Table 20.4).

Nursing Diagnoses

Analysis of the significance of findings collected during assessment leads to the establishment of nursing diagnoses. Possible nursing diagnoses *for the newborn* are as follows:

1. Ineffective breathing pattern related to obstructed airway
2. Alteration in comfort: pain related to circumcision
3. Impaired gas exchange related to hypothermia (cold stress)

Possible nursing diagnoses *for the parent or parents* are as follows:

1. Alteration in parenting related to knowledge deficit of newborn's social capabilities
2. Alterations in parenting related to knowledge deficit of newborn's dependency needs

Planning

Plans for care of the newborn reflect the rapid growth and development during the neonatal period. Changes in biologic and behavioral states are measured in minutes and hours since birth. The neonatal period extends through the first 28 days after birth. By that time the rate of change has slowed enough so that the child's appearance and needs can be referred to in terms of weeks and months.

The focus of care changes between birth and 28 days. During the first 2 hours of life the main focus is on the infant's physiologic adaptation. By the end of the neonatal period the infant's socialization needs assume equal importance with physiologic needs.

The care given the neonate during the *first 2 hours of life* is part of the care given parents and newborns in the fourth stage of labor (Chapter 18). Care related to *nutritional needs* of infants, including techniques of feeding, is presented in Chapter 21. *Parent-child interactions* are discussed in detail in Chapters 23 and 24.

The information in this section pertains to the maintenance of vital functions, the daily care of infants, and the forms of general therapy carried out routinely in newborn nurseries. Parental education before discharge from the hospital and at the well-baby visit is outlined.

Goals. The goals for newborn care relate to the infant and to the caretaker. The goals for the infant include the following:

1. To support the infant's transition from intrauterine to extrauterine life
2. To provide freedom from trauma such as injury and infection
3. To provide opportunities to continue the relationship with the primary caretakers begun in the prenatal period

Goals for the parents include the following:

1. To provide the client with knowledge, skill, and confidence relevant to child care activities
2. To provide opportunities that help parents recognize their knowledge of the infant's behavior begun prenatally, and
3. To provide opportunities to reorganize and intensify relationships with their newborn

Implementation

The nurse assumes various caretaking roles in the care of the newborn and his or her parents. The nurse can be support person, teacher/counselor/advocate, or technician. The roles may be assumed singly or in combination, depending upon client needs.

Much of the mother's knowledge concerning infant care stems directly from previous experience with infants, folkways learned from her ethnic or social group, and teaching by professionals during parent-craft classes. For the new parent with little skill in child care, these activities can cause much anxiety. Support from the nursing staff in the mother's beginning efforts can be an important factor in her seeking and accepting help in the future.

TECHNICIAN

The technical aspects of neonatal care include techniques for health maintenance, detection of disability, and institution of remedial measures. These techniques can be used for teaching purposes. Careful and concise recording of client responses or laboratory results contributes to the continuous supervision vital to mother and fetus.

Protective environment. The provision of a protective environment is basic to the care of the newborn. In hospitals the construction, maintenance, and operation of nurseries in accredited hospitals are directed by national professional organizations such as the American Academy of Pediatrics and local or state governing bodies. Detailed information concerning standards of care for newborn nurseries may be obtained from a number of sources (see Appendix B). Prescribed standards cover areas such as the following:

1. *Environmental factors:* provision of adequate lighting, elimination of potential fire hazards, safety of electric appliances, adequate ventilation, controlled temperature (warm and free of drafts) and humidity (lower than 50%).

2. *Measures to control infection:* adequate floor space

to permit positioning bassinets at least 60 cm (24 in) apart, hand-washing facilities, techniques for safe formula preparation and storage, and cleaning and sterilizing of equipment and supplies.

In addition, hospital personnel develop their own policies and procedures directed for protecting the newborns under their care. For instance:

1. Nursery personnel are restricted to those directly involved in the care of mothers or infants. This restriction minimizes the number of people to whom each infant is exposed, thereby reducing the introduction of pathogenic organisms. In this respect children born at home are at an advantage because other people who come in contact usually are family members. This home environment is somewhat duplicated in hospitals when the infant and mother "room together." The mother and father are active in the care, thereby reducing the number of nursing personnel involved. In many hospitals, nurseries are constructed with anterooms. Physicians carry out examinations here and procedures such as circumcisions. Parents may also come here to feed and hold their infants when the newborn must remain in the hospital for care.

2. Personnel assigned to the nursery wear special uniforms or cover gowns, and before beginning the care of infants, they carry out a *hand-washing technique*.

3. Anyone coming from "outside" is expected to gown and *wash his or her hands* before coming in contact with infants or equipment. Such people include nurses, physicians, parents, brothers and sisters, department supervisors, electricians, and housekeepers (Fig. 20.27, *A* to *C*).

4. Individuals with infectious conditions are excluded from contact with newborns; this includes people with upper respiratory tract infections, gastrointestinal tract infections, and infectious skin conditions. Most agencies have now coupled this day-to-day screening of personnel with yearly health examinations.

Routine assessment of the infant. Evaluation of the infant is a continuous process. Whenever any care is given to a newborn, observations and recordings of the child's progress are made. At the beginning of each 8-hour shift the following assessments are made, compared with the norm, and recorded:

1. Respiratory rate, rhythm, and effort
2. Breath sounds
3. Heart rate and rhythm
4. Skin color
5. Activity level and muscle tone
6. Feeding behavior

The nurse will be expected to perform or assist with assessment techniques such as obtaining specimens for laboratory analysis. Most of these techniques cause some discomfort or pain to the infant and therefore the infant may have to be restrained. The child needs to be held and comforted after completion of the procedures.

Restraining the infant. Reasons for restraining an infant include (1) protecting the infant from injury, (2) facilitating examinations, and (3) limiting discomfort during tests, procedures, and specimen collections. When restraining an infant, one must keep in mind special considerations:

1. Check the infant frequently.
2. Apply restraints, and check them frequently to prevent skin irritation and circulatory impairment.
3. Maintain proper body alignment.
4. Apply restraints without use of knots or pins if possible. If knots are necessary, make the kind that can be released quickly. Use pins with care to prevent puncture wounds and pressure areas—and to prevent the infant's swallowing one of them.
5. If the child is in an incubator, secure him or her to the mattress to protect the extremities, especially when the lid is raised or the mattress moved.

Mummy technique. The mummy technique is used with the stronger, more vigorous newborn. It is used during examinations, treatments, or specimen collections that involve the head and neck.

Equipment includes a blanket and one or two large safety pins (Fig. 20.28, *A*).

The procedure is as follows:

1. Spread blanket on flat surface; crib should suffice.
2. Fold over one corner (12 o'clock position).
3. Lay newborn on blanket so that neck is at fold.
4. Fold corner at 9 o'clock position over right shoulder; tuck this corner securely under infant's left side.
5. Bring corner at 6 o'clock position up over feet and tuck it either under infant's left side or, if long enough, fold it over blanket, crossing it under infant's chin.
6. Swing corner of 3 o'clock position snugly over infant and fold under infant's right side. Pin this corner into place.

Extremity restraints. This type of restraint is used to control movements of the infant's arms or legs. It is used during many procedures, such as intubating or gavage feedings.

Equipment includes gauze strips or wide strips of soft material and cotton wadding; pins are optional.

The procedure depends on which type of extremity restraints is used. Following are examples:

1. *Pad extremity with cotton wadding.* Fold one end of gauze strip over extremity and pin. Pin other end to mattress.
2. *Clove-hitch restraint.* Arrange a long strip of mate-

Fig. 20.27
Protection for the newborn. **A,** Brother prepares to meet his new sister by washing his hands and **B,** gowning. **C,** All family members wear gowns when coming close to baby in hospital. (Courtesy Marjorie Pyle, RNC, Life circle, Costa Mesa, California.)

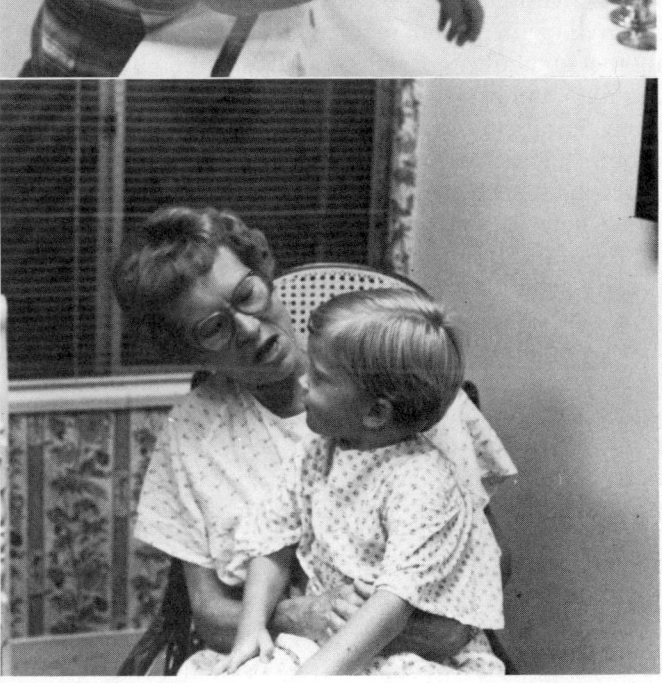

A

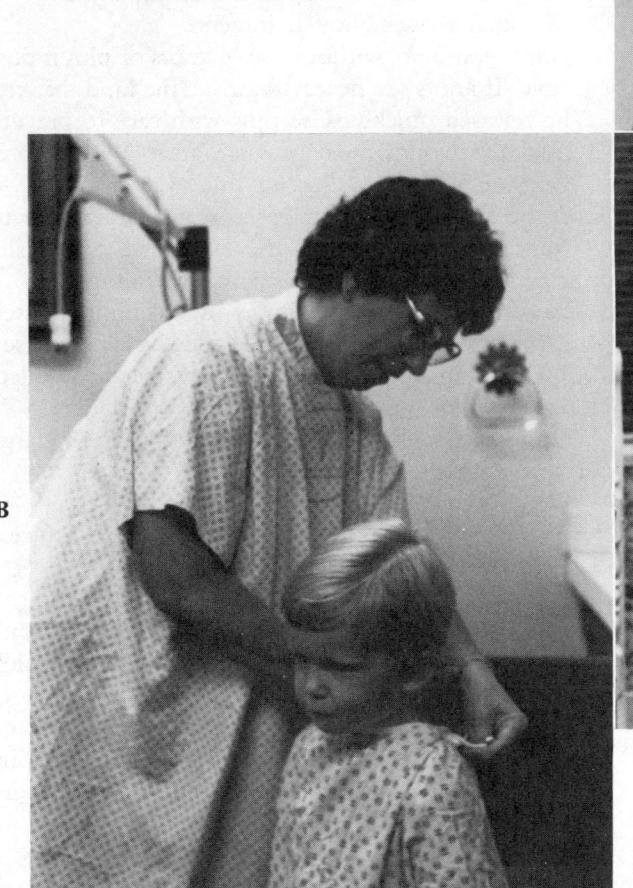

B

C

rial that is 5 cm (2 in) wide as shown in Fig. 20.28, *B* and *C*. Loop device over extremity, which has been padded with cotton; pin loose ends to mattress. Clove hitch does not tighten even if infant's movements tug on restraint.

Towel support. Although the towel support is not a true restraint, it controls the infant's position and movement. The towel may be rolled and placed at the infant's back or sides or folded and placed under the neck or upper back. A towel support has the following advantages:

1. It provides comfort and security by stabilizing the infant's position.
2. It maintains positioning to assist respiratory effort and gastrointestinal functions and prevent skin breakdown.
3. It prevents the infant from rolling against the incubator wall, where the child may lose heat by convection.
4. It prevents the infant from falling out of the incubator when the lid is lifted.

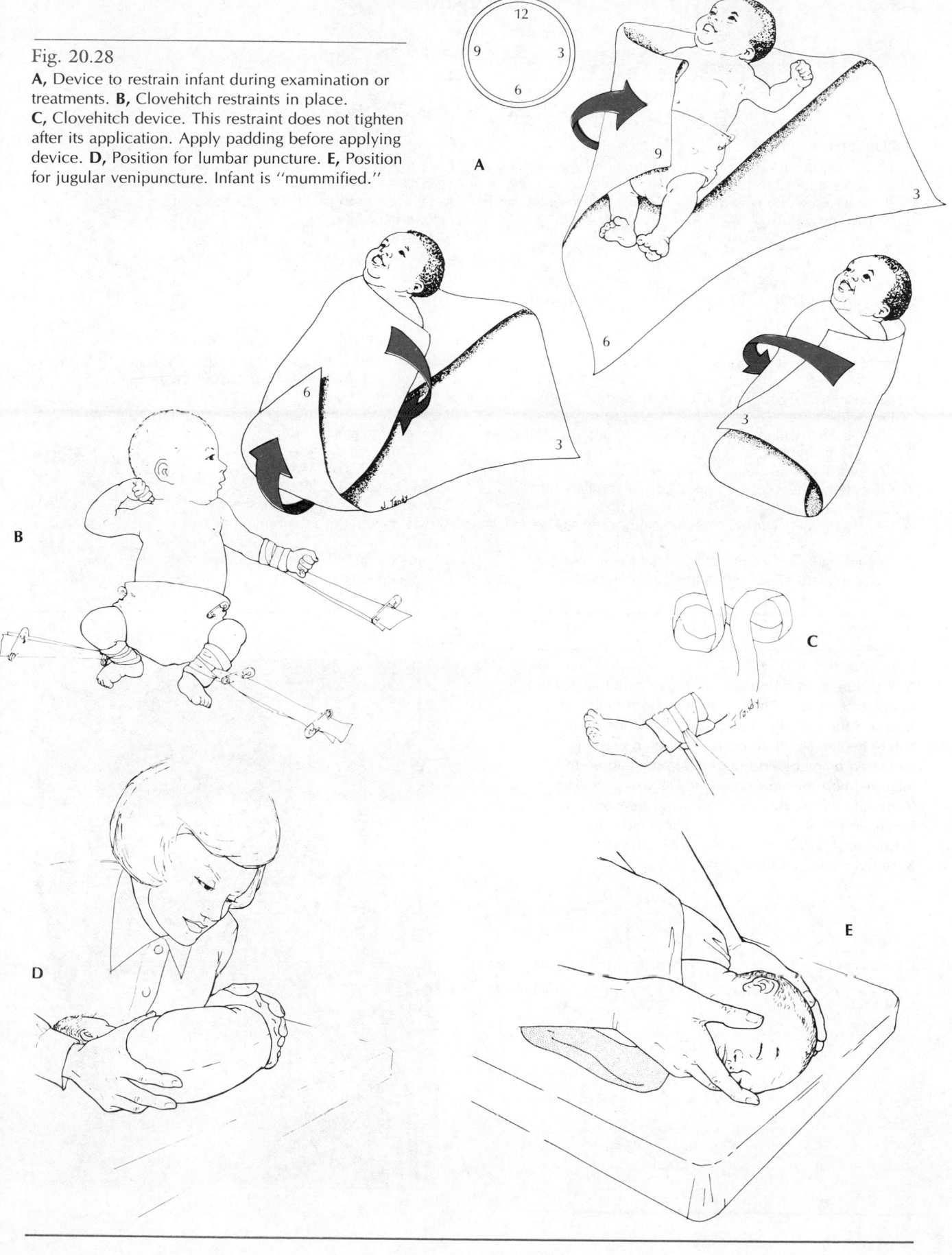

Fig. 20.28

A, Device to restrain infant during examination or treatments. **B,** Clovehitch restraints in place. **C,** Clovehitch device. This restraint does not tighten after its application. Apply padding before applying device. **D,** Position for lumbar puncture. **E,** Position for jugular venipuncture. Infant is "mummified."

Procedure 20.1

HEEL STICK (Fig. 20.29)

PURPOSE
1. To obtain blood for the determination of the infant's glucose level and hematocrit
2. To test for phenylketonuria (PKU), galactosemia, and hypothyroidism

EQUIPMENT
1. Bard-Parker No. 11 or Redi-Lance blade
2. 70% alcohol
3. Sterile cotton pledget or gauze square
4. Capillary tube
5. Plastic bandage
6. Laboratory slip and label

NURSING ACTION	RATIONALE
Identify infant.	Ensures procedure is done on correct infant.
Select correct site on heel (Fig. 20.29, *A*).	Residual scars and corn formation may result if procedure is not done in proper area of the heel.
Cleanse heel by rubbing with 70% alcohol.	Prevents infection.
Dry with sterile cotton pledget or gauze square.	Prevents introduction of contaminants into puncture.
Use blade to puncture heel deep enough to obtain free flow of blood.	Allows sufficient blood for test.
Discard first drop.	Minimizes contamination.
Quickly collect blood in appropriate capillary tubes.	Blood coagulates quickly.
Cover puncture area with plastic bandage.	Prevents bleeding or infection.
Send specimen with completed laboratory slip for analysis.	Allows ongoing evaluation and adjustment of care plans.
Record time, site of puncture, infant response	Ensures communication with other caretakers.
Cuddle infant when procedure is completed.	Prompts feeling of safety.

Fig. 20.29

A, Puncture sites (x) on sole of infant's foot for heel-stick samples of capillary blood. **B,** Newborn with foot wrapped for warmth to increase blood flow to extremity before heel stick. Note posture, linea nigra, and increased pigmentation of genital area caused by maternal hormones of pregnancy. Baby is smiling. (**A** modified from Babson, S.G., and Benson, R.C.: Management of high-risk pregnancy and intensive care of the neonate, ed. 3, St. Louis, 1975, The C.V. Mosby Co. **B,** photograph by I.M. Bobak.)

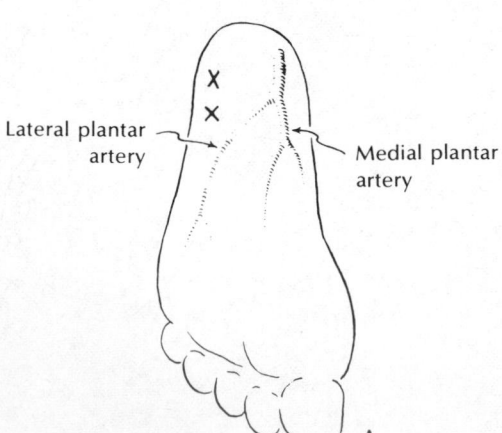

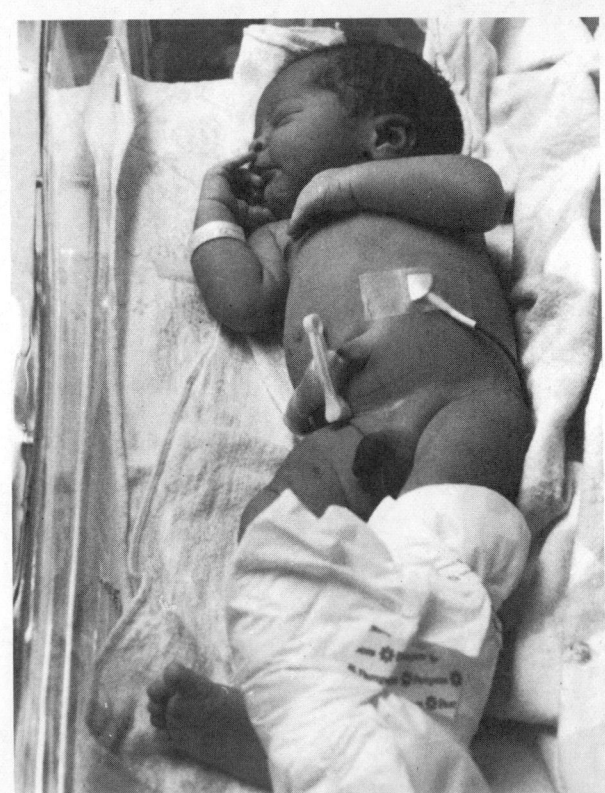

Procedure 20.2

ASSISTING WITH A VENIPUNCTURE

PURPOSE
To obtain blood specimen for laboratory analysis

EQUIPMENT
1. Restraint blanket
2. Sterile syringe and needles
3. Labeled specimen tubes
4. Laboratory slips
5. Sterile alcohol wipes

NURSING ACTION	RATIONALE
Identify infant.	Ensures procedure is done on correct infant.
Position and restrain infant	Facilitates venipuncture. Prevents tissue trauma.
Femoral venipuncture: Position child in frog posture; place hands over infant's knees. Avoid pressure of fingers over inner aspect of thigh because vein in this area may be occluded.	
External jugular venipuncture: (Fig. 20.28, *E*) "Mummy" infant as necessary. Lower infant's head over rolled towel, edge of table, or your knee, and stabilize.	
Handle infant gently; talk quietly to infant during procedure.	
After venipuncture, apply pressure over area with sterile gauze for 1 to 3 min.	Prevents leakage of additional blood into tissues or formation of hematoma (later this may result in hyperbilirubinemia). If infant is vigorous, direct pressure, restraint, and comforting prevent activity that could initiate or prolong bleeding.
Observe infant for 1 hour.	Facilitates detection of further bleeding (oozing, hematoma). Enclosed bleeding can lead to hypovolemic shock, hyperbilirubinemia, or both.
Send specimen with completed slip for analysis.	Allows ongoing evaluation and adjustment of care plan.
Record time, site, amount of blood taken, reason for specimen, infant's response.	Ensures communication with other caretakers.
Cuddle infant when procedure is completed.	Prompts feelings of safety.

Restraint without appliance. The nurse may restrain the infant by using the hands and body. Fig. 20.28, *D*, illustrates restraint of the infant in position for lumbar puncture.

Collection of specimens. Ongoing evaluation of a newborn requires obtaining blood and urine specimens. The following procedures are used for collecting those specimens.

Maintenance of an adequate oxygen supply. Four conditions are essential for maintenance of an adequate oxygen supply:

1. A clear airway, fundamental to adequate ventilation
2. Respiratory efforts, necessary to ensure continued ventilation
3. A functioning cardiopulmonary system, essential to maintain oxygen
4. Heat support, necessary because exposure to cold stress increases oxygen needs

Maintenance of clear airway. Generally the normal full-term infant born vaginally has little difficulty clearing the air passages. Most secretions are drained by gravity, propelled to the oropharynx by the cough reflex, to be drained or swallowed. The infant is maintained in a side-lying position with a rolled blanket at the back to facilitate drainage (Fig. 29.31). If excessive mucus is present, the foot of the crib is elevated and the oropharynx is suctioned with a bulb syringe or a catheter and DeLee mucus trap. The nurse's knowledge and skill in suctioning may be critical in helping both normal and distressed infants establish or maintain adequate respirations. "Milking" the trachea is ineffective. This procedure may injure cartilage and will often delay effective suctioning. During all procedures heat loss must be avoided or minimized for the infant. This is accomplished by drying, wrapping, and placing the infant in a warmed Kreisselmann or comparable

URINE SPECIMEN

PURPOSE
To obtain urine specimen for analysis

EQUIPMENT
A variety of urine specimen collection bags are available, usually with accompanying instruction. Although the following directions are specific to the U-bag (Hollister Inc., Chicago), they are generally applicable to many other types.

NURSING ACTION	RATIONALE
Identify infant.	Ensures procedure is done on correct infant.
Separate infant's legs. Make sure pubic and perineal area is clean, dry, and free of mucus. Do not apply powders, oils, or lotions to skin.	Ensures leak-proof seal. Decreases chance of contamination.
Remove protective paper, exposing hypoallergenic adhesive (Fig. 20.30, A).	Exposes adhesive. Decreases chance of allergic reaction.
For girls, stretch perineum to flatten skin folds. Press adhesive firmly to skin all around urinary meatus and vagina. (NOTE: start with narrow portion of butterfly-shaped adhesive patch). *Be sure to start at bridge of skin separating rectum from vagina and work upward.* (Fig. 20.30, B).	Ensures leak-proof seal. Decreases chance of contamination from urine and stool.
For boys, tuck penis and scrotum through aperture of collector before removing protective paper from adhesive. Fit bag over penis, and press flaps firmly to perineum, making sure entire adhesive coating is firmly attached to skin with no puckering of adhesive. (Fig. 20.30, C).	
To drain, hold bag in left hand. Tilt bag so urine is away from blue tab. Remove tab and drain into clean receptacle (Fig. 20.30, D).	Facilitates emptying without use of scissors, which can contaminate or be contaminated.
or	
Apply the 24-hour U-Bag in the manner just described; Direct the drainage into a receptacle. The collection tube can be shortened or capped (Fig. 20.30, E). See directions accompanying the bag.	
Send specimen with completed laboratory slip for analysis.	Allows ongoing evaluation.
Record time, reason for specimen to laboratory.	Ensures communication with other care givers.

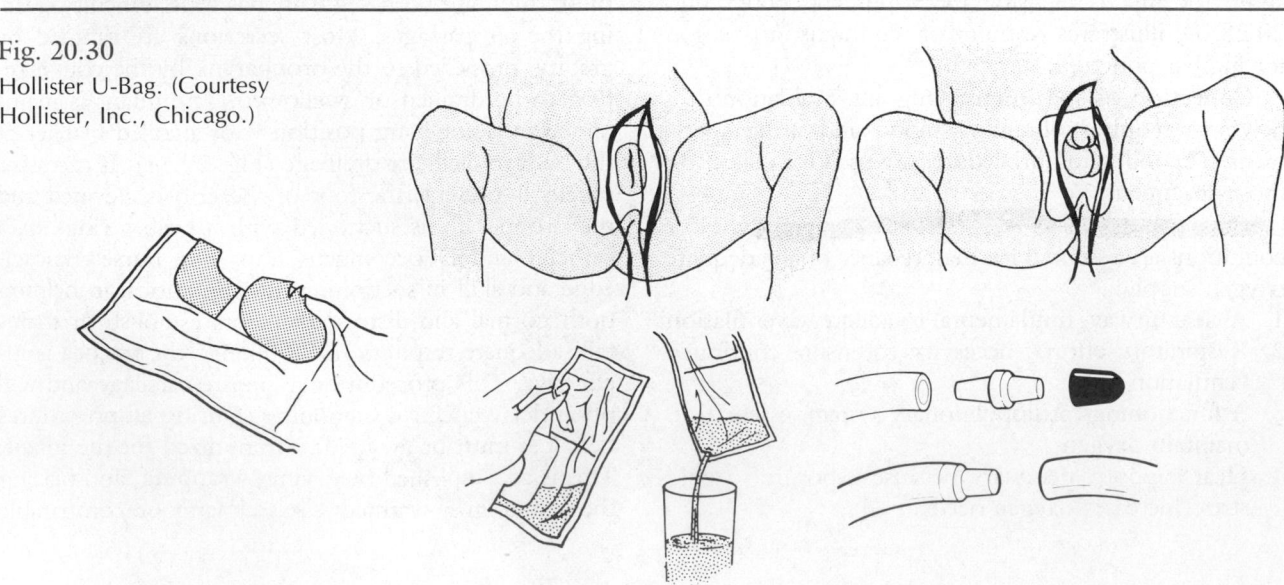

Fig. 20.30
Hollister U-Bag. (Courtesy Hollister, Inc., Chicago.)

Fig. 20.31
Infant is turned to right side and supported in this position to facilitate drainage from mouth.

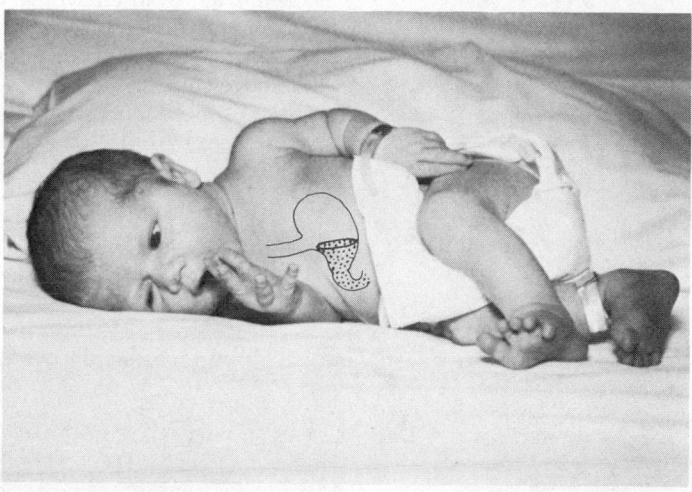

Procedure 20.4

SUCTIONING OF UPPER AIRWAY: ASPIRATION OF MOUTH AND NOSE (Fig. 20.32, *A-C*)

PURPOSE
To remove mucus from the mouth and nose

EQUIPMENT
Sterile bulb syringe (intact and fairly firm)

NURSING ACTION	RATIONALE
Position infant: Support the wrapped infant on the arm or on the hip (in a football hold), positioning the child's head downward. *Never* suspend infant by ankles in head-down position.	Assists gravity drainage. Raises cerebral venous pressure, increases the risk of accidently dropping the infant, hyperextends and stretches the spine, and is painful to the baby.
Suction mouth first.	Sensitive receptors around the nares respond to stimuli by initiating gasp. Any mucus present could be pulled into lower airway.
Compress the bulb *before* insertion, expelling air.	Prevents blowing secretions deeper into mouth and nose.
Insert syringe into space between cheek and gums, release compression gradually, and create suction (to suck out mucus).	Prevents tissue trauma and removes secretions.
Remove from mouth. Compress syringe to empty it and to create new vacuum to repeat procedure.	Prevents secretions being forced into respiratory tract.
Repeat steps 2 and 3 as needed in mouth, then in nose. Stop suctioning when cry is clear (infant cry does not sound as though there were mucus or a bubble in the mouth).	If cry is clear, infant's airway is patent.
Cuddle and reassure infant once episode is over.	Infant's feeling of discomfort and fear and subsequent crying increases need for oxygen.
Demonstrate care of gagging or choking infant to parents.	Learning to meet this emergency in the hospital increases parental self-confidence and self-esteem and prepares parents for this activity at home.
Supervise parents in the technique.	Permits correction of any parental errors.

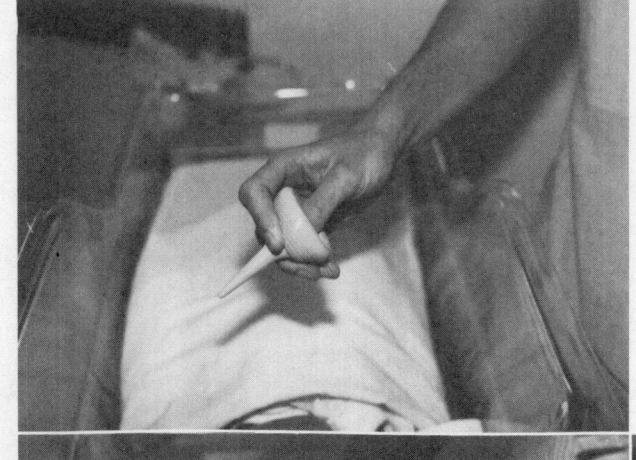

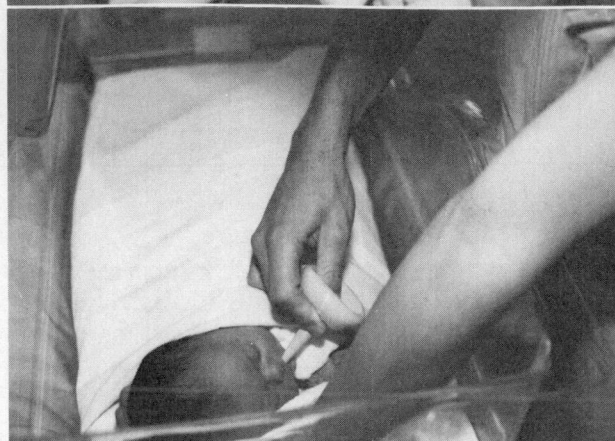

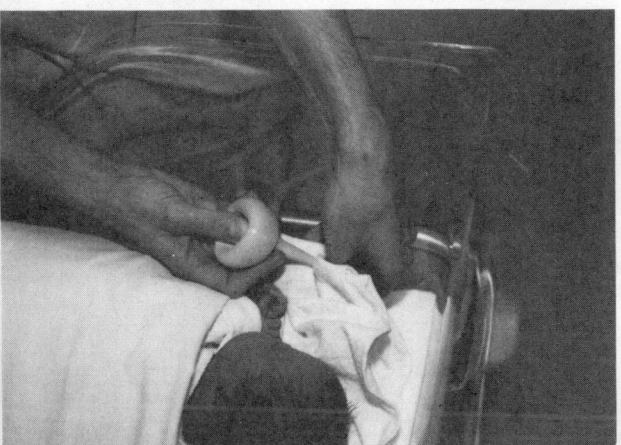

Fig. 20.32
Use of bulb syringe. **A,** Compress bulb before insertion, expelling air. **B,** Insert syringe into space between cheek and gum, and release compression gradually to create suction. **C,** Remove syringe from mouth, compress syringe to remove contents, and repeat procedure until airway is clear. **D,** DeLee mucus-trap catheter. (**A, B,** and **C,** photographs by I.M. Bobak.)

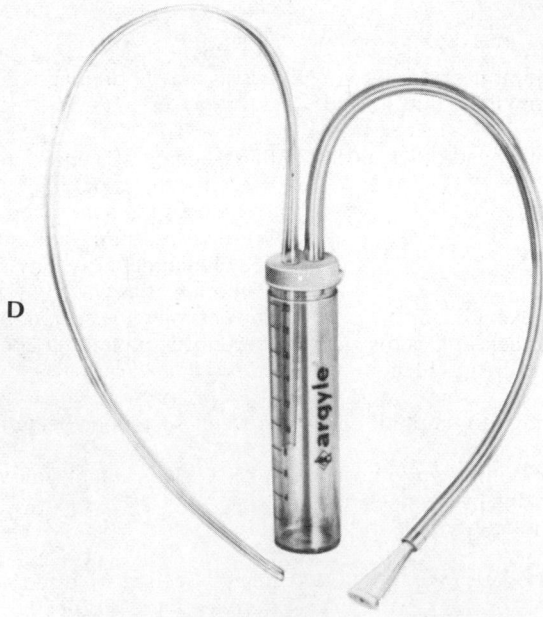

SUCTIONING OF MIDAIRWAY (NASOPHARYNX AND OROPHARYNX) AND STOMACH ASPIRATION USING THE DELEE MUCUS TRAP (Fig. 20.32, *D*)

PURPOSE

1. To remove mucus from the nasopharynx and oro-pharynx
2. To remove amniotic fluid from the stomach

EQUIPMENT

Sterile DeLee mucus trap catheter (available in reusable glass or disposable plastic), with two-hole tip

NURSING ACTION	RATIONALE
Position infant in supine position.	Facilitates suctioning.
Lubricate catheter in sterile water. A 120 ml (4 oz) bottle of sterile water for feeding is convenient, is already in sterile container, and decreases risk of contamination possible with large stock bottles.	Facilitates passage of tube and prevents infection.
Aspirate mouth and throat first, then the nose.	Prevents inhalation of pharyngeal contents.
Insert catheter:	Decreases risk of laryngeal spasm and reflex apnea.
Orally along base of tongue.	
Nasally horizontally into nares, then raising it to advance it beyond bend at back of nares.	
Avoid forcing catheter.	**Hazard:** direct tissue trauma or perforation in presence of congenital anomalies such as choanal, esophageal, or intestinal atresia.
Suction is supplied by operator.	Negative pressure obtained in mucus trap is sufficient to withdraw mucus or other substances.
Limit suctioning to 10 s or less.	Prolonged suctioning stimulates laryngospasm and reduces air (O_2) content in airway.
Apply suction only as tube is withdrawn.	Prevents direct tissue trauma.
Rotate catheter when suctioning.	Prevents tissue trauma consequent to tissue's being drawn into eye of catheter.
Discontinue suctioning when:	Gagging indicates entrance into esophagus; coughing indicates entrance into trachea.
The cry is clear.	
Air entry into lungs is heard by stethoscope.	
Cuddle infant.	Reassures infant.
Detach mucus trap and send the enclosed specimen to the laboratory for examination and culture as necessary.	Allows ongoing evaluation of infant's condition.
Cuddle infant and reassure.	Prompts feeling of safety.
Record the amount of mucus or amniotic fluid removed.	Ensures communication with other care givers.

crib or under overhead radiant heat or another source of heat. In addition a humidified oxygen source and equipment for the administration of oxygen must be readily available. The nurse must be prepared to carry out the following life-saving procedures if the need arises.

Maintenance of respiratory efforts. The normal term infant establishes respirations within minutes of birth, usually without undue difficulty. However, nursery personnel need to be skilled in the techniques for reestablishing respirations and providing increased oxygen in case the need arises.

Maintenance of cardiopulmonary function. Cardiac arrest can occur in term newborns who have experienced stress. Careful monitoring of infants is essential if treatment is to be instituted rapidly.

Maintenance of infant's temperature. Cold stress is detrimental to the newborn. It increases the need for oxygen and can upset the acid/base balance. The temperature may be taken either by axilla or rectum every hour until stabilized (Fig. 20.5). Initial temperatures as low as 36° C (96.8° F) are not uncommon. By the twelfth hour the temperature should stabilize at 36.5° C (97.6° F). The nurse can help stabilize the infant's

Text continued on p. 558.

Procedure 20.6

SUCTIONING OF MIDAIRWAY (NASOPHARYNX AND OROPHARYNX) USING A NASOPHARYNGEAL CATHETER WITH MECHANICAL SUCTION APPARATUS

PURPOSE

To remove excessive or tenacious mucus from the naso-pharynx and oropharynx in resuscitating an infant

EQUIPMENT

1. Catheters
   a. French, rubber (moderately firm); sizes 10, 12, and 14; whistle tip; two-hole tip
   b. French, plastic disposable: sizes 8, 10, and 12; finger control; two-hole tip
2. External suction source
3. Sterile water

NURSING ACTION	RATIONALE
Position the infant: 　Place the infant in the supine position. 　Place a folded towel under the head to move it slightly forward from the neck (as in sniffing). Adjust negative pressure on portable and wall gauges. Keep deep suctioning to a minimum.	To (a) separate tongue from pharyngeal wall and (b) prevent obstruction of newborn's normally low palate and macroglossia. (Some physicians prefer to work with the baby on a flat surface with no towel.) Prevents excessive suction. **Hazards:** Direct trauma to mucosa with edema formation, bleeding, or increased secretions. Stimulation of vagal reflex; bradycardia, cardiac arrhythmias, laryngospasm, and apnea, especially if this type of suctioning is done within first few minutes of infant's birth.
Limit each suctioning to 10 s or less. If infant is active, an attendant may be needed to stabilize infant's head. Or if there is time, restrain infant by mummy technique before this procedure. Lubricate catheter in sterile water. A 120 ml (4 oz) bottle of sterile water for feeding is convenient, is already in sterile container, and reduces risk of contamination possible with large stock bottles. Suction is *off* as tube is put into position. Avoid forcing catheter.	Prevents laryngospasm and oxygen depletion. Prevents trauma and affects suctioning. Both hands are needed to manipulate catheter and finger control of suction pressure. Facilitates passage of tube and prevents infection. Prevents direct tissue trauma. **Hazard:** direct tissue trauma or perforation in presence of congenital anomalies such as choanal, esophageal, or intestinal atresia. Decreases risk of laryngeal spasm and reflex apnea.
Insert catheter: 　Orally along base of tongue. 　Nasally horizontally into nares, then raising it to advance it beyond bend at back of nares. With catheter in place, place thumb over finger control to create suction. Rotate tubing between fingers while withdrawing catheter. Apply suction only as tube is withdrawn. Rotate catheter when suctioning.	Prevents direct trauma caused by drawing mucosa into eye of catheter. Prevents direct tissue trauma. Prevents tissue trauma consequent to tissue's being drawn into eye of catheter.
Observe infant's response. Withdraw tube to suction posterior nasopharynx. Comfort infant. Record procedure.	Gagging indicates entrance into esophagus; coughing indicates entrance into trachea. Prompts feelings of safety. Ensures communication with other care givers.

Procedure 20.7

MOUTH-TO-MOUTH RESUSCITATION

PURPOSE
To reestablish respiration

EQUIPMENT
None needed

NURSING ACTION	RATIONALE
Clear airway of any mucus or debris.	Prevents propelling debris down airway.
Position infant in "sniffing" position by putting rolled towel under head to move it slightly forward from neck, or leave baby on flat surface.	Opens airway by straightening trachea and permitting back of tongue to fall away from posterior pharynx.
Insert plastic airway if available.	Provides unobstructed airway (especially from tongue if infant is flaccid).
Place your mouth over infant's nose and mouth to create seal.	Permits insufflation under pressure.
Repeat the word *ho* as you gently puff volume of air *in your cheeks* into infant. *Do not* force air.	Prevents injury to lung tissue (e.g., pneumothorax, pneumomediastinum).
Repeat puffs at rate of 30/min.	Approximate normal respiratory rhythm.
Infant's chest should rise slightly with each puff; keep fingers on chest wall to sense air entry.	Determines if air is reaching alveolar level.
Allow chest to fall by passive recoil.	Allows removal of insufflated air.
If available, place tubing of oxygen in your mouth as you inhale quickly between puffs.	Increases O_2 content in insufflated air.
Consider airway obstruction. Prepare for laryngoscopy and endotracheal intubation aspiration. See hospital procedure manual.	Chest wall does not rise and the infant's vital responses do not improve in 30 s.
Record procedure.	Ensures communication with other care givers.

Procedure 20.8

OXYGEN THERAPY

PURPOSE
To increase level of O_2 in respired air and thereby increase level of arterial Po_2

EQUIPMENT
1. *Incubator.* The maintenance of a high and constant level of oxygen in an incubator is almost impossible because (1) the mechanism cannot achieve concentrations beyond 60% to 70% ambient oxygen and (2) oxygen rapidly dissipates into the room whenever the incubator's lid or portholes are opened.
    or
2. *Plastic hood.* The plastic hood is suitable for administering humidified oxygen warmed to 31° to 34° C (87.8°-93.2° F). It is also useful inside the incubator; the porthole or lid can be opened without affecting oxygen levels inside the hood (Fig. 31.5) Another advantage is that the plastic hood is practical outside the incubator when the infant is being treated. An overhead radiant heater maintains a thermoneutral environment for the infant at this time.

NURSING ACTION	RATIONALE
Assess infant for symptoms of hypoxemia, including cyanosis, the most frequent indication, indirect bradycardia (heart rate of less than 100 beats/min), hypothermia (temperature of less than 35.5° C [95.9° F]), prolonged periods of apnea (apnea episodes longer than 15 s), and anemia.	Oxygen is vital to an infant at birth for hypoxemia, to counteract acidosis, to promote pulmonary blood flow and closure of the ductus arteriosus, and to maintain capillary integrity.

Continued.

Procedure 20.8—cont'd

OXYGEN THERAPY

NURSING ACTION	RATIONALE
Send specimens for laboratory assessments of blood gases and acid-base status to determine oxygen needs.	Clinical measurements may be insufficient to determine oxygen need, since some noncyanotic (pink) infants are hypoxemic.
Individualize positioning of infant.	The infant's particular needs are considered: the amount of secretions; the maturity of gag, swallow, and cough reflexes; and the maturity of neuromuscular and skeletal systems.
Place infant on firm mattress.	There is no need to elevate the head. Abdominal contents in a normal abdomen offer no difficulty to diaphragmatic movement. Furthermore, with the head elevated, pulmonary secretions are more likely to pool if the head of the bed is elevated.
Flex and abduct infant's arms and place at sides.	Weight of arms is kept off chest. Facilitates greater thoracic expansion.
Avoid use of diapers, or pin diapers on loosely.	Assists infant's efforts to use abdominal muscles for respirations.
Extend neck slightly to "sniffing" position or leave infant flat.	Lessens tracheal obstruction by extending trachea. Prevents hyperextension obstruction from low palate or macroglossia. Overextension may make it difficult or impossible for infant to swallow secretions. Hyperextension also causes apposition of vocal cords so glottis is considerably smaller than otherwise. This impedes entry of air into larynx and from there to rest of respiratory tract.
Check towel placement frequently.	Obstruction may occur from flexion or overextension of neck (towel under head).
Turn infant from side to side every 1 to 2 hours.	Facilitates drainage of pulmonary secretions and prevents skin breakdown.
Monitor oxygen levels carefully to regulate oxygen dosage. Oxygen dosage should be sufficient to relieve cyanosis.	Oxygen overdosage results in tissue damage and can cause the following:
Administer 100% oxygen by mask or bag for short periods for cyanotic episodes.	**Hazards:** Bronchopulmonary dysplasia. This histologic change observed in pulmonary tissue is a thickening of the alveolar walls, epithelial lining, and basement membranes.
	Eyesight may be slightly to severely impaired, or total blindness (retrolental fibroplasia) may ensue. In the retina, oxygen overdose causes vasoconstriction and, later, ischemia. About 2 months after the cessation of oxygen therapy, these retinal vessels dilate, leading to edema, scarring, and detachment.
Send specimen of blood to laboratory for analysis. Laboratory values used to determine dosage are the following:	
■ Blood pH between 7.35 and 7.44	
■ Arterial Po_2 between 50 and 70 mm Hg (for the premature infant, 90 mm Hg may be too high and may expose the child to sequelae of oxygen overdosage. Although the precise figure is unknown, an arterial Po_2 of 65 mm Hg should be safer).	
■ Arterial hemoglobin saturation between 85% and 90% (based on fetal maturity).	
Newer methods of continuous monitoring of oxygen tension are available; these methods permit moment-to-moment changes in administration of oxygen.	Necrotizing enterocolitis (NEC) is a possible sequel if the infant survives.
Record procedure.	Ensures communication with other caregivers.

CARDIOPULMONARY RESUSCITATION (Fig. 20.33)

PURPOSE

To prevent cardiac arrest following cessation of respirations (apnea extending beyond 15 s)

EQUIPMENT

Resuscitation equipment should be readily available in areas in which respiratory arrest might take place, and the status of this resuscitation equipment should be checked regularly, at least once a day

NURSING ACTION	RATIONALE
Palpate peripheral pulses and quickly check heartbeat.	Absence of carotid or temporal pulse is considered sufficient indication to begin external cardiac massage.
Position infant. The infant's spine must be supported during compression of the sternum.	Prevents injury.
Restore patent airway (by removal of foreign material and secretions if indicated).	Permits restoration of breathing.
Initiate cardiac massage.	Restores cardiac function without injuring the infant.
External pressure must be forceful but not traumatic.	
Apply sternal compression to small infants with both thumbs on the midsternum while joining the fingers of both hands behind the infant's back. It is best applied from the superior direction with the operator at the infant's head. This minimizes the chance of damage that might occur to the liver or spleen if applied from an inferior position. The *depth of compression* is adapted to the size of the child—for infants, 1 to 1.5 cm (0.5 to 0.75 in) (Fig. 20.33) The *rate of administration* for external massage is 100 to 120 times per minute.	
Ventilate infant at a ratio of *one breath for five to eight compressions* by the mouth-to-mouth method or artificial ventilator.	Maintains arterial P_{O_2} level.
Continue massage until signs of recovery occur, as indicated by palpable peripheral pulses, return of pupils to normal size, and the disappearance of mottling and cyanosis.	Ensures recovery.
Record time and duration of procedure and effects of intervention.	Ensures communication with other caretakers.

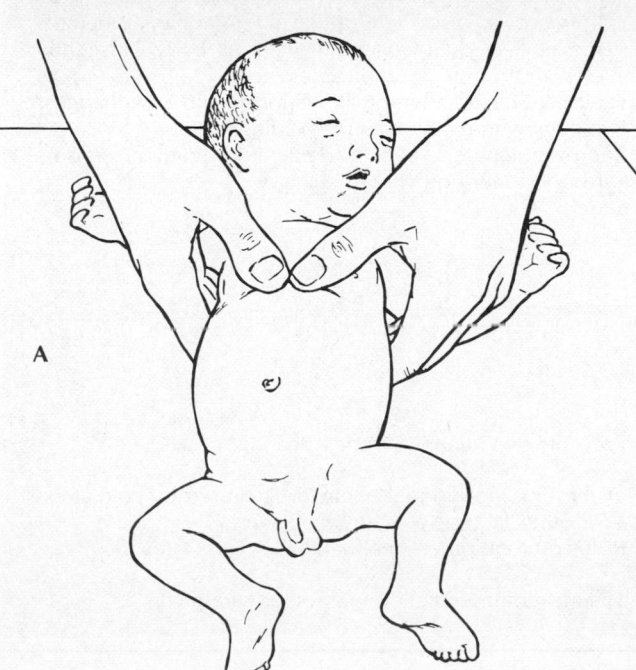
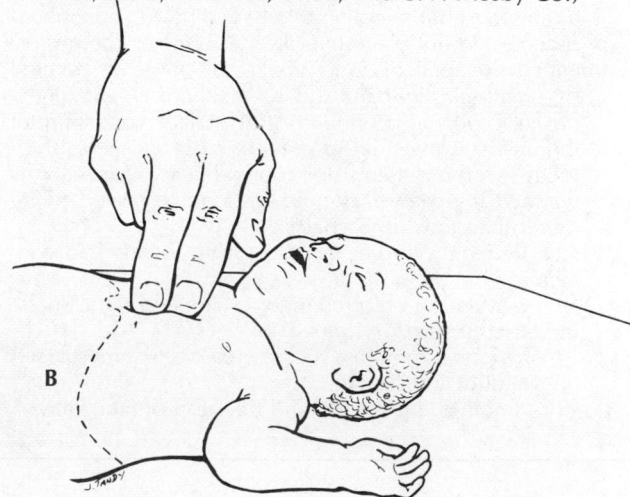

Fig. 20.33

A, Closed chest massage in small infant with thumbs superimposed over midsternum. **B,** Closed chest massage in infant with two fingers over midsternum. (From Whaley, L.F., and Wong, D.L.: Nursing care of infants and children, ed. 3, St. Louis, 1987, The C.V. Mosby Co.)

body temperature in one of the following ways:

1. Check the temperature in the nursery. (The ambient temperature of the nursery unit should be kept at 24° C [75° F].)
2. Keep the baby dry and wrapped in warmed blankets, taking care to keep the head well covered while the parent is holding the infant. (Check the baby's body temperature at least every hour until it is stabilized; this also helps prevent hyperthermia.)
3. Place the thoroughly dried, unclothed baby under a radiant heat panel until the body temperature is stabilized.
4. Perform examinations or other activities with the baby under a heat panel and postpone the initial bath until the newborn's temperature reaches 36.5° C (97.6° F). Minimize the heat loss.

Warming infant with hypothermia. Even a normal full-term baby in good health can become hypothermic. Birth in a car on the way to the hospital, a cold delivery room, or inadequate drying and wrapping immediately after birth may cause the infant's temperature to fall. Warming the hypothermic baby is accomplished with care. Rapid warming or cooling may cause apneic spells and acidosis in an infant. Therefore, the warming process is monitored to progress slowly over a period of 2 to 4 hours (Procedure 20.10).

Therapies. Certain techniques, such as administering vitamin K intramuscularly, are routine in newborn nurseries. Others, such as the therapy for treatment of hyperbilirubinemia and circumcision, are performed frequently. Nurses must become skilled in the use of therapies to ensure infant safety and therapeutic effec-

---

Procedure 20.10

WARMING INFANT USING OVERHEAD RADIANT HEATER

PURPOSE

To maintain or restore infant's body temperature.

EQUIPMENT

Overhead radiant heater. The heater thermostat must be kept plugged into an electric outlet at all times. It is set to maintain an abdominal skin temperature of 36.5° C (97.6° F). The set point of 36.4° C (97.5° F) is usually chosen for activation of the heater.

NURSING ACTION	RATIONALE
With warm, absorbent blanket, dry and place newborn under radiant heat shield.	Reduces heat loss by evaporation, conduction, convection, and radiation.
Adjust bassinet in head-down position (about 10 degrees).	Allows for gravity drainage of mucus in respiratory tract. If infant is suspected of having intracranial hemorrhage, keep head on same level as body or slightly elevated if mucus is not excessive.
Remove gross soiling (e.g., meconium, blood).	Facilitates observation of skin coloring and any changes.
Check thermostat setting for accuracy.	Prevents overheating or underheating.
Apply thermistor probe (metal side next to infant) with paper tape or nonirritating plastic tape (e.g., Hy-tape) to anterior abdominal wall between navel and xiphoid process; do not place over bony rib cage. Thermistor, after it is taped to abdominal wall, must be covered by small plastic-foam square insulator. Optimally it has a cover of aluminum foil. Foam insulation of thermistor is essential to prevent radiant heat from directly warming thermistor more quickly than baby is warmed (mechanism would respond to heated probe rather than to warmed baby).	Improves accuracy of skin temperature reading. Sensors respond more quickly to change.
Check frequently to ensure that probe retains skin contact.	Prevents overheating or underheating.
Observe infant for color change; crying and restlessness; increased respiratory rate.	Determine if abnormal behavior is caused by cold stress or other factors (e.g., debility, sepsis).
Note previous symptoms; recheck probe, thermostat setting, and heater contact.	Rules out equipment malfunction.
Record findings. Note time and duration of procedure.	Ensures communication with other care givers.

tiveness. Parents expect to be told the reasons for the particular therapy and what results to expect.

Therapy for hyperbilirubinemia. The goal of hyperbilirubinemia treatment is to help the newborn's body reduce serum levels of unconjugated bilirubin. The term infant may have trouble conjugating the increased amount of bilirubin derived from disintegrating fetal red blood cells; the serum levels of unconjugated bilirubin rise beyond the limits of normal 12 mg/dl. If untreated the levels can continue to rise and the risk of kernicterus increases (Chapter 31).

There are two principal methods for reducing serum bilirubin levels: exchange blood transfusion and phototherapy. Exchange transfusion is used to treat infants whose levels of bilirubin cannot be controlled by phototherapy (Chapter 31).

Phototherapy. Recent research (Speck, 1985) indicates that phototherapy causes a structural isomerization of bilirubin in the skin. During phototherapy infants form a substance called lumirubin, a water-soluble product. Lumirubin is formed slowly and excreted rapidly. Lumirubin is excreted both in the urine and feces. Since lumirubin is excreted efficiently by infants, increasing the formation of lumirubin improves the efficacy of phototherapy in the treatment of neonatal jaundice.

The effectiveness of phototherapy is increased by increasing the intensity of the light. An alternative method is to use *green* fluorescent light in place of *blue or white* light. Green fluorescent light does not appear to produce undesirable side effects (Speck, 1985). *Bronze baby syndrome* has occurred in some newborns

Procedure 20.11

WARMING INFANT USING SERVO-CONTROL INCUBATOR

PURPOSE

To maintain or restore infant's body temperature if it has not returned to normal within 2 hours using a radiant overhead heater.

EQUIPMENT

Servo-Control incubators or their equivalents employ the same principle as the thermostat in maintaining an even temperature in an oven or a room. The infant's skin temperature, rather than the circulating air, provides the point of control.

NURSING ACTION	RATIONALE
Set the incubator control panel at the predetermined physician-ordered level, usually between 36° and 37° C (96.8° and 98.6° F).	To maintain a skin temperature of 36.5° C (97.6 ° F).
Tape a thermistor probe (automatic sensor) from the control panel to the right upper quadrant of the abdomen immediately below the right infracostal margin.	Measurements of skin temperature provide a more reliable indicator of the energy exchange between the infant and the environment. The skin is an extremely sensitive indicator of the infant's thermal state. Receptors detect even minor changes resulting from peripheral vasoconstriction, dilatation, or increased metabolism long before a change in deep (core) body temperature develops. The abdominal skin temperature of 36.5° C (97.6 ° F) is considered optimum because at this temperature, oxygen consumption and metabolic rate are minimum. When the skin temperature is increased to 37.2° C (98.9° F), the oxygen consumption increases by 6%; a drop in skin temperature to 35.9° C (96.6° F) is accompanied by an increase in oxygen consumption by 10%.
Check the sensor periodically for its continued firm application to skin; check and record the core temperature (rectal) with a clinical thermometer; record incubator temperature readings.	Ensures proper functioning of the equipment.
Record skin temperature reading and the ambient temperature inside the incubator every 2 to 4 hours after the infant's temperature is stabilized.	Helps in assessing the maintenance of adequate body temperature.
Record the infant's general appearance and behavior.	Ensures communication with other caretakers.

Procedure 20.12

INTRAMUSCULAR INJECTION (Figs. 20.34 and 20.35)

PURPOSE
To administer medication

EQUIPMENT
1. Syringe and needle
2. Alcohol swab
3. Medication

NURSING ACTION	RATIONALE
Identify infant.	Ensures procedure is done on correct infant.
Restrain infant if necessary.	Infants offer little, if any, resistance to injections. Although they squirm and may be difficult to hold in position if they are awake, they can usually be restrained without assistance from a second person if the nurse is skilled.
Prepare medication (Fig. 20.34) (e.g., vitamin K [Aquamephyton, 0.5 mg]). Check physician's order. Check dosage and route of administration. Check medication.	Helps the newborn with clotting during the first week of life; vitamin K is administered to normal newborns as a routine measure.
Select site for injection.	Selection of the site for injection is important. Injections must be placed in muscles large enough to accommodate the medication, yet major nerves and blood vessels must be avoided. The muscles of newborns may not tolerate more than 0.5 ml. The preferred site for newborns is the vastus lateralis, although the rectus femoris muscle can also be used. These two muscles, except for the femoral artery on the medial aspect of the thigh, are free of important nerves and blood vessels. The vastus lateralis muscle is the larger of the two and is well developed in the newborn. NOTE: The posterior gluteal muscle is very small, poorly developed, and dangerously close to the sciatic nerve, which occupies a larger proportion of space in infants than in older children. Therefore it is not recommended as an injection site until the child has been walking for at least a year. The gluteal muscles develop with locomotion. Fig. 20.35, A, illustrates the location of the preferred intramuscular injection site for newborns.
Prepare injection site with alcohol cleansing.	Prevents infection.
Grasp the muscle mass of the thigh to be injected firmly in one hand and compress the muscle mass for injection with the other hand (Fig. 20.35, B).	Stabilizes the limb.
Inject the medication: Poise the needle just over the site (without touching the skin) and then insert the needle with a quick flexion of the wrist.	The dart method for injection is inappropriate when aiming at such a small target.
Comfort infant and settle in crib.	Allays tension.
Record medication, amount, route, and site of injection.	Ensures communication with other caretakers.

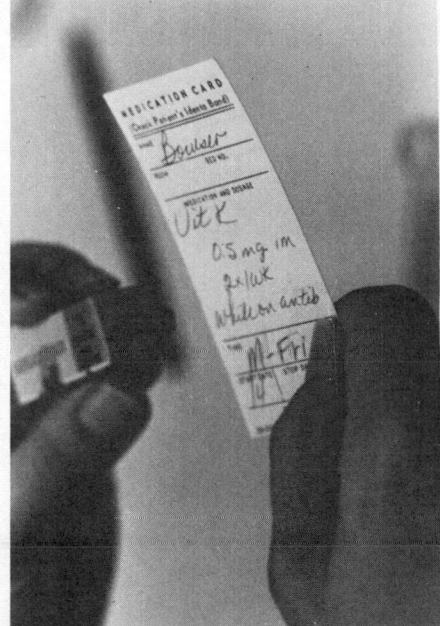

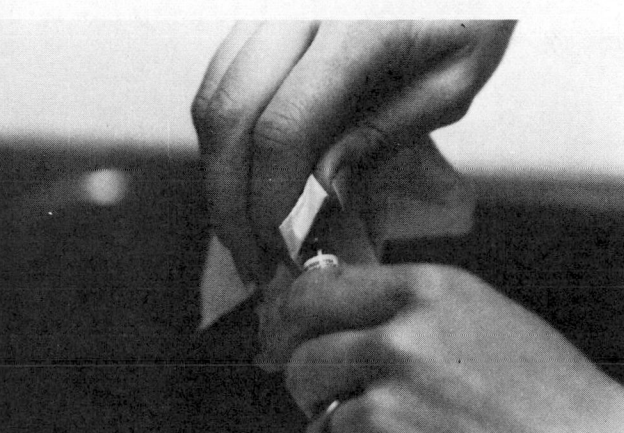

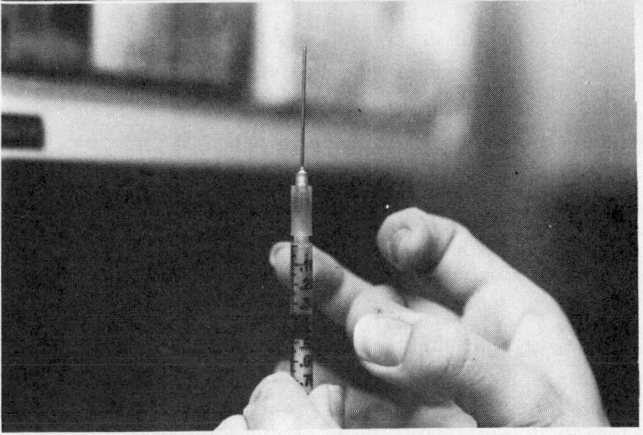

Fig. 20.34
A, Vitamin K$_1$ (Aquamephyton) container is checked against physician's order. **B,** Nurse has shaken medication to bottom of vial. She protects her fingers as she snaps off top with rapid wrist action. **C,** To avoid drawing small glass shards into syringe, nurse uses filter needle to withdraw medication. Nurse replaces filter needle with short, small-gauge tuberculin needle. Nurse records medication she has given on newborn's chart. (Photographs by I.M. Bobak.)

VASTUS LATERALIS MUSCLE
Landmarks
  1 Greater trochanter
  2 Knee
Injection site: lateral aspect of muscle mass in middle third of distance between landmarks; injected at 45 degree angle in direction of knee

Fig. 20.35
A, Acceptable intramuscular injection site for children, X, Injection site; Y, alternate injection site. **B,** Infant's leg stabilized for intramuscular injection. (From Whaley, L.F., and Wong, D.L.: Nursing care of infants and children, ed. 3, St. Louis, 1987, The C.V. Mosby Co.)

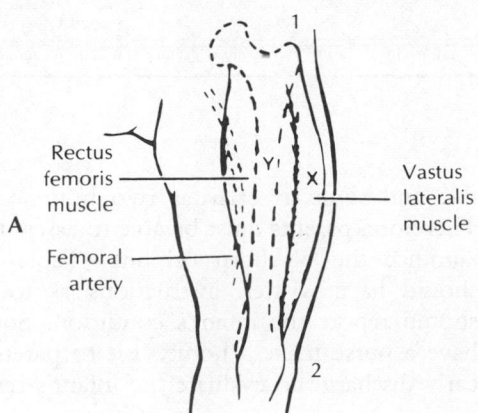

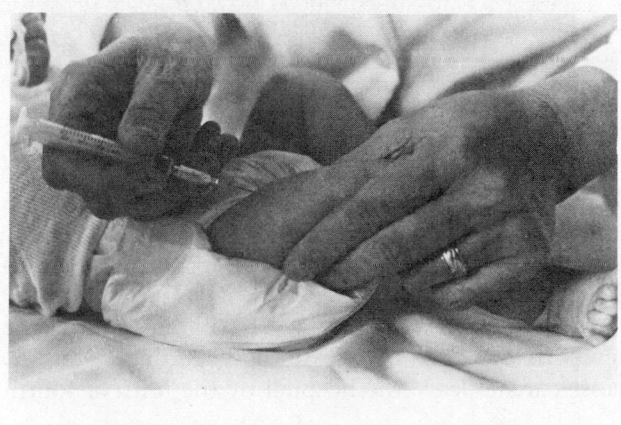

Procedure 20.13

PHOTOTHERAPY

PURPOSE

To reduce levels of unconjugated bilirubin

EQUIPMENT

1. Phototherapy unit (Fig. 20.36)
2. Eye patches (Fig. 20.36, A)
3. Diaper—a face mask with wire support removed works effectively (Fig. 20.36, B)

NURSING ACTION	RATIONALE
Identify infant.	Ensures procedure is done on correct infant.
Undress infant.	Expose as much skin area as possible to light.
Protect infant's eyes with eye patches (Fig. 20.36).	Prevents possible injury to conjunctiva or retina.
■ Be sure eyes are closed.	■ Prevents corneal abrasions.
■ Check eyes for drainage each shift.	■ Prevents or allows prompt treatment of purulent conjunctivitis, should it occur.
	■ Evidence suggests that exposure of the eyes to the bright lights of phototherapy units may injure the retina.
Cover head with stockinette.	This precaution is controversial and may differ from hospital to hospital.
For diapering, paper face mask may be used after removing metal nose strip (Fig. 20.36, B).	This "string bikini" is scanty enough to allow skin exposure, yet sufficient to protect genitals and bedding. Metal nose strip is heated by light and can burn baby's skin.
Monitor skin temperature. If infant is in incubator, temperature dial on control panel may need to be turned to maintain proper temperature.	Prevents hyperthermia or hypothermia. All electric equipment should be grounded, free of defects, and operationally sound to maximize therapeutic effectiveness and to prevent electric shock or burn to the baby or to the nurse.
Periodically, and especially for parents' visits, discontinue phototherapy for a few minutes and remove eye patches. Unwrap eyes and hold for feeding.	Necessary for normal psychosocial contact. Infant may visualize contact persons. Parent has opportunity to look into baby's eyes—a necessary activity to develop attachment to infant.
Observe infant's behavior:	Effect of phototherapy on biologic rhythms is uncertain.
Eating and sleep patterns	Data base is needed to differentiate common side effects (loose greenish stools or green urine) from other
Loose greenish stools, green urine.	problems that need appropriate treatment. Green color comes from end products of bilirubin.
Replace fluid losses by increasing fluid volume offered to infant by 25%.	Prevents dehydration; insensible and intestinal water loss is increased during phototherapy.
Protect skin from excoriation.	Prevents infection of broken-down skin areas.
Send serial bilirubins for analysis.	For evaluation of level of bilirubin and effectiveness of treatment.
Record time therapy began, note time removed for care, and if therapy discontinued. Record infant response, e.g., temperature, stools.	Ensures communication with other caretakers.

receiving phototherapy. The serum, urine, and skin turn bronze (brown-black). The cause is unclear. Almost all newborns recover from bronze baby syndrome without sequelae.

Parent education. Serum levels of bilirubin in the newborn continue to rise until the fifth day of life. Most parents leave the hospital by the third or fourth day and some as early as two hours after delivery. Therefore, parents must be able to assess the degree of jaundice the newborn exhibits (Table 19.3). They should have written instructions as to whom they should report the infant's condition. Some hospitals have a nurse make a home visit to parents who elect early discharge to evaluate the infant's responses. The

Fig. 20.36
A, Placement of eye patches for protection of eyes when infant is receiving phototherapy. Infant is undressed before being put under light. **B,** Under Bililite newborn wears face mask. Blanket draped over Bililite helps newborn maintain body temperature. (Courtesy Olympic Medical Corp., Seattle.)

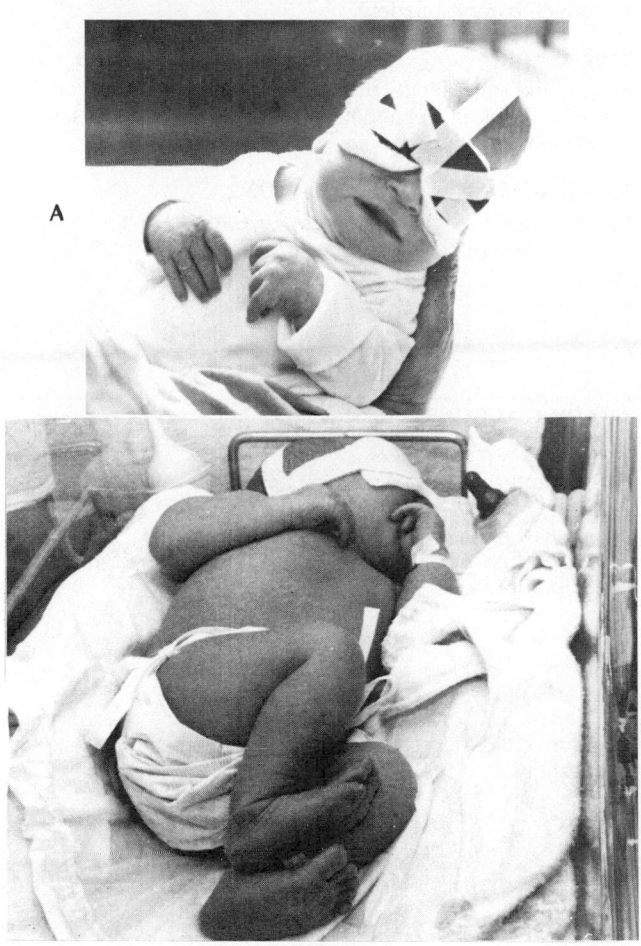

following guidelines provide a teaching tool to acquaint parents with the problem of hyperbilirubinemia and its treatment.

Circumcision

Historical perspective. Circumcision has been a rite in many cultures for centuries. It continues to be a ritual in religion, for example, the Jewish faith. Circumcision became a common practice in the United States in the early 1870s. From that time until the 1930s people thought masturbation was harmful and that removal of the foreskin would discourage it by making it less pleasurable. Circumcision was also credited with preventing or curing a number of conditions such as epilepsy, syphilis, asthma, mental illness, and tuberculosis. At present, about 25% of the world's population circumcise their males sometime between birth and young adulthood.

Current views. Recent studies (Pritchard, 1985; Witchell, 1985) do not support the connection between circumcision and penile or prostatic cancer and cervical cancer in the female partner. The coexistence of three noncircumcision-related factors is linked with cervical cancer: (1) the female who becomes sexually active before age 17 years, (2) the immature mucosal covering of the cervix of the female who is younger than 17 years that is exposed to sperm from a variety of different males, and (3) the cervix that has been infected with the herpes virus.

No evidence supports the claim that circumcision decreases the risk to the male for sexually transmitted diseases. Claims that circumcision facilitates hygiene can be refuted by teaching the young child daily cleansing of the penis. The use of circumcision for all males to prevent phimosis is unwarranted. Phimosis is a *rare* condition that can interfere with or impede the flow of urine (if the foreskin opening is tiny) and predispose to infection between the foreskin and glans.

It was thought that eliminating the foreskin would cure premature ejaculation because the foreskin contains numerous nerve endings that respond rapidly and intensely to sexual arousal. Premature ejaculation is now known to be primarily caused by emotional problems and not physical conditions.

Complications can occur with newborn circumcision. Possible difficulties include urethral fistulas and excessive removal of penile skin. Corrective measures have to be undertaken. They include grafting and the careful use of topical hemostatic agents (Gearhart and Callan, 1986).

Parental decision. Circumcision is an *elective* surgical procedure and as such is a matter of personal choice. The parents' decision to have their newborn circumcised is usually based on one or more of the following factors: hygiene, religious conviction, tradition, culture, or social norms. Some people do not like to touch their infant's genitals. For these parents, circumcision may be the wisest choice.

Regardless of the reason for the decision, it should be made only after parents have the available facts and sufficient time to review their options. The American Academy of Pediatrics (1975) reaffirmed its position that no medical indications for circumcision of the newborn are valid and that a program of good personal hygiene offers all the advantages of circumcision without the attendant surgical risks. The academy recommended that physicians provide parents with infor-

Guidelines for Client Teaching

HYPERBILIRUBINEMIA

ASSESSMENT

Infant, female term newborn, 7 lb 6 oz, 3 days old
Infant bilirubin level is 13 mg/dl
Physician orders:
    Serial total bilirubin levels
    Phototherapy
Parents unaware of causes of jaundice and what phototherapy is

NURSING DIAGNOSIS

Parental knowledge deficit related to hyperbilirubinemia and phototherapy

GOALS
Short term

To learn what hyperbilirubinemia is and why phototherapy is ordered

Intermediate

To increase parents' ability to evaluate newborn at home for hyperbilirubinemia
To reduce parent's anxiety

Long term

To provide knowledge of hyperbilirubinemia that can be used to prompt treatment for older infant or other family members

REFERENCES AND TEACHING AIDS

Charts, phototherapy equipment, eye masks, paper diaper (face mask with wire support removed)

CONTENT/RATIONALE	TEACHING ACTIONS
Review meaning of terms parents will hear: ■ Hyperbilirubinemia: higher levels of bilirubin than normal. ■ Bilirubin: end product of red blood cells when they grow old and break up. ■ Jaundice: yellow color of whites of eyes, skin, mucous membranes caused by circulating bilirubin. ■ Phototherapy: use of light (green) to break up bilirubin into substances that can be excreted in the feces (stool) or urine.	Seat parents where they can see charts and talk easily to the nurse. Have chart made with terms spelled out. If possible have mother and father hold wrapped infant for this part of class.
Review process of excreting bilirubin: when red blood cells (RBC) break up they release a material called bilirubin. Bilirubin circulates in the blood. In the liver it is combined with another substance. In the combined form it goes by way of the blood to the kidneys and the intestines. It gives the yellow color to the urine and the brown color to the stool.	Point to chart depicting process as you explain. Ask for questions.
Before the baby was born her RBCs were more numerous than ours. They also lived a shorter time, 70-90 days instead of 120 days. When they broke up, the baby's blood carried most of the bilirubin by way of the placenta to the mother's liver to be excreted.	Show picture of baby in utero. Trace route of blood from baby to mother's liver.
After the baby was born, her liver began to take care of all the bilirubin. Even though the baby's liver functions well, it cannot handle the whole load. Bilirubin seeps out of the blood and into the tissues, staining them yellow. The blood level of bilirubin rises quickly up to the fifth day, and then goes down; the jaundice clears up by the end of the week.	Point out yellowness of baby's skin. Show chart with approximate amounts of bilirubin and location of jaundice. Prepare graph illustrating rise and fall of bilirubin over first week.
Some babies seem to have extra bilirubin to excrete. The amount in the tissues becomes too great when the blood level reaches 12 mg/dl. There is a danger that the bilirubin at high levels will cause damage to the brain. So your doctor wants the baby to be placed under the Bililight for phototherapy. This will help the baby handle the extra bilirubin and prevent damage to the baby's brain.	Show Bililight equipment. Let parents feel warmth of light.
We put eye masks on the baby to keep the light from her eyes.	Demonstrate use of eye masks. Bring infant and place in crib away from Bililight. Apply eye masks.

Guidelines for Client Teaching—cont'd

HYPERBILIRUBINEMIA

CONTENT/RATIONALE	TEACHING ACTIONS
We keep the baby undressed so as much light as possible can reach her skin.	Undress baby. Place in crib under the Bililight.
We use the face mask as a small diaper.	Diaper infant.
We will take her temperature often so she will not become too hot or too cold.	Take and record temperature. Settle baby comfortably.
We will give her extra water to drink because she will have watery, green stools from the extra bilirubin broken up by the light.	Return to seats and review care. Show on chart.
We will be taking her out of the Bililight for feedings and cuddlings. We will let you know when to come for feedings and to hold her.	
We will be taking blood tests to check the amount of bilirubin and will let you know the results.	
If you have any questions, ask us anytime for answers. We know you will be anxious about Sally. It is hard not to take her home with you today.	Leave parents with infant. Tell them they can touch her, but not to shield her skin from the light. Demonstrate stroking baby's hand. Return in about 10 min to see if there are questions. Arrange feeding schedule with mother. Mother can breast feed the baby and bring breast milk for feedings she will miss (Chapter 21).

EVALUATION Woman or couple demonstrate degree to which the goals of care have been met.

---

mation about the risks of circumcision as well as options regarding this surgical procedure well in advance of delivery.

Parents need to begin learning about circumcision during the prenatal period (NAACOG, 1985a). However, circumcision often is not discussed with the parents before labor. In many instances, it is during admission to the hospital or labor unit that the mother confronts the decision regarding circumcision. The stress of the perinatal period makes this a difficult time for parental decision making. Although consenting to their boy's circumcision is ultimately the parents' personal choice, the fact that there are no medical indications for the procedure is emphasized.

Procedure. In circumcision the prepuce (foreskin) of the glans penis is excised to expose the glans. The operation is performed in the hospital before the infant's discharge. The procedure is no longer done immediately after birth because the amount of cold stress had proved detrimental to the infant. Clotting factors drop somewhat immediately after birth and return to prebirth levels by the end of the first week. Therefore performing the circumcision after the baby is a week old has a firmer physiologic basis. The circumcision of a Jewish male is performed on the eighth day after birth unless the infant is unwell.

For the circumcision procedure the infant is positioned on a plastic restraint form so that his movements are restricted (Fig. 20.37). The penis is cleansed

with soap and water. The infant is draped to provide warmth and a sterile field. The sterile equipment is readied for use.

Numerous instruments have been designed for circumcision (Figs. 20.38 and 20.39). The Yellen clamp, for instance, may make this an almost bloodless operation. Once the procedure, which takes only a few minutes, is completed, a small petrolatum gauze dressing may be applied for the first day to prevent a cloth diaper from adhering. (A cloth diaper is used because blood absorbed by cloth is easier to see than that absorbed by a disposable diaper.) The infant is then dressed.

Discomfort. If the infant has undergone this surgery without anesthesia, he is comforted until he is quieted. Then he is returned to his crib. These infants usually are fussy for about 2 to 3 hours and may refuse a feeding.

In the Jewish ritual, the newborn is given a few drops of wine to relax him in preparation for the surgery. In an article advocating dorsal block for the circumcision, Kirya and Werthmann (1978) wrote:

Anyone who circumcises a neonate using any of the available techniques, senses the pain and stress that the manipulative stages of this procedure generate. During the procedure when the prepuce is clamped with forceps, the infant cries vigorously, trembles, and tries to wiggle out of the restraint. He may eventually become plethoric (flushed), dusky, and mildly cyanotic because of prolonged crying. Oc-

Fig. 20.37
A, Proper positioning of infant in Circumstraint. **B,** Physician performing circumsion. Baby is completely covered to prevent cold stress. (Photographs by I.M. Bobak.)

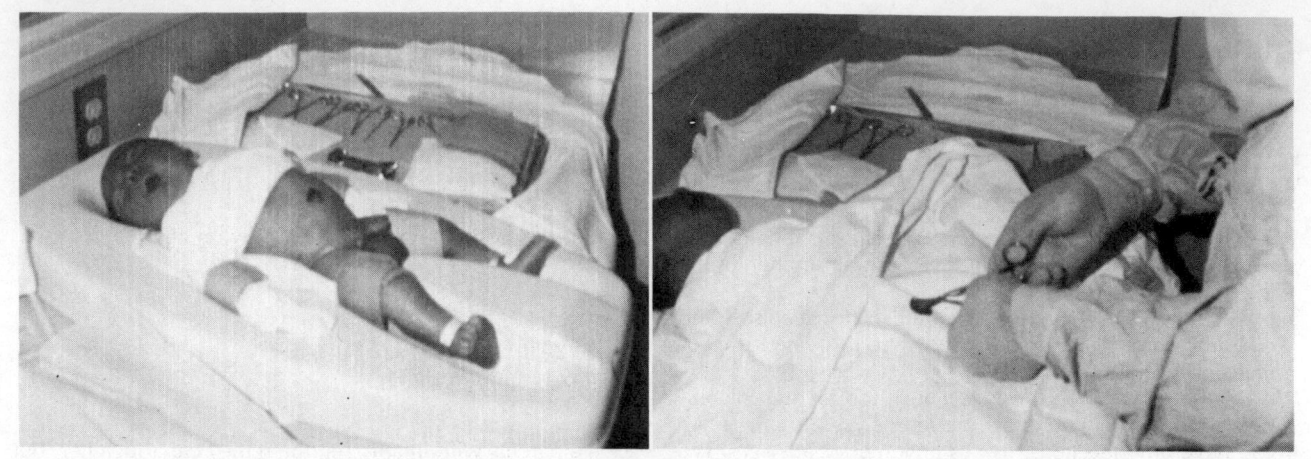

Fig. 20.38
Technique of circumcision. **A** to **D,** Prepuce is stripped and slit to facilitate its retraction behind glans penis. **E,** Prepuce is now clamped and excessive prepuce cut off. **F** and **G,** Suture material used is plain 00 or 000 catgut in very small needle, but some physicians prefer silk.

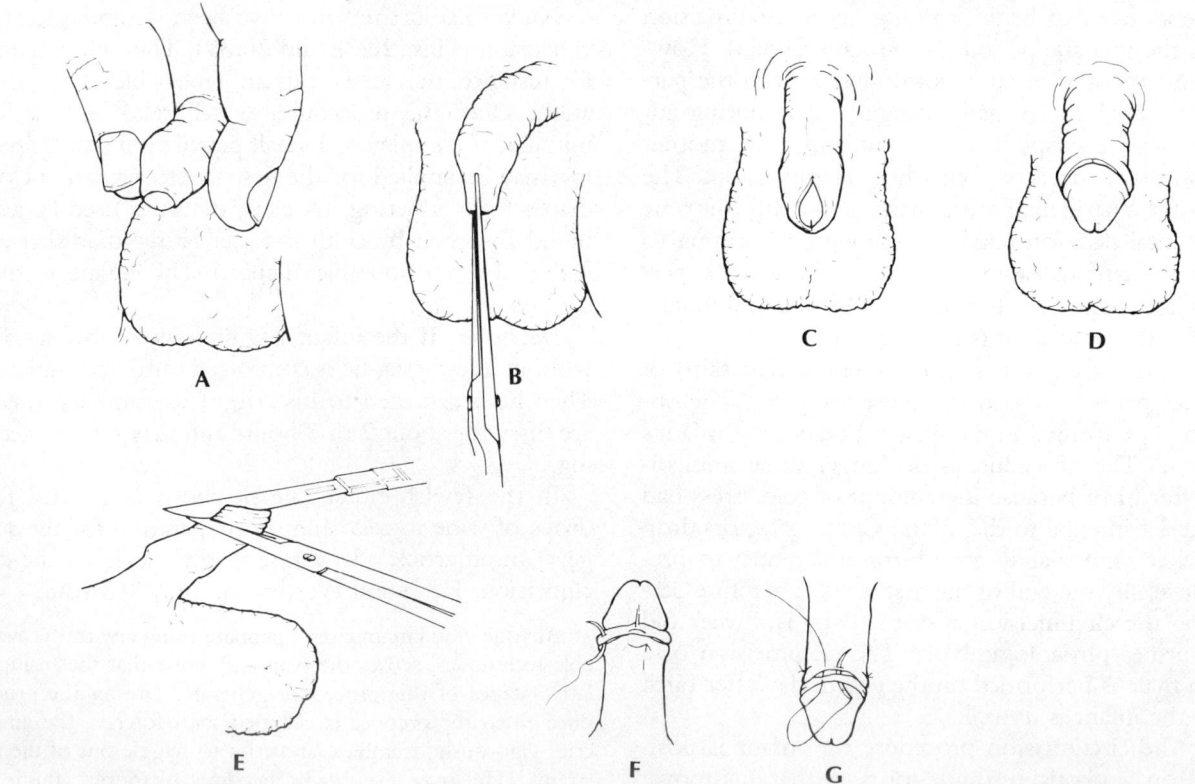

Fig. 20.39
Circumcision with Yellan clamp. **A,** Prepuce drawn over cone. **B,** Pressure on prepuce between cone and device for 3 to 5 minutes produces hemostasis. **C,** Prepuce (over cone) is cut away. **D,** Glans penis appears deep red during healing.

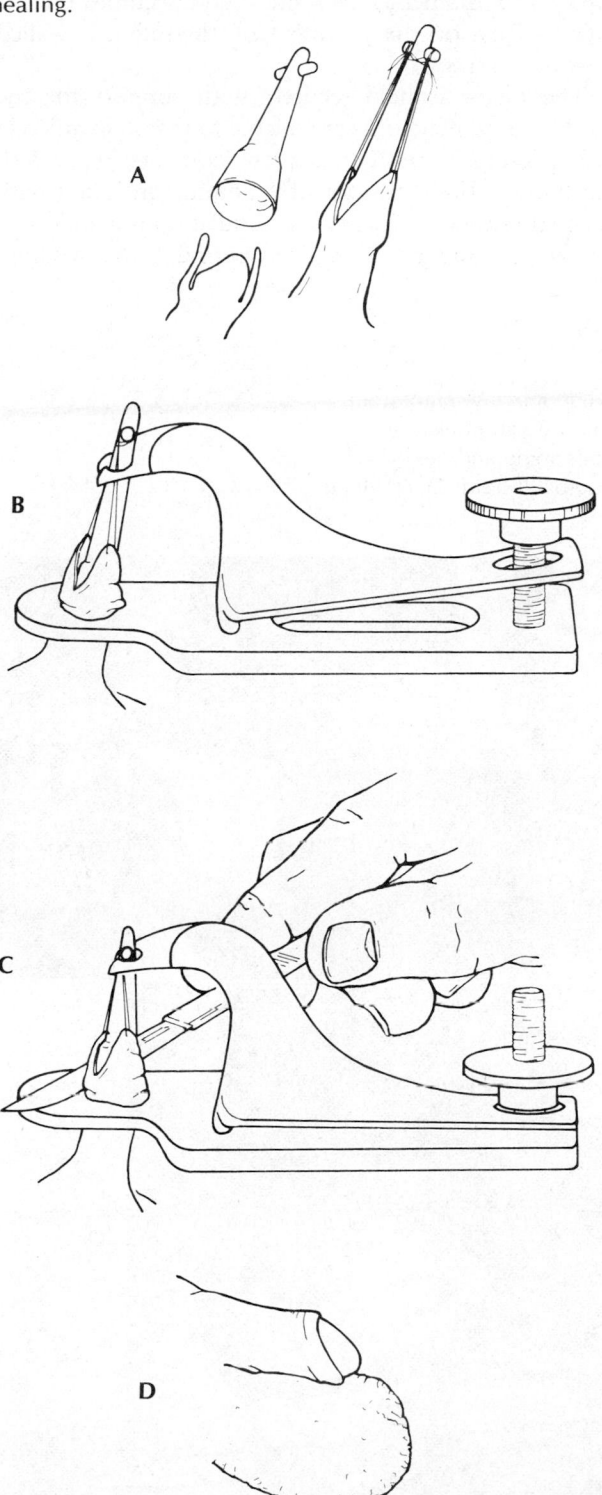

casionally this results in respiratory pauses or regurgitation of feeding.

Pain may not end when the operation is over because the wound requires as long as a week to heal.

Care of the newly circumcised penis. The nurse observes the infant for bleeding. If bleeding is noted from the circumcision, the nurse applies gentle pressure to the site of bleeding with a folded sterile gauze pad, 4 in × 4 in. If bleeding is not easily controlled, a blood vessel may need to be ligated. One nurse notifies the physician and prepares equipment (circumcision tray and suture) while the other nurse maintains pressure *intermittently* until the physician arrives. The penis is checked hourly for bleeding for 12 hours; if the parents take the baby home before the end of 12 hours, they have to be taught the actions described previously. Before discharge, the nurse checks to see that the parents have the physician's phone number.

Nursing actions are planned and implemented to prevent infection. The nurse washes the penis gently with water to remove urine and feces and reapplies a fresh (sterile) petrolatum gauze around the glans after each diaper change. The glans penis, normally dark red in appearance, becomes covered with a yellow exudate in 24 hours. This is part of the normal healing process, not an infective process. No attempt is made to remove the exudate, which persists for 2 to 3 days. Cloth diapers are applied loosely for 2 to 3 days because the incised area at the base of the glans penis remains tender. Cloth diapers are used for about a week or until the glans is completely healed.

If a plastic bell is used to cover the glans, petrolatum gauze is not needed. The plastic bell remains firmly applied to the glans, preventing hemorrhage and contamination. The bell falls off when the glans is healed.

TEACHER AND SUPPORT PERSON

Caretaking activities for the newborn are shared by the nurse and the mother. The nurse acts as teacher and support person. As soon as the mother feels physically able she is encouraged to participate in her child's care. The mother's need for knowledge and the factors that may impede her learning are determined through questioning and observation. The content taught and teaching aids used should reflect the mother's level of understanding. Films and tapes can be valuable time-savers in teaching. Most hospitals provide written instructions in infant care for parents. The care given the child is supervised and the parents are encouraged to ask questions.

Daily care activities. The daily care of infants includes such activities as positioning and holding the infant, clothing the infant, attending to the infant's need for socializing, care of infant linens, and daily hygiene. The techniques of feeding the infant are discussed in Chapter 21.

Positioning and holding the infant. Placing the infant in the crib in a side-lying position permits drainage of mucus from the mouth and applies no pressure to the cord or the sensitive circumcised penis (Fig. 20.31). The infant's position is changed from side to side to help develop even contours of the head and to ease pressure on other parts of the body.

Anatomically the infant's shape—barrel chest and flat, curveless spine—makes it easy for the child to roll.

A folded or rolled blanket against the spine will prevent rolling to the supine position and will promote a feeling of security. Care must be taken to prevent the infant from rolling off of flat, unguarded surfaces. The parent or nurse who must turn away from the infant even for a moment keeps one hand securely on the infant. If left on the parent's bed, the infant is walled in with pillows.

The infant is held securely with support for the head because newborns are unable to maintain an erect head posture for more than a few moments. Fig. 20.40 illustrates various positions for holding an infant with adequate support. Too much stimulation is avoided after feeding and before a sleep period. After feeding,

Fig. 20.40

Holding baby securely with support for head. **A,** Holding infant while moving infant from one place to another. Baby (whose temperature is well stabilized in a warm nursery) is undressed to show posture. Note lack of curvature in normal infant's spine and flexion of extremities. **B,** Holding baby upright in "burping" position. **C,** "Football" hold. **D,** Cradling hold. (Photographs by I.M. Bobak.)

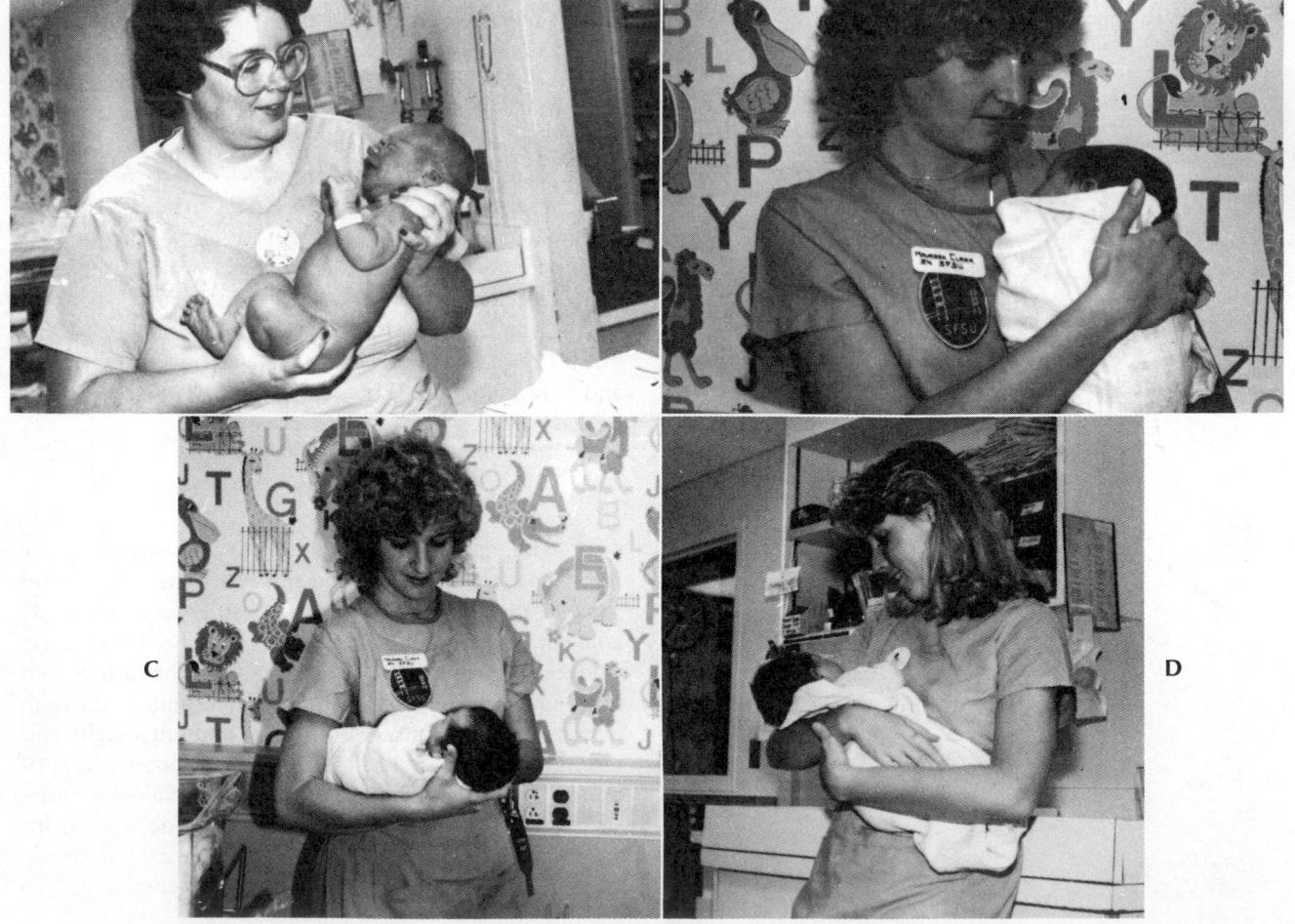

positioning the infant on the right side promotes gastric emptying into the small intestine (Fig. 21.3, *B*).

Umbilical cord care. The care of the umbilical cord is the same as that for any surgical wound. The goal of care is prevention and early identification of hemorrhage or infection. If bleeding from the blood vessels of the cord is noted, the nurse checks the clamp (or tie) and applies a second clamp next to the first one. If bleeding is not stopped immediately, the nurse calls for physician assistance at once.

Hospital protocol directs the time and technique for routine cord care. The nurse cleanses the cord and skin area around the base of the cord with the prescribed preparation (for example, erythromycin solution, triple blue dye, or alcohol) and checks daily for signs of infection. The cord clamp is removed after 24 hours (Fig. 20.41).

Diaper rash. Treatment of diaper rash involves exposing the rash to warmth and air. Immediately washing and drying the wet and soiled area and changing the diaper after voiding or defecating prevent and help treat diaper rash. The warmth can be achieved with a 25-watt bulb placed 45 cm (18 in) from the affected area.

Fig. 20.41
Removal of cord clamp when cord is dry. (Photograph by I.M. Bobak.)

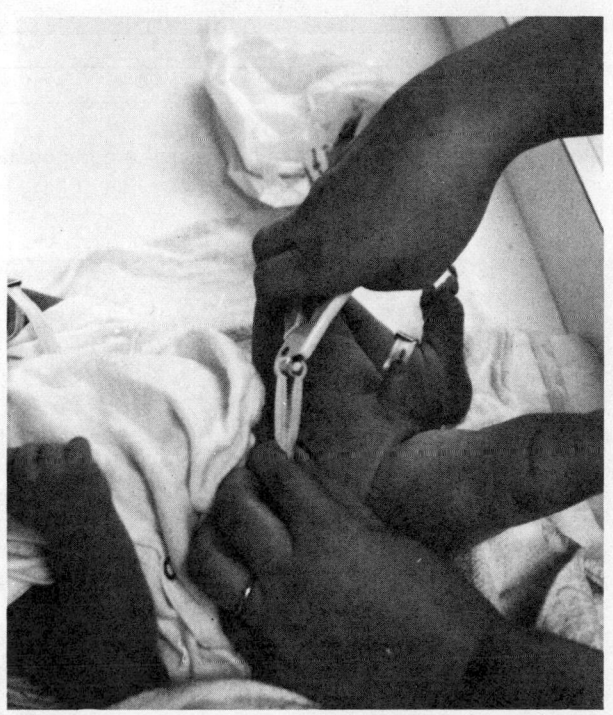

The most severe type of diaper rash occurs when the area becomes infected, indurated (hardened), and tender. Medical advice should be sought and a specifically ordered medication applied.

Other rashes. A rash on the face may result from the infant's scratching (excoriation) or from rubbing the face against the sheets, particularly if regurgitated stomach contents are not washed off promptly.

Clothing the infant. Parents frequently ask how warmly they should dress their infant. A simple rule of thumb for parents is to dress the child as they dress themselves, adding or subtracting clothes and wraps for the child as they do for themselves. A shirt or diaper may be sufficient clothing for the young infant. A bonnet is needed to protect the scalp and minimize heat loss if it is cool or to protect against sunburn and shade the eyes if it is sunny and hot. Wrapping the infant snugly in a blanket maintains body temperature and promotes a feeling of security. Overdressing in warm temperatures can cause discomfort and prickly heat; underdressing in cold weather can also cause discomfort. Cheeks, fingers, and toes can readily become frostbitten. The incident noted below shows the need for teaching a young parent.

■ A nurse was called to make a home visit to see an infant because the "baby just sleeps and sleeps and doesn't have any energy." In the apartment the thermostat was set for 33° C (92° F) because the mother "thought that babies need it warm." The mother was wearing a sleeveless dress because she could barely tolerate the extreme heat. The baby was found heavily wrapped in blankets. Lowering the thermostat and dressing the infant to match the temperature resulted in normal newborn behavior.

Care of the infant's linens. Care of the infant's clothes and bedding is directed toward minimizing cross infection and removing residues from soap, feces, or urine that may irritate the infant's skin. In the hospital, clothing and bedding are washed separately from other linens and are autoclaved. Some hospitals use disposable shirts and diapers. At home the baby's clothes should be washed separately, with a mild detergent or soap and hot water. A double rinse usually removes traces of the potentially irritating cleansing agent or acid residue from the urine or stool. If possible, dry the clothing and bedding in the sun to neutralize residues. Parents who have to use coin-operated machines to wash and dry clothes may find it expensive or almost impossible to wash and rinse the baby's clothes well.

Bedding requires frequent changing. The plastic-coated, firm mattress must be washed daily and the crib or bassinet damp dusted. The infant's toilet articles may be kept separate and convenient for use in a box or basket.

Infant's social needs. The sensitivity of the caretaker to the social responses of the infant is basic to the development of a mutually satisfying parent-child relationship. Sensitivity increases over time as parents' awareness of their infant's social capabilities becomes more acute.

Parental awareness. The "Mother's assessment of the behavior of her infant" (MABI) determines how mothers perceive their infants (Field and others, 1978). It was found that mothers perceived their infants in much the same way as the professional examiners did. For example, the mothers noted the postmature infants were not as adaptable or in tune rhythmically with parents. There was one notable exception: Mothers were not as aware of the social capabilities of their infants as were the examiners.

One way nurses can promote parental sensitivity is to share with the parents the process of the Brazelton assessment. Examples of comments of parents involved in such teaching about their infants include the following (Edelstein, 1985):

"After the examination I seemed to notice the various things that were pointed out. Also, I myself tested the baby once we were home. Through the testing I realize more so now that the baby is quite aware of what goes on around him, and since, I've noticed I talk to the baby more now."

"It helped me feel confident that she was a normal, healthy baby and that her reflexes and responses were good."

"The test examination in the hospital made me more aware of various responses to expect from my baby. It also made me more aware of just how much more an infant can do than I had ever known before."

"I was assured that my baby was normal and healthy. Also, it was fascinating to discover all the things he was already aware of. I learned more about him (and babies in general) from participating in the test."

Planning times for social interactions. The activities of daily care during the neonatal period offer the best times for infant and family interaction. While caring for their baby mother and father can talk to the infant, play baby games, and caress and cuddle the child. In Fig. 20.42, mother, father, and infant engage in arousal, imitation of facial expression, and finally smiling. Fig. 20.43 shows a sister kissing her new brother. Older children's contact with a newborn needs to be supervised for strength of hugs, exploring of eyes and nose, and attempts to feed the baby. Parents often keep baby books that record their infant's progress.

Bathing the infant. Bathing serves a number of purposes. It provides opportunities for (1) a complete

Fig. 20.42
Mother-father-baby interaction. Baby is in active alert state. Note parents' and baby's posture, especially hands and feet. Note eye contact. Mouth opens, hands move in rhythm to the father's voice, father's hands open, too. Mother moves close and imitates baby's mouth. (Courtesy Colleen Stainton.)

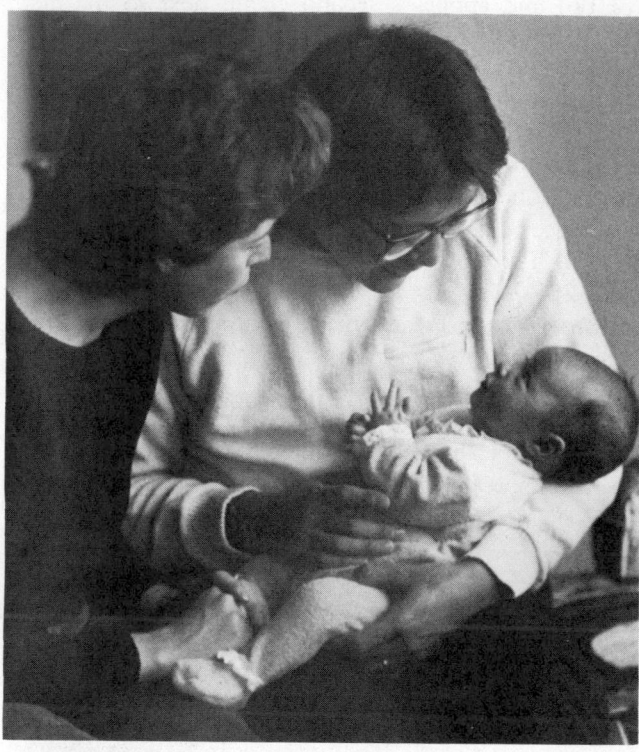

Fig. 20.43
Sister kisses her new brother. Family contacts are important for newborn and siblings. (Courtesy Marjorie Pyle, RNC, Lifecircle, Costa Mesa, California.)

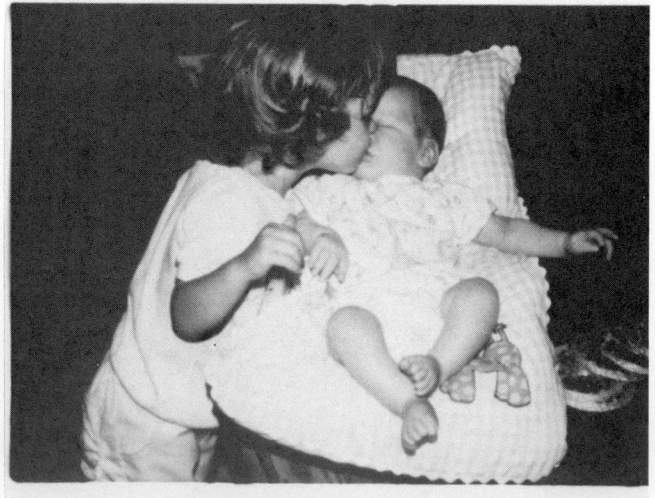

cleansing of the infant, (2) observing the infant's condition, (3) promoting comfort, and (4) parent-child-family socializing. The initial bath is postponed until the infant's temperature stabilizes at 36.5° C (97.6° F). In some hospitals the infant is given the initial bath, and then cleansing of the genitals as necessary is deemed sufficient for the first 3 to 4 days. Bathing with warm water is sufficient for the first week. Then a mild soap may be used (NAACOG, 1985b). If a documented staphylococcal skin infection outbreak occurs in a nursery, the newborn is bathed with dilute hexachlorophene detergent (pHisoHex) (less than 3%), followed by thorough rinsing of the skin. As pHisoHex is a potential neurotoxin, particularly for infants who weigh less than 2000 g, it is no longer used in many nurseries. Guidelines for client teaching are provided for use with mothers who need instruction in the bathing of their infants.

Guidelines for Client Teaching

BATHING AN INFANT

ASSESSMENT
Woman has delivered her first child, a boy.
She has had little experience with the care of children.

NURSING DIAGNOSIS
Knowledge deficit relating to bathing an infant

GOALS
Short term
To learn infant bathing technique

Intermediate
To become skilled in bathing an infant

Long term
To adjust bathing technique to developing child

REFERENCES AND TEACHING AIDS
Texts
Hospital or clinic prepared instructions
Film of parent bathing a baby

CONTENT/RATIONALE	TEACHING ACTIONS
Review the purposes for bathing. It provides opportunities for (1) a complete cleansing of the infant, (2) observing the infant's condition, (3) promoting comfort, and (4) parent-child-family socializing. Timing of baths. ■ Initial bath: The initial bath is postponed until the infant's temperature stabilizes at 36.5° C (97.6° F). ■ Daily bath: A daily bath may be given at any time convenient to the parent but not immediately after a feeding period, since the increased handling may cause regurgitation of the feeding. Prevention of heat loss: the temperature of the room should be 24° C (75° F), and the bathing area should be free of drafts to prevent heat loss. Heat loss in the infant is greater than heat loss in the adult because of the relatively large ratio of skin surface to body mass in the newborn. Heat loss must be controlled during the bath period to conserve the infant's energy. Bathing the infant quickly, exposing only a portion of the body at a time, and thorough drying are therefore part of the bathing technique. Prevention of skin trauma. The infant's fragile skin can be injured by too vigorous cleansing. Vernix, the white material that looks like cold cream is not removed vigorously as it is attached to the upper layer of the skin. Too vigorous removal results in removal of the protective skin layer. Vernix may be left on for 48 hours; if it persists beyond that time, it may be washed off gently. If stool or other debris has caked and dried on the skin, soak the area to remove it. Do not attempt to rub it off because abrasion may result. Gentleness, patting dry rather than rubbing, and use of a mild soap without perfume or coloring are recommended. Chemicals in the coloring and perfume can cause rashes in sensitive skin.	Introduction: Set tone for class. Have mother seated comfortably (she may need a pillow to sit on). Make sure she can see demonstration. Welcome father, if he is present, and include him in the process. Ask mother when father and siblings would be available for infant bath. Review material pertinent to care before beginning bath to prevent heat loss. Review material pertinent to care before beginning bath to prevent heat loss.

Continued.

Guidelines for Client Teaching—cont'd

CONTENT/RATIONALE	TEACHING ACTIONS
Supplies and clothing are made ready. ■ Clothing suitable for wearing indoors: diaper, shirt ■ Soap; unscented, mild ■ Baby lotion, not powder. Baby can inhale powder. ■ Pins, if needed for diaper, are placed well out of baby's reach. ■ Cotton balls. ■ Towels for drying infant and clean washcloth. ■ Receiving blanket.	Arrange work area while explaining process. Comment on equipment and clothing so that mother sees importance of preparing area before child is brought in.
Bring infant to bathing area when all supplies are ready. The infant is never left alone on the bath table or in the bath water, not even for a second. If the mother or nurse has to leave, the infant is taken along or put back into the crib.	Model holding of infant and protecting him with hand (Fig. 20.44).
Test temperature of water. It should feel pleasantly warm to the inner wrist (about 98-99° F).	Demonstrate testing water. Let mother feel.
The infant's head is washed before unwrapping and undressing to prevent heat loss. ■ Cleanse the *eyes* from the canthus outward, using a *clean* washcloth. For the first 2 to 3 days a discharge may result from the reaction of the conjunctiva to the substance (silver nitrate or erythromycin) used as a prophylactic measure against infection. Any discharge should be considered abnormal and reported to the physician. When removing eye discharge, avoid contamination of one eye with the discharge from the other by using a separate cotton swab and water source (running water from a tap is best) for each eye.	Explain that the infant is washed from head to toe starting with the eyes and ending with the genitals. ■ Demonstrate cleansing the eyes and washing the face (Fig. 20.44, A and B).
■ The *scalp* is washed daily with water and a mild soap. It must be rinsed well and dried thoroughly. Scalp desquamation, called *cradle cap,* can often be prevented by removing any scales with a fine-toothed comb or brush after washing. If the condition persists, the physician may order an ointment to massage into the skin.	■ Demonstrate washing and drying head. Use football hold (Fig. 20.44, C).
■ *Creases* under the chin and arms and in the groin need daily cleansing. The crease under the chin may be exposed by elevating the infant's shoulders 5 cm (2 in) and letting the head drop back.	■ Demonstrate washing creases.
■ Cleanse the *ears* and *nose* with twists made of moistened cotton.	■ Demonstrate cleaning ears and nose.
Undress baby and wash body and arms and legs. Pat dry gently. Baby may be tub-bathed after the cord drops off.	Demonstrate sponge bath of infant. Rinse well. Pat dry (Fig. 20.44, C to E).
Care of the cord. Use a Q-tip. Dip swabs into the solution your doctor ordered and cleanse around the base of the cord, where it joins the skin. Notify your physician of any odor, discharge, or skin inflammation around the cord. The clamp is removed when the cord is dry (about 24 hours) (Fig. 20.41). When you diaper the infant the diaper should not cover the cord. A wet or soiled diaper will slow or prevent drying and foster infection. When the cord drops off in a week to 10 days, small drops of blood can be seen when the baby cries. This will heal itself. It is not dangerous.	Demonstrate care of cord. Ask mother what she would report.
Wash and dry between the fingers and toes daily.	Check between fingers and toes. Show picture of mitts (Fig. 20.45).

Continued.

Fig. 20.44
Bathing baby. **A,** Eyes. **B,** Face. **C,** Head and hair. **D,** Sponge-bathing baby. **E,** Rinsing baby. **F,** Brushing hair. Mother in **A, B,** and **C** is being supervised. Note in **D, E,** and **F** that nurse keeps one hand on baby. (Courtesy Marjorie Pyle, RNC, Lifecircle, Costa Mesa, California.)

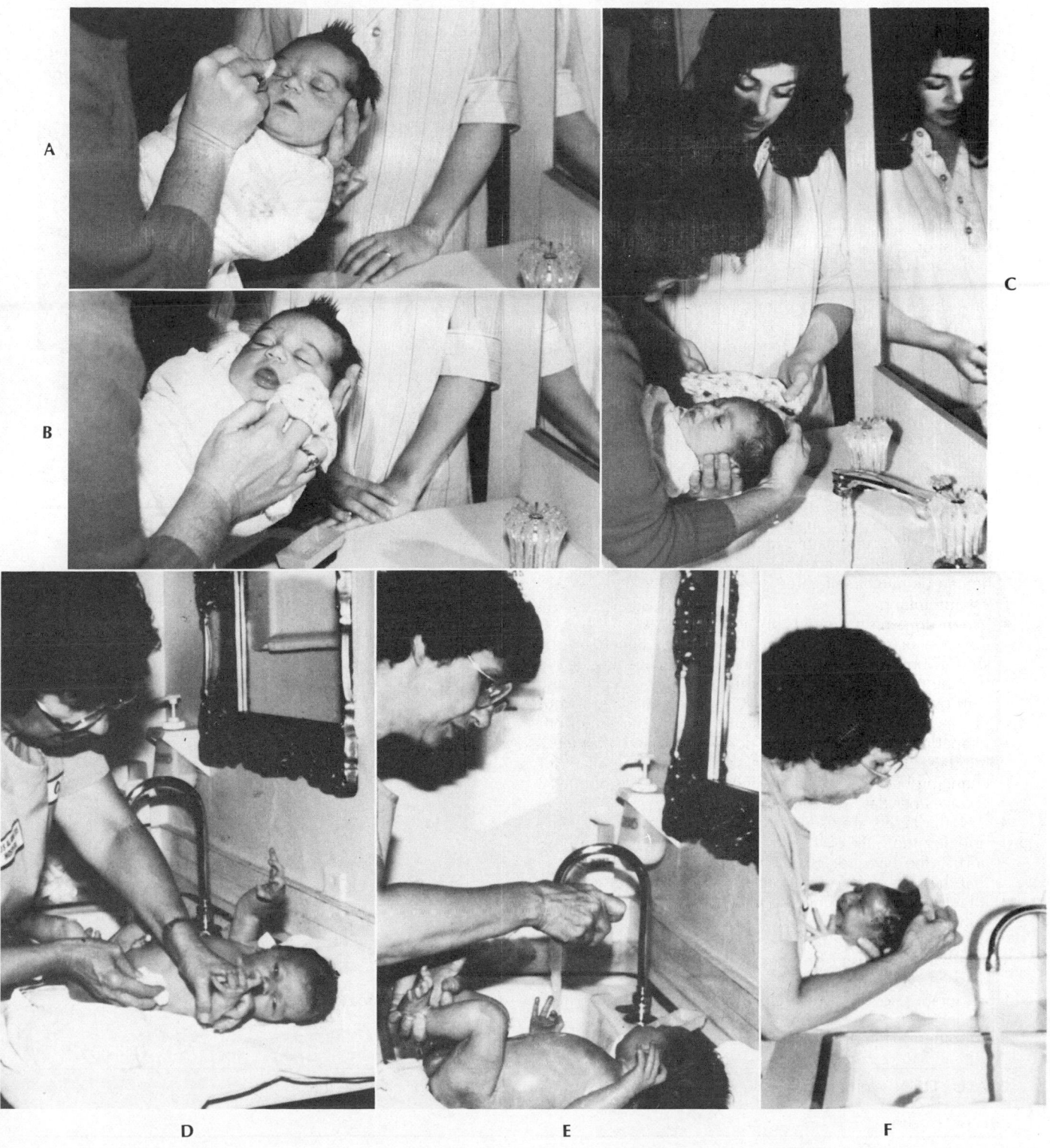

Guidelines for Client Teaching—cont'd

CONTENT/RATIONALE	TEACHING ACTION

Fingernails and toenails are not cut immediately after birth. The nails have to grow out far enough from the skin so that the skin is not cut by mistake. Before the nails can be cut, if the baby scratches himself, you can apply loosely fitted mitts over each hand. Placing mitts on the hands is done as a last resort because it interferes with the baby's ability to console herself or himself. When the nails have grown the *fingernails* and *toenails* can be cut more readily with manicure scissors (preferably with rounded tips) when the infant is asleep. Hold the skin back from the nail and cut straight across. The nails are kept short; otherwise, they can be snagged by clothing and can scratch the infant during normal random hand and leg movements.

Cleanse the *genitals* of both girl and boy infants daily and after voiding or defecating. For girls, cleansing of the genitals may be done by separating the labia and gently washing from the pubic area to the anus. For uncircumcised boys, gently pull back (retract) the foreskin. Stop when resistance is felt. Wash the tip (glans) with soap and warm water and replace the foreskin over the glans. The foreskin must be returned to its original position to prevent constriction and swelling. In the majority of newborns the inner layer of the foreskin adheres to the glans. By the age of 3 years, in 90% of boys the foreskin can be retracted easily without pain or trauma. For others, the foreskin is not retractable until the teens. As soon as the foreskin is partly retractable and the child is old enough, he can be taught self-care.

Dress the infant.

■ When dressing the child, do not pull shirts roughly over the face or catch fingers in shirt-sleeves. Bunch up the shirt in both hands and expand the neck opening before placing the neck opening over the face first. Then slip the shirt over the rest of the head. Or, form a mask with your fingers over the baby's face as you pull the shirt on or off.

■ Diapering the infant may be done before and after feeding (Fig. 20.47). It is not necessary to wake the infant for changing because the preceding routine means about 12 changes per day.

■ If cloth diapers are used, absorbency can be increased by bringing the bulk of the diaper to the front area for boys and to the back for girls. This will help absorb urine so that the skin surface is protected. The diaper between the infant's legs should not be bulky because it can cause outward displacement of the hips. A soaker pad can be placed under the infant as a protection for the blanket. The continued use of rubber or plastic pants may lead to diaper rash.

Store infant's towels, wash-cloth, and supplies apart from the family for 3 to 4 months to prevent infection.

Tell mother that you will watch her give the bath tomorrow.

Fig. 20.45
Note mitts on baby's hands to prevent her from scratching her face. Father enfolds her in his arms. (Courtesy Marjorie Pyle, RNC, Lifecircle, Costa Mesa, California.)

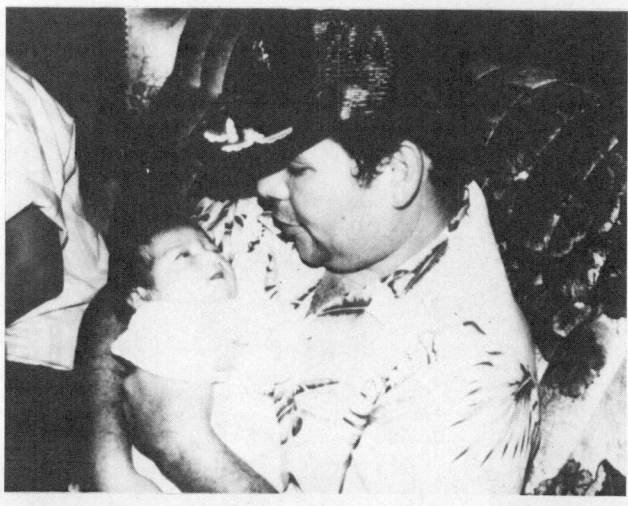

Demonstrate cleansing the genitals, in this case a boy.

Demonstrate technique and explain rationale while doing it (Fig. 20.46).

Clean and tidy area.

EVALUATION Woman or couple demonstrate degree to which the goals for care are met.

Fig. 20.46
A, Gathering up shirt to enlarge neck opening. **B,** Placing neck opening to avoid dragging it across face. **C,** Drawing shirt down over back of head, still avoiding face. **D,** Reaching into shirt sleeve to grasp baby's hand to pull arm through without snagging fingers. **E,** Pulling left arm through. **F,** Pulling shirt down to cover trunk. (Photograph by I.M. Bobak.)

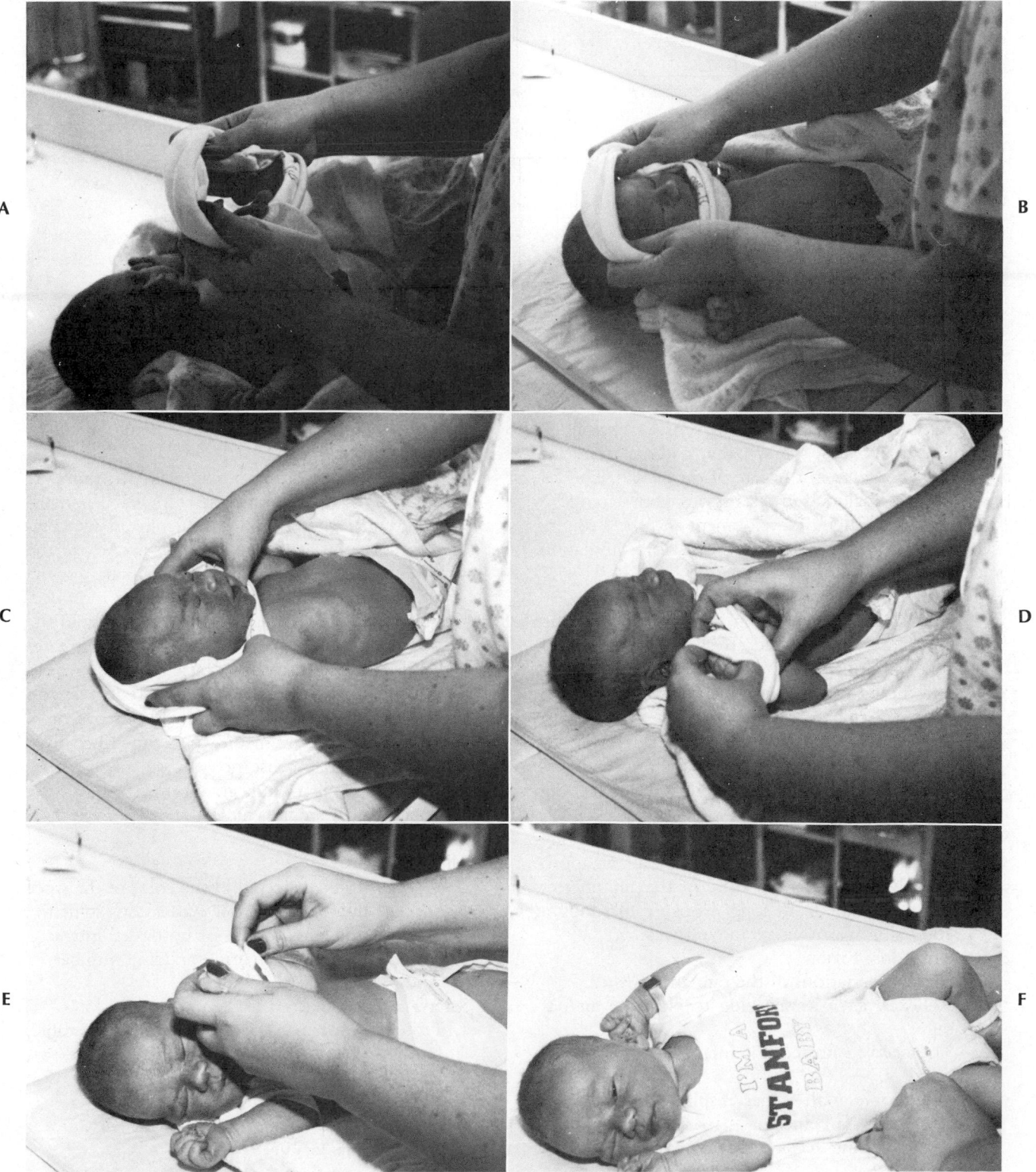

Fig. 20.47
Diapering infant. Dotted lines indicate folds. For kite type, start with large, regular diaper if single thickness is thin.

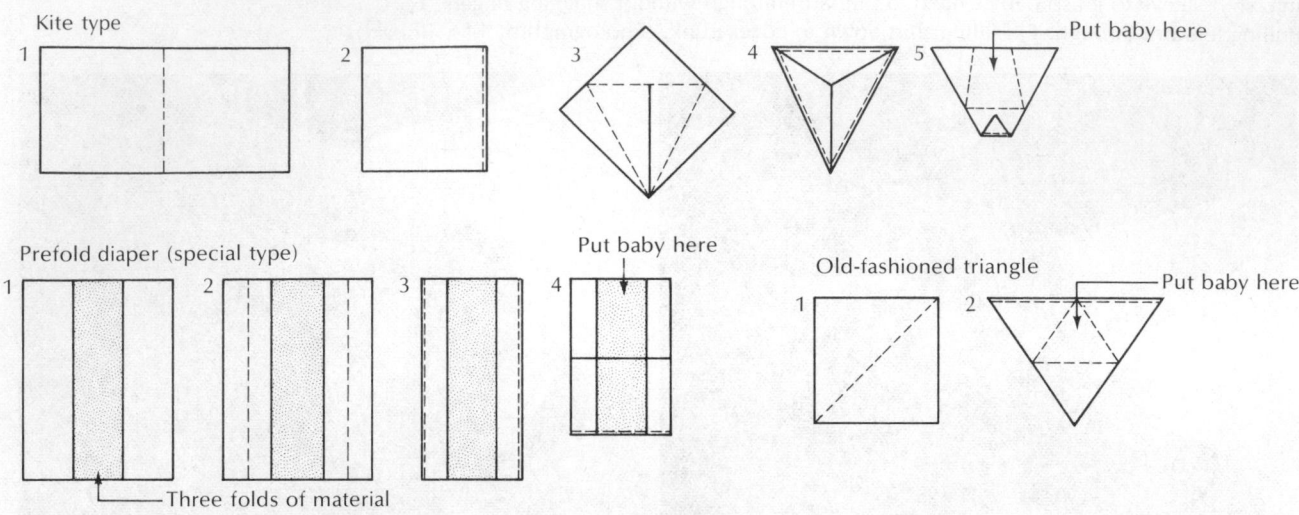

Anticipatory guidance for parents. Whether or not this is the couple's first baby, parents appreciate *anticipatory guidance* in the care of their child. The following can be included in discussions with parents.

1. Normal growth and development and the changing needs of the infant (for example, for stimulation, exercise, and social contacts).
2. Temperature: review
   a. The causes of elevation in body temperature (such as exercise, cold stress with resultant vasoconstriction, minimum response to infection) and the body's response to extremes in environmental temperature.
   b. Symptoms to be reported, such as high or low temperatures with accompanying fussiness, stuffy nose, lethargy, irritability, poor feeding, and crying.
   c. Ways to reduce body temperature, such as giving a cool tub bath, dressing the infant appropriately for the temperature of the air; protecting the infant from long exposure to sunlight, and using warm wraps in cold weather.
3. Respirations: review
   a. Normal variations in the rate and rhythm.
   b. Reflexes, such as sneezing to clear the air passage.
   c. The need to protect the infant from the following:
      (1) People with upper respiratory tract infections (an efficient mask can be made by wrapping toilet tissue around the head to cover the mouth and nose if the parent or another has a cold).
      (2) Pollution from a smoke-filled environment.
   d. Symptoms of the common cold: nasal congestion, coughing, sneezing, difficulty in swallowing (sore throat), low-grade fever. Advise the parents on measures to help the infant: for example, feed smaller amounts but feed more frequently to avoid overtiring the infant; hold the baby in an upright position to feed; offer extra sterile water; for sleeping, raise the infant's head and chest by raising the mattress 30 degrees (do not use pillow); avoid drafts; do not overdress the baby; use only medications prescribed by a physician (do not use nose drops, since aspiration may result in lung involvement); cover the upper lip with a light film of petrolatum to minimize excoriation.
4. Elimination: review
   a. Changes to be expected in the color of the stool and the number of bowel evacuations, plus the odor of stools for breast- or bottle-fed infants.
   b. The color of normal urine and the number of voidings to expect each day.
5. Safety: review the need for
   a. Protecting the infant from trauma; for example, keeping objects such as pins and scissors closed and well out of baby's reach.
   b. Preventing overheating or chilling.
   c. Care in transporting infants, particulary in automobiles (Fig. 20.48).

Fig. 20.48
Rearward-facing shell car seat. Infant is placed in car seat when going home from hospital. (From Whaley, L.F., and Wong, D.L.: Nursing care of infants and children, ed. 3, St. Louis, 1987, The C.V. Mosby Co.)

Fig. 20.49
Well-baby check. Notice how father holds and supports infant for examination. Baby is fascinated by physician (Sweden). (Courtesy Coleen Stainton.)

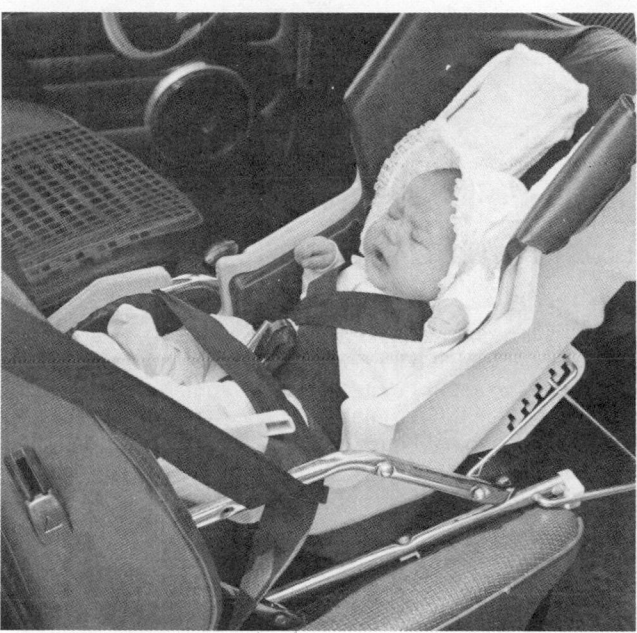

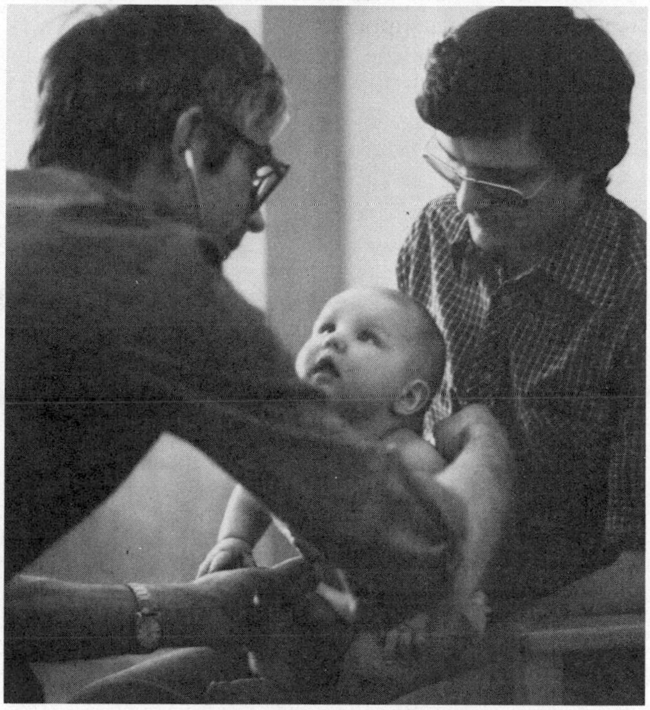

d. Supervising brothers' and sisters' attention to the new baby.

6. Review schedule for immunizations. The *ability* to protect against antigens by formation of antibodies *develops sequentially.* The fetus or infant must be developmentally capable of responding to antigens. This is the reason for planning sequential immunizations in infants. See Appendix L.

7. A form of passive immunity is present in colostrum and breast milk. It is specific for microbial agents present in the mother's own gastrointestinal tract. As the neonate is being freshly colonized, *these antibodies limit bacterial growth in the gastrointestinal tract and protect against overgrowth* (see also Chapter 5). This information helps health care professionals to plan for the use of polio vaccine in breast-fed infants. According to Korones (1981):

> Oral polio vaccine depends, for its effectiveness, on multiplication in the intestinal tract. The vaccine fails to immunize babies on breast milk from mothers with high antibody titers to poliovirus because vaccine virus is inactivated in the gut by secretory IgA from breast milk.

8. Plan for infant health supervision, that is, at 2 to 4 weeks of age, then every 2 months until 6 to 7 months of age, then every 3 months until 18 months, at 2 years, 3 years, preschool, and every 2 years thereafter (Fig. 20.49).

Evaluation

Evaluation is a continuous process. To be effective, it needs to be based on measurable criteria, which reflect the parameters used to measure the goals for care. Parental skill in infant caretaking techniques and their knowledge of their infant's needs and growth patterns form the context in which newborn care is given. The areas of parental competence as evaluated against normal infant response are presented as outcome criteria in the Summary of Nursing Actions. These criteria are the basis for selecting appropriate nursing actions and evaluating their effectiveness.

Summary

The care the newborn receives in the first months of life is reflected in the normal growth and development of a healthy infant. The nurse in the various roles as teacher/counselor, support person, and technician acts as an advocate for the vulnerable infant. Nurses are present during the formative stages of parent-child interactions. From their unique perspective they can do much to help both parents and child. A summary of the care needed by infant and parents can be found below, and application of the nursing process to nursing care of the newborn is presented on p. 590.

Summary of Nursing Actions

NURSING CARE OF THE NORMAL NEWBORN

GOALS

1. For the infant:
   a. To provide support for the infant's transition from intrauterine to extrauterine life
   b. To provide freedom from trauma such as injury and infection
   c. To provide opportunities to continue the relationship with the primary caretakers begun in the prenatal period
2. For the family:
   a. To provide opportunities to acquire knowledge, skill, and confidence relevant to child care activities
   b. To provide opportunities for parents to recognize their knowledge of their infant's behavior begun prenatally
   c. To provide opportunities for parents to reorganize and intensify relationships with their newborn

PRIORITIES

1. Establish and maintain respiration
2. Maintain stable body temperature
3. Protect infant from infection and trauma
4. Protect infant from injury
5. Provide optimal nutrition
6. Promote infant-family attachment

ASSESSMENT	EXAMPLES OF POTENTIAL NURSING DIAGNOSTIC CATEGORIES*
The first day of life **On admission to nursery 2 hours after birth** A. Check infant's identification with transfer nurse from delivery unit. B. Assess significance of the following: 　1. Gestational history (e.g., mother's age, any social problems, EDC, any physical problems) 　2. Labor and birth experience (e.g., whether labor was lengthy and difficult, what maternal medications and anesthesia were given, whether cord was wrapped around neck, type of delivery, Apgar score) 　3. Care at birth (e.g., if prophylaxis to eyes is completed) 　4. General condition and activity (e.g., infant is alert; respirations are normal; infant has voided; number of vessels in cord is normal) 　5. Color for signs of jaundice C. Physical assessment 　1. By physician or nurse practitioner before twenty-fourth hour of life 　2. By nursery personnel during caretaking activities	Potential for newborn compromise† Alteration in normal physiologic processes†

*Diagnoses approved by Seventh National Conference, 1986, except those indicated by a dagger.
†Not included by NANDA, 1986.

Summary of Nursing Actions—cont'd

ASSESSMENT	EXAMPLES OF POTENTIAL NURSING DIAGNOSTIC CATEGORIES*
D. Measure the following after temperature is stabilized: 1. Weight on admission and at 8 hours 2. Length 3. Chest circumference 4. Head circumference (repeat after molding and caput succedaneum are resolved)	
Respirations A. Check infant's respiratory effort every 15 min for 4 hours, then every hour until breathing is stable. Record findings every hour. 　1. Count respirations by observing chest wall. Note whether sternum retracts or nares flare and chin lags on inspiration. 　2. Note whether infant is normal nose breather (i.e., sleeps with mouth closed, does not have to interrupt feedings to breathe). 　3. Note abnormal sounds—grunting or wheezing—during inspiration or expiration. 　4. Assess breath sounds. 　5. Note efficiency of gagging, sneezing, and swallowing reflexes related to maintaining clear airway. B. Watch for bouts of rapid and irregular respirations, gagging, and regurgitation of mucus, etc., during "reactivity" periods: 　1. Following birth 　2. After 4 to 6 hours of life C. Assess infant's color for cyanosis. Color over head and trunk and mucous membrane is indicative of adequate oxygenation. Feet and hands may remain slightly cyanotic for 48 hours, especially when they are cold.	Alteration in respiratory function† Ineffective airway clearance Ineffective breathing pattern Impaired gas exchange Alteration in normal physiologic processes related to congenital anomalies†
Assess fluids and nutrients A. Feeding capability B. Intake	Alteration in normal physiologic processes related to maturity, sleep-wake cycle, congenital conditions, etc.† Parental knowledge deficit Ineffective airway clearance Fluid volume deficit Alteration in nutrition (calories): less than body requirements
Cardiovascular system Assess rate and rhythm of heartbeat every 4 hours. Note its regularity and presence of any heart murmurs. Assess blood pressure on admission and per hospital protocol.	Impaired gas exchange Alteration in cardiac output: decreased Alteration in normal physiologic processes related to congenital conditions
Temperature Take and record infant's temperature on admission to unit and then every hour until it is stabilized. After that, take infant's temperature every 4 hours for remainder of first 24 hours by one of the following methods: A. Rectal temperature (some hospital protocols require at least one to establish patency of anus) B. Axillary temperature C. Skin temperature by sensor	Ineffective thermal regulation related to: ■ Immaturity ■ Congenital disorder ■ Environmental factors ■ Disease process ■ Fluid deficit (hypovolemia)

Continued.

Summary of Nursing Actions—cont'd

ASSESSMENT	EXAMPLES OF POTENTIAL NURSING DIAGNOSTIC CATEGORIES*
Cord	Impairment of skin integrity
A. Check every 30 min for 4 hours for excessive bleeding.	Potential for infection
B. Check healing process. By 24 hours, cord appears dry (becomes black and stiff, like twig), with no bleeding or signs of inflammation (odor, discharge, reddened skin at base), and clamp or cord tie may be removed.	Alteration in comfort: pain
Urination	Alteration in patterns of urinary elimination
A. Note evidence of voiding before infant's admission to nursery (report of voiding at birth or wet diaper).	Alteration in normal physiologic processes related to congenital conditions†
B. Record voiding when noted. Some infants void as part of delivery process; most void by 12 hours; about 8% may not void for 2 to 3 days, depending on amount of fluid in bladder at birth and fluid intake.	
C. If infant has not voided after 24 hours, check bladder for distension and note whether infant is restless or appears in pain as pressure is applied to bladder; assess fluid intake and notify physician of findings. Physician may aspirate bladder to ascertain if urine is present. Position infant as for circumcision. Suprapubic area is exposed and cleansed. Physician will require sterile gloves, syringe (30 ml), and long needle.	
D. Note presence of urates, which appear as pink (copper dust) staining on diaper (these dissolve and disappear when diaper is placed in water and are not significant). Note also presence of blood, which does not disappear when diaper is soaked in water. Blood may result from pseudomenstruation in female or from circumcision in male. If blood on diaper is not from these sources, report it to physician.	
Meconium	Alteration in bowel elimination
A. Note evidence of meconium passage (vernix stained yellow, report of meconium-stained amniotic fluid, or passage of meconium at birth) before infant's admission to nursery.	Alteration in normal physiologic processes related to congenital conditions†
B. Record passage of meconium; may be anticipated by 4 to 6 hours or at beginning of waking periods and after feedings (gastrocolic reflex). Patency of lower (but not upper) gastrointestinal tract can then be assumed.	
C. If delay occurs in passage of meconium (24 hours or more), check for patency of anus, abdominal distension, and bowel sounds; assess amount of fluid intake and notify physician of findings. About 6% of healthy infants do not defecate for 48 hours.	
Integument (skin)	Potential for infection (transplacental, chorioamnionitis, birth canal, environmental hazards including people)
On admission and each time skin is exposed while giving care, assess for:	Impaired gas exchange
A. Rashes	Potential for injury (hyperbilirubinemia, fragility of skin)
B. Excoriations (e.g., from fingernails)	Alteration in parenting related to knowledge deficit
C. Color (e.g., petechiae, ecchymosis, jaundice, general color, mottling)	Fluid volume deficit
D. Dehydration	
E. Wounds (e.g., internal fetal monitoring, forceps, scalpel during cesarean birth, circumcision, cord, heel sticks, injections)	
F. Cleanliness	

Summary of Nursing Actions—cont'd

ASSESSMENT	EXAMPLES OF POTENTIAL NURSING DIAGNOSTIC CATEGORIES
Other physical findings Assess for other physical findings, e.g., head, eyes, ears, nose, mouth and throat, etc. (See Tables 20.1 and 20.2)	Alteration in normal physiologic processes related to congenital conditions Potential for infection
Behavioral characteristics Assess for behavioral characteristics, e.g., cuddliness, sleep-wake cycles, etc. (see Tables 20.1, 20.2, and Chapter 19)	Alteration in parenting, related to knowledge deficit Alteration in family processes Ineffective individual or family coping
Safety Assess family provisions for safety of infant in relation to: A. Caretaking activities B. Social interactions C. Transportation of infant D. Professional assistance for health maintenance or illness	Potential for newborn compromise† Potential for injury Alteration in normal physiologic processes† Alteration in health maintenance
Parental and family responses to and interactions with newborn (see also Tables 24.1, 24.2, and 24.3) A. Mother interactions: Note mother's responses as she examines and holds infant, and assess her knowledge of and skill in infant care. B. Father interactions: Note father's responses as he holds or cares for infant; assess his knowledge of and skill in infant care. C. Grandparent: Note whether grandmother and grandfather are pleased with newborn. D. Siblings: Note sibling interactions with infant, gentle or rough. Note whether mother is angry, depressed, or unaffected by sibling reactions to newborn.	Alteration in parenting related to knowledge deficit Alteration in family process Ineffective individual or family coping Grieving Impaired home maintenance management Disturbance in self-concept: body image, self-esteem, role performance, personal identity Anxiety Potential for injury

OUTCOME CRITERIA*	PLAN/IMPLEMENTATION
The first day of life **On admission** A. Report from labor nurse is complete and records are up-to-date. B. Newborn is admitted to unit per hospital protocol. C. Newborn is placed in crib and protected from cold stress. D. Assessment of newborn by twenty-fourth hour by professional personnel reveals satisfactory adjustment of newborn and a normal physical status. Newborn's appearance and activity (reflexes and behavior patterns) are within normal. E. Environment provides for protection and safety of infant.	**On admission** A. Receive reports of newborn progress to date. B. Maintain ambient temperature of nursery unit at 24° C (75° F). Make sure crib and area for bathing, changing, and examining are away from windows and drafts. C. Perform initial admission assessment per hospital protocol. D. Notify pediatrician of admission. E. Provide for: 1. Skilled personnel and adequate facilities to ensure continuous assessment, protection against infection or trauma, and care in case of emergency. 2. Consideration of needs of particular newborn with unique history, constitution, and membership in particular family group. 3. Complete medical and nursing records.

*Outcome criteria direct the selection of nursing actions (**plan/implementation**) and measure their effectiveness (**evaluation**).   *Continued.*

Summary of Nursing Actions—cont'd

OUTCOME CRITERIA	PLAN/IMPLEMENTATION

Respirations
 	
Airway is open and by 6 to 10 hours respirations are stabilized at 30 to 60/min with short periods of apnea (e.g., periodic breathing, apneic periods no longer than 15 s). Breathing is quiet (no grunting or wheezing). Chest and abdomen rise and fall in synchronized motions, and there is no sternal retraction. Infant breathes through nose; nares do not flare on inspiration. Cyanosis may be present in hands and feet.
	Respirations
	A. Perform procedures as necessary for clearing airway of mucus.
	  1. Position infant on side to facilitate drainage from mouth.
	  2. Hold infant face downward with head slightly lowered and aspirate mouth and nose with bulb syringe.
	  3. Clear airway of mucus with DeLee trap or nasal suction apparatus.
	  4. Empty stomach with DeLee trap if regurgitation of mucus is excessive.
	  5. Comfort infant after bout of gagging.
	B. If abnormal symptoms occur, institute intervention indicated (e.g., mouth-to-mouth resuscitation, oxygen therapy).
	C. Inform parents of infant's breathing pattern.

Feeding A. Initial feeding of newborn is done by the sixth hour. Mother begins breast feeding at birth (first wakeful period), or newborn is given water by nursery personnel. B. Acceptance and swallowing of nutrients and fluids (water, formula, or colostrum) are satisfactory by twelfth hour. Amount of regurgitation of mucus or nutrients and fluids is within normal limits by twenty-fourth hour.	*Feeding* A. Provide or supervise initial feeding before the sixth hour. Note newborn's feeding behavior. B. Inform parents as to newborn's feeding behavior. C. Assist with breast feeding or bottle feeding (Chapter 21). D. Demonstrate and supervise practicing of care that is required if newborn chokes or regurgitates at feeding time; demonstrate at first feeding.
Cardiovascular system A. Heart rate: heart rate (between 120 and 160 beats/min) and regularity in rhythm are stabilized by twelfth hour; rate may drop to 100 beats/min in deep sleep but returns immediately with activity. It increases with stress and activity. Most soft murmurs heard during neonatal period are functional and without pathologic significance. B. Blood pressure: Systolic pressure, 60-80 mm Hg; diastolic pressure, 40-50 mm Hg.	*Cardiovascular system* Prevent stress by providing warmth, fluids, nutrients and comfort as needed; protect newborn from infection and trauma.

Temperature
Newborn's axillary temperature is stabilized by twelfth hour and maintained between 36.5° and 37° C (97.6° to 98.6° F).
	Temperature
	A. Stabilize newborn's temperature by one of the following methods:
	  1. Remove blood and excessive vernix from newborn, dress in shirt and diaper, wrap snugly in blanket, and give to parent to hold.
	  2. Position newborn on side in bassinet, cover with light blanket, and then place infant under heat lamp until temperature is stabilized. Check body temperature every hour to prevent hyperthermia.
	  3. Place thoroughly dried infant under radiant panel without clothing until the temperature has stabilized. Check body temperature every hour to prevent hyperthermia. Then bathe newborn; if body temperature drops, place newborn under heat panel until temperature is stabilized.
	B. Minimize heat loss by performing examinations under heat panel and postpone initial bath (if given) until newborn's temperature reaches 36.5° C (97.6° F).

Summary of Nursing Actions—cont'd

OUTCOME CRITERIA	PLAN/IMPLEMENTATION
Cord Healing of cord is adequate (i.e., no oozing of blood or evidence of inflammation).	*Cord and circumcised penis* A. Administer prescribed dosage of vitamin K_1, (preparation Aqua-mephyton) intramuscularly.
Penis Healing of penis is adequate if circumcision was performed (i.e., no excessive bleeding or evidence of inflammation).	B. Position infant so no pressure is exerted on cord or circumcised penis. C. Clean routinely and as needed after soiling.
Urination Some infants void at birth; most void by twelfth to twenty-fourth hour after birth.	*Urination* A. Instruct parents as to number of times newborns void (6 to 10 per day), color of urine (pale, strawcolored), need for diaper changes. B. If urates or blood appear on diaper, tell parents of their source and significance.
Defecation Meconium stool may be passed at birth or any time thereafter until twenty-fourth hour.	*Defecation* A. Instruct parents as to characteristics of their newborn's stool and patterns of stooling. B. If necessary teach parents how to diaper their newborn.
Integument Initial bath given once newborn's temperature is stabilized. Routine of hygienic care is established.	*Integument* A. Bathe quickly to prevent loss of heat; use mild soap and water. B. Remove only surface excess vernix and blood (mats in the hair). C. Dress, diaper, and wrap snugly.
Infant-family relationship Parents interact with infant as soon as possible after birth. Parents' responses reflect their style of care, ethnic background, and energy level. Initial and subsequent contacts between parents and infant promote close parent-child ties.	*Infant-family relationship* A. Give infant to father or mother to hold as soon after birth as possible. B. Examine infant in parents' presence. Discuss normalcy of infant's condition, appearance, and behavior. C. Inform parents as to infant's progress (sleeping, waking, crying, feeding, urination, defecation, weight) and of characteristics, including cord, genitals, and appearance of stool. D. Discuss parental-family responses to child (see also Chapter 24). Review plans of care for infant.

ASSESSMENT	EXAMPLES OF POTENTIAL NURSING DIAGNOSTIC CATEGORIES
Days 2 to 14 *Respirations* Observe respirations and breath sounds and record every 8 hours while infant is in hospital.	Alteration in respiratory function† Ineffective airway clearance Ineffective breathing pattern Impaired gas exchange
Nutrition Observe and record feeding behavior, amount of formula, water taken, any regurgitations (see also Chapter 21).	Alteration in normal physiologic process† Parental knowledge deficit Ineffective airway clearance Alteration in nutrition: less than body requirements
Cardiovascular system Assess rate and rhythm of heartbeat (apical) every 4 hours. Note its regularity and presence of heart murmurs. Record findings while in hospital.	Impaired gas exchange Alteration in normal physiologic process, related to congenital disorder† Alteration in cardiac output: decrease

Continued.

Summary of Nursing Actions—cont'd

ASSESSMENT	EXAMPLES OF POTENTIAL NURSING DIAGNOSTIC CATEGORIES
Temperature Take and record body temperature every 8 hours while infant is in hospital.	Ineffective thermal regulation related to overdressing, or underdressing, exposure to heat, cold, inadequate fluid intake (inanition fever), disease process
Cord Note healing of cord. When cord drops off, (usually by tenth day) small beads of blood may appear for 1-2 days when infant cries or strains at stool. Navel may be protuberant.	Impairment of skin integrity Potential for infection Alteration in comfort: pain
Circumcised penis (third day) Check healing process. Incised area of penis should appear clean. Check for infection. No odor or discharge.	Impairment of skin integrity. Potential for excessive blood loss† Potential for infection Alteration in comfort: pain
Urination Record number of voidings. Note color and consistency of urine; record if abnormal.	Alteration in patterns of urinary elimination Alteration in normal physiologic process†
Defecation Note and record changes in stool color and consistency and in pattern infant establishes while in hospital.	Alteration in bowel elimination Alteration in normal physiologic process†
Integument Assess for: 1. Rashes 2. Excoriations 3. Color: by second day, jaundice 4. Dehydration, peeling and cracking, skin turgor 5. Wounds 6. Cleanliness	Potential for infection Potential for injury Knowledge deficit related to parenting Fluid volume deficit
Weight Weigh daily while infant is in hospital; weigh at end of second week.	Alteration in normal physiologic process†
Review findings of blood tests 1. Phenylketonuria test 48 hours after ingestion of protein—formula or breast milk 2. Galactosemia 3. Hypothyroidism	Potential newborn impairment† Knowledge deficit related to parents
Other physical findings Assess for other physical findings related to head, eyes, ears, nose, mouth, throat, reflexes (see Tables 20.1 and 20.2)	Alteration in normal physiologic process† Potential for injury Potential for infection
Behavioral characteristics Assess for behavioral characteristics, sleep and wake states, self-comforting ability (see Tables 20.3 and 20.4).	Alteration in parenting Knowledge deficit related to parenting Alteration in family process Ineffective individual coping
Safety Assess parental competence in caretaking activities, monitoring sibling activities with infant. Assess methods of transportation, knowledge of available assistance for health maintenance or illness.	Potential for newborn compromise† Potential for injury Alteration in normal physiologic process Alteration in health maintenance

Summary of Nursing Actions—cont'd

ASSESSMENT	EXAMPLES OF POTENTIAL NURSING DIAGNOSTIC CATEGORIES
Parent and family response to and interaction with newborn (see also Tables 24.1, 24.2 and 24.3)	
A. Mother interactions: Note mother's responses as she examines and holds infant, and assess her knowledge of and skill in infant care.	A. Alteration in parenting Knowledge deficit Alteration in family process
B. Father interactions: Note father's responses as he holds or cares for infant. Assess his knowledge of and skill in infant care.	B. Ineffective individual or family coping Grieving Impaired home maintenance management Disturbance in self-concept: body image, self-esteem, role performance, personal identity Anxiety
C. Grandparent: Note whether grandmother and grandfather are pleased with newborn. Are they prepared to help or "take over" the infant?	C. Alteration in family process
D. Siblings: Note sibling's interaction with infant, gentle or rough; note mother's and father's reaction to sibling response, i.e., angry, depressed, or unaffected.	D. Disturbance in self-concept: body image, self-esteem, role performance, personal identity Potential for injury Alteration in family process Anxiety Grieving

OUTCOME CRITERIA	PLAN/IMPLEMENTATION
Days 2 to 14	
Respirations	*Respirations*
Respirations are stabilized within normal limits (30 to 60/min). Mother is aware of normal variations in breathing rhythm and rate. Mother is able to keep infant's airway clear by positioning infant on side in bassinet or crib to facilitate drainage, or, if choking occurs, by turning infant onto abdomen with head down and removing mucus with bulb syringe.	Maintain open airway.
Feeding	*Feeding*
Newborn becomes adept in feeding techniques, breast or bottle, sleeps between feedings. Intake of nutrients and fluids is adequate for growth and hydration (Chapter 21).	Parent becomes adept at feeding infant and assessing fluid and nutritional needs (see also Chapter 21).
Cardiovascular system	*Cardiovascular system*
Heart rate and rhythm are normal.	Inform parents of normalcy.
Temperature	*Temperature*
Infant's temperature is maintained within normal limits. Mother becomes adept at using thermometer and is aware of influence of heat, cold, and dehydration on infant's temperature.	A. Dress infant in clothing suitable to maintain warmth in varying temperatures. B. If baby's temperature is elevated, rule out dehydration, fever, and overheating; give up to 120 ml (4 oz) of sterile water; remove some of infant's coverings. Recheck temperature in 1 hour. If elevated temperature persists, contact pediatrician.
Cord	*Cord*
Healing of cord continues; cord drops off within first 2 weeks. There is no evidence of inflammation. Mother adept at cleaning cord. Mother knows when cord drops off and what to expect.	A. Prevent infection and clean routinely every 8 hours. Notify physician of any odor or discharge and if skin around cord becomes inflamed. B. Remove cord clamp when cord is dried. C. Demonstrate care of cord. Supervise mother's care of cord.

Continued.

Summary of Nursing Actions—cont'd

OUTCOME CRITERIA	PLAN/IMPLEMENTATION
Circumcised penis Healing of circumcised penis continues. Yellowish exudate forms over glans penis; incised site remains tender for 2 or 3 days.	*Circumcised penis* Circumcision is a surgical procedure and requires routine measures related to postsurgical care. A. Control excessive bleeding by use of pressure (4- × 4-in gauze). If bleeding is not controlled, vessel may be ligated. Notify physician and prepare equipment (circumcision tray and suture). Maintain pressure intermittently until physician arrives. B. Prevent infection. Change soiled diapers and wash penis and glans with soap and water. C. Demonstrate care of circumcised penis. Supervise mother's care.
Genitalia A. Female: no excoriation, may be some mucus discharge. B. Male: clean; foreskin not retracted.	*Genitalia* A. Demonstrate care and supervise mother's efforts. B. Wash penis with soap and water. Do not attempt to retract foreskin with force. Replace after bathing if retracted. C. Instruct parents in care of diapers and how to recognize rashes. Supervise parents changing diapers.
Urination Infant voids 6 to 10 times in 24 hours; urine is pale, straw colored.	*Urination* Instruct mother that diapers need to be changed frequently but not to waken newborn for a diaper change.
Defecation Number of stools varies on basis of type of feeding—breast or bottle. Stools go through transitional process from meconium to greenish yellow, curdy stool, to yellow, more formed stool if mother is bottle feeding; or they remain golden yellow and loose if mother is breast feeding (Chapter 21).	*Defecation* Instruct parents on appearance of stool and changes to expect. Suggest they assess infant for pattern of stooling.
Weight Newborns lose up to 10% of birth weight in first few days (if birth weight was over 4256 g [9 lb 8 oz], infant may lose up to 15%). Birth weight is regained by end of second week.	*Weight* Report weight to physician if loss exceeds 10% of birth weight. Report weight to parents and its significance.
Integument A. Icterus neonatorum begins 24 hours or later after birth (in ≥ 50%), reaches peak on fourth or fifth day, then subsides and disappears within 7 days of onset. B. Melanin in skin responds to light, and color tone changes from ruddy tones at birth to black, yellow, brown, or pink, depending on amount of melanin present. C. Rashes are transitory; skin may appear dry and may peel, especially in skin folds.	*Integument* Inform parents of significance of jaundice and of tests if ordered. Perform heel sticks for blood specimen for bilirubin tests.
Appearance and behavior A. Molding of head lessens and head assumes more rounded contour by second or third day. B. Infant sleeps about 17 hours per day, wakens for feedings, and is alert and responsive. Cry is lusty, sustained, and demanding in tone. Smiles and moves arms and legs in response to human voice. Muscle tone is good.	*Appearance and behavior* Help parents become aware of infant's normal level of responses.

Summary of Nursing Actions—cont'd

OUTCOME CRITERIA	PLAN/IMPLEMENTATION

Daily hygiene
 	
 A. Parents are aware of and practice necessary activities of infant hygiene.
 B. Hygienic care and examination of infant are practiced as daily routine. Mother (father) is aware of normal characteristics and responses of infant.
 C. Parent practices safe techniques for bathing and changing infant, including care of scalp, eyes, nose, mouth, cord, nails, body creases, buttocks, and genitals.
 D. Parent is knowledgeable about dressing infant and care of infant's clothing.
 E. Parent is aware of measures used to control discomfort (e.g., diaper rash, prickly heat rash).
 F. Parents become adept at caretaking activities.
	Bathing
	
	 A. Give sponge bath as indicated. Wash scalp every day. If soap is used, use mild, nonperfumed variety. Baby lotion may be used, but do not use powder and oil.
	 B. Substitute tub bath for sponge bath when cord drops off.
	 C. Select area for bathing infant that is warm and free of drafts, with surface large enough so infant will not roll off.
	 D. Complete preparations for bathing before bringing infant to area; have clothing organized and available.
	 E. Form habit of keeping instruments, pins, scissors, and so on closed and well out of reach of infant.
	 F. Cut nails using a manicure or special infant scissors when infant is soundly asleep.
	 G. Provide care for genitals.
	    1. Change diapers when they are soiled, but do not rouse infant from sleep to change diapers.
	    2. Rashes over buttocks may appear by second or third day. Wash and dry area, expose buttocks to air, and use heat lamp if rash is severe. Position light source (25 watts) at least 45 cm (18 in) above infant; secure infant so that baby cannot move and come into direct contact with light source.

Infant-family relationships (Chapter 24) A. Parents become increasingly aware of infant's behavior as "cues" for type of care needed (food, fluids, easing of discomfort, reassurance, cuddling, exercise, changing, social contacts). B. Parents become knowledgeable as to "normal" versus "abnormal" responses of infant and where and how to seek assistance for infant problems and parenthood concerns. C. Brothers and sisters are helped to accept newborn. D. Grandparents are willing to act as assistants to parents, not take over.	*Infant-family relationships* Promote healthy infant family relationships (Chapter 24).

Safety
 	
 A. Sources of readily available emergency care are known to parents.
 B. Protection is continued against infection and trauma.
 C. Parents agree to tests for protection of infant.
    1. Phenylketonuria test 48 hours after ingestion of protein—formula or breast milk
    2. Galactosemia
    3. Hypothyroidism
 D. Plans are made for the fourth week infant checkup and for continued health supervision.
	Safety
	
	 A. Instruct parents in safety measures.
	 B. Provide parents with written information on where to call and what to report for newborn illness or other problems.
	 C. Perform heel stick on newborn to obtain blood specimen for the tests. Send for analysis.
	 D. Review purpose of test with parents. These tests are required by most states. If, on religious or moral grounds, parents object to tests, tests are not done. Parents are asked to sign statement relieving hospital and physicians of liability for damages resulting from lack of early detection and treatment for these disorders. Even if parents refuse tests while infant is in hospital, they can request them from physician or public health nurse at later date. However, serious damage can occur within first few weeks of life.

Summary of Nursing Actions—cont'd

ASSESSMENT	EXAMPLES OF POTENTIAL NURSING DIAGNOSTIC CATEGORIES
Days 14 to 28	
Assess general appearance of parent and child. Observe for signs of tension, fatigue, stress.	Anxiety Ineffective individual coping Alteration in parenting Potential newborn impairment†
Weigh infant. Measure infant's height and head circumference.	Potential newborn impairment†
Assess all body systems, using techniques of inspection, palpation, auscultation, and percussion.	Potential newborn impairment† Alteration in health maintenance
Assess infant's motor development: neurologic status (reflexes and behavior), including hearing and sight (follows moving object, raises head, looks about room).	Potential newborn impairment† Alteration in health maintenance Impairment in normal physiologic process†
Assess nutritional status.	Alteration in nutrition: less or more than body requirements.
Assess general condition of infant (alert; skin soft and clear; no rashes or evidences of trauma).	Alteration in health maintenance.
Laboratory tests (hemoglobin or hematocrit, urinalysis, intradermal tuberculin test) if needed. They are usually left until infant is 10 to 12 months of age.	Potential newborn impairment†
Assess parents' relationship with child and their knowledge of normal growth and development and symptoms of disease.	Alteration in parenting Ineffective family coping

OUTCOME CRITERIA	PLAN/IMPLEMENTATION
Days 14 to 28 A. Parent(s) brings infant for health supervision. B. Parent(s) participates in health supervision	A. Welcome parent and infant. B. Explain routine to be followed (e.g., physical assessment, discussion of changes to be expected, and assistance with problems). C. Have parent undress infant and help with examination (this provides opportunity to assess parental approach to infant).
Body systems are normal A. Respirations are stabilized within normal limits (30-60/min), and lungs sound normal. Parents are aware of signs and symptoms of respiratory distress, whom to call, and what to communicate. Family practices protective measures to minimize respiratory tract infections. B. Temperature: Infant's temperature is maintained within normal limits—36.5° to 37° (97.6° to 98.6° F). Parents are aware of signs and symptoms of fever, what measures to institute to reduce fever, and whom to contact for assistance. C. Heart rate: Stabilized at 100-120 beats/min. D. Defecation: Infant establishes pattern, varying from three to four times a day to once or twice a week. Stools are yellowish brown and soft. E. Urination: Voiding 6 to 10 times a day continues: urine is pale, straw colored. F. Nutrition: Infant establishes pattern; sucking and swallowing reflexes are normal. Appears satisfied with nutritional intake.	A. Explain significance of findings. B. Inquire about parental problems. C. Discuss solutions that are acceptable to parents. D. Review plan of well-baby supervision; that is, every 2 months until 6 to 7 months of age, then every 3 months until 18 months, at 2 years, 3 years, preschool, and every 2 years thereafter.
Appearance and behavior Assessment of infant reveals the following: A. Growth and weight are normal for infant's age and body structure. B. Vision and hearing are normal.	A. Explain significance of findings. B. Inquire about parental problems. C. Discuss solutions that are acceptable to parents. D. Give information about changes in growth and development to be expected over next 2 months.

Summary of Nursing Actions—cont'd

OUTCOME CRITERIA	PLAN/IMPLEMENTTION
C. Skin is soft with no evidence of bruising; there is no excoriation of buttocks or creases. Skin is in good condition.	E. Give information about disease processes and what to report to physician or health nurse.
D. Umbilicus: Umbilicus may protrude slightly; parents are aware of its cause and effect. No treatment is necessary; however, care learned as part of an ethnic group is accepted and supervised.	F. Review schedule for immunizations.
E. Muscle tone is good.	
F. There is no evidence of malformation of or injury to bones or joints.	
G. Infant is alert and responsive (smiles, may coo, follows people and objects with eyes, and enjoys stimulation and social contacts).	
H. Sleep pattern is established (infant is awake between one or two feedings; fussy period may be consistent).	
Parent has assumed responsibility for the following:	Help parent or parents in coping with problems. (General statement such as "Tell me how you and the baby spend your day" is preferable to "Are you having any problems?" which can be answered by a flat "No," or "Are you bathing the baby every day?" which can place parent on defensive.)
A. Plan for periodic assessment of infant, established with private physician or well-baby clinic.	
B. Continuing protection against infection or trauma.	
C. Learning about community sources of assistance for infant and for themselves.	
D. Routine observation of infant's growth and developmental needs is established as component of family's daily care of infant.	
E. Establishing a routine of care and using caretaking activities as modes of expression of parent-child relationships. There are opportunities for increasing socialization of infant with other family members and for verbal, tactile, and visual stimulation of infant.	
F. Parent-family-newborn relationships	
1. Child is accepted as a person with persisting infantile dependent needs.	
2. Child is accepted as integral part of family unit.	

NURSING CARE OF THE NORMAL NEWBORN

Ellen (19 years) and Bill (20 years) are a young couple with their first child. The baby was born 8 days ago and is a healthy term female infant. Ellen phoned the clinic to ask for help with two problems. She told the nurse the baby's cord had fallen off and the navel had blood on it. Also the baby had the sniffles. The nurse asked Ellen what the blood looked like and when did she notice it. Ellen states it bled more when the baby was crying. The blood was in little drops.

FUNCTIONAL HEALTH PATTERN: ASSESSMENT	NURSING DIAGNOSIS	RATIONALE: PLAN/IMPLEMENTATION	EVALUATION
HEALTH PERCEPTION– HEALTH MANAGEMENT Baby has sniffles.	Ineffective airway clearance.	*To increase parent's knowledge:* ■ Review symptoms of common cold: nasal congestion, coughing, sneezing, difficulty in swallowing (sore throat), low-grade fever. ■ Advise parents on ways to help infant: ● Feeding: feed smaller amounts but feed more frequently to avoid overtiring infant; hold baby in upright position to feed; offer extra sterile water. ● Sleeping: for sleeping, raise infant's head and chest by raising mattress 30 degrees *(do not use pillow);* avoid drafts; do not overdress. ● Medications: use only medications prescribed by physician; *do not use nose drops,* since aspiration may result in lung involvement. ● Cover lip with light film of petrolatum to minimize excoriation. ■ Ask Ellen to phone in 2 days and report on baby's condition.	Ellen states that measures helped. Ellen states that measures helped.

Application of the Nursing Process—cont'd

FUNCTIONAL HEALTH PATTERN: ASSESSMENT	NURSING DIAGNOSIS	RATIONALE: PLAN/IMPLEMENTATION	EVALUATION
HEALTH PERCEPTION– HEALTH MANAGEMENT Newborn's cord has fallen off on eighth day. Blood appears in the navel especially when infant cries.	Benign alteration in normal physiologic process related to increased abdominal pressure when infant cries. Knowledge deficit	*To reduce the mother's anxiety:* ■ Assure mother that bleeding from navel is not dangerous. *To increase mother's knowledge:* ■ Instruct the mother that the area under the cord is like the area under a scab. It can bleed when the scab (or cord) drops off. ■ When the baby cries, pressure in her abdomen increases. This is why it bleeds more when the baby cries.	Ellen expresses understanding.

References

American Academy of Pediatrics, Committee on Fetus and Newborn: Report of the Ad Hoc Task Force on Circumcision, Pediatrics 56:610, 1975.

Brazelton, T.B.: Infants and mothers, New York, 1969, Dell Publishing Co.

Brazelton, T.B.: Neonatal behavioral assessment scale, Philadelphia, 1973, J.B. Lippincott Co.

Coll, C.G., and others: Cultural and biomedical correlates of neonatal behavior, Dev. Psychobiol. 14:147, 1981.

Edelstein, J.: In Jensen, M.D., and Bobak, I.M.: Maternity and gynecologic care: the nurse and the family, ed. 3, St. Louis, 1985, The C.V. Mosby Co., p. 442.

Field, R., and others: Mother's assessments of the behavior of their infants, Infant Beh. Dev. 1:156, 1978.

Freedman, D.G.: Ethnic differences in babies, Hum. Nature, p. 4, Jan. 1979.

Freedman, D.G., and Freedman, N.: Behavioral differences between Chinese-American and European-American newborns, Nature 224:1227, 1969.

Gearhart, J., and Callan, N.: Complications of newborn circumcision, Contemp. OB/Gyn. 27:57, Jan. 1986.

Kirya, C., and Werthmann, M.: Neonatal circumcision and penile dorsal nerve block: a painless procedure, J. Pediatr. 92:998, June, 1978.

Korones, S.G.: High-risk newborn infants: the basis for intensive care, ed. 4, St. Louis, 1986, The C.V. Mosby Co.

Murray, A.D., and others: Effects of epidural anesthesia on newborns and their mothers, Child Dev. 52(1):71, 1981.

NAACOG: Nurses' role in neonatal circumcision, OGN Nursing Practice Resource 14:3, 1985a.

NAACOG: Neonatal skin care, OGN Nursing Practice Resource 12:3, March 1985b.

Nelson, N.M., and others: A randomized clinical trial of the Leboyer approach to childbirth, N. Engl. J. Med. 302(12):655, 1980.

Pritchard, J.A., and others: Williams obstetrics, ed. 17, New York, 1985, Appleton-Century-Crofts.

Saisal, S., and others: A comparison of infants delivered by the Leboyer and conventional methods, Am. J. Obstet. Gynecol. 139(6):715, 1981.

Speck, W.T.: Jaundice and phototherapy: Wonder where the yellow went? Paper presented at "The Fetus and the Newborn," Contemporary Forums, San Diego, 1985.

Witchell, M.: The circumcision decision and the role of the health provider, ICEA News 24(3):4, 1985.

Bibliography

Albright, G.: Neurobehavioral assessment—a prospective, J. Cal. Perinat. Assoc. 1(1):60, 1981.

Anderson, C.J.: Enhancing reciprocity between mother and neonate, Nurs. Res. 30(2):89, 1981.

Axnic, K., and Yarborough, M.: Infection control: an integrated approach, St. Louis, 1984, The C.V. Mosby Co.

Barnard, K.E., and others: Early parent-infant relationship, White Plains, N.Y., 1978, The National Foundation, March of Dimes.

Boyer, D.: Routine circumcision of the newborn: reasonable precaution or unnecessary risk? J. Nurse Midwife 25(6):27, 1980.

Crockenberg, S.B.: Infant irritability, mother responsiveness and social support influences on the security of infant-mother attachment, Child Dev. 52(3):857, 1981.

Davis, V.: The structure and function of brown adipose tissue in the neonate, J.O.G.N. Nurs. 9(6):368, 1980.

Edelstein, J.: The effect of nursing intervention with the Brazelton Neonatal Behavioral Assessment Scale on postpartum adjustment and maternal perception of the infant, unpublished masters thesis, 1975.

Ellison, S., and others: Sucking in the newborn infant during the first hour of life, J. Nurs. Midwife 24(6):18, 1979.

Eoff, M., and others: Temperature measurements in infants, Nurs. Res. 23:457, 1974.

Färdig, J.: A comparison of skin-to-skin contact and radiant heaters in promoting neonatal thermoregulation, J. Nurse Midwife 25(1):19, 1980.

Grimes, D.: Routine circumcision of the newborn infant: a reappraisal, Am. J. Obstet. Gynecol. 130:127, 1978.

Herrera, A.J., and others: Parental information and circumcision in highly motivated couples with higher education, Pediatrics 71:233, 1983.

Hutton, N., and Schreiner, R.: Urine collection in the neonate: effect of different methods on volume, specific gravity, and glucose, J.O.G.N. Nurs. 9(13):165, 1980.

Jaundiced babies bloom with home phototherapy, Clin. News 84(7):871, 1984.

Kaplan, L., and others: Circumcision: an overview, Curr. Prob. Pediatr. p. 1, March 1977.

Kesselman, S.: Circumcision reconsidered: neither harmless nor healthful, routine circumcision no longer seems justified, Childbirth Educator 1(3):43, 1982.

King, L., and others: Circumcision: rite, ritual or both? Patient Care 12:72, March 15, 1978.

Leijon, I., and Finnstrom, O.: Studies on the Brazelton neonatal behavioral assessment scale, Neuropediatrics 12(3):242, 1981.

Lovell, J., and Cox, J.: Maternal attitudes toward circumcision, J. Fam. Pract. 9:811, 1979.

Lowrey, G.: Growth and development in children, ed. 8, Chicago, 1986, Year Book Medical Publishers.

Maisals, M.J., and others: Circumcision: the effect of information on parental decision, Pediatrics 71:453, 1983.

McFadden, R.: Decreasing the infant's respiratory compromise during suctioning, Am. J. Nurs. 81(12):2148, 1981.

Pelosi, M.A., and Apuzzio, J.: Making circumcision safe and painless, Contemp. OB/Gyn. 24(1):42, 1984.

Perry, D.: The umbilical cord: transcultural care and custom, J. Nurse Midwife 27(4):25, 1982.

Reid, T.: Newborn cyanosis, Am. J. Nurs. 82(8):1230, 1982.

Rosner, B.S., and Doherty, N.E.: The response of neonates to intrauterine sounds, Dev. Med. Child Neurol. 21(6):723, 1979.

Saco-Pollitt, C.: Birth in the Peruvian Andes: physical and behavioral consequences in the neonate, Child Dev. 52(3):839, 1981.

Schachter, J., and others: Heart rate and blood pressure in black newborns and white newborns, Pediatrics 58:283, 1976.

Shearer, M.J., and others: Plasma vitamin K in mothers and their newborn babies, Lancet 2:460, 1982.

Simkin, P., and others: "Physiologic" jaundice of the newborn, Birth Fam. J. 6(1):23, 1979.

Slumek, M.: Screening infants for hearing loss, Nurs. Outlook 19:115, 1971.

Strohback, M.E., and Kratina, S.: Diaper versus bag specimens: a comparison of urine specific gravity values, M.C.N. 7(3):198, 1982.

Styer, G., and French, K.: Feeding infants with cleft lip and/or palate, J.O.G.N. Nurs. 10(5):329, 1981.

Tobiason, S.: Touching is for everyone, Am. J. Nurs. 81(4):728, 1981.

Vanderzanden, E.: Anticipatory guidance for the first two months of life, J. Nurse Midwife 24(5):28, 1979.

Wallerstein, E.: Circumcision: an American health fallacy, New York, 1980, Springer Publishing Co.

Wayland, J., and Higgins, P.: Neonatal circumcision: a teaching plan to better inform parents, Nurse Pract. 7(6):26, 1982.

Whaley, L.F., and Wong, D.L.: Nursing care of infants and children, ed. 3, St.Louis, 1987, The C.V. Mosby Co.

Whitner, W., and Thompson, M.: The influence of bathing on the infant's body temperature, Nurs. Res. 19:30, 1970.

Williams, C., and Oliver, T.: Nursery routines and staphylococcal colonization of the newborn, J. Pediatr. 44:640, 1969.

Wranesh, B.: The effect of sibling visitation on bacterial colonization rate in neonate, J.O.G.N. Nurs. 11(4):211, 1982.

Yu, V.: Body position and gastric emptying, Arch. Dis. Child. 50:500, 1975.

Newborn Nutrition and Feeding

The first year of life is a period of rapid growth and development. Physiologic growth and nutritional needs of an infant are interdependent. Therefore skillful health supervision of children requires knowledge of nutrition. The adage that "as the twig is bent the tree's inclined" is appropriate when one is considering nutrition experiences in infancy and possible health consequences in later life. The purpose of this chapter is to provide the nurse with specific information on nutrition for early infancy. It also gives more general information that will be useful for anticipatory guidance during the infant's first year of life.

Growth and Development

Growth and development represent a continuum of interactions between innate genetic potential and environmental factors. Although individual children have their own genetically predetermined growth patterns, growth proceeds in an orderly and predictable sequence. Discussion of the child's growth pattern is often the starting point for effective communication with parents.

Weight, length, and head circumference. The full-term infant will generally double the birth weight by the age of 5 months and triple it in 1 year. Most full-term infants regain their birth weight in 10 days after their initially small weight loss representing a loss of excessive body fluid. Weight loss of up to 10% is acceptable without concern, small infants losing proportionately less than larger ones.

Length increases about 50% during the first year, but doubling of birth length does not occur until about 4 years of age. Head circumference also increases rapidly during the first year in conjunction with rapid growth of the brain.

Body fat. Body composition gradually changes during the prenatal and postnatal periods. The fat content of the body increases slowly in the early fetal period and more rapidly in the last trimester. At birth the normal infant has a body composed of about 16% fat (by weight). Between 2 and 6 months of age, the increase in adipose tissue is more than twice as great as the increase in muscle mass; fat deposition occurs at a steady pace until about 9 months of age. Throughout infancy, girls add a greater percentage of weight as fat than boys; this trend continues throughout the remaining developmental years.

Growth charts. To assist in the clinical evaluation of physical growth of children in the United States, growth "standards," or "norms," have been developed for height or length, body weight, and head circumference.

Comparison of the measurements for an individual child against the National Center for Health Statistics (NCHS) percentiles indicates where the child ranks relative to all contemporary American children of the same age and sex (Hamill and others, 1979). Measurements outside the extreme percentiles may indicate nutritional problems sufficiently severe to affect growth. On the other hand, measurements within the control or intermediate percentiles indicate that growth is within normal limits by current standards (see Appendix J).

Developmental Readiness for Feeding

Healthy term neonates possess physical readiness for ingesting and digesting selected foods. They also possess the social capabilities necessary to elicit and maintain the mother's interest in feeding them.

Digestive system. All the secretions of the infant's digestive tract contain enzymes especially suited to the digestion of human milk. The ability to handle foods other than milk depends on the physiologic development of the infant. The capacities for salivary, gastric,

Table 21.1
Digestion in Infancy

Location	Function	Effect on Feeding
Birth to 3 months		
Salivary	Lactose is not produced in salivary secretions; amylase not available in significant quantities.	Salivary enzymes play no role in digestion of milk.
Gastric	Hydrochloric acid (HCl) and pepsin precipitate casein into curds; separate and acidify whey protein.	Protein digestion begins; lactose ($C_{12}H_{22}O_{11}$) digestion partly begins; fat is not digested in stomach.
Intestinal	Pancreatic and intestinal enzymes digest proteins into amino acids, reduce carbohydrate to monosaccharides, and split fatty acids from triglycerides in the small intestine.	Protein from human milk is 95% digested, and a similar percentage of protein is digested from commercial formulas that are heat treated and sufficiently dilute to produce a soft curd.
	Disaccharidases are present in border of the intestinal mucosa.	Lactose in human milk and lactose or other carbohydrates in commercial formulas are digested in intestinal mucosa.
	Pancreatic amylase is present in small quantities.	Complex carbohydrates are poorly used.
	Pancreatic lipase is present in sufficient quantity.	A total of 80% of human milk fat is digested at birth, and almost 95% is digested by 1 month.
	Lipase, naturally found in human milk, is activated by bile salts.	Digestion of fats from commercial formulas equals that of human milk; fat from other sources (butterfat) is poorly digested.

Modified from Willis, N.H.: Infant nutrition, birth to 3 months: a syllabus, Philadelphia, 1980, J.B. Lippincott Co.

pancreatic, and intestinal digestion increase with age, indicating what may be a natural pattern for introduction of various solid foods (Table 21.1).

Renal system. Kidney function of the full-term infant is not completely mature. Well-developed glomeruli filter the blood presented to the kidneys satisfactorily. The tubules, which are functionally less mature, are somewhat limited in their ability to resorb water and some solutes. Therefore it is important that the kidneys not be presented with excess solutes (renal solute load) to excrete. For this reason protein beyond that needed for growth and the extra sodium sometimes added to foods as sodium chloride (NaCl) should be avoided.

Neuromuscular system. The development of feeding behavior depends on the maturation of the central nervous system. The rooting, sucking, and swallowing reflexes are present in the term neonate. The infant also has an extrusion reflex that automatically pushes food out of the mouth when it is placed on the tongue.

Between 3 and 6 months the extrusion reflex becomes less pronounced. Sucking comes under voluntary control with lateral (sideward) movements of the jaw. This is the beginning of chewing action. At 4 to 6 months of age the infant will be able to sit with support and will have good neuromuscular control of the head and neck. The infant will be able to indicate a desire for food by opening the mouth and leaning forward. The infant will also be able to indicate disinterest or satiety by leaning back and turning around (Table 21.2).

Psychosocial development. Early emotional, psychologic, and social attachment of the mother to the infant may determine future aspects of the infant's personality. Feeding is the main means by which the newborn establishes a human relationship with the mother. Development of trust is built on the close relationship between mother and infant. If the infant's needs are satisfied through food and love, a sense of trust is developed between the child and the mother. Food becomes the infant's means of bringing his mother and his world together. The newborn communicates by vigorous and sustained crying to express hunger, thirst, pain, and discomfort.

The mother's feeding practices from birth, whether breast or bottle feeding, determine the infant's exposure to tactile stimulation. This stimulation is essential to the infant's physical and emotional growth (Table 21.2).

Nutrient Needs

The first year of life is a time of more rapid growth and development than any subsequent year. It depends on appropriate intake of calories and essential nutrients. The dietary allowances recommended by the National Academy of Sciences—National Research Council for infants during the first year of life are included in Table 21.3.

Energy (calories). The energy requirements of the infant may be considered in three areas: (1) the basal energy requirement that sustains organ metabolic

Table 21.2
Neuromuscular and Psychosocial Development: Birth to 3 Months

Neuromuscular	Psychosocial	Implication for Feeding
Month 1		
Sucking and swallowing reflexes are present at birth; stimulus in mouth leads to rhythmic sucking and swallowing pattern; tongue protrusion predominates.	Early emotional, psychologic, and social attachment of mother and infant may determine future aspects of infant's personality. Mother's feeding practices determine exposure to tactile stimulation, which is essential to infant's physical and emotional growth.	Oral reflex is a definite adaptive food-seeking reflex for survival. On reaching satiety, infant withdraws head from breast or bottle and falls asleep. If infant's needs are satisfied through food and love, trust is developed between child and mother. Feedings are main means by which infant establishes human relationship with mother.
Month 2		
Corners of mouth are well approximated but not active in sucking; open gap separates lateral portions of lips. Tonic grasp is disappearing.	Strong emotional bond develops between mother and infant and can be viewed as beginning of social interaction of infant.	Infant is individual who shapes his own behavior and feeding schedule. Infant learns to equate mother with food. Infant eats about five times each day and may sleep through night.
Month 3		
Lip movement begins to refine; lower lip pulls in; infant may smack lips. Tongue protrusion, still present, but infant may swallow with less protrusion. Infant can hold onto object without focusing on it. By end of third month, control of head and eyes is achieved.	More tactile stimulation exists with breast-fed infant. Basic trust factor (if established) is manifested in infant's responses to mother. Infant ceases to cry with hunger when mother approaches. Infant stares into mother's face while feeding and shows response to human voice.	Infant recognizes bottle or breast as source of food. Milk runs out of sides of mouth when nipple is withdrawn. Infant still does not readily accept cup.

Modified from Owen, A.L., and others: Infant feeding guide, Bloomfield, N.J., 1980, Health Learning Systems, Inc.

function, (2) the energy needed for physical activity, and (3) the energy needed for growth. During the first 4 months of life 50% of the infant's energy is expended for basal metabolism, 25% for physical activity and other maintenance functions, and 25% for growth.

During the first year energy allowances range from 120 kcal/kg at birth to 100 kcal/kg at the end of the year. The recommended daily dietary allowance (RDA) for energy is therefore stated as approximately 115 kcal/kg (52 kcal/lb) for the first 6 months and 105 kcal/kg (47 kcal/lb) for the second half of the year (Table 21.3). During the first 4 months about one third of the energy (calories) is used for growth. Both human milk and infant formulas supply approximately 67 kcal/dl (20 kcal/oz); thus 720 ml (24 oz) of human milk formula will supply about 480 kcal.

Water and fluid. The fluid requirement for normal infants is about 105 ml (3.5 oz)/kg/24 hours. This amount is usually consumed from the breast or in properly prepared formulas. Infants receiving this amount of water have approximately 100 ml/24 hours available for secretion of urine.

Water intoxication resulting in hyponatremia, weakness, restlessness, nausea, vomiting, diarrhea, polyuria or oliguria, and convulsions can result from excessive feeding of water to infants (David and others, 1981). This also may occur when water is fed as a replacement for milk (Partridge and others, 1981). In one reported case, water intoxication resulted from an infant swallowing too much water while swimming in the home pool (Knopp and Schwartz, 1982).

The percentage of body water decreases from 75% at birth to 60% at 1 year of age. This reduction is almost entirely in extracellular water. The ability to retain body water through kidney function improves in the early months of life. To the infant this means that risk of dehydration decreases as renal concentrating capacity becomes better.

Protein. The protein requirement is greater per unit of body weight in the newborn than at any other time of life. The recommended daily allowance (RDA) for protein decreases from 2.2 g/kg during the first 6 months to 2 g/kg for the second half of the first year.

The *protein* content of human milk, lower than that of cow's milk, is sufficient for the infant. Human milk

Table 21.3
Recommended Dietary Allowances for Infants

Nutrient	Age (0-6 months)
Kilocalories	wt (kg) × 115
Protein (g)	wt (kg) × 2.2
Calcium (g)	0.36
Iron (mg)	10.0
Iodine (μg)	40.0
Zinc (mg)	3.0
Magnesium (mg)	50.0
Vitamin A (μg RE*)	420.0
Vitamin D (mg)	10.0
Vitamin E (IU) (mg α-TE†)	3.0
Ascorbic acid (mg)	35.0
Folacin (μg)	35.0
Niacin (mg NE)‡	6.0
Riboflavin (mg)	0.4
Thiamin (mg)	0.3
Pyridoxine (mg)	0.3
Vitamin B_{12} (μg)	0.5

From Food and Nutrition Board: Recommended daily dietary allowances, ed. 8, Washington, D.C., 1980, National Academy of Sciences—National Research Council.
*Retinol equivalents (1 retinol equivalent = μg retinol or 6 μg carotene).
†α-tocopherol equivalents (1 mg D-α-tocopherol = 1 α-TE).
‡NE (niacin equivalent) is equal to 1 mg niacin or 60 mg dietary tryptophan.

contains far more lactalbumin in relation to casein, which reduces the amount of potential curd formation in the gut of the infant. The *amino acid* composition of human milk is ideally suited to the newborn infant's metabolic capabilities. For example, phenylalanine and methionine levels are low and cystine and taurine levels are high.

Fat. For infants to acquire adequate calories from the limited amount of milk or formula they are able to consume, at least 15% of the calories provided must come from fat. The fat must be easily digestible. Fecal loss of fat and therefore of energy may be excessive if whole or evaporated milk without added carbohydrate is fed to infants.

Fat in human milk is easier to digest and absorb than that in cow's milk. This is caused in part by the arrangement of fatty acids on the glycerol molecule. It also is related to the natural lipase activity present in non-heat-treated human milk.

Carbohydrate. Lactose is the primary carbohydrate of milk and is the most abundant carbohydrate in the diet of infants to 6 months of age. Lactose provides calories in an easily available form. Its slow breakdown and absorption probably benefit calcium absorption. The lactose content in human milk is significantly higher than that in cow's milk.

Honey is sometimes used as a sweetener for home-prepared infant foods or formula, and occasionally it is recommended for use on pacifiers to promote sucking in hypotonic babies. Use of honey for any of these purposes is currently discouraged because some sources contain spores of *Clostridium botulinum* (Arnon and others, 1979). These spores are extremely resistant to heat and therefore are not destroyed in the processing of honey. If ingested by a young infant, spores may germinate and lethal toxin may be released into the lumen of the bowel. Infant botulism may ultimately develop, and in some cases it is known to be fatal.

Major minerals
Iron. The RDA for iron for infants is 1.5 mg/kg body weight per day during the first year of life. Because both human and cow's milk are poor sources of iron, breast-fed infants and those receiving whole cow's milk formulas need the early introduction of a good bioavailable source of iron in their diets. Commercial infant formulas fortified with iron supply between 8 and 12mg/L and provide an adequate source of iron during the first 12 months. With the introduction of solid food at 6 months, iron-fortified infant cereal should be offered first.

Calcium, phosphorus, and magnesium. The RDA for calcium, phosphorus, and magnesium during the first year of life apply to bottle-fed infants. A calcium-phosphorus ratio similar to that of human milk (2:1) is more desirable for the infant than the calcium-phosphorus ratio (1.2:1) found in cow's milk. Hence levels of calcium and phosphorus in commercial formulas based on cow's milk protein have been adjusted to achieve a ratio comparable to that of human milk.

Fluoride. Fluoride assumes particular importance in the early feeding of infants with respect to the development of teeth resistant to decay. The amount of fluoride supplementation recommended from the second week through the second year of life for the breast-fed infant is 0.25 mg/24 hours. Similar levels should be provided for the formula-fed infant living in areas where the water supply contains less than 0.3 parts per million (ppm).

Trace minerals
Zinc. Human milk contains zinc at concentrations between 1 and 5 mg/L. Commercial formulas contain approximately 5 mg/L; it has been shown to be as well absorbed as that in human milk.

Iodine. There has been less concern over inadequate intakes of iodine for infants with the increase of iodine in food. Soy-based formulas for infants are fortified with iodine to counteract the effect of goitrogens (substances that cause the development of goiters, enlargement of the thyroid gland) found in soy products.

Other trace minerals. Estimates of intake of copper, chromium, cobalt, manganese, molybdenum, and selenium assumed to be required by the infant are based on amounts present in human milk. Since these amounts vary depending on the amount in the mother's diet and also vary with the same mother at different times, recommendations for intake can include only a range of values.

Fat-soluble vitamins

Vitamin A. The RDA for vitamin A is 1400 IU for the first 6 months and 2000 IU for infants aged 6 to 12 months. The human infant enters life with a reserve of fat-soluble vitamin A stored in the liver. This amount depends on the maternal vitamin A status.

Vitamin D. The need for vitamin D during infancy, when rapid calcification of bones and teeth occurs, is well documented. The ingestion of 400 IU/24 hours promotes good calcium absorption and skeletal growth. Since human milk supplies substantially less than this level of vitamin D, it is recommended that breast-fed infants be supplemented with 400 IU/24 hours from birth. Commercial formulas that are fortified provide adequate levels of vitamin D, assuming that the young infant receives adequate amounts of formula to meet energy needs.

Vitamin E. Human milk is higher in vitamin E and will meet the infant's requirement, whereas cow's milk is low and will not meet the RDA. Most commercial formulas have had vitamin E added to them and supply approximately 5 IU/L.

Vitamin K. It is recommended that every newborn infant receive a single parenteral dose of 0.5 to 1 mg of vitamin K soon after birth. This is especially important for breast-fed infants, since human milk provides much less vitamin K (15 μg/L) than does cow's milk (60 μg/L). Thus vitamin K deficiency in the newborn period is more likely to occur in breast-fed infants than in those fed on commercial formulas.

Water-soluble vitamins

Ascorbic acid. Ascorbic acid is a critical nutrient related to growth. The recommended amount of 35 mg/24 hours is easily met by human milk and by formula.

Folacin. The RDA for folacin during the first year is supplied by either human milk or cow's milk, both of which are relatively good sources of this nutrient. Folic acid has been added to several of the prepared commercial formulas in amounts to supply 30 to 50 μg/L.

Thiamine. The RDA for thiamine has been set at 0.5 mg/1000 kcal, although urinary excretion data indicate that the minimum requirement is 0.2 mg/1000 kcal.

Riboflavin. Infants up to 6 months of age need 0.4 mg of riboflavin and by 6 to 2 months need 0.6 mg. Human milk, with 0.4 mg/L, will provide slightly below this amount in the usual 850 ml consumed by the average 3-month-old infant.

Niacin. Human milk provides 0.17 mg of niacin, or a total of 0.5 mg niacin equivalents (NE) per deciliter of milk. The recommended intake of 5 to 8 mg NE can be met by human milk.

Pyridoxine (B_6). At birth the infant has a sufficient store of pyridoxine to protect against a diet practically devoid of this nutrient. The RDA recommends an intake of 0.3 mg up to 6 months of age and 0.4 mg from 6 to 12 months of age.

Vitamin B_{12}. Ordinarily there is little likelihood of vitamin B_{12} deficiency among breast-fed infants except those whose mothers are strict vegetarians. The RDA for B_{12} during the first year of life is 0.3 mg/24 hours.

Lactation

Successful lactation is the end result of numerous interacting factors, including the maturity and anatomy of the newborn, the health and nutrition of the mother, and the development of the mammary glands. Physiologically lactation is under the control of numerous endocrine glands, particularly the pituitary hormones prolactin and oxytocin. It is influenced by the suckling process and by maternal emotions. The establishment and maintenance of lactation in the human is determined by at least three factors:

1. The anatomic structure of the mammary gland and the development of alveoli, ducts, and nipples
2. The initiation and maintenance of milk secretion
3. The ejection or propulsion of milk from the alveoli to the nipple

Stages of breast development. The female human breast is a large exocrine gland that is largely quiescent during most of the woman's life span. It is composed of about 18 segments embedded in fat and connective tissues and lavishly supplied with blood vessels, lymphatic vessels, and nerves (Fig. 21.1). The size of the breast is largely related to the amount of fat present and gives no indication of functional capacity. The principal feature of mammary growth in pregnancy is a great increase in ducts and alveoli under the influence of many hormones (see Chapter 9). Late in pregnancy there is maximum development of the lobuloalveolar system and presumably a sensitization of glandular tissue for action by prolactin. Colostrum is secreted in small amounts during the last 3 months of pregnancy.

Fig. 21.1
A, General anatomic features of human breast showing its location on anterior region of thorax between sternum and anterior axillary line. **B,** Detailed structural features of human mammary gland showing terminal glandular (alveolar) tissue of each lobule leading into duct system, which eventually enlarges into lactiferous duct and lactiferous sinus. Lactiferous sinuses rest beneath areola and converge at nipple pore. (From Worthington-Roberts, B., Vermeersch, J., and Williams, S.R.: Nutrition in pregnancy and lactation, ed. 2, St. Louis, 1981, The C.V. Mosby Co.)

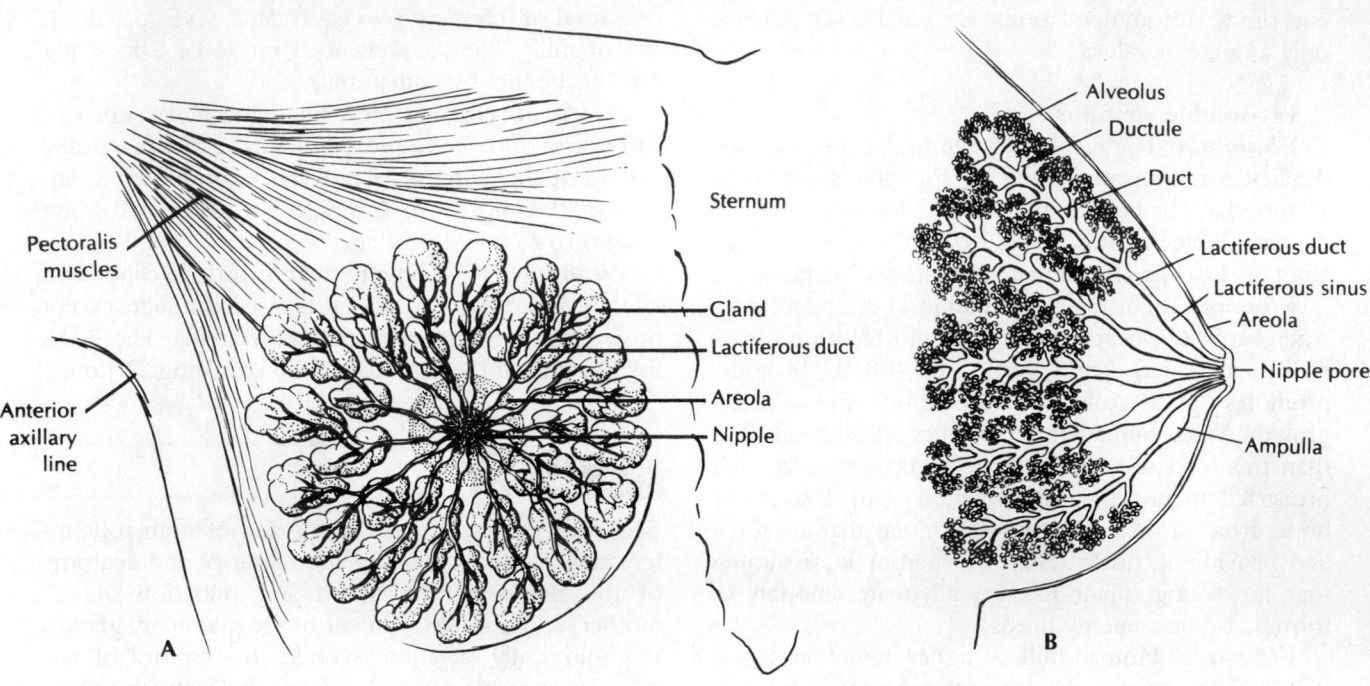

Stages of lactation. Lactation, or more properly the process of breast feeding, results from the interplay of (1) hormones and (2) instinctive reflexes and learned behavior of the mother and newborn.

Milk initiation (lactogenesis). Lactogenesis commences during the latter part of pregnancy, when secretion of colostrum occurs as a result of stimulation of the mammary alveolar cells by placental lactogen, a prolactin-like substance. It continues after birth as an automatic process.

Milk secretion. The continuing secretion of milk is mainly related to (1) sufficient production of the anterior pituitary hormone prolactin and (2) maternal nutrition. Milk secretion occurs by a process of extrusion from the cells.

Milk ejection. Movement of milk from alveoli, where it is secreted, to the mouth of the infant is an active process within the breast. This process is brought by the let-down, or milk-ejection, reflex.

Milk ingestion. The last stage of human lactation is the ingestion of milk by the suckling baby. The full-term, healthy newborn baby possess three instinctive reflexes needed for successful breast feeding: the rooting, sucking, and swallowing reflexes (see Chapter 20). Three major maternal reflexes involved in breast feeding include secretion of prolactin, nipple erection, and the let-down reflex.

Maternal breast-feeding reflexes

Prolactin reflex. Prolactin can be considered the key lactogenic hormone in initiating and maintaining milk secretion. Its production by the anterior pituitary is mainly the result of the prolactin reflex, resulting from the infant's sucking the breast (Fig. 21.2, *A*). The amount of prolactin secreted and hence the milk produced are related to the amount of sucking stimulus, that is, the frequency, intensity, and duration with which the baby nurses.

Nipple erection reflex. Stimulation of the breast nipple by the infant's mouth leads to nipple erection. The stimulation makes the nipple more prominent. This assists in the propulsion of milk through the lactiferous sinuses to the nipple pores.

Fig. 21.2

A, Diagrammatic representation of basic physiologic features of milk production. Sucking stimulus provided by baby sends message to hypothalamus. Hypothalamus stimulates anterior pituitary to release *prolactin,* hormone that promotes milk production by alveolar cells of mammary glands. **B,** Diagrammatic representation of basic features of *let-down reflex.* Sucking stimulus arrives at hypothalmus, which promotes release of *oxytocin* from posterior pituitary. Oxytocin stimulates contraction of myoepithelial cells around alveoli in mammary glands. Contraction of these musclelike cells causes milk to be propelled through duct system and into lactiferous sinuses, where it becomes available to nursing infants. (From Worthington-Roberts, B., Vermeersch, J., and Williams, S.R.: Nutrition in pregnancy and lactation, ed 2., St. Louis, 1981, The C.V. Mosby Co.)

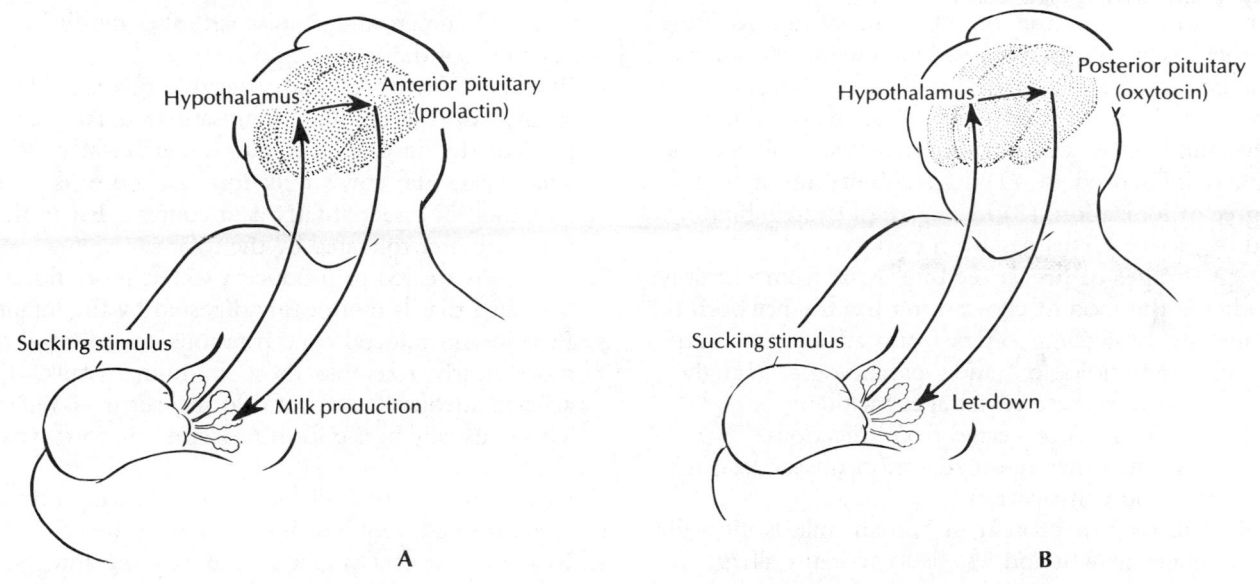

Let-down reflex. The ejection of milk from the alveoli and milk ducts occurs as a result of the let-down or milk ejection reflex. The let-down reflex is regulated in part by the central nervous system (Fig. 21.2, *B*). The primary stimulus is sucking on the nipple, which triggers the discharge of oxytocin from the posterior pituitary. Oxytocin is carried in the bloodstream to the myoepithelial cells around the alveoli, causing them to contract. The contraction forces or pushes milk out of the alveoli along the duct system, where it is easily available to the nursing infant.

The let-down reflex appears to be sensitive to small differences in circulating oxytocin levels. Minor emotional and psychologic disturbances may influence the ease with which breast milk is released to the baby. Signs of successful let-down are easily recognized by the nursing mother. Common and significant occurrences include milk dripping from the breasts before the baby starts nursing, milk dripping from the breast opposite to the one being nursed, and uterine cramps during nursing, caused by the action of oxytocin on the uterus. The attitude of the mother toward breast feeding (positive, doubtful, or negative) is a powerful factor in achieving successful lactation, influencing milk production, and facilitating the art of breast feeding.

Maternal nutrition needs during lactation. During lactation there is increased need for maternal energy, protein, minerals, and vitamins. This increase covers the cost of secreting milk, provides amounts secreted in milk for nourishment of the infant, and protects the mother's stores (see Chapter 12).

Immunologic considerations. There is evidence that the newborn infant acquires certain important elements of host resistance from breast milk while maturation of his own immune system is taking place. The human breast secretes antibodies to some intestinal microorganisms, which may help protect breast-fed infants from enteric infections. Immunologic benefits are primarily related to the effect on the intestinal flora. Immunoglobulins are believed to function directly in the infant's gastrointestinal tract by diminishing antigen contact with intestinal mucosa until the infant's own antibody responses are developed. Lactoferrin is secreted in human milk and is believed to play a role in controlling bacterial growth in the gastrointestinal tract. It works by competing with microorganisms that require iron for replication. The presence of these factors is believed to explain the reduced incidence of illness in breast-fed babies that has been reported not only in developing countries but also in the United States. (See also Chapter 8.)

Contaminants in human milk. Nonnutrients enter human milk from the bloodstream of the lactating mother. Such compounds include environmental pollutants, nicotine, marijuana, caffeine, and alcohol (see Appendix K and Chapter 28). The distribution of a compound across the membrane between plasma and milk is influenced by (1) its solubility in fat, (2) its degree of ionization, (3) its degree of protein binding, and (4) active versus passive transport.

Advantages of breast feeding. Milk from a healthy mother is the food of choice for a healthy newborn or infant. Breast feeding offers many advantages: nutritional, immunologic, and psychologic (Hughes, 1984). Some of these advantages include:

1. The infant is protected from infections.
2. The infant has fewer digestion upsets; less diarrhea, no constipation.
3. The type of protein in human milk is ideal for infant growth and less likely to cause allergic reactions.
4. The infant has fewer problems with overfeeding. The need to "empty the bottle" is eliminated.
5. Breast feeding is more convenient; no bottle washing, preparation of formula, or refrigeration are necessary.
6. Mother and child have an opportunity to develop an affectionate bonding relationship.
7. Breast feeding provides the infant with sensory stimulation—the touch and smell of the mother's body, taste of her milk, sound of her heartbeat.
8. Maternal organs return more quickly to their prepregnant condition.
9. The extra energy expended to breast feed (approximately 500 calories per day) may help quicken the return to prepregnant weight (Madgic, 1986).

Commercial Formulas

The Committee on Nutrition of the American Academy of Pediatrics proposed standards for infant formulas in 1976. Recommendations for minimum desirable concentrations of major nutrients were largely based on levels found in mature human milk.

Commercially manufactured formulas prepared from nonfat cow's milk are readily available and generally are used for feeding in early infancy. Most commercial formulas provide 20 kcal/oz. Several brands are marketed, with and without added iron. Composition of selected formula products, mature human milk, and cow's milk is shown in Table 21.4. A number of vitamins have been added to each different brand: almost all are fortified with vitamins A and D, ascorbic acid, and vitamin B_6; some also contain vitamin E, folic acid, and vitamin B_{12}; and others contain B-complex vitamins. Commercial formulas are also modified in one or more of the following ways:

1. Butterfat is removed and vegetable oils are added to increase the amount of unsaturated fatty acid, particularly linoleic acid, an essential fatty acid. This makes the cow's milk formula more like human milk in essential fatty acid content. Fat in this form is better tolerated by the infant.
2. Protein is treated to produce a softer, more flocculent curd that is more easily digested by the infant.
3. Protein and mineral concentrations are adjusted to more nearly resemble those in human milk. To achieve adequate levels of calories, sugar is added. This is usually in the form of lactose or corn syrup solids.

Most formulas are available in the following forms:

1. Concentrated: requires dilution with water
2. Ready-to-use (bulk): requires measuring into bottles
3. Ready-to-use (individual feedings): sold in disposable bottles
4. Dry powder form: requires mixing with water according to label instructions.

Advantages of formula feeding. Formula feeding has proven a successful substitute for breast feeding in certain instances. These include the following:

1. Some women and men are repulsed by the idea of breast feeding and are unwilling to breast feed their infant.
2. The mother may be physiologically unable to breast feed because of breast abnormalities or a disease process concomitant with pregnancy such as tuberculosis or cardiovascular disease.
3. The mother may have other commitments, for example, being the wage earner in the family.
4. The infant may be adopted.
5. The infant requires a special formula.

Assessment

Feeding an infant involves the infant and the primary caretaking parent, usually the mother. Therefore both need to be assessed.

Table 21.4
Composition of Milks and Formulas Commonly Fed to Infants

	Human Milk	Enfamil	Similac	SMA	Isomil	Nursoy	Prosobee	Whole Cow's Milk
Components								
Protein		Nonfat milk	Nonfat milk	Nonfat milk and dialyzed whey	Soy protein isolate	Soy protein	Soy protein isolate	
Fat (oils)		Soy and co-conut	Coconut and soy	Oleo, coconut, safflower, and soy	Coconut and soy	Oleo, soy, coconut safflower	Soy	
Carbohydrate		Lactose	Lactose	Lactose	Corn syrup solids and sucrose	Corn syrup solids and su-crose	Corn syrup solids and su-crose	
Constituents (per liter)								
Protein (g)	11.0	15.0	15.0	15.0	20.0	23.0	25.0	35.0
Fat (g)	38.0	37.0	36.0	36.0	36.0	36.0	34.0	37.0
Carbohydrate (g)	68.0	70.0	72.0	72.0	68.0	68.0	68.0	49.0
Vitamin A (IU)	1870.0	1664.0	2460.0	2600.0	2460.0	2600.0	1664.0	1024.0
Vitamin D (IU)	22.0	416.0	39.30	416.0	393.0	416.0	416.0	440.0
Vitamin E (IU)	1.8	12.5	14.6	9.4	14.8	9.4	14.6	1.6
Vitamin C (mg)	42.6	54.0	54.0	57.0	54.0	57.0	52.0	10.0
Thiamin (mg)	0.16	0.5	0.6	0.7	0.4	0.7	0.5	0.3
Riboflavin (mg)	0.35	0.6	0.9	1.0	0.6	1.0	0.6	1.8
Niacin (mg)	1.5	8.3	6.9	9.9	8.8	9.9	8.3	0.9
Pyridoxine (mg)	0.1	0.4	0.4	0.4	0.4	0.4	0.4	0.6
Pantothenate (μg)	1.8	3.1	2.9	2.0	5.0	3.0	3.0	3.4
Folacin (μg)	52.0	104.0	49.0	52.0	104.0	52.0	104.0	55.0
Vitamin B_{12} (μg)	29.0	2.0	1.5	1.0	3.0	2.0	2.0	4.0
Vitamin K (μg)	15.0			57.0	156.0	104.0	104.0	
Calcium (mg)	345.0	541.0	502.0	437.0	688.0	624.0	780.0	1168.0
Phosphorus (mg)	137.0	458.0	384.0	325.0	492.0	437.0	520.0	918.0
Sodium (mg)	158.0	276.0	215.0	148.0	311.0	198.0	416.0	505.0
Potassium (mg)	527.0	686.0	702.0	551.0	738.0	725.0	728.0	1360.0
Chloride (mg)	379.0		536.0	364.0	543.0	361.0	416.0	1028.0
Magnesium (mg)	40.0	47.0	41.0	52.0	49.0	68.0	73.0	120.0
Manganese (mg)	0.1	1.1	0.03	0.2	0.2	1.0	1.0	0.4
Copper (mg)	0.4	0.6	0.4	0.5	0.5	0.5	0.6	0.3
Zinc (mg)	4.1	4.2	4.7	3.6	5.0	3.6	5.0	4.0
Iodine (μg)	30.0	68.0	99.0	68.0	148.0	104.0	47.0	52.0
Iron	0.5	12.5	12.5	12.5	12.5	12.5	12.5	0.5

From Committee on Nutrition: Pediatrics **57**:281, Feb. 1976. Copyright American Academy of Pediatrics 1976.

Infant. The infant is assessed for developmental readiness for feeding, nutritional needs and success of the feeding program (Owen, 1980). Infant responses noted in Table 21.5 are assessed shortly after birth for the breast-fed and bottle-fed infant.

As the infant grows and matures, nutritional needs reflect the change. Table 21.6 illustrates the changing amounts of food intake and dietary supplements over the first 3 months of life.

The infant who is obtaining the necessary nutrients and fluid will exhibit a steady increase in weight, good skin and muscle tone, vigorous feeding behavior, and satisfaction. The satisfied neonate sleeps, cries in moderation, and is interested in socializing.

Mother. The mother (couple) is assessed as follows:

1. Physical ability and psychological readiness for feeding the newborn
2. Knowledge of the advantages of breast and bottle feeding so an informed choice of method can be made
3. Knowledge of the infant's nutritional needs and capabilities
4. Knowledge and skill in feeding methods

Table 21.5

Newborn Readiness for Feeding

Infant Response	Rationale
Newborn's age in hours or infant's age in days	During reactivity periods, excessive mucus with gagging may occur. Feeding increases the danger of aspiration. In general, reactivity times occur at birth and at 4 to 6 hours of age.
Condition at birth	Infants with Apgar scores of 6 or less (depressed) or the infant with low birth weight (2500 g or less) may display a delayed reactivity. This may occur after 12 to 18 hours of age.
Possibility of congenital anomalies of gastrointestinal or respiratory tract; incidence of congenital anomalies higher in preterm infants	With choanal atresia, the neonate is unable to breathe and feed simultaneously. With esophageal atresia, the infant will regurgitate and may aspirate. With tracheoesophageal fistula, feeding may enter trachea directly. With lower gastrointestinal tract obstruction (stenosis, atresia), regurgitation, vomiting, or abdominal distention may compromise respirations.
Gastric capacity	Limited stomach capacity dictates smaller feedings. To provide adequate nutrition, feedings are scheduled more frequently.
CNS maturity	Sucking and swallowing reflexes may not be well developed and synchronized (even in a term baby, the suck and swallow reflex may not be well coordinated during first few hours).
Energy level	Premature infant or infant with respiratory distress may not have sufficient energy to divert to the process of feeding.
Type of feeding; plain sterile water	Until infant's ability to feed is assessed, danger of aspiration exists. Plain sterile water is less irritating to the respiratory tract. Formula may cause aspiration pneumonia. Glucose water may cause inflammatory response in the respiratory tract similar to response to aspirated formula.

Table 21.6

Nutrition Profile: First 3 Months (Male Infant)

Age (mo)	Weight (kg)	Observed Range of Intake*		Suggested Intake of Food (Daily)	Supplements Required (Daily)	Feeding Schedule
		kcal/kg	kcal/24 hr			
0-1	3.3-4.3 (+1 kg)	(10th-90th)† 88-150	(10th-90th) 275-580	Human milk, 420-840 ml (14-28 oz) *or* Iron-fortified commercial formula, 420-840 ml (14-28 oz)	Iron, 7 mg Vitamin D, 400 IU Fluoride, 0.25 mg *or* Fluoride, 0.25 mg, if water supply contains less than 0.3 ppm	*Ad libitum*
1-2	4.3-5.2 (+0.9 kg)	(10th-90th) 108-157	(10th-90th) 465-680	Human milk, 690-1020 ml (23-34 oz) *or* Iron-fortified commercial formula, 690-1020 ml (23-34 oz)	Iron, 7 mg Vitamin D, 400 IU Fluoride, 0.25 mg *or* Fluoride, 0.25 mg (if applicable)	*Ad libitum*
2-3	5.2-6.0 (+0.8 kg)	(10th-90th) 93-139	(10th-90th) 505-795	Human milk, 750-1200 ml (25-40 oz) *or* Iron-fortified commercial formula, 750-1200 ml (25-40 oz)	Iron, 7 mg Vitamin D, 400 IU Fluoride, 0.25 mg *or* Fluoride, 0.25 mg (if applicable)	*Ad libitum*

Modified from Owen, A.L., and others: An infant feeding guide, Bloomfield, N.J., 1980, Health Learning Systems, Inc.;
*Data from Beal, V.A.: Nutritional intake. In McCammon, R.W.: Human growth and development, Springfield, Ill., 1970, Charles C Thomas, Publisher, p. 261.
†10th and 90th percentiles. Appendix J.

5. Knowledge of an adequate and safe diet during lactation

The techniques used to assess these areas include primarily interviews, discussions, and observation of skill in feeding methods.

Nursing Diagnoses

When dietary data have been collected and analyzed, nursing diagnoses relative to the infant nutritional status can be made. Examples include the following:
1. Knowledge deficit related to normal growth and development of the infant and his or her nutritional needs
2. Knowledge deficit related to feeding skills
3. Alteration in self-concept related to difficulties encountered in breast feeding

Plan

Teaching and counseling concerning the feeding of infants are part of the daily care plan for maternity clients. The benefits of both breast feeding and bottle feeding are presented so that the mother can make an intelligent choice as to how to feed her baby. Counseling begins in the first or second trimester of pregnancy when the mother is unrushed and has time to consider her choices (see Chapter 11). Women are encouraged to express their opinions and feelings so that they can be discussed and any misinformation can be corrected. During the last months of pregnancy, counseling on the process of lactation is made available to women who have decided to breast feed. Fathers are encouraged to participate in counseling sessions because their encouragement and emotional support contribute to successful lactation. Many mothers have never seen a woman nursing an infant; they therefore find it especially helpful to have a woman who has successfully nursed an infant available to answer questions and provide reinforcement.

With the birth of the infant, the decision of the parent to either breast or bottle feed is accepted and supported. Feeding is an emotionally charged area of infant care. Culturally, the size and growth of an infant are equated with excellence and evidence of mothering ability. The infant who is a fussy eater can serve to raise parental anxiety levels. The anxious parent appears to compound the problem, and a vicious cycle can develop. Relatives or friends can take over a feeding period or two. This seems to break the cycle so that the mother can view the feeding session in a more relaxed manner, not as a condemnation of her care.

Mothers need positive feedback to develop a feeling of confidence in their own ability. Often just listening and praising is the most effective intervention, as the following incident illustrates.

■ The mother reported her 6-day-old son (2604 g [5 lb, 13 oz]) had taken 90 ml (3 oz) at 11 PM, 45 ml (1.5 oz) at 3 AM, 30 ml (1 oz) at 6 AM, and now at the 10 AM feeding, "was sleepy and seemed to want only 45 ml (1.5 oz)." The nurse suggested she keep track of the total amount taken over 24 hours. The mother interrupted to say, "I know what is wrong—yesterday all the relatives visited and held him. I think he's tired out." The nurse agreed that this could be so. She also commented on how aware the mother was of her baby's intake.

    The next day the mother reported he was eating very well and noted, "I'm glad my instincts were right—it was just too busy a day for him."

Many mothers need considerable assistance with infant feeding. Both group and individual teaching are necessary. Hospitals usually provide excellent teaching aids.

Goals. The goals for the infant include the following:
1. To provide the levels and types of nutrients to support the infant's body composition, activity, and growth
2. To minimize the physiologic stress associated with digestion, metabolism, and excretion of nutrients
3. To supply sufficient water to maintain adequate body water control

The goals for the mother include the following:
1. To provide knowledge that can be used for sound nutritional selection and feeding practices
2. To assist her to become skilled in the feeding method of her choice
3. To foster mother-child closeness and pleasure

Implementation

Nurses act as teachers, counselors, and technicians in helping parents learn about feeding their infants. They act as change agents in motivating parents to adopt healthful eating behaviors for themselves and their families. In doing so they help parents clarify goals and make decisions. Parents need assistance in the techniques of breast and bottle feeding. They seek counseling for specific concerns and welcome anticipatory guidance. The first feeding method discussed is breast feeding, the second, bottle feeding. Anticipatory guidance is then reviewed.

Text continued on p. 608.

Guidelines for Client Teaching

BREAST FEEDING

ASSESSMENT

Primipara, planning to breast feed her infant girl, weight 3360 g (7½ lb).

NURSING DIAGNOSIS

Knowledge deficit related to breast feeding

GOALS

Short-term

To have infant breast feed successfully

Intermediate

To establish a feeding pattern satisfactory to infant and mother

Long-term

To be able to adjust feedings to needs of newborn by recognizing the infant's cues for hunger and satiety

REFERENCES AND TEACHING AIDS

Hospital pamphlets about infant nutrition, films on breast feeding, posters and booklets such as:

1. *Nutrition Notes for New Mothers* (1981) edited by D. Madgic, M.A., R.D., Department of Dietetrics, Stanford University Hospital, Standford CA 94305
2. *Breast Feeding, A Family Affair* (1985), by Marjorie Pyle, RNC, Lifecircle, Costa Mesa, CA 92626

CONTENT/RATIONALE	TEACHING ACTION
1. Before we put the baby to breast I will review some facts with you	
a. You can take any position you want that is comfortable for you. Let the breast fall forward without tension. Leave one hand free to guide the nipple into the child's mouth.	a. Have mother experiment with positions. Have her assume the one she feels is most comfortable (Fig. 21.3).
b. I'll review the structure of the breast. The nipple can be made more prominent by gently rolling it between your fingers. The areolar area will be put in the baby's mouth with the nipple. This prevents bruising the nipple.	b. Have woman expose her breast. Have woman prepare her nipple. Point out areolar tissue.
c. Colostrum is the yellow fluid you can express from your breasts now. It is good for the baby. It contains some fat and protein and helps the baby resist infections.	c. Demonstrate technique for expressing milk from her breast. Have her express some colostrum.
d. Milk may be expected to appear 48 to 96 hours after delivery. Before the milk comes in, the breasts feel soft to the touch. After the milk comes in, the breasts feel full and warmer.	d. Have her touch breasts to feel softness.
e. To put the baby to breast hold her so that her cheek touches the breasts. The pressure against the outer angle of the lip begins with the rooting reflex. She will turn toward the nipple. The baby can smell the colostrum and milk, and this also will make her turn toward the nipple.	e. Demonstrate rooting reflex by touching finger to infant's lips.
f. To put the baby to breast, the nipple and surrounding areolar tissue are guided into the infant's mouth and over the tongue. This is done by placing a finger on either side of the nipple and compressing the areolar area.	f. Have the mother practice (Fig. 21.4).
g. At first the baby sucks in short bursts of three to five sucks followed by single swallows. In 1 to 2 days a sucking pattern evolves. This consists of 10 to 30 sucks followed by swallowing. The infant's lips and jaws exert pressure on the areola and the tongue "cradles" the nipple so that the tip is not eroded. The pressure combined with negative intraoral pressure brings milk into the mouth (Fig. 21.5).	g. Bring infant to mother. Have her assess her baby's suck by placing her finger in the baby's mouth with the finger pad touching and stroking the palate. She should be able to feel the tongue cushioning the joint of her finger and stroking the finger, while keeping the gum covered. She should not feel an insecure or loose suction on the finger, a tapping of the gum on the finger alone, or combined with the tongue slipping back and forth across the gum (licking).
h. When the baby is sucking properly there is no "clicking" noise. This clicking noise means she is sucking on her own tongue in the back of the throat, past the	h. Have mother suck her own tongue at the back of the throat to hear the clicking sound.

Continued.

Fig. 21.3
Positioning the baby: series. **A,** Cradle hold. One arm and hand supports baby. Other hand supports breast (thumb above and fingers below). Breast is guided into baby's mouth. **B,** Side-lying position. Pillows support mother's head. Baby is turned toward mother. Mother depresses breast to facilitate baby's breathing. **C,** Variation on side-lying position. **D,** Football hold. Baby is held in one arm with hand supporting head. (Courtesy Marjorie Pyle, RNC, Lifecircle, Cost Mesa, California.)

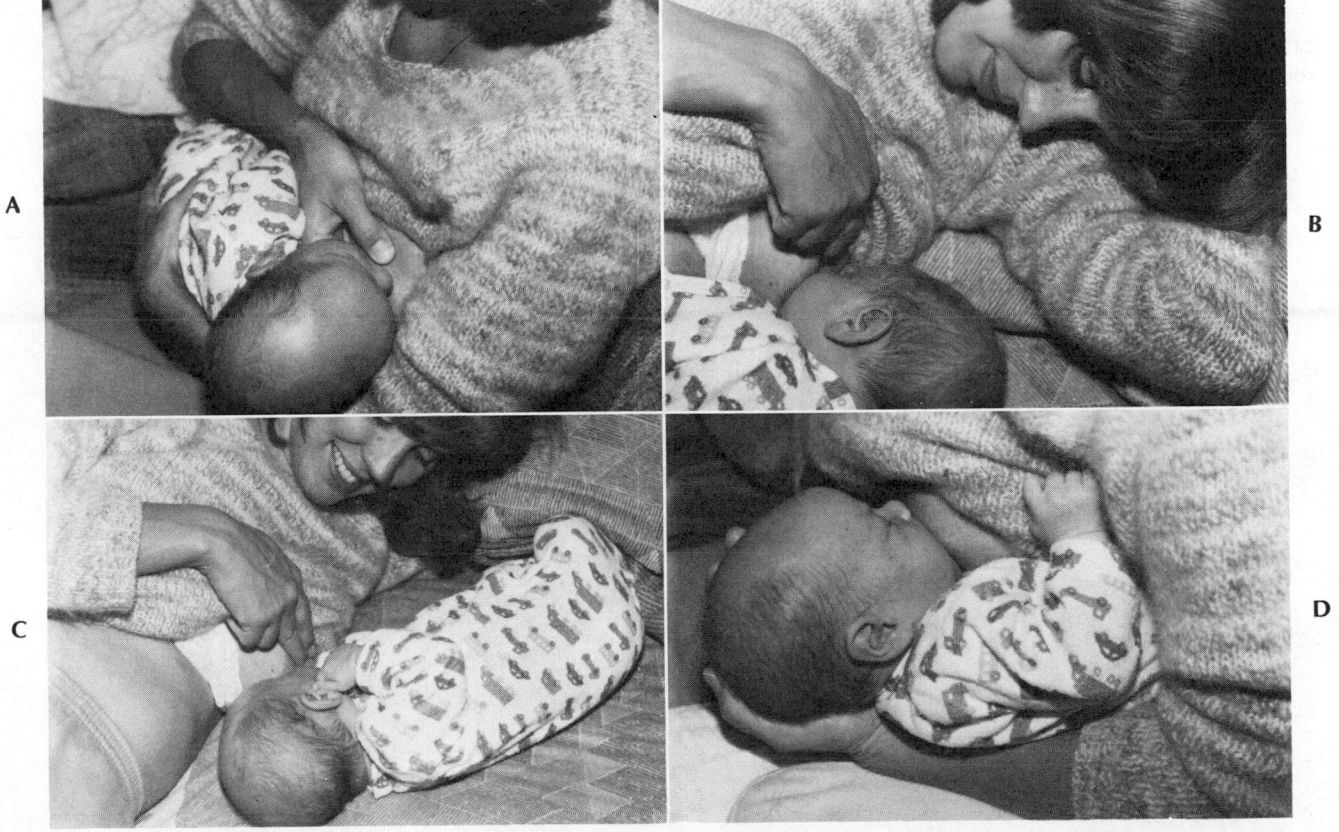

Fig. 21.4
Pointing nipple. (Courtesy Ross Laboratories, Columbus, Ohio.)

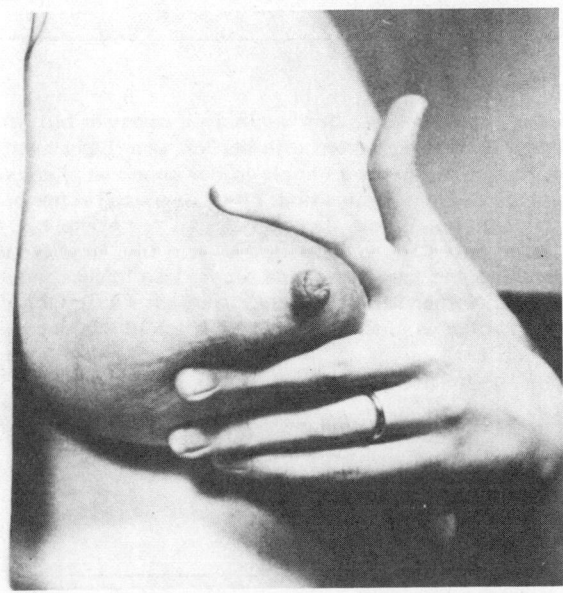

Fig. 21.5
Breast feeding. Sucking process: (1) Infant breathes
through nose. Tongue and palate meet closing
esophagus. (2) As infant takes nipple, tongue comes
forward and draws nipple and areola into mouth. (3)
Nipple is sucked to back of mouth. Areola is held in
place by gums. Tongue cradles nipple as it is pressed
against hard palate, forcing milk from sinuses. (4) Milk
flows because of negative intraoral pressure toward back
of mouth, and swallowing reflex is initiated. (5) Gums
relax, allowing nipple to refill, and cycle begins again.

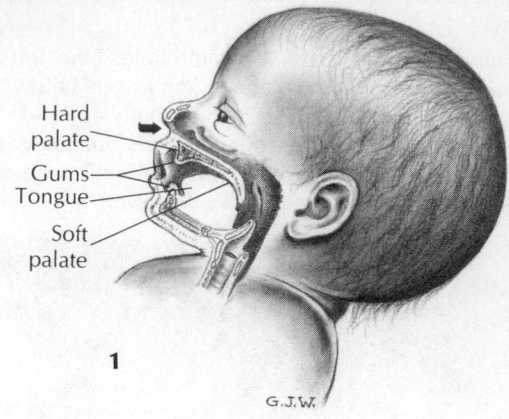

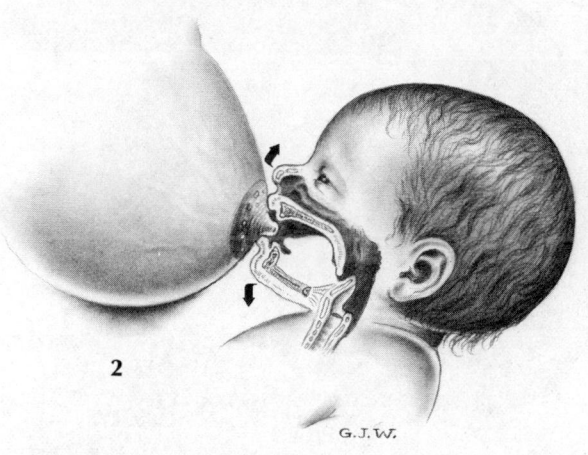

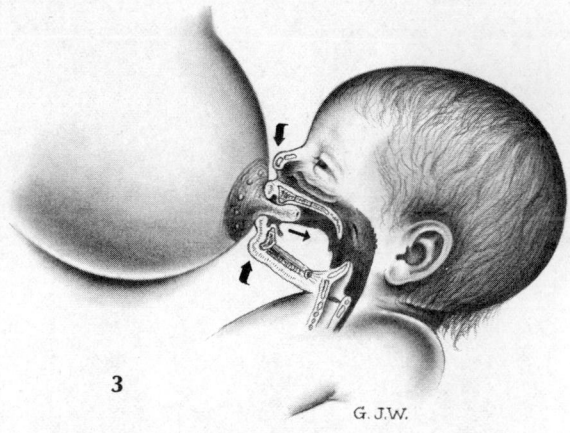

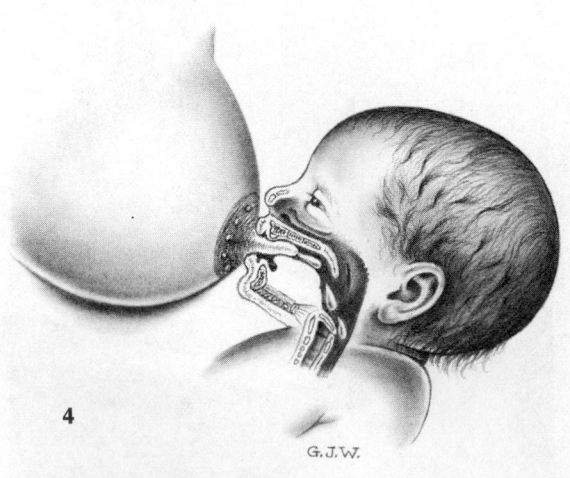

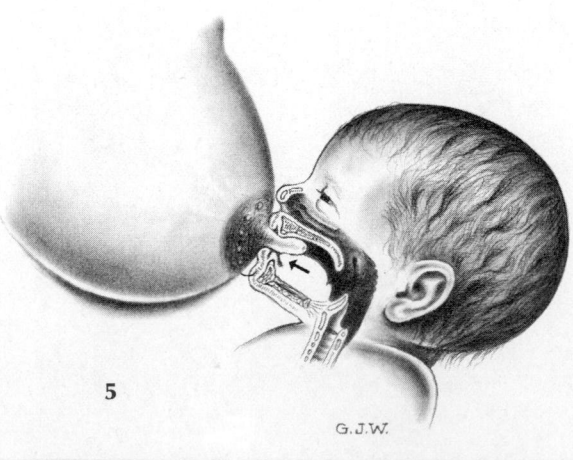

Guidelines for Client Teaching—cont'd

CONTENT/RATIONALE	TEACHING ACTION
nipple. You should hear the rhythmic suck-swallow breathing pattern that indicates milk is flowing. Some mothers can sense if the infant has drawn the areolar tissue into the mouth along with the nipple.	
2. Now let's get the baby ready and put her to breast. First we make sure she is awake.	2. If necessary waken the baby by stroking cheek, rubbing her feet, and talking to her.
3. Now put her to breast. Make dimple in breast to facilitate breathing (Fig. 21.3, *B*).	3. Help mother position baby so that the head is directly facing the breast and the nipple is not pulled to one side.
4. I will be back to help you put her to the other breast. It is best to use both breasts at each feeding. Once the milk has come in you can tell which breast to start with next time by feeling their weight. The heaviest one has the most milk, so start with that one.	
5. To remove the baby from the breast, place a finger in the corner of the baby's mouth until the suction is broken. The breast can then be comfortably removed. I will be back in about 5 minutes to help you. (Leave mother to enjoy her baby.)	5. Return in 5 mintues to supervise mother removing baby from the breast.
6. Before putting her to the other breast I will show you how to burp her. Some babies never burp, others do frequently. Gently rub the baby's back.	6. Demonstrate burping (Fig. 21.6). Supervise mother putting baby to other breast.
7. After feeding, place her on her right side. This allows any air in the stomach to come up and not bring the milk with it.	7. Show her a picture of an infant on right side (Fig. 20.31).

EVALUATION Mother demonstrates competency in breast feeding.

Fig. 21.6
Positions for burping a baby. **A,** Upright. **B,** Across the lap. **C,** Shoulder position. (Courtesy Marjorie Pyle, RNC, Lifecircle, Costa Mesa, California.)

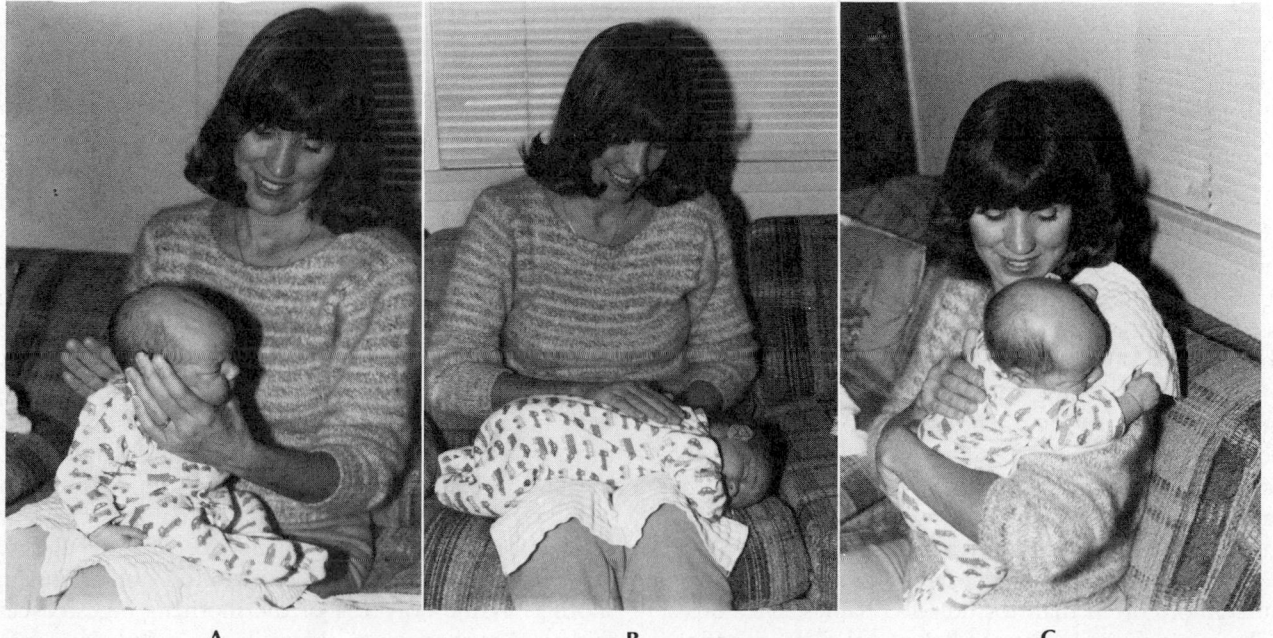

A   B   C

BREAST FEEDING

Breast feeding presents no problem for many women. Others require considerable assistance to become proficient (Riordan, 1983). They have had no contact with other mothers who breast feed and often little or no contact with newborns. They need patient support and encouragement. The Guidelines for Client Teaching outline a plan for helping an inexperienced mother with the first breast-feeding session with her baby.

Adjusting to breast feeding

Care of breasts. Daily washing of the breasts with water is sufficient for cleanliness. A lubricant such as liquid petrolatum or lanolin may then be massaged gently into the nipple area, and if feasible, the breasts can be exposed to the air for 20 to 30 minutes. The lubricant should not contain alcohol, since the drying effects of the alcohol tend to encourage cracking of the tissue. Some infants object to either the taste or smell of ointments and will refuse to nurse until the breast has been washed.

The nursing brassiere needs to be well-fitted, with broad shoulder straps and the flaps over the breasts large enough to release the breasts without discomfort. Milk leaking from the breasts, particulary just before the next feeding (ejection reflex), can be uncomfortable and embarrassing. Pad the brassiere with folded squares of soft cotton, a perineal pad cut in two, or commercially designed pads. A tingling sensation in the nipple area precedes leaking of the milk. Pressure with the heel of both hands over the nipple areas will often prevent the milk from forming so that leaking from the breasts is forestalled. Lining the brassiere cup with plastic material is not recommended, since moisture tends to soften the nipple and predispose it to erosion.

Diet and fluids. Certain *highly flavored foods* like garlic and onions may cause a flavoring of the milk. This is not sufficient reason for avoidance if the mother likes to eat them and they are taken in moderation. The important thing for the mother to remember is to eat a wide variety of foods and not to go "overboard" on any one particular food.

The breast feeding mother requires *extra fluids,* as much as 3 L per day. These can be taken routinely before each feeding. Glasses of water, fruit juices, decaffeinated tea, or milk can be alternated. The mother can keep a pitcher of water close by when breast feeding, as she often becomes very thirsty.

Infant responses. Breast-fed babies may wish to nurse more often than formula-fed babies, since breast milk is more easily digested than other foods. If the baby wants to nurse, there is no reason not to do so.

Breast-fed babies consume what they need and no more. Breast-feeding whenever the baby is hungry is easy to do because the milk is always ready. Some babies may be hungry as freqently as every hour or two on some days, on other days only every 4 hours. The more often the baby nurses, the more milk the breasts produce; thus whenever a woman's supply is low (e.g., during or after an illness), she should nurse more often. If the woman has too much milk, the baby may need to breast feed on only one side at a feeding for a while. This will reduce overall stimulation and reduce the milk supply.

Crying does not always mean that the baby is hungry. The baby may be physically uncomfortable or just want to be held, burped, or changed. Mother can be reassured that she is producing sufficient milk if the infant has 6 to 10 voidings of pale, straw-colored urine in 24 hours. In warm weather the baby may be thirsty. The mother can give the baby a bottle of sterile water (1 to 2 oz) or increase the number of breast feedings.

The *stools* of breast-fed babies are very loose. Some infants have a bowel movement at each feeding, whereas others may go up to 5 days without one. Babies who are fed only breast milk do not become constipated, although they may strain considerably in passing the stool. The stool is not irritating to the skin.

Tension tends to lessen milk production. The mother will require adequate rest. The first few days after the mother comes home with the new baby are often filled with excitement and anxiety about mothering activities. Entertaining company or undertaking extended family commitments may have to be restricted.

Secretion of drugs in maternal milk. If *oral contraceptives* are taken sooner than 6 weeks after delivery, the amount of milk a woman produces may be diminished. Experience indicates that most women will not have difficulty producing an adequate amount of milk if they do not use oral contraceptives until after weaning the infant.

Substance abuse poses significant concern for the nursing infant. Regular use of *alcohol* is common in our society. However, during both pregnancy and lactation, even moderate drinking can pose problems for the unborn child or infant. *Smoking* by the lactating woman can cause a decrease in her milk supply. Another reason not to smoke is the second-hand smoke in the baby's atmosphere. This smoke can aggravate or even trigger asthma symptoms, and babies of parents who smoke have a higher incidence of lung disease. *Caffeine* should be taken in moderation by the nursing mother. While only 1% of the mother's ingested caffeine passes through to the milk, the baby's immature system cannot get rid of the caffeine as effectively as an adult can. Some babies are very sensitive to even a small amount of caffeine. Caffeine is found in coffee, tea, chocolate, and some soft drinks. It is best to limit these drinks to no more than 24 oz per day total. If *cathartics* are taken, they may cause loose stools in the infant.

Effect of menstruation. If menstruation occurs, the mother can continue to breast-feed. Although some babies may act fussy, the quality and quantity of the milk are not affected.

Maternal commitments. On occasions when the mother needs to be away from the infant at the usual time of feeding, a bottle of breast milk, expressed earlier, can be substituted. If the mother returns to work, she can continue to breast feed (MacLaughlin and Strelnick, 1984; Price and Bamford, 1983). (See directions in the boxed material.) The length of time a woman breast-feeds her infant will depend on her own feelings and situation. Milk will continue to be produced as long as there is demand for it and it is taken from the breast.

Problems. The inexperienced nursing mother is likely to encounter major or minor problems in the course of adjusting to breast feeding. Success or failure at the breast-feeding effort may depend largely on the availability of help in the early weeks and the support of a clinician or friend who provides useful tips. Problems relating to the infant are presented in Table 21.7.

Women may encounter problems in relation to breast feeding (Chapman, 1985). Individual counsel-

---

How to Have a Totally Breast-fed Baby and Work Too! (Going Back to Work at Six Weeks Postpartum)

Starting out
 First 4 weeks breast feed only to establish your milk supply.
 Nurse your baby every 2 to 3 hours to build up your milk supply.
 RELAX AND ENJOY 6 weeks of nursing totally.
Establishing a home milk supply by pumping your breasts.
 Do NOT attempt to pump until the fifth week home from the hospital.
 Weeks 5 and 6 when baby doesn't nurse every 3 hours . . PUMP. This will mean you are either feeding or pumping every 3 hours.
 In the beginning you will only be able to pump approximately ½ to 1 ounce of breast milk . . DON'T PANIC . . after practicing *and* believing, you will be able to pump 1 to 3 ounces or more!
How to pump at home
 RELAX . . and drink plenty of fluids.
 Take a warm shower or use warm compresses on your breasts.
 Pump 15 minutes on each side . . or . . pump while nursing the baby by propping the baby on your lap with pillows on one side and pumping the other side. Baby feeding facilitates milk "let-down" and you will be able to obtain more breast milk while pumping. The baby will be well fed from one sided nursing.
 Pump at EVERY first morning feeding and you will get a good amount of breast milk for your reserve supply because baby has gone longer between feedings.
Pumping at work
 Pump every 3 to 4 hours to increase your milk supply . . or . . much easier
 Pump after 6 to 8 hours away from the baby or when engorgement is felt. This will give you 4 to 12 ounces of milk, enough to feed your baby the next day when added to your supply at home.
Storage
 Freeze IMMEDIATELY after pumping even at work. You can carry home the milk pumped at work in a small blue ice cooler . . remember that breast milk is now more precious than gold.
 Freeze in 1 to 2 ounce amounts In plastic baby bottle liners sealed with twist ties. Sit plastic bags in glass to freeze any spillage.
 Date milk and use oldest first.
Equipment
 Breast pads—Evenflo or Sears
 Handpump—Kaneson
 Electric pump—Eggnell (suggested that the equipment be rented). The cost is 80% to 100% covered by insurance if prescribed by your doctor. Have your doctor prescribe the pump in the hospital.
 Plastic baby bottles and nipples . . always use the same brand.
Preparation of frozen breast milk for feeding baby
 Hold plastic bag under hot running water until thawed and warm.
 Pour into plastic bottle and feed the baby.

Courtesy Fountain Valley Community Hospital, Fountain Valley, Calif., 1983, Childbirth education.

Table 21.7
Infant-related Problems in the Initiation of Breast Feeding

Problem	Nursing Action
The infant does not open wide enough to grasp the nipple.	Assist the mother to depress the infant's lower jaw with one finger as she guides the nipple into the mouth.
The infant grasps the nipple and areolar tissue correctly but will not suck.	Assist the mother to stimulate sucking motions by pressing upward under the baby's chin. Expression of colostrum results, and the infant is stimulated by the taste to begin sucking.
The infant makes frantic rooting, mouthing motions but will not grasp the nipple and eventually begins to cry and stiffen her or his body in apparent frustration.	Assist the mother to interrupt the feeding, comfort the infant, and take time to relax herself, and then she may begin again.
The infant may suck for a few minutes and then fall asleep.	Assist the mother to interrupt the feeding and take time to awaken the infant. Stimulation may include loosening the wraps, holding the baby upright, talking to the baby, or gently rubbing her or his back or the soles of the feet. A sleepy infant will not nurse satisfactorily. If it is impossible to wake the baby, it is better to postpone the feeding.
The infant starts by sucking vigorously and, as the milk flows freely, develops a long, slow, rhythmic sucking. The sucking then changes to a short, rapid sucking with frequent rest periods. This behavior indicates a slowing of the flow of milk.	Assist the mother to massage the breasts toward the nipple. This starts the milk flowing freely again, and the infant will revert to the slow, rhythmic sucking. As soon as sucking resumes, the massage is discontinued so that the infant will not be overwhelmed and choked by the milk flowing too rapidly.

Table 21.8
Mother-related Problems in Breast Feeding

Problem	Nursing Action
Engorged breasts	
If nursing has been on demand since birth, painful engorgement of the breasts is not likely to occur. However, because of the lag between the production of milk and the efficiency of the ejection reflexes, engorgement of the breasts may occur for up to 48 hours after the milk comes in. The mother often complains that the breast is tender and that the tenderness extends into the axilla. The breasts usually feel firm, tense, and warm as a result of the increased blood supply, and the skin may appear shiny and taut. The unyielding areolae makes it difficult for the infant to grasp the nipple. Nursing can be uncomfortable to the mother and frustrating for both mother and infant.	1. Applicaton of moist heat: Apply wet cloths as hot as can be endured to the whole breast and, at the same time, express milk from the nipple. As the wet cloth cools, replace with another one. Shower and direct the hot water to the breasts. 2. Breast massage: Put the thumbs together on top of the breast and the remaining fingers under the breast (Fig. 21.7). Gentle pressure is then exerted from around the breast toward the nipple. If the milk is to be used later, *it should be expressed into a sterile bottle and frozen.** Milk expression is not easy for some women at first, but persistence usually brings success if the mother takes the time. 3. Manual expression of milk: place the thumb and forefinger on opposite sides of the breast just outside the areola, press downward into the rib cage, and then squeeze together and downward; the nipple should not be pulled outward (Fig. 21.8). Repeat the procedure moving the thumb and forefinger around the nipple until as much milk as desired has been expressed.
Sore nipples	
The nipples may become sore during the early days of nursing. Soreness may be limited by using a correct nursing position and avoiding undue breast engorgement. If soreness occurs, it is always temporary until the nipples become accustomed to the baby's sucking (Borovies, 1984).	1. Expose the nipples to air. 2. Use a heat lamp to dry the nipples after the feeding (40-watt bulb in a desk lamp, positioned 45 cm [18 in] from breast). 3. Limit sucking time to 5 minutes on each breast, the time it takes to empty the breasts of milk. 4. Use a pacifier if the infant's sucking needs have not been met. 5. Use a nipple shield (Fig. 21.9).

*Freeze milk that will not be used within a few hours (see box, p. 609).

Table 21.8, cont'd
Mother-related Problems in Breast Feeding

Problem	Nursing Action
	6. Discontinue nursing for 48 hours. During this time the milk is expressed manually or with a breast pump, collected in a sterilized glass, and given to the baby by bottle. Precautions for maintaining the milk in a safe condition must be followed. Bottles and nipples must be sterilized by immersing them in water and boiling for 10 mintues; any milk not immediately consumed must be refrigerated or frozen.
Plugged ducts	
Occasionally a milk duct will become plugged, creating a tender spot on the breast, which may appear lumpy and hot. This might result from inadequate emptying of the milk ducts or from wearing a brassiere that is too tight.	1. Offer the sore breast first so that it will be emptied more completely. 2. Nurse longer and more often; if the breast gets too full, the plugged duct becomes worse and infection may develop. 3. Change positions at every feeding so that the pressure of the nursing will be applied to different places on the breast. 4. Apply warm compresses to the breasts between feedings to reduce the risk of infection by keeping the ducts open.

Fig. 21.7
Breast massage. **A,** Begin by placing one hand over the other above the breast. **B,** Gently, but firmly, exert pressure evenly with the thumbs across the top and fingers underneath the breast. **C,** Come together with the heel of the hand on each side and release at the areola, being careful not to touch the areola and nipple. **D,** Then gently lift the breast from beneath and drop lightly. Repeat 4 to 5 times with each breast. (Courtesy Marjorie Pyle, RNC, Lifecircle, Costa Mesa, California.)

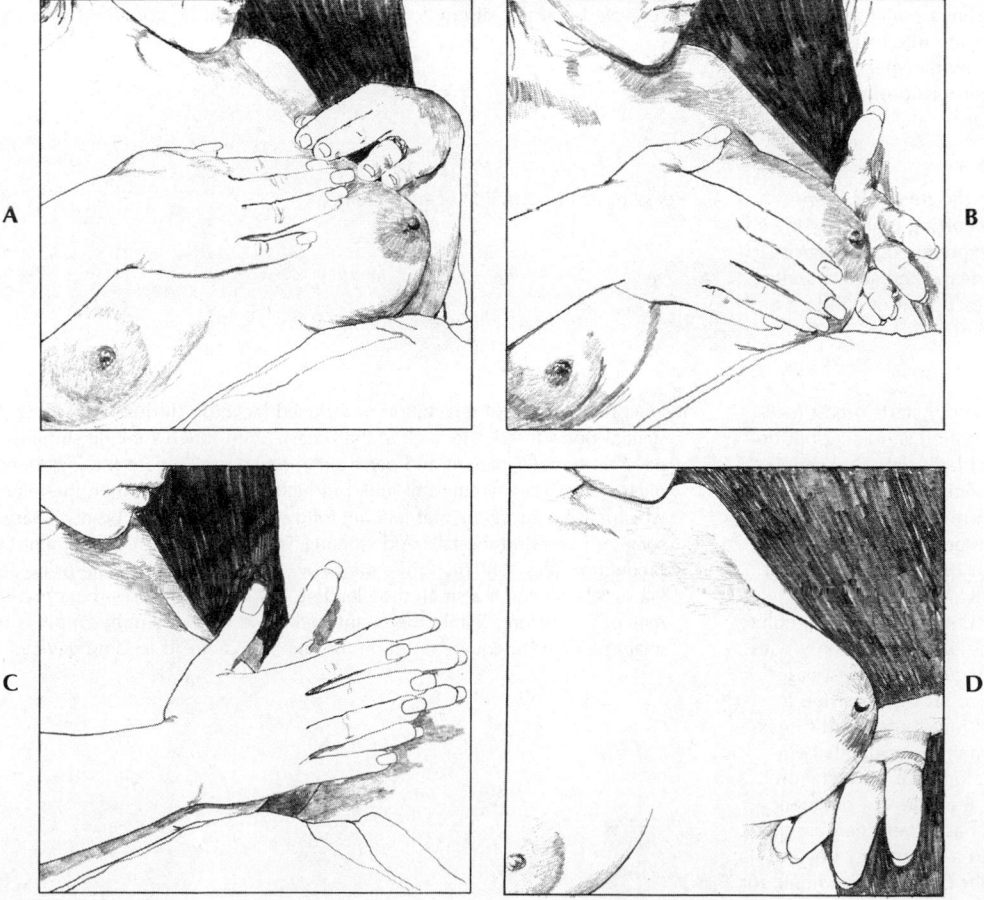

Continued.

Fig. 21.8
Manual expression of human milk. This is done by putting thumbs together on top of breast and remaining fingers under breast. Gentle pressure is exerted from around breast toward nipple. If milk is to be used later, it should be expressed into sterile bottle and refrigerated. (Courtesy Marjorie Pyle, RNC, Lifecircle, Costa Mesa, California.)

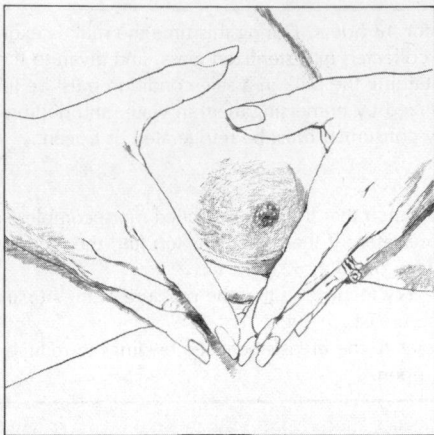 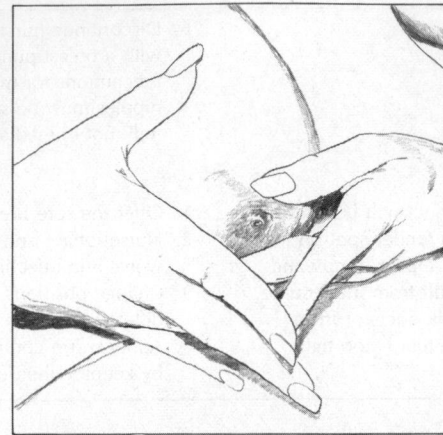

Table 21.8, cont'd
Mother-related Problems in Breast Feeding

Problem	Nursing Action
Increased lochial flow The nursing mother may note an increase in lochial flow once nursing begins. At times afterpains are intensified to such a degree that the mother becomes uncomfortable, and her tension interferes with nursing the infant.	Offer a mild analgesic for pain 40 minutes before the nursing period. The mother may be reassured that this discomfort is transitory and will be gone in 2 days.
Sexual sensations For some women the rhythmic uterine contractions occurring while nursing are akin to those experienced during orgasm. These unexpected sexual sensations within the context of child care may be disturbing.	Reassure as to normalcy of such feelings.
Relactation Occasionally a mother starts breast feeding late or discontinues nursing but decides at a much later date that she would like to begin again. After adopting an infant, a minority of women decide to attempt lactation even though they have never done so before or, at best, have breast fed a previous baby of their own. With much sucking stimulus, lactation can be induced but only with great perseverance and in most cases only if a woman has once carried a pregnancy well into the second trimester. Since the mammary glands complete their development for lactation during the first 6 months of pregnancy, a woman who has never been pregnant or never carried a pregnancy beyond the first trimester is a poor candidate for successful induction of lactation.	Instruct her to attempt relactation or induced lactation through providing the infant substantial opportunities to suck at the breast. With much sucking stimulus over several days' time many patient and persistent women can initiate the lactation process late or once again. Their volume of milk production may be less than the infant demands, in which case a supplemental feeding following nursing may be necessary. Alternatively, some women find the Lact-Aid Nursing Trainer to nicely complement their own milk production (Fig. 21.10). While the baby sucks at the breast she or he also obtains milk via suction through a small tube leading to a bag of fresh formula that is clipped to the mother's brassiere. While the infant sucks, the mother's milk supply is built up and the infant receives adequate nutrition through the Lact-Aid feeding device.

Fig. 21.9
Plastic breast cups of shells can also be used to continuously expose the nipple to air. *Avoid* use of *breast shields* as they do not prevent or help sore nipples and exert little pressure on milk ducts, which leads to decreased milk flow. (Courtesy Marjorie Pyle, RNC, Lifecircle, Costa Mesa, California.)

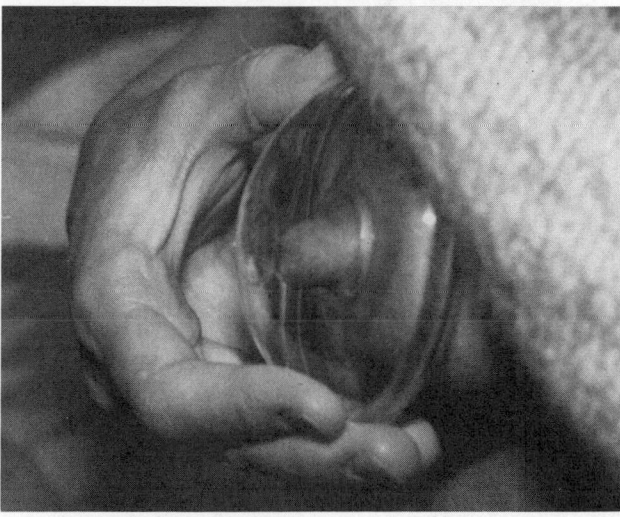

Fig. 21.10
Lact-Aid Nursing Trainer in use.

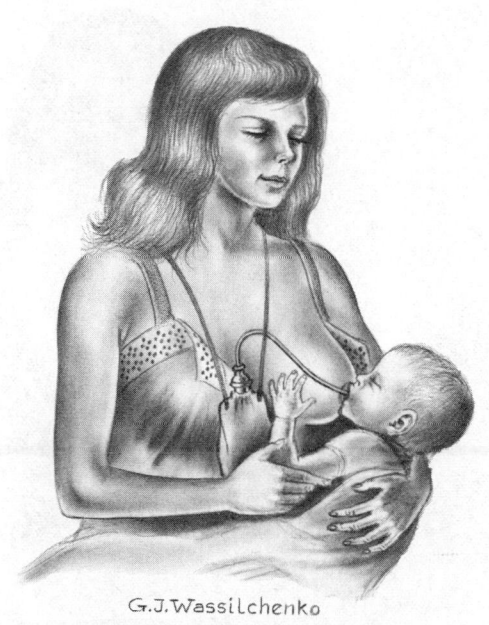

G.J.Wassilchenko

Table 21.8, cont'd
Mother-related Problems in Breast Feeding

Problem	Nursing Action
Breast pumping	
For a number of reasons, mothers may wish to remove milk from their breasts and save it for a later feeding, take it to their hospitalized newborn, or donate it to a milk bank. Under such circumstances, milk can be expressed by hand and for some women this method is satisfactory. For many women, however, a manual or electric breast pump provides a better stimulus for milk flow and a more efficient mode of milk collection.	Instruct the mother in the use of the breast pump (Fig. 21.11).
Failure of infant to thrive	
Insufficient milk supply is rarely a problem for the well-fed mother. Since sucking stimulates the flow of milk, feeding on demand for adequate duration should supply ample amounts of milk. Occasionally, however, an infant will fail to thrive while seemingly nursing properly.	1. Assist in the explanation of potential problems (Fig. 21.12). 2. Encourage mother to turn to commercial infant formula for at least partial nutritional support of the infant, if the cause of the problem cannot be identified or the defined problem cannot be corrected (Fig. 21.10).
Maternal infection	
If breast tenderness is accompanied by fever and a general flulike feeling, a breast infection is probably present (see Chapter 27).	Instruct the mother to notify her physician immediately.

Fig. 21.11
Commonly used breast pumps. **A,** Swedish pump. **B,** Syringe pump. **C,** Electric pump.

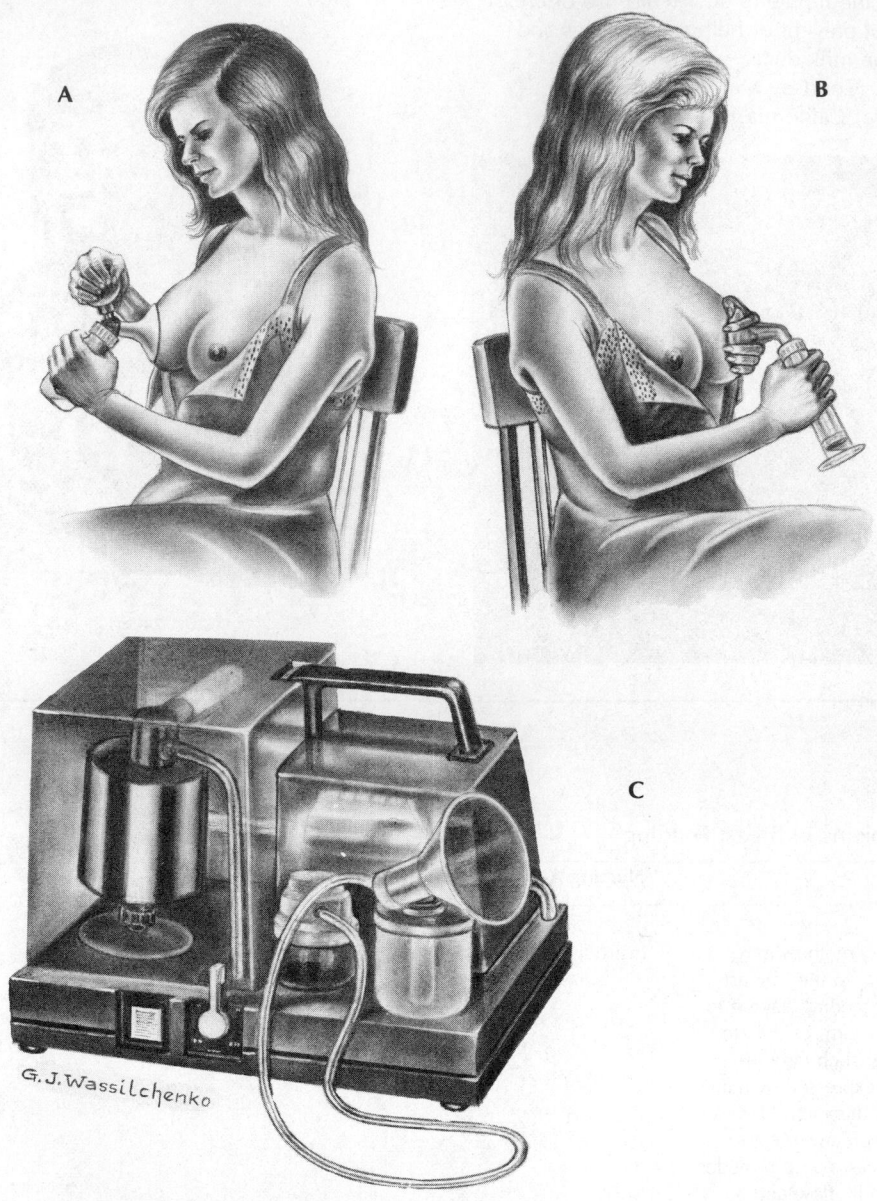

ing by a skilled clinician can greatly simplify the process of learning to cope with the problem. Table 21.8 presents mother-related problems in breast feeding.

BOTTLE FEEDING

Specific name brands of formulas are recommended by physicians. The choice of a particular brand is based on the infant's nutritional needs, cost, need for refrigeration, convenience, and the mother's ability to pre-

pare the formula accurately and safely. The physician provides written instructions as to the amounts of formula to be fed the infant over 24 hours and when to increase the amounts to ensure meeting the growing infant's nutritional needs.

Hospitals today use commercially prepared formula. It comes prepackaged and can be stored at room temperature. Many parents elect to use similar brands. Also there are a variety of nursing bottles and nipples from which to choose (Fig. 21.13).

Fig. 21.12
Diagnostic flow chart for failure to thrive. (From Lawrence, R.: Breast feeding: a guide for the medical profession, St. Louis, 1980, The C.V. Mosby Co.)

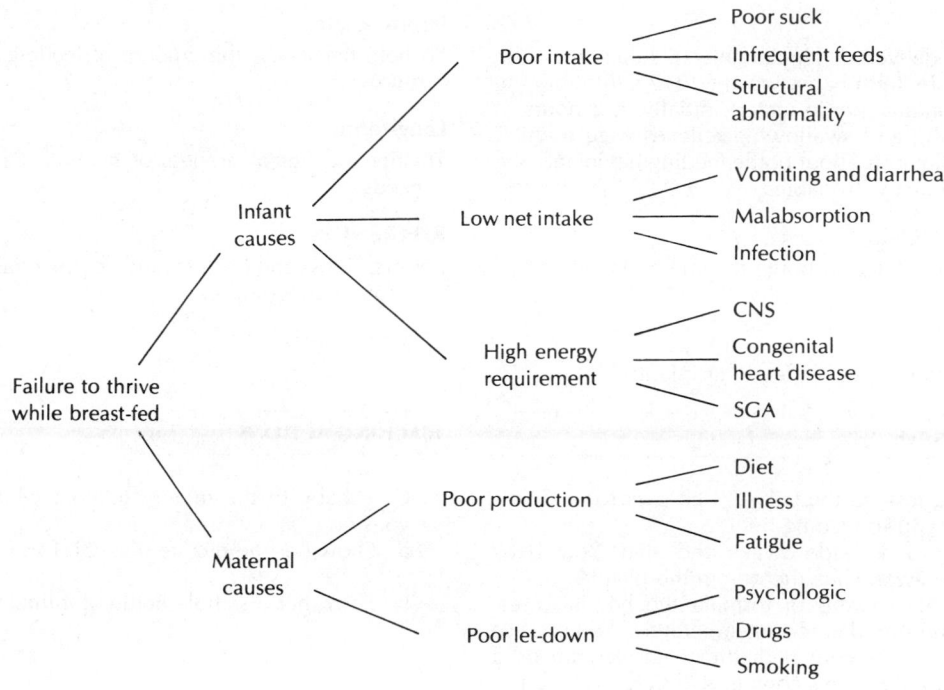

Feeding process. Inexperienced mothers who are bottle feeding their infants need the same teaching, counseling, and support as do the mothers who are breast feeding. They need assistance with the bottle-feeding process and with problems they experience. Some mothers who elect bottle feeding will express concern that the baby will suffer as a result of their decision. They need assurance that knowledge of their infant's nutritional needs and skill in use of formula feeding can be an acceptable substitute for breast feeding. Emphasis on the beneficial use of the feeding time for close contact with their infant can help relieve their tensions. The Guidelines for Client Teaching can be used to help an inexperienced woman bottle feed her infant.

Formulas. Some parents wish to prepare their own formulas. Knowledge of the following can help nurses answer client questions.

Types of formulas

Evaporated milk. Although home-prepared evaporated milk formula may be least expensive, it is not generally recommended because of the increased chance of improper measurement and bacterial con-

Fig. 21.13
Bottle feeding: types of bottles and nipples. (Courtesy Marjorie Pyle, RNC, Lifecircle, Costa Mesa, California.)

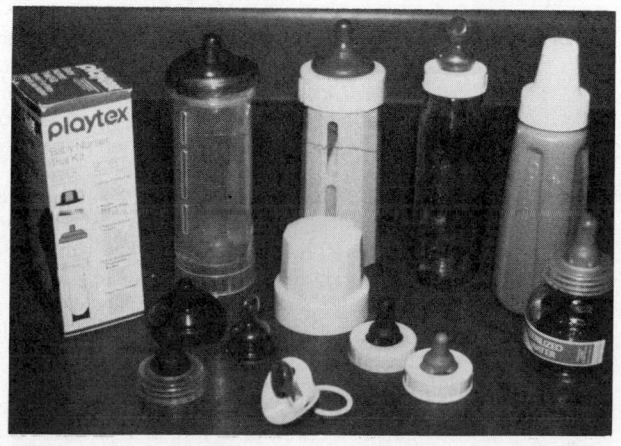

Guidelines for Client Teaching

BOTTLE FEEDING

ASSESSMENT

Jeanne, age 19, delivered her daughter 6 hours ago. The infant is a healthy term baby, weight 2912 g (6½ lb). The nurse fed the infant (sterile water) initially at 2 hours of age. Her sucking and swallowing reflexes were normal. The mother is anxious about bottle feeding her infant. She has had no contact with babies.

NURSING DIAGNOSIS

Knowledge deficit related to bottle feeding an infant.

GOALS
Short-term

To teach Jeanne how to bottle feed her infant.

Intermediate

To help her assess the amount of feeding her daughter requires.

Long-term

To increase her awareness of her infant's capabilities and needs.

REFERENCES

Posters, films, and hospital and commercial booklets related to formula feeding

---

CONTENT/RATIONALE	TEACHING ACTIONS
1. Before starting to feed the baby I'll go over some points that will help you in feeding her. a. She needs to be wide awake and alert. Your baby looks wide awake like the one in the picture. b. These are the bottles of formula the hospital uses. They can be stored at room temperature. You can use this brand or ask your pediatrician to recommend a type of formula. They contain 4 oz (120 ml) of formula. Your baby will probably drink 2 to 3 oz (60 to 90 ml) for a few days and then gradually increase. If you do not use all the formula, throw away what is left. It can spoil once it is opened. c. You can keep track of the number of ounces your baby has in one day by writing down the amount each time. When you take the baby for the well baby check they will ask you the amount of intake. d. Your baby will probably be hungry every 2½ to 3 hours. If she cries in between check her for voiding or the need to be picked up and cuddled. As she gets older she may be thirsty and you can give her 1 or 2 oz (30 or 60 ml) of sterile water. e. You can test the temperature of the formula by letting a few drops fall on the inside of the wrist. If the formula feels comfortably warm to you, it is the correct temperature. If you keep the formula in the refrigerator you can warm it by placing it in a pan of hot water. You can keep checking to see when it is warm enough. f. You can test the size of the holes in the nipple by holding the bottle and nipple upside down. The formula should drip from the nipple. If it runs in a stream, it is flowing too fast. It can make the baby choke. If it has to be shaken out the baby will have to expend too much energy to obtain enough formula "to grow on." To correct this you may try a softer nipple or may enlarge the holes in the nipple or both. To enlarge the holes, heat a needle stuck into a cork (use as a handle) and insert the hot needle into the nipple holes. New nipples may be softened by boiling 5 minutes before using. If the nipple collapses, the bottle lid can be unscrewed so air can enter the bottle and reinflate the nipple.	1. Give baby to the mother to hold while the discussion goes on. a. Show her the picture (Fig. 21.14). b. Show her a sample bottle of formula. c. Show her how to note time and amount on hospital record. e. Shake a few drops of formula on her inside wrist. Dry her wrist with a facial tissue. f. Demonstrate the procedure of testing the nipple. Demonstrate with needle embedded in a cork. Heat over match flame and enlarge holes on sample nipple.

Continued.

Fig. 21.14
Alert, wide-awake infant to be bottle fed. (Courtesy Fountain Valley Community Hospital, Fountain Valley, California; photograph by Nancy Newell.)

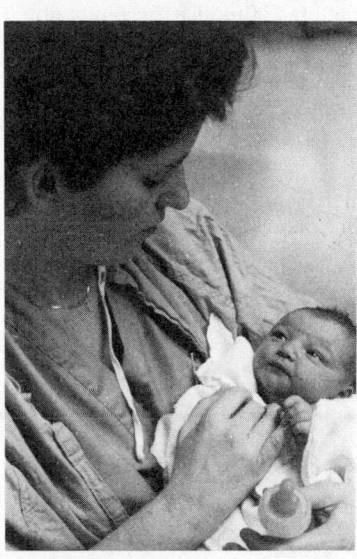

tamination during preparation of the formula. Often the families who could benefit most by savings are least able to understand the importance of sanitary precautions and accurate measurements in preparing the formula. Special counseling is needed for parents who choose to use evaporated milk formula.

To control growth of bacteria, single feedings should be prepared as needed rather than all feedings for a 24-hour period. A formula may be prepared as follows:

Evaporated milk: 3 oz. (90 ml)
Water: 4.5 oz (135 ml)
Corn syrup: 2 tsp

An opened can of evaporated milk should be covered and refrigerated. Evaporated milk is fortified with vitamin D and forms an easily digested curd because of the heat processing it undergoes. Supplements of vitamin C and iron are needed for the infant fed with evaporated milk formulas. Fluoride supplements may be needed also.

Cow's milk. Ingestion of whole cow's milk during the first 12 months places the infant at risk of developing deficiences of iron, vitamin C, and copper, as well as increased plasma osmolality and hyperphosphatemia.

Fig. 21.15
Bottle feeding. Bottle is held in hand like a pencil. Note milk covers nipple area so infant will not suck in air.

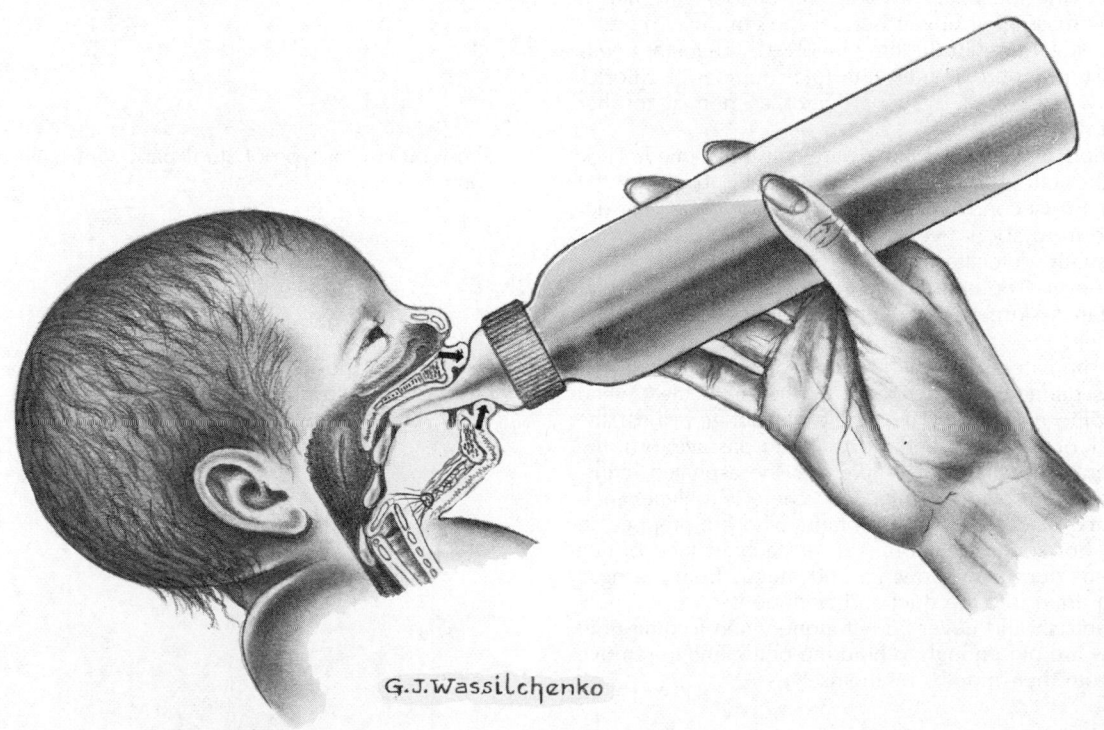

G.J.Wassilchenko

Guidelines for Client Teaching —cont'd

CONTENT/RATIONALE	TEACHING ACTIONS
g. Some babies need burping. They tend to swallow air when they are sucking. This is how you can burp her. The baby may be burped before beginning the feeding, especially if the baby has been crying, again after about 1 oz (30 ml) of formula has been taken, and at the end of the feeding. You will learn how often your baby needs burping after a few feedings.	g. Show pictures of mother burping baby (Fig. 21.6). Give inexperienced mother definite "time" instructions.
h. To feed the baby place the nipple in her mouth over the tongue. It should rest against the roof of her mouth. In that position her sucking reflex comes into play. You can practice the position by putting your fingertip, pad side up, into her mouth, over the tongue, and up against the roof. She has a powerful suck.	h. Show her picture (Fig. 21.15). Have her practice this.
i. You hold the bottle as you would a pencil. Keep the nipple covered with milk so the baby does not suck air.	i. Point out on picture (Fig. 21.15).
j. While the baby is learning about feeding, hold the baby away from you until the nipple is in her mouth. If you hold her close she will turn away from the bottle toward you. That is her rooting reflex.	j. Have her hold baby away from herself.
2. Now we can start her feeding from the bottle. After the baby begins sucking properly, you can hold her close so that the baby can relax against your warmth. Every infant needs physical contact with the mother, and the feeding period offers one of the most natural ways for infant and adult to share, to give, and to experience being cared for and loved.	2. Assist her to start feeding.
3. Some infants take "forever" to feed. This is not uncommon, particularly in smaller babies. Slow, patient feeding, keeping the infant awake, and encouraging her to suck by massaging upward under the chin may be necessary. Regardless of the time involved, the infant needs to consume approximately the total number of calories per day prescribed by your doctor as normal for her weight.	3. Reassure mother that this is a characteristic of infant feeding and does not indicate "poor mothering."
4. The stools of bottle-fed babies are soft but formed. They are light yellow and have a characteristic odor. By the end of the second week the number of stools has decreased from about five to one or two stools a day. She will usually defecate after a feeding, sometimes in the middle of it. The composition of the stool is irritating to the infant's skin; therefore the buttocks needs frequent cleansing.	4. Show picture of type of stool baby will have once meconium is passed.
5. While she is feeding, I will review some safety tips.	5. Use hospital poster to show dangers. Ask her to demonstrate what to do if the baby chokes. Place bulb syringe within reach.
a. It is dangerous practice to "prop the bottle" when feeding an infant. The nipple can lodge against the back of the throat and block the air passage; or if the infant regurgitates, the fluid may be aspirated, causing death or a lung infection. There is a higher incidence of otitis media in infants who are propped in the horizontal position. The eustachian tube orifice opens during swallowing, and mucus from the nose can drain into the duct and occlude it.	
b. Infants should never be left alone when feeding until they are old enough to hold the bottle and to remove it from their mouths by themselves.	

Guidelines for Client Teaching—cont'd

CONTENT/RATIONALE	TEACHING ACTIONS
c. Bottles at nap or bed time can lead to "baby bottle syndrome." This can be a cause of early dental problems in young children. d. Let's practice how to hold the baby and use the bulb syringe if she chokes. 6. I will be back in 10 minutes to see if you have any questions. 7. After the baby has finished her bottle, place her on her right side in the crib so any air can come up easily.	6. Check amount of formula taken for the baby's record. Supervise her burping the baby. 7. Show picture of baby (Fig. 20.31).

EVALUATION Mother demonstrates the knowledge and skill necessary to meet goals.

Guidelines for Client Teaching

PREPARATION OF FORMULA

ASSESSMENT

Jeanne, age 19, requests assistance in preparing formula for her newborn daughter. She intends to use a powdered commercial formula.

NURSING DIAGNOSIS

Knowledge deficit related to preparation of formula.

GOALS

Short-term

To teach the mother how to prepare formula for her newborn.

Intermediate

To help her plan for the changing nutritional needs of her infant.

Long-term

To promote optimal nutrition for the infant.

To teach a method of providing fluids that ensures the safety of the infant in case of events that contaminate water or food supplies.

REFERENCES

Commercial teaching materials available from suppliers.
Instructions on containers of formula mix.
Hospital-developed films.

CONTENT/RATIONALE	TEACHING ACTIONS

1. Collect equipment
  a. A regular bottle sterilizer, available at a baby-care store, or a large kettle with lid
  b. A wire rack (one should come with a commercial sterilizer) or a clean towel, which is used to separate bottles from the sterilizer or kettle bottom
  c. A can opener
  d. Tablespoon, slotted spoon, or eggbeater
  e. Seven nursing bottles, with nipples, caps, and collars (Fig. 21.13)
  f. Bottle and nipple brushes
  g. Tongs for sterile handling of bottles
  h. A can of the selected baby formula
2. Wash and rinse bottles and nipples to remove debris so that sterilization is facilitated.
  a. Scrub bottles, nipples, collars, and caps with the bottle brush, detergent, and hot water.
  b. Squeeze water through nipple holes during washing and rinsing.
  c. Rinse bottles and nipples with hot running water.
	1. Demonstrate equipment needed.
	
	2. Demonstrate technique.

Continued.

Guidelines for Client Teaching—cont'd

CONTENT/RATIONALE	TEACHING ACTIONS

3. Select technique for sterilizing formula preparations or drinking water for protection from infection.
  a. Terminal heating method
    (1) Fill the bottles with prescribed amount of formula, and loosely attach nipples, caps, and collars. Place the filled bottles on a wire rack or towel in a sterilizer or deep kettle.
    (2) Add water to sterilize to depth of 7.5 cm (3 in). When water in sterilizer starts to boil, cover and let boil for 25 minutes. Remove sterilizer from heat and leave covered until sterilizer has cooled to touch.
    (3) Check bottles to see if cool enough to handle. Remove them from sterilizer, tighten caps, and store in refrigerator.
  b. Aseptic method
    (1) Place bottles, nipples, collars, caps, mixing spoon, can opener, measuring pitcher, and tongs on a rack or towel in a sterilizer or deep kettle. Cover with water, and place over heat. Add the prescribed amount of water needed to make formula in a clean pan. Place over heat. When water in both sterilizer and pan comes to a boil, cover and boil 5 minutes.
    (2) Wash top of can of milk with soap and water, and dry. Shake can well. Make two puncture holes in the top with sterile can opener and mix prescribed amount of milk and boiled water.
    (3) Pour correct number of ounces of formula into each nursing bottle. Put nipples, collars, and caps on the bottles. Store in refrigerator until needed.
4. Review safety points
  a. Measure powdered formula carefully. *Do not* pack into spoon as concentration of formula can be increased. As a result infant cries from thirst. Mother assumes infant is hungry and feeds more formula. This can lead to dehydration, heavy renal solute load, and over-nutrition.
  b. Refrigerate formula.
  c. Throw away unused formula.
  d. Use sterile technique until physician advises use of tap water and clean technique.
	3. Demonstrate technique. Let mother practice measuring amount.
	
	4. Question mother about storage, use of clean technique.

EVALUATION Evaluation of the mother's knowledge and preparation is usually done at the first well baby check, unless follow-up home visits are part of postpartum care. Observe health of child and discuss feedings with the parent.

The high risk of dehydration and hypernatremia when febrile illnesses, diarrhea, or other conditions increase the demand for water.

Skim-Milk. Skim milk has about half the number of calories (10 kcal/oz) of breast milk, evaporated milk, or commercial infant formulas. They contain 20 kcal/oz. Research shows that infants fed skim milk have dif-

ficulty ingesting a volume sufficient to meet their energy needs (Foman, 1979).

Powders or concentrates. Instructions for mixing powdered or concentrated formulas should be followed accurately to prevent overdilution or underdilution. When formulas are underdiluted with water, the renal solute load is increased and may lead to dehydration of the infant. If overdilution occurs, inadequate calories and nutrients are provided, and failure to thrive may result. When the safety of the community or home water supply is in doubt, sterile water is recommended for diluting formulas.

Preparation of formula. Instruction in the preparation of formula includes methods for sterilizing and storing it. The guidelines for client teaching can be used as an instruction guide to help the inexperienced mother.

ANTICIPATORY GUIDANCE

Anticipatory guidance can be given before the mother leaves the hospital or at the well baby checkups if the mother elects early discharge. Knowledge such as the following is helpful to the parent (Pyle, 1985).

Frequency of feeding. During the daytime, awaken and feed the infant so that he or she is not sleeping more than 3 hours at a time. At night, let baby sleep and only feed if baby awakens. Make the night feedings very business-like so that baby learns that nights are not play time. At the beginning, most mothers prefer to take the baby to bed to nurse or bottle feed. Mothers also find that baby will sleep better if laid across her upper abdomen, so that baby hears her heartbeat and has the warm body contact.

For the newborn, a demand scheduling is ideal. The newborn will feed every 1½ to 3 hours during the daytime, and hopefully every 3 to 5 hours at night. Breast-fed infants need to nurse *at least every 3 hours* during the daytime. "Good" babies who rarely cry, sleep, and only awaken to nurse every 4 to 6 hours, usually do not have an adequate weight gain, and the mother may not maintain an adequate milk supply. Most babies will average 10 feedings during a 24-hour period. Table 21.9 provides a guide for bottle-fed infants' average intake of formula.

Appetite changes. Mothers will notice appetite spurts between 10 days and 2 weeks; 6 weeks and 9 weeks; and 3 months and 6 months. These appetite spurts correspond to growth spurts. The infant wants to nurse more frequently and for longer periods. For the breast-feeding baby, increasing the feedings results in a greater production of milk. The satisfied infant then tapers off his or her demands. For the bottle-fed baby, the amount of formula offered can be increased by 2 to 4 oz (60 to 120 ml).

Most 2- to 3-month old babies *may* lengthen the time between feedings to a 3- to 4-hour schedule during the daytime, and longer at night. By 4 to 6 months of age, some infants may sleep through the night without feeding.

Supplemental feeding for breast-fed babies. Do not offer a newborn a bottle until he or she is an accomplished breast feeder. Otherwise, it may interfere with the baby learning how to suckle. It also can reduce the milk supply. After the milk supply is established (usually at about 3 weeks), an occasional bottle will not affect breast feeding.

Weaning. Weaning may take place because the infant has signified a desire to drink from a cup or because the mother will be absent. Some infants wean themselves, gradually refusing more and more feedings until only the early morning and night feedings are left. Others resist attempts to wean them and mothers have to substitute other social times to compensate them for their loss. Ideally, the process is a gradual one extending over several weeks.

Introducing solid foods. The infant receives the right balance of nutrients from breast milk or formula during the first 4 to 6 months (Broussard, 1984). Introduction of solid foods too soon may result in the following problems (Madgic, 1986).

1. Overfeeding. The infant cannot communicate feeling full like an older child can by turning his or her head away.
2. Decreased intake of breast milk or formula. The proper balance of carbohydrate, protein, and fat for an infant to grow properly is in breast milk or formula.
3. Sleeping through the night. It is not true that when solids are given it will help the baby sleep through the night.
4. Readiness for solid foods. The infant's individual growth pattern should help determine just the right time to start solids. The physician will advise when to introduce solid foods.

The schedule for introducing solid foods is given in Table 21.10.

By 1 year a child is usually eating a variety of food from all the food groups. Cow's milk may also be introduced. Certain highly allergenic foods are *not* usually given during most of the first year. These foods include egg whites, tomato products, citrus fruits, and

Table 21.9
Guide for Formula Feeding

Age	Average Quantity Taken in Individual Feedings	Average Number of Feedings per 24 Hours
Birth to 3 weeks	2-3 oz (60-90 ml)	6-10
2 weeks to 2 months	5 oz (150 ml)	5-8
2-3 months	5-7 oz (150-210 ml)	5-6
3-4 months	6-8 oz (180-240 ml)	4-6
5-12 months	8 oz (240 ml)	3-4

Table 21.10
Introduction of Solids

Food	Age in Months
Cereal (iron-fortified infant rice)	4-6
Fruits (strained)	5-7
Vegetables (strained)	6-8
Meat (strained)	7-9
Egg yolk	10
Teething biscuits or dry toast	When teeth appear

berries. If either the mother or father of the infant has food allergies, parents may want to be especially cautious. Allergies should be discussed with the pediatrician (Madgic, 1986).

Referrals. Referral procedures provide an opportunity for individuals and groups to take advantage of services available from other sources. A properly coordinated health service delivery for infants and children can contribute to a sense of continuity and to consistency of care and advice. The mother is encouraged to contact the local association that assists with breast feeding (Appendix C).

Evaluation

The process of evaluation is continuous. As the infant matures, the norms for nutritional intake are adjusted to meet growth needs. The criteria are measureable in terms of the infant's growth, energy levels, and appearance. Parental knowledge is a key factor in infant nutrition and feeding. Parental knowledge and infant well-being and the findings that represent normal response are presented as outcome criteria in the Summary of Nursing Actions. These criteria are used as a basis for selecting appropriate nursing actions and evaluating their effectiveness.

Summary

Providing nutrition services to parents and their infants is a function of the health team. Physicians, nurses, nutritionists, social workers, and health educators are major contributors to the care. One of the most important contributors, the nurse, can assist with nutrition assessment and provide education and counseling. Nurses can help interpret dietary prescriptions and make appropriate referrals of more complicated problems to nutritional personnel. Following are a summary of nursing actions relating to newborn nutrition and a description of the application of the nursing process to a specific nutritional problem.

Summary of Nursing Actions

NEWBORN NUTRITION

GOALS

1. For the infant
   a. To provide the levels and types of nutrients to support the infant's body composition, activity, and growth.
   b. To minimize the physiologic stress associated with digestion, metabolism, and excretion of nutrients.
   c. To supply sufficient water to maintain adequate body water control.
2. For the mother
   a. To provide knowledge that can be used for sound nutritional selection and feeding practices.
   b. To assist her to become skilled in the feeding method of her choice.
   c. To foster mother-child closeness and pleasure.

PRIORITIES

1. Confirm newborn's ability to ingest nutrients (i.e., sucking, swallowing, gagging reflexes present, absence of structural abnormalities).
2. Confirm newborn's ability to digest nutrients (i.e., infant thrives).
3. Confirm newborn's ability to eliminate wastes.
4. Ensure mother (caretaker) has the necessary knowledge and skill to provide the nutrition needed for the infant.
5. Ensure mother has necessary income to obtain the needed nutrients for her infant and herself.

Summary of Nursing Actions—cont'd

ASSESSMENT	EXAMPLES OF POTENTIAL NURSING DIAGNOSTIC CATEGORIES*
First day of life	
A. Assess infant's ability to breast or bottle feed 1. Reflexes: sucking, swallowing, gagging 2. No structural abnormalities (e.g., choanal atresia)	Alteration in normal biologic processes† Ineffective airway clearance
B. Assess infant readiness for feeding (e.g., rooting reflex readily elicited, infant is alert and responsive).	Alteration in normal biologic processes†
C. Assess infant's ability to defecate, urinate	Alteration in bowel elimination
D. Assess mother's level of knowledge about feeding her infant and skills she possesses.	Knowledge deficit Impaired verbal communication Anxiety Alteration in comfort: pain
E. Assess condition of nipples if mother is to breast feed.	Impairment of skin integrity

*Diagnoses approved by the Seventh National Conference on Classification of Nursing Diagnosis held in 1986.
†Diagnosis not included by NANDA, 1986.

OUTCOME CRITERIA*	PLAN/IMPLEMENTATION
A. Reflexes (rooting, sucking, swallowing, gagging) are present and sufficiently developed to permit infant feeding by breast or bottle.	A. Test infant's ability. 1. Have infant suck on finger. 2. Remove excess mucus. 3. Feed infant sterile water. 4. Initiate feeding of infant by mother (breast or bottle) as soon as possible (e.g., put to breast at birth).
B. Periods of wakefulness when infant is alert and hungry are used to facilitate initiation of the feeding process and to promote a satisfying mother-child interaction.	B. Use wakeful periods for feeding infant. Wake infant before attempting to feed: otherwise baby may choke.
C. Mother begins feeding her infant by breast or bottle.	C. 1. Assist mother with feeding technique she has chosen. 2. Instruct as to nutritional needs of infant during first few days of life. 3. Instruct as to feeding abilities of infants (e.g., their sucking needs, how to burp them, that learning nursing process may require practice, and that there are variations in appetite).
D. Regurgitation or vomiting episodes are controlled, and the mother is able to care for the infant so that an open airway is maintained.	D. Demonstrate and supervise care needed if infant gags, chokes, or spits up during feeding process.
E. Infant accepts, swallows, retains, and assimilates feeding.	E. Record amounts of formula taken and times of breast or bottle feeding and response of infant.
F. Infant passes meconium and urinates.	F. Record character of stool and urine and time.
G. Mother is aware of care of breasts.	G. Instruct mother who is breast feeding in care of her breasts to prevent erosion of nipples, to augment supply of milk, and to prevent infection of breast or infant.

ASSESSMENT	EXAMPLES OF POTENTIAL NURSING DIAGNOSTIC CATEGORIES
Days 2 to 14	
A. Examine general condition of infant as part of routine care.	Alteration in neonatal health maintenance

*Outcome criteria direct the selection of nursing actions (**plan/implementation**) and measure their effectiveness (**evaluation**).
†Diagnosis not included by NANDA, 1986.

Summary of Nursing Actions—cont'd

B. Obtain reports from mother (family) concerning satisfaction of infant (e.g., whether infant sleeps soundly and then is hungry every 2 to 3 hours, and whether crying is appeased by nourishment).	Alteration in nutrition: less than body requirements or more than body requirements
C. Observe mother when she is engaged in feeding infant to determine skills and areas in which further assistance is needed.	Knowledge deficit Skill deficit Noncompliance Alteration in parenting Ineffective individual coping Alteration in normal physiologic processes†
D. Observe infant during and after feeding process to note ability to suck, swallow, and retain feedings. E. Assess condition of mother's breasts.	Alteration in health maintenance Alteration in normal physiologic processes†
F. Assess mother's knowledge of care of breasts if she is breast feeding. G. Assess mother's knowledge of diet for lactation and ability to obtain necessary nutrients.	Alteration in maternal health maintenance Health deficit† Alteration in health maintenance

OUTCOME CRITERIA*	PLAN/IMPLEMENTATION
A. Infant nutritional state is satisfactory. Evidence includes following: weight gain, adequate skin turgor, soft skin; fontanels not depressed; infant active and alert when awake; good muscle tone; infant sleeps contentedly 2 to 3 hours between feedings; crying from stress of hunger appeased by feeding; infant has soft stools and voids pale, straw-colored urine 6 to 10 times a day.	A. Share findings with parent.
B. Mother is aware of infant's nutritional needs for growth. C. Mother is adept at technique relative to breast or bottle feeding. *Breast feeding* ■ Initiating and terminating feeding session ■ Enhancing the supply of milk ■ Protecting her nipples from erosion and fissures ■ Adjusting the number of feedings to meet the infant's changing nutritional needs ■ Using alternative methods of feeding the infant to free her to take part in other activities *Bottle feeding* ■ Preparation of formula ■ Initiating and terminating feedings ■ Adjusting the schedule and formula to meet the infant's changing nutritional needs ■ Adopting practices that ensure infant-mother contact.	B and C. Continue instruction as to nutritional needs of infant. ■ Continue assistance with technique for breast feeding or bottle feeding. ■ Establish relaxed environment in which mother undertakes feeding process (free from pain, comfortable position, assistance from interested, supportive, and knowledgeable nurse, and privacy). ■ For breast-feeding mother, provide adequate diet (additional protein and fluids) and daily routine for care of breasts. ■ For bottle feeding mothers, provide information on preparation and storage of formulas
D. Mother and family express knowledge of meaning of baby's crying, hunger patterns, elimination patterns. E. Mother and family are aware of and using community resources for procuring adequate nutrients. F. Mother is aware of the symptoms indicative of gastrointestinal disturbances: depressed fontanels, dry skin, eyes lacking in luster, diarrhea with green, curdy stools, fever, refusal of feedings and fluids, lethargy, irritability, and a diminished number of voidings of urine. Mother	D. Assist mother (family) in recognizing cues infant uses and pattern of hunger and satiety each infant develops. ■ Assist mother in dealing with concern as to her ability to provide adequate nourishment for her child. E. Provide information regarding community resources. F. Instruct family as to symptoms indicating gastrointestinal disturbances. ■ Provide family with information as to whom to call for assistance and what symptoms to report.

*Outcome criteria direct the selection of nursing actions (**plan/implementation**) and measure their effectiveness (**evaluation**).

Summary of Nursing Actions—cont'd

is aware of the need to obtain medical care promptly to arrest lethal processes of dehydration and acid-base imbalance, as well as the procedure for obtaining assistance.

ASSESSMENT	EXAMPLES OF POTENTIAL NURSING DIAGNOSTIC CATEGORIES
Days 15 to 28	
A. Examination of infant by medical or nursing personnel reveals satisfactory nutritional status. Growth and development is normal for age.	Alteration in health maintenance Alteration in nutrition: less or more than body requirements
B. Assess mother's and family's knowledge of future nutritional needs of infant, process of weaning from breast or bottle, and introducing solid foods.	Knowledge deficit
C. Assess mother's and family's knowledge of symptoms of digestive problems requiring medical assistance.	Knowledge deficit

OUTCOME CRITERIA	PLAN/IMPLEMENTATION
A. Infant's nutritional status remains satisfactory; growth weight gain, and pattern of weight gain are within normal limits.	A. Share findings with parent(s). ■ Discuss any current problems
B. Mother is adept at adjusting feeding process to meet the infant's nutritional needs for growth, infant's need for socializing, and mother's need for widening scope of other activities.	B. Comment on successes. ■ Explore mutual solutions to problems.
C. Mother is aware of nutritional needs that may arise over next 2 months (addition of vitamins, minerals, solid foods).	C. Review changing nutritional needs of infant.
D. Breast-feeding mother is aware of use of alternative methods of feeding the infant to free her to take part in other activities.	D. Instruct mother regarding supplemental feedings. ■ Provide information about breast feeding and return to work.
E. Mother is aware of techniques of weaning the infant from breast or bottle and introduction of solid foods.	E. Provide information about weaning and introduction of solid foods.
F. Mother-infant relationship is positive as evidenced by her behavior toward the infant and the type of feeding and interactive processes instituted.	F. Encourage mother to discuss problems related to feeding her infant, explore methods of solution, and recognize and use measures instituted successfully in the past.
G. Mother is knowledgeable about signs and symptoms of gastrointestinal disturbances and what procedures to follow to obtain medical help.	G. Question mother about knowledge concerning gastrointestinal upsets.

Application of the Nursing Process

NEWBORN NUTRITION: NURSING MOTHER
WITH SORE NIPPLES

Andrea, age 27, delivered her first child, an 3584 g (8 lb) boy, 5 days ago. She is breast feeding. The nurse is making a home visit as follow-up for the hospital's early discharge program. Andrea reports the following. "My nipples are terribly sore. I can hardly bear to put Peter to breast. He sucks so hard. If this is what it is going to be like, I don't think I can stand it."

The nurse examined Andrea's nipples. They were reddened and excoriated. Her breasts were very firm with milk. Andrea went on to say, "The milk keeps leaking out. My bra is wet all the time." The nurse decides that as it is close to a feeding time, she will stay and help Andrea through the feeding.

FUNCTIONAL HEALTH PATTERN: ASSESSMENT	NURSING DIAGNOSIS	RATIONALE: PLAN/IMPLEMENTATION	EVALUATION
COGNITIVE-PERCEPTUAL ■ Complaints of pain throughout nursing period.	Alteration in comfort related to painful nipples	*To relieve discomfort, suggest:* ■ Manual expression of milk before feeding so infant can grasp nipple and areolar tissue. ■ Start with least sore nipple as infant sucks more vigorously at first.	At feeding session: 1. Have mother express milk manually. 2. Have mother change feeding positions.
HEALTH PERCEPTION–HEALTH MANAGEMENT ■ Nipples reddened and excoriated ■ Breast firm with milk ■ Infant sucking on nipple only	Injury to nipples related to vigorous sucking of infant, improper positioning of infant to breast feed	*To prevent injury, as above and:* ■ Change positions during feeding. Make sure baby is facing breast directly. ■ Skip use of sore nipple every other feeding; manually express milk so supply continues.	On return visit: 1. Examine nipples for healing. 2. Ask about any further problems.
HEALTH PERCEPTION–HEALTH MANAGEMENT ■ Milk leaking from breast ■ Bra wet	Potential for infection	*To promote healing review the following:* ■ Expose breast to air after feeding. ■ Use desk lamp to dry nipples. ■ Expose breast to sunlight. ■ Change bra often. ■ Wash breasts with warm water, *no* soap. ■ Use lanolin-based cream if not allergic to wool.	Have her set up desk lamp for use in drying nipples.

Application of the Nursing Process

NEWBORN NUTRITION: NURSING MOTHER WITH SORE NIPPLES

COGNITIVE-PERCEPTUAL			
"If this is what it is like, I don't think I can stand it."	Knowledge deficit related to length of time condition persists.	*To relieve tension, the nurse responds with the following:* ■ Sore nipples are worse about this time. ■ They should be improved in about 3 to 4 days. ■ Milk leaks out more at the beginning of breast feeding. You can help control it somewhat by pressing the heel of your hand against the nipple area. ■ I will be back in 3 days to see you, if that is convenient. ■ You have my number, phone me if you need to.	Phone Andrea in 3 days to check if the condition is improving.

References

Aberman, S., and others: Infant feeding practices, mother's decision-making, J.O.G.N. N. 14:394, Sept/Oct. 1985.

American Academy of Pediatrics, Committee on Nutrition: Commentary on breast-feeding and infant formulas, including proposed standards for formulas, Pediatrics 57:278, 1976.

Anderson, T.A.: Commercial infant foods: content and composition, Pediatr. Clin. North Am. 24:37, 1977.

Arnon, S.S., and others: Honey and other environmental risk factors for infant botulism, J. Pediatr. 95:331, 1979.

Borovies, D.: Assessing and managing pain in breast-feeding mothers, M.C.N. 9:272, July/Aug. 1984.

Broussard, A.: Anticipatory guidance: adding solids to the infant's diet. J.O.G.N. Nurs. 13:239, July/Aug. 1984.

Chapman, J., and others: Concerns of breast-feeding mothers from birth to 4 months, Nurs. Res. 34:374, Nov/Dec. 1985.

David, R., and others: Water intoxication in normal infants: role of antidiuretic hormone in pathogenesis, Pediatrics 68:349, 1981.

Fomon, S.J., and others: Recommendations for feeding normal infants, Pediatrics 63:152, 1979.

Food and Nutrition Board: Recommended dietary allowances, Washington, D.C., 1980, National Academy of Sciences.

Hamill, P.V.V., and others: Physical growth: National center for health statistics percentiles, Am. J. Clin. Nutr. 32:607, 1979. (Data from the Fels Research Institute, Wright State University School of Medicine, Yellow Springs, Ohio.)

Hughes, R.: Satisfaction with one's body and success in breast feeding, Issues in Comprehensive Pediatric Nursing 7:141, 1984.

Knopp, R.M., and Schwartz, J.F.: Water intoxication from swimming, J. Pediatr. 101:947, 1982.

Madgic, D.: Nutrition notes for new mothers, Stanford, Calif., 1986, Dept. of Dietetics, Stanford University Hospital.

MacLauglin, S., and Strelnick, E.: Breast feeding and working outside the home, Issues in Comprehensive Pediatric Nursing, 7:67, 1984.

Owen, A.L., and others: Infant feeding guide, Bloomfield, N.J., 1980, Health Learning System.

Parsons, L.: Weaning from the breast: for a happy ending to a satisfying experience, J.O.G.N. Nurs. 7:12, 1978.

Partridge, J.C., and others: Water intoxication secondary to feeding mismanagement, Am. J. Dis. Child, 135:38, 1981.

Price, A., and Bamford, N.: The breast feeding guide for the working woman, New York, 1983, Simon and Schuster.

Pyle, M.: Breast feeding is a family affair, Costa Mesa, Calif., 1985, Lifecircle.

Riordan, J.: A practical guide to breastfeeding, St. Louis, 1983, The C.V. Mosby Co.

Bibliography

American Academy of Pediatrics, Committee on Nutrition: Fluoride supplementation: revised dosage schedule, Pediatrics 63:150, 1979.

American Academy of Pediatrics, Committee on Nutrition: Iron supplementation for infants, Pediatrics 58:765, 1976.

Bachrach, S., and others: An outbreak of vitamin D deficiency rickets in a susceptible population, Pediatrics 64:871, 1979.

Blumenthal, S.: Infant nutrition and atherosclerosis. Dialogues in infant nutrition, vol. 1, no. 3, Bloomfield, N.J., 1977, Health Learning Systems.

Chase, H.P., and others: Kwashiorkor in the United States, Pediatrics 66:972, 1980.

Dallman, R.P., and others: Iron deficiency in infancy and childhood, Am. J. Clin. Nutr. 33:86, 1980.

Dwyer, J.T., and others: Risk of nutritional rickets among vegetarian children, Am. J. Dis. Child, 133:134, 1979.

Fomon, S.J., and Ziegler, E.: Skim milk in infant feeding, U.S. Department of Health, Education, and Welfare pub. no. (HSA) 77-5102, Washington, D.C., Aug. 1977, The Department.

Lakadawala, D.R., and Widdowson, E.M.: Vitamin D in human milk, Lancet 1:167, 1977.

McKay, S., and Mahan, C.: Ways to upgrade postpartal care, Contemp. OB/Gyn. 27:6:63, Nov. 1985.

Pipes, P.: Nutrition in infancy and childhood, ed. 2, St. Louis, 1981, The C.V. Mosby Co.

Saarinen, U.M.: Iron absorption in infants: high bioavailability of breast milk iron as indicated by the extrinsic tag method or iron absorption and by the concentration of serum ferritin, J. Pediatr. 91:36, 1977.

Willis, N.H.: Infant nutrition: birth to 6 months: a syllabus, Philadelphia, 1980, J.B. Lippincott Co.

Worthington-Roberts, B., Vermeersch, J., and Williams, S.R.: Nutrition in pregnancy and lactation, St. Louis, 1981, The C.V. Mosby Co.

Zmora, E., and others: Multiple nutritional deficiencies in infants from a strict vegetarian community, Am. J. Dis. Child. 133:141, 1979.

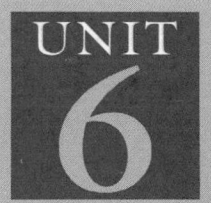

UNIT
6

Normal
Postpartum Period

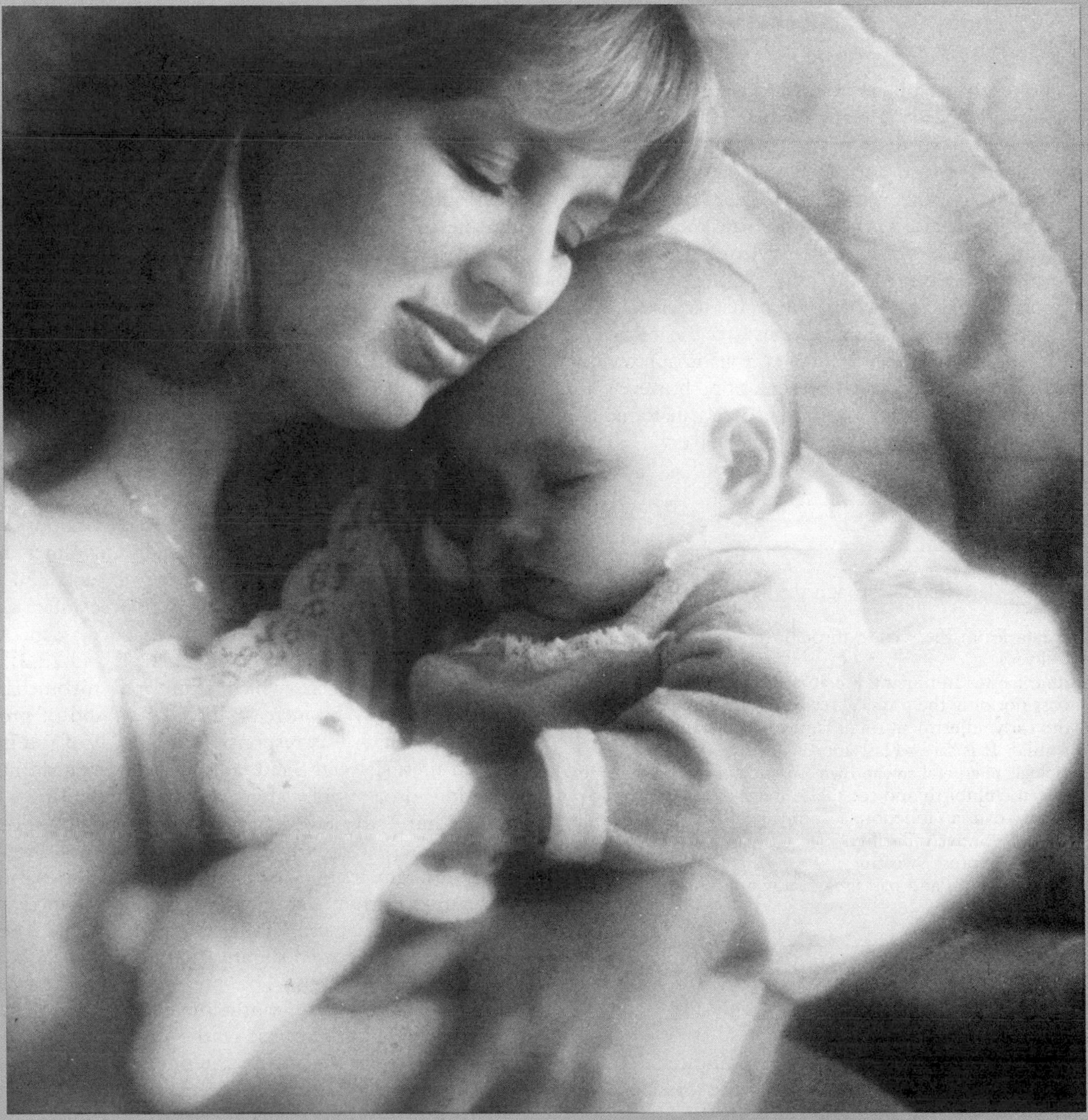

Maternal Physiology During the Postpartum Period

The responses of the mother to the birth of her infant are influenced by many factors. Her energy level, her freedom from discomfort, the health of her newborn, and the care and encouragement supplied by professional persons are contributing factors. To provide care beneficial to the mother, the infant, and the family, the nurse synthesizes knowledge from maternal anatomy and physiology of the recovery period, the newborn's physical and behavioral characteristics, child care activities, and family response to the birth of a child. The nurse, in short, uses a holistic approach to nursing care. For ease of presentation, however, the content of this chapter is limited to the anatomic and physiologic changes in women after delivery.

Definitions

puerperium
 p. early The second through the seventh day after delivery.
 p. late From the second through the sixth week after delivery.
fourth trimester In nursing literature the term used to encompass not only the physical recovery of the mother but also the early adjustment of all family members to the birth of a child. It is said to last approximately 3 months.
physiologic puerperal amenorrhea Absence of menstruation between childbirth and reestablishment of hypothalamic-pituitary-ovarian function, accompanied by genital hypoplasia and relative infertility.
diaphoresis Profuse sweating.
diuresis Secretion and passage of large amounts of urine.

Reproductive System and Associated Structures

Uterine corpus changes
Uterine involution. After the completion of the third stage of labor, the uterus is in the midline, about 2 cm *below* the level of unbilicus with the fundus rest-

ing on the sacral promontory. At this time, uterine size approximates the size at 16 weeks of gestation (about the size of a grapefruit). The uterus is about 14 cm (5½ in) long, 12 cm (4¾ in) wide, and 10 cm (4 in) thick and weighs about 1000 g (2 lb). When relaxed, the uterus is discoid; when contracted, its shape is globular.

Within 12 hours the fundus may be approximately 1 cm *above* the umbilicus (Fig. 22.1). From then on, involution progresses rapidly, and with the "take-up" and improved tone of the uterine supports, the fundus descends about 1 to 2 cm every 24 hours. By the sixth postpartum day the fundus normally will be half the distance from the symphysis pubis to the umbilicus. The uterus should not be palpable abdominally after the ninth postpartum day.

The uterus, which at full term weighs about 11 times its prepregnant weight, rapidly involutes to about 500 g (1 lb) 1 week after delivery and 350 g (11 to 12 oz) 2 weeks after delivery. A week after delivery the uterus lies in the true pelvis once again. At 6 weeks it weighs 50 to 60 g (Figs. 22.1, and 22.2).

Levels of estrogen, which stimulated myometrial growth primarily by increase in cell size, and of progesterone, which was responsible for much of the increased uterine weight and collagen formation during gestation, drop rapidly after delivery. Uterine involution within 4 to 6 weeks occurs principally by a decrease in the size of individual myometrial cells. However, the augmentation of connective tissue and elastin in the myometrium and blood vessels and the increase in the total uterine cell number are permanent. Hence uterine size is increased slightly after each pregnancy.

Uterine contractions. The intensity of uterine contractions increases significantly immediately after delivery, presumably in response to the greatly diminished intrauterine volume. During the first 1 to 2 postpartum hours, uterine activity decreases smoothly and progressively and stabilizes. Uterine contractions be-

Fig. 22.1

Assessment of involution of uterus after delivery. **A,** Days 1 through 9. **B,** Size and position of uterus 2 hours after delivery. Note extra hair, linea nigra, and striae gravidarum. **C,** Size and position of uterus 2 days after delivery. **D,** Size and position of uterus 4 days after delivery. (**B, C,** and **D** courtesy Marjorie Pyle, RNC, Lifecircle, Costa Mesa, California.)

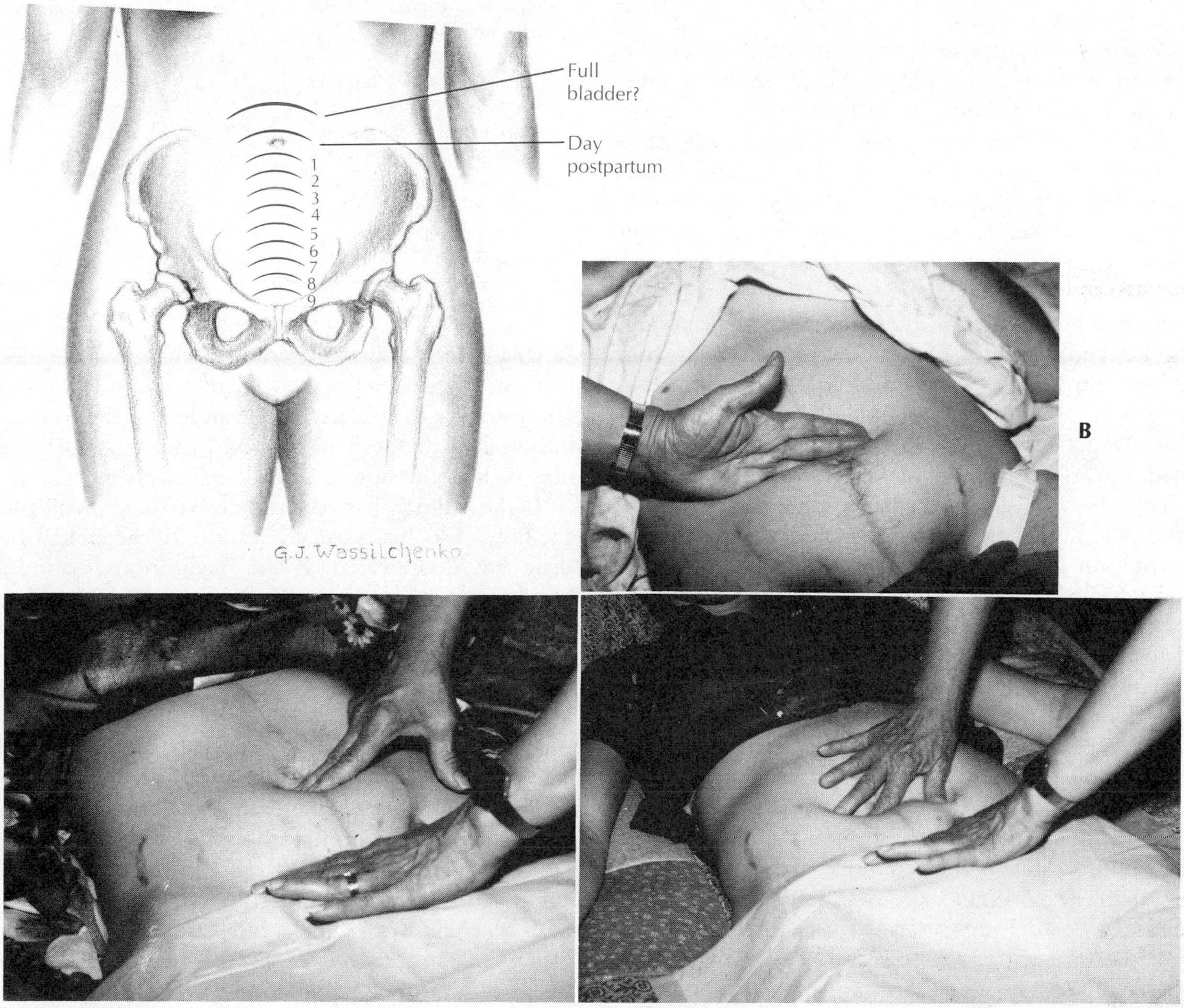

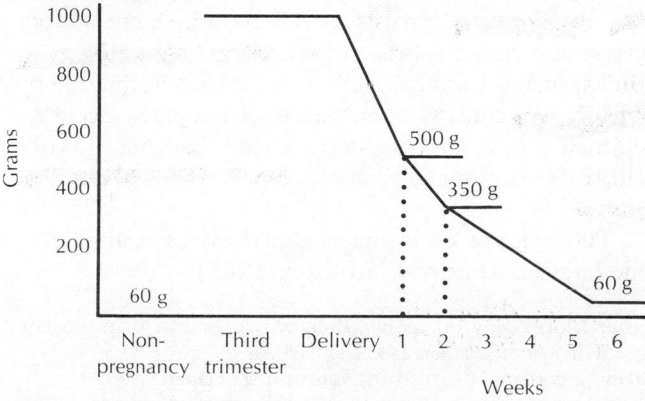

Fig. 22.2

Uterine weight before, during, and after pregnancy. Greatest change is in first week after childbirth. (Redrawn from Wiggins, J.D.: Childbearing: physiology, experiences, needs, St. Louis, 1979, The C.V. Mosby Co.)

come uncoordinated unless coordination is reestablished with exogenous (injected) oxytocin or endogenous oxytocin (released in response to nipple stimulation from suckling, for example). Uterine myometrial activity (tonus; the "living ligature" [see Fig. 5.16]) contributes to hemostasis by compressing the intramural blood vessels.

Afterpains. In primiparas the tone of the uterus is increased so that the fundus generally remains firm. Periodic relaxation and contraction are the rule for multiparas and may cause uncomfortable *afterpains* that persist throughout the early puerperium. Breast feeding frequently intensifies these afterpains because oxytocin is released by the posterior pituitary gland in response to stimulation of the nipple.

Placental site. Immediately after the placenta and membranes are delivered, the placental site is elevated, irregular, and partially obliterated by vascular constriction and thrombosis. According to Williams' classic description (Pritchard, MacDonald, and Gant, 1985), exfoliation (shedding) occurs because the site is undermined by an upward growth of endometrial tissue from the basal layer that remains after the separation of the placenta. Upward growth of the endometrium prevents scar formation that is characteristic of normal wound healing. This unique healing process enables the endometrium to resume its usual cycle of changes and to permit implantation and placentation in future pregnancies. Endometrial regeneration is completed by the end of the third postpartum week except at the placental site. Regeneration at the placental site usually is not complete until 6 weeks after delivery.

Failure of the placental site to heal completely is called *subinvolution of the placental site*. Women with this condition have persistent lochia and episodes of brisk, painless bleeding. Curettage usually is required.

Lochia. Postdelivery uterine discharge initially is bright red, changing to dark red or reddish brown (lochia rubra). *Lochia rubra* consists mainly of blood, and decidual and trophoblastic debris. The flow pales, becoming pink or brown after 3 to 4 days (lochia serosa). *Lochia serosa* consists of old blood, serum, leukocytes, and tissue debris. About 10 days after delivery, the drainage becomes yellow to white (lochia alba). *Lochia alba* consists of numerous leukocytes, decidua, epithelial cells, mucus, serum, and bacteria. Lochia alba may continue until about 2 to 6 weeks after delivery.

The amount of lochia is described as scant, light, moderate, and heavy (Jacobson, 1985):

scant Blood only on tissue when wiped or less than 2.5 cm (1 in) on a peripad (see Fig. 18.3).
light Less than 10 cm (4 in) stain on a peripad.
moderate Less than 15 cm (6 in) stain on peripad.
heavy Saturated peripad within 1 hour.

Table 22.1
Lochia and Nonlochia Bleeding

Lochia	Nonlochia Bleeding
Lochia usually trickles from the vaginal opening. The steady flow is greater as the uterus contracts.	If the bloody discharge spurts from the vagina, there may be cervical or vaginal tears in addition to the normal lochia.
A gush of lochia may result as the uterus is massaged. If it is dark in color, it has been pooled in the relaxed vagina, and the amount soon lessens to a trickle of bright red lochia (in the early puerperium).	If the amount of bleeding continues to be excessive and bright red, a tear may be the source.

Lochia refers only to uterine discharge. The blood seen on the peripad or bed linens may be from a different source (Table 22.1). Regardless of the source of bleeding, if the peripad is soaked through in 15 minutes or less, the flow is considered excessive.

If the woman has received an oxytocic medication, the flow of lochia is usually scant until the effect of the drug has disappeared. If the medication is administered intravenously, the effect persists for 30 minutes after the intravenous medication is discontinued; if the medication is administered intramuscularly, the effect persists for 30 to 60 minutes. If the woman is receiving ergonovine maleate (Ergotrate), 0.2 mg by mouth three to four times a day for 2 days, lochia is usually scant.

Persistence of lochia rubra early in the postpartum period suggests continued bleeding as a result of retained fragments of the placenta or membranes. Recurrence of bleeding about 10 days after delivery indicates bleeding from the placental site, which is healing. However, after 3 to 4 weeks bleeding may be caused by infection or subinvolution of the placental site. Continued lochia serosa or lochia alba may indicate endometritis, particularly if fever, pain, or tenderness is associated with the discharge. Lochia should smell like normal menstrual flow; an offensive odor usually indicates infection. Lochia clots, but normal menstrual blood does not.

Cervix. The cervix up to the lower uterine segment remains edematous, thin, and fragile for several days after delivery. The ectocervix (portion of the cervix that protrudes into the vagina) is soft, appears bruised, and has some small lacerations, optimum conditions for the development of infection. It remains easily distensible; two fingers may still be introduced for the first 4 to 6 days after delivery; only the smallest curette may be introduced by the end of 2 weeks. By the eighteenth hour the cervix has shortened, has a firm consistency, and has regained its form. By the end of the first week, recovery is almost complete. The external os, however, does not regain its prepregnant appearance; it is no longer shaped like a circle but appears as a jagged slit often described as "fish mouth" (see Fig. 5.18). Production of cervical and other estrogen-influenced mucus and mucosal characteristics may be delayed in the lactating woman.

Vagina and perineum. Postpartum estrogen deprivation is responsible for the thinness of the *vaginal mucosa* and the absence of rugae. The greatly distended, smooth-walled vagina gradually returns to its prepregnant size by 6 to 8 weeks after delivery. Rugae reappear by about the fourth week, although they are never as prominent as they are in the nulliparous woman. Most rugae may be permanently flattened. The mucosa remains atrophic in the lactating woman at least until menstruation begins again. Thickening of the vaginal mucosa occurs with the return of ovarian function. Profuse vaginal discharge is usually not present at 4 to 6 weeks after delivery unless there is an associated vaginitis. The hypoestrogenic condition of the vaginal epithelium is responsible for the decreased amount of vaginal mucus production and thinner vaginal mucosa. Local dryness and coital discomfort may persist until ovulation and menstruation resume.

Initially the *introitus* is erythematous and edematous, especially in the area of the episiotomy or laceration repair. Careful repair, prevention or early treatment of hematomas, and good hygiene during the first 2 weeks after delivery usually result in an introitus barely distinguishable from that of a nulliparous woman. The torn hymen heals with the development of fibrosed nodules of mucosa called *hymenal caruncles*.

Most *episiotomies* are visible only if the woman is lying on her side and her buttock is raised. A good light source is essential for visualization of some episiotomies. The healing process of an episiotomy is the same as for any surgical incision. Signs of infection (pain, redness, warmth, swelling, or discharge) or loss of approximation (separation) of the incision edges may occur.

Hemorrhoids (anal varicosities) are commonly seen. The women frequently experience associated symptoms such as itching, discomfort, and bright red bleeding with defecation.

Pelvic muscular support. Injury of the supporting structures of the uterus and vagina may occur during childbirth and may become gynecologic problems later in life. The term *relaxation* refers to the lengthening and weakening of the fascial supports of pelvic structures. These include the uterus, upper posterior vaginal wall, urethra, bladder, and rectum. Although relaxations can occur in any woman, most are direct but delayed sequelae to childbirth.

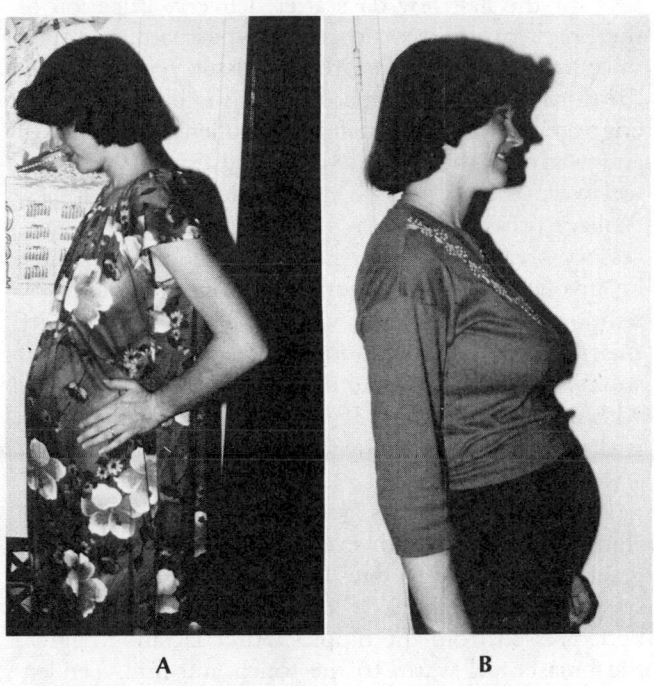

Fig. 22.3
Abdomen after delivery. **A,** Two hours after delivery. **B,** Eight days after delivery.

Abdominal wall. When the woman stands up during the first days after delivery, abdominal muscles cannot retain abdominal contents. The abdomen protrudes and gives her a still-pregnant appearance (Fig. 22.3). During the first 2 weeks after delivery the abdominal wall is relaxed. About 6 weeks are required before the abdominal wall almost returns to its nonparous state. The skin regains most of its previous elasticity, but some striae persist. The return of muscle tone depends on previous tone, proper exercise, and amount of adipose tissue. On occasion, with or without overdistention because of a large fetus or multiple fetuses, the abdominal wall muscles separate, a condition termed *diastasis recti abdominis*. Persistence of this defect may be disturbing to the woman, but surgical correction is rarely necessary. With time, the defect becomes less apparent.

Breasts. The concentrations of hormones that stimulated breast development during pregnancy (estrogen, progesterone, human chorionic gonadotropin, prolactin, cortisol, and insulin) decrease promptly after delivery. The time it takes for the return of these hormones to prepregnancy levels is determined in part by whether the mother breast feeds her infant.

Nonnursing mothers. The breasts feel generally nodular (in nonpregnant women they feel granular). The nodularity is bilateral and diffuse.

If the woman chooses not to breast feed and no antilactogenic medication is taken, prolactin levels drop rapidly. Colostrum secretion and excretion persists for the first few days after delivery. Palpation of the breast on the second or third postpartum day, as milk production begins, reveals tissue tenseness. On the third or fourth postpartum day the breasts become **engorged.** They are distended (swollen), firm, tender, and warm to the touch (vasocongestion makes them feel warm). Milk can be expressed from the nipples. Axillary breast tissue (the tail of Spence) and any accessory breast or nipple tissue along the milk line may be involved. Breast distention is primarily caused by temporary congestion of veins and lymphatics rather than from an accumulation of milk. Engorgement resolves spontaneously, and discomfort decreases usually within 24 to 36 hours. If suckling is never begun (or is discontinued), lactation ceases within a few days to a week.

Nursing mothers. As lactation is established, a mass (lump) may be felt; however, a filled milk sac will shift position from day to day. Before lactation begins, the breasts feel soft and a yellowish fluid, colostrum, can be expressed from the nipples. After lactation begins, the breasts feel warm to the touch and firm. Tenderness persists for about 48 hours. Bluish white milk (skim-milk appearance) can be expressed from the nipples. The nipples are examined for erectility as opposed to inversion and for cracks or fissures.

For a discussion of breast changes associated with lactation, see Chapter 21.

Endocrine System

Placental hormones. Plasma levels of placental hormones fall rapidly after delivery. *Human chorionic somatomammotropin* (HCS) (also known as human placental lactogen) reach undetectable levels within 24 hours (see also discussions of growth hormone and carbohydrate metabolism). *Human chorionic gonadotropin* (HCG) declines rapidly, so that standard urinary pregnancy tests are usually negative by the end of the first week.

Estrogen levels in plasma fall to 10% of the prenatal value within 3 hours after delivery; the lowest levels occur about day 7. The significant decline in estrogen is accompanied by the onset of breast engorgement on about postpartum day 3, a coincidence that supports the view that high estrogen levels suppress lactation despite elevated prolactin levels. Plasma levels of estrogen do not increase to follicular levels until 19 to 21 days after delivery. In lactating women, return to normal estrogen levels is somewhat delayed.

Progesterone levels in plasma fall below luteal levels by the third postpartum day and cannot be detected in serum after the first postdelivery week. Progesterone production begins with the first ovulation.

Pituitary hormones. *Prolactin* levels in blood rise progressively throughout pregnancy. After delivery, in nonlactating women, prolactin levels decline, reaching the prepregnant range within 2 weeks. Initially, suckling and lactation are accompanied by dramatic increases in prolactin concentration. Serum prolactin levels are influenced by the number of times per day breast feeding occurs. Normal basal values of prolactin are reached by 6 months if breast feeding occurs only 1 to 3 times per day. High prolactin levels persist for more than a year if suckling occurs more than 6 times per day.

Levels of *follicle-stimulating hormone* (FSH) and *luteinizing hormone* (LH) are very low in all women for 10 to 12 days after delivery.

Hypothalamic-pituitary-ovarian function. Little is known about the physiology of the hypothalamus, the pituitary gland, and the ovaries during the puerperium after term gestation. However, considerable information is available on the time of appearance of the first ovulation and the reestablishment of menstruation for lactating and nonlactating women. For all women, the first menses *usually* follows an *an*ovulatory cycle or a cycle associated with inadequate corpus luteum function (low LH and progesterone).

Among lactating women, 15% resume menstruation by 6 weeks, and 45% by 12 weeks. Among nonlactating women, 40% menstruate by 2 weeks, 65% by 12 weeks, and 90% by 24 weeks. For lactating women, 80% of first menstrual cycles are anovulatory; for nonlactating women 50% of first cycles are anovulatory.

Much of the variability in the reestablishment of menstruation and ovulation observed in lactating women way result from individual differences in the strength of the suckling stimulus. Partial weaning (formula supplementation) also may play a role. This emphasizes the fact that **suckling is not a reliable form of birth control.**

The first menstrual flow is usually heavier than normal. Within 3 to 4 cycles the amount of menstrual flow has returned to the woman's prepregnant volume.

Other endocrine changes. *Growth hormone* secretion remains depressed during late pregnancy and the early puerperium. The low level of growth hormone and the rapid decline in the hormones HCS, estrogens, and cortisol, and in the placental enzyme, insulinase, *reduce the anti-insulin factors* in the early puerperium. Therefore new mothers have low fasting plasma glucose levels, and insulin requirements for insulin-dependent diabetic women usually fall after delivery (see Chapter 28). Normal hormonal alterations render the early puerperium a transitional period for *carbohydrate metabolism* so that interpretation of glucose tolerance tests is difficult at this time.

Rapid fluctuations in many indices confound evaluation of *thyroid* function during the early puerperium. Postpartum hypothyroidism is suspected if the woman fails to lactate or recovery from childbirth is delayed.

A progressive increase of plasma levels of *corticosteroids* during pregnancy and labor is followed by a decline to nonpregnant values by the end of the first week after delivery. Within 2 hours after delivery, *plasma renin* and *angiotensin II* levels drop to within the normal nonpregnant range. This finding may indicate that the fetoplacental unit is one source of maternal plasma renin.

Basal metabolic rate. The basal metabolic rate remains elevated for 7 to 14 days after delivery. Normal nonpregnant values for respiratory system function are given in Appendix F.

Cardiovascular System

Blood volume. Changes in blood volume depend on several variable factors, for example, blood loss during delivery, and mobilization and subsequent excretion of extravascular water (physiologic edema). Blood loss results in immediate but limited decrease in total blood volume. Thereafter, normal shifts in body water result in a slow decline in blood volume. By the third to fourth week after delivery the blood volume usually has regressed to nonpregnant values (Fig. 22.4).

Maternal response to normal blood loss. Pregnancy-induced hypervolemia (increase of at least 40% from 1 to 2 liters near term) allows most women to tolerate a considerable blood loss at delivery. Many women lose 300 to 400 ml of blood during vaginal delivery of a single fetus and about twice this amount during cesarean delivery.

Retrogressive changes (readjustments) in the maternal vasculature after delivery are dramatic and rapid. The woman's response to blood loss during the early

Fig. 22.4
Rate of loss of 1500 ml in blood volume during first postdelivery month. Greatest change at delivery, then in week after childbirth. (From Wiggins, J.D.: Childbearing: physiology, experiences, needs, St. Louis, 1979, The C.V. Mosby Co.)

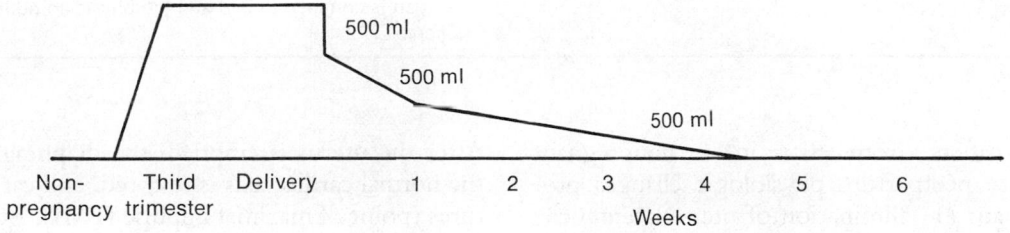

Fig. 22.5
Cardiac output. Work of heart increases during labor and decreases significantly immediately after birth of baby. (From Wiggins, J.D.: Childbearing: physiology, experiences, needs. St. Louis, 1979, The C.V. Mosby Co.)

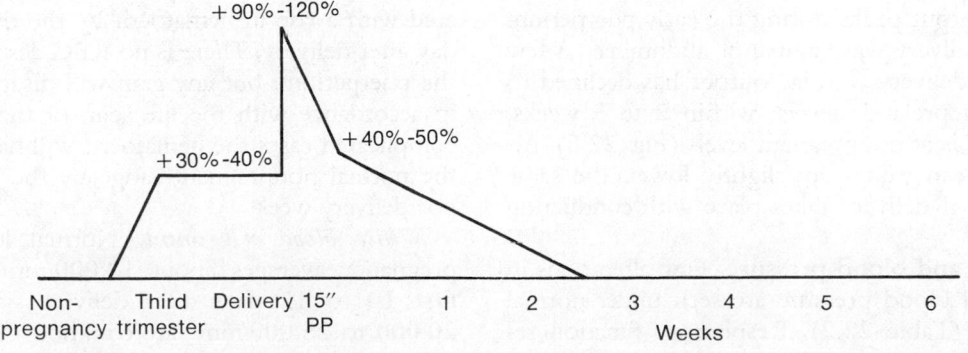

Table 22.2
Vital Signs and Blood Pressure After Delivery, Deviations From Normal Findings, and Probable Causes

Normal Findings	Deviations from Normal Findings and Probable Causes
Temperature	
During first 24 hours, may rise to 38° C (100.4° F) as a result of dehydrating effects of labor. Except for first 24 hours the woman should be afebrile.	A diagnosis of puerperal sepsis is suggested if a rise in maternal temperature to 38° C (100.4° F) is noted after the first 24 hours after delivery and recurs or persists for 2 days. Other possibilities are mastitis, endometritis, urinary tract infections, and other systemic infections.
Pulse	
Bradycardia is a common finding for the first 6 to 8 days after delivery. Bradycardia is a consequence of increased cardiac output and stroke volume. The pulse returns to nonpregnant levels by 3 months after delivery. A pulse rate of between 50 and 70 beats/min may be considered normal.	A rapid pulse rate or one that is increasing may indicate hypovolemia secondary to hemorrhage.
Respirations	
Respirations should fall within the woman's normal predelivery range.	Hypoventilation and hypotension may follow an unusually high subarachnoid (spinal) block.
Blood pressure	
Blood pressure is altered *slightly* if at all. Orthostatic hypotension, as indicated by feelings of faintness or dizziness immediately after standing up, can develop in the first 48 hours as a result of the splanchnic engorgement that may occur after delivery.	A low or falling blood pressure may reflect hypovolemia secondary to hemorrhage. However, it is a late sign, and other symptoms of hemorrhage usually alert the staff. An increased reading may result from excessive use of vasopressor drugs or oxytocic drugs. Since pregnancy-induced hypertension (PIH) can persist into or occur first in the postpartum period, routine evaluation of blood pressure is needed. If a woman complains of headache, hypertension must be ruled out as a cause before analgesics are administered. If the blood pressure is elevated, the woman is confined to bed and the physician notified. (See also Chapter 27.)

puerperium differs from that in a nonpregnant woman. Three postpartum physiologic changes protect the woman: (1) elimination of uteroplacental circulation reduces the size of the maternal vascular bed by 10% to 15%, (2) loss of placental endocrine function removes the stimulus for vasodilatation, and (3) mobilization of extravascular water stored during pregnancy occurs.

Cardiac output. The cardiac output continues to increase during the first and second stages of labor. The cardiac output peaks during the early puerperium whether the delivery was vaginal or abdominal. A few minutes after delivery, cardiac output has declined to about 50% of prelabor levels; within 2 to 3 weeks, cardiac output is at nonpregnant levels (Fig. 22.5). Although the mean values are slightly lower, the same changes occur if delivery takes place with conduction anesthesia.

Vital signs and blood pressure. Few alterations in vital signs and blood pressure are seen under normal circumstances (Table 22.2). Respiratory function returns to nonpregnant levels by 6 months after delivery.

After the uterus is emptied, the diaphragm descends, the normal cardiac axis is restored, and cardiologic features (point of maximal impulse [PMI], ECG) are normalized.

Blood constituents
Hematocrit. During the first 72 hours after delivery, there is a greater loss in plasma volume than in blood cells. The decrease in plasma volume plus the increase in red blood cell mass of pregnancy is associated with a rise in hematocrit by the third to seventh day after delivery. There is no RBC destruction during the puerperium, but any gain will disappear gradually in accordance with the life span of the RBC. In uncomplicated cases the hematocrit will have returned to the normal nonpregnant range by the fourth or fifth postdelivery week.

White blood cell count. Normal leukocytosis of pregnancy averages about 12,000/mm³. During the first 10 to 12 days after delivery, values between 20,000 to 25,000/mm³ are common. Neutrophils are the most numerous WBCs with a consequent shift to the left. Leukocytosis coupled with the normal increase in erythrocyte sedimentation rate may confuse the intrepretation of acute infections at this time.

Coagulation factors. An extensive activation of blood-clotting factors occurs after delivery. This activation, together with immobility, trauma, or sepsis, encourages thromboembolism. Factors, I, II, VIII, IX, and X decrease within a few days to prepregnant levels. The elevated levels of fibrin split products are probably the result of their release from the placental site.

Thromboembolism. The woman's legs are examined daily for signs of thrombosis (pain, warmth, and tenderness; swollen reddened vein that feels hard or solid to touch). There may or may not be a positive Homans' sign (dorsiflexion of foot [see Fig. 11.12], which causes calf muscles to compress tibial veins and produce pain if thrombosis is present). It is important to remember that deep venous thrombosis may be silent, that is, not give rise to pain.

Varicosities. Varicosities of the legs and around the anus (hemorrhoids) are common during pregnancy. Varices, even the less common vulvar varices, regress (empty) rapidly immediately after delivery. Surgical correction of varicosities is not considered during pregnancy. This is because of the likelihood of the total or the nearly total regression anticipated after delivery.

Urinary System

Renal function. The hormonal changes of pregnancy (high steroid levels) contribute to the increase in renal function, and conversely, the diminishing steroid levels after delivery may partly explain the reduced renal function during the puerperium. The renal glycosuria induced by pregnancy disappears. *Lactosuria* may be expected in lactating women. However, it cannot be detected by use of the Clinitest, since this test is specific for the presence of glucose, not lactose, in urine. The *blood urea nitrogen increases* during the puerperium as autolysis of the involuting uterus is accomplished. As a result of the catalytic processes of involution, *mild proteinuria* (+ 1) is a normal finding for 1 to 2 days after delivery in about 50% of women. *Acetonuria* may even occur in women with an uncomplicated delivery or after a prolonged labor with dehydration.

Kidney function returns to normal within a month after delivery. About 6 weeks are required for the pregnancy-induced hypotonia and dilation of the ureters and renal pelves to subside. In a small percentage of women, dilation of the urinary tract may persist for 3 months.

Reversal of water metabolism of pregnancy. **Profuse diaphoresis,** especially at night (night sweats), is not unusual for 2 to 3 days after delivery. Diaphoresis is a mechanism to reduce the retained fluids of pregnancy and usually is not a symptom of infection.

The renal plasma flow and glomerular filtration rate that increased by 25% to 50% during pregnancy remains elevated for at least the first postpartum week. Normally a **marked diuresis** begins within 12 hours after delivery. The volume of urinary output along with the insensible water loss through perspiration accounts for a large portion of the **weight loss** during the early puerperium. It is approximately 5.5 kg (12 lb) after delivery of the fetus, placenta, and amniotic fluid and an additional 4 kg (9 lb) during the puerperium because of excretion of fluids and electrolytes accumulated during pregnancy. The mechanism that facilitates elimination of the excess tissue fluid accumulated during pregnancy is often referred to as the *reversal of the water metabolism of pregnancy.*

Urethra and bladder. Trauma occurs to the urethra and bladder as the infant passes through the pelvis. The bladder wall is hyperemic and edematous, often with small areas of hemorrhage. Clean-catch or catheterized urine specimens after delivery often reveal hematuria from bladder trauma. Later in the puerperium, hematuria may be a sign of urinary tract infection. The urethra and urinary meatus may be edematous. Birth-induced trauma and the effects of analgesia, especially conduction anesthesia, cause relative insensitivity that depresses the urge to void. In addition, pelvic soreness caused by the forces of labor, vaginal lacerations, or the episiotomy reduces or alters the voiding reflex. This alteration, together with postpartum diuresis, may allow rapid filling of the bladder.

Distention of the bladder can readily occur as the water metabolism of pregnancy is reversed and fluids are mobilized in the elimination of end products of protein catabolism. Overdistention can make the bladder more susceptible to infection as well as impede the resumption of normal voiding. If prolonged bladder overdistention occurs, further damage to the bladder wall (atony) may result.

Gastrointestinal System

Appetite. The mother is usually hungry shortly after delivery and can tolerate a light diet. After full recovery from analgesia, anesthesia, and fatigue, most new mothers are ravenously hungry. Requests for double portions of food and frequent snacks are not uncommon. For a discussion of diet during lactation, see Chapter 21.

Motility. Typically, decreased muscle tone and motility of the gastrointestinal tract persists for only a short time after delivery. Excess analgesia and anesthesia could delay a return to normal tonicity and motility.

Bowel evacuation. A spontaneous bowel evacuation may be delayed until 2 to 3 days after delivery. This can be explained by decreased muscle tone (*adynamic ileus*) in the intestines during labor and the immediate puerperium, prelabor diarrhea or a predelivery enema, lack of food, dehydration, or perineal tenderness because of episiotomy, lacerations, or hemorrhoids. Regular bowel habits must be reestablished after delivery once bowel tone returns.

Neurologic System

Neurologic changes during the puerperium are those resulting from a reversal of maternal adaptations to pregnancy and those resulting from trauma during labor and delivery.

Pregnancy-induced neurologic discomforts abate after delivery. Elimination of physiologic edema through the diuresis that follows delivery relieves *carpal tunnel syndrome* by easing the compression of the median nerve. The periodic numbness and tingling of fingers that afflict 5% of gravidas usually disappear after delivery unless lifting and carrying the baby aggravates the condition. For a discussion of nerve injury incurred during childbirth, see Chapter 11. *Headache* requires careful assessment. Four types of headaches are compared in Table 22.3.

Musculoskeletal System

Adaptations in the mother's endocrine system are reversed in the puerperium. The adaptations include those that contribute to relaxation and subsequent hypermobility of the joints and in the change in the mother's center of gravity because of the enlarging uterus. *Stabilization of joints* is complete by 6 to 8 weeks after delivery. However, although all other joints return to their normal prepregnant position before restabilization, those in the parous woman's feet do not; the new mother may notice a permanent increase in shoe size.

Table 22.3
Comparison of Postpartum Headaches

	Postsubarachnoid Anesthesia	Stress Headache	Meningeal Irritation	Pregnancy-Induced Hypertension (PIH)
Cause	Leakage of cerebrospinal fluid through puncture in dura into extradural space	Anxiety, muscle tension especially in neck, shoulders,; fatigue, hunger	Aseptic chemical meningeal irritation	Etiologic factors of PIH (e.g., vasospasm)
Onset	Days 1-2	Variable		Late in the development of PIH; a frequent forerunner of eclampsia (convulsions)*
Location	Forehead, deep behind eyes; radiates to both temples and to occipital area	Band around head; occipital		Frontal or occipital, or generalized
Intensity	Severe to mild	More or less constant ache		Severe, constant throbbing or "splitting"
Modifiers	Increased intensity in sitting or standing position; eases in supine position	Relieved by physical and psychologic rest, food	Not relieved by lying down	Resistant to relief from analgesics
Duration	1-3 days to several weeks	Variable	1-3 days	Duration of severe PIH
Therapy	Increase oral fluids	Implement good communication techniques to help her identify concerns, to ventilate feelings regarding labor/ delivery experience; facilitate rest; offer food and fluids; administer medications as necessary; utilize comfort measures (e.g., back rubs, etc).	Administer analgesics, fluids, and other supportive measures	Treatment for PIH (see Chapter 27)
	Supplement oral fluids with at least 1000 ml 5% dextrose in normal saline solution			
	Administer analgesics			
	Assist physician in establishing extradural "blood patch" with client's own blood			
	Tight abdominal binder			

*Pritchard, MacDonald, and Gant, 1985.

Integumentary System

Chloasma of pregnancy usually disappears at the termination of pregnancy. *Hyperpigmentation* of the areolae and linea nigra may not regress completely after delivery.

Vascular abnormalities such as spider angiomas (nevi), palmar erythema, and epulis generally regress in response to the rapid decline in estrogens after termination of pregnancy. For some women, spider nevi persist indefinitely.

The abundance of fine *hair* seen during pregnancy usually disappears after delivery; however, any coarse or bristly hair that appears during pregnancy usually remains. *Fingernails* return to their prepregnant characteristics of consistency and strength.

Diaphoresis is the most noticeable change in the integumentary system (see reversal of water metabolism of pregnancy, p. 637).

Immune System

The mother's need for *rubella vaccination* or for prevention of Rh isoimmunization is determined.

Acquired immune deficiency syndrome. For discussion of acquired immune deficiency syndrome (AIDS) and other questions concerning immunology, see the section on immunology in Chapter 13.

Summary

The maternity nurse needs a solid understanding of normal physiologic responses during the postpartum period. This will enable the nurse to provide quality nursing care. Knowledge of normal findings will allow the nurse to plan for care and encourage client participation. Women and their families will be better able to anticipate and adjust to postpartum changes if they have been provided with adequate health information. The nurse is in a key role to provide health education to women and their families. The nurse can help to ease the transition from pregnancy to motherhood.

References

Jacobson, H.: A standard for assessing lochia volume, M.C.N. 10(3):174, May/June 1985.
Pritchard, J.A., MacDonald, P.C., and Gant, N.F.: Williams obstetrics, ed. 17, Norwalk, Conn., 1985, Appleton-Century-Crofts.

Bibliography

Danforth, D.N.: Textbook of obstetrics and gynecology, ed. 5, New York, 1982, Harper & Row, Publishers.
Jensen, M.D., and Bobak, I.M.: Maternity and gynecologic care: the nurse and the family, ed 3., St. Louis, 1985, The C.V. Mosby Co.
McKay, S., and Mahan, C.S.: Ways to upgrade postpartal care, Contemp OB/Gyn. 27:63, 1985.
Myles, M.F.: Textbook for midwives with modern concepts of obstetric and neonatal care, ed. 9, New York, 1981, Churchill Livingstone.
Oxorn, H.: Oxorn-Foote human labor and birth, ed. 5, Norwalk, Conn., 1986, Appleton-Century-Crofts.
Quistad, C.: How to smooth mom's postpartum path, R.N. 47:40, April 1984.
Wiggins, J.D.: Childbearing physiology, experiences, needs, St. Louis, 1979, The C.V. Mosby Co.
Willson, J.R., Carrington, E.R., and Ledger, W.J.: Obstetrics and gynecology, ed. 7, St. Louis, 1983, The C.V. Mosby Co.
Zuspan, F., and Quilligan, E.: Practical manual of obstetrical care, St. Louis, 1982, The C.V. Mosby Co.

Family Adjustment During the Postpartum Period

The birth of a child poses a fundamental challenge to the existing interactional structure of a family. The adults must change from an adult marital relationship between spouses to the establishment of a relationship between parents and child. In addition, the marital and parental relationships must be handled simultaneously (Kreppner and others, 1982). If there is another child (or children) in the family, the parent must adjust his or her own life space to include another child, and the firstborn children must adjust to another person's claim on parental time and love (Walz and Rich, 1983). This chapter reviews parenthood and parent, sibling, and grandparent adjustments to childbirth.

Parenthood

Biologic parenthood for both sexes begins with the union of ovum and sperm. During the prenatal period the mother is the primary agent in providing an environment in which the unborn child may develop and grow. This close symbiotic union of mother and child ends with birth. Others may then assume partial or complete involvement in the infant's care. Whoever— whether biologic or substitute parent, woman or man—assumes the parental role enters into a crucial relationship with a child that will persist throughout the life of each. Men and women, of course, may exist without a child; thus, in essence, parenthood is optional. Parenthood may serve as a maturation factor in the life of a man or woman regardless of whether it is biologically based. For children, parenthood is all important; their continued existence depends on the quality of care they receive.

Components. The tasks, responsibilities, and attitudes that make up parenting care have been designated by Steele and Pollock (1968) as the "mothering function." It is a process in which an adult (a mature, caring, capable, self-sufficient person) assumes the care

of an infant (a helpless, dependent, immature person). They describe parenting as one process with two components. The first, being practical or mechanical in nature, involves cognitive and motor skills; the second, emotional in nature, involves cognitive and affective skills. Both components are essential to the infant's well-being and future development.

Cognitive-motor skills. The first component in the process of parenting includes childcare activities such as "feeding, holding, clothing, and cleaning the infant, protecting it from harm, and providing motility for it" (Steele and Pollock, 1968). These task-oriented activities do not appear automatically as efficient caretaking behaviors at the birth of one's child. The parents' ability in these respects has been altered by the effects of cultural and personal experiences. Many parents have to learn how to do these tasks, and this learning process can be difficult. However, the majority of parents with the desire to learn and with the able and willing support of others become adept in caretaking activities.

Cognitive-affective skills. The psychologic component in child care, motherliness or fatherliness, appears to stem from the *parents'* earliest experiences with a loving, accepting mother figure. In this sense parents may be said to "inherit" the ability to show concern and tenderness and to pass on this ability to the next generation by repeating the kind of parent-child relationship they experienced. The cognitive-affective component of parenting includes attitudes of tenderness, awareness, and concern for the child's needs and desires. This component influences the environment of the child. It has a profound effect on the manner in which the practical aspects of child care are performed and on the emotional response of the child to the care. Benedek (1950) describes a positive parent-child relationship as mutually rewarding. This relationship is fundamental to a person's development of confidence in the expectations that others will be willing to help and that the person is worth helping. Erikson's concept (1959) of "basic trust" is similar. He postulates that such a psychologic entity forms the basis for the adult's eventual relationships with others and ability to trust others. Persons who experienced a positive parent-child relationship tend to be social or outgoing and able to seek and accept assistance from others. In contrast, those deficient in a sense of trust tend to be alienated and isolated. They are more likely to have crises because of their inability to make use of situational supports in times of stress.

Either parent may exhibit "motherliness." Motherliness is now recognized to be a non-gender-related ability. The ability to show gentleness, love, and understanding and to place another's welfare above one's own is not limited to women—it is a human characteristic.

Fig. 23.1
Hands. (Courtesy St. Luke's Hospital, Kansas City, Missouri.)

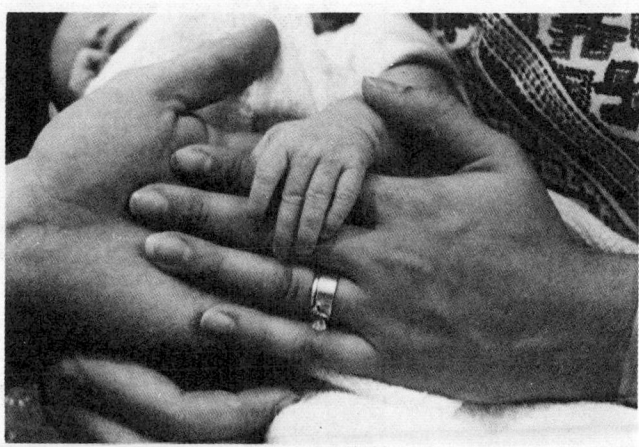

Attachment

Although much research has been directed toward unraveling the process by which a parent comes to love and accept a child and a child comes to love and accept a parent (Fig. 23.1), we still do not know what motivates and commits parent and child to decades of supportive and nurturing care of each other. We do know that it begins as a process of attachment. The attachment process has been described as linear, beginning during pregnancy, intensifying during the early post-delivery period, and being constant and consistent once established. It is critical to mental and physical health across the life span (Parkes and Stevenson-Hinde, 1982). According to Stainton (1983b), attachment is a mutual exchange of feelings predicated by attractiveness, responsiveness, and satisfaction and is subject to changes in intensity as circumstances change over time. Attachment is developed and maintained by proximity and interaction. As with any developmental process, it is characterized by periods of progress and regression, and temporary or permanent withdrawal from attachment figures can occur. Mercer (1982) notes that attachment is facilitated by *positive feedback*. "Positive feedback includes the social, verbal and nonverbal responses, either real or perceived, that indicate acceptance of one partner by the other." She goes on to say that attachment occurs through "a mutually satisfying experience."

Various theories have attempted to explain the basis for attachment. Freudian psychoanalytic theory emphasizes the development of a bond between child and mother as a result of the mother's satisfying the infant's innate needs. These needs are related to the human need to socialize with another and the physical needs for survival. Social learning theory contributed the principles of reinforcement to the attachment process. As discomfort is reduced or removed by the mother (or other caretaker) and pleasure substituted, the mother becomes associated with the pleasurable feeling of being satisfied. She becomes important to the infant, is loved, and can therefore act as a reinforcing agent or event. The mother becomes a *significant other* in the infant's life.

Bowlby (1958) and others (Ainsworth, 1969, 1970; Ainsworth and Bell, 1970; Brazelton, 1963, 1973) have extended the concept of attachment to include *mutuality;* that is, the infant's behaviors and characteristics call forth a corresponding set of maternal behaviors and characteristics. The infant possesses a repertoire of behaviors that serve to initiate and maintain contact with the mother. *Signaling* behaviors such as crying, smiling, and cooing bring the mother near the child. *Executive* behaviors such as rooting, suckling, grasping, and postural adjustments maintain the contact.

The *infant* influences the caretaker and plays an important role in creating a mutually satisfying experience. The caretaker is attracted to an alert, responsive, cuddly infant and repelled by an irritable, apparently disinterested infant. Attachment occurs more readily with the infant whose temperament, social capabilities, appearance, and gender fit the parent's expectations. If the child does not meet these expectations, resolution of disappointment can delay the attachment process. An important part of attachment is the family *identification of the new baby* (Fig. 23.2). The infant's identity gradually expands, beginning with the claiming pro-

Fig. 23.2
The family examines the new baby. They discuss her appearance and admire her.
(Courtesy Marjorie Pyle, RNC, Lifecircle, Costa Mesa, California.)

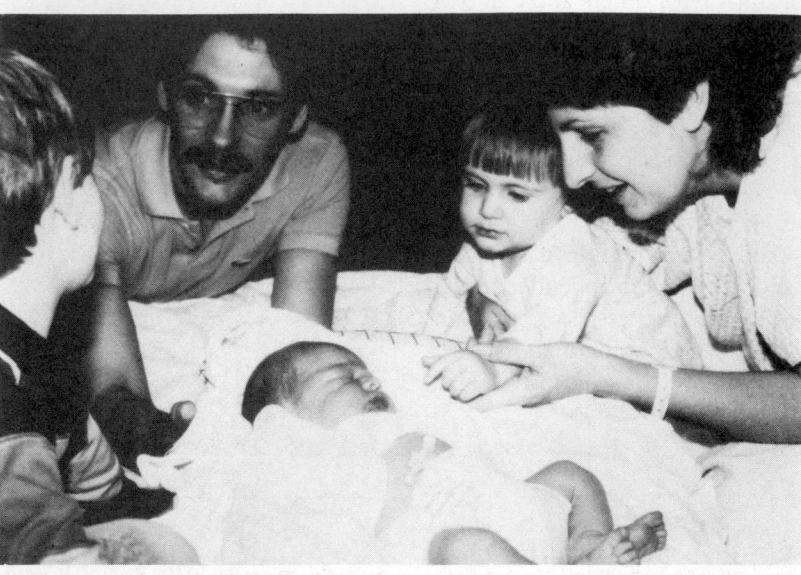

cess; that is, the child is first identified in terms of "likeness" to other family members, then in terms of "differences," and finally in terms of "uniqueness." The unique newcomer is thus *incorporated* into the family. Mothers and fathers scrutinize an infant very carefully. They point out characteristics that the child shares with other family members and indicate recognition of a relationship between them. Mothers make comments such as the following that reveal the claiming process: "Russ held him close and said, 'He's the image of his father,' but I found one part like me—his toes are shaped like mine. Look, he's smiling; he likes his mother's jokes."

On the other hand, some mothers react negatively. They "claim" the infant in terms of the discomfort or pain the baby causes the mother. The mother interprets the infant's normal responses as being derogatory to the mother. The mother reacts to her child with dislike or indifference. She does not hold the child close or touch the child to be comforting; for example, "The nurse put the baby into Marie's arms. She promptly laid him across her knees and glanced up at the television. 'Stay still 'til I finish watching—you've been enough trouble already.' "

Parental responses have direct implications for nursing. Nurses can establish an environment that enhances positive parent-child contacts. They can encourage parental awareness of infant responses and ability to communicate, provide support and encour-

agement as parents attempt to become competent and loving in their role, and enhance the attachment process.

Parental preconditions. Mercer (1982) lists five preconditions that influence attachment:
1. A parent's emotional health (including the ability to trust another person)
2. A social support system encompassing mate, friends, and family
3. A competent level of communication and caretaking skills
4. Parental proximity to the infant
5. Parent-infant fit (including infant state, temperament, and sex)

If any of these preconditions are not present or are distorted, skilled intervention is necessary to ensure the attachment process.

Sensual responses. Attachment is strengthened through the use of sensual responses or abilities by both partners in the parent-child interaction. The sensual responses and abilities include the following.

Touch. Touch or the tactile sense is used extensively by parents and other caretakers as a means of becoming acquainted with the newborn. The fingertip, one of the most touch sensitive areas of the body, is used to explore the infant's head, face, and body surfaces. The open palms and arms are used to handle the infant (Tulman, 1985). Many mothers reach out for their infants as soon as they are born and the cord is cut. They

Fig. 23.3
Mother interacts with daughter through touching Infant's head and feet. (Courtesy Judy Bamber, San Jose, California.)

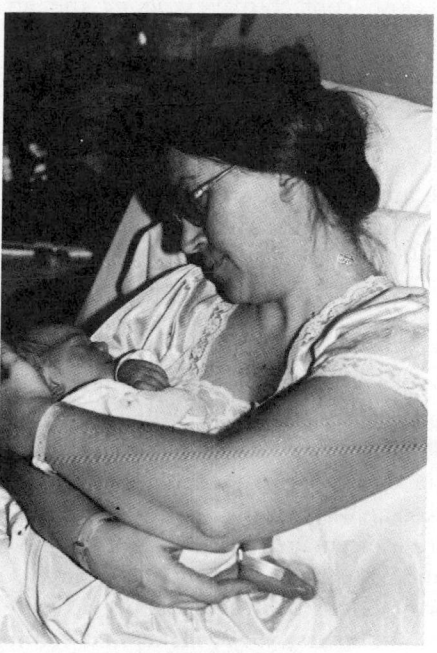

lift them to their breasts, enfold them in their arms, and cradle them. Once the child is close to them again they begin the exploration process with their fingertips. For some other mothers and other caretakers (fathers, nursing and medical students) studies have depicted a predictable pattern of touch behavior (Rubin, 1961; Klaus and others, 1982; Tulman, 1985). The caretaker begins with a fingertip exploration of the infant's head and extremities. Within a short time the caretaker uses the palm to caress the baby's trunk and eventually enfolds the infant in her or his arms. Gentle stroking motions are used to soothe and quiet the infant. Mothers pat or gently rub their infant's back after feedings. Infants pat the mother's breast as they nurse. Mothers and fathers want to touch, pick up, and hold their infant (Fig. 23.3). They comment on the softness of the baby's skin and are aware of milia and rashes.

Parents and child seem to enjoy sharing each other's body warmth. Mothers will say, "I love her warm little body against mine." Research has demonstrated that the newborn does not lose body heat if reasonable precautions are taken (e.g., if the infant is placed on the mother's abdomen after birth and dried thoroughly)

(Fardig, 1980). Infants sometimes relax completely against their mother's warm body.

The newborn infant grasps a finger or a strand of hair, becoming attached to the parent. A father commented on his son's grasp reflex, "I put my finger in his hand, and he grabbed right on. It is just a reflex, I know, but it felt good anyway."

Parents can be helped to recognize and respond to the similarities of responses of their unborn and born child. Parents are helped to come closer to their babies through recognition of the use of touch, both before and after birth, and increasing sensitivity to the infant's like or dislike of types of touch. Stainton (1983b) reports the following instances:

The unborn baby was perceived to be distressed at times and communicated this to the parents through excessive movement, especially kicking, indicating a need for, in their words, "calming down." One or both parents typically responded by rubbing the baby's body through the abdominal wall and all reported this resulted in a "settling" or "quieting." The majority stated the unborn baby liked to be rubbed. Mothers and fathers were observed rubbing or patting the abdomen.

Particularly, "when I am driving, there is some movement the baby does in the lower left side, so I assume it is with the hands. It won't stop until I reposition myself, so I assume he or she needs more room," reported one. Another described "wiggling its feet or pushing against my rib cage when I slouch until I straighten up."

Mothers also deal with discomfort caused by the unborn baby stretching or positioning. According to one woman, a verbal command such as "Hey, that's too high" resulted in the fetus's shifting position. Another unborn baby consistently moved enough to waken the mother at 4 AM but settled as soon as the mother emptied her bladder (Stainton, 1983b). The unborn comes "not as a stranger" but as one known to the parents and alert to the sound of their voices and their soothing actions.

Eye-to-eye contact. Interest in having eye contact is demonstrated again and again. Some mothers remark that once their babies have looked at them, they feel much closer to them (Klaus and others, 1982). Others have also noted this response: "I was a mother and looked into his eyes so clear; fell into his eyes, and in love" (Lang, 1972). Parents spend much time getting their babies to open their eyes and look at them. In our culture eye contact appears to have a cementing effect on the development of a beginning and trusting relationship and is an important factor in human relationships at all ages.

As newborns become functionally able to sustain eye contact, parents and child spend much time gazing at one another. We need to examine medical and nursing practices that thwart this exchange. Instillation of protective eye drops can be withheld until the infant and parents have some time together. Lights can be dimmed so that the child's eyes will open. Newborns can be held close enough to the parents' faces so that they can see the parents.

Voice. The shared response of parents and infant to each other's voice is also remarkable. Parents wait tensely for the first cry. Once it has reassured them of the baby's health, they begin comforting behaviors. As the parents talk in high-pitched voices, the infant is alerted and turns toward them.

Odor. Another behavior shared by parents and infant is responsiveness to each other's odor. Mothers comment on the smell of their babies when first born and have noted that each child has a unique odor. Infants learn rapidly to distinguish the odor of their own mother's breast milk (Stainton, 1985).

Entrainment. Newborns have been found to move in time with the structure of adult speech (Condon and Sander, 1974). They wave their arms, lift their heads, kick their legs, seemingly "dancing in tune" to their parent's voice. This means that the infant has developed *culturally determined rhythms* of speech long before using the spoken language in communicating. A *carryover* (entrainment) occurs once the child begins to talk. This shared rhythm also acts to give the parent positive feedback and to establish a positive setting for effective communication.

Biorhythmicity. The unborn child can be said to be in tune with the mother's natural rhythms, such as heartbeats. After birth one of the baby's tasks is to establish a personal rhythm. Parents can help in this process by giving consistent loving care and by using their infant's alert state to develop responsive behavior and thereby increase social interactions and opportunities for learning. The more quickly parents become competent in child-care activities, the more quickly their psychologic energy can be directed toward observing the communication cues the infant gives them.

Early contact. Research with mammals other than humans indicates that early contact between mother and offspring is important in developing future relationships. To date, no scientific evidence has demonstrated that immediate contact after birth is essential for the human parent-child relationship. According to Siegel (1982), findings from carefully controlled replicated investigations appear to document that—

Early contact, irrespective of its supplementation by extended contact, favorably affects maternal affectional behavior during the first postpartum days. The results are consistent across low and middle socioeconomic status mother-infant pairs as well as in developed and less developed countries.

He also notes that early contact has a positive effect on the duration of breast feeding. However, long-range effects of early contact have yet to be documented (Lamb, 1982).

Early close contact may *facilitate* the attachment process between parent and child. This is not to say a delay will negate this process (humans are too resilient for that), but additional psychologic energy may be needed to accomplish the same effect. For parents unable or unwilling to expend this energy the delay may affect the infant's future well-being.

In one of the first texts on newborn disorders, Budin (1907) notes that "mothers separated from their young soon lost all interest in those whom they were unable to nurse or cherish." Subsequent investigators have brought to light similar behaviors when interactions between parent and child meet interference. Bowlby's work (1958, 1969) emphasizes the attachment process between infant and mother and detailed the effects of loss of that attachment to the infant. Research in the area of child abuse documents the greater percentage of neglect, abuse, and failure to thrive among infants separated from parents for relatively long periods because of illness or preterm birth (Barnett, and others, 1970; Hefler and Kempe, 1965; Klaus and Kennell, 1982; Leifer and others, 1972).

Parents who desire but are unable to have early contact with their newborn infant *can be reassured that such contact is not essential for optimum parent-child interactions.* Otherwise, adopted infants would not form the usual affectional ties with their parents. Nor does the mode of infant-mother contact after delivery (skin-to-skin versus wrapped) appear to have any important effect. The mode of infant-mother contact after delivery is just one of many variables affecting mother-infant attachment (Curry, 1979). Nurses need to counsel mothers to allay fears that their emotional bond to their infant might be weaker because they missed early contact or because the contact was not skin to skin (Curry, 1979). The study by Klaus and co-workers (1982) has emphasized the need to respect the moments and hours after birth as a sensitive time for mother-infant interaction. Their study has been instrumental in facilitating the humanization of birthing practices. The physiologic benefits of early contact between mother and infant have been documented (Klaus and Kennell, 1982). For the mother, levels of oxytocin and prolactin rise; for the infant, sucking reflexes are employed early. The process of developing active immunity begins as the infant inhales flora from the mother's skin.

Consumer demands. The recent upsurge in demand by parents for home rather than hospital delivery is attributable in some measure to the parents' desire to share the birth process and to have immediate and continuous contact with their infant. The development in hospitals of family-centered maternity care units also reflects this demand. In December 1977 the American Medical Association adopted a policy on parent-newborn interaction that gives official medical sanction to efforts of groups identifying hospital practices that may frustrate family-oriented childbirth in the United States.

One widely used method of family-centered care is the provision of rooming-in facilities for the mother and her baby. The infant is transferred to the area from the transitional nursery after evidencing satisfactory postdelivery adjustment. The father is encouraged to visit and to participate in the care of the infant. Some hospitals have established alternative birth centers (Chapter 13). The mother is accompanied by the father during the delivery of the infant, and all three may remain together until discharged. Medical and nursing personnel are available for any care necessary for the mother and child. Other hospitals arrange for the discharge of mother and infant any time from 2 to 24 hours after delivery if the condition of the mother and that of the child warrants it. Follow-up care with nursing personnel from a health agency is part of this plan.

Until recently, in our efforts to physically safeguard mothers and babies, the obstetric client and her newborn were restricted in contact with family members. This practice served a useful purpose earlier when infection was a persistent threat to hospitalized women and their newborns. Unfortunately the practice persisted or was used inconsistently long after the need was no longer apparent. It took many years for professional workers to concede that a father could scrub, gown, and maintain good medical asepsis. As a result, much of the ritual of birth that acted as a ceremony to usher in parenthood and its many responsibilities was lost. Every child born depends for survival on the care given by concerned, loving adults. Any methods undertaken to enhance the nurturing quality of this care are worth serious consideration.

Parental Role After Childbirth

For the biologic parent the parental role does not begin at birth but rather enlarges and intensifies. Care and nurturing of the child is not initiated in the postdelivery period. Before birth the mother who carried out the dictates of health (e.g., diet, rest, exercise) for the "good of her baby," the father who supported and sheltered her, and the parents who became aware of and attached to their unborn child were functioning in the parental role.

During the postdelivery period, new tasks and responsibilities arise and old behaviors need to be modified or new ones added. Mothers' and fathers' responses to the parental role change over time and tend to follow a predictable course.

Early period. During the early period parents have to reorganize their relationship with their child. The child's needs for shelter, nourishment, protection, and socializing continue. What was accomplished through the biologic process of pregnancy now requires an array of caretaking activities. This period is characterized by intense learning and need for nurturing. The family structure and functioning as a system has been forever altered. The duration of this period varies with people but lasts about 4 weeks.

Consolidation period. The next period represents a time of drawing together and uniting the family unit. This period involves negotiations as to roles (wife-husband, mother-father, parent-child, sibling-sibling). It involves a stabilizing of tasks, a coming to terms with commitments. Parents demonstrate growing competence in child-care activities and become sensitive to the meaning of their infant's behavior. This period lasts approximately 2 months and in conjunction with the early period forms what is now termed the *fourth trimester*.

Growth period. Parents and children grow in their roles until separated by death. The most outstanding feature of the lifelong process of parent-child interaction is change, consistent evolution over time. The people involved deal not only with the present but also with the future. They need support and care in the here and now and anticipatory guidance for coming changes.

Parental tasks and responsibilities

1. Parents need to reconcile the actual child with the fantasy and dream child. This means coming to terms with the infant's physical appearance, sex, innate temperament, and physical status. If the real child differs greatly from the fantasy child, parents may delay acceptance for a period. In some instances they may never accept the child. Mothers describe the differences between the real and the imagined child as follows (Stainton, 1983a):

In the words of one mother, "I was surprised that she seemed to me to be a complete person with a personality of her own. I expected a blank tablet, a piece of clay for me to mold or a sponge for me to fill." Another, "I could not believe how determined and demanding he could be. I was going to control him and get him fitted into our life-style."

2. Parents need to establish the newborn as a person separate from themselves, that is, as someone hav-

Table 23.1
Infant Behaviors Affecting Parental Attachment

Facilitating Behaviors	Inhibiting Behaviors
Visually alert; eye-to-eye contact; tracking or following of parent's face	Sleepy; eyes closed most of the time; gaze aversion
Appealing facial appearance; randomness of body movements reflecting helplessness	Resemblance to person parent dislikes; hyperirritability or jerky body movements when touched
Smiles	Bland facial expression; infrequent smiles
Vocalization; crying only when hungry or wet	Crying for hours on end; colicky
Grasp reflex	Exaggerated motor reflex
	Feeds poorly; regurgitates; vomits often
	Resists holding and cuddling by crying, stiffening body
Anticipatory approach behaviors for feedings; sucks well; feeds easily	Inconsolable; unresponsive to parenting, caretaking tasks
Enjoys being cuddled, held	Unpredictable feeding and sleeping schedule
Easily consolable	Inability to attend to parent's face or offered stimulation
Activity and regularity somewhat predictable	Shows no preference for parents over others
Attention span sufficient to focus on parents	Unresponsive to parent's approaches
Differential crying, smiling, and vocalizing; recognizes and prefers parents	Seeks attention from any adult in room
Approaches through locomotion	Ignores parents
Clings to parent; puts arms around parent's neck	
Lifts arms to parents in greeting	

From Gerson, E.: Infant behavior in the first year of life, New York, 1973; Raven Press, Copyright © 1973. With permission.

ing many dependency needs and requiring much nurturing.

3. Parents need to become adept in the care of the infant. This includes the following:

a. Caretaking activities

b. Noting the communication cues given by the infant to indicate needs

c. Responding appropriately to the infant's needs

4. Parents need to establish reasonable evaluative criteria to use in assessing the success or failure of the care given the infant.

a. Infant responses. Parents are surprisingly sensitive to infant responses. One father told of his first attempt to give his child a kiss. At that moment the child turned her head. The father felt hurt, although he understood that the baby was totally unaware of her own movements. How the infant responds to the parental care and attention is interpreted by the parent as a comment on the quality of the care being given. These responses may include crying, weight gain or loss, or sleeping at a designated time. Continued responses deemed negative by the parent can result in alienation of parent and child to the infant's detriment (Table 23.1).

b. Competence in caretaking activities. Self-esteem grows with competence. Mothers of premature infants have noted that the adept handling of their infants by nurses was recognized as evidence of care yet at the same time was resented. It made *their* efforts to sustain their child appear inadequate. Mothers who have supplied breast milk for their infant comment that this makes them feel they are contributing in a unique way to the welfare of their child.

c. Opinion of significant others. Criticism, real or imagined, of new parents' ability to provide adequate physical care, nutrition, or social stimulation for their infant can prove devastating. These "critics" may need constructive direction. Assistance, including advice by husbands, wives, mothers, mothers-in-law, and professional workers, can be seen as supportive. Conversely, it can be seen as an indication of how inept these persons have judged the new parent to be.

5. Parents must establish a place for the newborn within the family group. Whether the infant is the first born or last born, all family members must adjust their roles to accommodate the newcomer. An only child needs support to accept a rival to parental affections. An older child needs support when losing a favored position. The parents are expected to negotiate these changes.

6. Parents need to establish the primacy of their adult relationships to maintain the family as a group. Since this includes reorganizing many roles, for example, sexual roles, child-care roles, career roles, and community roles, time and energy must be provided for this vital task.

Maternal adjustment. Three phases are discernible as the mother makes an adjustment to her version of the parental role. These phases are characterized by dependent behavior, dependent-independent behavior, and interdependent behavior.

Dependent phase. During the first 1 to 2 days after delivery, the mother's dependency needs predominate. To the extent that these needs are met by others, the mother is able to divert her psychologic energy to her child rather than to herself. She needs "mothering" to "mother." Rubin (1961) has aptly described these few days as the "taking-in phase": a time when nurturing and protective care are required by the new mother.

For a few days following birth, mature and apparently healthy women appear to suspend involvement in everyday responsibilities. They rely on others to respond to their needs for comfort, rest, nourishment, and closeness to their families and newborn.

This phase is a time of great excitement, and most parents are extremely talkative. They need to verbalize their experience of pregnancy and birth. Focusing on, analyzing, and accepting these experiences help the parents move on to the next phase. Some parents are able to use the staff or other mothers as an "audience." Others are unable to do this and need the opportunity to be with family or friends.

Since anxiety and preoccupation with her new role often narrow a mother's perceptual field, information may have to be repeated. The new mother may require reminders to rest, or conversely, to ambulate enough to promote recovery. Ward routine does not necessarily loom large in the new mother's order of priorities; showers are taken when examinations are scheduled, and telephone conversations preclude "being ready" for the baby. Regulations seem cumbersome, and sometimes mothers and their families have difficulty accepting rules that interfere with their needs to share reactions about their child.

Physical discomfort arising from an episiotomy, sore nipples, hemorrhoids, afterpains, and occasionally a sprained coccygeal joint can interfere with the mother's need for rest and relaxation. The judicious use of comfort measures and medication depends on the nurse. Many women hesitate to ask for medication, believing that any pain they experience is normal and to be expected; few have a knowledge of the use of heat or cold to relieve local pain.

Dependent-independent phase. If the mother has received adequate nurturing in the first few days, by the third day her desire for independent action reasserts itself. She alternates between a need for extensive nurturing and acceptance by others and the desire "to take charge" once again. She responds enthusiastically to opportunities to learn and practice the care of the baby or, if she is an accomplished mother, to carry out or direct this care.

The reality of parenthood must be experienced to be understood fully on a personal level regardless of the desire for a baby and the amount of prenatal preparation undertaken. One young mother expressed it as follows (Lang, 1972):

But then in my second week, as my strength began to return, my energies began to focus on the overwhelming task of motherhood that stood before me. And I realized then that I faced that task alone. Not that my husband wouldn't stand by me, not that my friends would not share experiences with me, but I stood alone with the realization that only I could be the child's mother.

In the period of 6 to 8 weeks after delivery the mastery of the tasks of parenthood are crucial. Realistic expectations facilitate the subsequent functioning of the family as a unit.

Some women adjust with considerable difficulty to the isolation of themselves with their babies and resent the endless coping with home and child-care responsibilities. The mothers who appear to need additional supportive counseling include:

1. Primiparas inexperienced in child care
2. Women whose careers had provided outside stimulation
3. Women who lack friends or family members with whom to share delights and concerns.

Depressive states are not uncommon during this phase. Feelings of extreme vulnerability may arise from a number of factors. Psychologically the mother may be overwhelmed by the actuality of parental responsibilities. She may feel deprived of the pregnant state, with its concomitant supportive care of family members and friends. Some mothers regret the loss of the mother-unborn child relationship and mourn its passing. Still others experience a letdown feeling when labor and birth are complete. They had girded themselves for an elemental experience, a walk "through the shadows," and now it is safely over.

Once immediate tasks and adjustments have been undertaken and brought under control, a plateau is reached. At this time the life-long effects of the parents' new responsibilities come into focus. Some parents experience a feeling of being trapped and wonder what life is all about.

Occasionally the mother becomes increasingly fatigued during the last month of pregnancy, when sleep is interrupted by shortness of breath and urinary frequency. Leg cramps, or inability to lie in a comfortable position can disturb sleep. Fatigue following delivery is compounded by around-the-clock demands of the new baby and can accentuate the feelings of depression. It has been suggested that a lowered level of circulating glucocorticoids or a condition of subclinical hypothyroidism may exist during the puerperium. This physiologic state could explain some minor degrees of depression.

Depressive reactions are not necessarily expressed verbally. A depressive state signified by typical behaviors (withdrawal, loss of interest in surroundings, and crying) can be manifested.

It is hoped that toward the end of the dependent-independent phase the tasks and adjustments of daily routine will begin to follow a pattern. The baby begins to take an established position in the family. Many of the feeding problems, whether related to breast feeding or bottle feeding, have been largely resolved. The mother's physical energy and strength return; the "taking-hold phase" (Rubin, 1961) is ending. By the fifth week the infant has been examined by the physician and the mother also has been examined or has made arrangements for a checkup. It is time to move on the the next phase of adjustment.

Interdependent phase. In this phase interdependent behavior reasserts itself, and the mother and her family move forward as a system with interacting members. The relationship of husband and wife, although altered by the introduction of a child, resumes many of its former characteristics. A primary need is to establish a lifestyle that includes but in some respects excludes the child. Husband and wife must share interest and activities that are adult in scope.

Most couples begin intercourse by the third or fourth week after the child is born; some begin earlier, as soon as it can be accomplished without discomfort for the woman. Sexual intimacy increases the man-woman aspect of the family, and the adult pair shares a closeness denied to other family members. Many new fathers speak of the alienation experienced when they observe the intimate mother-child relationship, and some are frank in expressing feelings of jealousy toward the interloper. The resumption of the marital relationship seems to bring the parents' relationship back into focus.

The interdependent phase is often one of stress for the parental pair. Career patterns of men from their 20s through their 40s show intense activity centering around advancement in their profession or job. This often necessitates long hours away from the home or moving from one locality to another. Meanwhile the women are engrossed in home activities directed toward the care of the young children. Interests and needs diverge, and there may be a gradual estrangement, which is glossed over for the time being because of the individual needs of each. A special effort must be undertaken to strengthen the adult-adult relationship as a basis for the family unit.

Paternal adjustment. During the last decade a growing interest in the relationship of the father and

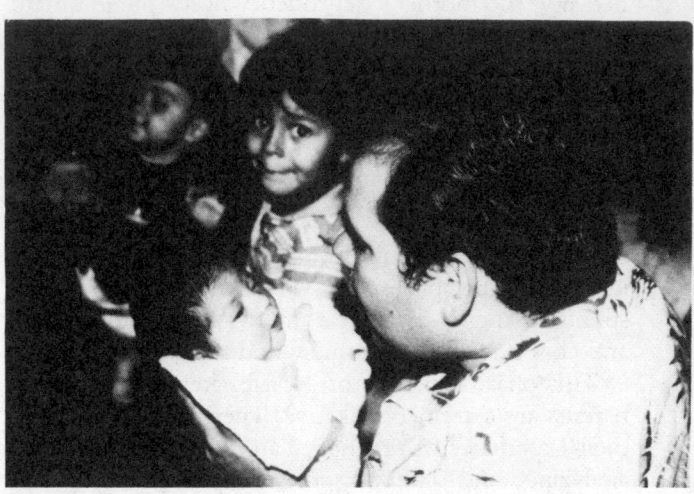

Fig. 23.4
Father and new baby make eye contact. (Courtesy Marjorie Pyle, RNC, Lifecircle, Costa Mesa, California.)

the child has become evident. It is now recognized that the mother-child relationship does not exist in a vacuum but within the context of the family system. Parent's attitudes toward and expectations of one another's parental behavior affects the behavior of each dyad. In our culture the newborn has been found to have a powerful impact on the father. Fathers have demonstrated intense involvement with their babies (Fig. 23.4). Greenberg and Morris (1976) named the father's absorption, preoccupation, and interest in the infant *engrossment*. These researchers delineate a number of characteristics of engrossment. Some of the sensual responses relating to touch and eye-to-eye contact are the same as discussed earlier. The father's keen awareness of features both unique and similar to himself is another characteristic related to the father's need to claim the infant. An outstanding response is one of *strong attraction* to the newborn. Much time is spent "communicating" with the infant and taking delight in the infant's response to the father. Fathers feel a sense of increased self-esteem, a sense of being "proud, bigger, more mature, and older" after seeing their baby for the first time. Studies have shown a difference in father-infant relationships. Fathers tend to take the lead in initiating play and other social situations. Mothers tend to take the lead in caretaking activities (Clarke-Stewart, 1978). The subtle and more overt differences in stimulation from two sources, mother and father, provide a wider social experience for the child. In addition the child has improved chances of developing at least one good parenting relationship (Kunst-Wilson and Cronenwett, 1981).

Fig. 23.5
Mother works to alert her daughter, 6 hours old. **A,** Infant is quiet and alert. **B,** Mother begins talking to daughter. Note frown of concentration. **C,** Infant responds, opens mouth like her mother. **D,** Infant gazes at her mother. **E,** Infant waves hand, opens mouth. **F,** Infant glances away, resting. Hand relaxes. (Courtesy Colleen Stainton.)

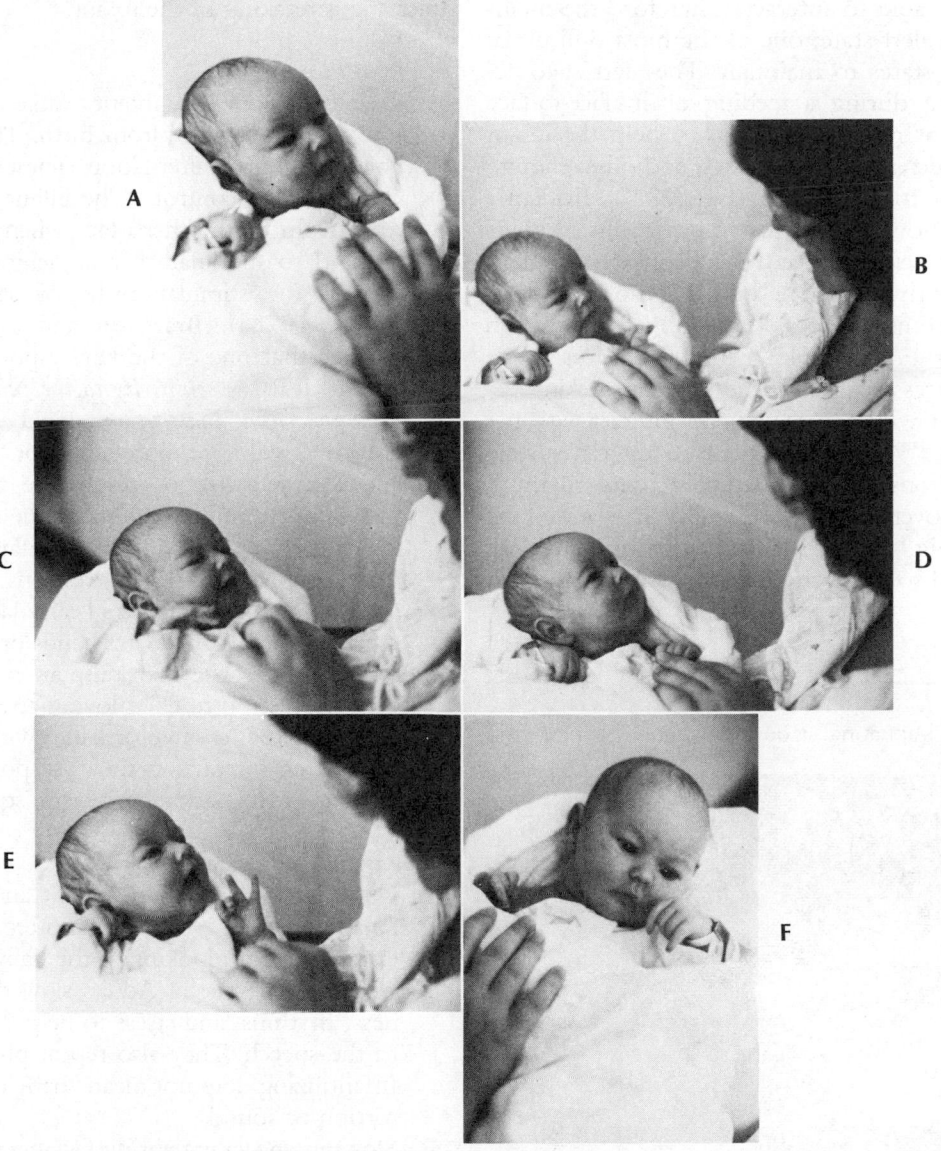

Much has still to be learned about the relationships between fathers and their offspring. The mother's biologic relationship with the child can be a basis for predicting behaviors in the mother-child relationship. But the knowledge that a man is the father of a child gives us no clues as to his relationships or behaviors with the child.

There is no evidence as yet as to what effect individual styles have on the father's actual experience with this child. Despite their active involvement in the perinatal period, fathers tend to gravitate toward more traditional roles as they become more involved in job-related activities and less in child-care activities. However, if the father does involve himself in caretaking, he responds much as the mother in talking to the infant (Field, 1978a).

Infant-parent adjustment. The infant-parent interaction is characterized by a "set of rhythms, behavioral repertoires, and responsivity or response styles" (Field, 1978a). These traits are unique to each partner. Interactions can be facilitated in any of three ways: (1) modulation of rhythm, (2) modification of behavioral repertoires, and (3) mutual responsivity.

Rhythm. To modulate the rhythm, both parent and infant must be able to interact. Therefore the infant must be in the alert state, one of the most difficult of the sleep-wake states to maintain. The alert state occurs most often during a feeding or in face-to-face play. The parent must work hard to help the infant maintain the alert state long enough and often enough for interactions to take place (Fig. 23.5). Evidently mothers learn how to do this: multiparous mothers show particular sensitivity and responsiveness to their infant's feeding rhythms. The mother who is sensitive to feeding rhythms reserves stimulation for pauses in sucking activity. For example, the mother learns not to talk or smile excessively while the infant is sucking because the infant will stop feeding to interact with her (Field, 1978b). With maturity the infant can sustain longer interactions by modulating activity rhythms, that is, limb movement, sucking, gaze alternation, and habituation (Fig. 23.6). "In the interim, the adult learns to attend to these rhythms, modulate his or her

own rhythms, and thereby facilitate a rhythmical turn-taking interaction" (Field, 1978a).

Repertoires. Both contributors to the infant-parent interaction have a repertoire of behaviors they can use to facilitate interactions. Fathers and mothers engage in these behaviors depending on the amount of contact and caretaking of the infant.

Infant's repertoire

1. Gaze behaviors. The infant is able to focus and follow the human face from birth. The infant is also able to use gaze alternation. These abilities are under voluntary control. "The infant appears to look away from the mother's face when under- or over-aroused to modulate his or her arousal level and process the stimulation he or she is receiving" (Field, 1978a). Brazelton and associates (1974) suggest that one of the key responses for the parents to learn is *sensitivity to the infant's capacity for attention and inattention.* Field (1978b) states, "Mothers who are more active or 'overstimulating' and less sensitive or responsive to their infant's pauses or turning away during the conversation are less able to elicit or hold their infants' gaze."
2. Vocalizing and facial expressions. Body gestures form a part of the infant's "early language." Babies greet parents with waving hands or with a reaching out of hands. They can raise an eyebrow or soften their expression to elicit loving attention. They can be stimulated to smile or laugh with game playing. To end an interaction they use pouting or crying, arching of the back, and general squirming.

Parents' repertoire

1. Constant looking at the infant and noting the infant's behavior. New parents often remark they are exhausted from looking at the baby and smiling.
2. Infantilizing speech. Adults slow the tempo, loudness, rhythms, and stress to help the infant "listen" to the speech. They also repeat phrases frequently. Infantilizing does not mean "baby talk" with its distortion of sounds.
3. Slowing and exaggerating facial expressions.
4. Game playing with the infant. "Peek-a-boo" is an example.
5. Imitating the infant's behaviors. For instance, if the baby frowns, the adult frowns.

Responsivity. Contingent responses that occur within a specific time and are similar in form to a stimulus behavior. They elicit a feeling in the person originating the behavior of having an influence on the interaction. In other words, they act as positive feedback. Adults view infant behaviors such as smiling, cooing, and sustained eye contact as contingent re-

Fig. 23.6
A, Alerting. **B,** Habituating. (Courtesy Colleen Stainton.)

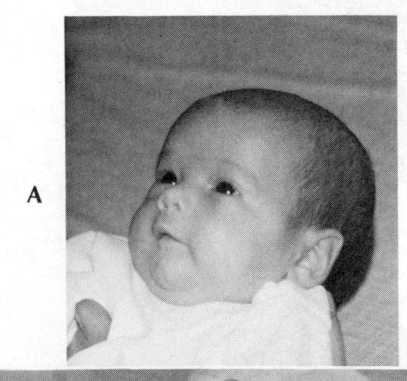

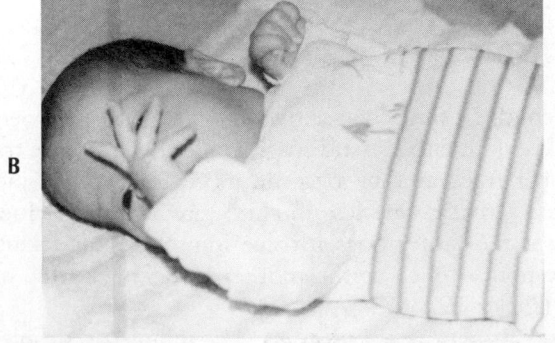

sponses. The adults are encouraged to continue the same game when the infant responds in such a way. These responses act as rewards to the initiator. When the adult imitates the infant, the infant appears to enjoy the responses. The infant in turn imitates behaviors of adults soon after birth. The parent shows progression in presenting behaviors for the baby to imitate; for example, in early interactions the parent will grimace rather than laugh, which is in keeping with the infant's developmental level. Such "turnabout" behaviors sustain interactions and promote harmony in the relationship.

Factors influencing parental responses

Physical condition of the mother. Women who have experienced a long and difficult labor often are too exhausted to respond other than in a perfunctory way to the newborn. They may welcome the attention of others and be grateful that the infant is healthy, but their primary need centers on recovery from a physical and emotional ordeal.

Physical condition of the infant. Infants born at risk as a result of either fetal or maternal disabilities usually are transferred to the intensive care nursery as quickly as possible. Concerns for their need for intensive medical and nursing care supersede concerns about providing close contact between the infant and the mother or father. Opportunities to be with the infant in the intensive care nursery, to touch or hold him if at all possible, and to receive reports of the infant's progress must be part of the nursing plan.

Parental expectations. Some parents are startled by the appearance of the infant—size, color, molding of the head, or bowed appearance of the legs (Chapter 19). Many parents have never seen or had contact with a newborn infant and find themselves disturbed by their feelings. Mothers and fathers may interpret the physical characteristics that are normal in all newborns as physical or mental deficiencies. Many fathers have commented that they thought the odd shape of the child's head (molding) meant the child would be mentally retarded.

Disappointment over the sex of the infant can take time to resolve. The mother or father may be able to give adequate physical mothering but may find it difficult to be sincerely involved with the infant until these feelings have been resolved. As one mother remarked:

■ I really wanted a boy. I know it is silly and irrational, but when they said, "She's a lovely little girl," I was so disappointed and angry—yes, angry—I could hardly look at her. Oh, I looked after her okay, her feedings and baths and things, but I couldn't feel excited. To tell the truth, I felt like a monster not liking my child. Then one day she was lying there and she turned her head and looked right at me. I felt a flooding of love for her come over me, and we looked at each other a long time. It's okay now. I wouldn't change her for all the boys in the world.

Nursing care plans need to include time for explanations about the child's appearance. Nurses need to provide opportunities for parents to discuss their lack of motherly feelings without fear of censure or ridicule. Often the expression of doubts and concerns provides relief and makes it easier for parents to accept help with such feelings.

Parenthood after 30 years. Maternal age has a definite effect on pregnancy outcome. The fetus and the mother are at highest risk when the mother is at either extreme of age and parity, although each age group has predominant problems (Table 23.2). The following discussion relates to the older client (over 30 years). Adolescent clients, both mother and father, are discussed in Chapter 30.

Two groups of older parents are now discernible in the population of women having a child late in their childbearing years. One group is made up of multiparous women who have many children or who have a child during the menopausal period. The other group of older parents includes relative newcomers to maternity care. These are persons who have deliberately delayed childbearing until their late 20s or early 30s.

The first group may have never used contraceptives either because of personal choice or lack of knowledge concerning contraceptives. Others may have used contraception successfully during the childbearing years. As menopause approaches they may cease to menstruate regularly, stop using contraception, and consequently become pregnant. Even after menstruation ceases, ovulation may continue for as long as a year. Therefore contraceptive techniques must be continued for this time. Hogan (1979) relates the response of older women to pregnancy. The older woman experiences a displaced feeling as pregnancy alienates her from her peer group and her age interferes with close associations with young mothers. Because the incidence of complicating conditions such as hypertension, preeclampsia-eclampsia, and hemorrhage increases in the mother of 40 years of age or older, many women do not view the pregnancy and childbirth as natural phenomena.

For some persons, amniotic fluid analysis or ultrasonography (Chapter 25) can allay anxiety concerning giving birth to an infant with a defect. Abortion is an option for mothers who learn they are carrying a fetus

Table 23.2
Age-related Pregnancy Problems

Age (years)	Maternal Problems	Fetal Problems
Less than 15	Nonsubstantial physical risk if care and nutrition are adequate, if there are no sexually transmitted diseases, and if life-style does not include harmful habits such as drugs. Psychosocial risk high	Highest incidence of growth retardation, immature-premature birth, perinatal morbidity and mortality
16–19	Ideal biologic time for childbearing if care and nutrition are adequate and life-style does not include harmful habits such as drugs. Psychosocial risk high	Healthy infants if prenatal care has been adequate and "mothering" sufficient
20–35	Few problems	Lowest perinatal morbidity and mortality Low-birth-weight newborns after excessive smoking or alcohol use Dizygous twins
35–40	Not substantial risk if care and nutrition are adequate Age-related medical disorders, e.g., diabetes mellitus, class E; infertility	More miscarriages Increased frequency of fetal anomalies and genetic disabilities
40–50	Cardiovascular and other medical-surgical disorders Diabetes mellitus, class F Uterine or ovarian neoplasms Premature separation of placenta Rupture of uterus Postdelivery hemorrhage	Higher perinatal morbidity and mortality Increased frequency of Down's syndrome and other congenital anomalies (e.g., hydrocephalus, trisomy, Klinefelter's syndrome)

with a defect. The percentage of older mothers who choose to terminate the pregnancy by abortion is relatively high. Many of these women, who had assumed they would never have to make such a choice, report depression.

Including the family in preparation for the birth is important. Because the other children in the family may be teenagers, women often welcome the professional person's support and suggestions concerning how to best involve them. Measures designed to assist the mother in regaining strength and muscle tone (e.g., prenatal and postdelivery exercises) are emphasized. Some older mothers may find that the care of the new infant exhausts their physical capabilities. If economic and social conditions are also adverse, they may neglect the child. Others welcome the unexpected infant as evidence of a maternal (and paternal) role still to be played. Because older siblings often assume aspects of the parental role, the child develops in a multiparent household.

The second group choose parenthood as opposed to the alternative, a child-free life-style. They often are successfully established in a career and a life-style with a partner that includes time for self-attention, establishment of a home with accumulated possessions, and freedom for travel. When questioned as to why they chose pregnancy late in life, many reply, "because time is running out." Sheehy (1977) points out that age 35 brings a biologic boundary into view. Deutch (1945) refers to the late desire for a child as a biologic "clos-

ing of the gates." Parents-to-be who belong to this emerging group are faced with having to resolve an important choice at a life stage when childbearing has increasing risks.

Women 35 years and older are at increased risk for diseases that complicate middle age, such as diabetes, class E. Some have difficulty in becoming pregnant, because of infertility. Cesarean deliveries are used more frequently in this age group. However, recent studies indicate that for those women who are in good physical health and who are able to obtain prenatal care and good nutrition, the physical risks of pregnancy may be no greater than those of younger women. The fetus is in increased jeopardy from congenital anomalies and genetic disabilities (Kirz, 1986).

The dilemma of choice includes recognition that being a parent will have both positive and negative consequences. Couples need to discuss the consequences of childbearing and child rearing before committing themselves to a lifelong venture. Partners in this group seem to share the preparation for parenthood, the planning for a family-centered birth, and the desire to be loving and competent parents. The reality of child care may prove difficult for these parents. The mother who is accustomed to the stimulation of and contact with other adults may find the isolation with her infant difficult to accept. Anger and resentment toward the father (or infant) can result. In the early infancy period this group needs careful follow-up and supportive care, including opportunities to discuss alternative parenting approaches. The nurse needs to be aware of community resources developed to meet the needs of this group.*

Social and economic conditions. Parents whose economic condition is made worse with the birth of each child and who are unable to use an acceptable method of family planning may find childbirth compounded by concern for their own health and a sense of helplessness. Mothers who are alone, deserted by husband, family, and friends, or who are in an untenable economic state may view the birth of the child with dread. The difficulties in which they find themselves may overcome any desire for mothering the infant (Chapter 28).

Nursing measures designed to help persons in these circumstances involve social and economic community agencies as well as health agencies. Satisfactory outcomes of such problems often require long-term commitments from both the woman or couple and the community. Adequate situational supports need to be instituted in the prenatal period.

Interference with personal aspirations. For some women parenthood interferes with or curtails their plans for personal freedom or advancement in their career. Resentment concerning their loss may not have been resolved during the prenatal period. If this resentment is not resolved, it will spill over into caretaking activities and may result in indifference and neglect. Or, conversely, it may result in oversolicitousness and the setting of impossibly high standards by the mother for her behavior or the child's performance (Shainess, 1970).

Nursing intervention includes providing opportunities for parents (1) to vent their feelings freely to an objective listener; (2) to discuss measures to permit personal growth of the parent, for example, by part-time employment, volunteer work, and use of agencies that provide babysitting care or mother substitutes during parents' vacations; and (3) to learn about the care of the child.

Sensory impairment. In the early dialogue between parent and child, all senses—sight, hearing, touch, taste, and smell—are used by both to initiate and sustain the attachment process. A parent who is deprived of one of the senses needs to develop an enriched use of the remaining sensory sources.

Blindness. Although mothers who are blind need the

presence as well as the support of another responsible person, they can become adept in some child-care activities, as the following report indicates:

■ We had always planned to have a child. My family and Dick's both wanted us to have the happiness of children and were willing to help us with the baby care. First I bathed and changed a doll; then I practiced caring for my sister's baby. I would feel in all the creases with my finger to see if they were clean and dry. We used disposable diapers that do not need pins. My mother made baby clothes with fastenings of press cloth (Velcro) so I would not have to fiddle with buttons. I feel really confident now. I know I can't do everything for her, but I can do enough to feel like a "mother," and I know she will have all the love she needs.

One of the major difficulties blind mothers experience is the skepticism, overt or covert, of the professional worker. Blind persons sense a reluctance on the part of others to concede that they have a right to be parents. One blind mother-to-be noted that the best approach by the nurse is for the nurse to assess the mother's capabilities. From that basis the nurse can make plans to assist the woman (i.e., the same as for a sighted mother). Another mother talked about the shyness, fear, or reluctance she sensed in nurses that resulted in her being left alone or being involved in awkward conversations:

■ I took it upon myself to put the nurses at ease. I was forthright about my condition and asked for specific help and supervision of my baby care efforts. Don't forget, I've had some 25 years' experience in dealing with the sighted public. I have considerable skill now in being blind.

Another mother expressed how sensitive the blind can become to other sensory output. She remarked that she could tell when her infant was facing her because she could feel his breath on her face.

Three mothers who are blind volunteered the following suggestions for providing care for the needs of women such as themselves during childbearing. The first mother noted that "sometimes they [health care providers] act like they're afraid they're going to catch our blindness" (example of avoidance). She offered the following suggestions:

1. Clients who are blind need verbal teaching from health care providers because maternity information is not accessible to blind people.
2. Clients need an orientation to the hospital room that allows the client to move about the room in-

---

*For example, Parenthood after Thirty is a project sponsored by the Foundation for Comprehensive Health Services and funded by grant no. 80-63575 from the Office of Family Planning, State of California Department of Health Services. For further information contact Parenthood after Thirty, 451 Vermont, Berkeley, CA. 94704 (415) 524-6635 (Lucy Scott, Ph.D., Project Director).

dependently. For example, "Go to the left of the bed and trail the wall until you feel the first door. That is the bathroom."

3. Clients need explanations of routines.
4. Clients need opportunities to feel devices (e.g., monitors, pelvic models) and to hear descriptions of the devices.
5. Clients need "a chance to ask questions!"
6. Clients need the opportunity to hold and touch their baby after delivery. "When they put him on my stomach he was warm; I could feel his heart going. That gave me the moment to see that he was really OK," and "Blind fathers like to cut cords, too."
7. Nurses need to demonstrate baby care by touch and to follow with, "Now let me see you do it."
8. Nurses need to give instructions such as "I'm going to give you the baby. The head is on the left side."

The second mother made the following observations:

■ We tend to respond as we're treated, as everyone does. If treated as inadequate, you can tend to overcompensate to try to prove you're adequate, or you can withdraw. People need to be recognized as people. I always tell people I'm not a blind person, I'm a person who happens to be blind. If you could take that one message to people, I know I shared something worthwhile.

I'm not saying blindness doesn't have its problems and adjustments, because it does. But I tend to think we do overemphasize blindness sometimes, especially when it comes to childbirth, pregnancy, and the basic delivery.

I can't think of a time when my hospital care wasn't good. People introduced themselves and said what they were about to do. I was assertive; I got what I wanted. I told the doctor during my prenatal visits about what kind of delivery I wanted. During delivery I put my hands down and felt the head of my child.

Her suggestion to promote attachment was to make certain the mother can "feel the head and face. Comb the hair with your fingers, kiss the cheeks. Breast feed right away if the baby wants to. Ask the nurse for help with positioning."

The third mother noted that "everyone is so visually oriented they can't see beyond their eyes. They don't think anything can be done without eyes." Her suggestions follow:
1. "Treat us like human beings. That's what we are!"
2. "Relate verbally. Explain! Don't say 'Do it like this' and assume we know what you're doing over there."

3. "Put bells on the baby's shoes to help keep track of them."
4. "Pull a stroller instead of pushing it."

Eye-to-eye contact is considered important in our culture. With a parent who is blind, this critical component in the parent-child attachment process is obviously missing. However, since the mother has no experience in using this strategy to promote relationships, she cannot be said to miss it. The infant will need other sensory input from the blind mother. Perhaps an infant looking into the eyes of a mother who is blind is not conscious that the eyes are unseeing. Other persons in the newborn's environment can participate in active eye-to-eye contact to supply this lack. Another problem may arise if the parent who is blind has an impassive facial expression. One observer noticed an infant making repeated attempts to engage in face play with his mother, who was blind. After repeated failure of his efforts, he abandoned the behavior with his mother and intensified it with his father. This problem might be overcome by the person's learning to accompany talking and cooing to the infant with head nodding and smiling.

Deafness. The mother who has a hearing impairment faces another set of problems, particularly if the deafness dates from birth or early childhood. About 2 of every 1000 Americans are deaf. An accepted definition for the deaf is persons who cannot hear or understand the spoken word with or without a hearing aid. The mother and her partner are likely to have established an independent household. A number of devices that transform sound into light flashes are now marketed.* The infant's room can be fitted with such a device to permit immediate detection of crying. Even if the parents are not speech trained, their vocalizing can serve as both stimulus and response to the infant's early vocalizing. Parents can provide additional vocal training by use of records and television so that from birth onward the child is aware of the full range of the human voice. Sign language is acquired readily by the young child, and the first sign used is as varied as the first word. One mother reported her child first signed "good boy," and another reported "candy" as her child's first effort.

Baranowski (1983) described childbirth education classes for expectant deaf parents: "The students were attentive, asked questions, and readily participated in discussions. Their regular attendance indicated that they were interested in the classes."

Section 504 of the Rehabilitation Act of 1973 re-

---

*A price list for the Crying Light and other useful visual alarms can be obtained from Applied Communication Corp., P.O. Box 555, Belmont, CA 94002.

quires that hospitals and other institutions receiving funds from the U.S. Department of Health and Human Services use various communication techniques and resources with the deaf, including staff members who are proficient in sign language. The nurse who is bilingual has an advantage in providing care for clients. Magilvy and co-workers (1979) point out that sign language is as complex as any spoken language and that deaf persons are linguistically and cognitively competent.

· · ·

Much more research in the areas of sensory impairment and the parent-child attachment process needs to be undertaken.*

Sibling Adjustment

Introduction of the infant into a family with one or more children may pose problems for the parents. They are faced with the task of caring for a new child while not neglecting the others. Parents need to distribute their attention in a manner that they consider fair.

Older children have to assume new positions within the family hierarchy. The older child's goal is to maintain a leading position. The child who is next in birth order to the infant has to gain a superior position over the newcomer (Kreppner and others, 1982). As the infant develops and begins to assert himself or herself, the older child works toward dominance. "He or she takes away toys and other objects the younger child is grasping for, thereby demonstrating that he or she has control over the situation. The older child also intervenes more openly when parents are interacting with the younger child" (Kreppner and others, 1982). One 3-year-old child encouraged his mother to put the new baby "out with the garbage because we've seen enough of her."

Regression to an infantile level of behavior may be seen in some children. They may revert to bed-wetting, whining, or refusal to feed themselves. An older child who is still young wavers between thinking "I'm big now" and thinking "I'm still a baby, so look after me." Jealous reactions are to be expected once the initial excitement of having a new baby in the home is over, since the baby absorbs the time and attention of the important persons in the other children's lives.

Parents, especially mothers, spend much time and

energy promoting sibling acceptance of a new baby. Other children are involved actively in preparation for the infant, and involvement intensifies after the birth of the child. Mother and father face a number of tasks related to sibling adjustment. The tasks include the following:

1. Making the older child feel loved and wanted.
2. Managing guilt arising from feelings that older children are being deprived of parental time and attention.
3. Developing feelings of confidence in her or his ability to nurture more than one child.
4. Adjusting time and space to accommodate the new baby.
5. Monitoring behavior of older children toward the more vulnerable infant and diverting aggressive behavior.

The new parent can learn many innovative techniques by listening to other parents describe their efforts to ease the older siblings' acceptance of the new child. Walz and Rich (1983) have described a number of creative parental interventions.

1. A mother took her firstborn on a tour of her hospital room and pointed out similarities to the first child. "This is the same room I was in with you, and I think the baby is in the same cot that you were in."
2. The newborn was described as a "special gift" for the older child.
3. The children were in the group (grandparents, sister) who were *first* to see the newborn.
4. Time was planned for both children. A mother remarked, "When I get home, I'll arrange my day so that I can have the baby's care done in the morning while Sam (first child) is at school. Maybe the baby will sleep part of the afternoon and I can spend some time with Sam." Another mother said, "When I'm breastfeeding I'll have one arm for the baby and one arm for my daughter (first child)."

Fathers were enlisted as the main support for mothers reallocating time to include older children. "My husband will take care of Becca (first child) and I will have the baby, because he can do things with Becca she will enjoy. I will give the baby things my husband can't." Other husbands were expected to help with the care of the newborn to permit the mother to spend more time with the older child. One mother said, "My husband took his vacation now. This will give me time to spend with my daughter (first child). I'll take her on the new swings we bought her and I'll read to her."

Many parents related difficulties with siblings when they are devoting attention to feeding the infant, either by breast or bottle. The other children seem to sense the closeness of the mother and child in this act

*We welcome information in this area. Address correspondence to I.M. Bobak, Department of Nursing, San Francisco State University, 1600 Holloway Ave., San Francisco, CA 94132.

Fig. 23.7
Older sister helps nurse assess new baby. (Courtesy Marjorie Pyle, RNC, Lifecircle, Costa Mesa, California.)

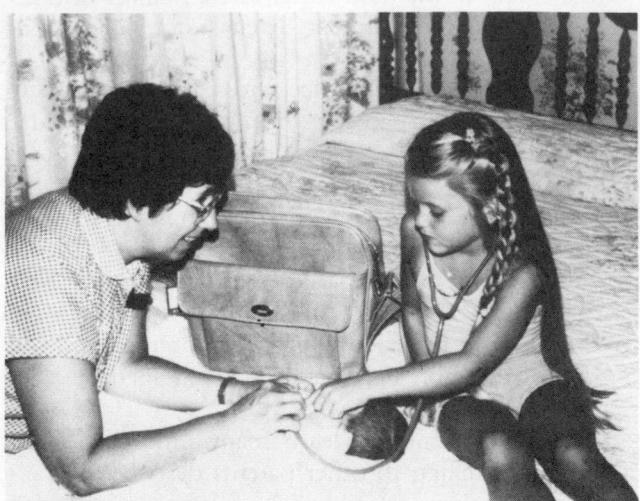

Fig. 23.8
Sister shares care of her new brother with her dolls. (Courtesy Marjorie Pyle, RNC, Lifecircle, Costa Mesa, California.)

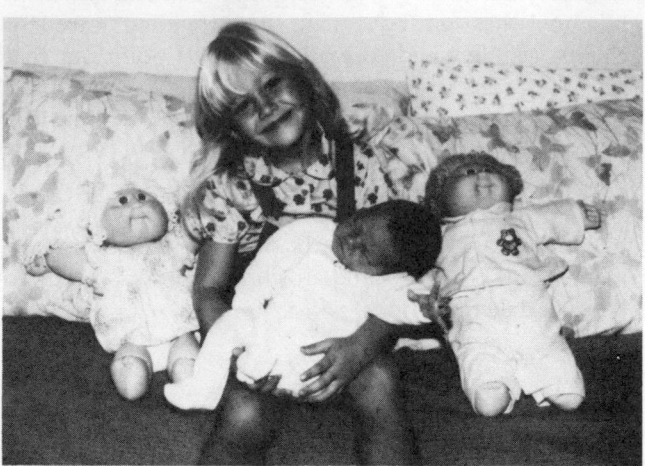

and resent it. To counter these reactions some mothers have let the older children drink from a bottle or breast, too. The tediousness and effort needed to obtain milk by this method often rapidly discourage them.

Both girls and boys seem to enjoy helping in the care of the baby or a substitute baby (doll) (Fig. 23.7). One mother reports that her young son routinely "breast fed" his doll while she breast fed the new baby. They had conversations at this time. She believed that sharing this experience seemed to give her son pride in his adult behavior of drinking from a cup. Children 6 years or older pose less of a problem than younger children. They have more significant others to turn to. They often assume "second parent" roles and boast about the new baby to friends and teachers (Fig. 23.8).

Another difficulty arises when well-meaning relatives or friends concentrate on the new baby to the exclusion of the older children. Thoughtful adults often bring gifts to the older children and shower attention on them as well as paying attention to the baby.

Many hospitals permit younger children to visit the mother and newborn. The early visits tend to reduce the older children's feelings of being deserted by the mother and help bring about faster integration of the neonate into the family. Studies (Umphenour, 1980; Kowba and others, 1985; and Wranesh, 1982) have demonstrated that healthy newborns who have direct sibling contact are not at risk for exposure to pathogenic organisms. Therefore separation of neonates and older siblings does not appear to be warranted.

The initial adjustment of older children to a newborn takes time. Parents will be faced with readjustments as the newborn matures and develops ability for more independent social and physical interactions (Kreppner and others, 1982). To expect a young child to accept and love a rival for the parents' affection assumes a too-mature response. Sibling love grows as does other love, that is, by being with another person and sharing experiences.

Grandparent Adjustment

The amount of involvement of grandparents in the care of the newborn depends on many factors, for example, willingness of the grandparents to become involved, proximity of the grandparents, and ethnic and cultural expectations of the role grandparents play (Grosso, 1981).

The woman's mother is an important model for childrearing practices (Rubin, 1975). She acts as a source of knowledge and as a support person (Fig. 23.9). Grandchildren are tangible evidence of continuity, of immortality. Often grandparents comment that the presence of grandchildren helps relieve loneliness and boredom.

Grandparents and the adult child. "There are many ways to encourage new parents to include the grandparents, enriching their child's life and benefiting from the extended family themselves" (Olson, 1981). As parents are assisted in working through differing opinions and unresolved conflicts (e.g., dependency,

Fig. 23.9
Grandmother holds new baby in sunlight to reduce bilirubin level. Older sibling looks on. (Courtesy Marjorie Pyle, RNC, Lifecircle, Costa Mesa, California.)

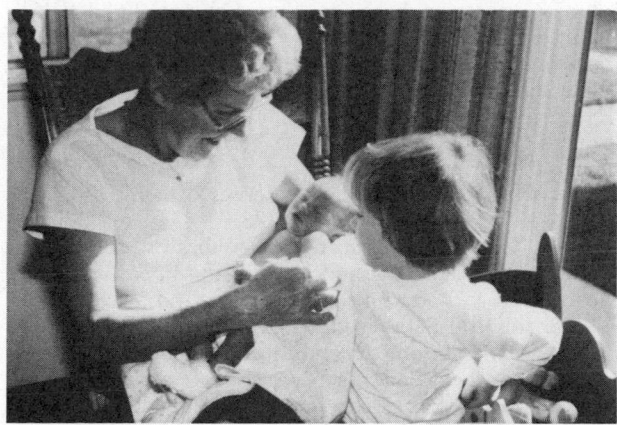

control) between themselves and their parents, they can move toward mastery of the developmental tasks of adulthood. Grandparental support can be a stabilizing influence for families undergoing developmental crises such as childbearing and new parenthood (Newell, 1984). Grandparents can foster the learning of parental skills and preserve tradition. One simple technique to help people span the generation gap is through a printed "letter to new parents." The letter can be included in prenatal kits distributed in childbirth preparation classes and can be made available to all family members on the postpartum unit (Olson, 1981). In the letter, feelings and needs of grandparents and parents are verbalized and foster open discussion between the generations.

Grandparents and the grandchild. "There are certain things that a grandmammy and granddaddy can do for a child that no one else can. It's sort of like stardust—the relationship between grandparents and children" (Haley, 1977). Grandparents who are free to love the grandchild crazily, blindly, lavishly, and without reservation (LeShan, 1975) can have a significant positive influence on the child's life. Praise and encouragement from a significant person fosters the development of a positive self-image and a sense of being worthy. Long-range effects include future relationships with others and preparation for the developmental tasks of adulthood: "With the removal of grandparents . . . from the world in which the child is reared, the child's experience of the future is shortened by a generation and his links to the past are weakened" (Mead, 1970).

Summary

The childbearing family faces a constant challenge of maintaining balance between the integration of new family members and changing established interaction patterns and problem-solving strategies. The family's ability to meet the challenge is critical for parents and children. Nursing actions designed to strengthen family bonds and facilitate the mother's and father's attainment of parental roles serve an important social purpose.

References

Ainsworth, M.D.: Object relations, dependency, and attachment: a theoretical review of the infant-mother relationship, Child. Dev. 40:969, 1969.

Ainsworth, M.D.: The development of infant-mother attachment. In Caldwell, B.M., and Reccurti, H.N., editors: Review of child development research, vol. 3, New York, 1970, Russell Sage Foundation.

Ainsworth, M.D., and Bell, S.M.: Attachment, exploration and separation: illustrated by the behavior of one-year-olds in a strange situation, Child Dev. 41:49, 1970.

American College of Obstetricians and Gyencologists: The development of family-centered maternity/newborn care in hospitals, Washington, D.C., 1978, The College.

Baranowski, E.: Childbirth education classes for expectant deaf parents, M.C.N. 8:143, 1983.

Barnett, C.R., and others: Neonatal separation: the maternal side of interactional deprivation, Pediatrics 54:197, 1970.

Benedek, T.: Adaptation to reality in early infancy, Psychoanal. Q. 7:200, 1950.

Bowlby, J.: The nature of the child's tie to his mother, Int. J. Psychoanal. 39:350, 1958.

Bowlby, J.: Attachment and loss, vol. 1: Attachment, New York, 1969, Basic Books, Inc., Publishers.

Brazelton, T.B.: The early mother-infant adjustment, Pediatrics 32: 931, 1963.

Brazelton, T.B.: Effect of maternal expectations on early infant behavior, Early Child Dev. Care 2:259, 1973.

Brazelton, T.B., and others: The origins of reciprocity: the early mother-infant interaction. In Lewis, M., and Rosenblum, L.A., editors: The effect of the infant on its caregiver, New York, 1974, John Wiley & Sons.

Budin, P.: The nursling, London, 1907, Caxton Publishing Co.

Clarke-Stewart, K.: And daddy makes three: the father's impact on mother and young child, Child Dev. 49:466, 1978.

Condon, W., and Sander, L.: Neonate movement is synchronized with adult speech: interactional participation and language acquisition, Science 183:99, 1974.

Curry, M.S.: Contact during the first hour with the wrapped or naked newborn: effect on maternal attachment behaviors at 36 hours and three months, Birth Fam. J. 6:4, Winter 1979.

Deutch, H.: The psychology of women: a psychoanalytic interpretation, vol. 2: Motherhood, New York, 1945, Grune & Stratton, p. 457.

Erikson, E.H.: Identity and the life cycle: selected papers. In Psychological issues, vol. 1, no. 1, New York, 1959, International Universities Press, Inc.

Erikson, E.H.: Childhood and society, New York, 1964, W.W. Norton & Co.

Fardig, J.A.: A comparison of skin-to-skin contact and radiant heaters in promoting neonatal thermoregulation, J. Nurse Midwife 25:19, Jan. Feb. 1980.

Field, T.: Maternal stimulation during infant feeding, Dev. Psychol. 13:539, 1977.

Field, T.: The three Rs of infant-adult interactions: rhythms, repertoires, and responsibility, J. Pediatr. Psychol. 3:131, 1978a

Field, T.: Visual and cardiac responses to animate and inanimate faces by young term and preterm infants, Child Dev. vol. 49, 1978b.

Greenberg, M., and Morris, N.: Engrossment: the newborn's impact on the father, Nurs. Digest 4:19, Jan. Feb. 1976.

Grosso, C., and others: The Vietnamese American family. . . and grandma makes three, M.C.N. 6:177, 1981.

Haley, A.: Haley's Rx: talk, write, reunite (interview), Time 109:72, Feb. 14, 1977.

Hefler, R.E., and Kempe, C.H.: The battered child, Chicago, 1965, University of Chicago Press.

Hogan, L.R.: Pregnant again—at 41, M.C.N. 4:174, 1979.

Howley, C.: The older primipara: implications for nurses, J.O.G.N. Nurs. 10:182, 1981.

Kirz, Donna S.: Report of study at Memorial Hospital, Medical Center at Long Beach, Calif: Pregnancy for older women, less of a risk, *San Francisco Chronicle*, April 24, 1986, p. 28.

Klaus, M.H., and Kennell, J.H.: Parent-infant bonding, ed. 2, St. Louis, 1982, The C.V. Mosby Co.

Klaus, M.H., and Robertson, M.: Birth, interaction and attachment, Pediatric Round Table 6, 1982, Johnson & Johnson Baby Products Co.

Klaus, M.H., and others: Maternal attachment and mothering disorders, Pediatric Round Table 1, 1982, Johnson & Johnson Baby Products Co.

Kowba, M.D. and others: Direct sibling contact and bacterial colonization in newborns, J.O.G.N. N. 14:412, Sept. Oct. 1985.

Kreppner, K., and others: Infant and family development: from triads to tetrads, Hum. Dev. 25:373, 1982.

Kunst-Wilson, W., and Cronenwett, L.: Nursing care for the emerging family: promoting paternal behavior, Res. Nurs. Health 4:201, 1981.

Lamb, M.: Early contact and maternal-infant bonding: one decade later, Pediatrics 70:325, 1982.

Lang, R.: Birth book, Ben Lomond, Calif. 1972, Genesis Press.

Leifer, A.D., and others: Effects of mother-infant separation on maternal attachment behavior, Child Dev. 43:1203, 1972.

LeShan, E.: The wonderful crisis of middle age, New York, 1975, Warner Books.

Magilvy, K., and others: Stereotyping, words, and concepts (letter), M.C.N. 4:254, 1979.

Mead, M.: Culture and commitment: a study of the generation gap, Garden City, New York, 1970, Doubleday & Co.

Mercer, R.T.: Parent-infant attachment. In Sonstegard, L.J., and others, editors: Women's health, vol. 2: Childbearing, New York, 1982, Grune & Stratton.

Newell, N.J.: Grandparents, the overlooked support system for new parents during the fourth trimester, NAACOG Update Series 1 (lesson 21), 1984.

Olson, M.L.: Fitting grandparents into new families, M.C.N. 6:419, 1981.

Parkes, C.M., and Stevenson-Hinde, J.: The place of attachment in human behavior, New York, 1982, Basic Books, Inc., Publishers.

Rubin, R.: Maternal behavior, Nurs. Outlook 9:682, 1961.

Rubin, R.: Maternal touch at first contact with the newborn infant, Nurs. Outlook 11:828, 1963.

Rubin, R.: Maternal tasks in pregnancy. Matern. Child. Nurs. J. 4:143, Fall 1975.

Shainess, N.: Abortion is no man's business, Psychology Today, p. 18, March 1970.

Sheehy, G.: Passages: predictable crises of adult life, New York, 1977, Bantam Books, p. 383.

Siegel, E.: A critical examination of studies of parent-infant bonding. In Klaus, M., and Robertson, M., editors: Birth, interaction and attachment, Evansville, Ind., 1982, Johnson & Johnson Baby Products Co.

Stainton, C.M.: A comparison of prenatal and postnatal perceptions of their babies by parents, paper presented to the First International Congress on Pre- and Para-natal Psychology, Toronto, July 8, 1983a.

Stainton, C.M.: Maternal newborn attachment origins and processes. III. Interactional synchrony: the prelude to attachment, doctoral thesis, University of California, San Francisco, 1983b.

Stainton, C.M.: Unpublished doctoral dissertation, University of California, 1985.

Steele, B., and Pollock, C.: A psychiatric study of parents who abuse infants and small children. In Helfer, R.E., and Kempe, C., editors: The battered child, Chicago, 1968, University of Chicago Press.

Tulman, L.: Mothers and unrelated persons' initial handling of newborn infants, Nurs. Res. 34:205, July Aug. 1985.

Umphenour, J.H.: Bacterial colonization in neonates with sibling visitation, J.O.G.N. Nurs. 9:73, 1980.

Walz, B., and Rich, O.: Maternal tasks of taking on a second child in the postpartum period, Matern. Child Nurs. J. 12:3, Fall 1983.

Wranesh, B.L.: The effect of sibling visitation on bacterial colonization rate in neonates, J.O.G.N. Nurs. 11:211, 1982.

Bibliography

Avanti, K.: anxiety as a potential factor affecting maternal attachment, J.O.G.N. Nurs. 10:416, 1981.

Brandon, H.K.: The blind mother, Am. J. Nurs. 75:414, 1975.

Celotta, B.: New motherhood: a time of crisis, Birth Fam. J. 9(1):21, 1982.

Craig, J.: Birth of a grandchild brings time of reflection, Menninger Perspect. 11:23, Autumn 1980.

deChateau, P.: The importance of the neonatal period for the development of synchrony in the mother-infant dyad: a review, Birth Fam. J. 10(4): 10, 1977.

deChateau, P.: Effects of hospital practices on synchrony in the development of the infant-parent relationship, Semin. Perinatol. 3:45, Jan. 1979.

deVore, N.: Parenthood postponed, Am. J. Nurs. 83:1160, 1983.

Dunn, J., and Kendrick C.: The arrival of a sibling, changes in patterns of interactions between mothers and first-born child, J. Child Psychol. Psychiatry 21:119, 1980.

Dunn, J., Kendrick, C., and McNamee, R.: The reaction of

first born children to the birth of a sibling: Mothers' reports, J. Child Psychol. Psychiatry 22(1):1, 1981.

Hans, A.: Postpartum assessment: The psychological component, J.O.G.N. N. 1511:49, Jan. Feb. 1986.

Jones, C.: Father to infant attachment: effects of early contact and characteristics of the infant, Res. Nurs. Health 4:193, 1981.

Kendrick, C., and Dunn, J.: Caring for a second baby: effects on interactions between mother and first child, Dev. Psychol. 16(4):303, 1980.

Korn, S.J.: The reality of difficult temperament, Merrill-Palmer Q. 28(1), Jan. 1982.

Lunch, A.: Maternal stress following the birth of a second child. In Klaus, M., and Robertson, M., editors: Birth, interaction and attachment, Evansville, Ind., 1982, Johnson & Johnson Baby Products Co.

May, K.A.: A typology of detachment/involvement styles adopted during pregnancy by first-time expectant fathers, West. J. Nurs. Res. 2:445, 1980.

McCrae, M.: Bonding in a sea of silence, M.C.N. 4:29, 1979.

McKay, V.: The decade of the eighties: significant trends and developments for hearing impaired individuals, Rehabil. Lit. 42:2, Jan. Feb. 1981.

McKay, V., and Hicks, D.: Relationship of rubella, herpes simplex, cytomegalovirus, and certain other viral disabilities, Am. Ann. Deaf 125:529, 1980.

Mercer, R.T., and Stainton, M.C.: Perceptions of the birth experience: a cross-cultural comparison, Health Care of Women International 5:29, 1984.

Morris, M.: Psychological miscarriage: an end to mother love, Transactions, p. 11, Jan. Feb. 1966.

Moss, J.R.: Concerns of multiparas on the third postpartum day, J.O.G.N. Nurs. 10:421, 1981.

Phillips, C.R., and Anzalone, J.T.: Fathering, participation in labor and birth, ed. 2, St. Louis, 1982, The C.V. Mosby Co.

Porter, R., and others: The importance of odors in mother-infant interactions, Matern. Child Nurs. J 12:147, Fall 1983.

Robertson, J.F.: Grandmotherhood: a study of role conception, J. Marriage Fam. 39:165, 1977.

Rutter, M.: Temperament: concepts, issues and problems, Ciba Foundation Symposium 89, Temperamental differences in infant and young children, London, 1982, Pitman.

Schiff, N.B.: Communication problems in hearing children of deaf parents, J. Speech Hear. Disord. 41:348, 1976.

Seitz, S., and Marcus, S.: Mother-child interactions: a foundation for language development, Except. Child. 42:445, 1976.

Smales, O.R., and Kime, R.: Thermoregulation in babies immediately after birth, Arch. Dis. Child. 53:58, Jan. 1978.

Sullivan, D., and Beeman, R.: Satisfaction with postpartum care: opportunities for bonding, reconstructing the birth and instruction, Birth Fam. J. 8:3, Fall 1981.

Stainton, C.M.: Parent-infant interaction: putting theory into practice, Calgary, Alta., Canada, 1981, University of Calgary Faculty of Nursing.

Sussman, A.E., and Steward, L.G.: Counseling with deaf people, New York, 1971, New York Deafness Research and Training Center.

Sweeney, A.: Genetic counseling in families with hearing impairment, J. Rehabil. Deaf 12:1, July 1978.

Sweet, P.T.: Prenatal classes especially for children, M.C.N. 4:82, 1979.

Tentoni, S., and High, J.: Culturally induced postpartum depression: a theoretical position, J.O.G.N. Nurs. 9:246, 1980.

Ventura, J., and Boss, P.: The family coping inventory applies to parents of new babies, J. Marriage Fam. 83:867, 1983.

Vernon, M., and Mindel, E.D.: Psychological and psychiatric aspects of profound hearing loss. In Rose, D., editor: Audiological assessments, Englewood Cliffs, N.J., 1971, Prentice-Hall.

Wilbur, R.: The linguistics of manual languages and manual systems. In Lloyd, L.L., editor: Communication, assessments and intervention strategies, Baltimore, 1976, University Park Press.

Nursing Care During the Postpartum Period

The approach to care of women during the postpartum (puerperal) period has changed from one modeled on the concept of sick care to one that is health oriented. Women are concerned about their comfort and recovery, desirous of having contact with their infants, motivated to learn about newborn care, and eager to share their experiences with their families and friends. Their health care is now a collaborative effort on the part of all involved—mother, nurse, physician, and family—to achieve certain goals.

Knowledge of physiologic changes in the mother and emotional changes in the entire family are essential in appropriately evaluating assessment findings. Nursing diagnoses, planning, and implementation consider the need of the mother and family to learn the essentials for self-care. Early discharge, within 24 hours after delivery, is the preference for some. For others, early discharge is a necessity for various reasons. Evaluation of ongoing learning is important. Effects of learning may not be evident because of the short-term contact with childbearing families after delivery. Long-term effects are yet to be identified through nursing research.

This chapter focuses both on the mother's physiologic needs and on the family's emotional needs. The first portion of the chapter provides the nurse with several procedures for care and guidelines for client teaching. The second portion addresses the emotional needs and care of the family. The nurse makes a significant contribution to providing total care to the woman and her family. Kunst-Wilson and Cronenwett (1981) make the following comment:

[Nurses'] unique ability to deal with both the physical and psychological spheres, and the interactions of each on the other, especially important in childbearing, makes nursing's potential contribution more comprehensive than that of related disciplines. The nurse has the professional skills to deliver services personally in the office, home, or hospital setting, depending on the family's needs. Thus, no major aspect

of the normal childbearing experience is beyond the bounds of the nurse's skills.

Physical Care: The Nurse as Technician and Teacher/Counselor/Advocate

Assessment. The initial assessment includes the report from the nurse in the labor unit. The admitting nurse is given a brief description of all pertinent information (see Table 18.4). The woman's record is reviewed for information from the prenatal and labor records that is necessary for her nursing care plan.

Interview. During the assessment the nurse can determine the mother's emotional status, energy level, degree and location of physical discomfort, hunger, and thirst. To some degree, her knowledge level concerning self-care and infant care can also be determined. If appropriate, ethnic and cultural expectations are assessed regarding postpartum recovery patterns. The nursing care plan must consider individual variations in maternal behaviors and degree of participation in self-care and in infant care.

Physical examination. Postpartum assessment is based on expected maternal changes. Progression of puerperal changes for the 72 hours after delivery is presented in Table 24.1.

The length of the fourth stage and the time of transfer to the postpartum unit varies. Therefore the schedule for assessment varies. To assist the nurse to plan assessments, a schedule starting with delivery is displayed in Table 24.2.

Laboratory tests. After normal childbirth, few laboratory tests are routine. Hemoglobin and hematocrit determinations are required. Clean catch or catheterized urine specimens are sent for culture, sensitivity, and routine analysis for some women. The prenatal record alerts the health care team to the woman's need for rubella vaccination and potential for Rh isoimmun-

Table 24.1
Progression of Puerperal Changes: Days 1 Through 3

Assessment	2-24 Hours	25-48 Hours	49-72 Hours
Temperature	Elevated (38° C [100.4° F])	Within normal range	Within normal range
Pulse	Bradycardia: 50-70 beats/min	Bradycardia may persist or rate may return to within normal range	Bradycardia may persist or rate may return to within normal range
Blood pressure	Within normal range	Within normal range	Within normal range
Energy level	Euphoric, happy, excited, or fatigued; may show need for sleep	Often tired, slow moving	Anxious to go home; level within normal range, but variable
Uterus	At umbilicus or just below	1 cm or more below umbilicus	2 cm or more below umbilicus
Lochia	Rubra; moderate; few clots, if any; fleshy odor of normal menstrual flow	Rubra to serosa; moderate to scant; odor continues to be "fleshy" or absent	Rubra to serosa; scant; odor continues to be "fleshy" or absent
Perineum	Edematous; clean, healing	Edema lessening; clean, healing	Edema lessening or absent; clean, healing
Legs	Pretibial or pedal edema; Homans' sign negative	Edema lessening; Homans' sign negative	Edema minimal or absent; Homans' sign negative
Breasts	Remain soft to palpation Colostrum can be expressed	Begin to feel firmer Occasionally feel lumpy	Increase in vascularity and initiation of swelling Feel firmer and warmer to touch Milk expected within 2-4 days after delivery
Appetite	Excellent; may ask for double helpings, snacks	Usually remains excellent	Varies; appetite may have returned to normal range or may lessen (especially if client is constipated)
Elimination			
Voiding	Up to 3000 ml	Large amounts	Amount/24 hours is lessening
Defecation	—	—	Usually defecates; may need enema, etc.
Discomfort	Generalized aching; perineal area: episiotomy, hemorrhoids	Muscle aches; perineal area: episiotomy, hemorrhoids	Possible tension headache, perineal area: usually lessening; breasts, nipples

Table 24.2
Minimal Schedule of Assessments After Delivery

Assessment Factor															
			1			2	3	4	5	6	7	8	24	48	72
	15"	15"	15"	15"	30"	30"	60"	60"	60"	60"	60"	60"	Every 8 Hours	Every 8 Hours	Every 8 Hours
Temperature				X				X				X	x3	x3	x3
Pulse, respirations, blood pressure	X	X	X	X	X	X	X	X				X	x3	x3	x3
Fundus, lochia	X	X	X	X	X	X	X	X				X	x3	x3	x3
Bladder	X	X	X	X	X	X	X	X				X	amount (ml)		
Perineum				X				X				X	x3	x3	x3
Breasts, legs												X	x3	x3	x3
Psychosocial factors	X	X	X	X				X				X	x3	x3	x3
Bowels													Daily	Daily	Daily

Fig. 24.1

Plan of nursing care for woman after normal delivery. (Adapted from Fountain Valley
Community Hospital, Fountain Valley California.)

Name:	Grav: Para: Ab: Stb:	Infant	Family:
	Marital status:	Sex: Wt: Length;	Adults:
Room:	Occupation:	Time: Day: Date:	
		Pediatrician: Feeding:	Siblings:
	Rh: Type:	Baby's Rh: Type: Coombs:	
		Condition of baby: Date:	
	Rubella antibody titer:		

| Short-term goal: | | Long-term goal: | |

| Emergency number: | Person: | Relationship: | Address: |

Date	Nursing diagnoses	Evaluative criteria	Nursing actions

Client teaching

Breast care	Infant care skills	Family planning options
Perineal care	Infant feeding techniques	Importance of follow-up care for self and infant
Lochia flow norms	Infant characteristics	Exercise/rest postpartum
Postpartum nutrition and fluid needs	Care of hemorrhoids	

Discharge planning

1. Mother will have follow-up care for self and infant arranged prior to discharge.
2. Mother has received and verbalized understanding of discharge instructions re: care of breasts, perineum, stitches, nutrition, rest/exercise, resumption of sexual activity, danger signals to report to physician.
3. Mother demonstrates comfort and competence in caregiver skills with own infant.

Return visit:
Referrals:　( ) social work
　　　　　　( ) home care

Date/ resolution	Client problem(s)	Expected outcome (short/long-term goals)	Date outcome to be reached	Nursing action	Signature
	Potential postpartum hemorrhage	Will verbalize lochia flow norms, how to report abnormals		Teach lochia flow norms: color, amount, odor, length of flow, and how to report to nurse/physician.	
				Assess fundal tone, height, position q15 min first hour postpartum, massage uterus prn.	
				Assess q½h x 2, then q shift and prn.	
				Teach mother how to massage fundus.	
	Potential infection	Will verbalize lochia flow norms, how to report abnormals.		Alert woman to report temp. of 100.4° F, foul-smelling lochia, abdominal pain, general feeling of not being well.	
		Will demonstrate appropriate hygiene and care of perineum, stitches.		Teach use of surgigator, squeeze bottle, sitz bath, avoidance of tampons, intercourse, swimming until postpartum checkup.	
	Potential anxiety secondary to lack of knowledge/experience in care taking of infant, feeding.	Will demonstrate competence in infant care taking and feeding techniques.		Provide early contact with infant and encourage eye-to-eye, skin-to-skin contact.	
				Assess readiness for learning, provide frequent opportunity for observing/practicing infant care skills, feedings.	
				Provide emotional support and positive reinforcement with learned skills.	

Fig. 24.2
Postpartum instruction.

Date	Area	Instructed	Demonstrated by mother	Nurse's signature
	Mother			
	Personal hygiene and care			
	Breast examination			
	Perineum			
	Lochia: amount, character			
	Comfort			
	Peri care			
	Tucks and Americaine			
	Peri lamp			
	Sitz bath			
	Sexual relations			
	Birth control			
	Nutrition			
	Exercise			
	Rest			
	Emotional adjustments			
	Cesarean delivery			
	Tubal occlusion			
	Infant			
	Bathing			
	Cord/circumcision care			
	Thermometer use			
	Bulb syringe			
	Safety/poison control			
	Car seats			
	Breast feeding			
	Breast pumping			
	Storage of milk			
	Formula feeding			
	Formula preparation			
	Positioning/handling			
	Diapering			
	Clothing			
	Signs of illness			
	Family schedules			
	Special situations			

ization. Postnatal assessment of fetal cord blood provides information about the woman's need for $Rh_0(D)$ immune globulin.

Nursing diagnoses. Although women experience similar problems during the postpartum period, certain factors act to make each woman's experience unique. The labor a woman experienced (whether it was long or short), whether she plans to bottle feed or breast feed, whether she had an episiotomy, and whether she has other children are some factors to consider. Nursing diagnoses lend direction to types of nursing actions needed to implement a plan of care. Examples of nursing diagnoses follow:

- Knowledge deficit related to importance of voiding as deterrent to hemorrhage.
- Sleep-pattern disturbance related to discomfort of breast engorgement, episiotomy, afterpains, and hemorrhoids.
- Self-care deficit related to knowledge deficit of perineal hygiene as promoter of healing during the puerperium.
- Potential for infection related to childbirth trauma to tissues.
- Alterations in bowel or urinary elimination related to post-childbirth discomfort.
- Disturbance in self-concept related to knowledge deficit of expected anatomic and physiologic changes during the puerperium.

Planning. The nursing plan is used for the care of women postpartum as it is for other clients. Once the nursing diagnoses are formulated, the nurse decides what nursing measures would be appropriate and which are to be given priority. The organization of care must take the newborn into consideration. The day actually revolves around the baby's feeding and care times.

The mother assumes increasing responsibility for her own self-care. The nurse is responsible for consistent assessment of actual or potential problems. In some areas "couple nursing" (mother and baby) has been introduced. The nurse acts as the primary nurse for both mother and infant even if the newborn is kept in the central nursery. This approach is a variation of rooming-in, in which mother and child room together and mother and nurse share the care of the infant.

The nursing care plan will include assessments to detect deviations from normal, comfort measures to relieve discomfort or pain and safety measures to prevent injury or infection. The nurse also will provide teaching and counseling measures designed to promote a mother's (and father's) feeling of competence in the care of herself and newly born child. The nurse evaluates continuously and is ready to change the plan if indicated. The nurse's ability to adapt the care plan

to specific medical and nursing diagnoses results in individualized care for the client.

Standardized care plans are used by almost all facilities and health care providers (Figs. 24.1 and 24.2) and are found in many nursing textbooks. A standard care plan is an aid for students and new graduates in grasping concepts or setting priorities and selecting appropriate actions for real or potential problems. In addition, it can be used as a checklist for giving general direction for implementing the nursing process with a client. Caution is advised against total reliance on a standardized plan: the uniqueness of the individual may be overlooked.

Goals

1. Prevent hemorrhage and other biophysical complications.
2. Promote involution and physiologic recovery from childbirth.
3. Promote physical comfort, rest, activity, and safety.
4. Facilitate return of woman's normal pattern of bowel and bladder elimination.
5. Meet learning needs for recovery from childbirth, normal involution, and self-care.
6. Enhance woman's self-concept by knowledgeable and caring application of the nursing process during the postpartum period.
7. Encourage continued health maintenance through self-care and use of home and community health care delivery systems.

Implementation

General precautions to ensure safety

Infection-free environment. Facilities (unit kitchens, bathroom, and bed units) and supplies (linens) must be kept scrupulously clean. Frequent changes of draw sheet and a daily change of linen are recommended. Supervision of use of facilities to prevent cross infection among women is necessary (e.g., common sitz bath must be scrubbed after each woman's use, ventilation system is monitored). Personnel must be conscientious about their hand-washing techniques to prevent cross infection. Im many institutions nurses are required to wear a face mask when carrying out perineal care. Personnel with colds, coughs, or skin infections (e.g., a cold sore on the lips [herpes simplex virus, type 1]) must not be in contact with women during the puerperium.

Client identification. The first step in providing individualized care is to confirm the client's correct identity by checking her arm band. At the same time, the infant's identification number is matched with the corresponding band on the mother's wrist. The nurse demonstrates caring and respect by determining how the mother wishes to be addressed and then notes her preference in her record and on the card index (Kardex).

Orientation to the environment. The woman and her family are oriented to their surroundings. Familiarity with the unit, routines, resources, and personnel reduces one potential source of anxiety—the unknown. The mother is reassured through knowing whom and how she can call for assistance and what she can expect in the way of supplies and services. If the woman's usual daily routine before admission differs from the facility's routine, the nurse works with the woman to develop a mutually acceptable and workable routine.

Ethnic and cultural variations in care of the woman after delivery can be discussed and plans for modifying nursing actions made. An example of a cultural variation follows:

■ A Vietnamese woman who had been in the United States for 4 years requested rooming-in facilities following delivery. Instead of participating in the care of her infant, she refused to do so, remained in bed, wore a woolen cap, and appeared distressed and angry. The staff were nonplussed by her behavior. One nurse decided to put newly learned concepts concerning cross-cultural nursing into effect. She began by praising the woman's ability to speak English and after eliciting a smile, remarked, "Every country has developed good ways to look after mothers and babies. Would you tell me about the care in Vietnam?" There was an immediate response. The woman explained that in her country women remained in bed for 10 days after delivery and the biggest danger to their health was getting a cold. The baby was kept in the room with his mother, but either a grandmother or nurse took complete charge of the care.

Evidently the woman was operating in tune with her cultural expectations, and the nurses were operating within theirs. This rather simple approach to resolving a nursing problem also proved successful in subsequent cases.

General care

Rest. The excitement and exhilaration experienced after the birth of the infant may make rest difficult. The new mother, who is often anxious about her ability to care for her infant or is uncomfortable, may also have difficulty sleeping. Backrubs, other comfort measures, and medication for sleep for the first few nights may be necessary.

Bed rest, ambulation, and exercise. Early ambulation has proved successful in reducing the incidence of

thromboembolism and in woman's more rapid recovery of strength. Most women can be ambulatory by at least 8 hours after normal delivery if a local or light general anesthetic agent was used.

Parturients who received *intrathecal subarachnoid spinal anesthesia* should remain flat in bed with one flat pillow to align the head with the shoulders for at least 8 hours before they are allowed to ambulate. This position prevents leakage of spinal fluid through the dural membrane at the site of the needle puncture (a potential fistula tract), which causes a severe *"spinal" headache*. Since mothers automatically raise their heads to view their infants, the nurse needs to warn the mother to remain flat in bed. The nurse then positions or holds the infant so that the mother can see the child. Bathroom privileges are curtailed, and infant feeding by the mother may be delayed until she can sit up (check hospital protocol).

Confinement to bed is not required for women who had *epidural* or *caudal anesthesia* or for women who had local anesthesia such as paracervical or pudendal block. Free movement is permitted once the anesthetic wears off unless an analgesic has been administered. After the first vital rest period is over (usually about 8 hours), the mother is encouraged to ambulate frequently.

Prevention of *thrombosis* is part of the nursing care plan. If a woman is confined to bed longer than 8 hours (e.g., after spinal anesthesia or cesarean birth), exercise to promote circulation in the legs is indicated:

1. Alternate flexion and extension of feet.
2. Rotate feet.
3. Alternate flexion and extension of legs.
4. Press back of knee to bed surface; relax.
5. Do straight-leg raises.

If the woman is susceptible to *thromboembolism* the physician may avoid use of estrogens to inhibit or suppress lactation. Women with varicosities are encouraged to wear support hose. The woman is encouraged to walk about actively for true ambulation, and she is discouraged from sitting immobile in a chair. If a thrombus is suspected, notify the physician immediately; meanwhile, the woman should be confined to bed, with the affected limb elevated on pillows.

Nursing care related to physiologic adaptations during the postpartum period. All nursing care given during the postpartum period is provided simultaneously with teaching. The rationale for each action can be provided and questions encouraged during each encounter with the new mother. The short span of time allotted the nurse to provide care necessitates that every opportunity for teaching must be used. The puerperium period is characterized by heightened interest in learning and readiness to change by the new

Table 24.3
Teaching the New Mother During the Early Postpartum Period

Assessment Findings	Nursing Actions	Teaching	Evaluation
Vital signs			
Temperature	Determine temperature. Assess for symptomatology of infection: ■ Mastitis ■ Urinary tract infection ■ Thrombophlebitis ■ Site of episiotomy/laceration ■ Endometritis ■ Other Report to physician. Initiate measures to lower temperature: ■ Fluids ■ Decrease environmental temperature, remove blankets or heavy clothing ■ Antipyretic medications	Normal ranges for values Causes of elevation **Symptomatology:** ■ Chills or fever, 100.4° F (38° C)+ ■ Localized redness, heat, pain ■ Urinary frequency, pain or burning with urination ■ Foul-smelling lochia Methods to lower temperature How to use and read a thermometer	Woman is aware of normal ranges. Mother learns methods to avoid or treat elevation. Mother reports any symptomatology she experiences immediately. Mother uses same temperature reduction measures after discharge home. Mother demonstrates appropriate technique for using and reading the thermometer.
Pulse Blood pressure	Assess pulse. Assess blood pressure. Assess complaint of headache (see Table 22.3)	Expected findings Expected findings Anticipatory guidance for prevention of hypertension Orthostatic hypotension related to splanchnic engorgement Causes of headaches Ways to decrease stress if headache is caused by stress	Woman knows normal range. Woman knows normal range. Woman implements preventive measures with self and family regarding diet, exercise. Woman takes precautions against fainting during first ambulation, e.g., calls for assistance. Woman knows and uses methods of relaxation and stress reduction. Woman does not develop hypertension during later life.
Uterus ■ Position, size, ■ Tone ■ Response to gentle massage ■ Afterpains ■ Rate of involution (about 1 cm/day)	Assess tone and response to gentle massage. Use nonpharmacologic or pharmacologic measures to maintain tone and relieve discomfort from afterpains (Procedure 24.1)	Location and feel of uterus Self-massage Medications: actions, purposes, effects (Table 24.4)	Mother understands purpose and follows through on self-massage.
Lochia ■ Color ■ Amount ■ Size, number of clots ■ Odor ("fleshy")	Assess amount and character (p. 698) Identify and report excessive or persistant lochia rubra or foul-smelling lochia.	Normal amount and characteristics through the puerperium Deviations from normal (e.g., foul-smelling lochia) is associated with endometritis. How and to whom to report suspicious findings A "small period" of painless bleeding is within normal at about 3 weeks	Infection does not occur in hospital or later at home. Woman reports STAT: ■ Foul-smelling lochia ■ Elevated temperature ■ Increased or bright red bleeding ■ Unusual pain in uterus/pelvis
Perineum ■ Healing of site of episiotomy/laceration ■ Size, number of hemorrhoids	Assess perineum. Provide comfort measures. Wash hands before and after care of perineum.	Description and opportunity to look at area of trauma/repair Measures for comfort/healing (Procedures 24.2 and 24.3) Expected healing of perineum and regression of hemorrhoids	Washes hands prior to and following care of perineum Utilizes comfort measures correctly Takes precautions to avoid contamination of vulva from anal area

Table 24.3, cont'd
Teaching the New Mother During the Early Postpartum Period

Assessment Findings	Nursing Actions	Teaching	Evaluation
■ Other trauma (e.g., swelling, bruising)			Perineum heals well Hemorrhoids regress
Musculoskeletal and integumentary systems ■ Pigmentation ■ Looseness or laxity of joints ■ Hair, fingernails, and skin changes	Assess woman for hyperpigmentation of integument. Inquire about changes experienced during pregnancy.	Regression of pregnancy-hormone-induced changes: Most of the adaptive changes to pregnancy—hyperpigmentation, changes in the hair and fingernails, the condition of the skin—will most likely return to their original prepregnant state. Striae gravidarum usually become lighter, silvery, and less noticeable. However, for most women, evidence of striae remain.	Woman understands expected changes and rate of regression.
Hemoglobin, hematocrit May be decreased at this time	Order lab work. Retrieve information and place in record. Alert physician and implement orders, as necessary.	Rationale for tests Range of normal values and where her values fit within that range Relationship to nutrition	Values are within normal limits. Woman learns self-care through nutrition. Woman prevents anemia in self and family.
Coagulation factors	Assess for symptomatology of thrombus formation, ambulation, exercise.	Rationale Measures to take should symptomatology of thrombus occur	No coagulation problems occur. Woman recognizes and seeks therapy for symptomatology of thrombus formation.
Varicosities Hemorrhoids ■ Location ■ Number, size	Assess for discomfort. Assess knowledge regarding self-care measures. Provide care for hemorrhoids (Procedure 24.3).	Return of muscle tone in blood vessel walls Preventive measures, good nutrition (which prevents obesity), avoidance of standing for long periods, exercise, avoidance of straining while defecating, and not wearing tight clothing.	Varicosities regress. Discomfort is minimized or is controlled. Continues with preventive measures.
Urinary tract ■ Symptomatology of infection ■ Distension ■ Completeness of emptying ■ Ability to void ■ Total amount at end of first 24 hours	Facilitate voiding: ■ Assist up to void ■ See Procedure 24.4 ■ Encourage oral fluids. ■ Catheterize as needed per physician's order.	See Procedure 24.4. Symptomatology of urinary tract infection.	Voids and empties bladder completely at least every 4 hours. Bladder distension does not occur. If catheterization was necessary, infection or loss of self-esteem does not occur. Woman knows symptomatology of urinary tract infection and reports them immediately.
Bowels ■ Bowel sounds ■ Passing flatus ■ Abdominal distension ■ Bowel movement ■ Constipation ■ Diarrhea ■ Hemorrhoids	Encourage and assist with early ambulation, fluids, foods with roughage. Encourage immediate response to urge to defecate. Administer stool softeners, enemas, as prescribed. Employ care of perineum (Procedure 24.2 and 24.3).	Counsel regarding: ■ Foods, fluids ■ Exercise ■ Bowel habits ■ Care of perineum (Procedures 24.2 and 24.3). ■ Hygiene after defecation.	Woman's bowel elimination pattern is restored. Woman has minimal discomfort. Woman continues to use preventive and comfort measures learned during hospitalization.

Continued.

Table 24.3, cont'd
Teaching the New Mother During the Early Postpartum Period

Assessment Findings	Nursing Actions	Teaching	Evaluation
Bowels—cont'd			
■ Labor record for last BM or enema			
NOTE: An enema or laxative suppository is contraindicated for a woman with a third- or fourth-degree laceration until the suture line has healed, since the tip of the enema tubing or hard suppository may rupture the sutures. Oral stool softeners and laxatives may be administered, however.			
Breasts			
■ Soft, filling, firm ■ Engorged ■ Painful ■ Mastitis	Assist with suppression of lactation (Procedure 24.5).	Newborn nutrition and feeding (see Chapter 21).	Lactation is suppressed with minimal discomfort.
	Assist with breast feeding (see Chapter 21).	Newborn nutrition and feeding (see Chapter 21). Preventive and comfort measures: ■ Hygiene: warm water, no soap; breasts washed first with fresh washcloth and towels ■ Supportive bra ■ Use of breast pump and manual expression	Lactation is initiated successfully. Woman is satisfied with breast feeding experience.
Nipples			
■ Protruding (everted), or ■ Inverted ■ Sore or tender ■ Cracked or bleeding	Assist with breast feeding (see Chapter 21).	Preventive and comfort measures: ■ Use Masse cream. ■ Rotate neonate's position at breast. ■ Correct latching-on. ■ Correct removal of baby from breast by breaking suction first.	Nipples are not injured or uncomfortable.

mother and often by her family as well. Table 24.3 outlines assessment findings, nursing actions, teaching, and evaluation. Evaluation of short-term goals that can be achieved during the hospital stay is readily done. However, it may not be possible to determine to what degree other goals have been met if the nurse has no further contact with the family after the woman returns home.

Procedures. The nurse's roles as technician, teacher, counselor, and advocate are highlighted in this section. To meet the physical care needs of the woman after childbirth, several procedures and guidelines for client teaching are helpful. Procedures for specific care needs include the following:

1. Nursing actions for a boggy uterus (See Table 24.4 also.)
2. Care following repair of episiotomy or laceration
3. Care of hemorrhoids

4. Nursing actions for full urinary bladder
5. Suppression of lactation

Guidelines for client teaching. Several guidelines for client teaching have been developed to assist the nurse to fulfill the role of teacher. These guidelines include the following:

1. Breast self-examination (BSE)
2. Postpartum exercises
3. Resumption of sexual intercourse
4. Postdelivery contraception

Immune system. Rubella vaccination and Rh_0 (D) immune globulin are administered during the puerperium as necessary. For a detailed discussion of the Rh factor and isoimmunization, see Chapter 31; for a general discussion of the immune system, see Chapter 5.

During the puerperium the nurse apprises the mother of the recommended schedule of immunizations for the infant (Appendix L).

Procedure 24.1

NURSING ACTIONS FOR BOGGY UTERUS

PURPOSE
To prevent hemorrhage by maintaining uterine muscle tone.

EQUIPMENT
None required

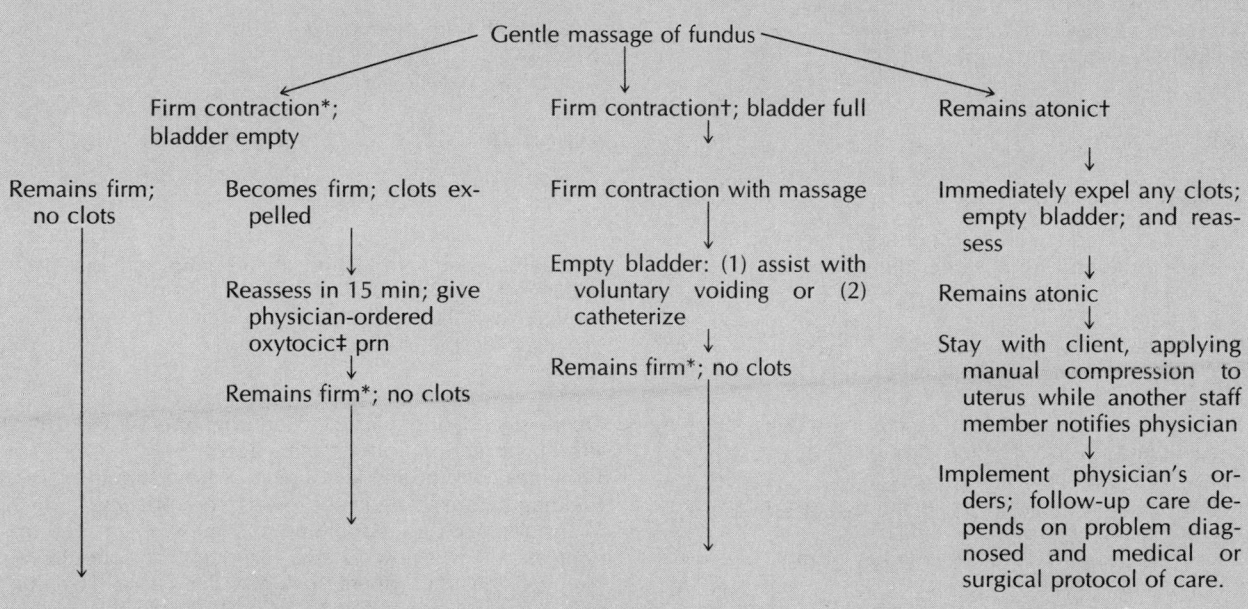

Gentle massage of fundus

Firm contraction*; bladder empty

- Remains firm; no clots
- Becomes firm; clots expelled → Reassess in 15 min; give physician-ordered oxytocic‡ prn → Remains firm*; no clots

Firm contraction†; bladder full
Firm contraction with massage → Empty bladder: (1) assist with voluntary voiding or (2) catheterize → Remains firm*; no clots

Remains atonic†
Immediately expel any clots; empty bladder; and reassess → Remains atonic → Stay with client, applying manual compression to uterus while another staff member notifies physician → Implement physician's orders; follow-up care depends on problem diagnosed and medical or surgical protocol of care.

> No further physical action is needed.
> Teach client importance of voiding and emptying bladder completely at least every 3 to 4 hours.

*Fundus is in midline, at level appropriate for time since delivery.

†Fundus is above umbilicus or at level higher than appropriate for time since delivery; uterus may or may not be displaced to right (usually by full bladder or full rectum).

‡See Table 24.4.

NURSING ACTION	RATIONALE
Massage gently.	Stimulates muscle contraction without causing muscle fatigue.
Teach woman to locate and massage uterus.	Encourages self-care.
Expel clots; reassess in 15 min.	Empties uterus so that "living ligature" can function. Verifies cessation of bleeding.
Prevent bladder distension: ■ Encourage spontaneous voiding; give rationale	Distended bladder can cause uterine relaxation: ■ Spontaneous voiding assists woman to maintain sense of control over her body. Knowing why bladder needs to be emptied completely adds to her knowledge base and encourages self-care.
■ Catheterize as needed; give rationale for need to catheterize vs. inability to void and need for bladder emptying.	■ Knowing rationale may decrease her sense of powerlessness over her body functions.
Put baby to suckle at breast.	Suckling stimulates release of oxytocin from posterior pituitary gland.
If uterus is not maintaining tone, stay with woman and call for assistance.	Continuous manual compression until intravenous infusion is started with pitocin decreases blood loss and is reassuring to woman.
Maintain a calm manner, provide explanations. Implement physician's orders to maintain uterine tone.	Uterus may need temporary stimulation from exogenous source of oxytocin to maintain tone.

Procedure 24.2

CARE AFTER REPAIR OF EPISIOTOMY OR LACERATION

PURPOSE
1. Promote healing.
2. Increase comfort.
3. Teach mother self-care techniques.
4. Identify and treat complications.

EQUIPMENT
1. Ice pack with cover
2. Squeeze bottle
3. Sitz bath with thermometer
4. Surgi-gator
5. Towels, as necessary

NURSING ACTION	RATIONALE
Ice Pack Apply a covered ice pack to perineum (see Fig. 18.5).	
■ During the first 2 hours after delivery.	Decreases edema formation at this time and increases comfort later. Provides anesthetic effect.
■ After the first 2 hours.	Provides anesthetic effect.
Sitz Bath (Fig. 24.3) Prepare bath by thoroughly scrubbing with cleaning agent and rinsing.	Decreases possibility of infection from another woman. Prevents irritation from cleaning agent.
Pad with towels before filling.	Promotes comfort and keeps woman from slipping. Padding before filling keeps towels from floating.
Fill ½ to ⅓ full with water of correct temperature (100.4°-105° F [38°-40.6° C]).*	Warm temperature is soothing to some women. The increased blood flow to area is thought by some to facilitate healing; others think that this causes swelling and adds to discomfort.*
Encourage woman to use twice a day or more often once she is ambulating.	
Place call bell within easy reach.	The warm water and other factors may cause her to feel faint and need assistance.
Teach her to enter bath by tightening gluteal muscles and keeping them tightened and then relaxing them after she is in bath.	Decreases perineal discomfort while sitting down. Allows water to reach perineum.
Place dry towels within reach.	

*Other authors propose cool sitz baths (Droegemueller, 1980).
†Peri-lights are still used in some hospitals. Care must be taken to prevent burns.

Fig. 24.3
Sitz bath. (Courtesy Marjorie Pyle, RNC. Lifecircle, Costa Mesa, California.)

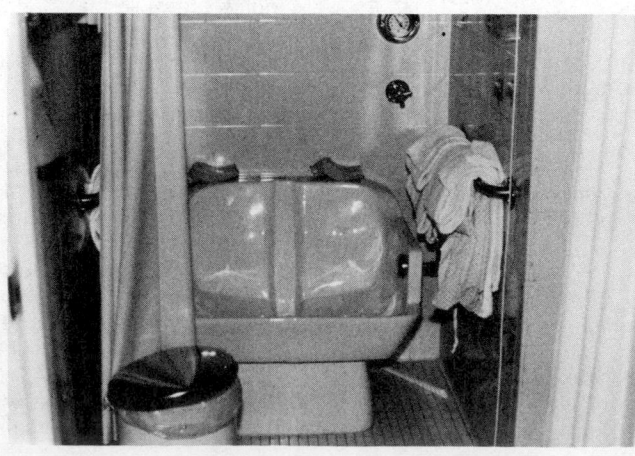

Procedure 24.2—cont'd

NURSING ACTION	RATIONALE
Squeeze Bottle	
Demonstrate for and assist woman; explain rationale.	Cleanses perineum after voiding. Encourages self-care.
Fill bottle with tap water warmed to approximately 100° F (38° C) (comfortably warm on the wrist).	Provides comfortable temperatures.
Instruct woman to position nozzle between her legs so that squirts of water reach perineum as she sits on toilet seat.	Cleanses and soothes perineum.
Explain that it will take several squirts of water over perineum.	Perineum needs to be cleansed well.
Remind her to blot dry with toilet paper or clean wipes (provided by the agency).	Blotting avoids tissue trauma and promotes comfort.
Remind her to avoid contamination from anal area.	Prevents infection.
Surgi-Gator	
Assemble Surgi-gator	Cleanses and provides comfort to perineum.
Instruct woman regarding use and rationale.	Encourages self-care.
Explain that each woman is issued her own applicator.	Prevents infection.
Follow package directions.	Promotes maximum benefit of appliance.
Instruct her to sit on toilet with legs apart and to put nozzle so tip is just past the perineum, adjusting placement as needed.	Provides the jets of water to the perineal area.
Remind her to return her applicator to her bedside stand.	Prevents loss or cross infection.
Dry Heat†	
Inspect lamp for defects.	Prevents fires or burns.
Cover lamp with towels.	Prevents burns if lamp touches skin.
Position lamp 50 cm (20 in) from perineum; use three times a day for 20 min periods.	Provides comfortable warmth. Promotes comfort. For some women, keeps area dry and thereby promotes healing.
Teach regarding use of 40-watt bulb at home.	Provides effective "heat" lamp in the home.
Provide privacy by careful draping over woman since knees must be kept up and separated for benefit.	Promotes privacy. Demonstrates respect and caring.
If same lamp is being used by several women, clean it carefully between uses.	Prevents cross infection.
Topical Applications	
Teach regarding use of sprays, ointments, or witch hazel pads (e.g., Tucks) that are applied directly to sutured area.	Adds to woman's knowledge base and encourages self-care.
Cleansing/Shower	
■ Wash perineum with mild soap and warm water at least once daily.	Fear of "breaking the stitches" or pain deters women from washing perineum.
■ Cleanse from symphysis pubis to anal area.	Prevents contamination of the vagina and urethra with fecal material.
■ Apply peripad from front to back, protecting inner surface of pad from contamination.	Prevents infection from contamination.
■ Wrap soiled pad and place in covered waste container.	
■ Change pad every time she voids or defecates or at least four times per day.	Prevents infection.
■ Wash hands before and after changing pads.	Prevents infection.
■ Assess amount and character of lochia with each pad change.	Identifies possible complications early.

Procedure 24.3

CARE OF HEMORRHOIDS

PURPOSE

1. Reduce hemorrhoidal swelling.
2. Promote comfort and eliminate or reduce itching.
3. Teach mother self-care techniques.

EQUIPMENT

1. Ice pack with cover
2. Sitz bath with thermometer
3. Cold witch hazel compresses (e.g., Tucks)
4. Ointments prescribed by the physician
5. Finger cot or rubber glove

NURSING ACTION	RATIONALE
Apply a covered ice pack (see Fig. 18.5) to hemorrhoids. Leave pack in position 20 min; repeat q4h.	Assists in reduction of hemorrhoidal swelling. Cover on ice pack minimizes possibility of a cold "burn." Provides anesthetic effect.
Provide sitz bath (see Procedure 24.2). Show woman how to apply cold witch hazel pads to hemorrhoids.	Encourages self-care. Adds to woman's knowledge base. Promotes comfort.
Instruct woman how to replace the hemorrhoid in the anorectal canal by using a lubricated finger cot or rubber glove.	Encourages self-care. Adds to woman's knowledge base.
Instruct woman that once the hemorrhoid is reduced, she needs to maintain digital pressure for 1-2 min.	Procedure may increase comfort for varying periods of time, depending on whether the hemorrhoid stays reduced.
Instruct woman that hemorrhoid may be extruded with a bowel movement and reduction may be necessary again.	Anal reflex will extrude the hemorrhoid.
Inform woman that unless the rectal condition was present before pregnancy, it will most likely correct itself once the increased blood supply and pressure symptoms of pregnancy are diminished and regular bowel habits are reestablished.	Adds to knowledge base. May decrease potential anxiety if hemorrhoids appear again. May reassure woman that the condition is temporary.
Instruct woman on ways to prevent constipation and straining at stool (see Chapter 11).	Encourages self-care. Increases knowledge base.

Rubella vaccination. For women who have not had rubella (10% to 20% of all women) or women who are serologically negative (i.e., titer of 1:8 or less) rubella virus vaccine is recommended in the immediate postdelivery period to prevent fetal anomalies in future pregnancies. Seroconversion occurs in approximately 90% of women vaccinated after delivery. The live attenuated rubella virus is not communicable; therefore nursing mothers can be vaccinated. However, the live attenuated rubella vaccine is made from duck eggs, and so women who have allergies to these eggs may develop a hypersensitivity reaction to the vaccine, for which they will need adrenalin. A transient arthralgia or rash is common in vaccinated women but is benign. Since the vaccine may be teratogenic the client should sign an informed consent and should receive written information about the vaccine, its side effects and risks, and the necessity for practicing contraception for a period of 2 to 3 months after vaccination.

Prevention of Rh isoimmunization. Injection of $Rh_0(D)$ immune globulin within 72 hours of delivery will prevent sensitization in the Rh-negative woman who has had a fetomaternal transfusion of Rh-positive fetal RBCs. The administration of 300 μg of $Rh_0(D)$ immune globulin is usually sufficient to prevent maternal sensitization. $Rh_0(D)$ immune globulin promotes lysis of fetal Rh-positive RBCs circulating in the maternal bloodstream before the mother forms her own antibodies against them. If a large fetomaternal transfusion is suspected, the dose needed can be assessed by either the Kleihauer-Betke smear or the D^u test, which detects 20 ml or more of Rh-positive fetal blood in the maternal circulation. The $Rh_0(D)$ immune globulin is administered after all known abortions (gestational age

Procedure 24.4

NURSING ACTIONS FOR FULL URINARY BLADDER

PURPOSE

To prevent bladder distension to decrease potential for bladder wall atony, infection, and uterine hemorrhage

EQUIPMENT

Catheter tray, as needed

Inform client that she needs to empty bladder

Able to void voluntarily; empties urinary bladder

Able to void voluntarily; does not empty bladder completely

If perineal discomfort is a factor, employ comfort measures and administer prescribed medications

Able to void voluntarily; empties bladder completely

Unable to void or does not empty bladder completely

If postanalgesia or postanesthesia effect is a factor, try spirits of peppermint; if unsuccessful, catheterize

Unable to void voluntarily or cannot empty bladder completely when distended again; insert closed system retention catheter or institute other action per physician's order

No further physical action is needed.
Teach client importance of voiding and emptying bladder completely at least every 3 to 4 hours.

NURSING ACTION	RATIONALE
Facilitate Spontaneous Voiding	
If she is ambulatory, assist her to bathroom.	Verifies woman's ability to walk without difficulty.
Assist her onto bedpan; provide privacy, pour warm water over the vulva, sound of running water, and provide call bell.	Facilitates spontaneous voiding.
Provide ordered medications if discomfort of the perineum is hindering spontaneous voiding.	Discomfort increases difficulty of spontaneous voiding.
Some women can void spontaneously if they know it is permissible to void in the sitz bath (then follow the bath with a shower) or while squirting water over perineum (see Procedure 24.2).	Water is relaxing and dilutes the urine.
Teach techniques to facilitate spontaneous voiding (e.g., void immediately when the urge is present; straddle the toilet seat facing the tank or sit on toilet in regular fashion and lean forward; push all the urine out even if it "makes noise").	Natural response to physiologic event. Directs the flow of urine away from repair of episiotomy and lacerations. Gives woman permission to "make noise" (many learned to "pee quietly" as little girls to be more "ladylike"). Urinating with force is more likely to empty the bladder completely.
Expose the urinary meatus to fumes from peppermint spirits.	Assists woman to void spontaneously if at all possible to decrease possibility of infection from catheterization and to give her a sense of control over her body functions.
Verify that she knows rationale for need to empty bladder.	Adds to her knowledge base and encourages self-care.

Continued.

Procedure 24.4 —cont'd

NURSING ACTION	RATIONALE
Catheterize, If Needed, Per Physician's Order	Swelling, pain, and residual effects of analgesia/anesthesia may prevent spontaneous voiding.
If spontaneous voiding has not occurred by 6 hours after delivery, catheterization is usually ordered.	Ensures emptying of the bladder.
Use aseptic technique.	Minimizes infection.
If urinary meatus is difficult to visualize because of swelling, with a dry sterile swab, gently brush upward from the vagina to the clitoris.	Causes the meatus to gape so that catheter can be inserted with the least amount of trauma.
Observe for symptomatology of infection: pain or burning on voiding, fever.	
Provide catheter care.	Minimizes infection.
Obtain urine specimen to send for culture, sensitivity, and routine urinalysis.	Identifies infection or other complication early.
If urinary antibiotic is started, counsel woman to continue to take antibiotic for the full time it is prescribed (usually 1 week).	If antibiotic is stopped too early, infection may flare up again and symptomatology will return.
If a drug such as sulfisoxazole (Gantrisin) is ordered, caution woman to avoid drinking cranberry juice.	Cranberry juice and sulfisoxazole (Gantrisin) combine to form a precipitate that causes considerable discomfort and requires therapy for about a week to clear out of the urinary tract.
After catheterization, assess for adequacy of spontaneous voiding, e.g., record times and amounts.	Ensure bladder functioning and adequacy of emptying.
Report retention with overflow.	
Teach mother symptomatology of urinary tract infection.	Early identification and therapy reduce morbidity. Bladder infections reduce the body's ability to fight other infections.

of 8 weeks or more), since the risk of sensitization after abortion is about half the risk after a full-term pregnancy.* It is administered after delivery to any woman who meets the following three criteria: (1) the mother must be $Rh_0(D)$ negative with no Rh antibodies (i.e., indirect Coombs' test is negative), (2) the infant must be $Rh_0(D)$- or D^u-positive, and (3) results of direct Coombs' test on the cord blood must be negative. If she meets these criteria, a 1:1000 dilution of $Rh_0(D)$ immune globulin† is cross-matched to the mother's red cells to ensure compatibility. The same precautions are followed when administering a blood transfusion to ensure that the immune globulin is administered to the correct woman. *If administered to an Rh-positive person, immune globulin will act to promote lysis of the Rh-positive RBCs.* The dose is administered to the mother intramuscularly (*never* intravenously or to the infant).

Cultural aspects of postdelivery care. The greatest conflict between Western and non-Western beliefs and practices in childbearing occurs in the postdelivery period. If a woman delivers in the hospital, she and her family are directly confronted with culturally related problems that are not as easily resolved as those encountered in the prenatal and labor and delivery stages. Moreover, nurses caring for these mothers may view the woman's behavior as totally incomprehensible since it varies so dramatically from Western health care provider's expectations.

The behavior patterns for many cultures include a period of seclusion for women lasting from 7 to 40 days with a minimum of activity allowed for mothers. These practices are based on two beliefs previously mentioned in this chapter: that delivery has upset the balance of the mother's body and that the mother, infant, and those caring for them are in a state of pollution.

Maintenance of a state of balance. Cultures that subscribe to a belief in the necessity of body balance believe that the body has lost a great deal of heat during the labor and delivery process and that the mother is therefore subject to a number of illnesses. Thus certain practices must be followed to restore the balance of heat and cold. Adherents of both humoral and yin and yang theories have prescriptions and proscriptions for restoration of balance of heat and cold (Currier, 1978).

---

*For prenatal prophylaxis, see Chapter 31.
†A blood product. Certain religions proscribe use of blood or blood products.

Procedure 24.5

SUPPRESSION OF LACTATION

PURPOSE
1. Discourage lactation by:
   a. Mechanical suppression
   b. Pharmacologic suppression
2. Increase comfort.
3. Teach mother self-care techniques.

EQUIPMENT
1. Tight compression "uplift" breast binder.
2. Covered ice packs.

MEDICATIONS
1. Analgesics
2. Bromocriptine mesylate (Parlodel)
3. Other antilactogenics and consent forms

NURSING ACTION	RATIONALE
Mechanical Suppression	Treatment of choice.
Apply a tight compression "uplift" binder for about 72 hours; advise woman to use a snug brassiere after 72 hours.	Backpressure gives body message that milk production is not needed. Stimulus for lactation and discomfort usually ease after 72 hours.
Avoid any stimulus that could support lactation, e.g., nursing the infant, expression of colostrum, pumping of the breast, using warm water on the breasts.	Nipple stimulation releases prolactin from posterior pituitary. Emptying breast is the primary stimulus for lactation.
Use covered ice packs or analgesics as necessary.	Promotes comfort.
Do *not* restrict fluid intake or use diuretics.	These methods do not suppress lactation.
Remind mother that breast firmness, tenderness, and distension are temporary.	Symptomatology usually decreases starting about the third day.
Administration of Bromocriptine Mesylate (Parlodel):	Bromocriptine mesylate (Parlodel) is a specific peptide ergot alkaloid derivative, a potent dopamine receptor agonist. This nonhormonal, nonestrogenic agent does not act on mammary tissues. Bromocriptine mesylate acts to suppress lactation by preventing the secretion of prolactin.
Confirm physician's explanation of drug to woman.	
Begin medication after vital signs and BP have stabilized but no sooner than 4 hours after delivery.	*One side effect is hypotension in some women.*
Remain with woman when she ambulates for first time.	Precautionary measure against injury from fainting.
Assess BP q4h for 72 hours.	Identifies hypotension.
Instruct woman:	Encourages self-care.
■ Recommended therapeutic dosage is one 2.5 mg tablet twice daily with meals.	Teaches accepted method of taking medication.
■ Medication is continued for 14 days, or if necessary, for 21 days.	
■ A rebound of breast secretion, congestion, or engorgement is experienced by 18%–40% of women.	Prepares woman for possible breast tenderness and need to start mechanical suppression of lactation.
■ Breast symptoms are usually only mild to moderate in severity.	May relieve anxiety by knowing that this occurrence is normal.
■ Mechanical suppression method to suppress symptomatology.	Encourages self-care. Adds to woman's knowledge base.
Administration of Other Antilactogenics	The administration of estrogens or androgens is not used often today and is not recommended to suppress lactation. Recent research has implicated the use of estrogen or other hormones as lactation-suppressant drugs in the cause of endometrial cancer. The woman must give informed consent to the use of these drugs. Estrogens have also been implicated in the occurrence of thromboembolism after delivery, particularly after cesarean delivery or a complicated vaginal delivery.
Follow hospital protocol for obtaining an informed consent.	
Administer medication per physician's directives.	
Observe woman for thrombus formation as per schedule (Table 24.2).	

Table 24.4
Summary of Measures to Stimulate Uterine Tone

Nonpharmacologic Measures	Rationale
Massage	Causes reflex contraction of muscles. Overstimulation could lead to muscle fatigue and atony.
Remove clots, if present	Keeps uterus empty to allow muscle fibers to contract completely.
Keep bladder empty	Prevents bladder distension, which elevates and displaces uterus, resulting in uterine atony.
Stimulate breasts or nipples (manually or by suckling infant)	Causes release of oxytocin from posterior pituitary.

Pharmacologic Interventions	Action, Uses During Puerperium	Onset of Effect, Duration, Usual Dose	Contraindications, Precautions	Comments
Oxytocin injection, USP (10 U/ml) (Pitocin, Syntocinon, Uteracon), oxytocic, synthetic posterior pituitary hormone	Stimulates phasic uterine muscle contraction, promotes milk ejection (let-down) reflex, facilitates flow of milk during engorgement.	IV injection, 10 U; onset in 1 min. IV infusion, 10-40 U/1000 ml 5% dextrose or physiologic electrolyte solution. IM injection, 3-10 U; onset in 3-7 min; duration 30-60 min	Hypersensitivity; return of atony when effect wears off. May cause severe hypertension if client is also receiving ephedrine, methoxamine, or other vasopressors.	**Alert:** Assess for return of atony; store in cool place.
Ergonovine maleate, USP, NF (Ergotrate maleate); oxytocic, ergot alkaloid	Stimulates prolonged, nonphasic uterine contractions.	Oral: 0.2-0.4 mg every 6-12 h for 48 h; onset in 6-15 min. IM injection: 0.2 mg (1 ml) if nausea precludes oral preparation, onset "in a few minutes." Initial response: firm, titanic contraction. Subsequent response: alternating minor relaxations and contractions for 1½ h; then vigorous rhythmic contractions for 3-4 h after injection.	Severe hypertensive episodes may occur if given to hypertensive clients or those receiving vasoconstrictors; hypersensitivity; nausea, vomiting; sudden change in blood pressure or pulse.	**Alert:** Assess for changes in blood pressure, pulse; store in cool place.
Methylergonovine maleate, NF (Methergine); oxytocic, ergot alkaloid and congener of lysergic acid (LSD)	Stimulates rapid, sustained titanic uterine contractions; used in treatment of subinvolution; has only minimum vasoconstrictive effect.	Oral: 0.2 mg tab, every 6-8 h for maximum of 1 wk; onset in 5-10 min. IM injection 0.2 mg (1 ml) every 2-4 h; onset in 2-5 min. IV infusion (emergency only): 0.2 mg (1 ml) slowly over 60 s; onset immediate.	Nausea, vomiting; transient hypertension; dizziness, headache; tinnitus; diaphoresis; palpitations; temporary chest pains.	**Alert:** Do not administer with Percodan—may result in hallucinations; assess blood pressure; store in cold place, away from light.

Food is one way in which heat can be restored and cold diminished. The classic Chinese diet (Campbell and Chang, 1973) represents an effort to decrease yin forces, which are cold. Included are an abundance of hot foods. The quality of heat and cold cannot always be measured by actual temperature. The essence of cold might be in a food even if the food is heated.

Pillsbury (1978) notes that some foods are considered cold because they are grown in the damp earth or in watery places. Green vegetables, fruits, meats, and fish are frequently considered cold foods. For Asians, rice, eggs, and chicken soup are foods high in quality of hotness and should be eaten frequently. For many cultures, chicken surpasses all other foods as a desirable

Guidelines for Client Teaching

BREAST SELF-EXAMINATION (BSE)

ASSESSMENT

Woman states she does not know how to examine her breasts.

NURSING DIAGNOSIS

Knowledge deficit related to self-care: breast self-examination.

GOALS
Short-term

Woman will verbalize steps of BSE and rationale.
Woman will demonstrate procedure correctly.

Intermediate 1 (by first postpartum check-up)

Woman verbalizes steps of BSE and rationale.
Woman states she has examined her breasts once.
After weaning: woman will be familiar with the normal feel and appearance of her breasts.

Long-term

Woman performs BSE every month.

REFERENCES AND TEACHING AIDS

American Cancer Society's pamphlet: *How to examine your breasts**
Mirror
Model for practicing palpation and recognition of masses

CONTENT/RATIONALE

TEACHING ACTION

HOW TO EXAMINE YOUR BREASTS*

This simple 3-step procedure could save your life by finding breast cancer early when it is most curable.

Provide pamphlet, mirror, and model for practice.

In the shower

Examine your breasts during bath or shower; hands glide easier over wet skin. Fingers flat, move gently over every part of each breast. Use right hand to examine left breast, left hand for right breast. Check for any lump, hard knot, or thickening.

Guide woman through steps outlined in the pamphlet.
Encourage questions.
Give answers honestly and simply.

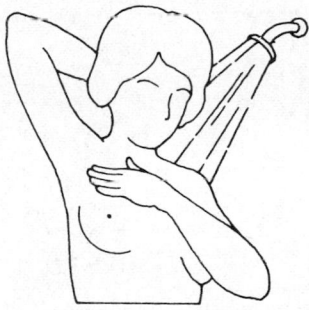

Before a mirror

Inspect your breasts with arms at your sides. Next, raise your arms high overhead. Look for any changes in contour of each breast, a swelling, dimpling of skin, or changes in the nipple.
Then, rest palms on hips and press down firmly to flex your chest muscles. Left and right breast will not exactly match—few women's breasts do.
Regular inspection shows what is normal for you and will give you confidence in your examination.

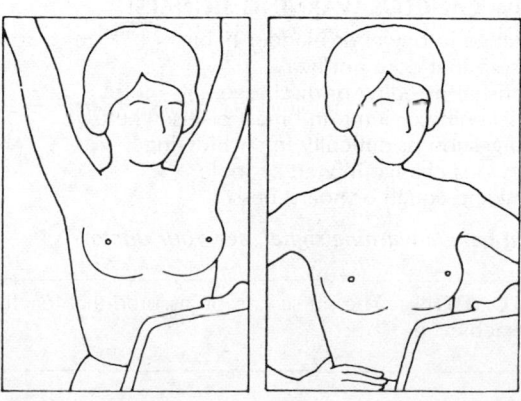

---

*From American Cancer Society: How to examine your breasts, Pamphlet no. 2088-LE, June 1978, The Society.

Continued.

Guidelines for Client Teaching—cont'd

CONTENT/RATIONALE	TEACHING ACTION

Lying down

To examine your right breast, put a pillow or folded towel under your right shoulder. Place right hand behind your head—this distributes breast tissue more evenly on the chest. With left hand, fingers flat, press gently in small circular motions around an imaginary clock face. Begin at outermost top of your right breast for 12 o'clock, then move to 1 o'clock, and so on around the circle back to 12. A ridge of firm tissue in the lower curve of each breast is normal. Then move in an inch, toward the nipple, keep circling to examine *every part of your breast,* including nipple. This requires at least three more circles. Now slowly repeat procedure on your left breast with a pillow under your left shoulder and left hand behind head. Notice how your breast structure feels.

Finally squeeze the nipple of each breast gently between thumb and index finger. Any discharge, clear or bloody, should be reported to your doctor immediately.

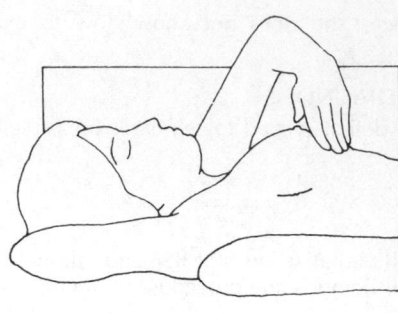

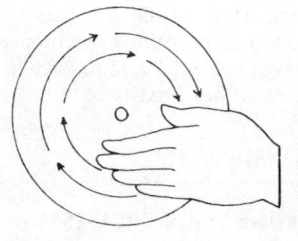

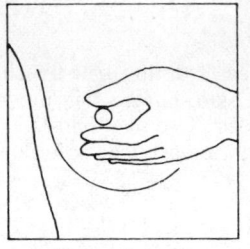

Why you should examine your breasts monthly

Most breast cancers are first discovered by women themselves. Since breast cancers found early and treated promptly have excellent chances for cure, learning how to examine your breasts properly can help save your life. Use the simple 3-step breast self-examination (BSE) procedure shown here.

For the best time to examine your breasts

Follow the same procedure once a month about a week after your period, when breasts are usually not tender or swollen (Fig. 5.28). After menopause, check breasts on the first day of each month. After hysterectomy, check your doctor or clinic for an appropriate time of the month. Doing BSE will give you monthly peace of mind, and seeing your doctor once a year will reassure you there is nothing wrong.

What you should do if you find a lump or thickening

If a lump or dimple or discharge is discovered during BSE, it is important to see your doctor as soon as possible. Don't be frightened. Most breast lumps or changes are not cancer, but only your doctor can make the diagnosis.

KNOW CANCER'S WARNING SIGNALS!

Change in bowel or bladder habits
A sore that does not heal
Unusual bleeding or discharge
Thickening or lump in breast or elsewhere
Indigestion or difficulty in swallowing
Obvious change in wart or mole
Nagging cough or hoarseness

If you have a warning signal, see your doctor.

EVALUATION   The nurse can be assured that teaching has been effective when all the goals have been achieved.

Guidelines for Client Teaching

POSTPARTUM EXERCISES

ASSESSMENT
Woman has just completed a full-term pregnancy.

NURSING DIAGNOSES
Knowledge deficit related to postpartum exercises.
Knowledge deficit related to diastasis of rectus abdominis muscle.
Potential for disturbance in self-concept related to change in body image.

GOALS
Short-term
Woman verbalized understanding of exercise program.
Woman begins exercise recommended for the first postpartum day.

Intermediate
Woman follows exercise program without untoward responses (e.g., fatigue).

Long-term
Woman continues with a balance between rest and exercise or activity.
Woman verbalizes satisfaction with the way she feels and looks.

REFERENCES AND TEACHING AIDS
Handout with illustrations and description of exercise program.

CONTENT/RATIONALE	TEACHING ACTION
Rigorous exercise may initiate uterine bleeding or fatigue and discomfort.	Caution woman against too rigorous and taxing exercises, regardless of the physical fitness of the woman.
Toning of the abdominal muscles takes time.	
Program progresses slowly from easy to more demanding exercises.	Review exercise program (pp. 677 and 678).
Girdles or other abdominal supports tend to make the woman "forget" to keep abdominal muscles contracted and thus delay regaining tone.	Discourage woman from wearing girdles or other abdominal supports.
Fatigue or discomfort drain energy needed for recovery and care of newborn and of self.	Remind her to stop exercise if she becomes fatigued.
Kegel exercises begun soon after delivery, or as soon as anesthesia has worn off, aid in the recovery of the pubococcygeal muscle, which is stretched during vaginal delivery. These exercises help restore muscle tone and function and facilitate healing during the puerperium by increasing circulation to this area. Kegel (1948) demonstrated that a strong pubococcygeal muscle is important in preventing and treating urinary stress incontinence and pelvic relaxation as well as in achieving and maintaining vaginal orgasm.	Assess woman's knowledge of Kegel exercises and review as needed.
There is no known therapy to prevent or treat diastasis (separation) of the rectus abdominis muscle.	If the woman has diastasis (separation) of the rectus abdominis muscle. ■ Share with her that the separation usually lessens with time, but that if separation is quite wide, it may not return to prepregnant state. ■ Share with her that exercise or girdles have not been known to speed the rate of recovery.

EVALUATION   The nurse can be assured that care was effective when the goals have been met.

hot food. Chicken soup is also believed important in the production of a nursing mother's milk. It is obvious that many, if not most, of the foods served on hospital trays, such as meats, vegetables, fruits, and fruit juices, are considered cold. These will probably not be eaten by many Asian, Southeast Asian, and Spanish-speaking women.

In addition to food, contact with air and wind is proscribed by Asians, Filipinos, Mexican-Americans, and southern blacks. Cold must be prevented from entering the body, to counteract further imbalance. Air is considered cold, whatever the temperature, and thus windows and doors must be kept closed. The Chinese belief that a woman's pores are open for 30 days after

Fig. 24.4
Postpartum exercise program.

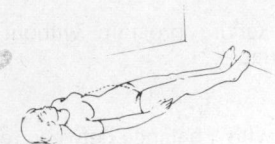

1st day: Raise abdomen while inhaling deeply. Slowly exhale through pursed lips while contracting abdominal muscle forcibly.

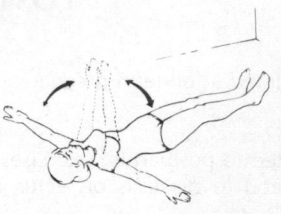

2nd day: Lying on your back with your legs slightly parted, place your arms at right angles to your body and slowly raise them, keeping your elbows stiff. When your hands touch, lower your arms gradually.

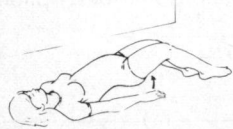

3rd day: Lying with your arms at your sides, draw your knees up slightly, arch your back.

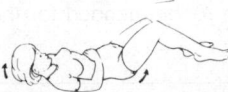

4th day: Lying with your knees and hips flexed, tilt your pelvis inward and tightly contract your buttocks as you lift your head.

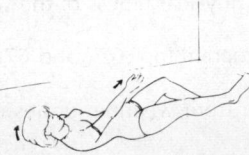

5th day: Lying with your legs straight, raise your head and left knee slightly, then reach for (but do not touch) your left knee with your right hand. Repeat using your right knee and left hand.

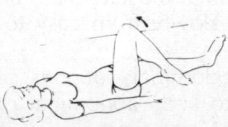

6th day: Lying on your back, slowly flex the knee and then the thigh toward the abdomen, lower your foot toward your buttock, then straighten and lower your leg.

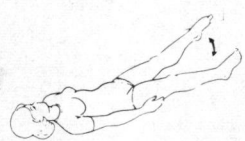

7th day: Lying on your back, toes pointed and knees straight, raise one leg and then the other as high as possible, using your abdominal muscles but not your hands to lower your legs slowly.

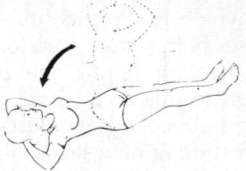

10th day: Lying on your back with your arms clasped behind your head, sit up and lie back slowly. At first you may have to hook your feet under furniture.

delivering a baby coincides with the period in which they believe the mother has an excess of cold (Campbell and Chang, 1973; Pillsbury, 1978). Air conditioners are a source of fear for women in the hospital. Fans are to be avoided. New mothers will keep themslves totally covered with blankets despite how hot the temperature of the room may be.

Water is considered cold at all times, even if it is heated. Therefore not bathing for a period of time is a widely held belief. Some mothers will take all kinds of measures to avoid the daily shower but will not directly refuse, complying by going to the shower room, turning on the water, and remaining in such a position that the water will not touch them. Pillsbury (1978) notes that Chinese women who have been westernized in so many ways still adhere to the postpartal practice of avoiding water. They must not wash themselves, their dishes, or their clothes. To the Chinese and other Asians, contact with water, considered cold, causes wind to enter the body and will result in future years in asthma, arthritis, and chronic aches and pains. However, if a hot substance is added to boiled water, it may counteract the coldness. For example, the chicken soup is so powerful that the cold quality of the

Guidelines for Client Teaching

RESUMPTION OF SEXUAL INTERCOURSE

ASSESSMENT

Couple state they wish to resume sexual intercourse by the third or fourth postdelivery week if bleeding has stopped and the episiotomy is healed.

Couple has heard that the first intercourse following delivery may be painful.

Couple has heard that reactions to sexual stimulation may be altered for a short time after delivery.

NURSING DIAGNOSES

Knowledge deficit related to resumption of sexual intercourse following delivery:

1. Timing of first intercourse.
2. Need for contraception if pregnancy is not desired.

Anxiety related to insufficient knowledge of postdelivery physiology and healing.

Alteration in comfort related to dryness of vaginal mucosa.

Ineffective family coping related to lack of knowledge of:

1. Timing for resumption of sexual intercourse.
2. Measures needed to promote comfort.
3. Precautions to prevent unplanned pregnancy (see Guidelines for Client Teaching: Postdelivery Contraception, p. 683).

GOALS

Short-term (within 3 to 4 weeks)

Woman or couple verbalize understanding of content.

Couple discuss subject between them and mutually agree to a course of action.

Intermediate

Couple resume sexual intercourse by mutual agreement.

Experience is without discomfort.

No pregnancy results.

Long-term

Couple maintain open lines of communication.

Couple mutually agree on choice of family planning methods.

REFERENCES AND TEACHING AIDS

Printed instructions from agency

Illustrations

Bing, E., and Colman, L.: Making love during pregnancy, New York, 1977, Bantam Books

---

CONTENT/RATIONALE

Information about postdelivery physiology and its effects on resumption of sexual intercourse:

The couple can safely resume sexual intercourse by the third or fourth postdelivery week if bleeding has stopped and the episiotomy has healed. For the first 6 weeks to 6 months the vagina does not lubricate well because steroid depletion inhibits the vasocongestive response to sexual tension.

Physiologic reactions to sexual stimulation for the first 3 postdelivery months are marked by a reduction in both rapidity and intensity of response. Vasocongestion of the labia majora and minora is delayed well into the plateau phase. The walls of the vagina are thin and pink, a condition similar to senile vaginitis. This results from the hormonal starvation of the involutional period. Finally, the size of the orgasmic platform and strength of orgasmic contractions are reduced.

A water-soluble gel, cocoa butter, or a contraceptive cream or jelly might be recommended for lubrication. If some vaginal tenderness is present, the partner can be instructed to insert one or two fingers into the vagina and rotate them within the vagina to help relax it and to identify possible areas of discomfort. A coital position in which the woman has control of the depth of penile penetration is also useful. The side-by-side or female-superior position often is recommended.

The presence of the baby influences postdelivery love-making. Parents hear every sound made by the baby; conversely they may be concerned that the baby hears every sound they make. In either case any phase of the sexual response cycle may be interrupted by hearing the baby cry or move, leaving one or both of the couple frustrated

TEACHING ACTIONS

Share information with woman and couple.

Encourage questions. Encourage open discussion between couple. Encourage couple to problem-solve the situation together.

Provide as many alternatives as possible to serve as a basis for discussion and to provide choices.

Acknowledge that this may be a difficult area for some people to talk about.

Validate that although these responses are within normal expectations, it still may be difficult to deal with frustration at times.

Continued.

Guidelines for Client Teaching—cont'd

CONTENT/RATIONALE	TEACHING ACTIONS
and unsatisfied. The amount of psychologic and physiologic energy expended by the parents in child care activities may lead to fatigue. One newborn requires a great deal of attention and time; imagine caring for twins, triplets, or older children as well!	
Some women have reported sexual stimulation to plateau and orgasmic levels when nursing their babies. It is interesting to note that although nursing mothers have a longer delay in ovarian steroid production, they are often interested in returning to sexual activity before nonnursing mothers. Nursing mothers also report higher levels of postdelivery eroticism.	Suggest that the woman take a rest during the day when the baby sleeps.
In the event of fetal or newborn death or the birth of an infant who is small, sick, or deformed, the emotional energy required of the woman and her partner, the mother's depleted physical state, and the stress of burying the dead child or of visiting the hospitalized child strain all relationships. Because little definitive data are available, professional caregivers can only speculate about the effect on sexual relationships during these stressful periods.	Help parents cope with grief (see Chapter 26).
The woman should be instructed to follow the Kegel exercises to strengthen her pubococcygeal muscle. The pubococcygeal muscle is the major sphincter of the pelvis. It is associated with bowel and bladder function and with vaginal perception and response during intercourse.	Teach Kegel exercises (see Chapter 11).

EVALUATION   The nurse can be assured that the care was effective when the goals have been met.

---

water with which it is made is counteracted. Ginger added to very hot water that has been boiled may cause the same effect. It is obvious then, that ice water, used frequently in hospitals, is forbidden.

Pollution state. In addition to an imbalance of hot and cold, several cultures consider that the mother and infant are in a state of pollution after delivery. A certain time must elapse and certain rituals must be performed before purity is restored. A state of seclusion is frequently compulsory, during which time the mother is encouraged to limit her activities. This is in contrast to the hospital practice of early ambulation following delivery, early infant care responsibilities, and early discharge from the hospital. Mexican-Americans may observe *la cuarentina* for 40 days after birth of babies (Clark, 1970). For the Chinese mother, going out during the first month after birth will offend the gods because dirty birth blood remains throughout the month (Pillsbury, 1978). The Filipino mother (Stern and others, 1980) is frequently misunderstood as lazy and not caring when she refuses to do what is requested in the hospital and at home. Recently, in a personal communication from a group of Cambodian women, concern was expressed about how they will

manage after the baby is born because they do not have an extended family to assist during the required time of seclusion and limited activity. The fear of subsequent illness, especially arthritis, in later years is very real to them. Homemaker services are not available to them because according to the Western view, they are able bodied and assistance cannot be justified. Their hope for the future is based on the belief that counteracting the bad effects of not carrying out cultural prescriptions for the postpartal period can be accomplished only by going through a follow-up pregnancy correctly. Their chances of doing future pregnancies "correctly" is remote, however. The cultural quandary for these women is clear.

Snow (1974) described the view of southern blacks that blood is a pollutant that carries contaminants from the body. Southern blacks and others believe that an adequate lochia flow is essential and going outside in the wind or air could thicken and halt the flow of blood, extending the time of pollution. Some Filipino mothers may remain bedfast for 2 weeks, after which time a special bath is taken to further remove the debris of pregnancy believed to be found in perspiration. According to Stern and co-workers (1980), "roasting,"

Guidelines for Client Teaching

POSTDELIVERY CONTRACEPTION

ASSESSMENT

Woman or couple request information regarding contraception after delivery.

Woman has heard that women cannot become pregnant while breast feeding.

NURSING DIAGNOSES

Ineffective family coping related to unplanned pregnancy.

Potential for disruption in lactation related to resumption of hormonal contraception.*

GOALS

Short-term

Woman or couple verbalize understanding of content.

Couple discuss postdelivery contraception.

Intermediate

Couple mutually agree on and employ contraceptive gels or foams, diaphragms, and condoms.

Long-term

Couple maintain open lines of communication.

Couple mutually agree on choice of family planning method.

CONTENT/RATIONALE

Content about contraception (see Chapter 7).

Women neither menstruate nor conceive while they successfully nurse their infant because all ovarian functions are suppressed by a high level of serum prolactin. This hormone, which is responsible for milk production, rises slowly during pregnancy and increases rapidly to a plateau with suckling. Prolactin blocks the production of pituitary gonadotropin; hence the ovaries become inactive. Follicle formation is suspended, and ovulation does not occur. Consequently the secretion of estrogen is minimal, and no progesterone is produced. However, women who do not nurse frequently or on demand (e.g., every 3 to 4 hours) or *who supplement the infant's feeding* do not maintain an effectively high level of serum prolactin; follicle-stimulating hormone (FSH), luteinizing hormone (LH), and estrogen are secreted once more, and ovulation and menstruation resume. If these women do not employ contraceptives, they may conceive again, sometimes without having a period following the prior pregnancy.

If the mother is not nursing, she may resume use of oral contraceptives (after delivery) under the physician's direction. If she is nursing, contraception, such as a diaphragm, condom, gel, or foam, should be provided until the first postdelivery examination, at which time the desired method can be instituted (see Chapter 7).

TEACHING ACTION

Discuss and outline a tentative program within the first week after delivery.

Share information with woman and couple.

Encourage questions. Encourage open discussion between couple. Encourage couple to problem-solve the situation together.

Provide as many alternatives as possible to serve as a basis for discussion and to provide choices.

Acknowledge that this may be a difficult area for some people to talk about.

EVALUATION   The nurse can be assured that care was effective when the goals have been achieved.

---

*Diagnosis not included by NANDA, 1986.

---

or sitting on a slotted chair over a small fire, is practiced by Filipinos in the most remote provinces only. The purpose of this is to hasten the healing process, much like perineal heat lamps used in recent times.

Horn (1982) supplies a recent example of acculturated behavior. After the birth of her first child, a Greek-American mother followed the ancient proscription of participation in church activities for 40 days.

While her husband attended the church wedding of a friend, this woman did her weekly shopping at the local supermarket. In most cultural groups sexual relations are prohibited until after the seclusion period and sometimes throughout lactation.

Some cultural groups have unique practices. For example, the women of Northern Thailand bind their wrists with string. The purpose of wrist binding is to prevent the loss of the soul, which may lead to wind disease, a specific complex of symptoms indicating a state of humoral imbalance characterized by weakness, nausea, and hypersensitivity to odors (Kundstadter, 1978). Northern Thai women giving birth will most likely have their wrists bound and would be extremely frightened and upset if the strings were removed.

The preceding examples indicate that, from the time of delivery to a certain designated time afterward, mothers in many cultures are considered highly susceptible to ensuing illness, either immediately or at an unspecified time in the future. Furthermore, their state of pollution requires that only certain persons contact them during the specified time they remain in seclusion. Most of their activities are carried on by others, usually members of the extended family or friends. The end of the time of seclusion is often marked by a ceremony and includes ritual cleansing of the woman, child, and place of seclusion (Brownlee, 1978). It is important for nurses to understand these factors, assist women in carrying out their beliefs and practices insofar as is possible, and assist them with necessary adjustments when their expectations are not feasible.

Evaluation. Evaluation is a continuous process. To be effective, evaluation is based on measurable criteria. The criteria reflect the parameters used to measure attainment of goals. The mother's recovery from childbirth is marked by definitive signs and symptoms. These signs and symptoms form the basis for continued evaluation of the involutionary process. The nurse's role as support person in providing emotional care to the new mother and family is as vital as the roles of technician, teacher/advocate/counselor. The discussion of the nurse's role as support person follows.

Emotional Care: The Nurse as Support Person

Nurses have played a leadership role in efforts to provide holistic client care in the postpartum period. Interventions aimed at establishing healthy early family relationships can be the unique contribution of nursing. Healthy family relationships promote the growth potential of the newborn and other family members. The care described in this part of the chapter is based on careful assessment and formulation of nursing diagnoses. It includes planning for and implementing appropriate nursing actions and evaluating their effectiveness.

Assessment of parental responses. Parental responses to the birth of a child include behaviors that are either adaptive or maladaptive. Both mother and father exhibit these behaviors, although to date most research has centered on the mother. Parents who are faced with a severe life stress may not be able to provide supportive parenting for their child. Life stress reduces both psychologic well-being and physical health. These are two important factors in establishing and maintaining relationships with others (Tansig, 1982; Thoits, 1983). Another critical factor is a feeling of personal control. Personal control is a "key element in the attitudes toward self and the world that are characteristic of the competent self" (Turner and Avison, 1985). Those people who do not possess a sense of control seem less able to make the purposive decisions that are necessary to plan for the future of their families (Turner and Avison, 1985).

The quality of motherliness or fatherliness in parent's behavior prompts nurturing and protection as opposed to neglect or abuse of their child. Cues indicating the presence or absence of this quality appear early in the postdelivery period as parents react to the newborn child and continue the process of establishing a relationship (Table 24.5).

Adaptive behavior. Adaptive behaviors stem from the parent's realistic perception and acceptance of their newborn's needs and his or her limited abilities, immature social responses, and helplessness (Steele and Pollock, 1968). According to Morris (1966):

Mother-infant unity can be said to be satisfactory when a mother can find pleasure in her infant and in the tasks for and with him; understand his emotional states and comfort him; read his cues for new experience, and sense his fatigue points.

Maladaptive behavior. Maladaptive behavior is exhibited when parents respond inappropriately to the needs of their infant. They expect responses from the infant far in excess of the infant's ability to perform. They interpret inadequate responses as defiance or as negative judgment of parental capabilities. They obtain no pleasure from physical contact with their child. Such infants tend to be handled roughly. They are held in a manner that allows the head to dangle without support, and are not cuddled. The parents see the child as unattractive. The child caring tasks of bathing and changing are viewed with disgust or annoyance. There is a lack of discrimination in responding to the infant's signals relative to hunger, fatigue, need for soothing or stimulating speech, and need for comforting body or eye contact. The parents of these infants often show excessive concern over the health of their child and cannot distinguish between the expected minor illnesses of childhood and serious disabilities. It appears difficult for them to accept their child as healthy and happy.

Table 24.5
Mothering Behaviors

Adaptive Behaviors	Maladaptive Behaviors
Feeding	
Offers appropriate amount and/or type of food to infant	Provides inadequate type or amount of food for infant
Holds infant in comfortable position during feeding	Does not hold infant, or holds in uncomfortable position during feeding
Burps baby during and/or after feeding	Does not burp infant
Prepares food appropriately	Prepares food inappropriately
Offers food at comfortable pace for infant	Offers food at pace too rapid or slow for infant's comfort
Infant stimulation	
Provides appropriate verbal stimulation for infant during visit	Provides no, or only aggressive, verbal stimulation for infant during visit
Provides tactile stimulation for infant at times other than during feeding or moving infant away from danger	Does not provide tactile stimulation or only that of aggressive handling of infant
Provides age-appropriate toys	No evidence of age-appropriate toys
Interacts with infant in a way that provides for infant's satisfaction	Frustrates infant during interactions
Infant rest	
Provides quiet or relaxed environment for infant's rest, including scheduled rest periods	Does not provide quiet environment or consistent schedule for rest periods
Ensures that infant's needs for food, warmth, and/or dryness are met before sleep	Does not attend to infant's needs for food, warmth, and/or dryness before sleep
Perception	
Demonstrates realistic perception of infant's condition in accordance with medical and/or nursing diagnosis	Shows unrealistic perception of infant's condition
Has realistic expectations for infant	Demonstrates unrealistic expectations of infant
Recognizes infant's unfolding skills or behavior	Has no awareness of infant's development
Shows realistic perception of own mothering behavior	Shows unrealistic perception of own mothering
Initiative	
Shows initiative in attempts to manage infant's problems, including actively seeking information about infants	Shows no initiative in attempts to meet infant's needs or to manage problems; does not follow through with plans
Recreation	
Provides positive outlets for own recreation or relaxation	Does not provide positive outlets for own recreation or relaxation
Interaction with other children	
Demonstrates positive interaction with other children in home	Demonstrates hostile-aggressive interaction with other children in home
Mothering role	
Expresses satisfaction with mothering	Expresses dissatisfaction with mothering

Reprinted by permission from Mercer, R.T.: In Sonstegard, L.J., and others, editors: Women's health: childbearing vol. 2, New York, 1982, Grune & Stratton, p. 30.

Response to the infant. The parents' response is profoundly affected by their interpretation of the infant's response. Feedback is an important component in any relationship. Mothers and fathers make value judgments about their infant's behavior and respond as though the baby had either "praised" or "criticized" them. Table 24.6 provides a listing of infant behaviors and their evaluation by parents as either adaptive (positive feedback) or maladaptive (negative feedback) (Mercer, 1982).

Many new mothers will experience *parenting diffi-* *culties* until their skills become established. Once they feel confidence in their skills, the increase in self-esteem promotes a positive affective response to the child. However, some parents will exhibit *parenting disorders* (a matter of degree) that place the child in jeopardy and at risk. Protocols for the physical screening of high-risk mothers and infants have been developed and confirmed. However, tools predicting high-risk parenting behaviors require more replication over larger population samples before they can be used with the same precision (see Table 11.9).

Table 24.6
Infant Behaviors

Adaptive Behaviors	Maladaptive Behaviors
Sleeping	
Receives adequate sleep for normal growth—at least 17 hours each day without restless sleep patterns or prolonged crying at nap or bedtime after other needs have been met	Receives inadequate sleep for normal growth—less than 16 hours each day; shows restless sleep patterns and/or prolonged crying at nap or bedtime.
Feeding	
Actively seeks food offered	Resists food offered
Actively sucks and swallows food	Does not suck effectively
Demonstrates pleasurable relief after eating	Remains fussy after adequate amount of feeding—no pleasurable relief
Response to environment	
Demonstrates active response to environment by ignoring or reaching-out behavior	Seems apathetic to environment
Vocalizing	
Demonstrates vocalizations when alert if developmentally ready	Makes infrequent or no vocalizations during visit although developmentally ready
Smiling	
Demonstrates smiling behavior if older than 2 months	Does not demonstrate smiling behavior during visit
Cuddling	
Cuddles when held	Resists being held or stiffens when held

Reprinted by permission from Mercer, R.T.: In Sonstegard, L.J., and others, editors: Women's health: childbearing vol. 2, New York, 1982 Grune & Stratton, Inc., p. 31.

Response to family and friends. The families and friends of the parents and their newborn child form an important dimension of the parent's social network. Social networks provide a support system on which parents can rely for assistance (Cronenwett, 1985a and b; Crawford, 1985). Positive emotional and affectional relationships appear critical to the enhancement of parenting skills and nurturance of children (Gottlieb, 1980; Schronkoff, 1984). Social networks function to promote the growth potential of children and the prevention of their maltreatment. Mercer (1982) and Crawford (1985) found that social networks provided support but were also a source of conflict. Parents or in-laws who assisted with household responsibilities and who did not intrude into the parent's privacy or critically judge them were most appreciated. Too large a network caused problems in that it generated conflicting advice to the new parents. Caretakers need to be alert to parents who have positive family circumstances, as well as to those who exhibit warning signs during the postdelivery period (Table 24.7).

Assessment strategies. Observing and interviewing provide much of the information needed to assess parent and child relationships and competency in child care. The nurse observes parental attitudes toward themselves and their responsibilities. She or he assesses the mother's perceptual acuity and the amount of physical and psychic energy the mother possesses. Cultural or ethnic variations in maternal and paternal roles are also noted. This information provides the context within which the parents will give care to their child. Competency in child care can be determined during feeding periods or when the mother or father is giving general care to the infant (Fig. 24.5).

Stainton (1981) has devised scoring tools for assessing parent-child interaction for use in the postdelivery period (Box, p. 689). The tools reflect the change in the mother's and father's responses as they move from first contact after delivery through the early puerperium. The tools are concise enough for easy application. They can assist the nurse to assess behaviors that may indicate adaptation or maladaptation to the parental role.

Recent studies (Bampton, 1981; Dunn and White, 1981; Tulman, 1985) relative to the sequencing of mothers' first touching and handling their newborn have revealed that they hold and manipulate their newborn using hands, arms, and trunk. They explore the details of their infant's body using their fingertips. The fingertip touch may be related to an instinctive use of highly sensitive areas to explore surfaces. The sequence of fingers, palms, arms, and trunk first proposed by

Table 24.7
Family Behaviors

Adaptive Behaviors	Maladaptive Behaviors
Marriage is stable.	Husband's or family's reactions to the baby have been negative or nonsupportive.
Father has stable job.	Mother is receiving little or no meaningful support from anyone.
Mother's intelligence and health are good.	There are sibling rivalry problems or a complete lack of understanding of this possibility.
Parents have their own home and stable living conditions.	Husband is jealous of the baby's drain on mother's time, energy, and affection.
Parents can have fun together and enjoy personal interests or hobbies.	Parents have expectations of development far beyond the child's capabilities.
Parents had helpful role models when growing up.	Parents remain disappointed over the sex of the child.
Parents have a good friend or relative to turn to, a sound "need-meeting" system.	Negative identification of the child: significance of name, who he or she looks like or acts like.
Parents exhibit coping abilities, i.e., capacity to plan and understand need for adjustments because of new baby.	Mother doesn't have fun with the baby.
Baby was planned or wanted.	Mother avoids eye contact with the baby and avoids the direct en face position.*
Parents see likable attributes in baby, see baby as separate individual.	Verbalizations to the infant are negative, demanding, harsh, etc.
Father is supportive to mother and involved in care of baby.	Most of mother's verbalizations to others about the child are negative.
Baby is healthy and not too disruptive to parents' life-style.	Mother is bothered by crying; it makes her feel hopeless, helpless, or like crying herself.
Either parent can rescue the child or relieve the other in crisis.	Mother does not comfort the baby when he or she cries.
Future birth control is planned.	Feedings: the mother sees the baby as too demanding; she is repulsed by his or her messiness or ignores his or her demands.
	Changing diapers is seen as a negative, repulsive task.
	Mother lacks control over the situation.
	She is not involved, nor does she respond to the baby's needs, but relinquishes control to the doctors or nurses.
	When attention is focused on the child in her presence, mother does not see this as something positive for herself.
	Mother makes complaints about the baby that cannot be verified.

Reproduced by permission and adapted from Gray, J.D., Christy, A.C., Dean, G.D., and Kempe, C.H.: Prediction and prevention of child abuse, Semin. Perinatol. 3:35, Jan. 1979.

*Eye contact is an important facet of attachment in our culture; however, it is not seen as important universally.

Fig. 24.5
Father bathes his infant with support of nursing student. (Courtesy Colleen Stainton.)

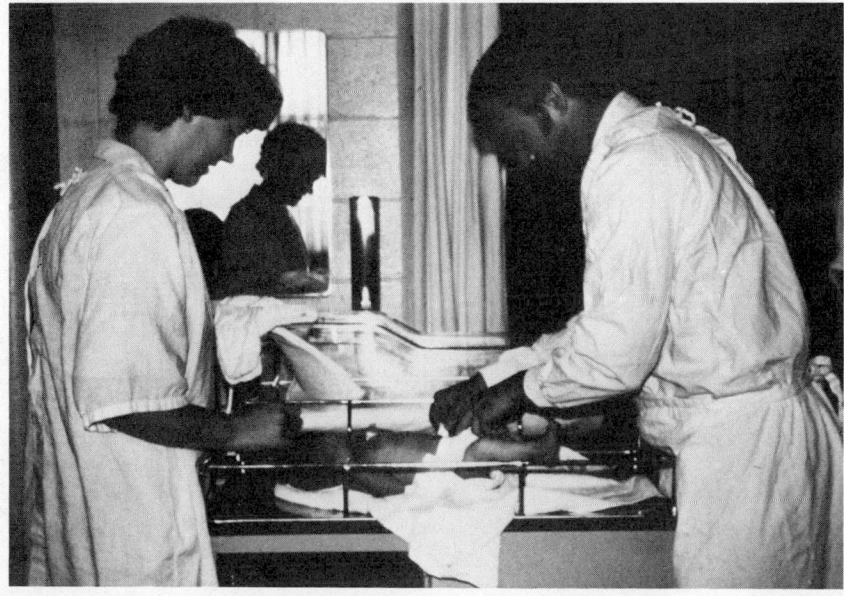

Rubin (1963) is seen in caretakers other than mothers; that is, fathers, nursing, and medical students (Rödholm, 1981). Therefore the pattern of handling may not be a valid criterion of maternal attachment (Tulman, 1985).

Nursing diagnoses. After analyzing the data obtained from assessment, the nurse establishes nursing diagnoses that will act as guides to action. The following are examples of diagnoses made for specific clients:

1. Alteration in family processes related to unexpected birth of twins
2. Impaired verbal communication related to client's deafness
3. Alteration in parenting related to long, difficult labor

Planning. The postnatal period is a crucial one for the family. It contains the potential for crisis in family adjustment. Developing a plan of care that recognizes family strengths and provides support for family weaknesses does much to assist family members to take on new tasks and responsibilities.

Goals. The goals for care include the following:

1. Promotion of healthy parent-child relationships
2. Increase in parents' participation in successful care of their newborn, themselves, and other family members

Implementation. In helping parents adapt to the parental role, nurses act as support persons, teachers/counselors/advocates, and technicians. Through the loving and attentive manner they exhibit while providing physical care to the newborn and to the mother, they act as role models. As one nurse described it:

■ I found the mother crying and distraught as she wrapped and unwrapped her baby. She said, "I don't seem to be able to do anything right." I took the baby from her and talked to him. "What are you doing to your mother? You've got her all upset!" The baby alerted to my voice and looked at me. Then I said to the mother, "Now, you talk to him." She said, "You're a big lovely boy, don't cry so much." The baby hearing her voice promptly turned his head from me to look at her. I said, "You see, he knows his mother's voice and prefers it to mine." The mother was surprised and seemed very pleased and excited. We then reviewed how to wrap a baby snugly.

Feelings of self-esteem in the mother are increased through positive feedback. Fig. 24.6 shows a feedback circle in which the left side presents an example of a positive mother-infant interaction based on the sequence outlined on the right side.

Fig. 24.6
Maternal-infant feedback mechanisms. (From Stainton, M.C.: Assessment and support of healthy parent-child relationships, Proceedings of POGP: Pediatrics, Obstetrics and Gynecology Workshop for Nurses, Saskatoon, 1977, University of Saskatchewan.)

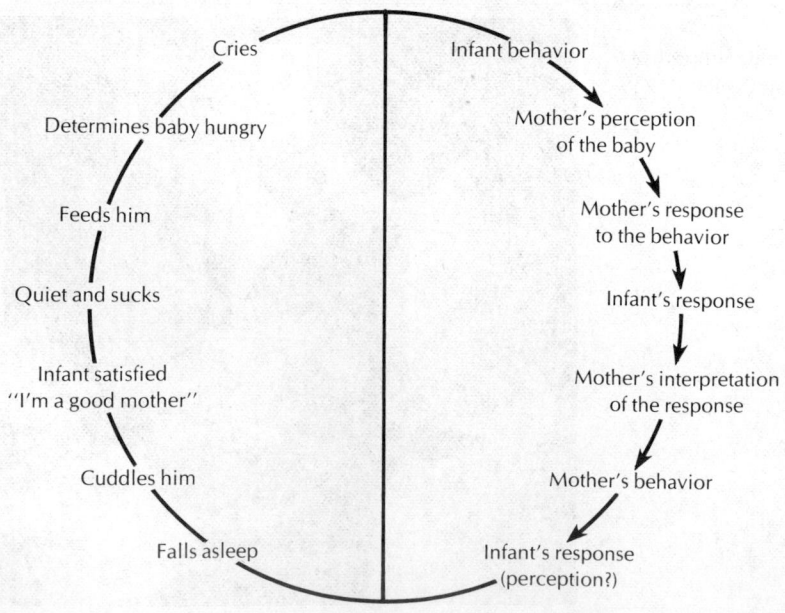

Parent-Baby Interaction

Type of delivery: Vaginal ☐ Time after birth _____ hours Para ☐☐☐☐ Gravida ☐☐☐
Cesarean ☐ Marital status _____ Age of mother _____
Father present for delivery of ☐ Yes ☐ No

Circle "M" and "F" for the best description in each of the five behavioral categories, to achieve a total score for Mother and Father: 8-10 requires *usual* nursing support for bonding; 5-7 requires *extra* nursing support for bonding; 0-4 requires *intensive* nursing support for bonding.

First contact

Two (2) points		One (1) point		Zero (0) points	
Asks for information about baby, e.g. condition, sex, appearance	M F	Listens to information given about baby without comment	M F	Express concern for self only	M F
Reaches out to baby, touching baby if possible	M F	Looks toward baby without reaching out or touching	M F	Does not look toward or touch baby	M F
Spontaneously speaks to baby in affectionate terms or tone	M F	Speaks to baby when prompted to do so	M F	Does not speak to baby (state reason why, if known)	M F
Holds baby in "en face" position and makes eye contact when possible	M F	Holds baby without maintaining "en face" or eye contact	M F	Does not hold baby (state reason why, if known)	M F
Expresses generally positive feelings about the labor and delivery experience	M F	Expresses dissatisfaction or anger at outcome of labor	M F	Even with assistance, expresses no feelings about outcome of labor	M F

Mother's total score _____ Father's total score _____
Other observations _____

Day 2

Seeks contact with baby	M F	Accepts contact with baby	M F	Avoids contact with baby	M F
With assistance, explores baby's whole skin surface	M F	Explores baby's body, avoiding some areas, e.g., genital area, back	M F	Avoids touching baby's skin	M F
Asks for interpretation of baby's appearance and behavior	M F	Interested when baby's appearance or behavior is interpreted but does not ask questions	M F	Shows little interest in baby's appearance or behavior	M F
Consistently positions baby in "en face" position and seeks eye contact with baby	M F	Positions baby in "en face" position and makes intermittent eye contact	M F	Does not hold baby in "en face" position	M F
Describe feelings about infant and her or his responses	M F	Needs assistance in describing feelings about infant and her or his responses	M F	Does not express feelings about infant or her or his responses	M F

Mother's total score _____ Father's total score _____
Other observations _____

Day 3

Holds baby close to body when feeding or cuddling, using both hands and arms	M F	Holds baby with a space between own and baby's body	M F	Unable, reluctant, or refusing to hold baby	M F
Spontaneously talks to baby, using name, "son," or endearing terms or tones	M F	Speaks about baby but does not speak directly to baby	M F	Does not speak to baby	M F
Consistently positions baby in "en face" position and maintains eye contact	M F	Positions baby in "en face" position and makes intermittent eye contact	M F	Does not make eye contact with baby	M F
Describes some infant's characteristics to listener; e.g., "He's strong"	M F	Responds with interest when infant's characteristics are pointed out	M F	Does not express any interest in infant characteristics	M F
Seeks opportunities to carry out care taking of baby	M F	Needs prompting with all caretaking of baby	M F	Unable, reluctant, or refusing to care for infant	M F

Mother's total score _____ Father's total score _____
Other observations _____

_____
Signature

Adapted from Stainton, C.M.: Parent-infant interaction: putting theory into practice, Calgary, Alta., Canada, 1981, The University of Calgary Faculty of Nursing.

Crisis prevention. Nursing is directed toward increasing the mother's mastery of the "art of motherhood," thereby increasing or sustaining her self-esteem. Nursing care encompasses measures that encourage assertive, self-reliant behaviors in family members. Research by Sullivan and Beeman (1981) indicates that parents express satisfaction with postpartum nursing care if efforts are made to facilitate parent-child relationships. This includes being willing to listen to parental review of the birth process, and to provide instruction in the care of self and infant.

Nursing interventions may be grouped under those pertaining to the crisis intervention theory: perception, situational supports, and coping mechanisms (see Chapter 1).

Perception. One of the main concepts to be stressed repeatedly is that parenthood is a learned role. As with any other learned role, it takes time to master, improves with experience, and evolves gradually and continually as the needs of the parents and child change. Rubin (1961) proposed that for 2 or 3 days after the birth of a child, a mother is receptive to learning about her new role. Rubin termed this the "taking in phase."

Caplan (1957) noted that intervention during the early peurperium had a much greater effect on influencing the attitudes of family members than it did at periods of stability of emotional functioning. Care during the early puerperium needs to reflect the mother's and father's psychological readiness for learning new skills. Table 24.8 outlines strategies the nurse can use to help the father adjust to his new role.

Mothers have been found to be receptive to information regarding their infants' interactive capabilities during the early puerperium. During this time mothers' awareness of their own behavioral responses toward their infants can be enhanced. The mother's anxiety level distorts her ability to learn.

Care of the newborn may be limited to feeding during the first few days. When the mother's strength returns, she also may wish to bathe and change the infant. Demonstrations of these techniques and supervision of her efforts are incorporated into the nursing care. Recognition and praise of her successes increase the mother's feeling of security in her ability to mother. Discussions with other mothers are very helpful. The multiparous mother provides practical advice for the primiparous mother.

Researchers in their studies of mother-infant interactions have used various techniques to promote the mother's awareness of the behavioral and social capabilities of their newborns. In one of Field's early studies (1977) mothers were asked to imitate their babies rather than attempt to keep their babies' attention. By doing this the mothers decreased their activities and increased responsiveness to infant behavior. By advising mothers to repeat phrases and to be silent during gaze aversion, Field noted mothers were increasingly sensitive to their infants' behavioral cues and responsive to their signals. Anderson (1981) combined providing information to the mother about neonatal behavior with a demonstration of the infant's behavior as a means of enhancing the quality of mother-infant in-

Table 24.8
Strategies to Support and Promote the Role of the Father, by Stages of Pregnancy

Antepartum	Intrapartum	Postpartum
Include father in initial antepartum visit and encourage his participation in all subsequent visits.	Encourage father's presence during labor and delivery. Support his planned role in labor, if appropriate.	Encourage father to come to follow-up pediatric visits.
Encourage father's involvement in birthing and parenting classes.	Allow time for father to hold and fondle newborn.	Conduct postpartum classes for both parents to discuss infant care and related issues.
Include educational materials that portray "active" father and joint parental involvement in infant care.	Allow time for father and mother to be alone with newborn after delivery.	Raise specific questions about difficulties experienced in sharing infant care responsibilities. Offer to help parents renegotiate a plan for sharing infant care, if appropriate.
Raise questions directly related to concerns fathers are likely to experience around childbirth and infant care.	Encourage father to "room in" with mother during hospitalization, if appropriate.	
Host one session for fathers only. Invite "highly involved" fathers to come and discuss parenting issues.	Support father's active involvement with infant during hospitalization (feeding, holding, changing the infant, etc.).	Support formation of father, mother, or joint postpartum lay support groups. Offer to provide consultation to support group or to individuals, as needed.
Encourage parents to negotiate parenting "roles" and infant care issues. Offer to serve as a facilitator of those discussions.		

From Kunst-Wilson, W., and Cronenwett, L.: Res. Nurs. Health 4:201, 1981.

teraction. Riesch and Munns (1985) provided an audiotape with accompanying text for the mothers to listen to privately. They reported the following:

Mothers who received the intervention to inform them of the neonate's social capabilities and of the maternal behaviors to enhance and support their infants reported significantly more of their own behavior than did mothers who did not receive the treatment. Awareness of one's own behavior undoubtedly was a significant factor in the mother's reporting of her own behavior that her infant noticed. The new mother is concerned about how she will perform her new role; she needs to meet her own expectations and those of others in the performance of her maternal role (Rubin, 1961). The mother's expectations may or may not be realistic. Unrealistic expectations may serve as a detriment to a mother's accomplishments. Informing the mother of the responses she can initiate in order to enhance or support her particular infant may relieve some of her role uncertainty, thus allowing her to interact freely with her infant (Riesch and Munns, 1985).

Because of the sheltered environment provided after delivery, women may misjudge the actual amount of physical and psychic energy they possess. They may expect to resume tasks too soon and then feel discouraged when they are not able to do so. In addition, the baby's behavior does not always meet expectations. Sore nipples, worry about adequate milk supply, or even lack of sensations anticipated with breast feeding can lead to a mother's disappointment. Some babies cry more than expected or do not seem satisfied with their feedings. Many babies have fussy periods that do not respond to any ministrations:

■ But my husband, too, was disconcerted at first, for the intense, unending plaintive cries of our firstborn reached to the very depths of our hearts. And, we both had really believed that, somehow, a baby born naturally at home and never separated from its mother would not be so fretful. However, it becomes apparent that all babies cry (Lang, 1972).

Depressive reactions after delivery, often called "the baby blues," are not dismissed lightly. Their prevalence has deprived many women of the support they need. Recognition of the state, helping the woman to verbalize her feelings, and conveying warmth in touch and tone of voice are helpful actions. Setting up tasks she can accomplish easily and successfully are interventions that also can assist to counteract the feelings of depression.

Mothers also are faced with the need to help siblings adjust to the new brother or sister. Sibling rivalry may require parental time and attention to be handled successfully. Even if the children have participated in planning for the new baby, they may be unable to accept the reality of diminished parental attention. Their behavior may reflect their feelings of frustration.

Forewarning about the possibility of such happenings even in the best regulated homes permits the parents to judge themselves less harshly. They are better prepared to seek assistance, change routine, or accept the happening as a passing phase.

Support systems. The U.S. culture has emphasized the instinctual components of motherhood. As a result, many parents hesitate to seek help from nurses, physicians, family, and friends. Long-term support by nurses or physicians is a positive factor in the ultimate adjustment of the family. Parents need to be encouraged to communicate openly with each other regarding their stresses. Relatives or friends can assist with housework and baby-sitting with older children and, eventually, the new baby. Being able to share experiences verbally with others who are interested and experienced also tends to reassure the new mother.

A mother, in discussing visits by the family to see the new baby, commented as follows:

■ I want the family to come. Your people praise him so and think he is the most wonderful baby. All my friends have their own babies and are too busy trying to get compliments for them to give us any. All babies need aunties and grandmothers!

Being given information about the availability of health facilities and how to get in touch with the nurse or physician relieves new parents of feeling total responsibility for the health of the new baby. A physician reported one aspect of his plan for new mothers as follows:

■ I make sure they have my phone number and ask them to call me day or night if they are worried. Since I've done this, the frantic calls have decreased to almost nothing. Knowing they can call seems to take the "steam" out of their concern. I feel it has worked both ways, for their benefit and mine.

Visits by nurses to the home may be spaced to take into account potential stress times, such as 2 or 3 days after coming home from the hospital and the third and sixth weeks at home (Fig. 24.7).

The supportive care given at such times includes care for the entire family. Parents are as concerned with the ups and downs of other family members as they are with those of mother and child. The nurse may give supportive care by listening to (1) accounts of successes and failures, (2) individuals' feelings about

Fig. 24.7
A, Nurse-midwife assesses newborn with mother watching. **B,** Nurse-midwife reviews assessment of newborn for older sister using sister's doll. (Courtesy Marjorie Pyle, RNC, Lifecircle, Costa Mesa, California.)

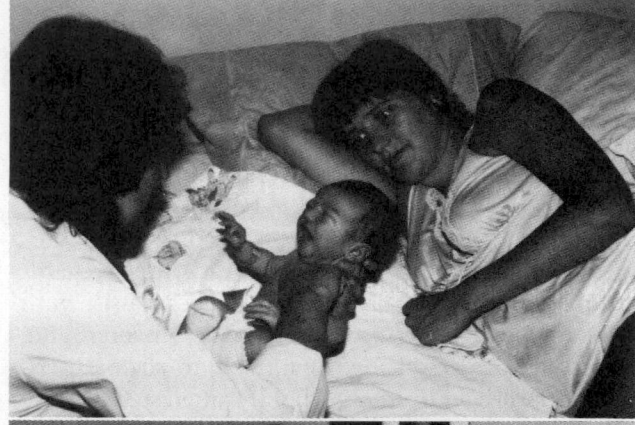

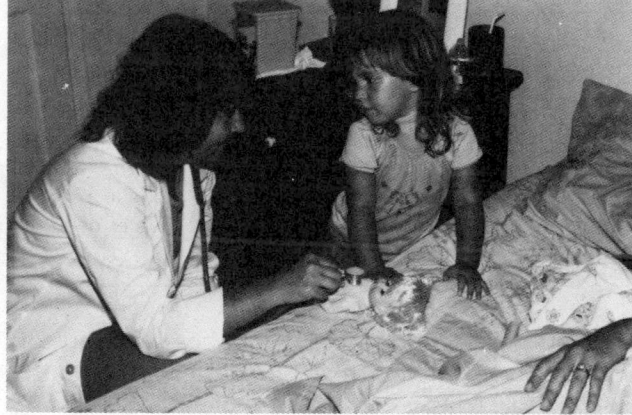

the new baby, and (3) individuals' comments about what they expect of others (e.g., the new parents) in their new roles. One prime requisite is to set up a climate for the safe expression of doubts and anger, as well as happiness. The family will test the nurse's intent and knowledge, and the nurse must recognize and accept this.

Coping mechanisms. Family commitments involve having both time and energy for individual family members—mother, father, and children. In addition to new parents' learning the techniques for care of themselves and their babies, other suggestions have proved helpful to parents in coping with readjusting their lives. A list of these suggestions can be given to new parents, but discussion of specific ways of handling them is also necessary. Discussion with the parents should include the following points.

1. Set priorities for tasks. Many tasks can be left for a later period or done by others. Be adamant about not taking on extra tasks for family, friends, or community. Try not to schedule a move to a new location soon after giving birth.

2. Do not become overly concerned with appearances—tidiness in the home is not as important as time spent with the family. Taking up the role of "super housekeeper" can be postponed until other adjustments are made.

Sometimes new mothers become overburdened with visits from relatives eager "to take over the baby." The husband can help his wife redirect these well-meaning people toward helping with housework and cooking. This leaves the parent free to interact with the child.

3. Get plenty of rest and sleep; rearrange schedules if necessary. Since naps may not be possible if there are other children in the family, going to bed early is recommended; let friends know when to visit.

4. Do not undertake the care of another incapacitated relative at this point; such responsibilities should be undertaken by other family members.

5. Arrange for some time away from the baby; enlist the help of friends, family, or others for baby-sitting. Relaxation for both husband and wife is necessary. Baby-sitting, if at all possible, must be planned and a regular schedule developed. This includes time off for the mother during the day so that she can get away from the home and its responsibilities. In some localities, churches or other agencies have developed programs attuned to the needs of mothers. The young children are cared for while the mothers take part in activities with other mothers. This serves to help them establish relationships with others who are also involved in the care of young children. A mutual sharing of successes and failures in this regard helps the new mother maintain a feeling of equilibrium.

At the very least the mother needs to plan to get out of the house at least once each day. Access to a car and being able to drive are assets. Taking the baby out for a walk or shopping helps to break up the daily routine.

6. Begin family planning before intercourse is resumed and the possibility of pregnancy arises.

7. Be open in your communication with others. Share incidents of delight or of worry with others. Be open in your requests for support.

8. Learn what health facilities are available and how to get in touch with the physician or nurse. If you have questions, remember that the hospital is open all day and night and you can call the emergency department at any time.

9. Prepare for returning to work. Most women are

physically able to return to work by the end of the sixth week. If a woman plans to return to work, certain adjustments for child care must be made. Ideally a substitute parent would be one who could come to the home and provide love, as well as care, for the child. Some parents are fortunate enough to have grandparents or other relatives to fill such a role. Others must take the child to another person's home or a day-care center early in the morning and pick the child up at night. The care provided by day-care centers is needed by some children whose mothers must work to help support them or who are the sole support of the child. For families who require this type of service, assistance in locating such help can be obtained from the local health department. Unfortunately there are not enough quality places available for all children requiring day care.

Ideally parents make plans for care before the birth of the baby. However, if plans have not been made, health personnel should be cognizant of the sources of assistance on a local level. They must make sure that parents are aware of them also. There are many health services available to parents in most communities (e.g., well-baby centers and immunization clinics).

10. Include the father in caretaking activities. Research shows that most fathers participate to the extent that the mother allows (Stainton, 1985). Table 24.8 outlines strategies that the nurse can use to help the father to promote growth in his role as parent.

Adapting nursing care to meet changing family needs. Nursing care during the postpartum period reflects the changing needs of parents, infant, and family. Parents become more knowledgeable of the infant, proficient in child care, a skillful in negotiating a place for the newborn in the family unit. Table 24.9 reviews nursing strategies specific to the early, consolidation, and growth periods of parent-infant-family relationships.

Discharge from Hospital

Discharge planning. Discharge planning begins with the first contact with the client, when the client's physical, emotional, social, and economic profiles start to emerge. The goals listed on pp. 664 and 688 in the Guidelines for Client Teaching and in the Summary of Nursing Actions serve as guidelines for assessing the client's needs at discharge. In the preparation of a client for discharge, the nurse does the following:

1. Identifies gaps in knowledge and reviews these points, if necessary:

Table 24.9

Adapting Nursing Care to Meet Changing Parental Needs

Early Period	Consolidation Period	Growth Period
Infant		
The contacts between parents and infant are as follows:	The nurse and clients discuss the normal rhythms of the child and the parents' awareness of how the child communicates needs. The parents are advised to take time to study their infant and discover what different types of crying mean and when wakeful periods occur—morning, afternoon, or evening. The nurse identifies problems (e.g., infant crying, sleeping) and assists with solutions. Together, nurse and clients note successes and failures in caretaking activities, and the nurse helps the parents with accumulating successful coping mechanisms and discarding unsuccessful ones (see Table 24.3).	The infant is examined at the time of the postbirth examination of mother or at 4 weeks of age. The findings are reviewed with the mother and father. The nurse reviews and assesses parental knowledge of the following:
1. Timed to make use of infant's normal patterns of sleeping and waking; at birth, at about 4 to 6 hours, and every 2 to 5 hours thereafter.		1. The signs and symptoms of illness and measures instituted to effect a cure or obtain medical assistance.
2. Provided at important times for parental attachment to take place (preferably at birth or as soon thereafter as the infant's and mother's conditions permit).		2. The infant's developmental needs:
3. Long and often enough to permit parents to hold, examine, care for, and enjoy their child.		a. Accommodation to physical growth (e.g., introduction of solid foods into diet or weaning).
4. The nurse reviews the normal characteristics of the newborn and gives the parent a report on the infant's initial physical examination. Later the nurse examines the infant in the parents' presence and reviews findings with them. Written instructions as to feeding, medications, and so on are provided. A daily report on the infant's progress and behaviors (e.g., eating, sleeping, voiding, defecating) is given.		b. Use of longer wakeful periods to increase stimulation of infant and social interaction with siblings and other family members.
		c. Adaptation to infant's persisting dependency, as well as ability to conform socially or show awareness of others' needs.
		d. The need for establishing routine pediatric care.

Continued.

Table 24.9, cont'd
Adapting Nursing Care to Meet Changing Parental Needs

Early Period	Consolidation Period	Growth Period
Parents		
The nurse provides a demonstration of infant care and explains hospital routines. When the infant goes from nursery area to mother's bedside, the nurse discusses and demonstrates identification of infant, emergency care of infant if gagging or choking occurs, and protective measures used to minimize the possibility of cross infection.	The nurse and clients discuss the normal responses of parents to the complex role of being a parent. The nurse provides an opportunity for safe revelation of feelings. Nurse and client discuss parental criteria for success in parenting skills (i.e., infant responses, competence in caretaking activities, and opinions of significant others).	The nurse provides the opportunity for mother and family to discuss problems such as the parents' reactions to the infant and the infant's needs and demands. Discussion of feelings of depression or helplessness and how such feelings affect care the parents can give the child can be helpful. The nurse gives recognition to parental success in nurturing their child. If necessary, the family is helped to obtain further assistance from public health agency personnel or social workers to help them develop more adequate coping mechanisms.
Nursing personnel are available to give infant care or assist with caretaking activities and infant feeding techniques. Parents are encouraged to participate in infant care and, whenever possible, to use techniques developed by themselves.	Success is praised, and parents are encouraged to be open-minded about expectations of their role and that of others (siblings, grandparents). They are encouraged to make realistic assessment of their infant's needs and abilities. The mother is helped to conserve her energy (e.g., resting when the infant sleeps, lying down while feeding the infant).	Some communities have established a round-the-clock telephone centers where parents can obtain help for emotionally based problems with the child.
	For some parents whose behavior indicates consistent rejection of the child's infancy and dependency needs, intensive nursing support is needed as follows:	These centers are in addition to emergency medical services. If parenting disorders are noted, the parents are referred to follow-up agencies such as the county public health department.
	1. Plan and implement repeated contacts with parents, i.e.,:	
	a. Contact the mother by telephone on the second day after discharge.	
	b. Provide more frequent office visits.	
	c. Accept phone calls at home.	
	d. Provide regular home visits by public health nurse or nurse visitor.	
	2. Provide additional attention to the mother, i.e.:	
	a. Use compliments rather than criticism.	
	b. Promote maternal attachment to the newborn.	
	c. Emphasize accident prevention.	
	3. Enlist the help of other supportive personnel, such as a social worker.	
Family		
Infant is introduced to the family. Young siblings may need reassurance that their mother will not leave them again, and they may respond to their loss by withdrawing from the mother for a short time. Older children are usually excited and pleased and are eager to take on the care of the baby.	The nurse discusses typical reactions of siblings to the newcomer to the family. She encourages parents to share with other parents their successful techniques of helping siblings adjust (Fig. 24.8). She encourages a return of family involvement in their community and going beyond family boundaries for support and encouragement.	The nurse discusses balancing the infant's needs with those of other family members (e.g., jealousy of siblings, husband's or wife's feelings of alienation), the parents' need to modify infant's behavior to meet their expectations (e.g., toilet training, sleeping patterns, stopping crying when admonished), and the infant's relative ability to conform.

Fig. 24.8
Mother shares feeding time of newborn with older sibling. Baby is supported on an adjustable pad (Keiki Designs). (Courtesy Marjorie Pyle, RNC. Lifecircle, Costa Mesa, California.)

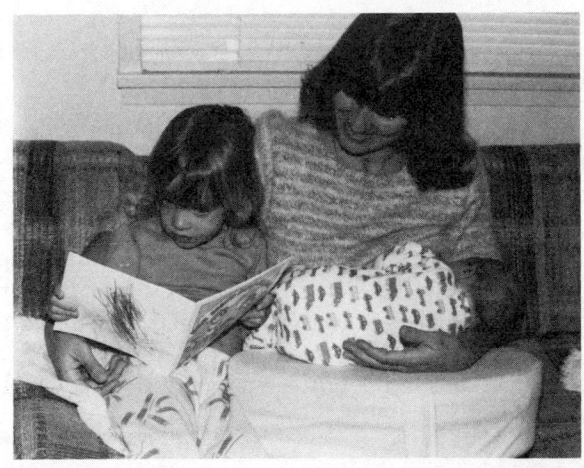

a. Self-care activities, e.g., general hygiene and comfort measures, perineal care, breast care, nutrition and elimination, rest and activity, including exercise
b. Signs of possible complications, e.g., fever with or without chills, foul-smelling lochia, excessive lochia or vaginal discharge, bright-red vaginal bleeding, pelvic or perineal pain, mastitis
c. Return of ovulation and menstruation
d. Lactation and weaning or suppression of lactation
e. Resumption of sexual intercourse and family planning
f. Medications that have been prescribed for the client
2. Assists the client to develop a support system for help with cooking, cleaning, child care, shopping, and so on
3. Identifies the need for referral to community resources (e.g., homemaker or child care services, food stamps) and offers suggestions, when appropriate
4. Provides the client with a printed instruction sheet
Early discharge. The duration of hospitalization and the subsequent convalescence at home are still under debate. Most women who do not experience complications can return home on the third postdelivery day. Some women who are carefully screened by the obstetrician and pediatrician leave much earlier—anywhere from 12 to 24 hours after delivery. Because these clients are in particular need of follow-up care for

themselves and their infants, hospitals have established early discharge programs to assist with such care. These programs provide an alternative mode of mother-infant care.

Planning for early discharge begins in the prenatal period. The families who participate should meet the following criteria: (1) live within a reasonable distance of the hospital, (2) have taken preparation-for-parenthood classes that include content related to assessment of the mother's recovery, care of the mother during the puerperium, and identification and reporting of possible complications, (3) have someone at home to assist in the care of the infant and mother, and (4) have no major medical problems. If a family is interested in early discharge, they are asked to notify the attending physician and nursing staff at the beginning of prenatal care. Opportunities are provided to meet the nurse who will be making home visits during the puerperium for health assessment and any teaching that is necessary. Women with complications, however, should be asymptomatic for at least 24 hours and capable of personal care before leaving the hospital.

Return visit. Since biblical times, the puerperium has been considered to last 6 weeks. Hence a return visit and examination have been scheduled traditionally 6 weeks after delivery. This is illogical because many problems, such as leukorrhea, may be identified and successfully treated earlier. Individualization is important, therefore, but a more logical date for return to the physician or clinic would be 3 or 4 weeks after delivery. See Summary of Nursing Actions: Nursing Care During the Postpartum Period.

Closing the client's chart. Just before the time when the client would be leaving the maternity unit, the nurse reviews the client's chart (audits the chart) to see that laboratory reports, medications, signatures, and so on are in order. Some hospitals have a checklist to follow before the client's discharge. The nurse verifies that medications, if ordered, have arrived on the unit, that any valuables kept secured during the client's stay have been returned to her and that she has signed a receipt for them, and that the infant is ready to be discharged.

Escorting the client from the hospital. The nurse is careful not to administer any medication that would make the mother sleepy if she is the one who will be holding the baby on the way out of the hospital. The woman is seated safely in a wheelchair and is usually given the baby to hold. Her possessions are gathered and taken out with her and her family; usually they are placed on some type of cart or carried by family members. Of course, the woman's and the baby's identification bands have been carefully checked. As the client and the baby are assisted into the car, the nurse should make sure that there is a car seat in which to secure the baby. If there is not, the nurse should return both to the unit and arrange with a social worker, if necessary, to provide one for the trip home.

CAUTION: Whether or not the woman and her family have chosen early discharge, the nurse and the physician are held responsible if the woman is discharged before her condition has stabilized within normal limits. If complications occur, the medical and nursing staff could be sued for "abandonment."

Evaluation

Evaluation is a continuous process. Parental, infant, and family relationships are consistently assessed as indicators of healthy family adjustments after the birth of a child. The clinical findings that represent normal responses are presented as outcome criteria in the Summary of Nursing Actions: Nursing Care During the Postpartum Period. These criteria are used as a basis for selecting appropriate nursing actions and evaluating their effectiveness.

Summary

The normal postpartum period is a time of rapid change. Change takes place in the physiologic and psychologic dimensions of the woman, the newborn, and their family. The nurse who makes pertinent assessments, plans and implements client-centered care, and evaluates the effectiveness of the care is enacting an important role in the health of the child-bearing family. An application of the nursing process to the care of a woman during the postpartum period is provided.

Summary of Nursing Actions

NURSING CARE DURING THE POSTPARTUM PERIOD

GOALS

1. For the mother: a successful physical recovery from childbirth and establishment of mother-child relationship.
2. For the newborn: an uncompromised adjustment to extrauterine existence and a successful incorporation into the family system.
3. For the family: a satisfying family-newborn relationship, an appropriate family participation in healthy care of themselves and the newborn, and a return to mutually satisfying family commitments.

PRIORITIES

Immediate and early postpartum

1. Prevent hemorrhage and infection.
2. Promote comfort.
3. Promote involution and return of nonpregnant physiologic functioning.
4. Encourage self-care.
5. Provide rubella vaccination and $Rh_0(D)$ immune globulin as needed.
6. Promote mother-father-infant relationships.
7. Promote sibling and grandparent and infant relationships.

Late postpartum

1. Identify any present or potential problems and initiate therapy.
2. Meet woman's knowledge needs.
3. Promote growth in family relationships.

ASSESSMENT	EXAMPLES OF POTENTIAL NURSING DIAGNOSTIC CATEGORIES*
PHYSICAL CARE: IMMEDIATE (FIRST 24 HOURS) AND EARLY (DAYS 2 THROUGH 7) POSTPARTUM	
Interview	
A. Ethnic or cultural variations and nursing actions desired	Noncompliance related to ethnic/cultural influences
B. Knowledge of hygiene	Knowledge deficit
C. Nutrition: amounts taken, food preferences, knowledge of, for self and family	Alteration in nutrition: more (or less) than body requirements
	Impaired verbal communication
D. Readiness for discharge from hospital:	
1. Extent of skill in self-care.	Knowledge deficit

*Diagnoses approved by NANDA at the Seventh National Conference (1986) except for those indicated by a dagger.
†Diagnosis not included by NANDA, 1986.
‡Outcome criteria direct the selection of nursing actions (**plan/implementation**) and measure their effectiveness (**evaluation**).

Summary of Nursing Actions—cont'd

ASSESSMENT	EXAMPLES OF POTENTIAL NURSING DIAGNOSTIC CATEGORIES*
2. Clients' need for knowledge of:	
a. Breast self-examination	Noncompliance
b. Resumption of sexual intercourse	Alteration in health maintenance
c. Contraception	
3. Client's need for help at home, acquisition of car seat for newborn, social assistance (e.g., food stamps).	Alteration in health maintenance
4. Client's knowledge of:	Potential for maternal compromise†
a. Danger signs and symptoms for which to call the physician	Knowledge deficit
	Alteration in health maintenance
b. Resources for assistance (e.g., hemorrhage, infection, information such as Tel-Med)	Potential for alteration in normal physiologic processes†
	Powerlessness

Physical examination

A. Receive report from nurse in labor unit and review prenatal record	Potential for alteration in normal physiologic processes†
	Spiritual distress
B. Assess physical recovery	
1. Vital signs and blood pressure	
2. Involution: fundus, lochia, perineum	Potential for hemorrhage†
3. Legs: Homan's sign, edema	Potential for infection
4. Breasts and nipples	Impairment of skin integrity
5. Elimination: urinary, bowel	Knowledge deficit
C. Assess for comfort	Alteration in bowel or urinary elimination
1. General comfort and energy level	Alteration in comfort: pain
2. Breasts: engorgement, nipples	Sleep pattern disturbance
3. Afterpains	Disturbance in self-concept: body image, self-esteem, role performance, personal identity
4. Perineum: episiotomy and laceration repair sites	Impairment of skin integrity
	Knowledge deficit
	Actual impairment of skin integrity
	Potential for infection
	Self-care deficit: bathing/hygiene, toileting
	Alteration in comfort: pain
5. Bladder and voiding	Potential for infection
	Knowledge deficit
	Alteration in patterns of urinary elimination
6. Hemorrhoids	Alteration in comfort: pain
	Knowledge deficit
7. Bowel evacuation	Alteration in comfort: pain
	Knowledge deficit
8. Legs	Alteration in tissue perfusion: peripheral, related to thrombosis
D. Assess ambulation: amount, tolerance for, knowledge of need for; plans for exercise and rest at home	Impaired physical mobility (e.g., especially after cesarean delivery)
	Noncompliance
	Alteration in comfort: pain
	Alteration in energy level
	Potential for injury
	Knowledge deficit

Laboratory tests

A. Hematocrit (Hct) or packed cell volume (PCV)	Alteration in tissue perfusion
B. Complete blood count (CBC) if needed	Potential for maternal compromise†
C. Urinalysis if needed	Potential alteration in normal physiologic processes†
D. Need for rubella vaccination	Potential for fetal compromise†: next pregnancy
E. Need for Rh₀(D) immune globulin	Knowledge deficit

Summary of Nursing Actions—cont'd

OUTCOME CRITERIA‡	PLAN/IMPLEMENTATION
Woman, family, and personnel establish a therapeutic relationship.	Welcome and greet by name. Orient to personnel, unit, and procedures as necessary: ■ Check woman's understanding of use of call bell. ■ Review routine of care: infant feeding and rooming-in, visiting regulations, ordering diets, etc. ■ Arrange for interpreter or translator as necessary. Record. Report as necessary. Teach mother normal limits. Implement therapy for emergent problems: infection, hemorrhage, PIH.
Vital signs and blood pressure are within normal limits: ■ In first 24 hours, temperature does not exceed 38° C (100.4° F); after 24 hours, temperature is within normal limits and there are no signs of infection. ■ Pulse rate may be within normal limits for woman or may be bradycardic between 50-70 beats/min for 6 to 8 days even in the absence of stress. ■ Respiratory rate remains within normal limits. ■ Blood pressure remains in accord with previous normal readings. Early ambulation is achieved without incident relative to hypotension or residual effects of analgesia or anesthesia.	Assist woman with first ambulation after delivery; explain reason (e.g., splanchnic engorgement) so that woman and family remember to call for assistance to ambulate.
Findings from laboratory assessments of blood and urine are within normal limits by the third postdelivery day: ■ **Hematocrit:** 42% ± 5%. ■ **White cell mass** within first 10-14 days may be 20,000 to 25,000/mm³. ■ **Proteinuria** may be present during first week.	Notify physician if findings are outside of normal range. Institute prescribed therapy if needed. Continue to monitor for symptomatology that would indicate infection or pregnancy-induced hypertension (PIH).
Woman receives correct medications and dosages by the correct route. Medication is effective. Woman knows medication, its purpose, and expected results. Woman experiences no allergic or other untoward responses.	Check with woman and her record regarding known allergies. Implement nonpharmacologic interventions first (e.g., for comfort) before using medications. Inform woman of medication and its expected effects if she does not know this. Chart medications; assess and record woman's response.
Involution: uterus ■ Involution progresses normally. ■ Size of uterus diminishes. ■ Uterine tone is maintained by contraction and retraction of uterine muscles. Uterus feels firm and contracts readily after massage. During the first 12 hours after delivery, contractions are strong, regular, and coordinated. Thereafter intensity, frequency, and regularity decrease. Afterpains occur for 2 to 3 days and are more noticeable in multipara than in primipara and during suckling of infant.	Meet woman's knowledge needs regarding involution: describe and give rationale for procedures to be used in assessing woman's recovery from childbirth and return of reproductive organs to nonpregnant state. Repeat and reinforce during hospital stay.
Involution: lochia ■ Lochia rubra contains blood, placental and decidual debris, and clots and is dark red. It persists from delivery through third day. ■ Lochia serosa is thin, serous, and brownish and lasts from fourth to tenth day. ■ Lochia alba, a yellowish white discharge, contains an increased number of leukocytes and lasts from tenth day to as long as sixth week. ■ Odor remains characteristically "fleshy" rather than foul. ■ Amount of discharge is moderate for first 2-3 days and then is scant. Some women may have none after 2 weeks; in, others discharge persists until sixth week.	Keep uterus empty and contracted. Implement physician's orders regarding low hematocrit (e.g., blood replacement, nutrition counseling). Implement physician's orders regarding infection (e.g., intravenous fluids, antimicrobial medications). Teach woman and family regarding reportable findings after discharge (e.g., return of lochia rubra, foul odor to lochia, uterine tenderness, fever, and chills). Offer printed instructions regarding reportable symptomatology and appropriate phone numbers. Teach regarding expected return of menstruation. Institute comfort measures for woman's discomfort and teach her self-care for afterpains.
Cervix regains its shape in a few days, external os is contracted by 2 weeks, and cervical mucosa is restored. **Vagina** remains distensible. Introitus gapes when intraabdominal pressure is increased by bearing-down effort or by coughing.	Discuss with woman and husband the resumption of sexual intercourse after healing occurs and discomfort eases. Explain external changes in appearance of vaginal introitus.

Summary of Nursing Actions—cont'd

OUTCOME CRITERIA‡	PLAN/IMPLEMENTATION
Perineum remains free of infection and signs of childbirth trauma. Episiotomy or laceration repair heals well. Hemorrhoids resolve.	Institute hygienic and comfort measures.
Breasts and **nipples** remain free of infection. Engorgement is prevented or minimized.	Meet woman's knowledge needs regarding breast and nipple care, techniques of infant feeding, support of breasts, and lactation. (See Chapter 21 for newborn nutrition and feeding.)
Mother learns to assist infant to nurse at the breast or from the bottle.	
Lactation begins:	
■ For 2 to 3 days after delivery breasts secrete colostrum in increasing amounts.	
■ By second day in multiparas and by third day in primiparas, breasts become engorged, firm, tense, and tender. This is caused by venous or lymphatic stasis. In 36 to 48 hours pain disappears as swelling spontaneously subsides. Fever does not accompany this process.	
■ Soon after onset of this engorgement, true milk is formed and let-down reflex in response to suckling of infant or manual manipulation causes expression of milk (see also Chapter 21).	
Bottle feeding is begun.	Meet woman's knowledge needs regarding suppression of lactation.
■ Suppression of lactation is successful.	Institute measures to suppress lactation per physician's directives, e.g., administer bromocriptine mesylate (Parlodel).
■ Engorgement is prevented or minimized.	Minimize engorgement by:
	■ Application of supportive bra
	■ Avoidance of breast stimulation, e.g., manual expression, warm water to breasts
Legs remain free of evidence of thrombus formation (e.g., there is no pain, warmth, localized tenderness, swollen, reddened vein that feels hard to touch). Homan's sign remains negative. If varicosities are present, they diminish in size.	Meet woman's knowledge needs regarding thrombus formation, prevention, and symptomatology, and urgency in notifying physician.
	Encourage leg exercises and ambulation.
	If symptomatology occurs, immobilize and elevate leg, avoid massage, and report to physican immediately.
	Apply supportive stockings per physician's directives.
Urinary system	
Most women void spontaneously by 8 hours following delivery and thereafter void copious amounts frequently for 48 hours as retained tissue fluids are released.	Meet woman's knowledge needs for fluid intake and emptying of bladder and reporting of symptomatology of infection to physician.
■ Complete emptying of bladder occurs. Nurse palpates empty bladder and well-contracted involuting uterus in midline.	Encourage adequate fluid intake and emptying of bladder, at least every 4 hours.
■ Urination occurs without symptomatology of urinary tract infection, e.g., frequency, urgency, sensations of burning (dysuria).	Provide and teach woman hygienic care.
■ Urine is straw-colored and clear; odor is not foul.	
Defecation occurs spontaneously or with the aid of laxatives, stool softeners, or enemas by the third day. Defecation occurs with minimal or no discomfort	Meet knowledge needs regarding defecation during postpartum period.
	Encourage use of fluids, food with roughage, and exercise to promote regular bowel habits.
	Avoid use of enemas for women whose deliveries were complicated by 4-degree lacerations or if episiotomy extended through the rectum.
	Counsel regarding expected spontaneous reduction of hemorrhoids during the puerperium and the continued avoidance of constipation with straining at stool.
Woman is **comfortable.** Woman is aware of and uses comfort measures.	Meet woman's knowledge needs.

Summary of Nursing Actions—cont'd

OUTCOME CRITERIA‡	PLAN/IMPLEMENTATION
■ General comfort and energy level reestablished.	Implement comfort measures: ■ Give back and foot massage. ■ Arrange for periods of rest without interruption. ■ Control environment: temperature, light, ventilation, privacy, and cleanliness. ■ Meet fluid and nutrient needs. ■ Promote rest and activity; teach exercises ■ Encourage talking about woman's or couple's experience. ■ Administer analgesia per physician order.
■ Woman states breasts feel comfortable.	Implement comfort measures: ■ Use of supportive bra ■ Applications of heat or cold
■ Woman states she understands and can cope with afterpains using general comfort measures or medications.	Meet mother's need for knowledge concerning physiologic basis for keeping bladder empty Provide a warmed, rolled towel over abdomen Administer analgesics per physician's directives
■ Woman states she understands reason for discomfort, uses appropriate method for sitting down and standing up, uses good hygiene, and achieves comfort through general measures or medications.	Meet mother's knowledge and skill needs for: ■ Physiologic basis for discomfort ■ Proper method to sit down and get up ■ General hygiene of area ■ Use of topical products, e.g., sprays, cold applications, medicated pads ■ Use of sitz bath, Surgi-gator Administer analgesics per physician's directives.
■ Woman states she has no difficulty voiding.	Meet mother's knowledge and skill needs regarding: ■ Need to empty bladder completely ■ Diuresis ■ General hygiene Assist with urination as needed, e.g., privacy, sound of running water, analgesics; catheterization.
■ Woman states her hemorrhoids are causing minimal or no discomfort as a result of intervention.	Meet mother's knowledge and skill needs regarding: ■ Etiology of hemorrhoids ■ Prevention of hemorrhoids through avoidance of constipation or straining at stool, standing for long periods of time, and excessive weight gain Administer stool softeners, enemas, as ordered by physician. Provide sitz bath Provide topical products per physician's directions, e.g., medicated pads, ointments.
■ Woman experiences no discomfort in her legs.	Meet mother's knowledge and skill needs regarding: ■ Preventing leg cramps, e.g., avoid pointing the toes ■ Treating leg cramps, e.g., stretch the affected muscle ■ Ambulation ■ Leg exercises while in bed ■ Thrombus formation
Abdominal wall is lax and weak in midline, where abdominal muscles may be widely separated. Muscles feel like masses on either side of abdomen and are not to be confused with fundus of uterus.	Meet mother's knowledge needs regarding abdominal muscles and appropriate exercises.
Approximately half the average 11.2 kg (25 lb) weight gain of pregnancy is lost at delivery. During the initial days of the puerperium, largely as a result of diuresis, an additional 2.5 to 3.5 kg (6 to 8 lb) *weight loss* can be expected.	Meet mother's knowledge needs regarding expected diuresis and weight loss. Remind woman and family that she is still not able to wear prepregnant clothes and that some people might think she is still pregnant in early days after delivery.
Woman follows good handwashing technique, cleanses her perineum, and changes her pads appropriately; cleanses her breasts and nipples appropriately.	Assure adequate supply of soap, towels, etc. Assure cleanliness of bath, showers, sitz rooms, and basins. Assist with hygienic measures

Summary of Nursing Actions—cont'd

OUTCOME CRITERIA‡	PLAN/IMPLEMENTATION
Woman's nutritional needs are met and she is comfortable with type and amount of prescribed diet. Woman states she can and will continue to maintain good nutrition.	Provide woman with choice of foods (if possible) in amounts desired, taking into consideration personal, cultural, ethnic, and religious variations. Refer to social service if family needs financial assistance for food. Offer and provide written information. Refer to nutritionist.
Woman and family indicate understanding of health maintenance activities: ■ Couple is aware of contraception techniques available and their questions are answered to their satisfaction. ■ Woman and family are aware of continued need for rest, exercise, and nutrition. ■ Postdelivery immunization is completed, e.g., rubella vaccination and prevention of Rh isoimmunization, if appropriate.	Meet woman's and family's knowledge and skill needs through: ■ Discussion with her and with family members ■ Formalized classes in hospital ■ Illustrations and photographs ■ Printed material and instructions ■ Asking her and them to write down notes and questions Reinforce physician's explanation for need for vaccination and precautions against pregnancy within 3 months. Administer per hospital protocol. Fill out card for $Rh_0(D)$ immune globulin (RhoGAM) and give to mother. May consider using this opportunity to discuss vaccination schedule for infant.
■ Couple is aware of danger signals, safety measures, and phone numbers of whom to contact for: Hemorrhage Infection Thrombolism Hypertension or hypotension Depressive states ■ Couple is aware of need for medical examination in 4 to 6 weeks for mother. ■ Family has an approved car seat for transporting infant home.	
	Determine that family has infant seat by checking car when discharging mother and infant. Return mother and infant to unit if there is no infant seat. Call social worker for loan of infant seat, if needed.
■ Family has list of phone numbers of community resources. Records are complete. Discharge summary is available for the 4 to 6 week examination.	Complete recording and close the chart.

ASSESSMENT	EXAMPLES OF POTENTIAL NURSING DIAGNOSTIC CATEGORIES*

PHYSICAL CARE: LATE POSTPARTUM (WEEKS 2 THROUGH 6)

Interview A. Review record to date. B. Inquire concerning vaginal discharge, urinary problems, bowel action, condition of breasts and nipples, resumption of sexual intercourse. C. Assess need for contraception information. If method is being used: what is it, how satisfactory is it, what additional information is desired? D. Assess for problems related to self, infant, or family (e.g., fatigue, insomnia, depression, lack of or excessive appetite, dyspareunia or other sexual concern).	Potential knowledge deficit Potential for anxiety, fear, or guilt† Potential for alteration in bowel or urinary elimination Potential alteration in comfort: pain Potential for impaired verbal communication Potential for ineffective individual or family coping Potential alteration in family processes Potential alteration in health maintenance Potential for injury Noncompliance

Summary of Nursing Actions—cont'd

ASSESSMENT	EXAMPLES OF POTENTIAL NURSING DIAGNOSTIC CATEGORIES*
E. Inquire regarding need for referrals (e.g., food stamps, medicaid, home health care, Parental Stress Line, vocational guidance, school [finish high school, etc.], child care [if woman is returning to work, etc.]). F. Assess for need for nutritional counseling (see Chapters 12 and 21).	Potential alteration in nutrition: less (or more) than body requirements Potential for powerlessness
Physical examination A. Obtain blood pressure, pulse, respirations, temperature, and weight. B. Assess woman's perception of her weight; is she satisfied, frustrated? C. Assist examiner or examine breasts, abdomen, uterus, adnexa, cervix, vagina, perineum, and rectum.	Potential alteration in normal physiologic processes† Potential disturbance in self-concept Potential for sexual dysfunction Potential impairment of skin integrity Potential for sleep pattern disturbance Potential for spiritual distress
Laboratory tests A. Obtain blood for analysis: CBC, Hct, Hgb. B. Obtain clean-catch urine sample for analysis and culture. C. Obtain cervical (Papanicolaou) smear for cytology.	Potential alterations in normal processes†

OUTCOME CRITERIA‡	PLAN/IMPLEMENTATION
Woman appears relaxed during interview. Vital signs and blood pressure are within normal limits. Weight is within normal limits. ■ Woman is satisfied with weight. ■ If weight is excessive or too low, woman makes an informed decision for either weight loss or gain and accepts nutrition counseling.	Welcome woman. Provide quiet space and relaxed environment for interview. Inquire concerning her general health and that of child and father. Share findings with woman and family. Record. Report any deviations to physician. Meet woman's knowledge needs regarding weight loss following pregnancy: ■ Further decrease occurs as uterus involutes and plasma volume contracts. ■ Most women lose the remaining weight gained at pregnancy over the ensuing weeks, returning to the nonpregnant weight within several months. ■ Parity alone has very little effect on weight. ■ Woman will retain about 60% of weight gained in excess of 11kg (24 lb). Encourage woman to talk about her weight if she is unsatisfied with present weight. Implement nutrition counseling or refer to registered dietitian. Refer her to social services if in financial need for food.
Abdomen and perineum: ■ Muscles of abdomen reveal some degree of laxity, but tone is returning to prepregnant level (Fig. 22.3). ■ Uterus is only slightly larger than in prepregnant state and anteverted. If retroverted, it has developed free mobility. ■ Uterine bleeding (lochia) had decreased until about third or fourth week and then ceased; vaginal discharge is minimum; small period (menstruation) may have occurred during fourth or fifth week after delivery. ■ Cervix is healed; external os has assumed typical transverse slit of parous woman. Occasionally glandular epithelium lining cervical canal can be visualized as bright red area surrounding external os.	Ensure privacy and have woman undress and put on examining gown. Assist client to position herself on table for examination of breasts, abdomen, and legs; explain rationale for examinations; answer questions. Position woman for pelvic examination, instruct her about how to relax. Acquaint examiner with information obtained during interview and assist with examination: provide mirror for her to watch examination, explanations, and descriptions of what is felt and seen.

Summary of Nursing Actions—cont'd

OUTCOME CRITERIA‡	PLAN/IMPLEMENTATION
■ Pelvic floor has essentially regained its tone, permitting only a mild degree of uterine prolapse, cystocele, or rectocele. Vulva and perineal area show no evidence of infection. Episiotomy or laceration usually is healed without undue contraction, and introitus remains adequate to permit coitus without discomfort. ■ Hemorrhoids are reduced. Breasts do not reveal soreness, tenderness, or masses. If woman is not breast feeding, no milk or only a small amount of milk may be expressed. If woman is breast feeding, lactation is well established. Nipples are intact. Legs remain free of evidence of thrombus formation, and varicosities are minimal or absent. Woman wears support hose as prescribed, as needed.	Engage woman in assisting with breast examination and discuss breast self-examination on routine basis. Instruct her concerning need for breast examination for males, too. Meet mother's learning needs regarding: ■ Recognition of thrombus formation and need for immediate notification of physician ■ Prevention of varicosities, e.g., by avoidance of constrictive articles of clothing (garters, thigh-high stockings), standing for long periods of time, and excessive weight gain ■ Proper application of support hose
No symptoms of urinary tract infection are present. Mother knows reportable symptomatology. Appetite is good. Diet is adjusted for weight maintenance or weight loss (average 2000-2500 cal/day). If woman is breast feeding, caloric intake is increased by 500 cal and fluid increased to about 3 L per day. Regular bowel habits are reestablished without fecal incontinence or fistula formation. Rectal examination reveals intact and healthy tissue. Woman states she feels comfortable, rested, and returned to prepregnancy energy level. Woman has established schedule for adequate rest and exercise. Woman and family indicate an understanding of health maintenance activities: ■ Couple has begun practicing their chosen method of family planning. ■ Woman is aware of need for a medical reexamination in 6 months. ■ Parents have chosen health care supervision for infant and have arranged for first examination.	Meet mother's knowledge needs regarding prevention of infection and reportable symptomatology. Meet mother's knowledge needs regarding nutrition. (See *weight* above.) Meet mother's knowledge needs regarding bowel elimination and reportable symptomatology. Discuss how she feels. Compliment her on achievements. After woman is dressed and upright, discuss and answer questions concerning: ■ Pelvic examination and findings ■ Family planning and birth control methods ■ Importance of 6-month reexamination ■ Other client-centered problems: continued lactation, weaning, etc. Assure woman that she is welcome to call back if she has questions and urge her to call if she notices any danger signs or symptoms. Provide woman and family with phone numbers of clinic, community resources. Encourage her to have emergency phone numbers (911 in some areas) readily on hand.
Laboratory findings are within normal limits: ■ Hemoglobin level is 12g/dl or greater, and hematocrit level is 42% ± 5%. ■ Urinalysis reveals normal findings, proteinuria has disappeared. Lactose may be present if woman is breast feeding, but no pus cells are present. Culture reveals no organisms. Record keeping is completed to date.	Meet mother's knowledge needs regarding blood and urine tests. Reinforce need for routine Papanicolaou smears as directed by her physician. Meet mother's learning needs regarding prevention of anemia and urinary tract infections. Schedule next appointment. Complete the record.

Summary of Nursing Actions—cont'd

ASSESSMENT	EXAMPLES OF POTENTIAL NURSING DIAGNOSTIC CATEGORIES*
EMOTIONAL CARE: EARLY PERIOD	
A. Assess maternal emotional response to birth of the child	Anxiety Alteration in comfort: pain Impaired verbal communication Ineffective individual or family coping Alteration in energy levels† Alteration in family processes Grieving Knowledge deficit Alteration in parenting
B. Assess paternal emotional response to birth of the child	Anxiety Alteration in comfort: pain Impaired verbal communication Ineffective individual or family coping Alteration in energy levels† Alteration in family process Grieving Knowledge deficit Alteration in parenting

C. Assess newborn's ability to respond to parent's repertoire of behaviors, for example:
  1. Gazing
  2. Habituation
  3. Hand and face movements
	Anxiety
	Alteration in comfort: pain
	Impaired verbal communication
	Ineffective individual or family coping
	Alteration in energy levels†
	Alteration in family process
	Grieving
	Knowledge deficit
	Alteration in parenting

D. Assess parental behaviors for cues as to needs for learning and teaching, for support to reduce tension levels, and for counseling with reference to presence or absence of motherliness or fatherliness for example:
  1. Parental contact with infant includes the following:
    a. Enfolding, massaging, and exploring with fingertips
    b. Scrutinizing infant's body carefully, noting variations in what parents deem normal and looking for reassurance
    c. Seeking eye contact
  2. Parents react in personal manner to emotional excitement (e.g., they may cry, laugh, talk, or remain silent).
  3. Parents show level of competence in handling and holding child consonant with their previous experience and level of anxiety.
  4. Parents respond to infant's going to sleep, stopping crying, etc. with lessening of tension and increasing relaxation.
  5. Parents respond to cues of newborn for rest or socializing.
	Anxiety
	Alteration in comfort: pain
	Impaired verbal communication
	Ineffective individual or family coping
	Alteration in energy levels†
	Alteration in family process
	Grieving
	Knowledge deficit
	Alteration in parenting

E. Assess sibling and grandparent behaviors for cues as to need for support
  1. Siblings' need for supervision in handling, examining newborn
  2. Siblings show regressive tendencies (e.g., bed wetting)
  3. Siblings dependency needs increase.
	Anxiety
	Alteration in comfort: pain
	Impaired verbal communication
	Ineffective individual or family coping
	Alteration in energy levels†
	Alteration in family processes
	Grieving

Summary of Nursing Actions—cont'd

ASSESSMENT	EXAMPLES OF POTENTIAL NURSING DIAGNOSTIC CATEGORIES*
4. Grandparents accept supportive, not dominant, role in care of newborn. 5. Grandparents express delight and love for mother/father and newborn.	Knowledge deficit Alteration in parenting

OUTCOME CRITERIA‡	PLAN/IMPLEMENTATION
Emotional response of parents A. Mothers exhibit typical dependent behaviors for 24-48 hours. These usually are superseded by mixutre of dependent-independent behaviors. Depressive reactions may begin by end of second postdelivery day and persist for 1 to 3 days. Mother-child relationships may be positive immediately or show a "maternal lag" that may not interfere unduly with child-care activities. Mother talks freely about her birthing experience (see also Chapter 23). B. Fathers exhibit typical behaviors (e.g., engrossment) (see also Chapter 23).	A. Correlate maternal behaviors with mother's lack of physical and psychic energy, anxiety level, freedom from discomfort, ethnic and cultural identity. Provide for rest. Provide comfort measures. Encourage mother to talk about her anxieties and need for support. Review her birthing experience. Join in family's pleasure with their newborn. B. Correlate paternal bahaviors with father's level of fatigue, anxiety, and ethnic and cultural diversity. Encourage father to talk about his reactions to the birth and his newborn.

Infant growth and development
Parents are reassured of normalcy of infant's characteristics.
  1. Appearance (e.g., molding of head, milia, lanugo, forceps marks)
  2. Behavior (e.g., sleeping, waking, crying, and sensory capabilities)
  3. Responses (e.g., eating, regurgitating, defecating, voiding, gaining weight)
	Meet parental knowledge needs in relation to infant growth and development. Examine or have infant examined in mother's presence and review findings with mother.
	Provide written instructions as to feeding, medications, etc.
	Give daily report on infant's progress and behaviors (e.g., eating, sleeping, voiding, defecating).

Attachment process Parents behave toward infant with love, for example, parents enfold infant in their arms, use repertoire of behaviors to communicate with infant, express pleasure with infant.	Assure parents of opportunity for attachment (bonding) with their infant (e.g., holding, touching, examining, establishing eye contact as soon after birth as possible, and either continuous contact [rooming-in or home birth] or protracted contact thereafter while in hospital). Correlate maternal behaviors with mother's level of physical and psychic energy, anxiety level, freedom from discomfort, and ethnic and cultural identity.
Infant identity A. Infant's identity is established. B. Identifying wristband is checked with mother's. C. Claiming process: parents look for similarities or differences between their infant and other family members regarding size, weight, sex, appearance, behavior, and responses. D. Child is recognized as person separate from the mother.	Arrange for time for parent and family interactions with infant while in hospital. Encourage claiming process (e.g., who does she look like?)
Parental criteria Parents are aware of criteria they will use in assessing success or failure of care they give their child.	Discuss parental criteria for success in parenting skills (i.e., infant responses, competence in caretaking activities, and opinions of significant others); point out behavior noted; praise successes.

Summary of Nursing Actions—cont'd

OUTCOME CRITERIA‡	PLAN/IMPLEMENTATION
1. Infant responses: parents may feel successful if infant snuggles against them, looks at them, stops crying when they hold him, or burps when feeding; they may feel unsuccessful if child persists in crying, is unable to breast feed, "frowns" at them, or will not wake up.	1. Encourage awareness by pointing out examples (e.g., "When she snuggles up, it makes me feel I'm doing what she wants" or "When babies cry, parents can think they are not giving the right care").
2. Parental competence in caretaking activities: parents may feel inadequate to extent that they feel incompetent in handling or holding child.	2. Demonstrate and supervise infant care activities—bathing, changing, and holding infant—and provide continued assistance with feeling. Encourage parents to participate in infant care and, whenever possible, to use techniques developed by mother or father. Provide infant care as needed. Reassure parents regarding normalcy of their infant (e.g., crying, Moro reflex).
3. Opinions of significant others: parents may expect that others will be supportive and accepting of their beginning attempts or critical and intolerant of their less-than-perfect efforts; these expectations can prompt them to seek assistance or to avoid it.	3. Encourage discussion of support from significant others. Comment on remarks such as "My mother makes me feel all thumbs" with statements such as "We all have to learn how to care for a baby. You will become skilled yourself in a little while. What does your mother say or do?"
Family relationships A. Newborn is introduced to family members; claiming process is positive.	Meet the mother's and family's learning needs concerning changes in family roles and integration of child into family unit.
B. Mother and father begin process of integrating newborn into family unit.	Recognize mother's needs for support in negotiating role change.
C. Mother and father recognize older siblings' feelings of excitement and rejection.	Encourage the mother and father to talk about problems with siblings and grandparents.
D. Mother and father state they are accepting or satisfied with siblings' and grandparents' behavior.	Suggest techniques the parents have found helpful in acquainting siblings with newborn.
E. Family roles are in the process of change through negotiation.	

ASSESSMENT	EXAMPLES OF POTENTIAL NURSING DIAGNOSTIC CATEGORIES*
CONSOLIDATION PERIOD	
A. Assess maternal response: happy, depressed; coping, disorganized; independent and interdependent behaviors, accepting of father's need for learning about newborn.	Anxiety Alteration in comfort: pain Impaired verbal communication Ineffective individual or family coping Alteration in energy levels† Alteration in family process Alteration in health maintenance Potential for injury Knowledge deficit Alteration in parenting Disturbance in self-concept: body image, self-esteem, role performance, personal identity
B. Assess paternal response: pleased, preoccupied with work; coping, disorganized; accepting of maternal dependency needs, impatient with family commitments.	Anxiety Alteration in comfort: pain Impaired verbal communication Ineffective individual or family coping Alteration in energy levels† Alteration in family process

Summary of Nursing Actions—cont'd

ASSESSMENT	EXAMPLES OF POTENTIAL NURSING DIAGNOSTIC CATEGORIES*
	Alteration in health maintenance Potential for injury Alteration in parenting Disturbance in self-concept: body image, self-esteem, role performance, personal identity
C. Assess newborn's ability to respond to parent, siblings and grandparents (e.g., gazing, following another's activities, reaching out with arms, hands, imitating others' facial movements).	Anxiety Alteration in comfort: pain Impaired verbal communication Ineffective individual or family coping Alteration in energy levels† Alteration in family process Alteration in health maintenance Potential for injury Knowledge deficit Alteration in parenting Disturbance in self-concept: body image, self-esteem, role performance, personal identity
D. Assess parental behaviors during feeding periods and when parent is giving care to infant for cues as to needs for learning and teaching, for support to reduce tension levels, and for counseling with reference to presence or absence of motherliness or fatherliness, for example: 1. Do parents seem to enjoy handling and touching, stroking and patting infant, or do they minimize any body contact? Is their touch gentle or rough? Personal or impersonal?	Anxiety Alteration in comfort: pain Impaired verbal communication Ineffective individual or family coping Alteration in energy level† Alteration in family processes Alteration in health maintenance Potential for injury Knowledge deficit Alteration in parenting Disturbance in self-concept: body image, self-esteem, role performance, personal identity
2. Although it is difficult to assess modes of address used by parents to their infants, does parents' tone of voice indicate acceptance or rejection of infant? 3. Do parents seek and maintain eye contact? Do they stare fixedly into infant's eyes? 4. Are parents able to overcome natural reluctance to handle excrement of infant? 5. Do parents have rigid plans for infant routines and expectations of infant's fitting into these plans? 6. Do parents respond to infant's cues for rest or socializing? 7. Do parents provide reasonably competent care to infant?	Anxiety Alteration in comfort: pain Impaired verbal communication Ineffective individual or family coping Alteration in energy levels† Alteration in family process Alteration in health maintenance Potential for injury Knowledge deficit Alteration in parenting Disturbance in self-concept: body image, self-esteem, role performance, personal identity
E. Assess sibling and grandparent behaviors for cues as to need for teaching or support. 1. Have earlier problems disappeared or become worse? 2. Have older child or children regained feeling of dominant position(s)? 3. Is newborn recognized as a part of the family system?	Anxiety Alteration in comfort: pain Impaired verbal communication Ineffective individual or family coping Alteration in energy levels† Alteration in family process Alteration in health maintenance Potential for injury Knowledge deficit Alteration in parenting Disturbance in self-concept: body image, self-esteem, role performance, personal identity

Summary of Nursing Actions—cont'd

OUTCOME CRITERIA‡	PLAN/IMPLEMENTATION

Emotional response of parents
A. *Mother* perceives herself positively.
  1. Is more competent, able to handle sibling rivalry, less fatigued.
  2. Mutually dependent with husband.
  3. Independence asserting itself.
  4. Coping with care of newborn (and other children). Making good use of support system.
 	
B. *Father* perceives himself as functioning well in his version of the parental role.
	A. Encourage mother to talk about herself, e.g., the relationships of siblings and newborn; her general health and energy level; how she is managing at home, at work.
	Discuss normal responses of parents to complex role of being parent.
	Correlate parental behaviors with parents' shared cultural and personal concepts of roles and previous experience with infants.
	Correlate both parental patterns against data collected earlier to establish evidence of consistent pattern of reaction to child and to parental role.
	B. Inquire as to how he is adjusting to newborn, what ways husband and wife share care of infant, how he is coping with sleep deprivation (night feedings of infant, crying). Comment on successes.

Infant growth and development A. Parents recognize infant's cues for interactions, meaning of types of cries; need for rest and privacy. B. Parents can assess infant temperature and respirations, feeding, waking, and sleep patterns for normalcy.	A. Meet parental knowledge needs relating to infant growth and development. B. Discuss normal rhythms of child and parents' awareness of how child communicates his needs.
Attachment process A. Parents recognize dual nature of parent-child relationship. B. Parents plan socializing periods with infant. C. Parents develop a satisfactory level of competence in physical caretaking activities of bathing, feeding, holding, and clothing infant. D. Parents find pleasure in being with their infant. E. Parents demonstrate cue sensitivity to their child's needs.	Meet parental knowledge needs relating to the growing attachment to their child. Correlate parental behaviors with energy levels, ethnic and cultural identity, other commitments.
Infant identity Infant's identity expands with parents' awareness of child's particular rhythms of sleeping, waking, hunger, and satiety, as well as child's cues for expressing the need for sleep, food, soothing, stimulation, socializing, and relief from pain or discomfort. Infant recognized as a separate person with her or his own rights.	Encourage parents to verbalize their knowledge of their infant. Comment on successes, mutually explore other areas.

Parental criteria
Parents establish realistic criteria for use in evaluating their efforts in parenting relative to the following:
A. Infant responses: they accept a mixture of success and failure in control they can exert over such infant behaviors as crying, fussing, eating, sleeping, waking, growing, and gaining weight.
B. Parental competence in caretaking activities:
  1. Self-esteem grows as skill in caretaking activities increases.
  2. Recognition develops as to what care is essential for well-being of infant as opposed to prior expectations of parents.
	Meet parental knowledge needs in relation to infant responses, caretaking activities, support systems.
	A. Help them identify areas of concern, (e.g., infant crying, sleeping) and assist with solutions.
	
	B. Discuss successes and failure in caretaking activities, and help parents with accumulating successful coping mechanisms and discarding unsuccessful ones.

Summary of Nursing Actions—cont'd

OUTCOME CRITERIA‡	PLAN/IMPLEMENTATION
3. Flexible schedule for infant care is accepted. 4. Parents seek assistance for health maintenance from community caretakers (e.g., nurses, physicians). C. Opinions of significant others: assistance from others is accepted or rejected as knowledge and skill grow; parent is aware of vulnerability to praise or criticism of significant others (e.g., own mother, spouse, close relatives).	Encourage parents to establish routine health checkup for mother, newborn, and other family members. C. Encourage parents to identify their strengths. Encourage parents to expand supportive network.
Family relationships A. Parents continue to negotiate change of roles and assist siblings with role adjustments; mother and father state newborn accepted as part of the family, newborn assumes place in family hierarachy. B. Parents set up their own intimate marital relationship.	Meet parental knowledge needs in relation to role changes needed and sibling rivalry. Encourage parents to discuss problems with siblings or grandparents. Explore solutions to problems. Comment on successes.

ASSESSMENT	EXAMPLES OF POTENTIAL NURSING DIAGNOSTIC CATEGORIES*
GROWTH PERIOD	
A. Assess maternal response to parenthood: her perceptions, coping mechanisms, support systems, for example: 1. **Mother's concern** with responsibilities is noted. How does mother manage child's crying? Household chores? Isolation from community? Keeping up her career? Repetitive nature of child care? Her inability to obtain unbroken rest? 2. Maternal coping mechanisms are noted. Does mother get away from home responsibilities occasionally? Can she express her feelings about her new responsibilities freely? Does she allow expression only of idealized mothering feeling? 3. Family members' assistance is noted. Do other family members help? Is there someone she can talk to?	Anxiety Alteration in comfort: pain Impaired verbal communication Ineffective individual or family coping Alteration in energy levels† Alteration in family process Alteration in health maintenance Potential for injury Knowledge deficit Alteration in parenting Disturbance in self-concept: body image, self-esteem, role performance, personal identity
B. Assess paternal responses to parenthood: his perceptions, coping mechanisms, support systems, for example: 1. **Father's concern** with responsibilities is noted. Does father help with childcare activities or care of older children? 2. Paternal coping mechanisms are noted. Does he feel lack of wife's interest and support? Is he able to express himself freely? Is there a family member or friend he can talk to?	Anxiety Alteration in comfort: pain Impaired verbal communication Ineffective individual or family coping Alteration in energy levels† Alteration in family process Alteration in health maintenance Potential for injury Knowledge deficit Alteration in parenting Disturbance in self-concept: body image, self-esteem, role performance, personal identity
C. Assess **parental behaviors** for cues as to needs for learning and teaching, for support to reduce tensions and for counseling with reference to presence or absence of motherliness or fatherliness. 1. Parental behaviors are assessed during hospital stay, during postdelivery visits to home, and during fourth-week checkup of infant at pediatrician's office or well-baby clinic. How is child held by mother (or	Anxiety Alteration in comfort: pain Impaired verbal communication Ineffective individual or family coping Alteration in energy levels† Alteration in family processes Alteration in health maintenance Potential for injury

Summary of Nursing Actions—cont'd

ASSESSMENT	EXAMPLES OF POTENTIAL NURSING DIAGNOSTIC CATEGORIES*
father)? Are her hand grasp and touch gentle? Does she look at child's face or at examiner? Does she participate in restraining and comforting child? Is she overly concerned about child's health? Is child isolated except for necessary caretaking activities? 2. Physical examination shows a healthy, developing child or evidence of neglect or abuse. 3. Information regarding physical responses of child (e.g., appetite, bowel movements, voiding, rashes) is elicited. D. Assess other family member's relationship to infant: 1. *Sibling* problems are resolved. 2. *Grandparents* are integrated into their grandparent role.	Knowledge deficit Alteration in parenting Disturbance in self-concept: body image, self-esteem, role performance, personal identity Anxiety Alteration in comfort: pain Impaired verbal communication Ineffective individual or family coping Alteration in energy levels Alteration in family processes Alteration in health maintenance Potential for injury Knowledge deficit Alteration in parenting Disturbance in self-concept: body image, self-esteem, role performance, personal identity

OUTCOME CRITERIA‡	PLAN/IMPLEMENTATION
Emotional responses of parents A. Mother and father feel comfortable in their new roles. B. Couple can discuss own needs and seek support of partner. C. Couple recognizes and accepts changing of roles as child matures.	Encourage parents to discuss their concerns. Help parents identify coping mechanisms that are applicable to their problems. Recognize success of parental efforts to nurture child.
Infant growth and development A. Parents become more knowledgeable about abnormal responses of infant and those responses for which professional consultation is required. B. Knowledge of normal growth and development of infant increases. C. Parents can anticipate change in infant's needs.	Examine infant and review findings with parents. Discuss infant's developmental needs. Provide opportunity for mother and family to discuss problems. Discuss balancing infant's needs with those of other family members. Discuss signs and symptoms of illness and measures instituted to effect a cure or obtain medical assistance.
Attachment process A. Parents share time and activity with the infant. B. Parents can adapt to the child to meet changing circumstances. C. Tension and the necessity for rigid schedules lessens as competency increases. D. Parents' pride in and love for their child is expressed.	Meet parental knowledge needs relating to the growing attachment to their child. Correlate parental behaviors with energy levels, ethnic and cultural identity, and other commitments.
Infant identity A. Infant recognized as a separate person with his or her own rights. B. Infant's identity continues to expand as he or she becomes part of a family group (e.g., interacts with siblings).	Encourage parents to recognize uniqueness of infant's responses. Explore problem areas mutually (e.g., negative comparisons of infant and other siblings).

Summary of Nursing Actions—cont'd

OUTCOME CRITERIA‡	PLAN/IMPLEMENTATION
Parental criteria: criteria for success in parenting are flexible	
A. Infant responses	A. Meet parental knowledge needs in relation to infant's responses, caretaking activities, and support systems. Encourage parents to verbalize success. Help them to identify areas of concern and solutions to problems.
1. Infant's dependency needs are recognized and accepted as a beginning level of development.	
2. Parents are aware of parental actions as an important factor in behavior exhibited by infant.	
3. Adaptation of parents' and infant's normal rhythms and responses begins as a process of mutual behavior modification.	
B. Parental competence in caretaking activities:	B. Plan for continuing care by other persons or facilities.
1. Parents recognize that skills required will change with child's growth and development and that it is reasonable to seek guidance and support as new needs arise.	1. Help family obtain further assistance, if needed.
2. Health care includes preventive as well as curative elements.	2. Plan for next routine visit.
3. Involvement goes beyond immediate family to include community.	3. Refer parents to other agencies for assistance with severe problems.
C. Opinions of significant others: parents recognize that this dependency will continue; but in its negative sense, it can be countered with mastery of parental tasks and growing self-esteem as a parent.	
Family relationships	Meet parental knowledge needs as indicated.
A. Family unit reestablished.	Encourage interfamily discussions of concerns and solutions to problems.
B. Parental roles are recognized and accepted.	Refer clients, if necessary, for additional support with parenting.
C. Parents resume intimate marital relations.	Recognize parental, sibling, and grandparent successes.
D. Siblings interact satisfactorily.	

Application of the Nursing Process

NURSING CARE DURING THE POSTPARTUM PERIOD

Marianne and Bill had their second child, a girl, 4 days ago. The first child, John, is now 3 years old. Marianne chose early discharge from the hospital. The hospital has an early discharge program with home health nurses. The home health nurses have standing orders from the affiliated physicians. Marianne phoned the hospital to report two problems:

1. She was having trouble with her first bowel movement. She had had an episiotomy and has hemorrhoids and she is concerned about being hurt and uncomfortable.
2. The 3-year-old son, John, was jealous of the new baby. He was whiny and fretful. He had begun to wet his pants again.

Bill's mother was staying with them to help out. She was very cross with John. She said, "He is very spoiled. If he were mine, I would spank his bottom."

When the nurse arrived, assessment findings included intact and healing episiotomy and three moderate-sized hemorrhoids. The grandmother had taken John with her to the grocery store. The infant was asleep. Marianne has been taking fluids well and had eaten well-balanced meals with plenty of fresh fruits and vegetables. She confided that she was "just afraid to be alone" while having the bowel movement.

Continued.

Application of the Nursing Process—cont'd

FUNCTIONAL HEALTH PATTERN: ASSESSMENT	NURSING DIAGNOSIS	RATIONALE: PLAN/ IMPLEMENTATION	EVALUATION
ELIMINATION Gave birth 4 days ago. Had an episiotomy that is now intact and healing. Has three moderate-sized hemorrhoids that hurt and itch. Last bowel movement was the day of delivery.	Alteration in bowel elimination: constipation related to fear of injury and pain at episiotomy site. Alteration in comfort: pain related to constipation, episiotomy, and hemorrhoids.	*To stimulate bowel elimination and minimize discomfort* ■ Share assessment data. ■ Prepare her for and administer a commercially available physiologic enema solution. ■ Stay within shouting distance as enema is expelled. ■ Note results. ■ Reassess perineum and share findings. ■ Review care of hemorrhoids with her (Procedure 24.3).	Woman states she feels so much better having a nurse available for her first bowel movement. Woman states the enema was not as uncomfortable as she had imagined it would be. Woman states she is glad to have had a chance to see her ''bottom'' with the nurse there to ''explain things.'' Woman verbalizes understanding of care of hemorrhoids. Woman states she will call in her progress regarding self-care of hemorrhoids and bowel elimination.
COPING–STRESS TOLERANCE Three-year-old sibling is jealous of new baby and has begun to wet his pants again.	Anxiety related to fear of losing his mother's attention.	*To relieve 3-year-old's stress:* ■ Plan time with child alone. ■ Plan playing ''older-level'' games with child. ■ Involve father with son (e.g., take to park).	Three-year-old's anxiety lessens as shown by his returning to his pattern of remaining dry, and he can be away from his mother for longer periods.
Grandmother is intolerant of older sibling's response to new sister.	Ineffective family coping related to conflict in method of supporting and disciplining child.	*To relieve stress-provoking situation:* ■ Have grandmother care for newborn during time older child is usually fretful. ■ Take over care of older child, changing pants, etc. ■ Praise grandmother for help she is giving (e.g., care of newborn, cooking, and cleaning). ■ Plan outing for father, grandmother, and 3-year-old son.	Grandmother becomes more understanding of older child's acting out. Grandmother verbalizes pleasure with outing and this time to get better acquainted with the men or boys in her life.

References
Physical Care

American Cancer Society, How to examine your breasts, Pamphlet no. 2088-LE, June 1978, The Society.

Bing, E., and Colman, L.: Making love during pregnancy, New York, 1977, Bantam Books.

Brownlee, A.T.: Community, culture, and care: a cross-cultural guide for health workers, St. Louis, 1978, The C.V. Mosby Co.

Campbell, T., and Chang, B.: Health care of the Chinese in America, Nurs. Outlook 21:245, 1973.

Clark, M.: Health in the Mexican-American culture: a community study, Berkeley, 1970, University of California Press.

Currier, R.L.: The hot-cold syndrome and symbolic balance in Mexican and Spanish-American folk medicine. In Martinez, R.A., editor: Hispanic culture and health care: fact, fiction, folklore, St. Louis, 1978, The C.V. Mosby Co.

Droegemueller, W.: Cold sitz bath for relief of postpartum perineal pain, Clin. Obstet. Gynecol. 23:1039, 1980.

Horn, B.M.: Northwest coast Indians: the Muckleshoot. In Kay, M.A., editor: Anthropology of human birth, Philadelphia, 1982, F.A. Davis Co.

Kegel, A.H.: Progressive resistance exercise in the functional restoration of the perineal muscles, Am. J. Obstet. Gynecol. 56:238, 1948.

Kundstadter, P.: Do cultural differences make any difference? Choice points in medical systems available in Northwestern Thailand. In Kleinman, A., and others, editors: Culture and healing in Asian societies, Cambridge, Mass., 1978, Schenkman Publishing Co.

Kunst-Wilson, W., and Cronenwett, L.R.: Nursery care for the emerging family: promoting paternal behavior, Res. Nurs. Health 4:201, 1981.

Pillsbury, B.L.K.: "Doing the month": confinement and convalescence of Chinese women after childbirth, Soc. Sci. Med. 12:11, 1978.

Snow, L.: folk medical beliefs and their implications for care of patients, Ann. Intern. Med. 81:82, 1974.

Stern, P.N., and others: Culturally induced stress during childbearing: the Filipino-American experience, Issues Health Care Women 2(3-4):67, 1980.

Emotional Care

Anderson, C.J.: Enhancing reciprocity between mother and neonate, Nurs. Res. 30:89, 1981.

Bampton, B., Jones, J., and Mancini, J.: Initial mothering patterns of low-income black primiparas, J.O.G.N. Nurs. 10:174, 1981.

Caplan, G.: Psychological aspects of maternity care, Am. J. Public Health 47:25, 1957.

Crawford, J.: A theoretical model of support network conflict experienced by new mothers. Nurs. Res. 34:100, March/April 1985

Cronenwett, L.R.: Network structure, social support, and psychological outcomes of pregnancy, Nurs. Res. 34:93, March/April 1985a.

Cronenwett, L.R.: Parental network structured and perceived support after birth of first child, Nurs. Res. 34:347, Nov./Dec. 1985b.

Dunn, D.M., and White, D.G.: Interactions of mothers with their newborns in the first half-hour of life, J. Adv. Nurs. 6:271, 1981.

Field, T.M.: Effects of early separation, interactive deficits, and experimental manipulation on infant-mother face-to-face interaction, Child Dev. 48:763, 1977.

Gottlieb, B.H.: The role of individual and social support in preventing child maltreatment. In Garbarino, J., and Stocking, S., editors: Protecting children from abuse/neglect, San Francisco, 1980, Jossey Bass.

Kunst-Wilson, W., and Cronenwett, L.R.: Nursery care for the emerging family: promoting paternal behavior, Res. Nurs. Health 4:201, 1981.

Lang, R.: Birth book, Ben Lomond, Calif., 1972, Genesis Press.

Mercer, R.T.: Parent-infant attachment. In Sonstegard, L.J., and others, editors: Women's health, vol. 2, Childbearing, New York, 1982, Grune & Stratton.

Morris, M.: Psychological miscarriage: an end to mother love, Transactions, p. 11, Jan./Feb. 1966.

Riesch, S., and Munns, S.: Promoting awareness: the mother and her baby, Nurs. Res. 33:271, Sept./Oct. 1985.

Rödholm, M.: The behavior of human male adults at their first contact with a newborn. Unpublished doctoral dissertation. Department of Psychology, University of Goteberg, Goteberg, Sweden, 1981.

Rödholm, M., and Larsson, K.: Father-infant interaction at the first contact after delivery, Early Hum. Dev. 3:21, 1979.

Rubin, R.: Puerperal change, Nurs. Outlook 9:753, 1961.

Rubin, R.: Maternal touch, Nurs. Outlook 11:828, 1963.

Schornkoff, J.P.: Social support and the development of vulnerable children, Am. J. Public Health 74:310.

Stainton, C.M.: Parent-infant interaction: putting theory into practice, Calgary, Alberta, Canada, 1981, University of Calgary Faculty of Nursing.

Stainton, C.M.: Maternal newborn attachment origins and processes. III. Interactional synchrony: the prelude to attachment, doctoral thesis, University of California, San Francisco, 1985.

Steele, B., and Pollock, C.: A psychiatric study of parents who abuse infants and small children. In Helfer, R.E., and Kempe, C., editors: The battered child, Chicago, 1968, University of Chicago Press.

Sullivan, D., and Beeman, R.: Satisfaction with postpartum care: opportunities for bonding, reconstructing the birth and instruction, Birth Fam. J. 8:3, Fall 1981.

Tansig, M.: Measuring life events, J. Health Soc. Behav. 23:52, Jan. 1982.

Thoits, P.A.: Dimensions of life events that influence psychological distress: an evaluation and synthesis of literature. In Kaplan, H.B., editor: Psychosocial stress: trends in theory and research, New York, 1983, Academic Press.

Tulman, L.: Mothers and unrelated persons initial handling of newborn infants, Nurs. Res. 34:205, July/Aug. 1985.

Turner, R.J., and Avison, W.R.: Assessing risk factors for problem parenting: the significance of social support, J. Mar. Fam. 47:881, Nov. 1985.

Bibliography

Avery, M., and others: An early postpartum hospital discharge program: implementation and evaluation, J.O.G.N. Nurs. 11:200, 1982.

Balkam, J.A.: Guidelines for drug therapy during lactation, J.O.G.N. N. 15:65, Jan./Feb. 1986.

Brooten, D.A., and others: A comparison of four treatments

to prevent and control breast pain and engorgement in nonnursing mothers, Nurs. Res. 32:225, 1983.

Bull, M., and Lawrence, D.: Mother's use of knowledge during the first postpartum weeks, J.O.G.N. N. 14:315, July/Aug. 1985.

Carr, K.C., and Walton, V.E.: Early postpartum discharge, J.O.G.N. Nurs. 11:29, 1982.

Claypool, J.M.: Rubella protection for maternal child health care providers, M.C.N. 6:53, 1981.

Croog, E.H., and Zigrossi, S.T.: Parenting luncheons on the postpartum unit, M.C.N. 8:277, 1983.

Danforth, D.N.: Textbook of obstetrics and gynecology, ed. 5, New York, 1982, Harper & Row, Publishers.

Devaney, S.W., and Lavery, S.F.: Nursing care for the relinquishing mother, J.O.G.N. Nurs. 9:375, 1980.

Donaldson, N.E.: The postpartum follow-up nurse clinician, J.O.G.N. Nurs. 4:249, 1981.

Edwards, M.: The crises of fourth trimester, Birth Fam. J. 1:19, Winter 1973-1974.

Fischman, S.H., and others: Changes in sexual relationships in postpartum couples, J.O.G.N. N. 15:58, Jan./Feb. 1986.

Goebel, J.B., and others: Infant car seat usage; effectiveness of a postpartum education program, J.O.G.N. Nurs. 13:33, 1984.

Goodlin, R.C., and Frederick, I.B.: Postpartum vulvar edema associated with the birthing chair, Am. J. Obstet. Gynecol. 146:334, 1983.

Gorrie, T.M.: Postpartal nursing diagnoses, J.O.G.N. N. 15:52, Jan./Feb. 1986.

Gosha, J., and Brucker, M.C.: A self-help group for new mothers: an evaluation, M.C.N. 11:20, Jan./Feb. 1986.

Hans, A.: Postpartum assessment: the psychological component, J.O.G.N. N. 15:49, Jan./Feb. 1986.

Harr, B., and Hastings, J.: Parturition care planning, J.O.G.N. Nurs. 10:54, 1981.

Harvey, K.: Mother-baby nursing, Nurs. Management 13(7):22, 1982.

Henderson, J.S.: Effects of a prenatal teaching program on postpartum regeneration of the pubococcygeal muscle, J.O.G.N. Nurs. 12:403, 1983.

Hensleigh, P.A.: Preventing rhesus isoimmunization, Am. J. Obstet. Gynecol. 146:749, 1983.

Horn, M., and Manion, J.: Creative grandparenting: bonding the generations, J.O.G.N. N. 14(3):233, May/June 1985.

Jacobson, H.: A standard for assessing lochia volume, M.C.N. 10:174, May/June 1985.

Jensen, M.D., and Bobak, I.M.: Maternity and gynecologic care: the nurse and the family, ed. 3, St. Louis, 1985, The C.V. Mosby Co.

Jiminez, M.H., and Niles, N.: Activity and work during pregnancy and the postpartum period: a cross cultural study of 202 societies, Am. J. Obstet. Gynecol. 135:198, 1979.

Ketter, D.E., and Shelton, B.J.: In-hospital exercises for the postpartal woman, M.C.N. 8:120, 1983.

Kowba, M.D., and Schwirian, P.M.: Direct sibling contact and bacterial colonization in newborns. J.O.G.N. N. 14:412, Sept./Oct. 1985.

Leininger, M.: Transcultural nursing: an essential knowledge and practice field for today, Can. Nurse 80:41, Dec. 1984.

Malinowski, J.: Bladder assessment in the postpartum patient, J.O.G.N. Nurs. 7(4):14, 1978.

Mansell, K.A.: Mother-baby units: the concept works, M.C.N. 9:132, 1984.

Marecki, M.P.: Postpartum follow-up goals and assessment, J.O.G.N. Nurs. 8:214, 1979.

Marecki, M., and others: Early sibling attachment, J.O.G.N. N. 14:418, Sept./Oct. 1985.

McCary, J.L., and McCary, S.P.: McCary's human sexuality, ed. 4, Belmont, Calif., 1982, Wadsworth Publishing Co.

McKay, S., and Mahan, C.S.: Ways to upgrade postpartal care, Contemp. OB/Gyn. 27:63, Nov. 1985.

McKenzie, C.A., and others: Comprehensive care during the postpartum period, Nurs. Clin. North Am. 17:23, 1982.

Mercer, R.T.: The nurse and maternal tasks of early postpartum, M.C.N. 6:341, Sept./Oct. 1981.

Mercer, R.T.: The relationship of developmental variables to maternal behavior, Res. Nurs. Health, 9:25-33, 1986.

Mercer, R.T.: Relationship of the birth experience to later mothering behaviors, J. Nurs. Midw. 30:204, July/Aug. 1985.

Mercer, R.T.: The relationship of age and other variables to gratification in mothering, Health Care Women Internat. 6:295, 1985.

Mercer, R.T., and Stainton, M.C.: Perceptions of the birth experience: a cross-cultural comparison, Health Care Women Internat. 5:29, 1984.

Myles, M.F.: Textbook for midwives with modern concepts of obstetric and neonatal care, ed. 9, New York, 1981, Churchill Livingstone.

Mynick, A.: Instituting a postpartum self-medication program, M.C.N. 6:419, 1981.

Newell, N.J.: Grandparents: the overlooked support system for new parents during the fourth trimester, NAACOG Update Series, 1(lesson 21), Washington, D.C., 1984, The Association.

Nurses Association of the American College of Obstetricians and Gynecologists: Standards for obstetric gynecologic and neonatal nursing, ed. 3, Washington, D.C., 1986, The Association.

Olson, M.L.: Fitting grandparents into new families, M.C.N. 6:419, 1981.

Petrowski, D.D.: Effectiveness of prenatal and postnatal instruction in postpartum care, J.O.G.N. Nurs. 10:386, 1981.

Pritchard, J.A., MacDonald, P.C., and Gant, N.F.: Williams obstetrics, ed. 17, Norwalk, Conn., 1985, Appleton-Century-Crofts.

Quistad, C.: How to smooth mom's postpartum path, R.N. 47:40, April 1984.

Rubin, R.: Basic maternal behaviors, Paper presented at the National League for Nursing Biennial Convention, Cleveland, Ohio, 1961.

Russell, T.R.: Managing hemorrhoids during and after pregnancy, Contemp. OB/Gyn. 21(special issue), March 1983.

Strang, V.R., and Sullivan, P.L.: Body image attitudes during pregnancy and the postpartum period, J.O.G.N. N. 14:332, July/Aug. 1985.

Strelinck, E.G.: Postpartum care: an opportunity to reinforce breast self-examination, M.C.N. 7(4):249, 1982.

Tilkian, S.M.: Clinical implication of laboratory tests, ed. 3, St. Louis, 1983, The C.V. Mosby Co.

Tucker, S.M., and others: Patient care standards, ed. 3, St. Louis, 1984, The C.V. Mosby Co.

Vestal, K.W.: A proposal: primary nursing for the mother-baby dyad, Nurs. Clin. North Am. 17:3, 1982.

Wadd, L.: Vietnamese postpartum practices: implication for nursing in the hospital setting, J.O.G.N. Nurs. 12:252, 1983.

Willson, J.R., Carrington, E.R., and Ledger, W.J.: Obstetrics and gynecology, ed. 7, St. Louis, 1983, The C.V. Mosby Co.

Wong, S., and Stepp-Gilbert, E.: Lactation suppression: nonpharmaceutical versus pharmaceutical method, J.O.G.N. N. 14(4):302, July/Aug. 1985.

Woods, N.F.: Human sexuality in health and illness, ed. 3, St. Louis, 1984, The C.V. Mosby Co.

Varney, H.: Nurse midwifery. 1980. Blackwell Scientific Publication, distributed by The C.V. Mosby Co., St. Louis.

Zalar, M.K.: Human sexuality: a component of total patient care, Nurs. Digest. 3:40, 1975.

Zalar, M.K.: Sexual counseling for pregnant couples, M.C.N. 1:176, 1976.

Zuspan, F., and Quilligan, E., editors: Practical manual of obstetrical care, St. Louis, 1982, The C.V. Mosby Co.

UNIT 7

The High-Risk Family

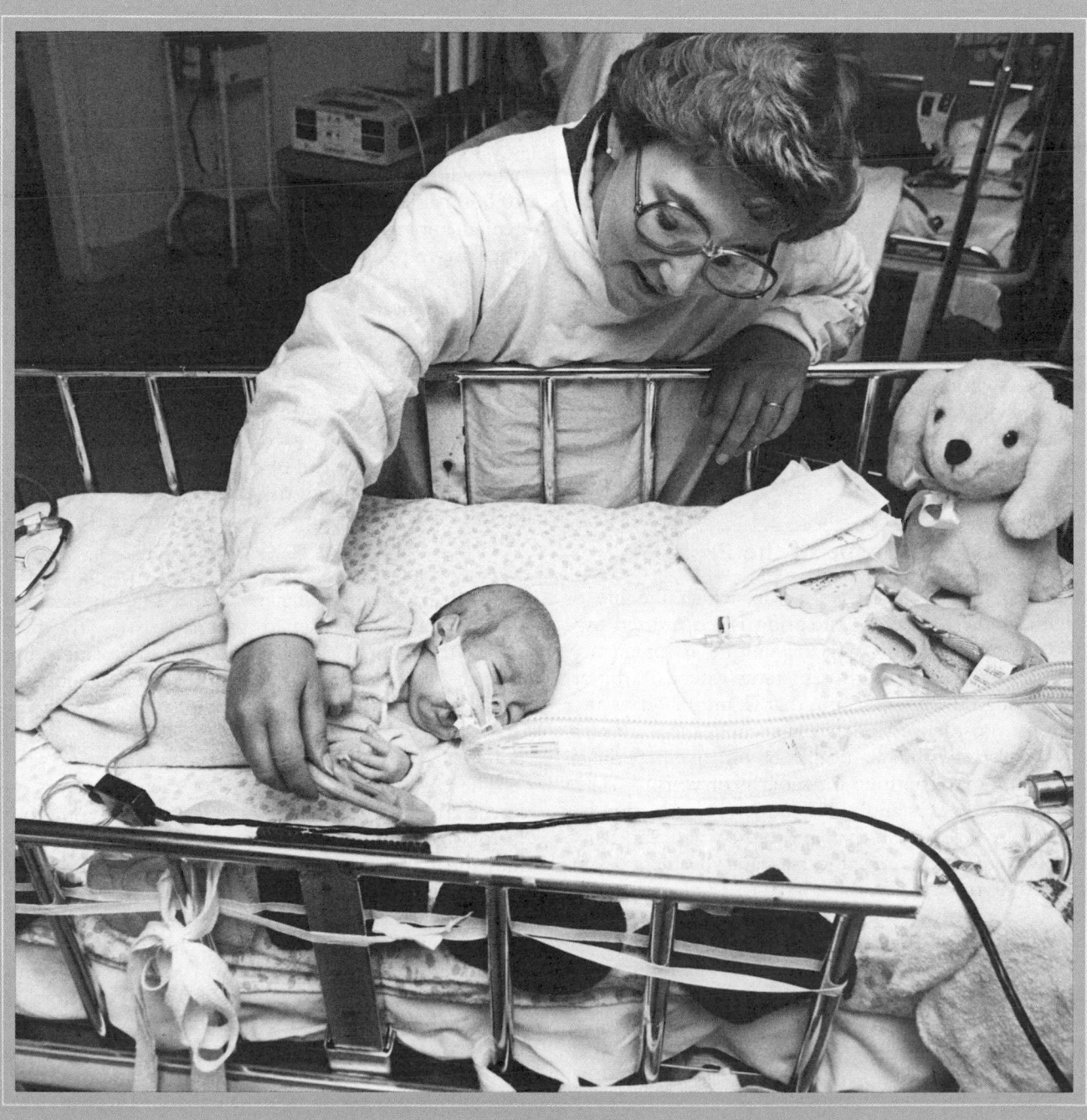

Maternal and Neonatal Risk and the Compromised Neonate

Of the approximately 3 million births that occur in the United States each year, 500,000 will be categorized as high risk because of maternal or fetal complications. The united efforts of all members of the obstetric team and close collaboration with other medical personnel are required to adequately care for the high-risk client. In this chapter the high-risk client and the factors associated with diagnosis of high risk are identified. Techniques of biophysical monitoring of fetal health are emphasized. General care of the compromised newborn is presented. Techniques inherent in the nursing care of infants, for example, maintenance of respirations, oxygen therapy, and feeding measures, are included.

Definition and Scope of the Problem

A high-risk pregnancy is one in which the life or health of the mother or offspring is jeopardized by a disorder coincidental with or unique to pregnancy. For the mother the high-risk status extends (arbitrarily) through the puerperium, that is, until 29 days after delivery. Postdelivery maternal complications are usually resolved within a month of birth, but perinatal morbidity may continue for months or years.

A better understanding of human reproduction has greatly reduced maternal morbidity and mortality. Knowledge of the fetus and neonatal disorders has increased dramatically in the last 10 to 15 years. This has led to a gratifying drop in perinatal morbidity and mortality during this period.

Of the 5 to 10 million pregnancies that occur in the United States each year, 2 to 3 million terminate as spontaneous abortions. Many of the abortions are caused by genetic faults or infection. About 1 million early gestations end as elective abortions. Approximately 3.5 million pregnancies reach viability (24 to 28 weeks' gestational age), but of these at least 45,000 fetuses fail to survive. About the same number of neonates die during the first month of life. Another 40,000 babies have severe but perhaps correctable congenital anomalies. Pregnancy and delivery complications are responsible in part at least for approximately 90,000 mentally retarded individuals. In addition, these complications have partially handicapped more than 150,000 persons, who have difficulty coping in our complex society (see Statistical picture and definitions, Chapter 2).

Even considering fetuses who have reached viability, perinatal mortality exceeds that of all other causes of death combined until 65 years of age. When viewed in this perspective, high-risk pregnancy presents one of the most critical and urgent problems of modern medicine.

A new social emphasis on the quality of life has developed. Family planning has reduced family size and the number of unwanted pregnancies. With these trends the wanted child has become increasingly important. As a consequence, periodic maternal and perinatal assessment is essential to emphasize safe delivery of normal infants who can develop to their maximal potential.

The experience of childbirth for each woman is influenced by many factors. Interaction of the various factors results in a holistic experience unique to each individual. At the start of this holistic view of the childbearing experience is the culture into which the woman was born (Fig. 25.1). As the young girl matures, she integrates cultural expectations (occasionally couched in folklore) and adds to these societal norms to which she is exposed. Her family and peers further direct and influence her expectations of herself as a member of the family, society, and community. Onto this structure of role definitions and expectations is the physiologic process of pregnancy that begins with conception and ends at childbirth. Between these two points there is an expected length of time—9 months—during which predictable events occur. Under optimal circumstances, even a normal pregnancy brings profound psychologic as well as physiologic changes. Even a normal pregnancy is a time of transient ego vulnerability for the woman and anticipated changes in the family unit.

It is well known that pregnancy is a **maturational crisis** in both the physiologic and psychologic sense. The diagnosis of high risk imposes another crisis, a **situational crisis** (e.g., the pregnancy terminates before the anticipated date; the woman develops gestational diabetes mellitus with its potential complications; a neonate is born who does not meet cultural, societal, or familial norms and expectations). Understanding of the high-risk client will allow the nurse to provide therapeutic nursing care.

Maternal health problems. Different parts of the world have different leading causes of maternal death attributable to pregnancy. In general three major causes have persisted for the last 35 years: hypertensive disorders, infection, and hemorrhage.

Causes of Mortality	Percent
Hypertensive disorders	21
Infection	18
Hemorrhage	14
Other (cardiac, diabetes mellitus)	46

In the United States, maternal mortality among white women and all other women still differs, although the gap that existed 30 years ago has been narrowed dramatically. Today the mortality ratio for white women and all others is 2:3. This decline is attributed to changes in social and economic factors and availability of health care.

Many factors have contributed to the decrease in maternal mortality:

1. Advances in medical management
2. Expansion of knowledge and capability to apply knowledge
3. Emergence of a philosophy of maternity care that recognizes the advantages of client participation in health care and focuses on childbirth as a healthy event
4. Acceptance of prenatal care

Fetal and neonatal health problems

Fetal death. Fetal death (demise) is defined as the death in utero before complete expulsion of the product of human conception irrespective of the duration of pregnancy. It does not result from therapeutic or elective abortion. It is also called intrauterine death.

Fig. 25.1
Psychosocial expectations originating from every level are integrated by each woman into a unique pattern that individualizes her childbearing experience.

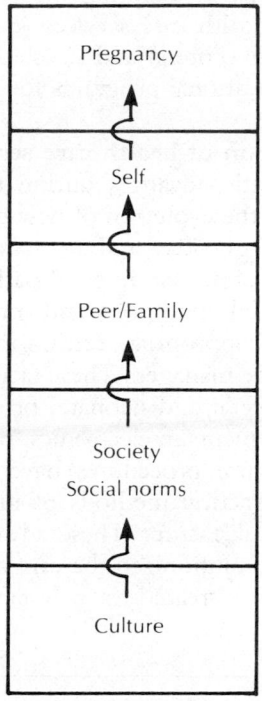

Neonatal death. Neonatal death is the death of a liveborn neonate at 20 weeks' gestation or more. A liveborn neonate is one who shows any evidence of life after birth, even if only momentary (respiration, heartbeat, voluntary muscle movement, or pulsation within the umbilical cord), and who dies at 28 days or less.

Perinatal death rate. Perinatal death rate is defined as the sum of fetal and neonatal death rates. This statistic is considered the most sensitive indicator of the effectiveness of perinatal care.

The incidence of each cause of **infant mortality** (Chapter 2) is expressed as the number of deaths per 100,000 live births. For 1979, the leading causes in the United States were congenital anomalies (257.7), respiratory distress syndrome (155.8), disorders related to preterm birth and low birth weight (100.5), intrauterine hypoxia and birth asphyxia (48.4), pneumonia and influenza (33.1), and birth trauma (31.7). Infant mortality includes the neonatal death rate. Problems related to low birth weight and preterm birth are chiefly responsible for deaths during the first 4 weeks of life.

These statistics are used to determine health care needs for the general population. Resources such as funds and facilities are allocated to those segments of the population within a community or to the geographic location of the United States where the needs are the greatest. In addition, the identified causes of mortality are used in planning for (1) the type and distribution of health care services (e.g., research, location or regional centers) and (2) the development of curricula for educational programs for health care providers.

Regionalization of health care services. Diagnostic and therapeutic advances during the past decade have resulted in the evolution of new types of facilities for the care of gravidas and neonates at high risk. Newly acquired understandings of pathophysiology of pregnancy-induced conditions and intercurrent disorders required an appropriate setting in which severely ill clients could be managed. These facilities would also need to handle fetal and neonatal problems. Simultaneously, developments in electronics, biochemistry, genetics, and surgical procedures have resulted in the availability of practical methods of identification and monitoring of risk factors. These advances and developments have revolutionized the care of clients at high risk. The need was created for new facilities, reorganization of services, and specially trained personnel in several disciplines. These health care providers must learn to function together collaboratively if lives are to be saved.

There is excellent evidence that mortality decreases when high risk is identified and intensive care applied. In addition, follow-up studies have shown that serious residual handicaps (physical and mental) of surviving infants have been dramatically reduced.

It is not feasible nor reasonable for each hospital to develop and maintain the full spectrum of medical and nursing specialists, laboratory capabilities, and facilities with equipment. As a consequence, care is being regionalized; that is, all levels of care will be available within a given area, but facilities will be organized to provide different levels of care. A coordinated system within a region first requires the designation of certain hospitals for provision of levels of care based on their capacity to provide the care required. To provide appropriate services and continuity of care for each client, an effective pattern of communication for consultation and for transport of clients is mandatory. Fundamental to all these activities is a regional program for continuing education of personnel.

Fig. 25.2
Summary of risk factors that may affect pregnancy outcome. (From Fogel C.I., and Woods, D.F.: Health care of women, St. Louis, 1981, The C.V. Mosby Co.)

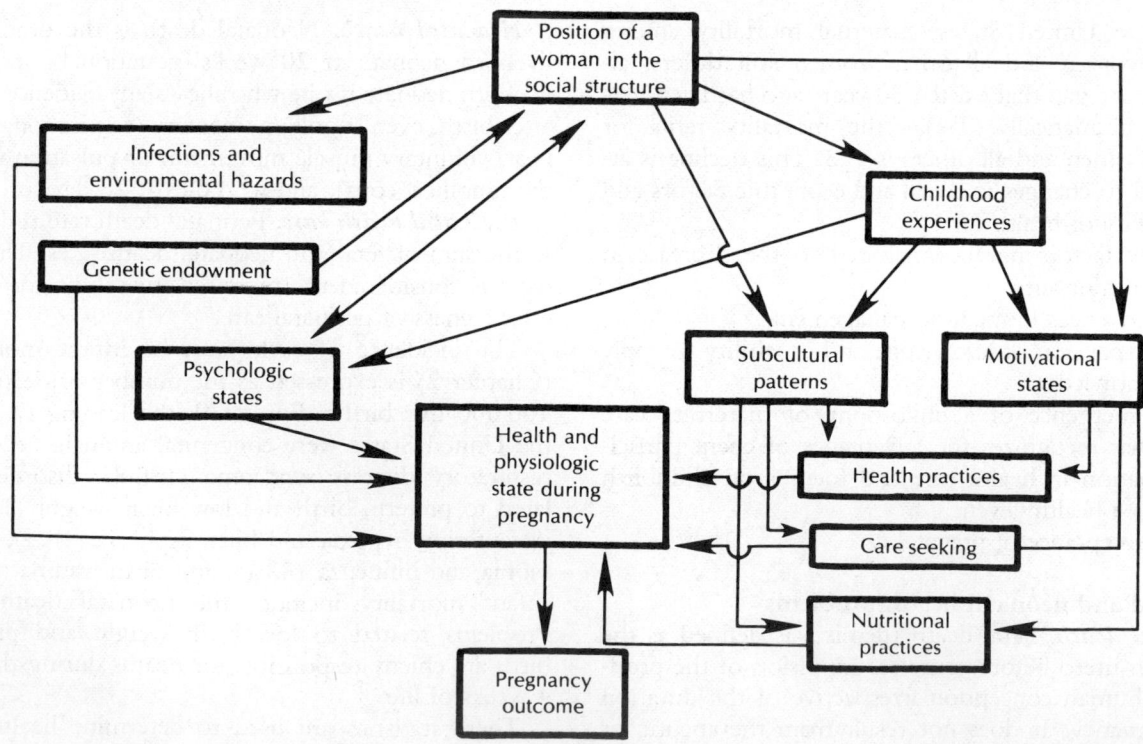

Ideally, a regionalized system includes primary care and three levels of facilities within a designated geographic area. Level I facilities have three main functions: (1) the management of normal pregnancy, labor, and delivery, (2) the earliest possible identification of high-risk pregnancy and high-risk neonates, and (3) the provision of competent care in the event of unanticipated obstetric or neonatal emergencies.

Level II facilities provide care for a number of maternal and neonatal complications as well as offer a full range of maternity and neonatal care in uncomplicated cases.

Level III facilities, the **regional centers,** have the capacity to manage uncomplicated maternity and neonatal cases and the most complex disorders. In addition, the regional centers provide outreach services; for example, consultation and continuing education for obstetricians, pediatricians, and nurses within the region.

Assessment for Risk Factors

Interview and physical examination. Serious biologic handicaps, health problems, obstetric disorders, and social deprivation may compromise the mother and the infant in subtle or more obvious ways. Early or late fetal damage may occur. The baby may be small for gestational age (SGA), preterm, or postterm. Occasionally the infant may be preterm but of excessive size; that is, large for gestational age (LGA). In other instances the postterm infant is large. Such hazards and their management are unique perinatal problems.

Research and experience have led to the identification of factors that jeopardize the pregnant and postdelivery woman and the fetus-neonate. This knowledge has permitted the development of increasingly effective preventive and therapeutic measures that could minimize the incidence of morbidity, disability, and death of the mother or infant. Frequently it is the alert nurse, conversant and familiar with deviations from normal, who notes and reports potential or real high-risk factors (Tables 25.1 and 25.2 and Boxes, p. 722 and p. 724). The interrelationship of risk factors that influence pregnancy outcome are summarized schematically in Fig. 25.2.

BIOPHYSICAL MONITORING

Ultrasonography
Definitions

static Stationary.
dynamic Moving.

real time Dynamic imaging (limb and respiratory movements), as well as static images (biparietal diameter [BPD], placental location).
hertz (Hz) Frequency of sound; 1 Hz equals 1 cycle per second or 1 oscillation/s (1 kHz = 1000 Hz; 1 MHz = 1,000,000 Hz).
transmitter Device that emits or transmits energy.
receiver Device that receives or detects energy.
transceiver Device that is both a transmitter and a receiver.
transducer Transceiver that also changes electrical signals into mechanical motion so that it is displayed on a screen or traced on graph paper.
piezoelectric crystal Active element in the transducer; the substance that emits sound at megahertz level (e.g., crystalline quartz, lithium sulfate, barium lead zirconate, barium lead titanate).
pulsed wave Sound emitted at intervals.
continuous wave Sound emitted continuously.
A mode One-dimensional image that appears as spikes on a horizontal base; distance between spikes can be measured (e.g., BPD).
B mode (gray scale) Rough, two-dimensional image of various tissue densities for visualizing tissue texture and contour.
M mode Time-related tracings showing straight lines for motionless structures and wiggly lines for structural motion (e.g., atrial septal defects and patent ductus arteriosus).
10 mW/cm² (milliwatts per square centimeter) Emission of sound frequencies at the *intensity* of 10 mW/cm² by 2.25 MHz crystal transducer; diagnostic ultrasound.
Doppler effect Detection of change in frequency (wavelength) of structures in motion (e.g., blood flow in umbilical cord and placenta, closure of fetal cardiac valves).

General comments. When directional beams of sound strike an object, an echo is returned. The time delay between the emission of the sound and the return of the echo is noted, as well as the direction from which the echo comes. From these data, the object's distance and location can be calculated. Sonar (underwater) and radar (air) are familiar uses of very high frequency sound.

First introduced in the 1960s, diagnostic ultrasound has developed rapidly to enjoy a principal position in medical imaging today. Ultrasound is sound having a frequency higher than that of normal human hearing. The range of human hearing extends from 20 Hz to 20 kHz (20,000 Hz). Bats and some insects use ultrasound in the range of about 100 kHz to navigate. Diagnostic ultrasound is beyond audible range but well below that used by sonar and radar. Medical diagnostic ultrasound covers the range from approximately 1 to 10 MHz; 2.25 MHz (2,250,000 Hz) is generally used in obstetric and gynecologic imaging.

The biophysical principles of diagnostic ultrasound are beyond the scope of this text, but several excellent resources are available in the references and bibliography at the end of this chapter.

Operational modes. Table 25.3 presents a summary of modalities, imaging, and principal uses of diagnos-

Categories of High-Risk Pregnancy

1. Maternal age and parity factors
a. Age 16 years or under
b. Nullipara 35 years or over
c. Multipara 40 years or over
d. Interval of 8 years or more since last pregnancy
e. High parity (5 or more)
f. Pregnancy occurring 3 months or less after last delivery

2. Nonmarital pregnancy

3. PIH, hypertension, kidney disease
a. Preeclampsia with hospitalization before labor
b. Eclampsia
c. Kidney disease—pyelonephritis, nephritis, nephrosis, etc.
d. Chronic hypertension, severe (160/100 mm Hg or over)
e. Blood pressure 140/90 mm Hg or above on two readings 30 minutes apart

4. Anemia and hemorrhage
a. Hematocrit 30% or below in pregnancy
b. Hemorrhage (previous pregnancy)—severe, requiring transfusion
c. Hemorrhage (present pregnancy)
d. Anemia (hemoglobin below 10 g) for which treatment other than oral iron preparations is required (hemolytic, macrocytic, etc.)
e. Sickle cell trait or disease
f. History of bleeding or clotting disorder at any time

5. Fetal factors
a. Two or more previous premature deliveries (twins = one delivery)
b. Two or more consecutive spontaneous abortions (miscarriages)
c. One or more stillbirths at term
d. One or more gross anomalies
e. Rh incompatibility or ABO immunization problems
f. History of previous birth defects—cerebral palsy, brain damage, mental retardation, metabolic disorders such as phenylketonuria (PKU)
g. History of large infants (over 4032 g [9 lb])

6. Paternal age (?) and other factors (?)

7. Dystocia (history of or anticipated)
a. Contracted pelvis or cephalopelvic disproportion (CPD)
b. Multiple pregnancy in current pregnancy
c. Two or more breech deliveries
d. Previous operative deliveries, e.g., cesarean or midforceps delivery
e. History of prolonged labor (more than 18 hours for nullipara; more than 12 hours for multipara)
f. Previously diagnosed genital tract anomalies (incompetent cervix, cervical or uterine malformation, solitary ovary or tube) or problem (ovarian mass, endometriosis)
g. Short stature (1.5 m [60 in] or less)

8. History of or concurrent conditions
a. Diabetes mellitus; gestational diabetes
b. Hyperemesis gravidarum
c. Thyroid disease (hypothyroidism or hyperthyroidism)
d. Malnutrition or extreme obesity (20% over ideal weight for height; 15% under ideal weight for height)
e. Organic heart disease
f. Syphilis and TORCH infections: toxoplasmosis, rubella in first 10 weeks of *this* pregnancy, cytomegalovirus (CMV), and herpes simplex; AIDS
g. Tuberculosis or other serious pulmonary pathologic condition (e.g., emphysema, asthma)
h. Malignant or premalignant tumors (including hydatidiform mole)
i. Alcoholism, drug addiction
j. Psychiatric disease or epilepsy (documented)
k. Mental retardation

9. Those with previous history of
a. Late registration
b. Poor clinic attendance
c. Home situation making clinic attendance and hospitalization difficult
d. Mothers, including minors, without family resources (includes desertions, adoptions, injuries, separations, family withdrawals, sole support)

Modified from Fogel, C.I., and Woods, N.F.: Health care of women: a nursing perspective, St. Louis, 1981, The C.V. Mosby Co.

Table 25.1
Factors that Place the Pregnancy and Fetus-neonate at High Risk by Trimester and During Labor

Category	Factors that Result in Risk	Category	Factors that Result in Risk
First trimester		**Third trimester**	
Anatomic	Maternal	Anatomic	Malpresentation
	Ectopic pregnancy		Cord complications
	Uterine abnormality		Placenta previa*
	Retroversion of uterus	Maternal complications	Hypertensive disease*
Physiologic	Fetal		Rh incompatibilities
	Gross chromosomal defect		Diabetes
	Hydatidiform mole		Thryotoxicosis
	Multiple pregnancy	Infections	Viral infection*
	Poor trophoblast invasiveness		Pneumonia
	Folate deficiency	Nutritional	Protein lack
	Endocrine deficiency		Iron deficiencies
	Hyperemesis gravidarum		Abruptio placentae*
	Defective sperm		Antibacterial drugs
Psychologic	Psychologic shock	Therapeutic to mother	Tetracycline
	Drugs		Antithyroid drugs
Therapeutic	Social abortion (aspiration, saline		Corticosteroids
	solution, prostaglandin)		Anticonvulsants
	Drug therapy		Anticoagulants
	X-ray therapy	Fetal complications	Premature rupture of membranes
Infection	Viral infection		Preterm labor, postmaturity
Genetic	Sporadic mutation		Hydramnios or oligohydramnios
	Inherited characteristics		Multiple gestation
	Sex-linked disease		Poverty
Environmental	Poverty	Environmental	Drugs, tobacco, alcohol
	Drugs, tobacco, alcohol		Nutrition, inadequate
	Nutrition, inadequate		
Second trimester		**Labor**	
Anatomic	Maternal	Anatomic	Fetal head compression
	Uterine abnormality		Malpresentation
	Incompetent cervical os		Umbilical cord prolapse
	Fetal		Breech presentation
	Gross abnormality		Placenta previa, abruptio placentae
	Acute hydramnios		Rigid soft tissues
	Multiple pregnancy		Multiple gestation
	Poor implantation		Fetal hemorrhage
Maternal complications	Rh incompatibility		Placental or umbilical cord compression
	Cyanotic heart disease		Excessive or inadequate or fetal size
	Hypertension	Physiologic	Dehydration
	Renal disease		Ketosis
	Urinary tract infections		Fetal acidosis (pH 7.25 or less in the
	Accidents		first stage of labor)
	Anoxia of eclampsia or epilepsy		Meconium staining of amniotic fluid
Infections	Viral-polio, syphilis, hepatitis,		Fetal bradycardia or tachycardia
	TORCH,† AIDS		(longer than 30 minutes)
Genetic	Amniocentesis		Abnormal nonstress test or oxytocin
Idiopathic	Genetic death		challenge test
Environmental	Poverty		Falling urinary estriol levels
	Drugs, tobacco, alcohol		Immature fetal lungs
	Nutrition, inadequate	Maternal complications, iatrogenic	Severe preeclampsia-eclampsia
			Sedative depression
			Hypotension; anesthesia; supine position
			Oxytocin (Pitocin) augmentation or induction of labor
			Prolonged labor; precipitous labor (less than 3 hours)
			Operative delivery: cesarean, forceps, vacuum extraction
		Uterine and placental	Uterine hypotonicity, hypertonicity, inertia
			Placental insufficiency

Modified from Fogel, C.I., and Woods, N.F.: Health care of women: a nursing perspective, St. Louis, 1981, The C.V. Mosby Co.
*Associated with intrauterine growth retardation (IUGR).
†Toxoplasmosis, rubella, cytomegalovirus, and herpes simplex.

Factors that Place the Postpartum Woman and Neonate at High Risk

Specific factors that place **mother in high-risk** category:
1. Hemorrhage
2. Infection
3. Abnormal vital signs
4. Traumatic labor or delivery
5. Psychosocial factors

Criteria for selection of high-risk infants for admission to neonatal intensive care units:

1. Specific factors that place **infant in high-risk** category:
    a. Infants continuing or developing signs of respiratory distress syndrome (RDS) or other respiratory distress
    b. Asphyxiated infants (Apgar score of less than 6 at 5 minutes); resuscitation required at birth
    c. Preterm infants; dysmature infants
    d. Infants with cyanosis or suspected cardiovascular disease; persistent cyanosis
    e. Infants with major congenital malformations requiring surgery; chromosomal anomalies
    f. Infants with convulsions, sepsis, hemorrhagic diathesis, or shock
    g. Meconium aspiration syndrome
    h. Central nervous system (CNS) depression for longer than 24 hours
    i. Hypoglycemia
    j. Hypocalcemia
    k. Hyperbilirubinemia

2. Factors indicating **moderate-risk:**
    a. Dysmaturity
    b. Prematurity (weight between 2000 and 2500 g)
    c. Apgar score of less than 5 at 1 minute
    d. Feeding problems
    e. Multiple birth
    f. Transient tachypnea
    g. Hypomagnesemia or hypermagnesemia
    h. Hypoparathyroidism
    i. Failure to gain weight
    j. Jitteriness or hyperactivity
    k. Cardiac anomalies not requiring immediate catheterization
    l. Heart murmur
    m. Anemia
    n. CNS depression for less than 24 hours

---

tic ultrasound. Dynamic image scanners are well suited for obstetric work; static image scanners are useful for gynecologic diagnosis. Dynamic image scanners provide direct visualization of indicators of fetal viability—fetal cardiac and body movement. The usual examination takes only about 5 minutes. Since the scanner can be moved about, it can be taken directly into labor and delivery rooms for directing amniocentesis or evaluating the source of vaginal bleeding.

Current applications in pregnancy. Major indications for obstetric sonography by trimester appear in Table 25.4. During the **first trimester,** ultrasound examination is performed to obtain the following information: (1) number, size, and location of gestational sacs (Fig. 25.3), (2) presence or absence of fetal cardiac and body movement, (3) presence or absence of uterine abnormalities (e.g., bicornuate uterus, fibroids) or adnexal masses (e.g., ovarian cysts, ectopic pregnancy), (4) pregnancy dating (e.g., BPD, crown-rump length), and (5) coexistence and location of an intrauterine device (IUD).

During the **second** and **third trimesters,** the following information is sought: (1) fetal viability, number, position, gestational age, growth pattern, and anomalies, (2) amniotic fluid volume, (3) placental location and maturity, (4) uterine fibroids and anomalies, and (5) adnexal masses. An example of the appli-

cation of the findings is presented in Table 25.5. In general, the use of ultrasound has hastened diagnoses so that appropriate therapy can be instituted early in the pregnancy. Early therapy may decrease the severity and duration of morbidity, both physical and emotional, of the mother (family). Early diagnosis of fetal anomaly, for instance, makes possible choices such as (1) intrauterine surgery or other therapy for the fetus, (2) discontinuation of the pregnancy, and (3) preparation of the family for the care of a child with a disorder or planning for placement of child after birth.

Findings

Fetal viability. Fetal heart activity can be demonstrated as early as 6 to 7 weeks by real-time echo scanners and at 10 to 12 weeks by Doppler ultrasound. This information assists in management when the woman experiences vaginal bleeding; incomplete, complete, and missed abortion can be differentiated. By 9 to 10 weeks, molar pregnancy can be diagnosed as a missed abortion (Fig. 25.4).

Gestational age. Not all women are candidates for the use of ultrasound to determine gestational age. Several indicators have been established for need. Indications for ultrasonographic estimation of fetal age include (1) uncertain dates for the last menstrual period or last normal menstrual period, (2) recent discontinuation of

Table 25.2
Psychosocial Factors: Child Abuse, Neglect, and Abnormal Parenting Practices: Perinatal Warning Indicators for Families at Risk*

Indicator	Pregnancy	Labor and Delivery	Post Partum
Parents' physical and psychological well-being	Pregnancy is perceived as very difficult or burdensome Mother feels her health will suffer from childbearing or child rearing Mother intellectually subnormal Mother shows great depression over pregnancy Mother remains feeling frightened and alone, especially before delivery. Careful explanations do not dissipate the fear Excessive visits for health care or expresses multiple psychosomatic complains Evidence of emotional instability or mental illness History of drug or alcohol abuse Child wanted in order to fill unmet need in parents' lives Evidence of low self-esteem ("I'm no good"), particularly re parenting ability Mother aged under 20 years Previous pregnancy has resulted in abortion, fetal or neonatal death, or birth of a damaged child History of previous child's death or removal from home because of abuse and/or neglect	Mother experiencing excessive discomfort, fatigue, drug effects, or physical complications immediately following delivery Mother and/or father perceive labor and/or delivery as very traumatic or unsatisfactory Obvious lack of supportive interaction between couple Hostile interaction between couple	Mother does not see attention focused on infant as something positive for herself Mother bothered by infant's crying; makes her feel helpless, hopeless, or unloved Mother relinquishes control to doctors and nurses for meeting needs of infant Evidence of low self-esteem ("I'm no good"), especially re parenting ability Parents express excessive feelings of failure re performance during labor and/or delivery Parents express resentment and/or anger toward infant over childbirth experience Express excessive doubt re ability to care for infant
Characteristics of child		Premature Physically or mentally defective Immature or defective reflex behaviors Unresponsive Condition necessitates separation from parents "Wrong" sex Looks and/or behavior perceived in negative way by parents	As in column 3 Perceived by parent as being different or "not normal" despite normal findings Sex of infant remains unacceptable to parent Denies or exaggerates handicapped infant's capabilities Difficult feeder Unresponsive, i.e., sleepy baby Irritable or difficult to console Hyperreflexive infant Rigid or noncuddly infant
Parent-child attachment	Pregnancy unplanned or unwanted Parents considered abortion or relinquishment Denial of pregnancy, i.e., unwilling to gain weight, refusal to talk about pregnancy	Mother looks distressed, disappointed Does not talk to infant in affectionate terms Makes negative or hostile remarks to infant Expresses disappointment with sex of infant	Does not comfort infant when crying and does not heed physical needs Appears apathetic toward or disinterested in infant Expresses excessive doubt about ability to care for infant Remains disappointed over sex of infant

From Ledger, K.E., and Williams, D.L.: Parents at risk: an instructional program for perinatal assessment and preventive intervention, Victoria, B.C., Canada, 1981, Ministry of Health and Queen Alexandra Solarium for Crippled Children Society.

*It must be noted that it is not merely the presence or number of warning indicators that signify a high-risk situation. It is the unique combination of these indicators and their degree of expression in each individual family situation that is of importance. Factors such as culture, educational level, age of parents, receptiveness to change, etc. *must* be taken into consideration.

Continued.

Table 25.2, cont'd
Psychosocial Factors: Child Abuse, Neglect, and Abnormal Parenting Practices: Perinatal Warning Indicators for Families at Risk*

Indicator	Pregnancy	Labor and Delivery	Post Partum
Parent-child attach- ment—cont'd	In advanced pregnancy, mother dresses and acts as though she is not pregnant Absent or disturbed response to quickening Mother perceives fetal movement as abusive or aggressive actions Mother reports an experience she fears will damage baby (i.e., a "scare," accident, etc.) Undue concern re infant's sex or performance Absence of any fantasies about what baby will be like or predominantly negative fantasies Mother attributes negative characteristics to fetus Apparent lack of concern for physical well-being of unborn fetus, as evidenced by refusal to make health and life-style changes (i.e., poor nutrition, excessive use of drugs and/or alcohol, etc.) Absence of "nesting" behavior in the third trimester (i.e., preparation of clothing, equipment, space for infant)	Mother makes inappropriate verbalizations, glances, or disparaging remarks about or toward infant Avoids eye contact and direct "en face" position Mother does not hold, touch, or examine infant Mother handles infant in rough manner	Frequently voices negative feelings about or toward infant Repelled by messiness and diaper changing Negative identification of infant by name or association with someone disliked No feelings of attachment toward infant after 1 month Mother does not appear to enjoy playing with infant
Parenting knowledge beliefs, and expectations	Perceive own upbringing as abusive or neglectful Experienced harsh physical punishment during childhood Express belief that physical force is necessary in rearing and discipling children Express a strong desire to parent in manner different from own parents Express inaccurate knowledge of infant care and development Express rigid or unrealistic expectations for infant re physical characteristics, behavior, development, etc.		As in column 2 Unaware of infant's characteristics and ability See infant as demanding or manipulative Inadequate preparation for child rearing Express expectations developmentally far beyond infant's capabilities Express fear of "spoiling" the infant
Support systems	No spouse, mate, or significant other Express dissatisfaction with spouse or mate relationship Chronic marital discord, especially if focus of conflict is around childbearing or child rearing Chronic conflict with or alienation from one's own mother and/or other female relatives History of loss of mother's own mother before her own puberty	Mother expresses hostility toward father, who "put her through all this" As in column 2	As in column 2

Table 25.2, cont'd
Psychosocial Factors: Child Abuse, Neglect, and Abnormal Parenting Practices: Perinatal Warning Indicators for Families at Risk*

Indicator	Pregnancy	Labor and Delivery	Post Partum
Family circumstances	Mate and/or family's reaction to pregnancy is negative or non-supportive Lack or loss of support systems, i.e., no supportive friends or relatives nearby Show evidence of social isolation, i.e., no phone, outside interests, use of community resources Parent seems unaware or denies impact of new baby on relationship with mate, own time, other siblings Express concern that this child is going to be "one too many" Inadequate housing for family's needs Children too closely spaced Recent death or loss of loved one Have recently moved Financial, health, social, or interpersonal problems in the family Parents describe stresses of chaotic nature (i.e., physical fights, heavy drinking, and arguments among immediate family members, abandonment by mate, etc.) Parents exhibit few skills for dealing with stress Express inability to cope with present life circumstances Dissatisfied with career or career change	As in column 2	As in column 2

Table 25.3
Diagnostic Ultrasound: Operational Modes

Modality	Product	Principal Use
Pulsed ultrasound		
A mode	Static image	Diagnostic evaluation of brain
B mode (gray scale)*	Static image	Imaging of abdominal and pelvic structures
M mode	Dynamic imaging	Monitoring of heart and measuring of heart wall displacement
Real time*	Dynamic imaging	Provides moving dynamic images
Continuous wave		
Doppler mode*	Ranging mode	Fetal heart monitoring

*Used extensively in obstetrics and gynecology.

Table 25.4
Major Indications for Obstetric Sonography

First Trimester	Second Trimester	Third Trimester
Confirm pregnancy	Establish or confirm dates†	If no fetal heart tones
Confirm viability	If no fetal heart tones	Clarify dates/size discrepancy
Rule out ectopic pregnancy	Clarify dates/size discrepancy	Large for dates—rule out
Confirm gestational age*	Large for dates—rule out	Macrosomia (diabetes mellitus)
Birth control use	Poor estimate of dates	Multiple gestation
Irregular menses	Molar pregnancy	Polyhydramnios
No dates	Multiple gestation	Congenital anomalies
Postpartum pregnancy	Leiomyomata	Poor estimate of dates‡
Previous complicated pregnancy	Polyhydramnios	Small for dates—rule out
Caesarean delivery	Congenital anomalies	Fetal growth retardation
Rh incompatibility	Small for dates—rule out	Oligohydramnios
Diabetes mellitus	Poor estimate of dates	Congenital anomalies
Fetal growth retardation	Fetal growth retardation	Poor estimate of dates‡
Clarify dates/sizes discrepancy	Congenital anomalies	Determine fetal position—rule out
Large for dates—rule out	Oligohydramnios	Breech
Leiomyomata	If history of bleeding—rule out total placenta previa	Transverse lie
Bicornuate uterus	If Rh incompatibility—rule out fetal hydrops	If history of bleeding—rule out
Adnexal mass		Placenta previa
Multiple gestation		Abruptio placentae
Poor dates		Determine fetal lung maturity
Molar pregnancy		Amniocentesis for lecithin/sphingomyelin ratio
Small for dates—rule out		Placental maturity (grade 0-3)
Poor dates		If Rh incompatibility—rule out fetal hydrops
Missed abortion		
Blighted ovum		

From Athey, P.A., and Hadlock, F.P.: Ultrasound in obstetrics and gynecology, ed. 2, St. Louis, 1985, The C.V. Mosby Co.
*Accuracy ± 3 days.
†Accuracy ± 1 to 1½ weeks.
‡Accuracy only ± 3 weeks.

Table 25.5
Application of Sonography During Pregnancy

Condition	Sonographic Evidence	Intervention
Impending abortion (prior to eighth menstrual week)	Poorly formed or "sagging" gestational sac	Eliminate time trying to save pregnancy; possibly decrease blood loss and sequelae of blood loss or of treatment for blood loss
Fetal death (after eighth menstrual week)	No cardiac activity	Empty uterus prior to development of retained dead fetus syndrome
Ectopic pregnancy	Adnexal mass	Early surgical intervention to prevent emergency situation
Molar pregnancy	"Snow storm" appearance within enlarged uterus (Fig. 25.4)	Terminate pregnancy to decrease morbidity from preeclampsia and begin surveillance of HCG* levels
Developmental uterine abnormalities	Resembles coexistent solid neoplasm; variable appearance	Avoid misdiagnosis with inappropriate therapy; provide time to consider type of delivery
Intrauterine device (IUD) (not a rare occurrence)	Locate site	
	Imbedded in myometrial wall apart from gestational sac and placenta	Pregnancy usually goes to term with no IUD-related problem
	Located partially or totally within gestational sac or within placenta	Pregnancy usually ends in spontaneous abortion and may be associated with generalized sepsis

*Human chorionic gonadotropin.

Fig. 25.3
A, Transverse static image scan demonstrates three well-formed gestational sacs. **B,** Subsequent static image scan demonstrates three well-defined fetal heads in this woman carrying triplets. (From Athey, P.A., and Hadlock, F.P.: Ultrasound in obstetrics and gynecology, ed. 2, St. Louis, 1985, The C.V. Mosby Co.)

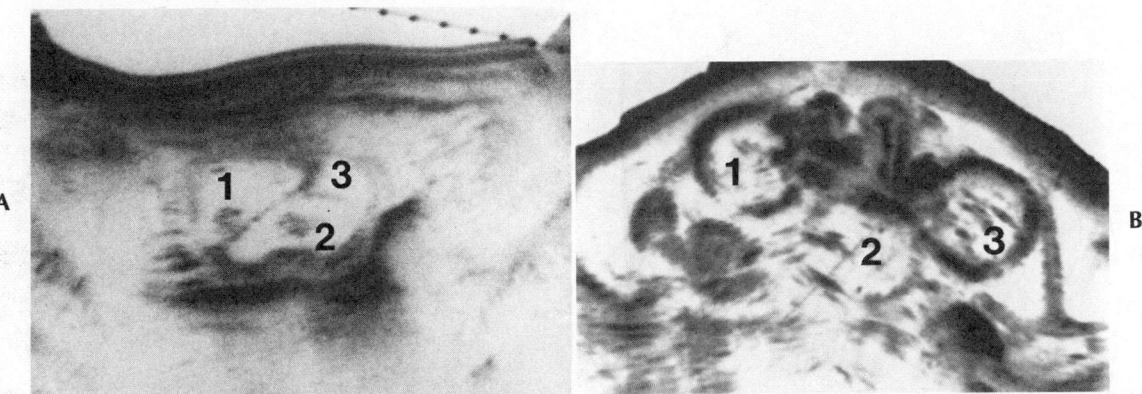

Fig. 25.4
A, Longitudinal and **B,** transverse scans of molar pregnancy *(m)*. Note typical vesicular (grapelike) pattern. Also demonstrated are multiloculated lutein ovarian cysts *(c)* in cul-de-sac. (From Athey, P.A., and Hadlock, F.P.: Ultrasound in obstetrics and gynecology, ed. 2, St. Louis, 1985, The C.V. Mosby Co.)

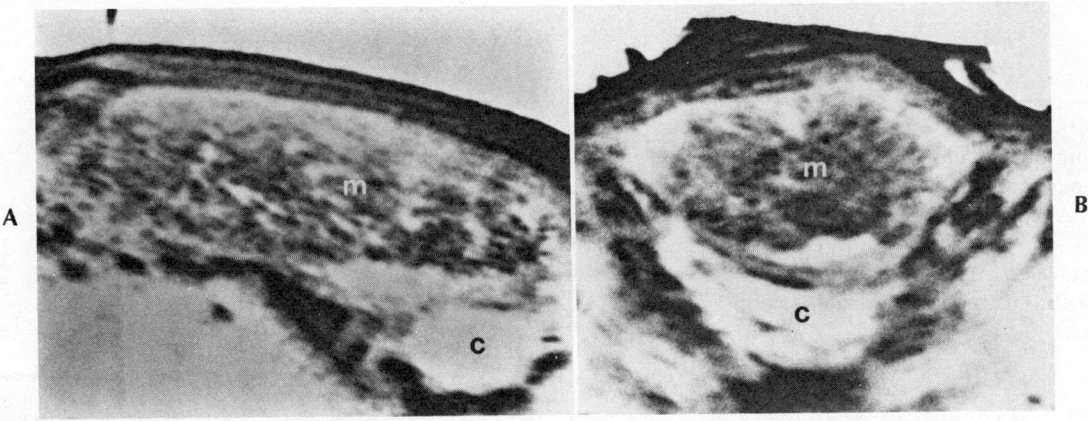

oral hormonal suppression of ovulation (birth control pills), (3) bleeding episode during the first trimester, (4) amenorrhea of at least 3 months' duration, (5) uterine size that does not agree with dates, (6) previous cesarean birth, and (7) other high-risk conditions. Four methods of estimation of fetal age are used: (1) determination of gestational sac dimensions (about 8 weeks), (2) measurement of crown-rump length (between 7 and 14 weeks), (3) measurement of femur length (after 12 weeks), and (4) measurement of the BPD (starting at about 12 weeks).

Fetal BPD at 36 weeks should be approximately 8.7 cm. Term pregnancy and fetal maturity can be diagnosed with considerable confidence if the biparietal cephalometry by ultrasonography is greater than 9.8 cm (Fig. 25.5 and Table 25.6).

Fetal growth. Fetal growth may be jeopardized under certain conditions. Some of the conditions that serve as indicators for ultrasound assessment of fetal growth include the following: poor maternal weight gain or pattern of weight gain; previous **intrauterine growth retardation (IUGR)**; chronic infections (es-

Fig. 25.5

A, Biparietal cephalometry by ultrasound. **B,** Linear-array, real-time image demonstrates fetal BPD *(arrow)* at 18 weeks. **B,** From Athey, P.A., and Hadlock, F.P.: Ultrasound in obstetrics and gynecology, ed. 2, St. Louis, 1985, The C.V. Mosby Co.

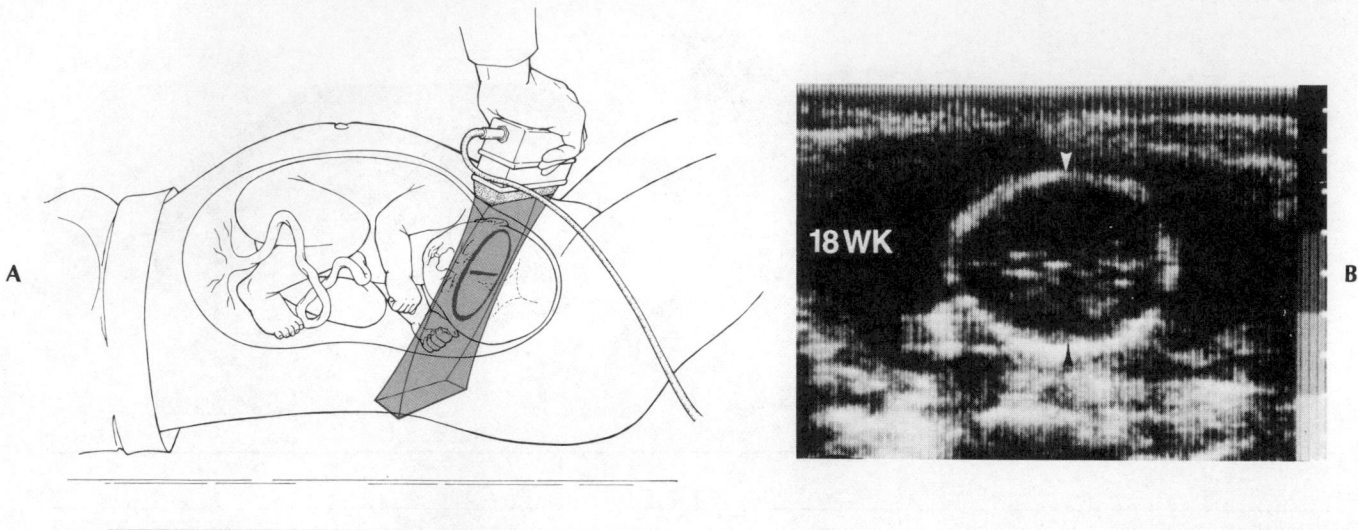

Fig. 25.6

A, Schematic presentation of appropriate planes of sections *(dotted lines)* for BPD, head circumference *(HC),* and abdominal circumference *(AC).* **B,** Real-time ultrasound image demonstrates typical head and body images that correspond to planes in **A.** Using these two images, one can determine BPD (7.9 cm), HC (30 cm), AC (28 cm), and estimated fetal weight. *(EFW)* (1840 g) in this normal 32-week fetus. (From Athey, P.A., and Hadlock, F.P.: Ultrasound in obstetrics and gynecology, ed. 2, St. Louis, 1985, The C.V. Mosby Co.).

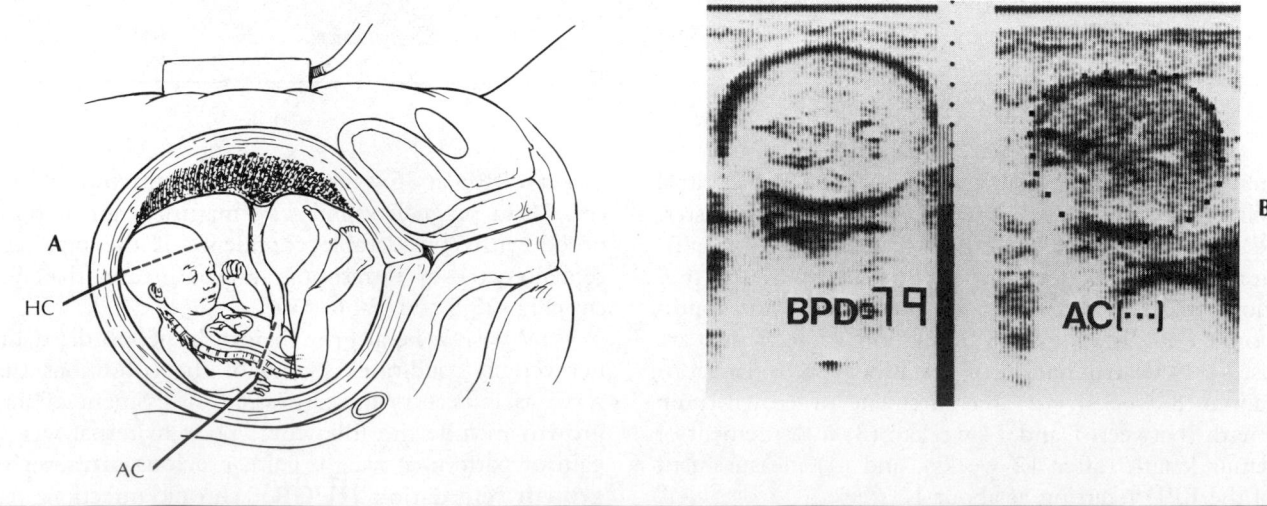

Table 25.6
Correlation of Fetal Weight and BPD

BPD (cm)	Estimated Fetal Weight
8.2	2290 g (5 lb, 1 oz)
8.5	2500 g (5 lb, 8 oz)
8.8	2730 g (6 lb, 0 oz)
9.4	3180 g (7 lb, 0 oz)
10.0	3630 g (8 lb, 0 oz)
10.6	4070 g (9 lb, 0 oz)

pecially urinary tract infections); ingestion of drugs such as anticonvulsants or heroin; maternal diabetes mellitus, pregnancy-induced or other hypertension; multiple pregnancy; and other medical and/or surgical complications. Serial evaluations of BPD and limb length can differentiate between wrong dates and true IUGR. IUGR may be symmetric (the fetus is small in all parameters) or asymmetric (head and body growth vary). Symmetric IUGR may be due to low genetic growth potential, intrauterine infection, maternal undernutrition and/or heavy smoking, or chromosomal aberration. Asymmetric IUGR may reflect placental insufficiency secondary to hypertension, renal disease, or cardiovascular disease. Therapy varies with the probable cause.

The BPD, head circumference, abdominal circumference, and estimated fetal weight for a normal 32-week fetus are illustrated in Fig. 25.6.

Adjunct to amniocentesis. The safety of amniocentesis is increased when the physician knows the exact position of the fetus, placenta, and pockets of amniotic fluid. Ultrasonography has greatly reduced previous risks associated with amniocentesis.

Fetal anatomy. Depending on the gestational age, the following structures may be identified: head (including ventricles and blood vessels), neck, spine, heart, stomach, small bowel, liver, kidneys, bladder and limbs. Structural defects may be identified prior to delivery. Advances in technology may make fetal surgery and genetic engineering a reality for many conditions in the next few years.

Placental position and function. The pattern of uterine and placental growth and the fullness of the bladder influence the apparent location of the placenta. During the first trimester, differentiation of the endometrium and the small placenta is difficult and adds to the difficulty of performing an amniocentesis. During the middle of the second trimester the placenta can be clearly defined, but if it is seen to be low lying, its relationship to the internal cervical os can sometimes be altered dramatically by changing the degree of fullness of the maternal bladder. In approximately 15% to 20% of all pregnancies in which ultrasound scanning

is done in the second trimester, the placenta seems to be overlying the os; at term the incidence of placenta previa is only 0.5%. Three factors may be responsible for the seeming "migration" of the placenta: (1) the maternal bladder can distort the uterine cavity, (2) the lower uterine segment elongates as pregnancy progresses, and (3) poor imaging or misinterpretation of the image can result in an inappropriate diagnosis. The diagnosis of placenta previa can seldom be confirmed until the third trimester.

Fetal well-being. Among the many physiologic measurements that can be accomplished with ultrasound are the following: heart motion, beat-to-beat variability, fetal breathing movements (FBM), urine production (following serial measurements of bladder volume), fetal limb and head movements, and analysis of vascular waveforms from the fetal circulation (McCallum, 1984). It has been noted that FBM are decreased with maternal smoking and alcohol ingestion and increased with hyperglycemia. Fetal limb and head movements serve as an index of neurologic development.

Preparation of the woman. The woman is directed to come for the examination (Fig. 25.7) with a full bladder. The full bladder supports the uterus in position for the imaging. If her bladder is empty, the test may be delayed for about 1 hour until she is able to fill her bladder; it takes only a few moments to empty the bladder if this is needed for the examination.

Safety of the diagnostic ultrasound. Biologic effects of extremely high intensities of sound persisting over long periods of time can result in (1) *thermal* changes within the cells, (2) *cavitation,* or formation of tiny gas bubbles that can lead to rupture of cell membranes, and (3) *viscous* stresses. However, no biologic damage has been measured at ultrasonic intensity of less than 100 mW/cm^2, even for extended periods of exposure time. Diagnostic ultrasonic beams all have intensities less than 10 mW/cm^2 and are applied for relatively short periods of time (Athey and Hadlock, 1985).

There is no conclusive evidence that humans have been harmed by diagnostic ultrasound during the 20 years it has been used. No detrimental effects have been observed to date on the fetus or mother either histologically, functionally, or embryologically in experimental work; however, there is a hypothetical risk that cannot be ignored or overlooked. Benefit must be weighed against hypothetical risk. Gravidas should be informed of the clinical indication for ultrasound, specific benefit, potential risk, and alternatives, if any. In addition, a record should be kept of the exposure time, mode, and ultrasound frequency.

Magnetic resonance imaging. Magnetic resonance imaging (MRI; also known as nuclear magnetic reso-

Fig. 25.7
Ultrasonography. Woman is positioned comfortably with a small pillow under her head and under her knees. Display panel is positioned so that she can observe images on screen if she wishes (some woman do *not* want to watch). (Courtesy March of Dimes).

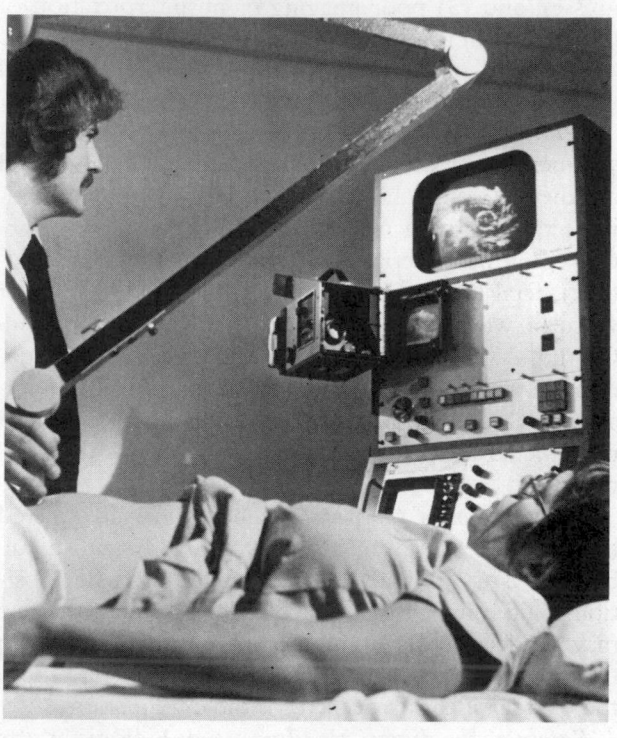

nance), a noninvasive tool for obstetric and gynecologic imaging, has recently been approved by the Food and Drug Administration. This tool tracks the distribution and motion of the body's hydrogen nuclei in cellular water and lipids to obtain detailed cross-sectional images. Like computerized tomography (CT), MRI provides excellent pictures of soft tissue; unlike CT, ionizing radiation is not used.

The MRI scanners contain a transmitter, receiver coils, and a magnetic coil that localizes the signal from the part to be imaged. After MRI signals are generated and analyzed, they are displayed on an oscilloscope screen. At present, MRI is particularly good for evaluating pelvic masses and assessing blood flow. The technique has not been evaluated for fetal imaging at present. However, it is likely that MRI has considerable potential for the accurate localization of the fetus and placenta and for the identification of placental infarction.

Fetoscopy. Direct visualization of the fetus is possible via a tiny telescope-like instrument with the caliber of a large hypodermic needle. The fetoscope is introduced into the uterus through the abdominal wall with the woman under local anesthesia. This method is not used extensively at this time because there is a risk of causing premature labor. The fetoscope is more often used to obtain fetal blood samples directly for biochemical analysis. It is especially useful for diagnosing serious hereditary blood disorders (e.g., sickle cell anemia). Risks to the fetus from fetoscopy range from 3% to 5%.

Amnioscopy. Fetal hypoxia is known to result in meconium passage by the mature fetus. Transcervical visualization of greenish amniotic fluid through the intact membranes indicates fetal asphyxia. Unfortunately, since the cervix must be more than 1 cm dilated and special equipment (amnioscope with tungsten lamp) is needed, this technique is used rarely.

Roentgenography. Bone abnormalities can be detected by simple x-ray studies, although the bone structure is at a very early stage of development at about 16 weeks gestation. Most bone defects are not apparent until a later stage. A special x-ray technique, termed *amniography* or *fetography,* allows visualization of gross structural abnormalities, although there has been little experience with its use in early pregnancy. The procedure involves the instillation of a contrast medium into the amniotic fluid. The medium adheres to fetal skin to produce a clear fetal silhouette on the x-ray film.

The presence of distal femoral ossification centers indicates a fetal age of 36 weeks. If the proximal tibial centers are present, the fetus has reached 40 weeks' gestational age. X-ray visualization of the distal femoral and proximal tibial epiphyseal centers also indicates term pregnancy. This procedure is used with great caution because of the danger of fetal and maternal gonadal damage. In addition, there is growing concern over the use of ionizing radiation because of potential carcinogenic, teratogenic, and mutagenic effects on developing embryonic or fetal tissues.

Chorionic villi sampling. Chorionic villi sampling (CVS) could partially replace amniocentesis for genetic diagnosis. Although there are risks to the fetus, the greatest advantage in this new technique is that genetic diagnosis can be moved ahead from the second to the first trimester—as early as the eighth week—and can produce results rapidly. Earlier diagnosis reduces a couple's waiting period, imposes less social and psychologic stress, permits the couple "privacy" because the pregnancy is not obvious as yet, and allows for an earlier and safer abortion if the couple so chooses.

This procedure involves the removal of a small tissue specimen from the fetal portion of the placenta. Since chorionic villi originate in the zygote, that tissue reflects the genetic makeup of the fetus. The specimen is removed either from the chorion frondosum or the chorion laeve.

Real-time ultrasound is used to guide the procedure. The aspiration cannula and obturator must negotiate the cervical canal, must be placed at a suitable site, and must avoid rupturing the amniotic sac. The magnitude of the risk in CVS is unknown, but the types of complications (e.g., spontaneous abortion, infection, hematoma, intrauterine death, growth retardation, and trauma) are predictable. At present, if the risk of a fetal genetic disorder (e.g., hemoglobinopathies) is 25% or more, CVS is one possible diagnostic alternative.

BIOCHEMICAL MONITORING

Maternal urine assessments

Glucosuria, acetonuria, and proteinuria. See index for the pages in which these findings are discussed. See Appendix E for laboratory values.

Infection. See Chapters 27 and 31 for content regarding maternal and neonatal infection.

Maternal urinary estriol determinations. The steroid precursor produced by the fetal adrenals is synthesized into estriols in the placenta and is excreted by the mother's healthy kidneys. Maternal estriol level in maternal urine (24-hour specimen) is an indicator of the normalcy of the fetoplacental unit. Estriol levels are elevated in multiple pregnancy, but they are extremely low in the presence of a failing pregnancy, anencephaly, or fetal death. Estriol levels fall in dysmaturity, preeclampsia-eclampsia (PIH), complicated diabetes mellitus, and partial separation of the placenta. Serial estriol determinations (never a single estimate) are essential to establish a trend to justify delivery of fetus.

Correct estimates of the estimated date of confinement (EDC) based on estriol levels in maternal urine are unlikely with obesity, multiple pregnancy, or pelvic tumors, because the EDC will often be an early estimate. Growth retardation of the fetus, oligohydramnios, or fetal death may suggest a false later EDC.

Purpose. The woman is told the purpose of the urine tests; that is, "to assess the health of your developing baby."

Preparation. The woman is provided with written directions for obtaining the specimens.

Procedure

1. Printed instructions are given to the woman, to void and discard the first morning urine; to collect all urine for the next 24 hours, storing it in the refrigerator; and then to bring it to the laboratory.

2. The following equipment is needed: two collection bottles, one sieve, and a preservative solution.

Timing of serial determinations

1. Determinations are possible by 20 weeks.
2. A more reliable baseline is possible after 28 weeks.
3. Best results are obtained after 32 weeks.

Factors altering results

1. Closely spaced serial evaluations are required to get the slope of increase or decrease. One reading at one point is useless.
2. The same technician should do all the tests for a particular woman to increase reliability of the results.
3. A false reading is likely if the woman is taking any of the following medications: corticosteroids, ampicillin, methenamine mandelate (e.g., Mandelamine) for urinary tract infection.
4. The methods of specimen collection and preservation are also factors.

Results (Table 25.7)

1. High estriol levels with a rising slope are associated with a good prognosis for the fetus.
2. Low estriol levels *may* be associated with a compromised fetus. NOTE: Factors not strictly related to fetal health may be associated with abnormal values (e.g., if a true 24-hour specimen is not collected, gestational age is overestimated, or if there is a high level of urinary glucose).
3. If the woman's kidney clearance ability is questioned, the woman has diabetes mellitus, or the woman is unable to give a true 24-hour urinary specimen, plasma estriol may be assayed.

Maternal blood assessments

Plasma estriols. Plasma estriols may be assayed as either unconjugated, or free, estriol (8% to 10% of total estriol) or as total estriol. Plasma assays *do* reflect the fetal-placental production and secretion of estriols, and 24-hour urine specimens do not have to be collected. Plasma estriols are less affected by disorders of the mother's liver or kidneys.

Human placental lactogen. Human placental lactogen (HPL), also called human chorionic somatomammotropin (HCS), is produced by the syncytiotrophoblast. However, assay for this hormone is of little value in assessing placental integrity. Other, more accurate and reliable tests, have replaced the routine assessment for HPL levels.

Table 25.7
Summary of Biochemical Monitoring Techniques

Test	Results	Significance of Findings
Maternal urine estriols	High and rising levels	General fetal well-being
	Low and falling levels	Possible fetal jeopardy
Maternal blood		
Human placental lactogen	High levels	Large fetus; multiple gestation
	Low levels	Threatened abortion, IUGR, postmaturity
Unconjugated and plasma estriol	High and rising levels	General fetal well-being
	Low and falling levels	Possible fetal jeopardy
Heat-stable alkaline phosphatase	Normally elevated during pregnancy	Poor correlation with fetal outcome
Oxytocinase	200-400 U at term	General fetal well-being
	Low levels	Associated with fetal death, postmaturity, IUGR
Coombs' test	Titer of 1:8 and rising	Significant Rh sensitization
Alpha-fetoprotein	See below	
Amniotic fluid analysis		
Color	Meconium	Possible hypoxia or asphyxia
Lung profile		Fetal lung maturity
L/S ratio	>2	
PGL*	Present	
Creatinine	>2/dl	Gestational age > 36 weeks
Billirubin (ΔOD† 450/nm)	<0.015	Gestational age > 36 weeks, normal pregnancy
	High levels	Fetal hemolytic disease in isoimmunized pregnancies
Lipid cells	>10%	Gestational age > 35 weeks
Alpha-fetoprotein	High levels after 15-week gestation	Open neural tube defect
Osmolality	Decline after 20-week gestation	Advancing nonspecific gestational age
Genetic disorders	Dependent on cultured cells for karyotype and enzymatic activity	
Sex-linked		
Chromosomal		
Metabolic		

From Tucker, S.M.: Fetal monitoring and fetal assessment in high-risk pregnancy, St. Louis, 1978, The C.V. Mosby Co. In an effort to summarize these studies in tabular form, generalization must be made.
*Phosphatidylglycerol.
†Delta optical density.

Coombs' test. Coombs' test for Rh incompatibility is discussed at length in Chapter 31.

Amniotic fluid assessment
Amniocentesis. Amniocentesis is possible after the fourteenth week, when the uterus becomes an abdominal organ and when there is sufficient amniotic fluid for this procedure (Table 25.8 and Fig. 25.8).

Indications
1. Prenatal diagnosis of genetic problems (Chapter 31).
   a. Karyotype from a cell culture indicating chromosomal aberrations, which appear in fetuses of 1% to 2% of women between 35 and 38 years of age, 2% of women between 39 and 40 years of age, and 10% of women over 45 years of age.

   b. Sex chromatin in fetal cells (no culturing needed) if a sex-linked disorder (especially in the male fetus) is suspected.
   c. Biochemical analysis of enzymes produced from a cell culture to detect inborn errors of metabolism (over 60 types are possible now)
   d. Determination of alpha-fetoprotein (AFP) levels

Table 25.8
Typical Amniotic Fluid Increase During Pregnancy

Weeks' Gestation	Amniotic Fluid Volume (ml)
12	50
14	100
16	175
18	250
20	325

From Queenan, J.T.: Contemp. OB/Gyn. 15:61, Feb. 1980.

Fig. 25.8

A, Amniocentesis and laboratory utilization of amniotic fluid aspirant. **B,** Transabdominal amniocentesis. (**A** from Whaley, L.F.: Understanding inherited disorders, St. Louis, 1974, The C.V. Mosby Co. **B** courtesy March of Dimes.)

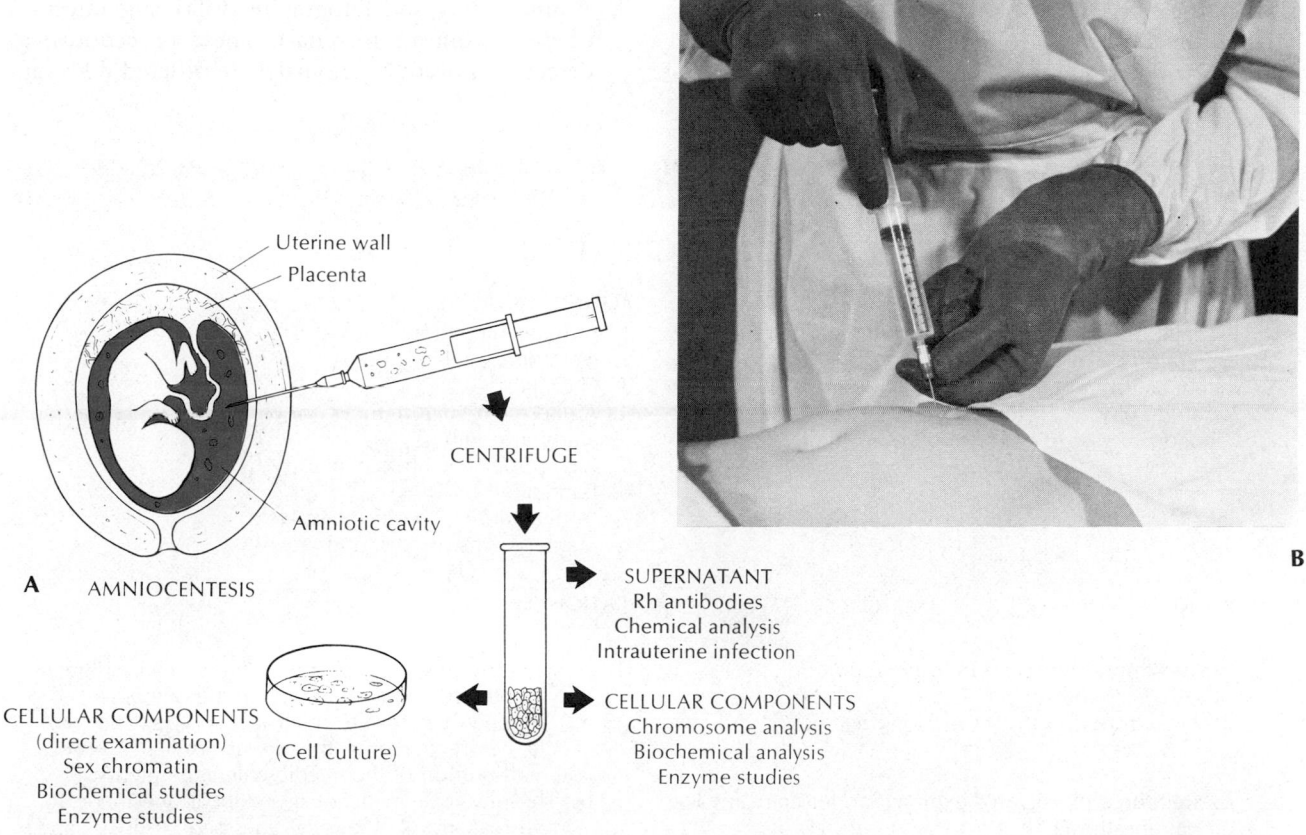

in supernatant fluid to detect neural tube defects, such as spina bifida and anencephaly. It may also be elevated with severe fetohemolytic disease, esophageal atresia, congenital nephrosis, omphalocele, fetal demise, and fetal hemorrhage into amniotic fluid. The amount of AFP should decrease to 18.5 μg/ml at 15 weeks and to 0.26 μg/ml at term. The recurrence rate of neural tube defects is 5%.

2. Gestational age. Greater accuracy in estimating fetal maturity is now possible through use of amniotic fluid or its exfoliated cellular content. Technically, term pregnancy and fetal maturity have been reached if more than one of the following are properly demonstrated by laboratory studies:

   a. A **lecithin/sphingomyelin ratio (L/S ratio)** that is greater than 2 indicates adequate lung maturity for extrauterine life (Chapter 8). This will be achieved if the fetus is older than 36 weeks' gestational age. A practical variation of

the L/S ratio is the rapid surfactant test, also known as the **shake test** or bubble test. Equal parts of fresh amniotic fluid and normal saline solution are added to two parts 95% ethyl alcohol. The mixture is shaken vigorously for 30 seconds. If bubbles are still present at meniscus 15 minutes after shaking, fetal lung is judged to be mature. See Chapters 8 and 31 for discussion of other phospholipids and lung maturity.

   b. When the delta optical density of *bilirubinoid pigments* is 450 nm <0.01, this indicates a gestational age of greater than 38 weeks. Bilirubin disappears after 36 weeks.

   c. When the *creatinine* (estimate of renal maturity) value is greater than 1.8 mg/dl, the gestational age is greater than 36 weeks in the absence of maternal renal disease and dehydration or of fetal anomaly.

   d. After *fetal lipid-containing exfoliated cells* are stained with Nile blue sulfate, a finding of more than 20% orange-staining cells indicates a gestational age of greater than 35 weeks; the fetus probably weighs 2500 g. (For information regarding the use of amniocentesis in estimating fetal health, see Procedure 25.1.)

3. Identification and follow-up of isoimmune disease (Chapter 31).
   a. First determination is postponed until 24 to 25

weeks, since intrauterine transfusion of packed, Rh-negative, type O red blood cells is not possible before that time.
   b. Transfusion is usually indicated if Coombs' titer is above 1:8 to 1:16.

4. Amniography and fetography (following infection of radio contrast material). These procedures, to detect fetal death or anomaly, are ordered with cau-

Procedure 25.1

AMNIOCENTESIS

PURPOSE

1. Prenatal diagnosis of genetic problems
2. Estimation of gestational age
3. Identification and follow-up of isoimmune disease
4. Amniography and fetography
5. Second-trimester elective abortion (Chapter 7)

EQUIPMENT

1. Amniocentesis tray
2. Electronic fetal monitor
3. Flashlight
4. Amber-colored test tubes (or test tubes wrapped in aluminum foil)
5. Razor (to shave abdomen)
6. Bandage
7. Antibacterial cleanser (pHisoHex)
8. Sterile gowns, masks, and gloves

NURSING ACTION	RATIONALE
1. Act as support person during procedure: a. Explain reason for such a long needle. b. Reinforce physician's explanation for not using local anesthesia.	1. As with any surgical procedure, the woman and family will be tense and anxious as to the outcome. a. The needle passes through layers of fat and muscle before reaching the uterus. Actually only a small portion of the needle enters the uterus. b. The physician will not use a local anesthetic for two reasons: (1) the local anesthetic "stings" and (2) it would mean two needles. Once the skin is pierced, there is a sensation of pressure, but not pain.
2. Implement technician role: a. Take baseline vital signs and the FHR. b. Premedicate (if ordered). c. Place the woman in a supine position with her hands under her head. d. Prepare the abdomen with a shave and scrub with povidone-iodine (Betadine). e. Draw a blood sample.	2. Collaborative effort facilitates procedure. a. To assess against subsequent values. b. To assist woman in relaxing. c. To position in her a way that facilitates procedure. d. To minimize possibility for infection. e. To compare with a postprocedure blood sample for assessing probable fetomaternal hemorrhage.
3. Assist the physician, monitor and support the mother, assess FHR as indicated, assist with the specimens, and record the procedure. a. Label three sterile tubes. b. If a bilirubin determination is needed, darken the room, use a flashlight, and immediately cover the filled aluminum foil–wrapped tube. c. After fluid is withdrawn, wash all povidone-iodine off the abdomen and apply a bandage. d. Assist with or draw a blood sample. e. Continue monitoring the FHR for 30 minutes and assess for uterine contractions.	3. To collaborate in the completion of the procedure accurately and with least potential for injury to maternal-placental-fetal unit. a. To identify specimen. b. To prevent light from altering bilirubin, since a true reading cannot be obtained if the fluid is exposed to light. c. To prevent skin burn. d. To assess for the presence of fetomaternal hemorrhage. e. To identify complications.

tion because of concern regarding carcinogenic, teratogenic, and mutagenic effects on future generations.

5. Second-trimester elective abortion (Chapter 7).
6. Hydramnios. This is treated by aspiration of amniotic fluid.

Preparation. An amniocentesis is performed when there is indication of problems with the pregnancy or the fetus. The mother and family are informed of the need for the surgical procedure and appraised of the risks. An informed consent statement and a surgical permit are signed by the woman (Chapter 3). Ultrasonography is performed to locate the placenta. If the pregnancy is less than 20 weeks, a full bladder helps to brace the uterus (see bladder preparation under Ultrasonography, p. 731).

Risks

1. Overall complications are less than 1% for both mother and fetus.
2. Maternal: hemorrhage, fetomaternal hemorrhage with possible maternal Rh isoimmunization, infection, labor, abruptio placentae, inadvertent damage to the intestines or bladder, amniotic fluid embolism.
3. Fetal: death, hemorrhage, infection (amnionitis), direct injury from the needle, abortion or premature labor, leakage of amniotic fluid.

Procedure. During the amniocentesis (Procedure 25.1) the nurse implements roles of teacher/counselor/advocate, technician, and support person. The content of Procedure 25.1 can be used as a basis for teaching the woman and her family.

Rupture of membranes

Tests for rupture of membranes. Tests for rupture of membranes and assessment of the color, character, and amount of amniotic fluid are discussed at length in Chapter 15.

Apt test. The Apt test is used to differentiate maternal and fetal blood when there is vaginal bleeding. It is performed as follows: Add 0.5 ml bloody fluid to 4.5 ml distilled water. Shake. Add 1 ml 0.25N sodium hydroxide. Fetal and cord blood remain pink for 1 or 2 minutes. Maternal blood becomes brown in 30 seconds.

Significance of meconium in amniotic fluid: a reappraisal

Antenatal period. Antenatal amniotic fluid meconium may be just physiologic passage without association with poor fetal status or outcome. With the advent of more sophisticated, noninvasive tools to assess fetal health, the clinical significance of amniotic fluid meconium has been reduced (Danforth, 1982, p. 810).

Intrapartum period. Intranatal amniotic fluid meconium is an indication for more careful evaluation. The recent trend is *not* to rely on the presence of meconium as an indication for intervention (Danforth, 1982, p. 810); now there is increased reliance on electronic fetal monitoring and fetal scalp blood sampling for evaluation of fetal status.

There are three possible reasons for the passage of meconium during the intrapartum period: (1) it is a normal physiologic function that occurs with maturity; (2) it is the result of hypoxia-induced peristalsis and sphincter relaxation, and (3) it may be a sequela to umbilical cord compression–induced vagal stimulation in mature fetuses (meconium passage is infrequent before weeks 32 to 34, with an increased incidence after 38 weeks).

The following new criteria are proposed for evaluating meconium passage during the intranatal period (Danforth, 1982, p. 811):

1. Consistency: "old and thin" versus "new and thick." A new and thick consistency is more likely to be the result of fetal stress.
2. Timing: early in labor versus late in labor. Meconium passage is associated with severe variable or late fetal heart rate (FHR) decelerations and is an ominous sign.
3. Relationship to FHR.

ANTEPARTUM TESTING: FHR AND FETAL MOVEMENT

Evaluation of fetal well-being and maturity is essential in the management of the high-risk pregnancy. The nonstress test (NST), or fetal activity determination (FAD), and the contraction stress test (CST) have been widely employed for the determination of fetal well-being. In addition, daily fetal movement count (DFMC), as recorded by the expectant mother, has proved to be an additional method of assessing fetal well-being.

The desired goals of antepartum monitoring are to prevent intrauterine fetal death and avoid unnecessary premature intervention.

Indications for both the NST and the CST are the following:

1. Maternal diabetes mellitus
2. Chronic hypertension
3. Hypertensive disorders in pregnancy
4. Intrauterine growth retardation
5. Sickle cell disease
6. Maternal cyanotic heart disease
7. Suspected postmaturity
8. History of previous stillbirth
9. Rh sensitization (isoimmunization)

10. Meconium-stained amniotic fluid (at amniocentesis)
11. Abnormal estriol excretion pattern
12. Hyperthyroidism
13. Collagen diseases
14. Older gravida (≥40 weeks' gestation)
15. Chronic renal disease

There are no contraindications for the NST. Absolute contraindications for the CST are rupture of membranes and previous classical cesarean delivery. The following are considered relative contraindications for the CST: multiple pregnancy, previous premature labor, placenta previa, hydramnios, and previous low transverse cesarean delivery.

Nonstress test (fetal activity determination). The basis for the NST, or FAD, is that the normal fetus will produce characteristic heart rate patterns. Acceleration of FHR in response to fetal movement is the desired outcome of the NST. This then allows most high-risk pregnancies to continue, with the test being repeated twice a week. A **reactive pattern suggests fetal well-being** with an associated good perinatal outcome.

The nurse observes the strip chart for signs of fetal movement and a concurrent acceleration of FHR. If evidence of fetal movement is not apparent on the chart paper, the woman is asked to depress a button on a handheld event marker that is connected into the appropriate outlet on the monitor when she feels fetal movement. The "event" of fetal movement is then noted by a spike or arrow printed by the stylus on the uterine activity panel of the strip chart. The test usually takes 20 to 30 minutes but may take longer if the fetus needs to be moved or awakened because of a sleep state (Fig. 25.9).

A guide for interpretation of the NST follows:

Result	Interpretation
Reactive	Two or more accelerations of FHR of 15 beat/min lasting 15 seconds or more, associated with each fetal movement in a 20-minute period
Nonreactive	Any tracing with either no FHR accelerations or accelerations less than 15 beats/min or lasting less than 15 seconds throughout any fetal movement during testing period
Unsatisfactory	Quality of FHR recording not adequate for interpretation

Fig. 25.9

Nonstress test. **A,** Decreased variability caused by fetal sleep cycle. **B,** Reactive nonstress test, indicative of fetal well-being, 15 minutes later. (From Perez, R.H.: Protocols for perinatal nursing practice, St. Louis, 1981, The C.V. Mosby Co.)

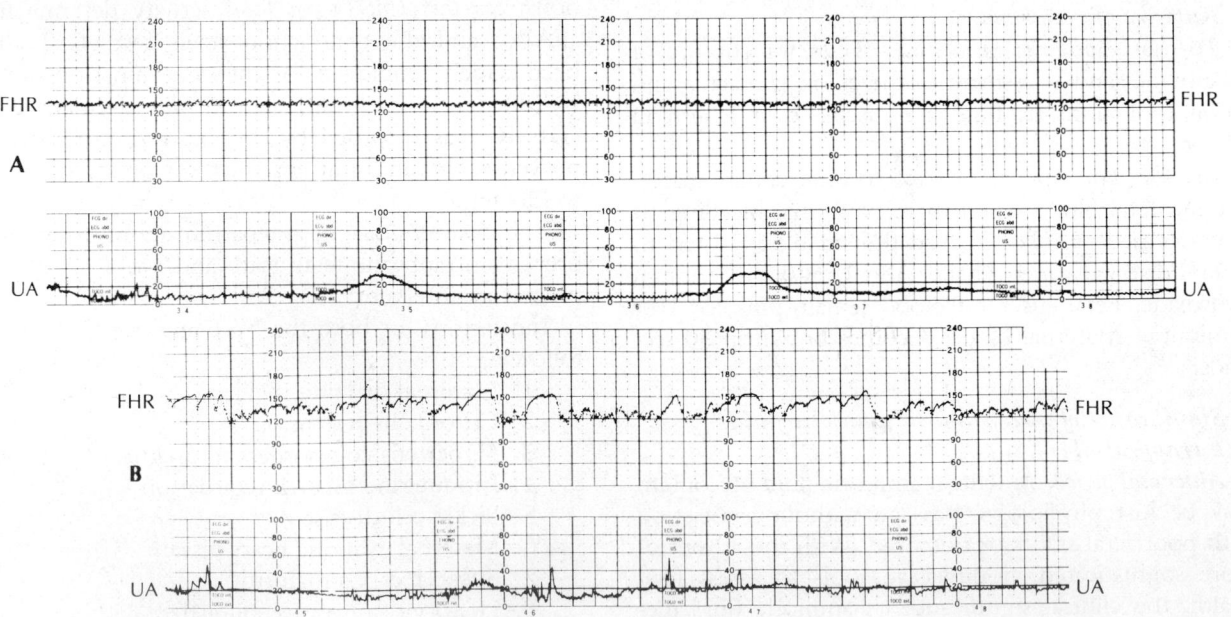

The clinical significance of the interpretation of the NST is as follows:

Reactive NST	As long as twice weekly NSTs remain reactive, most high-risk pregnancies are allowed to continue.
Nonreactive NST	Further indirect monitoring may be attempted with abdominal fetal electrocardiography in an effort to clarify FHR pattern and quantitate variability. External monitoring should continue, and a CST should be done.
Unsatisfactory	Test is repeated in 24 hours, or a CST is done, depending on the clinical situation.

The acoustic stimulation test is another method of testing antepartum FHR response. The test takes approximately 10 minutes to complete, with the fetus monitored for 5 minutes before fetal acoustic stimulation to obtain a baseline FHR. The sound source is then applied on the maternal abdomen over the fetal head. Monitoring continues for another 5 minutes, and the strip chart is assessed.

A guide for interpretation of the acoustic stimulation test follows:

Reactive acoustic stimulation test	FHR acceleration of at least 15 beats/min for at least 120 seconds or two accelerations of at least 15 beats/min for at least 15 seconds within 5 minutes of stimulus
Nonreactive acoustic stimulation test	Inability to fulfill either criterion for reactivity as described above within 5 minutes

Contraction stress test. The basis for the CST is that a healthy fetus can withstand a decreased oxygen supply during the physiologic stress of an oxytocin-stimulated contraction, whereas a compromised fetus will demonstrate late decelerations that are nonreassuring and indicative of uteroplacental insufficiency. **A negative test suggests fetal well-being.**

Nipple-stimulated contraction stress test. The woman is monitored indirectly, and the nurse observes the strip chart for 10 minutes before initiating nipple-stimulated contractions. If the woman has three or more spontaneous contractions within a 10-minute period, the nipple-stimulated contractions need not be initiated. If less than three spontaneous contractions occur within the period, and if late decelerations do not occur with intermittent spontaneous contractions, nipple stimulation can be initiated. The nurse explains the procedure to the woman and then proceeds by applying warm, moist washcloths to both breasts for several minutes. The woman is instructed to massage or roll the nipple of one breast for 10 minutes. If uterine contractions do not occur, both breasts should be stimulated for 10 minutes. The breasts should be restimulated intermittently as needed to maintain uterine contractions. If nipple stimulation does not produce the desire uterine activity, the nurse should proceed with an oxytocin-stimulated CST.

Oxytocin-stimulated contraction stress test. The physician orders the dosage, which usually starts at 0.5mU/min.* The oxytocin is always diluted in an IV solution and piggybacked into the tubing of the main IV. The infusion is usually delivered by an infusion pump or controller to ensure accurate dosage. The oxytocin infusion is usually increased by 0.5mU/min at 15- to 20-minute intervals until three uterine contractions of good quality are observed within a 10-minute period. The FHR pattern is then interpreted. The oxytocin infusion is discontinued and the maintenance IV solution infused until such time as uterine activity has returned to the preoxytocin infusion level. The IV is then removed, and the fetal monitor is discontinued. The woman can be sent home on the physician's orders.

A guide for the interpretation of the CST follows:

Result	Interpretation
Negative	No late decelerations with a minimum of three uterine contractions lasting 40 to 60 seconds within a 10-minute period (Fig. 25.10)
Positive	Persistent and consistent late decelerations occurring with more than half the contractions (Fig. 25.11)
Suspicious	Late decelerations occurring with less than half the uterine contractions once an adequate contraction pattern has been established
Hyperstimulation	Late decelerations occurring with excessive uterine activity (contractions more often than every 2 minutes or lasting longer than 90 seconds) or a persistent increase in uterine tone
Unsatisfactory	Inadequate uterine contraction pattern or tracing too poor to interpret

*See Tables 29.5 and 29.6 for calculating dosage of oxytocin (Pitocin) and drops per minute.

Fig. 25.10
Negative CST: fetal well-being.

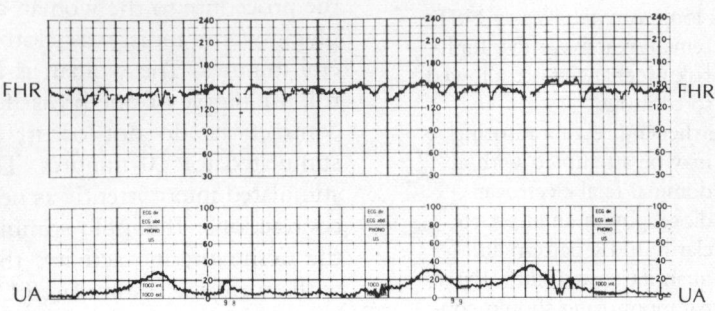

Fig. 25.11
Positive CST: compromised fetus. (From Perez, R.H.: Protocols for perinatal nursing practice, St. Louis, 1981, The C.V. Mosby Co.)

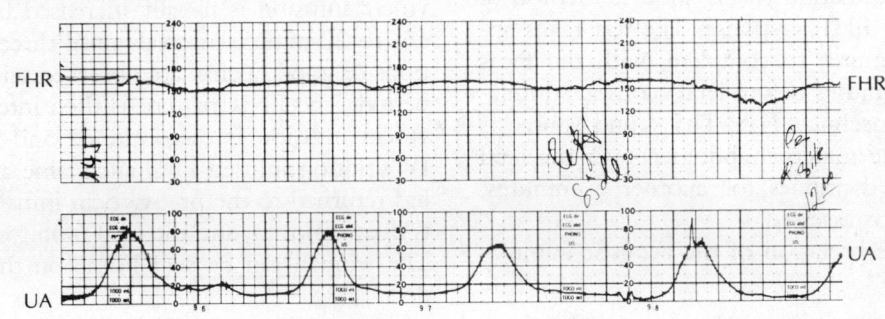

The clinical significance of the CST is as follows:

Result	Interpretation
Negative CST	Reassurance that the fetus is likely to survive labor, should it occur within 1 week; more frequent testing may be indicated by the clinical situation.
Positive CST	Management lies between use of other tools of fetal assessment and termination of pregnancy. A positive test indicates that the fetus is at increased risk for perinatal morbidity and mortality. The physician may perform an expeditious vaginal delivery following a successful induction or may proceed directly to cesarean delivery.
Suspicious, hyperstimulation, or unsatisfactory	NST and CST should be repeated within 24 hours. If interpretable data cannot be achieved, other methods of fetal assessment must be used.

Daily fetal movement count. Frequent movements of the fetus, as perceived by the mother, have been reassuring signs for centuries. Various investigators have recently reported a marked decrease in fetal movement before an episode of fetal distress or fetal death.

DFMCs, as reported by the mother, have been compared with movements recorded electronically, revealing that almost 90% of all fetal movements can be identified by the mother. This simple, inexpensive, readily applied "test" is continuously available away from the clinical area and relatively easy for the woman to do accurately.

Should a woman complain of decreased fetal movement, she may be asked by the physician to lie down for a period of 1 hour and count all the fetal movements. If she feels three or more during that time, she can be reassured. However, she is cautioned to continue to be aware of fetal movements and report the hourly observations should the problem recur. An immediate NST is usually performed if only one or two movements are felt. If the NST is reactive, no further testing is done unless there are some other risk factors. A nonreactive NST would be followed by a CST, the potential outcomes and significance of which have been previously described.

General Care of Compromised Neonate

The high-risk infant is a sick baby whose intact survival is in jeopardy at the moment he is being considered high risk. Health care must support the high-risk newborn's basic functioning while compensating for inadequacies and weaknesses. "Normal" values and parameters vary with the infant's level of maturity and developmental problems. Assessment and therefore supportive care are complicated further by the infant's inability to speak and by nonspecific, generalized responses to dysfunctional problems. Assessment rests heavily on historical data provided by the mother and obstetric team and on current levels of knowledge related to gestational age and disorders of the neonate. Plan and implementation of the nursing process with the high-risk infant focus on the physiologic maintenance of warmth, respiration, and nutrition.

The care of the infant at risk has become highly specialized and beyond the scope of this text.* The following discussion presents general content relevant to the care of the high-risk infant. Care of infants with selected risk factors is discussed in greater detail in Chapter 31.

Transport to a regional center. Hospitals that are not staffed or equipped to care for the mother and fetus or newborn at high risk arrange for their immediate transfer to a specialized perinatal or tertiary care center. If a compromised newborn is expected to be born, a maternal transport is arranged, if possible; that is, the anticipated compromised newborn is transported in utero. In utero transport has two distinct advantages: (1) the mother and newborn are not separated so that attachment is facilitated, and (2) neonatal morbidity and mortality are decreased. It is not always possible to transport the mother before delivery for a variety of reasons (e.g., imminent delivery, lack of prior diagnosis). Therefore it is necessary for physicians and nurses to have the necessary skills and equipment for accurate diagnosis and emergency intervention to stabilize the client's physical condition and to maintain it until transport can be effected. (For surgical emergencies of the newborn, see Chapter 31; for specific maternal conditions, see Index.)

During transport to a regional perinatal center, the following general categories of supplies, equipment, and medications are needed*:
Needed by both mother and fetus/newborn
  Oxygen and equipment for maintaining a clear airway and adequate gas exchange
  Intravenous equipment and solutions for meeting hydration needs, for administering medications, for transfusion of blood or blood products, and for obtaining blood samples
  Equipment for monitoring of vital signs and blood pressure
  Blood-drawing supplies
  Supplemental electric source
Additional supplies for the mother
  Stretcher with approved restraints or safety belts; linen.
  Eclamptic tray: supplies, medications, and equipment
  Delivery pack
  Emesis basin
  FHR monitor
Additional supplies for the newborn
  Transport unit with total life support and monitoring capacity
  Thoracotomy tray and thoracentesis set
The transport vehicle should have the capacity for safety precautions:
1. Ground transport: money (change) for telephone call; restraints.
2. Air transport: in-flight turbulence precautions (restraints, intravenous fluids in plastic bags, etc.) and precautions against changes in atmospheric pressure.

Nursing the newborn with respiratory distress. Any newborn with respiratory difficulty is in jeopardy.† The infant's response to prompt, appropriate treatment bears a direct relationship to the cause, degree of maturity, and other medical problems.

Breathing is a new experience for the infant. In priority of care, it ranks second only to massive hemorrhage. Because of its high priority and its challenging nursing aspects, considerable space in the delivery room is devoted to the initiation and maintenance of respirations.

The alert nurse often is the pivotal point between functional and dysfunctional survival for the infant in

---

*See References and Bibliography. Most facilities have developed modular study guides and manuals for procedures and for laboratory values and their management.

*Carefully outlined and specific guidelines are provided in NAACOG-OGN Nursing Practice Resource, Maternal-Neonatal Transport, No. 8, June 1983. (The Nurses Association of the American College of Obstetricians and Gynecologists, 600 Maryland Avenue, S.W., Suite 200, Washington, D.C., 20024, 202/638-0026.)
†See discussion on techniques for suctioning the newborn, oxygen therapy, and resuscitation in Chapter 20.

respiratory distress. The nurse's alertness and informed observations place the nurse in a preventive, curative, and rehabilitative role.

Assessment. The infant in distress at birth is immediately identifiable. In addition, some infants who at birth appear pink and vigorous, with good muscle tone and respiratory rates and rhythms within normal range, become distressed soon afterward. Respiratory difficulty, with cyanosis and retractions such as occur after aspiration or tension pneumothorax, may appear suddenly. More commonly, respiratory difficulty follows a progressive sequential pattern:

1. The **respiratory rate** initially may increase without a change in rhythm. Flaring of the nares and expiratory grunt are also early signs of respiratory distress.
2. The **apical pulse** increases in rate.
3. **Retractions,** depending on the cause, may begin as subcostal and xiphoid and then progress upward to intercostal, suprasternal, and clavicular retractions (Fig. 25.12).
4. The **color** changes from pink to circumoral pallor, to circumoral cyanosis, and then to generalized cyanosis; acrocyanosis deepens.
5. **Respiratory effort** and deepening distress are indicated by the following (Fig. 25.13)
   a. Chin tug (Chin is pulled down [and mouth opens wider] as auxiliary muscles of respiration are activated.)
   b. Abdominal seesaw breathing patterns (Figs. 19.3, 19.4, and 25.13).
   c. Increased number of apneic episodes
6. If the newborn is hypoxic, the **temperature** may begin to drop. (Avoid rapid warming of the newborn; it may evoke apneic episodes; see Chapter 20.)

Nursing diagnosis. Examples of nursing diagnoses for the newborn with respiratory distress include the following:

1. Alteration in respiratory function* related to:
   a. Immaturity
   b. Cold stress
2. Ineffective airway clearance related to:
   a. Newborn anatomy
   b. Meconium aspiration
   c. Immaturity or congenital disorder
   d. Respiratory depression secondary to narcosis or acidosis
3. Impaired gas exchange related to immaturity (e.g., insufficient surfactant)

Planning. During the important planning step, goals are set to meet the unique needs of the high-risk

---

*Diagnosis not included by NANDA, 1986.

Fig. 25.12
Retraction: substernal, subcostal, and intercostal retractions are evident. (Courtesy Ross Laboratories, Columbus, Ohio.)

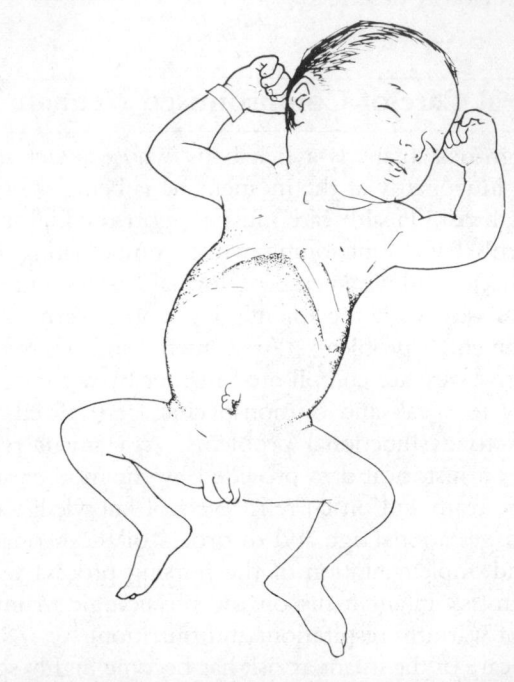

neonate. The goals are prioritized. Nursing actions are selected to meet the goals. Before nursing care is implemented, the nurse plans carefully to assure that the care provided is goal directed.

Goals
1. Respirations are maintained.
2. Bronchopulmonary dysplasia and retrolental fibroplasia do not develop.
3. Metabolism meets needs of repair, maintenance, and growth.
4. Respiratory needs of all tissues are met, (e.g., blood gases and acid-base balance are maintained within normal limits).
5. Congenital dysfunctions or anomalies are recognized early, and appropriate treatment is initiated.
6. Parents are supported in coping constructively with the situation and relating to the infant as a person.

Implementation
Positioning. The newborn's respiratory efforts must be supported by careful positioning.

When the infant is supine, the arms will be at the sides, flexed and slightly abducted. Diapers, if used, must be pinned loosely. (For more detail, see Chapter 20.)

Fig. 25.13
Observation of retractions. Silverman-Anderson index of respiratory distress is determined by grading each of five arbitrary criteria: *grade 0* indicates no difficulty; *grade 1*, moderate difficulty; and *grade 2*, maximal respiratory difficulty. Retraction score is sum of these values; total score of 0 indicates no dyspnea, whereas total score of 10 denotes maximal respiratory distress. (Modified from Silverman, W., and Anderson, D.: Pediatrics **17:**1, 1956.)

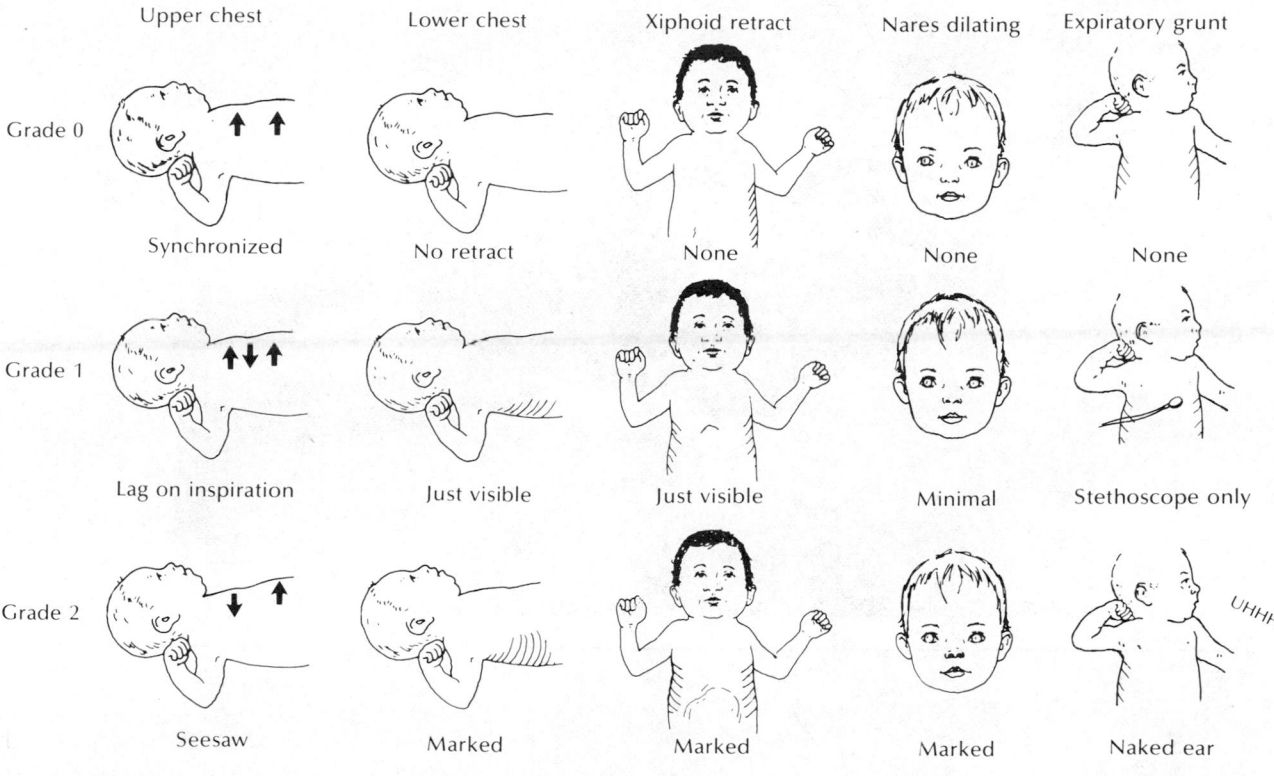

The prone position recently has been shown to improve respiratory effort, increase Pao$_2$, and diminish the work of respiration.

Suctioning. An open airway usually decreases the newborn's labored breathing by improving ventilation. (See discussion of suctioning procedures in Chapter 20.)

Oxygen needs and administration. Oxygen therapy may be lifesaving, but its administration must be carefully monitored as with any drug. Indiscriminate use of oxygen may be hazardous, resulting in retrolental fibroplasia and bronchopulmonary dysplasia. See the discussion on oxygen therapy (Chapter 20), retrolental fibroplasia, and pulmonary dysplasia (Chapter 29).

Warmth. A thermoneutral environment is essential for metabolic homeostasis. Cold stress is detrimental to the well-being of any infant but especially the infant at risk. For a discussion of thermogenesis and the prevention of cold stress, see Chapter 20.

Nutrition. Nutrition and feeding of the infant in respiratory distress is as much a challenge for the nurse as for the infant. The extra work of breathing taxes the infant's energy reserves and demands greater caloric input. Breast feeding and bottle feeding are not appropriate for the newborn in distress. The newborn in severe distress may require gavage feeding exclusively. Parenteral fluids or total parenteral nutrition (TPN) may be required for the newborn who cannot tolerate gavage feedings.

For the convalescent infant in no respiratory distress who can bottle feed, a softer nipple with an adequate opening is used (e.g., when the bottle is inverted, fluid should drip at 1 drop per second). The airway must be cleared before and during feeding as necessary. Moreover, the infant is "bubbled" before feedings.

If the convalescent infant is feeding at the breast, the nurse remains at the bedside with a bulb syringe at

Fig. 25.14
High-risk newborn (under heat panel not shown). Note CPAP, eye patches (infant is receiving phototherapy), probe *(left)* for heartbeat, probe *(right)* for respirations, umbilical catheter from three-way stopcock, and syringe filled with heparinized saline. Note enlarged labia characteristic of premature newborn. Thermistor probe shown should not be near right shoulder. Thermistor probes for Servo-Control should be placed properly in right upper quadrant of abdomen just below inferior costal margin. (Photograph by I.M. Bobak.)

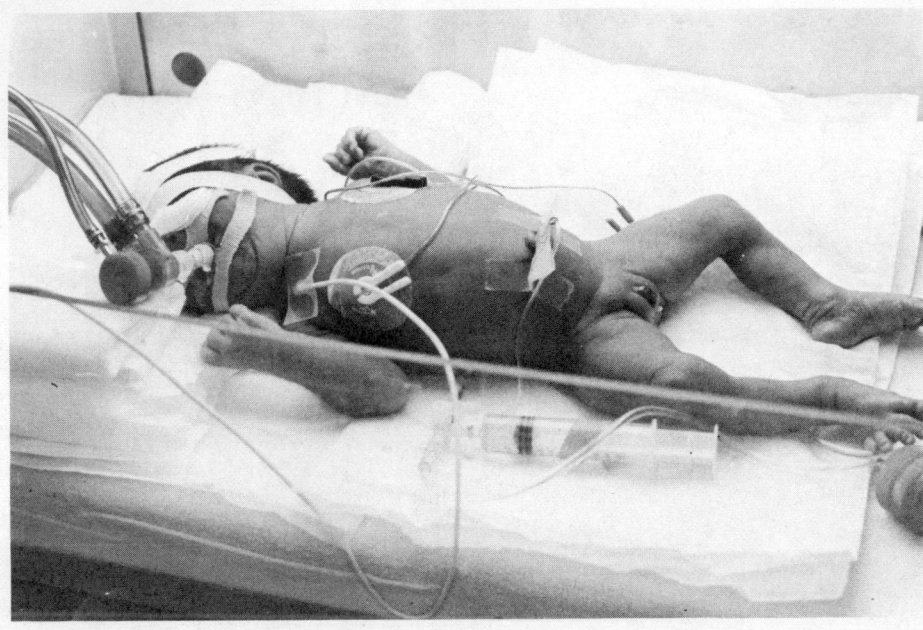

hand. This provides reassurance for the mother and avoids a buildup of tension, which might be transferred from mother to infant. Should the infant gag or choke, the nurse can show the mother how to manage such a situation.

Evaluation. The nurse is assured that care was effective if the selected goals of care are met.

Oxygen therapy. Oxygen therapy, seen frequently in the normal newborn nursery, is discussed in Chapter 20.

Continuous positive airway pressure. Continuous positive airway pressure (CPAP) is most commonly administered through nasal prongs or an endotracheal tube (oral or nasal) (Fig. 25.14). The purposes of this technique include the following:

1. Employs same principle as the expiratory grunt (The expiratory grunt is a physiologic adaptation to trap air within the lungs, keeping alveoli open to prevent atelectasis on expiration.)
2. Increases functional residual capacity
3. Improves oxygenation
4. Decreases pulmonary shunting

Transcutaneous oxygen tension monitoring. Older methods of monitoring arterial oxygenation in the ill newborn involved such invasive techniques as umbilical artery catheterization and radial and temporal artery puncture or catheterization. Oxygen electrodes placed intravascularly to achieve continuous monitoring of arterial oxygenation did not meet with success in recent years.

Today accurate noninvasive transcutaneous (tc) oxygen tension (tcPo$_2$) monitoring is feasible on a continuous basis. The tcPo$_2$ electrode is applied according to the manufacturer's instructions. However, all electrodes are applied to a hairless and greaseless site, and an airtight contact with the skin is secured. The electrode application site is changed every 4 hours to avoid burns. The distinct advantage of this method is that the data are available on a moment-to-moment basis; for example, complications can be identified

Procedure 25.2

WEANING FROM OXYGEN THERAPY

PURPOSE

Prepare infant to breathe room air.

EQUIPMENT

1. Equipment already in use by the infant being weaned
2. Regular bassinet, blankets, linens as needed after infant is weaned.

NURSING ACTION	RATIONALE
1. Weaning process is gradual.	1. The hazards of sudden cyanosis and respiratory collapse become greater with increased time that infant has received oxygen therapy.
2. Decrease oxygen by 10% every 30 to 60 minutes (or 2 to 4 hours) as child improves.	2. Too rapid weaning with hypoxia can re-open right-to-left shunts: foramen ovale, ductus arteriosus.
3. Monitor laboratory values simultaneously: blood pH, PaO_2,* $PaCO_2$ arterial hemoglobin concentration.	3. This provides data for modifying rate of weaning process.

4. Observe infant closely for the following:
  a. Pulse
  b. Respiratory effort
  c. Skin color
If symptoms occur, increase oxygen and proceed with slower weaning schedule
	4. Monitoring avoids adverse reactions to weaning.
	  a. Pulse elevation
	  b. Respiratory distress
	  c. Cyanosis

*Blood gas values are given in Appendix I. Hospital intensive care units have protocols for care based on blood gas findings.

early. The efficiency of respiratory therapy can be evaluated readily.

Determining blood pressure. Blood pressure readings are obtained by the Doppler method or electronic monitor. A blood pressure cuff of appropriate size must be used. A too wide cuff results in a false low reading; an overly narrow cuff will give a false elevated reading. For the newborn a cuff of about 2.5 to 3 cm (1 in) width and 7.5 cm (3 in) length is usually adequate (Fig. 25.15).

The stethoscope should have a pediatric-sized diaphragm for maximum skin contact and localization of sounds. The stethoscope is applied with firm pressure but not so much pressure that transmission of sound and vibrations is compromised.

The Doppler instrument and electronic monitoring device (on a biometic console) (see Fig. 25.22, C) are more accurate methods for determining blood pressure. However, these types of equipment are not available in all hospitals or community health settings.

The monitor displays the systolic and diastolic value, the mean systolic/diastolic pressure (the reading is midway between the diastolic and systolic pressures), and the newborn's heart rate. An accurate and timely blood pressure reading can assist in the early detection and proper treatment of the high-risk infant. The existing standard normal range for the mean pressure for infants weighing 2500 g (5½ lb) or more is 30 to 60 mm Hg.

Temperature support and regulation
Assessment
1. Monitor infant's temperature (see Chapter 20)
   a. Overhead radiant heat source with thermistor probe to skin

---

Fig. 25.15
Preparing to assess a newborn's blood pressure electronically. (Photograph by I.M. Bobak).

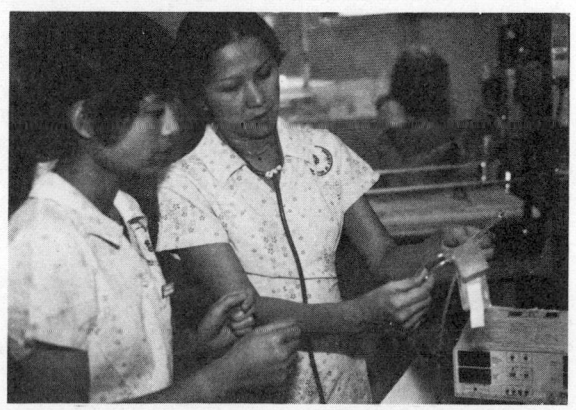

b. Servo-Control incubator
  (1) Thermistor probe taped to skin
  (2) Thermometer on incubator wall
c. Anal (core) temperature
d. Axillary temperature
e. Coolness or warmth to touch of infant's body and extremities
2. Observe for physiologic signs of cold stress
  a. In stronger, more mature infant: increased physical activity, crying
  b. Increased respiratory rate
  c. Color change
    (1) Deepening acrocyanosis
    (2) Appearance of generalized cyanosis
    (3) Mottling of skin (cutis marmorata)
  d. In boy with descended testes, activated cremasteric reflex (On exposure to cold, testes are pulled up into inguinal canal.)

Nursing diagnosis. Examples of nursing diagnoses related to temperature support and regulation include the following:
1. Ineffective thermoregulation, related to:
  a. Immaturity
  b. Congenital disorder
2. Alteration in body temperature related to:
  a. Environmental factors leading to hypothermia or hyperthermia
  b. Disease processes such as infection
  c. Fluid deficit secondary to hypovolemia
3. Potential for cold stress related to physiologic immaturity of newborn*

Planning. During the important planning step, goals are set in client-centered terms. The goals are prioritized. Nursing actions are selected to meet the goals. The speed and accuracy with which planning is accomplished depends on the nurse's level of competence (Chapter 2).

Goals
1. Skin temperature is maintained between 36.1° and 36.7° C (97° to 98° F).†
2. No apneic spells occur.
3. Adequate weight is gained.
4. Sequelae of cold stress (i.e., sclerema, oxygen deprivation to tissues, metabolic acidosis, hypoglycemia, abnormal blood gases, and dysfunction of CNS) do not develop.

---

*Diagnosis not included by NANDA, 1986.
†See discussions on techniques for regulating warmth and humidity in infant's environment and for maintaining thermoneutral environment in Chapter 20.

Implementation
1. Nursing care should be planned and implemented to prevent or minimize cold stress.
  a. Quickly dry newborn infant in warm, absorbent blanket, taking particular care to dry and cover head (one fourth of body length). (If infant is of good weight and in good condition, he or she may be given to mother to hold.) Prevent cold air from blowing over face; receptors in facial skin are extremely sensitive to cold.
  b. Place wrapped infant in warm incubator, Kreisselmann, or other heated carrier. Infant may be placed unwrapped under radiant heat source.
  c. All procedures and observations when infant is unwrapped are done in incubator, under radiant heat, on warm surface, etc.
  d. All surfaces and materials touching infant are warm.
  e. Caretakers' hands should be warm when handling neonate.
  f. O_2 or air administered to infant is warmed.
2. Maintain equipment in excellent operative condition. Know procedures and rationale for procedures.
  a. Maintain abdominal skin temperatures at 36.1° to 36.7° (97° to 98° F), axillary temperature at 36.5° C (97.8° F). Report any rise in temperature over 37.3° C (99° F) or a drop of 0.6° to 1° C (1° to 2° F).
  b. Equipment is plugged in and operative. Thermostat is set on control panel. Probe is in contact with skin. Portholes and lid are closed. Incubator is placed away from windows, air-conditioning units, etc.
  c. Know procedures for anal and axillary temperature taking (see Chapter 20).
  d. Place bassinet away from drafts or sources of heat or cold. Take temperatures by thermometer periodically to check accuracy of equipment.
3. Alter environment to return infant to desired body temperature if infant's temperature is too low or too high.
  a. Check and readjust thermostat setting as necessary. Is equipment plugged into electrical outlet?
  b. Check and reapply probe as necessary. Wet or detached probe may lead to hyperthermia.
  c. Are portholes closed? open? Is sleeve off track (on incubators with plastic sleeve covers)?
  d. Increase or decrease amount of clothing and blankets as necessary.
  e. Lighting: if gooseneck lamp is directly over infant, it may increase the temperature.

f. Check placement of incubators, cribs, etc.

g. Use different thermometer.

Evaluation. The nurse can be assured that care was effective if the goals of care are met and nursing diagnoses are resolved. A new plan of care is designed to meet the changing needs of the high-risk infant.

Warming the hypothermic infant. Rapid warming or cooling may produce apneic spells and acidosis in an infant. Therefore the warming process is increased slowly over a period of 2 to 4 hours.*

The nurse places the infant in a Servo-Control incubator and proceeds as follows:

1. Set incubator temperature on control panel at 1.2°C (2° F) above skin temperature even if lower than normal.
2. Tape thermistor probe to skin of anterior abdominal wall.
3. When skin temperature reaches predetermined temperature, set incubator temperature, repeat process until abdominal skin temperature of 36.5° C (97.7° F) is achieved.

Weaning infant from Servo-Control incubator. The weaning process is accomplished slowly over a period of hours or days or as follows:

1. Dress the infant in diaper and shirt.
2. Lower incubator temperature; record temperatures of infant and incubator.
3. Assess baby's response.
4. Repeat steps 2 and 3 until incubator temperature equals room temperature, and infant's abdominal skin temperature is 36.5° C (97.7° F).
5. Wrap infant in blanket, open incubator portholes, and assess infant's response.
6. Remove baby to open crib if axillary temperature is adequate.

Nutrition and elimination. Low-birth-weight newborns make up the largest number of high-risk infants. Of these, about one third are small for gestational age (SGA) regardless of maturity. About two thirds are preterm and appropriate for gestational age (AGA). SGA newborns may also be preterm.

The feeding and nutrition of the high-risk infant warrant careful consideration. The extent to which nutritional needs are met is directly related to the infant's immediate and long-range well-being. For example, if the low-birth-weight infant with low glycogen stores is not fed promptly, the resultant symptomatic or asymptomatic hypoglycemia may seriously damage carbohydrate-dependent brain cells (see Chapter 31).

Early feeding. Early feeding is feeding within 6 to 8 hours after birth. For the term, nonstressed newborn, early oral or parenteral feeding is necessary for the following reasons:

- To prevent dehydration
- To spare the available stores of glycogen
- To maintain blood glucose levels
- To lessen initial weight loss
- To keep serum bilirubin levels within normal limits
- To curtail protein catabolism that would result in metabolic acidosis, hyperkalemia, or elevated BUN levels
- To conserve energy for growth
- To stimulate sucking response

Early feeding is avoided if the newborn had low Apgar scores. Early feeding of asphyxiated newborns may be an important cause of necrotizing enterocolitis (NEC) (see Chapter 29).

Nutritional requisites. Caloric, nutrient, and fluid requirements of the infant at risk may be greater for many reasons, some of which follow:

1. Limited stores: preterm or dysmature (malnourished) newborn
2. Depleted stores: newborn who is stressed by one or a combination of the following factors:
   a. Birth asphyxia
   b. Increased respirations or respiratory effort
   c. Insensible fluid loss by evaporation when infant is under radiant heat or during phototherapy
   d. Hypothermic environment
3. Immature systems
   a. Gastrointestinal tract: losses through vomiting, diarrhea, dysfunctional absorption
   b. Kidneys: losses caused by inability to concentrate urine and maintain an adequate rate of urea excretion and by an inadequate response to antidiuretic hormone (ADH)
4. Growth demands: preterm newborn's growth rate approximates fetal growth rate during the last trimester, which is two or more times that of an infant after delivery at term

Weight and fluid loss. As much as 80% to 85% of the preterm (28 to 34 weeks) newborn's body weight consists of water as compared to 70% in the term infant. Most of this water occupies the extracellular fluid compartment. Even with the early fluid and nutritional intake, the preterm infant's weight and fluid losses seem exaggerated. Factors predisposing to weight and fluid losses include the following:

1. Inadequate fluid intake (e.g., from delayed administration or insufficient volume) predisposes the infant to weight loss.

---

*Rapid warming is elected by some authors: Kaplan and Eidelman (1984).

2. Insensible water loss (IWL) represents evaporative losses that occur largely through the skin. Approximately 30% of this IWL is from the respiratory tract and most of this is prevented by humidified oxygen—enriched gases that are used for respiratory support in sick infants. Total IWL ranges anywhere from 1.75 to 3.6 ml/kg/hour. The quantity is influenced by gestational age, postnatal age, weight, and use of radiant warmer or incubator and other factors.

3. Greater fluid demands to meet increased cellular metabolic processes (e.g., from stress, repair, or growth) predispose the newborn to weight and fluid losses.

The limits of acceptable weight loss are as follows: During the newborn's first 3 days of extrauterine life, the preterm infant can lose 12% or less of birth weight. For the term infant, a weight loss of 10% or less is acceptable for newborns of normal weight for gestational age; weight loss of 15% or less is acceptable for infants weighing 4500 g (9 lb 14 oz) or more. For dysmature SGA infants, a loss of 5% or less of birth weight is acceptable.

After the first 3 days, a preterm newborn's loss or gain during each 24-hour period should not exceed 2% of the previous day's weight.

The following examples illustrate how to calculate weight loss and gain, suggesting causes and nursing actions for each case.

EXAMPLE 1

Day 4 1750 g
Day 5 1730 g
———
20 g loss

$$\frac{20}{1750} = \frac{x\%}{100\%}$$
$$1750x = 2000$$
$$1750\sqrt{2000.00} \quad 1.1\%$$
$$x = 1.1\% \text{ weight loss}$$

Probable causes: Stool passage
Inadequate fluid: amount and type
Nursing actions: Record and report.
Observe infant.
Perform Dextrostix test.

EXAMPLE 2

Day 4 1750 g
Day 5 1790 g
———
40 g gain

$$\frac{40}{1750} = \frac{x\%}{100\%}$$
$$1750x = 4000$$
$$1750\sqrt{4000.0} \quad 2.3$$
$$x = 2.3\% \text{ gain}$$

Probable causes: Overfeeding
Fluid retention
Nursing actions: Record and report.
Observe newborn for other symptoms.
Collect urine in bag: check amount, specific gravity.
Perform Dextrostix test.

EXAMPLE 3

Day 4 1750 g
Day 5 1715 g
———
35 g loss

$$\frac{35}{1750} = \frac{x\%}{100\%}$$
$$1750x = 3500$$
$$1750\sqrt{3500.0} \quad 2.0$$
$$x = 2\% \text{ weight loss}$$

Probable causes: Excessive stooling, voiding
Excessive evaporative losses
Inadequate amount and type of fluid
Malabsorption problem
Nursing actions: Record and report.
Check incubator and infant for temperature; check incubator for humidity.
Observe newborn for other symptoms.
Collect urine in bag: check urine for amount and specific gravity; use Clinistix.
Perform Dextrostix test.

Formula and feeding schedules. The formula and feeding schedule of the infant at risk are based on the following criteria:

1. Infant's birth weight and pattern of weight gain or loss
2. Estimated gestational age
3. Physical condition: pharyngeal coordination (sucking, swallowing reflexes are present and coordinated), fatigability, malformations, amount of urine excreted per hour
4. Laboratory values: nitrogen balance, electrolyte imbalance, glucose level, serum bilirubin level, and other results

The following variants influence the feeding of the infant at risk:

1. Fluid volume given
2. Caloric requirements
3. Mode of feeding
4. Formula: breast milk, predigested formula, and calories per ounce.

Parenteral fluids and total parenteral nutrition. The very small newborn or the newborn who is unable to suck because of developmental or respiratory problems (especially the infant on assisted ventilation) is sustained by parenteral infusions. The electrolytes and nutrients per milliliter, as well as the milliliters of fluid per kilogram of body weight per hour, are carefully calculated by the physician. The nurse monitors the functioning of infusion equipment (tubing, infusion pump), ensures asepsis, secures and protects the needle (catheter) at the insertion site, and assesses and records the newborn's responses.

WEANING FROM PARENTERAL THERAPY. As the infant's condition improves, the infant may be offered fluids by nipple. As the amount of feeding given orally is increased and tolerated, the amount given by infusion is decreased.

Oral preparations. The nurse assists in assessing the newborn's tolerance for oral feeding by noting the following:

- Pharyngeal coordination (suck and swallow reflexes present and synchronized)
- Presence and degree of respiratory distress or apneic episodes, if any
- Presence of bowel sounds and absence of abdominal distension
- Gastric residual of 2 ml or less before feeding

Various milk formulas are available. These formulas vary in calories, protein, and mineral content (see Chapter 21). Breast milk or formula may be fed by continuous flow with a pump and feeding tube inserted into the stomach or jejunum or by intermittent gavage or nipple. During the transition to nipple it may be necessary to use both nipple and gavage to ensure the prescribed intake. Each newborn must be evaluated for ability to handle solute and fluid load.

Oral feedings begin with sterile water. Feedings are advanced by increasing the amount of fluid *or* the number of calories per 30 ml (1 oz) at any one feeding. The maximum number of calories per ounce is 24. During the feeding the newborn's tolerance is observed. For infants weighing less than approximately

1800 g (4 lb) the feedings are advanced more slowly. Too rapid advancement may lead to the following:

1. Vomiting, diarrhea, abdominal distension
2. Apneic episodes
3. Residual feeding of 2 ml or more at the time of the next feeding
4. Retention of fluid with cardiopulmonary embarrassment or marked diuresis with loss of sodium (Na^+), leading to hyponatremia
5. Regurgitation—aspiration pneumonia

Feeding the high-risk infant
Assessment
1. Weight plotted on growth grid
   a. On admission
   b. Daily: weight loss or rate of weight gain
2. Elimination patterns
   a. Frequency of urination
   b. Amount, frequency, and character of stool
      (1) Obstipation or constipation or both
      (2) Diarrhea
      (3) Loss of fats (steatorrhea)
      (4) Guaiac
      (5) pH
3. Oral feedings*
   a. Type of formula; calories/30 ml (1 oz)
   b. Volume
   c. Behavior during feeding
      (1) Attempts at sucking
      (2) Abdominal distension (Fig. 25.16)
      (3) Vomiting, regurgitation
      (4) Cyanosis
      (5) Amount of mucus
   d. Time necessary to feed
4. Gavage feedings*
   a. As for oral feedings
   b. Feeding tube of correct size; use nasogastric or orogastric route
5. Abdominal distension
   a. Time, degree, and effect on respiratory system
   b. X-ray examination
6. Vomiting or regurgitation or both
   a. Color, amount, time in relation to feeding, and character (e.g., forceful? spill over?)
   b. Pass nasogastric tube for diagnosis as necessary
7. Parenteral fluids: type, rate per minute, infusion site
8. TPN (alimentation): assess per hospital protocol

Nursing diagnoses. Examples of nursing diagnoses related to nutrition and elimination include the following:

Fig. 25.16
Sudden abdominal distension. (Courtesy Ross Laboratories, Columbus, Ohio.)

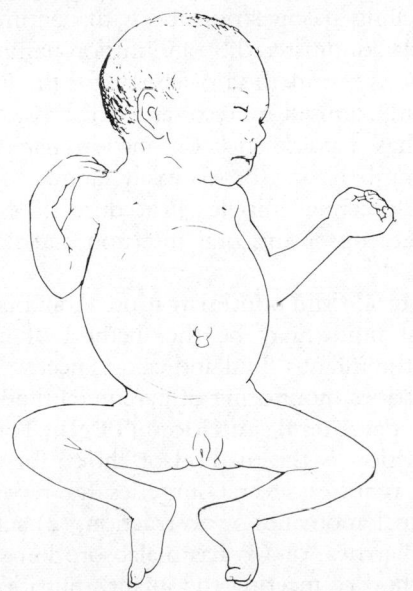

---

*See discussions relevent to feeding, nutrition, and elimination in Chapter 21.

1. Alteration in nutrition: less than body requirements, related to problems of immaturity.
2. Alteration in fluid volume: deficit or overload related to immaturity or neonatal disorder
3. Ineffective breathing pattern related to sudden abdominal distension

Planning. During the important planning step, goals are set in client-centered terms. The goals are prioritized. Nursing actions are selected to meet the goals. The speed and accuracy with which planning is accomplished depends on the nurse's level of competence (Chapter 2).

Goals

1. Feeding and nutrition of the high-risk newborn are accomplished with the following results:
   a. Minimal respiratory distress; no aspiration or aspiration pneumonia
   b. Minimal expenditure of energy
   c. Hypoglycemic reactions avoided
   d. Acceptable fluid-electrolyte balance
   e. No abdominal distension
   f. No trauma to tissues of the gastrointestinal tract
   g. No diarrhea
2. Sucking satisfaction is maximized.
3. Nutrition is sufficient to accomplish the following:
   a. Meet resting metabolic requirements
   b. Provide sufficient energy to perform physical activity
   c. Counter losses through gastrointestinal and urinary tracts
   d. Supply constituents for growth (The infant establishes a steady pattern of appropriate weight gain.)
4. Parent-child relationship is fostered in the following ways:
   a. Parent begins to participate in the feeding process in light of the infant's physical capabilities and the parent's desired degree of involvement
   b. Infant begins to associate feeding and eating with pleasure as she or he develops a sense of trust
   c. At discharge parents are comfortable with the feeding method needed by the infant, whether feeding is by breast, bottle, gavage, or gastrostomy

Implementation

1. Readjust feeding (or infusion) to achieve acceptable weight gain.
2. Record observations accurately. Deviations from normal range in weight losses or gains guide future diagnostic evaluations to determine cause and treatment.

3. Readjust nursing care regarding continuation of gavage feedings, attempting oral feedings, providing simultaneous sucking satisfaction as soon as possible (before tenth day of life, gavage through nipple if necessary), type and amount of formula, and frequency of feedings.
4. If infant is taking oral feeding, readjust nursing care regarding type of nipple ("preemie," regular, breast).
5. Avoid overfeeding: evaluate by checking amount of residual before subsequent feeding; refeed residual and subtract this amount from this feeding; decrease amount of feeding; feed more frequently.
6. Burp or "bubble" infant as necessary; readjust positioning during feeding.
7. Determine when to involve parents in actual feeding or when to teach parents how to give gavage feedings if child will need them after going home.

Evaluation. Nursing care is evaluated to determine if the nursing goals have been met. Care is adjusted to accomplish the goals, and assessment continues as the nursing process is repeated.

Feeding newborn with cleft lip and palate. The baby born with a cleft lip and palate may be normal in every other way. Surgical repair on the lip is usually done soon after birth if possible to assist parents in the attachment process with their newborn. The palate is usually repaired some months later. The nurse may be called to feed the newborn during the early neonatal period or to teach the parent to do so. The following procedure is presented to assist the nurse in feeding the newborn with cleft lip and palate and to serve as a guide for teaching the parent(s).

Gavage feeding. Gavage feedings are supplied by an indwelling nasogastric tube with continuous flow of formula administered by an infusion pump. Feeding by gavage is the method of choice for the infant who is (1) compromised by respiratory distress, (2) immature or has a weak suck or uncoordinated sucking-swallowing behavior, or (3) easily fatigued even when using a "preemie" nipple. Procedure 25.4 describes gavage feedings using oral insertion and nasal insertion.

Parenteral fluid administration. Administration of parenteral fluids may be the method of choice for meeting the infant's fluid and caloric needs. Procedure 25.5 describes monitoring of parenteral fluid therapy.

Total parenteral nutrition (TPN). Total parenteral nutrition is the method of choice for the infant who (1) requires several surgeries for repair of gastrointestinal anomalies or obstruction, (2) suffers from chronic diarrhea, or (3) has malabsorption syndrome. This method of meeting the infant's nutritional needs is described in Procedure 25.6.

Text continued on p. 757.

Procedure 25.3

FEEDING NEWBORN WITH CLEFT LIP AND PALATE

PURPOSE

1. Facilitate feeding when infant has difficulty creating a vacuum and sucking.
2. Prevent aspiration of feeding.
3. Prevent discomfort from increased amount of swallowed air.

EQUIPMENT (Fig. 25.17)

1. Lamb's nipple
2. Duckey nipple with flange to fit over defect
3. Brecht feeder
4. Rubber-tipped Asepto syringe

NURSING ACTION	RATIONALE
1. Prepare thickened formula as ordered, usually with dried rice cereal.	1. Thickened formula increases gravity flow of fluid into stomach and prevents aspiration.
2. Enlarge the hole in the nipple as needed.	2. Larger hole permits passage of thickened feeding.
3. During feeding, observe for the following signs: aspiration—choking and cyanosis; swallowed air—abdominal distension.	3. The defect prevents formation of vacuum and normal sucking pattern. Abdominal distension and aspiration can compromise respirations.
4. Check infant for clear airway.	4. This minimizes possibility of aspiration.
5. Hold infant in upright position.	5. Upright position minimizes possibility of aspiration and return of fluid through nose and aids swallowing.
6. Interact with infant: talk to infant and so on.	6. Interaction is important for psychosocial development. If mother sees nurse doing this, it may facilitate her acceptance of the child.
7. Burp or bubble infant frequently.	7. More air is swallowed when there is unnatural passage between nose and mouth. Technique increases infant's comfort and minimizes regurgitation and aspiration.
8. When feeding infant with a rubber tipped Asepto syringe, place rubber tip on top of and to side of infant's tongue.	8. Facilitates feeding. Prevents tip of syringe from entering cleft in palate.
9. Offer feeding slowly.	9. Allows infant time to swallow.
NOTE: The child with a cleft lip only may be able to feed well with a regular or "preemie" nipple.	

Fig. 25.17
Cleft palate nipples. **A,** Side view and, **B,** front view of rubber flange that covers defect during feeding. Flange can be cut to fit. **C,** Lamb's nipple. Nipple carries formula beyond defect.

Fig. 25.18
Indwelling gavage tube: nasal route. Infant is propped on right side to facilitate emptying of stomach into small intestine. Note rolled towel for support. (See also Fig. 20.31.)

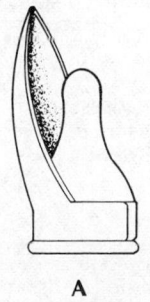
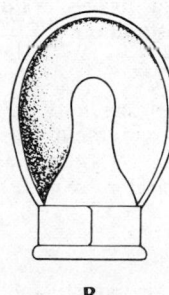
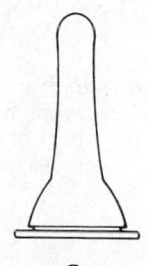

A   B   C

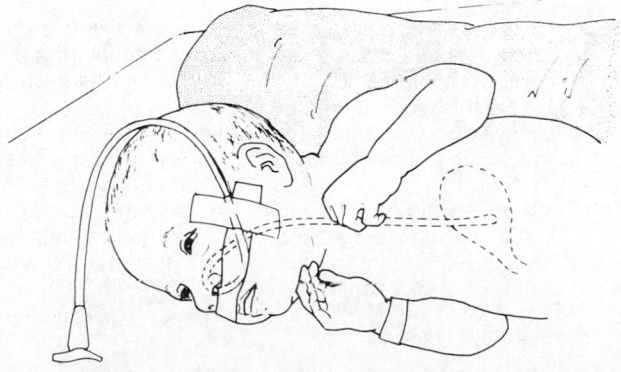

Procedure 25.4

GAVAGE FEEDING

PURPOSE

Meet the nutritional and fluid needs of the infant who cannot suck.

EQUIPMENT

1. Sterile feeding tube: rubber or plastic, rounded tips, sizes 5 to 10, infant lengths
2. Clearly calibrated syringe for feeding
3. Stethoscope and sterile medication syringe without needle
4. Sterile water for lubrication
5. Feeding formula
6. Medications

NURSING ACTION

The infant's anatomy makes it difficult to enter the trachea. One or more of the following tests are done to determine correct stomach placement.
1. Use sterile syringe to inject 0.5 cc of air through catheter into stomach. Simultaneously, listen for sound of air bubbling or "growling" in stomach with stethoscope over epigastric region.
2. The most complete procedure involves listening with stethoscope first over the epigastrium and then on each side of the anterior chest.
3. Aspirate small amount of stomach contents.

4. Fill tube with stomach contents, and pinch off tube; add syringe containing feeding.

Oral Insertion: Intermittent or Indwelling Catheter
1. Position infant: head of mattress up one notch, folded towel under shoulders to slightly extend neck.
2. Select size 8 French feeding tube.

3. Measure distance between bridge of nose and lower end of xiphoid process. Mark distance with 5 cm (2 in) thin strip of paper tape. Fold tape over tube, leaving two long ends with which to secure tube when it is in place.
4. Lubricate tube in sterile water.
5. Pass tube along base of tongue, advancing it into esophagus as infant swallows.

6. Test placement of tube.

7. Aspirate and measure any residual feeding in stomach. If 1 ml or less, substract same amount from this feeding. If more than 1 ml, physician may wish to have this feeding skipped.
8. Slowly pour warmed formula into syringe barrel and allow it to flow by gravity into stomach. Hold reservoir 15 to 20 cm (6 to 8 in) above infant's head. If gravity flow is too rapid, lower syringe, or insert plunger into syringe, and inject *slowly*. Feeding time should approximate that of nipple feedings (20 minutes or about 1 ml/min).
9. Do not allow level of formula to go below neck of syringe.

RATIONALE

These tests assure paper placement of the nasal or oral tube for gavage feedings.

1. Sound of air bubbling confirms tube placement in stomach.

2. The sound of rushing air heard over the anterior chest should be of considerably diminished intensity compared to that heard over the epigastrium.
3. Aspiration of stomach contents confirms proper placement of tube.
4. This avoids allowing air into stomach with feeding.

1. Opens oropharynx. Extends and straightens esophagus.

2. Is adequate size for feeding. Less apt to fold over or curl up.
3. Determines length necessary to reach into stomach without folding back on itself. Facilitates anchoring tubing, if it is to be indwelling. Paper tape is usually less irritating to skin.

4. Prevents trauma and infection.
5. Offers less risk of vagal stimulation or of accidental entry into trachea. Stimulates esophageal peristalsis and opens cardiac sphincter.
6. Avoids introduction of formula, vitamins, and medicines into trachea or esophagus.
7. Avoids overfeeding. Excessive fluid in stomach suggests intestinal obstruction.

8. Rapid entry of formula into stomach causes rapid rebound response with regurgitation, thus increasing danger of aspiration or abdominal distension, which compromises respiratory effort.

9. Prevents entry of air into stomach to minimize risks of regurgitation and distension.

Procedure 25.4 —cont'd

NURSING ACTION	RATIONALE
10. Observe infant's response.	10. Prevents respiratory distress. Assists gastrointestinal functioning.
11. Follow formula with specified amount of sterile water.	11. Gets all formula into stomach and clears tubing of formula.
12. Pinch tubing (or clamp it off) and withdraw it rapidly.	12. Prevents entry of air into stomach. Creates vacuum to hold fluid in tubing to prevent dripping it into trachea on withdrawal.
13. Burp or bubble infant. With left hand, support infant's head and shoulders. Raise to a sitting position and lean infant onto right hand. Right hand supports infant's chest with palm and infant's jaw with thumb and forefinger. Gently rub back with left hand.	13. Increases comfort. Prevents regurgitation.
14. Position on right side with small rolled drape or towel.	14. Facilitates stomach emptying.

15. Record the following:
  a. Amount of residual
  b. Type and amount of feeding, medicine
  c. Time of feeding
  d. Infant response: fatigue, peaceful sleep, abdominal distention, respiratory distress, type and amount of vomiting or regurgitation; heart and respiratory rate
	15. Provides basis for evaluation and readjustment of feeding regimen. Facilitates communication among personnel.

Nasal Route: Intermittent or Indwelling Catheter

1. Position as for oral route (Fig. 25.18).	1. Opens oropharynx. Extends and straightens esophagus.
2. Select size 3½ to 5 French feeding tube.	2. Is adequate size for feeding and small enough to allow breathing space around it, since neonates are obligate nose breathers.
a. If indwelling, change every 2 or 3 days (48 to 72 hours) or more frequently if otitis is present, alternating sides of nares.	a. Prevents infection, irritation; excess mucus, ulceration, bleeding.
b. Observe infant for respiratory distress.	b. If tube causes distress, remove it. Use oral route.
c. May be preferred route for indwelling tube for continuous drip feeding.	c. Very small preterm infant often tolerates feeding better by continuous drip; stomach is not overloaded.
3. Measure distance from bridge of nose to xiphoid process (just beyond tip of sternum). Mark spot with 5 cm (2 in) thin strip of paper tape, and overlap tube, leaving ends free	3. Provides adequate length to reach stomach without curling. Facilitates anchoring of tubing. Decreases risk of skin irritation from tape.
4. Lubricate with sterile water.	4. Prevents tissue trauma.
5. Insert tube, holding it horizontally until it reaches back of nares; then lift tubing slightly and continue to advance. Allow infant to swallow tube while it is being advanced.	5. Accommodates to bend in back of nares and minimizes direct tissue damage. Stimulates peristalsis and opens cardiac sphincter.
6 to 15. Same as for oral route.	6 to 15. Same as for oral route.

Nursing Care After Feedings

1. Burp infant gently after feedings.	1. Promotes comfort and prevents vomiting.
2. Turn infant's head or position the infant on right side after feeding and burping.	2. Protects against aspiration of stomach contents if vomiting occurs. Allows release of air from baby's stomach (Fig. 20.31).
3. Postpone postural drainage and percussion for a minimum of 1 hour after feeding.	3. Promotes retention of feeding.
4. Avoid feeding the infant within an hour before a laboratory test for blood glucose.	4. Promotes accurate reading in laboratory tests.

Procedure 25.5

MONITORING PARENTERAL FLUID ADMINISTRATION

PURPOSE

Meet the newborn infant's fluid needs

EQUIPMENT

1. Supplies to start or maintain intravenous therapy by way of a peripheral vein, venous cutdown, or umbilical catheter
2. Supplies to prevent accidental overhydration:
   a. Bottles containing 250 ml of infusion fluid
   b. Administration sets with enclosed reservoirs and minidropper
   c. Infusion pump with automatic alarm to signal an empty fluid chamber
   d. Medicine cup (paper) or other appliance to protect insertion site (Fig. 25.19)

NURSING ACTION	RATIONALE
1. Prepare equipment.	1. Avoids searching for missing articles after procedure has begun.
2. Restrain infant.	2. Provides for infant's safety and increased ease of starting parenteral fluids.
3. Provide pacifier to infant if appropriate.	3. Provides comfort for the infant who can handle a pacifier.
4. Continue care of intravenous infusion. Regulate rate of flow.	4. Provides for adequate infusion.
a. Infusion pump: check setting; double-check by counting drops per minute every hour, and note amount infused every 4 hours.	a. Assures a more accurate and constant flow rate. Double-checks for equipment malfunction.
b. Reposition extremity or infant's head.	b. Assures proper body alignment and prevents breakdown of skin. Protects infusion site.
c. *Do not* make up deficiency or excess by changing rate of flow without consulting physician.	c. Fluid may overload infant's system. An infant who has received more than prescribed amount for period must be assessed for overhydration and cardiac decompensation.
5. Check infusion site every hour.	5. Prevents trauma to tissues. Assures adequate hydration. Possible complications:
a. Check for tissue infiltration (swelling).	a. Infection
b. Check for tissue trauma: color, temperature.	b. Thrombophlebitis
c. If needle is in extremity, compare and contrast with other extremity.	c. Tissue and vein trauma (Fig. 25.20)
d. If needle is in scalp vein, check head and face for symmetry of contour and movement.	d. Needle out of vein with injection of fluid into surrounding tissues and possible tissue breakdown
6. Evaluate infant's hydration every hour.	6. Determines adequate rate of flow.
a. Urinary ouput: collect or weigh diapers.	a. Assesses amount of urine excreted.
b. Specific gravity of urine (see Appendix I and Procedure 20.3 for use of urine collectors).	b. Assists in assessing appropriate solute or fluid infant needs and kidney function.
c. Weight: infant may be weighed every 8, 12, or 24 hours.	c. Weight gain or loss greater than 2% of body weight within a 24-hour period is cause for concern.
d. Urine: check for glucose every 8 to 24 hours.	d. Presence of excess glucose in the urine would indicate an excessive glucose load in the intravenous fluid.
e. Other: tissue turgor; fever; sunken fontanels; soft, sunken eyeballs; or behavior changes may be present.	e. Assesses state of hydration.

Procedure 25.5—cont'd

NURSING ACTION	RATIONALE

7. Record the following:
  a. Type of fluid being used.
  b. Amount of fluid absorbed every hour and amount scheduled to have been absorbed.
  c. Amount of fluid in bottle or fluid chamber.
 	
  d. Flow rate.
 	
  e. Infant's condition.
 	
8. Change intravenous tubing and bottle every 24 hours.
9. Irrigate intravenously.
  a. Three-way stopcock may be used to connect tubing to needle.
 	
  b. Without three-way stopcock, clamp intravenous tubing and disconnect at junction with needle. Keep tubing end sterile. Attach syringe containing 1 to 3 ml of normal saline solution or heparinized saline solution to needle.
  c. *Slowly* inject fluid into vein. Disconnect syringe and reconnect to intravenous tubing. Unclamp intravenous tubing and regulate flow of infusion.
10. After intravenous fluid is discontinued:
  a. Observe infant for hypoglycemia for 24 hours.
 	
  b. Observe infant for adequacy of nutrition and hydration.
  c. Continue to assess infant for thrombophlebitis at previous insertion site and sloughing.
	7. Provides complete data.
	  a. Evaluates treatment.
	  b. Meets infant's changing needs.
	
	  c. Identifies possible cause of any existing or new problem.
	  d. Provides base line for continuation at present rate or change in rate.
	  e. Indicates infant's response to this regimen and readiness for progression.
	8. Decreases possibility of infection.
	
	9. Maintains patency of system.
	  a. Facilitates flushing needle while decreasing chance of contamination and loss of blood during procedure.
	  b. Clears out small occluding clots; prevents formation of clots.
	
	  c. Prevents trauma to vein or dislodging the needle.
	
	10. Ensures adequate nutrition and hydration.
	  a. Hypoglycemia often is seen after discontinuation of parenteral therapy.
	  b. Assesses infant's ability to take and utilize nutrients and fluids by mouth or gavage.
	  c. Begins definitive treatment and prevents tissue damage.

Fig. 25.19

A, Venipuncture of scalp vein. **B,** Paper cup protecting venipuncture site.

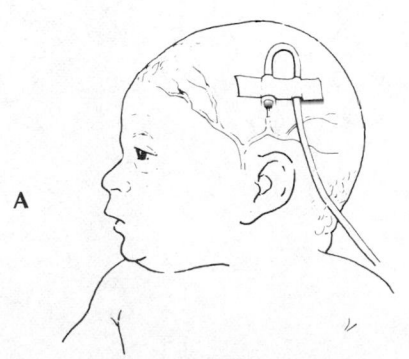
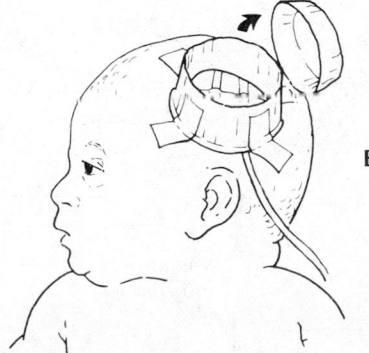

Fig. 25.20

A, Intravenous infiltration in small infant can cause severe ischemia. **B,** Fortunately, preterm infant has remarkable regeneration abilities (same hand 1 week later). (Courtesy Mount Zion Hospital and Medical Center, San Francisco.)

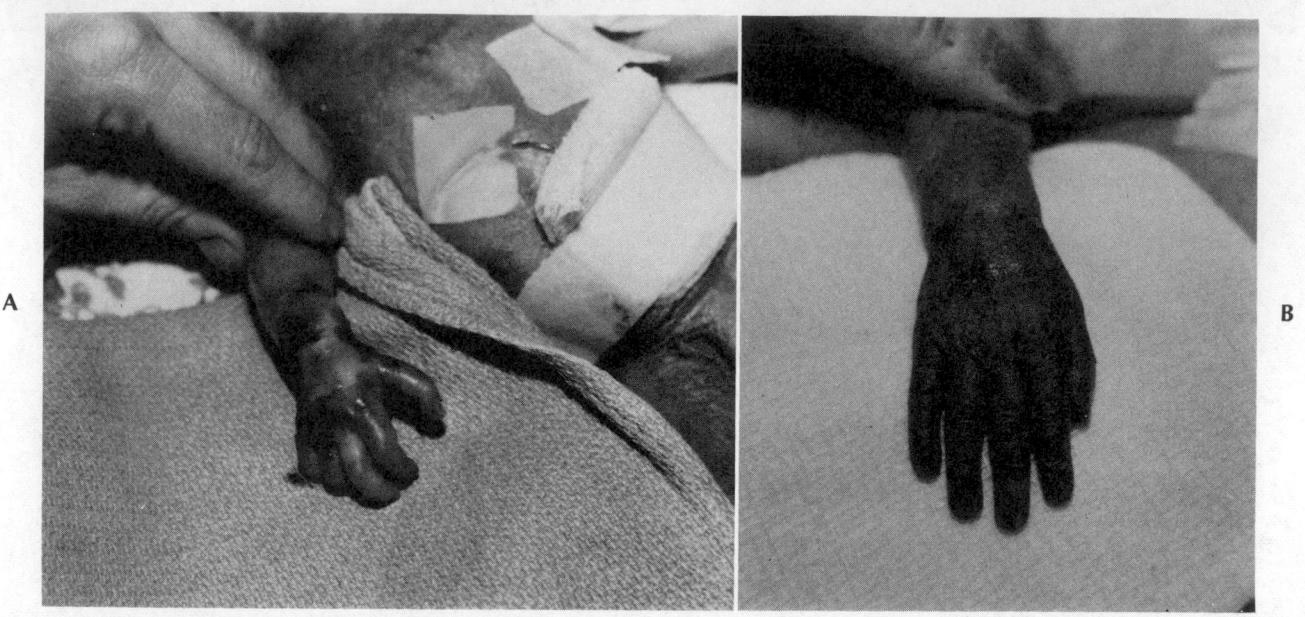

Fig. 25.21

A, Total parenteral nutrition (TPN). **B,** Close-up to show infusion site and internal placement of catheter into the descending vena cava. Parenteral nutrition is often used in conjunction with other forms of feeding, particularly when weaning to oral feedings.

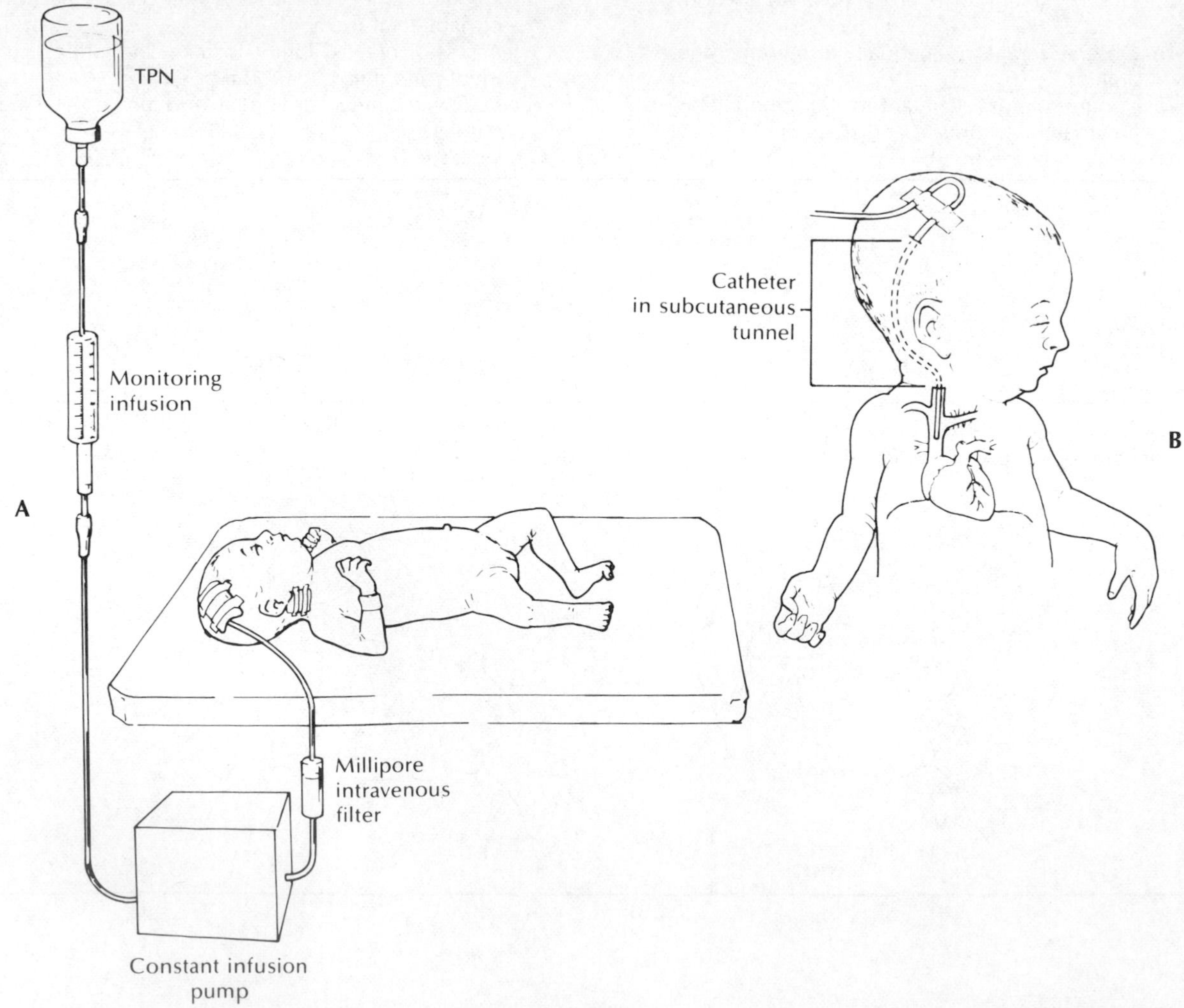

TPN

Monitoring
infusion

Catheter
in subcutaneous
tunnel

A

B

Millipore
intravenous
filter

Constant infusion
pump

Procedure 25.6

TOTAL PARENTERAL NUTRITION (TPN)

PURPOSE

Provide complete continuous nutrition at a prescribed rate for extended periods of time through an indwelling catheter threaded into the vena cava (Fig. 25.21). Infusion solutions used are protein hydrolysate, glucose, electrolytes, minerals, and vitamins.

EQUIPMENT

1. Instruments for starting intravenous infusion or a cut-down
2. Silastic catheter of appropriate size
3. Millipore intravenous filter
4. Constant infusion pump (Holter or other)
5. TPN solution (infusion fluid)
6. Pacifier and mobiles
7. Restraints as necessary

NURSING ACTION	RATIONALE
The procedure may be done in the operating room. Nursing actions are the same as those for care of an infant receiving intravenous fluid therapy, except for the following notable additions:	Maintain strict aseptic technique.
1. Avoid using the catheter for purposes other than the infusion solution (e.g., not used for blood or medications).	1. Maintain patency; avoid mixing incompatible fluids.
2. Avoid making up excess or deficit by altering the drip rate without consulting the physician.	2. Avoid fluid overload or deficit.
3. Order prescribed mixture from pharmacy or mix under aseptic conditions.	3. Ensures accuracy of amounts. Prevents microbial contamination.
4. Check on rate of flow.	4. Avoids overfeeding or underfeeding. Checks equipment for malfunction.
a. Check pump setting.	
b. Check amount given from calibrated, enclosed reservoir every 2 to 4 hours.	
5. Change bottle, tubing, and Millipore filter every 1 or 2 days. Culture filter after use.	5. Decreases risk of microbial contamination.
6. Change dressing around catheter.	6. Prevents infection and allows observation of area of needle insertion.
7. Monitor infant's weight daily at same times on same scales.	7. Provides index of response to this form of therapy.
8. Provide pacifier and mobiles.	8. Provides sucking satisfaction and some visual stimulation.
9. Observe infant for complications associated with TPN.	9. Facilitates prompt identification and treatment of problems.
a. Catheter and its insertion: local skin infection, septicemia, blood vessel thrombosis, obstruction or dislodgment of catheter, cardiac symptoms such as arrhythmia. *Candida* septicemia is quite common.	a. Fifty percent of complications from sepsis
b. Infusion solution—type and amount: glucosuria, dehydration, acidosis, amino acid imbalance.	b. Metabolic complications

Emotional aspects of care

Newborn's emotional needs. Premature and sick infants who are not in acute distress or who are convalescing have at least the same emotional and developmental needs that the normal term infant has. It may be difficult to meet the needs of the infant at risk. The sick infant who needs intravenous therapy, nasogastric feedings, heel-stick samples, oxygen by plastic hood, or continuous positive airway pressure cannot be cuddled, fondled, or played with as can the term infant. Instead she or he must experience many painful stimuli, including numerous intrusive procedures, such as having electronic leads taped to and removed from the chest wall. The view through the plastic walls of the incubator is blurred, a cacophony of sounds (e.g., motors, hiss of oxygen) penetrates the infant's closed-in world, and overhead bright lights deny diurnal and nocturnal rhythms.

Without adequate attention to emotional and developmental needs, the premature and sick infant may begin to show signs of great anxiety and tension, including the following:

- Failure to thrive (slow or absent recovery, growth, weight gain)
- Looking away from or to the side of the people who are caring for her or him
- Absent, weak, or infrequent crying (as if to say, "What's the use?")

These are a result of being exposed to life-support measures while being separated from the constant presence of one mothering and comforting person.

Communication patterns. Babies communicate with the world around them in various ways (Cole, no date). Developing skill in reading these cues is essential for the nurse to individualize a plan of care that maximizes the neonate's potential for healing and growth. Most full-term babies thrive on stimulation. However, the compromised neonate may be overwhelmed by too much stimulation. *Cues of a baby who is ready for interaction* include an overall appearance of relaxation. The neonate looks at the caregiver's face and appears to listen.

Cues of a baby who is overstimulated and needs time-out from interaction include color changes (e.g., pale or flushed). The infant may hiccough, gag, or spit up. The breathing pattern changes. Muscle tone changes. Frequent startles and tremors may be seen. The baby uses several methods to cope with overstimulation. Nurses and parents alike benefit from being on the alert for these cues. The coping strategies include ways to decrease the intensity of incoming cues (avoiding eye contact), to take time away from interaction (yawning, becoming drowsy, and sneezing), and to provide self-gratification (thumb sucking). These strategies allow the child to avoid overload and loss of energy, (Cole, no date).

Several methods are available to the nurse to *reduce* the neonate's *incoming stimuli.* Swaddling the infant (when possible), propping the neonate with rolled diapers, covering the crib with a blanket, and organizing care to allow for long stretches of rest in between treatments are a few. Do Not Disturb signs on the crib remind people to give the infant time to rest.

Infant stimulation. The infant's sense of trust develops when she or he learns the feel, sound, and smell of the same mothering person who comforts her or him and who removes uncomfortable stimuli (e.g., hunger, wet or soiled clothing). The infant even learns to anticipate these happenings and soon learns that cries bring this mothering person. These conditions cannot be duplicated in the nursery, but some modifications often can be made in the nursing care plan. In the technologic environment of a premature or sick baby nursery (Fig. 25.22), nursing's focus must be on people, not on equipment. The possibilities are limited only by the parameters of human creativity.

When the baby is ready for stimulation, the nurse has many options. Some suggestions follow:

1. Schedule time from treatments to stroke the infant's skin. The parents may touch the infant through portholes.

2. Insert mobiles and decals that can be changed frequently inside the incubator.

3. Respond to the infant's efforts to cry by reassuring her or him and offering a pacifier while stroking the skin and talking to the infant.

4. When the infant can tolerate being out of the incubator, even for short periods of time, remove, cuddle and rock, and sing to the infant, especially during feedings—even when feeding by gavage or gastrostomy. If possible, take the infant out and hold her or him while helping raise bubbles of air from the stomach. If the mother or father is able to visit frequently, both parent and infant will benefit immeasurably from this activity.

5. If the infant must have feedings by gavage or gastrostomy, offer a pacifier during the feeding process (in the absence of respiratory distress). This will provide sucking satisfaction, and the infant will begin to associate this pleasant, self-gratifying, and self-initiated activity with the comforting feeling of a filling stomach.

6. Talk, sing, and hum to the infant whenever possible. Avoid loud talking and excessive discordant noise. Some nurseries permit the placement of windup musical toys in the incubator or crib.

7. Hold the newborn so that she or he can see your face. Establish eye contact as you talk or sing to the infant.

8. Even if the infant is undergoing phototherapy, there can be some periods when she or he is not under the lamp. Remove the blindfold so that she or he can see your face or the parent's face during periodic, short comforting sessions.

Technologic versus human incubator: "kangaroo method"

Vivian Wahlberg

In Western countries and cultures, preterm infants are usually cared for in a technically advanced environment—an incubator—to conserve warmth and energy for repair, maintenance, and growth. Thus, these infants are separated from their mothers. They are faced with many technologic treatments and procedures, such as gavage feedings and biometric monitoring.

Fig. 25.22
Mother in special care nursery. A, Mother listens intently as physician keeps her informed of her baby's condition and progress. Nurse stands by for support. Note bulb syringe at foot of bed. **B,** Newborn in special care nursery. **C,** Nurse encourages mother to touch her baby. Mother is speaking to child as she prepares to touch. Note Servo-Control panel and biometric monitor. **D,** Note mother's tentative, tender fingertip touch as she begins to explore her baby. Nurse is offering encouragement. Mother is not talking during touching experience. (Courtesy Nanci Newell, Fountain Valley Community Hospital, Fountain Valley, California.)

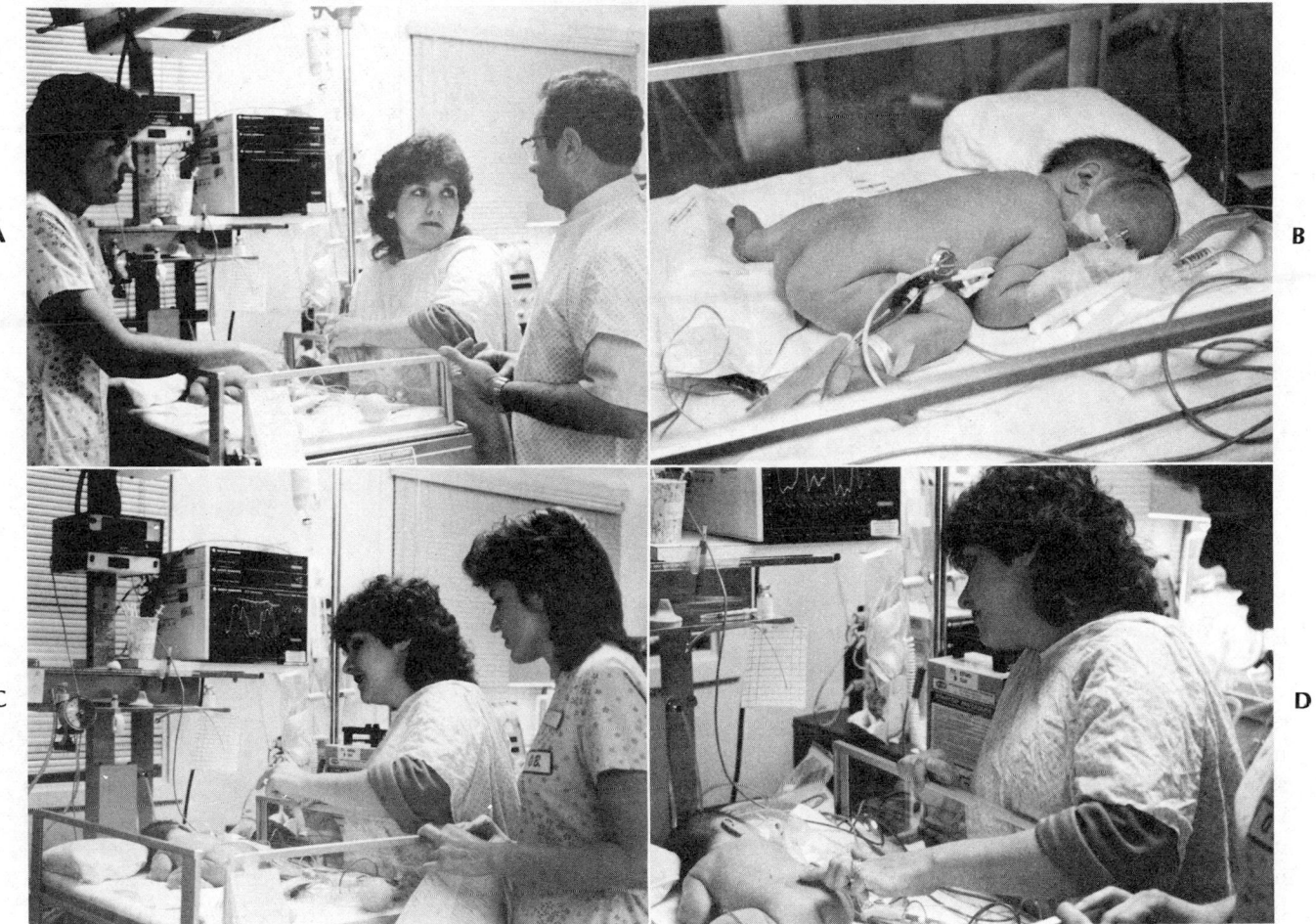

However, in Colombia, South America, it has been possible for recently born healthy preterm infants to be cared for by their mothers. The babies are tucked inside their mother's blouses in a head-up position and are breastfed as soon as their condition is stable (Ress, 1984; Anderson, Marks, and Wahlberg, 1986). Here, in the "human incubator," the infants have all they need in a natural way: skin-to-skin contact, humidity, nourishment, warmth, and love. Because of its marsupial nature, this initial care of the preterm infant by the mother has become known around the world as the "kangaroo method" (Fig. 25.23). It originated in 1979 in Bogota, Colombia. This method is in sharp contrast to the care of preterm infants in North America and Europe.

History of the method. The Instituto Materno Infantil at San Juan de Dios Hospital in Bogota is a large maternity hospital with an average of 12,000 deliveries a year. It serves the low-income population of the city and has a large number of high-risk pregnancies. The

Fig. 25.23
The kangaroo method. **A,** Infant snuggled inside wrap. **B,** Infant inside mother's blouse in skin-to-skin contact. (Bogota, Colombia, S.A.). (Courtesy Vivian Wahlberg, R.N., C.M., Dr. Med. Sc., Karolinska, Stockholm.)

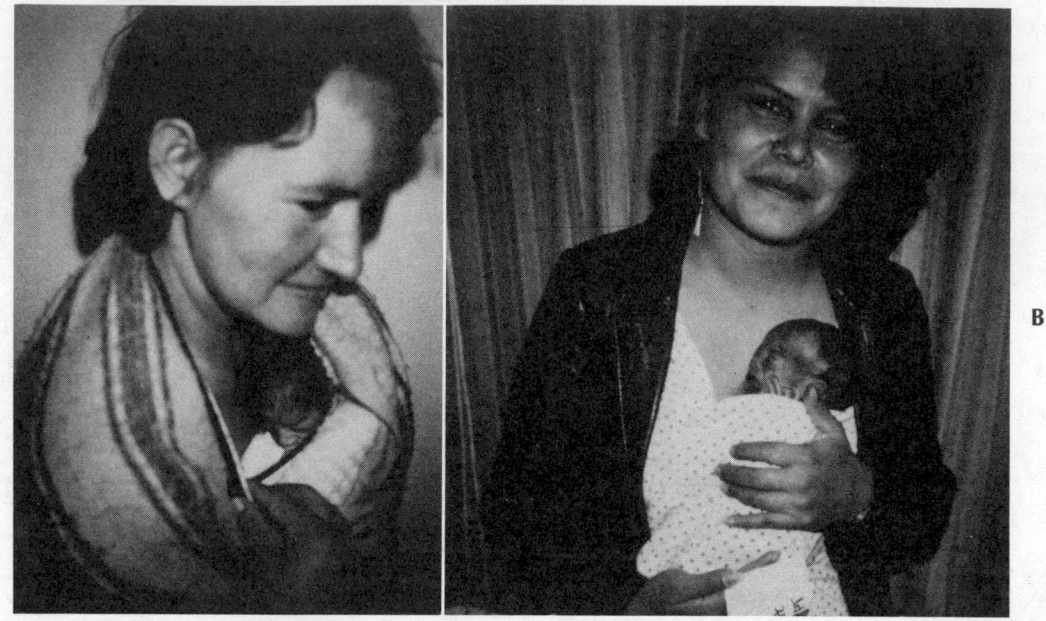

lack of resources motivated Dr. Rey and Dr. Martinez, two pediatricians working at the hospital, to devise the alternative approach.

The Programma Ambulatorio de Prematuros arose out of severe economic restraints and problems with nosocomial and cross-infections but is based on a deep respect for natural processes. Premature infants in satisfactory clinical condition, no matter how small, are not kept in intensive care units. Instead they go directly to their mothers as early as 2 to 3 hours after birth and are mostly discharged within 12 to 24 hours after birth. Mother and infant remain together 24 hours a day.

Mothers are requested to breast feed their infants in self-regulatory fashion. The babies are to feed on demand to satiety. The mothers carry the babies skin-to-skin to maintain their warmth. Reports in 1983 by the founders of the program showed dramatic decreases in mortality, morbidity, and parental abandonment.

The "kangaroo method" (K-method), in a modified form, has now also been introduced in many European neonatal units: Hammersmiths Hospital in London (Whitelow and Sleath, 1985) and Karolinska Hospital in Stockholm. Low-birth-weight (LBW) or preterm infants who are AGA and who no longer require oxygen or intensive care can be nursed by their mothers in the "kangaroo position" with skin-to-skin contact without untoward results.

It has been observed in Columbia, Sweden, and England that the continuity of closeness and mutual stimulation between the mother and preterm infant has reciprocal effects. Mothers reported feelings of emotional harmony and a psychologic sense of oneness with their infants. Because the infant's head is in an upright position, the risk of a "pathologic flat" head (seen in many preterm infants) was not observed. In this upright position the risk of regurgitation and aspiration is minimized.

Summary. The kangaroo method of caring for the compromised newborn promotes early emotional attachment between mother and infant. Normal growth of the cranium is facilitated. Natural methods of meeting the infant's needs replace technologic means. For infants who are in a stable physical condition, the K-method may also shorten the length of care in the incubator and the hospital and thus decrease cost for care. The experience increases the mothers' sense of comfort and confidence in providing care for their premature infants.

Discharge planning. Adequate discharge planning for the high-risk infant and follow-up arrangements should include general pediatric care, visiting nurse service, and parenting classes. This is especially true for young or psychosocially high-risk parents (Merenstein and Gardner, 1985). Referrals to county social service departments should be made for single mothers who are eligible for Aid to Families of Dependent Children and Medicaid. For infants with special problems (spina bifida, cerebral palsy, or Down syndrome), referrals should be made for special programs. These programs provide services for the infants and support groups for parents. Parents whose infants have special medical needs (gavage feedings, tracheostomy or colostomy care, or oxygen) should be evaluated by the medical and nursing personnel. This evaluation will help to determine community resources (equipment, supplies, or emergency care) and to make appropriate referrals. Home nursing care and homemaker services are sometimes covered by medical insurance. Home visits may be necessary to provide actual nursing activities and to relieve parents from the emotional burden inherent in caring for an infant with medical problems. For infants who are developmentally disabled, infant stimulation programs and follow-up programs provided by many hospitals that have NICUs are extremely valuable. Locating babysitters who will care for a child with special problems can be an overwhelming task for parents. Cultivating a resource list for parents and suggesting that parents exchange services with each other can be helpful. Graduate parents and neonatal nurses can provide a useful service to parents in this situation. Lastly, parents should be referred to appropriate funding agencies (Handicapped or Crippled Children's Program, Medicaid, or Social Security Disability) that provide financial assistance.

Postmortem care: stillbirth

Definition of fetal death. According to Civil Code Section 1798.9 (California), fetal death is defined as follows:

1. Fetal death is death before the complete expulsion or extraction from its mother of a product of conception (irrespective of the duration of pregnancy); the death is indicated by the fact that after such separation the fetus does not breathe or show any other evidence of life, such as beating of the heart, pulsation of the umbilical cord, or definite movement of voluntary muscles.

2. Fetal death is required to be registered if the twentieth week of gestation has been reached.

Parents and family. The death of any infant can prove very disturbing to the parents. The concerns expressed include both emotional responses and informational requests. The three questions most often raised by families pertain to feelings of personal guilt, uncertainty about heredity and its possible effect on the infant, and apprehension about the cause of death. These questions can be dealt with reasonably successfully on an informational level in the postmortem counseling session. The emotional problems of loneliness and depression seem less amenable to amelioration by counseling, however.

When an infant has been transferred to an intensive care unit many miles from the home or hospital of delivery, parents can feel isolated and uninformed. Parents who experience the death of an infant who has been transferred derive benefit from a follow-up phone call from the neonatologist.

Care of the child

1. Remove the baby to a work area.
2. Remove all instruments from the baby. Occlude the cord with a tie or plastic clamp.
3. Baptize the baby if so requested by parents or if not explicitly denied by parents.
4. Measure baby.
5. Weigh baby.
6. Identify baby with one baby band. Place other band on mother's wrist.
7. Attach completed stillborn card to baby.
8. Wrap baby in shroud.
9. Pin the second copy of stillborn card to shroud.
10. Take baby and placenta to designated area in the hospital.

Parents may request to see and hold their baby (see Chapter 26). Follow hospital or community protocol for care of the stillborn and for legal requirements for filing certificate of death.

Baptism. The rite of baptism is particularly significant to Roman Catholic, some Episcopalian, and Greek Orthodox religious groups. If death appears inevitable, the clergy should be notified according to the family's wishes. If death is imminent, any adult, preferably of the same faith, may baptize the infant. Water is poured down the head or other skin surface and the following words spoken: "I baptize you, in the name of the Father, of the Son, and of the Holy Spirit." If an abortion or fetal death occurs, the expelled products of conception are baptized. The parents and the priest or minister should be notified of the baptism and a notation made on the record.

Legal requirements for filing certificate of death (California). California requires that each death shall be registered with the local registrar of birth and death registration in the district in which the death was officially pronounced or the body was found, within 5 days after death and before any disposition of the human remains.

The medical and health section data and the time of death shall be completed and attested to by the physician last in attendance, provided such physician is legally authorized to certify and attest to these facts or by the coroner in those cases in which he is required to complete the medical and health section data and certify and attest to these facts.

The medical and health section data and the physician's or coroner's certification shall be completed by the attending physician within 15 hours after the death. It should also be completed by the coroner within 3 days after examination of the body.

Summary

The woman, her family, and the compromised neonate are highly vulnerable. Protection of the neonate by maintenance of a warm environment, adequate oxygen, and safety is an important part of the nurse's care. The neonate's nutrition, fluid, and elimination needs must be monitored and met carefully. The family of the woman experiencing a high-risk pregnancy, labor, and delivery and the sick neonate require skilled nursing care. The manner in which parents are counseled and supported initially and subsequently influences parental adjustment and parent-child interactions. The nurse needs to examine her or his own feelings about high-risk pregnancy, compromised neonates, and neonatal death. Coming to terms with these feelings increases the nurse's ability to assist grieving families and parents. The result can be a rewarding and fulfilling experience for the nurse.

References

Anderson, G.C., Marks, E.A., and Wahlberg, V.: Programma ambulatorio de prematuros, Am. J. Nurs. In press, 1986.

Athey, P.A., and Hadlock, E.P.: Ultrasound in obstetrics and gynecology, ed. 2, St. Louis, 1985, The C.V. Mosby Co.

Cole, J.G.: The competent preemie: a guide for parents, Project WELCOME, Children's Hopsital, Wheelock College, 200 the Riverway, Boston, MA 02215 (no date given).

Danforth, D.N., editor: Obstetrics and gynecology, ed. 4, New York, 1982, Harper & Row, Publishers.

Kaplan, M., and Eidelman, A.T.: Improved prognosis in severely hypothermic newborn infants treated by rapid rewarming, J. Pediatr. 105:468, 1984.

McCallum, W.D.: Ultrasound applications in pregnancy, Midcoastal California Perinatal Outreach Program, Jan. 1984.

Merenstein, G.B., and Gardner, S.L.: Handbook of neonatal intensive care, St. Louis, 1985, The C.V. Mosby Co.

Ress, P.E.: Saving underweight babies in Bogota, Secretariat News 39(13): 7, 1984. (United Nations Headquarters, New York).

Wahlberg, V.: Technologic versus human incubator: "kangaroo method," Personal correspondence and consultation.

Whitelaw, A., and Sleath, K.: Myth of the marsupial mother: home care of very low birth weight babies in Bogota, Colobmia, Lancet 1(8439):1206-1208, 1985.

Bibliography

Aberman, S., and Kirchoff, K.T.: Infant-feeding practices: mothers' decision making, J.O.G.N. N. 14:394, Sept./Oct. 1985.

Barnico, L.M., and Cullinane, M.M.: Maternal phenylketonuria: an unexpected challenge, M.C.N. 10:108, Mar./Apr. 1985.

Bernbaum, J.C., et al. Non-nutritive sucking during gavage feeding enhances growth and maturation in premature infants, Pediatrics 71, 41, 1983.

Blackburn, S., and Lowen, L.: Impact of an infant's premature birth on the grandparents and parents, J.O.G.N. N. 15(2):173, Mar./Apr. 1986.

Bobak, I.M., and Jensen, M.D.: A modular study guide to maternity care, St. Louis, 1983, The C.V. Mosby Co.

Bowen, P.A.: Regional centers. I. A comparison of nursing responsibilities in level II and level III centers, Issues Health Care Women 2(5-6):1, 1980.

Bowen, P.A.: Regional centers. II. The newborn transport system, Issues Health Care Women 2(5-6):5, 1980.

Bowen, P.A.: Regional centers. III. Three regions' educational efforts and infant mortality rates, Issues Health Care Women 2(5-6):19, 1980.

Boynton, B.R., and Boynton, C.A.: Discharge planning for high-risk infants, J. Perinatol. 5:44, Fall 1985.

Bracero, L.A., Schulman, H., and Baxi, L.V.: Fetal heart rate characteristics that provide confidence in the diagnosis of fetal well-being, Clin. Obstet. Gynecol., 19:3, March 1986.

Carey, J., Seamonds, J.A., and Galligan, M.: Infant-death rate: rise linked to health-care cuts, U.S. News & World Report, Feb. 24, 1986, p. 67.

Censullo, M.: Home care of the high-risk newborn, J.O.G.N. N. 15:146, Mar./Apr. 1986.

Chatterjee, M.S.: Paternal age and Down's syndrome, Contemp. OB/Gyn. 21(5):171, 1983.

Consolvo, C.A.: Relieving parental anxiety in the care-by-parent unit. J.O.G.N. Nurs. 15:154, Mar./Apr. 1986.

Douvas, S.G., and others: Intrapartum fetal heart rate monitoring as a predictor of fetal distress and immediate neonatal condition in low-birth-weight (under 1,800 grams) infants, Am. J. Obstet. Gynecol. 148:300, 1984.

EFM today, Contemp. OB/Gyn. 22(4):15, 1983.

Elliot, J.P., and others: Helicopter transportation of patients with obstetric emergencies in an urban area, Am. J. Obstet. Gynecol. 143(2):157, 1982.

Elsea, S.F.: Ethics in maternal-child nursing, M.C.N. 10:303, Sept./Oct. 1985.

Ferrara, A., and Harin, A.: Emergency transfer of the high-risk neonate: a working manual for medical nursing and administrative personnel, St. Louis, 1980, The C.V. Mosby Co.

Fogel, C.I., and Woods, N.F.: Health care of women: a nursing perspective, St. Louis, 1981, The C.V. Mosby Co.

Gaffney, S.E.: Intrauterine fetal surgery: the ramifications for nurses, M.C.N. 10:250, July/Aug. 1985.

Gennaro, S.: Anxiety and problem-solving ability in mothers of premature infants, J.O.G.N. N. 15:160, Mar./Apr. 1986.

Hammer, R.M., and Tufts, M.A.: 11:29, Chorionic villi sampling for detecting fetal disorders, M.C.N. Jan./Feb. 1986.

Harrison, L.L., and Twardosz, S.: Teaching mothers about their preterm infants, J.O.G.N. N. 15:165, Mar./Apr. 1986.

Hattner, J.A.: Personal communicaton regarding nutrition, 1985.

Holtzman, N.A.: Prenatal screening for neural tube defects, Pediatrics 71:658, 1983.

Horwell, D.H., et al.: Assessment of transcervical aspiration technique to chorionic villus biopsy in the first trimester of pregnancy, Br. J. Obstet. Gynaecol. 90:196, 1983.

Jenkins, R.L., and Tock, M.K.: Helping parents bond to their premature infant, M.C.N. 11:32, Jan./Feb. 1986.

Jensen, M.D., and Bobak, I.M.: Maternity and gynecologic care: the nurse and the family, ed. 3, St. Louis, 1985, The C.V. Mosby Co.

Johnson, S.H.: Nursing assessment and strategies for the family at risk: high-risk parenting, ed. 2, Philadelphia, 1986, J.B. Lippincott Co.

Korones, S.B.: High-risk newborn infants: the basis for intensive nursing care, ed. 4, St. Louis, 1986, The C.V. Mosby Co.

Korones, S.B.: Personal correspondence, 1982.

Kremkau, F.W.: How safe is obstetric ultrasound? Contemp. OB/Gyn. 20(6):182, 1982.

Ledger, K.E., and Williams, D.L.: Parents at risk: an instructional program for perinatal assessment and preventive intervention, Victoria, B.C., Canada, 1981, Ministry of Health, Province of British Columbia, and Queen Alexandra Solarium for Crippled Children Society (Queen Alexandra Hospital, 2400 Arbutus Rd., Victoria, B.C., Canada V8N 1V7).

McCluggage, N.A.: Nursing interventions: nipple stimulation contraction stress test, J. Perinatol. 5:56, Summer 1985.

Mina, C.F.: A program for helping grieving parents, MCN 10(2):118, 1985.

NAACOG–OGN Nursing Resource: Maternal neonatal transport, Washington, D.C., 1983, The Association. (The Nurses Association of the American College of Obstetricians and Gynecologists, 600 Maryland Avenue, S.W., Suite 200, Washington, D.C., 20024, 202/638-0026).

Nursing photobook: managing I.V. therapy, Nursing '82 books. Springhouse, Pa., 1982, Intermed Communications, Inc.

Nursing photobook: using monitors, Nursing '81 books, Horsham, Pa., 1981 Intermed Communications, Inc.

Oehler, J.M.: Family-centered neonatal nursing care, Philadelphia, 1981, J.B. Lippincott Co.

Oki, E.: A protocol for the nipple-stimulation CST, Contemp. Obstet. Gynecol. 22(4):157, 1983.

Perez, R.H.: Protocols for perinatal nursing practice, St. Louis, 1981, The C.V. Mosby Co.

Petrie, R.H.: Intrapartum fetal monitoring, Clin. Obstet. Gynecol. 19:1, March 1986.

Platt, L.D., and DeVore, G.R.: Detecting fetal malformations, Contemp. OB/Gyn. 21(1):203, 1983.

Queenan, J.T.: OB ultrasound in the office, Contemp. OB/Gyn. 22:134, 1984. (Technology symposium.)

Queenan, J.T.: Old questions about a new procedure (chorionic villi sampling) (editorial), Contemp. OB/Gyn. 22:3, 1984. (Technology symposium.)

Quimette, J.: Perinatal nursing: care of the high-risk mother and infant, Boston, 1986, Jones and Bartlett Publishers.

Quirk, J.G., and Miller, F.C.: FHR tracing characteristics that jeopardize the diagnosis of fetal well-being, Clin. Obstet. Gynecol. 19:12, March 1986.

Raff, B.S.: Nursing care of high-risk infants and their families: introduction, J.O.G.N. N. 15:141, Mar./Apr. 1986.

Raff, B.S.: The use of homemaker-home health aides' perinatal care of high-risk infants, J.O.G.N. N. 15:142, Mar./Apr. 1986.

Ream, S., and others: Infant nutrition and supplements, J.O.G.N. N. 14:371, Sept./Oct. 1985.

Richardson, B.S.: Fetal activity: measure of well-being, Contemp. Obstet. Gynecol. 22(3):211, 1983.

Sahler, O.J., editor: The child and death, St. Louis, 1978, The C.V. Mosby Co.

Serafini, P., and others: Antepartum fetal heart rate response to sound stimulation: the acoustic stimulation test, Am. J. Obstet. Gynecol. 148:41, 1984.

Simpson, J.L.: Advances in prenatal genetics: past, present, and future, Contemp. OB/Gyn. 21(1):193, 1983.

Styer, G.W., and Freeh, K.: Feeding infants with cleft lip and/or palate, J.O.G.N. Nurs. 10:329, 1981.

Tucker, S.M.: Fetal monitoring and fetal assessment in high-risk pregnancy, St. Louis, 1978, The C.V. Mosby Co.

U.S. National Center for Health Statistics: Vital Statistics of the United States, 1980, Washington, D.C., 1982, U.S. Government Printing Office.

Ward, R.H.: Chorionic villi sampling: its promise and its problems, Contemp. OB/Gyn. 22:31, 1984. (Technology symposium.)

Weil, S.G.: The unspoken needs of families during high risk pregnancies, Am. J. Nurs. 81(11):2047, 1980.

Whaley, L.F., and Wong, D.L.: Nursing care of infants and children, ed. 3, St. Louis, 1987, The C.V. Mosby Co.

Who's afraid of a hundred milliwatts per square centimeter (100 mW/cm²) SPTA? (brochure), Washington, D.C., 1979, American Institute of Ultrasound in Medicine

Loss and Grief

H ow often one hears that the "maternity ward is the happiest place in the whole hospital." This type of comment is most often expressed by those with no experience on a maternity service. However, experienced maternity nurses recognize the need to be prepared to meet the grief and grieving needs of women and their families.

Pregnancy and birth constitute an identity crisis situation in which everything is expected to proceed normally. During this natural transition in the woman's life cycle, she examines and actively relates to her femininity, sexuality, and capacity for motherhood. An unnatural or unexpected interruption in the process poses a potential threat to a woman's self-esteem and femininity. Possible threats to maternal health include abortion (spontaneous, elective, or therapeutic), non-marital pregnancy, premature or postmature delivery, birth trauma, placing the baby for adoption, stillbirth, neonatal death, or the birth of a child with a defect.

The death of a mother during the perinatal period is an unexpected tragedy. Even if the mother had been designated as "high risk," maternal death sends ripples of shock throughout the maternity unit. "Death of the mother completely disrupts the family structure and often leaves the father with the care of a baby at a time when his emotional reserves are lowest" (Johnson, 1986). For the family the sense of loss and grief is enormous.

When expectations of birth and joy are replaced by loss, the nurse's role is critical. The nurse must be able to cope constructively with her or his own response to loss and grief to meet the woman's needs. As in any crisis situation, the nurse's problems may be reactivated by those presented by the woman and her family. The nurse also becomes vulnerable as these internal conflicts emerge while she or he helps with the woman's problems. An understanding of loss and the normal grieving process is fundamental to the implementation of the nursing process.

The Grieving Process

When anticipating a loss or threat of a loss, the person's reactions usually follow a predictable pattern. Effects of maternal analgesia or general anesthesia may affect her grieving process. Phases of mourning have been described by Lindemann (1944) and Kübler-Ross (1969) and may be compared as follows:

Lindemann (Three Phases)	Kübler-Ross (Five Stages)
1. Shock and disbelief	1. Denial and isolation: "No, not me!"
2. Developing awareness and acute mourning	2. Anger: "Why me?"
3. Resolution or acceptance	3. Bargaining: "If I . . ."
	4. Depression and acute grief: "How can I . . ."
	5. Acceptance: "I can, I must."

The phases of mourning according to Lindemann are explained further.

Shock and disbelief. During the period immediately after the loss the person struggles with the reality of the event and may even deny its existence. Mental symptoms may include restlessness, confusion, and apathy. The following somatic manifestations are common: dizziness, lightheadedness or syncope, pallor, perspiration, tachycardia, palpitations, nausea, and other gastrointestinal tract symptoms.

Developing awareness and acute mourning. Reality of the loss begins to penetrate awareness; interest in daily affairs and activity diminishes. Feelings of sadness, self-depreciation, depression, guilt, helplessness, and hopelessness surface. Intense feelings of loneliness or emptiness, a strong urge to cry, and preoccupation with the loss are common. Blame may be internalized or projected onto others. Anger is a common characteristic in this phase. Exhaustion and shortness of breath may occur occasionally.

Resolution or acceptance. Recovering from grief may take a year or longer, although the acute period lasts approximately 6 weeks. With resolution of the mourning process, the person gradually resumes daily activities, reestablishes precrisis relationships in light of the crisis event, forms new relationships, and becomes less preoccupied with the loss.

Pathologic mourning. The critical period for intervention is in the immediate crisis period. The goal of crisis intervention is to assist the woman and her family to begin *now* to mourn appropriately. The following signs *may* signal pathologic mourning:

1. Cheerfulness
2. Avoidance of the topic
3. Marked or persistent hostility toward the staff, her husband, or the maternal or parental family
4. Marked or persistent guilt feelings regarding the event
5. Viewing the sick or premature infant or the infant with a disorder as normal or deceased

The nurse must be aware of possible individual differences and cultural prescriptions for mourning and the expression of grief when assessing the appropriateness of the grief response.

Loss, Grief, and Maternity Nursing

The intent of this chapter is to present the nurse with quick complete reference packets for specific maternity problems; therefore repetition of some content is unavoidable. Each packet can be used to add to the nurse's confidence and ability in initiating pertinent psychosocial care of the family immediately. This is possible without the need to read extensively for general concepts and specific interventions.

Assessment

1. Assess woman's and family's responses to the loss, both verbal and nonverbal.
2. Assess woman's and family's external support system—who they are, their availability, their effect on her and her family (i.e., does she seem comforted by them).
3. Assess woman's and family's desire for spiritual support (e.g., baptism of the conceptus or newborn).
4. In the case of maternal death, assess the spouse in the same manner as in numbers 1 through 3.

Nursing diagnosis

1. Anxiety, or potential loss of self-esteem related to lack of understanding of the grieving process.
2. Coping, ineffective individual (or family), re-

lated to perinatal death of fetus or newborn or mother.
3. Family processes, alterations in, related to loss of a family member or birth of a child with a disorder.
4. Knowledge deficit related to loss and grieving process.
5. Parenting, alterations in, related to loss of a family member, maternal morbidity, or birth of a child with a disorder.
6. Powerlessness related to loss and grief.
7. Sleep pattern disturbance related to grieving process.
8. Spiritual distress related to loss and grieving process.

Planning. During this important step, goals are set in client-centered terms. The goals are prioritized. Nursing actions are selected to meet the goals. The speed and accuracy with which planning is accomplished depends on the nurse's level of competence (see Chapter 2).

Goals

1. The woman retains a positive sense of self-esteem and self-worth as a woman, mother, and sexual being.
2. The woman and family appraise the situation realistically (e.g., ambivalent or negative feelings toward the pregnancy did not cause the loss).
3. The woman and family receive anticipatory guidance regarding components of the grieving process and possible reactions of family and friends.

Implementation. Implementation of nursing actions are individualized. General actions to assist the nurse who is helping families to cope with loss related to childbearing are presented in the tables that follow. The most commonly encountered situations are:

1. Spontaneous abortion
2. Fetal death (before admission to hospital for delivery)
3. Intranatal death (stillbirth) or neonatal death
4. Premature labor
5. Birth of a newborn with a defect or disorder

Maternal death is rarely encountered. Suggestions for nursing actions with her family are discussed in some detail.

Evaluation. Evaluation of the effectiveness of nursing actions is somewhat more difficult when working with loss and grief. The grieving response takes a considerable period of time. The nurse's contact with the family may be limited. The nurse must rely on the knowledge that supportive and understanding care is significant to the family's successful resolution of their loss.

Loss of the Fetus or Newborn

Conditions

Spontaneous abortion and ectopic pregnancy: psychologic aspects. Conception affirms the woman's ability to initiate her biologic role. Any event that interferes with her ability to carry a normal fetus to term causes her to question her biologic intactness. The event may be perceived as an assault to the woman's self-concept and feelings of self worth. She may feel cheated. Many women experience ambivalent feelings toward the idea of pregnancy; many harbor thoughts of self-abortion. Coincident loss of the pregnancy may precipitate a guilt reaction for real or imagined negative thoughts or actions.

For the woman who has a history of difficulty in conceiving and carrying a pregnancy to viability (about 24 weeks), negative feelings about herself as a complete woman may be expected. Nursing care of such a woman and her family should focus on helping them verbalize their feelings openly and honestly. Sympathetic, active listening by the nurse may assist the women in retaining or regaining her self-esteem and feelings of self worth (Table 26.1).

One woman who suffered spontaneous abortion submitted these "thoughts on being a habitual aborter" (Zlomke, 1986):

The term "habitual aborter" is an insidious one, and one which I believe no woman should ever hear. It is a phrase which implies that she could have control over her life if she would only exert herself, as though she were a smoker or a nail biter. The truth is that she has lost all control over her life. With the death of each baby a little more of her future dies until she finally can bear it no longer and gives up. The pain is so great that even after having had a healthy baby since my last miscarriage, I notice that I wrote this whole paragraph in the third person.

Fetal death: psychologic aspects. Fetal movements may cease before the onset of labor, that is, between 20 weeks and term. The mother may deny a lack of fetal activity: "Maybe he's just asleep . . . he's quiet sometimes." She may call the physician for reassurance that everything is all right. Subsequently she may be admitted to the hospital for tests of fetal status. Even in light of evidence from the tests and clinical symptoms, some women cling tenaciously to the hope that the infant will be born alive and well.

Other women acknowledge fetal death by a change in their behavior. One woman arrived on a maternity unit in active labor. A review of her chart showed that she had kept all her clinic appointments until 4 weeks before labor. She stated she was feeling well and described her labor so far. She said nothing as the nurse checked for the fetal heart rate (FHR). When none were heard, the nurse inquired about fetal activity. Quietly and unemotionally, the mother replied, "They stopped a month ago."

Occasionally it is the nurse who responds with denial. The nurse may rationalize the absence of FHR

Table 26.1
Psychosocial Role of Nurse in Care of Parents Experiencing Spontaneous Abortion or Ectopic Pregnancy

Assessment	Plan/Implementation	Rationale

1. Assess woman's behavior:
  a. Euphoric, talkative
  b. Quiet, nonverbal
  c. Denial or acknowledgment
2. Review her obstetric history:
  a. Was there difficulty conceiving?*
  b. Any previous abortions?†
  c. Was anything done to initiate abortion?
3. Assess family's reponse.
	1. Be available and indicate willingness to sit and listen to woman and family.
	2. Encourage and assist verbalization of:
	  a. Feelings of loss, of being cheated
	  b. Woman's fear of not being able to ever carry to term, of having something wrong with her
	  c. Any feelings, actions, or lack of action that woman or family may believe caused this
	  d. Reflections on previous pregnancies, labors, etc.
	3. Act as advocate to physician in regard to woman's questions concerning cause and her biologic functioning capacity.
	4. Make appropriate referrals: family planning, psychiatric social worker, genetic counselor, etc.
		1. Verbal repetition of experience helps one cope with a situation and integrate experience into one's perception of self in nonthreatening manner.
		2. People experiencing loss may need to ask same questions repeatedly from same or other people. Answers may need to be given frequently, with patience and understanding.
		3. People experiencing grief feel alienated from others, lonely, and helpless; they may exhibit anger in presence of or toward accepting, understanding, and caring other, such as nurse.

*For a discussion of the grief response and infertility, see Chapter 7.
†For a discussion of the nurse's response and the woman's response to elective abortion, see Chapter 7.

and funic and uterine souffles as "positional," "too much noise in the room," "defective fetoscope," and the like. The nurse may choose to avoid the woman or to avoid open communication on the subject. The nurse has several therapeutic alternatives available, however (Table 26.2).

Intranatal fetal or newborn death: psychologic aspects. FHR may be lost late in the first stage of labor or during the second stage. The atmosphere in the labor unit becomes tense and subdued. There is a sudden change from joyful anticipation to dread. Silence accompanies the birth. Resuscitative measures are attempted. All persons present focus on the newborn. Shock and disbelief are experienced by parents and staff alike.

The supportive role of the nurse in the care of parents who experience the death of their infant during labor and delivery is presented in Table 26.3.

The nurse. The nurse may undergo a period of self-recrimination relevant to her own behavior surrounding the incident, for example: Could the physician have been called earlier? Were the fetal heart tones really there and was the rate normal when they were last checked? Was it judicious to give that last medication at the time it was given? Were there any clues earlier? Did the nursing care (ability to assess labor and the maternal-fetal condition during labor, ability to resuscitate) cause the fetal or neonatal death? The nurse's self-examination can undermine self-confidence as a nurse. In their search for answers and to vent angry feelings, the mother and family may also probe. The nurse may perceive the questioning as challenges to her capabilities as a nurse. At times like this even the most competent and self-assured nurse may need peer or other support to identify feelings and verbalize them and to regain perspective.

Table 26.2
Psychosocial Role of Nurse in Care of Parents Experiencing Fetal Death

Assessment	Plan/Implementation	Rationale
Prenatal		

1. Detection by gravida
  a. Determine time interval between first suspicion of cessation of fetal movements and calling physician.
  b. Note time when she stopped keeping appointments.
2. Detection by physician
  a. Pattern of increase in fundal height and weight gain not consistent with normal pregnancy.
  b. Tests for fetal status: estriol levels, sonography, amniocentesis, others.
  c. Test for maternal platelet levels.
3. Obstetric history
  a. Previous spontaneous abortion or fetal loss?
  b. Was she in high-risk category?
  c. Did she have any recent experiences with or is she now experiencing loss (other than this fetus)?
	1. Arrange for immediate appointment.
	  a. Call gravida who misses appointments.
	  b. Schedule sufficient time to meet with physician or nurse, if situation is suspicious.
	2. Help woman to express feelings of guilt or self-blame for any perceived acts of commission or omission.
	  a. "Many women are unhappy when they first learn they are pregnant and wish they were not pregnant."
	  b. "Are you thinking you may have done something to cause this?"
	  c. "You are trying to find reasons . . .?"
	3. Help woman to express her feelings about carrying dead baby.
	  a. "It isn't easy to know the baby is dead."
	  b. "Do you wonder if you can stand it until delivery?"
	  c. "Do you wonder if you will be hurt somehow?"
	  d. "Are you wondering how to tell the other children, husband, grandparents, etc.?"
	4. Fill in gaps in information and clarify misconceptions. Help woman formulate questions for physician; help her understand what physician tells her.
	5. Prepare woman and family for procedures, tests for fetal status.
		1. After mothers feel life, or quickening, most mothers begin to relate differently to child. Child is now real; there is, at least in fantasy, promise of child.
		2. Generally, people feel uneasy about death. It is difficult for the woman to realize that she is carrying within her something that is dead.
		3. When medical and nursing staff are able to communicate comfortably and openly about fetal death and woman's possible reactions and feelings, she may be better able to face and cope with situation.
		4. Knowledge about any situation helps dispel fear of unknown, misconceptions, fantasy. Knowledge supports ego strength. Woman needs to know following:
		  a. When to expect labor and delivery. (Will it be induced, when, and how?)
		  b. What to expect of her labor.
		  c. What physiologic effect this may have on her.
		  d. What may have caused fetal death. She has had sole responsibility for care and nurturance of embryo-fetus. She needs to be advised of possible causes well beyond her control.
		  e. How to tell other children at home.
		  f. What reactions she may expect from others and some help with how to handle these.

Continued.

Table 26.2, cont'd
Psychosocial Role of Nurse in Care of Parents Experiencing Fetal Death

Assessment	Plan/Implementation	Rationale

1. Assess maternal emotional response.
  a. Quiet, composed.
  b. Denial: "I just don't believe it"; euphoric, animated.
  c. Overtly upset, crying.
  d. Angry toward staff, others; "Why do I have to feel anything? Give me something now"; "If the doctor had only . . ."; "If I had only . . ."; sad, tearful.
2. Assess woman's external support system.
  a. Presence of relatives.
  b. Behavior of relatives. (Does she seem reassured by their presence and actions?)
  c. Family's interest and ability to stay with her, to provide comfort measures, etc.
3. Assess for desire to have fetus baptized.
	1. Do not do Leopold's maneuvers or listen for FHR. Focus on woman (and family).
	2. Introduce yourself and immediately indicate your awareness of situation.
	  a. "This is a very difficult and sad time for you."
	  b. If possible, keep father close by; he may feel awkward in "Dad's room." "This is hard for you, too. One feels so helpless. Can I help you?"
	3. Respect woman's choice of anesthesia. If she wishes to be awake or if couple wishes father to be present at birth, prepare them for following:
	  a. Silence and tension at delivery.
	  b. Sight of still, pale, or reddish infant; infant's peeling skin, and markedly molded head.
	4. If mother, spouse, or relatives wish to see or hold infant:
	  a. Prepare family for sight of infant and tell them you will stay with them as long as they desire.
	  b. Prepare infant: bathe and wrap.
	  c. Provide private space; physician, member of clergy, nurse, or other may stay close by for support.
	  d. Give permission to cry by your actions, by giving tissues, by saying, "It's worth crying over."
	5. Be cognizant of own nonverbal messages.
	6. Arrange for baptism and record event in progress notes.
		1. Focus remains on the woman and family.
		2. Open communication and being available physically and psychologically helps in following ways:
		  a. It fosters open communication between mother and significant others and between mother and staff. Energy does not have to be diverted to keeping up a front.
		  b. It gives permission to grieve, validates appropriateness of grieving here and now in a manner acceptable to them, and gives permission to speak of death.
		3. General anesthesia may keep experience unreal, dreamlike, thereby complicating efficient grieving.
		4. Seeing and holding infant is useful in following ways:
		  a. It validates reality of event.
		  b. It allows identification of infant and eliminates fantasy of what woman or couple thought infant looked like (fantasy is frequently more horrifying than reality).
		  c. It permits grieving process to begin. Even if event was anticipated, reality reactivates entire grief process. Usually takes less time when death has been diagnosed before beginning of labor.

The nurse may be unaware of personal struggles with reactions to grief. The nurse may resort to reassuring and comforting the grieving individual or individuals in a manner that does not foster a healthy grieving response. Some commonly heard *responses* given by physicians, nurses, and well-meaning friends should be avoided:

- "There was a reason why God wanted this baby. Have faith."
- "It's God's will. We have to have faith that it was for the best."
- "It's probably better this way. This often happens when the baby has something wrong with it."
- "You are so young. There's time for more."
- "Be thankful you have those other lovely children at home. They'll be a solace and comfort to you."

This baby is important *now*. The mother needs to talk about *this* baby. She does not want or need to focus on her other children or any suggestions for substitutes for her loss.

The parents. Certain behaviors give the message that to face grief is "bad" for a person and to avoid facing it is better for all concerned. An example might be avoiding talking about the infant, quelling tears, and forbidding the mother to see and hold the infant.

Somehow it is thought that to avoid an issue is the healthiest and easiest way. It does prevent "scenes." Out of sight is out of mind. But out of sight is not out of the mother's mind. The mother has felt life. She has developed a relationship with the infant through shared internal physical sensation and fantasy. If the child lives for a few hours or days after birth, the

Table 26.3
Psychosocial Role of Nurse in Care of Parents Whose Baby Dies During the Intrapartum Period

Assessment	Plan/Implementation	Rationale
1. Assess mother's response: Does she show appropriate signs and symptoms of grieving process? (Her cultural background and past experiences with grief and the grieving process influence how she progresses through the grieving process.) a. Shock, disbelief, and anger. b. Developing awareness. c. Occasionally mother must withdraw for a short while as if to take experience a small piece at a time. Signs that she is withdrawing are closing her eyes, drawing curtains around her bed (or shutting door), changing subject. 2. Assess mother's support system: husband, family, friends, culture, or religion. 3. Note mother's age—adolescent's needs are different from those of middle-aged woman. 4. Are there definite cultural (or religious) influences that help mother define death and direct her grieving process? 5. If possible, assess the older child's (children's) reactions. Assess the parent's reactions as they face the need to tell the older child or children, other family members, and friends. 6. If older child is an adolescent, assess family's knowledge of adolescent's needs regarding developing sexuality and sexual awareness.	1. Provide physical care and meet dependency needs in thoughtful and unhurried manner. 2. Make infant as attractive as possible, for example, clean her or him up, wrap her or him in pretty blanket. Allow time for the mother or couple to caress their dead infant if they choose to do so. Stay with mother or couple during this time. 3. Arrange time for mother to talk over labor and delivery, to accomplish the following: a. Validate and assimilate experience. b. Work through shock and disbelief. c. Clarify events. d. Ease her need to search for reasons. 4. Assist woman (couple) to identify and verbalize feelings: a. "You must feel like you were cheated." b. "Somehow it just doesn't seem fair." c. "You seem so angry." d. "One feels so helpless, so powerless, in this type of situation." e. "There are times when your feelings may seem strange to you." 5. Do *not* minimize event with comments such as "You are still young" or "You'll have others." 6. Let mother (couple) share her (their) feelings without giving scientific reasons, referring to logic, and so on. 7. Encourage mother (couple) to verbalize concerns perhaps to role-play different approaches regarding ways to inform siblings, other family members, friends. 8. Encourage family to discuss event openly with adolescent.	1. Mother's postdelivery physical needs must be met. a. To revitalize after pregnancy and labor. b. To release energy for emotional work. 2. In her search for causes, mother reviews and rehashes events leading up to stillbirth. a. It is normal to look for answers. Nurses should not feel they must have all answers at their fingertips. b. Focusing in on an event to exclusion of all other activities of daily living and interaction with other family members is normal now. c. It is normal to feel confused, indecisive, and a sense of unreality. Some grieving persons fearfully confide, "I think I must be going crazy." 3. Adolescent needs: a. Reassurance of her femininity. Adolescent who is unwed may have become pregnant to prove to herself her femininity and reproductive capacity. b. Reassurance that her conversations with nurse are confidential. c. "Safe" authority to whom to vent angry feelings. Bravado, defensiveness, and withdrawal may be signs of immaturity and struggles with autonomy, or she may use these behaviors to cover feelings that the stillbirth occurred as punishment for out-of-wedlock pregnancy. d. Support and empathy. Self-esteem and a sense of worth can be generated by including woman in planning for her care after discharge, providing information regarding her body after delivery, referring her to teenage rap sessions at family planning and adolescent clinics or other groups in area. 4. Needs of older woman: a. Support and empathy. If this is the first child, the woman's responses may be compounded by several factors. Among these factors may be feelings about having waited too long to get pregnant and concerns about diminishing time available for "trying again." b. Reassurance of her femininity. Woman may interpret the event as a sign that her youth is slipping away.

mother's relationship with the child has progressed even further. Even after delivery the hormones that sustain an attachment between mother and child are still present. The physical signs and discomforts that occur during the normal postpartum period also exist. At home are the baby clothes and furniture, family, and friends, awaiting the hoped-for new arrival. Resolution of grief is important *now* and can be a healthy growth-inducing process.

Mothers and families look to the hospital staff to meet their needs. Having had an unfortunate maternity experience, these mothers may suffer a severe blow to their sense of worth associated with the ability to give life. Their role concept, self-esteem, and femininity may be diminished. Nursing interventions that assist the grieving family in coping with this ego-threatening experience may foster a healthy mourning process and can be incorporated easily within the busiest nursing assignment (Table 26.3).

Death is often equated with powerlessness, an end, and failure. However, the nurse need not be professionally and personally helpless. Preventive mental health measures are well within the scope of the nurse. Some therapeutic nursing interventions are as follows:

1. Parents need an objective listener, one who is genuinely interested and willing to face true feelings and will not try to "talk them out of it." The nurse acts as a role model for open communication in facing grief and for feeling safe and comfortable in dealing with an unpleasant situation.

2. Parents need to feel that those around them know that it is natural for them to feel sad, weepy, and easily distracted.

3. Nurses should convey to parents that grieving takes time and that they may never really "get over it," although the pain does ease with time; good memories then tend to persist.

4. Nurses should be prepared for the anger and self-blame parents may feel and assist the parents to identify these feelings: "You may be wondering if you did or did not do something to cause this." Parents may not be able to work through their anger before discharge; some parents return or write many months later to apologize for their behavior and to thank those who were able to see beyond their anger and help them with their needs.

5. Coping with grief and recovering from childbirth exact a heavy toll on the mother's resources. Although the grieving process often makes sleep difficult and appetite nonexistent, adequate rest and diet must be assured to replenish the mother's vitality. Thoughtful nursing actions (e.g., back rubs, just sitting quietly with her) can meet very real, critical needs. Sleeping pills may delay the grieving process.

6. The nurse should prepare the parents for returning home, for example, what to expect of themselves emotionally and physically and what they can expect from the older children. Siblings may feel that the parent or parents lied to them about the coming of a new baby. The older child may feel that it is his or her fault that the baby died because he or she may not have wanted a new sibling now, or wanted a boy but got a girl, so that the girl then died. Older siblings may act out their feelings in other ways.

Physical symptoms that parents may experience include sleep problems with fatigue, anorexia, muscle aches and "knots," gastrointestinal symptoms, and palpitations.

Psychologic or emotional symptoms that parents may experience include an inability to concentrate for long on any one activity (i.e., their minds may wander or they may feel everything is whirling around in their heads) and pressure in the head. People frequently express the fear of "going crazy" when they experience reactions that they do not expect or understand. The mother may hold her abdomen and state she feels "empty" and that her arms "ache to hold a baby." Parents may fear being alone, wish to go away somewhere, or become overconcerned about or disinterested in their other children. Irritability with or disinterest in the other children may compound guilt feelings.

Birth of a Compromised Newborn

Conditions

Premature labor and delivery: psychologic aspects. Prematurity puts the infant and the family at risk (see Chapters 29 and 31).

Psychosocial role of nurse in care of parents after birth of child with disorder. The birth of a child with an obvious defect is a shattering experience for parents and a disturbing experience for those who attended the birth. Parents feel devastated and inadequate; anticipated joy ends in despair and confusion. A flurry of activity often follows such a birth. The child may then be examined by specialists, often at a facility far from the mother's hospital. Physicians and others (e.g., clergy) may talk with the parents. The natural order of postdelivery psychologic tasks is disrupted, and the new parents are in crisis. The nurse is in a unique and critical position. Of all the members of the health team, the nurse alone can be available 24 hours a day. A nurse can help plan for discharge and postdischarge care. Although clinical intervention will vary with each situation, in every case the nurse must establish herself or himself as a caring, knowledgeable, resourceful person.

Whether the child is premature, ill, or has a defect, the parental responses and needs are similar in many respects. In general, the couple's needs can be summarized to include (1) mourning the loss of the fantasized perfect baby, (2) immediate diagnosis and management of the newborn, (3) clinical evaluation and diagnosis of the causes of the infant's disorder, (4) when appropriate, preparation and planning for the continued care of the affected newborn, (5) redefinition of the parental role in their social network (i.e., reentrance into their society), and (6) family planning and genetic counseling. Nursing management is planned to help parents meet these needs.

Mourning loss of perfect child. Grieving is the first difficult task of the new parents of a child with a malformation or disorder. Psychologic shock, frequently coupled with the necessity of physical separation from the infant, makes this period trying. The parents are vulnerable. Resolution of grief for the lost, assumed-perfect child precedes the development of acceptance or attachment to the real imperfect child or any decisions regarding her or his placement. The period of acute grief is usually about 6 weeks; however, in the continued presence of a child with a defect, grief may become chronic and persist for a lifetime.

The parents are profoundly affected by the manner and attitudes of those around them, especially the medical and nursing personnel. Parents are sensitive to and respond quickly to nonverbal cues from others that may connote nonacceptance, revulsion, or blame. Voice inflections, facial expressions, or the posture of the nurse who witnesses parental grief reactions or views the infant is quickly noted and internalized. Nurses also are representatives of society and may reflect society's reactions to them as parents of a child who is less than perfect.

Early parent-child relationship. Interaction between parent and child in the immediate postdelivery period is important in the development of potential maternal feelings. If a parent does not have the opportunity to see, hold, and fondle the child early and often after birth, parental feelings and the development of parenting skills are adversely affected. The very small premature infant, the sick infant, or a child with a serious congenital disorder may have to be taken to another institution immediately after birth. This event can cause the mother to feel psychologically estranged from her infant.

Continuing parent-child relationship. The skilled medical and nursing care required by the infant in this period, which the parents cannot provide, may be overwhelming. In fact, they may focus on the gadgetry—the machines, tubes, and bottles—associated with the infant's care rather than on the infant.

Parents need to "keep in touch" with the infant somehow. This may be accomplished by viewing the infant frequently and at close range and hearing frequent progress reports and answers to their questions. At other times, parents may be permitted to touch, fondle, and stroke the infant when it is still not practical to involve them in actual feeding and bathing. During these initial contacts, and until parents gain self-confidence, the nurse should remain nearby, offering support as needed.

If the infant's hospitalization is prolonged, the nursing staff should keep the parents informed of the infant's progress. This can be accomplished with telephone calls and notes "from the baby."

The parents and nurse may feel frustrated, uncomfortable, and even helpless when faced with the birth of a child with a defect. However, the parents and nurse can grow from a mutually shared experience. Touching and sharing another's experience of loss can be threatening but also rewarding.

Families' grief reactions. Grandparents may take this opportunity to blame the other parent's family, with remarks such as, "We've never had this happen in *our* family before—ever." Other comments that are frequently heard include, "The women in *our* family have never had problems having babies" and "I told him [her] that nothing good would come of this marriage [relationship]."

Comments such as these from members of the parents' families may mask hidden feelings. Such feelings might include inadequacy about themselves, a deep concern for the young mother or couple, feelings of helplessness in the situation, concern by the grandparents that there may be no grandchild and therefore no "immortality" for them. Many other emotional reactions are possible.

The nurse must avoid the pitfall of taking sides. The nurse provides patience, tact, and warm sympathy. This is coupled with efforts to help family members identify and explore feelings, clarify misconceptions, and provide simple, cogent explanations that may contribute to the comfort, strength, and unity of the entire family.

Immediate diagnosis and management of child. Diagnosing the disorder and initiating appropriate therapy is the physician's responsibility; however, the nurse must be conversant with diagnostic techniques and rationale for therapy to reinforce and clarify the physician's explanations. If possible, the nurse should sit in with the parents and physician during their sessions to know what is being said. Open lines of communication between physician and nurse, always essential, are vital now. One nursing function is to assist parents to identify and verbalize their questions as well as their misgivings and fears. The nurse must deal with those questions and concerns within her realm of expertise and channel others to appropriate health care team members.

The history taking and diagnostic procedures necessary to uncover the etiology are exacting. One is asked to look for disorders in ancestors, to explore prenatal acts of omission and commission (e.g., nutrition, drugs), and to seek out other environmental factors.

Parents may express feelings of shame and embarrassment lest they be carrying a "bad" gene or be responsible for exposure to a devastating environmental agent. Others are anxious to fix the blame somewhere. Many women remember transient (or persistent) negative feelings about the pregnancy or baby and interpret these feelings as punishment for their real or imagined transgressions.

The nurse's role must be supportive. This includes preparing parents for what to expect and allowing for anticipatory worry, listening actively, and assisting with the formulation of questions and the ventilation of feelings.

Long-term management of child. Long-term management of a child with a disorder necessitates multidisciplinary planning and cooperation. A coordinated program of continual guidance and counseling of the parents is essential. The emotional, physical, and financial status of the parents, available community resources, and the child's condition must be evaluated.

The nurse's role varies with the situation: Is the defect obvious? Is it curable? Is it treatable? How do parents perceive the disorder? Skillfully executed, the nurse's supportive function aids parents in decision making and in self-acceptance regarding their decisions (e.g., surgical procedures, institutionalization).

If the child requires medications, diet, or physical manipulation, the nurse should assist in teaching how, when, and why. Parents will benefit from supervised practice before discharge and frequent positive reinforcement of their ability to perform necessary tasks.

Community resources should be tapped to assist with the financial burden, equipment, drugs, and psychologic support (see Appendix C). For example, in the San Francisco Bay area, there is a group of parents of children with cleft lip and palate who meet to share feelings, problems, techniques, and new developments. A social worker may have the prime responsibility in this area of management, but the nurse should be cognizant of resources also. Visiting nurse associations may be involved in the follow-up care in the home.

Continued guidance and counseling are essential in helping the family and its members to live in harmony with each other, increasing their comfort and strengthening their unity. The child with a defect needs love, affection, and social and physical stimulation as much as or more than any other child. At the same time, the child's special needs and reactions must be considered. Other family members also need love, a sense of fulfillment, and recognition as worthwhile persons. Meeting all these needs requires much energy from each family member. The nurse can help family members understand the special dynamics of their situation and cope with the inevitable tensions and resentments that arise.

Redefinition of parental role and social network. A society expects adults to produce healthy children to perpetuate that society. A social stigma is attached to bearing a defective child, a reality with which the parents must learn to cope.

After parents grieve and come to terms with their failure to produce a healthy offspring, they still face several hurdles. One is to make a decision regarding the disposition of the child—institution or home. If the child comes home, they must learn to meet her or his special needs and introduce the child to society.

Another hurdle is facing others—the other children, family, friends, and strangers. Even during the hospital stay, parents experience society's adverse reaction. Subtle or blatant expressions of social isolation are evident. The cards, flowers, and other gifts of congratulation are sparse. Frequently the cheery forms of congratulations come only from those unaware of the "situation." Telephone conversations are guarded. Even medical personnel, unhappily, may shun these parents. Families may be insinuating blame on each other. At home, callers do not ask to see the baby. If they do, verbal response may be stilted, although nonverbal response is poignant.

The entire health team and community resources such as clergy must accept the task of helping parents reenter the outside world. Several of the techniques already discussed are helpful, but others also may prove helpful.

One simple technique is **role playing.** The anticipated meetings with the other children, family, and friends are acted out. Another approach is to discuss how parents will handle the curiosity of friends, acquaintances, and strangers. These techniques help in several ways. First, by anticipating the words and reactions of others, they verbalize their own. Second, the practice augments their store of coping strategies. Both techniques may uncover feelings that can be dealt with here and now, although resolution of these feelings may not come until much later. Each encounter may serve to strengthen coping mechanisms and bring the resolution of feelings a step closer.

Response of family members to birth of high-risk infant

Siblings' reactions. As discussed earlier, preparation of parents of a high-risk infant begins long before the infant is discharged from the hospital. Preparation of the older children also needs to be undertaken before the infant's coming home. The very young child can easily "forget" the existence of a brother or sister in the hospital. If possible, visits to see the new baby should be encouraged. For the older child the idea of an imperfect baby can be clarified by seeing him and having a chance to discuss fears and misconceptions. One 8-year-old boy was given the job of "explaining" all about his premature sister to the visiting grandparents. He discussed the care of the baby and use of supportive equipment surprisingly well.

If, however, the infant dies, the older children will be affected as well as the parents. A small child who cannot understand verbal explanations needs demonstrations of love and affection to provide reassurance and security. He may be unable to express frightening thoughts that he is experiencing. Occasionally the small child may resort to misbehavior to draw attention or may cling excessively to his parents.

Older children may need verbal explanations as well as assistance in voicing feelings and thoughts. Discussion about the fetal or newborn death as well as death in general should be an open subject in the family. The cause of the death should be openly presented so that the child may cope with any existing feelings of guilt.

Avoid references such as, "The baby went away (or to sleep)" or "God took him." These euphemisms are usually meant to help the child, but more often they can be threatening. Regardless of the way parents handle the reaction to the death, some children may manifest their inner disturbance in nightmares, bed-wetting, school problems, or other ways.

Grandparents' responses. Grandparents are also touched by the birth of an infant at risk. Grandparents can be very supportive to the young family. For some, there is a natural response to protect their offspring. Producing a child who is less than perfect seems to lower the grandparents' own self-esteem. They may resort to blaming the young parents or their child's spouse for acts of omission or commission in precipitating the problem. A nursing care plan is incomplete without an assessment and plan for action regarding grandparental responses.

Loss of the Mother

Maternal death: psychologic aspects. Childbirth is viewed as a normal physiologic event. The survivors may respond in a wide variety of ways. The newborn infant may be targeted as the cause of the mother's death. Family members who feel that the newborn is somehow responsible may find it difficult to develop a positive, caring relationship with the child. The loss leaves the father emotionally drained at this time when the newborn and older children need him most. In the back of his mind, he may experience guilt for his role in family planning. He may wonder how the family can manage financially whether or not the wife had contributed to the family income.

Families have a need to know why the event occurred. Consent for autopsy is usually given. The physician may gain more information with which to discuss the maternal death with the family.

Older children and grandparents feel the loss intensely as well. The older child is discussed later in this chapter. Parents, including grandparents, expect that their children will survive them in the "natural order" of things. The death of their daughter is a break in the continuity. Furthermore the maternal grandparents may be faced with the possibility that the husband will remarry and thus create a distance between them and their grandchild. Working with the family who suffers this type of loss is very challenging but also potentially very rewarding (Table 26.4).

Children under 5 years of age. There is a special necessity for preventive work with children under 5 when a parent dies. Children under 5 form the most vulnerable age group (Sahler, 1978). Such children depend solely on parental support for their ego development and mastery of the instinctual drives. Their reality testing is limited. They are easily overwhelmed with anxiety. Their capacity to verbalize affects is not fully developed. They need adult help in identifying feelings. Symptoms of anxiety and inner stress are prone to take the form of physical activity, e.g., regression behaviors, over or under activity, or psychosomatic symptoms.

The time to offer counseling is at the time when a death occurs, before conflicts and anxieties have resulted in behavior difficulties or symptom formation. Important areas involve helping the bereaved around burial services. This includes clarifying with the parent the importance of discussing the nature of the illness so that the child can achieve his own differentiation and supporting the bereaved in their grief so that they in turn can allow the expression of grief in their children (Sahler, 1978).

Children of any age. Denial is the prominent defense mechanism used intermittently by children of all ages. Denial is used even though intellectually death is comprehended. The pain of coming to grips with the loss extends over a long period of time. For varying

Table 26.4
Psychosocial Role of Nurse in Care of Family After Maternal Death

Assessment	Plan/Implementation	Rationale

1. Assess husband's and family's emotional response:
  a. Quiet, composed.
  b. Denial: "I just don't believe it"; euphoric, animated.
  c. Overtly upset, crying.
  d. Angry toward staff, others; "If only the doctor had . . ."; "If I had only . . ."; sad, tearful.
  e. Responses toward newborn and older children
2. Assess external support system.
  a. Presence of relatives.
  b. Behavior of relatives. Do husband and children seem reassured by their presence and actions?
  c. Family's interest and ability to stay with husband or siblings.
  d. Ask if they wish to contact clergy or members of their church.
3. Young children (under 5 years):
  a. Concept of death
  b. Behavioral responses
4. Children of any age:
  a. Use of denial
  b. Concept of death
5. Adolescent:
  a. Level of maturity
  b. Prominant developmental tasks: Identity, including sexual identity; moving toward independence.
  c. Assess for suicidal ideation.
	1. Be available and indicate willingness to sit and listen.
	2. Encourage and assist verbalization of:
	  a. Feelings of loss, of being cheated.
	  b. Any feelings, actions, or lack of action that family may believe caused this.
	3. Act as advocate of family with physician regarding questions concerning cause.
	4. Fill in gaps in information and clarify misconceptions. Help family formulate questions for physician; help them understand what physician tells them.
	5. Alert family to characteristics of grieving process:
	  a. Personal responses.
	  b. Variations in responses to be expected at different developmental levels.
	  c. Duration for child versus adult.
	6. Assist family with concerns such as, "Are you wondering how to tell the other children, the grandparents, etc.?"
	7. Make appropriate referrals: Home health care, child care, psychiatric social worker, homemaker service.
		1. Verbal repetition of experience helps one cope with a situation and integrate experience into one's perception of self in nonthreatening manner.
		2. People experiencing loss may need to ask same questions repeatedly from same or other people. Answers may need to be given frequently, with patience and understanding.
		3. People experiencing grief may feel alienated from others, lonely, and helpless; they may exhibit anger in presence or toward accepting, understanding, and caring other, such as nurse.
		4. Response to loss and grief is influenced by a number of factors, some of which are:
		  a. Age, developmental level of survivor.
		  b. Events leading up to her death.
		  c. Circumstances related to social aspects of this pregnancy.
		5. When medical and nursing staff are able to communicate comfortably and openly about death and grief reactions and feelings, the family may be better able to face and cope with situation. Knowledge about any situation helps dispel fear of unknown, misconceptions, fantasy. Knowledge supports ego strength.
		Open communication and being available physically and psychologically helps in following ways:
		  a. It fosters open communicaton between husband and significant others and between family and staff. Energy does not have to be diverted to keeping up a front.
		  b. It gives permission to grieve, validates appropriateness of grieving here and now in a manner acceptable to them, and gives permission to speak of death.

lengths of time there is hope and expectation that the loved one will return.

Adolescent reactions. Because of greater ego maturity the normal adolescent is better able to cope with the finality of death. The predominant task of adolescence is to move toward independence, to free oneself from close dependence on parents. Adolescents need repeated attempts to break away, to try various activities outside the family. Although critical of and hostile to parents at times, adolescents have an option to re-

turn and be cared for. When one parent is no longer available to meet this need for comfort and care, the struggle toward independence may be disrupted. Guilt is common. The child wonders if the parent might have lived if they had done something different (e.g., been nicer, not rebelled so much).

The relationship between the adolescent and the surviving parent needs consideraton. The living parent may be preoccupied with his own grief. Thus the adolescent is doubly deprived. Attempts to console the father may be met with anger and irritation. The adolescent may turn away with a sense of being a failure. The potential for suicide often arises in the adolescent group. Many develop a renewed interest in immortality. Deutsch (1967) has made the point that as the adolescent struggles with intense anxieties, he or she is confronted with one of life's sharpest paradoxes—namely, that on the threshold of a new life, he or she feels the threat of death.

Adolescents are struggling with their sexual identity as well. The death of their mother during childbirth can have a negative effect on both the female and male adolescent. Open communication is essential in helping the adolescent identify these feelings and differentiate herself or himself from the deceased (Sahler, 1978).

Adults often mourn at a faster pace than children. When the two generations are out of phase in their grieving, a sensitive nurse is aware that children may be confused, especially if the father remarries. The nurse can play a supportive role by alerting the family to expect this reaction. The adolescent needs much emotional support and opportunities to verbalize her or his concerns so that misconceptions about death can be clarified.

Summary

Stuart and Sundeen (1983) summarize the nurse's role in loss and grief as follows. Although death is the most certain aspect of life, fear of it is universal. Because of this and because of their proximity to the situation of dying, death is a necessary concern for nurses. Attitudes toward death are culturally learned. Personal reactions have their basis in the psychologic maturity and personality characteristics of the individual. The individual's own values, beliefs and experiences influence the cognitive aspects of dying.

The nurse needs to have a cognitive grasp of the developmental aspects of the concept of death, the stages and processes associated with grief, and resources available to the individual and family. It is important to assess one's own viewpoints and attitudes toward death, since these often transfer over into the caregiving situation.

Understanding of the dying process is closely linked to the level of maturity and cognitive abilities of the child and adults involved. Assisting children and adults to learn to express their fears about death can help diminish some of the emotional strain of grief work. Adaptation to changes within the existing family structure and interactions are invariably necessary. Change is difficult. The family may require support from com-

munity resources. The death of a newborn or the mother is a shattering experience.

Nurses are expected to provide physical care, comfort, understanding, and emotional support to the individual and family. However, nurses must recognize that there are limitations and immense emotional strains that pervade the caregiving situation. Nurses caring for the bereaved need a professional support system of their own.

References

Deutsch, H.: Selected problems of adolescence, Monogr. Ser. Psychoanal. Study Child No. 3, 1967, International University Press.

Johnson, S.H.: Nursing assessment and strategies for the family at risk: high-risk parenting, ed. 2, Philadelphia, 1986, J.B. Lippincott Co.

Kübler-Ross, E.: On death and dying, New York, 1969, Macmillan Publishing Co.

Lindemann, E.: Symptomatology and management of acute grief, Am. J. Psychol. **101**:141, 1944.

Sahler, O.J., editor: The child and death, St. Louis, 1978, The C.V. Mosby Co.

Stuart, G.W., and Sundeen, S.J.: Principles and practice of psychiatric nursing, ed. 2, St. Louis, 1983, The C.V. Mosby Co.

Zlomke, E.: Personal correspondence, Spring, 1986.

Bibliography

Backer, B., and others: Death and dying: individuals and institutions, New York, 1982, Wiley Medical Publication.

Barnes, J.: Reactions to the death of a mother, Psychoanal. Study Child. 19:334, 1964

Beckey, R.D., and others: Development of a perinatal grief checklist, J.O.G.N. N. 14:194, May/June, 1985.

Bethea, S.W.: Primary nursing in the infant special care unit, J.O.G.N. Nurs. 13:202, May/June 1985.

Blackburn, S., and Lowen, L.: Impact of an infant's premature birth on the grandparents and parents, J.O.G.N. N. 15:173, Mar./Apr. 1986.

Carr, D., and Knupp, S.F.: Grief and perinatal loss: a community hospital approach to support, J.O.G.N. N. 15:173, Mar./Apr. 1986

Cefalo, R.C.: Managing missed abortion and antepartum fetal death, Contemp. OB/Gyn. 22(3):17, 1983.

Consolvo, C.A.: Relieving parental anxiety in the care-by-parent unit, J.O.G.N. N. 15:154, Mar./Apr. 1986.

Cordell, A., and Apolito, R.: Family support in infant death, J.O.G.N. Nurs. 10(4):281, 1981.

Drane, J.F.: The defective child: ethical guidelines for painful dilemmas, J.O.G.N. Nurs. 13(1):42, 1984.

Eager, M., and Exoo, R.: Parents visiting parents for unequaled support, J. Matern. Child. Nurs. 5:35, 1980.

Ehrenkranz, R.A.: Neonatal death: caring for parents, Contemp. OB/Gyn. 22(3):24, 1983.

Elsea, S.F.: Ethics in maternal-child nursing, M.C.N. 10:303, Sept./Oct. 1985.

Estok, P., and Lehman, A.: Perinatal death: grief support for families, Birth 10(1):17, 1983.

Field, T., and Goldson, E.: Pacifying effects of nonnutritive sucking on term and preterm neonates during heelstick procedures, Pediatrics 74:1012, 1984.

Field, T., and others: Nonnutritive sucking during tube feedings: effects on preterm neonates in an intensive care unit, Pediatrics 70:381, 1982.

Furlong, R.M., and Hobbins, J.C.: Grief in the perinatal period, Obstet. Gynecol. 61:497, 1983.

Furman, E.: A child's parent dies; studies in childhood bereavement, New Haven, 1974, Yale University Press.

Hawkins-Walsh, E.: Diminishing anxiety in parents of sick newborns, Am. J. Matern. Child Nurs. 5:20, 1980.

Helping patients and doctors cope with perinatal death (symposium), Contemp. OB/Gyn. 20(2):98, 1981.

Jensen, M.D., and Bobak, I.M.: Maternity and gynecologic care: the nurse and the family, ed. 3., St. Louis, 1985, The C.V. Mosby Co.

Kaplan, D.M., and Mason, E.A.: Maternal reactions to premature birth viewed as an acute emotional disorder, Am. J. Orthopsychiatry 30:118, July 1960.

Klaus, M.H., and Fanaroff, A.A.: Care of the high-risk neonate, ed. 2, Philadelphia, 1979, W.B. Saunders Co.

Laufer, M.: Object loss and mourning during adolescence, Psychoanal. Study Child. 21:269, 1966.

Ledger, K.E., and Williams, D.L.: Parents at risk: an instructional program for perinatal assessment and preventive intervention, Funded by Ministry of Health, Province of British Columbia and Queen Alexandra Solarium for Crippled Children Society, Canada. (Queen Alexandra Hospital, 2040 Arbutus Road, Victoria, B.C., Canada, V8N 1V7).

Luske, M.P.: The effect of group counseling on the frequency of grief reported by infertile couples, J.O.G.N. N. 14:67s. Nov./Dec. 1985.

Marino, B.L.: When nurses compete with parents, J.A.C.C.H. 8:94-98, 1980.

Merenstein, G.B. and Gardner, S.L.: Handbook of neonatal intensive care, St. Louis, 1986, The C.V. Mosby Co.

Mina, C.F.: A program for helping grieving parents, F.M.C.N. 10:118, Mar./Apr. 1985.

Quimette, J.: Perinatal nursing: care of the high-risk mother and infant, Boston, 1986, Jones and Bartlett Publishers.

Raff, B.S. Nursing care of high-risk infants and their families: introduction, J.O.G.N. N. 15:141, Mar./Apr. 1986.

Raff, B.S.: The use of homemaker-home health aides' perinatal care of high-risk infants, J.O.G.N. N. 15:142, Mar./Apr. 1986.

Rothenberg, L.S.: Down's syndrome babies: decisions not to feed and the letter from Washington, J. Calif. Perinatal Assoc. 2(1):73, 1982.

Schwab, F., and others: Sibling visiting in a neonatal intensive care unit, Pediatrics 71:835, 1983.

Stewart, D.: Spiritual care of the neonate, Periscope (published by the California Perinatal Association), pp. 1-2, June 1980.

Veach, S.A.: Down's syndrome: helping the parents of a special infant, Nurs. '83, 13(9):42, 1983.

Wessel, M.: Death of an adult—and its impact upon the child, Clin. Pediatr. 2:28, 1973.

Wessel, M.: The adolescent and death of a parent. In Gallagher, R., Heald, F., and Garrelagher, D., editors: Medical care of the adolescent, New York, 1976, Appleton-Century-Crofts.

Whaley, L.F.: Genetic counseling in maternity nursing. In Mcnall, L.K., and Galeener, J.T., editors: Current practice in obstetric and gynecologic nursing, vol. I, St. Louis, 1976, The C.V. Mosby Co.

Whaley, L.F., and Wong, D.L.: Nursing care of infants and children, ed. 3, St. Louis, 1987, The C.V. Mosby Co.

Whitaker, C.M.: Death before birth, Am. J. Nurs. 86:156, Feb. 1986.

Hypertensive States in Pregnancy, Infection, and Hemorrhage

Adequate care of the high-risk client requires the united efforts of all members of the health care team and close collaboration with other medical personnel. This chapter reviews major maternal conditions that predispose or commit the client to an abnormal response to pregnancy. The three major maternal conditions are hypertensive states, infection, and hemorrhage.

Hypertensive States in Pregnancy

Hypertension usually of vasospastic origin may complicate pregnancy. Hypertension may first appear during a well-established pregnancy (pregnancy-induced hypertension), or it may predate the pregnancy and be a manifestation of cardiovascular or renal disease. Both mother and infant are adversely affected by maternal hypertension. Pregnancy-induced hypertension is recognized as the leading cause of maternal mortality. The joint efforts of physicians and nurses can do much to prevent and treat the condition and thereby promote satisfactory outcomes for mother and baby.

PREGNANCY-INDUCED HYPERTENSION (PIH)

The syndrome pregnancy-induced hypertension (PIH) is characterized by **hypertension** and **proteinuria** often accompanied by **edema.** It develops only during pregnancy or in the early puerperium. The syndrome usually appears between the twentieth and twenty-fourth weeks of gestation and disappears after the tenth postpartum day.

Definitions
Gestational hypertension. Gestational hypertension during pregnancy is defined as an elevation of systolic

and diastolic pressure equal to or exceeding 140/90 mm Hg. An alternative definition that is more sensitive to individual variations is a rise in systolic pressure of 30 mm Hg or a rise in diastolic pressure of 15 mm Hg above the woman's baseline values. The latter definition is useful because blood pressure varies with age, race, physiologic state, dietary habits, and heredity.

The blood pressure elevation must be present on two occasions 6 hours apart. Techniques of measurement must be standardized, for instance, always taken with the woman sitting *or* supine *or* in a lateral position. The technique used must be noted in the client's record to provide data to guide interpretation of previous, present, and future readings.

Gestational proteinuria. Gestational proteinuria is the occurrence of proteinuria during pregnancy or in the early puerperium. The protein must be in amounts greater than 300 mg/L (+ 1) in a 24-hour specimen or greater than 1 g/L (+ 2) in a random daytime urine collection on two or more occasions at least 6 hours apart (Table 27.1). The urine must be a midstream clean-catch or catheter-derived specimen.

Gestational edema. Gestational edema is a generalized accumulation of interstitial fluid (face, hands, abdomen, sacrum, tibia, ankles) after 12 hours of bed

Table 27.1
Protein Readings

Code	Milligrams per Deciliter
0	
Trace	
+ 1	30 mg/dl (equivalent to 300 mg/L)
+ 2	100 mg/dl
+ 3	300 mg/dl
+ 4	Over 1000 mg (1 g)/dl

Fig. 27.1
Assessment of pitting edema: **A,** +1; **B,** +2; **C,** +3; **D,** +4.

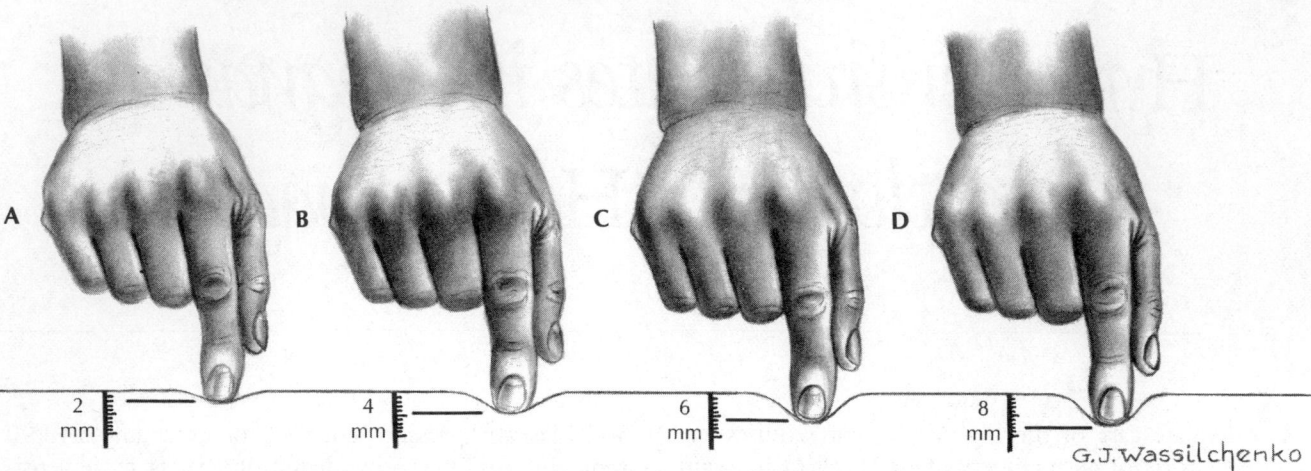

rest or a *weight gain* of more than 2 kg (4 to 4½ lb) per week. The presence of edema is less significant than the rapidity of weight gain.

Edema may be described as dependent, pitting, or nonpitting (Kozier and Erb, 1983).

Dependent edema (edema of the lowest or most dependent parts of the body, where hydrostatic pressure is greatest). If a person is ambulatory, this edema may first be evident in the feet and ankles. If the person is confined to bed, the edema is more likely to occur in the sacral region.

Pitting edema (edema that leaves a small depression or pit after finger pressure is applied to the swollen area). The pit is caused by movement of fluid to adjacent tissue, away from the point of pressure. Within 10 to 30 seconds the pit normally disappears. Pitting may be slight (+1) as in Fig. 27.1, *A*, or increase up to +4 as in Fig. 27.1, *D*.

Nonpitting edema. In nonpitting edema the fluid in edematous tissues cannot be moved to adjacent spaces by finger pressure. Nonpitting edema is not a sign of extracellular fluid excess but often accompanies infections and traumas that cause fluid to collect and coagulate in tissue spaces. The coagulation prevents displacement of fluid to other areas by pressure.

Although the amount of edema is difficult to quantitate, the following method may be used to record relative degrees of edema formation:

+1 Minimum edema of the pedal and pretibial areas
+2 Marked edema of the lower extremities
+3 Edema of the face and hands, lower abdominal walls, and sacrum
+4 Anasarca (generalized massive edema) with ascites

Preeclampsia. Preeclampsia is another term for the syndrome of hypertension with proteinuria or edema or both during pregnancy or within 48 hours of delivery. It is now thought that preeclampsia is a progressive process. Preeclampsia may be divided into mild or severe degrees for treatment purposes. Mild preeclampsia may be treated at home; severe preeclampsia needs to be treated in the hospital with modern technology.

Eclampsia. Eclampsia includes the symptoms of severe preeclampsia and one or more of the following: (1) tonic and clonic **convulsions or coma,** with the coma possibly following an unobserved seizure related to other seizure disorders, or (2) **hypertensive crisis or shock.**

The sensory symptomatology of preeclampsia-eclampsia (headache, epigastric pain, blurring of vision, lowered affect) may be caused by generalized edema of the brain. It may also be a result of ischemia of the brain following vasoconstriction.

Classification. Pregnancy-induced hypertension is classified as follows (Pritchard and others, 1985):
1. Hypertension alone.
2. Preeclampsia with proteinuria or generalized edema. It may be *mild* or *severe.*
3. Eclampsia with proteinuria, generalized edema, and convulsions. "Eclampsia" is derived from the Greek word meaning "shining forth," used to describe convulsions.

Incidence. About 5% of pregnant women in North America experience PIH, and approximately 5% of these develop eclampsia.

The following conditions are associated with PIH:

1. Primigravidity. Approximately 65% of cases of PIH occur with first pregnancies, especially if the primigravida is under 17 or over 35 years of age.
2. Multiple pregnancies. The incidence of PIH increases progressively with the number of fetuses (twins, triplets).
3. Vascular disease. PIH is most common in women with essential hypertension, hypertensive renal diseases, or diabetes mellitus.
4. Hydatidiform mole (molar pregnancy). This condition predisposes to development of PIH. *The disease often becomes manifest before week 20 of pregnancy.*
5. Dietary deficiencies, severe malnutrition. Protein deficiencies and probably a deficiency in water-soluble vitamins may be associated with increased incidence of PIH.
6. Familial tendency. The family history may reveal relatives who had the disease.

Theories of cause of pregnancy-induced hypertension. Pregnancy-induced hypertension is defined in empirical clinical terms because its cause and pathogenesis are still unknown. It has always been a subject of much speculation and has been called "the disease of theories." No known theory as yet accounts for all symptoms. Evidently PIH is somehow related to the physiologic changes of pregnancy because it disappears after the termination of pregnancy. Therefore, the gravid uterus, placenta, or fetus could be the central factor in the condition. Pritchard and associates (1985), note that

Any satisfactory theory must take into account that pregnancy-induced or aggravated hypertension is very much more likely to develop in the woman who (1) is exposed to chorionic villi for the first time, (2) is exposed to superabundance of chorionic villi, as with twins or hydatidiform mole, (3) has preexisting vascular disease, or (4) is genetically predisposed to the development of hypertension during pregnancy. While chorionic villi are essential, they need not support a fetus nor need they be located within the uterus. The possibility that immunologic as well as endocrine and genetic mechanisms are involved in the genesis of PIH is intriguing.

Pathologic findings. General arteriolar spasm is characteristic of PIH. Whether this is a primary or secondary reaction is uncertain, however. In any event the arterial system becomes hyper-responsive to vasopressor drugs such as vasopressin and angiotensin II. The general arteriolar spasm and the consequent increased peripheral resistance results in hypertension. **Every organ in the body is affected** (Pritchard and others, 1985). The characteristic symptoms of PIH occur as a result of changes in the functioning of body organs. Table 27.2 presents a description of organ changes and the symptomatology present.

Table 27.2

Responses of Body Systems to PIH and the Resulting Symptomatology

System	Symptomatology
Cardiovascular system	
Cardiac output does not decrease with arteriolar constriction and increased peripheral resistance.	Blood pressure rises
Blood volume expansion is extravascular not intravascular. As a result of decreased celloid osmotic pressure (see renal system) fluid leaves the intravascular space and accumulates in interstitial tissues.	Hematocrit rises (hemoconcentration)
	Generalized edema
	Sudden weight gain (>2 lb[1 kg]/week or >6 lb[2.5 kg]/ month
Coagulation (intravascular) is a sequelae to PIH.	Platelets decrease
Renal system	
Renal perfusion and glomerular filtration rate (GFR) decreases.	Levels of creatinine and urea increase
	Oliguria (<100 ml/ 4 hours)
Degenerative changes in renal glomeruli occur. Protein is lost in urine. Colloid oncotic pressure decreases.	Proteinuria increases
	Generalized edema occurs, including periorbital, finger, sacral.
	Sudden weight gain (as above)
Central nervous system	
Lesions and edema occur.	Headaches
	Convulsions
	Hyperreflexia
	LOC changes
Hepatic system	
Hepatic cellular lesions occur with edema, hemorrhage rarely occurs; there is a stretching of the hepatic capsule.	Epigastric or right upper quadrant pain
	Nausea and vomiting
Visual system	
Ischemia and edema occur. Retinal detachment can occur.	Blurring, double vision
	Blindness
Respiratory system	
Edema occurs.	Presence of rales
Placenta	
Placental perfusion is reduced.	Fetal growth is retarded (SGA)
	Fetal stress, late decelerations in FHR.

Effects on the mother. Pregnancy-induced hypertension is one of the three *major* causes of maternal morbidity and mortality. About 8% of women with eclampsia die of the disease or its complications. The most common causes of death are intracranial hemorrhage and congestive heart failure. Placental abruption with or without hypofibrinogenemia or disseminated intravascular coagulation (DIC) may occur. In addition, a woman who sustains eclamptic convulsions may bite her tongue or lips. Ribs or vertebrae may be fractured while the woman flails about during a convulsion. Retinal detachments may ensue.

With good therapy most women improve significantly in 24 to 48 hours. Rapid improvement follows early termination of pregnancy.

Effects on the fetus and newborn. Perinatal *morbidity* is high, because most women with pregnancy-induced hypertension deliver before the thirty-seventh week of gestation. The fetal outcome of maternal hypertension is questionable because of placental insufficiency. Generally the fetus is small for gestational age. However, these infants generally do better than other preterm infants of the same weight and gestational age born of nonhypertensive mothers. This is probably because of intrauterine stress that increases the rapidity of fetal lung maturation.

The perinatal *mortality* is at least 20% with eclampsia in many parts of North America. This is mainly because of the effects of hypoxia, prematurity, or acidosis during maternal convulsions. A single, maternal convulsion increases the prospect of perinatal death at least fivefold.

Course of the disease. The disease can occur without warning or with the gradual development of symptoms. The caretaker needs to be alert to the signs

Fig. 27.2
Funduscopic examination is performed daily to detect arteriospasm, edema, hemorrhages, arteriovenous nicking, and exudates.

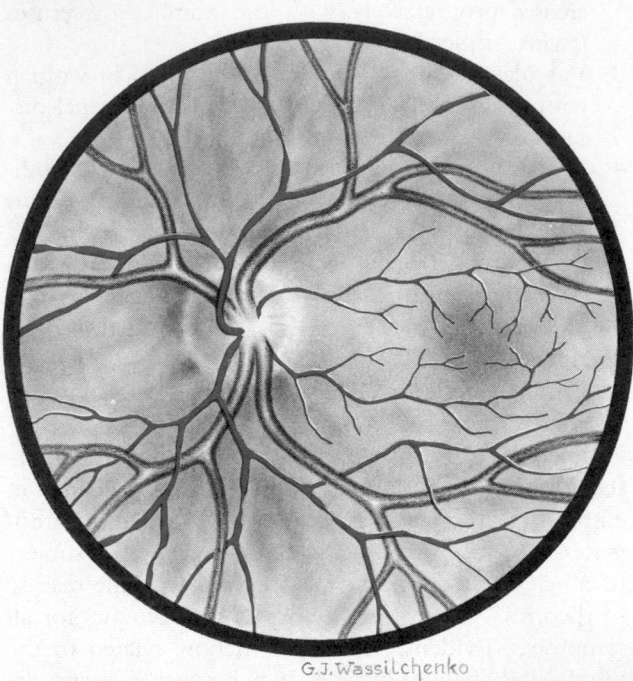

G.J.Wassilchenko

and symptoms of PIH (Table 27.2 and box below) so that prompt remedial therapy can be instituted. Differentiation of mild and severe preeclampsia is presented in Table 27.3.

Management of PIH. The management of the woman with PIH requires the coordinated efforts of medical and nursing personnel. The first requisite of a successful health service is to make contact with childbearing families. Pregnant women who do not receive regular prenatal care and consequent monitoring of their unborn child's condition are particulary vulnerable to the complications of PIH.

Goals. The overall goals for care during the maternity cycle are as follows:

1. Provision of early adequate prenatal care, including adequate nutrition, specific to the needs of each women to protect against PIH.
2. Prompt intensive therapy for preeclampsia to drastically reduce the incidence of eclampsia and the severity of its complications.
3. Prompt initiation of corrective therapy for eclamptic convulsions to reduce maternal and perinatal morbidity and mortality.

Home management. The most effective therapy for PIH is preventing progression of the condition. Man-

Symptomatology of Pregnancy-Induced Hypertension (To Be Reported Immediately)

1. A rapid rise in blood pressure
2. A rapid gain in weight
3. Generalized edema
4. A quantitative increase in proteinuria
5. Epigastric gain
6. Marked hyperreflexia and especially, transient or sustained ankle clonus
7. Severe headache
8. Visual disturbances
9. Oliguria, with urinary output of less than 100 ml in 4 hours
10. Drowsiness, listlessness (dulled sensorium)
11. Nausea and vomiting

Table 27.3
Differentiation of Mild and Severe Preeclampsia

	Mild Preeclampsia	Severe Preeclampsia
Maternal effects		
Blood pressure	Rise in systolic blood pressure of 30 mm Hg or more. A rise in diastolic blood pressure of 15 mm Hg or more or a reading of 140/90 mm Hg 6 hours apart.	Rise to 160/110 mm Hg or more on two separate occasions 6 hours apart with pregnant woman on bed rest.
Weight gain	Weight gain of more than 1.4 kg (3 lb)/month during the second trimester, more than 0.5 kg (1 lb)/week during the third trimester, or a sudden weight gain of 2 kg (4-4½ lb)/week at any time.	Same.
Proteinura Qualitative dipstick Quantative 24-hour analysis	Proteinuria of 300 mg/L in a 24-hour specimen or greater than 1 g/L in a random daytime specimen on two or more occasions 6 hours apart as protein loss is variable. With dipstick varies from 1+ to 2+.	Proteinuria of 5-10 g/L in 24 hours or 3+ to 4+ protein on dipstick.
Edema	Dependent edema, some puffiness of eyes, face, fingers; pulmonary rales absent.	Generalized edema, noticeable puffiness of eyes, face, fingers. Pulmonary edema → rales.
Reflexes	Hyperreflexia 3+. No clonus.	Hyperreflexia 3+ or 4+. Clonus.
Oliguria	Output matches intake.	Oliguria: less than 100 ml/4 h output.
Headache	Transient.	Severe.
Visual problems	Absent.	Blurred, photophobia, blind spots on funduscopy. Retinal arterial spasm (Fig. 27.2).
Irritability	Transient.	Severe.
Fetal effects		
Placental perfusion	Reduced.	Total growth retardation. FHR: late decelerations.
Premature placental aging	Not apparent.	At birth placenta appears smaller than normal for the duration of the pregnancy. Premature aging is apparent with numerous areas of broken syncytia. Ischemic necrosis (white infarcts) are numerous, and intervellous fibrin deposition (red infarcts) may be recorded.

agement at home can be satisfactory if the preeclampsia is mild and fetal growth retardation is not a problem. Home therapy includes twice-weekly medical and nursing assessment, encouraging the client to participate in the care, dietary modifications, and bed rest. Application of the nursing process to at-home care of a woman with mild preeclampsia is presented on pp. 782-784. This care is given in addition to the general care needed in pregnancy (Chapter 11).

Hospital management. If the woman's condition becomes increasingly severe, hospitalization is recommended. Following are criteria for hospitalization:

1. Hypertension of 150/100 mm Hg or more or proteinuria of 5 g/24 h or more *or* 3+ to 4+ protein on dipstick.
2. Lesser degrees of hypertension but with any of the following:
   a. Proteinuria of 1+ or more
   b. Increasing edema

   c. Oliguria or anuria
   d. Persistent or severe headache
   e. Blurred vision
   f. Nausea and vomiting
   g. Epigastric pain

The medical therapy includes the following (Pritchard, 1985):

1. An appropriate history and general physical examination followed by daily assessment for the development of such signs and symptoms as headache, visual disturbances, epigastric pain, and rapid weight gain
2. Weight measured on admittance and every 2 days thereafter
3. Urine screened for protein on admittance and subsequently at least every 2 days
4. Blood pressure readings with an appropriate-size cuff every 4 hours (except between midnight and morning, unless the midnight pressure has risen)

Application of the Nursing Process

HOME MANAGEMENT OF MILD PREECLAMPSIA

Renee, age 34, is pregnant for the third time. Both Renee and her husband, Bruce, are pleased about the pregnancy. The doctor has diagnosed twins. The course of Renee's pregnancy has been uneventful until the thirty-third week. At her regular checkup her physical assessment revealed the following:

BP: 140/90
Edema: Dependent edema and puffiness of eyes and fingers
Urinalysis: Protein + 2

Her physician recommended the following regimen:

1. Bed rest at home
2. Weighing herself daily
3. Diet of 70-80 g of protein, up to 6 g sodium chloride
4. Return visits Fridays and Tuesdays

The nurse's interview revealed the following:

1. There were two preschoolers at home, ages 2 and 4.
2. Bruce's mother would be willing to help.
3. Renee knew little of what PIH meant to her and her baby's health.
4. She thought bed rest meant lying down a few times a day when the children were asleep.
5. She felt that the family's diet was adequate. She did not know food equivalents for 70-80 g of protein *or* 3 g NaCl.

The nurse developed the following plan for nursing care:

FUNCTIONAL HEALTH PATTERN: ASSESSMENT	NURSING DIAGNOSIS	RATIONALE: PLAN/ IMPLEMENTATION	EVALUATION
HEALTH PERCEPTION– HEALTH MANAGEMENT ■ BP 140/90 ■ Edema generalized; eyes puffy, fingers swollen ■ Proteinuria +2	Potential maternal and fetal compromise* related to edema, proteinuria, hypertension	*To monitor severity of maternal response to PIH,* assess at least twice a week to note any change in the following: ■ Vital signs and BP ■ Extent of edema ■ Weight gain 1 kg (2 lb)/week ■ Amount of protein in the urine ■ CNS symptomatology ■ Hepatic symptoms ■ Urinary output *To monitor severity of fetal responses to PIH:* ■ Assess FHR biweekly ■ Instruct mother to assess fetal activity daily ■ Plan for NST and ultrasonography *To prepare for further complications:* ■ Have family plan for early delivery and possible hospital confinement for management of care.	Symptoms of complications subside and remain within normal ranges. Fetal health remains satisfactory as measured by FHR and activity. Family is able to review plans for emergencies with the nurse.

*Diagnosis not included by NANDA, 1986.

Application of the Nursing Process—cont'd

FUNCTIONAL HEALTH PATTERN: ASSESSMENT	NURSING DIAGNOSIS	RATIONALE: PLAN/ IMPLEMENTATION	EVALUATION
COGNITIVE-PERCEPTUAL Mother has little understanding of complications of PIH	Knowledge deficit related to the following:	*To increase Renee's understanding of PIH and encourage her and her family's participation in the care:*	
	■ PIH and its effects on mother and baby	■ Ensure that the woman and other family members are able to recognize danger symptoms that require prompt reporting (Box, p. 780)	■ The woman can describe the signs and symptoms requiring immediate care and how to report them. Family reports any symptomatology immediately if it occurs.
	■ How to obtain assistance	■ Instruct Renee how to obtain treatment and advice.	■ Family places emergency phone numbers near telephone.
	■ How to assess blood pressure	■ Instruct her how to assess blood pressure if the equipment is available (Rayburn and others, 1984)	■ Woman and family demonstrate competency in assessing BP.
	■ How to assess for edema	■ Instruct her to keep a daily record of her weight (expect a 2 kg [4 to 4½ lb] loss in 3 days as a result of diuresis) • Instruct her how to assess intake and output • Instruct her how to assess for presence of edema	■ Woman and family maintain accurate record of weight.
COGNITIVE-PERCEPTUAL Mother does not understand diet as prescribed	Knowledge deficit related to diet required in PIH ■ Protein intake	*To maintain an adequate protein intake:* ■ Instruct woman as to dietary food groups that are equivalent to 70 to 80 g of protein (Chapter 12) ■ Provide rationale for diet: • Helps to reduce edema and BP • Helps baby grow	Woman complies with diet. Dietary history demonstrates knowledge.
	■ Sodium intake	*To maintain adequate but not excessive sodium intake:* • Instruct woman as to amounts of salt to use in preparing or serving foods • Advise her to refrain from salty foods, e.g., potato chips	As above.

Continued.

FUNCTIONAL HEALTH PATTERN: ASSESSMENT	NURSING DIAGNOSIS	RATIONALE: PLAN/ IMPLEMENTATION	EVALUATION
	■ Roughage and fluids	■ Advise about including ample roughage and fluids; restricted exercise (bed rest) can compound problems with constipation	Constipation does not occur.
COGNITIVE-PERCEPTUAL Mother does not understand what is meant by bed rest and the significance of bed rest to her care	Knowledge deficit related to the meaning of bed rest and its significance to her and her infant's condition	*To maintain adequate rest:* ■ Instruct the woman and her family on what is meant by bed rest— she is to spend most of the day in bed, preferably lying on her left side (p. 375 and Fig. 15.14) (she may be up for meals and to use the bathroom). She should not go up and down stairs. Outings are restricted to visits to the physician's office.	The woman complies with the regimen for rest and exercise.
ACTIVITY-EXERCISE Mother states she has young children at home, feels she will be up and down with them	Activity intolerance related to minimizing effects of PIH Diversional activity deficit related to activity restriction Impaired home maintenance management related to activity restriction	*To maintain adequate rest and activity:* ■ Include the family in the plan of care, as the regimen can be boring and stressful. Care of children and the house must be undertaken by another family member ■ Discuss need to plan diversion for both mother and younger children in the family ■ Instruct her in breathing and leg exercises	The woman is able to maintain a positive outlook about herself and her baby.
COPING–STRESS TOLERANCE Mother wonders how she will manage; thinks husband's mother would come to help out	Ineffective individual and family coping related to mother's restricted activity and concern over a complicated pregnancy	*To reduce tension:* ■ Encourage family to use network support; for instance, family and relatives can help by assuming the children's care for part of each day and arranging for outdoor activity during this period ■ Encourage open discussion of problems ■ Help family seek solutions to problems, e.g., community agency support for homemakers	Woman and family accept woman's temporary disability.

5. Measurements of plasma creatinine
6. Measurements of hematocrit, platelets, and serum SGOT
7. Frequent evaluation of fetal size by the same experienced examiner and by serial sonography if remote from term

The therapy and subsequent treatment are then evaluated. Improvement is evidenced by:

1. Diuresis in 24 to 48 hours
2. Decrease in blood pressure
3. Weight loss of more than 2 kg

If improvement occurs therapy is continued until labor begins spontaneously. If the fetal age is greater than 38 weeks with a lecithin/sphingomyelin (L/S) ratio of 2:1 and other indications of fetal maturity, labor may be induced (Chapters 25 and 29). If improvement does not occur or the fetus shows signs of stress, the care for severe preeclampsia/eclampsia is initiated.

Severe preeclampsia/eclampsia. Severe preeclampsia represents an obstetric emergency. Immediate and continuous care by the obstetric team is mandatory to prevent maternal and fetal morbidity or mortality.

Goals. The goals of therapy are as follows:

1. Prevention of convulsions (eclampsia)
2. Survival of mother with minimum morbidity (e.g., stroke)
3. Birth of an infant as mature as possible without significant postdelivery complications
4. Therapy that benefits mother and fetus and minimizes danger to each.

Medical management. Medical management will include directives relative to the following, in addition to those necessary for normal labor and delivery:

- Absolute bed rest
- Electronic monitoring of mother and fetus
- Convulsion precautions
- Precipitate delivery precautions
- Elective delivery preparations: induction, cesarean delivery (Chapter 29)
- Medications (see Table 27.4)
- Evaluation according to hospital and physician protocol for the following:
  BP
  Weight
  Edema
  Urine screened for protein
  Symptoms (Table 27.2)
  Reflexes
  Funduscopic examination (Fig. 27.2)
  Measurement of plasma, creatinine, hematocrit, platelets, and SGOT

Nursing care. The development of severe preeclampsia causes anxiety in the woman and her family; there is a threat to the well-being of the mother and her unborn child, and the family's expectations about pregnancy and delivery must be altered. Such disruption in a family constitutes a crisis. The physical nature of the crisis requires the beneficial use of modern technology. The woman and her family's perception of the disease process, the reasons for it and the care received will affect their compliance with and participation in therapy. The family will need to use coping mechanisms and support systems to help them through the experience. A plan of care for the woman suffering from severe PIH is presented on p. 789. The care is superimposed on the nursing care all women need during labor and delivery.

Convulsion control. One of the important goals of care for the woman with severe PIH is preventing or controlling convulsions. Emergency equipment and drugs are kept in the room. These include a plastic airway or tongue depressor bite-stick, a padded tongue blade, oxygen and suction equipment, and an ophthalmoscope. Medications include magnesium sulfate, calcium gluconate, cardiac stimulants, and hypertensive controls such as hydralazine and 50% glucose (p. 792). An emergency delivery pack is also kept in the room. The nurse maintains a matter-of-fact and calm attitude and approach and briefly explains the rationale of

Drugs and Equipment for Preventive Treatment of Convulsions of Eclampsia

Drugs

Magnesium sulfate: 2 ampules, 10 ml/ampule (5 g 50%); 500 mg (4 mEq)/ml
Sodium bicarbonate: 50 ml (7.5%) (44.6 mEq)
Hydralazine: 5 ampules, 20 mg/ampule
Heparin sodium: 10 ml, 5000 USP units/ml
Diazepam: 2 ml, 5 mg/ml
Chlordiazepoxide: 5 ml, 20 mg/ml
Epinephrine: 2:1000, 1 mg/ml
Atropisol, 1% (mydriatic)
Atropine sulfate: 0.4 mg/0.5 ml
Sterile water ampules
Sterile normal saline ampules
Calcium gluconate: 10%, 1 g/10 ml; 97 mg (4.8 mEq)/10 ml Ca ++
Phenytoin: 2 ml, 50 mg/ml
Propranolol: tablets 40 mg
Intravenous barbiturates

Supplies

Emergency delivery pack
Ophthalmoscope
Reflex hammer
Fetal monitor
Padded tongue blade
Plastic airway
Oxygen and suction
Tourniquets
Syringes: 2, 10, and 50 ml
Cutdown tray

Table 27.4
Pharmacologic Control of Hypertension and Its Sequelae in Pregnancy and Labor

Medication	Target Tissue	Effects of Medication		Nursing Actions
		Maternal	Fetal/Neonatal	
Anticonvulsants				
Magnesium sulfate IV or IM Dosage: Pritchard (1980)—first dose: 4 g 20% IV at 1g/min and 10 g 50% IM, subsequently: 5 g 50% IM q4 h; Zuspan (1966)—first dose: 6 g 20% IV, subsequently: 10-24 g/L of 5% D/W at 1 g/h (or see p. 792)	Myoneural junction: decreases acetylcholine, thereby depressing neuromuscular transmission Thyroid: decreases parathormone secretion, resulting in increased urinary excretion of calcium Placental perfusion dynamics not altered	Minimum hypotensive effect Minimum if any direct effect on CNS because of blood-brain barrier to magnesium Hypocalcemia CAUTION: Do not give excessive dosages that tend to decrease urinary output to depress deep tendon reflexes (DTRs) DANGER: Muscular paralysis (cardiopulmonary) **Antidotes: calcium gluconate,** neostigmine, pentylenetetrazol (Metrazo)	Mild depression in small number (6%) Neonatal hypermagnesemia easily treated: calcium; exchange transfusion with citrated blood	Notify perinatal staff Decrease CNS irritability Arrange environment to promote rest Provide continuous nursing care Encourage kidney perfusion with left side-lying position and insert indwelling urinary catheter; monitor urinary output every hour Under 25 ml/h—do not repeat dose Diuresis—good prognostic sign Repeat dose per order if: DTRs present (Fig. 27.3) Respirations of 12/min or more Urinary output over 1 dl/4 h Assess maternal condition Hydration Affect Other signs or symptoms of preeclampsia Keep 20 ml of 10% calcium gluconate at bedside; with linen/equipment for delivery, eclamptic tray, oxygen, and suction equipment
Diazepam (Valium)	Thalamus and hypothalamus: direct depressant effect	Effective in initial management of eclamptic convulsions	Flattens fetal heart rate (FHR) base line (loss of beat-to-beat variability), an important criterion in assessing fetal oxygenation High levels in newborn: Depressed sucking ability Hypotonia Temperature instability (decrease) Decreased respiratory rate	Notify perinatal staff Assess DTRs, respirations, signs of labor Monitor labor; see Normal labor

*By midpregnancy, diastolic and systolic blood pressure normally falls by 10-15 mm Hg. If diastolic blood pressure is 75 mm Hg or more in second trimester and 85 mm Hg or more in third trimester, statistical increase in fetal mortality occurs.

NOTE: For obese woman, use thigh cuff or ultrasound to obtain accurate readings.

†For control of chronic hypertension, pulmonary edema, renal oliguria, acute renal failure, chronic nephrotic syndrome. If used, physician must be ready to justify action.

‡May not be appropriate for woman with severe preeclampsia-eclampsia.

Table 27.4, cont'd
Pharmacologic Control of Hypertension and Its Sequelae in Pregnancy and Labor

Medication	Target Tissue	Effects of Medication		Nursing Actions
		Maternal	**Fetal/Neonatal**	
Barbiturates (rapid-acting) Phenobarbital sodium: 0.2-0.3 mg IV Amobarbital sodium: 0.25-0.5 g IV	CNS: depressant effect	Controls seizures	Depressant effect on fetus May minimize hyperbili-rubinemia	See Diazepam
Antihypertensive*				
Hydralazine (Apresoline, Neopresol)	Peripheral arterioles: decreases muscle tone, thereby decreasing peripheral resistance Hypothalamus and medullary vasomotor center; minor decrease in sympathetic tone	Headache Flushing Palpitation Tachycardia Some decrease in utero-placental blood flow	Minimum effects; some decrease in Po$_2$	Assess for effects of medications Alert mother (family) to expected effects of medications Assess blood pressure (precipitous drop can lead to shock and perhaps to abruptio placentae) and urinary output Maintain bed rest with side rails for safety
Methyldopa (Aldomet) (used if maintenance therapy is needed): 250-500 mg orally every 8 h	Postganglionic nerve endings: interferes with chemical neurotransmission to reduce peripheral vascular resistance CNS: sedation	Sleepiness Postural hypotension Constipation Rare: drug-induced fever in 1% of women and positive Coombs' test in 20%	After 4 mo of maternal therapy, positive Coombs' test in infant	See Hydralazine
Diuretics†				
Thiazides	Arteriolar smooth muscels: reduces responsiveness to cathecholamines	Ineffective in preventing preeclampsia Further reduces already-present decreased plasma volume of preeclampsia Complications Fluid and electrolyte imbalance Pancreatitis Decrease in CHO intolerance Hyperuricemia	Hyponatremia Thrombocytopenia	Arrange to have blood drawn to measure levels of Na, Cl, H$_2$O, K, and H+ to prevent hyponatremia, hypokalemia, hypochloremia, metabolic acidosis
Furosemide (Lasix): 40 mg IV	Loop of Henle	Relieves pulmonary edema Excessive use results in hypokalemia and hyponatremia	No abnormalities noted	See Thiazides
Ethacrynic acid (Edecrin)	Similar to furosemide	Similar to furosemide	Deafness	See Thiazides
Mannitol (for impending renal failure, oliguria, DIC): 12.5-25 mg IV	Osmotic diuretic: pulls fluid into vascular bed (therefore not recommended for persons with congestive heart failure)	Increases renal plasma flow and urinary output Flushes out kidneys Reduces swelling in ischemic cells in kidney and myocardium	No known effect	See Thiazides
Blood volume expanders				
Salt-poor, serum albumin‡	Intravascular volume	Increases blood volume		

Fig. 27.3

A, (1) Elicitaton of biceps reflex. Downward blow is struck over thumb, which is situated over biceps tendon. Normal response is flexion of arm at elbow. (2) Elicitaton of patellar reflex with client's legs hanging freely over end of examining table, (3) with client in supine position. Blow with percussion hammer is dealt directly to patellar tendon, inferior to patella. Normal response is extension or kicking out of leg. **B,** (1) Assessment for hyperactive reflexes (clonus) at ankle joint. Support leg with knee flexed. With one hand, sharply dorsiflex foot, and maintain dorsiflexed position for a moment, then release foot. (2) Normal (negative clonus) response. While foot is held in dorsiflexion, no rhythmic oscillations (jerking) are felt. When foot is released, no oscillations are seen as foot drops to plantar flexed position. (3) Abnormal (positive clonus) response. Rhythmic oscillations are felt when foot is in dorsiflexion and are seen as foot drops to plantar flexed position.

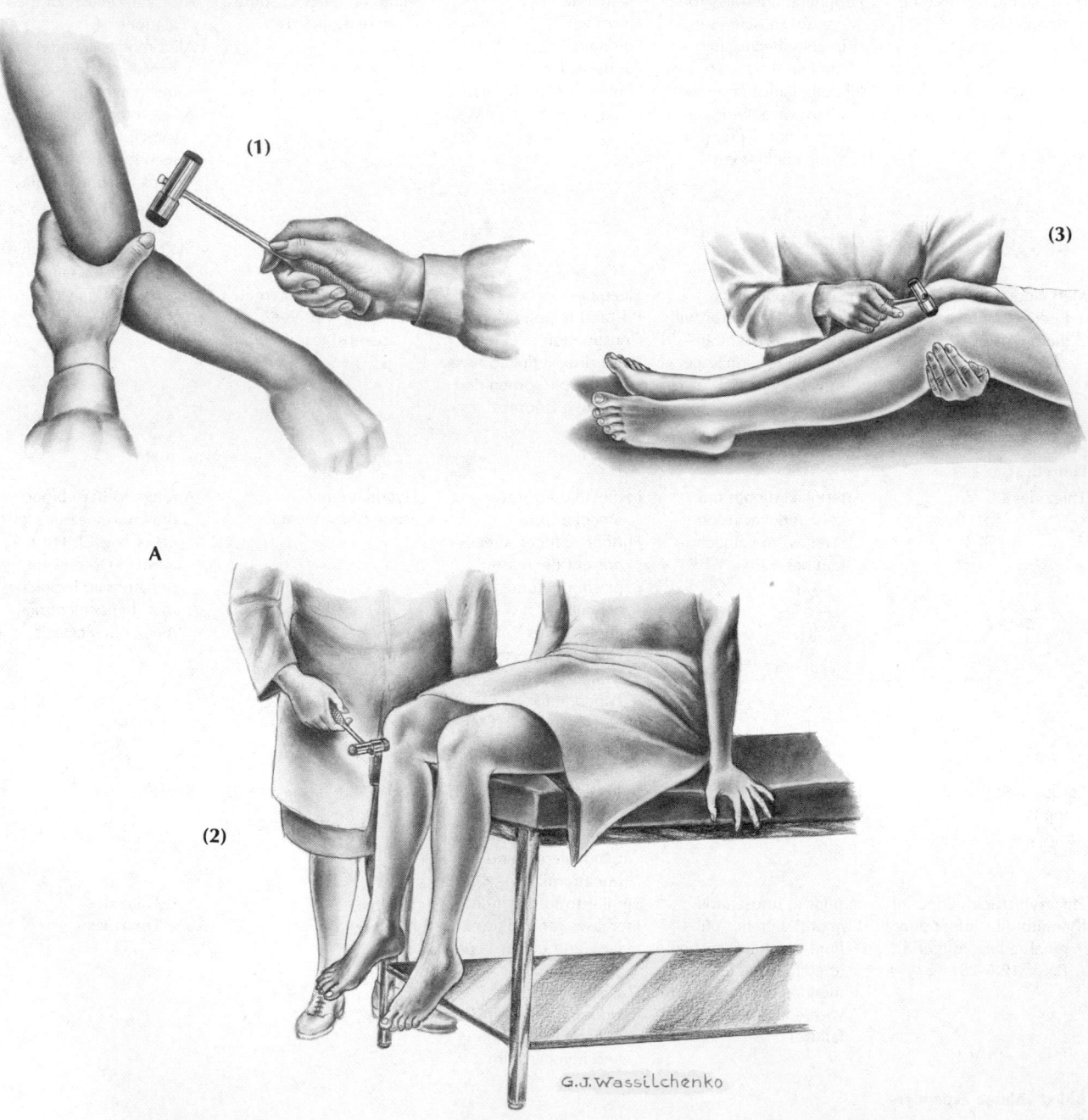

Fig. 27-3, cont'd

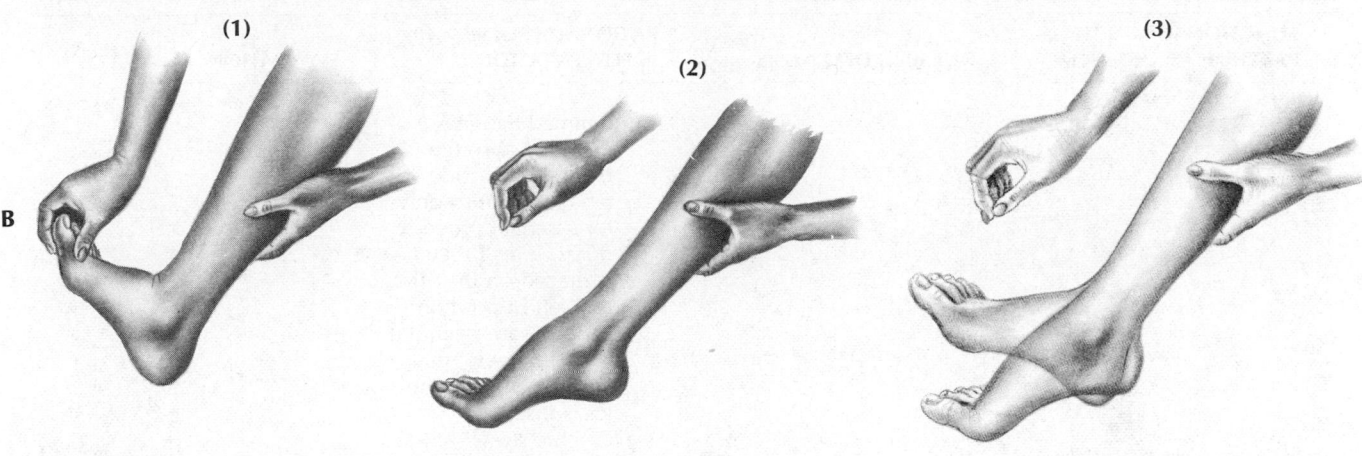

Application of the Nursing Process

HOSPITAL MANAGEMENT OF SEVERE PREECLAMPSIA

Patricia (age 19) and Jim (age 24) are expecting their first child. Patricia's pregnancy has presented few problems. She had a urinary infection that responded well to treatment. In her thirty-fifth week, on a Friday, Patricia noticed that her face "felt tight" and her fingers were swollen. She had gained 2 kg (4 lb) in 1 week. She did not phone her doctor since she "felt okay" and was going for her regular thirty-sixth week checkup on Tuesday. By the thirty-sixth week examination she was found to have

    BP 160/110
    Generalized edema +4
    Proteinuria +3
    Severe headache

Her doctor arranged for her to be admitted to the hospital immediately, and treatment for severe PIH with seizure precautions was begun. Patricia and Jim were anxious and upset over the sudden change in her condition. She worried about not reporting her symptoms immediately and was concerned that she had hurt her baby.

FUNCTIONAL HEALTH PATTERN: ASSESSMENT	NURSING DIAGNOSIS	RATIONALE: PLAN/ IMPLEMENTATION	EVALUATION
HEALTH PERCEPTION– HEALTH MANAGEMENT			
BP 160/110 Proteinuria 3+ Edema 4 I Urinary output, scant dark color Weight gain, 2kg (4 lb) in 2 days	Maternal/fetal compromise* related to edema, proteinuria, hypertension Sensory-perceptual alteration related to body response to stress	*To minimize effects of edema, proteinuria, and hypertension on the following systems:* **Central nervous system** ■ Control amount of stimulation: • External stimuli: keep nurse/client ratio 1:1; place in quiet, private room with	Woman remains quiet, anxiety level under control.

---

*Diagnosis not included by NANDA, 1986.

Continued.

Application of the Nursing Process—cont'd

FUNCTIONAL HEALTH PATTERN: ASSESSMENT	NURSING DIAGNOSIS	RATIONALE: PLAN/ IMPLEMENTATION	EVALUATION
		dimmed lighting; maintain absolute bed rest with side rails up; disturb only for essential procedures, e.g., BP cuff is placed on the arm and left in position; IV fluids are begun at a "keep open" rate; an indwelling catheter is inserted • Psychic stress: have the woman select the people she wishes to stay with her; limit other visitors; assure her her family will be kept informed; explain rationale for care; maintain calm, unhurried approach; report on progress, labor, and FHR	
	Alteration in comfort: pain Sensory-perceptual alteration related to edema, proteinuria, hypertension	■ Monitor symptomatology: (p. 779, Table 27.2) • Level of consciousness (LOC) • Headaches • Visual disturbances • Irritability • **Epigastric or right upper quadrant pain** • Hyperreflexia	
	Potential for injury related to effects of MgSO₄ Potential for injury related to body's response to CNS seizure	Follow protocol for care of MgSO₄ therapy p. 792 Follow protocol for prevention and care of seizures p. 785	
	Alteration in tissue perfusion related to edema, proteinuria, hypertension	**Cardiovascular system** ■ Monitor symptomatology: • BP at least q1 h or more often • Check for generalized edema • Weigh daily • Record findings of daily funduscopic examination	Symptoms improve.

Application of the Nursing Process—cont'd

FUNCTIONAL HEALTH PATTERN: ASSESSMENT	NURSING DIAGNOSIS	RATIONALE: PLAN/ IMPLEMENTATION	EVALUATION
	Potential injury to mother and fetus related to undetected hemoconcentration, clotting disturbances (DIC), hepatic problems	Send blood specimens for measurement of hematocrit, platelets, and SGOT daily; check results against normal values and report deviations immediately	Woman does not develop complications.
	Potential injury to fetus related to alteration in tissue perfusion of placenta	Prevent supine hypotension: woman is placed on her left side; if she insists on lying on her back, the headrest is raised and a wedge (rolled towel) is placed under her right hip to prevent supine hypotension syndrome	FHR remains stable.
		Pulmonary system	
	Alteration in respiratory function related to edema, proteinuria, and hypertension	Check for pulmonary edema, rales	Respiratory function remains within normal limits.
		Urinary system	
	Alteration in patterns of urinary elimination related to edema, proteinuria, and hypertension	■ Check urinary output q1h ■ Report output of less than 100 ml/4 h ■ Check input q8h ■ Check urine for protein q8h ■ Send blood specimen to laboratory for measurement of creatinine; check results against normal values and report deviations immediately	Urinary elimination pattern remains within normal limits. Diuresis occurs. Proteinuria decreases or ceases.
COPING STRESS– INTOLERANCE Woman and husband appear anxious and upset over suddenness of change; they are anxious about the baby's health	Ineffective individual and family coping related to stress of experiencing a major complication of pregnancy	*To monitor coping mechanisms:* ■ Assess affect, restlessness, anxiety • Response to support person • Response to labor contractions ■ Keep woman informed of progress	Woman feels free to express worries and concerns. Support person's anxiety does not prevent support to woman.

Continued.

Application of the Nursing Process—cont'd

FUNCTIONAL HEALTH PATTERN: ASSESSMENT	NURSING DIAGNOSIS	RATIONALE: PLAN/ IMPLEMENTATION	EVALUATION
HEALTH PERCEPTION– HEALTH MANAGEMENT Labor contractions begin before due date	Alteration in normal physiologic process* related to type of delivery	*To monitor labor and delivery:* ■ Monitor woman for signs of progress in labor and for complications, such as prolapsed cord. ■ Prepare for precipitous labor; have delivery pack available in room. ■ Prepare for elective delivery if ordered, e.g., cesarean delivery, order type and cross-match and 2 units of blood	Labor progresses normally *or* ■ If precipitate delivery occurs, safety of mother and baby is safeguarded. ■ If elective delivery is ordered, care is given promptly and skillfully to safe-guard health of mother and infant.

*Diagnosis not included by NANDA, 1986.

treatment. NOTE: A plastic airway is preferred over a padded tongue blade because it permits passage of a tube for suction and for administering oxygen.

PREVENTION OF CONVULSIONS AND USE OF MAGNE-SIUM SULFATE. To prevent convulsions, various drugs may be used in conjunction with medical and nursing care (Table 27.4). The one most commonly used is magnesium sulfate, a CNS depressant.

1. *Administration.* Magnesium sulfate may be given intravenously or intramuscularly. Various dosage schedules are used. For example, an initial dose of 4 g of magnesium sulfate in 250 ml of 5% dextrose in water may be given intravenously (injected *slowly* at a rate of 5 ml/30 s). Four to five grams may then be given intramuscularly in each buttock (1% procaine can be added to the solution to reduce the pain of injection). The intramuscular dose can be followed at 4-hour intervals with intramuscular doses of 4 to 5 g. When magnesium sulfate is given intravenously, the effect is immediate and lasts for about 30 minutes. When it is given intramuscularly, the onset of action occurs in 1 hour and the effect lasts 3 to 4 hours.
2. *Monitoring for toxicity.*
   a. *Blood pressure.* Magnesium sulfate has a CNS-depressant effect. It reduces blood pressure by splanchnic vasodilation; therefore severe hypotension can occur. The woman's blood pressure should be monitored continuously while the

drug is being administered intravenously and every 15 minutes at other times.

   b. *Urinary output.* The drug also increases the retention of sodium. The drug is excreted by the kidneys. The woman's urinary output must total 100 ml or more every 4 hours. If the urinary output is less than 25 ml/h and the doses of magnesium sulfate are repeated, toxic levels of the drug can occur. There can be severe diminution or absence of the patellar reflex and respiratory depression. An indwelling catheter is inserted, and an hourly urometer is attached to ensure careful monitoring of urinary output and to minimize stress to the woman. If the output is not maintained, the drug should not be repeated.

   c. *Respirations.* Adverse effects of magnesium sulfate also include respiratory paralysis. *Maternal toxicity has been reached when respirations are fewer than 12/min.* The drug is withheld if respirations are fewer than 12/min. The woman receiving magnesium sulfate therapy **should never be left unattended** because MgSO₄ toxicity with respiratory arrest may occur.

   d. *Reflex activity.* Maternal toxicity has been reached when reflex activity is absent. It is imperative that the reflexes be checked before and after each injection of magnesium sulfate (Table 27.5 and Fig. 27.3).

Table 27.5
Assessing Deep Tendon Reflexes (DTRs)

Degree	Grading	Clinical Significance and Nursing Actions
Hyperactive re-sponse	4+	Woman not responding to medications as desired; may be accompanied by apprehension, restless-ness, excitability; notify physician
More than normal	3+	Woman responding; however, important to assess frequently
Normal	2+	Safe dosage level, therapeutic effect
Low response	1+	Notify physician for medical directives
No response	0	Turn off magnesium sulfate drip; change to "keep open" solution; notify physician for immediate care; prepare antidote (20 ml vial of 10% calcium gluconate) for injection

e. *Serum levels.* A response to rise in serum levels of magnesium occurs:

4 mg/dl or more: Convulsions are prevented

10-12 mg/dl: Reflexes disappear

12-15 mg/dl: Respirations slow (below 12) or respiratory arrest

15+ mg/dl: Cardiac arrest is possible

3. *Fetus.* Toxic levels in the fetus cause marked slow-ing of respirations and hyporeflexia after birth. The danger signals for both fetus and mother that are associated with magnesium sulfate toxicity are sum-marized below.

4. *Antidote.* The antidote for magnesium sulfate tox-icity is a calcium salt such as calcium gluconate. A 20 ml vial of a 10% aqueous solution of calcium gluconate should be kept at the bedside. If needed, it is administered slowly intravenously and repeated every hour until the respiratory, urinary, and neu-rologic depression has been alleviated. *The maxi-mum number of injections of a calcium salt is 8 injec-tions in a 24-hour period.*

Because magnesium salts cross the placenta, the fe-tus may be affected. The drug should not be adminis-tered intravenously in the 2 hours preceding delivery (intramuscular magnesium does not seem to have ad-verse effects on the neonate), and the newborn should be assessed for hyporeflexia and for respiratory prob-lems.

Danger Signals MgSO₄ Toxicity

Assess	Indications of Toxicity
Blood pressure	Sudden hypotension
Urinary output	Less than 25 ml/h
Respiration	Less than 12/min
Reflexes	Hyperreflexia, hyporeflexia, absence
Serum levels	10-12 mg/dl: reflexes absent
	12-15 mg/dl: cardiorespira-tory arrest
Fetal heart rate	Sudden decrease

IMMEDIATE CARE OF CONVULSIONS. The convulsions that occur in eclampsia make eclampsia an awesome, frightening sequence to observe. Increased hyperten-sion precedes the tonic-clonic convulsions; hypoten-sion and collapse follow. Stertorous breathing and coma are the aftermath of a seizure. Nystagmus and muscular twitching persist for a time. Disorientation and amnesia cloud the immediate recovery. Oliguria and anuria are notable. A more detailed description of tonic-clonic convulsions is given below.

The immediate care during a convulsion is to ensure a patent airway. Once this has been attained adequate oxygenation must be provided.

1. *Immediate care of convulsions*

a. If convulsions occur, turn woman onto left side to prevent aspiration of vomitus and supine hy-potension syndrome.

b. Insert folded towel, plastic airway, or padded tongue blade into side of mouth to prevent bit-ing of lips or tongue and to maintain airway. Do not put fingers into woman's mouth; she may bite them involuntarily.

c. Aspirate food and fluid from glottis or trachea.

d. Give magnesium sulfate as ordered.

e. Administer oxygen by means of face cone or tent after convulsion ceases (masks and nasal catheters cause excessive stimulation). Oxygen

Tonic-Clonic Convulsions

Stage of invasion: 2 to 3 seconds; eyes fixed; twitching of facial muscles.

Stage of contraction: 15 to 20 seconds; eyes protrude and are bloodshot; all body muscles in tonic contraction (e.g., arms flexed, hands clenched, legs inverted).

Stage of convulsion: Muscles relax and contract alterna-tively. Respirations are halted and then begin again with long, deep stertorous inhalation. Coma ensues (2 to 3 minutes to hours).

Occurrence: During prenatal, intranatal, or postdelivery pe-riod.

Recurrence: Within minutes of first convulsion or never.

rate may be up to 10 L/min (as opposed to 3 L/min advocated for continuous O_2 in chronic conditions).

 f. Record time and duration of convulsions; include description.

 g. Note any urinary or fecal incontinence.

2. *Transfusion.* Have the woman's blood typed and matched. Keep the blood available for emergency transfusion; women with eclampsia often develop premature separation of the placenta, hemorrhage, and shock.

3. *Fluids.* Give fluids as directed; record the time, the amount and the woman's response. Hospital protocols vary.

 a. Permit nothing by mouth if woman is convulsing.

 b. Insert retention catheter for accurate measurement of urinary output.

 c. Assist physician with intravenous infusion of 200 to 300 ml of 20% glucose solution, two to three times a day during critical period to support liver function, aid nutrition, and replace fluid; 50% glucose is rarely used, since it often scleroses veins.

 d. To correct hypovolemia, crystalloids (0.9% saline or Ringer's lactated solution) are infused intravenously.

 e. If woman is oliguric or if serum protein level is low, physician may order salt-poor albumin (25 to 50 ml) or 250 to 500 ml of plasma or serum to be administered intravenously.

 f. Note and record maternal response.

4. *Medications.* Give medications as directed; monitor and record the woman's response. Record drugs, dosages, and times given.

 a. Diuretics are *no longer* advocated (see Table 27.4).

 b. Sedatives such as phenobarbital, 0.05 g, are given orally or intramuscularly on admission to the hospital and repeated to maintain moderate sedation until the woman's condition improves. Monitor for start of labor, since woman may be unaware of sensation.

 c. Magnesium sulfate (intravenous or intramuscular) may be ordered as necessary. Before administering magnesium sulfate, check the following:

  (1) DTRs present

  (2) Respirations at least 12/min

  (3) Urinary output at least 100 ml/4 h

5. *Hygiene.* Maintain body hygiene. The vulvar area may be washed with warm, soapy water.

6. *Psychologic support.* The physician or nurse explains procedures briefly and quietly. The woman is never left alone if the condition is severe or if she is receiving magnesium sulfate therapy. The family is also kept informed of management, rationale, and the woman's progress.

7. *Delivery.* Preeclampsia-eclampsia and severe hypertensive or renal disease are intensified by the continuation of pregnancy. Termination of gestation is the only practical treatment. The fetus may therefore be premature or otherwise compromised.

 a. Eclampsia is controlled before induction of labor is attempted; then labor is induced by amniotomy.

 b. Oxytocin may be used cautiously to stimulate labor.

 c. Nitrous oxide (70%) and oxygen (30%) may be given with contractions, but 100% oxygen should be given between contractions.

 d. Vaginal delivery with pudendal block anesthesia is preferred. However, if labor cannot be induced readily, if woman is bleeding, or if there is fetal distress, cesarean delivery should be effected, preferably with procaine (or equivalent) local infiltration of abdominal wall. Thiopental (Pentothal) may be given after delivery of infant for incisional closure.

 e. Pediatrician and pediatric (intensive care nursery) nurse are present to provide immediate care for the newborn.

8. Evaluation

 a. Within 24 to 48 hours:

  (1) Condition improves.

   (a) CNS irritability is reduced.

   (b) Convulsions (if any) are terminated.

   (c) Hypertension is reduced (normal values usually return by 10 days after delivery).

   (d) Water imbalance, acid-base imbalance, and other electrolyte imbalances are corrected.

   (e) Proteinuria is reduced, and serum protein level is increased.

   (f) Fetal well-being continues.

   (g) Placental complications are absent or controlled, and delivery can proceed as previously planned whether vaginal, induced, or cesarean.

  (2) If condition does not improve, nurse assists in care for elective delivery, that is, induction of labor or cesarean birth (Chapter 29).

 b. Woman and family are aware of need for care, cause of symptoms, and prognosis. Informed consent forms are completed.

 c. Records are complete at all times.

Postdelivery nursing care. The nursing care of the woman who experiences PIH differs from that required in a normal postpartum period in a number of respects. The following content emphasizes the specific nursing strategies needed by these women.

Assessment

1. Check blood pressure every 4 hours for 48 hours or more frequently as woman's condition warrants. Even if no convulsions occurred before delivery, they may occur within this period.
2. Ask woman to report headaches, blurred vision, etc. Assess affect, alertness, or dullness. Check blood pressure before giving analgesic for headache. NOTE: No ergot products are given because they increase blood pressure.
3. Assess woman's and family's response to labor.
4. Continue regular assessment.

Nursing diagnoses. Examples might include the following:

1. Disturbance of self-concept related to inability to accept high-risk nature of delivery experience.
2. Potential compromise of mother related to initial occurrence of hypertension during puerperium.
3. Potential disturbances in family processes related to stress during high-risk prenatal, intranatal, and postdelivery periods.

Plan/implementation. Postpartum care for the woman with PIH includes care related to normal involution. In addition the woman and her family need opportunities to discuss their emotional response to complications. The nurse also provides information concerning the following:

1. Prognosis (i.e., preeclampsia-eclampsia does not necessarily recur in subsequent pregnancies, but careful prenatal care is essential).
2. Evaluation must be thorough during the postdelivery examination to rule out chronic hypertension.
3. Family planning information (the next pregnancy should be delayed for 2 years; the woman is not a candidate for oral contraceptive use) (Chapter 7).

Evaluation. The nurse uses the following criteria to evaluate the plan of care:

1. Recovery from PIH is complete *or* woman begins therapy for underlying cause of hypertension not related to pregnancy.
2. Woman's self-concept is not impaired.
3. Infant is healthy *or* has minimal impairment.

HYPERTENSIVE CARDIOVASCULAR DISEASE

Hypertension is considered to be present in women during the childbearing years when the blood pressure is maintained at or above 140/90 at rest. Hypertensive disorders during pregnancy make up an extremely important group that accounts for a high maternal and perinatal morbidity and mortality. The vascular complications of hypertension, such as intracranial hemorrhage (stroke and cardiovascular accident), are the consequence of increased arterial pressure and related ateriosclerosis.

Primary (essential) hypertensive disease, in which no cause can be determined, is the diagnosis in about 85% of nonpregnant, premenopausal hypertensive women. The remaining 15% of women with hypertension have secondary hypertensive vascular disease, caused by disorders such as chronic pyelonephritis or

Table 27.6
Differential Diagnosis of Essential Hypertension and Preeclampsia

Features	Essential Hypertension	Preeclampsia
Onset of hypertension	Before pregnancy; during first 20 weeks of pregnancy	After 20 weeks of pregnancy (exception: trophoblastic tumors*)
Duration of hypertension	Permanent; hypertension beyond 3 months after delivery	Hypertension absent 10 days after delivery
Family history	Often positive	Usually negative, may be positive
Past history	Recurrent "toxemia"	Psychosexual problems common
Age	Usually older	Generally teenaged or in early 20s
Parity	Usually multigravida	Usually primigravida
Habitus	May be thin or brachymorphic	Usually eumorphic
Retinal findings	Often arteriovenous nicking, tortuous arterioles, cotton-wool exudates, hemorrhages	Vascular spasm, retinal edema; rarely, protein extravasations
Proteinuria	Often none	Usually present; absent at 6 weeks after delivery

Reproduced with permission, from Benson, R.C., editor: Current obstetric and gynecologic diagnosis and treatment, ed. 5. Copyright 1984 by Lange Medical Publications, Los Altos, Calif.

*Hydatidiform mole (molar pregnancy).

Table 27.7
Differential Diagnosis of Nephrosis and Preeclampsia

	Nephrosis	Preeclampsia
Onset	Any trimester	After 20 weeks (exception: tropho-blastic tumors)
Proteinuria	Massive	Variable (as defined)
Edema	Usually marked	Variable
Hypertension	Commonly absent	Present
Hematuria	Usually microscopic	Absent
Serum cholesterol	Greatly elevated	Same as normal pregnancy
Hypoproteinemia	Marked	Decreased below normal pregnancy
α- and β-globulins	Decreased	Increased
Glomerular filtration rate	Decreased, normal, or increased	Decreased
Urinary sediment	Usually oval, doubly refractile fat bodies, fatty casts, waxy casts	Absent

Reproduced with permission, from Benson, R.C., editor: Current obstetric and gynecologic diagnosis and treatment, ed. 5. Copyright 1984 by Lange Medical Publications, Los Altos, Calif.

glomerulonephritis, renal artery stenosis, or coarctation of the aorta.

Differential diagnosis. The differential diagnosis of hypertension begins with the past history of disease, for example, nephritis. The woman's health and progress over the years may disclose advancing symptoms of hypertensive disease, perhaps worsened by pregnancy. Careful evaluation of the woman's endocrine and cardiovascular-renal systems, as well as other possible causes of hypertension, may disclose the cause, independent of PIH. Occasionally, when the hypertensive woman is seen initially late in pregnancy, studies after the puerperium may be required before the cause of hypertension can be determined. Often the etiologic factors are obscure and the tentative impression may be one of "essential hypertension" (see Tables 27.6 and 27.7).

Prognosis. The prognosis for the pregnant woman with hypertension depends on the cause, the degree of hypertension, the woman's symptoms, and her response to treatment. Whatever the cause, the fetus may be severely affected by hypertension and its sequelae. Early delivery may be lifesaving for the mother and fetus.

Medical and nursing management. With chronic hypertensive disease, the physician treats the symptomatology during pregnancy. The pregnancy is usually permitted to continue if the woman responds to therapy. Frequent estriol determinations after the thirty-second week will be ordered in an attempt to allow the woman to carry the fetus to 34 to 36 weeks (Chapter 25). Protracted or maternal CNS, cardiac, or renal complications may develop. If the woman's blood pressure reaches 200/110, immediate medical attention is necessary. The physician will usually order antihypertensive drugs such as hydralazine (see Table 27.4)

and assess the need for a prompt delivery.

The nursing care of women with chronic hypertensive disease is the same as that of women with hypertension attributable to pregnancy. If and when cardiac involvement is diagnosed, the nursing care of the woman with cardiac disease is superimposed on the original plan (see Chapter 28). The woman and her family must be aware of the possibility of premature delivery and of the need for careful and continuous supervision during the prenatal, intranatal, and postdelivery periods.

Maternal Infection

Infection in the prenatal period. Pregnancy confers no immunity against infection and both mother and fetus must be considered when the pregnant woman contracts an infection. In some disorders, such as tuberculosis, the fetus is almost always spared, even though the mother may be dying. In other diseases, such as rubella, the fetus may be critically compromised, whereas the mother may be only slightly ill.

Preventive medicine is particularly important in obstetrics. Many tragedies can be averted by informed anticipation. For example, vaccination against rubella before pregnancy currently is the only means to control this disorder. No cure is available for rubella. Women are becoming more knowledgeable about factors such as infections, which can jeopardize fetal development. The large number of infections, the varying responses of the fetus or newborn, and the range of nursing and medical actions necessitate a readily available resource. The box on p. 797 and Tables 27.8 to 27.10 provide this information. Examples of antimicrobial therapy are presented in Table 27.11.

Sexually Transmitted Disease (STD)

Historically defined venereal diseases

Syphilis: acquired, congenital (annual worldwide incidence is estimated at 50 million people, with 400,000 in the United States)

Gonorrhea (annual worldwide incidence is estimated at 250 million people, with 3 million in the United States)

Chancroid

Lymphogranuloma venereum

Granuloma inguinale

Newly defined STDs

Hepatitis B (serum hepatitis)

Genital and anorectal herpes

Balanoposthitis; balanitis

Proctitis

Genital warts

Genital candidiasis

Nonspecific sexually transmitted infection (e.g., nonspecific urethritis)

Chlamydial infection (?)

AIDS

Enteric diseases that may be sexually transmitted

Salmonellosis

Amebiasis

Typhoid

Giardiasis

Shigellosis

Diseases spread by body contact but not necessarily by coitus

Pediculosis

Molluscum contagiosum

Scabies

Sexually transmitted diseases (STD). Venereal diseases (named after Venus, the goddess of love), now termed *sexually transmitted diseases* (STD), often share common characteristics. They have a predilection for genital and perigenital sites, perhaps because of genital pH, temperature, moisture, and hormonal influences. The causative organisms are relatively unstable when removed from their natural habitat. They are either completely or predominantly transferred from one person to another sexually (see box above).

Herpesvirus hominis infections. Genital herpesvirus hominis infections are caused by herpes simplex type 2 virus (Table 27.8). Recurrences are sometimes preceded by itching, a burning sensation in the genital area, tingling in the legs, or a slight increase in vaginal discharge. Symptomatic therapy alone is available (p. 805). No specific cure has been identified.

Condylomata acuminata. Condylomata acuminata are sexually transmitted lesions caused by a virus as yet unidentified. The lesions grow rapidly during pregnancy

and may involve the cervix, vagina, and vulva, so that vaginal delivery is impossible and a cesarean delivery is necessary.

The huge growths on the vulva may be excised by cautery without scarring or deformity. However, since the vaginal and cervical growths are multiple and small, cauterization cannot be used, because it would result in necrosis and scarring.

Placentitis and chorioamnionitis. Placentitis, or infection of the placenta, may be bacterial, viral, rickettsial, or protozoal in origin. The most common agents are bacterial, which cause the greatest changes in the placenta. Bacterial infections may result in fatal fetal and even maternal septicemia.

Chorioamnionitis may be the cause or the result of premature rupture of the membranes (PROM). Chorioamnionitis may be followed by placentitis and fetal congenital pneumonia, omphalitis, or septicemia. These conditions often are caused by enteric streptococci, an aerogenic type of colon bacteria. Placentitis and chorioamnionitis may be followed by endometritis and parametritis. The result is serious puerperal sepsis.

Infection in the postnatal period

Puerperal infection. Puerperal infection (puerperal sepsis or "childbed fever") is any clinical infection of the genital canal that occurs within 28 days after abortion or delivery. Infections may result from bacteria commonly found within the vagina *(endogenous)* or from the introduction of pathogens from outside the vagina *(exogenous).* An episiotomy or lacerations of the vagina or cervix may open avenues for sepsis. Even more formidable, however, may be the large placental site. Here the denuded endometrium (decidua basalis) and residual blood after parturition make the uterus an ideal site for a wound infection. The virulence of infecting organisms, the woman's resistance to them, and the rapidity and specificity of therapy determine the efficacy of treatment. Puerperal sepsis occurs after about 6% of deliveries in the United States. Fortunately body defenses generally limit the disease in most instances. Puerperal infection probably is the major cause of maternal morbidity and mortality throughout the world.

The most common infecting organisms are the numerous streptococcal and anaerobic organisms. Fulminating epidemic puerperal sepsis classically is caused by the hemolytic streptococcus. The less virulent anaerobic streptococci may be responsible for other puerperal infections, however, *Staphylococcus aureus,* gonococci, coliform bacteria, and clostridia are less common but serious pathogenic organisms causing puerperal infection.

Frequently the infection is complicated by medical

Table 27.8
Maternal Infections: Effects in Pregnancy and Fetus or Newborn

Infection	Maternal Effects	Fetal or Neonatal Effects	Counseling: Prevention, Identification, and Management
Chlamydia trachomatis (**intra**cellular bacterium)	Mild infection usually Cervix: asymptomatic; or congestion, edema, mucopurulent discharge may be asymptomatic; symptoms similar to gonorrhea: discharge and bleeding from or an infection of the cervix Lymphogranuloma venereum Urethritis Acute salpingitis Conjunctivitis Sore throat	Stillbirth and neonatal death 10 times more common than in noninfected women; preterm birth Newborns: asymptomatic, or pneumonia; **inclusion conjunctivitis** occurs in one-third of exposed newborns; conjunctivitis appears after 3 to 4 days; chronic follicular conjunctivitis (with conjunctival scarring and corneal neovascularization) About 25% of newborns with chlamydia **pneumonia** can present with serious tachypnea, dyspnea, or apnea that require hospitalization (Schachter, 1986).	STD; three times more common than gonorrhea; high incidence in teenage girls; usually controlled with antibiotics, but *not* by penicillin; **erythromycin** is the drug of choice; untreated, can lead to pelvic inflammatory disease (PID), with painful infection of uterine tubes; in men it is linked to nongonococcal urethritis (NGU); newborn may acquire disease by direct contact with infected birth canal; transmitted through sexual contact (?), and genitals-to-hand-to-eye contact (oculogenital).
Chicken pox (varicella) (a herpes virus)	Herpes zoster (shingles)	Abortion; fetal death; defects of skin, bone, and muscle; chorioretinitis; hydrocephalus	Severe disseminated epidemic type of varicella during pregnancy may be fatal for mother (and fetus) because of necrotizing angitis (inflammation of blood and lymph vessels); zoster immune globulin (IM) may be given prophylactically to exposed gravidas.
Coxsackie B virus	Mild illness	Fetal death; cardiovascular anomalies; myocarditis; meningoencephalitis	
Gardnerella (*Hemophilus vaginalis* vaginitis) (bacterium)	Low virulence; mild illness Milklike discharge characteristic of bacterial vaginitis; foul, fishy odor; itching, burning, pain may be present	Chorioamnionitis; septicemia; fetal or neonatal death	Counsel regarding transmission through sexual contact, especially when estrogen levels are high; often occurs along with other infections of vagina. Because therapy is often a sulpha-based medication (suppository, cream, etc.) assess for sensitivity to sulfanamide. Best results if partner is treated at same time.
Gonorrhea ("clap, drip") *Neisseria gonorrhoeae* (gonococcus diplococci bacterium) Gram-negative; paired; bean-shaped Genitourinary Anorectal Oropharyngeal Systemic	Lower urogenital tract (early stage): dysuria, frequency, heavy purulent vaginal discharge; cervical tenderness; vulvovaginitis; bartholinitis Upper urogenital tract (later stage) (10%-15% of cases): lower abdominal pain, cervical tenderness; fever, nausea, vomiting; adnexal abscess, tenderness (PID); ectopic pregnancy; chronic pelvic pain Anorectal: inflammation, burning, pruritis Oropharyngeal: asymptomatic or inflammation, sore throat Systemic: gonococcemia, skin rashes, arthritis, pericarditis, meningitis	Gonococcal **ophthalmia neonatorum,** pneumonia; neonatal sepsis with temperature instability, hypotonia, poor feeding, and jaundice	Most common contagious bacterial disease in North America Transmitted by sexual contact and fomites such as underwear, bedding, towels Both (all) partners treated to prevent reinfection (the ping-pong effect); couple should use condoms and avoid orogenital sex until posttreatment cultures are negative at two consecutive follow-up visits Incubation period: 2-5 days; in females, early stage may be asymptomatic 5% of clients also have syphilis Gravid women allergic to penicillin can be given erythromycin or spectinomycin; nongravid clients

Table 27.8, cont'd
Maternal Infections: Effects in Pregnancy and Fetus or Newborn

Infection	Maternal Effects	Fetal or Neonatal Effects	Counseling: Prevention, Identification, and Management
			can be given the cephalosporins and kanamycin During postnatal period, infection may reappear as gonococcal endometritis; acute salpingitis, dermatitis, or arthritis. Penicillin G, 4.8 million units intramuscularly, is the therapy recommended by the Food and Drug Administration for the treatment of gonorrhea in women. It is interesting and important that this dosage is the same for the treatment of both gonorrhea and syphilis. Spectinomycin, erythromycin, tetracycline, the cephalosporins, and kanamycin (in adequate doses) can be given to women sensitive to penicillin.
Group B β-hemolytic streptococcus (bacterium)	Septicemia; cellulitis (erysipelas); fever; puerperal infection; impetigo; scarlet fever; abortion	Neonatal death within 2-12 hours; blindness, deafness, spinal meningitis, mental retardation, learning or behavior problems in survivors	See Table 27.11 for antimicrobial therapy. Penicillin is the drug of choice.
Influenza (virus)	Serious prognosis if complicated by pneumonia; abortion; premature labor	Abortion; fetal death; prematurity; occasionally anencephaly or meningomyelocele	Polyvalent influenza virus (attenuated live virus) vaccine contraindicated for pregnant women.
Listeriosis (Gram + bacterium, *Listeria monocytogenes*)	Harbored in vagina and/or cervix by 4% of pregnant women; may exhibit influenza-like symptoms, most commonly in summer or fall; vaginitis; urinary tract infection (UTI); enteritis	Abortion; amnionitis or placentitis Amniotic fluid may appear dirty brown in color Neonatal infection: generalized skin rash, meningitis, pneumonia (50% mortality) Meningitis (most often in term boys) may appear later in neonatal period High rate of morbidity and mortality	Treatment with penicillin or erythromycin usually successful; unfortunately diagnosis of listeriosis often is obscure or delayed; hence prognosis for fetus generally is poor.
Malaria (*Plasmodium falciparum*, protozoan)	Chills and fever; infertility; abortion, premature labor; labor may be prolonged, hazardous; fatiguing, and end in cesarean birth; recurrence in puerperium	Malarial infection in 10% of newborns of infected women Extensive involvement of placenta; small-for-gestational-age (SGA) neonates, stillbirth, abortion	Quinine (chloroquine phosphate; Aralen) may be fetotoxic; in severe cases of malaria, however, employment of appropriate medications may be an acceptable calculated risk.
Mumps (virus)	Parotitis (rare); abortion; premature labor	Fetal death; congenital malformation (e.g., endorcardial fibroelastosis [?])	Prophylaxis of epidemic parotitis possible with administration of hyperimmune mumps γ-globulin
Poliomyelitis (virus)	Increased susceptibility to poliomyelitis during pregnancy; if paralyzed, labor progresses normally; increased mortality	First trimester: abortion, possible anomalies, intrauterine growth retardation (IUGR) Flaccid paralysis; may contract poliomyelitis during passage through birth canal	Prophylaxis for poliomyelitis (polio) has almost eradicated this disorder in some countries; however, it is still prevalent and potentially devastating in parts of Asia and Africa. Prophylaxis for pregnant women possible with Salk vaccine (killed virus) but *not* Sabin vaccine (attenuated live virus); Salk vaccine confers an immunity of about 2

Table 27.8, cont'd
Maternal Infections: Effects in Pregnancy and Fetus or Newborn

Infection	Maternal Effects	Fetal or Neonatal Effects	Counseling: Prevention, Identification, and Management
			years; Sabin vaccination is followed by permanent immunization.
Pyelonephritis (bacteria)	Acute UTI: frequency, urgency, dysuria, chills, fever, backache, tenderness over affected kidney May be asymptomatic	Prematurity with its hazards; sulfonamides may cause icterus, hemolytic anemia, kernicterus, growth retardation (?), or thrombocytopenia Nitrofurantoin therapy for mother may lead to megaloblastic anemia, G6PD deficiency in newborn	Most vulnerable are primigravidas; women with difficult labors; women with diabetes or sickle cell disease.
Rubeola (2-week measles, virus)	Rubeola uncommon during pregnancy because most women have had the disease and are immune	Abortion or premature labor; newborn may be born with a rash but generally survives without developmental anomalies	Prophylactic γ-globulin may prevent disease; measles vaccination of susceptible women before (but never during) pregnancy is recommended.

Syphilis ("lues")
Treponema pallidum (spirochete)
 	
Chancre
Condylomata lata
"The great imitator"
Cardiovascular disease
Neurologic disease
Congenital syphilis
	Incubation period: several weeks—asymptomatic
	Primary stage: chancre (red base with firm, rolled edges); painless; local lymphadenopathy clears without treatment in 4-6 weeks
	Secondary Stage: symmetric, nontender rash anywhere over body, including palms of hands and soles of feet; on scalp, causes loss of hair
	Moist papular lesions, condylomata, on any moist skin surface
	Systemic: malaise, fever, headache
	Clears without treatment in 2-6 weeks
	Latent stages:
	  Early: up to 4 years after infection, lesions reappear
	  Late: for 50% to 70%, lasts a
		Syphilis probably continues to be major cause of late abortion throughout the world, despite widespread success of diagnosis and treatment of this disease.
		Primary and secondary stages of untreated syphilis lead to stillbirth
		Latent, tertiary stages of untreated syphilis lead to secondary syphilis (congenital syphilis) in neonate
		Congenital syphilis: spirochetes cross placenta after sixteenth to eighteenth week of gestation with the following sequelae: snuffles (rhinitis), rhagades (scars around mouth), hydrocephaly, and corneal opacity; later: saddle nose, saber shin, Hutchinson's teeth
			Transmitted through sexual contact from infected lesion of one person through intact mucosa or break in skin of other person, into blood and lymphatic systems to all parts of the body within a few hours.
			Spirochetes are numerous in lesions in primary, secondary, and early latent stages, and in blood during late latent and tertiary stages.
			If the gravida is treated with penicillin by the fifth month of gestation, congenital syphilis; woman with untreated syphilis in labor should receive 3 million units intramuscularly and 2 million units every other day for a total of 7 million units; infant should be treated also.*

*Several methods of assessment of syphilis are available: (1) dark-field microscopic examination or direct fluorescent antibody staining of material from lesions or umbilical cord, (2) assessment of clinical signs, (3) roentgenographic evidence of characteristic bone involvement, and (4) serologic testing for antibodies known as reagins. Any test for antibodies may be negative in the presence of active infection because it takes time for the body's immune system to develop antibodies to any antigen. NONSPECIFIC SEROLOGIC TESTS. Nonspecific serologic tests for nontreponemal antigens used for screening purposes are of two types: complement fixation (Kolmer, Wasserman) and flocculation (Kahn, RPR, [rapid plasma reagin] VDRL [Venereal Disease Research Laboratories]). The VDRL test is positive in 10-90 days after infection; that is, 50% are positive in 3 weeks, 90% in 6 weeks, and 100% in 13 weeks. Therefore infection may exist in the presence of a negative result from the VDRL test. If the antibodies have been acquired from the mother, titers should drop to zero by 3 months. False-positive results may occur if the newborn has an acute infection of any kind or a collagen disease. Even in the presence of a syphilitic infection a false-negative result may occur, for example, if the mother became infected late in pregnancy. A false-positive result may occur in the presence of heroin dependence. SPECIFIC TESTS FOR SYPHILIS. Specific tests for treponemal antigen are more expensive, require special laboratory equipment, and are therefore used for differential diagnosis. These tests include TPI (*Treponema pallidum* immobilization), FTA-ABS (fluorescent treponemal antibody absorption), and FTA-ABS IgM. The FTA-ABS IgM is most specific for neonatal syphilis; a positive result is especially valuable in diagnosis of the condition in the asymptomatic child. Results of the FTA-ABS IgM test may be negative, however, in the presence of active disease if infection occurred late in pregnancy and the fetus or newborn had insufficient time for an IgM response. In questionable cases the test is repeated.

Table 27.8, cont'd
Maternal Infections: Effects in Pregnancy and Fetus or Newborn

Infection	Maternal Effects	Fetal or Neonatal Effects	Counseling: Prevention, Identification, and Management
	Late: for 50% to 70%, lasts a lifetime, no outward evidence of disease Tertiary: clincial evidence of disease seen throughout body; obliterative endarteritis leading to cell damage and death and to gumma nodules of dead tissue. The acronym "paresis" summarizes possible sequelae seen in changes in the following: Personality Affect Reflexes Eye function Sensorium Intellect Speech	(notched, tapered canines), and diabetes; no residual fetal-newborn effects if mother is treated adequately before fifth month.	NOTE: Yaws, a nonvenereal, contagious disease, is caused by the spirochete *Treponema pertenue*, closely related to the causative organism of syphilis; yaws is spread by contact with secretions or sores from an infected person; both syphilis and yaws give a positive result in the STS tests; yaws is a common disease in equatorial Africa, Hawaii, South America, and the East and West Indies; it is effectively treated with antibiotics, especially penicillin.
Tuberculosis (gram-negative, acid-fast bacillus)	Pulmonary tuberculosis does not jeopardize pregnancy, although urinary and CNS tuberculosis may. Pregnancy does not affect pulmonary tuberculosis adversely Genital infection: 20% end in spontaneous abortion; many pregnancies are ectopic.	Outcome depends on stage of tuberculous infection Congenital tuberculosis rare Streptomycin may result in congenital nerve deafness	Contraception is most important for women with active tuberculosis; pregnancy is contraindicated until woman has been free of the disease for 1½-2 years. All pregnant women should be evaluated for tuberculosis (tine test or PPD) early in pregnancy and again later if suspicion of disease exists. Once infant has been delivered she or he should have no intimate contact with mother or others who may have the disease until contagion is no longer a problem. Therapeutic abortion rarely is indicated; cesarean delivery is warranted only for obstetric indications.
Typhoid fever			Intrauterine fetal death: abortion; premature birth

disorders such as anemia, malnutrition, or diabetes mellitus. Obstetric problems, including premature rupture of the membranes (PROM), a long, exhausting labor, instrument delivery, hemorrhage, and retention of the products of conception, increase the likelihood and severity of puerperal sepsis.

An endometritis, usually at the placental site, permits infection to begin. Localized infection may be followed by salpingitis, peritonitis, and pelvic abscess formation. (Tubal occlusion after salpingitis is a common cause of infertility.) Septicemia may develop. Secondary abscesses may arise in distant sites such as the lungs or liver. Pulmonary embolism or septic shock, often with disseminated intravascular coagulation (DIC),

from any serious genital infection may prove fatal. Postdelivery femoral thrombophlebitis ("milk leg") may result in a swollen, painful leg.

Clinical findings. The symptomatology of puerperal infection may be mild or fulminating. Any fever, that is, **a temperature of 38° C (100.4° F) or more on 2 successive days, not counting the first 24 hours after delivery,** must be considered caused by puerperal infection in the absence of convincing proof of another cause.

General malaise, anorexia, chills, or fever may begin as early as the second postdelivery day. Perineal discomfort or lower abdominal distress, nausea, and vomiting may soon develop. Foul or profuse lochia, hectic

Table 27.9
Maternal Infection: TORCH

Infection	Maternal Effects	Fetal or Neonatal Effects	Counseling: Prevention, Identification, and Management
Toxoplasmosis (protozoa)	Acute infection: similar to influenza; lymphadenopathy	With maternal acute infection: parasitemia Less likely to occur with maternal chronic infection Abortion likely with acute infection early in pregnancy (see Table 31.17)	Avoid eating raw meat and exposure to litter used by infected cats; if cats in house, have toxoplasma titer checked If titer is rising during early pregnancy, abortion may be given to the mother as an option
Other: Hepatitis A (virus)	Abortion—cause of liver failure during pregnancy	Exposure during first trimester; fetal anomalies; fetal or neonatal hepatitis; premature birth; intrauterine fetal death	Usually spread by droplet or hand contact especially by culinary workers; γ-globulin can be given as prophylaxis for hepatitis A
Hepatitis B (serum hepatitis) (virus)	May be transmitted sexually Symptomatology variable: fever, rash, ar1hralgia, depressed appetite, dyspepsia, abdominal pain, generalized aching, malaise, weakness, jaundice, tender and enlarged liver	Infection occurs during birth See Table 31.17 Maternal vaccination during pregnancy should present no risk for fetus; however, data are not available. See Chapter 31 for information about vaccination of children at risk for hepatitis B.	Generally passed by contaminated needles, syringes, or blood transfusions; can also be transmitted orally or by coitus, however, but incubation period is longer; hepatitis B immune globulin can be given prophylactically after exposure Hepatitis B vaccine recommended for populations at risk; vaccine consists of series of 3 IM doses Populations at risk: women from Asia, Pacific islands, Haiti, sub-Africa, Alaska (women of Eskimo descent) Other women at risk include health care providers
Rubella (3-day German measles, virus)	Rash, fever, mild symptoms; suboccipital lymph nodes may be swollen; some photophobia Occasionally arthritis or encephalitis Abortion	Incidence of congenital anomalies; first month, 50%; second month, 25%, third month, 10%, fourth month, 4% Exposure during first 2 months: malformations of heart, eyes, ears, or brain, abnormal dermatoglyphics Exposure after fourth month: systemic infection, hepatosplenomegaly, IUGR, rash At 15-20 years of age, may experience deterioration of intellect and development or develop epilepsy	Vaccination of pregnant women contraindicated, **pregnancy should be prevented for 2 months after vaccination;** hemagglutinin-inhibition-antigen-negative parturients can be safely vaccinated after delivery
Cytomegalovirus (CMV) (a herpes virus)	Respiratory or sexually transmitted asymptomatic illness or mononucleosis-like syndrome; may have cervical discharge	Fetal or neonatal death or severe, generalized disease—hemolytic anemia and jaundice; hydrocephaly or microcephaly; pneumonitis; hepatosplenomegaly	Virus may be reactivated and cause disease in utero or during delivery in subsequent pregnancies; fetal infection may occur during passage through infected birth canal; disease is frequently progressive through infancy and childhood
Herpes genitalis (herpex simplex virus; HSV II)—poses same threat to newborn as does HSV I	Symptomatology more pronounced with first infection; painful blisters that rupture, leaving shallow ulcers that crust over and disappear after 2-6 weeks; vaginal discharge if cervix or vaginal mucosa involved; fever, malaise, anorexia; painful inguinal lymphadenopathy	Abortion; premature birth Transplacental infection (rare): microcephaly; mental retardation; retinal dysplasia; patent ductus arteriosus; intracranial calcification; with intranatal infection, symptoms appear in 4-7 days: lethargy, poor feeding; jaundice; bleeding; pneumonia; convulsions; opisthotonus; bulging fontanels; skin, mouth lesions	If cervical lesions are acquired, infection initiates chain of events that leads to invasive carcinoma in middle age (cervical cells are more vulnerable just after puberty, when they change from columnar to squamous); age 17 years; frequency of intercourse, and number of different partners are factors.

Table 27.9, cont'd
Maternal Infection: TORCH

Infection	Maternal Effects	Fetal or Neonatal Effects	Counseling: Prevention, Identification, and Management
Scrapings of open lesions stained by Giemsa or other appropriate stain reveal intranuclear inclusion bodies (virus aggregations)	Ascending infection of fetus may occur from lesions in birth canal after rupture of fetal membranes; therefore abdominal delivery is indicated before rupture of membranes	Neonatal infection with disseminated disease results in 82% mortality; survivors suffer central nervous system (CNS) or ocular sequelae and face recurrence in first 5 years of life According to the CDC* (1986) substantial numbers of intrauterine or postpartum infections occur and cannot be prevented by cesarean delivery	Transmitted primarily by sexual contact but also possibly by fomites. Incubation period: 2-4 weeks. Remains in body cells indefinitely; therefore infection recurs throughout lifetime—triggered by infection, fever, menstruation, emotional upset; lies dormant in sensory nerve ganglia; more severe during pregnancy. **Drug therapy: acyclovir** (Zovirax) is first FDA drug approved for treatment of HSV II infection; effective in selected cases (see current literature); researchers are seeking a herpes vaccine. For symptomatic therapy, see Guidelines for Client Teaching, p. 805.

*Centers for Disease Control, Atlanta, Ga.

Table 27.10
Other Infections of the Vulva and Vagina

Clinical Situation	Clinical Symptoms and Gross Findings	Nursing Actions and Management
Vulvar dermatitis	Pain; pruritus; formication*; ulceration exudation	
Eczema	Moist dermatitis	Remove antigen or irritant
Psoriasis	Red, slightly elevated flat lesions (in body folds)	Dermatologist; topical steroid
Viral infections		
Herpes genitalis	See Table 27.9	
Herpes zoster (shingles)	Burning, pain, along sensory nerves	Analgesic, bed rest, compresses (Burrow's solution of aluminum acetate)
Warts (verruca vulgaris or plana)	On skin or mucosa	May not respond to treatment, surgery, cryotherapy
Other infections		
Impetigo—hemolytic *Staphylococcus aureus* or streptococcus	Pruritus, formication, vesicles and bullae	Isolate; topical antibiotic
Furunculosis—staphylococcus	Perifollicular abscesses, pain	Incision and drainage (I and D); isolate; systemic antibiotics
Erysipelas—β-hemolytic streptococcus	Red, raised, confluent induration; pain, fever, burning, aching, chronic exudative sores	Isolate; systemic antibiotics; hot, wet compresses (Burow's solution of aluminum acetate)
Tuberculosis—*Mycobacterium tuberculosis*		Systemic antituberculosis chemotherapy with vitamin B$_6$ replacement

*Abnormal skin sensation.

Table 27.11
Antimicrobial Therapy

Medication	Indications	Nursing Actions
Combination antibiotic therapy: penicillin, amnioglycosides (kanamycin or gentamicin and clindamycin)	Acute endometritis—most common: aerobic and anaerobic microorganisms	Counsel regarding administration of medications and need for follow-up: creatinine determination every 48 hours to assess for renal and ototoxicity.
Erythromycin	Penicillin-sensitive people; chlamydial infections	Assess for drug allergies.
Clindamycin IV	If above therapy is not effective	Assist with administration.
Procaine penicillin G with Probenecid, 1 g (0) to delay excretion of penicillin	Endometritis associated with gonorrhea	Assess for side effects.
Tetracyline (or, doxycycline)	Treat gonorrhea in penicillin-sensitive people *Chlamydia trachomatis; Mycoplasma hominis*	Counsel regarding prescribed treatment regimen, possible side effects, and necessity for prescribed follow-up, CBC, sedimentation rates,* endometrial or other specimen cultures, and biopsy as circumstances require.
Single broad-spectrum antibiotic (e.g., cephalothin)		If oral ingestion is prescribed for any antibiotic, suggest that client take acidophilus (Lactinex) to reduce or prevent the gastrointestinal upset that often accompanies antibiotic therapy.
γ-Benzene hexachloride 1% shampoo, cream or lotion	Lice infestation ("crabs") Pediculosis pubis *Phthirus pubis* (a parasite)	Counsel regarding transmission: direct contact with infected person; fomite spread: apart from human body (in clothes, linen) eggs may live 6 days; live, 24 hours partners and any or all family members must be involved with treatment. Counsel regarding therapy: remove all visible lice with medication ordered; massage cream or lotion over infected areas; leave on for 24 hours, then bathe; change clothing and linen; launder; kerosene—apply to infected area for 30 min; wash with soap and water.
γ-Benzene hexachloride 1%	Scabies *Sarcoptes scabiei* (a parasite)	Counsel regarding transmission: direct contact with infected person; all contacts require treatment. Counsel regarding therapy: apply for 3 consecutive nights, bathing between applications.

*Sedimentation rate determination is unreliable for differential diagnosis during pregnancy. During pregnancy the sedimentation rate is normally elevated.

fever, tachycardia, ileus, pelvic pain, and tenderness characterize critical puerperal sepsis. Without improvement, bacteremic shock or death may ensue.

Laboratory findings. Considerable **leukocytosis, a shift to the left** of the differential WBC count and a markedly increased red blood cell (RBC) sedimentation rate are typical of puerperal infections. Anemia, often an accompaniment, is evidenced by reduced RBC, hemoglobin, and hematocrit values. Intracervical or intrauterine bacterial cultures (aerobic and anerobic) should reveal the offending pathogens within 36 to 48 hours.

The physician must distinguish nongenital from genital sepsis. Mastitis, respiratory and urinary tract infections, and enteritis are considered in that order of probability.

Management. The most effective and cheapest treatment of puerperal infection is prevention. Preventive measures might include good prenatal nutrition to control anemia and intranatal control of hemorrhage. Good maternal hygiene is essential. Strict adherence by all medical personnel to the best aseptic techniques during the entire hospital and delivery period is mandatory. Coitus after rupture of membranes is contraindicated. Dystocia or prolonged labor should be avoided, especially after leaking of amniotic fluid.

Guidelines for Client Teaching

GENITAL HERPES

ASSESSMENT

Woman has genital herpes.

NURSING DIAGNOSES

Knowledge deficit related to symptomatic therapy for and prevention of recurrence of genital herpes.

Alterations in comfort: pain related to genital herpes.

GOALS

Short-term

Relief from discomfort.

Intermediate

Preventive measures are instituted.

Long-term

Recurrence of genital herpes does not occur.

REFERENCES AND TEACHING AIDS

Printed instructions

CONTENT/RATIONALE	TEACHING ACTION
Printed instructions provide information such as the following: ■ Take warm sitz bath for 15 minutes at a time with a drying agent such as Domeboro (two packets or tablets to a shallow tub of warm water) three to five times daily. Keep the genital area dry and clean. Drying the genital area with a blow dryer after showering is useful. ■ Avoid strong deodorant soaps, creams, and ointments. ■ Wash hands after using the toilet, and do not touch face after genital contact. Urinating through an empty toilet paper tube is helpful in preventing pain during urination. ■ Avoid *any* sexual contact during the entire time that lesions are present. Using condoms and spermicides will help prevent the spread of herpes. ■ Wear 100% cotton underwear. ■ Avoid tight-fitting jeans, pants, and pantyhose with nylon inserts. ■ Taking care of one's physical and mental health is important. Being run down makes the woman more vulnerable to infection. ■ Yearly Papanicolaou smears are advisable. ■ If the woman becomes pregnant, she should inform the physician that she has herpes.	Provide printed instructions. Encourage discussions of feelings regarding infection and its therapy. Describe purpose of each measure that ■ Provides comfort. ■ Prevents inoculation of self or other. ■ Prevents recurrence. ■ Screens for tissue dysplasia (Table 27.9).

EVALUATION The nurse can be assured that teaching was effective when the goals of care have been met.

Traumatic vaginal delivery must be avoided, blood loss replaced, and fluid-electrolyte balance maintained.

Infection measures for cure and comfort are instituted. Fluid and electrolyte balance is vital. Broad-spectrum antibiotics are administered intravenously until the infecting organism is identified. Then organism-specific antibiotic therapy is begun. The mother and infant are separated during the febrile period. Other members of the family are encouraged to nurture the newborn. The mother is positioned in high-Fowler's to facilitate gravity drainage of discharge from the uterus and vagina. Isolation protocol of the agency is warranted.

Surgical measures may be required. These include surgical procedures such as dilation and curettage (D & C) to remove the retained products of conception, hysterectomy (if the uterus is ruptured), colpotomy to drain a pelvic abscess or ligation or clipping of the vena cava and ovarian veins to prevent septic embolism.

The virulence of the organisms, the resistance of the woman, and her likely response to treatment are the intangibles of prognosis. Prevention, supportive therapy, and prompt massive antibiotic administration have reduced the maternal mortality in the United States to less than 0.4%. Regrettably, in underdeveloped countries the death rate may be more than 10 to 20 times this figure.

Toxic shock syndrome. Toxic shock syndrome (TSS) is a potentially life-threatening systemic disorder that has three principal clinical manifestations: **fever of sudden onset, hypotension,** and **rash.** The acute phase of TSS lasts about 4 to 5 days; the convalescent phase, about 1 to 2 weeks.

The Centers for Disease Control (1982) have established diagnostic criteria for TSS that include the above signs plus the following manifestations.

1. Involvement of three or more other organ systems:

System/Area	Manifestations
Gastrointestinal	Nausea; vomiting; diarrhea
Renal	Decreased urinary output; pyuria
Hepatic	Jaundice; abnormal values (increased transaminase)
CNS	Altered sensorium (decreased LOC); headache
Respiratory	Adult respiratory distress syndrome (ARDS)
Mucous membranes	Inflammation of vaginal, oropharyngeal, and conjunctival membranes
Muscular	Myalgia
Hematologic	Thrombocytopenia; disseminated intravascular coagulation (DIC)
Cardiac	Ischemic changes on ECG; decreased left ventricular contractility

2. Laboratory tests are *negative:* cultures of blood and cerebrospinal fluid; serologic tests for Rocky Mountain spotted fever, leptospirosis, measles.

A toxin (pyrogenic exotoxin C [PEC] or enterotoxin F) that is secreted by strains of *Staphylococcus aureus* is the causative factor in TSS. About 9% of women harbor the organism normally in their vaginas; about 1% to 5% of sexually active males have urethral cultures that are positive for *S. aureus* without having

---

Emergency Toxic Shock Syndrome

Signs
Fever of sudden onset: over 38.9° C (102° F)
Hypotension: systolic pressure under 90 mm Hg; orthostatic dizziness; disorientation
Rash: diffuse, macular erythrodema

First priority of therapy: Fluid resuscitation

---

the disease. Commonly associated conditions that may predispose the person to TSS by providing a portal of entry into systemic circulation include the following:

1. Menstruation
2. Puerperal endometritis
3. Incisional abscess
4. Soft tissue abscess
5. Skin infection following a bee sting
6. IV injection of heroin
7. Use of high-absorbency tampons or diaphragms
8. Neonatal infection concurrent with maternal infection.

The population at greatest risk is females between the ages of 15 and 24 who use tampons during menstruation.

Pathophysiology. The toxins may suppress synthesis of IgM antibodies. Toxin-induced injury to capillary endothelium alters capillary permeability. Fluid leaks out, and the volume of venous blood returning to the heart is diminished. Impaired tissue perfusion results in tissue hypoxia and renal and CNS abnormalities. Other problems arise from the toxin's direct damage to target organs. Tissue damage releases thromboplastin, which initiates the coagulation cascade. Thrombocytopenia and coagulopathy (for example, DIC) are potential hazardous sequelae. In some people, impaired tissue perfusion, with its sequelae, has resulted in loss of toes and fingers following gangrene.

Prognosis. Mortality is associated with TSS. In order of incidence the three causes of mortality are (1) ARDS (Adult respiratory distress syndrome [see Chapter 28]), (2) uncontrollable hypotension, and (3) DIC.

Although most affected women have an uneventful recovery with no recurrence, some suffer adverse sequelae. Infection is likely to recur, often with the next menstrual cycle. Recurrence is most likely if the woman had not been treated with beta lactamase-resistant antibiotics. Some women have persistent abnormalities in intellectual function. Persistent problems include impaired memory, concentration, and calculation, abnormal ECG, and impaired cerebellar function (hyperreflexia). For a few women sequelae are more serious. Impaired renal function, neuromuscular function (vocal cord paralysis), and peripheral perfusion, especially of the hands and feet may persist after the infection is cured.

Management. Early identification of TSS is essential so that appropriate therapy can be initiated. Nurses must be on the alert for this syndrome because of the increased likelihood of its occurrence in obstetric and gynecologic settings. Nursing actions for TSS are summarized in Procedure 27.1.

Procedure 27.1

NURSING CARE FOR TOXIC SHOCK SYNDROME

PURPOSE

Early identification and prompt treatment of TSS.
Prevention of complications of TSS and its therapy.
Teach mother self-care techniques.

EQUIPMENT

Equipment and infusates for initiating and monitoring
   parenteral therapy
Medications, as ordered
Materials for good oral hygiene
Oxygen
Restraints, as necessary
Antishock garments, as necessary

NURSING ACTION

Combat Hypotension and Maintain Blood Pressure

A. First priority: fluid resuscitation
1. Assist with the use of central venous pressure (CVP) or pulmonary artery wedge pressure (PAWP) balloon flotation catheter monitoring devices; assess MAP, pulse, jugular vein pulse, and urinary output.
2. Insert intravenous infusion line with a large bore needle; be prepared to administer fluids that may include packed red blood cells or coagulation factors, isotonic crystalloids (normal saline, lactated Ringer's solution), or colloids (plasmanate, salt-poor albumin).
3. Assess for signs of fluid overload: flushed skin, headache, increased pulse, venous distention, coughing (sign of pulmonary edema), and shortness of breath; if noted, change the infusion rate to "keep open" and place the person in high-Fowler's position immediately.
4. Assess for signs of fluid deficit: thready pulse, clammy skin, and increased capillary refilling time following pressure on nail beds; increase infusion rate.
5. Insert a urinary retention catheter to monitor output: oliguria, equal to input, greater than input.

6. If nausea and vomiting complicate therapy, a nasogastric tube and prochlorperazine (Compazine) are usually ordered.
   a. Provide good mouth care.

   b. Apply lidocaine (Xylocaine) or anesthetic spray.
   c. Provide hydrogen peroxide, sips of cold water, or ice chips, or apply petrolatum salve to lips.
   d. Apply nystatin (Mycostatin or Nilstat) to affected mucosa; the infection may occur on any mucosa—oropharyngeal, vaginal, or conjunctival.
B. Use antishock garments, per hospital protocol.

C. Institute vasopressor therapy.
1. Administer dopamine (IV) in low doses, per order.

RATIONALE

A. Combat hypotension.
1. Monitor intravenous fluid infusion. PAWP gives the mean arterial pressure (MAP).

2. In the event that blood or blood products must be used to treat coagulopathy.
Combat hypotension.

3. Fluid overload requires immediate therapy to correct the condition.

4. Combat hypotension.

5. Ensure accurate assessment of output; output below 20 ml/h may indicate impending kidney shutdown.
6. Prevent further disturbance of fluid and electrolyte balance.

   a. Prevent stomatitis that often accompanies TSS and the irritation that occurs from the nasogastric tube.
   b. Relieve oropharyngeal pain from dryness and NG tube irritation.
   c. Add to comfort by relieving dry mucosa and lip dryness.
   d. Prevent further debilitation; TSS and antibiotic therapy put the sufferer at great risk for fungal infection.

B. Used by some hospitals to help raise blood pressure until the fluid therapy is successful (Gunning, 1983).
C. Maintain blood pressure.
1. Dopamine has a weak beta-mimetic effect that increases myocardial contractility and heart rate without a disproportionate rise in myocardial oxygen consumption; dopamine also exerts a vasoconstrictive action on skeletal muscle.

Continued.

Procedure 27.1—cont'd

NURSING ACTION	RATIONALE
2. Administer naloxone (Narcan), per order.	2. Naloxone is used to counter the effect of stress-induced elevated levels of endorphins that depress the cardiovascular system and lower blood pressure.

Cure Infection

A. Per order, administer beta lactamase-resistant antibiotics such as methicillin (Staphcillin), nafcillin (Nafcil, Unipen), and oxacillin (Prostaphlin). In penicillin-sensitive persons the following drugs are used: vancomycin HCl (Vancocin), gentamicin SO₄ (Garamycin, Gentamicin), and clindamycin HCl (Cleocin).

A. Effective against the staphylococcal organism only; there is no effect on the toxins already in the bloodstream; most *S. aureus* strains are penicillin-resistant. Prevents anaphylactic shock secondary to penicillin sensitivity (allergy).

B. Assist with surgical intervention for the removal of infection (drainage of an abscess, removal of fetus in a septic pregnancy [septic abortion]).

B. Removes causative factor.

Prevent ARDS

Represents one cause of mortality.

A. Administer oxygen with mechanical ventilation as necessary and monitor by arterial blood gases (ABGs).

A. Meets oxygenation needs.

B. Prevent fluid overload and shock lung.

B. Increases risk for and severity of ARDS.

Ensure Safety

A. Provide appropriate restraints or constant bedside attendance.

A. May be necessary to prevent injury from falls, pulling out IV lines, etc.; confusion, combativeness, and restlessness characterize the acute phase of this disorder.

B. Reposition the woman frequently and encourage to cough and breathe deeply as often as possible.

B. Prevent problems of immobility—pneumonia, thrombus formation, and embolism.

Plan for Discharge

Prevent recurrence through:

A. If woman had experienced menstruation-related TSS:
  1. Instruct about good hygiene practices, such as washing hands before inserting tampons and changing tampons frequently.
  2. Caution against the use of tampons for at least 3 months or until cultures for *S. aureus* are negative.
  3. Advise regarding use of tampons:
    a. Use tampons only during the period of heavy flow, changing tampons at least every 1 to 4 hours.
    b. During time of moderate flow, use tampons during the day and pads at night, changing them every 4 to 8 hours.
    c. During the period of light flow, use pads only.
B. If the woman has never had TSS:
  1. Counsel to use tampons during the period of heavy and moderate flow and to change them according to the schedule already noted.
  2. During light flow, use tampons or pads during the day and pads at night.
  3. Caution all women against using high-absorbency tampons at any time.

A. Avoiding predisposing conditions.
B. Using good hygiene practices.

High-absorbency tampons and the diaphragm are thought to provide a portal of entry by causing microulcerations in the vaginal mucosa. In addition, superabsorbent tampons contain more oxygen and are retained for a longer time than less absorbent tampons.

Mastitis. Mastitis, or breast infection, affects about 1% of recently delivered women, most of whom are primiparas who are nursing. Mastitis is almost always unilateral and develops well after the flow of milk has been established. The infecting organism generally is the hemolytic *Staphylococcus aureus*. An infected nipple fissure usually is the initial lesion, but the ductal system is involved next. Inflammatory edema and engorgement of the breasts soon obstruct the flow of milk in a lobe; regional, then generalized mastitis follows. If prompt resolution of the septic process does not occur, a breast abscess is virtually inevitable.

Chills, fever, malaise, and local breast tenderness are noted first. Eventual localization of sepsis and axillary adenopathy are delayed developments.

Intensive antibiotic therapy (such as cephalosporin and vancomycin, which are particularly useful in staphylococcal infections), support of breasts, local heat (or cold), and analgesics are required. Lactation is maintained (if desired) by emptying the breasts every 4 hours by manual expression or breast pump. If an abscess develops, wide incision and drainage must be effected. Most women respond to treatment, and an abscess can be prevented.

Almost all instances of acute mastitis can be avoided by proper nursing technique (see Chapter 21) to prevent cracked nipples. Missed feedings, waiting too long between feedings, and abrupt weaning may lead to clogged nipples and mastitis. Cleanliness practiced by all who have contact with the newborn and new mother also reduces the incidence of mastitis.

Urinary tract infections. Postdelivery urinary tract infections (UTIs) are usually caused by coliform bacteria. UTIs are common because of trauma to the base of the bladder and urethra and catheterization during or after labor.

Suprapubic or costovertebral angle pain, fever, urinary retention, hematuria, dysuria, or urinary frequency often signifies urinary tract infection. This symptomatology indicates the need for urinalysis, urine culture, bacterial sensitivity tests, and probable wide-spectrum antibiotic therapy. Substitution of a specific antibacterial drug must await an assessment of the woman's history, response to initial therapy, and the sensitivity report.

Prompt treatment of definite urinary tract infections is indicated. However, prophylactic therapy rarely is warranted. Most cases yield to treatment within a week. Urologic consultation is indicated if symptoms persist. Prevention of recurrence of UTI is an important part of therapy. See Chapter 11 for information on teaching UTI prevention.

Vaginal infections. Any irritating vaginal discharge should be evaluated promptly and appropriate treatment initiated immediately for maternal and fetal well-being.

Management of vaginal infections becomes more complicated if multiple organisms or agents are involved. Pediculosis pubis, threadworm, varicosities, and allergic response to perineal deodorants may obstruct the differential diagnosis and management. The discomforts imposed by these conditions challenge the woman's emotional as well as her physical well-being.

Infections must be distinguished from the normal vaginal discharge, leukorrhea. *Leukorrhea* is a whitish discharge. It consists of mucus and exfoliated vaginal epithelial cells secondary to hyperplasia of the vaginal mucosa such as occurs during pregnancy, at the time of ovulation, and just before menstruation. If it is copious, it can cause discomfort from maceration.

Vaginal infections may be sexually transmitted. *Trichomonas vaginitis* and *monilial vaginitis* are considered to be sexually transmitted in most, but not all cases. Simple vaginitis may be attributed to faulty hygiene, tight clothing, or emotional stress.

Simple vaginitis. Infectious organisms such as *Escherichia coli*, staphylococci, and streptococci change the normal acidity of the vagina. A pH of 3.5 to 4.5 is needed to support Döderlein's bacilli, the vagina's main line of defense. The proximity of the urethra to the vagina predisposes the woman with vaginitis to a concurrent urethritis.

Burning, pruritus (itching), redness, and edema of surrounding tissues are characteristic of simple vaginitis. The symptoms are particularly discomforting during voiding and defecating.

Objectives of management of simple vaginitis are to relieve discomfort, to foster growth of Döderlein's bacilli, to eradicate offending organisms, and to prevent recurrence. Interventions include the following:

1. Maintain scrupulous cleanliness, especially after elimination.
2. Douche with a weakly acid solution such as 15 ml (1 tbsp) white vinegar to 1000 ml (1 qt) water.
3. Insert a β-lactose suppository (to enhance growth of Döderlein's bacilli).
4. Observe chemotherapy regimen specific for organisms by inserting suppository into the vagina with an applicator or applying cream locally to the area as directed.

Atrophic vaginitis. Low estrogen levels, such as that which occurs during preadolescence and lactation and after menopause, result in a thin vaginal lining. Infection may occur from the normal vaginal flora. Antibiotics and hormone replacement therapy comprise this therapy.

Cervicitis. Abnormal discharge may be caused by an infection of the cervix and not to vaginitis. Spotting of blood between periods or after intercourse, and cramping during intercourse are characteristic. Sexually transmitted gonorrhea, chlamydia, trichomoniasis or, herpetic infections are the usual infection implicated. Therapy is specific to the causative microbe.

Monilial vaginitis. Candida albicans, a fungus (yeast) normally found in the intestinal tract, contaminates and infects the vagina. Infection with *C. albicans* is also known as moniliasis, thrush, or candidiasis. This infection is seen commonly in women with poorly controlled diabetes mellitus, since the organism thrives in a carbohydrate-rich milieu. Antibiotic or steroid therapy may be a causative factor by reducing the number of Döderlein's bacilli. Döderlein's bacilli help to maintain an acidic pH.

The thick vaginal discharge is irritating and pruritic. Frequently dysuria and dyspareunia are common complaints. Speculum examination reveals thick, white, tenacious cheeselike patches adhering to the pale, dry and sometimes cyanotic vaginal mucosa.

Objectives of treatment are the same as for simple vaginitis with one exception: women with recurrent infection should be checked for diabetes mellitus, and control of diabetes should be instituted if required (see Chapter 28).

Candida albicans also causes thrush in the newborn. Infection may occur by direct contact with an infected birth canal or from the contaminated hands of those who take care of the infant.

Guidelines for Client Teaching

MONILIAL INFECTIONS

ASSESSMENT
Woman has been diagnosed as having a monilial vaginal infection.

NURSING DIAGNOSES
Knowledge deficit related to care and prevention of monilial vaginal infection

GOALS
Short-term
Woman verbalizes understanding of measures to care for and prevent monilial vaginal infections.

Intermediate
Woman implements measures to care for present monilial infection.
Infection is cured.

Long-term
Woman does not have a recurrence of monilial vaginal infection.

REFERENCES AND TEACHING AIDS
Printed instructions

CONTENT/RATIONALE

Causative agent: *Candida albicans*
Predisposing and aggravating conditions
Prescribed therapy for this episode:
1. Maintain scrupulous cleanliness, especially after elimination.
2. Observe chemotherapy regimen; for example:
   a. Clotrimazole (Gyne-lotrimin). Use as directed.
   b. Nystatin (Mycostatin) vaginal tablets, 100,000 units twice each day for 14 days, or suppositories, 0.5 g twice each day for 10 days, should be inserted.
   c. Gentian violet (2%) swabs may be administered to the vaginal mucosa with an applicator every 2 to 3 days until the vaginitis is cured. (The woman should wear a perineal pad to prevent permanent staining of clothing.)
3. Abstain from intercourse or use a condom until the infection is cured.
4. Gently bathe the vulva with a weak solution of sodium bicarbonate to relieve discomfort.

TEACHING ACTION

Determine woman's knowledge of condition.
Discuss feelings about having the infection.
Identify emotional stressors that may predispose to or aggravate the condition.
Review diet (e.g., sugar intake), hygiene, preference for type of clothing.
Determine her knowledge of need to include sexual partner; discuss partner's willingness to comply.

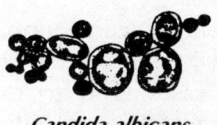

Candida albicans

EVALUATION The nurse can be assured that teaching was effective if the goals for care have been met.

Trichomonas vaginitis. *Trichomonas vaginalis* (trichomoniasis) is a hearty protozoan that thrives in an alkaline milieu. Of all pregnant women, 20% to 30% harbor this organism, usually with no symptoms. In symptom-free individuals, the infection may be identified during a routine examination or with a Papanicolaou smear.

The profuse, bubbly (foamy), white leukorrhea characteristic of this infection causes irritation, hyperemia, edema of the vulva, and dyspareunia (painful intercourse). Urinary frequency and dysuria may occur.

In the male partner the protozoan may be harbored in the urogenital tract (without symptoms) and remain a source of reinfection for his mate.

Guidelines for Client Teaching are presented below.

Vaginal douche. A vaginal douche is used to cleanse the vagina and to apply local medication or heat (Fig. 27.4 and p. 812).*

---

*Douching is not recommended during pregnancy.

Guidelines for Client Teaching

TRICHOMONAL INFECTION

ASSESSMENT
Woman has been diagnosed as having a trichomonal vaginal infection.

NURSING DIAGNOSIS
Knowledge deficit related to care and prevention of trichomonal vaginal infections

GOALS
Short-term
Woman verbalizes understanding of measures to care for and prevent trichomonal vaginal infections.

Intermediate
Woman implements measures to care for present trichomonal vaginal infection.
Infection is cured.

Long-term
Woman does not have a recurrence of trichomonal vaginal infection.

REFERENCES AND TEACHING AIDS
Printed instructions

CONTENT/RATIONALE

Causative agent: *Trichomonas vaginalis*
A. Predisposing and aggravating conditions
B. Prescribed therapy for this episode:
  1. Maintain scrupulous cleanliness, especially after elimination.
  2. Douche with a weak acid solution (the same as for simple vaginitis).
  3. Observe chemotherapy regimen as follows:
    a. Metronidazole (Flagyl), one dose of 2 g (Metronidazole is contraindicated during the first half of gestation even though there is no evidence of fetotoxicity.)
    b. If metronidazole is not well tolerated by mouth, vaginal suppositories such as furazolidone (Tricofuron) or Vagisec should be used.
    c. To prevent ping-pong reinfection, the male partner should be treated with metronidazole and informed that intercourse should be avoided until the infection is cured.
C. Relief should be noted in 1 to 2 weeks. Rarely is a second course of treatment necessary.

TEACHING ACTION

Determine woman's knowledge of condition.
Discuss feelings about having the infection.
Identify emotional stressors that may predispose to or aggravate the condition.
Review hygiene, preference for type of clothing.
Determine her knowledge of need to include sexual partner; discuss partner's willingness to comply.

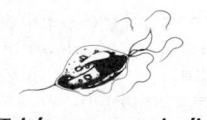

Trichomonas vaginalis

EVALUATION The nurse can be assured that teaching was effective if the goals for care have been met.

Guidelines for Client Teaching

VAGINAL DOUCHING

ASSESSMENT

Vaginal douching has been prescribed by the physician.

NURSING DIAGNOSIS

Knowledge deficit related to vaginal douching.

GOALS
Short-term

Woman verbalizes understanding of vaginal douching.

Intermediate

Woman implements vaginal douching per physician's orders.

Infection is cured.

Long-term

Woman does not have recurrence of condition that required vaginal douching.

REFERENCES AND TEACHING AIDS

Printed instructions
Douche equipment

CONTENT/RATIONALE

A. Reasons for douching
B. Method of douching safely:
   1. Void and wash hands before douching.
   2. Use the following position:
      a. The optimal position is semirecumbent in a clean tub (after a bath) or in bed. A douche pan may be used in the tub as well.
      b. The woman can douche while seated on the toilet; however, the labia should be held together to permit solution to fill the entire vaginal vault.
   3. Prepare solution. The temperature should be 40° to 43° C (105° to 110° F), comfortably warm to the inner aspect of the wrist. Allow some solution to flow out of nozzle to lubricate tip, or lubricate with K-Y jelly or other water-soluble lubricant.
   4. Hold or place solution container 60 cm (2 ft) above the hips (avoid greater heights, which increase the pressure of the flow). Do *not* use a bulb syringe; water or air embolus and death may ensue.
   5. Insert nozzle upward and backward for 7.6 cm (3 in).
      a. Rotate nozzle so that fluid flushes entire mucosa, including that of the posterior fornix. Rotation of nozzle also reduces the chance of forcing fluid into the cervix.
      b. When douching seated on a toilet, hold labia together to fill vaginal vault, then allow fluid to exit rapidly to flush out debris. Repeat until solution is used up.
      c. Hold labia together for specified period of time if the objective of the douche is to expose the mucosa to medication or moist heat.
   6. If the woman is in the semirecumbent position for douching, sitting up and leaning forward aid in emptying the vagina.
   7. Wash douche equipment with warm soap and water, dry, and store in well-ventilated place away from extremes of temperature.
   8. Wash hands!

TEACHING ACTION

Demonstrate technique to woman.
Watch woman give a return demonstration.
Read over instructions on package of douche medication, answer questions, clarify, etc.
Discuss how she will implement method at home; for example, does she have a bathtub, storage space for equipment?

Fig. 27.4
Vaginal douche should be done with woman lying in bathtub. Douche pan may be placed under woman if desired. Douching is not recommended during pregancy.

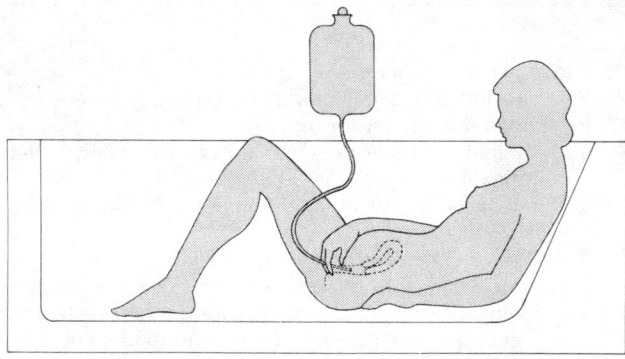

EVALUATION The nurse can be assured that teaching was effective when the goals of care have been met.

Bacteremic shock. Critical infections, particularly by bacteria that liberate endotoxin, such as enteric gram-negative bacilli, may cause bacteremic (septic) shock. Pregnant women, especially those with diabetes mellitus, or women who are receiving immunosuppressive drugs are at increased risk of having this disorder.

High spiking fever and chills are evidence of serious sepsis. Anxiety is followed by apathy. Concomitantly the temperature often falls to slightly subnormal levels. The skin then becomes pale, cool, and moist. The pulse will be rapid and thready. Marked hypotension and peripheral cyanosis develop. Oliguria occurs.

Laboratory studies reveal marked evidence of infection (blood culture may reveal bacteremia later). Hemoconcentration, acidosis, and DIC may develop. Central venous pressure (CVP) generally is low. Electrocardiogram (ECG) may reveal changes indicative of myocardial insufficiency. Evidence of cardiac, pulmonary, and renal failure will be notable. Hypoxia is the major problem, however. Hypoxia is especially noxious to the CNS, myocardium, and lungs.

The physician will initiate antishock therapy. Massive doses of antibiotics and corticosteroids are given intravenously if possible. The woman may be given digitalis. Heart function and urinary output are monitored closely. The infected area is drained or the focus of infection is removed (for example, by hysterectomy or abortion) if the woman's condition will permit.

Prompt diagnosis and intensive treatment afford a fairly good prognosis. Encouraging signs include increasing alertness and the establishment of good urinary flow.

Summary. Infections during the childbearing cycle are potentially hazardous to the fetus or newborn. The discomfort of the infections compromise the woman's ability to meet the physical and emotional demands during this time. The knowledgeable nurse can help the woman prevent or treat infections successfully. Overall therapeutic measures include educating the general public regarding immunization for nonimmune people. Many states are introducing or passing laws requiring screening for rubella titer. Tests for exposure to syphilis are routine. Easily accessible and person-oriented (nonjudgmental) clinics should be available to all, so that people are encouraged to use them for diagnosis and treatment.

Summary of Nursing Actions

NURSING CARE FOR MATERNAL INFECTIONS

GOALS

1. For the mother: freedom from infection.
2. For the fetus and newborn: freedom from infection and the adverse effects of infection on fetal development and neonatal well-being.
3. For the family: knowledge of methods to avoid infection and to treat it appropriately if infection occurs.

PRIORITIES

1. Prompt identification of infection and initiation of therapy.
2. Education of the woman and her family for the prevention of infection.
3. Encouragement of self-care.

ASSESSMENT	EXAMPLES OF POTENTIAL NURSING DIAGNOSTIC CATEGORIES
PRENATAL **Interview** A. General malaise, fever, rashes, gland enlargement, etc. B. History of UTIs, vaginal infections C. Population at risk **Physical examination** A. Fever B. General affect C. Signs and symptoms of infection **Laboratory tests** A. Urinalysis B. Blood tests: Hgb, HCT, antibody titers, syphilis, AIDS, diabetes C. Cultures: gonorrhea, etc.	Knowledge deficit Potential for injury Noncompliance Potential disturbance in family process related to interruption of sexual relations Spiritual distress Disturbance in self-concept: body images, self-esteem, role performance, personal identity Anxiety Fear Alteration in patterns of urinary elimination

Continued.

Summary of Nursing Actions—cont'd

ASSESSMENT	EXAMPLES OF POTENTIAL NURSING DIAGNOSTIC CATEGORIES
POSTNATAL **Record, interview** A. Prenatal data B. Intrapartal data **Physical examination** A. Newborn: assess for symptomatology of infection (Chapter 31) B. Mother: vital signs, general affect, malaise, rash, gland enlargement; redness, tenderness, warmth, pain over a specific area **Laboratory tests** A. Cultures of any exudate B. Blood tests for infection C. Urinalysis	Knowledge deficit Potential for injury Potential alteration in parenting related to infection Alteration in patterns of urinary elimination

OUTCOME CRITERIA*	PLAN/IMPLEMENTATION
Infection is prevented. Infection is treated promptly with no or minimal sequelae for mother and infant. Parent or parents learn about prevention, identification, and management of infection.	**PRENATAL** Viral infections are treated symptomatically. Prophylactic antibiotic therapy may be instituted to prevent secondary infection. If woman is to be treated at home, assist her and family in planning how she will implement prescribed care. Assist physician and support woman and family during tests and when hearing results. Assist with counseling before proposed therapeutic abortion. If genital lesions are found (herpesvirus type 2) prepare woman for elective cesarean delivery. Isolation techniques (institute and prepare woman for this situation). Reinforce physician's explanations of cause, management, possible outcomes. General care: ■ Adequate hydration. ■ Rest. ■ Adherence to medication regimen (if on oral antibiotics, woman may prevent gastrointestinal upset by taking Lactinex or eating yogurt between doses). ■ Temperature should be kept down with acetaminophen (Tylenol), fluids, cool sponge baths. **POSTNATAL** Provide nursing-medical care for high-risk infant (Chapter 31). Isolate infant and mother if indicated. Assist woman and family with grieving if indicated. Ensure bed rest and proper diet. Answer questions regarding infection, cause, management, expected prognosis.

EVALUATION The nurse can be assured that care was effective if the goals of care have been met.

*Outcome criteria direct the selection of nursing actions (**plan/implementation**) and measure their effectiveness (**evaluation**).

Maternal Hemorrhage

Hemorrhagic disorders in pregnancy are medical emergencies. They require expert teamwork on the part of physician and nurse to minimize the deleterious effects.

The nurse must be alert to the symptoms of hemorrhage and shock and be prepared to obtain necessary blood replacement and complete laboratory orders. (If there is no time for typing and matching of blood, group O Rh-negative blood may be ordered.) The pregnant woman and her family need much supportive care during these times of stress. Support includes prompt attention to needs, competent technical care, and information regarding the rationale for care and the progress of treatment. The woman's inability to carry a pregnancy to term or to maintain a normal sequence of development to delivery often causes her to question her femininity and capabilities as a woman.

Early in pregnancy, abortion or ectopic pregnancy is the most common cause of excessive bleeding. Later, premature separation of the normally implanted placenta or placenta previa may be the cause of hemorrhage.

Postdelivery hemorrhage is a possibility during any childbirth experience. Specific problems that result in hemorrhage are uterine atony, lacerations of the birth canal, hematomas, episiotomy dehiscence, retained placenta, inversion of the uterus, and subinvolution of the uterus. Postdelivery anterior pituitary necrosis (Sheehan's syndrome) secondary to hypovolemic shock is also discussed.

Summaries of nursing actions for various hemorrhagic conditions have been developed and follow the discussion of each condition. However, several nursing actions are common to all of the hemorrhagic conditions. Discussion of hemorrhagic conditions follows the definition of terms and a summary of general nursing care of pregnancy-related hemorrhage.

DEFINITIONS

benign Noncancerous; not an immediate threat. Compare with malignant.

cerclage Band of homologous fascia, or nonabsorbable ribbon (Mersilene), placed around the cervix beneath the mucosa to constrict the cervix near the internal os.

choriocarcinoma Malignancy (cancer) that develops from the chorionic portion of the products of conception (placenta).

Cullen's sign An ecchymotic blueness of the umbilicus that is indicative of hematoperitoneum. Bleeding into the peritoneum may occur in a neglected ruptured intraabdominal ectopic pregnancy.

dissemination Spreading throughout the body; generalization.

ectopic Situated in an unusual place, away from its normal location.

incompetent cervix Condition characterized by dilatation of the cervical os of the uterus before term without labor or contractions of the uterus.

malignant Virulent; tending to become worse and cause death. Descriptive of cancer.

metastatic Pathologic process by which a tumor is spread to distant parts of the body.

referred pain Pain felt at a site different from that of an injured or diseased organ or part of the body.

spontaneous abortion A termination of pregnancy before the twentieth week of gestation as a result of abnormalities of the conceptus or maternal environment. Compare with induced abortion.

trophoblastic disease A malignant neoplastic disease of the uterus derived from the chorion of the placenta, characterized by a high level of human chorionic gonadotropin (HCG).

recurrent (habitual) spontaneous abortion The loss of three or more previable pregnancies.

uterine lithopedion ("womb stone") Failure to abort a pregnancy after the embryo or fetus has died; missed abortion. A missed abortion that is retained for months or years, during which time the products of conception have calcified.

GENERAL NURSING CARE OF PREGNANCY-RELATED HEMORRHAGE

GOALS

1. For the mother: A physiologically and emotionally safe experience.
2. For the lost embryo: Baptism, as necessary.
3. For the viable fetus: A safe passage from intrauterine to extrauterine existence as close to term gestation as possible.
4. For the family: Successful coping with the experience.

PRIORITIES

1. Identify hemorrhage and treat appropriately.
   a. Replace blood, blood products, fluids, and electrolytes immediately.
   b. Monitor therapy carefully to prevent complications such as fluid overload, shock lung.
   c. Correct the underlying problem.
2. Manage discomfort:
   a. Administer analgesics per physician's orders.
   b. Keep woman informed regarding her condition and its management.
3. Provide emotional support:
   a. Implement care for individuals experiencing loss (Chapter 26).
   b. Keep woman and family informed.
   c. Summon clergy or other support persons per woman's or family's request.

ASSESSMENT

Interview

A. Time in childbearing cycle:
   1. Prenatal: duration since LMP.
   2. Postnatal: duration since delivery.
B. Events preceding symptomatology, e.g., falls, vaginal examination, coitus; childbirth.
C. Previous obstetric history: past, current.
D. Amount of bleeding, presence and size of clots.
E. Associated discomfort: amount and location, e.g., uterine, referred pain, bladder.
F. Passage of tissue.

Physical examination

A. Vital signs and blood pressure.
B. Affect/LOC, e.g., anxious, agitated, uncomfortable, dull.
C. Tenderness, e.g., uterine, abdominal, cervical, perineal.
D. Integument, e.g., color, warmth, moisture, turgor.

Laboratory tests

A. Blood
   1. Rh and blood group; type and cross match as necessary
   2. Hgb, HCT
   3. CBC: WBC, platelets
B. Urine
   1. Pregnancy test, e.g., if woman is suspected of being in early pregnancy
   2. UTI
C. Chest x-ray: if extrapelvic infection is suspected, or if surgery is anticipated

EXAMPLES OF POTENTIAL NURSING DIAGNOSTIC CATEGORIES

Hemorrhage
Potential for infection
Anxiety
Fear
Alteration in cardiac output decreased
Alteration in comfort: pain
Ineffective individual or family coping
Fluid volume deficit secondary to hemorrhage
Alteration in fluid volume: excess secondary to blood and fluid replacement therapy
Grieving
Potential for injury
Knowledge deficit
Powerlessness
Impaired gas exchange secondary to hemorrhage or its therapy
Spiritual distress
Alteration in tissue perfusion, secondary to hemorrhage
Potential for impaired home maintenance management
Disturbance in self-concept: body image, self-esteem, role performance, personal identity

Summary of Nursing Actions—cont'd

OUTCOME CRITERIA*	PLAN/IMPLEMENTATION

Condition is identified promptly, and appropriate therapy is instituted.
Blood loss is minimized.
    Vital signs and BP remain within normal limits.
    DIC does not occur.
    Complications of blood, fluid, and electrolyte replacement are averted.
    Fluid-electrolyte balance is maintained.
    Woman's reproductive capability is maintained.
    Surgical intervention is successful with no adverse sequelae.
    Comfort is maximized.
Woman and family come to terms with loss in a positive manner (Chapter 26).
    Guilt or blame is averted.
    Self-concept is not disturbed.
    Spiritual distress is averted.
    Sense of power is retained, e.g., participates in own care.
Woman and family verbalize understanding of the condition and its management.
Knowledge needs are met.
	Implement nurse's roles as:
	
	Technician
	Report and record findings promptly.
	Save all peripads, linens soaked with blood, clots, and tissue.
	Obtain specimen collection, e.g., blood, urine, culture.
	Administer medications, as ordered, e.g., analgesics, oxytocics, antibiotics.
	Start IV infusion using large bore needle in the event blood transfusion is needed.
	Monitor vital signs, BP, LOC, CVP, integument.
	Insert retention urinary catheter.
	Provide pre- and postoperative care as needed.
	Hang appropriate blood product.
	
	Support person
	Implement care for woman and family experiencing loss (Chapter 26).
	If possible, give couples opportunity to see fetus or inform them of sex.
	Explain procedure, sensations, expected outcomes; answer questions.
	Assist woman and family with emotional reactions.
	Involve family in planning and care.
	Baptize products of conception or newborn, or summon clergy.
	
	Teacher/counselor/advocate
	Carefully explain known etiologies, management, and expected outcomes.
	Counsel regarding antibiotic therapy.
	Assist with identifying questions for the physician.
	Refer for social services, e.g., home health care, homemaker service, etc.
	Counsel regarding nutrition to prevent anemia.
	Teach woman about danger signs and symptoms (bleeding, fever, cramping, pain) and whom to call should they occur.
	Provide information regarding contraceptives as appropriate.

EVALUATION The nurse can be assured that nursing care was effective when the goals for care have been met.

*Outcome criteria direct the selection of nursing actions (**plan/implementation**) and measure their effectiveness (**evaluation**).

EARLY PREGNANCY

Spontaneous abortion. Abortion is the termination of pregnancy before viability of the fetus. The abortion may be spontaneous, resulting from natural causes, or the pregnancy may be interrupted deliberately for medical reasons (therapeutic abortion) or for social reasons (elective abortion) (see Chapter 7).

Viability is reached at about 24 weeks' gestation, when the fetus weighs 600 g or more. With excellent newborn care, such an infant has at least a chance to survive. An **early spontaneous abortion,** or miscarriage, is one that occurs before 16 weeks' gestation; a **late abortion** is one occurring between 16 and 24 weeks' gestation. About three fourths of these abortions occur before the sixteenth week of pregnancy, and the majority of these take place before the eighth week. More than half of all spontaneous abortions are caused by fetoplacental development defects. Most of the other spontaneous abortions result from maternal causes; the reasons for the remainder are speculative. Many very early pregnancies are lost for unknown reasons before the diagnosis of pregnancy is even made. The diagnosis of the type of abortion a woman is experiencing is based on the signs and symptoms present (Table 27.12).

Little can be done to avoid genetic causes of pregnancy loss, but prepregnancy correction of maternal disorders, immunization against infectious diseases, proper early prenatal care, and treatment of pregnancy complications will do much to prevent abortion. Cervical incompetence, a cause of second-trimester abortion, can be surgically corrected before or even during pregnancy in the majority of cases.

Management (Table 27.13) depends on the classification of spontaneous abortion. Therefore an early accurate diagnosis of spontaneous abortion is vital.

A summary of nursing actions for the woman and family experiencing spontaneous abortion, recurrent abortion, or incompetent cervix begins on p. 819.

Ectopic pregnancy. Ectopic pregnancy is one in which the fetus is implanted outside the uterine cavity (Fig. 27.6). The vast majority (90%) of ectopic pregnancies occur in the uterine (fallopian) tube, most of these on the right side, for undetermined reasons. Approximately 1 of every 200 pregnancies is ectopic. At least three fourths of ectopic pregnancies become

Table 27.12
Assessing Abortion

Type of Abortion	Amount of Bleeding	Uterine Cramping	Passage of Tissue	Tissue in Vagina	Internal Cervical Os	Size of Uterus
Threatened	Slight	Mild	No	No	Closed	Agrees with length of pregnancy
Inevitable	Moderate	Moderate	No	No	Open	Agrees with length of pregnancy
Incomplete	Heavy	Severe	Yes	Possible	Open with tissue in cervix	Smaller than expected for length of pregnancy
Complete	Slight	Mild	Yes	Possible	Closed	Smaller than expected for length of pregnancy
Septic	Varies; usually malodorous; fever present	Varies; fever present	Varies; fever present	Varies; fever present	Usually open; fever present	Any of the above with tenderness
Missed	Slight	No	No	No	Closed	Smaller than expected for length of pregnancy

From Gordon, R.T.: Emergencies in obstetrics and gynecology. In Warner, C.G., editor: Emergency care: assessment and intervention, ed. 3, St. Louis, 1983, The C.V. Mosby Co.

Table 27.13
Types of Spontaneous Abortion and Usual Management

Type of Abortion	Management
Threatened	Bed rest, sedation, and avoidance of stress and orgasm are recommended. Further treatment will depend on client's course.
Inevitable and incomplete	Prompt termination of pregnancy is accomplished usually by dilation and curettage (D & C).*
Complete	No further intervention may be needed if uterine contractions are adequate to prevent hemorrhage and if there is no infection.
Septic	Immediate termination of pregnancy by method appropriate to duration of pregnancy (see Table 7.12). Cervical cultures and sensitivity studies are done and broad-spectrum antibiotic therapy (e.g., ampicillin) is started. Treatment for septic shock is initiated if necessary.
Missed	If spontaneous evacuation of the uterus does not occur within 1 month, however, pregnancy is terminated by method appropriate to duration of pregnancy (see Table 7.12). Blood clotting factors are monitored until uterus is empty. Disseminated intravascular coagulation (DIC) and incoagulability of blood with uncontrolled hemorrhage may develop in cases of fetal death after twelfth week if products of conception are retained for longer than 5 weeks (see pp. 835 to 838 for discussion of DIC).

*For a discussion of dilation and curettage, see Chapter 7.

Summary of Nursing Actions

SPONTANEOUS ABORTION, RECURRENT ABORTION, AND INCOMPETENT CERVIX*

GOALS

1. For the mother: Prevent or control hemorrhage and provide appropriate therapy.
2. For the fetus or newborn: Sustain the pregnancy if possible or feasible, or treat the compromised infant, whether preterm or full term.
3. For the family: Help family manage grief resulting from the loss of the infant or mother.

PRIORITIES

1. Establish the diagnosis.
2. Prevent hypovolemia and hemorrhagic shock.
3. Institute appropriate therapy for the specific diagnosis.

ASSESSMENT	EXAMPLES OF POTENTIAL NURSING DIAGNOSTIC CATEGORIES
SPONTANEOUS ABORTION A. Vital signs and blood pressure. B. Symptomatology of hemorrhagic shock: skin color, warmth, and moisture; LOC. C. Uterine cramping D. Passage of tissue E. Counseling needed regarding etiology and management. F. Blood tests for blood group, Rh, Hgb, HCT, CBC (WBCs, platelets). G. Urine tests for pregnancy, evidence of infection.	Hemorrhage† Alteration in comfort: pain Anxiety Fear Grieving Potential for infection Powerlessness Spiritual distress Potential for disturbance in self-concept: body image, self-esteem, role performance, personal identity Potential for injury related to surgical interventions, septicemia, or septic emboli Potential for infertility†, related to septic abortion

OUTCOME CRITERIA‡	PLAN/IMPLEMENTATION
Pregnancy is saved. Comfort is maximized. If pregnancy is lost: ■ Uterus is emptied completely spontaneously or by D & C. ■ No hemorrhage occurs. ■ No sepsis occurs. ■ Woman and family come to terms with loss (Chapter 26). Physiologic condition remains stable: ■ Vital signs and BP remain stable within normal limits. ■ Blood loss is minimized. ■ Fluid-electrolyte balance is maintained.	Implement nursing actions relevant to type and usual management of abortion (Table 27.13). Provide pre- and post-DIC care. Monitor oxytocin induction, if used. Provide post delivery care: ■ Monitor involution ■ Prevent hemorrhage ■ Prevent sepsis ■ Counsel regarding convalescent care Administer medications are ordered: ■ Oxytocics ■ Analgesics ■ Antibiotics ■ Rh$_0$(D) immune globulin, if indicated

ASSESSMENT	EXAMPLES OF POTENTIAL NURSING DIAGNOSTIC CATEGORIES
RECURRENT ABORTION A. Spontaneous loss of three or more previable pregnancies.	Potential disturbance in self-concept: body image, self-esteem, role performance, personal identity

*See p. 816 for general nursing care for pregnancy-related hemorrhage.
†Diagnosis not included by NANDA, 1986.
‡Outcome criteria direct the selection of nursing actions (**plan/implementation**) and measure their effectiveness (**evaluation**).

Continued.

Summary of Nursing Actions—cont'd

ASSESSMENT	EXAMPLES OF POTENTIAL NURSING DIAGNOSTIC CATEGORIES

B. Presence of one or more of the following possible etiologic factors:
  1. Anomalies of the reproductive tract
  2. Endocrine imbalance (e.g., hypothyroidism, diabetes mellitus)
  3. Infections (e.g., syphilis, *Chlamydia trachomatis*)
  4. Systemic disorders (e.g., lupus erythematosus)
  5. Genetic factors (about 60% of early abortions display an abnormal chromosomal makeup)
	Anxiety
	Ineffective individual or family coping
	Alteration in family process
	Grieving
	Potential for injury related to repeated spontaneous abortions
	Powerlessness

OUTCOME CRITERIA	PLAN/IMPLEMENTATION
Etiology is identified. Existing problem is corrected. Subsequent pregnancy is achieved and carried to term; or woman (couple) make alternative plans (e.g., adoption, remain childless). Self-concept is maintained or strengthened.	Be available to listen; provide emotional support. Refer to appropriate services: ■ Genetic counseling ■ Family planning or adoption agency ■ Infertility clinic ■ Registered dietitian Administer postabortal medications: same as for spontaneous abortion.

ASSESSMENT	EXAMPLES OF POTENTIAL NURSING DIAGNOSTIC CATEGORIES

INCOMPETENT CERVIX
A. Obstetric history may reveal a prior traumatic delivery or forceful dilation and curettage (D & C).
B. History may be nonremarkable.
C. In current pregnancy:
  1. Membranes are intact.
  2. Cervix is not more than 3 cm dilated or not more than 50% effaced.
	Potential disturbance in self-concept: body image, self-esteem, role performance, personal identity
	Spiritual distress
	Anxiety
	Ineffective individual or family coping
	Alteration in family process
	Potential for grieving related to adverse sequelae to cerclage procedure
	Powerlessness

OUTCOME CRITERIA	PLAN/IMPLEMENTATION
Self-concept is maintained or strengthened. Problem is identified in time for cerclage procedure. Cerclage (Fig. 27.5) is accomplished without adverse sequelae, e.g., preterm labor, hemorrhage, sepsis. Pregnancy continues to full term.	Be available to listen. Discuss meaning of "incompetent cervix,"§ that the term is not a reflection on her competency as a person or woman. Answer questions woman may have about the physician's description of the procedure; assist with the procedure. Monitor the fetus during and following the procedure. Monitor for uterine contractions and rupture of membranes. Administer medications as ordered, e.g., antibiotics. Teach woman about danger signs and symptoms, e.g., uterine contractions, rupture of membranes, bleeding, fever, pain and whom to call should they occur.

EVALUATION The nurse can be assured that care was effective when the goals for care have been met.

---

§The word "incompetent" is unfortunate. It connotes that the person with an "incompetent" os is deficient. This label can lead to a loss in self-esteem. A better designation may be "premature dilation of the cervix."

Fig. 27.5
Correction of incompetent cervical os: McDonald operation. Cross-section view of closed internal os.

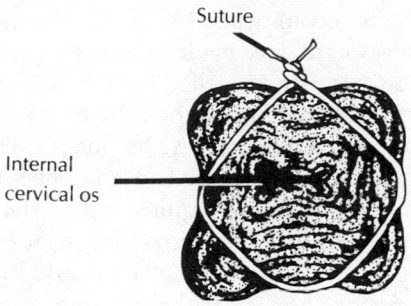

Fig. 27.6
Sites of implantation of ectopic pregnancies. Order of frequency of occurrence is ampulla, isthmus, interstitium, fimbria, tubo-ovarian ligament, ovary, abdominal cavity, and cervix (external os).

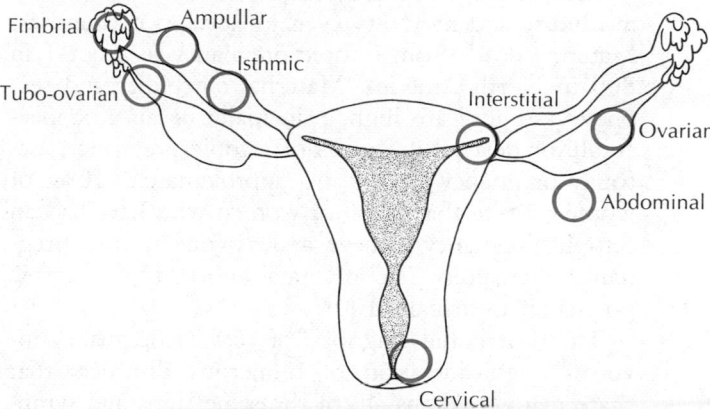

Table 27.14
Differential Diagnosis of Ectopic Pregnancy

	Ectopic Pregnancy	Appendicitis	Salpingitis	Ruptured Corpus Luteum Cyst	Uterine Abortion
Pain	Unilateral cramps and tenderness before rupture	Epigastric, periumbilical, then right lower quadrant pain; tenderness localizing at McBurney's point; rebound tenderness	Usually in both lower quadrants with or without rebound	Unilateral, becoming general with progressive bleeding	Midline cramps
Nausea and vomiting	Occasionally before, frequently after rupture	Usual; precedes shift of pain to right lower quadrant	Infrequent	Rare	Almost never
Menstruation	Some aberration; missed period, spotting	Unrelated to menses	Hypermenorrhea or metrorrhagia or both	Period delayed, then bleeding, often with pain	Amenorrhea, then spotting, then brisk bleeding
Temperature and pulse	37.2°-37.8° C (99°-100° F); pulse variable; normal before, rapid after rupture	37.2°-37.8° C (99°-100° F); Pulse rapid: 99-100	37.2°-40° C (99°-104° F); pulse elevated in proportion to fever	Not over 37.2° C (99° F); pulse normal unless blood loss marked, then rapid	To 37.2° C (99° F) if spontaneous; to 40° C (104° F) if induced (infected)
Pelvic examination	Unilateral tenderness, especially on movement of cervix; crepitant mass on one side or in cul-de-sac	No masses; rectal tenderness high on right side	Bilateral tenderness on movement of cervix; masses only when pyosalpinx or hydrosalpinx present	Tenderness over affected ovary; no masses	Cervix slightly patulous; uterus slightly enlarged, irregularly softened; tender with infection
Laboratory findings	WBC to 15,000/μl; RBC strikingly low if blood loss large; sedimentation rate slightly elevated	WBC: 10,000-18,000/μl (rarely normal); RBC normal; sedimentation rate slightly elevated	WBC: 15,000-30,000/μl; RBC normal; sedimentation rate markedly elevated	WBC normal to 10,000/μl; RBC normal; sedimentation rate normal	WBC: 15,000/μl if spontaneous; to 30,000/μl if induced (infection); RBC normal; sedimentation rate slightly to moderately elevated

symptomatic and are diagnosed during the first trimester. The uterus is the only organ capable of containing and sustaining a term pregnancy. However, the rare abdominal pregnancy, with delivery by laparotomy, may result in a living infant.

Ectopic pregnancy is a significant cause of maternal morbidity and mortality even in developed countries. Maternal death from ectopic pregnancy is about 1 in 800 in North America. Maternal morbidity and secondary surgery are high, principally because of inaccurate or delayed diagnosis of ectopic pregnancy. Ectopic pregnancy recurs in approximately 10% of women. More than 50% of women who have had an ectopic pregnancy achieve at least one normal pregnancy thereafter. The perinatal mortality in ectopic pregnancy is virtually 100%.

The differential diagnosis of ectopic pregnancy involves a consideration of numerous disorders that share many, perhaps all, of the same signs and symptoms. The physician must consider several possibilities (Table 27.14).

The major **management** problem in ectopic pregnancy is hemorrhage. Bleeding must be controlled quickly and effectively. Blood transfusions must be available. Immediate laparotomy is done. Blood and clots are evacuated and bleeding vessels are controlled. Hysterectomy usually is necessary for ruptured cornual or interstitial pregnancy. Excision of the cornua and uterine tube is recommended if the tube is grossly involved. Ultrasound has made it possible to identify uterine tube pregnancy earlier than in the past. Because of this early diagnosis, the tube may be saved. A linear incision, salpingostomy, is made. The small tubal pregnancy is removed and the tube repaired. Ovarian pregnancy always requires loss of the ovary.

Advanced **ectopic abdominal pregnancy** requires laparotomy for delivery of the fetus as soon as the woman is fit for surgery. If the placenta of a second- or third-trimester abdominal pregnancy is attached to a vital organ, such as the liver, no attempt at separation and removal should be made. The cord is cut flush with the placenta and the afterbirth left in situ. Degeneration and absorption of the placenta usually occur without complications.

Interview and observational skills enable the knowledgeable nurse to identify the woman who is experiencing an ectopic pregnancy. A summary of nursing actions related to ectopic pregnancy is provided below.

Summary of Nursing Actions

ECTOPIC PREGNANCY*

GOALS
1. For the mother: a safe resolution of the ectopic pregnancy.
2. For future pregnancy: normal implantation of conceptus.
3. For the family: successful resolution of the emotional responses to an ectopic pregnancy.

PRIORITIES
1. Control of hemorrhage.
2. Replacement of blood and blood products.
3. Removal of the ectopic pregnancy with as little damage as possible to maternal organs.
4. Support of emotional responses to the experience.

ASSESSMENT	EXAMPLES OF POTENTIAL NURSING DIAGNOSTIC CATEGORIES

A. History of conditions that could prevent the transit of the fertilized ovum through the uterine tube, e.g., pelvic inflammatory disease (PID), salpingitis, adhesions secondary to prior abdominal surgery.
B. Presence of the three findings that are associated with **early** ruptured ectopic pregnancy in almost 50% of cases:
  1. Amenorrhea or an abnormal menstrual period followed by slight uterine bleeding
  2. Adnexal or cul-de-sac mass
  3. Unilateral pelvic pain over the mass
C. Additional findings of **acute** rupture may include shock, referred shoulder pain, or evidence of acute blood loss.
D. In **chronic** ruptured tubal pregnancy, which represents slightly more than half the total of ectopic pregnancies, internal bleeding usually has been slow and the symptoms atypical or inconclusive:
	Hemorrhage
	Anxiety
	Fear
	Ineffective individual or family coping
	Fluid volume deficit
	Knowledge deficit
	Powerlessness
	Disturbance in self-concept: body image, self-esteem, role performance, personal identity
	Spiritual distress

*See p. 816 for a summary of nursing care for pregnancy-related hemorrhage.

Summary of Nursing Actions—cont'd

ASSESSMENT	EXAMPLES OF POTENTIAL NURSING DIAGNOSTIC CATEGORIES

1. Slight, dark vaginal bleeding
2. Sense of pelvic pressure or fullness
3. Lower abdominal tenderness
4. Slight fever
5. Leukocytosis
6. Falling HCT and Hgb
7. Cullen's sign
E. Findings of diagnostic activities:
  1. Culdocentesis may yield free blood that will not clot or is already clotted.
  2. Culdotomy may release gross clotted blood, perhaps including the aborted products of an extrauterine pregnancy.
  3. Laparoscopy may disclose an extrauterine pregnancy.
  4. Laparotomy will reveal the correct diagnosis and provide the best opportunity for treatment.
  5. Ultrasound may reveal the site of the ectopic pregnancy.
F. Postsurgery:
  1. Assess woman's physiologic response: vital signs, bleeding, reaction to therapy, elimination, etc.
  2. Assess woman's and family's emotional reactions to experience.	

OUTCOME CRITERIA*	PLAN/IMPLEMENTATION
The woman's physiologic functions are restored; shock is controlled. The woman understands the anatomic and physiologic alterations in reproductive capacity resulting from the surgical intervention. Sequelae (e.g., infection) are prevented or promptly diagnosed and treated; Rh isoimmunization is prevented; anemia is treated. The woman retains a positive sense of self-esteem and self-worth. The woman returns for follow-up care. No adverse sequelae to the ectopic pregnancy are found.	**Before surgery** Refer woman to physician immediately; alert physician that woman is coming to hospital. Alert laboratory and request blood work; type, cross match. Set up for administration of intravenous fluids (use large-bore needle to accommodate blood if necessary), oxygen, and emergency medications, with appropriate equipment. (Frequently, women are admitted directly to surgery by way of emergency room.) Carry out preoperative procedures. Inform woman and family briefly of happenings. Reexplain (clarify, simplify) physician explanations regarding cause, management, and postoperative recovery, including chances for subsequent pregnancies. Arrange for conceptus to be baptized (or perform the rite). **After surgery** Administer and monitor fluids, medications, treatments, and diet per physician's order and woman's preference and tolerance. Inform woman and family if baptism was done (also record on nurses' notes). Notify clergy member to visit if woman and family desire. Facilitate grieving process. Give $Rh_0(D)$ immune globulin, if indicated. Acquaint woman with what to expect during recovery. Alert woman to symptoms to report to physician immediately. Reinform woman regarding physician's explanations. Encourage woman to return for follow-up care.

EVALUATION The nurse can be assured that care was effective when the goals for care have been met.

---

*Outcome criteria direct the selection of nursing actions (**plan/implementation**) and measure their effectiveness (**evaluation**).

Hydatidiform mole (trophoblastic disease). Hydatidiform (hydatid) mole is a **developmental anomaly of the placenta;** the fetus usually is absent. The fertilized ovum deteriorates, and the **chorionic villi** convert into a mass of clear, grapelike vesicles of tapioca consistency (Fig. 27.7).

The cause of hydatidiform mole is unknown. This type of mole occurs in about 1 in 2000 pregnancies. It is much more common in the Orient, for unexplained reasons. Hydatidiform mole is more frequent after induction of ovulation by clomiphene. It is also more common in older women. No prevention of hydatidiform mole is known.

The clinical classification of a hydatidiform mole reflects its localization or dissemination. A benign mole is well localized in the uterus. A metastatic mole must be considered malignant.

Management of hydatidiform mole involves evacuation of the uterus by carefully induced abortion or performance of a hysterectomy. Induced abortion may be followed by D and C in a few days after the friable (easily torn or perforated) uterine wall becomes firmer. Curetted tissue is examined for residual or proliferative trophoblastic tissue. Hysterectomy is often the procedure of choice, especially if the woman is 45 years of age or older or if the uterus appears to be ready to rupture. Blood loss is replaced.

Fig. 27.7

Hydatidiform mole. **1,** Expulsion of mole through cervix. **2,** Rupture of uterus and spillage of mole into peritoneal cavity (rare).

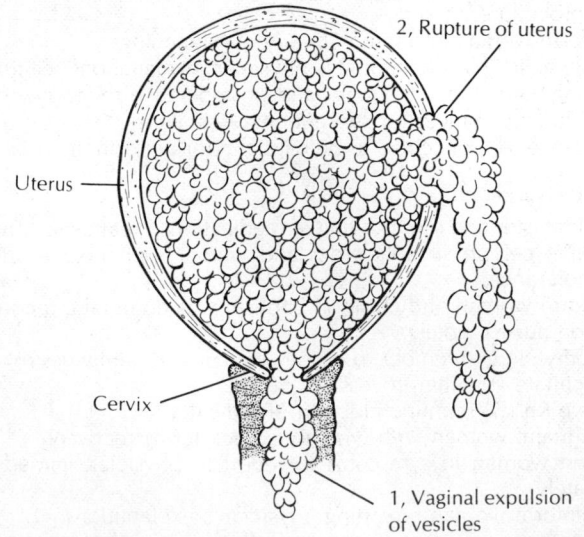

2, Rupture of uterus

Uterus

Cervix

1, Vaginal expulsion of vesicles

Follow-up supervision for 1 year includes the following:

1. **Human chorionic gonadotropin (HCG)** is measured (a) once weekly until HCG titers are negative for 3 consecutive weeks, then (b) once monthly for 6 months, then (c) every 2 months for 6 months, and (d) every 6 months.

2. Continued high titers or rising titers of HCG indicate a pathologic condition. D and C is done if the uterus is intact, and the tissue is examined. If malignant cells are found, chemotherapy for **choriocarcinoma** is begun: methotrexate and dactinomycin are the drugs of choice. Chemotherapy (methotrexate or dactinomycin or a combination of drugs) is administered if (a) HCG titers plateau for 3 consecutive weeks or double at any time, or (b) HCG titers remain elevated at any level 3 to 4 months after termination of pregnancy. If chemotherapy is ineffective, the choriocarcinoma has a tendency toward rapid and widespread metastasis. Death results.

3. Chest x-ray studies to detect metastases are done every month until HCG titers are negative and then every 2 months for 1 year.

4. Oral contraceptive use is advocated to prevent another pregnancy (which would distort HCG titers) and to suppress endogenous pituitary luteinizing hormone (LH), which could distort HCG titer assays.

5. Another pregnancy is not advised until 1 year after tests are negative.

Pregnancy is discouraged because HCG is used as the biologic marker for detecting the trophoblastic disease. If HCG is noted, chemotherapy for choriocarcinoma is initiated. If the HCG is due to pregnancy, the products of conception would be destroyed by the anti-carcinogenic medications. If HCG levels remain within normal limits for a year, the physician may assure the woman or couple that normal pregnancy can be anticipated. However, there is a low probability of recurrence of hydatidiform mole if the woman is 40 years of age or younger.

The **prognosis** for hydatidiform mole is favorable if the chorionic gonadotropin titer does not persist at elevated levels or recur after elimination of the mole. The prognosis is unfavorable if a malignant mole is discovered and is untreated.

A summary of nursing actions related to hydatidiform mole is presented on pp. 825 to 826. The summary can be used both as a guide to studying the disorder and as a guide for teaching clients about trophoblastic disease and its management.

Summary of Nursing Actions

HYDATIDIFORM MOLE*

GOALS

1. For the woman: correct diagnosis of hydatidiform mole and eradication of trophoblastic disease.
2. For the family: successful coping with the experience.

PRIORITIES

1. Identify presence of molar pregnancy through interview, physical examination, and diagnostic techniques such as ultrasound.
2. Initiate appropriate therapy to empty the uterus.
3. Assist woman and family with emotional responses to the condition.
4. Engage woman's and family's cooperation in follow-up care.

ASSESSMENT	EXAMPLES OF POTENTIAL NURSING DIAGNOSTIC CATEGORIES

Diagnostic activities
A. No FHR can be heard, nor can fetal parts be discerned on abdominal palpation.
B. Ultrasonography (the most useful tool) may identify molar pregnancy by the third month (Fig. 25.4). No fetal skeleton is revealed.
 	
Interview and physical examination
A. The uterus becomes enlarged out of proportion to the duration of pregnancy. At 3 months it may be the size expected with a 5-month pregnancy.
B. Excessive nausea and vomiting (hyperemesis gravidarum) occur (see Chapter 28).
C. By the twelfth week an intermittent or continuous brownish-red discharge is present.
D. Uterine discomfort from overstretching may be reported. Rarely the uterus may rupture (Fig. 27.7).
E. Fullness, softness, and thinning of the lower uterine segment can be detected.
F. In addition, symptoms of true preeclampsia-eclampsia may occur even though it is well before the twentieth week of pregnancy.
 	
Laboratory findings
A. Routine urinalysis may reveal protein. Pregnancy-induced hypertension [PIH] may occur in the *first* trimester as a result of this complication.
B. Blood values:
  1. Hematocrit and Hemoglobin values as well as the red blood count (RBC) decrease as a result of bleeding and infection.
  2. The sedimentation rate and WBC increase as a result of infection.
  3. HCG titers are elevated up to 1 to 2 million IU in 24 hours. (Normal HCG titer at 10 weeks is approximately 400,000 IU.)
 	
During surgery
Observe woman's response to medical induction of labor or surgical intervention: vital signs, pain, etc.
 	
After surgery
Observe for signs of grief and grieving by woman and family. Assess woman's support system.
	Anxiety
	Fear
	Grieving
	Ineffective individual or family coping
	Knowledge deficit
	Potential for injury
	  a. Woman related to trophoblastic disease and its treatment
	  b. Subsequent pregnancy if one should occur sooner than one year following evacuation of molar pregnancy from uterus.
	Powerlessness
	Spiritual distress
	Disturbance in self-concept: body image, self-esteem, role-performance, personal identity

*See p. 816 for general nursing care for pregnancy-related hemorrhage.   *Continued.*

Summary of Nursing Actions—cont'd

OUTCOME CRITERIA*	PLAN/IMPLEMENTATION
Pregnancy is terminated in a manner most conducive to the woman's health.	Refer woman immediately to physician; alert physician to findings.
If invasive mole or choriocarcinoma develops, control and treatment with chemotherapy are successful.	Prepare woman for diagnostic activities; sonography, serum HCG determination, induced abortion, possible D & C or hysterectomy.
The woman and family appreciate the seriousness of the condition and adhere to the treatment schedule; the couple postpones another pregnancy until a safe date.	Assist physician with induction or other procedures.
The woman and family realize that the prognosis is excellent (almost 100%) if treatment is undertaken.	Encourage woman and family to grieve by assisting them in the following ways:
	■ To cry and act out their grief
	■ To identify and explore feelings (inadequacy, guilt) regarding this event, responsibility for it, or delay in seeking treatment (should this exist)
	■ To talk of fears for future childbearing, possible surgery, and death from cancer
	Provide simple, cogent explanations to woman and family, reemphasizing or repeating what physician has told her (them) regarding the following:
	■ Etiology
	■ Course of treatment of hydatidiform mole and any coexisting problems (e.g., hemorrhage, D & C, hysterectomy)
	■ Follow-up supervision for 1 year
	■ Need for contraception for 1 year

EVALUATION The nurse can be assured that care has been effective if the goals of care are met.

*Outcome criteria direct the selection of nursing actions **(plan/implementation)** and measure their effectiveness **(evaluation).**

LATE PREGNANCY

Premature separation of the placenta. Premature separation of the placenta, also termed *abruptio placentae,* is the separation of part or all of the placenta from its implantation site. Separation occurs in the area of the decidua basalis after the twentieth week of pregnancy, before the birth of the baby.

Premature separation of the placenta is a serious disorder and accounts for about 15% of all perinatal deaths. Approximately one third of infants of women with premature separation of the placenta die. More than 50% of these die as a result of preterm delivery, and many others die of intrauterine hypoxia. Queenan and Hobbin (1982) state that rapid correction of resultant problems of abruptio placentae can decrease perinatal mortality from a high between 35% and 60% to a low of 3.6%.

The separation may be partial or complete, or only the margin of the placenta may be involved. Bleeding from the placental site may dissect (separate) the membranes from the decidua basalis and flow out through the vagina; it may remain concealed (retroplacental hemorrhage); or it may do both (Fig. 27.8 and Table 27.15).

Most of the following **complications** accompany moderate to severe abruptio placentae:

1. Hypovolemic shock
   a. Pituitary necrosis (Sheehan's syndrome)
   b. Renal failure
2. Fetal hypoxia, or anoxia with possible fetal death
3. Coagulopathy; disseminated intravascular coagulation (DIC)
4. **Couvelaire uterus** (bleeding into the myometrium resulting in boardlike rigidity of the uterus)
5. Hepatitis
   a. Sequal to blood transfusion
   b. Sequal to fibrinogen replacement

Hypovolemic shock may result from loss of blood from the maternal circulation. Prolonged hypovolemia results in ischemia (and hypoxia). Ischemia of the pituitary gland causes pituitary necrosis (see p. 844). Ischemia of the kidneys leads to renal failure: acute tubular necrosis that may be reversible or acute cortical necrosis that is not reversible.

Continued bleeding that cannot exit easily may rupture through the fetal membranes or spread between the muscle fibers of the myometrium. Pressure from

Fig. 27.8
Abruptio placentae. Premature separation of normally implanted placenta. (Courtesy Ross Laboratories, Columbus, Ohio.)

Abruptio placentae (premature separation)

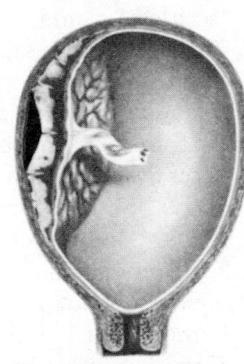   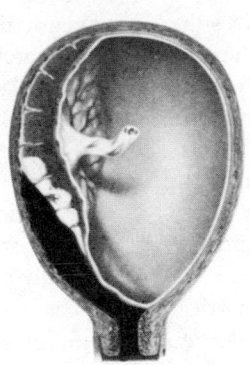   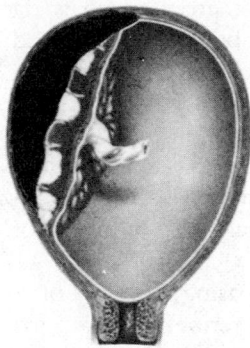

Partial separation   Partial separation   Complete separation
(concealed hemorrhage)   (apparent hemorrhage)   (concealed hemorrhage)

Table 27.15
Summary of Findings: Abruptio Placentae and Placenta Previa

	Abruptio Placentae			
	Marginal Separation	**Moderate Separation**	**Severe Separation* (More Than 66%)**	**Placenta Previa**
Bleeding: external, vaginal	Minimal	Absent to moderate	Absent to moderate	Minimal to severe and life threatening
Color of blood	Dark red	Dark red	Dark red	Bright red
Shock	Absent	Frequent	Very common; often sudden	Occasional
Coagulopathy	Rare	Occasional	Common	Rare
Uterine tonicity	Normal	Increased—may be localized to one region or diffuse over uterus; uterus fails to relax between contractions	Tetanic, persistent uterine contraction; board-like uterus	Normal
Tenderness	Usually absent; if present, is localized	Increased—usually diffuse over uterus	Agonizing, unremitting uterine pain	Absent
Ultrasonographic findings				
Location of placenta	Normal—upper uterine segment	Normal—upper uterine segment	Normal—upper uterine segment	Abnormal—lower uterine segment
Station of presenting part	Variable to engaged	Variable to engaged	Variable to engaged	High—not engaged
Fetal position	Usual distribution†	Usual distribution	Usual distribution	Frequently transverse, breech, or oblique
Concurrent hypertensive state	Usual distribution	Frequently present	Frequently present	Usual distribution

*Onset is usually abrupt; fetus usually dies.
†Usual distribution refers to the usual variations or incidence seen when there is no concurrent problem.

the confined expanding volume of blood may rupture the amniotic sac; the blood imparts a port-wine color to the amniotic fluid.

Extravasation of blood into the myometrium has several sequelae:

1. Myometrial tissue is damaged, necrosis results, and thromboplastin is released, thus initiating the clotting mechanism (see p. 835). Fibrinogen and platelet levels fall as these clotting factors are used to form the retroplacental clot, and coagulopathy results.

2. Small amounts of blood in the myometrium cause ecchymosis and a localized increase in tonicity. The woman may or may not experience uterine tenderness.

3. Increasing amounts of blood in the myometrium increase uterine tonicity, irritability, and tenderness that spread over the entire uterus; the ability of the uterus to relax between contractions diminishes or is lost. Electronic fetal monitoring reflects the increasing fetal distress that may finally end in fetal death.

4. After delivery, the uterus may feel firm because of the blood between the muscle fibers in the myometrium. However, uterine contractile efficiency and therefore its ability to close off bleeding sinuses are diminished or absent (Couvelaire uterus). Serious postpartum hemorrhage is a life-threatening sequel. Hysterectomy may be necessary to control bleeding.

Maternal mortality approaches 1% in premature separation of the placenta; this condition remains a leading cause of maternal death. The **mother's prognosis** depends on the extent of the placental detachment, overall blood loss, degree of DIC, and time between the placental "accident" and delivery. Fortunately, 80% to 90% of all premature separations of the placenta only involve two or three cotyledons, and therefore the prognosis is generally not grave.

Fetal prognosis is poor. At least 25% of babies of mothers with premature placental separation die before, during, or soon after birth. Of those who survive, there is an increase in the absolute numbers of neurologically damaged infants. Fetal depression occurs with at least twice the normal frequency. If the Apgar score at 5 minutes is less than 3, the infant may have sustained neurologic damage. If the 5-minute Apgar score is 7 or greater, there is about a 90% chance of normal growth and development. Infants involved in premature separation of the placenta who weigh more than 2500 g and who have good Apgar scores usually develop normally. About 60% of infants involved in premature separation of the placenta who weigh less than 2500 g at birth develop normally.

Summary of Nursing Actions

ABRUPTIO PLACENTAE (PREMATURE SEPARATION OF THE PLACENTA)

OBJECTIVES
1. For the mother: Prevention of predisposing factors *or* prompt identification and appropriate therapy to prevent serious sequelae to hemorrhage or its therapy.
2. For the fetus or newborn: Prevention of preterm birth and hypoxia.
3. For the family: A healthy mother and newborn.

PRIORITIES
1. Prevent causative factors.
2. Identify and treat abruptio placenta promptly.
3. Prevent sequelae to hemorrhage and to therapy for hemorrhagic shock.

ASSESSMENT	EXAMPLES OF POTENTIAL NURSING DIAGNOSTIC CATEGORIES

PRIOR TO ABRUPTION
Interview and record
 	
A. Predisposing factors:
  1. Hypertension of any cause
  2. Multiple gestation
  3. Multiparity
  4. Advanced maternal age
  5. History of reproductive loss (abortion, premature labor, prenatal hemorrhage, stillbirth, or neonatal death)
  6. Previous premature separation of the placenta
	Hemorrhage*
	Potential for injury related to DIC
	Potential for shock* related to hemorrhage
	Anxiety
	Fear
	Alteration in comfort: pain
	Grieving
	Fluid volume deficit related to hemorrhage
	Alteration in fluid volume: excess related to therapy for hemorrhage

*Diagnosis not included by NANDA, 1986.

Summary of Nursing Actions—cont'd

ASSESSMENT	EXAMPLES OF POTENTIAL NURSING DIAGNOSTIC CATEGORIES

7. Diabetes mellitus
8. Hypotensive syndrome
9. Rare: abdominal trauma (5% of cases); short cord (1% of cases)
 	
Physical examination
Clinical symptoms vary with the degree of separation (Table 27.15):
A. **Uterine bleeding** with small to moderate amount of dark red vaginal bleeding in 80% to 85% of cases
  1. Hypovolemia: shock; oliguria, anuria
  2. Coagulopathy
  3. Port-wine-colored amniotic fluid
B. **Uterine tone**
  1. During labor, uterus may not contract evenly or relax between contractions.
  2. Hypertonicity (mild to severe).
  3. Abdomen may or may not be rigid (if blood can exit, uterus is not rigid); myometrium becomes boardlike (Couvelaire uterus).
C. **Pain**
  1. Mild to severe, localized over one region of the uterus or diffuse over uterus with a boardlike abdomen.
  2. Uterine pain may be severe and sudden (if retroplacental) or painless (if separation is marginal and blood drains out through the vagina).
  3. Hyperactivity of fetus with onset of pain may be followed by loss of FHR. Use electronic monitor if available.
D. **Fetal position** and station: within normal distribution.
E. **Ultrasonography**
  1. Implantation site of placenta: normal
  2. Retroplacental blood clot may not be visible initially, but enlarging clot may be seen when sonogram is repeated.
 	
Laboratory findings
A. Apt test (see Chapter 25) of amniotic fluid: indicates presence of maternal blood
B. Fall in hemoglobin and hematocrit: may appear later
C. Fall in coagulation factors: from 10% to 30% of clients will develop DIC coagulopathies, the majority within 8 hours of hospital admission.
D. Clot retraction increased
 	
POSTDELIVERY OR POSTSURGERY
A. Determine:
  1. If hysterectomy was performed
  2. If fetus died
  3. If newborn is alive, her or his condition
B. Assess woman's physiologic response: amount and source of bleeding, vital signs, gastrointestinal functioning, renal function. If uterus was retained, check height of fundus and its contractility; hemorrhage may occur in presence of "firm" fundus (Couvelaire uterus).
C. Observe for any reaction to cryoprecipitate, if this was given.
	Ineffective individual or family coping related to loss or threat of loss of mother or fetus
	Knowledge deficit
	Powerlessness
	Spiritual distress
	Alteration in tissue perfusion related to hemorrhage or DIC
	
	Hemorrhage*
	Potential for injury related to DIC
	Potential for shock* related to hemorrhage
	Anxiety
	Fear
	Alteration in comfort: pain
	Grieving
	Fluid volume deficit related to hemorrhage
	Alteration in fluid volume: excess related to therapy for hemorrhage

Continued.

Summary of Nursing Actions—cont'd

ASSESSMENT	EXAMPLES OF POTENTIAL NURSING DIAGNOSTIC CATEGORIES
D. Assess for puerperal infection. E. Assess for onset of lactation (a sign of pituitary function). F. Assess woman's and family's emotional response to experience.	Ineffective individual or family coping related to loss or threat of loss of mother or fetus Knowledge deficit Powerlessness Spiritual distress Alteration in tissue perfusion related to hemorrhage or DIC

OUTCOME CRITERIA*	PLAN/IMPLEMENTATION

Blood loss is minimized, and lost blood is replaced to prevent ischemic necrosis of distal organs, including kidneys.
DIC is prevented or successfully treated.
Normal reproductive functioning is retained.
The fetus is safely delivered.
The woman retains a positive sense of self-esteem and self-worth.
	1. Encourage left-lateral position during labor to avoid compressing the vena cava. Instruct the couple in breathing and other techniques while the woman is in this position.
	2. If symptoms are noted:
	  a. Send for physician.
	  b. Turn woman onto her side; administer oxygen at 10 to 12 L/min by means of face mask; start intravenous infusion or increase flow (if intravenous fluid does not have oxytocin in it).
	  c. Do not leave woman.
	  d. Anticipate coagulopathy. Have someone request laboratory work: blood type and cross match, platelets, prothrombin time (PT), and partial thromboplastin time (PTT) (Table 27.16).
	  e. Monitor fetal status.
	  f. Prepare for double setup examination to rule out placenta previa and for induction or augmentation of labor (e.g., amniotomy), abdominal surgery (cesarean birth, hysterectomy), or immediate vaginal delivery if cervix is dilated and presenting part is low.
	3. The nurse assists the physician in implementing the following therapeutic measures:
	  a. Restore blood loss.
	    (1) If shock is present or appears imminent *and* clotting mechanism is intact, central venous pressure (CVP) or pulmonary artery wedge pressure (PAWP) monitoring is started to monitor blood and fluid replacement accurately.
	    (2) A retention catheter is placed to monitor urinary output accurately for volume and proteinuria (oliguria and proteinuria are ominous signs).
	  b. Deliver the fetus.
	    (1) Fetal membranes are ruptured.
	    (2) Oxytocin infusion is begun if labor does not start spontaneously or if labor must be augmented.
	    (3) Cesarean delivery may be performed.
	  c. Perform hysterectomy if Couvelaire uterus occurs.
	  d. Provide emotional support for the woman and her family.
	4. Alert pediatrician and supporting nursing staff to be present for delivery. Infant may require attention for prematurity, hypoxia, or birth injury caused by interventions.
	
	POSTDELIVERY OR POSTSURGERY
	Institute care following cesarean or vaginal birth.
	Administer medications per physician's order for discomfort, infection, anemia, or uterine atony. Monitor intravenous fluids.

*Outcome criteria direct the selection of nursing actions (**plan/implementation**) and measure their effectiveness (**evaluation**).

Summary of Nursing Actions—cont'd

ASSESSMENT	EXAMPLES OF POTENTIAL NURSING DIAGNOSTIC CATEGORIES
	Report oliguria, hematuria, or proteinuria so that therapy for acute renal tubular necrosis (may be reversible) or bilateral renal cortical necrosis (may be fatal) can be started promptly if either of these diagnoses is made. Assist woman and family with grieving process. Reinforce physician's explanation regarding cause, management, and prognosis.

EVALUATION The nurse is assured that care was effective if the goals of care are met.

Placenta previa. In placenta previa the placenta is implanted in the lower uterine segment. The degree to which the internal cervical os is covered by the placenta determines how placenta previa is classified. Placenta previa (Fig. 27.9) often is described as **complete, total, or central** if the internal os is entirely covered by the placenta, when the cervix is fully dilated. **Partial placenta previa** implies incomplete coverage. **Marginal placenta previa** indicates that only an edge of the placenta approaches the internal os. The term **low-lying (low) implantation** is used when the placenta is situated in the lower uterine segment but away from the os. Gestational age and cervical dilation and effacement affect the extent of coverage of the internal os. The cause of placenta previa is uncertain.

In the second trimester approximately 45% of all placentas are implanted in the lower uterine segment.

As the lower uterine segment elongates, the placenta seems to move upward. By term only 1 placenta in 150 is still a previa. Those placentas most likely to remain unchanged are the ones classified as central (complete).

The site of implantation and size of the placenta are related. Specifically, because the circulation of the lower uterine segment is less favorable than that of the fundus, placenta previa may need to cover a larger area for adequate efficiency. In placenta previa the surface area may be at least 30% greater than the average placenta implanted in the fundus.

The location of the placental site close to the cervical os renders it more accessible to ascending infection from the vagina. Hemorrhage and anemia increase the predisposition to antenatal infection (placentitis) and postpartum (puerperal) infection.

Fig. 27.9

Types of placenta previa after onset of labor. **A,** Complete, or total. **B,** Incomplete or partial. **C,** Marginal, or low lying.

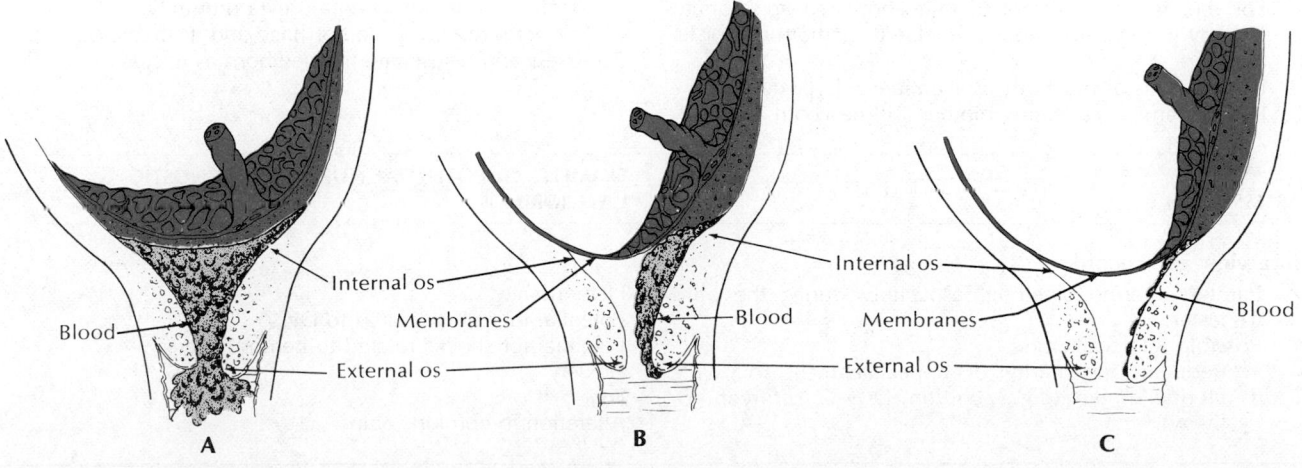

Blood loss may not cease with the delivery of the infant. The large vascular channels in the lower uterine segment may continue to bleed because of the diminished muscle content of the lower uterine segment. The natural mechanism to control bleeding—the interlacing muscle bundles (the "living ligature") contracting around open vessels—so characteristic of the upper part of the uterus is absent in the lower part of the uterus. Therefore postpartum hemorrhage may occur even if the fundus is contracted firmly. If uterine bleeding cannot be controlled with oxytocic drugs, ligation of the internal iliac arteries or even hysterectomy may be necessary.

Maternal morbidity may occur from the placenta previa itself, from the management, or from the birth. Antenatal hemorrhage may be fatal or nearly fatal. Prolonged hypovolemia and hypotension, more frequently associated with abruptio placentae, lead to cerebral or renal damage.

Complications associated with the management of placenta previa include sepsis, surgery-related trauma to structures adjacent to the uterus, anesthesia complications, blood transfusion reactions, or overinfusion of fluids.

Maternal mortality in placenta previa has dropped almost 50%, to about 0.6%, during the past decade in larger centers in North America because of conservative therapy. Regrettably, however, the perinatal mortality (resulting primarily from prematurity) still approaches 20% in most hospitals. This figure undoubtedly can be reduced by half with better management. Currently, placenta previa increases the likelihood of death of the newborn by about 10 times.

Vaginal examination. A sterile vaginal speculum examination by the physician for diagnosing placenta previa may be performed after the ultrasound report is available. The vaginal examination, known as the **double-setup procedure,** is a serious undertaking; it is attempted only if the physician is prepared for delivery.

In a double setup a sterile vaginal examination is performed in an operating room with staff and equipment ready to effect an immediate vaginal or cesarean delivery. Since manipulation of the lower uterine segment or cervix may result in profound hemorrhage, preparation for immediate delivery is essential. Readiness implies an intravenous unit in place with a needle large enough to accommodate blood transfusion, two units of matched blood for the mother, sterile tables set up and open, anesthetist present, at least one physician and one nurse scrubbed, and a pediatrician present. Amniotomy for anticipated vaginal delivery (if placenta is low lying, cervix is favorable, and presenting part is low) or cesarean delivery (if placenta encroaches on or covers cervical os or fetus is in oblique or transverse lie) should be performed.

Amniocentesis. If 35 to 36 weeks' gestation is reached, ultrasound-guided amniocentesis for assessing fetal lung maturity (lecithin/sphingomyelin [LS] ratio or presence of phosphatidyglycerol) is warranted (see Chapter 25). Immediate delivery by cesarean surgery is recommended if fetal lungs are mature. (A major problem related to placenta previa is preterm delivery.)

Summary of Nursing Actions

PLACENTA PREVIA

OBJECTIVES
1. For the woman: Prompt identification and appropriate therapy to prevent serious sequelae to hemorrhage or its therapy.
2. For the fetus or newborn: Prevention of hypoxia.
3. For the family: A healthy mother and newborn.

PRIORITIES
1. Identify and treat placenta previa promptly.
2. Prevent sequelae to hemorrhage and its therapy.
3. Assess and resuscitate the newborn as necessary.

ASSESSMENT	EXAMPLES OF POTENTIAL NURSING DIAGNOSTIC CATEGORIES
Interview and record A. Painless uterine bleeding, especially during the third trimester. B. Possible related factors: 1. Reduced vascularity of upper segment following uterine surgery (e.g., abortion, D & C, cesarean delivery).	Hemorrhage* Potential for injury related to DIC Potential for shock* related to hemorrhage Anxiety Fear Alteration in comfort: pain

*Diagnosis not included by NANDA, 1986.

Summary of Nursing Actions—cont'd

ASSESSMENT	EXAMPLES OF POTENTIAL NURSING DIAGNOSTIC CATEGORIES
2. Altered vascularity of upper segment following previous pregnancies. 3. Tumor (myomas) necessitating lower implantation of the placenta. 4. Multiple gestation that requires a larger surface area for placental implantation.	Grieving Fluid volume deficit related to hemorrhage Alteration in fluid volume: excess related to therapy for hemorrhage Ineffective individual or family coping related to loss or threat of loss of mother or fetus

Physical examination

A. **Uterine bleeding**
1. First episode is rarely life threatening or a cause of hypovolemic shock.
2. May be intermittent, occur in gushes, or rarely, may be continuous.
3. Woman will describe amount of blood as a "cupful" or a "tablespoonful," or that it was enough so that it "ran down" her legs; count pads and weigh pads and linen.

B. **Uterine tone**
1. Normal tone.
2. Relaxes completely between contractions.

C. **Pain**
1. Painless bleeding; nontender uterus.
2. Woman may be experiencing labor contractions at the same time, however.

D. **Fetal position:** If the fetus is in a longitudinal lie, the fundal height is usually greater than expected for gestational age because the low placenta hinders descent of the presenting fetal part. Leopold's maneuvers may reveal a fetus in an oblique or breech position or transverse lie because of the abnormal site of placental implantation.

E. **Ultrasonography.** Obstetric ultrasound, with either real-time (linear or sector) or static imaging, is the diagnostic method of choice (see Chapter 25). If ultrasound reveals a normally implanted placenta, a speculum examination is performed to rule out local causes of bleeding (e.g., cervicitis, polyps, or carcinoma of the cervix) and a coagulation profile is obtained to rule out other causes of bleeding.

F. As a rule, fetal distress or fetal death occurs only if a significant portion of the placenta previa becomes detached from the decidua basalis or if the mother suffers hypovolemic shock.

Knowledge deficit
Powerlessness
Spiritual distress
Alteration in tissue perfusion related to hemorrhage or DIC

Laboratory tests

Hemoglobin and hematocrit values, Rh factor, urinalysis

POSTDELIVERY AND POSTSURGERY

A. Assess surgical response (if birth was cesarean).
B. Monitor height of fundus, uterine contractility, and amount of bleeding. (Lower uterine segment does not contract well; myometrial trauma may predispose it to atony.)
C. Observe woman for signs of infection. Woman is at increased risk for infection because abnormal placental site is slower to heal and closer to the vagina, and hemorrhage predisposes her to infection.

Hemorrhage*
Potential for infection
Potential for injury related to DIC
Potential for shock* related to hemorrhage
Anxiety
Fear
Alteration in comfort: pain
Grieving
Fluid volume deficit related to hemorrhage

Continued.

Summary of Nursing Actions—cont'd

ASSESSMENT	EXAMPLES OF POTENTIAL NURSING DIAGNOSTIC CATEGORIES
	Alteration in fluid volume: excess related to therapy for hemorrhage
	Ineffective individual or family coping related to loss or threat of loss of mother or fetus
	Knowledge deficit
	Powerlessness
	Spiritual distress
	Alteration in tissue perfusion related to hemorrhage or DIC

OUTCOME CRITERIA*	PLAN/IMPLEMENTATION
A viable newborn is delivered, or if the infant dies, adequate emotional support is provided.	**Do *not* perform rectal or vaginal examination; do *not* give enema.**

OUTCOME CRITERIA*

A viable newborn is delivered, or if the infant dies, adequate emotional support is provided.
The woman sustains minimum hemorrhage or hypovolemia, and anemia is rectified.
The woman and family understand the cause of, management of, and expected recovery from the experience.
The woman maintains a positive sense of self-worth and self-esteem.

PLAN/IMPLEMENTATION

Do *not* perform rectal or vaginal examination; do *not* give enema.

PRIOR TO DELIVERY

When fetal maturity is near, conservative management (e.g., bed rest in the hospital to extend the period of gestation) is usually possible because initial spontaneous critical bleeding almost never occurs in placenta previa. When fetal lung maturity is achieved and survival is likely, then elective termination of pregnancy can be carried out.

Keep woman on NPO regimen.

Maintain bed rest with head of bed elevated 20 to 30 degrees (semi-Fowler's position). (This encourages fetal body to act as tamponade.)

Start intravenous fluid administration with large-bore needle (Ringer's lactated solution is a better volume expander than 5% dextrose in water.) Monitor drip rate. At least two units of blood, typed and cross matched, must be available for emergency use.

If the woman has greater than a 30% placenta previa or if bleeding is excessive, **cesarean delivery** is indicated, preferably with the woman under light general inhalation anesthesia.

If hemorrhage is in progress and **vaginal delivery** is planned, the membranes are ruptured, if this can be done easily, permitting the presenting part to tamponade the edge of an incomplete placenta previa, thus checking brisk bleeding. If there is less than a 30% placenta previa, cautious stimulation of labor by continuous intravenous oxytocin drip is permissible unless bleeding is aggravated. If labor does not ensue within about 6 hours and if progress is not rapid, cesarean delivery is indicated.

Throughout management, encourage verbalization of concerns and questions. Explain procedures to woman and family.

If FHR is being monitored electronically and is good, turn audio on so couple can listen if they wish.

Alert pediatrician and nursery staff to be present for delivery.

FOLLOWING DELIVERY

After vaginal delivery, give usual postdelivery care, monitor blood transfusion, and administer antibiotics, oxytocics, and analgesics as ordered.

*Outcome criteria direct the selection of nursing actions (**plan/implementation**) and measure their effectiveness (**evaluation**).

Summary of Nursing Actions—cont'd

OUTCOME CRITERIA	PLAN/IMPLEMENTATION
	After cesarean birth, give postoperative care. If infant has died or is ill, provide emotional support. Encourage verbalization and questions about this experience. Reaffirm physician's explanations regarding cause, management, and expected recovery.

EVALUATION The nurse can be assured that care was effective if the goals of care have been met.

Placental variations. A velamentous insertion of the cord is a rare placental anomaly in which the cord vessels begin to branch at the membranes and then course onto the placenta. Rupture of the membranes or traction on the cord may tear one or more of the fetal vessels. As a result the fetus may quickly exsanguinate (bleed to death). On rare occasions, when slight antenatal bleeding occurs and fetal red blood cells or hemoglobin is identified, prompt rescue of the offspring, usually by cesarean delivery, may be feasible.

Rarely, the placenta may be divided into two or more separate lobes. Each lobe has a distinct circulation; the vessels collect at the periphery, and the main trunks unite eventually to form the vessels of the cord. Blood vessels joining the lobes may be supported only by the fetal membranes and are therefore in danger of tearing during labor or during the birth of the baby or of the placenta. During delivery of the placenta, one or more of the separate lobes may remain attached to the decidua basalis, preventing the uterus from contracting. Bleeding and infection are possible consequences. Therefore the margins of the placenta are always examined for torn vessels, and if the latter are found, the retained lobes are manually removed.

CLOTTING DISORDERS IN PREGNANCY

Normal clotting. Normally there is a delicate balance (homeostasis) maintained between two opposing systems, the hemostatic system and the fibrinolytic system. The hemostatic system is involved in the life-saving process; this system stops the flow of blood from injured vessels, in part through the formation of insoluble fibrin that acts as a *hemostatic* plug. The phases of the coagulation process involve an interaction of the coagulation factors (see box) in which each factor sequentially activates the factor next in line in the so-called cascade effect sequence.

The *fibrinolytic* system refers to the process by which the fibrin is split into fibrinolytic degradation products (FDP) and circulation is restored.

Clotting problems. A history of abnormal bleeding, inheritance of unusual bleeding tendencies, and a report of significant aberrations of laboratory findings indicate a bleeding or clotting problem (Table 27.16). The comprehension of useful tests of hemostasis is based on the usual mechanisms for the control of bleeding, that is, the function of platelets and the necessary clotting factors. Aspirin inhibits platelet aggregation.

Disseminated intravascular coagulation. Disseminated intravascular coagulation (DIC, defibrination syndrome, defibrination coagulopathy), a pathologic form of clotting, (1) is diffuse rather than localized, (2) injures rather than protects the necessary site of coagulation, and (3) consumes clotting factors, such as fibrinogen, so avidly that widespread external and internal bleeding follows. Multiple factors are involved,

Blood Clotting Factors

Factor	Synonyms
I	Fibrinogen
II	Prothrombin
III	Platelet factor 3, thromboplastin
IV	Calcium
V	Labile factor, proaccelerin, AC globulin (ACG)
VI	Synonymous terms no longer used
VII	Serum prothrombin conversion accelerator (SPCA), proconvertin, autoprothrombin
VIII	Antihemotrophic factor (AHF), antihemophilic globulin
IX	Plasma thromboplastin component (PTC), Christmas factor, autoprothrombin II
X	Stuart-Prower factor, Stuart factor, Prower factor
XI	Plasma thromboplastin antecedent (PTA)
XII	Hagemen factor
XIII	Fibrin (protein) stabilizing factor

Table 27.16
Coagulation Tests

Test	Comments
Activated partial thromboplastin time (PTT; measures intrinsic system): 25-36 s	Screening test of choice: very sensitive, relatively easy to perform, inexpensive. All coagulation factors except proconvertin are measured.
One-stage prothrombin time (PT; Quick test; measures extrinsic system); 9.5-11.3 s	Test for proconvertin (VII), proaccelerin (V), Stuart-Prower factor (X), prothrombin (II), and fibrinogen deficiencies. Unfortunately, it does not measure factors necessary for earlier stages of coagulation.
Thrombin time (plasma): 10-15 s	Test measures conversion of fibrinogen to fibrin and depends on concentration of fibrinogen or inhibitors such as fibrin split-products, antithrombins, and heparin.
Platelet count: 130,000-370,000/mm^3	Most reliable index for DIC.
Specific factor assays (e.g., plasma fibrinogen): 195-365 mg/dl	Each of coagulation factors can be assessed by indirect clotting method using natural or synthetic factor-deficient substrates and compared to activity of normal plasma (100%). However, fibrinogen is only factor that can be measured directly by chemical method.
Bleeding time Template: 2-8 min Ivy: 1-7 min Duke: 1-3 min	Finger or earlobe puncture 5 mm deep and 2 mm wide (Bard-Parker blade no. 11) is made after antiseptic preparation of skin. Note time of puncture; touch bleeding point gently with sterile filter paper to absorb blood every 30 s until bleeding stops.

including platelet and coagulation dysfunction. DIC in pregnancy may occur insidiously or with dramatic suddenness. Constant vigilance on the part of the obstetric team is necessary. Unless DIC is treated immediately and effectively, death often results.

Stimuli likely to initiate DIC. The general categories of stimuli to initiate DIC include infusion of tissue extract, endothelial damage, anoxia, bacterial debris or endotoxins (bacteremic or septic shock), chemical and physical agents, hemolytic processes, immune reactions, and thrombocytopenia. **DIC occurs in critical obstetric problems:**

1. Abruptio placentae
2. Intrauterine dead fetus syndrome
3. Amniotic fluid embolism
4. Preeclampsia-eclampsia
5. Hemorrhagic shock
6. Saline abortion
7. Hydatidiform mole
8. Ruptured uterus
9. Sepsis
10. Tumultuous or hypertonic labor
11. Difficult delivery
12. Oxytocin (Pitocin) induction

The prognosis is guarded. It depends on the degree and extent of the underlying disorder as well as the response of the woman to proper treatment.

Summary of Nursing Actions

DISSEMINATED INTRAVASCULAR COAGULATION

OBJECTIVES
1. For the mother: prompt identification and appropriate therapy to prevent serious sequelae to hemorrhage or its therapy.
2. For the fetus or newborn: prevention of hypoxia.
3. For the family: a healthy mother and newborn.

PRIORITIES
1. Identify and treat disseminated intravascular coagulation promptly.
2. Prevent sequelae to disseminated intravascular coagulation.

ASSESSMENT	EXAMPLES OF POTENTIAL NURSING DIAGNOSTIC CATEGORIES
Interview and record The woman is experiencing one or more predisposing conditions.	Potential for injury Potential for shock* related to hemorrhage

*Diagnosis not included by NANDA, 1986.

Summary of Nursing Actions—cont'd

ASSESSMENT	EXAMPLES OF POTENTIAL NURSING DIAGNOSTIC CATEGORIES

Physical examination
A. Spontaneous bleeding from gums or nose.
B. Excessive bleeding from site of slight trauma (e.g., venipuncture sites, intramuscular or subcutaneous injection sites, nicks from shaving of perineum or abdomen, injury from insertion of urinary catheter).
C. Sudden tachycardia, diaphoresis or restlessness with anxiety.
D. Sequelae:
   1. Acute renal failure.
   2. Pituitary insufficiency (Sheehan's syndrome [see p. 844]).
 	
Laboratory tests
A. **Platelet count (the most reliable index) shows a decreased number.**
B. In the presence of a healthy liver, low coagulation factors are not a reliable index, since increased consumption of these factors is matched by increased production.
C. Bleeding time is normal; coagulation time shows no clot; prothrombin time is increased; and partial thromboplastin time (PTT) is increased.
	Anxiety
	Fear
	Alteration in comfort: pain
	Grieving
	Fluid volume deficit related to hemorrhage
	Alteration in fluid volume: excess related to therapy for hemorrhage
	Ineffective individual or family coping related to loss or threat of loss of mother or fetus
	Knowledge deficit
	Powerlessness
	Spiritual distress
	Alteration in tissue perfusion related to intravascular clots and subsequent hemorrhage

OUTCOME CRITERIA*	PLAN/IMPLEMENTATION

The woman survives the disease with minimum or no damage to body organs or systems.
The woman's blood-clotting mechanism returns to normal.
The woman and her family understand the disease process and its management.
The newborn survives with no adverse sequelae.
	The nurse assists the physician in the treatment of DIC, which includes the following measures:
	1. Removal of causative factor, for example, delivery of dead fetus; treatment of existing infection or eclampsia; or delivery of fetus by cesarean birth and removal of abrupted placenta.
	2. Establishment of support mechanisms (see Management of hemorrhagic shock, p. 844).
	  a. Woman's right hip elevated to prevent hypotensive syndrome.
	  b. Oxygen administered by tight-fitting mask at 10 to 12 L/min.
	  c. Parenteral therapy begun (e.g., Ringer's lactated solution).
	  d. CVP monitoring begun with attempt to maintain CVP within normal limits: 6 to 12 cm H_2O (Table 27.17).
	3. Treatment of the condition.
	  a. Administer whole blood as needed at rate sufficient to maintain hematocrit (HCT) at 30% and urinary output at 30 to 60 ml/h.
	  b. Administer blood components as needed.
	    (1) One unit of platelets raises adult level by 5000.
	    (2) One unit of cryoprecipitate (fibrinogen and factor VIII) replaces depleted coagulation factors. Cryoprecipitate is more effective in restoring normal coagulation than lyophilized fibrinogen. In addition, it has the advantage of minimizing transmission of serum hepatitis (about 20% of people who receive fibrinogen acquire homologous serum hepatitis), *or*

*Outcome criteria direct the selection of nursing actions (**plan/implementation**) and measure their effectiveness (**evaluation**).

Summary of Nursing Actions—cont'd

OUTCOME CRITERIA	PLAN/IMPLEMENTATION
	(3) Two units of fresh frozen plasma replace coagulation factors and fibrinogen. The frozen plasma is thawed in the laboratory. It should be administered within 15 to 20 minutes, since the factors disintegrate as the plasma warms. c. Heparin may be ordered.* This is administered by constant infusion pump at 12.5 U/kg/hr to arrest coagulation and fibrinolysis. 4. Diagnosis and treatment of sequelae; minor or major hemorrhagic diathesis, acute renal failure, pituitary insufficiency (Sheehan's syndrome), compromised newborn (usually not affected, except indirectly through hypoxia). 5. Explain disease process and its management to woman and family. 6. Assist woman and family with grieving process.

EVALUATION The nurse can be assured that nursing care is effective if the goals of care are met.

*Paradoxically, cautious intravenous heparin administration may stop the abdominal clotting and check bleeding. Heparin should be administered only after appropriate investigative studies, however, and usually in consultation with a hematologist.

Idiopathic thrombocytopenic purpura. Idiopathic thrombocytopenic purpura (ITP) is an autoimmune disorder in which antiplatelet antibodies decrease the life span of the platelets. The following results of tests are diagnostic: (1) thrombocytopenia, (2) capillary fragility, (3) increased bleeding time, and (4) a bone marrow smear showing a normal or increased megalocyte count with many young forms.

ITP may result in severe hemorrhage following cesarean delivery or from cervical or vaginal lacerations. The incidence of postdelivery uterine bleeding or vaginal hematomas is also increased in ITP. Neonatal thrombocytopenia occurs in about 50% of the cases and is associated with a high mortality. Platelet transfusions are given to maintain the platelet count as 100,000/cu mm. Corticosteroids are given if the diagnosis is made before or during pregnancy. (Splenectomy is deferred until after the puerperium.)

Hemophilia. At least nine types of congenital disorders of the clotting mechanism have been identified. These include hemophilia A, hemophilia A and C, and von Willebrand's disease. About 75% of hemophiliacs have the A variety, and about 15% have the B variety. These two types represent about 90% of all congenital hemorrhagic diseases caused by defective formation of a fibrin clot.

Classic hemophilia (A) is a bleeding disorder typified by a deficiency of factor VIII antihemophilic factor (AHF), an antihemophilic globulin that is essential in thromboplastin formation in phase 1 of blood coagulation. The source of factor VIII in the body is unknown. All degrees of severity of the disease have been reported. Bleeding occurs most often from the nasal or oral mucosa or from contusions or lacerations. Bleeding into the skin, muscles, or joints may also ensue. Hemophilia B, or Christmas disease, is caused by a genetically determined deficiency of factor IX and is clinically indistinguishable from hemophilia A.

Both hemophilia A and hemophilia B are transmitted as sex-linked recessive traits by the mother. Because they are expressed predominantly in the son and only rarely in the daughter (only in homozygous females), the major problem arising with pregnancy is the birth of an affected infant. Hematomas after injections and bleeding from circumcision are common. However, most affected newborns exhibit no clinical abnormalities. Recording and reporting of such incidences, if they occur, will aid in diagnosis at a later date.

The affected woman requires treatment with cryoprecipitate or fresh frozen plasma to replace factor VIII or factor IX. This treatment prevents hemorrhage during and after childbirth.

von Willebrand's disease. One type of hemophilia is von Willebrand's disease. It results from a factor VIII deficiency and platelet dysfunction. It is transmitted as an incomplete autosomal-dominant trait to both sexes. Although von Willebrand's disease is rare, it is one of the most common congenital clotting defects in American women of childbearing age. The symptoms include a familial bleeding tendency, previous bleeding episodes, prolonged bleeding time (most important test), factor VIII deficiency (mild to moderate), and bleeding from mucous membranes. Since factor VIII increases during pregnancy, this increase may be sufficient to offset danger from hemorrhage during childbirth.

Treatment of von Willebrand's disease consists of replacement of factor VIII, if it is less than 30%. Administration of cryoprecipitate of fresh frozen plasma is the usual treatment.

POSTDELIVERY HEMORRHAGE

Hemorrhage is a leading cause of maternal death worldwide. Postdelivery hemorrhage, traditionally the loss of 500 ml of blood or more after delivery, is the most common and most serious type of excessive obstetric blood loss. At least 5% of women suffer postdelivery hemorrhage.

A small woman is less able to withstand the loss of blood than a larger one. It has been noted that the average maternal blood loss can be as much as 10% of the woman's blood volume without immediate critical consequence. Therefore a more meaningful definition of postdelivery hemorrhage is the loss of 1% or more of body weight, a figure easily referable to blood volume because 1 ml of blood weighs 1 g.

Postdelivery hemorrhage may be sudden and even exsanguinating. Moderate but persistent bleeding may continue for days or weeks. Postdelivery hemorrhage may be early, within the first 24 hours after delivery, or late, from 24 hours after delivery until the twenty-eighth day.

Control of bleeding from the placental site is accomplished by prolonged contraction and retraction of interlacing strands of myometrium, the **living ligature.** A firm or contracted uterus does not normally bleed after delivery unless placenta previa had existed. Therefore careful assessment of uterine tone and the maintenance of uterine contractions through manual massage or oxytocic stimulation are important parts of postdelivery care.

Etiology. The causes of postdelivery hemorrhage, in approximate order of frequency, are as follows:

1. Mismanagement of the third stage of labor (e.g., incomplete placental separation)
2. Uterine atony caused by excessive analgesia or anesthesia, prolonged labor, overdistention of the uterus or urinary bladder
3. Lacerations of the birth canal
4. Hematologic disorders (e.g., DIC)
5. Complications of pregnancy (e.g., inversion of the uterus, placenta accreta)

6. Tumors of the cervix or uterus
7. Medical complications of pregnancy (e.g., hyperthyroidism, vitamin K deficiency)
8. Infections of the genital tract (e.g., endometritis)

Early postdelivery hemorrhage almost invariably is caused by uterine atony, lacerations of the birth canal, or DIC. **Late postdelivery hemorrhage** most commonly is the result of subinvolution of the placental site, retained placental tissue, or infection.

Clinical findings and differential diagnosis. It is helpful to consider the problem of excessive bleeding with reference to the stages of labor. From delivery of the fetus until separation of the placenta, the character and quantity of blood passed may suggest excessive bleeding. For example, dark blood is probably of venous origin, perhaps from varices or superficial lacerations of the birth canal. Bright blood is arterial and indicates, for example, deep lacerations of the cervix. Spurts of blood with clots may indicate partial placental separation. Failure of blood to clot or remain clotted is indicative of coagulopathy.

The period from the separation of the placenta to its delivery may be when excessive bleeding occurs. Frequently this is the result of incomplete placental separation, often caused by poor management of the third stage of labor (e.g., undue manipulation of the fundus). After the placenta has been recovered, persistent or excessive blood loss usually is the result of atony of the uterus (i.e., its failure to contract well or maintain its contraction) or prolapse of the uterus into the pelvis. Late hemorrhage may be the result of partial involution of the uterus and unrecognized lacerations of the birth canal.

Complications of postdelivery hemorrhage are either immediate or delayed. Hemorrhagic (hypovolemic) shock (p. 844) and death may occur from sudden, exsanguinating hemorrhage. Delayed complications provoked by postdelivery hemorrhage include anemia, puerperal infection, and thromboembolism.

Specific problems

Uterine atony. Uterine atony is marked hypotonia of the uterus. Uterine atony occurs in at least 5% of deliveries, particularly when the woman is a grand multipara; with hydramnios; when the fetus is large; or after the delivery of twins or triplets. In such conditions, the uterus is "overstretched" and is poorly contractile. Uterine atony is the principal cause of postdelivery hemorrhage.

Placental separation and expulsion are facilitated by contraction of the uterus, which also prevents hemorrhage from the placental site. The corpus is, in essence, a basketwork of strong, interdigitating, smooth muscle bundles through which pass many large maternal blood vessels. If the uterus is flaccid after detachment of all or part of the afterbirth, brisk venous bleeding will occur and normal coagulation of the open vasculature will be impaired. In contrast, a firm, contracted uterus will not bleed because the myometrium will compress the vasculature and resolution of the placental site can occur.

Numerous preventable problems may be responsible for uterine atony. For example, undesirable side effects may follow the administration of ill-chosen drugs, of very potent analgesic agents (e.g., morphine) late in the first stage of labor, and of certain anesthetics (e.g., ethyl ether) that are especially efficient smooth muscle-relaxing drugs. Mismanagement of the third stage of labor, allowing only partial separation of the placenta or retention of placental fragments, may be associated with uterine atony. Moreover, the poorly contracting uterus may have slipped deep into the true pelvis to cause chronic passive congestion of the organ, an added cause of abnormal bleeding.

The first step in the treatment of uterine bleeding is to elevate and hold the uterus out of the pelvis and to massage the corpus to initiate and maintain a firmly contracted organ (Fig. 18.3). The physician orders oxytocin, 10 U administered intravenously (well diluted), or its equivalent. Moreover, continuous intravenous administration of oxytocin solution (5 U/500 ml of 5% dextrose in water) should run for 3 or 4 hours. Blood transfusion for the treatment of shock and blood replacement may be urgently needed.

The accoucheur should hasten to palpate the interior of the uterus so that retained products of conception can be removed and possible rupture of the uterus diagnosed. Lacerations of the **cervix** or of the birth canal should be repaired promptly. If the blood being lost fails to clot, a coagulopathy (e.g., DIC) may have developed, and prompt appropriate treatment may be lifesaving.

If the procedures outlined are ineffectual and normal clotting of blood is ensured, bilateral ligation of the internal iliac arteries will usually stop the bleeding. Thus the uterus will be preserved for future childbearing. If this is not a serious consideration, if rupture of the uterus is confirmed, or if hemorrhage from uterine atony persists, hysterectomy may be required.

Lacerations of the birth canal. Lacerations of the birth canal are second only to uterine atony as a major cause of postdelivery hemorrhage. Therefore prevention, recognition, and prompt, effective treatment of birth canal lacerations are vitally important.

Continued bleeding despite efficient postdelivery uterine contractions demands inspection or reinspection of the birth passage. Continuous bleeding from so-called minor sources may be just as dangerous as a sudden loss of a large amount of blood, although often it is ignored until shock develops. Birth canal lacerations may include injuries to the labia, perineum, vagina, and cervix.

Factors that influence the causes and incidence of obstetric lacerations of the lower genital tract encompass several conditions:
1. Operative delivery
2. Aseptic or unattended spontaneous delivery
3. Congenital abnormalities of the maternal soft parts
4. Contracted pelvis
5. Size, presentation, and position of the fetus
6. Relative size of the presenting part and the birth canal
7. Prior scarring from infection, injury, or surgery
8. Vulvar perineal and vaginal varices
9. Abnormalities of uterine action, for example, precipitate delivery

Other associated problems may be abnormal tissue elasticity or friability, the presence of tumors, the general condition of the mother (e.g., exhaustion, dehydration), and the presence of complicating diseases. All these factors may exist alone or in combination.

The diagnosis of birth canal lacerations requires (1) an inherent awareness of their possible occurrence and (2) an immediate routine, meticulous inspection of the entire lower birth canal after each delivery. Prerequisites for an adequate appraisal include aseptic technique (the woman for whom labor and birth has been precipitate must be prepared and draped), standard instruments for surgical repair, an assistant to provide exposure by retraction, and appropriate lighting.

Upward displacement of the cervix after its inspection by means of a "tailed" or "tagged" vaginal pack will greatly facilitate the inspection of the entire vaginal tract. Hence lacerations may be seen and repaired, and hematomas may be identified and treated before they reach serious proportions. A vaginal pack also serves to elevate the uterus, enhancing its contractility and limiting blood loss during repair.

Proper anatomic reapproximation of all tissues is performed immediately after delivery for the following reasons:
1. To ensure hemostasis and to prevent hematomas
2. To eliminate open sources of puerperal infection
3. To correct problems (e.g., a poorly repaired old laceration of the rectal sphincter may be revised when increased vascularity and physiologic hypertrophy of pregnancy may favorably influence healing)

Blood replacement and the administration of appropriate antibiotic agents, when indicated, are important. A retention urinary catheter may be required in specific cases.

Labial lacerations. Extreme vascularity in the labial and periclitoral areas often results in profuse bleeding. Immediate repair, by means of fine catgut such as no. 4-0 on an atraumatic needle, is required. Counterpressure with a gauze pad and a T binder may be required.

Perineal lacerations. Lacerations of the perineum are the most common of all injuries in the lower genital tract. These are classified as follows:

first degree Involves the mucosa and skin with some fibers of the superficial musculature.
second degree Includes the above and deeper structures of the perineum as well.
third degree Involves all the structures of the vaginal wall, and the sphincter ani muscles are severed.
fourth degree Involves all the aforementioned and the anal wall, so that the anus is laid open.

An episiotomy may extend to become either a third- or fourth-degree laceration.

The care of the woman who has suffered lacerations of the perineum is similar to that advocated for episiotomies, that is, analgesia as needed for pain, and heat or cold applications as necessary. To avoid injury to the suture line, a woman with third- or fourth-degree lacerations is not given routine postdelivery rectal suppositories or enemas. Attention to diet and intake of fluids is emphasized, as well as oral stool softeners to assist her in reestablishing bowel habits.

Vaginal lacerations and hematomas. Prolonged pressure of the fetal head on the vaginal mucosa ultimately will interfere with the circulation and may produce ischemic or pressure necrosis. The state of the tissues, therefore, together with the type of delivery, may result in deep vaginal lacerations and may predispose to vaginal hematomas.

Vaginal hematomas occur more frequently in association with forceps rotation of a fetus in an occipitoposterior (OP) position. They are often found on the same side as the occiput, perhaps because of long-continued pressure of the fetal head in one posterior quadrant of the vagina.

A vaginal hematoma should be diagnosed at the incipient, or early stage. Most hematomas can usually be detected by routine inspection after delivery. Many vaginal hematomas occur beneath the mucosa opposite the ischial spines in the plane of the midpelvis. Therefore the physician will palpate the vaginal walls to detect a full, crepitant, or fluctuant area that may not have become visible. The large masses will be purple, in contrast to the dark red of the remainder of the vaginal mucosa.

Many small hematomas undoubtedly go undetected and may even be self-limiting. Because all hematomas have a small start, the underlying principle of treatment is the prevention of a large hematoma. The sequelae may include tissue devitalization, serious blood loss, shock, and infection.

During the postdelivery period, if the woman complains of persistent perineal pain or a feeling of fullness in the vagina, a careful inspection of the vulva is made. The woman assumes a side-lying position, the upper buttock is raised, and she is asked to bear down. A large purplish mass may be seen at the introitus.

Once the hematoma is diagnosed, treatment is initiated. The woman is returned to the delivery unit, where (after a suitable anesthetic has been administered) the hematoma is incised and evacuated and deep sutures are placed for control of the bleeding.

If the hematoma is larger than 5 cm in diameter, a catheter is placed in the urinary bladder and a moderately tight vaginal pack inserted. A vaginal pack must be inserted carefully to avoid traumatizing the tissues. To facilitate insertion of the pack, an antibiotic ointment may be spread on the pack or applied within the vagina. The catheter and pack may be removed in 6 to 8 hours. Antimicrobial agents for systemic action are not routinely required.

Episiotomy dehiscence. An episiotomy dehiscence or hematoma in the absence of infection suggests coagulopathy. Abnormal coagulation factors can cause either poor wound healing or bleeding into the tissues. Any surgical procedure should be delayed until routinely available coagulation tests have been performed and results are within normal limits.

Retained placenta

Nonadherent placenta. The obstetrician must recognize the normal completion of the third stage of labor, or complications may result. If the operator is hasty, for example, the placenta may not have an adequate opportunity to separate. If one waits too long, needless loss of blood may occur.

In the period after birth of the baby but before recovery of the placenta, some women may have only slight bleeding, but others may have considerable blood loss. If no significant bleeding occurs and with proper management, the normally implanted placenta separates with the first or second strong uterine contraction after delivery of the infant. Placental separation occurs within 15 minutes in about 90% of women. Within 30 minutes after birth, an additional 5% of women will have a separated placenta. If one waits 45 minutes after delivery, only another 1% or 2% will achieve placental separation. Hence there is little to be gained by an extended wait-and-see attitude. If the placenta has not been recovered within 30 minutes of delivery, manual removal should be attempted.

If overly generous analgesia, such as morphine sulfate within 1 or 2 hours of delivery, or third-plane anesthesia with halothane or ether is given, prompt resumption of potent uterine contractions after the birth of the infant may be suppressed. Avoidance of sedation, administration of oxytocin intravenously (slowly) or intramuscularly immediately after delivery, and elevation of the uterus without manual stimulation should aid separation of the placenta and reduce blood loss. If excessive bleeding develops, manual separation and removal of the placenta are carried out immediately.

Some obstetricians practice elective manual separation and extraction of the placenta to expedite the delivery sequence or to avoid abnormal bleeding, for example, after twin delivery. No supplementary anesthesia will be needed for parturients who have had block anesthesia for delivery. For other women, administration of light nitrous oxide and oxygen inhalation anesthesia or intravenous thiopental (Pentothal) will suffice for intrauterine exploration, placental separation, and recovery of the placenta.

If delivery occurs early (fifth or sixth month), either spontaneously or by induced abortion, placental retention is the rule because of poor separation of the afterbirth. This may be caused by an immature zone of separation, weak uterine contractions, or a relatively large placenta.

Retained placenta may be the result of one of the following:

1. Partial separation of a normal placenta.
2. Entrapment of the partially or completely separated placenta by an hourglass constriction ring of the uterus.
3. Mismanagement of the third stage of labor, for example, massage of the uterus (Credé's method) before separation of the placenta or ill-timed administration of ergot products.
4. Abnormal adherence of the entire placenta or a portion of the placenta to the uterine wall.

In all instances postdelivery hemorrhage or infection may be a critical complicating factor.

Because of the possible complications, ergot preparations should be given only *after* recovery of the placenta. They should always be given intramuscularly or orally, never intravenously.

Adherent placenta. Abnormal adherence of the placenta occurs for reasons unknown, but it is thought to be the result of zygote implantation in a zone of defective endometrium. Abnormal adherence of the placenta is diagnosed in only about 1 of every 12,000 deliveries. Approximately 90% of the mothers are multiparous, and many of them have also had abortions. The mother with an abnormally attached placenta is jeopardized mainly by postdelivery hemor-

rhage leading to hypovolemic shock. Firm placental attachment is associated with increased maternal morbidity and mortality. Moreover, premature birth caused by associated problems such as placenta previa accounts for increased perinatal loss.

Factors that predispose to abnormally firm placental attachment are (1) scarring of the uterus such as occurs after cesarean delivery, myomectomy, or vigorous curettage; (2) endometritis, associated with tuberculosis; (3) abnormal site of implantation, such as the cervix or lower uterine segment; or (4) malformation of the placenta, for example, extrachorial placenta.

Unusual placental adherence may be partial or complete, and the following degrees of attachment are recognized.

- Placenta accreta (vera): slight penetration of myometrium by placental trophoblast (rare)
- Placenta increta: deep penetration by placenta (very rare)
- Placenta percreta (destruans): perforation of uterus by placenta (exceptional)

More cases of partial than complete placenta accreta occur.

In all types of abnormal adherence, placentation occurs in an area of deficient, sparse, or absent decidua. Thus the placenta develops on a surface partially or completely devoid of decidua (basalis). The uterine muscle is exposed, and invasion of the trophoblast and chorionic villi of the myometrium soon occurs. A dense fibrous area develops, together with hyalinization of neighboring uterine muscle. **There is no zone of separation:** no cleavage plane can be developed between the placenta and the uterine wall. Attempts to remove the placenta in the usual manner are therefore unsuccessful, and laceration or perforation of the uterine wall may result.

At least 15% of cases of abnormally adherent placenta (all types) are associated with placenta previa. Stated another way, about 3% of all cases of placenta previa are accompanied by placenta accreta, increta, or percreta. There are no sure signs of an abnormally adherent placenta during pregnancy.

Bleeding with complete or total placenta accreta does not occur unless separation of the placenta is attempted. Partial placenta accreta invariably is associated with excessive intranatal or postdelivery bleeding. The reason is that vessels adjacent to the adherent placenta remain open, and free bleeding prevents clotting.

When manual removal of a placenta accreta is attempted, damage to placental tissue and decidua, both rich in thromboplastin, occurs. When this substance is released in quantity into the circulation, DIC may develop.

At vaginal delivery the diagnosis of an abnormally

adherent placenta generally is made when manual separation of a retained placenta is attempted. If the placenta will not separate readily (even a portion), immediate abdominal hysterectomy may be indicated. Persistent attempts at placental removal rarely will be successful, and fatal hemorrhage may result.

Placenta accreta or increta usually is diagnosed at cesarean delivery when an abnormally adherent placenta is discovered. In such cases, especially when surgery was indicated because of placenta previa, total hysterectomy may be the best treatment. If the woman wants to have another child and is in good condition, and if hemorrhage can be controlled, the risk of not removing the uterus may be justifiable. Small retained portions of the placenta may separate or be absorbed, but infection often is an added late complication. A second operation may be necessary because of later hemorrhage. After a subsequent viable pregnancy, elective repeat cesarean delivery will be mandatory because another placenta accreta or increta is likely. Delivery should be followed immediately by total abdominal hysterectomy.

Inversion of the uterus. Inversion of the uterus (turning inside out) after delivery is a critical obstetric complication. The inversion may be complete or partial. Traction applied to the fundus, especially when the uterus is flaccid, may result in inversion. More specifically, the causes include straining (Valsalva's maneuver); traction on the cord before the placenta has separated; Credé's method, that is, kneading the uterine fundus in an attempt to separate an adherent placenta; and placental extraction under deep relaxing anesthesia. Occasionally a large uterine tumor may be responsible for inversion.

Profound shock follows complete inversion; postdelivery hemorrhage accompanies partial uterine inversion. Prompt assistance is imperative because maternal mortality may reach 30% without immediate corrective therapy.

Prevention. Prevention—always the easiest, cheapest, and most effective therapy—is especially appropriate in the avoidance of puerperal uterine inversion. *One must not pull on the umbilical cord unless the placenta has definitely separated.* The fundus should never be used as a piston to "push the placenta out." Credé's method is not used; it is harmful and not useful. Regional anesthsia is employed when feasible. An experienced attendant remains with the woman until the uterus is firm and rounded.

Physical findings. Complete inversion of the uterus is obvious; a large, red, rounded mass (perhaps with the placenta attached) protrudes 20 to 30 cm outside the introitus. Incomplete inversion cannot be seen but must be felt; a smooth mass will be palpated through the dilated cervix, reducing the size of the uterine cavity by at least half.

Medical treatment. The nurse assists the physician in implementing the following:

1. Combat shock, which invariably is out of proportion to the blood loss. Give oxytocin intravenously to contract the uterus. (Ergot products are strictly contraindicated because the cervix, as well as the uterus, will contract, and replacement may be difficult unless the cervix is severed.)

2. Replace the uterus, after the woman is under deep ether or halothane anesthesia, by inserting and "working" first the lower uterine segment and then, finally, the fundus upward while applying traction to the cervix. Leave the placenta attached if it has not yet separated, and then manually free the placenta. Give the oxytocic as ordered. As the uterus and cervix contract, withdraw the placenta with the hand. Pack the uterus if inversion seems about to recur.

3. Abdominal or vaginal surgery may be necessary to reposition the uterus if successful manual replacement fails.

4. Give the woman a transfusion; initiate broad-spectrum antibiotic therapy; and insert a nasogastric tube to decompress the stomach and to minimize adynamic (paralytic) ileus, a frequent sequela.

Prognosis. Successful, prompt vaginal replacement is likely in about 75% of women. Uterine invasion may occasionally recur in a subsequent delivery.

Subinvolution of uterus. Late postdelivery bleeding may occur as a result of subinvolution of the uterus. Subinvolution is defined as the delayed return of the enlarged puerperal corpus to normal size and function. The causes of subinvolution include reduced circulation because of malposition, myomas, retained products of conception, and infection.

Subinvolution may complicate the puerperium because of such symptoms as pelvic discomfort or backache, or there may be signs of abnormality such as leukorrhea or bleeding from an enlarged, boggy, perhaps tender utcrus.

In the absence of frank bleeding, treatment is with ergonovine, 0.2 mg/4 h for 2 or 3 days, antibiotic therapy, and warm acetic douches. With hemorrhage, D and C to remove stained placental secundines and to freshen the placental site for adequate healing generally is required, together with oxytocics and antibiotics.

The woman needs to be instructed to report symptoms to the physician. Although many women experience a short bleeding episode of up to 3 weeks after delivery, prolonged bleeding must be reported. After 3 to 4 weeks, bleeding may be caused by infection or subinvolution of the placental site.

POSTDELIVERY ANTERIOR PITUITARY NECROSIS

Postdelivery anterior pituitary necrosis (Sheehan's syndrome) follows hypovolemic shock and DIC in about 15% of survivors of severe postdelivery hemorrhage. Infarction of much or all of the anterior hypophysis causes partial or total loss of thyroid, adrenocortical, and gonadal functions. The degree of hormonal deficiency depends on the extent of gland destruction.

Women with Sheehan's syndrome fail to lactate and have a decrease in breast size. Loss of axillary and pubic hair, genital atrophy, and amenorrhea are the rule. Such women are apathetic and easily suffer fatigue.

The prognosis of Sheehan's syndrome depends on the degree of residual anterior pituitary function and the supplementary therapy required. Minimum treatment requires thyroid hormone, cortisone, and estrogen replacement. Infertility, reduced resistance to infection, proneness to shock, and premature aging are problems of women with pituitary cachexia.

HEMORRHAGIC SHOCK

Hemorrhage is a major threat to the mother during the childbearing cycle. Shock may result. Shock is an emergency situation in which the perfusion of body organs may become severely compromised and death may ensue. Vigorous treatment is necessary to prevent adverse sequelae (e.g., cellular death, fluid overload, shock lung, and oxygen toxicity). A brief explanation of the physiologic mechanisms is provided to assist the nurse in implementing appropriate actions.

Physiologic mechanisms. Physiologic compensatory mechanisms are activated in response to hemorrhage (or other trauma such as cardiac arrest). The adrenals release catecholamines, causing arterioles and venules in the skin, lungs, gastrointestinal tract, liver, and kidney to constrict. The available blood flow is diverted to the brain and heart and away from other organs, including the uterus. If shock is prolonged, the continued reduction in cellular oxygenation results in an accumulation of lactic acid and acidosis (from anaerobic glucose metabolism). Acidosis (lowered serum pH) causes arteriole vasodilation; venule vasoconstriction persists. A circular pattern is established: decreased perfusion, increased tissue anoxia and acidosis, edema formation, and pooling of blood further decrease the perfusion. Cellular death occurs. Table 27.17 is an assessment guide to assist the nurse in the observation and evaluation of the degree of shock.

Assessment and management. The following nursing interventions should be considered (Royce, 1973):

1. Stay with the woman. Send others to alert the physician and to obtain needed equipment. An emergency cart should be well supplied and available at all times. It should include equipment to start intravenous fluid, to give oxygen, to suction, a retention catheter with urinometer, and blood pressure and CVP or PAWP apparatus.

Nurses should have standing orders to start intravenous fluids and know the type of infusion fluid to use and laboratory tests to order.

2. While waiting for the physician, the nurse should perform the following procedures:

Table 27.17
Symptoms of Shock

	Mild	Moderate	Severe	Irreversible
Respirations	Rapid, deep	Rapid, becoming shallow	Rapid, shallow, may be irregular	Irregular, or barely perceptible
Pulse	Rapid, tone normal	Rapid, tone may be normal but is becoming weaker	Very rapid, easily collapsible, may be irregular	Irregular apical pulse
Blood pressure	Normal or hypertensive	60-90 mm Hg systolic	Below 60 mm Hg systolic	None palpable
Skin	Cool and pale	Cool, pale, moist, knees cyanotic	Cold, clammy, cyanosis of lips and fingernails	Cold, clammy, cyanotic
Urinary output	No change	Decreasing to 10-22 ml/h (adult)	Oliguric (less than 10 ml) to anuric	Anuric
Level of consciousness (LOC)	Alert, oriented, diffuse anxiety	Oriented, mental cloudiness or increasing restlessness	Lethargy, reacts to noxious stimuli, comatose	Does not respond to noxious stimuli
CVP	May be normal (6-12 cm H_2O)	3 cm H_2O	0-3 cm H_2O	

Modified from Royce, J.A.: Nurs. Clin. North Am. **8:**377, 1973; and Wagner, M.M., Clinical Nursing Specialist, University of Iowa Hospitals and Clinics.

a. Insert an airway to facilitate oxygen administration and suction.

b. Start intravenous administration of 5% dextose in water or 0.45% or 0.2% normal saline solution to maintain peripheral vascular circulation.

c. Elevate the right hip (if woman cannot be in left side-lying position) to avoid vena cava syndrome. *Trendelenburg's position* (with head down and feet elevated) *is not advised.* This position may interfere with cardiac function. Use this position on physician request only.

3. Assist physician in instituting and monitoring measures to increase tissue perfusion. Monitor intravenous fluids. Too slow a rate (caused by a slowing of drip rate or kinking or occlusion of tubing) may be inadequate to dilute blood viscosity or to maintain peripheral circulation. Too rapid a rate may result in fluid overload and pulmonary edema.

Fluids to increase blood volume include whole fresh blood, plasma, and albumin. Fluids to dilute hemoconcentration (viscosity) are dextrose in water and Ringer's lactated solution.

4. Monitor, assess, and record respirations, pulse, blood pressure, skin condition, urinary output, level of consciousness, and CVP (Fig. 27.10) to evaluate effectivenss of management (Table 27.17):

a. **Respirations.** The body rids itself of excess acids by increasing the respiratory rate. Ventilatory assistance with oxygen or respirator or both may be needed.

b. **Pulse.** The pulse rate increases and becomes irregular as shock progresses in severity.

c. **Blood pressure.** In later stages of shock the systolic pressure decreases.

d. **Skin.** Perfusion of the skin is sacrificed in the body's attempt to maintain blood flow to the

Fig. 27.10
Measurement of CVP with manometer.

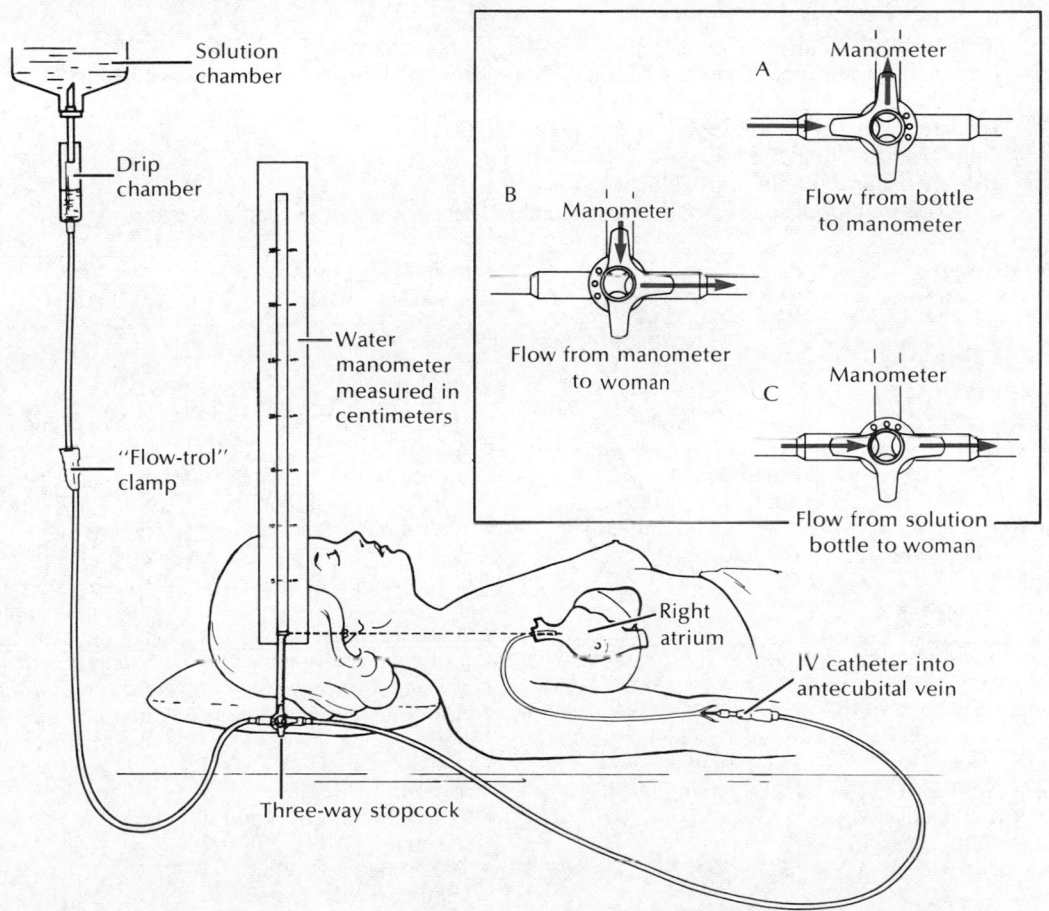

heart and brain. Therefore the condition of the skin is a valuable index to the severity of shock. The nurse assesses the degree of ischemia or cyanosis of the nail beds, eyelids, and skin inside the mouth (buccal mucosa, gums, tongue). The nurse notes the degree of coolness and clamminess.

e. **Urinary output.** Measure hourly output. Oliguria may indicate worsening of shock or inadequate fluid therapy; an increased output indicates improvement in the woman's condition.

f. **Level of consciousness.** The adequacy of cerebral perfusion may be estimated by an evaluation of the woman's level of consciousness. In early stages of decreased blood flow the woman may complain of "seeing stars," feeling dizzy, or feeling nauseous. She may become restless and orthopneic. As cerebral hypoxia increases, the woman may become confused and react slowly or not at all to stimuli. An improved sensorium is an indicator of improvement.

Application of the Nursing Process

MATERNAL HEMORRHAGE AND INFECTION

Mindy is a 26-year-old, married G_2,P_2. She had a normal, healthy, full-term pregnancy. Two days ago she gave birth to a 3360 g (7½ lb) girl after an 8-hour labor. Her only medication for pain was a local anesthetic for repair of the episiotomy. During delivery delayed placental separation resulted in an estimated blood loss of 750 ml of blood. Mindy states she does not understand why she has an infection when her pregnancy was so normal.

Assessment findings on postpartum day 2:

HCT 27%
T   38.4° C for last 6 hours
R   16
BP   118/74
Fundus: firm after massage at 1 cm below umbilicus; slightly tender; persistence of lochia rubra
Episiotomy, breasts and nipples: within normal limits
Legs: Homan's negative
Urinary pattern: within normal limits
Results from blood, urine, and lochia culture and sensitivity: not available as yet.

FUNCTIONAL HEALTH PATTERN: ASSESSMENT	NURSING DIAGNOSIS	RATIONALE: PLAN/ IMPLEMENTATION	EVALUATION
HEALTH PERCEPTION– HEALTH MAINTENANCE ■ HCT 27% ■ T 38.4° C or past 6 hours ■ Fundus: firm after massage at 1 cm below umbilicus; slightly tender ■ Persistance of lochia rubra	Potential for infection secondary to anemia Potential for knowledge deficit related to prevention and treatment of infection.	*To treat low HCT:* ■ Administer therapy per orders: blood transfusion, iron preparation. ■ Advise regarding nutrition. *To treat puerperal infection:* ■ Administer IV fluids and antibiotics per physician order. ■ Advise regarding nutrition.	Hematocrit increases. Temperature returns to normal range. Uterine involution progresses normally. Woman learns relationship between prevention of anemia (nutrition) and susceptibility to infection.
COGNITIVE-PERCEPTUAL ■ Mindy states she does not understand why she has an infection when her pregnancy was so normal.	Knowledge deficit related to connection between anemia and infection	*To prevent spread of infection:* ■ Teach methods of good hygiene. ■ Teach methods of preventing spread to newborn.	Newborn does not acquire an infection from the mother.

g. **Heart function***
   (1) CVP: CVP readings measure the function (e.g., blood pressure) of the right side of the heart. Normal values range between 6 and 12 cm H_2O. A low or falling value indicates inadequate blood volume or hypovolemia. A high or rising value indicates impaired contractility of the heart.
   (2) PA catheter: A multiple-lumen pulmonary artery (PA) catheter is used to measure both right and left-side heart functions.
   (3) PAWP: A PA catheter, when properly placed and when its flexible latex balloon is inflated, is used to measure the pulmonary artery wedge pressure (PAWP), an indicator of left-side heart function.

Anxiety is contagious. The nurse's calm, confident manner, coupled with brief, simple explanations, is an important adjunct to the interventions just discussed.

Hazards of therapy. The 24 hours after the shock period are critical. Observe the woman for fluid overload, shock lung, and oxygen toxicity. **Fluid overload** results in pulmonary and peripheral edema. Alert the physician and decrease the drip rate if moist respirations, stridor, or dyspnea occurs. **Shock lung** may develop after the woman receives mechanical ventilatory assistance, especially if the ventilator is not maintained between 50 and 70 mm Hg. Tachypnea, dyspnea, anxiety, a rise in blood pressure, cyanosis, and harsh loud breaths follow alveolar capillary damage. **High concentrations of oxygen** are toxic to the adult as well as the newborn. Irritation of mucous membranes of the upper respiratory tract, substernal pain, and cough may occur. The first sign may be muscular twitching about the face, followed by convulsions resembling grand mal seizures. Later neurologic symptoms include tinnitus, euphoria, confusion, and respiratory arrest.

The nurse-physician team's quick response and coordinated efforts are essential to institute, monitor, and continuously readjust therapy to the woman's changing needs. This collaboration, given the essential emergency apparatus and supportive services (e.g., laboratory tests), is requisite to meeting client care objectives.

An example of the application of the nursing process related to hemorrhage and infection is presented on p. 846.

---

*Techniques for measuring hemodynamic pressure are beyond the scope of this text. An excellent reference is *Nursing PhotoBook: Using Monitors,* Nurs. '81 Books, Horsham, Pa., 1981, Intermed Communications.

Summary

We have presented the pathophysiology, medical management, and nursing care for hypertension, infection, and hemorrhage in pregnancy. The potential for any of these complications, singly or in combination, exists for any gravida or new mother. The observant, knowledgable nurse plays a significant role in preventing or promptly identifying these complications. Should they occur, the nurse's skill as technician, advocate/counselor/teacher, and support person are of paramount importance to the family.

References

Centers for Disease Control: Hepatitis B virus and vaccine, Hepatitis Branch, Center for Prevention Services, CDC, Atlanta, Ga., 1986.

Centers for Disease Control: Toxic shock syndrome, Center for Prevention Services, CDC, Atlanta, Ga., 1982.

Gunning, J.E.: For controlling intractable hemorrhage: the gravity suit, Contemp. OB/Gyn. 22:22, July, 1983.

Kozier, B., and Erb, G.: Fundamentals of nursing, ed. 2, Menlo Park, Calif., 1983, Addison-Wesley Publishing Co.

Pritchard, J.A.: Management of preeclampsia and eclampsia, Kidney Int. 18:259, Aug. 1980.

Pritchard, J., and others: Williams obstetrics, ed. 17, New York, 1985, Appleton-Century-Crofts.

Queenan, J.T., and Hobbin, J.C., editors: Protocols for high-risk pregnancies, Oradell, N.J., 1982, Medical Economics Books, Medical Economics Co.

Rayburn, W., Zuspan, F., and Piehl, E.: Self-monitoring of blood pressure during pregnancy, Am. J. Obstet. Gynecol. 148:159, 1984.

Royce, J.A.: Shock emergency nursing implications, Nurs. Clin. North Am. 8:377, 1973.

Schachter, J., and others: Erythromycin in the routine treatment of chlamydial infections in pregnancy, N. Engl. J. Med. 314:276, Jan. 30, 1986.

Zuspan, F.P.: Treatment of severe preeclampsia and eclampsia, Clin. Obstet. Gynecol. 9:954, 1986.

Bibliography
Hypertensive States in Pregnancy

Aladjem, S., and others: Experimental induction of a toxemia like syndrome in the pregnant beagle, Am. J. Obstet. Gynecol. 145(1):27, 1983.

Beer, A.E.: Possible immunologic bases of preeclampsia/eclampsia, Semin. Perinatol. 2:39, Jan. 1978.

Brewer, T.: Role of malnutrition in preeclampsia and eclampsia, Am. J. Obstet. Gynecol. 125:281, May 15, 1976.

Brewer, G.S., and Brewer, T.: What every pregnant woman should know, New York, 1977, Random House.

Cavanagh, D., and Knuppel, R.A.: Preeclampsia and eclampsia. In Iffy, L., and Kaminetzky, H.A., editors: Principles and practice of obstetrics and perinatology, New York, 1981, John Wiley & Sons.

Curet, L.B., and Olson, R.W.: Evaluation of a program of bed rest in the treatment of chronic hypertension in pregnancy, Obstet. Gynecol. 53:336, 1979.

Danforth, D., editor: Obstetrics and gynecology, ed. 4, New York, 1982, Harper & Row, Publishers.

de Alvarez, R.R.: Preeclampsia-eclampsia and other gestational edema-proteinuria-hypertension disorders (GEPH). In Benson, R.C., editor: Current obstetrical and gynecologic diagnosis and treatment, ed. 4, Palo Alto, Calif., 1982, Lange Medical Publications.

Dennis, E.J., and others: The preeclampsia-eclampsia syndrome. In Danforth, D., editor: Obstetrics and gynecology, ed. 4, New York, 1982, Harper & Row, Publishers.

Friedman, E.A., and Neff, R.k.: Pregnancy hypertension: a systematic evaluation of clinical diagnosis criteria, Littleton, Mass., 1977, John Wright, Publisher.

Gant, N.F., and Worley, R.J.: Hypertension in pregnancy: concepts and management, New York, 1980, Appleton-Century-Crofts.

Gant, N.F., and others: Clinical management of pregnancy-induced hypertension, Clin. Obstet. Gynecol. 21:397, 1978.

Hill, M.N.: Hypertension: what can go wrong when you measure blood pressure, Am. J. Nurs. 80:942, 1980.

Hoffmaster, J.: Detecting and treating pregnancy-induced hypertension, M.C.N. 8:398, 1983.

Kasser, N.S., and others: Roll over test, Obstet. Gynecol. 54:411, 1980.

Kelley, M.: Maternal position and blood pressure during pregnancy and delivery, Am. J. Nurs. 82:809, 1982.

Kelley, M., and Mongiello, P.: Hypertension in pregnancy, labor, delivery and postpartum, Am. J. Nurs. 82:813, 1982.

Kotchen, J.M., and others: Blood pressure of young mothers and their children after hypertension in adolescent pregnancy: six-to-nine year follow-up, Am. J. Epidemiol. 115:861, 1982.

McKay, D.G.: Chronic intravascular coagulation in normal pregnancy and preeclampsia, Contrib. Nephrol. 25:108, 1981.

Moore, L.G., and others: The incidence of pregnancy induced hypertension is increased among Colorado residents at high altitude, Am. J. Obstet. Gynecol. 144(14):423, 1982.

Nursing photobook: Dealing with emergencies. In Nursing '81 Books, Horsham, Pa., 1981, Intermed Communications.

Nursing photobook: Managing I.V. therapy. In Nursing '82 Books, Springhouse, Pa., 1982, Intermed Communications.

Nursing skillbook. Giving emergency care competently. In Nursing '78 Books, Horsham, Pa., 1978, Intermed Communications.

Infection

Axnick, K.J., and Yarbrough, M., editors: Infection control: an integrated approach, S. Louis, 1984, The C.V. Mosby Co.

Bettoli, E.J.: Herpes: facts and fallacies, Am. J. Nurs. 82:924, 1982.

Brunham, R.C.: Therapy for acute pelvic inflammatory disease: a critique of recent treatment trials, Am. J. Obstet. Gynecol. 148:235, 1984.

Cabral, G.A.,: Expression of herpes simplex virus type 2 antigens in premalignant and malignant vulvar cells, Am. J. Obstet. Gynecol. 143:611, 1982.

California Nurses Association: UC sets guide on AIDS, Calif. Nurse 79:1, July/August 1983.

Can AIDS be a threat to your patients? Contemp. OB/Gyn. 23:163, 1984.

Charles, D., and Larsen, B.: How pregnancy alters infection defenses, Contemp. OB/Gyn. 23(6):96, 1984.

Cohen, M., and Cohen, H.: Viral hepatitis during pregnancy, Contemp. OB/Gyn. 22:29, 1983.

Curran, W., and others: Acquired immunodeficiency syndrome (AIDS) associated with transfusions, N. Engl. J. Med. 310:69, 1984.

Deresinski, S.C., and others: AIDS transmission via transfusion therapy, Lancet no. 8368, p. 102, Jan. 14, 1984.

Dowdle, Walter R.: The epidemiology of AIDS, Public Health Rep. 98:308, 1983.

Ezrati, J.B., and Gordon, H.: Puerperal mastitis: causes, prevention, and management, J. Nurs. Midwife. 24:3, 1979.

Fish, E.N., and others: Update on the relation of herpesvirus hominis Type II to carcinoma of the cervix, Obstet. Gynecol. 59:220, 1982.

Haggerty, L.: TORCH: a literature review and implications for practice, J.O.G.N. N. 14:124, Mar./Apr. 1985.

King, J.: Vaginitis. J.O.G.N. Nurs. 13:41s, 1984.

Larson, E.: Intransigent genital infection? suspect chlamydiae, RN 47:42, 1984.

Loveman, A., Colburn, V., and Dobin, A.: AIDS in pregnancy, J.O.G.N. N. 15:91, Mar./Apr. 1986.

Miles, P.A.: Sexually transmitted diseases, J.O.G.N. Nurs. 13:102s, 1984.

Nurses Association of the American College of Obstetricians and Gynecologists: Erythromycin, tetracycline equally effective against chlamydia, NAACOG Newsletter 10:7, 1983.

Nurses Association of the American College of Obstetricians and Gynecologists: Toxoplasmosis during pregnancy threatens fetal health, NAACOG Newsletter 11:1, 1984.

Nursing photobook: Controlling infection. In Nursing '82 Books, Springhouse, Pa., 1982, Intermed Communications.

Nurses's Reference Library: Assessment. In Nursing '82 Books, Springhouse, Pa., 1982, Intermed Communications.

Olsen, T.G.: Your pregnant patient's rash: is it PUPP syndrome? Contemp. OB/Gyn. 22:151, 1983.

Osborne, N.G., and Pratson, L.: Sexually transmitted diseases and pregnancy, J.O.G.N. Nurs. 13:9, 1984.

Ouimette, J.: Perinatal nursing: care of the high-risk mother and infant, Boston, 1986, Jones & Bartlett Publishers.

Ritter, S.E., and Vermund, S.H.: Congenital toxoplasmosis. J.O.G.N. N. 14:435, Nov./Dec. 1985.

Romanowski, B., and Harris, J.R.: Sexually transmitted diseases, Clinical Symposia 36:1, 1984.

Shaw, F.E., and Maynard, J.E.: Hepatitis B: still a concern for you and your patients, Contemp. OB/Gyn. 27(special issue):27, March 1986.

Stango, S. and Whitley, R.J.: Current concepts: herpesvirus infections of pregnancy. II. Herpes simplex virus and varicella-zoster virus infections, N. Engl. J. Med. 313:1327, Nov. 21, 1985.

Symposium: Establishing bacterial vaginosis, Contemp. OB/Gyn. 27:186, Feb. 1986.

Torrington, J.: Pelvic inflammatory disease, J.O.G.N. N. 14:21s, Nov./Dec. 1985.

USPHS AIDS information hotline: 800/342-AIDS.

Vaginitis: common and curable. I. Harv. Med. School Health Let. 9(4), 1984.

Vaginitis. II. Harv. Med. School Health Let. 9(5), 1984.

Witter, F.R.: Pharmacology: TB regimens during pregnancy, Contemp. OB/Gyn. 23:101, 1984.

Hemorrhage

Acker, D., and others: Abruptio placentae associated with cocaine use, Am. J. Obstet. Gynecol. 146:220, 1983.

Appelman, Z., and Golbus, M.S.: Screening for hemoglobinopathies before delivery, Contemp. OB/Gyn. 27:129, April 1986.

Beeman, P.B.: Peers, parents, and partners: determining the needs of the suppport person in an abortion clinic, J.O.G.N. N. 14:54, Jan./Feb. 1985.

Benson, R.C., editor: Current obstetric and gynecologic diagnosis and treatment, ed. 3, Los Altos, Calif., 1980, Lange Medical Publications.

Berkowitz, R.S., and Goldstein, D.P.: Complications of molar pregnancy, Contemp. OB/Gyn. 24:57, 1984.

Celeste, S.M., and Smith, M.D.: Gestational trophoblastic neoplasms, J.O.G.N. N. 15:11, Jan./Feb. 1986.

Clark, S.L., and Phelan, J.P.: Surgical control of obstetrical hemorrhage, Contemp. OB/Gyn. 24:70, 1984.

Danforth, D.: Obstetrics and gynecology, ed. 4, New York, 1982. Harper & Row, Publishers.

Dreyfus, T.M., and others: Management of immune thrombocytopenia in pregnancy: response to infusions of immunoglobins, Am. J. Obstet. Gynecol. 148:225, 1984.

Duff, P.: Defusing the dangers of amniotic fluid embolism, Contempt. OB/Gyn. 24:127, 1984.

Gordon, R.T.: Emergencies in obstetrics and gynecology. In Warner, C.G., editor: Emergency care: assessment and intervention, ed. 3, St. Louis, 1983, The C.V. Mosby Co.

Hayashi, R.H.: Heading off disaster in postpartum hemorrhage, Contemp. OB/Gyn. 20:90, 1982.

Higgins, S.D.: Essentials of fluid resuscitation and blood transfusion, Contemp. OB/Gyn. 24:102, 1984.

Huff, R.W.: How to handle third-trimester bleeding, Contemp. OB/Gyn. 20:39, 1982.

Jennings, B.M.: Improving your management of DIC, Nurs. '79 9(5):60, 1979.

Jensen, M.D., and Bobak, I.M.: Maternity and gynecologic care: the nurse and the family, ed. 3, St. Louis, 1985, The C.V. Mosby Co.

Kajii, T., and Omaha, K.: Androgenic origin of hydatidiform mole, Nature 286:633, 1977.

Nursing photobook: Dealing with emergencies. In Nursing '81 Books, Horsham, Pa., 1981, Intermed Communications.

Nursing photobook: Managing I.V. therapy. In nursing '82 Books, Springhouse, Pa., 1982, Intermed Communications.

Nursing Photobook: Using monitors. In Nursing '81 Books, Horsham, Pa., 1981, Intermed Communications.

Nursing skillbook: Giving emergency care competently. In Nursing '78 Books, Horsham, Pa., 1978, Intermed Communications.

Nursing skillbook: Monitoring fluid and electrolytes precisely. In Nursing '79 Books, Horsham, Pa., 1979, Intermed Communications.

Problem-patient conference: habitual aborters, Contemp. OB/Gyn. 27:147, Feb. 1986.

Programmed instruction. Nursing care of patients in shock. I. Pharmacotherapy, Am. J. Nurs. 82:943, 1982.

Programmed instruction. Nursing care and the intra-aortic baloon pump, Am. J. Nurs. 82:1401, 1982.

Programmed instruction. Nursing care of patients in shock. III. Evaluating the patient, Am. J. Nurs. 82:1723, 1982.

Purcell, J.A.: Shock drugs: standardized guidelines, Am. J. Nurs. 82:965, 1982.

Querin, J.J., and Stahl, L.D.: Twelve simple, sensible steps for successful blood transfusions, Nurs. '83 13(11):34, 1983.

Siskind, J.: Handling hemorrhage wisely, Nurs. '84 14(1):34, 1984.

Wall-Haas, C.L.: Women's perceptions of first trimester spontaneous abortion, J.O.G.N. N. 14:50, Jan./Feb. 1985.

CHAPTER 28

Endocrine, Cardiovascular, and Psychosocial Disorders

Some complications of pregnancy stem from the pregnant condition. Others are preexisting or represent pathologic conditions that affect the population in general. In this chapter the pathologic basis for understanding the effects of selected clinical complications on pregnancy and the medical and nursing care that can lead to early detection and effective management are presented.

Several conditions are discussed in this chapter. The following disorders may coexist with or complicate pregnancy:

Endocrine disorders
Cardiovascular disorders
Pulmonary disorders
Gastrointestinal disorders
Integumentary disorders
Neurologic disorders
Autoimmune diseases

Surgical conditions coincident with pregnancy
Battered pregnant woman
Malignant disease and pregnancy
Emotional disturbance associated with childbearing
Substance abuse
Poverty

Endocrine Disorders

DIABETES MELLITUS

Definitions

diabetes mellitus A complex disorder of carbohydrate, fat, and protein metabolism caused primarily by a relative or complete lack of insulin secretion by the beta cells of the pancreas.

overt diabetes Elevation of plasma glucose (hyperglycemia) and presence of classic symptoms (polyuria, polydipsia, polyphagia, nocturia, weight loss).

type I diabetes mellitus Formerly called juvenile-onset diabetes or insulin-dependent diabetes; onset in people 40 years or *younger* etiology: genetic, immunologic, viral.

type II diabetes mellitus Formerly called maturity-onset diabetes or non–insulin-dependent diabetes; onset in people 40 years or *older;* etiology: primarily genetic.

type III diabetes mellitus Formerly called gestational diabetes; intolerance to glucose with onset during pregnancy with return to normal glucose tolerance after delivery.

type IV diabetes mellitus Formerly called secondary diabetes; refers to abnormalities in glucose tolerance following pancreatic disease, endocrine disorders (Cushing's syndrome), drug ingestion (oral contraceptives), cirrhosis, and the like.

impaired glucose tolerance Formerly known as chemical diabetes, this type of disorder is characterized by a normal fasting blood glucose, but an abnormally elevated blood glucose following food intake or injection of glucose.

glucose intolerance Inability of the body to metabolize carbohydrates resulting in high plasma (and urine) levels of glucose.

endogenous insulin Insulin produced by the person's own pancreas.

exogenous insulin Insulin injected into the body.

insulin reserve Ability of the pancreas to increase supply of insulin as needed. In type I there is little or no insulin reserve; in type II there is some insulin reserve.

excursion Movement or range in levels from one moment to another, that is, blood glucose levels or changing insulin requirements.

macrovascular disease Vascular disease resulting in problems such as myocardial infarction, angina, vascular accidents (stroke), and peripheral vascular disease of large and small vessels.

microvascular disease Renal and ophthalmologic complications caused by thickening of the lining of blood vessels.

glucose tolerance test (GTT) A test to see how well the pancreas can respond to a load of glucose.

glycohemoglobin (HbA$_{1c}$) The hemoglobin to which glucose attaches. If the person is producing and breaking down RBCs at a normal rate, the percent of HbA$_{1c}$ at the time the blood is drawn for this test accurately reflects the average level of blood glucose *over the preceding 4 to 8 weeks;* normal values are between 6% and 8.8%.

Classification. To reduce confusion and facilitate communication among health professionals and facilitate communication among health professionals a revised classification of diabetes mellitus was issued in

1979 by the National Diabetes Data Group. This classification incorporates newer concepts into the terminology. The new terms are found in the definitions above. Older literature refers to White's terminology (1978). White's classification of pregnant diabetic women considers age at onset, duration, and vascular or renal changes, if any.

1. *Class A:* abnormal GTT caused by diabetes mellitus. This class includes gestational diabetes.
2. *Class B:* frank (overt) diabetes with onset over 20 years of age; duration, 0 to 9 years; no vascular disease.
3. *Class C:* onset of diabetes between 10 to 19 years of age; duration, 10 to 19 years; no vascular disease.
4. *Class D:* onset under 10 years of age; duration, 20 years or more; vascular disease (retinitis; calcification in leg muscles).
5. *Class E:* diabetes with calcified pelvic vessels.
6. Class F: same as class E plus retinopathy and nephropathy (often Kimmelstiel-Wilson intercapillary nephrosclerosis).

Although even milder forms of diabetes pose a threat to mother and infant, the incidence of perinatal death increases with the presence and degree of vascular or renal pathologic changes (classes D, E, and F).

Significance. Diabetes mellitus as a complication of pregnancy was a rare occurrence before the discovery of insulin. Before insulin therapy was available many diabetic girls died before or during puberty; many were amenorrheic and therefore infertile or sterile. When pregnancy did occur, the maternal mortality was 25%; fetal-neonatal loss was 50%. Today the incidence of insulin-dependent diabetes mellitus among school children is increasing, affecting approximately 1 in 600 (American Diabetes Association, 1979). Improved techniques for diagnosing and managing this disorder in children have increased the numbers of women who reach childbearing age and who have normal ovulatory menstrual cycles. As a result the number of pregnancies complicated by type I diabetes is expected to increase yearly. Only 25% of all diabetic persons develop the condition before the age of 40; however, the disorder is far more serious for this group.

Incidence. Diabetes mellitus is a complication in about 1 to 2 in 100 pregnant women. It has been found that 1 in 4 families has a history of diabetes. The incidence of diabetes mellitus increases with age. About 3.8 in every 100 women will eventually become diabetic. Many of these cases will be diagnosed during pregnancy. There is a 30% to 40% chance for the gestational diabetic woman to develop diabetes mellitus within 1 to 25 years. To prevent potential damage to the mother and fetus, investigation for defective carbohydrate metabolism is an essential part of good medical and nursing management of every mother and her child from the embryo stage through birth. Although there is an overall improvement in the perinatal outcome of the well-managed *diabetic* pregnancy, there is still a significant risk for neonatal morbidity.

Pathogenesis. Diabetes mellitus is regarded primarily as a genetically determined syndrome. It is usually inherited as a recessive trait but occurs as a dominant trait in some families. If the beta cells of the islets of Langerhans (pancreas) are deficient either in number or in function, the production of endogenous insulin falls short of the need. As a result, glucose is poorly used, and abnormalities of carbohydrate, protein, and fat metabolism appear.

When glucose is poorly used it accumulates in the blood (hyperglycemia). This results in a hyperosmolarity of the blood. The body compensates by attempting to dilute the heavy concentration of carbohydrates by transferring fluids from the cellular and interstitial compartments into the vascular compartment. Thus, the person becomes *dehydrated* at the cellular and tissue level while having an excess volume in the vascular compartment. The kidneys then function to excrete large volumes of urine *(polyuria)* in an attempt to regulate the excess vascular volume and to excrete the unusable glucose. Hypertonic glucose serves as a diuretic and results in even more body dehydration with excessive thirst *(polydipsia)*.

In the absence of sufficient insulin, the body compensates for its inability to convert carbohydrate into energy by burning proteins and fats. Unfortunately the end products of this metabolism are ketones and fatty acids, which in excess quantity produce *acidosis* and *acetonuria*.

Inheritance of the genetic trait (genotype) for diabetes mellitus does not necessarily mean that the individual will demonstrate diabetic glucose intolerance (phenotype). Many people with the genotype do not show any evidence of diabetes until they experience one or more of a variety of *precipitating factors*. Examples of stressors include the following:

1. Increase in chronologic age
2. Normal developmental periods of rapid hormonal change (Rapid normal hormonal changes occur during menarche, pregnancy, and menopause.)
3. Obesity
4. Infection
5. Surgery
6. Pregnancy
7. Emotional factors
8. Tumor or infection of the pancreas (Tumor or infection may damage the beta cells so that diabetes occurs secondary to the trauma.)

Pregnancy. Among the normal adaptations to pregnancy are alterations in metabolism. Metabolic changes must occur so that (1) the conceptus will have an adequate supply of glucose, its main energy fuel, for development and growth; and (2) the woman can meet her own energy needs for pregnancy and lactation.

Normal pregnancy: insulin resistance. The placenta is developed by the eighth to the tenth week of gestation. As it continues to develop and increase in size, there is a gradual increase in the production of placental hormones: **human chorionic somatomammotropin (HCS), estrogen, progesterone,** and the placental enzyme **insulinase.** HCS and estrogen gradually cause maternal tissue to become resistant to insulin. Insulin resistance is defined as the inability of tissue to use glucose at the cellular level. Insulin resistance is further increased as the woman's adrenal cortex increases its production of **cortisol.** Insulin resistance reaches its peak between weeks 18 and 20, when the levels of estrogen, HCS, and cortisol reach their peaks. Insulinase breaks down maternal insulin.

Normal pregnancy: changing insulin needs (Fig. 28.1)

First trimester. During the first trimester, the developing embryo-fetus siphons (moves by active transport) glucose across the placenta from the mother; **maternal insulin does not cross the placenta.** By the eighth week of gestation, the conceptus secretes its own insulin at levels adequate to use the glucose obtained from the mother. As maternal glucose is used by the fetus, maternal glucose level drops, and therefore insulin production decreases (Fig. 28.1, *A*).

Second and third trimesters. The development of maternal resistance to insulin keeps pace with the increasing levels of placental hormones, insulinase, and cortisol. Insulin resistance is a glucose-sparing mechanism that assures an abundant supply of glucose to the fetus. The mother responds by increased gluconeogenesis and production of insulin (Fig. 28.1, *B* to *C*). The size and number of islets of Langerhans in the normal, healthy pancreas increase to meet increased maternal demands. Fetal insulin production matches the amount of glucose received from the mother.

Postnatal period. Delivery of the placenta brings about an abrupt drop in levels of circulating placental hormones, insulinase, and cortisol. Maternal tissues quickly regain their prepregnancy sensitivity to insulin, and the maternal pancreas rapidly decreases its production of insulin (Fig. 28.1, *C* to *D* or *E* to *F*) and returns to the prepregnant state.

Gestational diabetes mellitus. When the mother's pancreas is challenged by the normal adaptations to pregnancy and the pancreas cannot respond appropriately to the increased demands for insulin, gestational diabetes mellitus* results. The following discussion de-

---

*Pregnancy-induced glucose intolerance.

Fig. 28.1

Changing insulin needs during pregnancy caused by properties of placental hormones and enzyme (insulinase) and cortisol. **A,** gestational period characterized by nausea, vomiting, and often, decreased food intake by mother while glucose use of embryo-fetus increases. **B,** Increase in peripheral resistance to insulin (mother becomes less sensitive to insulin). **C,** Day of delivery: maternal insulin requirements drop dramatically to about prepregnancy levels; she is now very sensitive to insulin. **D,** For nonnursing mother prepregnancy insulin-carbohydrate balance usually returns in about 7 to 10 days. **E,** For nursing mother, her insulin requirements will remain low for up to 6 to 9 months. **F,** At weaning, woman's prepregnancy carbohydrate metabolism is reestablished.

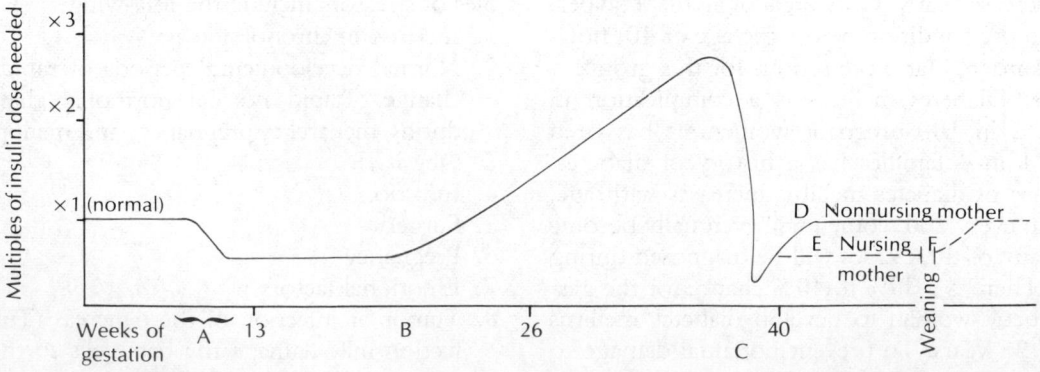

scribes the process leading to the exposure of pancreatic inadequacy during pregnancy.

First trimester. During the first trimester, maternal insulin needs decrease so that the mother's diabetic state remains hidden to routine surveillance.

Second and third trimesters. Between weeks 18 and 20, the maternal insulin requirements return to the prepregnancy level. Starting about weeks 18 to 20, the maternal pancreas is challenged to increase (endogenous) insulin production; pancreatic response is sluggish or incapable of meeting the challenge. Signs (e.g., glucosuria) and symptoms (e.g., thirst) of the developing diabetic condition appear. Exogenous insulin therapy may need to be started at or soon after the twentieth week.

Insulin-dependent diabetes mellitus. Many insulin-dependent women are capable of conceiving and maintaining a pregnancy today (as opposed to the low fertility of diabetic women in preinsulin days). They too must make the normal maternal adaptations to pregnancy. The following discussion describes the changes that occur during a pregnancy that are complicated by insulin-dependent diabetes mellitus.

First trimester. During the first trimester, maternal insulin needs decrease. The woman must *decrease* the dosage of exogenous insulin to prevent episodes of hypoglycemia and the resultant ketoacidosis.

Second and third trimesters. Starting about week 20, maternal insulin needs *increase* progressively to term. Throughout the pregnancy, the woman is supervised closely to prevent wide fluctuations in blood glucose—hypoglycemia and hyperglycemia. Carbohydrate and insulin balance is maintained in the following ways:

1. Careful assessment of blood and urine glucose
2. Management of woman's diet, exercise, insulin dosage, and avoidance of other stressors, for example, infections, and emotional upheaval

Oral hypoglycemic agents, for example, tolbutamide (Orinase) and chlorpropamide (Diabinese), *are never used in pregnancy.* These drugs (1) may be teratogenic, (2) stimulate increased production of insulin by the fetus, and (3) exaggerate neonatal hypoglycemia. **A decrease in insulin requirements in later weeks of pregnancy is a grave prognostic sign for the fetus; the decreasing need reflects decreasing placental function.**

Effects of diabetes on pregnancy

Associated risk factors. Conditions associated with diabetes increase maternal morbidity and mortality. Associated conditions vary slightly with the class of diabetes. In the presence of mild diabetes in which there *is no* associated vascular disease there is a greater incidence of the following:

1. Intensification of preexisting diabetic condition
2. Pregnancy-induced hypertension (PIH; preeclampsia)
3. Hydramnios
4. Intranatal fetal death
5. Macrosomia (large for gestational age [LGA])
6. Large placenta

In the presence of more advanced diabetes in which there *is associated vascular disease* there is a greater incidence of the following:

1. Spontaneous abortions
2. Intrauterine growth retardation (small for gestational age [SGA])
3. Intrauterine fetal deaths and neonatal deaths
4. Complications associated with mild diabetes (above) occur but are less common

Insulin dosage per day does not reflect the severity of diabetes. The age of onset and the duration of diabetes are more important to pregnancy outcome.

Dystocia. Dystocia (Chapter 29) is a possible complication because of hydramnios or macrosomia.

Hydramnios. Hydramnios (polyhydramnios) occurs about 10 times as often in pregnancies of diabetic women as in pregnancies of nondiabetic women. Hydramnios (amniotic fluid in excess of 2000 ml) increases the possibility of compression of abdominal blood vessels (vena cava and aorta), causing supine hypotension. Hydramnios also causes maternal dyspnea because of upward pressure on the diaphragm. Hydramnios has been associated with premature labor perhaps because of overstretching of the uterus.

Macrosomia. There is a greater likelihood of large fetuses (macrosomia). Large fetuses are associated with dystocia (difficult labor and delivery), often resulting in the following (Chapter 29):

1. Operative vaginal delivery (episiotomy and forceps)
2. Trauma to the mother's soft tissues or to the baby
3. Cesarean delivery

Infections. Infections are much more common and serious in diabetic women who are pregnant (e.g., pyelonephritis, monilial vaginitis). Disorders in carbohydrate metabolism alter the body's normal resistance to infection. The inflammatory response, leukocyte function, and vaginal pH are all affected. Pregnancy changes predispose any woman to urinary tract infection. Infection results in increased insulin resistance and ketoacidosis. Unless recognized and treated promptly, ketoacidosis adversely affects the fetus. Ketoacidosis is poorly tolerated by the fetus. Fetal death may occur.

Vascular damage. In the presence of type I diabetes mellitus, vascular lesions are of great concern. During pregnancy, preexisting vascular lesions may cause angina (followed by myocardial infarction) or other vascular lesions throughout the body, including the retina. A retinal examination should be done routinely. Fetal-neonatal (perinatal) mortality is related directly to the amount of vascular damage. During pregnancy, especially if diabetes is poorly controlled, there is a rapid progression in vascular damage that results in increasing retinopathy, uremia (nitrogen retention), and ketoacidosis. The severity of preeclampsia (occurring in 10% to 20% of pregnant diabetic women) is associated directly with the degree of renal vascular involvement. Severe vascular involvement has the following results:

1. Deterioration of the placenta and intrauterine growth retardation or death
2. The need to deliver the baby prematurely because of the risk to the mother in continuing the pregnancy
3. Possible abruptio placentae (premature separation of the normally implanted placenta, Chapter 27)

Prognosis. The outcome for both the mother and her child from the embryo stage through birth is determined in large measure by the degree to which diabetes is controlled. If there are no complicatons of pregnancy, and diabetes is well controlled, mortality for the woman with diabetes is about the same as that for any other woman.

Prognostically poor signs in pregnancy of diabetic woman. Perinatal mortality increases by threefold to fourfold for the pregnancy of a diabetic woman, during which the following conditions become evident: pyelonephritis, severe acidosis, PIH, poor compliance by the woman, or poor diabetic control. Perinatal mortality of 50% follows an acute onset of hydramnios or a rapid drop in insulin requirements.

Gestational diabetes mellitus. The gestational diabetic woman's GTT typically returns to within normal range 3 to 5 weeks after delivery. About 30% of these women will develop diabetes within 5 years; and about 60%, within 2 to 15 years. Only 4% of nondiabetic pregnant women would become diabetic within this same period. For infants of diabetic mothers, 7% will become diabetic by the age of 20 years.

Management
Goals. The goals of management are several:
1. Minimize the risk to the mother
2. Minimize the need for antepartum hospitalization to maintain or restore diabetic control
3. Educate the woman and her family about diabetes mellitus and its control
4. Prevent perinatal morbidity and mortality
5. Help the mother maintain her self-esteem

Euglycemia. Euglycemia (blood sugars within normal range) is the key to achieving the goals of management for the following reasons:

1. Maternal hyperglycemia early in pregnancy adversely influences embryogenesis resulting in major congenital anomalies such as caudal regression syndrome.
2. Fetal hyperglycemia and hyperinsulinism later in pregnancy are associated with (a) intrauterine fetal death; (b) delayed pulmonary maturation leading to respiratory distress syndrome in the newborn; and (c) neonatal illness, regardless of gestational age, such as hypoglycemia, hypocalcemia, and nonhemolytic hyperbilirubinemia.
3. Poorly controlled diabetes places the woman at increased risk for (a) pregnancy complications such as preeclampsia-eclampsia (and therefore abruptio placentae) and pyelonephritis and (b) permanent vascular damage. To achieve the primary focus of management—euglycemia—the woman needs to become a member of the health team.

The diabetic gravida as a member of the health care team. As an active participant, the woman maintains or enhances her self-esteem, and her self-confidence in being able to care for herself and for her baby is developed. The responsive, reliable, self-assured woman, who has learned to assess her own blood glucose and maintain euglycemia and who communicates openly and frequently with the physician and nurse, often can be seen at the clinic or the office on the same schedule as the nondiabetic gravida (i.e., once per month until week 32; every 2 weeks until week 36; and then every week until labor begins). Open communication is encouraged to facilitate client participation in self-care. The need for hospitalization during pregnancy to control diabetes and the need for early delivery are minimized. Under this type of team management the nurse-clinician or nurse-practitioner is the primary educator for the woman and her family.

Prenatal period
Diagnosis of diabetes mellitus. Early identification of glucose intolerance is essential so that prompt appropriate therapy can be initiated. Factors in a woman's *history* that are associated with the risk of pregnancy-induced glucose intolerance include:

1. Family history of diabetes (first-degree relatives only [i.e., parents, siblings])
2. Poor obstetric history (e.g., spontaneous abortion, unexplained stillbirth, hydramnios, unexplained prematurity or low birth weight)
3. Birth of a previous newborn weighing 4000 g or more
4. Previous newborn with major congenital anomalies.

Findings in the current pregnancy that alert the physician to the possibility of gestation-onset diabetes include:

1. Maternal age of 25 years or older
2. Obesity (weight of 90.7 kg [200 lb] or more)
3. Recurrent monilial (*Candida albicans* or "yeast") vaginitis that is not responding to therapy
4. Glycosuria
5. Hydramnios
6. Fetus that is LGA

Glycosuria can be diagnosed with Tes-Tape or Clinistix, both of which depend on enzyme reactions *specific for glucose*, without confusion with fructosuria and lactosuria.

Laboratory tests are required to establish the diagnosis of diabetes mellitus. Two types of laboratory tests are available: tests to identify levels of glucose in blood (Table 28.1) and a test to determine the percent of hemoglobin that is glycosylated (HbA$_{1c}$). A decreased incidence of congenital anomalies is associated with HbA$_{1c}$ values that are within normal limits.

Some physicians suggest that *all* pregnant women should be screened for blood glucose using the *1-hour glucose screen* during the first prenatal visit. This test can be accomplished in a clinic or office setting on a woman who is not fasting. It is unfortunate that the test is not accurate before the seventh week of gestation when malformation from any preexisting abnor-

Table 28.1
Blood Tests for Diabetes Mellitus in Pregnancy

Test	Instructions	Technique	Findings	Precautions
Fasting blood sugar (FBS): measures amount of glucose in blood when woman is fasting	No food for 12 h before test, e.g., 8 PM to 8 AM; water is only fluid allowed	Blood drawn by venipuncture and sent to laboratory	Normal: 80-120 mg/dl serum Abnormal: 220 mg/dl or more, diagnostic of diabetes mellitus	None
Postprandial blood sugar: measures blood sugar following meal	None	Woman eats meal containing 100 g of carbohydrate; blood drawn by venipuncture 2 h after meal and sent to laboratory	Normal: 80-120 mg/dl serum	None
Oral glucose tolerance test (GTT): measures woman's response to measured dose of glucose	High-carbohydrate diet (300 g of carbohydrates per day) for 3 days preceding test; no food for 12 h before test or during test; no smoking, tea, coffee during test (alter body's response to carbohydrate); minimize activity (alters glucose metabolism); minimize stress (epinephrine and cortisone raise glucose levels by promoting gluconeogenesis)	Weigh woman, obtain fasting blood and urine specimens; administer 100 g of glucose orally in lemon juice; collect blood samples at 1, 2, and 3 h; mark each specimen with time obtained and send to laboratory	Plasma glucose level*: Normal fasting: <100 mg/dl 1 h: <200 mg/dl 2 h: <150 mg/dl 3 h: <120 mg/dl Abnormal fasting: elevated or two other values lie outside normal range (p. 856)	Caution woman she may experience dizziness, sweating, weakness, nausea, vomiting, or diarrhea during second and third hour Diuretics, glucocorticoids, oral contraceptives may distort findings; do not use if FBS over 200 mg/dl
Intravenous glucose tolerance test: preferred test in pregnancy since absorption of glucose from intestinal tract is variable and may result in distorted findings in oral GTT	Same as oral GTT	Weigh woman; obtain fasting blood and urine specimen: administer 50 ml of 50% glucose in distilled water IV over a 4 min period and serial blood specimens obtained until 2 h is reached, labeled as to time obtained, and sent to laboratory	Plasma glucose level Normal fasting: <100 mg/dl 2 h: level not higher than fasting level	Caution woman she may experience facial flushing and dizziness as glucose is being administered Other precautions: same as for GTT
Tolbutamide response test not used since tolbutamide may have teratogenic effect on fetus				

*Blood glucose readings lower.

Table 28.2
Properties of Insulin Preparations

Type of Insulin	Activity and Time of Onset	Peak Activity and Time When Hypoglycemia Most Likely to Occur*
Regular, crystalline	Short: 15-45 min	2-4 h; before lunch
Semilente	Short: 45-60 min	6-10 h; afternoon
Globin	Medium: 2-3 h	6-10 h; afternoon
NPH (neutral-protamine-Hagedorn)	Medium: 2-3 h	8-12 h; 3 PM to dinner
Lente (a combination 30% semilente and 70% ultralente)	Medium: 2-3 h	8-12 h; 3 PM to dinner
PZI (protamine zinc insulin)	Long: 4-6 h	16-24 h; 11 PM to 7 AM
Ultralente	Very long: 8 h	16-24 h; 11 PM to 7 AM

From Jensen, M.D., and Bobak, I.M.: Handbook of maternity care: a guide for nursing practice, St. Louis, 1980, The C.V. Mosby Co.
*When administered approximately at 7 A.M.

malities of the carbohydrate metabolic state occurs. If the value is greater than or equal to 140 mg/dl, the 3-hour GTT is performed.

The *GTT* is abnormal if two or more of the following values are found.

	Serum (mg/dl)	Venous Whole Blood (mg/dl)
Fasting blood sugar (FBS)	≥105	≥90
One hour	≥190	≥170
Two hours	≥165	≥145
Three hours	≥145	≥125

The above criteria are the same regardless of age, duration of pregnancy, or obesity.

Diet. Dietary or insulin management must be based on blood glucose (not urinary glucose) values. The diet is individualized to allow for increased maternal and fetal metabolic requirements: calories, 35 to 40 kcal/kg ideal body weight*; protein, 1.5 g/kg ideal body weight; carbohydrates, 30% of total calories; fat to make up the remainder. Distribution should be two sevenths for each of three meals and one seventh for an evening snack. Women with brittle diabetes may require six small meals a day. The obese woman may need more food to prevent ketoacidosis. Sodium is not restricted; however, excesses are discouraged. An average weight gain of 27.5 lb (12.5 kg) is associated with the lowest incidence of preeclampsia and perinatal mortality.

Exercise. Exercise must be regular. The woman must be capable of making necessary adjustments to diet and insulin intake if the exercise pattern alters.

Insulin (Table 28.2). Prenatal insulin requirements increase after the eighteenth to twentieth week. Before that time hypoglycemic episodes may occur because of fetal drain and the low level of hormone antagonists to insulin. Insulin reactions are therefore common.

Monitoring blood glucose. The woman requires instruction as to the relevance of testing urine for glucose levels in pregnancy. By midpregnancy, trace to 1+ glucose is acceptable. Blood glucose levels need monitoring by fasting blood sugar (FBS) and 2-hour postprandial tests (Table 28.1).

A recently developed technique using a color-graph machine (glucose reflectance meter) reduces or eliminates the necessity of obtaining venous blood samples and thereby "saves" accessible veins. The woman can perform the test at home (Fig. 28.2). Using a micro lance,* the woman obtains a blood sample from the side of a finger (all the fingers are used in rotation). The drop of blood is placed on a glucose reagent strip. After the strip is rinsed in water and placed in the machine, the color graph is read. The results are recorded and reported to the physician. If blood glucose levels measure less than 100 mg/dl, it has been found that the infant is normosomic and has few hypoglycemic problems after delivery.

The advent of glucose reflectance meters has been credited with increasing the person's feeling of control over self, and decreasing or eliminating hospitalizations and therefore separation from family.

Continuous insulin infusion. Continuous insulin infusion systems (Fig. 28.3) simplify insulin administration for women who need multiple injections per day. The system infuses insulin at a set basal rate with a bolus dose to cover meals. The infusion tubing from this portable, battery-operated pump can be left in place for several weeks without local complications. Several biochemicals in addition to glucose are also maintained within normal limits, thus decreasing the risk of developing diabetes-related complications.

Supervision. If there is a question about the woman's ability to maintain euglycemia, visits are scheduled

---

*The actual number of kilocalories the individual woman should receive varies. The woman needs sufficient kilocalories to achieve optimal weight gain and to prevent acidosis.

*The Autolet facilitates finger sticks. It consists of a disposable lancet on a springboard arm.

Fig. 28.2
Nurse whose responsibility is to provide primary care for women whose pregnancies are complicated by diabetes mellitus is teaching family and nursing student home monitoring for blood glucose. After return demonstration, nurse proceeded to review with woman how to balance insulin doses with findings. (Courtesy Stanford University Medical Center, Stanford, California.)

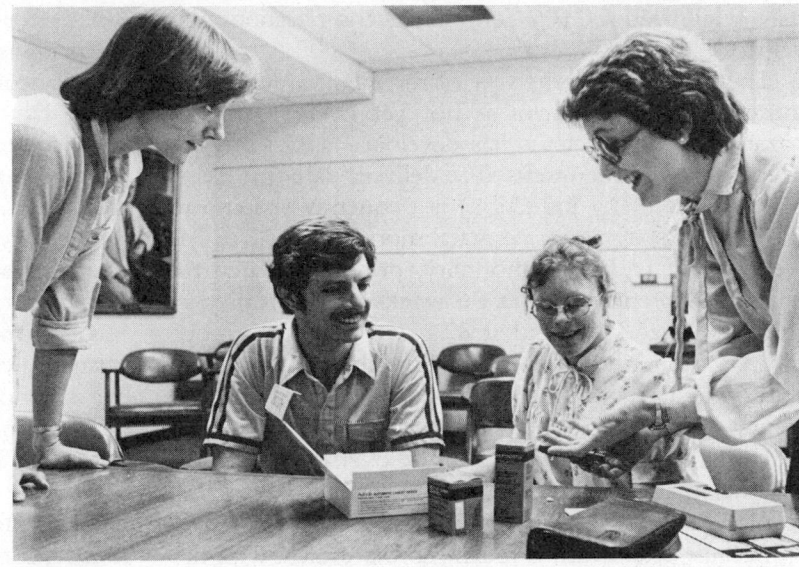

a minimum of every 2 weeks for the first 32 weeks and then weekly until delivery. A urine sample is checked at each visit throughout pregnancy for blood, glucose, ketones, protein, bilirubin, pH, and *microscopic examination;* asymptomatic urinary tract infections are frequent and can cause fetal demise.

Fetal well-being is monitored closely. For example, after week 32, three estriol determinations per week and one fetal activity determination per week may be scheduled (see Chapter 25). Procedures for estimating gestational age, fetal lung maturity, and fetal response to labor contractions (nonstress tests and stress tests) are appropriate.

Hospitalization. The woman may require regulation of insulin. Before pregnancy she may have been taking tolbutamide, and during pregnancy she must change to regular insulin. She may have poor control ("brittle diabetes") so that daily evaluation is necessary. If she develops an infection, intravenous antibiotic therapy may be indicated. Close monitoring of fetal health may be required as a basis for early termination of the pregnancy.

Complications. The diabetic pregnant woman is provided with written instructions as to the need for **prompt reporting of nausea, vomiting,** and **infections.** Women having poor control need to be carefully assessed for infection; for example, asymptomatic urinary tract infections may significantly change a woman's insulin requirements. Mycotic vaginitis in the diabetic pregnant woman is more common and difficult to control.

Intranatal period

Determination of delivery date. The infants of class A diabetic women generally do well. These mothers

Fig. 28.3
Continuous insulin infusion regulated closely with home monitoring of glucose makes tighter control of diabetes mellitus possible. (Photograph by I.M. Bobak.)

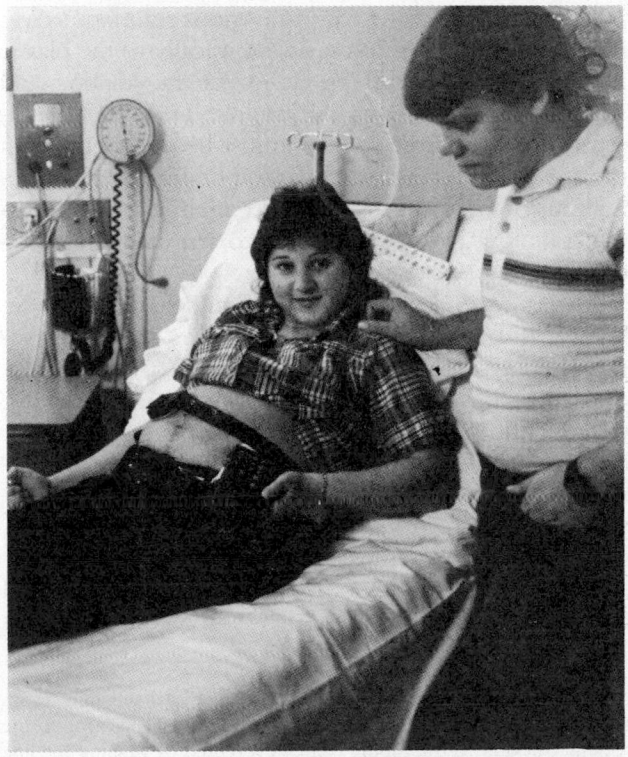

may be allowed to go to term unless complications develop.

The best time for delivery of the infant is when the intrauterine environment is not yet overwhelmingly hazardous and the fetus has developed sufficiently to exist outside of the uterus. The delivery date (by cesarean delivery or by induction) is frequently chosen on the basis of statistics of perinatal mortality: at 32 to 34 weeks there is a 19% mortality, primarily related to hazards of prematurity; **at 36 weeks the mortality is the lowest,** at 11%; and at 37 to 40 weeks, the mortality is the highest, at 26%, primarily because of intrauterine death from acidosis or placental insufficiency. It is unclear whether the placenta is inadequate to meet the nurturing needs of the oversized infant or whether diabetes-induced vascular changes contribute to placental dysfunction.

Because fetal death is much more prevalent with diabetic women in classes B through F, planned delivery about the thirty-seventh week has become accepted policy in most maternity centers. However, estimation of the gestational age is always subject to error. Monitoring the maternal serum or urinary estriol level during the last trimester provides some indication of developing placental insufficiency. A *steady decline in estriol level* (see Chapter 25) is one indication for termination of the pregnancy.

Insulin therapy. Intranatal insulin requirements involve a prescribed dose of insulin added to 100 ml of 10% dextrose in water for intravenous solution. NOTE: Insulin, a protein, is attracted chemically to the plastic in the intravenous tubing. It leaves the solution and adheres to the lining of the tubing. Therefore a sufficient quantity of the solution must be cleared through the tubing to completely coat the lining. Then the remaining solution of insulin will remain stable. (A protein [albumin]* may be added to the solution; however, it is more expensive.)

General care. The mother should assume a side-lying position during bed rest in labor to prevent supine hypotension because of a large fetus or polyhydramnios. If strong labor and good progress do not ensue within 6 to 8 hours, cesarean delivery should be carried out. Poorly controlled diabetes or obstetric indications such as fetopelvic disproportion, positive oxytocin challenge test (OCT), change in estriol levels, or preeclampsia-eclampsia are also indications for a cesarean delivery. The woman is observed and treated for diabetic complications such as hyperglycemia, ke-

tosis, ketoacidosis, and glycosuria (Table 28.3). A pediatrician should be present at delivery to initiate proper neonatal care.

Postnatal period
Insulin requirements. The woman must be closely monitored. She may require only one half to two thirds of her prenatal dosage on the first postnatal day if she is eating a full diet. It takes several days after delivery to reestablish carbohydrate homeostasis.

Complications. Possible complications include preeclampsia-eclampsia, hemorrhage, and infection. *Preeclampsia* occurs in one fourth of all diabetic new mothers and in one third of all diabetic new mothers, class C or D. *Hemorrhage* is a possibility if the mother's uterus had been overdistended (hydramnios, macrosomic fetus), or overstimulated (oxytocin induction). Monilial *infection* of the vagina or nipples or other infections are more likely to occur in a woman suffering from diabetes.

Breast feeding. Breast feeding is encouraged. Advantages of breast feeding include (1) maternal satisfaction and pleasure and (2) its antidiabetogenic effect. Breast feeding decreases the dosage for insulin-dependent women. The insulin dosage must be readjusted at the time of weaning (Fig. 28.1, *E* to *F*).

Counseling: family planning and contraception. The insulin-dependent woman must realize that *she must eat on time.* This is true even if the baby needs feeding or other pressing demands exist.

The new mother needs information for *family planning* and *contraception.* To assist in their decision making, couples need to be informed that if the mother has type I diabetes, the offspring have a 22% chance of developing diabetes; if she has type II diabetes, the offspring have a 4% chance. Nearly 100% of offspring of parents who both have noninsulin-dependent diabetes develop that type of diabetes. Only 45% to 60% of the offspring of both parents who have insulin-dependent diabetes will develop the syndrome.* The risk of diabetes doubles with every 20% of excess weight, and this figure applies to the young as well as to the older diabetic person. Diabetes is now the sixth leading cause of death by disease in adults and the first leading cause of new cases of blindness between the ages of 20 and 75. If contraception is chosen, the woman is advised to use the *diaphragm with spermicide.* Oral hormonal contraceptives are contraindicated because of their effect on carbohydrate metabolism. IUDs are associated with an increased risk of infection. In the presence of severe renal disease and proliferative retinopathy, sterilization may be advised.

---

*Insulin does not have to be mixed with expensive albumin (more than $50 per bottle) to prevent loss of insulin by its adhering to the tubing. Sticking to the tubing can be prevented by flushing the line first with 100 ml of normal saline and 10 units of insulin.

*Prediction of risk varies from author to author.

Table 28.3
Differentiation of Hypoglycemia, Ketoacidosis, and Hyperglycemic Hyperosmolar Nonketotic Coma (HHNK)

GOAL: Prevention or early recognition of these complications to establish and maintain good control in diabetic woman

	Hypoglycemia (Insulin Reaction)	Ketoacidosis (Diabetic Coma)	HHNK
Causes	Too much insulin Not enough food (delayed or missed meals) Excessive exercise or work Indigestion, diarrhea, vomiting	Too little insulin Too much or wrong kind of food Infection, injuries, illness Insufficient exercise	Abnormally high glucose levels without ketoacidosis in mild or suspected diabetic—pancreatic disorders that lower production of insulin Complication of extensive burns, excess steroids (i.e., with steroid therapy), acute stress, TPN,* hemodialysis, peritoneal dialysis
Onset	Sudden (regular insulin) Gradual (modified insulin or oral agents)	Slow (days)	Rapid if woman dehydrated

Symptomatology	Hunger
	Sweating
	Nervousness
	Weakness
	Fatigue
	Blurred or double vision
	Dizziness
	Headache (especially with NPH or PZI insulin)
	Pallor, clammy skin
	Shallow respirations
	Normal pulse
	Laboratory values
	   Urine: negative for sugar and acetone
	   Blood glucose: 60 mg/dl or less
		Thirst
		Nausea or vomiting
		Abdominal pain
		Constipation
		Drowsiness
		Dim vision
		Increased urination
		Headache
		Flushed, dry skin
		Rapid breathing
		Weak, rapid pulse
		Acetone (fruity) breath odor
		Laboratory values
		   Urine: positive for sugar and acetone
		   Blood glucose: 250 mg/dl
			Polyuria
			Thirst (intracellular dehydration)
			Hypovolemia
			Blood serum levels
			   Fasting blood sugar (FBS): 600-3000 mg/dl
			   Acetone level: normal or slightly elevated
			Dry skin
			Coma, death

Nursing actions	Notify physician Give orange juice Obtain blood and urine specimens for laboratory testing	Notify physician Keep woman flat in bed and warm Record intake and output Check and record vital signs	Administer insulin in line with blood glucose levels Monitor IV therapy (sodium and water deficits corrected without extreme shift of fluid into intracellular compartment with no reduction of hyperosmolarity of blood) Monitor woman for dehydration; record intake and output Check and record vital signs Notify physician of changes in symptomatology

Modified from form used at Santa Clara Valley Medical Center, San Jose, Calif.
*TPN (total parenteral nutrition) replaces the term hyperalimentation.

Summary of Nursing Actions

DIABETES MELLITUS

GOALS

1. For the mother: the woman and pregnancy suffer no adverse sequelae to diabetes mellitus.
2. For the fetus or newborn: the fetus or newborn suffers no adverse sequelae to diabetes mellitus.
3. For the family: the family copes with the complication successfully and learns ways to prevent progression of the disease. If the fetus or newborn is lost, the family copes successfully with the loss.

PRIORITIES

1. The woman and family become active participants in self-care.
2. Gestational diabetes mellitus is identified and treatment begun promptly.
3. Euglycemia is maintained.

ASSESSMENT	EXAMPLES OF POTENTIAL NURSING DIAGNOSTIC CATEGORIES
ANTEPARTUM PERIOD **Interview/record** A. Existence of insulin-dependent diabetes mellitus B. Presence of factors suggesting pregnancy at risk for gestational diabetes mellitus C. Knowledge of disease and its management D. Woman's and family's response to disease and its management E. Woman's and family's need for referral to social services (housekeeping aid, financial assistance, peer support group) F. Success with home monitoring and management of the condition **Physical examination** A. Symptomatology of diabetes mellitus and its sequelae B. Diabetic complications, e.g., hypoglycemia, hyperglycemia, ketosis, ketoacidosis, glycosuria (Table 28.3) C. Obstetric conditions complicating diabetes, e.g., nausea or vomiting, PIH D. Associated conditions complicating pregnancy, e.g., infection E. Fetal well-being: fundal height, nonstress test ([NST], fetal activity determination [FAD]), and contraction stress test (CST) **Laboratory tests** A. Blood tests (Table 28.1) B. Urine tests for diabetic status, urinary traction infections (UTIs), fetal well-being (estriols)	Anxiety Fear Ineffective individual or family coping Grieving Alteration in family processes Alteration in health maintenance Potential for injury Knowledge deficit Noncompliance related to insufficient funds or lack of transportation to grocery store, etc. Alteration in nutrition: less or more than body requirements Powerlessness Self-care deficit: feeding, bathing/hygiene, dressing/grooming, toileting Disturbance in self-concept: body image, self-esteem, role performance, personal identity Spiritual distress

---

OUTCOME CRITERIA*	PLAN/IMPLEMENTATION
General *Ability to cope with diagnosis* Verbalizes reaction to diagnosis and expectations and verbalizes level of comprehension about diabetes *Pathophysiology of disease; urine testing* Verbalizes knowledge of normal and altered use of insulin and glucose in body Verbalizes reasons for testing and significance of results	**General** Ascertain level of understanding and knowledge of client and family and receptiveness to teaching Assess feelings about diabetes Have client fill out client information sheet Discuss pathophysiology with client or significant other Check with physician about S/A method client will do at home ☐ Clinitest ☐ Acetest ☐ Ketodiastix ☐ Other _____

Adapted from Stanford University Hospital, Stanford University Medical Center, Stanford California.
*Outcome criteria direct the selection of nursing actions (**plan/implementation**) and measure their effectiveness (**evaluation**).

Summary of Nursing Actions—cont'd

OUTCOME CRITERIA*	PLAN/IMPLEMENTATION

Demonstrates accurate testing of urine ac and hs or as ordered (second voiding)
Records results and interprets each test; follows urine testing schedule without being reminded (keep at bedside)
Demonstrates correct care of equipment
	Teach, demonstrate techniques, interpret results (second voiding), and record results
	Supervise client or significant other
	Clinitest tablets—emphasize the following:
	    Pass-through phase: 20 ml (4 tsp)—orange→muddy brown→orange
	    Wait 15 s before shaking for final reading
	    Do not touch tablets
	    Store tablets in cool, dark place
	Ketodiastix—emphasize the following:
	    Read acetone after 15 s
	    Read sugar after 30 s

Insulin administration (if appropriate)
Defines insulin and states its action on body function
States peak action of insulin
Verbalizes importance of using correctly calibrated syringe with correct strength of insulin; e.g., U100 insulin with U100 syringe
Demonstrates correct withdrawal and administration of insulin to self
Verbalizes importance of site rotation and identifies sites used
Verbalizes proper techniques of insulin storage
 	
Woman gives own injection daily with RN supervision
	Determine correct injection technique (check angle used)
	    □ 45-degree angle
	    □ 90-degree angle
	Teach strict aseptic technique for withdrawal and administration of insulin
	Stress importance of giving and drawing up accurate dose
	Stress importance of using correct syringe with correct insulin
	
	Have client or significant other practice drawing up with normal saline and giving injection to an orange for a day
	Teach importance of rotation and sites available
	Woman to give own injection with RN supervision remainder of hospital stay
	Use U100 insulin unless ordered otherwise
	Stress that current bottle of insulin being used can be stored at room temperature; unused bottle in refrigerator

Hyperglycemia and ketoacidosis Lists four precipitating factors causing ketosis Describes potential signs and symptoms of ketoacidosis Verbalizes rationale for seeking medical attention for illness, infection Verbalizes need to continue testing urine and taking insulin during periods of illness	Stress sick day rules: take insulin, do S/A, notify physician if urine sugar levels run 4+ for 2 days or if vomiting Point out that *illness, especially infection, vomiting and diarrhea, may precipitate ketoacidosis*
Hypoglycemia Explains causes and dangers of insulin (hypoglycemia) reaction Lists signs and symptoms of insulin reaction Describes care and treatment of and prevention of insulin reaction; verbalizes importance of treating immediately Lists foods to take during insulin reaction and amount to take Significant other verbalizes what to do in case of insulin coma (e.g., glucagon injection) Verbalizes that increased exercise may induce hypoglycemia Relates importance of carrying diabetic identification	Review causes and dangers of insulin reaction with client or significant other Stress importance of carrying fast-acting sugar and consuming extra carbohydrate before exercise and importance of bedtime snacks Stress relationship of exercise and diet Stress seeking medical care immediately with onset of hypoglycemic reaction Stress importance of client or significant other to learn to recognize signs and symptoms of precipitating factors leading to hypoglycemic reaction Discuss glucagon action and injection technique with client or significant other Give Medic-Alert information

Continued.

Summary of Nursing Actions—cont'd

OUTCOME CRITERIA*	PLAN/IMPLEMENTATION
Diet management	
Calorie count; other restrictions; type of diet ordered for discharge	Ascertain type of diet client is to follow at home
Verbalizes what is meant by carbohydrate, fat, protein, and nutrient needs for basic good nutrition	RN informs dietitian that client is on diabetic protocol
Verbalizes interrelationship of energy expenditure, food intake, and weight control	Dietitian (with reinforcement from nurse) performs the following:
Correctly selects foods and exchanges for three meals for 2 days (to be done with dietitian)	Teaches role diet plays in disease management
Verbalizes need to maintain or achieve normal body weight	Assesses client's dietary habits and develops prescribed diet management within this framework
	Provides resource material to show equivalent food values
	RN to check with dietitian to see if client selects correct foods
Susceptibility to multiple system complications	
Skin; feet	Discuss with client importance of good foot and skin care
Arteriosclerosis; neurologic changes	Washing daily and drying
Sick day rules	Avoidance of temperature extremes
Verbalizes understanding of good skin and foot care	Good-fitting shoes
Demonstrates proper care of skin and feet	Inspection of feet and skin daily
Verbalizes potential changes in sensation and circulation and appropriate action	Trim toenails straight across
Importance of exercise	Discuss possible complications of diabetes
Avoidance of restrictive clothing	Neurologic changes
Extremes in temperature	Arteriosclerosis and importance of observing for and reporting symptoms to physician
Verbalizes what to do on sick days and why	Discourage use of heating pads and hot water bottles if complications are already present
	Stress sick day rules: take insulin, do S/A, notify physician
	Stress that blood glucose is elevated with fever, chills, etc.
Exercise	
Verbalizes understanding of relationship between exercise, insulin, and glucose use	Stress that exercise enhances use of glucose and decreases need for insulin
Discusses realistically exercise and activities to be maintained and reason for regular exercise	Stress importance of regular exercise of any kind within client's limits
Demonstrates ability to perform toe and ankle exercises	Teach toe and foot exercises that help to increase peripheral circulation
Verbalizes understanding reason for eating extra carbohydrate before strenuous exercise and need to carry fast-acting sugars	Stress importance of eating a little extra carbohydrate before engaging in strenuous exercise and stress that fast-acting sugars should be carried
Travel	
Verbalizes importance of consultation with a physician before travel and obtaining necessary supplies	Stress importance of seeing physician before traveling for prescriptions for insulin syringes, where to seek medical assistance, and a written statement that client is a diabetic
Verbalizes reason for carrying insulin on self	*Stress carrying of insulin, syringes, and fast-acting sugars on self, not in glove compartments or nonpressurized cabins of planes or trains*
	Stress carrying an exchange list for dietary needs; call airlines, etc., to arrange for necessary meals
	Stress wearing ID bracelet, learn how to say "diabetes" in foreign language
	Provide pamphlets: (1) *A Guide for the Diabetic* (Lilly), (2) *What is Diabetes?* (Lilly), (3) *An Instructional Aid on Juvenile Diabetes* (Travis). Assign reading as appropriate.

Summary of Nursing Actions—cont'd

OUTCOME CRITERIA*	PLAN/IMPLEMENTATION
Prenatal The woman and family understand the disease process and are informed about and willing to participate actively in its management. Adverse effects of associated problems (i.e., changes in glucose tolerance, alterations in insulin metabolism, and use and increased tendency to ketosis) have a minimal effect on the mother and fetus. The woman suffers no sequelae of diabetes (e.g., nephropathy, retinopathy) or worsening of preexisting complications. The woman suffers no related complications during pregnancy: hyperemesis gravidarum, preeclampsia-eclampsia, hydramnios. Through home monitoring of blood glucose and management of diet, exercise, and insulin, the woman maintains euglycemia.	**Prenatal** *First half of pregnancy* Elicit woman's and family's cooperation in management of diabetes and pregnancy; make sure she keeps appointments and follows up on missed appointments, performs daily urine tests and/or blood glucose determinations accurately, maintains strict dietary control, gets adequate rest and exercise, and receives early treatment for infection and symptoms of insulin shock (reaction). Reinforce need for keeping the urine test at 1+ sugar level (to be assured of mild hyperglycemia and therefore of a control over hypoglycemia and hyperinsulinemia, which are very dangerous to the embryo and fetus). (Urine should be freshly voided.) If complications develop, refer woman to physician. Encourage woman to join community diabetic groups to help maintain motivation and follow diet. *Second half of pregnancy* Encourage visits every week to supervise management. Keep woman and family informed; reinforce physician's explanations (e.g., that insulin needs are usually higher during the third trimester). ■ Maintenance: NPH until delivery. ■ Fractional urine specimens tested four times daily as necessary. Woman's diet may need adjustment for rapid growth needs of fetus. Prepare for tests (Table 28.1). Observe the woman closely during teaching sessions to see how well she is dealing with what is being taught. Encourage woman's and family's expression of feelings regarding self and infant. If the woman is hospitalized, provide care as appropriate for hospitalization (e.g., NST). Provide diversional activities for woman if appropriate.
ASSESSMENT	EXAMPLES OF POTENTIAL NURSING DIAGNOSTIC CATEGORIES

INTRANATAL PERIOD
A. Observe woman for hypoglycemia: palpitation, tachycardia, hunger, weakness, sweating, tremor, pallor.
B. Observe woman for preeclampsia (see Chapter 27 for symptomatology).
C. Monitor urine for amount and presence of protein and glucose.
D. Monitor intravenous infusions: insulin, oxytocin.
E. Culture urine following clean-catch collection for asymptomatic urinary tract infection
F. Monitor labor.
  1. Monitor induction: maternal/fetal responses.
  2. Use electronic fetal monitor if available.
  3. Assess amount and character of amniotic fluid.
	Anxiety
	Fear
	Ineffective individual or family coping
	Potential for injury
	Knowledge deficit
	Powerlessness
	Disturbance in self-concept: body image, self-esteem, role performance, personal identity
	Spiritual distress
	Alteration in nutrition: less or more than body requirements.

Summary of Nursing Actions—cont'd

OUTCOME CRITERIA*	PLAN/IMPLEMENTATION
Woman suffers no related complications during labor, e.g., vena cava hypotensive syndrome, dystocia, energy/insulin imbalance. Parent-newborn attachment occurs; or if newborn exhibits a disorder or dies, the grieving process is initiated (Chapter 26).	The physician and nurse keep woman and family informed of treatment and fetal status. Do not allow woman to consume anything by mouth. Monitor intravenous fluids per order for the following: ■ For induction (with oxytocin [Pitocin]). ■ 10% dextrose in water and insulin to meet woman's caloric and insulin needs for work of labor. Provide supportive labor nursing, which is especially important to prevent hypoglycemia and acidosis from anxiety. Prepare for induction or cesarean birth (e.g., in case of fetal distress, fetopelvic disproportion, or lack of response to induction). Alert pediatrician and nursery personnel.

ASSESSMENT	EXAMPLES OF POTENTIAL NURSING DIAGNOSTIC CATEGORIES

POSTNATAL PERIOD
A. During first 24 to 48 hours after delivery insulin requirements fluctuate rapidly. Termination of pregnancy reverses gestation-induced endocrine changes: high serum blood glucose level, elevated levels of human growth hormone (HGH) and its potentiator, human placental lactogen (HPL).
  1. Do frequent fractional urine tests.
  2. Monitor foods and fluids taken.
  3. Assess woman for clinical manifestations of high or low serum glucose levels.
B. Monitor vital signs, amount of bleeding, uterine contractility, output, and so on as per usual postdelivery routine.
C. Assess woman's and family's reaction to experience, especially if fetal-neonatal death occurs or infant is malformed or at risk.
	Anxiety
	Fear
	Ineffective individual or family coping
	Potential for injury
	Knowledge deficit
	Powerlessness
	Alteration in nutrition: less or more than body requirements
	Disturbance in self-concept: body image, self-esteem, role performance, personal identity
	Spiritual distress
	Potential for grieving

OUTCOME CRITERIA*	PLAN/IMPLEMENTATION
Woman suffers no related complications during the early postpartum period, e.g., wide variations in blood glucose, PIH, hemorrhage (especially after delivery of large baby or polyhydramnios). Parent-child attachment occurs; or if newborn exhibits a disorder or dies, the grieving process is initiated (Chapter 26).	Adjust insulin intake (usually regular insulin) according to protocol ordered. Woman may need no insulin for first 24 hours to 48 hours. Progress to NPH according to physician's orders. Allow woman to take over insulin injections when she desires. Provide postdelivery nursing care (after vaginal or cesarean birth) according to routine. Provide supportive care for woman and family after fetal-neonatal death or if neonate is malformed or at risk (see Chapter 26). Keep woman and family informed of her status and infant's condition. Give instructions on breast-feeding: ■ Caloric intake and insulin requirements will need adjusting; for example, women requiring large doses of insulin may need to triple caloric intake and decrease insulin by

Summary of Nursing Actions—cont'd

OUTCOME CRITERIA*	PLAN/IMPLEMENTATION
	one half because of antidiabetogenic action (free glucose is used in production of lactose).
	■ If mother develops acetonuria, discontinue breast-feeding (pump breasts and discard milk) and contact physician for supervision.
	■ If mother becomes hypoglycemic from lack of food or anxiety or other reason, her epinephrine level increases, which decreases her milk supply and inhibits the letdown reflex.
	Counsel woman regarding personal care: she *must* eat on time even if it means that others must wait; it will take more energy to add care of the new baby to her previous routine.
	Couple may request genetic counseling. Infant will not necessarily acquire the disease.
	Counsel couple on contraception, sterilization, and planning for future pregnancies (see Chapter 7).

EVALUATION The nurse can be assured that care and teaching were effective when the goals of care have been met.

HYPEREMESIS GRAVIDARUM

Hyperemesis gravidarum (pernicious vomiting of pregnancy) is defined as excessive vomiting during pregnancy, leading to dehydration and starvation. Many pregnant women suffer nausea and vomiting at some time during early gestation. The indisposition is mild in most cases, but in about 1 of every 1000 pregnant women, severe intractable emesis will require hospitalization and perhaps even therapeutic abortion.

The *etiology* of hyperemesis during pregnancy is still debated. Psychologically unstable women whose established reaction patterns to stress involve gastrointestinal disturbances often are affected. In some women, however, psychologic etiology cannot be elicited. Other causes could be multiple pregnancy, hormonal abnormalities (elevated T_4), or trophoblastic disease (hydatidiform mole).

In extreme cases *dehydration* leads to fluid-electrolyte complications, particularly acidosis. Rarely does vomitus contain only gastric acid fluids. Most vomiting involves loss of contents (alkali) from deeper within the gastrointestinal tract. This leads to the development of metabolic acidosis. *Starvation* causes hypoproteinemia and hypovitaminosis. Degenerative changes produce characteristic symptomatology. Jaundice and hemorrhage secondary to vitamin C and B-complex deficiency and hypothrombinemia lead to bleeding from mucosal surfaces. The embryo or fetus may die, and the mother may die from irreversible metabolic alterations. In most cases hyperemesis gravidarum will respond to therapy; hence the prognosis is good. The woman is discharged home when fluid and electrolyte balance is restored and weight gain begins. A summary of nursing actions for hyperemesis gravidarum is presented on p. 866.

Summary of Nursing Actions

HYPEREMESIS GRAVIDARUM

GOALS

1. For the mother: a physiologically safe and psychologically satisfying pregnancy.
2. For the fetus: a physiologically safe intrauterine environment.
3. For the family: effective family coping with the condition.

PRIORITIES

1. Prevention of dehydration and starvation.
2. Support of family coping.

ASSESSMENT	EXAMPLES OF POTENTIAL NURSING DIAGNOSTIC CATEGORIES
Amount of vomiting. Dietary progress and daily weight, fluid intake, and urinary output. Woman's affect and response to home environment and pregnancy. Fetal heart rate and growth of fetus. Jaundice (a rare occurrence). Abnormal bleeding, for example, from mucosal surfaces (a rare occurrence). Intravenous line for infiltration, etc.	Anxiety Fear Ineffective individual or family coping Alteration in family process Fluid volume deficit related to vomiting Alteration in fluid volume: excess related to therapy Grieving Knowledge deficit Alteration in nutrition: less than body requirements Powerlessness Disturbance in self-concept: body image, self-esteem, role performance, personal identity Spiritual distress

OUTCOME CRITERIA*	PLAN/IMPLEMENTATION
Severe vomiting episodes are resolved; fluid and electrolyte homeostasis is achieved, and weight gain occurs. No adverse sequelae, maternal or fetal, develop as a result of condition. If medical treatment is unsuccessful, surgical intervention to terminate pregnancy is undertaken. Woman comes to terms with self, pregnancy, and life situation.	Management of hyperemesis gravidarum includes hospitalization in a pleasant, well-ventilated room. Parenteral fluids, electrolytes, sedatives, and vitamins will be required. For the first 48 hours parenteral fluids are used to maintain hydration and restore fluid and electrolyte balance. Cautious resumption of a dry diet in six small feedings with clear liquids an hour after meals generally is acceptable. Accept woman's behavior in gentle, nonjudgmental manner. Encourage woman to discuss her feelings, emphasizing her complete recovery. Keep conversational topics pleasant. Keep family informed as to progress. (Family may feel anger or hurt at being excluded from visiting, as well as contempt for wife and mother.) Maintain excellent daily hygiene. If additional psychotherapy is indicated, the physician will give woman referrals. Report and record FHR abnormalities, maternal jaundice, and bleeding from mucosal surfaces. Change intravenous tubing per hospital protocol to prevent infection. Reinsert intravenous line at another site if infiltration or venous thrombosis occurs.

EVALUATION The nurse can be assured that care was effective when the goals of care have been met.

*Outcome criteria direct the selection of nursing actions (**plan/implementation**) and measure their effectiveness (**evaluation**).

DISORDERS OF THE THYROID GLAND

Hyperthyroidism. Hyperthyroidism, which affects about 1 of every 1500 pregnant women, may seriously complicate gestation or endanger the fetus. Hyperthyroidism may be responsible for anovulation and amenorrhea, but the disease is not a cause of abortion or fetal anomaly. Hyperthyroidism is associated with an increased incidence of premature labor and delivery. Symptoms include weakness, sweating, weight loss (or poor gain), nervousness, loose stools, and heat intolerance. Warm, soft, moist skin, tachycardia, stare with exophthalmos, tremor, and goiter (enlarged gland) with a bruit are characteristic. Enlargement of the thyroid gland is symmetric. Laboratory findings, particularly the basal metabolic rate and the free T_4 index, will be elevated.

Radioactive iodine must not be used in testing or in therapy because it may destroy or compromise the fetal thyroid. Other antithyroid drugs such as iodine or the thiouracils may be employed to control the overactive maternal thyroid, provided the free T_4 index remains normal and that leukopenia does not develop.

Partial thyroidectomy, also an acceptable treatment for toxic goiter, requires preoperative preparation by antithyroid medication, usually Lugol's solution. Hypothyroidism, which occurs in at least 20% of hyperthyroid women postoperatively, must be treated promptly to spare the fetus. A free T_4 index determination on the cord blood at birth should be run to aid in determining the status of the infant.

Any maternal therapy for thyroid dysfunction may induce fetal thyroid insult. Determination of free thyroxine index in cord blood of such an infant is necessary.

Hypothyroidism. Hypothyroidism may be responsible for anovulation in the infertile woman. Moreover, thyroid deficiency may cause spontaneous abortion, fetal maldevelopment, or fetal goiter. Mild degrees of hypothyroidism in women may go unrecognized or may suggest a disease process of another system, or example, menorrhagia. In the latter instance diagnosis depends largely on laboratory tests. Simple goiter generally is caused by iodine lack, and the woman is only slightly thyroid deficient.

Clinical early hypothyroidism is characterized by easy fatigability, cold intolerance, lethargy, constipation, dry skin, or headache. Thin brittle nails, dry skin, alopecia, poor skin turgor, and delayed deep tendon reflexes are typical. During pregnancy, normal or reduced protein-bound iodine (PBI), reduced thyroxine (T_4) (column or D), reduced triiodothyronine (T_3) (resin), and a reduced T_4 index (normal range is 0.75 to 2.5 units if T_4 by column is used; 1.3 to 5 units if T_4[D] is used with resin T_3 uptake).

Malignant disease of the thyroid. Surgical treatment rather than use of radioisotopes is preferred when malignant thyroid disease complicates pregnancy. It is permissible to follow with well-shielded radiation therapy. Hill and associates (1966) found that pregnancy subsequent to the diagnosis of thyroid malignancy seems to have no effect on the outcome of this disease.

DISORDERS OF THE ADRENAL GLAND

Hyperadrenocorticism. Hyperfunction of the adrenal cortex occurs in Cushing's syndrome, Cushing's disease, adrenogenital syndrome, hyperaldosteronism, and pheochromocytoma. The individual's principal problem in all these disorders is abnormal loss of salt, as well as hypertension and its related complications. Pregnancy is not easily achieved in such women because of amenorrhea and anovulation. A tumor (e.g., pituitary, adrenal) should be identified if present and removed if feasible. Adrenocortical hyperplasia and hyperfunction may be controlled with one of the cortisones. Preeclampsia-eclampsia, infection, osteoporosis, and shock may be associated problems. The frequency of fetal anomaly is not increased in hyperadrenocorticism, but there is a risk of premature delivery.

Hypoadrenocorticism (Addison's disease). Hypoadrenocorticism, idiopathic in more than 50% of cases and caused by tuberculosis in most of the rest, is an uncommon complication of pregnancy. These women, whose fluid-electrolyte balance may be precarious, especially after pernicious nausea and vomiting of pregnancy, are susceptible to infection and especially to shock. A low plasma sodium chloride level, reduced 17-ketosteroid and 17 hydroxycorticoid levels, a low or absent plasma cortisol level, together with eosinophilia and lymphocytosis, are diagnostic laboratory findings in Addison's disease. With cortisone replacement therapy, electrolyte supplementation, and the avoidance of hemorrhage, the woman usually can go through pregnancy successfully. Therapeutic abortion rarely is indicated; vaginal delivery is desirable. Whether cortisone is teratogenic in humans is still debated.

People with Addison's disease display easy fatigability, anorexia, and frequent episodes of nausea, vomiting, and diarrhea. They also have sparse axillary hair and increased skin pigmentation and suffer hypotension.

■ ■ ■

Other endocrine disorders, for example, hypoparathyroidism and hyperparathyroidism, are rarely encountered during pregnancy. The student is referred to medical texts and the references at the end of this chapter.

Cardiovascular Disorders

Every pregnancy taxes the cardiovascular system. The strain is present during pregnancy and is maintained for a few weeks after delivery. An increase in blood volume begins by the tenth or twelfth week of gestation, reaches a maximum of 30% to 50% at 20 to 26 weeks, and levels off after the thirtieth week. Blood volume returns to nonpregnant levels within the first 2 to 3 weeks after delivery. The increase in blood volume is correlated with birth weight and thus tends to be greater in multigravidas and women with multiple pregnancies. The cardiac output and stroke volume at rest show a corresponding increase in the blood volume but return to normal by 6 weeks after delivery. The heart rate is accelerated by a maximum of 15 to 20 beats/min in the last trimester. With delivery of the placenta and closure of the placental vascular shunt, venous hypertension occurs during the first 24 hours after childbirth.

The normal heart can compensate for these and associated burdens so that pregnancy and delivery are generally well tolerated. If myocardial or valvular disease develops, or if a congenital heart defect is large, cardiac decompensation is likely.

Incidence and characteristics. Heart disease affects 0.5% to 2% of pregnant women. Currently in North America congenital heart disease occurs more frequently with pregnancy than does rheumatic carditis. Syphilis, arteriosclerosis, and pulmonary and renal disorders are responsible for cardiac complications, some of which develop during pregnancy. Heart disease is of considerable importance for the expectant woman because a maternal mortality of 1% to 3% is likely with severe heart disease. It ranks fourth as a cause of maternal death. A perinatal mortality of up to 50% must be expected with persistent cardiac decompensation.

Rheumatic fever attacks the mitral, aortic, or tricuspid valve. Congenital maldevelopment involves the septa, valves, and conduction system. Persistently patent fetal cardiovascular communications may reduce the efficiency of the heart. Syphilis and arteriosclerosis principally alter the aortic valves and the conduction system.

Effects of pregnancy on heart disease. The effects of pregnancy on heart disease result from the maternal cardiovascular adaptations during pregnancy. The stress these place on an already weakened heart may cause cardiac decompensation. Cardiac failure can develop during the last few weeks of pregnancy, during labor, and during the postdelivery period (Pritchard, McDonald, and Gant, 1985).

Effects of heart disease on pregnancy. Spontaneous abortion is increased, and premature labor and delivery are more prevalent with heart disease. Probably because of the low P_{O_2} level, fetal growth retardation frequently occurs during gestation in the pregnant woman with cardiac problems.

Symptoms. Symptoms of cardiac decompensation may appear abruptly or gradually. Medical intervention must be instituted immediately to correct cardiac status.

The *pregnant woman* notes the following *subjective symptoms:* increasing fatigue or dyspnea or both with her usual exertion, a feeling of smothering or difficulty in breathing, the need to cough frequently (coughing may be accompanied by hemoptysis), and periods of palpitations and tachycardia. Unfortunately dyspnea, chest pain, palpitations, and syncope occur commonly in pregnant women and can mask the symptoms of a developing cardiovascular disorder.

The *examiner* observes the following *objective symptoms:* progressive, generalized edema; rales at the base of the lungs; and pulse irregularity. The clinical findings are summarized in the emergency box below.

Diagnosis. The differential diagnosis of heart disease involves ruling out respiratory problems, primarily arrhythmias. The diagnosis of heart disease depends on the history, physical examination, x-ray films, and ultrasonograms when required.

Classification. The degree of dysfunction (disability) of the woman with cardiac disease often is more important in the treatment and prognosis of cardiac disease complicating pregnancy than the diagnosis of the valvular lesion per se. The New York Heart Association's functional classification of organic heart disease, a widely accepted standard, is as follows:
1. Class I: persons with cardiac disease who have no limitation of physical activity

---

Danger Signals: Cardiovascular Disease

Increasing fatigue
Increasing dyspnea
Frequent cough
Irregular rapid pulse 100/min
Rapid respirations 25/min
Generalized edema
Rales at base of lung

2. Class II: persons with cardiac disease who have a slight limitation of physical activity
3. Class III: persons with cardiac disease who have considerable limitation of activity, with even ordinary activity producing symptoms
4. Class IV: persons with cardiac disease who are unable to undertake any physical activity without discomfort and who have symptoms of cardiac insufficiency even at rest

No classification of heart disease can be considered rigid or absolute, but this one offers a basic practical guide for treatment, assuming frequent prenatal visits, good client cooperation, and proper obstetric care.

Medical management. Medical therapy is conducted as a team approach with a cardiologist. The functional class of the disease is determined at 3 months and again at 7 or 8 months. The therapy includes the following:

1. Treatment of anemia, hyperthyroidism, or obesity as necessary to reduce risk factors that increase the work load of the cardiovascular circulation
2. Treatment of any infections promptly, since respiratory, urinary, or gastrointestinal tract infections can complicate the condition by accelerating heart rate and by direct spread of organisms (e.g., *Streptococcus*) to the heart structure
3. Restriction of sodium intake with careful monitoring for hyponatremia. The sodium ion, with its ability to attract and hold fluid, affects the quality and the amount of the circulating volume
4. Monitoring the woman's intake of potassium to prevent hypokalemia. It is associated with heart and other muscular weakness and dysfunction
5. Monitoring anticoagulant therapy, if used

Other therapy is directly related to the functional classification of heart disease.

Class I. The pregnant woman with class I heart disease should limit stress to protect against cardiac decompensation. Additional rest at night and after meals, frequent evaluations, and the early and effective treatment of respiratory and other infections should be stressed. Therapeutic abortion is never medically warranted. If there are no obstetric problems, vaginal delivery is recommended. This is accomplished using pudendal block anesthesia with forceps for shortening of the second stage of labor.

Class II. A program similar to that for class I should be followed for the pregnant woman with class II heart disease. However, the woman should be admitted to the hospital near term (if signs of cardiac overload or arrhythmia develop) for evaluation and treatment.

Penicillin prophylaxis of nonsensitized pregnant women against bacterial endocarditis in labor and during the early puerperium is advised. Mask oxygen and pudendal block anesthesia are important. Ergot products should not be used because of increases in blood pressure. Dilute intravenous oxytocin immediately after delivery may be employed to prevent postdelivery hemorrhage. Tubal sterilization may be performed, but surgery should be delayed several days at least to ensure homeostasis. If sterilization is not achieved, effective contraception must be provided.

Class III. Bed rest for much of each day is necessary for pregnant women with class III cardiac disease. Cardiac decompensation occurs during pregnancy in about 30% of class III women. With this possibility, hospitalization of the woman for the remainder of pregnancy and the early puerperium is advised. Early therapeutic abortion may be warranted, particularly after a previous episode of cardiac failure. Therapeutic abortion and elective sterilization may be feasible. Breast feeding is contraindicated. Sterilization should be postponed until a later date, but explicit contraceptive advice must be given.

Class IV. Because persons with class IV cardiac disease have decompensation even at rest, a major initial effort must be made to improve the cardiac status of pregnant women in this category. Early therapeutic abortion, although not innocuous, may be feasible with regional anesthesia in some cases. Prophylactic antibiotic therapy should be used with the procedure. Vaginal delivery of women with class IV lesions is the safest approach if abortion is not done. Maternal mortality approaches 50% in class IV heart disease; the perinatal mortality is even higher.

Operative care. Operations for the correction of congenital or acquired heart disease should be done before pregnancy if possible. Closed cardiac surgery such as release of a stenotic mitral orifice can be accomplished with little risk to mother or fetus. On the other hand, open heart surgery requires extracorporeal circulation, and under these circumstances, hypoxia may develop. As a consequence the risk of fetal damage or loss rises to almost 30%. If anticoagulant therapy is required during pregnancy, heparin should be used because this large molecular drug does not cross the placenta. Oral anticoagulants, such as warfarin (Coumadin) compounds, cross to the fetus and may cause anomalies or hemorrhage in the infant. However, valvuloplasty clients should receive penicillin or other antibiotic prophylaxis against bacterial endocarditis during gestation.

Nursing care. The nursing care of a woman with cardiac disease spans the maternity cycle. It includes careful assessment and analysis of the data collected as a basis for formulating nursing diagnoses. The nursing diagnoses focus attention on the plan and implementation of care. The nursing process is applied to the three pregnancy periods—prenatal, intranatal, and postdelivery. The evaluation of care is presented at the end of the sequence.

The goals for care of the woman whose pregnancy is complicated by a cardiac problem are (1) minimize stress associated with pregnancy and (2) support cardiac function. The care begins in the prenatal period and continues until the mother has recovered from the birth.

Prenatal care

Assessment. The woman is examined at weekly intervals at home or on a continuous basis if hospitalized. The nurse assesses for factors that would increase stress on the heart, such as anemia, infection, or a home situation that includes responsibility for the house, other children, or extended family members. The client is observed for signs of *cardiac decompensation,* that is, *progressive generalized edema, rales at the base of the lungs,* or *pulse irregularity.* The routine monitoring continues for the prenatal period, including monitoring weight gain and pattern of weight gain, edema, vital signs, discomforts of pregnancy, urinalysis, and blood work. The nurse keeps careful check of the side effects and interactions of all medicatons—including supplemental iron—that the woman is taking and reports them to the physician. Their use also is documented on the client's record. For example, if a woman is receiving anticoagulant therapy with dicumarol, the drug will need to be changed to heparin because dicumarol causes fetal hemorrhage.

Nursing diagnoses. Examples of nursing diagnoses might include the following:
1. Fear related to increased peripartum risk
2. Potential alteration in tissue perfusion of placenta related to hypotensive syndrome
3. Impaired home maintenance management related to mother's confinement to bed

Plan and implementation. The plan of care takes into consideration the women's social situation. The woman may be concerned with the welfare of other family members at the expense of her own welfare and that of the fetus. The care includes the following:
1. Reinforcing the physician's explanation for need for close medical supervision.
2. Reviewing symptoms of cardiac decompensation: increasing fatigue or dyspnea with the woman's usual exertion, feeling of smothering, need to cough frequently (hemoptysis at times), periods of palpitations and tachycardia. Give the woman written as well as verbal instructions.

3. Promoting adequate rest: The woman should sleep 8 to 10 hours every day and ½ hour after meals. Activities are restricted; for example, if the woman is at home, she is to do no housework, no shopping, and no laundry.
4. Teaching regarding nutrition (especially difficult when someone else shops and cooks): The woman needs a diet high in iron and protein and adequate calories to gain 10.8 kg (24 lb) during pregnancy. To prevent pyrosis (heartburn) the woman is advised to assume a semi- or low-Fowler's position after eating.
5. Teaching the woman to give herself heparin, if heparin is ordered in place of dicumarol. If she is taking heparin, she is cautioned to avoid foods high in vitamin K, such as raw, deep green, leafy vegetables. Vitamin K counteracts the effects of heparin. Therefore she will require a substitute source of folic acid.
6. Teaching regarding the danger of infection: The woman should notify the physician at the first sign of infection or when she is exposed to infection.
7. Reviewing the information pertaining to management of the woman's labor and her early postdelivery period. The woman and her family will need time to plan for the necessary extra care the mother will require.

Intranatal care

Assessment. The assessment includes the routine assessments for all laboring women as well as assessments for cardiac decompensation. The latter include taking vital signs at least every 10 to 30 minutes. The physician is alerted if the pulse rate is 100/min or greater or if respirations are 25/min or greater. Respiratory status is checked constantly for developing dyspnea, coughing, or rales at the base of the lungs. The color and temperature of the skin are noted. Pallor, cooling, and sweating may indicate cardiac shock. The woman is carefully watched for symptoms of emotional stress.

Nursing diagnoses. Examples of nursing diagnoses might include:
1. Anxiety related to fear for infant's safety
2. Fear of dying related to perceived inability to control stress of labor

Plan and implementation. These clients require a one-to-one staff ratio. The collaborating internist is notified of the woman's labor. Close cooperation between members of the obstetric team is mandatory. A pediatrician and nurse from the intensive care unit are present at the birth for the immediate care of the newborn infant.

Nursing actions include the following:
1. Making sure the woman does not take dicumarol if receiving anticoagulant therapy.
2. Administering prophylactic antibiotics as ordered to prevent infection that could cause further valvular damage.
3. Promoting cardiac function by the following measures:
   a. Alleviating anxiety through maintaining a calm atmosphere and keeping the woman and her family informed.
   b. Placing the woman in a side-lying position with her head and shoulders elevated and body parts supported (with pillows, etc.).
   c. Medicating for discomfort and sedating as needed.
   d. Assisting the physician with anesthesia—saddle block (low spinal), caudal, or lumbar epidural—to minimize discomfort, eliminate bearing-down reflex, and decrease peripheral resistance, venous return, and cardiac output. Prevent, recognize, and report and treat hypotension, which may follow anesthesia.
4. Assisting the physician if evidence of cardiac decompensation appears *(pulse rate is 100/min or greater; respirations are 25/min or greater; dyspnea)*. Administer medications and record what has been given. These may include the following:
   a. Deslanoside (Cedilanid-D) (fast acting, for digitalization).
   b. Oxygen by intermittent positive pressure (decreases chance of pulmonary edema).
   c. Diuretics (furosemide [Lasix] is potent and fast acting).
5. Informing family members of the woman's progress.

Delivery is accomplished with the woman in the left side-lying position, or if placed in the supine position, a pad is positioned under the left hip to minimize the danger of supine hypotension. The knees are flexed, and the feet are flat on the bed. Stirrups are not used to prevent compression of popliteal veins and an increase in blood volume in the chest and trunk as a result of the effects of gravity. An episiotomy and the use of outlet forceps also decrease the work of the heart.

Postdelivery care. The immediate postdelivery period is hazardous for a woman with a compromised heart. Cardiac output increases rapidly as extravascular fluid is remobilized into the vascular compartment.

At the moment of delivery, intraabdominal pressure is reduced drastically; pressure on veins is removed, the splanchnic vessels engorge, and blood flow to the heart is increased. Fluid begins to move from the extravascular spaces into the bloodstream. Some physicians favor the application of the abdominal binder or alternating tourniquets on the extremities to minimize the effects of this rapid change in intraabdominal pressure.

Assessment. Cardiac monitoring for decompensation continues through the first weeks after delivery because it has been known to occur as late as the sixth postpartum day. Routine assessment as for any newly delivered woman is instituted, for example, vital signs, bleeding, uterine contractility, urinary output, pain, rest, diet, and daily weight. Laboratory (e.g., hemoglobin, hematocrit, and urinalysis) results are noted and reported if indicated to the physician. It is important to assess the woman's support systems, since activity will be curtailed until the cardiac system is recovered. The family response to the birth and infant need to be observed because the mother may not be directly involved in the infant's care for a period of time (prematurity of infant, health of mother).

Nursing diagnoses. The nursing diagnoses derived from analyses of clinical findings act as guides to develop care. This care addresses the specific needs of the client. The mother who has cardiovascular problems faces curtailment of her activities. The restrictions can have physical and emotional implications. Diagnoses such as the following might be made.
1. Self-care deficit related to need for bed rest
2. Disturbance in self-concept related to restrictions placed on involvement in care of infant

Plan and implementation. The woman's hospital stay is extended to 7 days or more to permit continuous assessment for cardiac decompensation and to support cardiac and respiratory function. The latter is achieved by the following measures:
1. Providing proper positioning in bed with the same position as for labor; that is, elevate the head of the bed and encourage the woman to lie on her side.
2. Providing bed rest with bathroom privileges as tolerated. The nurse meets the woman's grooming and hygiene needs and may even assist her with turning in bed, eating, and other activities.
3. Assisting with progressive ambulation as tolerated. The nurse assesses the woman's pulse, skin, and affect before and after walking.
4. Promoting bowel movements without stress or strain. Stool softeners, diet, and fluids plus mild analgesia and local anesthetic spray applied to the episiotomy may facilitate the process.
5. Preventing overdistension of bladder (more than 1000 ml) because:
   a. A distended bladder prevents contraction of the uterus (Chapters 18 and 24), and this predisposes to hemorrhage.

b. Rapid emptying of the distended bladder results in a precipitous drop in intraabdominal pressure, leading to splanchic engorgement and generalized hypotension. The nurse institutes intake and output recording.
6. Isolating the woman from sources of infection such as people and objects. A private room is appropriate for this client.
7. Initiating prevention or prompt and efficient treatment of hemorrhage or infection.
8. Facilitating mother-infant interactions that do not stress the mother. The mother may direct care of the infant by a designated family member. The mother may nurse if her condition warrants; that is, classes I and II may nurse (for classes III and IV, nursing is not advised). The fed baby can be brought regularly to the mother, held at her eye level and by her lips, and brought to her fingers so that she can establish an emotional bond with her baby with a low expenditure of her energy. At the same time, involving the mother passively in her infant's care helps the mother feel vitally important—as she is—to the infant's well-being (e.g., "You can do something no one else can: provide your baby with your sounds, touch, and rhythms that are so comforting"). Perhaps the mother can be encouraged to make a tape recording of her talking, singing, or whispering, to be played for the baby in the nursery, to help the infant feel her presence and be in contact with her voice.

Before discharge the nurse assesses the home support for the woman and infant. Preparation for discharge is carefully planned with the woman and family as follows:
1. Provision of help in the home for the mother by relatives, friends, and others. If necessary, the nurse refers the family to community resources (e.g., for homemaking services).
2. Planning of rest and sleep periods, activity, and diet by the mother.
3. Provision of information to the couple regarding reestablishment of sexual relations, contraception, sterilization of the man or the woman (usually advocated for women in classes II, III, and IV), and medical supervision.

Evaluation. The nurse uses the following criteria as *overall indications* for the success of therapy:
1. The woman is able to tolerate the stresses imposed by pregnancy. These include increase in cardiac output by more than one third, increase in pulse rate by 10 beats/min, expansion of blood volume by 25%, and psychologic stress common to pregnancy and related to the heart condition.

2. Congestive heart failure, the primary cause of maternal mortality in women with cardiac disease, is prevented.
3. The home situation is controlled, with assistance provided as necessary.
4. The mother and family accept the limitations imposed on the woman by the presence of heart disease.
5. The parent and child relationship is fostered by the family.

Peripartum cardiomyopathies*
Definition. Peripartum cardiomyopathies comprise a syndrome of cardiac failure (1) occurring during the peripartum period, (2) with no previous history of heart disease, and (3) with no specific etiologic factors (Demakis and Rahimtoola, 1971). When not associated with pregnancy the disorder is known by an array of names: hypertrophic cardiomyopathy (HCM), idiopathic hypertrophic subaortic stenosis, and asymmetric septal hypertrophy. It is a commonly diagnosed disease of the heart muscle. Its exact cause is unknown, although it may be genetically transmitted.

Symptomatology. Most clients are asymptomatic until late adolescence or early adulthood (childbearing years) or more rarely middle age. Symptoms include angina pectoris, exertional dyspnea, supraventricular and ventricular arrhythmias, dizziness and syncope. Most deaths associated with HCM are sudden, unexpected, and unrelated to functional status. HCM may be precipitated by physical or emotional stress, and the myocardial ischemia resulting from stress may promote ventricular fibrillation.

Incidence and characteristics. The incidence of peripartum cardiomyopathies has been reported as 1 in 3000 to 4000 pregnancies. It occurs more often in the multiparous woman. The maternal mortality has been estimated in the range of 30% to 60%, the infant mortality approximately 10%.

Clinical findings are those of congestive heart failure (left ventricular failure). Findings include breathlessness, tachyarrhythmias, and edema (Fig. 28.4) with radiologic findings of cardiomegaly.

The *prognosis* is good if cardiomegaly is not persistent after 6 months. The prognosis for women whose hearts remain enlarged is not as favorable.

Future pregnancies usually result in some cardiac failure (50% to 88%). Mortality has been estimated as high as 60%.

Treatment. Bed rest is advocated up to 7 months, with some women requiring 20 to 22 months. The

---
*For a more intensive discussion see Bohachick and Rongaus (1984) and Veille (1984).

Fig. 28.4
Summary of course of peripartum cardiomyopathy. (From Veille, J.C.: Am. J. Obstet. Gynecol. 148:805, 1984.)

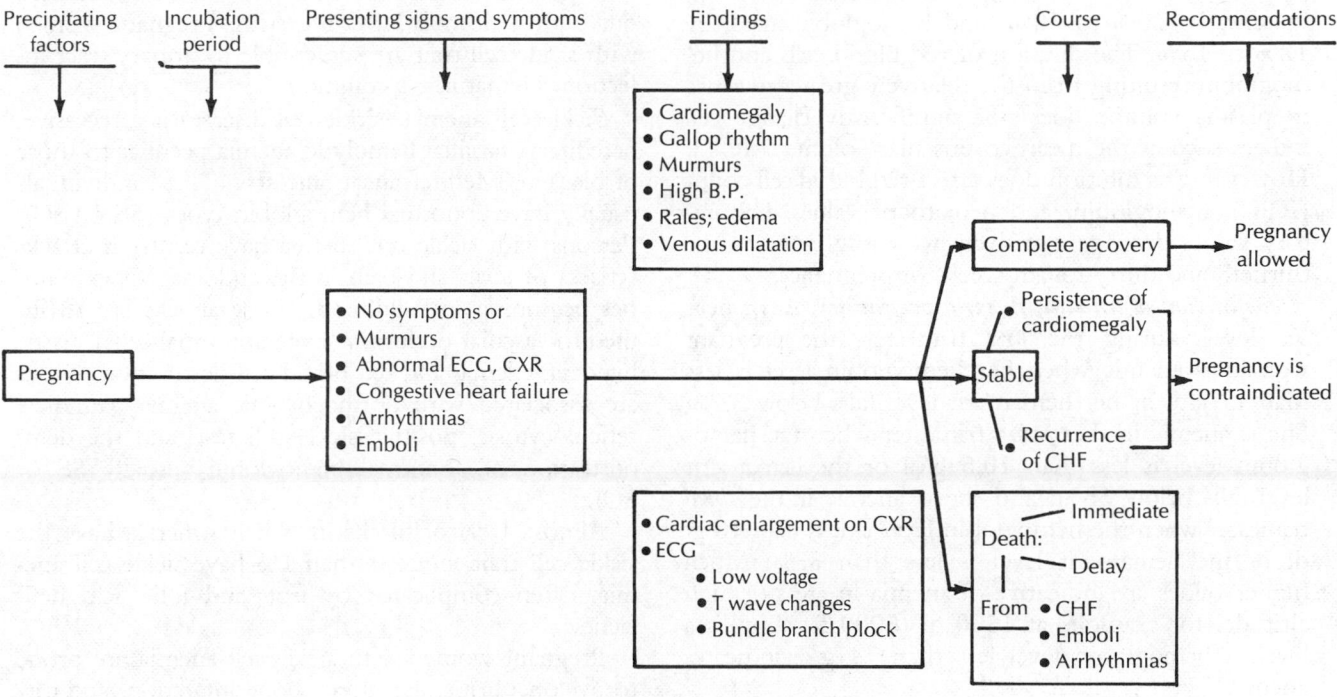

rationale for instituting bed rest is to decrease the heart rate, stroke volume, and arterial pressure.

Low sodium intake (1.5 to 2 g/day) is ordered for women with severe congestive failure. The use of diuretics, digitalis, and anticoagulants requires close medical supervision to detect toxicity. Suppression of lactation is often recommended with no particular rationale other than to minimize stress. (All women experience some rise in blood pressure at the onset of lactation.)

Nursing care. The nursing care of clients with peripartum cardiomyopathies is essentially the same as for those with other types of cardiac problems. The use of Trendelenburg's position for relief of syncope has been demonstrated. The necessity for prolonged bed rest can pose social and economic hardships for a family; therefore referral to community resources for assistance may be necessary. Because sudden death is a feature of this condition, the family needs to be trained in cardiopulmonary resuscitation. Clients need to have ready access to emergency care. (Some hospitals provide special numbers to dial for immediate dispatch of a medically staffed ambulance.)

Anemia

Anemia, the most common medical disorder of pregnancy, affects at least 20% of pregnant women. These women have a higher incidence of puerperal complications such as infection than do pregnant women with normal hematologic values.

Anemia results in reduction of the oxygen-carrying capacity of the blood. An indirect index of the oxygen-carrying capacity is the packed red blood cell volume (PCV), or hematocrit level. The normal hematocrit range in nonpregnant women is 38% to 45%. However, normal values for pregnant women with adequate iron stores may be as low as 34%. This has been explained by hydremia (dilution of blood), or the **physiologic anemia of pregnancy.**

About 90% of cases of anemia in pregnancy are of the iron deficiency type. The remaining 10% of cases embrace a considerable variety of acquired and hereditary anemias, including folic acid deficiency and hemoglobinopathies.

Normal values during pregnancy. Normal and abnormal changes confuse the hematologic profile during pregnancy. The blood values of pregnant women differ significantly from those of nonpregnant women. All the constituents of blood normally increase during pregnancy: plasma volume, by 30% to 35%; red cell volume, by 20% to 30%; and hemoglobin mass, by 12% to 15%. The dilution of red blood cells and hemoglobin resulting from the relatively greater increase in plasma volume does not significantly change cell indices such as the mean corpuscular volume (MCV). However, this dilution does affect red blood cell count (RBC), hemoglobin, and hematocrit values. Laboratory values drop progressively to a low between the thirtieth and thirty-fourth weeks of pregnancy.

Definition of anemia during pregnancy. At or near sea level, during the *first* trimester, the pregnant woman is anemic when her hemoglobin level is less than 11 g/dl or her hematocrit level falls below 37%. She is anemic in the *second* trimester when the hemoglobin level is less than 10.5 g/dl or the hematocrit level falls below 35%; and she is anemic in the *third* trimester when the hemoglobin level is less than 10 g/dl or the hematocrit level is less than 33%. Much higher values are indicative of anemia in areas of high altitude; for example, at 1500 m (5000 ft) above sea level, a hemoglobin level less than 14 g/dl indicates anemia.

Iron deficiency anemia. Without iron therapy even pregnant women who enjoy excellent nutrition will conclude pregnancy with an iron deficit. Diet alone cannot replace gestational iron losses. Inadequate nutrition without therapy will certainly mean iron deficiency anemia during late pregnancy and the puerperium.

Successful iron therapy during pregnancy can be carried out in the vast majority of cases with oral iron supplements (e.g., ferrous sulfate, 0.3 g three times a day). Some pregnant women cannot tolerate or fail to take the prescribed oral iron. In such cases the woman should receive parenteral iron such as the iron-dextran complex (Imferon).

Folic acid deficiency anemia. Folic acid deficiency anemia occurs in at least 2% of pregnant women in North America, an incidence much higher than that suspected even 5 years ago. Many of these women have urinary tract infections because of their anemia.

Poor diet, cooking with large volumes of water, or canning of food may lead to folate deficiency. Also, malabsorption or increased folate use may play a part in the development of anemia caused by a lack of folic acid.

During pregnancy the recommended daily intake is 150 μg of folic acid. In folate deficiency a dosage of about 5 mg per day orally for several weeks should ensure a remission. A generous maintenance dose each day should prevent a relapse. Because iron deficiency anemia may also accompany folate deficiency, augmented iron intake should also be provided.

Sickle cell hemoglobinopathy. Sickle cell trait (SA hemoglobin pattern) is sickling of the red blood cells but with a normal RBC life span. Pregnant women with sickle cell trait are susceptible to urinary tract infection. Hematuria is common.

Sickle cell anemia (sickle cell disease) is a recessive, hereditary, familial hemolytic anemia peculiar to those of black or Mediterranean ancestry. These individuals usually have abnormal hemoglobin types (SS or SC). Persons with sickle cell anemia have recurrent attacks (crises) of fever and pain in the abdomen or extremities beginning in childhood. These attacks are attributed to vascular occlusion (from abnormal cells), tissue hypoxia, edema, and red blood cell destruction. Crises are associated with normochromic anemia, jaundice, reticulocytosis, positive sickle cell test, and the demonstration of abnormal hemoglobin (usually SS or SC).

Almost 10% of blacks in North America have the sickle cell trait, but less than 1% have sickle cell anemia, often complicated by iron and folic acid deficiency.

Pregnant women with sickle cell anemia are prone to pyelonephritis, leg ulcers, bone infarction, and cardiopathy. (Oral contraceptives are contraindicated.) An aplastic crisis may follow serious infection. Medical therapy, including transfusions to maintain the hematocrit level at at least 30% is essential. Cesarean delivery is warranted only on obstetric indications.

Pregnancy may impose critical complications in sickle cell disease. Maternal mortality often ranges between 5% and 10%, and the perinatal mortality may reach 30%. Therapeutic abortion is not medically indicated.

Thalassemia. Thalassemia (Mediterranean or Cooley's anemia) is a relatively common anemia in which an insufficient amount of hemoglobin is produced to fill the red blood cells. Thalassemia is a hereditary disorder that involves the abnormal synthesis of the α-or β-chains of hemoglobin. β-thalassemia is the more common variety in the United States and is often diagnosed in individuals of Italian, Greek, or southern Chinese descent. The unbalanced synthesis of hemoglobin leads to premature red blood cell death resulting in severe anemia. Thalassemia major is the homozygous form of the disorder, thalassemia minor is the heterozygous form.

Thalassemia major may complicate pregnancy. Preeclampsia is more frequent in women with thalassemia major. Thalassemia major may be associated with low—birth weight infants and increased fetal wastage. Placental weight often is increased, perhaps secondary to maternal anemia. The frequency of fetal distress from hypoxia is greater than in control women. Therefore pregnant women with thalassemia major should be monitored more closely than normal pregnant women.

Regular transfusion may be necessary. Folic acid should be given to avoid folate deficiency. Partial exchange transfusion may be warranted in severe thalassemia. Splenectomy may be necessary if enlargement and pain occur. Women with thalassemia major may die of chronic infection or progressive hepatic or cardiac failure, the result of excessive iron deposition.

Persons with *thalassemia minor* have a mild persistent anemia, but the RBC may be normal or even elevated. However, no systemic problems are caused by the anemia that is a part of the minor form of the disease. Thalassemia minor must be distinguished principally from iron deficiency anemia.

Pregnancy will neither worsen thalassemia minor nor will it be compromised by the disease. The anemia will not respond to iron therapy. Prolonged parenteral iron can lead to harmful, excessive iron storage. Infants born to parents with thalassemia will inherit the disorder. Persons with thalassemia minor should have a normal life span despite a moderately reduced hemoglobin level.

Pulmonary Disorders

Bronchial asthma. Bronchial asthma is an acute, dramatic respiratory illness caused by allergens, marked change in ambient temperature, or emotional tension. In many cases the actual cause may be unknown. A family history of allergy is likely in about 50% of all persons with asthma. Almost 2% of individuals in the United States have bronchial asthma, but less than 1% of pregnant women suffer from this disorder. The effect of pregnancy on asthma is unpredictable. Psychologic alterations induced by pregnancy do not make the pregnant women more prone to asthmatic attacks. Asthma increases the incidence of abortion and premature labor, but the fetus per se is unaffected. In severe cases, asthma may be life threatening for the gravida. The prognosis for both mother and fetus will be good in most cases.

Therapy for bronchial asthma has two objectives: (1) release of the acute attack and (2) prevention or limitation of later attacks. In all asthmatics, known allergens should be eliminated and a comfortable home temperature maintained. Tranquilizers (but not sedatives) should be given to relieve apprehension. Respiratory infections should be treated and mist or steam inhalation employed to aid expectoration of mucus. The outline below details treatment of asthma and

pregnancy, providing a basis from which to develop a nursing care plan:

1. Treatment of acute bronchial asthma
   a. Administer hydrocortisone sodium succinate and aminophylline as ordered.
   b. Employ oxygen freely by mask.
   c. Correct fluid-electrolyte imbalance.
2. Treatment of mild or moderate bronchial asthma
   a. Administer epinephrine (1:1000).
   b. Offer isoproterenol inhalation (1:200 aqueous solution) by nebulizer for one or two inhalations.
   c. Give phenobarbital, 30 mg orally three times daily, if necessary to counteract overstimulation by bronchodilator drugs. Except for this purpose, sedatives should be avoided in the treatment of persons with asthma.
3. Interim therapy of bronchial asthma
   a. Diagnose offending antigens and treat allergy properly—by desensitization, if feasible.
   b. Reduce emotional tension; avoid respiratory infections or treat if they occur.
4. Management of pregnancy
   a. Consider therapeutic abortion only in extremely severe cases of asthma recurrent during pregnancies.
   b. Do not use morphine in labor, since it may cause bronchospasm. Meperidine (Demerol) usually will relieve bronchospasm.
   c. Avoid or limit ephedrine and corticotropins (pressor drugs) in preeclampsia-eclampsia.
   d. Opt for vaginal delivery using local or regional anesthesia, whenever possible.

Adult respiratory distress sydrome. (ARDS, shock lung) occurs when the lungs are unable to maintain levels of oxygen and carbon dioxide within normal limits. Marked tachycardia, dyspnea, and cyanosis that does not respond to nasal oxygen or intermittent positive pressure breathing are the most noted signs. This condition may occur in women who have given birth vaginally or by cesarean delivery. ARDS also may occur after spontaneous or medically induced abortion. The chance of developing ARDS increases with the amount of trauma experienced during pregnancy or delivery. ARDS is not a condition specific to pregnancy; it can also result from chest trauma, drug ingestion, or pneumonia. When ARDS is associated with pregnancy, pulmonary embolism, disseminated intravascular coagulation (DIC) (see Chapter 27), and aspiration pneumonia are the precipitators.

It has been noted that during pregnancy there is an increase in some of the coagulation factors. This increase in coagulation results in shortening of the partial thromboplastin time (PTT). This state predisposes the woman to an increase in rapidity of blood clotting and an increased tendency to form blood clots (hypercoagulability).

Laboratory reports are important in identifying the origin of acute pulmonary problems. The important observations for the nurse to note are vital signs, signs of thrombophlebitis, and hemorrhage.

Vital signs. Temperature elevation may indicate the development of thrombophlebitis. The pulse rate increases to compensate for respiratory insufficiency of any origin. The severity of the pulmonary problem increases as the pulse rate rises. An initial rise in blood pressure occurs as cardiac output increases to try to supply the body tissue with oxygen. When lung damage is severe, the blood pressure drops. The most important indicator of ARDS is respiratory changes. The rate, depth, respiratory pattern, symmetry of chest movement, and use of accessory muscles should be noted; therefore observation of respiratory characteristics after activity is important. If there is any indication of abnormality, count respirations for a full minute; an error of plus or minus four may be highly significant. During the postdelivery period, apprehension, distended neck veins, cyanosis, diaphoresis, or pallor may be clues to watch for. Also mental confusion or disorientation may be noted.

On auscultation of the lungs, rales, rhonchi, wheezes, or a pleural friction rub need to be reported, especially when they have occurred since an earlier normal assessment. The pregnant woman should be positioned for breathing comfort. Oxygen and emergency equipment should be available while the physician is notified. Reassure the woman so that her anxiety is lessened.

Thrombophlebitis. The lower extremities need to be checked for swelling, pain, inflammation, venous distention, and Homans' sign. If thrombophlebitis is suspected, the woman should be kept on bed rest until the physician can be notified. Sudden movement or straining can dislodge a clot and lead to pulmonary embolism.

Postdelivery hemorrhage. Petechiae, ecchymosis, hematuria, and epistaxis are important indications of DIC. Replacement of clotting factors and heparin therapy may be required for DIC. Sources of trauma should be identified and eliminated so that outside causes of hemorrhage are avoided.

Pulmonary embolus. Pregnancy also brings about changes in the vascular system. Alterations in vein distensibility have been noted, possibly because of softening of collagen induced by humoral influences. The combination of vein distensibility and obstruction of venous blood return from the lower extremities (caused by fetal pressure on veins, especially in the last

trimester) predisposes a woman to pooling of blood. In addition, hypercoagulation and pooling may lead to thrombophlebitis. Thrombophlebitis can result in ARDS (emboli from thromboembolism cause obstruction in the pulmonary circulation).

Aspiration pneumonia. Aspiration pneumonia can be caused by changes in the gastrointestinal system during pregnancy. Progesterone has been known to relax smooth muscles. When the resting tone is lowered, the cardiac sphincter becomes weak and reflux of the stomach contents can easily occur. Increased intraabdominal pressure (because of fetal growth) further predisposes the mother to gastric reflux. Food eaten as long as 24 to 48 hours before labor can be vomited and then aspirated. Aspiration of solid foods and liquids may cause bronchial obstruction leading to bronchoconstriction, which in turn can result in ARDS. Large particles can be removed by coughing, suctioning, or bronchoscopy, but liquids are harder to remove. The hydrochloric acid in the aspirated stomach contents may cause an asthmatic-like syndrome with necrotizing bronchitis. For this reason an antacid is given preoperatively to women who are to have cesarean delivery as a prophylactic measure.

Gastrointestinal Disorders

Compromise of gastrointestinal function during pregnancy is apparent to all concerned. There are psychogenic overtones generally admitted in nausea and vomiting of pregnancy. However, a capricious food choice is observed in many women during pregnancy. In addition, obvious physiologic alterations, such as the greatly enlarged uterus, and less apparent changes, such as hypochlorhydria, require understanding for proper diagnosis and treatment.

Peptic ulcer. Peptic ulcer is less common in women than in men, and this problem is even more uncommon during pregnancy. Moreover, women with a diagnosed peptic ulcer generally improve during gestation. Therefore hemorrhage and perforation are unlikely. Fortunately emergency surgery for peptic ulcer complications rarely jeopardizes the pregnancy. Postdelivery reactivation of the ulcer may occur. Medical therapy is similar to that recommended for nonpregnant individuals.

Cholelithiasis and cholecystitis. Women are more likely to have cholelithiasis (gallstones) than are men, and pregnancy seems to play a part in its development. It is known that gallstones are more frequently diagnosed in women of advanced parity than in nulliparas of the same age and background. Increased biliary cholesterol and biliary stasis are probable causes. Cholecystitis does not commonly occur during pregnancy.

Generally, gallbladder surgery should be postponed until the puerperium. Impaction of a stone in the cystic or common duct during pregnancy may require cholelithotomy or cholecystectomy. Meperidine (Demerol) or atropine alleviates ductal spasm and pain. Morphine may be given also.

Ulcerative colitis. The cause of ulcerative colitis is unknown. Its effect on pregnancy is minimal unless there is marked debilitation, whereupon spontaneous abortion, fetal death, or premature delivery may occur. In general, when pregnancy coincides with active ulcerative colitis, the great majority of women will experience a severe exacerbation of the disease. When pregnancy occurs during a period of inactivity of the disorder, a flare-up is unlikely. There is no specific therapy for ulcerative colitis, but adrenocorticosteroids and antibiotics may be beneficial.

Inborn error of metabolism: maternal phenylketonuria. Phenylketonuria (PKU) is an inborn error of metabolism caused by an autosomal recessive trait that creates a deficiency in the enzyme phenylalanine hydroxylase. Absence of this enzyme results in the inability to metabolize phenylalanine to tyrosine. Prompt diagnosis of this disorder in the newborn and subsequent dietary intervention has made it possible for individuals to live a productive life with exception of reproduction. Homozygosity for this disorder in a woman whose fetus is heterozygous produces disastrous fetal results.

Elevated maternal blood phenylalanine levels during pregnancy result in fetal hyperphenylalaninemia (p. 310). Maternal risk in this disorder is not a factor; however, for the fetus, intrauterine and postnatal growth retardation, including mental retardation, is almost universal. About one quarter of fetuses are malformed. Apparently, a maternal diet low in phenylalanine has questionable preventive value unless followed before conception. A simple urine test (Phenostix) is available and is usually applied routinely to every woman in early pregnancy.

Integumentary Disorders

Dermatologic disorders induced by pregnancy (see Table 11.7) include melasma (chloasma), herpes gestationis, noninflammatory pruritus of pregnancy, vascular spiders, palmar erythema, and pregnancy granulomas (including epulides). Skin problems generally aggravated by pregnancy are acne vulgaris (in the first trimester), erythema multiforme, herpetiform dermatitis, granuloma inguinale, condylomata acuminata, neurofibromatosis, and pemphigus. Dermato-

logic disorders usually improved by pregnancy include acne vulgaris (in the third trimester), seborrhea dermatitis, and psoriasis. An unpredictable course during pregnancy may be expected in atopic dermatitis, lupus erythematosus, and herpes simplex.

Therapeutic abortion or early delivery may be justified for some dermatologic conditions. These conditions include herpes gestationis, disseminated lupus erythematosus, and neurofibromatosis (von Recklinghausen's disease).

Explanation, reassurance, and common sense measures should suffice for normal skin changes (see Table 11.7). In contrast, disease processes during and soon after pregnancy may be extremely difficult to diagnose and treat.

Neurologic Disorders

Epilepsy. Epilepsy may result from developmental abnormalities or injury. Epilepsy seriously complicates about 1 of every 1000 gestations. Convulsive seizures may be more frequent or severe during complications of pregnancy, such as edema, alkylosis, fluid-electrolyte imbalance, cerebral hypoxia, hypoglycemia, and hypocalcemia. On the other hand, the effects of pregnancy on epilepsy are unpredictable.

The differential diagnosis of epilepsy vs. eclampsia may pose a problem. Epilepsy and eclampsia can coexist. However, a past history of seizures, the absence of hypertension, generalized edema or proteinuria, and a normal plasma uric acid level point to epilepsy. Electroencephalography (EEG) rarely is diagnostic.

Grand mal seizures can be controlled by intravenous sodium amobarbital or magnesium sulfate. Phenytoin (Dilantin) and its analogues may be fetotoxic. Diazepam (Valium) or chlordiazepoxide (Librium) are safe analeptic drugs. Epilepsy is not an indication for therapeutic abortion or cesarean delivery. Diazepam and chlordiazepoxide affect the newly delivered infant.

Multiple sclerosis. Multiple sclerosis, a patchy demyelinization of the spinal cord and CNS, may be a viral disorder. Multiple sclerosis frequently develops initially after a pregnancy and is more common during the childbearing years. Multiple sclerosis may occasionally complicate pregnancy, but exacerbations and remissions are unrelated to the pregnant state. For this reason medically indicated therapeutic abortion is illogical. The burden of pregnancy and subsequent care of the child may warrant early interruption of pregnancy and sterilization in extreme cases. Women with multiple sclerosis occasionally may have an almost painless labor. The character of uterine contractions is unaffected by the disease, however.

Myasthenia gravis. Myasthenia gravis, a motor (muscle) end plate disorder that involves acetylcholine use, affects the motor function at the myoneural junction. Muscle weakness, particularly of the eyes, face, tongue, neck, limbs, and respiratory muscles results. The peak prevalence of myasthenia gravis is about 25 years of age. Pregnancy may complicate the disorder, although some women experience a remission during gestation. Pregnancies in women with this disease can be carried to safe delivery if certain precautions are taken. Moreover, congenital myasthenia gravis is rare. Therefore the disorder is not an indication for therapeutic abortion.

The nurse and physician should be alert to symptomatology, which includes easy fatigue, intermittent double vision, upper eyelid drooping, and facial muscle weakness. In more serious cases, upper arm weakness and breathing difficulty are seen. Infections may precipitate the onset or relapse and must be treated aggressively during pregnancy.

Parturients with myasthenia gravis usually tolerate labor well, because they already have some degree of muscle relaxation. Meperidine is the obstetric analgesic of choice. Local anesthesia is preferred. If a general anesthetic is required, a combination of nitrous oxide, oxygen, and cyclopropane generally is best. Oxytocin may be given, but scopolamine and muscle relaxants are contraindicated. After delivery, women must be carefully supervised, because relapses often occur during the puerperium.

Occasionally an infant born to a mother with severe myasthenia gravis also shows myasthenic signs sufficient to require neostigmine treatment for 1 to 2 months. Complete recovery of the infant is the rule. However, infants born with the disorder do not have as good a prognosis as infants born without the disorder.

Bell's palsy. An association between idiopathic facial paralysis and pregnancy was first cited by Bell in 1830, but it was not until 1975, that Hilsinger and colleagues proved this association. Not all neurologists agree with this association, however (Aminoff, 1978). There does not seem to be any causative relationship between the appearance of Bell's palsy and any of the complications of pregnancy.

No effects of maternal Bell's palsy have been observed in infants. Maternal outcome is generally good. Electromyography and nerve conduction velocity studies are useful in predicting the outcome. Evidence of a complete block in conduction carries a worse prognosis. Loss of taste also carries a less favorable prognosis. Steroids are sometimes prescribed for the condition. In most affected women, 90% or more return of facial function can be expected.

Autoimmune Diseases

Autoimmune disorders (see Chapter 5) have a predilection for women in their reproductive years; therefore associations with pregnancy are not uncommon. Pregnancy may affect the disease process. Some disorders adversely affect the course of pregnancy or are detrimental to the fetus. Autoimmune disorders include rheumatoid arthritis, systemic lupus erythematosus, hyperthyroidism, myasthenia gravis, and immunologic thrombocytopenic purpura. Autoantibodies from rheumatoid arthritis do *not* cross the placenta; those of the other disorders do. The woman with immunologic thrombocytopenic purpura may deliver a child who demonstrates thrombocytopenia. Petechiae and bleeding into the gastrointestinal and genitourinary tracts and into the brain may be evident. If the mother has myasthenia gravis, the newborn may exhibit a weak cry, sucking mechanism, and facial muscles and may have respiratory problems. Thyrotoxicosis is probable in the newborn of the mother with hyperthyroidism.

Rheumatoid arthritis. Approximately three of every four women with rheumatoid arthritis (RA) find that the severity of symptoms decreases during pregnancy (Cecere and Persellin, 1981). For this reason many affected women attempt to become pregnant as often as possible; however, many are subfertile because of the RA. During normal pregnancy an increase in α_2-glycoprotein surpasses 40 mg/dl in about 75% of women (Cecere and Persellin, 1981). In addition, total plasma and free cortisol (especially estrogens and progesterones) show an increase (Nolten and Reuckert, 1981). This combination apparently leads to depressed cellular immunity (Persellin, 1981). Women in whom the rheumatoid factor (autoantibodies found in the synovial fluid) decreases during pregnancy report improvement in their symptoms. Researchers are now investigating the possibility of a positive effect on RA associated with the use of oral contraceptives (see also Table 5.12).

The woman with RA needs to be informed of the positive and negative aspects that accompany pregnancy. She must be cautioned that, although symptoms may subside during pregnancy, she should anticipate a return of her symptoms after delivery. Exacerbations often recur about a month after delivery. "In short, she will be trading off a 75% chance that she will feel better against the strong possibility that she could 'crash' when the infant is about a month old" (Baum, 1984).

During pregnancy, the woman must be informed that medications she needs to treat RA may be unsafe for her fetus. As yet, information on the effects of nonsteroidal antiinflammatory drugs on pregnant women is insufficient. There is evidence that these medications may delay closure of the ductus arteriosus in the newborn. Medications have a tendency to increase gastrointestinal toxicity during the last trimester. Therefore medications are discontinued during the last trimester. Aspirin not only has an irreversible effect on the platelets, it also is likely to increase blood loss during parturition. The neonate may have similar bleeding tendencies.

Although proof that the nursing infant can be harmed is lacking, nonsteroidal antiinflammatory medications are not recommended for mothers who breast feed. These drugs have been demonstrated in breast milk.

Systemic lupus erythematosus. One of the most common serious disorders of childbearing age, systemic lupus erythematosus (SLE), is a chronic multisystem inflammatory disease. The condition is not rare; more than 250,000 persons are known to have SLE, with an estimated 50,000 new cases per year. Although the antibody may be formed in response to a virus, a familial tendency seems to be involved (see also Table 5.12).

The vague early symptoms, such as fatigue, may be overlooked. Eventually all organs become involved. The condition is characterized by a series of exacerbations and remissions. A subcommittee of the American Rheumatism Association has proposed an extensive set of criteria to standardize the diagnosis.

If the diagnosis has been established and the woman desires a child, she is advised to wait for 2 years. At that time, if the disease has been controlled well on low doses of corticosteroids, pregnancy may be reasonably considered (Danforth, 1982). Oral contraceptives are contraindicated; diaphragms, condoms, and IUDs are the preferred methods of birth control if pregnancy is desired, but sterilization is suggested if no more children are desired. The outlook for persons with SLE has improved markedly in the past few years. The survival rate is now more than 90% for 5 years and more than 80% for those who survive for 10 years after diagnosis.

Although the effect of pregnancy on SLE seems inconsistent, most maternal deaths occur during the puerperium or after abortion (Danforth, 1982). The rate of spontaneous abortion is high. Maternal complications correlate with the degree of cardiac or renal involvement. Renal failure, hypertension, and death are associated with diffuse proliferative lupus glomerulonephritis. When the kidneys are involved, gravidas are subject to superimposed preeclampsia, stillbirths, preterm delivery, and small-for-gestational age infants. However, if the disease is stable during pregnancy, the risk that the disease will worsen with gestation is only slight.

Obstetric management includes surveillance of the woman's renal and cardiovascular status and determination of fetal status. Corticosteroid (prednisone) therapy is maintained throughout pregnancy; hydrocortisone is administered intravenously during labor and delivery. Corticosteroid therapy is continued for about 2 months after delivery.

Although the antibodies cross the placenta, their amount varies so that the effect on the fetus also varies. The most severely affected newborns suffer from discoid lupus, anemia, neutropenia, thrombocytopenia, and congenital heart block. Great strides in diagnosis, drug therapy, and knowledge about the immune system provide hope for the future.

Surgical Conditions Coincident with Pregnancy

The need for immediate abdominal surgery occurs as frequently among pregnant women as among nonpregnant women of comparable age. Diagnosis is more difficult in the pregnant woman, however. An enlarged uterus and displaced internal organs may prevent adequate palpation and alter the position of the surgical procedure.

Differential diagnosis includes consideration of obstetric complications (e.g., ectopic pregnancy and premature separation of the placenta) and the onset of labor. Mild leukocytosis and increased serum values of alkaline phosphatase and amylase are characteristic of pregnancy, as well as surgical intraperitoneal processes. Rising or abnormally high laboratory values are suspect, however. X-ray evaluation, a valuable adjunct to diagnosis, is contraindicated, particularly in the first trimester, except in extreme cases. The surgeon is confronted with both a surgical and an obstetric problem.

Laparotomy or laparoscopy may be required. Hazards of these procedures include abortion and premature labor. But surgical or anesthetic intervention does not affect the incidence of congenital malformations.

Principles of maternity nursing are added to those of nursing care of the surgical client. The preoperative and postoperative plan of care incorporates consideration for the woman's concern for her infant as well as for herself. Fetal vital signs and activity and uterine contractility (labor may have begun) are monitored, and constant vigilance for symptoms of impending obstetric complications is maintained. The woman and her family may have heightened concerns regarding effects of the procedure and medication on fetal wellbeing and the course of pregnancy.

Fig. 28.5
Change in position of appendix during pregnancy.

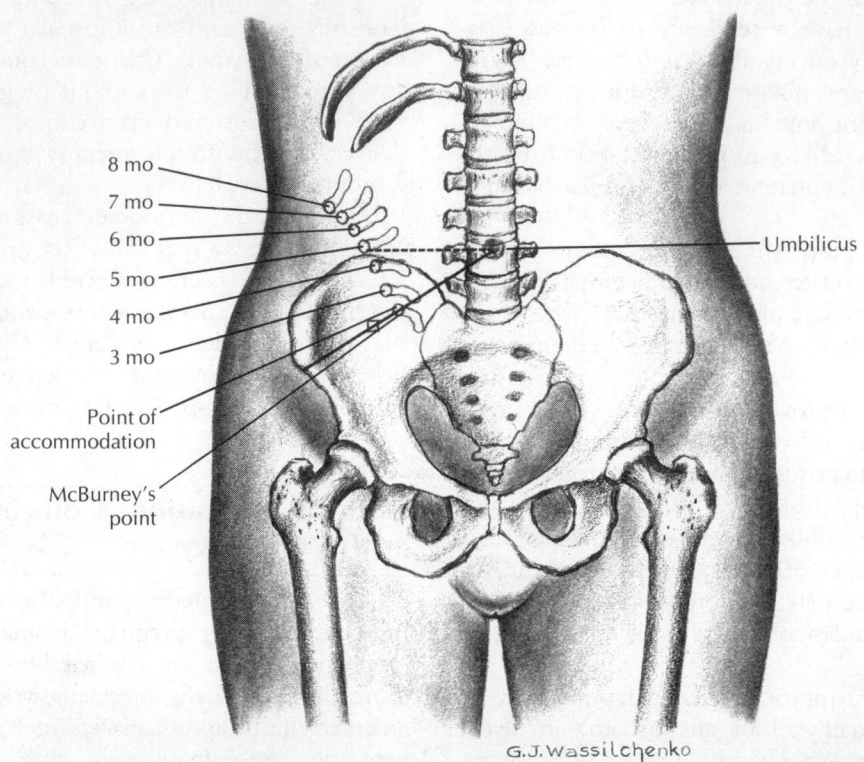

G.J.Wassilchenko

Appendicitis. Acute suppurative appendicitis complicates about 1 in every 1000 pregnancies. This disorder poses the following special problems during gestation:

1. Appendicitis is more difficult to diagnose during pregnancy. The appendix is carried high and to the right, away from McBurney's point, by the enlarged uterus (Fig. 28.5).
2. Appendiceal rupture and peritonitis occur two to three times more often in pregnant women than in nonpregnant women.
3. Maternal and perinatal morbidity and mortality are greatly increased when appendicitis occurs during pregnancy.

Most cases of acute appendicitis occurring during the first 6 months of gestation, with decreasing frequency through the third trimester, labor, and puerperium. The differential diagnosis of appendicitis during pregnancy is also difficult because of gastrointestinal or genitourinary problems that may be confused with appendicitis. A high level of suspicion is important in the diagnosis of appendicitis.

Management. Appendectomy before rupture is extremely important. Antibiotic therapy before rupture is of questionable value; after rupture it may be lifesaving. Therapeutic abortion is never indicated in appendicitis. Cesarean delivery at or near term may be justified in association with appendectomy.

Prognosis. Maternal mortality increases to about 10% in the third trimester and is about 15% when appendicitis develops during labor. Perinatal mortality is approximately 10% with unruptured appendicitis but is at least 35% with peritonitis.

Intestinal obstruction. Although intestinal obstruction (dynamic ileus) is not common during pregnancy, any woman with a laparotomy scar is more likely to suffer intestinal obstruction during gestation. Adhesions, an enlarging uterus, and displacement of the intestines are etiologic factors.

Persistent, abdominal, cramplike pain, vomiting, auscultatory rushes within the abdomen, and "laddering" of the intestinal shadows on x-ray films aid in the diagnosis of intestinal obstruction. Immediate surgical intervention is required for release of the obstruction. Pregnancy is rarely affected by the surgery, assuming the absence of complications such as peritonitis. Cesarean delivery is not indicated in intestinal obstruction.

Abdominal hernias. The incidence of abdominal

hernias and related incarceration of the bowel is reduced during pregnancy despite permanent enlargement of umbilical or incisional hernial rings. Displacement of nonadherent bowel by the enlarging uterus and its shielding of so-called weak areas of the abdominal wall are fortuitous. In fact, temporary spontaneous reduction of some abdominal wall hernias occurs during gestation. In contrast, however, the uncommon irreducible or adherent hernias may become incarcerated as pregnancy progresses.

Women with hernias should not strain or bear down during the second stage of labor. Therefore low forceps delivery should be planned. Abdominal hernia is not an indication for cesarean delivery; herniorrhaphy should be done as an interval procedure (i.e., between pregnancies).

Gynecologic problems. Ovarian cysts and twisting of ovarian cysts or adnexal tissues may occur. Pregnancy predisposes a woman to ovarian pathoses, especially during the first trimester. Pathoses include retained or enlarged cystic corpus luteum of pregnancy, ovarian cyst, and bacterial invasion of reproductive or other intraperitoneal organs.

Laparotomy or laparoscopy is required to discriminate between ovarian pathoses and early ectopic pregnancy, appendicitis, or other infectious processes. See Chapter 27 for a discussion of common vaginitis.

Battered Pregnant Woman

The battered pregnant woman should be treated as a high-risk obstetric client because she often has medical, social, and psychologic needs (Mercer, 1977) that require special attention. She is at additional risk for repeated physical trauma and for psychologic trauma because of a deficient support system.

Pregnancy is a time of increased battering episodes (Walker, 1979) for a variety of reasons: (1) The biopsychosocial stresses of pregnancy may strain the relationship beyond the couple's ability to cope; frustration is followed by violence. (2) The man may be jealous of the fetus, resenting its intrusion into the couple's relationship. As one expectant father succinctly stated, "I don't get the TLC I got before that thing came along." (3) The beating may be the man's conscious or subconscious attempt to end the pregnancy. After delivery the mother may be so physically and emotionally drained that she may have difficulty bonding with her infant. She is considered at risk of becoming an abusive mother whether she chooses to stay in the abusive relationship or not. If she remains with her husband, the chances are 1 in 3 or 4 that he will batter the child as well.

When the woman is asked why she remains with a battering mate, she may say that there are times when their relationship is fine. Walker (1979) identified a cyclic pattern to the battering behavior. There is a period of increasing tension leading to the battery, followed by an aftermath characterized by kind, loving behavior and a plea for forgiveness by the husband.

Other women in this type of relationship verbalize many reasons for remaining with the husband. Many women retain the hope that he will change. Other reasons include the following: feelings of love for him, fear of reprisals from him, wanting the children to be with their father, lack of a place to go, lack of financial or emotional support, their or others' negative feelings about divorce, low self-esteem, and an immobilizing sense of lack of control over their lives.

Whichever way the battered woman turns, she usually undergoes a grief reaction for her losses—her lost fantasies of marriage, of being a wife in a trusting relationship, of choosing the perfect mate, and often of financial security.

Malignant Disease and Pregnancy

Extrapelvic malignant disease. Fortunately the peak incidence for most malignant diseases does not occur during the reproductive years (DiSaia, 1983). The most common cancers reported during pregnancy in order of frequency are breast cancer, leukemia and lymphoma, melanoma, various gynecologic cancers, and bone tumor. A brief discussion follows.

Cancer of the breast. Cancer of the breast during pregnancy is extremely serious. Fortunately, breast cancer is rare before the age of 35, which is beyond the age of reproductive activity for most women. Approximately 1% to 2% of women are pregnant at the time of diagnosis. Apparently abortion does not improve the prognosis. However, termination of pregnancy is recommended if diagnosis is made during the first trimester because there is a high probability that the malignancy may be estrogen or progesterone-dependent. Estrogen-binding tests are now available to aid in this diagnosis.

A second- or third-trimester abortion is not recommended because there is no clear evidence that it would improve survival. Radical mastectomy is well tolerated during pregnancy. After delivery, if distant metastases appear, oophorectomy produces remission in 50% of affected women.

Breast feeding is contraindicated on two counts: (1) if one of the oncogens for breast cancer is a virus, as many have postulated, then the remaining breast may be contaminated and the virus may be passed to the newborn and may act as a latent inducer of breast carcinoma, and (2) lactation increases vascularity in the remaining breast, which may contain a neoplasm.

For advanced disease in the second or third trimester, alkylating agents, 5-fluorouracil, and vincristine are relatively safe for the fetus (DiSaia, 1983). Chemotherapy may significantly improve the survival of these women.

Leukemia. The average age for gravidas with acute leukemia is 28. The incidence during pregnancy is not specified, but the incidence in the general population in the United States is 10 in 100,000.

Pregnancy seems to have no specific effect on the course of the disease, except that vigorous therapy is detrimental to early gestation. Premature labor and postpartum hemorrhage are associated with acute leukemia. Acute myelocytic leukemia (90% of cases) has a more fulminant course and requires immediate therapy. In the presence of chronic myelocytic leukemia, therapy can be delayed somewhat. Some gravidas with the chronic form of the disease who had chemotherapy and radiotherapy directed at the spleen have delivered apparently healthy infants. The decision to terminate the pregnancy rests with the woman and her family; however, prompt, aggressive therapy is always advisable if remission is to be achieved.

Hodgkin's disease (lymphoreticuloma). Hodgkin's disease is a malignant lymphoma that affects many younger people and complicates about one in 6,000 pregnancies. Younger women (under 40) have a better prognosis.

Although pregnancy in the early stages does not appear to affect the course of the disease adversely, aggressive therapy has improved overall survival considerably. Radiotherapy and chemotherapy are now responsible for the care or control of Hodgkin's disease for long periods of time. Unless gestation is well into the third trimester, delay in initiating therapy should be minimal. Radiotherapy to diseased areas above the diaphragm can be initiated during the third trimester with proper shielding of the fetus. Chemotherapy is strongly indicated during the first trimester and is relatively contraindicated in the second and third trimesters.

If the gravida and her family refuses any therapy until pregnancy terminates naturally, the physician has no choice. However, termination of the pregnancy before initiating radiotherapy or chemotherapy is most desirable (DiSaia, 1983).

Melanoma. Malignant melanoma may be one of the rare cancers that can be affected adversely by pregnancy. Maternal adaptations to pregnancy (Chapter 9) are implicated:

1. Melanocyte-stimulating hormone (MSH) increases after 8 weeks gestation.

2. Adrenocorticotropic hormone (ACTH) production increases also and ACTH heightens MSH activity. Although pregnancy has been implicated in the more rapid metastases to regional lymph nodes, stage for stage, there does not seem to be a significant difference in the survivial of gravid and nongravid women. Diagnosis is established by biopsy. Therapy consists of radical local excision.

For most other malignancies, the placenta is unexplainably resistant to invasion by maternal cancer. Though melanoma accounts for few cases of malignant disease during pregnancy, almost 50% of the *placental metastases* and almost 90% of *fetal metastases* occur from maternal melanoma.

Bone tumors. Ewing's sarcoma and osteogenic sarcoma are the most frequent primary malignant bone tumors seen in pregnancy. Usually the areas involved are the clavicle, sternum, spine, humerus, and femur. A lump or mass, local pain, and disability are characteristic manifestations.

Osteogenic sarcoma affects areas of high bone turnover (during growth spurts especially); Ewing's sarcoma is a rare condition that develops within bone marrow. Pregnancy does not affect nor is affected by the disease.

Surgical excision is usually well tolerated during pregnancy. Adjuvant chemotherapy is delayed until after delivery if the cancer is diagnosed near term. With prompt chemotherapy (within a few weeks of diagnosis), 50% to 70% (compared to 5% before the advent of chemotherapy) of affected women are disease-free at 5 years. If the disease recurs, it usually does so within 3 years. Therefore women are counseled to defer pregnancy during this time.

Gestational trophoblastic disease (GTD)

Description. GTD is a morphologic continuum with the first deviation from normal implantation at one end, followed by hydatidiform mole (a benign condition), (see Chapter 27). GTD may evolve into invasive mole. The disease may end as choriocarcinoma, the most proliferative and aggressive stage. Trophoblastic disease follows pregnancy (ectopic or intrauterine). In choriocarcinoma, the villi are absent and the neoplasm is composed of sheets of malignant trophoblast. Hemorrhage and necrosis, common in choriocarcinoma, result from the lack of vascular supply.

Before 1956, metastatic GTD had a short clinical course and was fatal. In 1956, complete remission with methotrexate in some women was reported (Li, Hertz, and Spencer). In 1960, actinomycin-D (Dactinomycin), when given sequentially with methotrexate, increased the remission rate from 50% to approximately 75%. These drugs remain the drugs of choice.

Hertz is credited with conceptualizing GTD as a

disease continuum. Recognition that the benign hydatidiform mole has the potential to persist or recur as a proliferative and highly metastatic malignancy has improved cure rates by improving diagnosis.

Diagnosis. Clinical manifestations of molar pregnancy are discussed in Chapter 27. Sonographic characteristics are discussed in Chapter 25.

Radioimmunoassay based on the β-subunit of human chorionic gonadotropin (HCG) permits detection of a very low level of HCG. This test identifies those who need chemotherapy or those in whom persistent neoplasia mandates further therapy.

Treatment. Evacuation of the intact mole is the initial therapy. The uterus is evacuated with a cervical dilation and curettage (D & C) accompanied by oxytocin infusion to stimulate uterine contractions that facilitate emptying of the uterus. Hysterectomy is an option if retention of reproductive capacity is not an issue. This procedure results in a cure rate of 90%.

Chemotherapy is begun if the HCG level rises, plateaus, or persists. Following evacuation of a mole, the woman is monitored with radioimmunoassay for HCG at weekly intervals.

Some women are at greater risk for malignancy: the woman whose molar disease is complicated by excessive bleeding after evacuation or by pulmonary symptoms, the older woman, and the woman with high parity. Women are categorized to be at low, moderate, or high risk based on limitation of metastasis to lungs and pelvis, metastasis to brain or liver, and level of HCG.

Drug toxicity. The woman receiving combination drug therapy must be monitored for white blood cell and platelet counts. The regimen is withheld if absolute polymorphonuclear leukocyte counts drop below 1500/mm^3, the platelet count goes below 100,000/mm^3, or if there is evidence of hepatic or renal impairment. The intravenous infusion must be inspected frequently for extravascular infiltration. Infiltration results in tissue necrosis and sloughing.

Follow-up. Each woman is followed until three consecutive HCG β-subunit of HCG radioimmunoassay tests are negative. Women are counseled to avoid pregnancy for 1 year so the HCG levels, if found, are not confused with pregnancy. Long-term follow-up is warranted.

Pelvic malignancies
Cancer of the vulva. The diagnosis of preinvasive (vulvar intraepithelial neoplasia) disease during pregnancy is not uncommon. Therapy is postponed until the postpartum period.

If invasive disease is diagnosed during the first trimester, vulvectomy with bilateral groin dissection may be done after the fourteenth week. When it is di-

agnosed in the third trimester, local wide excision is done, deferring definitive surgery until after delivery. Pregnancy does not alter the course of the disease.

After radical vulvectomy and bilateral inguinal lymphectomy, several women have become pregnant again. These women have carried the pregnancies to term and delivered vaginally. If local fibrosis is present and could impede delivery, abdominal delivery is advisable.

Cancer of the vagina. Except for clear-cell adenocarcinoma of DES-exposed women, cancer of the vagina is not common. If clear-cell adenocarcinoma of the cervix and vagina or sarcoma are found in the upper vagina, the preferred surgery is radical hysterectomy, upper vaginectomy, and bilateral pelvic lymphadenectomy, followed by chemotherapy. If disease is advanced, the preferred treatment is to empty the uterus and begin radiotherapy.

Cancer of the cervix. A diversity of opinion abounds in the literature concerning the cause and effect of carcinoma of the cervix in the gravida (DiSaia and Creasman, 1981). Overall incidence ranges from 1 to 13 per 10,000 pregnancies (approximately 0.01% of gravidas). Carcinoma of the cervix is curable if diagnosed and treated in its early stages. Diagnosis and therapy is the same whether or not the woman is pregnant. Further diagnosis and treatment for carcinoma in situ and dysplasia are deferred until the puerperium. Therapy for invasive disease depends on the length of gestation, the religious conviction of the woman and her family, and the desire of the mother and the family for the child. The cancer itself does not harm the pregnancy; stage for stage, the outcome for the gravida with cervical cancer is roughly the same as for the nonpregnant woman (DiSaia and Creasman, 1981).

For the pregnancy at 24 weeks gestation or more, therapy is usually delayed until fetal viability is achieved. For the pregnancy that is less than 24 weeks, the proposed treatment is based on the disease, and the pregnancy is disregarded, except when the woman refuses this approach. In the presence of invasive carcinoma, abdominal surgical delivery is preferred; vaginal delivery seems to lower the cure rate. If cervical lesions are large, serious bleeding and infection may be sequelae to vaginal delivery.

Cancer of the uterus. Endometrial carcinoma during pregnancy is rare; only a few cases have been documented since 1900. Diagnosis was usually an incidental finding after therapeutic abortion or surgery and the lesions were minimally or not invasive. Recommended therapy is total abdominal hysterectomy and bilateral salpingo-oophorectomy and adjuvant radiotherapy.

Cancer of the uterine (fallopian) tube. With a peak incidence between 50 and 55 years, concurrent pregnancy is only a remote possibility. Should it occur, the recommended therapy (total abdominal hysterectomy and bilateral salpingo-oophorectomy with postoperative radiotherapy or chemotherapy) is the same as for the nongravid woman. A few cases have been first diagnosed following tubal ligation during routine histologic evaluation of the small resected segment.

Cancer of the ovary. Ovarian tumors are infrequent complications during pregnancy. Serious complications may develop: pelvic impaction, obstructed labor, torsion of the ovarian pedicle, hemorrhage into the tumor, rupture of a cyst, and infection; or they may be malignant (only 2% to 5% of all ovarian neoplasms are found during pregnancy). The peak incidence of cancer of the ovary is over 50, therefore it is less likely to be seen during a pregnancy.

Differential diagnosis, especially during the second half of pregnancy, is difficult. Abdominal palpation and ultrasonography are the tools. The most common complication is torsion, which occurs most often when the uterus is rising rapidly (8 to 16 weeks) or involuting during the puerperium. Indicators of torsion are lower abdominal pain, tense and tender abdomen with guarding, nausea, vomiting, and shock-like symptoms.

An ovarian tumor may be first diagnosed at delivery because the enlarged uterus obscured its presence. If it falls back into the cul-de-sac, it may obstruct the birth canal and during labor may be traumatized. Hemorrhage into the tumor is followed by necrosis and suppuration (pus formation).

Malignancy of the ovary occurs approximately once in 8,000 to 20,000 deliveries. The pregnancy does not alter the woman's prognosis if an aggressive therapeutic approach is taken. Fortunately, ovarian germ cell neoplasms occurring in pregnancy are usually benign (DiSaia and Creasman, 1981).

Chemotherapy during pregnancy. Many cytotoxic agents are teratogenic early in pregnancy and would result in either spontaneous abortion or fetal abnormality. In addition, these drugs theoretically are mutogenic, abortifactants, and lethal to the fetus at any time. Nothing is known about the long-term effects of in utero exposure should the child survive. Chemotherapy with some drugs (aminopterin and methotrexate) in the second and third trimesters may not cause observable harm to the fetus.

Radiotherapy during pregnancy. During embryonic development, tissues are extremely radiosensitive. If cells are genetically altered or killed during this time, the child either will fail to survive or will be deformed. From a radiologic stance there are three significant periods in embryonic development (see Chapter 8):

1. *Preimplantation:* If irradiation does not destroy the fertilized egg, it probably does not affect it significantly.

2. *Critical period of organogenesis:* During this period, especially between days 18 and 38, the organism is most vulnerable; microcephaly, anencephaly, eye damage, growth retardation, spina bifida and foot damage may occur.

3. *After day 40:* Large doses may still cause observable malformation and damage to the central nervous system.

Irradiation of gonads involves genetic damage— gene mutation and chromosome breakage—even at relatively low doses. Most mutations are recessive so that mutant effects may not surface for many generations.

Emotional Disturbance Associated With Childbearing

Postpartum mental illness ranges from a transitory depression to severe postpartum emotional disturbances. The transitory depression, "maternity blues," may occur in 30% to 80% of all childbirths, whereas the severe postpartum emotional disturbance is noted in only 1% to 2% of all normal childbirths.

Transitory depression begins the second or third day after birth, and the symptoms include anxiety, poor concentration, tearfulness, and despondency. The symptoms usually subside within the first week. However, approximately 40% of women with mild depression have symptoms that persist as long as 1 year (Gelder, 1978; Tentoni and High, 1980). For the more severe conditions, 2% to 9% of women admitted to mental hospitals are admitted for conditions related to childbearing (Stevens, 1970; Weiner, 1982). The disorder may be acute or chronic in nature and appears cross-culturally.

Etiology. No one single factor has been isolated as responsible for precipitating an episode of postpartum mental illness. Predisposing factors have been categorized by Herzog and Detre (1976) as follows: (1) genetic-constitutional, (2) social-environmental, and (3) physiologic-endocrine.

Pregnancy per se is not a cause of psychiatric illness. The psychologic and physical stresses relating to pregnancy or to the formidable new obligations of motherhood may, however, precipitate an emotional crisis (Affonso, 1984). The principal emotional disturbances complicating gestation are affective disorders and schizophrenia. The affective disturbances include depression or depression with manic episodes. Toxic delirium associated with drug addiction, excessive analgesia, or serious metabolic disorders are not common. Rarely, psychosis secondary to alcoholism or syphilis may complicate both prenatal and postdelivery progress.

Affective disorders. Although the etiology of affective depressive disorders is unknown, the family history may record one or more adults who have had this problem. Moreover, women who have psychiatric complications during the course of pregnancy often have had similar crises previously.

Over 50% of pregnancy-related mental illnesses are affective reactions. Of these, about 10% are predelivery manic or depressive states; the remainder disturb the postdelivery period. Younger women seem more prone to manic reactions, but depression is the more common problem for most women.

Rejection of the infant, often caused by abnormal jealousy, is a prominent feature of affective disorders. The mother may be obsessed by the notion that the offspring may supplant her in her husband's affections. In other instances, guilt regarding aversion to pregnancy, attempted abortion, or other personal conflicts may be the basic problem.

Depressive reactions, far more common than manic reactions, may begin as a mild feeling of discouragement (the "baby blues") during the first week after delivery. However, anxiety, anorexia, and exaggerated fatigue soon color the despondency. The woman seems helpless; she is self-accusatory and often expresses strange or inappropriate thoughts or feelings. Occasionally a disconsolate mother may kill her infant and herself.

Depression may continue for weeks or months. Amphetamines are not helpful and may add to agitation. However, a tranquilizer with a prominent stimulatory effect, such as trifluoperazine (Stelazine), may be beneficial. Psychotherapy must be intensive and often prolonged. Meanwhile, separation of mother and infant will be necessary. If the depression lifts within several weeks, the prognosis is good. However, women who have been depressed previously, especially those who have had even longer depressions, have a poor prognosis.

Manic reactions often occur during the first or second week of the puerperium, perhaps after a brief depression. Agitation, excitement, and volubility, often with rhyming or punning, develop. The woman becomes disinterested in personal care and food. Because dehydration or exhaustion may ensue, prompt and effective supportive treatment is essential.

Psychiatric therapy may include a tranquilizer with a prominent sedative effect, for example, promethazine hydrochloride (Phenergan). Lithium carbonate may be given later for more prolonged control. Psychotherapy is essential. The usual duration of the manic state is 1 to 3 weeks. The prognosis for mother and infant is good after initial separation and gradual reunion.

Schizophrenia. Schizophrenic reactions, now suspected of being a disorder of cerebral metabolism, affect adolescents and younger adults rather than older persons. Abnormal personality features are common. Unusually shy, retiring, hypersensitive, or overly suspicious women are prone to schizophrenic break. A sudden onset of delusions or hallucinations may alter a seemingly well-accepted normal pregnancy. The symptoms indicate the woman's inability to adjust to and cope with her new obligations as a mother.

The husband and infant are totally rejected. Hostility toward the spouse and the medical staff is obvious. Often the excited, confused woman believes hers to have been an immaculate conception, or she may believe that she is being influenced by the Deity. The woman abandons reality and retreats completely into her own world of unreality. The mother totally neglects her infant but rarely harms it. Suicide is unlikely. A phenothiazine type of tranquilizer, for example, chlorpromazine (Thorazine), will be useful. Transfer of the woman to a psychiatric hospital usually is necessary. Electroshock therapy and psychotherapy usually are effective.

A good prognosis is likely with the first psychotic episode, especially if it occurs unexpectedly during the puerperium. The child probably will never suffer from schizophrenia, despite speculation regarding hereditary tendencies.

Substance Abuse

The adverse effects of exposure of the fetus to drugs are variable. They include transient behavioral changes such as fetal breathing movements or irreversible effects such as fetal death, intrauterine growth retardation, structure malformations, or mental retardation. Maternal use of drugs may be for the pharmacologic control of disease process (e.g., insulin) or for symptomatic relief of benign problems (e.g., aspirin). It has been shown that 92% to 100% of all obstetric clients took at least one physician-prescribed drug, and 65% to 80% also took self-prescribed drugs. In addition to the therapeutic use of drugs the nontherapeutic use of drugs, such as alcohol, nicotine, or narcotics, poses threats to fetal well-being (Zacharias, 1983). Critical determinants of the effect of the drug on the fetus include the specific drug, the dosage, the route of administration, the genotype of the mother or fetus, and the timing of the drug exposure. Figs. 28.6 and 8.11 show critical periods in human embryogenesis and the teratogenic effects of drugs.

Fetal alcohol syndrome. Reference to the association between fetal malformation and maternal alcoholism can be found in Greek and Roman mythology. Laws in Carthage and Sparta forbade consumption of alcohol by couples on their wedding night to prevent

Fig. 28.6
Critical periods in human embryogenesis. (From Fanaroff, A., and Martin, R., editors:
Behrman's neonatal-perinatal medicine: diseases of the fetus and infant, St. Louis, 1983,
The C.V. Mosby Co.)

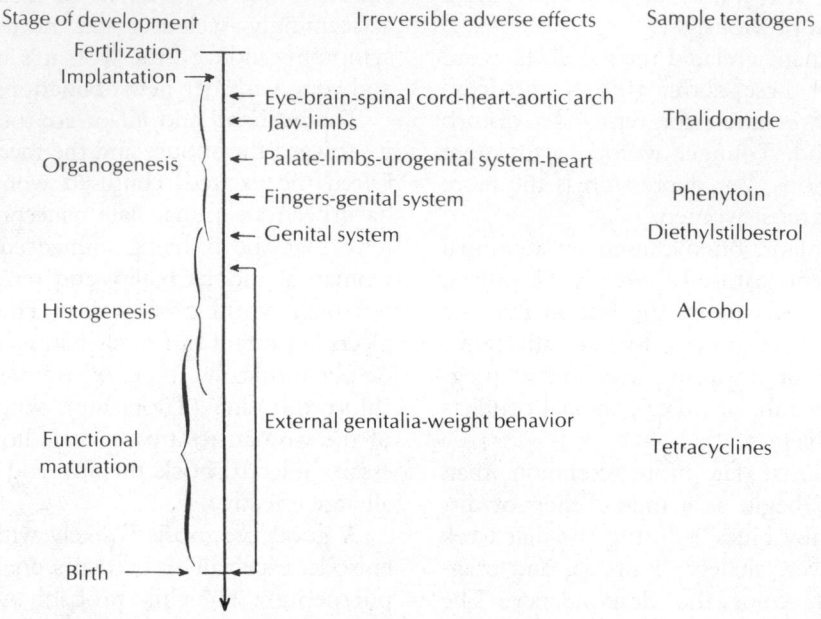

the conception of children with defects. Documentation of the fetal alcohol syndrome can be found in the literature since the early part of the eighteenth century.

Predictable patterns of fetal and neonatal dysmorphogenesis are attributed to severe, chronic alcoholism in women who continue to drink heavily during pregnancy (Davis and Keith, 1983). The pattern of growth deficiency begun in prenatal life persists after delivery, especially in the linear growth rate, rate of weight

gain, and growth of head circumferences (Zuspan, 1984). The box below, left, summarizes the risks associated with maternal alcohol ingestion.

Ocular structural anomalies are frequent findings (Fig. 28.7). Limb anomalies, a variety of cardiocirculatory anomalies, especially ventricular septal defects, pose problems for the child. Mental retardation (IQ of 79 or below at 7 years of age), and fine motor dysfunction (poor hand-to-mouth coordination, weak grasp) add to the handicapping problems that maternal alcoholism can impose. Genital abnormalities are seen in daughters of alcoholic mothers. Two thirds of newborns with fetal alcohol syndrome are girls; the cause of this altered sex birth ratio is unknown. Severe and chronic alcoholism (ethanol toxicity), not maternal malnutrition, is responsible for the severity and consistency of postdelivery performance problems. High alcohol levels are lethal to the developing embryo. Lower levels cause brain and other malformations (McCarthy, 1983). Long-term prognosis (no studies are available as yet) is discouraging even in an optimum psychosocial environment, when one considers the combination of growth failure and mental retardation. The box on p. 888 summarizes the clinical findings.

The infant of a mother who abuses alcohol is faced with a number of clinical problems. Identification of

Risks Associated with Maternal Alcohol Ingestion

	Risks
Two or more drinks daily Includes:	Intrauterine growth retardation
2 mixed drinks, 1 oz. liquor each	Immature motor activity
2 glasses of wine, 5 oz. each	Increased rate of anomalies
	Decreased muscle tone
2 beers, 12 oz. each	Poor sucking pressure
	Increased rate of stillbirths
	Decreased placental weight
Five or more drinks on occasion	Increased risk of structural brain abnormalities
Six or more drinks daily	FAS

From McCarthy, P.: Am. J. Primary Health Care 8:34, 1983. Copyright the Nurse Practitioner: The American Journal of Primary Health Care.

Fig. 28.7

Fetal alcohol syndrome (FAS). **A,** One-year-old American Indian girl. Note short palpebral fissures and maxillary hypoplasia. **B,** Three-year-old black girl. Note short palpebral fissures, bilateral ptosis, and strabismus on left. **C,** Two-year-old white boy. Note short palpebral fissures and maxillary hypoplasia. (From Rementeria, J.L., editor: Drug abuse in pregnancy and neonatal effects, St. Louis, 1977, The C.V. Mosby Co.)

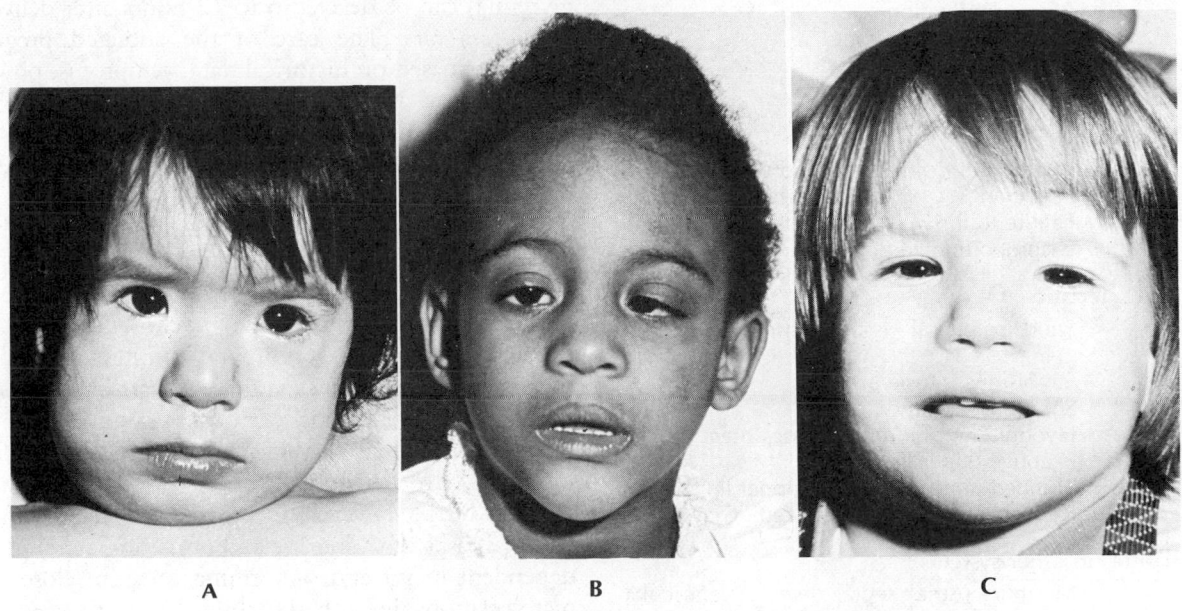

A   B   C

the problems leads to the medical diagnosis of fetal alcohol syndrome. Table 28.4 summarizes the clinical problems and their physiologic bases.

Nursing care. Nursing care involves many of the same strategies used for the care of preterm infants (Chapter 29). Special efforts are made to involve the parents in their child's care and encourage opportunities for parent-child attachment. The application of the nursing process to the care of an infant with fetal alcohol syndrome is presented on p. 888.

Narcotic drug dependence. Drug abuse implicates many chemical preparations. However, the morphine derivatives or synthetic opium derivatives are the most serious for the newborn whose mother is narcotic dependent. The perinatal mortality of newborns whose mothers are dependent on narcotics is six to eight times higher than that of a control group. Abortion, premature birth, stillbirth, and neonatal complications are the major reasons.

The mother. The number of pregnant narcotic addicts has increased considerably over the last decade. Early recognition of the addict, awareness of potential problems, and institution of care for the woman and her unborn infant are of great importance.

Many addicts are poorly nourished, consume excessive alcohol, and frequently have sexually-transmitted diseases, all factors that have a deleterious effect on the developing fetus. These women are particularly prone to cellulitis, superficial abcesses, and septic phlebitis. Pulmonary disease with acute pulmonary edema is a frequently encountered complication.

Table 28.4

Fetal Alcohol Syndrome: Clinical Problems and Physiologic Bases

Clinical Problem	Physiologic Basis for Problem

Respiratory distress	Related to
	  Prematurity
	  Neurologic damage
	  "Floppy" epiglottis and small trachea

Cardiopulmonary arrest	Related to tracheal-epiglottal anomalies

Feeding difficulties	Related to
	  Prematurity
	  Cleft palate
	  Poor sucking ability

Anomalies	Related to
	  Brain dysfunction
	  Microcephaly
	  Grand mal seizures

Manifestations of the Principal Features of Fetal Alcohol Syndrome

Central nervous system dysfunction

Intellectual	Mild to moderate mental retardation
Neurologic	Microcephaly (small head size)
	Poor coordination
	Decreased muscle tone
Behavioral	Irritability in infancy
	Hyperactivity in childhood

Growth deficiency

Prenatal	Less than 3% for length and weight
Postnatal	Less than 3% for length and weight
	Failure to thrive
	Disproportionate-diminished adipose tissue

Facial characteristics

Eyes	Short palpebral fissures (small eye openings)
	Strabismus, ptosis, myopia
Nose	Short and upturned
	Hypoplastic philtrum (flat or absent groove above upper lip)
Mouth	Thinned upper vermilion (upper lip)
	Retrognathia in infancy (receding jaw)

Abnormalities in other systems

Cardiac	Murmurs (Atrial septal defects, ventricular septal defects, great-vessel anomalies, tetralogy of Fallot)
Skeletal	Limited joint movements (especially fingers and elbows and hip dislocations)
	Aberrant palmar creases
	Pectus excavatum
Renogenital	Kidney defects
	Labial hypoplasia
Cutaneous	Hemangiomas

From McCarthy, P.: Am. J. Primary Health Care 8:34, 1983. Copyright The Nurse Practitioner: The American Journal of Primary Health Care.

It has been estimated that 75% of pregnant addicts do not seek prenatal care until labor begins (Finnegan and Macnew, 1974). They will take the drug of addiction just before seeking admission, therefore withdrawal symptoms (anxiety, nervousness, jittery behavior, anorexia, rhinorrhea, hypotension and hypoglycemia) can be delayed 6 to 12 hours after delivery.

Nursing care. The care of the addicted pregnant woman is based on historical data, symptoms, physical findings, and laboratory results. As a result of the woman's defensiveness and frequent denial, history taking has to be done in a sensitive and competent manner (Bodendorfer and others, 1979).

The woman addicted to a drug tends to exhibit a passive response to life and its responsibilities. She may show a high degree of depression. Drug use has meant a way for her to relieve psychologic distress, to encourage social interaction, and to blunt the feelings of loneliness and emptiness that are part of depression. Pregnancy is not planned, it occurs as an "accidental" phenomena. It may serve as a positive event, confirming her worth as a woman.

After birth, however, the woman is faced with the parental tasks of caring for and nurturing a completely dependent infant and of forming a warm, close, intimate relationship with the child. Care of the woman addicted to a drug offers a tremendous challenge to nursing.

Realization of the difficulty of the nursing challenge becomes very apparent. The demands of motherhood are being made of a person who is herself dependent and arrested at the stage of taking and receiving rather than giving. Most addicts are unable to establish positive intimate relationships and lack a meaningful support system. The mother's ability to care for her infant

Application of the Nursing Process

FETAL ALCOHOL SYNDROME

Bobby Albert was born 3 hours ago. His birth weight was 2464 g (5½ lb). His mother, age 24, drank heavily during pregnancy. Bobby exhibits the typical clinical problems of fetal alcohol syndrome. Both his mother and father are anxious to care for their baby.

FUNCTIONAL HEALTH PATTERN: ASSESSMENT	NURSING DIAGNOSIS	RATIONALE: PLAN/ IMPLEMENTATION	EVALUATION
ACTIVITY-EXERCISE			
Monitor for ■ Increased respiratory distress	Alteration in respiratory function*	*To prevent respiratory distress* ■ Place on cardiac monitor.	Respiratory distress does not occur or is relieved.

*Diagnosis not included by NANDA, 1986.
†Abnormal acuteness of the sense of hearing.

Application of the Nursing Process—cont'd

FUNCTIONAL HEALTH PATTERN: ASSESSMENT	NURSING DIAGNOSIS	RATIONALE: PLAN/ IMPLEMENTATION	EVALUATION
■ Development of bronchopulmonary dysplasia (BPD) ■ Apnea of prematurity with associated bradycardia ■ Seizure activity		■ Position on side with neck slightly extended using roll behind back and under shoulders. ■ Have suction and O_2 (bag and mask) at bedside.	
Monitor cardiopulmonary response	Alteration in cardiac output: decreased	*To prevent cardiopulmonary arrest or effect recovery* ■ Have resuscitation equipment at bedside (suction, bag, and mask, O_2, endotracheal tube, etc.). ■ Initiate CPR, "Stat," and "Code" call. ■ Inform anesthesiology of anomalies that have been encountered with previous intubations.	Cardiac arrest does not occur or infant recovers with no sequelae.
Observe cyanosis, potential aspiration, gagging, and choking episodes.	Alteration in nutrition: less than body requirements related to inability to feed	*To minimize feeding difficulties* ■ Gavage orally in upright position. ■ Burp well after meals. Increase amounts of feedings slowly as condition permits, maintaining adequate calories and hydration. ■ Keep suction ready for use; aspirate nares as circumstances require.	Infant takes and retains feedings.
COGNITIVE-PERCEPTUAL Observe for indications of brain dysfunction, tremulousness, irritability, hyperacusis,† poor suck.	Alteration in family process related to need to care for and love a child with a handicap.	*To promote functioning on the best possible level* ■ Encourage parental visits and physical contact with infant. ■ Assist parents to verbalize their concerns regarding anomalies. ■ Be realistic when discussing infant's potential for survival and future physical, neurologic, and emotional development. ■ Involve the parents in baby's care (diapering, holding after meals). ■ Offer appropriate auditory and sensory stimulation—do not overstimulate.	Parents recognize and accept infant's handicaps.

after discharge from the hospital should be assessed by frequent observations, including some in the home setting.

The *goals* for her care would include the following:
1. Provide the pregnant addict with optimum and comprehensive antenatal care.
2. Prevent premature delivery, perinatal loss, and neonatal drug dependence.
3. Involve the pregnant addict in long-term medical, social, psychiatric, and vocational rehabilitation.

The newborn. The nurse is frequently the first to observe the symptoms of drug dependence in the newborn. The nurse's observations serve to assist the physician in differentiation between drug dependence and other conditions: tracheoesophageal fistula, CNS disorder, sepsis, hypoglycemia, and electrolyte imbalance.

Typical signs, which are caused by withdrawal rather than narcosis, appear soon after birth or after several hours. The signs depend on the length of maternal addiction, the amount of drug taken, and the time of injection before birth. The newborn may be depressed initially. The onset of withdrawal signs in the newborn generally begins within 24 hours after birth. The infant whose mother is on methadone may not demonstrate signs of withdrawal until a week or so after birth. The symptoms of infants whose mothers used heroin or methadone are similar in nature. The newborn may be jittery and hyperactive. Table 28.5 gives a comparison between neonatal jitteriness and seizures. Frequently the infant's cry is shrill and persistent. The infant may yawn or sneeze frequently. The tendon reflexes are increased, but the Moro reflex is decreased (Bartlett and Davis, 1980; Merker, Higgins, and Kinnard, 1985). If withdrawal is not treated, the infant may develop fever, vomiting, diarrhea, dehydration, apnea, and convulsions and die.

The long-term effect on these newborns is now being studied. Researchers have found that "many serious" mental and physical problems are evident in the child's first few months of life, as well as "numerous indications . . . [of] serious abnormalities in the brain

structure that will not be revealed until later years" (Howard, 1986). The infants exposed to PCP (phencyclidine) appear to be alert, active babies. "Their mothers often think they are smarter. They hold their heads up faster. . . . But, in fact, it is abnormal behavior. Although we aren't sure why, the tone of the muscles in the head is of the kind that we see in [children with] cerebral palsy," a disorder of the central nervous system characterized by spastic paralysis or other forms of defective motor ability (Bean, 1986). The infants exposed to cocaine are typically lethargic, almost catatonic. They have visual attention problems in that they are unable to focus on their parents's face. These children often have been subjected to numerous small strokes because of abrupt changes in their mothers' blood pressure during pregnancy (Howard, 1986).

Treatment. Therapeutic programs that have been effective include the following:
1. Phenobarbital, 6 mg/kg/24 h intramuscularly or 2 mg orally four times a day for 3 or 4 days; the dose is reduced by one third every 2 days for about 2 weeks, at which time treatment is discontinued.
2. Compound tincture of opium (paregoric), 2 to 4 drops/kg orally every 4 to 6 hours initially to as much as 20 to 30 drops/kg orally every 4 to 6 hours, depending on the symptomatology.

Methadone should not be given to the newborn, even if the mother is on methadone maintenance, because of possible addiction.

Reports on observations of methadone-dependent newborns indicate that withdrawal symptoms may occur more frequently and be more prolonged than in heroin-dependent newborns. Most infants are asymptomatic and normal by 10 days of age. Crib death has been linked to methadone dependence. Further study of the short-term and long-term effects of methadone on the newborn and young child is needed.

With treatment the prognosis for the newborn is good. Without treatment at least one third of infants of narcotic addicts will die.

Nursing care. Nursing care of the drug-dependent newborn involves supportive therapy for fluid balance, infection control, and respiratory care. Early recogniton of symptoms and initiation of remedial measures has improved the outcome of these infants.

Drug dependence in the newborn is physiologic, not psychologic, so there is no predisposition to dependence later in life. However, the psychosocial environment in which the infant is raised may predispose to addiction.

Fetal tobacco syndrome. Cigarette smoking in pregnancy has been found to be associated with birth weight deficits of up to 250 g for a full-term neonate (Stein and Sussler, 1984). Maternal cigarette smoking

Table 28.5
Comparison of Newborn Jitteriness and Seizures

Normal Newborn Jitteriness	Newborn Seizure
Dominant movement tremor	Clonic jerking that cannot be stopped by flexing the affected limbs
No ocular movement	Ocular movement
Highly sensitive to stimulation	Not sensitive to stimulation
Persists for about 4 days after birth	Persists beyond 4 days after birth

Application of the Nursing Process

INFANT DEPENDENT ON NARCOTICS

Sharon West was born 24 hours ago. The nurse noted that she exhibited the symptoms of drug withdrawal. She was jittery and hyperactive; her cry was shrill and persistent. She was diagnosed as having withdrawal syndrome. Her mother used heroin on a regular basis.

FUNCTIONAL HEALTH PATTERN: ASSESSMENT	NURSING DIAGNOSIS	RATIONALE: PLAN/ IMPLEMENTATION	EVALUATION
SLEEP-REST **High-pitched cry** ■ When does it occur? ■ How long does it last? ■ Does the infant appear to be in pain? ■ Are there CNS signs?* Bulging fontanel when infant is at rest? Increasing head circumference? Widely spaced cranial sutures? Fixation of gaze without blinking? ■ Does crying stop or increase with soothing?	Alterations in comfort related to withdrawal effects	*To promote comfort:* ■ Reduce environmental stimuli (e.g., shield infant's eyes from bright lights). ■ Swaddle infant with blankets, cuddle, and hold close.	Infant relaxes. Crying diminishes.
Inability to sleep for other than short intervals ■ Note pattern—how long asleep, awake, when does sleep occur? ■ Assess effects of medications (e.g., effective = more sleep, overdose = lethargy). ■ Note yawning—onset and frequency.	Sleep pattern disturbance related to withdrawal effects	*To promote rest:* ■ Reduce environmental stimuli (e.g., organize care so rest periods are lengthened). Try holding for a period, wrap securely, place rolled blanket at back for support.	Infant goes to sleep and remains asleep for 3 to 4 hours.
NUTRITIONAL-METABOLIC **Feeding ability** ■ Note sucking pattern—can infant coordinate sucking and swallowing? ■ Note frantic sucking (prominent symptom of withdrawal). ■ Note onset and frequency. ■ Note if sucking on converted nipple helps. ■ Watch for sucking blisters and infection.	Alterations in nutrition: less than body requirements related to inability to ingest and retain food	*To maintain nutritional intake:* ■ Feed small amounts often. ■ Position nipple in mouth so sucking is effective. ■ Protect hands and wrists with shirts with cover sleeves. ■ Provide safe sucking nipple. ■ Use aseptic technique, keep skin clean. ■ Notify physician of results of glucose tests, feedings, responses, etc.	Infant ingests and retains sufficient nutrients. Infant gains weight.

*Signs of **increased intracranial pressure**.

Continued.

Application of the Nursing Process—cont'd

FUNCTIONAL HEALTH PATTERN: ASSESSMENT	NURSING DIAGNOSIS	RATIONALE: PLAN/ IMPLEMENTATION	EVALUATION
■ Assess for other causes of poor feeding (e.g., esophageal atresia, immaturity, hypoglycemia, sepsis). **Regurgitation** ■ Note occurrence (e.g., after manipulation, feeding, medication). ■ Note character and amount of regurgitated material. ■ Measure intake and output.		■ Avoid handling after feeding: medicate between feedings, if possible. ■ Correlate nutritional intake with infant's general condition, growth, and therapy.	
Vomiting and diarrhea ■ Note signs of dehydration, weight loss, sunken fontanels, poor skin turgor. ■ Note characteristics— estimate fluid loss, color.	Fluid volume deficit related to inability to retain fluids	*To maintain fluid and electrolyte balance* ■ Weigh every 8 hours or more often if vomiting and diarrhea continue. ■ Give supplementary fluids if indicated for dehydration. ■ Maintain intravenous therapy as ordered.	Infant ingests and retains sufficient fluids *or* parenteral infusions provide sufficient fluids.
Note reddened areas over bony prominences. Note skin scratches on face.	Impairment of skin integrity related to excessive movement or pressure areas	*To maintain skin integrity* ■ Use careful skin care. ■ Change position frequently. ■ If skin is excoriated, treat for possible infection.	
ACTIVITY-EXERCISE Assess patency of respiratory system ■ Note sneezing and nasal stuffiness, note amount of mucus. ■ Assess other possible causes (e.g., esophageal atresia).	Ineffective airway clearance related to mucus obstruction or anatomic obstruction	*To maintain respirations* ■ Aspirate nasopharynx as indicated. ■ Feed slowly and in small amounts. ■ Support infant with head elevated while feeding. ■ Give careful skin care to excoriated area. ■ Notify physician of any abnormal symptoms.	Infant breathes more easily.
Assess for respiratory distress. ■ Note onset of tachypnea (respiratory rate over 60/min) ■ If tachypnea persists, note heart rate. ■ Note presence of respiratory difficulties, (e.g., retraction, flaring of nostrils, apnea).	Impaired gas exchange related to withdrawal effects	*To maintain oxygen intake* ■ Place infant on cardiopulmonary monitor. ■ Position for respiratory distress. ■ Provide O_2 therapy. ■ Provide monitoring of blood gases, etc. ■ Resuscitate if needed.	Infant able to maintain O_2 intake by own efforts

Application of the Nursing Process—cont'd

FUNCTIONAL HEALTH PATTERN: ASSESSMENT	NURSING DIAGNOSIS	RATIONALE: PLAN/ IMPLEMENTATION	EVALUATION
■ Note infant's color—pallor or cyanosis (where, how extensive). ■ Note mottling: is it intensified by handling? ■ Note any symptoms indicating pathology (e.g., heart disease).			
COGNITIVE-PERCEPTUAL Note hyperactive Moro's reflex. ■ Is reflex symmetric or asymmetric, moderately or markedly exaggerated? ■ Has medication affected reflex (absent or diminished)?	Sensory impairment related to increased sensitivity to stimuli secondary to withdrawal symptoms	*To maintain normal functioning of CNS* ■ Assess infant during caretaking activities to minimize stimulation. ■ Decrease environmental stimuli.	Infant relaxes.
Note hypertonicity and degree of muscle tonus	Sensory impairment related to CNS impairment, secondary to withdrawal symptoms	*To assess for hypertonicity and degree of muscle tonus* ■ Straighten arm and leg. Note degree of resistance. ■ Raise infant by hands. Pull to sit or traction reflex. Note body rigidity and degree of head lag. (Withdrawal = body rigidity, maintenance of alignment of head and body. There is no normal head lag.) ■ Stand infant upright. (Withdrawal = leg rigidity supports infant in standing position longer than normal.)	Degree of CNS involvement is ascertained.
Note tremors, convulsions. ■ Note occurrence with stimuli. ■ Note location of tremors (e.g., upper extremities, lower extremities, generalized). ■ Note degree of tremor: slight, moderate, marked. ■ Observe for seizures; onset; origin; body involvement; clonic, tonic, or both; eye deviation; skin color.	Sensory impairment related to CNS, impairment secondary to increased intracranial pressure.	If infant convulses, maintain patent airway and prevent trauma. If infant has respiratory difficulty, begin resuscitation.	Infant recovers from seizure with minimal or no sequelae.

Continued.

Application of the Nursing Process—cont'd

FUNCTIONAL HEALTH PATTERN: ASSESSMENT	NURSING DIAGNOSIS	RATIONALE: PLAN/ IMPLEMENTATION	EVALUATION
Correlate mother's history with infant's condition and watch for complications—hypoglycemia, meningitis, intracranial hemorrhage, pyrexia.	Potential fetal complications related to mother's condition	Assess temperature, pulse, and respirations every 4 hours; decrease environmental temperature if infant develops pyrexia.	Infant responds well to therapy.

is implicated in 21% to 39% of low-birth-weight infants. The rate of preterm birth is increased, and the Apgar scores of infants are significantly lower (Department of Health and Human Services [DHHS], 1983). Nicotine and cotinine, the two pharmacologically active substances in tobacco, are found in higher concentrations in infants whose mothers smoke (Luck and others, 1982). These substances can be secreted in breast milk for up to 2 hours after the mother has smoked. Long-term studies show residual effects beyond the neonatal period. Deficits in growth, intellectual and emotional development, and behavior have been documented (DHHS 1983, Naeye and Peters, 1984).

The *fetal tobacco syndrome* is a diagnostic term applicable to infants who fit the following criteria (Nieberg and others, 1985):

1. The mother smoked five or more cigarettes a day throughout pregnancy.
2. The mother had no evidence of hypertension during pregnancy, specifically: (a) no preeclampsia and (b) documentation of normal blood pressure at least once after the first trimester.
3. The newborn has symmetric growth retardation at term (up to or greater than 37 weeks), defined as (a) a birth weight less than 2500 g and (b) a ponderal index ([weight in g] / [length in m]) greater than 2.32.
4. There is no other obvious cause of intrauterine growth retardation (e.g., congenital infection or anomaly).

Pregnant women need to be aware of the deleterious effects of smoking on their unborn baby's health. Mothers need to refrain from smoking while near their newborn infant or before breast feeding the child.

Poverty

The differences in pregnancy outcomes related to socioeconomic class have been well documented for over half a century (Fig. 28.8). Studies have consistently demonstrated a relationship between economic class and maternal and infant morbidity and mortality. These discrepancies have been of major concern to nursing groups as they have attempted to improve the health and well-being of all individuals in society. Researchers have repeatedly identified two recurrent factors that predispose low-income women to poor pregnancy outcomes (Osofsky and Kendall, 1973). The first relates to reproductive experience of the women and the second to the specific obstetric and neonatal complications involved.

Reproductive experience. Low-income individuals tend to begin reproducing at an earlier age and to end at a later age than other women. In addition, they have many pregnancies and these are adversely affected by the close spacing of the gestations. Birch and Gussons (1970) describes this phenomenon as "too young, too old, and too often." Maternal age and parity are implicated in perinatal mortality. There is increased risk to

Fig. 28.8

Poverty influences on pregnancy outcomes. (From Fogel, C.I., and Woods, N.F.: Health care of women, St. Louis, 1983, The C.V. Mosby Co.)

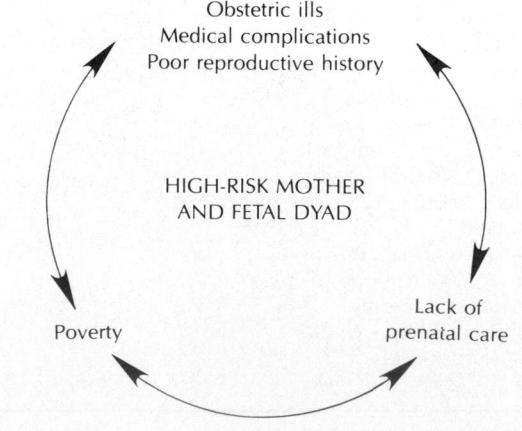

the fetus, infant, and mother when the mother is at either extreme of age or parity (see Table 23.2). Prematurity and its complications remain the chief causes in perinatal mortality. Low-income mothers are more likely to give birth to premature infants than are mothers in the population at large.

Complications. Low-income mothers are more predisposed to intercurrent illness and obstetric complications during pregnancy. Obstetric complications such as placenta previa, abruptio placentae, and placental insufficiency often result in preterm births or small-for-gestational-age babies and subsequent infant difficulties. Many obstetric complications have life-threatening consequences for the mother as well as for the infant. Examples of complications include hemorrhage, cardiac disease, or uncontrolled infection.

The problems faced by low-income mothers have direct implication for nursing service. At present much of our current knowledge could be used to ameliorate or prevent the occurrence of the problems. One of the prerequisites to providing assistance to the low-income mother is to bring her into the health care system.

Availability of services. The vulnerability of economically and socially deprived persons in our society to health problems is apparent across the spectrum of health care from prevention to rehabilitation. Preventive health is more than the prevention of disease states. It involves those factors in an individual's life that protect the individual and allow for growth and development of potential. Adequate clothing and shelter, proper nutrition, education, a safe environment, are noticeably lacking in the health experience of many low-income groups.

The concept of preventive health is often missing. The development of a concept of preventive health begins in childhood as the child is directed and encouraged to "eat your dinner and grow up to be a strong boy," "clean your teeth," "go to the doctor for a checkup," and "get enough sleep." These repeated admonitions eventually result in a concept of health care that includes prevention as well as cure. For women who have experienced this indoctrination, acceptance of the necessity for prenatal care comes more readily. For those women who have only gone to a physician when they were very ill, the relative health of the pregnant state precludes full use of care available. For some low-income women a choice between prenatal care (preparation for birth) and providing their families with necessities results in their foregoing prenatal care.

In some communities clinics have been established specifically for high-risk mothers and their infants. Adolescent mothers and prematurely born infants make up a large part of the client population at these clinics. Although prevention of the problem is probably the best approach, follow-up care is of great importance. Helping mothers to develop parenting skills will do much to promote the optimal growth and development of these disadvantaged children. Nursing and nursing researchers are in the forefront of efforts to provide care for childbearing families.

Summary

Pathophysiology, medical treatment, and nursing care of several disorders are presented in this chapter. The chapter discusses the knowledge base for understanding various disorders to assist the nurse in implementing the nursing process with diabetes mellitus and the less commonly seen problems that occur during pregnancy. A general knowledge of medical-surgical and mental health nursing is invaluable to the maternity nurse. As always, sensitivity to the woman and her family during the childbearing experience that is complicated by a physical or psychosocial disorder is as important as expert technologic assistance.

References
Endocrine Disorders

American Diabetes Association: Principles of nutrition and dietary recommendations for individuals with diabetes mellitus, Diabetes Care 2:520, 1979.
Hill, C.S., Jr. and others: Effect of pregnancy after thyroid carcinoma, Surg. Gynecol. Obstet. 122:1219, 1966.
National Diabetes Data Group: Classification and diagnosis of diabetes mellitus and other categories of glucose intolerance, Diabetes 28:1039, 1979.
White, P.: Classification of obstetric diabetes. Am. J. Obstet. Gynecol. 130:228, 1978.

Cardiovascular Disorders

Bohachick, P., and Rongaus, A.: Hypertrophic cardiomyopathy, Am. J. Nurs. 84:321, 1984.
Demakis, J.G., and Rahimtoola, S.H.: Peripartum cardiomyopathy, Circulation 44:964, 1971.
Pritchard, J., McDonald, P., and Gant, N., Williams Obstetrics, ed. 17, New York, 1985, Appleton-Century-Croft.
Veille, J.C.: Peripartum cardiomyopathies: a review, Am. J. Obstet. Gynecol. 148:805, 1984.

Neurologic Disorders

Aminoff, M.J.: Neurological disorders and pregnancy, Am. J. Obstet. Gynecol. 132:325, 1978.
Hilsinger, R.L., and others: Idiopathic facial paralysis, pregnancy, and the menstrual cycle, Ann. Otol. Rhinol. Laryngol. 84:433, 1975.

Autoimmune Diseases

Baum, J.: Arthritis and pregnancy, Contemp. OB/Gyn. 23(3):97, 1984.
Cecere, F.A., and Persellin, R.H.: The interaction of pregnancy and the rheumatic diseases, Clin. Rheum. Dis. 7:747, 1981.
Danforth, D.N., editor: Obstetrics and gynecology, ed. 4, Philadelphia, 1982, Harper & Row, Publishers.

Nolten, W.E., and Rueckert, P.A.: Elevated free cortisol index in pregnancy: possible regulatory mechanism, Am. J. Obstet. Gynecol. 139:492, 1981.

Persellin, R.H.: Inhibitors of inflammatory and immune responses in pregnancy serum, Clin. Rheum. Dis. 7:769, 1981.

Battered Pregnant Woman

Mercer, R.T.: Nursing care for parents at risk, Thorofare, N.J., 1977, Charles B. Slack.

Walker, L.E.: The battered woman, New York, 1979, Harper & Row, Publishers.

Malignant Disease and Pregnancy

DiSaia, P.J.: When extrapelvic malignant disease strikes in pregnancy, Contemp. OB/Gyn. 21:109, 1983.

DiSaia, P.J., and Creasman, W.T.: Clinical gynecologic oncology, St. Louis, 1981, The C.V. Mosby Co.

Li, M., Hertz, R., and Spencer, D.B.: Effects of methotrexate therapy upon choriocarcinoma and chorioadenoma, Proc. Soc. Exp. Biol. Med. 93:361, 1956.

Emotional Disturbance

Affonso, D.: Postpartum depression . In Fields, P., editor: Recent advances in perinatal nursing, New York, 1984, Churchhill Liomyston.

Gelder, M.: Hormones and postpartum depression. In Sandler, M., editor: Mental illness in pregnancy and the puerperium, New York, 1978, Oxford University Press.

Herzog, A., and Detre, T.: Psychotic reactions associated with childbirth, Dis. Nerv. Sys. 37:229, 1976.

Stevens, B.: Postpartum psychoses: a changing pattern, Nursing Times 66:1257, 1970.

Tentoni, S., and High, K.: Culturally induced postpartum depression, J.O.G.N. Nurs. 9:246, July/Aug. 1980.

Weiner, A.: Childbirth related psychiatric illness, Compr. Psychiatry 25:143, 1982.

Substance Abuse

Bartlett, D., and Davis, A.: Recognizing fetal alcohol syndrome in the nursery, J.O.G.N. Nurs. 9:23, 1980.

Bean, Y.: Report of ongoing research on the infants of mothers using cocaine and PCP, Los Angeles Times, January 1986.

Bodendorfer, T.W., and others: Obtaining drug exposure histories during pregnancy, Am. J. Obstet. Gynecol. 135:490, 1979.

Davis, R.P., and Keith, L.: Fetal alcohol syndrome: incurable but preventable, Contemp. OB/Gyn. 21(3):57, 1983.

Finnegan, L.P., and Macnew, B.A.: Nursing care of the addicted infant, Am. J. Nurs. 74:685, 1974.

Howard, J.: report of ongoing research on the infants of mothers using cocaine and PCP, Los Angeles Times, January 1986.

Luck, W., and others: Nicotine and cotinine: two pharmacologically active substances as parameters for the strain on fetuses and babies of mothers who smoke, J. Perinatal Med. 10:107, 1982.

McCarthy, P.: Fetal alcohol syndrome, Nurse Practitioner: Am. J. Primary Health Care 8:34, 1983.

Merker, L., Higgins, P., and Kinnard, E.: Assessing narcotic addiction in neonates, Pediatr. Nurs. 11:177, 1985.

Naeye, R.L., and Peters, E.C.: Mental development of children whose mothers smoked during pregnancy, Obstet. Gynecol. 64:60, 1984.

Nieberg, L., and others: The fetal tobacco syndrome (commentary), J.A.M.A. 253:2998, 1985.

Stein, Z.A., and Sussler, M.: Intrauterine growth retardation: epidemiological issues and public health significance, Semin. Perinatol. 8:5, 1984.

The health consequences of smoking for women: a report of the Surgeon General, Pub. No. 410-889/1284, Washington, D.C., 1983, Department of Health and Human Services.

Zacharias, J.: A rational approach to drug use in pregnancy, J.O.G.N. Nurs. 12(3):183, 1983.

Zuspan, F.P.: When drugs and alcohol complicate pregnancy, Contemp. OB/Gyn. 24(1):35, 1984.

Poverty

Birch, H.G., and Gussons, J.D.: Disadvantaged children: health, nutrition, and failure, New York, 1970, Harcourt Brace & World.

Osofsky, H.J., and Kendall, N.: Poverty as a criterion of risk, Clin. Obstet. Gynecol. 16:103, 1973.

Bibliography
Endocrine Disorders

Coustan, D.R., and Carpenter, M.W.: Detection and treatment of gestational diabetes, Clin. Obstet. Gynecol. 28:507, Sept. 1985.

Coustan, D.R.: Home glucose monitoring becomes more sophisticated, Contemp. OB/Gyn. 20:7, Oct. 1982. (Special issue, Technology 1983.)

Danforth, D.N., editor: Obstetrics and gynecology, ed. 4, Philadelphia, 1982, Harper & Row, Publishers.

Fredholm, N.Z.: The insulin pump: new method of insulin delivery, Am. J. Nurs. 81(11):2024, 1981.

Gabbe, S.G.: Diabetes in pregnancy, Clin. Obstet. Gynecol. 28:455, Sept. 1985.

Golde, S., and Platt, L.: Antepartum testing in diabetes, Clin. Obstet. Gynecol. 28:516, Sept. 1985.

Hare, J.W.: Diabetes control to reduce congenital malformations, Contemp. OB/Gyn. 20:(2):85, 1982.

Hay, W.W., and Sparks, J.W.: Placental, fetal, and neonatal carbohydrate metabolism, Clin. Obstet. Gynecol. 28:473, Sept. 1985.

Hollingsworth, D.R.: Maternal metabolism in normal pregnancy and pregnancy complicated by diabetes mellitus, Clin. Obstet. Gynecol. 28:457, Sept. 1985.

Jensen, M.D., and Bobak, I.M.: Handbook of maternity care: a guide for nursing practice, St. Louis, 1980, The C.V. Mosby Co.

Jovanovic, L., and others: The clinical utility of glycosylated hemoglobin, Am. J. Med. 70:331, 1981.

Jovanovic, L., and others: Effect of euglycemia on the outcome of pregnancy in insulin-dependent women as compared with normal control subjects, Am. J. Med. 71:921, 1981.

Kivelowitz, T.: Diabetes: a guide to self-management for patients and their families (client handbook), Englewood Cliffs, N.J., 1981, Prentice-Hall.

Landon, M.B., and Gabbe, S.G.: Glucose monitoring and insulin administration in the pregnant diabetic patient, Clin. Obstet. Gynecol. 28:496, Sept. 1985.

Lenke, R.R., and Levy H.L.: Maternal phenylketonuria and hyperphenylalaninemia: an international survey of the outcome of untreated and treated pregnancies, N. Engl. J. Med. 303:1202, 1980.

Lipman, A.G.: Drugs that interfere with urine glucose tests, Mod. Med., Aug. 15-Sept. 15, p. 195, 1978.

Miller, E., and others: Elevated maternal Hb_{Alc} in early pregnancy and major congenital anomalies in infants of diabetic mothers, N. Engle. J. Med. 304:891, 1981.

Mennuti, M.T.: Teratology and genetic counseling in the diabetic pregnancy, Clin. Obstet. Gynecol. 28:486, Sept 1985.

Moore, D.S., and others: Nursing care of the pregnant woman with diabetes mellitus, J.O.G.N. Nurs. 10:188, 1981.

Nemchik, R.: Diabetes today: the news about insulin (the latest in insulins, plus self-injection tips), R.N. 45:49, 1982.

Nesler, C.L., and others: Diabetic nephropathy in pregnancy, Clin. Obstet. Gynecol. 28:528, Sept. 1985.

Nurses Association of the American College of Obstetricians and Gynecologists: Care of the infant of the diabetic mother, N.A.A.C.O.G. Tech. Bull. No. 11, Sept. 1981.

Nurses Association of the American College of Obstetricians and Gynecologists: A sample teaching guide for the pregnant diabetic, N.A.A.C.O.G. O.G.N. Nurs. Pract. Resource, no. 5, Sept. 1981.

Penticuff, J.H.: Psychologic implications in high-risk pregnancy, Nurs. Clin. North Am. 17:69, 1982.

Plasse, N.J.: Monitoring blood glucose at home: a comparison of three products, Am. J. Nurs. 81:2028, 1981.

Queenan, J.T.: Managing polyhydramnios, Contemp. OB/Gyn. 22:17, Aug. 1983.

Sinclair, S.H., Nesler C.L., and Schwartz, S.S.: Retinopathy in the pregnant diabetic, Clin. Obstet. Gynecol. 28:536, Sept. 1985.

Steel, J.M.: Prepregnancy counseling and contraception in the insulin-dependent diabetic patient, Clin. Obstet. Gynecol. 28:553, Sept. 1985.

Stevens, D.: Monitoring blood glucose at home: who should do it and how, Am. J.. Nurs. 81:2026, 1981.

Surr, C.W.: Teaching patients to use the new blood-glucose monitoring products, Nurs. '83 13:42, 1983.

Cardiovascular Disorders

Baandrup, U., and Olsen, E.G.J.: Critical analysis of endomyocardial biopsy from patients suspected of having cardiomyopathy I. Morphological and morphometric aspects, Br. Heart J. 45:475, 1981.

Birch, E.G.: Heart disease and pregnancy, Am. Heart J. 93:104, 1977.

Danforth, D., editor: Obstetrics and gynecology, ed. 4, New York, 1982, Harper & Row, Publishers, p. 506.

Eikayam, U., and others: Interface: treating arrhythmias of pregnancy, Contemp. OB/Gyn. 23(6):55, 1984.

Eilen, B., and others: Aortic valve replacement in the third trimester of pregnancy: case report and reviews of the literature, Obstet. Gynecol. 57:119, 1981.

Glick, G., and Braunwald, E.: The cardiomyopathies and myocarditides. In Isselbacher, K.J., and others, editors: Harrison's principles of internal medicine, ed. 9, New York, 1980, McGraw-Hill Book Co.

Gothard, J.W.W.: Heart disease in pregnancy: the anesthetic management of a patient with prosthetic heart valves, Anaesthesia 33:523, 1978.

Higgard, L.T.: Maternal mortality due to cardiac disease, Clin. Obstet. Gynecol. 18:27, 1975.

Hodgman, M.T., and others: Cerebral embolism as the initial manifestation of peripartum cardiomyopathy, Neurology 32:668, 1982.

Laird-Meeter, K., and others: Cardiocirculatory adjustments during pregnancy: an echocardiographic study, Clin. Cardiol. 2:328, 1979.

Hankins, G.D.: Invasive cardiovascular monitoring: an update. Contemp. OB/Gyn. 27:114, Nov. 1985.

Masoorli, S.T., and Piercy, S.: A step-by-step guide to trouble-free transfusions, R.N. 47(5):34, 1984.

Richardson, E.A.; and Milne, L.S.: Sickle-cell disease and the childbearing family: an update, M.C.N. 8:417, 1983.

Ship-Horowitz, T.: Nursing care of the sickle cell anemic patient in labor, J.O.G.N. Nurs. 12(6):381, 1983.

Pulmonary Disorders

Holbreich, M.: Care of the asthmatic during pregnancy, Contemp. OB Gyn. 21(4):155, 1983.

Wotring, K.E.: Adult respiratory distress syndrome as a complication of pregnancy, M.C.N. 4:314, 1979.

Neurologic Disorders

Weisz, R.R.: Facial paralysis in a pregnant woman, Clini-Pearls 7(1):5, 1984.

Autoimmune Diseases

Chez, R.A., and Rizzuto, R.S.: When your patient develops rheumatoid arthritis, Contemp. OB/Gyn. 23(3)77, 1984.

Latman, N.S.: Relation of menstrual cycle phase to symptoms of rheumatoid arthritis, Am. J. Med. 74:957, 1983.

Linos, A., and others: Case-control study of rheumatoid arthritis and prior use of oral contraceptives, Lancet 1:1299, 1983.

General

Babaknia, A., and others: Appendicitis during pregnancy, Obstet. Gynecol. 50:40, 1977.

Berkow, R., editor: The Merck manual of diagnosis and therapy, ed. 14, Rahway, N.J., 1982, Merck & Co.

Phipps, W.J., and others: Medical-surgical nursing: concepts and clinical practice, ed. 3, St. Louis, 1987, The C.V. Mosby Co.

Tucker, S.M., and others, editors: Patient care standards, ed. 3, St. Louis, 1984, The C.V. Mosby Co.

Battered Pregnant Woman

Greany, G.D.: Is she a battered woman? A guide for E.R. response, Am. J. Nurs. 84:724, 1984.

Loraine, K.: Battered women: the ways you can help: R.N. 44:22, 1981.

Matteson, P.S.: Pregnant and battered, Am. Baby's Childbirth Educ. p. 46, Winter 1985/1986.

Sammons, L.N.: Battered and pregnant, M.C.N. 6:246, July/Aug. 1981.

Malignant Disease and Pregnancy

Breast cancer articles (treatment factor, hormone factor, sensations after mastectomy, stress points, prognosis with pregnancy): Am. J. Nurs. 84(9):1109, 1984.

Davis, S.R.: The breast lumps that aren't cancer, R.N. 46:30, 1983.

Greiner, L., and Weiler, C.: Early-stage breast cancer: what do women know about treatment choices? Am. J. Nurs. 83:1570, 1983.

Hassey, K.M., and others: Radiation: alternative to mastectomy, Am. J. Nurs. 83:1567, 1983.

Holden, L.S.: Helping your patient through her hysterectomy, R.N. 46:42, 1983.

Emotional Disturbance

Ballinger, B.C., and others: Emotional disturbance following childbirth: clinical findings and urinary excretion of cyclic AMP, Psychol. Med. 9:293, 1979.

Braverman, J., and Roux, J.F.: Screening for the patient at risk for postpartum depression, Obstet. Gynecol. 52:731, 1978.

Carmack, B.J., and Corwin, T.A.: Nursing care of the schizophrenic maternity patient during labor, M.C.N. 5:107, 1980.

Cox, J.L.: some sociocultural determinants of psychiatric morbidity associated with childbearing. In Sandler, M., editor: Mental illness in pregnancy and the puerperium, New York, 1978, Oxford University Press.

Devore, N.E.: The relationship between previous elective abortions and postpartum depressive reactions, J.O.G.N. Nurs. 8:237, 1979.

Fisher, L.Y.: Care of the pregnant psychotic patient, CNA Calif. Nurse 82:4, April 1986.

Focusing on today's issues in perinatal care: postpartum depression (commentary by Niles Newton), I.C.E.A. Rev. 4:2, 1980.

Malasanos, L., and others: Assessment of mental status. In Health assessment, ed. 3, St. Louis, 1987, The C.V. Mosby Co.

Petrick, J.: Postpartum depression: identification of high-risk mothers, J.O.G.N. Nurs. 13(1):37, 1984.

Spitzer, R.L.: Diagnostic and statistical manual of mental disorders, ed. 3, Washington, D.C., 1980, American Psychiatric Association.

Stuart, G., and Sundeen, S.: Principles and practice of psychiatric nursing, St. Louis, 1983, The C.V. Mosby Co.

Tentoni, S., and High, K.: Culturally induced postpartum depression, J.O.G.N. Nurs. 9:246, 1980.

True-Soderstrom, B., and others: Postpartum depression, Matern. Child Nurs. J. 3:109, 1983.

Uddenberg, N., and Englesson, I.: Prognosis of postpartum mental disturbance: a prospective study of primiparous women and their 4- and 5-year-old children, Acta Psychiatr. Scand. 58:201, 1978.

Weinberg, P.C., and Turnbull, J.M.: When to refer psychiatric problems, Contemp. OB/Gyn. 22:249, 1983.

Substance Abuse

Berman, S.M., Hogue, C.J.R., and Marks, J.S.: Maternal cigarette smoking: effect on infant birth weight (Letter), J.A.M.A. 253:911, 1984.

Bureau, M.A., and others: Maternal cigarette smoking and fetal oxygen transport: a study of P50, 2,3-diphosphoglycerate, total hemoglobin, hematocrit, and type F hemoglobin in fetal blood, Pediatrics 72:22, 1983.

Etzel, R.A., and others: Urine cotinine excretion in neonates exposed to tobacco smoke products in utero, J. Pediatr. 107:146, 1985.

Green, M., and Suffett, F.: The neonatal narcotic withdrawal index: a device for the improvement of care in the abstinence syndrome, Am. J. Drug Alcohol Abuse, 8:203, 1981.

Householder, J., and others: Infants born to narcotic-addicted mothers, Psychol. Bull. 92:383, 1980.

Lemons, P.M.: Prenatal addiction: a dual tragedy, Crit. Care Q. 4(1):79, 1981.

Lemons, P.K.M.: Victims of addiction, Crit. Care Update 10(5):12, 1983.

Lindor, E., and others: Fetal alcohol syndrome, J.O.G.N. Nurs. 9:222, 1980.

Sexton, M., and Hebel, J.R.: A clinical trial of change in maternal smoking and its effect on birth weight, J.A.M.A. 251:911, 1984.

Sweet, A.Y.: Narcotic withdrawal syndrome in the newborn, Pediatr. Rev. 3:285, 1982.

Streissguth, A.P., Barr, H.M., and Martin, D.C.: Effects of maternal alcohol, nicotine, and caffeine use during pregnancy on infant development at eight months, Alcoholism (NY) 4:152, 1980.

Whaley, L., and Wong, D.: Nursing care of infants and children, ed. 3, St. Louis, 1987, The C.V. Mosby Co.

Wilcox, A.J.: Intrauterine growth retardation: beyond birth weight criteria, Early Hum. Dev. 8:189, 1983.

Poverty

Curry, M.A.: Nurses study effects of cuts on access to prenatal care, Am. Nurs. 15:1, 1983.

Fogel, C.T., and Woods, N.F.: Health care of women, St. Louis, 1983, The C.V. Mosby Co.

Griffith-Kenney, J.: Contemporary women's health, Menlo Park, Calif., 1986, Addison Wesley Publishing Co.

Jensen, M.D., and Bobak, I.M.: Maternity and gynecologic care: the nurse and the family, ed. 3, St. Louis, 1985, The C.V. Mosby Co.

Johnson, S.H.: Nursing assessment and strategies for the family at risk: high-risk parenting, ed. 2, Philadelphia, 1986, J.B. Lippincott Co.

Kotelchuck, M.: W.I.C. participation and pregnancy outcomes: Massachusetts Statewide Evaluation Project, Am. J. Pub. Health 74:10, Oct. 1984.

Marieskind, H.: Women in the health system: patients, providers, and programs, St. Louis, 1980, The C.V. Mosby Co.

Swartz, J., and Schwartz, L.: Vulnerable infants, New York, 1977, McGraw-Hill Book Co.

Resources

American Cancer Society, Inc.
National Headquarters
777 Third Ave.
New York, NY 10017

Ca—A Cancer Journal for Clinicians
777 Third Avenue
New York, NY 10017

For additional information and answers to questions you have about breast lumps, call the following toll-free telephone number and you will be automatically connected to the Cancer Information Service office serving your area: 1-800-4-Cancer. In Alaska, call 1-800-638-6070; in Washington, D.C. (and suburbs in Maryland and Virginia) call 636-5700; on Oahu call 524-1234 (Neighbor Islands call collect). Spanish-speaking staff members are available to callers from the following areas (daytime hours only): California (area codes 213, 714, 619, and 805), Florida, Georgia, Illinois, Northern New Jersey, New York City, and Texas.

The American Society of Plastic and Reconstructive Surgeons, Inc.
Patient Referral Service
233 North Michigan Avenue, Suite 1900
Chicago, IL 60601

Dystocia and Preterm and Postterm Labor

Complications during the birth period can cause death or injury to both mother and infant. Prevention and detection of complications and consequent institution of remedial measures require the concerted efforts of the obstetric team. Many of the complications can be diagnosed before the beginning of labor, and preparation can limit their effects. Others arise suddenly, thus only the critical judgment of those present safeguards the mother or infant. The care afforded the expectant mother through normal labor must be adjusted to meet additional needs (Fig. 29.1).

Dystocia

Dystocia is defined as difficult birth as opposed to easy (normal) birth, or eutocia. Dystocia results from differences in the normal relationships between any of the five essential factors of labor (see Chapter 14). The five factors are as follows:

1. Passenger
   a. Fetus: gestational age, size, attitude, presentation, and position of the fetus; number of fetuses
   b. Placenta: type, sufficiency of, and site of insertion
2. Passageway
   a. Configuration and diameters of the maternal pelvis
   b. Distensibility of the lower uterine segment, cervical dilation, and capacity for distension of the vaginal canal and introitus
3. Powers
   a. Primary powers: intensity, duration, and frequency of uterine contractions
   b. Secondary powers: bearing-down efforts
4. Position of the mother: standing, walking, side-lying, squatting, hands and knees
5. Psychologic response: previous experiences, emotional readiness, preparation, cultural-ethnic heritage, support systems, and environment

The differences between dystocia and eutocia relate to **changes in the pattern of progress in labor.** Changes in the pattern of progress are reflected in the following aspects:
1. Alterations in the characteristics of uterine contractions

Fig. 29.1
Labor room. Equipment necessary for high-risk pregnancy: labor bed with side rails, oxygen flowmeter, call bell, blood pressure apparatus on wall behind bed, fetal monitoring equipment to left of bed, intravenous stand and drip meter to right of bed, and stethoscopes on overhead table. Clients and support persons need careful explanation of use of this equipment to reduce anxiety when seeing it for first time.

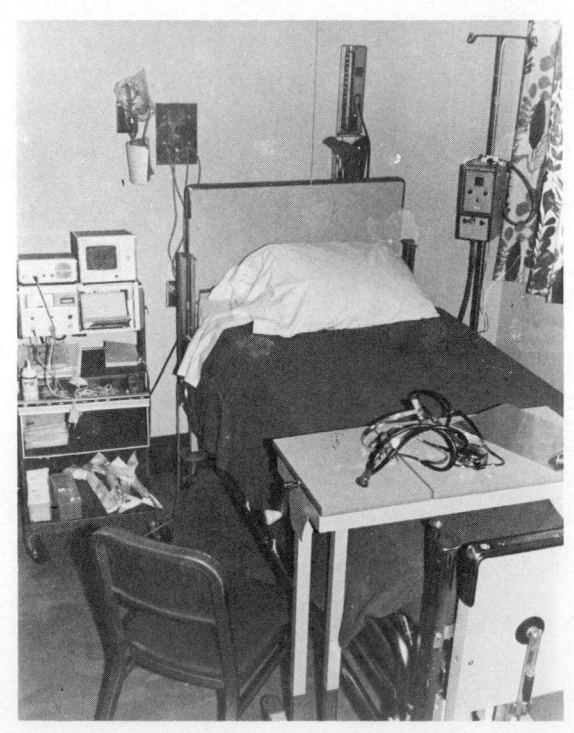

2. Lack of progress in effacement or dilation of the cervix
3. Lack of progress in descent and expulsion of the fetus

Dystocia is classified according to the area or tissue of the birth canal that is involved. The condition may occur singly or in combination with another. Tables 29.1 to 29.3 present descriptions of the various types of conditions that cause dystocia. They include a description of the condition of dystocia, changes in the pattern of labor, potential maternal and fetal effects, and the medical management. The nursing care of the woman with any type of dystocia is similar to that associated with prolonged labor.

PELVIC DYSTOCIA

Pelvic dystocia may occur with significant shortening of one or more of the internal diameters of the bony pelvis. Such diminution in capacity is termed *pelvic contracture*. The *mechanism* of labor depends on the configuration of the interior of the pelvis (see Chapter 14). However, the *outcome of labor* is affected more by the size of the pelvis than by pelvic configuration. Table 29.1 presents an overview of the various types of pelvic contracture.

DYSFUNCTIONAL LABOR

Dysfunctional labor is defined as an abnormality of the contractile pattern of the uterine muscles. The abnormality prevents normal progress in labor. The uterine contractions may be too weak, too short, irregular, or infrequent (Figs. 29.2 and 29.3). Therefore progressive cervical dilatation and effacement and descent of the presenting part do not occur.

Uterine dysfunction complicates almost 5% of all labors at term, and approximately 90% of the women

Table 29.1
Pelvic Dystocia

Assessment	Inlet Contracture	Midpelvic Contracture	Outlet Contracture
Description	Diagonal conjugate less than 11.5 cm (see Fig. 14.9)	Sum of interischial spinous and posterior sagittal diameters of midpelvis 13.5 cm or less (see Fig. 14.10) Interischial spinous diameter less than 9 cm (see Fig. 14.10)	Interischial spinous diameter 8 cm or less Outlet contraction alone, without midplane contraction, rare
Change in pattern of labor	**Rupture of membranes, early, spontaneous** **Dilation of cervix slows or ceases** **Descent does not occur**	**Descent arrested (transverse arrest of the fetal head); fetal head cannot undergo internal rotation and descend** **Contractions decrease in frequency and intensity** **Dilation of cervix slows**	**Descent arrested**
Potential maternal effects	Intrauterine infection Rupture of abnormally thinned lower segment of uterus (see Fig. 14.13). Pathologic retraction ring develops. Formation of fistulas Psychologic trauma from difficult delivery	Rupture of uterus Exhaustion Psychologic trauma from difficult delivery	Extensive perineal lacerations Exhaustion
Potential fetal effects	Fetal asphyxia Fetal and neonatal death Excessive molding of fetal head Prolapse of cord	Fetal asphyxia Fetal death Excessive molding of head	Fetal asphyxia Fetal death
Medical management	Cesarean delivery if safe vaginal delivery not possible	Cesarean delivery if fetal head cannot pass obstruction Forceps delivery if fetal head passes obstruction (head descends, perineum bulges, vertex is visible) Vacuum extractor when cervix fully dilated	Extensive mediolateral episiotomy

Fig. 29.2
Uterine contractility patterns in labor. **A,** Typical normal labor. **B,** Subnormal intensity, with frequency greater than needed for optimal performance. **C,** Normal contractions, but too infrequent for efficient labor. **D,** Incoordinate activity. **E,** Hypercontractility.

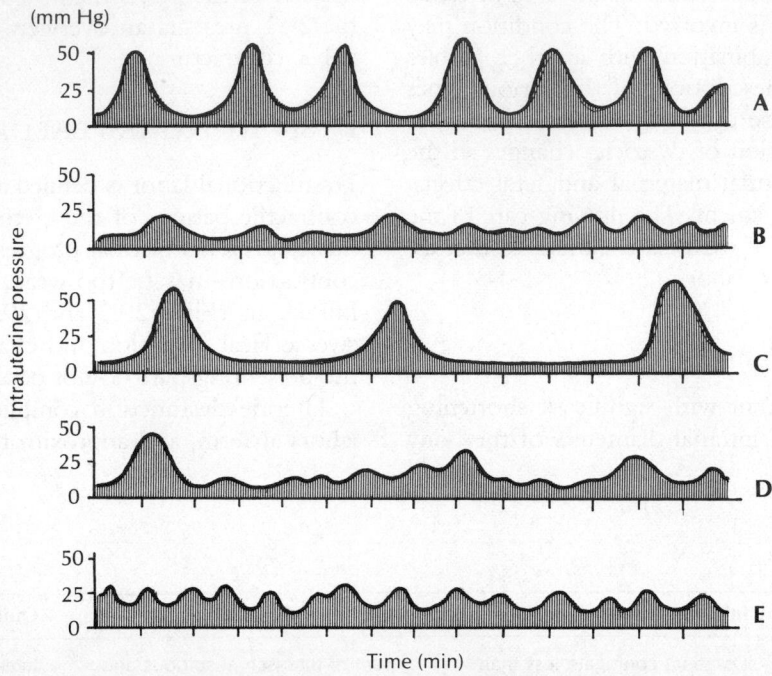

Fig. 29.3
Normal and dysfunctional uterine contraction types. *Black area,* strong contraction; *shaded area,* slight contraction, *white area,* atonic areas.

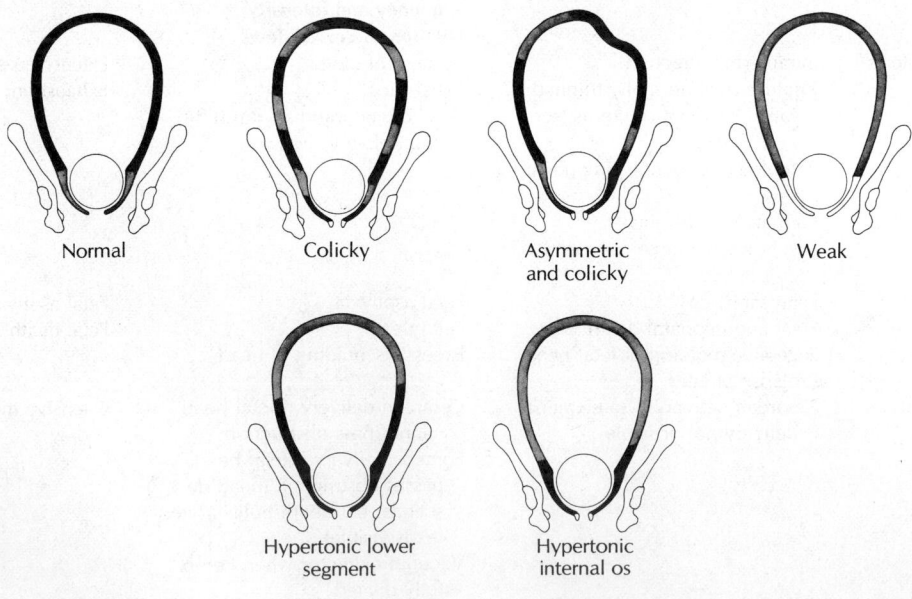

Table 29.2
Dysfunctional Labor: Primary and Secondary Powers

Assessment	Hypotonic Uterine Dysfunction	Hypertonic Uterine Dysfunction	Inadequate Voluntary Expulsive Forces
Description	Cause may be contracture and fetal malposition, overextension of uterus (twins), or unknown (primary powers) (Figs. 29.2 and 29.3)	Usually occurs before 4 cm dilation; cause not yet known, may be related to fear and tension (primary powers) (Figs. 29.2 and 29.3)	Involves abdominal and levator ani muscles Occurs in second stage of labor; cause may be related to conduction anesthesia, heavy analgesia, paralysis or intense pain with contractions (secondary powers)
Change in pattern of progress	**Contractions decrease in frequency and intensity** **Uterus easily indentable even at peak of contraction** **Uterus relaxed between contractions (normal)**	**Pain out of proportion to intensity of contraction** **Pain out of proportion to effectiveness of contraction in effacing and dilating the cervix** **Contractions increase in frequency** **Contractions uncoordinated** **Uterus is contracted between contraction (basal hypertonus), cannot be indented.**	**No voluntary urge to push or bear down**
Potential maternal effects	Infection Exhaustion Psychologic trauma	Loss of control related to intensity of pain and lack of progress Exhaustion	Spontaneous vaginal delivery prevented
Potential fetal effects	Fetal infection Fetal and neonatal death	Fetal asphyxia with meconium aspiration	Fetal asphyxia
Medical management	Oxytocic stimulation of labor (p. 917) Prostaglandin stimulation of labor (p. 917)	Analgesic (morphine, meperidine) if membranes not ruptured or fetopelvic disproportion not present Relief of pain permits mother to rest; when she awakens, normal uterine activity may begin	Coach mother in bearing down with contractions Analgesia to counteract pain Cesarean delivery only if fetal distress

are nulliparas. It is classified as follows:

1. Primary uterine inertia: inefficient contractions persist from the onset of labor.
2. Secondary uterine inertia: well-established, efficient contractions become weak and inefficient or stop altogether.

Table 29.2 presents a summary of dysfunctional labor.

DYSTOCIA OF FETAL ORIGIN

Dystocia may be caused by fetal anomalies, excessive size, or malpresentation or malposition of the fetus. Although these conditions are uncommon, they constitute obstetric emergencies.

Fetal dystocia may be classified according to the cause of the abnormality as follows:

Fetopelvic disproportion. Excessive *fetal size* is arbitrarily 4000 g (8 lb, 13½ oz) or more in North America. Such large fetuses represent about 5% of term births. Frequently, excessive size is a result of di-

abetes mellitus, obesity, maternal multiparity, or the large size of one or both parents.

The *fetal anomalies* include twins, gross ascites or abdominal tumor, and myelomeningocele.

Table 29.3 presents a summary of fetopelvic disproportion.

Fetal malposition. The most common fetal malposition is *persistent occiput posterior position*. Other fetal malpositions are encountered rarely, for example, *transverse lie* (see Fig. 14.5, *D*). Table 29.2 presents a summary of persistent occiput posterior position.

Fetal malpresentation. *Breech presentation* is the most common example of malpresentation. Table 29.3 presents a summary of breech presentations. The table also includes the nursing care required during labor as the labor may or may not be prolonged.

Multiple pregnancy. Multiple pregnancy is the gestation of twins, triplets, quadruplets, or more infants. Twins produced from a single ovum are termed monozygotic, or identical, and the sibling is always of the

Table 29.3
Summary: Dystocia of Fetal Origin

	Fetopelvic Disproportion	Malposition	Malpresentation: Breech
Description	Fetal macrosomia with normal or small pelvis Fetal anomaly	Persistent occiput posterior positions Leopold's manuevers reveal small parts against abdominal wall Abdominal contours differ (Fig. 29.4) Vaginal examination: the cervix must be fully dilated before the diagnosis can be made; if fetus is in an occiput posterior position, examiner will be able to feel four suture lines that enter anterior fontanel	Related to prematurity; most infants assume a longitudinal lie with vertex presenting at term Related to multiple fetuses, hydramnios, oligohydramnios, fetal or maternal anomalies Breech presentations revealed by abdominal and vaginal examinations, x-ray films, and sonography Breech presentation occurs in four types (Fig. 29.5)
Change in pattern of progress	**Engagement does not occur** **Descent does not occur** **Uterus unusual size or contour** **Membranes rupture early** **Cervical dilation slows** **Contractions decrease in frequency and intensity**	**Contractions are diminished in frequency and intensity** **Backache is accentuated** **Cervical dilation slows** **Descent is delayed** **Second stage of labor may be prolonged**	**Heart sounds loudest slightly above the umbilicus (Fig. 15.5)** **Labor not unduly prolonged** **Spontaneous complete expulsion seldom successfully accomplished** **Aftercoming head does not have time to mold during descent and therefore expulsion may be prevented**
Potential maternal effects	Infection Development of pathologic ring Rupture of uterus Vaginal fistulas	Exhaustion Increased sensitivity to pain Extension of episiotomy Psychologic trauma from prolonged labor	Morbidity and mortality increased as result of operative delivery including cesarean delivery
Potential fetal effects	Infection Prolapse of cord Excessive molding of the head; may result in intracranial hemorrhage	Fetal asphyxia	Prematurity Congenital anomalies Birth trauma, asphyxia from cord compression Fetal death Infant has little molding of the head If frank breech, infant resting posture is not flexion. Legs are extended straight up over abdomen.
Medical management	Cesarean delivery if vaginal delivery poses a potential threat to mother or fetus	Conservative approach followed as most of fetuses (70%) in occiput posterior position: ■ Rotate spontaneously to an anterior position and deliver spontaneously ■ May deliver in the face-to-pubes position if posterior position persists **Care during labor** Hydration is maintained with intravenous infusion. Electronic fetal monitoring is initiated (see Chapter 16) Medications for pain relief and relaxation are ordered (see Chapter 16)	External version may be attempted after 34 weeks gestation (Fig. 29.6) Vaginal delivery is done as soon as umbilicus comes into view to prevent compression of cord between fetal head and pelvis or traction on cord—a possible cause of bleeding or placental separation (Fig. 29.7) Cesarean delivery is commonly used in nulliparas and in multiparas with fetuses estimated to be larger than 3360 g (7¼ lb) if labor is ineffective or when hazardous complications arise. (Research related to safe method of delivery,

Continued.

Fig. 29.4
Comparison of abdominal contours with fetus in occiput anterior position, **A,** and occiput posterior position, **B.** The indentation between the fetal chin and small parts forms a concavity above the level of the symphysis (may be obscured by a full bladder).

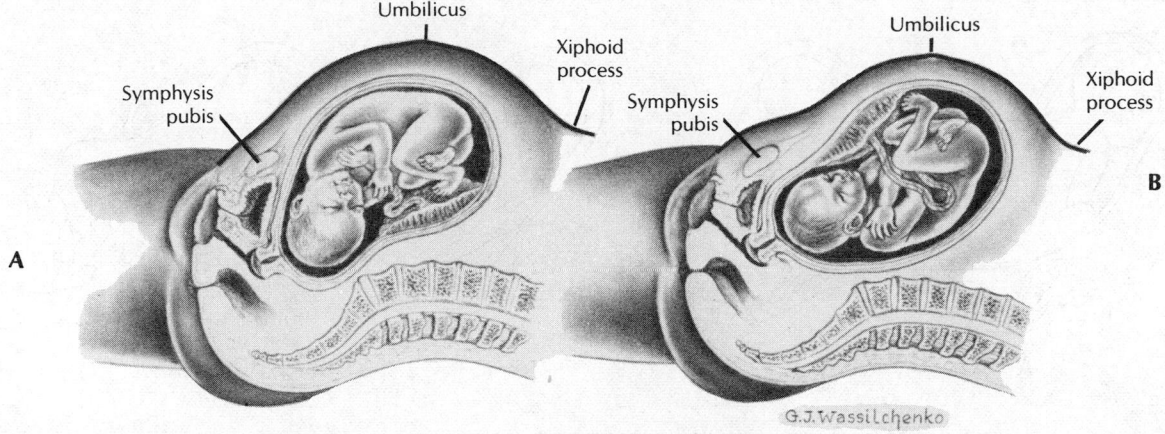

Fig. 29.5
Types of breech presentation. **A,** Frank breech: thighs are flexed on hips; knees are extended. **B,** Complete breech: thighs and knees are flexed. **C,** Incomplete breech: foot extends below buttocks. **D,** Incomplete breech: knee extends below buttocks.

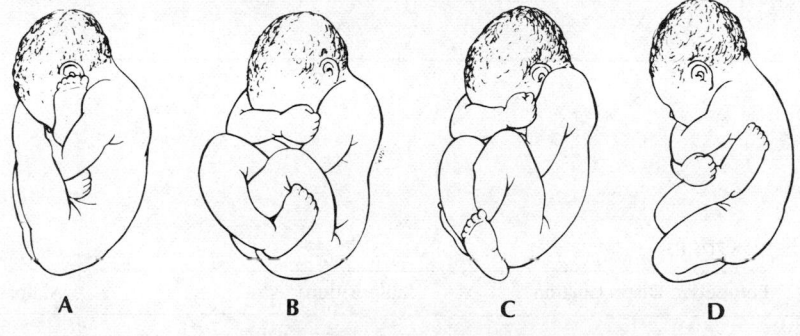

Fig. 29.6
External version of fetus from breech to vertex presentation. This must be achieved without force. **A,** Breech is pushed up out of pelvic inlet while head is pulled toward inlet. **B,** Head is pushed toward inlet while breech is pulled upward.

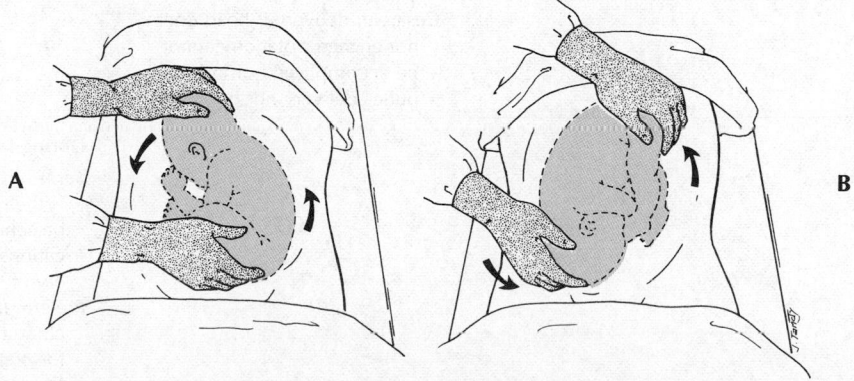

Fig. 29.7
Mechanism of labor in breech position. **A,** Breech before onset of labor. **B,** Engagement and internal rotation. **C,** Lateral flexion. **D,** External rotation or restitution. **E,** Internal rotation of shoulders and head. **F,** Face rotates to sacrum when occiput is anterior. **G,** Head is delivered by gradual flexion during elevation of fetal body.

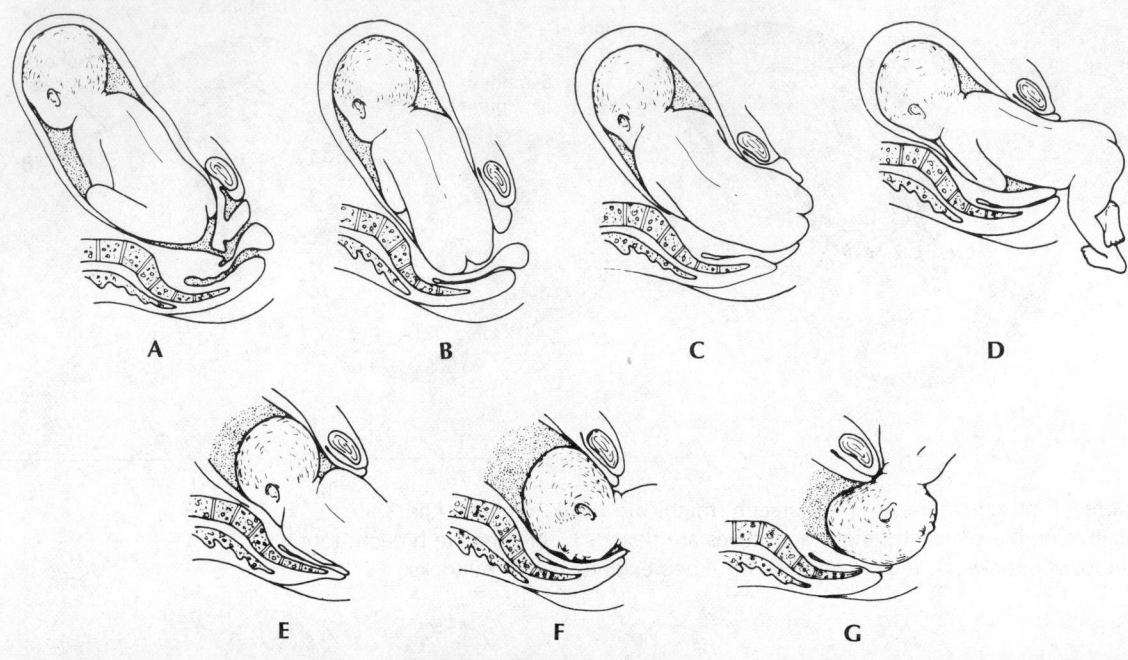

Table 29.3, cont'd
Summary: Dystocia of Fetal Origin

	Fetopelvic Disproportion	Malposition	Malpresentation: Breech
		Care during delivery	i.e., vaginal versus cesarean delivery continues)
		Anesthesia administered	
		Mediolateral episiotomy done to permit manual or forceps rotation	
		Low forceps delivery of vertex may be needed	
		Cesarean delivery if head does not engage, rotation cannot be accomplished or face-to-pubes delivery not possible	
			During labor
Nursing care			*Term birth.* Routine nursing care is the same as that for vertex presentation because complications arise as part of delivery of the infant
			Preterm birth. Care would include routine care and care for preterm birth discussed later in this chapter

Table 29.3, cont'd
Summary: Dystocia of Fetal Origin

	Fetopelvic Disproportion	Malposition	Malpresentation: Breech
Nursing care—cont'd			Parental anxiety is increased by awareness of possible injury to infant; parents will need supportive care from attending nurses and physicians. Use of cesarean delivery as mode of delivery for breech presentations has lessened fear for infant survival; mothers in this situation will need care outlined for cesarean delivery described later in this chapter
			For vaginal delivery
			Extra sterile towels and Piper forceps (Fig. 29.14) are added to routine supplies and equipment on delivery table
			Resuscitation equipment and supplies are readied for use
			Pediatricians and nursing staff from intensive care nursery are notified and present for delivery
			Postpartum
			Care will depend on method of delivery; in event of vaginal delivery, care is same for all mothers (see Unit 6); care for cesarean delivery is discussed later in this chapter; Care of infants will be dictated by their gestational age (see Chapter 31) and by whether trauma or hypoxia were sustained; if healthy and at term, infants are cared for as any normal infants (see Unit 5). Resting posture of infant who was frank breech is explained to parents; some may think the infant has a hip deformity

same sex (Fig. 29.8). Those produced from separate ova are dizygotic, or fraternal, and may be of the same or opposite sex (Fig. 29.9). Monozygotic twinning is a random occurrence. Dizygotic twinning (multiple ovulation), on the other hand, is an autosomal-recessive trait carried by the daughters of mothers of twins. It occurs more frequently as maternal age at conception increases. Triplets can develop from one, two, or three ova (Fig. 29.10).

Infants of multiple pregnancies account for 2% to 3% of all viable births. Of twins, more than 15% weigh less than 2500 g. Most of these are preterm. Twins occur in about 1 in 99 conceptions; triplets and quadruplets occur much less frequently. Multiple pregnancy is most common in blacks, least common in Orientals, and of intermediate occurrence in whites. Almost 30% of twins are monozygotic; nearly 70% are dizygotic. Fewer males than females are born in multiple pregnancies. Maternal morbidity and mortality are greatly increased in multiple pregnancy because of medical and obstetric complications. The prenatal diagnosis of multiple pregnancy is made in only about

Fig. 29.8
Formation of monozygotic twins. **A,** One fertilization: blastomeres separate, resulting in two implantations, two placentas, and two sets of membranes. **B,** One blastomere with two inner cell masses, one fused placenta, one chorion, and separate amnions. **C,** Later separation of inner cell masses, with fused placenta and single amnion and chorion. (From Whaley, L.F.: Understanding inherited disorders, St. Louis, 1974, The C.V. Mosby Co.)

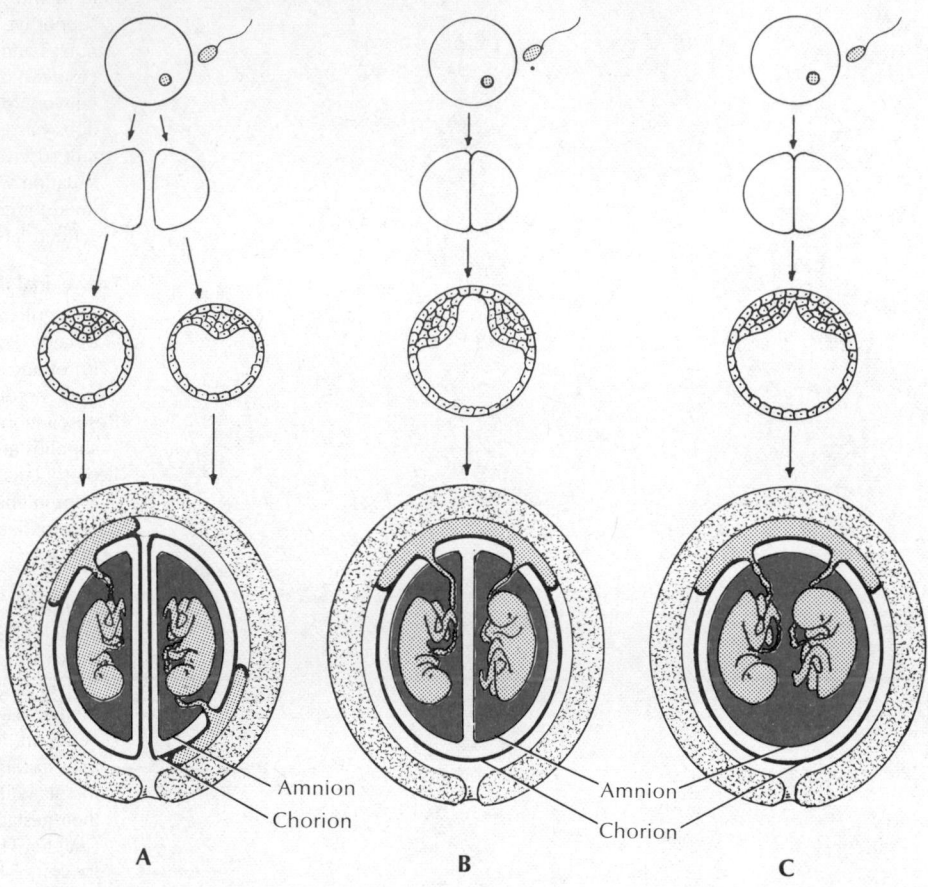

75% of cases and often late in gestation. This is regrettable, since much can be done for the mother and her infants if treatment is instituted early.

Maternal problems

1. Maternal blood volume is increased in multiple gestations. As a result there is increased strain on the maternal cardiovascular system.
2. Anemia often develops because of a greater demand for iron by the fetuses.
3. Marked uterine distension and increased pressure on the adjacent viscera and pelvic vasculature occur in multiple pregnancy. Diastasis of the two recti abdominis muscles (in the midline) may occur.
4. Placenta previa develops more frequently in multiple pregnancies because of the large size or placement of the placentas (see Fig. 29.8, *A*, and note

placement of placentas). Premature separation of the placenta may occur before the second and subsequent fetuses are born.

Fetal problems

1. Weight of each twin and her or his placenta usually is less than an infant and placenta of a singleton pregnancy after the thirtieth week. However, the aggregate weight is almost twice that of a singleton near term. The mean weight of twins in the United States is more than 2270 g (5 lb).
2. Congenital malformations are twice as frequent in monozygotic twins as in singletons. There is no increase in the incidence of congenital anomalies in dizygotic twins.
3. Two-vessel cords, that is, cords with a single umbilical artery, occur more often in twins than in sin-

Fig. 29.9
Formation of dizygotic twins. There is fertilization of two ova, two implantations, two placentas, two chorions, and two amnions. (From Whaley, L.F.: Understanding inherited disorders, St. Louis, 1974, The C.V. Mosby Co.)

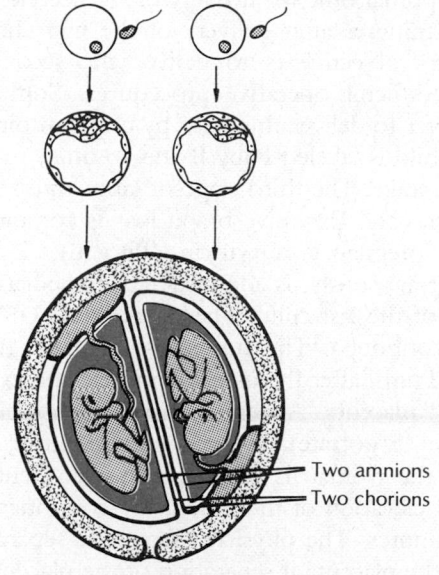

Two amnions
Two chorions

gletons, and this abnormality is most common in monozygotic twins.

4. The most serious problem for the fetus is the local shunting of blood between placentas (twin-to-twin transfusion). The *recipient* twin is larger. However, this twin may develop congenital heart failure during the first 24 hours after birth. The *donor* twin will be small, pallid, dehydrated, malnourished, and hypovolemic.

5. Prematurity is a serious problem for the newborns.

Medical diagnosis. Clinical diagnosis of multiple pregnancy is accurate in only about three fourths of cases. A correct diagnosis of twins may be possible in most instances by the twenty-fourth to twenty-sixth week based on the following:

1. History of dizygous twins in the female lineage
2. Abnormally large maternal weight gain (inconsistent with diet or edema)
3. Polyhydramnios
4. Palpation of excessive number of small or large parts
5. Asynchronous fetal heart beats or more than one fetal electrocardiographic (EEG) tracing.
6. Radiographic or ultrasonographic (B-scan) evidence of more than one fetus (Chapter 25).

In twin pregnancy, both fetuses will present by the vertex in about one half of cases; one will present by the vertex and one by the breech in approximately one

Fig. 29.10
Formation of triplets and quadruplets indicating variety of mechanisms that can produce multiple births. Quadruplets can be formed from one to four ova. (From Whaley, L.F.: Understanding inherited disorders, St. Louis, 1974, The C.V. Mosby Co.)

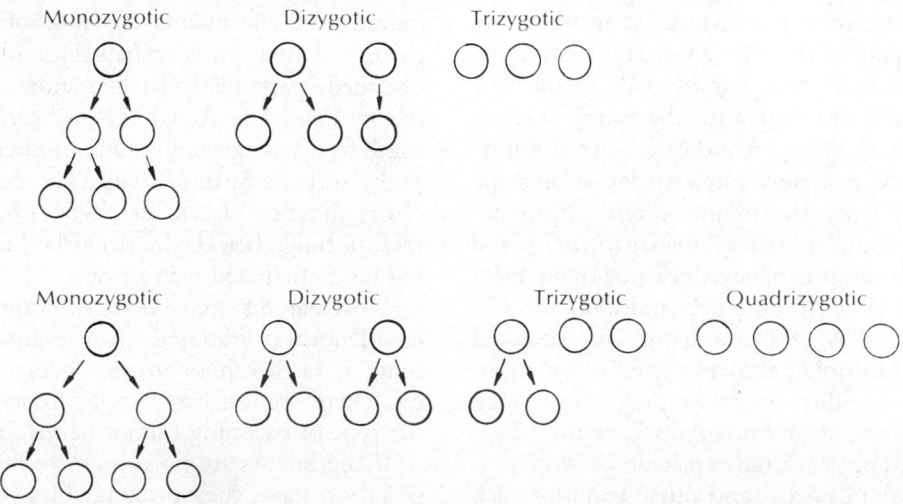

third of the total births. Other combinations are un-common.

Prenatal care. Prenatal care will include changes in the pattern of care and modifications in other aspects such as weight gain and diet. Prenatal visits by the mother with multiple pregnancy are scheduled at least every 2 weeks in the second trimester and weekly thereafter.

Diet and weight control are supervised to allow weight gain of about 50% or more than the average woman with a singleton pregnancy (as much as 18 kg [40 lb] above the woman's ideal nonpregnant weight). Iron and vitamin supplementation is desirable. Attempts are made to prevent preeclampsia-eclampsia and vaginitis; if they do develop, they are treated early and properly.

Support from a well-fitted maternity girdle may be welcomed. The considerable uterine distension can cause increase in backache. Elastic stockings or tights may control leg varices.

Abstinence from coitus or masturbation to the point of orgasm during the last trimester is recommended. This may help prevent preterm labor.

Enforced rest periods, begun as soon as pregnancy is diagnosed, may help to avoid untimely early labor. The mother needs to assume the left lateral position.

Untimely early labor should be avoided. Delivery after the thirty-sixth week increases the likelihood of survival of the newborns.

Intranatal care. Delivery in a maternity center where specialty care is always available is advisable when there is a multiple pregnancy. The woman is admitted to the hospital at the first sign of labor.

First stage. The woman is placed on bed rest in a left lateral position. Her blood is typed and cross matched, and several units of bank blood are kept available in the delivery room for emergency transfusion. Parenteral infusion of 5% dextrose in water (or other infusate) is started through a no. 16 or 18 needle (that can accommodate blood if needed) in the first stage of labor and continued until the fourth stage is completed. Blood or drugs, if indicated, are administered intravenously at a slow rate. Analgesia must be limited drastically since the infants often are premature. If no complications occur, management of the first stage in multiple pregnancy does not differ from the single pregnancy with same presentation.

Cesarean delivery is performed only for accepted obstetric reason. Multiple pregnancy itself is not an indication. However, disproportion (e.g., conjoined twins), fetal distress, or monoamniotic twins (diagnosed by amniography) warrant cesarean delivery.

Second stage. A physician and nurse team for each newborn is scrubbed, gowned, and gloved for the multiple birth delivery. After the first twin is born the cord is clamped promptly to prevent the second twin of a monozygotic pregnancy from partially exsanguinating through the first cord. The time of birth is noted, and the infant is labeled as Baby A.

The optimal time for delivery of the second child is 5 to 20 minutes after delivery of the first child. The physician's objective is to deliver the second child without difficult operative procedures. Some physicians prefer to deliver this fetus by cesarean birth. The second child is labeled Baby B and so on.

Third stage. The third stage of labor must be managed with care. Excessive blood loss is common with multiple pregnancy. Oxytocin (Pitocin), 1 ml (10 units) intravenously, is administered immediately after delivery of the last child. The intravenous D5W infusion is continued. The fundus is elevated. It is not massaged until after the uterus contracts and expels the separated placenta. An ergot preparation such as ergonovine (Ergotrate), 0.1 mg intravenously, is then given if the woman is not hypertensive. Gentle massage and elevation of the fundus are continued for 15 to 30 minutes. The physician manually separates and extracts the placenta if separation of the placenta is delayed or bleeding is brisk.

Postpartum care. The mother with multiple pregnancy requires the same physical care as any other parturient. She is more prone to develop postdelivery hemorrhage because of excessive uterine distension. Therefore she must be carefully assessed.

Psychologically, however, even the most willing of mothers can find their coping mechanisms overwhelmed by both the idea and reality of caring for two or more infants. Mother-child attachment takes longer because the mother attaches first to one newborn and then to the other. Parents must organize simplified and flexible plans of care. The almost constant attention required until the infants' schedule of care can be synchronized may prove exhausting. If possible, help is obtained, particularly to guarantee sufficient rest for the mother. The added expense can also be burdensome to a young family. One mother expressed anger at the surprise birth of twins. The explanation of such errors did not placate her. She needed time to vent these feelings before she could be helped with changing her anticipated plan of care.

Most parents are anxious to know if their children are identical or fraternal. Gross examination of the placenta at birth cannot prove whether twins are identical. Therefore it is best to tell parents differentiation in the type of twinning cannot be made at this time.

If the infants are born prematurely or are small for gestational age, their prolonged hospital stay can cause parental separation anxiety. If this is the case, the mother may be encouraged to visit or care for the infants in the hospital. She can use this waiting time to recover as much physical strength as possible. It provides time for the family to prepare for the infant's homecoming. Introduction of multiple siblings into a family also can result in intense rivalry. All children compete for the mother's attention. Substitute mothering by interested relatives can do much to ease the strain.

Nursing twins takes planning and patience. If the mother elects the rooming-in regimen, the added care of two infants may prove too taxing to her strength. However, many mothers have stated that the early adjustment made going home easier. It is suggested that these mothers remain longer in the hospital unless there is help at home. It is important to establish a feeding schedule as soon as possible. The mother may use a modified demand schedule. She can feed the first baby who wakes up, then wake up the second baby. She may decide to nurse them simultaneously (Fig. 29.11).

A record of the feeding times, which breast was used by which baby, and which side was used first is essential during the early weeks. If one twin nurses more readily than the other, an effort should be made to have that twin nurse on alternate breasts to equalize stimulation. If feeding simultaneously, the mother should experiment with positions. Each baby may be supported on pillows and in the football hold. One may be held in the football hold and the other in the cradle hold. Obviously the mother with twins will need extra assistance from her family, extra nourishment, and extra rest. She will need sufficient energy not only to care for and nurse each baby but also to provide the mothering each child needs.

Having twins or triplets can be a most rewarding experience. As the children develop, they experience a closeness unique for siblings. One twin, when asked how many brothers and sisters she had, answered, "three sisters and Pam (her twin)."

SOFT TISSUE DYSTOCIA

Soft tissue dystocia results from obstruction of the birth passage by an anatomic abnormality other than that of the bony pelvis. The obstruction may result from placenta previa (low-lying placenta), that partially or completely obstructs the internal os of the cervix. Care relative to placenta previa is discussed in Chapter 27. Other causes include congenital anomalies, tumors, or infection. Some may arise during labor. A **full bladder** may fill the pelvic inlet and prevent descent of the presenting part as the cervix dilates. Occasionally, **cervical edema** occurs in labor when the

Fig. 29.11
Breast-feeding twins. Note support with pillows. Infants in "football hold" position. If one twin nurses vigorously, change sides for each feeding. (Courtesy Colleen Stainton.)

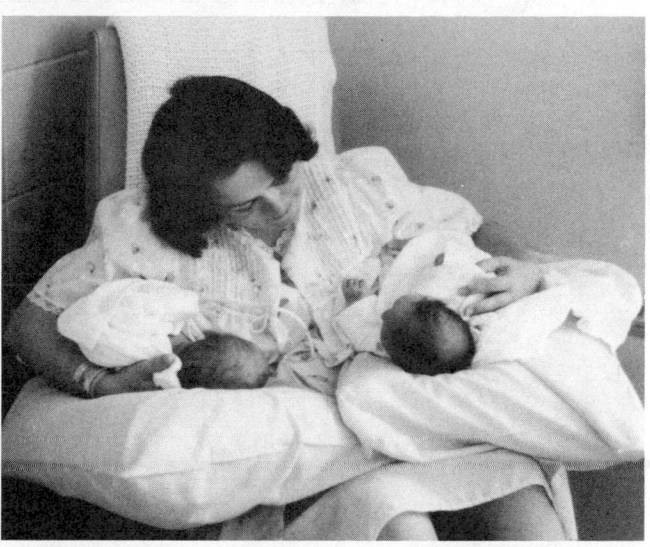

cervix is caught between the presenting part and the symphysis. Cervical edema prevents complete dilation of the cervix.

PROLONGED LABOR

Prolonged labor is true, clinically evident labor that lasts more than 18 hours (Danforth, 1982). It may result from varying causes. Pelvic contractures, fetopelvic disproportion, or inadequate uterine contractions can occur singly or in combination. The cervix may be *unripe*, that is, not relaxed and partially dilated in preparation for labor. Progress in either the first or second stage is delayed or protracted. Fig. 29.12 compares and contrasts the partogram of a normal labor with major types of deviation from normal progress of labor.

The partogram in Fig. 29.12, *A,* is a graphic appraisal of the time factor in normal labor for a primigravida. The *latent phase* includes that portion of the first stage between the onset of labor contractions and the acceleration in rate of cervical dilation. The upswing in the curve denotes the onset of the *active phase* of the first stage of labor, which includes the *acceleration phase,* the *phase of maximal slope,* and the *deceleration phase.* Compare this with Fig. 29.12, *B,* which are major types of deviation from normal progress of labor. These can be detected by noting the dilation of the cervix at various intervals after labor begins. If a woman exhibits an abnormal labor pattern as depicted

Fig. 29.12
A, Partogram of a normal labor. **B,** Arrest of descent in the active phase: no progress for 1 hour or more in the nullipara and 30 minutes in the parous woman.

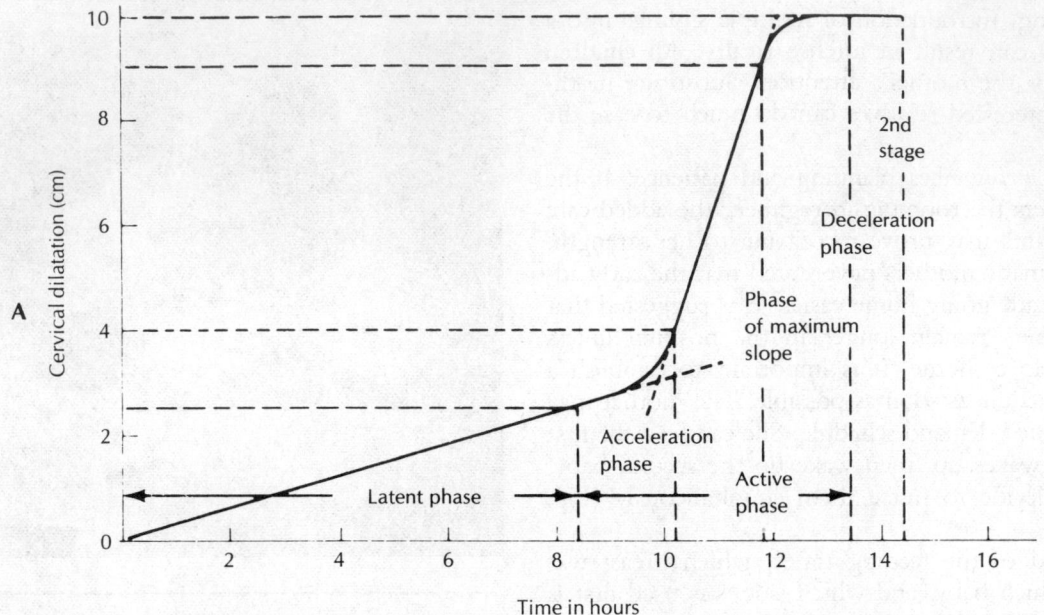

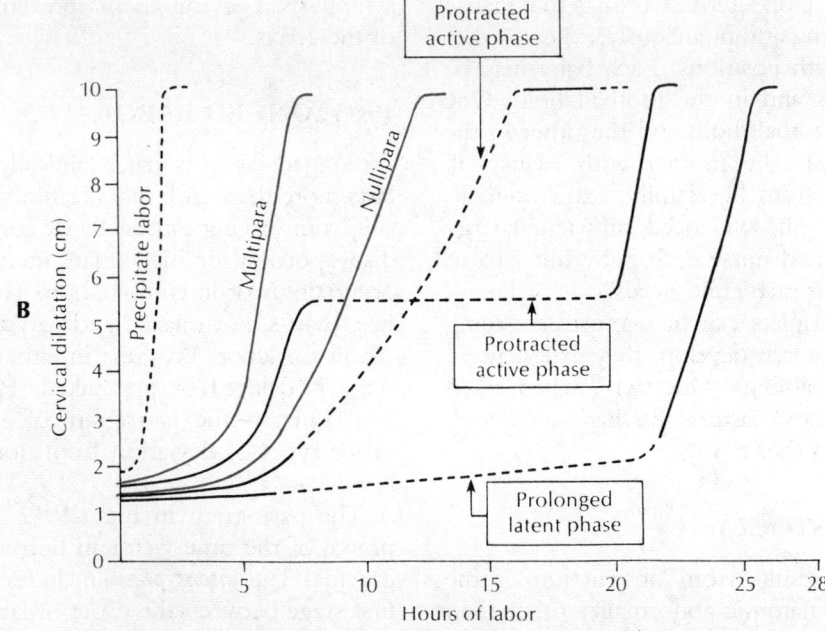

by the broken lines, the physician should be notified immediately!

1. Cervical dilation patterns: report to physician
   a. Prolonged latent phase: 20 hours or longer in the nullipara and 14 hours or longer in the parous woman
   b. Protracted active phase: cervical dilation of less than 1.2 cm/h in the nullipara and less than 1.5 cm/h in the parous woman
   c. Arrest of the active phase: no progress in the active phase for more than 2 to 4 hours
   d. Precipitate labor: labor of less than 3 hours.

1. D, A
2. D
3. B
4. D
5. C
6. B
7. B
8. A
9. C
10. A, C
11. D
12. C, D
13. D
14. D
15. D
16. B, D
17. C
18. B
19. A
20.

thank
you

OUR RETURN AND EXCHANGE POLICY

GENERAL

ALL MERCHANDISE TO BE RETURNED MUST BE:

1. RETURNED WITHIN 10 DAYS OF PURCHASE.
2. ACCOMPANIED BY SALES RECEIPT.
3. RETURNED IN ORIGINAL CARTON AND PACKING.
4. UNUSED AND SHOW NO EVIDENCE OF WEAR.
5. REGULAR MERCHANDISE AND NOT A SPECIAL ORDER.
6. A STANDARD SIZE (NOT SIZED OR FITTED).
7. UNCUSTOMIZED (FOR EXAMPLE, NOT ENGRAVED).

EXCEPTIONS

NO REFUNDS, EXCHANGES OR RETURNS ON FIREARMS AND AMMUNITION, LAWN AND GARDEN EQUIPMENT, CLEARANCE MERCHANDISE AND CERTAIN VACUUM CLEANERS AS SPECIFIED UNDER THE TERMS OF THE MANUFACTURER'S WARRANTY.

WARRANTIES

IT IS THE CUSTOMER'S RESPONSIBILITY TO COMPLY WITH THE TERMS OF ANY APPLICABLE MANUFACTURER'S WARRANTY. MERCHANDISE IN NEED OF REPAIR SHOULD BE RETURNED TO THE MANUFACTURER OR ITS AUTHORIZED SERVICE CENTER AS SPECIFIED UNDER THE TERMS OF THE WARRANTY. THE MANUFACTURER'S WARRANTY APPLICABLE TO A PARTICULAR PRODUCT IS THAT PRODUCTS ONLY WARRANTY. SERVICE MERCHANDISE MAKES NO WARRANTY, EXPRESS OR IMPLIED, EXCEPT AS MAY BE SPECIFICALLY REQUIRED BY APPLICABLE STATUTE.

GENERAL

ALL MERCHANDISE TO BE RETURNED MUST BE:

1. RETURNED WITHIN 10 DAYS OF PURCHASE.
2. ACCOMPANIED BY SALES RECEIPT.
3. RETURNED IN ORIGINAL CARTON AND PACKING.
4. UNUSED AND SHOW NO EVIDENCE OF WEAR.
5. REGULAR MERCHANDISE AND NOT A SPECIAL ORDER.
6. A STANDARD SIZE (NOT SIZED OR FITTED).
7. UNCUSTOMIZED (FOR EXAMPLE, NOT ENGRAVED).

Labor Patterns in Normal and Prolonged Labor

Normal labor
1. Dilatation: continues
   a. Latent phase: <4 cm and low slope
   b. Active phase: >5 cm or high slope
   c. Deceleration phase: ≥9 cm
2. Descent: active at ≥9 cm dilatation
3. Normal labor progresses rapidly; multiparas faster than nulliparas

Prolonged labor patterns	Nulliparas	Multiparas
1. Prolonged latent phase	>21 h	>14 h
2. Protracted active-phase dilatation	<1.2 cm/h	<1.5 cm/h
3. Secondary arrest: no change for	≥2 h	≥2 h
4. Prolonged deceleration phase	>3 h	>1 h
5. Protracted descent	<1 cm/h	<2 cm/h
6. Arrest of descent	≥1 h	≥½ h

2. Descent patterns: report to physician
   a. Protracted descent pattern in the active phase: rate of descent less than 1 cm/h in the nullipara and less than 2 cm/h in the parous woman
   b. Arrest of descent in the active phase: no progress for 1 hour or more in the nullipara and 30 minutes in the parous woman

The labor patterns in normal and prolonged labor are given in the box above.

Fetal mortality rate increases sharply after 15 hours of the active first stage of labor. Maternal morbidity and mortality may occur as a result of uterine rupture, infection, serious dehydration, and postpartum hemorrhage. A long difficult labor can have an adverse psychologic effect on the mother, father, and family. The application of the nursing process presented below relates specifically to the care of a woman with prolonged dysfunctional labor. The facets of her care that are the same as for normal labor are not repeated (see Chapter 15).

Application of the Nursing Process

PROLONGED DYSFUNCTIONAL LABOR

Susan and Andrew, age 31 and 35 respectively, are expecting the birth of their second child. Susan's prenatal course has been uneventful. The pelvic measurements revealed a slightly contracted midplane as a result of protruding spinous processes. The fetal weight has been estimated at 3584 g (8 lb). Their first child, born 5 years ago, weighed 2912 g (6½ lb). Both parents attended prenatal review classes. Susan's contractions began at 12 midnight. By 5 AM the contractions were coming every 5 minutes. Susan was admitted to the hospital at 5:30 AM following the labor room nurse's instructions.
1. Assessment on admission to the labor suite; 6 AM:
   TPR: 98.2° F, 84, 16
   BP: 120/80
   Contractions: q 5 min, 20 s, regular, mild intensity
   Presentation: vertex
   Position: LOA
   Station: floating
   Cervix: soft, dilated 2 cm
   Membranes: intact
   Bloody show: scant
   FHR: regular —|₁₂₀
2. Susan was encouraged to ambulate or assume any position in bed in which she felt comfortable. She was reminded to assume a left lateral position when she was lying down.

Continued.

Application of the Nursing Process—cont'd

3. Routine assessment was carried out (see Chapter 15).
4. 10 AM—progress in labor was as follows:
   Contractions: q 5-7 min, 20-40 s, mild intensity
   Station: −2
   Cervix: dilated 3 cm, 40% effaced
   Bloody show: scant
   FHR: regular $-\frac{}{120}$
5. The physician felt that the slow descent and dilation of the cervix was related to incomplete flexion of the fetal head (see Fig. 14.3, *B*). The incomplete flexion was related to hypotonic contractions. The physician ordered:
   a. Oxytocin stimulation of labor (see p. 917)
   b. Electronic fetal monitoring (see Chapter 16)
   c. Nurse/client ratio 1:1
6. 1 PM—progress in labor was as follows:
   Contractions: q 5 min, 40 s, moderate intensity
   Station: −1
   Cervix: dilated 4 cm, 60% effaced
   Mother apprehensive, circumoral pallor, crying with each contraction, says she "feels exhausted."
7. 1:25 PM—spontaneous rupture of membranes with meconium staining
   FHR: $-\frac{}{105}$, irregular, late decelerations
8. The physician ordered an immediate cesarean delivery (pp. 922 to 924). Susan was experiencing prolonged labor secondary to dysfunctional uterine contractions.

FUNCTIONAL HEALTH PATTERN: ASSESSMENT	NURSING	RATIONALE: PLAN/ IMPLEMENTATION	EVALUATION
HEALTH PERCEPTION– HEALTH MAINTENANCE			
Assess progress of labor (see Chapters 14 and 15) for alteration in patterns of progress	Alteration in comfort: pain	*To reduce* **pain** *and induce relaxation:* ■ Use analgesics ordered ■ Encourage use of relaxation techniques (see Chapter 15) ■ Use techniques to minimize discomfort • Cool, wet cloth to brow • Back massage (see Fig. 15.16) ■ Assist her to assume most comfortable position	Mother rests between contractions.
	Maternal compromise related to exhaustion	*To relieve* **exhaustion:** ■ Encourage rest between contractions ■ Encourage use of glucose suckers ■ Use psychologic nurturing such as acceptance of her behavior ■ Plan care to minimize disturbing her	Mother appears less tired.
Assess for fetal health status (see Chapter 16)	Potential for injury related to decrease in perfusion of placenta	*To maintain* **continuous assessment** *of the fetus:* ■ Initiate electronic fetal monitoring	Electronic monitoring is continuous.

Application of the Nursing Process—cont'd

FUNCTIONAL HEALTH PATTERN: ASSESSMENT	NURSING	RATIONALE: PLAN/ IMPLEMENTATION	EVALUATION
		To facilitate perfusion of placenta: ■ Maintain maternal positions that prevent hypotensive syndrome, that is: • Ambulation • Sitting • Side lying position	FHR remains within normal limits.
Assess for prolapse of cord (see Chapter 15)	Potential for injury related to prolapse of cord	*To prevent **prolapse of the cord:*** ■ Maintain bed rest after membranes rupture and engagement is absent	FHR remains within normal limits. Cord does not prolapse.
Assess intake and output	Alteration in fluid volume: excess related to IV infusion with oxytocin	*To prevent fluid overload:* ■ Maintain amount of fluid per hour per physician's order ■ *DO NOT* speed up infusion to catch up ■ Report imbalance of intake and output to physician	Fluid overload does not occur.
Assess bladder distension and pressure and amount of stool in rectum	Alteration in normal physiologic process related to obstruction of birth canal secondary to full bladder or full rectum	*To prevent **obstruction** of the birth canal:* ■ Encourage her to void every 2 hours ■ Catheterize as necessary per physician's order ■ Give enema as necessary per physician's order	Obstruction of birth canal does not occur.
SELF-PERCEPTION			
Assess psychologic status and support: ■ Preparation for childbirth ■ Expectations of woman and family ■ Response to first stage	Powerlessness related to loss of control	*To minimize woman's concern for loss of control:* ■ Explain treatment and rationale ■ Let her choose position in labor ■ Maintain husband coaching in labor	Mother assumes some responsibility for choice of position, makes needs known to staff.
	Fear of injury to baby related to changes in expected pattern of labor	*To encourage expression of fears:* ■ Explain significance of clinical findings	Mother questions nurse freely.
	Ineffective individual coping related to disappointment, pain, fear, or exhaustion	*To increase her self-esteem:* ■ Comment on how well she is doing ■ Accept her expressions of anger or disappointment	Mother turns to coach/ nurse for support.

Continued.

Application of the Nursing Process—cont'd

FUNCTIONAL HEALTH PATTERN: ASSESSMENT	NURSING	RATIONALE: PLAN/ IMPLEMENTATION	EVALUATION
	Alteration in self-concept related to inability to give birth to baby as expected	*To increase her self-esteem:* ■ Comment on successful prenatal period ■ Comment on her mothering ability with older child ■ Listen to her complaints	Mother relates instances of her "good mothering"
	Knowledge deficit related to dystocia	*To increase her knowledge:* ■ Keep her informed of progress ■ Describe condition (e.g., "baby's head needs to flex more").	Mother can describe labor process when visited the following day by nurse or feels free to ask the nurse what happened.

PRECIPITATE LABOR

Precipitate labor lasts less than 3 hours. It is characterized by tetanic-type contractions. If the birth canal is in a relaxed state, effects on the mother can be minimal. However, if the birth canal is not readily distensible, uterine rupture or lacerations of the birth canal can occur. Pritchard (1985) notes **"The uterus that contracts with unusual vigor before delivery is likely to be hypotonic after delivery with hemorrhage from the placental implantation site as the consequence."** The fetus may suffer from hypoxia as a result of diminished placental perfusion secondary to tetanic-type contraction.

THERAPIES FOR DYSTOCIA

Modern maternity care continues to increase the margin of safety and comfort for both the mother and the infant. Improved methods for monitoring and assessing fetal and maternal well-being have contributed to more effective prevention and treatment of medical and surgical complications of childbirth. The use of antibiotics and blood products has reduced the morbidity and mortality associated with infection and hemorrhage. The judicious use of prostaglandins or injectable oxytocin for the stimulation or augmentation of labor has been lifesaving at times. Preventive surgical procedures (episiotomy, forceps delivery, and birth by cesarean delivery) have helped reduce the risk to the mother and infant.

Some procedures in operative obstetrics are complicated, whereas others are so frequently used that they are considered adjuncts or aids to normal delivery. Episiotomy and outlet forceps delivery are included in such a category. Cesarean delivery is used with increasing frequency because the problems that indicate the need for nonvaginal delivery can be detected earlier and with greater accuracy.

Trial of labor. If the fetus is clinically large and at term or past due or the mother has a "questionable pelvis," x-ray pelvimetry and fetal sonography are used to assess the possibility of a vaginal delivery. If there is no demonstrable fetopelvic disproportion and the cervix is soft and dilatable, a *trial of labor* may be instituted. A trial of labor is a reasonable period (4 to 6 hours) of active labor. Active labor includes adequate contractions, engagement and descent of the presenting part, and progressive effacement and dilatation of the cervix. Trial of labor is seldom induced artificially. During this period it is essential to assess the following carefully:

1. Strength, frequency, and character of uterine contractions
2. Progressive effacement and dilatation of cervix
3. Descent of head
4. Fetal well-being

Induction of labor. Induction of labor is the deliberate initiation of uterine contractions before their spontaneous onset. The need for initiating labor may arise from maternal or fetal sources, for instance, severe pregnancy-induced hypertension or postterm pregnancy. Such conditions may harm the mother or infant if birth does not occur. Elective induction may be indicated for the woman who has a history of precipitous labors (less than 3 hours). Labor is induced under controlled conditions to avoid an unexpected out-of-hospital birth.

There are a number of medically approved methods to induce labor. They include chemical inductions of labor, with prostaglandins (PGE) and oxytocins, and mechanical methods, such as rupture of membranes (amniotomy).

Prostaglandin. A prostaglandin gel for local application to the cervix has been formulated. The gel is used to soften or prime the cervix and induce labor. The cervix is assessed using the Bishop score (Table 29.4). For those women whose cervix is unfavorable, induction using prostaglandins is more effective than using oxytocin.

Procedure. The client is admitted to the labor suite, and routine assessments are completed. The dilation and effacement of the cervix is determined. A Bishop score of 5 or less is required. A 30-minute electronic monitoring of the FHR and uterine contractions is done to establish baseline data. The physician instills 0.5 mg of PGE gel intracervically, using a plastic catheter. The catheter is then removed. The woman remains in bed for 30 minutes; then she may ambulate. The FHR, blood pressure, and pulse are monitored at least every 30 minutes. Ideally the monitoring is done electronically. Contractions usually begin a half-hour after administration of the gel. The time of the beginning of contractions is recorded. An amniotomy is performed at 4 cm cervical dilation, and internal fetal monitoring is applied. Progress of labor is then recorded as it is for all clients.

The local application of prostaglandins appears to minimize side effects. Any hypertonic contractions of the uterus are reported immediately. If the woman does not deliver within 24 hours, the cervix is reassessed using the Bishop score, and an induction using oxytocin is done if indicated (Table 29.4).

Oxytocin. Oxytocic stimulation of labor may be used either to induce the labor process or to augment a labor that is progressing slowly because of inadequate uterine contractions. It can also be used to assess fetal response to the stress of labor contractions (oxytocin challenge test [OCT]; see Chapter 25).

Indications. The indications for oxytocin induction of labor include the following:

1. Slowing of progress of labor
2. Management of abortion, to stimulate the uterus to pass the conceptus
3. Prolonged rupture of the membranes
4. Prolonged pregnancy (42 to 43 weeks)
5. Preterm delivery in diabetic mother or infant with severe isoimmunization
6. Severe preeclampsia, abruptio placentae, or fetal death necessitating termination of the pregnancy artificially
7. Multigravidas with a history of precipitate labor who live a long distance from the hospital

The management of stimulation of labor is the same regardless of indication. Because of the potential dangers associated with the use of injectable oxytocin in the prenatal and natal periods, the Food and Drug Administration has issued new restrictions on its use (*FDA Drug Bulletin,* 1978).

Contraindications. Contraindications to oxytocic stimulation of labor include the following:

1. Fetopelvic disproportion
2. Fetal distress
3. Previous uterine surgery (e.g., cesarean birth)
4. Overdistended uterus (hydramnios, multiple birth)
5. Grand multiparity (over four)

Hazards. Hazards of oxytocin stimulation to both mother and infant include the following:

1. Maternal
   a. Tumultuous labor and tetanic contractions, which may cause premature separation of the placenta, rupture of the uterus, laceration of the cervix, or postdelivery hemorrhage
   b. Sequelae to above complications: infection, disseminated intravascular coagulation (DIC), amniotic fluid embolism
   c. Fear or anxiety: may be compounded if the procedure is not successful (the woman must be aware of this possibility and of what other techniques can be used)
2. Fetal
   a. Fetal asphyxia and neonatal hypoxia from too frequent and prolonged uterine contractions
   b. Physical injury
   c. Prematurity, if the estimated date of confinement (EDC) has been estimated inaccurately.

Table 29.4
Bishop's Scale for Assessing Candidates for Induction of Labor

	Score*			
	0	1	2	3
Dilation (cm)	0	1-2	3-4	5-6
Effacement (%)	0-30	40-50	60-70	80
Station (cm)	−3	−2	−1	+1
Cervical Consistency	Firm	Medium	Soft	
Fetal position	Posterior	Midline	Anterior	

*Parous woman can be induced at score of 5; nulliparous woman, at score of 7.

Table 29.5
Oxytocin Administration by Size of Tubing

Drops per Minute (gtt/min)	10 U Oxytocin in 1000 ml Fluid (mU/min)	5 U Oxytocin in 1000 ml Fluid (mU/min)
15 gtt/ml tubing		
15	10.00	5.00
14	9.33	4.67
13	8.67	4.33
12	8.00	4.00
11	7.33	3.67
10	6.67	3.33
9	6.00	3.00
8	5.33	2.67
7	4.67	2.33
6	4.00	2.00
5	3.33	1.67
4	2.67	1.33
3	2.00	1.00
2	1.33	0.67
1	0.66	0.33
10 gtt/ml tubing		
10	10	5.0
9	9	4.5
8	8	4.0
7	7	3.5
6	6	3.0
5	5	2.5
4	4	2.0
3	3	1.5
2	2	1.0
1	1	0.5

From Tucker, S.M.: Fetal monitoring and fetal assessment in high-risk pregnancy, St. Louis, 1978, The C.V. Mosby Co.

Table 29.6
Oxytocin Administration by Volumetric Infusion Pump

Milliliters per Hour (ml/h)	Dilution of Oxytocin in IV Fluid (mU/min)		
	5 U Oxytocin in 1000 ml Fluid	10 U Oxytocin in 1000 ml Fluid	20 U Oxytocin in 1000 ml Fluid
1.5	0.125	0.25	0.5
3	0.25	0.5	1
9	1.5	1.0	2
12	0.75	1.5	3
15	1.0	2.0	4
18	1.25	2.5	5
21	1.5	3.0	6
24	1.75	3.5	7
27	2.0	4.0	8
30	2.25	4.5	9
33	2.50	5.0	10
36	2.75	5.5	11
39	3.0	6.0	12
42	3.25	6.5	13
45	3.5	7.0	14
48	3.75	7.5	15
51	4.0	8.0	16
54	4.25	8.5	17
57	4.5	9.0	18
60	4.75	9.5	19
63	5.0	10.0	20
66	5.25	10.5	21
69	5.5	11.0	22
72	5.75	11.5	23
75	6.0	12.0	24
78	6.25	12.5	25
81	6.5	13.0	
84	6.75	13.5	
87	7.0	14.0	
90	7.25	14.5	
93	7.5	15.0	
96	7.75	15.5	
99	8.0	16.0	
102	8.25	16.5	
105	8.5	17.0	
108	8.75	17.5	
112	9.0	18.0	
115	9.25	18.5	
118	9.50	19.0	
119	9.75	19.5	
	10.0	20.0	

Induction process. The responsibility for initiating oxytocin stimulation of labor belongs to the physician, although the procedure is often administered by the nurse. The physician must determine the correct amount of oxytocin to be added to the infusion bottle, together with the number of drops per minute that will deliver a specific oxytocin dose in milliunits per minute (Tables 29.5 and 29.6).

Procedure 29.1, specific to induction of labor, is added to the care of the woman with dystocia (see also Application of Nursing Process, pp. 913 to 916).

Transcervical amniotomy or artificial rupture of membranes. Transcervical amniotomy or artificial rupture of the membranes can be used to stimulate labor. The cervix should be soft, partially effaced, and slightly dilated, preferably with the presenting part engaged or engaging. Simple rupture of the membranes using a hook or other sharp instrument passed over a finger into the cervix will allow the drainage of amniotic fluid. The mother can be assured that neither she nor the infant will feel any pain from the amniotomy. Within 6 to 8 hours, labor may be under way. Some obstetricians prefer to first stimulate the uterus with intravenous oxytocin and, as soon as good contractions are evident, rupture the membranes. Others prefer merely to rupture the membranes, knowing that oxytocin stimulation often is unnecessary.

Methods not recommended for stimulation of labor. The following methods are not recommended for stimulation of labor:

Procedure 29.1

INDUCTION OF LABOR

PURPOSE

To initiate or augment the uterine contractions of labor.

EQUIPMENT

1. Oxytocin (Pitocin) or synthetic oxytocin (Syntocinon)
2. Container of 1000 ml 5% dextrose in water for oxytocin solution
3. Container of 1000 ml 5% destrose in water for piggyback set-up (maintenance IV)
4. Infusion pump (IVAC) or standard pump (Harvard)

NURSING ACTIONS	RATIONALE
Apply fetal and maternal electronic monitor before beginning induction	To obtain constant, accurate recording of FHR and contractions To obtain baseline reading
Explain technique, rationale, and reactions to expect: Route and rate: what "piggyback" is for Reasons for use: ■ Induce labor ■ Improve labor	To promote cooperation of woman and family To lessen anxiety over technique To assure woman and family of careful monitoring To prepare woman and family for chances of success
Reactions to expect—nature of contractions: "Intensity of contraction increases more rapidly, holds the peak longer, and ends more quickly. The contractions will begin to come regularly and more often." Monitoring to anticipate: ■ Maternal: BP, P, uterine contractions, uterine tone ■ Fetal: heart rate, activity Success to expect: reaffirm physician's explanation that if inertia is not overcome in 8 hours or less (using 5 U of Oxytocin), the chance of success is minimal	
Position woman in left lateral position	To maximize placental perfusion and oxygenation of fetus
Prepare solutions and administer according to prescribed orders with pump delivery system: ■ Infusion pump and solution is set up ■ Solution with oxytocin (Pitocin) is flagged with a red label ■ Piggyback solution is connected to IV line	To promote safety a piggyback setup is used; this permits the induction solution to be stopped while the vein remains open with the second solution
Begin induction at 1 mU/min (Tables 29.5 and 29.6)	To ensure that only amount of medication necessary for success is used
Increase dose arithmetically by 2 mU increments (e.g., 1, 3, and 5 mU/min at 15 min intervals) (Tables 29.5 and 29.6)	To determine minimun amount of medication necessary for success
Maintain dose when: ■ Intensity of contraction results in intrauterine pressures of 50 to 75 mm Hg (by internal monitor) ■ Duration of contraction is 40 to 60 seconds ■ Frequency of contractions is 2½ to 4-minute intervals	To maintain needed stimulation and avoid overstimulation
Discontinue use of oxytocin as per hospital protocol; keep line open with nonmedicated solution	Woman, is in active labor; further stimulation is not required
Keep woman and family informed of progress	To reduce anxiety
Discontinue infusion of oxytocin and keep vein open with plain solution if **danger signs** occur: ■ **Contractions:** excessive intrauterine pressure above 75 mm Hg, duration over 60 seconds, and frequency more often than every 2 or 3 minutes ■ **Fetal stress:** fetal bradycardia, tachycardia, or heart irregularity (Oxytocin is stopped and 5% dextrose in water is infused.)	To prevent further complication

Continued.

Procedure 29.1—cont'd

NURSING ACTIONS	RATIONALE
■ Other **complications** such as boardlike abdomen or cessation of labor require cessation of oxytocin infusion	
Report danger signs to physician immediately	To permit immediate initiation of remedial care for safety of mother and of child
Make preparations for emergency delivery, vaginal or cesarean	To be ready for change in management plans
Charting	To provide data base against which to compare future findings
■ *Medication:* kind, amount, time of beginning, increasing dose, maintaining dose, and discontinuing medication in client record and on monitoring strip	To provide data base for implementation
■ *Reactions of mother and fetus:*	To promote collaboration with other members of health care team
• Pattern of labor	
• Progress in labor	
• FHR	
■ *Signs of maternal or fetal stress*	

1. Intramuscular or intranasal oxytocin is condemned because of the physician's inability to control the effects of the drug, that is, tetanic, prolonged uterine contractions.
2. "Stripping of the membranes" before or instead of rupture of the membranes is a dangerous procedure. It consists of the physician's inserting a finger through the soft, dilatable cervix at term and stripping the fetal membranes off the uterine wall in and around the internal os. It may cause rupture of the membranes, displacement of the presenting part, or prolapse of the cord, or it may initiate bleeding or sepsis. Rarely it may predispose the mother to amniotic fluid embolism.
3. Insertion of a bougie or packing the cervix may result in labor. However, these procedures are condemned because of the dangers of trauma, bleeding, and infection.
4. Intraamniotic injection of hypertonic sodium chloride is lethal for the infant and cannot be employed for induction of labor unless the fetus is dead.

Operative Obstetrics

Episiotomy. An episiotomy is an incision made in the perineum to enlarge the vaginal outlet. Episiotomies are performed more frequently in the United States and Canada than in Europe. The use of the side-lying position for delivery is routinely used in Europe. The position with legs in stirrups is more commonly used in the United States and Canada. With the side-lying position there is less tension on the perineum, and a gradual stretching of the perineum is possible. As a result the indications for use of episiotomies are less.

The proponents of use of the episiotomy maintain it serves the following purposes:
1. Prevents tearing of the perineum: The clean and properly placed incision heals more promptly than does a ragged tear. Some conditions predispose a woman to perineal tearing. They include a large infant, a rapid labor in which there is not sufficient time for stretching of the perineum to take place, a narrow suprapubic arch with a constricted outlet, and malpresentations of the fetus (e.g., face). Such conditions are indications for episiotomy.
2. Minimizes prolonged and severe stretching of the muscles supporting the bladder or rectum, which may later lead to stress incontinence or vaginal prolapse.
3. Reduces duration of the second stage, which may be important for maternal reasons (e.g., a hypertensive state) or fetal reasons (e.g., persistent bradycardia).
4. Enlarges the vagina in case manipulation is needed to deliver an infant, for example, in a breech presentation or for application of forceps.

Those who are opposed to the *routine* use of episiotomies maintain that:
1. The perineum can be prepared for delivery through use of the Kegel exercises. Use of the exercises in the postpartum period improves and restores the tone of the perineal muscles.
2. Lacerations may occur even with the use of an episiotomy. Studies indicate a 13% to 22% occur-

rence of lacerations after episiotomies (Benyon, 1974).

3. Pain and discomfort from episiotomies can interfere with mother-infant interactions and the reestablishment of parental intercourse.
4. Episiotomies *are indicated* (a) if the well-being of the mother or fetus is in jeopardy to shorten the second stage of labor, (b) if the infant is preterm and cerebral hemorrhage is a possibility because of capillary fragility, or (c) if the infant is large (greater than 4000 g [9 lb]).

Types of episiotomies. The type of episiotomy is designated by site and direction of the incision (Fig. 29.13). The types are lateral, median, and mediolateral episiotomy. For nursing care related to episiotomies, see Chapter 24.

Median episiotomy. Median episiotomy is the one most commonly employed. It is effective, easily repaired, and generally the least painful. Occasionally there may be an extension through the rectal sphincter (third-degree laceration) or even into the anal canal (fourth-degree laceration). Fortunately primary healing and a good repair usually will be followed by good sphincter tone.

Mediolateral episiotomy. Mediolateral episiotomy is used in an operative delivery when posterior extension is likely. Although a fourth-degree laceration may thus be avoided, a third-degree laceration may occur. Compared with a median episiotomy, the blood loss is greater, the repair more difficult, and the healing more painful.

Forceps delivery. Obstetric forceps are made from two double-curved, spoonlike articulated blades. They are used to assist in the expulsion of the fetal head. This instrument, regarded by many as one of the greatest inventions of all time, was devised by Peter Chamberlen about 1625. The commonly employed forceps have a cephalic curve shaped similarly to that of the fetal head. A pelvic curve of the blades conforms to the pelvic axis (Fig. 29.14). The blades are joined by a pin, screw, or groove arrangement (Fig. 29.15). These locks prevent the forceps from compressing the fetal skull. Indications for the use of forceps include the following:

1. Maternal: to shorten the second stage in dystocia (difficult labor), or when the mother's expulsive efforts are deficient (e.g., she is tired or she has been given spinal anesthesia), or when the woman is endangered (e.g., cardiac decompensation).
2. Fetal: to rescue a jeopardized fetus (e.g., premature labor or fetal distress close to delivery).

Prerequisites for forceps operations. The following conditions must apply for successful forceps delivery:

1. *Fully dilated cervix.* Severe lacerations and hemorrhage may ensue if a rim of cervical tissue remains.
2. *Head engaged.* The extraction of a mature fetus with a "high" (unengaged) head usually is disastrous.
3. *Vertex presentation or face presentation* (mentum anterior). Other presentations require wider-than-average pelvic diameters.
4. *Membranes ruptured* to ensure a firm grasp of the forceps on the fetal head.
5. *No cephalopelvic disproportion.* If there is engagement, there must be no outlet contracture or gross sacral deformity.
6. *Empty bladder and bowel* to avoid visceral laceration and fistula formation.

Level of forceps application. The station of the head determines the level of forceps application and, generally, the relative difficulty to be expected in forceps operations.

High forceps. The biparietal diameter of the vertex is above the ischial spines when the forceps are applied. Most hospitals have policies against high-forceps application.

Midforceps. The vertex is at the ischial spines, almost to the ischial tuberosities on application of the forceps. The delivery often is difficult, depending on the size of the vertex, its position, and the pelvic architecture and diameters.

Low forceps. The vertex is distending the introitus with outlet forceps. This should be an "easy" forceps delivery. The blades are applied principally to provide control and guidance of the head.

Nursing care. Nursing responsibilities include the following:

Fig. 29.13
Types of episiotomies.

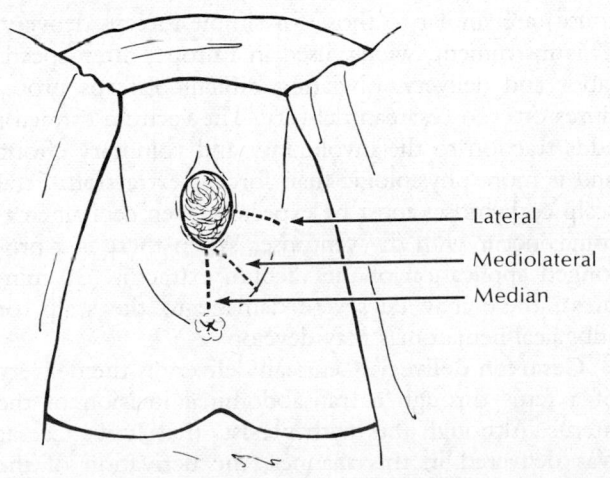

- Lateral
- Mediolateral
- Median

Fig. 29.14
Types of forceps.

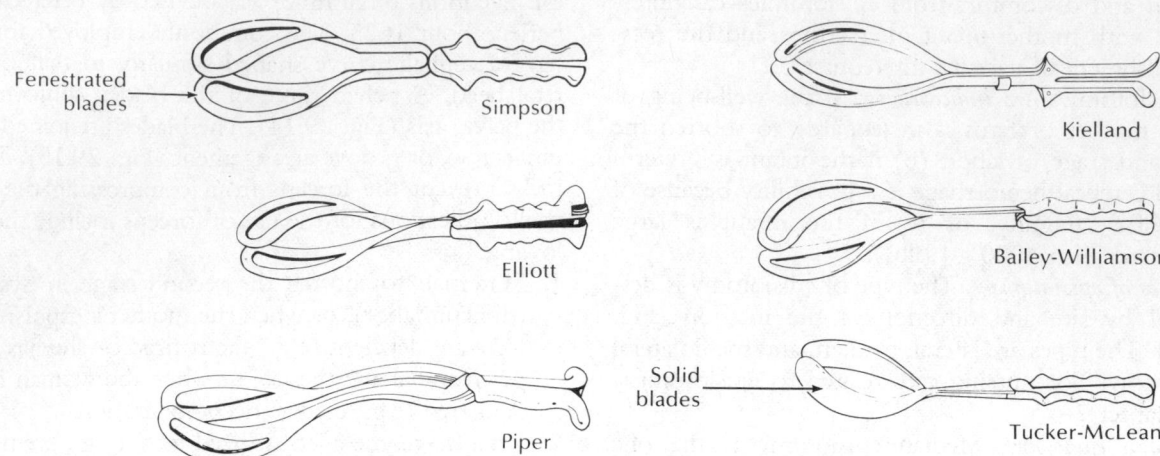

Fenestrated blades — Simpson

Kielland

Elliott

Bailey-Williamson

Piper

Solid blades — Tucker-McLean

Fig. 29.15
Types of forceps locks.

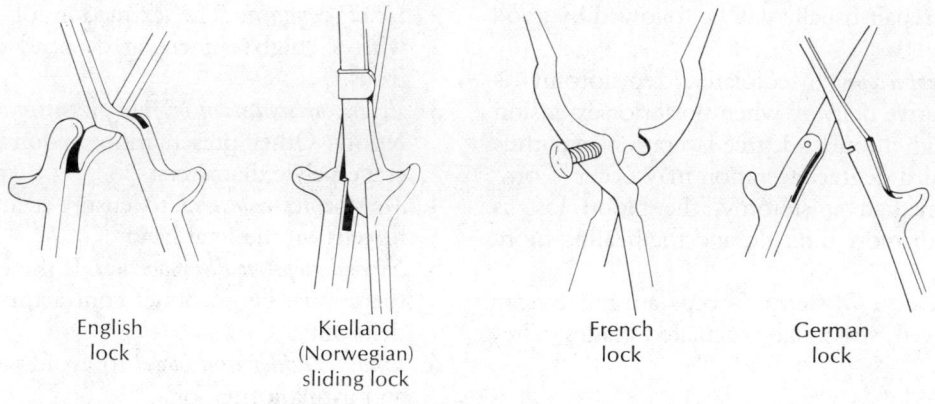

English lock

Kielland (Norwegian) sliding lock

French lock

German lock

1. Obtain forceps designated by physician (Fig. 29.14).
2. Check report and record FHR *before* forceps are *applied*.
3. Inform the mother that the forceps blades fit like two tablespoons around an egg. The blades come over the baby's ears.
4. Recheck report and record FHR *before traction* is applied after application of forceps. Compression of the cord between the fetal head and the forceps would cause a drop in FHR. The physician would then remove and reapply the forceps.

Vacuum extraction. Vacuum extraction is delivery of a fetus in *vertex* presentation with the use of a cup-suction device that is applied to the fetal scalp for traction. Indications for use of the vacuum extractor (ven-

touse) are similar to those for simple forceps delivery. This instrument, widely used in Europe, often speeds labor and delivery, obviating difficult forceps procedures or even cesarean delivery. The vacuum extractor adds traction to the involuntary and voluntary efforts and is more physiologic than forceps extraction. Fetal scalp ecchymoses must be expected; even cephalhematomas occur with the ventouse. When there is a prolonged application of the vacuum extractor (30 minutes), there may be severe damage to the scalp, or subgaleal hematomas may develop.

Cesarean delivery. Cesarean delivery is the delivery of a fetus through a transabdominal incision of the uterus. Although the myth persists that Julius Caesar was delivered in this manner, the derivation of the term is more likely from the Latin word *caedo* meaning

Cesarean Delivery: Indications, Maternal and Fetal Effects, and Types of Uterine Incisions

Indications for Cesarean Delivery	Effects of Cesarean Delivery	Type of Uterine Incisions
Maternal	**Maternal**	**Classic cesarean incision**

1. Fetopelvic disproportion
2. Previous cesarean delivery
3. Breech presentation
4. Medical complications (e.g., PIH)
5. Placental abnormalities (i.e., placenta previa, premature separation of the placenta)
6. Infections (e.g., herpes virus, type 2)
7. Trauma to the pelvis
	1. Mortality (1:1000) from
	  a. Anesthesia
	  b. Severe sepsis
	  c. Thromboembolic episodes
	2. Morbidity higher than with vaginal delivery because of:
	  a. Infection
	  b. Injury to the urinary tract
		Incision is vertical through skin and vertical through contractile portion of uterus (Fig. 29.16, *A*). It is used when rapid delivery is necessary, in shoulder presentation, and in placenta previa when the placenta is implanted on the anterior wall. Classic cesarean delivery is useful when general anesthesia is unavailable, since this operation can be carried out with local infiltration anesthesia. The potential for rupture of the scar (1% to 2%) with a subsequent pregnancy and the frequent occurrence of small bowel adhesions to the anterior suture line have limited the use of this type of cesarean delivery.

Fetal	**Fetal**	**Lower segment cesarean incision**

1. Fetal hypoxia
2. Prolapse of cord
3. Breech presentations
4. Malpresentations (e.g., shoulder)
5. Fetal anomalies (e.g., hydrocephalus)
	1. Mortality has declined where cesarean delivery is used in conjunction with improved perinatal care
	2. Morbidity
	  a. Birth trauma is reduced
	  b. Reduced morbidity in breech deliveries, transverse lie of the fetus, and placenta previa
		Lower segment cesarean delivery is possible by means of a vertical incision (Fig. 29.16, *B*) or a transverse incision (Fig. 29.16, *C*). The transverse incision is the preferred method. It "(1) results in less blood loss, (2) is easier to repair, (3) is located at a site least likely to rupture with extrusion of the fetus into the abdominal cavity during a subsequent pregnancy, and (4) does not promote adherence of bowel or omentum to the incisional line" (Pritchard, McDonald, and Gant, 1985).

"to cut." Whether cesarean delivery is planned (elective) or unplanned (emergency), the loss of the experience of delivering a child in the traditional manner may have a negative effect on a woman's self-concept. In an effort to maintain the focus on the *birth* of a child rather than the operative procedure, the term *cesarean delivery* or *cesarean birth* has come into common usage. The mother experiences abdominal rather than vaginal birth.

The basic purpose or use of cesarean delivery is to preserve the life or health of the mother and her fetus. The use of cesarean delivery is based on evidence of maternal or fetal stress. Maternal and fetal morbidity and mortality have decreased since the advent of modern surgical methods and care. However, cesarean delivery still poses threats to the health of both mother and infant. The technique of cesarean surgery has changed. Today incisions into the lower uterine segment rather than into the muscular body of the uterus permit a more effective healing. These findings are presented in the box above.

Cesarean delivery rates. The rate for cesarean delivery has increased dramatically. From the mid-1960s to the early 1980s the cesarean delivery rate has increased from less than 5% to more than 15% (Morrison and others, 1982). Concern about the rising cesarean delivery rates in the United States prompted the National Institute of Health to convene a Consensus Development Conference in 1980 (Petitti, 1985). Recommendations included the following:

1. "Women with low transverse incision be permitted a trial of labor in properly equipped hospitals and in the absence of other indications for a repeat cesarean" (Petitti, 1985).
2. The category "dystocia" as an indication for cesarean delivery be investigated further.
3. Vaginal delivery of the *term breech* be considered an acceptable alternative in carefully selected cases.

In spite of these recommendations and support from the American College of Obstetricians and Gynecologists, rates have not declined (Gleichner, 1984).

There is considerable disagreement as to whether the decrease in perinatal mortality is a direct result of the use of cesarean delivery. Some researchers contend that recent advances in perinatal care have an equal or greater effect (O'Driscoll and Foley, 1983). Pritchard, McDonald and Gant (1985) note that "final answers with respect to the frequency, indications, results in

Fig. 29.16
Cesarean delivery: skin and uterine incisions. **A,** Classic: vertical incisions of skin and uterus. **B,** Low cervical: horizontal incision of skin; vertical incision of uterus. **C,** Low cervical: horizontal incisions of skin and uterus.

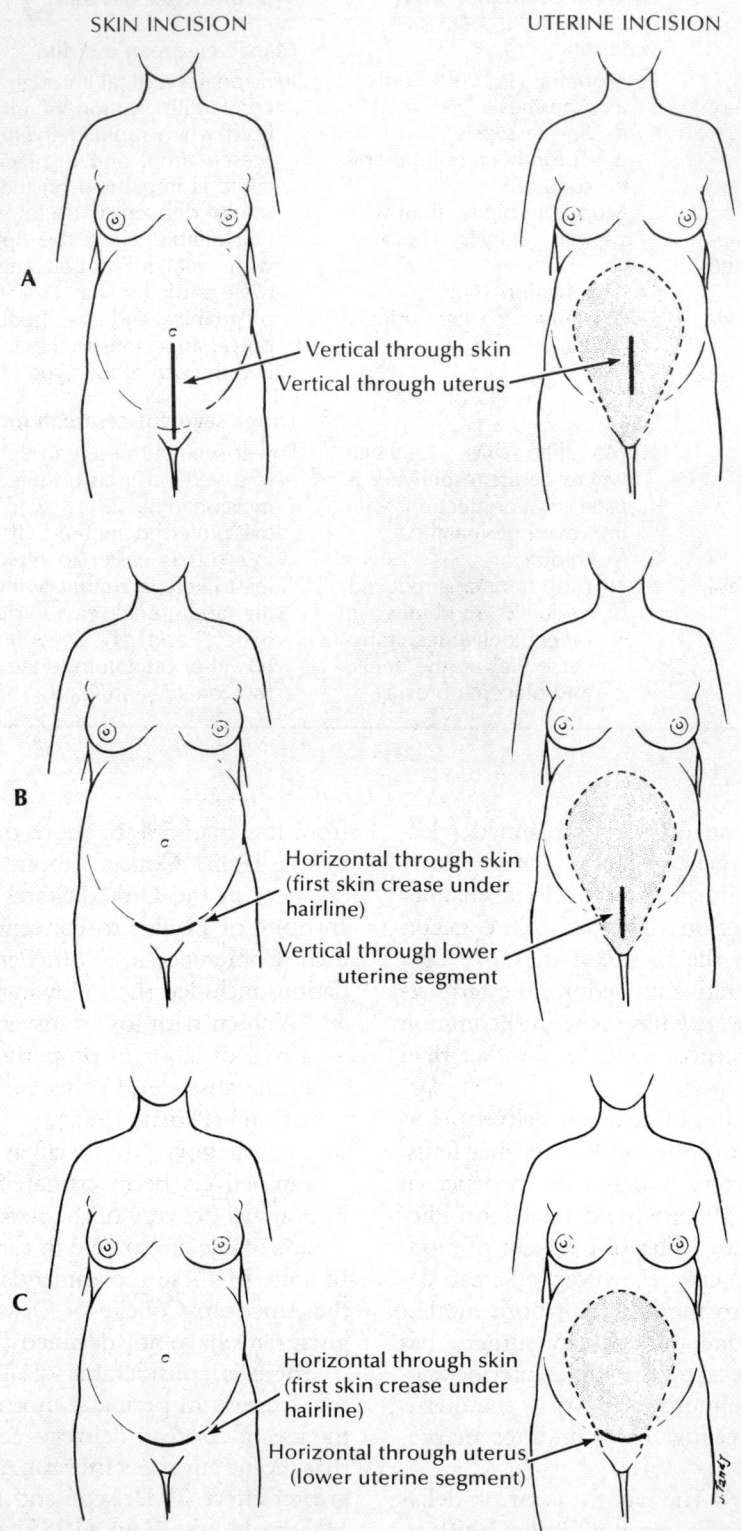

SKIN INCISION   UTERINE INCISION

A

Vertical through skin
Vertical through uterus

B

Horizontal through skin
(first skin crease under
hairline)

Vertical through lower
uterine segment

C

Horizontal through skin
(first skin crease under
hairline)

Horizontal through uterus
(lower uterine segment)

terms of safety to the mother and fetus, and the legal, ethical, and economic consequences of cesarean section are unlikely to become apparent for several years."

Vaginal birth following cesarean. Data are gradually accumulating concerning the safety of vaginal delivery after cesarean delivery (Meier and Parreco, 1982; Gellman and others, 1983). In the past, once a woman had a cesarean delivery, all future deliveries were elective cesarean deliveries. Often the woman was counseled to limit the number of pregnancies to three. Today the type of subsequent delivery is a decision to be made by the woman after full consultation with her physician. Danforth (1982) states that in general, suitable candidates for future vaginal deliveries are (1) those women whose operation was of the low cervical (not classic) type, (2) those women who begin labor before the EDC, and (3) those women who enter the labor suite with the fetal head well-engaged and the cervix soft, anterior, effaced, and dilated at least 3 cm.

If the original indication for the cesarean delivery is still present in a subsequent pregnancy, for example, a grossly contracted pelvis, repeat cesarean delivery is indicated. Moreover, a cesarean delivery is recommended for women who had a classic cesarean incision or any cesarean delivery marred by a septic course wherein questionable healing of the scar may result in rupture during labor.

When the *original complication* for which a cesarean delivery was initially done *has not recurred* (e.g., fetal distress caused by cord compression at term during labor), a trial of labor is recommended. Trial labor occurs under close observation with equipment for immediate cesarean delivery available in an emergency. Equipment for an elective low forceps delivery is available if full dilatation is achieved. The alternative would be another cesarean delivery because of concern for the strength of the uterine scar. A trial of labor and vaginal delivery are considered to be too great a risk for mother and fetus unless the woman is in a center where facilities are available for emergency surgery, anesthesia, continuous electronic monitoring of FHR and uterine activity, and blood transfusion. A major physical hazard in performing elective repeat cesarean delivery is miscalculating the EDC and the consequent delivery of a premature infant.

Nursing care. Women who must undergo cesarean delivery as the mode of delivery may be categorized in three groups. The first group is made up of women who will have elective cesarean deliveries. The second group is made up of those women who face an emergency cesarean delivery as a result of unexpected fetal or maternal stress. The third group are women who are candidates for vaginal birth after cesarean (VBAC).

Elective cesarean delivery. These women have time for psychologic preparation. The psychic response of

women in these groups may differ. Those women scheduled for repeat surgery may have disturbing memories of the conditions preceding the initial surgical delivery and their experiences in the postoperative recovery period. The added burden of care of an infant while recovering from a surgical operation may be faced with great concern. Women who face elective cesarean delivery for the first time share with other surgical clients the same apprehensions concerning surgery. These anxieties are coupled with the uncertainty of being able to cope with child care after a major operation.

Emergency cesarean delivery. Women in this group share with their families abrupt changes in their expectations for birth, postdelivery care, and the care of the new baby at home. This may be an extremely traumatic experience. The woman approaches surgery usually tired and discouraged from a fruitless labor. She is worried and fretful about her own and the child's condition. She may be dehydrated, with low glycogen reserves. All preoperative procedures must be done quickly and competently. The time for explanation of procedures and of operation is short. Since maternal and family anxiety levels are high, much of what is said is forgotten or perhaps misconstrued. Postoperatively, time must be spent reviewing the events preceding the operation and the operation itself to ensure that the woman understands what has happened. Fatigue is often noticeable in these women. They need much supportive care.

Many women who experience a cesarean birth speak of the feelings that interfere with their maintaining an adequate self-concept. These feelings include fear, disappointment, frustration at losing control, anger (the "why me" syndrome), and loss of self-esteem as their body image is not sustained. Success in mothering activities and in the recovery process can do much to restore these women's self-esteem. Some women see the scar as mutilating, and worries concerning sexual attractiveness may surface. Some men are fearful of resuming intercourse because of the fear of hurting their mates.

The separation of mother and child may prove detrimental to the establishment of parent-child bonds, particularly if other negative factors are present. They need to view their mothering ability positively. One mother expressed her feelings about the impact of an unexpected cesarean delivery regarding her self-concept as follows:

■ At first I was despondent over not being able to deliver vaginally, but then I comforted myself with the thought, you were a good mother for 9 months, no 12-hour period (delivery) can alter that. My baby and I have our whole lives to be mother and daughter.

Professional staff can expect some anger directed toward them. Parents will wonder if it was absolutely necessary for them to have a cesarean delivery. Such feelings may surface even years later.

Vaginal birth after cesarean. The women who come into this category fulfill the physiologic requirements noted earlier. If the physiologic requirements are met, the woman and her family make the choice between vaginal or repeat cesarean birth. Some women elect the repeat cesarean birth because they can exert more *control* over events. Others have such negative feelings concerning the previous birth experience that they recognize they should not attempt a vaginal birth (Lipson, 1984). The expectant woman and her family need positive reinforcement that whatever decision they make is acceptable. Contact with mothers who have experienced vaginal birth after cesarean can provide role models for these women.

The attitude of the physician presenting options to the woman is important (Lipson, 1984). The emphasis, currently, is placed on "a vaginal is the best way to go." The care of the woman who elects vaginal birth after cesarean includes a trial of labor.

Community support. Concerned professional and lay groups in the community have established councils for cesarean birth in an attempt to meet the needs of these women and their families. Such groups advocate including preparation for cesarean birth in all parenthood preparation classes. No woman can be guaranteed a vaginal delivery, even if she is in good health and there is no indication of danger to the fetus before the onset of labor. Every woman needs to be aware of and prepared for this eventuality. The unknown and unexpected are ego weakening. Each woman or couple needs accurate data to build new coping abilities or to strengthen old ones. "Walking through," role playing, or worry work before a crisis situation increases one's sense of control in that situation and serves to minimize the sense of loss experienced.

Childbirth educators stress the importance of emphasizing the similarities as well as differences between cesarean and vaginal birth. Also, in support of the phi-

Table 29.7
Meeting the Challenge

Objectives	Nursing Approaches
1. *All* couples will receive preparation for the possibility of a cesarean birth.	1. Routinely include content on cesarean deliveries in prenatal classes. 2. Encourage discussion of cesarean deliveries with the physician early in the pregnancy.
2. Couples anticipating a cesarean birth will be provided with special preparation.	1. Include cesarean delivery room (or operating room) in hospital tours. 2. Review specific procedures for the father as a participant in the cesarean birth at the time of the hospital tour.
3. Cesarean deliveries will be viewed as alternative methods of birthing.	1. Avoid any practices that unnecessarily discriminate cesarean from vaginal births. 2. Be selective in choosing terminology that projects a positive view.
4. The loss, implicit in a cesarean delivery, will be acknowledged and accepted.	1. Assess the impact of emotional conflicts imposed by the cesarean birth. 2. Facilitate resolution of conflict, e.g., by empathetic listening and promotion of problem-solving.
5. Birthing options to facilitate a family-centered approach will be available.	1. Be aware of the options that are available. 2. Assist couples in the choice of options that meet *their* needs.
6. Nurses will accept the responsibility for client advocacy in order to attain positive changes in cesarean birthing experiences that meet consumer needs.	1. Encourage consumers to assert their rights to make choices before the birth. 2. Following the birth, assess the level of consumer satisfaction; encourage parents to evaluate their experiences in terms of the options available. 3. Channel feedback and suggestions for change from parents and consumer groups to decision-making bodies with power to initiate change. 4. Gain a voice in policy change through representation on committees that plan and implement policies and procedures. 5. Collaborate with physicians who support changes to facilitate family-centered cesarean births.

From Leach, L., and Sproule, V.: Meeting the challenge of cesarean birth, J.O.G.N. Nurs. 13:194, May/June 1984.

losophy of family-centered birth, many hospitals have changed policies to permit fathers to share in these births as they have in vaginal ones. Women undergoing cesarean birth agree that the continued presence and support of their partners have helped them to experience a positive response to the whole process:

■ Knowing that he would be there and that he would be among the first to hold and nurture our baby made a tremendous difference to me. Even though "I" as the woman couldn't participate as directly as I had anticipated, "we" as the family could. I felt a sense of control, not a sense of being a passive . . . well . . . organ.

Table 29.7 reviews the supportive care that can be offered families in meeting the challenge of cesarean birth.

Care during cesarean delivery. The goal for the woman and her family is family-centered care for a cesarean delivery. Facing cesarean delivery relates to (1) the option for father to be present at the birth, (2)

availability of regional as well as general anesthesia, and (3) receiving support from the health care staff. The box below reviews the options that can be made available to couples.

Preparation for surgery. The preparation of the woman for cesarean birth is the same for either elective or emergency surgery. The obstetrician discusses the need for the cesarean delivery and the prognosis for mother and infant with the woman and her family. The anesthesiologist assesses the woman's cardiopulmonary system and presents the options for anesthesia. Informed consent is obtained for the procedures. Procedure 29.2 contains the nursing care necessary in preparation for surgery.

Operative process. Once the woman has been taken to surgery her care becomes the responsibility of the obstetric team, surgeon, anesthesiologist, pediatrician, and nursing staff (Figs. 29.17 and 29.18). If possible, the father, gowned appropriately, accompanies the mother to the surgical unit and remains close to her.

Care of the infant. Care of the infant is delegated to a pediatrician and a nurse because these infants are

Options to Facilitate Family-centered Cesarean Births*

1. Admission to the hospital on the morning of the birth for elective cesareans so that parents can spend the previous night together (provided they have had previous orientation).
2. Father to remain with the mother during the physical preparation, e.g., shave, catheterization.
3. The choice of regional anesthesia where possible, and explanation of the differences between regional and general anesthesia.
4. Father in the delivery room when either regional or general anesthesia is the choice.
5. Mirror and/or ongoing commentary from a staff member for mother and/or father.
6. Photographs or video taken in the delivery room—if even one parent is unable to witness the birth.
7. Mother's hand freed from restraint for contact with husband and baby.
8. Opportunity for both parents to interact with the baby in the delivery room and/or postanesthetic recovery room.
9. Opportunity for breast feeding in the delivery room or postanesthetic recovery room.
10. Modified Leboyer practices, e.g., father to submerge baby in warm water until relaxed and alert in the delivery room or in the nursery, if available for vaginal delivery.
11. Delayed antimicrobials in baby's eyes.
12. If father not in the delivery room:
    a. A support person should replace him at the mother's side;
    b. Father to be given baby to hold en route to nursery;
    c. Father to have the birth experience relayed to him by a staff member.
13. Father to accompany baby to the nursery and remain with infant until both are reunited with the mother.
14. Family reunited in postanesthetic recovery room if possible.
15. Father to be in postanesthetic recovery room to tell his wife about the birth if she has had a general anesthetic.
16. If it is difficult to reunite the family in postanesthetic recovery room, the mother's condition should be judged individually to allow the family to be reunited as soon as possible.
17. Baby's condition to be judged individually so that time alone in an incubator in the nursery can be avoided if possible.
18. Provision of time alone for the family in those first critical hours.
19. Rooming-in as soon as possible, i.e., if mother feels well enough she may be able to manage rooming-in on the first day.
20. Father to be included in the teaching of caregiving skills.
21. Siblings to be included where possible.

From Leach, L., and Sproule, V.: Meeting the challenge of cesarean birth, J.O.G.N. Nurs. 13:193, May/June 1984.
*In an effort to make the cesarean delivery more family-centered, the following options should be available where safety permits.

Procedure 29.2

CESAREAN DELIVERY: PREPARATION

PURPOSE
1. To complete the preparation for surgery as competently and quickly as possible.
2. To provide emotional support through a caring attitude, calm manner, and technical competence.

EQUIPMENT
1. Skin preparation kit
2. Retention (Foley) catheter kit
3. Intravenous infusions (as ordered)
4. Medications (as ordered)

NURSING ACTION	RATIONALE
Explain procedures to be carried out.	To keep the family informed
Complete preoperative preparation of the abdomen. The abdomen is shaved beginning at the level of the xiphoid process and extending to the flank on both sides and down to the pubic area.	To minimize potential for infection
Insert a retention catheter (Foley). It is attached to a continuous drainage system. Care must be taken to see that the catheter is properly placed within the bladder and is draining adequately	To ensure that the bladder remains empty during the operation
Administer preoperative medications as ordered, e.g.:	To promote relaxation before surgery
■ Analgesia	To minimize amount of secretion in bronchial secretion in bronchial tree
■ Atropine	
■ Antacid	To prevent irritative pneumonia if aspiration of gastric juice from stomach occurs
Begin intravenous infusion, e.g., 1000 ml Ringer's lactate solution or 5% dextrose in water.	To maintain hydration
	To have a line open for administration of blood, medications, etc. if needed.
Send specimens to laboratory for analysis.	
■ Blood is sent for typing and cross matching. Two units of matched blood are kept in reserve for 48 hours after surgery.	To replace blood loss during surgery or postpartum if excessive
■ Urine is sent for routine analysis.	To establish baseline data
■ Blood is analyzed for CBC and chemistry	
Take and record vital signs, BP, FHR.	To establish baseline data
Complete routine preoperative care including removal of dentures, contact lenses, rings, and fingernail polish. Valuables are put into safekeeping.	To protect client
Ready the woman's chart for use in surgery and to see whether permission forms for care of the mother and infant are signed. If the woman has received analgesia or anesthesia, the responsible adult accompanying the woman signs the necessary forms.	To provide data base against which to compare findings To provide data base for implementation of the next steps in the nursing process To promote collaboration with other members of the health care team.
Provide as much information as possible to the woman and her family while carrying out the necessary care.	To relieve apprehension and promote understanding.

---

considered to be at risk until there is evidence of physiologic stability after delivery (Fig. 29.19). A crib with resuscitative equipment is readied before surgery. Those responsible for care are expert in resuscitative techniques, as well as in observational skills for detecting normal infant responses. After birth, if the infant's condition permits, she or he is given to the father to hold and to show to the mother (Fig. 29.20). The attachment process can continue uninterrupted. Some mothers are able to nurse the infant in the recovery room area. However, many are not ready for this direct participation. They need to be reassured that the parent-child attachment process will not be impaired.

If compromised, the infant is transported immediately to the infant intensive care unit. Personnel keep the family informed of the infant's progress. Father-child contacts are initiated as soon as possible.

If the family-oriented approach is not feasible, the family is directed to the surgical waiting room. The physician reviews with the family members the condi-

Fig. 29.17
A, Preparation for cesarean birth. Pad under hip tilts
abdomen and prevents supine hypotension. **B,** Scrub nurse
prepares abdomen for surgery. (Courtesy Judy Bamber, San
Jose, California.)

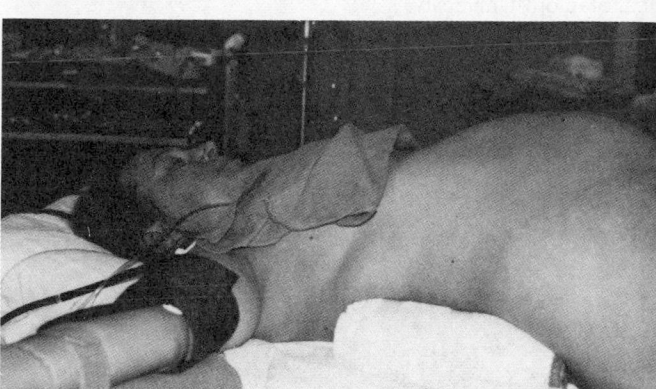
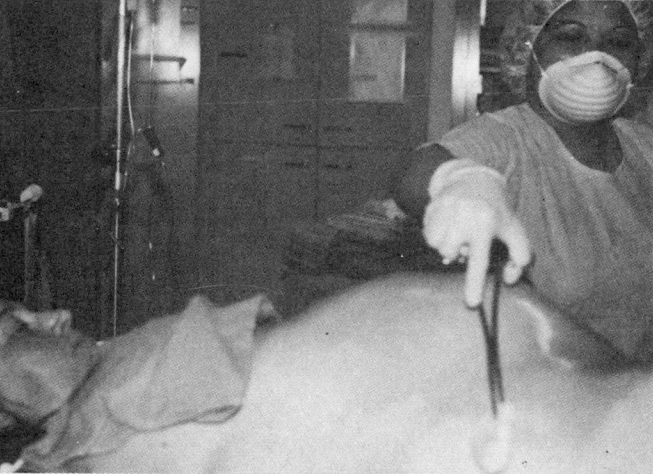

Fig. 29.18
A, Surgical team continues preparing woman for surgery. Note father, wearing checked
cap, at lower right. **B,** Surgery in progress. **C,** A time to be born: by cesarean birth. (**A** and
B courtesy Jose Mercado. From News and Publication Service, Stanford University,
Stanford, California. **C** courtesy Marjorie Pyle, RNC, Lifecircle, Costa Mesa, California.)

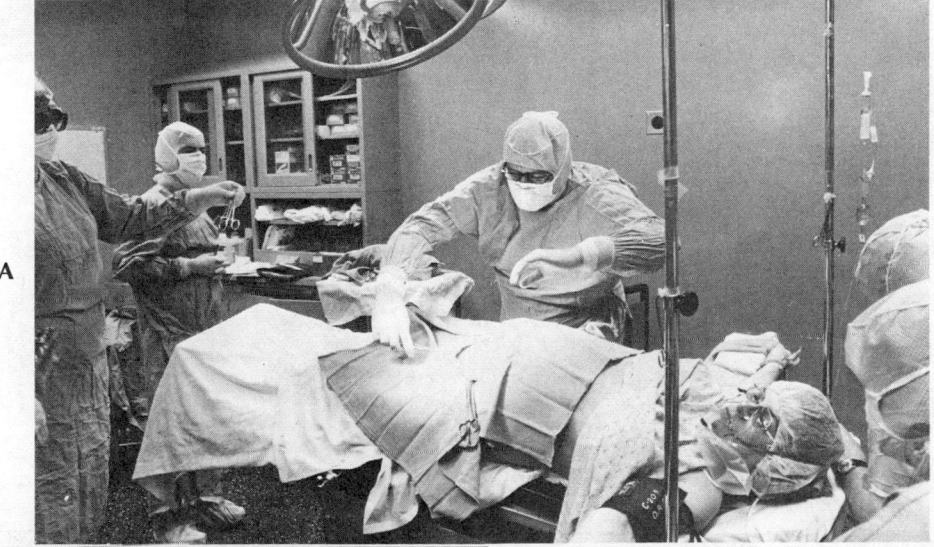
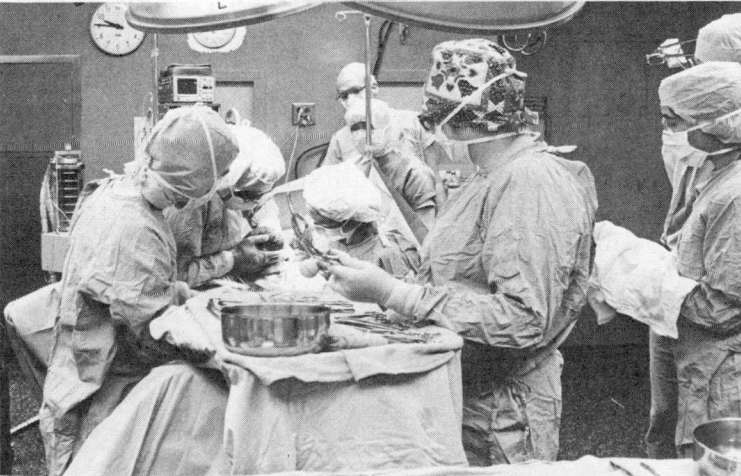
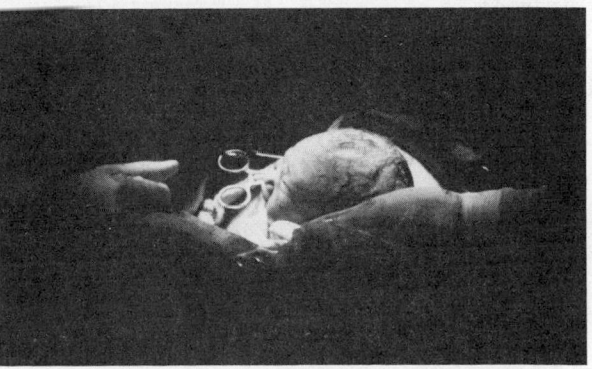

Fig. 29.19
A, Care of newborn: pediatrician and nurse give immediate care to newborn.
B, Pediatrician administers oxygen. Note mask is held above infant's face; oxygen is heavier than air and will sink to face level. Nurse is assessing fetal heart rate. Infant is crying; note muscle tone now. Arms and legs are flexed and not resting on bed.
(**A** courtesy Jose Mercado. From News and Publications Service, Stanford University, Stanford, California. **B** courtesy Judy Bamber, San Jose, California.)

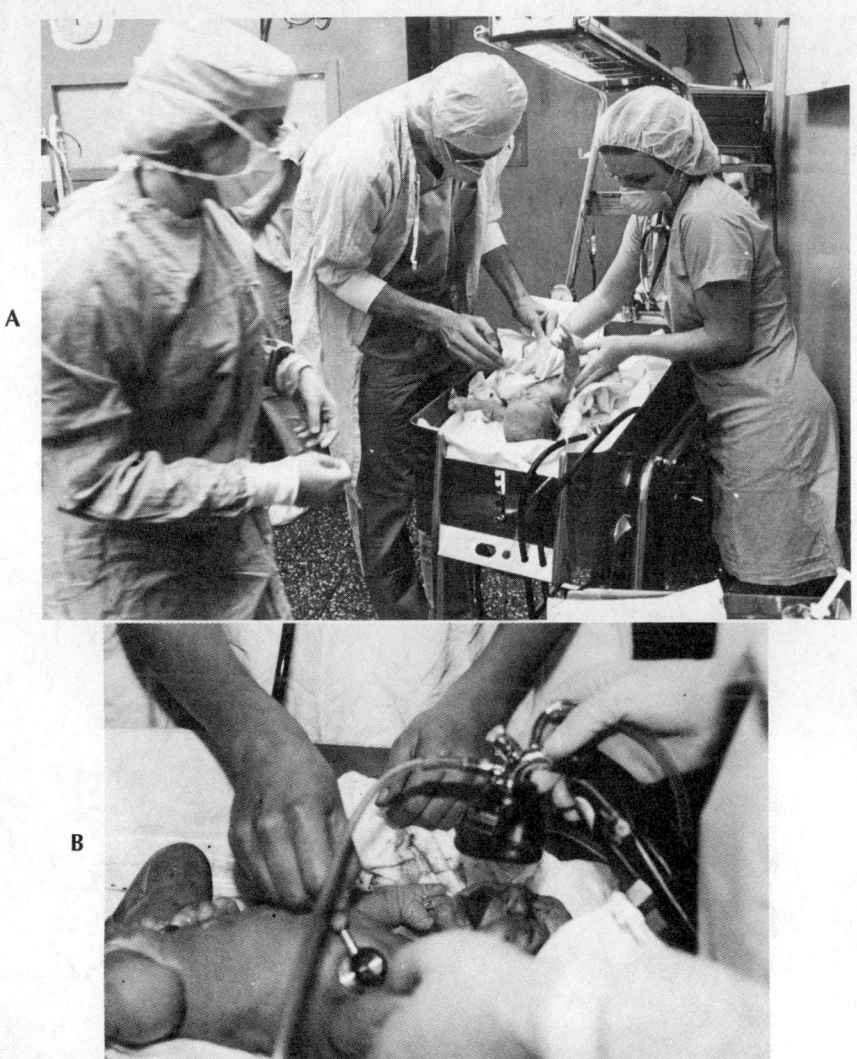

tion of the mother and child after the birth is completed. Family members may accompany the infant as he or she is transferred to the nursery. This gives the family opportunity to see and admire the infant.

Postpartum period. The care of the woman after cesarean delivery combines surgical and obstetric nursing. Once surgery is completed, the mother is trans-

ferred to the recovery room for intensive care until her condition stabilizes. Then she is moved to the postdelivery unit. The following goals are associated with the mother who has had a cesarean delivery:
1. For the mother
   a. Prevention of hemorrhage
   b. Prevention of infection

Fig. 29.20
A, Parents and their newborn. Father holds child. **B,** Father shows infant to mother.
C, Mother holds and examines infant. (Courtesy Jose Mercado. From News and
Publications Service, Stanford University, Stanford, California.)

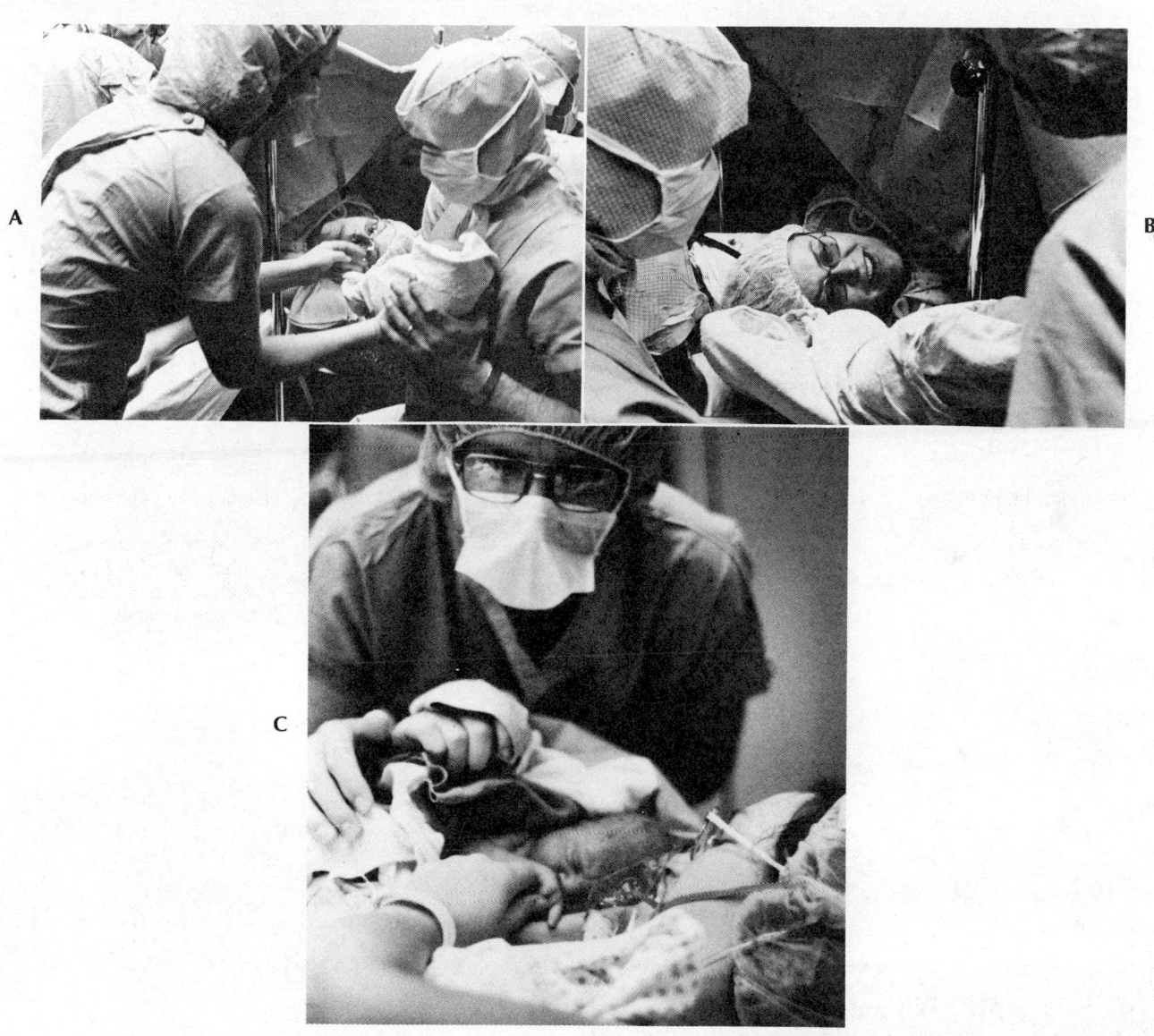

c. Prevention of embolytic complications
d. Control of pain
e. Promotion of feelings of self-esteem
2. For the infant
   a. Healthy adjustment to extrauterine life, see Chapter 20
   b. With complications, see Chapter 31

3. For the family
   Promotion of positive mother-family-infant relationships.

The application of the nursing process for a mother and her family following a cesarean delivery is presented below.

Application of the Nursing Process

CARE FOLLOWING CESAREAN DELIVERY

Susan was transferred from the recovery room at 5:30 PM. The recovery room nurse reported that she was conscious. Susan had a spinal anesthetic. Her vital signs were stable before transfer. At transfer the IV solution was infusing well. The catheter was draining satisfactorily, and the output was 850 ml in 4 hours. Susan was transferred to her bed and placed in a supine position, head flat, and knees slightly elevated with a pillow.

1. Assessment revealed the following:
   - *Fundus:* firm
   - *Lochia:* less than moderate
   - *Dressing:* dry and intact
   - *BP:* 120/80
   - *TPR:* 98°, 90, 16
   - Complaining of pain at incision site
2. Standard postoperative orders per hospital policy or physician

FUNCTIONAL HEALTH PATTERN: ASSESSMENT	NURSING DIAGNOSIS	RATIONALE: PLAN/ IMPLEMENTATION	EVALUATION
NUTRITIONAL-METABOLIC Assess for hemorrhage.	Fluid deficit related to loss of blood	*To prevent undue loss of blood:* ■ Check the fundus gently but firmly. Since the uterus is sutured securely, the procedure may cause discomfort but will not rupture the incised uterus (Fig. 29.21). ■ Check amount and character of lochia (see Chapters 18 and 24). Discharge and lochia will follow the same pattern as for vaginally delivered woman. ■ Check the skin incision for signs of excessive bleeding or formation of hematomas. ■ Check vital signs for evidence of shock. A woman who has had a cesarean delivery can lose a considerable quantity of blood before signs or symptoms of shock appear. ■ Administer oxytocin per physician orders, e.g., by IV infusion for 4 hours or longer. ■ Record findings.	Hemorrhage does not occur. If hemorrhage occurs, physician is notified and remedial treatment begun immediately (see Chapter 27)

Fig. 29.21
Typical incision for cesarean birth. Note "skin clips" used to suture incision.

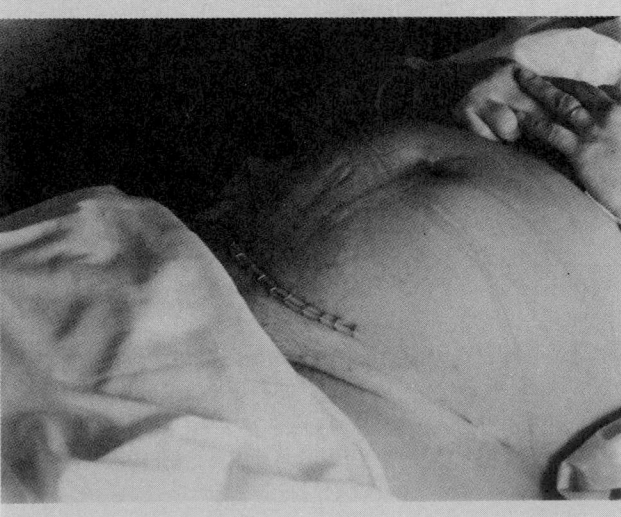

Application of the Nursing Process—cont'd

FUNCTIONAL HEALTH PATTERN: ASSESSMENT	NURSING DIAGNOSIS	RATIONALE: PLAN/ IMPLEMENTATION	EVALUATION
ELIMINATION Assess urinary elimination.	Alteration in patterns of urinary elimination related to dehydration, anesthesia	*To prevent urinary complications:* ■ Record intake and output. IV infusion used until water by mouth tolerated. ■ Note whether catheter is draining properly. Palpate gently for bladder fullness. ■ Note character of drainage. ■ Administer fluid by infusion per physician's order. ■ Record findings.	Urinary complications such as infections or inability to void after catheter is removed *do not occur.*
COGNITIVE-PERCEPTUAL Assess mother's need for pain medication and comfort measures.	Alteration in pain	*To detect and initiate remedial measures for pain:* ■ Note facial expression, rigidity of body, uncomfortable-appearing posture, circumoral pallor. ■ Question woman about nature of pain and where it is located. Client problems most frequently noted by the nurse related to: • Discomfort from the incisional site • Flank pain from manipulation of the incision and stretching of abdominal muscles with retractors during the surgery. • Muscle fatigue and ache resulting from immobility • "Gas pains" because of decreased or absent gastric intestinal peristalsis related to anesthesia, manipulation of abdominal organs during surgery, immobilization, and restricted diet • Pain from a distended urinary bladder	Woman remains comfortable or is able to cope with discomfort

Continued.

Application of the Nursing Process—cont'd

FUNCTIONAL HEALTH PATTERN: ASSESSMENT	NURSING DIAGNOSIS	RATIONALE: PLAN/ IMPLEMENTATION	EVALUATION
		• Afterpains (particularly if the woman is a multipara) ■ Administer medication per physician's order. ■ Institute comfort measures, e.g., positioning the woman in bed, splinting incision while she does deep breathing exercises. ■ Ambulate for relief of gas pains. If gas pains are not relieved by increased ambulation, a Harris flush may be ordered to relieve the flatulence. With the Harris flush or return-flow enema the intestine is alternately filled with normal saline or water and drained to help remove flatus by stimulation of peristalsis.	
	Knowledge deficit related to source of pain after abdominal surgery	*To allay apprehension:* ■ Inform her that pain arises from the stretching of uterine musculature and supporting tissues, as well as from the incision site.	Woman states she understands source of pain, that pain does not mean "complications."
HEALTH PERCEPTION– HEALTH MANAGEMENT Assess for signs of infection.	Infection related to contamination of incision, urinary tract, genital tract, respiratory tract	*To prevent infection:* ■ Incision: maintain aseptic technique. ■ Urinary tract: maintain fluid intake. ■ Genital tract: prophylactic antibiotic therapy usually is ordered for administration via infusion. ■ Respiratory tract: institute coughing and deep breathing exercises.	Infection does not develop. Vital signs remain normal.
ACTIVITY-EXERCISE Assess for signs of embolitic complications.	Impaired physical mobility related to postsurgical condition	*To detect and prevent complications related to immobility:* ■ Assess for thromboembolism. ■ Counteract effects of bed rest first postopera-	Complications related to immobility do not occur.

Application of the Nursing Process—cont'd

FUNCTIONAL HEALTH PATTERN: ASSESSMENT	NURSING DIAGNOSIS	RATIONALE: PLAN/ IMPLEMENTATION	EVALUATION
		tive day by instituting bed exercise routines, e.g., turning routines, paddling feet. ■ Ambulate as soon as possible, e.g., after 8 hours or after anesthesia has completely worn off. The woman must be carefully watched for fainting episodes as a result of hypotension and use of analgesic drugs.	
NUTRITIONAL-METABOLIC Assess for signs of degree of hydration. Postsurgery wound healing requires adequate nutrition and hydration. Assess for return of bowel sounds.	Alterations in nutrition related to postoperative condition.	*To maintain nutrition and hydration:* ■ Give surgical liquids within 4 to 6 hours orally as tolerated. ■ Maintain intravenous infusion (1000 ml/8 h) at least 24 hours until liquids are tolerated and bowel sounds are heard. ■ Increase diet gradually once bowel sounds are heard. ■ Instruct regarding roughage in diet and in bowel elimination.	Nutrition and hydration are maintained. Wound healing progresses adequately.
HEALTH PERCEPTION–HEALTH MAINTENANCE Routine postpartum assessment (see Chapter 24).	Alteration in normal physiologic process related to recovery from childbirth and initiation of infant feeding	*To promote recovery:* ■ Maintain routine postpartum care including sedation for afterpains or engorged breasts, breast care, perineal care for cleanliness, and temperature and blood pressure taken every 4 hours ■ Encourage woman to shower by the second postoperative day if a spray dressing is used.	Recovery is uneventful: see Chapters 23 and 24.
ROLE-RELATIONSHIP Assess response to newborn.	Alteration in parenting related to condition of mother or condition of infant	*To promote attachment:* ■ Show the mother her infant as soon as possible and give her time to handle and examine the child. If the infant	Mother responds positively to infant.

Continued.

FUNCTIONAL HEALTH PATTERN: ASSESSMENT	NURSING DIAGNOSIS	RATIONALE: PLAN/ IMPLEMENTATION	EVALUATION
		is in the intensive care unit, the mother may be taken by wheel-chair. ■ Encourage participation in infant care as soon as mother feels able (often after 24 hours). If feeding is attempted, the infant can be supported on pillows to relieve pressure on the mother's abdomen. Some mothers find the side-lying position most comfortable (Fig. 21.3).	
SELF-PERCEPTION, SELF-CONCEPT Assess mother's feelings about giving birth by cesarean.	Disturbance in self-concept related to mother's inability to give birth vaginally	*To promote feelings of self-esteem:* ■ Encourage mother to express her feelings. ■ Review her care of herself during pregnancy. Comment on when parenting begins. ■ Praise child care efforts.	Mother talks freely about her birth experience.
COGNITIVE-PERCEPTUAL Assess woman's and family's understanding of care needed.	Knowledge deficit related to reactions and to care needed after discharge from hospital	*To provide knowledge that enables the woman and her family to provide care needed:* ■ *Discomfort.* Analgesics may be taken that do not adversely affect the nursing infant. ■ *Exercise.* Progressive exercises may be started after abdominal discomfort has eased. Lifting objects heavier than the infant should be avoided for about 2 weeks. ■ *Complications.* Immediately report fever, dysuria, and frequency suggestive of urinary tract infection (may be secondary to use of catheters).	Woman asks questions about her care. Woman relates knowledge of the care needed.

Application of the Nursing Process—cont'd

FUNCTIONAL HEALTH PATTERN: ASSESSMENT	NURSING DIAGNOSIS	RATIONALE: PLAN/ IMPLEMENTATION	EVALUATION
		■ *Intercourse.* Intercourse may be resumed as soon as it is comfortable for the woman. Contraceptive information is provided as needed. ■ *Return examination.* This examination is planned for the third week; by that time the physical findings should be comparable to those of women who deliver vaginally.	

Preterm Birth

Preterm birth is traumatic for both child and parent. The infant is faced with adjustment to extrauterine existence before final readiness for the event. Parents are faced with an unexpected emotional crisis as a result of the natural process of pregnancy and birth being altered. Parents and child often are separated. The separation extends over a period of time. Death or disability of the infant is a possibility that must be faced. The elements that foster parent-child attachment, that is, closeness, positive perception of the self and the child, and infant responsiveness, are radically changed. Child and parents experiencing the crisis of premature birth need the concerted support of all members of the health care team.

Definition. Preterm birth is that which occurs after the twentieth but before the end of the thirty-seventh week of gestation. It results in the birth of a premature infant usually weighing less than 2400 g. The overall incidence of premature birth in the United States is 6% to 7%; in blacks the incidence is 10% to 11%. *Premature birth is responsible for almost two-thirds of infant deaths.* The infant born prematurely does not possess the growth and development necessary for uncomplicated adjustment to extrauterine life. Hence its prospects for survival or good health may be severely compromised.

Causes
Maternal and fetal causes
Maternal problems. Debilitating disorders, trauma, abdominal surgery, maternal injury, preeclampsia-eclampsia, uterine anomalies or tumors, cervical incompetence, and sepsis often are preludes to premature labor.

Placental disorders. Gross placental abnormalities such as placental separation or extrachorial placenta are associated with premature labor.

Fetal abnormalities. Transplacental infections such as rubella, toxoplasmosis, or syphilis may be responsible for premature labor. Multiple pregnancy, hydramnios, and premature rupture of the membranes are also notable. Congenital adrenal hyperplasia is usually associated with premature labor.

Iatrogenic causes. Premature labor can result from elective delivery because of misjudgment of fetal maturity or miscalculation of the EDC. Iatrogenic prematurity accounts for slightly less than 10% of preterm babies.

Unknown causes. In approximately two-thirds of cases, no definite cause can be identified. Thirty to fifty percent of premature labors occur after premature rupture of the membranes.

Medical diagnosis. The diagnosis of preterm labor contractions may be difficult to distinguish from painful Braxton Hicks contractions or false labor. True labor is progressive and associated with cervical dilatation, effacement, or both. It may be helpful to use external monitoring to record the frequency and intensity of contractions to be certain that labor is underway. Fetal well-being is monitored by the FHR.

Infant mortality and morbidity. Infants weighing more than 2500 g (5½ lb) and delivered after 37 weeks of pregnancy have the best prospects of survival. There is a dramatic reduction in mortality in infants,

Preterm Birth Risk Factors

Health history

Pyelonephritis: History of one or more episodes of kidney infection at any time in the past.
Cone biopsy: History of the removal of the lower portion of the cervical canal and outer surface of the cervix.
Uterine anomaly: Any malformation of the uterus such as a bicornuate or T-shaped uterus or a uterine septum, etc.
DES exposure: Exposure to diethylstilbestrol in utero.

Obstetric history

First-trimester abortion: Abortions, spontaneous or induced, at less than 13 weeks of gestation. These do not include ectopic pregancies. (If a woman has had more than three first-trimester abortions, she is given a maximum score of three).
Second-trimester abortion: Spontaneous abortions at 13 to 19 weeks and induced abortions at 13 weeks or more.
Less than 1 year since last birth: Less than 1 year from last birth to the time of conception of this pregnancy. Does not include abortions or ectopic pregnancies.
Preterm delivery: Spontaneous labor and delivery or delivery indicated by premature rupture of the membranes occurring before 37 completed weeks of pregnancy during any previous pregnancies.
Preterm labor: Spontaneous labor or premature rupture of the membranes occurring before 37 completed weeks of any previous pregnancy, leading to hospitalization and resulting in delivery after the thirty-seventh completed week of gestation.

Psychosocial history

Two children at home: Two or more children at home under 6 years of age.
Single parent: Limited social network.
Socioeconomic status I: Mother has completed 9 to 11 years of education.
Socioeconomic status II: Mother has completed 8 years or less of education.
Smoking: More than 10 cigarettes per day.
Work outside home: Any work outside the home or in the home for pay, full-time or part-time, not included under heavy work.
Heavy work: Work involving strenuous physical effort, standing, or continuous nervous tension, such as managerial positions, nurses, physicians, dentists, sales staff, cleaning staff, hairdressers, babysitters, laborers, and farmers.
Long tiring commute: 1 hour or more of continuous riding to or from work.

Current pregnancy

Less than 152 cm: Less than 5 feet in height.
Less than 45.5 kg: Less than 100 pounds at time of conception.
Maternal age: Less than 18 years or more than 40 years of age at first prenatal visit.
Less than 3.3 kg by 22 weeks: Weight gain of less than 7 pounds by 22 weeks of gestation.
Albuminuria: Proteinuria of 1 + or greater.
Hypertension: A rise in systolic pressure of at least 30 mm Hg, or a rise in diastolic pressure of at least 15 mm Hg; the presence of a systolic pressure of at least 140 mm Hg, or a diastolic pressure of at least 90 mm Hg; currently receiving antihypertensive therapy.
Bacteriuria: Symptomatic or asymptomatic, diagnosed by urine culture with colony count of 100,000 or more.
Fibroids: Myomas diagnosed before or during pregnancy.
Febrile illness: Systemtic illness with temperature of 38.3° C (101.0° F) or greater, such as pyelonephritis, influenza, determined by thermometer reading on two or more occasions.
Head engaged at 32 weeks: Presenting part engaged at or before 32 weeks of gestation.
Metrorrhagia: Vaginal bleeding or spotting after 12 weeks of pregnancy of any amount, duration, frequency, which is obviously not due to cervical contact.
Effacement greater than 50%: Cervical length of less than 1 cm at less than 34 weeks of gestation.
Dilation: Cervical dilation of the internal os of 1 cm or more at less than 34 weeks of gestation.
Uterine irritability: Uterine contractions of greater than five in 1 hour at rest perceived by the woman or documented by the provider at less than 34 weeks of gestation.
Placenta previa: Placenta covering all or part of the internal cervical os, documented by ultrasound at 26 weeks or later.
Hydramnios: Either oligohydramnios (insufficient guantity of amniotic fluid) or polyhydramnios (excessive quantity of amniotic fluid) at less than 34 weeks of pregnancy confirmed by ultrasound.
Twins: Diagnosis of multiple pregnancy (twin, triplets, etc.) by ultrasound.
Abdominal surgery: Any abdominal surgery performed at 18 or more weeks of gestation.
Cervical surgery: Cervical cerclage at any time during current pregnancy.

Adapted from Creasy, R., and others: System for predicting spontaneous preterm birth, Obstet. Gynecol. 55:6, 692, 1980.

regardless of weight, who are delivered after the thirty-sixth week of gestation. The prognosis for low-birth-weight infants weighing more than 1800 g (4 lb) is more favorable than for those weighing 1500 to 1800 g (3 to 4 lb). The mortality is less than 5% if the pregnancy has progressed to 35 weeks and the fetus weighs more than 2000 g (4½ lb). With these guidelines it is illogical to try to stop labor if the duration of pregnancy is 37 weeks or longer. The hazardous zone is 34 to 37 weeks, and the fetus should weigh more than 1800 g.

Management of preterm birth. Obstetric management of prematurity involves (1) early detection of preterm labor, (2) suppressing uterine activity, and (3) improving intrapartum care of the fetus destined to be born early.

Over the past 25 years, little if any progress has been made in preventing preterm birth, and the incidence of low-birth-weight babies has remained unchanged. At present the United States ranks sixteenth among industrialized nations in perinatal mortality, mainly because of the high incidence of preterm birth. Consequently it is unlikely that this ranking will improve substantially unless this high incidence is lowered.

Prevention has played a minor role because the mechanisms responsible for the majority of cases of preterm labor are unknown. However, certain conditions predisposing women to preterm birth are recognized. The presence of these conditions places the woman at risk for preterm birth (box, p. 938).

Client education program. Many women are unaware of the danger of preterm delivery and need to be informed of how they might reduce the risk. Client education programs have been established by concerned professional groups for the purpose of early detection of preterm labor. If preterm labor can be detected, early preventive therapy can be initiated. Research indicates treatment needs to be started in the early latent phase of labor to be successful (Spisso, Harbert, and Thiagarajah, 1982; Pritchard, McDonald, and Gant, 1985). One such program was developed by the nursing staff in a perinatal nursing program (Herron and Dulock, 1982). An outline of the preterm birth prevention programs follows. All pregnant women are screened according to risk factors associated with preterm labor at their initial prenatal visit (Table 29.8). They are assessed at 22 to 26 weeks of gestation. Women with a score of 10 or more, at

Table 29.8
Screening Tool for Risk of Preterm Birth

Score	Socioeconomic	Past History	Daily Habits	Current Pregnancy
1	2 Children at home Low socioeconomic status	⚠ Abortion × 1 Less than 1 year last birth	Work outside home	
2	Less than 20 years Low socioeconomic status More than 40 years Single parent	⚠ Abortion × 2	More than 10 cigarettes per day	Less then 3.3 kg by 22 weeks. Albuminuria Hypertension Bacteriuria
3	Less than 152 cm Less than 45.5 kg	⚠ Abortion × 3	Heavy work Long, tiring commute	Fibroids Weight loss of 2.3 kg Febrile illness Head engaged 32 weeks
4	Less than 18 years	Pyelonephritis		Metrorrhagia after 12 weeks Effacement > 50% Dilation Uterine Irritability
5		Cone biopsy Uterine anomaly ⚠ Abortion × 1		Placenta previa Hydramnios
10		DES exposure Preterm delivery ⚠ Abortion × 2 Preterm labor		Twins Abdominal surgery Cervical surgery

From Herron, M., and Dulock, H.L. Preterm labor: a staff development program in perinatal nursing care, 1982, March of Dimes, White Plain, N.Y.

Recognizing Premature Labor*

Definition

Premature labor occurs after the 20th week but before the 37th week of pregnancy. It is a condition in which uterine contractions (tightenings of the womb) cause the cervix (mouth of the womb) to open earlier than normal. It could result in the birth of a premature baby. Babies born before 37 weeks may have problems breathing, eating, and keeping warm.

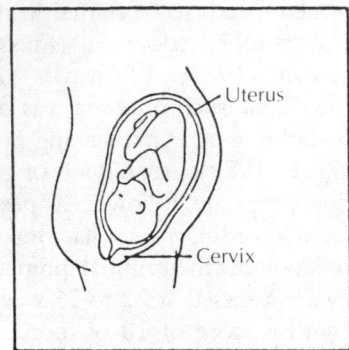

Cause

Although certain factors or reasons may increase a woman's chances of having premature labor, such as carrying twins, the specific cause or causes of premature labor are not known. Sometimes a woman may have premature labor for no apparent reason.

Prevention

It may be possible to prevent a premature birth by knowing the warning signs of premature labor and by seeking care early if these warning signs should occur.

Uterine contractions

It is *normal* to have some uterine contractions throughout the day. They usually occur when a woman changes positions, such as from sitting to lying down.

It is *not normal* to have frequent uterine contractions (every ten minutes or more often for one hour). Frequent uterine contractions or tightenings may cause the cervix to begin to open.

Self-detection of uterine contractions

Since the onset of premature labor is very subtle and often hard to recognize, it is important to know how to feel your abdomen for uterine contractions. You can feel for contractions this way:

1. While lying down, place your fingertips on the top of your uterus like this—

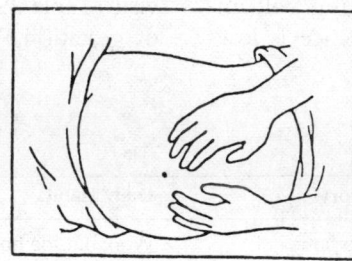

2. A contraction is the periodic "tightening" or "hardening" of your uterus. If your uterus is contracting, you will actually feel your abdomen get tight or hard, and then feel it relax or soften when the contraction is over.

Warning signs and symptoms

- *Uterine contractions* that happen every 10 minutes or more often, with or without any other warning sign
- *Menstrual-like cramps* felt in lower abdomen: may come and go or be constant
- *Low dull backache* felt below the waistline; may come and go or be constant
- *Pelvic pressure* feels like baby is pushing down; pressure comes and goes
- *Abdominal cramping* with or without diarrhea
- *Increase or change in vaginal discharge;* more vaginal discharge than usual, or change into a mucousy, watery or light bloody discharge

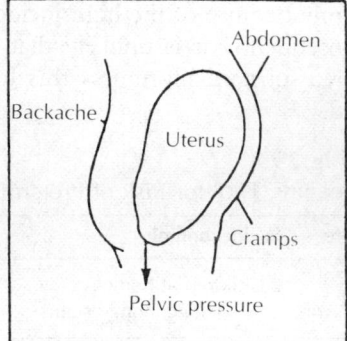

---

*Written by Marie Herron, R.N. With acknowledgement to Robert K. Creasy, M.D., of UCSF for his assistance and to the March of Dimes Birth defects Foundation for their support. Adapted from Papiernik, E., *Seminars in Perinatology*, 1981. Copyright 1983 by The Regents of the University of California. Published by the University of California, San Francisco, California 94143.

Recognizing Premature Labor—cont'd

What should you do . . .

If you think you are having uterine contractions or any of the other signs and symptoms of premature labor:

1. Lie down tilted towards your side. Place a pillow at your back for support.
   - Sometimes lying down for an hour may slow down or stop the signs and symptoms
   - Do not lie flat on your back, because lying flat may cause the contractions to occur more often
   - Do not turn completely on your side because you may not be able to feel the contractions
2. Check for contractions for 1 hour.
   - To tell how often contractions are occurring, check the minutes that elapse from the beginning of one contraction to the beginning of the next.

3. Call your doctor, clinic, or delivery room, or go to the hospital if:
   - You have uterine contractions every 10 minutes or more often for 1 hour (more than five contractions in 1 hour)
     or
   - You have any of the other signs and symptoms for 1 hour
     or
   - You have any spotting or leaking of fluid from your vagina

REMEMBER: Uterine contractions that happen every ten minutes or more often for one hour may cause the cervix to open

REMEMBER: Do not wait for signs and symptoms to disappear. The symptoms may not go away, and waiting to call for help could result in the birth of a premature baby

REMEMBER: Medication is available to help stop premature labor if it is recognized early!

---

any screening, are considered as being at high risk for preterm labor and are followed in the preterm labor clinic.

Women in the high-risk group for preterm labor are seen weekly and receive the following:

1. Education in the symptoms of preterm labor (box, pp. 940-941).
2. Instruction in palpation and timing of uterine contractions.
3. Education regarding notification of health care provider if symptoms of preterm labor are experienced.
4. Routine prenatal care and weekly cervical evaluations.

Therapy for prevention of preterm birth. Attempts to arrest labor are justified if the following conditions are present.

1. Labor is diagnosed. There are three or more contractions of moderate intensity and duration per 20 minutes; the cervix is dilated no more than 4 cm or effaced no more than 50%; but the membranes must be intact with no bulging.
2. The fetus must be live and viable (some hospitals specify 20 to 36 weeks; others, 27 to 37 weeks' inclusive gestation). Estimation of gestational age by ultrasonagraphy is the preferred technique.
3. There are no signs of fetal distress or disease.
4. There must be no medical or obstetric disorder or

clinically significant abnormalities in laboratory findings that are a contraindication to the continuation of pregnancy.

5. The woman is both willing and capable of giving an informed consent. She should be able to comply with the prescribed regimen of medication (on an out-of-hospital basis) and weekly visits until delivery and to return for the 6-week postdelivery examination.

Home management. Preterm labor may be treated by bed rest in the home.

1. Bed rest is intended to keep the pressure of the fetus off the cervix and to enhance uterine perfusion. Kneeling or sitting in bed does not keep the fetus from pressing on the cervix. The woman is advised to lie on her left side with her head flat or raised on a small pillow. Physical rest is facilitated by peace of mind. Someone other than the mother must assume care of older children, cooking, and cleaning. Many women are allowed out of bed only for use of the bathroom.
2. Medications are reviewed and the woman is given written instructions regarding care.
   a. If the woman is being maintained at home on an *oral* dose of tocolytic medication (ritodrine hydrochloride), she is informed about the action and side effects of the drug. She is instructed to take her pulse and report any rate greater than

120 beats/min to her physician. She also is taught to report symptoms, including palpitations, tremors, agitation, and nervousness. The client is not to use ritodrine with any over-the-counter drugs unless the physician approves. Some over-the-counter drugs may cause deleterious effects. Oral administration may be better tolerated when taken with food.
  b. Sedation is often ordered to facilitate relaxation and rest. The woman is instructed and given written instructions (for herself and her family) regarding the medication. This includes the prescription for sedation, dosage, times for administration, and side effects.
3. Sexual stimulation is contraindicated because (1) prostaglandins in semen can stimulate labor in a susceptible woman and (2) touching the cervix may stimulate Ferguson's reflex (the increase in myometrial contractility that follows mechanical stretching or touching of the cervix). Nipple stimulation may induce oxytocin production that can cause recurrence of uterine activity.
4. **Hazards** are reviewed. The woman is given written instructions regarding:
  a. What to do and whom to notify in case of onset of labor or rupture of membranes
  b. Maintaining personal hygiene if membranes have ruptured earlier
  c. Assessing for signs of infection (e.g., odor of vaginal discharge, increase in body temperature).
5. Social service consultation may be helpful if the woman has to be transported into a center from an outlying area. Living arrangements, meals, transportation, and financial assistance may be needed for some families.

In-hospital suppression. Various drugs have been used to suppress labor. They are known as tocolytic drugs. *Toko-* or *toco-* are Greek roots referring to obstetrics; *-lytic* means "to break down or stop."

Ritodrine hydrochloride (Yutopar) (Ueland, 1981; Pritchard, McDonald, and Gant, 1985) is the first β-sympathomimetic drug approved in the United States for use in preterm labor. The administration of ritodrine must be closely supervised by persons having knowledge of the pharmacology of the drug. They must be qualified to identify and manage complications of drug administration or pregnancy.
1. Drug action. Ritodrine hydrochloride stimulates type II β-adrenergic receptors. These cause uterine muscle relaxation, vasodilation, bronchodilation, and muscle glycogenolysis. Decrease in serum potassium levels may cause arrhythmias.
2. Contraindications for use. Not all fetuses can ben-

efit from prolonging intrauterine life. An adverse uterine environment may be more detrimental than premature birth. Contraindications to inhibition of labor include the following conditions (NAACOG, 1984):
  a. Fetal death confirmed by ultrasound
  b. Antepartum hemorrhage, which requires immediate delivery
  c. Pregnancy-induced hypertension (degree to be evaluated individually)
  d. Dilation more than 3 to 4 cm (tertiary consultation should be attained if dilation greater than 4 cm)
  e. Maternal cardiac pathology (β-mimetics contraindicated)
  f. Insulin-dependent diabetes
  g. Maternal hyperthyroidism
  h. Gestational age less than 20 weeks, confirmed by ultrasound
  i. Ruptured fetal membranes, afebrile mother (controversy; some physicians delay delivery to mature fetal lungs)
  j. Chorioamnionitis
  k. Mother already taking β-mimetics for a previously existing medical condition; should not be receiving additional β-mimetic therapy.
3. Beneficial effects of women in premature labor may be prevented from delivering for at least 48 hours by treatment with tocolytic drugs. A delay of premature delivery is potentially beneficial to the fetus. In addition the tocolytic agents currently available are usually able to delay delivery long enough for the use of glucocorticoids to effect fetal pulmonary maturation.
4. Toxic effects. Cardiopulmonary complications are possible. Therefore careful assessment and monitoring are essential. Because of the possible cardiopulmonary effects an electrocardiogram may be ordered before the treatment. A cardiac monitor for the mother may be indicated to maintain continuous assessment for *tachycardia* and *arrhythmia*. See Procedure 29.3 for a summary of the hazardous complications and the care required for a client receiving ritodrine hydrochloride.
5. Administration and dosage. The drug may be administered either intravenously or orally. Intravenous administration precedes the oral administration. The dosage is determined by the physician.

Magnesium sulfate in sufficiently high concentrations can suppress uterine contractions (Spisso and others, 1982). The *precautions* taken during administration of magnesium sulfate are *the same* regardless of whether the rationale for therapy is the suppression of labor or the prevention of eclampsia (see Chapter 27).

NURSING CARE OF A WOMAN RECEIVING RITODRINE HYDROCHLORIDE

PURPOSE

Suppression of premature labor.

EQUIPMENT

1. IV infusion equipment
2. Sphygmomanometer
3. Stethoscope
4. Equipment for cardiopulmonary arrest
5. Fetal monitoring equipment

HAZARDOUS SYMPTOMS

Cardiovascular

1. Hypotension
2. Tachycardia 110 beats/min or greater
3. Arrhythmia
4. Chest pains or tightness

Pulmonary

Chest discomfort, dyspnea, slight recurring cough

Other

Tremors	Nausea	Headache
Anxiety	Vomiting	Erythema

NURSING ACTION	RATIONALE
Assessment	To obtain baseline data
Monitor vital signs and blood pressure every 15 minutes until stable and then follow hospital protocol.	To detect complications
■ Maternal pulse should not exceed 140 beats/min for more than 10 minutes. Note regularity and quality. Prepare mother for use of cardiac monitor.	
■ Breath sounds are noted when counting respiratory rate.	
Monitor fetal heart rate, which should not exceed 180 beats/min. Intermittent evaluation should continue during oral therapy.	
Observe for symptoms.	
Ask woman to report symptoms.	
Send blood samples to laboratory for analysis of levels of glucose, potassium, and hematocrit.	As glucose moves intracellularly, potassium is similarly shifted from the extracellular to the intracellular space, resulting in hypokalemia and acidosis. Several of the well-recognized complications of β-adrenergic therapy such as cardiac arrhythmias and maternal tremors may be explained on this basis (Gross and Sokol, 1980)
Prevent hypotension	
Maintain absolute bed rest during IV infusion	To minimize stress and reduce pressure on cervix
Keep woman in left-lateral position or place wedge under right hip if in supine position	To maintain placental perfusion
Apply antiembolism stockings. Do not use under knees. Encourage passive leg exercise.	To prevent pooling of blood in lower extremities
Maintain adequate hydration, 2000 to 3000 ml daily.	To maintain cardiac output
Prevent overhydration	
Measure intake and output.	To detect complications
Weigh daily.	To detect complications
Prevent undue stress	To promote relaxation.
Prepare woman for potential side effects, i.e., agitation, palpitations, nervousness, tremors, tachycardia.	
Instruct her to report symptoms.	
Treat for complications	
Hold medication. If IV, keep line open with unmedicated solution.	To minimize effects of medication
Notify physician.	To initiate immediate therapy
Prepare antidote as ordered.	
Maintain woman in high Fowler's position.	To minimize effects of pulmonary edema (Philipsen and others, 1981)
Administer oxygen.	To maintain sufficient oxygenation
Initiate CPR for cardiopulmonary arrest if necessary.	To maintain oxygenation

Pharmacologic stimulation of fetal lung maturity. Respiratory distress syndrome (RDS) was formerly known as hyaline membrane disease of the newborn (HMD). It is common in small premature infants who have fetal lung immaturity. The incidence and severity of RDS has been found to be reduced if glucocorticoids are administered to the mother at least 24 to 48 hours before the delivery. The fetus must be less than 34 weeks gestation. The administration must be made at least 24 hours before delivery and no longer than 7 days before delivery (Liggins and Howie, 1974; Brown and others, 1979). Children who have been exposed to the stated levels of glucocorticoids in utero appear to grow and develop normally during the early years of life (Liggins, 1976, 1982). Hence some authorities consider that the chance of benefit to the fetus far outweighs the chance of harm. Pritchard, McDonald, and Gant (1985) note that controversy still exists over the efficacy of glucocorticoid prophylaxis. The following are recognized as contraindications for glucocorticoid therapy:

1. Multiple pregnancy
2. Maternal infection, such as tuberculosis
3. Complications of pregnancy, such as PIH
4. Imminent delivery

Care during irreversible or acceptable preterm birth. The labor is conducted according to the principles that apply to a low-birth-weight (easily compromised) fetus. If vaginal delivery is chosen, the analgesia is limited, and continuous FHR monitoring is applied. Artificial rupture of membranes (ARM) is delayed until the cervix is more than 6 cm dilated, and there is sufficient descent of the presenting part to avoid prolapse of the cord.

If the augmentation of labor is advisable, a low concentration of oxytocin is infused continuously. Pudendal block anesthesia is desirable. An episiotomy is done to limit the length of the second stage and excessive pressure on the fragile fetal head. Outlet forceps are used for delivery unless easy spontaneous birth is likely. A pediatrician and a nurse from the infant intensive care unit are present at the birth so that resuscitative and supportive care for the infant can be initiated immediately if necessary (see Chapters 25 and 31). The newborn is permitted several breaths before clamping the cord; if resuscitation is required, however, the cord is clamped and cut immediately.

Parental concern for the well-being of the infant is apparent during labor. Parents need to be aware of the interest and support of the staff. However, false assurance of fetal health must be avoided. For some parents the reality of the situation is not appreciated until they see their son or daughter in the intensive care unit. For others who experience fetal or neonatal death, the loss intensifies once the stress of labor and delivery is over (see Chapter 26).

During the postpartum period physical care of the mother is similar to that required for any vaginal delivery. However, the family will be very anxious concerning the health and prognosis of their infant. Nursing care of the preterm infant involves not only medical and nursing personnel but also the participation of the parents (see Chapter 31).

Postterm Birth

The postterm pregnancy persists beyond the end of the forty-second week, 2 weeks beyond the EDC figured from Naegele's rule. The infant whose gestational age is beyond 42 weeks is referred to as "postterm" if healthy and "dysmature" if adversely affected by the delayed birth (see Chapter 31).

Maternal risks are related to the delivery of an excessively sized infant. Fetal risks appear to be twofold. The first is related to the possibility of birth trauma and asphyxia through fetopelvic disproportion. The second risk is felt to result from the compromising effects on the fetus of an "aging" placenta. Danforth (1982) notes "the normal life span of the placenta is about 40 weeks; after this time, its capacity and reserve are progressively reduced in the face of increasing demands by the growing fetus." Oligohydramnios and consequent cord compression are also suspected to affect fetal well-being (Leveno and others, 1984). There is still considerable controversy over the predominant cause of postterm fetal effects (Shearer and Estes, 1985).

The decision whether to initiate labor is difficult. Pritchard, McDonald, and Gant (1985) report five problems that can affect the decision:

1. Gestational age is not always precisely known. Thus the fetus may actually be less mature than thought.
2. Precise identification of those fetuses who are likely to die or develop serious morbidity if left in utero is difficult.
3. Most fetuses fare rather well.
4. Induction of labor is not always successful.
5. Cesarean delivery appreciably increases the risk of serious maternal morbidity not only in this pregnancy but also to a degree in subsequent ones.

Summary

Complications during birth have both physical and emotional sequelae. The mother faces hazards to her life. Prolonged and difficult labor can be physically debilitating. The consequent fatigue may interfere with the initial interactions with her newborn. Memories of a difficult birth can resurface years later as a stress factor in subsequent births. The family will be faced with long-term grief reaction if the infant suffers disability. If death of either mother or infant occurs, the family, as it was, no longer exists. Parents, during this time of crisis, need the best possible medical and nursing care that our technically and psychologically knowledgeable society can offer.

References

Dystocia

Benyon, C.: Midline episiotomy as a routine procedure, J. Obstet. Gynaecol. Br. Commonw. 81:126, 1974.

Danforth, D.: Obstetrics and gynecology, Philadelphia, 1982, Harper & Row, Publishers.

Gellman, E., and others: Vaginal delivery after cesarean section, J.A.M.A. 249: 2935, 1983.

Gleichner, N.: Cesarean section rates in the United States: the short-term failure of the National Consensus Development Conference in 1980, J.A.M.A., 252:3273, 1984.

Lipson, J.: Repeat cesarean birth, social and psychological issues, J.O.G.N. Nurs. 13:157, May/June 1984.

Meier, P.R., and Parreco, R.P.: Trial of labor following cesarean section: a two-year experience, Am. J. Obstet. Gynecol. 144:671, 1982.

Morrison, and others: Cesarean section: what's behind the dramatic rise? Perinatal Neonatal. 6:87, 1982.

O'Driscoll, K., and Foley, M.: Correlation of decrease in perinatal mortality and increase in cesarean section rates, Obstet. Gynecol. 61:1, 1983.

Petitti, E.: Recent trends in cesarean delivery rates in California, Birth 12:25, Spring 1985.

Pritchard, J., McDonald, P., and Gant, N.: Williams obstetrics, ed. 17, New York, 1985, Appleton-Century Croft.

U.S. Department of Health and Human Services: Cesarean childbirth, Report of a consensus development conference, Sept. 22-24, 1980, Oct. 1981, NIH pub. no. 82-2967.

Preterm and Postterm

Brown, E.R., and others: Reversible induction of surfactant production in fetal lambs treated with glucocorticoids, Pediatr. Res. 13:491, 1979.

Danforth, D.: Obstetrics and gynecology, Philadelphia, 1982, Harper & Row, Publishers.

Gross, T.L. and Sokol, R.J.: Severe hypokalemia and acidosis: a potential complication of beta-adrenergic treatment, Am. J. Obstet. Gynecol. 138:1225, Dec. 15, 1980.

Herron, M.A., and Dulock, H.L.: Preterm labor: a staff development program in perinatal nursing care, 1982, March of Dimes Birth Defects Foundation.

Leveno, K.J. and others: Prolonged pregnancy. 1. Observations concerning the causes of fetal distress, Am. J. Obstet. Gynecol. 150:465, 1984.

Liggins, G.C.: The prevention of RDS by maternal betamethasone administration. In Lung maturation and the prevention of hyaline membrane disease. Report of the Seventieth Ross Conference on Pediatric Research, Columbus, Ohio, 1976, Ross Laboratories.

Liggins, G.C.: Report on children exposed to steroids in utero. Contemp. OB/Gyn. 19:205, 1982.

Liggins, G.C., and Howie, R.N.: The prevention of RDS by maternal steroid therapy. In Gluck, L. editor: Modern perinatal medicine, Chicago, 1974, Year Book Publications.

Philipsen, T., and others: Pulmonary edema following ritodrine-saline infusion in premature labor, Obstet. Gynecol. 58:304, Sept. 1981.

Pritchard, J., McDonald, P., and Gant, N.: Williams obstetrics, ed. 17, New York, 1985, Appleton-Century Croft.

Shearer, M., and Estes, M.: A critical review of the recent literature on posterm pregnancy and a look at women's experience, Birth 12:95, Summer 1985.

Spisso, K.R., Harbert, G.M., Jr., and Thiagarajah, S.: The use of magnesium sulfate as the primary tocolytic agent to prevent premature delivery, Am. J. Obstet. Gynecol. 142:840, 1982.

Veland, K.: Ritodrine hydrochloride (Yutopar) for treatment of preterm labor, Periscope, p. 4, April 1981.

Bibliography

Dystocia

Banta, D., and Thacker, S.: The risks and benefits of episiotomy: review, Birth 9:25, 1982.

Buchan, P.C., and Nicholls, J.A.J.: Pain after episiotomy—a comparison of two methods of repair, J.R. Coll. Gen. Pract. 30:297, 1980.

Cranley, M., and others: Women's perceptions of vaginal and cesarean deliveries, Nurs. Res. 32:11, 1983.

Hott, J.: Best laid plans: pre- and postpartum comparisons of self and spouse in primiparous Lamaze couples who share delivery and those who do not, Nurs. Res. p. 20, Jan/Feb 1980.

Leach, L., and Sproule, V.: Meeting the challenge of cesarean birth. J.O.G.N. Nurs. 13:19, May/June, 1984.

Oakley, A.: Social consequence of obstetric technology: the importance of measuring soft outcomes, Birth 10:99, Summer 1983.

Queenan, J., and Hobbins, J., editors: Protocols for high-risk pregnancies, Oradell, N.J., 1982, Medical Economics Co.

Preterm and Postterm

Creasy, R.K., Gummer, B.A., and Liggins, G.C.: System for predicting spontaneous preterm birth, Obstet. Gynecol. 55:692, 1980.

Creasy, R.K., & Herron, M.A.: Prevention of preterm birth, Semin. Perinatol. 5:295-302, 1981.

Herron, M.A., Katz, M., & Crease, R.K.: Evaluation of preterm birth prevention program: a preliminary report, Obstet. Gynecol. 59:452, 1982.

Herron, M.A.: Preterm labor. I. Preventing preterm births, N.A.A.C.O.G. update series, lesson 2, vol. 1983.

Morrison, J.C.: Forum on prematurity, Contemporary OB/Gyn. 20.182, Oct. 1982.

N.A.A.C.O.G.: Preterm labor and tocolytics, Nurs. Pract. Res. 10:1, Sept. 1984.

Newton, R., and others: Psychosocial stress in pregnancy and its relation to the onset of premature labor, Br. Med. J. 2:411, 1979.

Shortridge, L.: Using ritodrine hydrochloride to inhibit preterm labor, M.C.N. 8:58, Jan./Feb. 1983.

Adolescent Pregnancy and Parenthood

Adolescent pregnancy, a worldwide phenomenon, represents one of the most critical problems for persons engaged in maternity care. Although the period of adolescence varies somewhat depending on the culture, the World Health Organization (1975) defines it as follows:

1. The person progresses from the point of the initial appearance of the secondary sex characteristics to that of sexual maturity.
2. The individual's psychologic processes and patterns of identification develop from those of a child to those of an adult.
3. A transition is made from the state of total socioeconomic dependence to one of relative independence.

Adolescent Mother

In an assessment of the biopsychosocial risks faced by the adolescent mother and her offspring, it is necessary to distinguish age groups within the adolescent range: early adolescence, 10 to 14 years; middle adolescence, 14 to 17 years; and late adolescence, 17 to 20 years. Each age group responds to pregnancy and the care of infants in ways characteristic of its particular developmental level and personal abilities.

Trends. The following trends (MacDonnell, 1981) have been identified in adolescent pregnancy and childbearing in the United States and Canada. Proportionately fewer adolescents are bearing children; however, of all children born, a greater percentage of the infants are being born to adolescent mothers. Birth to an adolescent is more likely to be out of wedlock, to a mother who has less than a high school education and who received inadequate prenatal care. Young single mothers are choosing to keep and raise their children. They are making this choice without seeking advice or help from any of the traditional agencies, for example,

children's aid societies or maternity homes. To a great degree these young mothers are dependent on public services and welfare agencies for financial support.

Factors. Factors contributing to adolescent pregnancy are physically and culturally interrelated. Sexual maturity is now occurring at an earlier age, although marriage is taking place at a later age. The now-traditional patterns of sexual activity, ranging from dating in the early teens to living together in late adolescence, lack the stabilizing effect of known expectations or norms. Studies indicate that although teenagers with unplanned pregnancies have an adequate level of knowledge of contraceptives, they do not practice contraception consistently (Chapter 7 and Baldwin, 1981). There is a lack of explicit education in sexuality both in the home and at school.

Efforts have been made to predict which teenagers are at risk of becoming pregnant. However, "no combination of demographic factors and attitudes could be found that identified the majority of pregnant teenagers without incurring unacceptable overreferral" (Vernon and others, 1983). Evidently teenage pregnancy occurs for multiple reasons.

Physical consequences. The adolescent mother today is at risk of having an adverse pregnancy and an unfavorable neonatal outcome. Research indicates a *greater incidence* of complications of pregnancy, such as pregnancy-induced hypertension, and of low-birthweight infants, either at term or prematurely.

At present, however, considerable disagreement exists as to the significance of research findings into the *causes* of unfavorable pregnancy. Research is also not conclusive on neonatal outcomes associated with teenage pregnancies, particularly those of mothers under 15 years of age.

It is found that very young adolescents who bear children experienced an early menarche. It may be that at the time the very young adolescent becomes pregnant, there is an incomplete maturation of the endometrial and hypothalamic-pituitary axis (Chapter 5). Her gynecologic age may be low. Gynecologic age is defined as the difference between the mother's age at conception or delivery and her age at menarche. Earlier studies reported that mothers who delivered more than 2 years after menarche had fewer low-birth-weight infants (Erkan and others, 1971). More recent studies, however, did not find the same correlation between gynecologic age and poor neonatal outcome (Forbes, 1981; Hollingsworth and Kotchen, 1981). "Childbirth at a low gynecologic age or early chronologic age does not appear to have adverse effects when *prepregnancy health and nutrition are good and excellent prenatal care is readily available*" (Hollingsworth and others, 1983).

In a 1979 statement the Committee on Adolescence of the American Academy of Pediatrics attributed a greater *incidence* of low-birth-weight infants to adolescent mothers. In the preamble to an amendment to Public Law 95-626 (1981) on Adolescent Family Life, the previous findings of a high incidence of low-birth-weight infants to adolescent mothers were reaffirmed. Other researchers, although agreeing on the incidence, concluded that factors *other than maternal age* were responsible. Factors such as inadequate prenatal care and life-style (use of drugs, smoking, drinking, exposure to sexually transmitted disease), which are known contributors to poor perinatal income, are implicated (Baldwin, 1981; Merritt and others, 1980a, b; Miller and Merritt, 1979; Perkins and others, 1978; Zuckerman and others, 1983).

Adolescents, even those in early adolescence, who receive excellent prenatal care, including nutritional guidance, have been found not to be at greater obstetric (biologic) risk than older adolescents or adult women who are of similar socioeconomic status, wedded status, and race. It is of interest that new data suggest that the ideal biologic ages for women to bear children are between 16 and 19 years (Merritt and others, 1980a).

In a review of research in 1981, Lawrence and Merritt summarized the state of our knowledge: "It is yet to be determined whether biologic or social inadequacies best explain the apparent reproductive disadvantage of the American teenager and the well-being of their babies."

Psychosocial consequences. Adolescent pregnancy has direct implications, however, for the psychosocial well-being of the young parent, her child, and society. Although teenage pregnancy is better accepted today than it was in the past, it still remains a problem for all concerned. The pregnancy comes at a time that is outside of the recognized social norms for childbearing. It introduces situational stresses—pregnancy, parenthood, and marriage—at a period when the young person is trying to cope with the maturational stresses of adolescence.

In a highly technical society such as ours, educational attainment is the basis for vocational choice and success. Women who delay childbearing have a greater level of educational achievement than women who begin childbearing at an early age. One study reported that, whereas only 50% of adolescent mothers completed high school, 97% of mothers who had delayed childbearing were high school graduates (Card and Wise, 1978). The adolescent mother may, in fact, be relegated to a low socioeconomic job with a lower income and less prestige. Many adolescent parents are dependent on families or on government social programs for financial support.

Dynamics

Psychosocial development. The psychosocial development of the teenager reflects the three stages (early, middle, and late) of adolescence. These stages roughly approximate chronologic age but more precisely are characterized by predominate drives, moods, and abilities (Sahler, 1983). Hatcher (1976) described five aspects of personality development that have proved to be good indicators of the adolescent's overall developmental level. The five aspects were as follows:

1. The identity of the parent most related to conflicts
2. The quality and style of her relationships with others
3. Her view of herself
4. Her major defense mechanisms
5. Her goals and interests

Sahler (1983) applied these findings to readiness for the task of childbearing. Her discussion is summarized in Table 30.1.

Adolescent choices. The adolescent is faced with making decisions about sexuality in the early teens. Sexual intercourse leading to pregnancy is not "an accident," in spite of youthful protestations. The adolescent must assume responsibilities for her actions in a sphere that poses both physical and psychologic consequences for the teenager, her infant, and her family.

The decision-making ability of the teenager will change with maturity; however, all age groups need factual information relative to sexuality, intercourse, and parenthood on which to base decisions. Fig. 30.1 represents a process of sexual decision making. Unfortunately very young teenagers use "denial" as a coping mechanism. They can *deny* the significance of what they hear (Table 30.1).

Sexual activity. The pressure of the peer group on the adolescent to initiate sexual activity is very strong in present-day teen culture. It can supersede the influence

Table 30.1
Adolescent Development and Readiness for Child Bearing

	Early Adolescence	Middle Adolescence	Late Adolescence
Parent most related to conflicts	Beginning to loosen ties with her mother. Vacillates between wanting to be closer, i.e., a mother herself, and wanting to be babied, i.e., cannot conceive of herself as a mother.	Struggling to break from both parents and become autonomous.	Personal identity stronger; some emotional independence from parents; ready for outside love interest.
Quality and style of relationships with others	Strong relationships with other girls. Experiences crushes on safe, i.e., unattainable, adults.	Relationship with peers intense; parents replaced with peers; difficulty with authority figures, cannot either accept or compromise. Friends are heterosexual but self-identity needs (who am I), not intimacy needs, are uppermost.	Conflict with parents lessens, nurturant feelings for others emerge, wants to share love and commitment.
View of herself	Self-concept inconsistent and fluctuating; parallels rapid physical changes and capability changes. Vague sense of self as female.	Self-involvement a critical need. Ambivalence and uncertainty predominate. Senses her femininity and has a beginning awareness of responsibility for actions. Definitive commitments not yet necessary. Unresolved dependency needs preclude her wanting to accept dependency of others.	More realistic about who and what she is. Behaviors and responses more predictable. Capable of personal reflections, more in touch with her own feelings.
Defense mechanisms	Primary defense is denial, manifested by unwillingness to hear pertinent information (e.g., almost never protected by contraception during sexual experimentation).	Magical thinking and feelings of greater power pervade fantasy, mood swings experienced, any nonsuccess is a tragedy. Exaggeration of response prevents an accurate assessment of real tragedy.	Uses reality-based strategies to cope with stress. Can think through problems, uses rational thought.
Goals and interests	Is "now" oriented. The immediacy of her needs requires instant gratification. Operates by fixed rules and authority, little ability to "give and take," therefore rigid and punitive.	Goals and interest reflect growing ability to problem solve. Dependency-independency needs make her inconsistent in approach. Intensely narcissistic (self-centered). Generally unempathetic and unable to tolerate others' demands that detract from her self-focus.	Goals and interests reflect longer-range view. More ready to accept responsibility for self and others. Recognizes need to develop educational or vocational skills. Approximates the adult in being able to provide warm, nurturing care for a child.

Modified from Sahler, O.J.: In McAnarney, E.R., editor: Premature adolescent pregnancy and parenthood, New York, 1983, Grune & Stratton. Reprinted by permission.

of parents or older friends. Often teenagers feel that once virginity has been lost, they have nothing more to lose. Abstinence needs positive reinforcement, but if abstinence is not to be, the next decision for the teenager is whether to use birth control.

Birth control. Many teenagers have been sexually active for 6 months before seeking birth control measures (Zelnik, 1983). The techniques of birth control are the same as those advocated for adults (Chapter 7). Teenagers often need help in taking the step to use contraceptives. They may object that the "obvious planning" presumes eventual intercourse or that "it's against their religious scruples." Open discussion of

the issues surrounding birth control and the availability of contraceptives are key components in the decisions that are made relative to the use of birth-control measures.

Abortion. Once pregnancy occurs, the adolescent is faced with the choice of abortion or carrying the pregnancy. The teenager who delays telling parents about the pregnancy or who vacillates regarding abortion, often makes a decision to have her baby in a roundabout way. Options need to be presented in a nonjudgmental manner to ensure the young person's freedom of choice (Chapter 7). Fewer teenagers are electing abortion today than in the 1970s.

Fig. 30.1
Decision tree for adolescent sexual decision making. (From Kreipe, R.E. In McAnarney, E., editor: Premature adolescent pregnancy and parenthood, New York, 1983, Grune & Stratton. Reprinted by permission.)

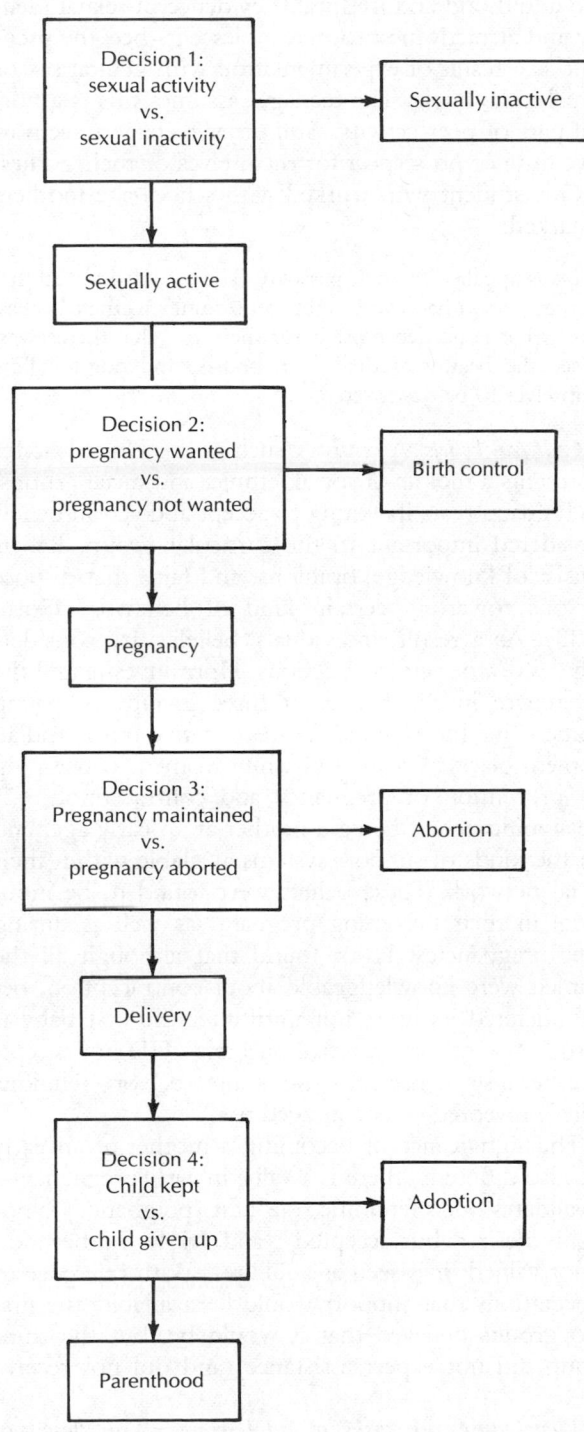

Adoption. If the adolescent mother opts to have her child, she can either keep the baby or place the child for adoption. The majority of teenagers are electing to keep their infants. If, however, adoption is contemplated, discussion of the adoption process begins in the prenatal period. The adolescent is encouraged to talk freely of her feelings, both for and against the process. If possible, the girl's family and boyfriend are part of the group that help the teenager with her decision. The adolescent needs to be assured that what she is doing is positive in nature and that feelings of sadness and of frustration are bound to occur.

After the baby is born, the young mother may or may not wish to see the baby or to know its sex. It is generally agreed that releasing a child is facilitated if one grieves for an *actual loss* rather than a *fantasy* one; however, the mother has the right to make her own choice. She can be given the information about the infant's health (e.g., "your baby is healthy and strong"), since it may affect her response to her own feelings of self-worth.

Placing an infant for adoption may be accepted by some young parents with varying emotional responses. For some, it may be another episode in a "bad" experience. On the other hand, giving a baby up for adoption may be attended by all the symptoms of grief one would expect at the death of a newborn: "She is only 15 years old, but she loves the baby. Her parents won't take it, so she has to give it up. Her grief was heartbreaking. On the day she went home she came into the nursery to hold her baby for one last time."

It is essential to help the young woman to cultivate a positive attitude toward potential future pregnancies. "Subconsciously, she may compensate for the loss of this infant by producing another as soon as possible, by carelessly entering into new relationships while seeking support during her grief, by making unreasonable demands on subsequent children, or by becoming overly protective of subsequent offspring" (Sorosky and others, 1978).

Today the teenager and her parent need to be informed of the possibility that the infant given for adoption may, as an adult, seek to identify his or her biologic parents. It is now a recognized practice to provide adoptive parents with all pertinent biologic knowledge that may affect the infant. It is also helpful for the child to know of psychosocial "successes" in his or her biologic family—musical ability, sports prowess, scientific success—all of which can be part of the adopted baby's history and a source of pride.

The grief of the young parent at her loss has to be balanced with the need of her infant for continued care and nurturing. The experience of relinquishing her child "for the child's good" may be the young woman's first major autonomous decision in her life and as such is an important step toward maturity.

Motivation. On a personal level the reasons adolescents give for becoming pregnant vary widely. They include the effect of family relationships, use of coping mechanisms, love and commitment to one another, the enhancement of self-concept, and cultural beliefs.

Family relationships. For some adolescents there may be faulty relationships within the family. It may be that in mother-daughter conflicts the daughter uses pregnancy to act out her rebellion or as a statement of her growing sexuality as opposed to her mother's declining sexuality. For others there may be a search for nurturance from a mother or father who failed to provide it.

Some adolescents living in certain ethnic and multigenerational families know that their offspring will become family members. In a few instances the pattern for early adolescent pregnancy out of wedlock is a familiar and accepted one. There appears to be a warm, supportive relationship that, once the initial shock to the family system is resolved, results in supportive and nurturing care for the adolescent and her infant.

Coping mechanisms. If human behavior is purposeful (even if the purpose is obscure), cues to the young girl's behavior may sometimes be gained by having her assess where she is now and where she was before pregnancy. Pregnancy may function as a coping mechanism. For young girls living in poverty, having babies is one form of economic survival. The allotments of money, food stamps, medical and dental care, and special schooling provided by the government establish their economic as well as personal independence. In reality, however, the adolescent's concept of wealth is usually distorted, and a cycle of poverty can be established or perpetuated.

Sometimes an unwanted partner is removed or tested: "Somehow I sensed that if I got pregnant, he wouldn't stand by me. Was I ever right! He abandoned me in a foreign country—just took off. I'm glad I found out his true colors."

Some adolescents view the child to be born as an ally for themselves, someone who will love them in spite of adversity and who will act as a supportive person. The infant's need to be dependent, to be nurtured, and to be viewed as a person apart is not recognized. The young mother's disappointment and bewilderment over her infant's normal behavior can lead to bitterness and eventual neglect.

Love and commitment. Researchers have found a significant love relationship in some teenage couples (Elster and Panzarine, 1981). They report that a crisis during the pregnancy often arose in the relationship between the putative father and the girl's parents. Of those adolescents who keep their children, a substantial number eventually marry; the premarital sexual relationship was part of a longer commitment to one another.

Self-concept. Pregnancy can serve as a rite of passage into adulthood and irrefutable evidence of sexual identity and attractiveness. Some adolescents become pregnant as a result of experimentation with genital sex or sexual intercourse. The teenager assumes this is a normal part of peer activity. Still other teenagers seem to have little or no respect for themselves or their bodies.

One student who worked with school-age mothers remarked:

I was appalled by their passivity. They seemed to feel that another person had every right to do things to their bodies. I feel what is needed most is for them to value themselves, to see the beauty of their own bodies, and not to allow themselves to be destroyed.

Cultural beliefs. A country such as the United States represents a mosaic of social, ethnic, and racial groups. Each group rears its young to accept and act on beliefs considered important to the particular group. Beliefs consist of knowledge, opinions, and faith that dispose persons toward a certain kind of behavior (Horn, 1983). As a result, individuals' beliefs vary considerably, as do the resulting actions. Horn investigated the differences in the beliefs of three groups of young women in the United States (native-born Indian women, black women, and white women) concerning (1) prevention of pregnancy and contraception, (2) the significance of being a mother at an early age, and (3) the kinds of support systems available within their social network. These beliefs were found to be influential in their becoming pregnant, as well as during their pregnancies. Horn found that although all the women were knowledgeable about contraception, beliefs dictated its use: "not until after the first baby is born," "use of birth control pills and IUD not acceptable because menstrual cycle is altered," or "religious belief prevented or encouraged use."

The significance of becoming a mother at an early age also differed: "there is a value in early pregnancy—it validates one's feminine role"; "it [pregnancy] is not highly desired but accepted"; and "early motherhood is not valued; it is seen as a failure." With reference to expectations that support would be available, the first two groups believed that it would be, but the third group did not expect assistance (and did not receive it).

Developmental tasks of adolescence. The developmental tasks of adolescents are interrupted by pregnancy. As with other developmental sequences, there are critical periods when interference can have traumatic effects. Obviously the younger the adolescent, the greater will be the effects. For the 12- to 14-year-old girl, pregnancy can be a fearful experience. Because of the extreme youth of these younger adolescents, society tends to respond in a more protective way, and there seems to be a generalized effort to minimize the trauma. The 15- to 17-year-old girl, with her mixture of childlike and adult behavior and her more overt conflicts with parents, seems to arouse more societal anger and resentment, perhaps because both family and society must respond in a responsible way to behavior they are at a loss to control. The 18- to 20-year-old girl is viewed somewhat as an adult who, with a modicum of support, can fend more adequately and who can assume the major responsiblity for her offspring.

The following developmental tasks may be interrupted by pregnancy in adolescence:

1. *Achievement of new and more mature relations with age mates of both sexes*

The pregnant adolescent may find herself isolated from her peer group. Within some social groups, parents will try to prevent contact between their teenagers and the one who has become pregnant—an attempt to proclaim societal condemnation of adolescent behavior. In some areas regular school attendance must be discontinued, which effectively limits meetings with peers. The pregnant adolescent has contact largely with other pregnant teenagers, her boyfriend if he remains faithful, and relatives. Thus the practice time for developing social relationships is curtailed.

2. *Achievement of a feminine social role*

In one sense pregnancy confers overt adult sexuality on the teenager, but in another sense it limits the feminine role to one of procreation. Opportunities for social development of feminine potential are either abandoned or are set aside until early or middle adulthood.

3. *Acceptance of her physique and effective use of the body*

Adolescents are experiencing a period of rapid change in physical growth and become acutely conscious of their bodies and body sensations. The symptoms of pregnancy can cause the teenager much dismay. Elimination, for example, is not necessarily talked about openly, and the need for care related to this area is equated with being infantile or elderly. The frequent urination of early and late pregnancy may be "treated" by restricting fluid intake. This restriction increases the likelihood of severe constipation or bladder infections.

The increase in melanin causes deepening of color in the areolar tissue of the breasts, the formation of the mask of pregnancy, and the appearance of the linea nigra. These changes may be viewed by the adolescent as stigmas. The increased mucoid vaginal secretions may be thought to be caused by infection, and if the adolescent resists care, they may increase her anxiety and fear. Increased sensitivity of the breasts can be a source of discomfort and anxiety. The fatigue of early pregnancy, compounding the fatigue experienced by many adolescents, can cause the adolescent to assume that she is ill.

Until late adolescence, body image is still formative. By midpregnancy the enlarging abdomen and the increasing size of breasts and buttocks may prompt the teenager to try to control her appearance by dieting, with adverse consequences for fetal health and her own growth needs. The shift in the center of gravity as body posture changes to accommodate the protuberant abdomen causes back strain and lack of balance. These are aggravated by the disparity between the rate of growth of the skeleton and the muscles supporting it; the muscles are not strong enough (even in the nonpregnant state) to maintain correct posture. The effects may be severe if the teenager feels compelled to compete in strenuous activities (including dancing) or to wear nonsupportive shoes because of her need to belong to her peer group. Symptoms of abnormalities, vaginal bleeding, and dizziness are sometimes concealed until serious conditions develop.

It is one thing for a woman who is knowledgeable and secure to accept and cope with the symptoms of pregnancy. She may feel compensated by the feeling that the child she is creating will be wanted and loved. For the adolescent whose pregnancy is condemned and whose baby most often will not be welcomed, the discomforts of pregnancy can assume major proportions. Unfortunately to some they are seen as punishment for their illicit or "sinful" behavior.

4. *Achievement of independence from parents and other adults*

For the teenager who becomes pregnant, her move toward independence comes to an end, and she is compelled to turn to her family for nurturance just as she did as a young child. Even with the support provided by social agencies, the school-age mother-to-be finds it almost impossible to separate herself from her family. With that support comes a reestablishment of family dominance and dependency.

For example, a 15-year-old-girl cannot make a decision relative to the continuing care of her infant without family concurrence. She is not able to provide such care for her child unless some adult is willing to provide shelter and assistance for them both. If this support is not forthcoming, the young teenager must examine other options (e.g., foster care or giving the child up for adoption). The pregnancy may, however, serve as a catalyst to force the family to examine its relationships. In many instances the pregnancy has been a means of resolving parent-child conflicts in a more growth-responsive way.

Although certain areas of independence are curtailed, others may be substituted. The teenager who assumes responsibility may emerge from this life experience as one who can function in an interdependent manner with adults. These responsibilities include attendance at prenatal care classes, following an adequate dietary regimen, and participating in parent-craft groups.

For some adolescents the forced contact with a caring health professional during pregnancy may have a dramatic effect and provide a role model. As one 16-year-old girl expressed it:

■ The only thing that was okay with it all was that I met F _____ (nursing counselor). She likes me—well, I know she does. Even when I got rough, she'd be there. I never knew grown people were like that, that they cared about me. I would like to be like her, not a nurse, but like someone who loves people.

---

5. *Establishment of a life-style that is personally and socially satisfying*

A prerequisite of a satisfying life-style is the opportunity to make thoughtful and informed choices in the areas of career, sexual relationships, marriage, family interdependence, and parenthood.

Because of interruptions in schooling, many teenagers who might realistically have had other career goals are relegated to occupations that are not commensurate with their capabilities and temperament. Some never overcome this disadvantage; others must postpone any formal preparations until much later in life.

Precipitate marriage by the older adolescent does not have a good success rate. This results because the adolescent is unprepared for the give-and-take of such a close relationship, beset by economic problems, and living in inadequate housing (often with inlaws). Often the adolescent has no time for the "fun" of growing up. Thus participants in early marriage tend to experience desertion or divorce, intensifying their sense of alienation and defeat. For the early adolescent, pregnancy and parenthood seem not to be recognized as possible consequences of sexual behavior. Pregnancy comes as a surprise. Parenthood is something that happens to parents, from whom the younger teenager is seeking to establish independence, not a state in which giving of oneself to another will be required.

The older adolescent, being less egocentric and more capable of problem solving, often is able to face the reality of pregnancy and parenthood in an adult manner. She can seek assistance from social agencies in her own right. She may find, however, that the care of a child without the emotional and economic support of another caring adult means altering career plans.

6. *Acquisition of a set of values (an ethical system) that will serve as a guide to socially responsible behavior*

Becoming pregnant and producing a child who will not receive the concerned parenting that is due cannot be said to be socially responsible behavior. However, by assuming adult responsibilities associated with pregnancy and parenthood, some adolescents emerge as stronger, other-centered individuals. For those who are unable to be helped or who are not helped to use this experience as a time of maturation, pregnancy may become a coping mechanism, albeit an inadequate one, to solve the problems of the moment. For this group recidivism is more prevalent, and the adolescent who sought to become independent through sexual activity remains a dependent person.

Developmental tasks of pregnancy. In common with the older pregnant woman, the adolescent faces certain developmental tasks directly related to becoming a parent. Her response to the implications and challenges of these tasks reflects her cognitive level (Chapter 6). Adolescents are in the period of transition between the inductive reasoning of late childhood (concrete operations) and the deductive reasoning of the older individual (formal operations). For an adolescent whose thoughts are circumscribed by the "here and now" and "seeing is believing," movement toward the "there and then" and predictions of the future may be very limited. The old saying that "you cannot put an old head on young shoulders" holds true.

1. *Accepting the biologic reality of pregnancy*

The usual response of the adolescent is denial. Anxiety about the response of her family or boyfriend will often delay the seeking of outside support. Adolescents have reported that sharing their suspicions of pregnancy with their parents was the most difficult part of their pregnancy and assumed crisis proportions. Many parents also have reported how emotionally distraught their daughter became. Evidently the idea of being pregnant comes with a sense of surprise and belief: "I can't believe it is happening to me," "I didn't think I could get pregnant; I'm too young," "I keep thinking it is some awful dream and I will wake up." The sense of denial is so profound that the girl experiences genuine shock at the consequences of her sexual behavior.

Suspicions of pregnancy may first be discussed with a girlfriend, and fantasies about what will happen when the mother is told will be reviewed. Some adolescents leave clues that they hope will by noticed by their mothers. Containers of pills are left in accessible places, diaries previously locked and secreted are left open, or letters to girlfriends are placed so they can easily be read. The parent is expected to note the repetitive nausea, vomiting, and weight loss in early pregnancy and the changing body shape of mid-pregnancy. It is hoped the parent will bring up the subject of possible pregnancy. The girl expects anger, recriminations, and, depending on the family culture, perhaps physical abuse. She is surprised by the support and nurturing that are often forthcoming. If the pregancy were not such a tragic event, the components of the drama resemble many adolescent-adult confrontations. The girl speaks in her adolescent language and expects the all-wise and all-knowing adult to understand.

The end result of the denial of the reality of pregnancy is the postponement of medical care, to the detriment of both the adolescent and her fetus. Abortion as an option may have to be ruled out because of the advanced stage of pregnancy. Infection, drug ingestion, and inadequate nutrition may have already traumatized the fetus. Those who have contact with school-age adolescents need to be particularly alert to changes in their behavior patterns. Often the teacher, school counselor, or school nurse is the first to note symptoms suggestive of pregnancy and to broach the possibility of pregnancy to the girl. In many instances the professional acts as the girl's support in telling her parents of her condition and in initiating medical and social care. The older adolescent will often seek professional confirmation of pregnancy before seeking parental or societal help. Once the pregnancy is confirmed and care has been initiated, the adolescent, whatever her age, needs help in assuming the responsibility for continuing the care.

2. *Accepting the reality of the unborn child*

The second task relating to acceptance of the reality of the unborn child develops in the same manner with the adolescent as with the older women. The idea of a happy, cuddly baby who will love and obey the parent seems a common fantasy. The young adolescent can be enthusiastic about how she will dress her baby, take her baby out for walks, and bathe and play with the baby. In fantasy the infant acquires a doll-like form. The realities of infant caretaking and the problems with alleviating crying, feeding the infant, and washing clothes are not faced. The concept of the infant's growth and development into first a toddler, then a preschooler, next a school-age child, and an adolescent does not occur to them. They tend to be centered in the present.

3. *Accepting the reality of parenthood.*

Being a parent implies being loving, concerned, and capable of providing the nurturing care an infant needs. It is the most difficult task for adolescents, as it is for many adult pregnant women. The desire for

knowledge about child-care activities, nutritional needs of infants, and infant growth and development is evidenced in this group as in any other. One is impressed by the *desire* of the adolescent to be a good mother. The young adolescent is limited in her ability to fulfill the commitment to her child. This results from her meager life experiences, her own need to grow and develop, and her inability to cope with abstractions and to solve problems on the basis of inference and projection.

The older adolescent, being able to project herself into the future, can see herself and her infant more readily as separate entities with differing needs. She is more able to fantasize about her child as a preschooler or even a teenager. However, in spite of her greater ability to propose solutions to problems and follow through on suggestions, the family she will create will remain one of the most vulnerable in our society.

Developmental tasks of parenthood. The developmental tasks of parenthood include, reconciling the imagined with the actual child, becoming adept in caretaking activities, being aware of the infant's needs, and establishing oneself and one's infant as a family. These tasks will be as important to the new adolescent parent's schema as to the adult's (see also Chapters 23 and 24).

Parenting abilities. Studies to date have not produced conclusive evidence to show there are major attitudinal differences between adolescent and adult mothers. However, some differences in parenting behaviors are beginning to be documented. For example, adolescents, although providing warm and attentive physical care, appear to use less verbal interaction than do older parents.

Development of cognitive ability appears to be related to the amount of exposure of the infant to verbal communication—the more verbal exchanges, the greater the development of cognitive ability. Jones and others (1980) found that adult mothers were significantly more responsive to their newborn infants than were younger mothers, regardless of race or of socioeconomic or marital status. Other researchers have confirmed clinical observations that some adolescents use aggressive, inappropriate behaviors, for example, poking and pinching their infants. These behaviors are rarely seen in adult mothers (Lawrence and others, 1981). The negative attitudes may reflect the adolescent's self-centeredness and level of cognitive development. Excessive child abuse by adolescent mothers has not been substantiated by research. It may be that neglect is a more pronounced feature of parenting disorders in the adolescent.

Parenting ability is based on a parent's sensitivity to the infant's needs. Many factors can affect sensitivity, including stress, developmental level, knowledge, infant responses, and support systems.

Stress. The adolescent's ability to function in a mothering role is affected by the level of stress she is experiencing. Adolescents are exposed to many stresses as they undertake the tasks and responsibilities of parenthood, a role that in our culture is traditionally reserved for adults who are financially and educationally secure. Stress can affect the quality of a person's functioning, making her insensitive to other needs.

Developmental level. The level of cognitive development of the younger adolescent affects her ability to view her problems realistically and plan for the future. The care of a baby cannot be set aside as can the care of a doll. The all-consuming nature of child care can prove frustrating and may result in nonnurturing behavior toward the child. Adolescents' reactions to perceived stress depend on the quality of their support systems, their self-esteem, and their ability to solve problems directly.

Knowledge. The adolescent's knowledge of child development is usually limited. This lack may directly affect parental sensitivity by influencing the mother's perception, interpretation, and responsiveness to infant cues (Elster and others, 1983).

Teenage parents have been found to expect too much of their children too soon. A study of adolescent couples revealed that they consistently overestimated the age at which their child could accomplish certain behaviors, for example, sitting alone at 12 weeks (mothers) or at 6 weeks (fathers) (DeLissovoy, 1973). Jarrett (1982) found a similar lack of knowledge (Table 30.2). In addition, teenage parents were found to possess inaccurate knowledge of their offspring's cognitive, social and language development.

Infant responsiveness. The responses of teenage mothers to their infant's responses parallel those of the adult mother (Chapter 23). Adolescents certainly respond to positive feedback from their infants. They are pleased when their infants recognize them and prefer them

over others. However, studies do indicate that adolescents perceive their infants as more temperamentally difficult than do adult mothers (Field, et al, 1980).

Support systems. There appears to be a direct relationship between the amount of social support and evidence of appropriate maternal behavior (Mercer, 1985). Emotional support is seen by the young mothers as being the most important type of support, especially if provided by the mother's family of origin (Colletta and Gregg, 1981).

Nutritional needs. Adolescence (ages 13 to 18 years) presents its own special nutritional problems. Most adolescent girls attain physiologic maturity at 17 years of age; pregnancy before that age presents certain biologic hazards if optimal care is not used. The course and outcome of pregnancy of women between 18 and 20 years of age are comparable to those of mature women 20 to 24 years of age.

The orderly sequence of growth and skeletal maturation is related to sexual maturation. Sexual maturity may be attained before musculoskeletal maturation is complete. Dietary surveys among adolescents have revealed that this group receives less than two thirds of the recommended daily intake of iron, calcium, and vitamins A and C (Food and Nutrition Board, 1970). About one in ten adolescents who become pregnant is obese. Since weight-conscious adolescents may consume less than 2000 calories per day, the recommended allowance of iron (18 mg/24 h) is deficient. Female adolescents who are anemic and underweight at a time when their body growth needs are at a peak (17 years of age or younger) are more vulnerable to skeletal problems, communicable diseases, and infections. Pregnancy at this time superimposes metabolic demands for nutrients on the dietary requirements for the adolescent's own growth. Weight gain during pregnancy must be evaluated in light of her normal growth (anabolism) during this period. (Tables 30.3 and 30.4). The pregnant adolescent's need for increased protein, calories, and iron will exceed that of

Table 30.2
Ages at Which Mothers Expect Children to Accomplish Specific Behaviors

Behavior	Norm for Mastery	Mother's Expectations (%)			
		<12 Months	12-18 Months	18-24 Months	>36 Months
Bladder control	18-24	43	43	14	0
Bowel control	14-36	26	30	30	14
Obedience training	>24	80	14	6	0
Recognition of right from wrong	30-36	78	20	2	0

From Jarret, E.: M.C.N. 7:119, 1982.

the pregnant woman over 20 years of age, as shown by Frank's calculation (1981) of calorie requirements for pregnant adolescents below.

The outcome for the fetus may not be reflected in lowered birth weight alone. Research indicates that brain growth takes place in an orderly sequence, as does growth of other organs. The first-phase hyperplasia (growth by increase in the number of cells) takes place prenatally. The second-phase hypertrophy (growth by increase in cell size), in combination with hyperplasia, is the growth pattern noted in the first 6 months of life. Maternal malnutrition may therefore contribute to a reduced complement of brain cells in the fetus, and the mother's lack of knowledge of the nutritional requirements of her newborn compounds the problem.

Calorie Requirements and Sample Menus for Pregnant Adolescents

Calculating calorie requirements*

1. Allow calories for maximal daily growth needs:	123 calories
2. Add RDA† of calories for pregnancy:	300 calories
3. Add average RDA† of calories for age and growth percentile for nonpregnant female:	2100 calories
	2523 total daily calories
4. *Underweight:* Add 500 additional calories per day, 16% of which should be protein (20 g):	3023 total daily calories

5. *Overweight:* Use lower range of "normal" suggested values or 38 calories/kg or 17 calories/lb pregnancy weight.

Sample menus

	Day 1	Day 2
Breakfast	Egg and ham on English muffin (fast food) 1 cup milk 1 glass orange juice (6 oz; 180 ml)	1 cup cornflakes with 1 cup milk 2 T raisins 1 glass orange juice (6 oz; 180 ml)
Snack	1 pkg peanut butter crackers 1 can apple juice (6 oz; 180 ml)	1 pkg nuts 1 carton chocolate milk (8 oz; 240 ml)
Lunch	Cheeseburger on bun with lettuce and tomato 1 carton chocolate milk (8 oz; 240 ml) 1 slice watermelon	"Sub"—1 slice each ham, salami, and cheese with lettuce, tomato, onion, green pepper, 1 T dressing 1 can apple juice (6 oz; 180 ml)
Snack	Ice cream cone	1 cup buttered popcorn
Dinner	Baked chicken leg and thigh ½ cup rice ½ cup string beans 1 cup milk ½ cup fruit cocktail	2 cups spaghetti and meatballs 1 slice Italian bread Tossed salad—lettuce, tomato, onion 1 T dressing 1tsp margarine
Snack	1 slice pizza	Milkshake, vanilla

Calories	Protein (g)	Fat (g)	Cholesterol (g)	Calories	Protein (g)	Fat (g)	Cholesterol (g)
2604	119	132	286	2857	115	147	248
Underweight: replace cheeseburger with extra-large hamburger deluxe; add 1 cup orange juice to evening snack.				*Underweight:* add 1 carton chocolate milk to afternoon snack, extra cheese or cold cuts to lunch, 2 T dressing for salad.			
3149	133	155	334	3353	137	172	278
Overweight: replace ice cream cone with 1 can apple juice (6 oz; 180 ml)				*Overweight:* replace milkshake with 1 cup skim milk			
2354	111	114	270	2400	112	131	196

From Frank, D., and others: J. Calif. Perinatal Assoc. 3(1):21, 1981.

*These calculations are based on the maximum calorie allowance for growth. The best indication of whether a pregnant female is getting sufficient calories is to monitor her growth. If inadequate or excess weight gain occurs, consultation with a nutritionist is recommended.

†Recommended daily dietary allowance.

Table 30.3
Recommended Daily Dietary Allowances for Calories*

Growth Percentile	Nonpregnant (by Age in Years)				Added Pregnancy Allowance
	11-14	15-18	19-22	23-50	
50	2200	2100	2100	1000	300
10	1500	1200	1700	1600	300
90	3000	3000	2500	2400	300

From Frank, D., and others: J. Calif. Perinatal Assoc. 3(1):21, 1981; based on National Center for Health Statistics weight-for-length data and recommendations of the Committee on Maternal Nutrition.
*The allowance for energy is established at the lowest value corresponding to good health. No extra allowance is included.

Table 30.4
Adolescent Protein Requirements for Pregnancy*

Age (Years)	Protein
15-18	1.5 g/kg pregnant body weight
<15	1.7 g/kg pregnant body weight

From Food and Nutrition Board: Recommended daily dietary allowances, Washington, D.C., 1970, National Academy of Sciences—National Research Council.
*Adequate calories need to be provided for optimum utilization of protein.

Community support for care of the adolescent mother. Before 1960 the care of adolescent parents was centered in maternity residences for unmarried mothers, operated in many cases by either the Salvation Army or the Florence Crittendon organizations (Appendix C). In the 1960s and 1970s the age of the mother, rather than the legitimacy aspects of the parenthood, became the focus of attention. As a result, community programs with a triad of services—medical, social, and educational—were established. In 1978 Congress passed Public Law 95-625 to improve coordination and linkage between community agencies working with pregnant or parenting adolescents. In 1982 the Act was incorporated into the Maternal and Child Services Block Grant. The 1982 Act placed more emphasis on families, adoption alternatives, research, and evaluation. Federal funding for the various projects is currently being curtailed. Budget cuts may also reduce public health nursing services from health departments, social workers in hospitals and clinics, and Medicaid for prenatal care during a first pregnancy. Child care programs are also vulnerable to budget cuts.

Adolescent clinics. Because of the circumstances of adolescent pregnancy, programs specifically addressing the problems of the adolescent are being developed across the country (Appendix C). Clinics for adolescents are better equipped to provide health care ser-vices that are responsive to the teenager's unique needs. They also provide for supportive associations with the father of the child and with the girl's parents or other authority figures. They utilize a multidisciplinary team of nurse-midwives, physicians, nurses, nutritionists, and social workers. The outcomes of lower recidivism and increased birth weights are two indicators of their effectiveness (Chanis and others, 1979; Doyle and Widhalm, 1979; Peoples and Barrett, 1979; Neeson and others: 1983; Osofsky, 1985).

Nursing Care: The Nursing Process

Many interacting biologic and social factors affect the quality of human reproduction, and these in turn are influenced by the preconceptional, maternity, and neonatal care that is made available. The adolescent and her offspring are particularly vulnerable to the risks inherent in pregnancy and parenthood. This is a result of circumstances characteristic of her age group, such as psychologic immaturity, economic dependency, poor nutritional status, lack of education, inadequate or delayed medical care, and political ineffectiveness. For these reasons the care of the adolescent parent requires the concerted effort of physicians, nurses, nutritionists, and social workers. The team approach has proved to be effective in the care of young teenage mothers (Osofsky, 1985). The nursing process—assessment, formulation of nursing diagnoses, plan, implementation, and evaluation—reflects the particular needs of the adolescent client.

Assessment. Assessment of the adolescent mother parallels that of the older woman. Assessment is individualized to meet the needs of the pregnant teenager in areas in which she is particularly vulnerable.

Physical complications of the mother and child. Teenage mothers appear to be at higher risk than the older woman for anemia, abruptio placenta, and pregnancy-induced hypertension. Careful determination of baseline blood pressure is necessary since teenagers have lower systolic and diastolic pressures than older women. A teenager could be in serious jeopardy for eclampsia with a BP reading of 140/90.

During labor and delivery the young teenager suffers from dystocia more frequently than the older teenager or woman. Therefore the incidence of cesarean delivery is higher. Prematurity, SGA, and perinatal mortality are also increased. The risk of maternal mortality is 60—higher for pregnant teenagers under age 15 than for women in their early 20s (Carey and others, 1983).

Life style. The life style of many pregnant teenagers includes abuse of alcohol, smoking, and substance abuse (Chapter 28). The sexually transmitted diseases—gonorrhea, syphilis, genital herpes, and chlamydia—are common risks in this group. Nutritional problems stemming from the current "in" diet for teenagers can compromise both the mother and fetus (Osofsky, 1985).

Socioeconomic problems. Many teenage mothers come from a socially and economically deprived group. Use of health care facilities and compliance with health care measures may not be part of their perception of what health is or of how to maintain health.

Self-concept problems. The pregnant adolescent and mother is particularly sensitive to the attitudes and actions of persons in her support system (Mercer, 1985). These people include parents, boyfriends, or husbands, and health personnel. Mercer (1985) notes that assessment of the following can provide a basis for supportive care:

1. How the mother perceives her role
2. Who is helpful to her
3. How she views her infant

Nursing diagnoses. The information gathered during physical examinations, interviews, and laboratory analysis of specimens is analyzed, and nursing diagnoses are formulated. Nursing diagnoses relevant to the adolescent parent might include:

1. Potential fetal compromise* related to inadequate placental perfusion secondary to pregnancy-induced hypertension (PIH).
2. Knowledge deficit related to nutritional needs of the mother and baby during pregnancy
3. Potential noncompliance with care related to substance abuse
4. Potential infant care deficit* related to ignorance of infant's growth and developmental needs
5. Disturbance in self-concept related to inability to relate to own mother

Plan. The plan of care reflects the adolescent mother's need for increased surveillance, complying with health care measures, and feelings of positive self-worth. The care begins as early as possible in the prenatal period and extends through the formative period of the new family.

Goals. The goals for care of pregnant adolescents parallel those for care of all pregnant women: to assist them in experiencing a physically safe and emotionally satisfying pregnancy and to promote optimum health in their offspring. Care of teenage mothers also includes the following goals:

1. Encourage early prenatal care.
2. Provide comprehensive obstetric, psychosocial, and outreach services in one setting.

---

*Diagnosis not included by NANDA, 1986.

3. Use creative forms of health care delivery to maximize services to all pregnant adolescents and their families.

Implementation. Nurses assume various roles during their contacts with the adolescent client. They act as support persons, teachers/counselors/advocates, and technicians.

Nursing roles

Support person. The characteristics of persons who work with pregnant adolescents are very important. They need to have come to terms with their own sexuality to be able to maintain a nonjudgmental approach. They must be genuinely interested in the adolescent, as well as being enthusiastic, warm, caring individuals able to view adolescents as young persons involved in an exciting growth period. They need to accept the adolescent as someone willing to respond to a concerned adult and who basically wants to be accepted and successful. Nurses need to be able to listen and to respond with honest answers, to be available when needed, and to be capable of accepting repeated "testing" by the adolescent. They need to be able to create a safe and stable environment that engenders trust. Such an environment will enable the professional to determine the adolescent's real problems and to set realistic goals.

Teacher/counselor/advocate. Nurses who work with pregnant adolescents need to be knowledgeable concerning (1) the physical attributes of the adolescent and her developmental needs, (2) the adolescent's maturational level relative to personality and cognitive development, (3) maternal responses to pregnancy and the adolescent's interpretation of them, and (4) the cues that indicate stress in the adolescent and difficulties in parenting.

Nurses working with adolescents need to be adept in using a variety of teaching strategies. Group discussions are effective because adolescents have a strong need for peer contact and acceptance. However, because of the immaturity of the participants the nurse will often need to act as leader. Question boxes and anonymous pretests are devices that reveal gaps in knowledge or belief in myths. Demonstrations by the nurse, with group members exhibiting the same skill, are an effective means of assessing the teenager's abilities.

As counselors and advocates, nurses are concerned with the adolescent's ability to make decisions, to explore the risks and consequences of her actions, and to assume responsibility for her behavior. Some of the techniques used to encourage growth in these areas include having the adolescent set up a discussion group, decorate a child care space, select a menu, plan a day for herself and her infant, and talk over solutions to problems. Independent function is encouraged; the nurse acts as a catalyst in solving problems, but the problem solving belongs to the adolescent.

Another area in which the adolescent requires assistance is in helping her separate herself from her baby so that she can see the child's unique needs. Information relative to child development and to infant caretaking activities is basic to this goal.

Technician. Nurses can act as role models for adolescent parents in the care of themselves and their infants. Areas that are particularly important to the mother are emphasis on healthy life styles, cleanliness, and good eating habits. The nurse can help the young mother become skillful in taking care of the daily needs of her infant. The nurse's physical assessment skills can be taught to the parent so that she becomes more knowledgeable about her child's needs.

Prenatal period. The adolescent is considered to be at risk during her pregnancy. There is an increase in scheduled prenatal visits. Effort is expended to encourage prompt attendance at the clinic; lapses in attendance are followed up by telephone calls or personal contacts.

Prenatal classes. The content of prenatal classes is chosen with the adolescent's needs in mind. Content relating to maternal adaptations during pregnancy should be presented in terms of how the adolescent can adjust to changes. For example, exercises to promote posture, the care of skin, hair, and nails, and hygiene for increased perspiration and vaginal secretions are discussed. Concrete examples of "what to do" and "what not to do" are needed.

Information about what happens during labor and delivery and how pain is controlled requires considerable emphasis. Opportunities to discuss feelings and fears with other adolescents who have experienced birth are welcome. Basic information about sex and reproduction is needed to ensure accuracy of the adolescent's knowledge in this area. Birth control information should be included in prenatal classes and presented realistically and nonjudgmentally. Adolescents welcome information about infant care but need help to see the usefulness of information given about child growth and development.

Nutritional counseling. Adolescence is a period of developing independence. Symbols of home—milk, fresh fruits and vegetables, and a "square meal"—if these were present, are associated with dependency and as such may be threatening (e.g., "peanut butter is for children"). Often there is the desire to "be free" to choose "forbidden" foods. Peers congregate at the hamburger stand; soda, hamburgers, and french fries may be supplemented with candy bars.

The young married adolescent may have just learned how to cook. This achievement, as well as her desire to please her husband and meet his preferences, must be considered in nutrition counseling. Supporting her inner desire to assert independence during nutrition counseling sessions lends support to the overall developmental task of this period: movement from the role of child to that of adult. Listen and allow her to talk. Build on what she and her family already know and practice. Reinforce sound dietary patterns and acknowledge adaptations that are willingly made. In planning a teaching strategy to meet the objectives of nutrition counseling, the nurse must first set realistic goals such as the following:

1. To support the pregnant adolescent's psychosocial move toward independence
2. To increase her knowledge of nutrients and daily allowances
3. To teach her how to plan diets for herself and her family
4. To teach her how to select foods to meet nutritional needs, personal preferences, budget requirements, and seasonal availability
5. To teach her how to prepare foods to ensure optimum nutritive value

Of necessity these goals go beyond the immediate objectives of a healthy pregnancy, an uneventful labor, and a full-term, healthy infant whose weight and maturity are appropriate for gestational age. Subsequently, the infant grows and develops normally. Recent animal research has disclosed that two generations are required to counteract the mental and physical retardation resulting from protein deficiency during pregnancy. The young mother who improves her own and her family's dietary patterns is building the foundation for a healthier beginning for generations to follow.

The relationship between sound nutrition and physical appearance can be used to gain the attention of adolescents (and perhaps older women as well) for nutrition education. Frequently the condition and appearance of the skin, hair, and nails are uppermost in the minds of adolescents. Body contours in both the male and female adolescent and muscular development in the male teenager are selling points for good nutrition.

Labor period. The adolescent in labor should have the support of a knowledgeable coach, whether husband, boyfriend, parent, or nurse. Many teenagers come to labor lacking preparation; they are fearful and often alone. If they are admitted early in the first stage, teaching about relaxation with contractions, ambulation, side-lying positions, and comfort measures can be accomplished (Unit 4). According to Mercer (1979) the teenager's rights to grant informed consent and to refuse treatments must be continually acknowledged. This is also true of her right to be informed of her progress and of both her own and her infant's health status. Recognizing the rights of youthful parents fosters their self-esteem and personal development.

Today most adolescents keep their infants and are responsive to the staff's sharing in their delight and joy. For these young parents, efforts to promote parent-child attachment are particularly important.

Postdelivery period. Physically the adolescent mother will require the same care as any woman who has delivered an infant. Increased emphasis on teaching self-care and breast examination is warranted. Explicit directions as to follow-up care for herself and her infant are required. The need for continued assessment of her parenting abilities during the postdelivery period is essential if needed support is to be forthcoming. Although the nurse may be responsive to cues of parenting ability evidenced in the prenatal period, these findings are not as predictive as the cues noted during the reality phase of parenthood.

If possible the young mother and child are placed in a rooming-in accommodation so that the process of mothering the child can be started as early as possible. This support needs to be sustained after the mother and child return home. The process of continued care should include home visit and group sessions for discussion of infant care or parenting problems. Research indicates that outreach programs that are concerned with parent-child interactions, child injuries, and instances of failure to thrive and that provide prompt and effective community intervention do prevent more serious subsequent problems (Gray and others, 1979).

The adolescent who has an infant who was born prematurely or who is small-for-gestational-age (SGA) may find it extremely difficult to reconcile this tiny, scrawny infant with her fantasized baby. Her feelings of helplessness when she contemplates the care of a healthy term infant are compounded when she is introduced to her child in the intensive care unit. It may be impossible for her to perceive herself as mothering such an infant. The additional care needed by the infant can overwhelm the coping mechanisms she had built up so trustingly in the prenatal period. The consequent alienation of mother and infant may never be overcome. Intensive teaching and continuous support programs are essential if both the young mother and her vulnerable infant are not to be overwhelmed.

As noted earlier the young adolescent is not able to establish a family unit for herself or her child. The interdependence possible in such a unit is denied her. If the young mother and her child are incorporated into the older family unit, the process in which she was

moving from dependent to interdependent behavior must be adjusted to accommodate an essentially dependent individual. Persons who provide counseling that involves the parents of the young mother seek to set realistic goals for developing the independence of the adolescent. Topics for open discussions among all persons concerned should include infant care responsibilities, the teenager's need to continue her education, and her need to work toward maturity. The adolescent's parents will need support as well, since they face a new set of responsibilities and tasks. They, too, in a sense, must adjust a fantasy to an actual child.

When assistance is given to a young mother, efforts are made to determine her feelings toward her infant, the quality of the interaction between mother and infant, her knowledge of and attitude toward infant caretaking activities, and her understanding of her infant's growth and developmental needs. Many young mothers pattern their practice on what they themselves experienced. It is vital, therefore, to determine the kind of support that those close to these young mothers are able or prepared to give and the kinds of community aid that can supplement this support. The sample interview questions developed by Poole (1976) help the nurse to obtain information (box, p. 960). The information can serve as the data base for the supportive care needed by the adolescent parent and her child.

Evaluation. The maternity nurse needs to evaluate the care she provides to the adolescent client to see how effective her nursing actions have been. As with all pregnant women, the plan of care will have to be redesigned to meet the unique needs of the individual adolescent client. The maternity nurse has the responsibility of becoming involved in the increasing health needs of the teenage mother.

The following descriptions of three 17-year-old girls illustrate the differences in attitude, acceptance of the pregnancy, readiness for parenthood, and amount and kind of outside support available.

■ Case 1. Sharon, 17 years old and with an attractive, outgoing personality, was married 3 months before the birth of her baby. She was enthusiastic about attending parent-craft classes, and her husband, Bob, came to those relating to support in labor. She stated that he was to finish high school in June, 2 months before the baby was born, and she expected him to go to work immediately in a local gas station. Their parents were going to help them for 6 months by paying the rent on a small, three-room apartment, but they were expected to provide for other necessities. Bob made a cradle for the baby, and she made most of the baby clothes. They were using old furniture, but the baby had a new crib. Both families were excited about the baby and

Sample Interview Questions

Often girls your age, when they become mothers, find their lives to be different from what they had planned for themselves. They sometimes must drop out of school, and it may be hard for them to find a job they like. Plans they once had for themselves may just seem like unreachable dreams. Let's talk about how you feel regarding these things.

1. Are you going to school now? What do you feel about that?
    If necessary: Are you glad that you are? or Do you wish that you were?
2. Do you have any kind of job right now? What do you feel about it?
    If necessary: Do you like your job? Does it seem adequate to meet your needs? or Do you wish you were working?
3. What would you most like to be doing with your life right now if you could do anything that you wished?
4. What would you most like to do in the future if you had the choice of doing anything that you wanted to do? Is this a possible goal for you? What do you feel about that?

Young mothers often find their lives totally filled with school, job, and caring for their babies. Often they do not have time to do the things they like to do, such as visit with their friends, make new friends, or be with their husband or boyfriend. Sometimes their own mothers seem to use the baby as a means of controlling what their daughters do and do not do. This can sometimes be very frustrating.

5. Do you seem to be able to find time to be by yourself? What do you feel about that? What do you usually do when you have free time for yourself? What would you most like to do during this time?
6. Do you find time to be with your friends? Are you able to see them as often as you would like? What do you feel about that? Have you made any new friends since you had the baby?
    If unmarried: Have you been able to be with your boyfriend or meet and date new guys since you had the baby? What do you feel about that?
7. Do you feel that your mother puts a lot of pressure on you to do things that you should do? What do you feel about that?

Husbands or boyfriends sometimes get involved with the baby, and sometimes they do not. Young mothers often feel isolated and alone and resent the fact that the father is not helping much with the baby. Sometimes mothers feel that they do not get along with the husband or boyfriend as well as they did before the baby came.

8. Does your baby's father seem to enjoy the baby? What type of things does he do with him (her)? Change diapers? Bathe? Feed? Play? Other? Do you get enough help from him? What do you feel about that? Do you seem to be closer, less close, or about the same as you were before the baby was born? What do you feel about that?

It is important what some people think about us, but with other people we do not really care what they think. I'm going to give you a list of people and I want you to tell me whether or not they would agree with the way you take care of your baby and how you feel about whether they agree or not.

9. Mother   Social worker
   Father   Nurse
   Baby's father   Doctor
   Baby's father's parents   Church members
   Teacher   Minister or priest
   Employer   Neighbors
   Friends   Relatives
   Nutritionist

Some things about caring for the baby are fun, but others may be very irritating to a mother. I'm going to ask you about different things you do in caring for your baby and about what your baby does. Tell me what you feel about them.

10. First, feeding your baby. What do you feel about this? How much time does it usually take? Does it seem to take a lot out of you?
11. Now let's consider changing your baby's diapers. What do you feel about that?
12. How about bathing your baby?
13. How about playing with your baby? What do you feel about that? Do you find time to play with your baby often? Do you feel that it is important for you to play with her [or him]?
14. Does your baby try to annoy you sometimes? What does the baby do that really annoys you? What do you feel about that? What do you usually do about it? Do you ever find that you need to punish your baby? What types of things does your baby do that need punishment? How do you usually punish your baby when this is necessary?

Reprinted with permission of the publisher of Pediatric Nursing. From Poole, C.J.: Pediatr. Nurs. 2:7, Mar. Apr. 1976.

nonjudgmental in their attitudes toward Sharon and her husband.

Sharon had a normal pregnancy and delivery. She was pleased and happy with her baby and found caring for the child rewarding. Bob did well in his job and accepted his new responsibilities. When they began to feel too confined to home and child care, the young couple decided that Sharon could supplement the family income by caring for the neighbors' children,

rather than Bob's getting a second nighttime job, since they needed the time to be together. The additional money would be spent on recreation for themselves.

■ Case 2. Mary Lou, 17 years old, was a small, fragile-looking young woman. Mary Lou was the youngest of four sisters, all of whom were married and away from home. She had numerous relatives—aunts, uncles, and cousins—in the vicinity. Both her mother and father worked.

Mary Lou never divulged the name of the father of her child. She had no intention of giving the baby up for adoption, she intended to stay home and care for it herself. She refused to attend group classes but was eager and willing for the nurse to teach her individually. When she was taken on a tour of the hospital facilities, she clung to the nurse and needed much reassurance and mothering. The birth was normal, and Mary Lou had a baby boy. This was an occasion for great family rejoicing, since there had not been a boy for three generations, and her sisters had had girls. Mary Lou came to the hospital with a suitcase containing pretty clothes for herself and lovely baby clothes. The extended family accompanied her to the hospital and were there to greet the new baby. On the first visit to the home, the nurse was extremely aware of the overwhelming presence of the family, particularly Mary Lou's father. Mary Lou was feeding the baby his bottle in a correct but perfunctory manner. Subsequent visits found her increasingly trying to isolate herself. The nurse encouraged Mary Lou to seek additional counseling because she was concerned with Mary Lou's lack of affective response. Mary Lou refused, and within a week ran away from home, leaving the baby boy behind.

■ Case 3. Betty, 17 years old, was an overweight young woman. She refused to wear maternity clothes and bought herself an overlarge dress in a dark-brown material with small red flowers. She took no other interest in her appearance. She talked repeatedly about how the father of the child had taken advantage of her, that she was a good girl, and that "he was bad." The baby was to be put up for adoption. She refused to discuss her relationships with her parents, who lived in another city.

Betty had a long, difficult labor. At one time she struck the nurse who was caring for her and screamed for the nurse to "get this monster out of me." She refused to see the baby or to talk about the child. She appeared to deny the whole experience. When the time came for her to return to her home, the nurse accompanied her to the bus. She boarded the bus, an overweight girl in an unattractive, dark-brown dress. The bus pulled away; the nurse waved, but Betty did not look back.

It is obvious that to each of these teenagers, pregnancy had a different meaning; their perceptions of themselves varied, as did their needs. A stereotyped approach to the young pregnant woman is no more successful than a similar approach to the older one.

Adolescent Father

Trends. The National Center for Health Statistics reported that in 1979, of the infants born to adolescent mothers, 20% had fathers under 20 years of age. Of all infants born in the United States in 1979, 135,581 infants had fathers less than 20 years of age. The majority of these were in their late teens. Most fathers are in the older age brackets.

Factors. The effect of pregnancy and parenthood on adolescent fathers has recently become an area of nursing concern. Three major factors have prompted interest in the problems of these young parents.

1. The critical role of the father in the development of a child has been demonstrated (Frodi and Lamb, 1978; Lamb, 1976; Lamb, 1981; Parke and O'Leary, 1975; Parke and others, 1980).

2. Health programs have been developed that consider the needs of both the adolescent mother and the adolescent father.

3. The role of the father in the birth process has changed. Fathers are now encouraged to be participants in birth. Responsibilities and rights of fathers are more accepted. For example, the federal government expects the unwed mother to attempt to gain child support from the father of the child before it will grant financial assistance (Moore, 1981). A father has the legal right to petition for custody of his child if the mother wishes to place the baby for adoption (Panner and Evans, 1975).

Nursing care. The adolescent father, as well as the adolescent mother, is faced with immediate developmental crises, that is, completing the developmental tasks of adolescence and making a transition to parenthood. If the young couple marry, a third stress is added—transition to marriage. The long-range effects of premature parenthood are related to delayed educational and vocational attainment and to lack of stability in marriage.

If at all possible, the father is approached through his pregnant partner. Some clinics make clear that the pregnant adolescent will bring her partner to the clinic and that he will take an active interest in the birth process. At other times the father needs to be contacted directly. Data needed for inclusion of the young father in all aspects of the care are based on the assessment of four areas; (1) the future of the couple together, (2) the adequacy of coping, (3) educational and vocational goals, and (4) the adequacy of health education knowledge (Elster, 1982 a, and b).

Adolescent fathers (as all fathers) need support to discuss their emotional responses to the pregnancy. These may include pleasure, ambivalence, or anger. Counseling needs to be reality oriented. Topics such as child care and expense, parenting skills, and the father's role in the birth experience need to be explored. Teenage fathers also need knowledge of reproductive physiology and birth control options.

The adolescent mother's boyfriend, as well as her family, have an impact on how she will deal with her pregnancy, labor and delivery, and subsequent parenthood. The adolescent partner has usually been involved in an ongoing relationship with the young mother. In many instances he plays an important role in the decisions she faces in pregnancy. He may influence her decision to continue the pregnancy or have an abortion and to keep the child or place the child for adoption.

The nurse supports the young father by helping him develop realistic perceptions of his role as "father to a child." The nurse encourages his use of coping mechanisms that are not detrimental to his, his partner's, and his child's well-being. The nurse enlists support systems, parents, and professional agencies on his behalf.

Summary

Much has still to be done before the problem of adolescent pregnancy and its sequelae for infant, mother, family, and society in general is solved. Cooperative effort on personal, local, and national levels is mandatory. In spite of the development of many successful programs, adolescent pregnancy remains the most pressing problem in maternity nursing care today.

References

Adolescent Family Life Act of 1982, Title XX, Section 2001(b)3.

Baldwin, W.: Adolescent pregnancy and childbearing: an overview, Semin. Perinatol. 5:1, Jan. 1981.

Card, J.J., and Wise, L.L.: Teenage mothers and teenage fathers: the impact of early childbearing on the parents' personal and professional lives, Fam. Plann. Perspect. 10:299, 1978.

Carey, W., McCann-Sanford, T., and Davidson, E., Jr.: Adolescent age and obstetric risk. In McAnarney, E., editor: Premature adolescent pregnancy and parenthood, New York, 1983, Grune & Stratton.

Chanis, M., and others: Adolescent pregnancy, J. Nurse Midwife, 24:18, May/June 1979.

Colletta,N.D., and Gregg, C.H.: Adolescent mothers' vulnerability to stress, J. Nerv. Ment. Dis. 169:50, 1981.

Committee on Adolescence, American Academy of Pediatrics: Statement on teenage pregnancy, Pediatrics 63:795, 1979.

DeLissovoy, V.: Child care by adolescent parents, Child Today 2:23, 1973.

Doyle, M.B., and Widhalm, M.V.: Midwifing the adolescent at Lincoln's Hospital's teenage clinics, J. Nurse Midwife. 24:27, July/Aug. 1979.

Elster, A.B., and Panzarine, S.: Teenage fathers: a trajectory of stress over time. Presented at the Society for Adolescent Medicine, New Orleans, Oct. 29, 1983.

Elster, A.B.: Effects of pregnancy and parenthood on adolescent fathers and implications for clinical intervention, J. Calif. Perinatal Assoc. 2(2):44, 1982a.

Elster, A.B., and Lamb, M.E.: Adolescent fathers: a group potentially at risk for parenting failure, Infant Ment. Health J. 3:148, 1982b.

Elster, A.B., and others: Parental behavior of adolescent mothers, Pediatrics 71:494, 1983.

Erkan, K.A., and others: Juvenile pregnancy role of physiologic maturity, Md. State Med. J. 20:50, 1971.

Field, T.M., and others: Teenage, lower-class black mothers and their preterm infants: an intervention of developmental follow-up, Child Dev. 51:426, 1980.

Food and Nutrition Board: Recommended daily dietary allowances, Washington, D.C., 1970, National Academy of Science–National Research Council.

Forbes, G.B.: Pregnancy in the teenager: biologic aspects. In McAnarney, E.R., and Stickle, G., editors: Pregnancy and childbearing during adolescence: research priorities for the 1980s, New York, 1981, Alan R. Liss.

Frank, D., and others: Nutrition in adolescent pregnancy, J. Calif. Perinatal Assoc. 3(1):21, 1981.

Frodi, A.M., and Lamb, M.E.: Fathers' and mothers' responses to the faces and cries of normal and premature infants, Dev. Psychol. 14:490, 1978.

Gray, J.D., and others: Prediction and prevention of child abuse, Semin. Perinatol. 3(1):85, 1979.

Hatcher, S.L.: Understanding adolescent pregnancy and abortion, Primary Care 3:407, 1976.

Hollingsworth, D., and Kotchen, J.: Gynecologic age and its relation to neonatal outcome. In McAnarney, E.R., and Stickle, G., editors: Pregnancy and childbearing during adolescence: research priorities for the 1980s, New York, 1981, Alan R. Liss.

Hollingsworth, D., and others: Impact of gynecologic age on outcome of adolescent pregnancy. In McAnarney, E.R., editor: Premature adolescent pregnancy and parenthood, New York, 1983, Grune & Stratton.

Horn, B.: Cultural beliefs and teenage pregnancy, The Nurse Practitioner 8:35, Sept. 1983.

Jarrett, G.E.: Childrearing patterns of young mothers: expectations, knowledge, and practices, M.C.N. 7(2):119, 1982.

Jones, F.A., and others: Maternal responsiveness of primiparous mothers during the postpartum period: age differences, Pediatrics 65:579, 1980.

Lamb, M.E.: Interaction between two-year-olds and their mothers and fathers, Psychol. Rep. 38:447, 1976.

Lamb, M.E.: Fathers and child development: an integrative overview. In Lamb, M.E., editor: The role of the father in child development, New York, 1981, Wiley-Interscience.

Lawrence, R.A., and Merritt, T.A.: Infants of adolescent mothers: perinatal, neonatal, and infancy outcome, Semin. Perinatol. 5(1):19, 1981.

Lawrence, R.A., and others: Aggressive behaviors in young mothers: markers of future morbidity? Pediatr. Res. 15:443, 1981.

MacDonnell, S.: Vulnerable mothers, vulnerable children: a follow-up study of unmarried mothers who kept their children, Halifax, Nova Scotia, 1981, Policy Planning and Research Division, Nova Scotia Department of Social Services.

Mercer, R.T.: The adolescent experience in labor, delivery, and early postpartum. In Mercer, R.T., editors: Perspectives on adolescent health care, New York, 1979, J.B. Lippincott Co.

Mercer, R.: Relationship of birth experience to later mothering behaviors, J. Nurse Midwife. 30:204, July/Aug. 1985.

Merritt, T., and others: The infants of adolescent mothers, Pediatr. Ann. 9:32, 1980a.

Merritt, T., and others: The infants of adolescent mothers, Pediatr. Ann. 9:100, 1980b.

Miller, H., and Merritt, A.: Fetal growth in humans, Chicago, 1979, Year Book Medical Publishers.

Moore, K.A.: Government policies related to teenage family formation and functioning: an inventory. In Ooms, T., editor: Teenage pregnancy in a family context: implications for policy, Philadelphia, 1981, Temple University Press.

National Center for Health Statistics, U.S. Department of Health and Human Services: Final natality statistics, 1978, Monthly Vital Stat. Rep. 29:1, 1980.

Neeson, J.D. and others: Pregnancy outcome for adolescents receiving prenatal care by nurse practitioners in extended roles, J. Adolesc. Health 4:94, June 1983.

Osofsky, H.: Mitigating the adverse effects of early parenthood, Contemp. OB/Gyn. 25:57, Jan. 1985.

Panner, R., and Evans, B.W.: The unmarried father revisited, J. School Health 45(5):271, 1975.

Parke, R.D., and O'Leary, L.: Father-mother-infant interaction in the newborn period: some findings, some observations, and some unresolved issues. In Riegel, K.F., and Meacham, J., editors: The developing individual in a changing world, vol. 2, The Hague, 1975, Mouton.

Parke, R.D., and others: The adolescent father's impact on the mother and child, J. Soc. Issues 36:88, 1980.

Peoples, M.D., and Barrett, A.E.: A model for the delivery of health care to pregnant adolescents, J.O.G.N. Nurs. 8(6):339, 1979.

Perkins, R.P., and others: Intensive care in adolescent pregnancy, Clin. Obstet. Gynecol. 52:179, 1978.

Poole, C.: Adolescent mothers: can they be helped? Pediatr. Nurs. 2:7, Mar./Apr. 1976.

Public Law 95-626: Amendment to Public Health Service Act, 1981.

Sahler, O.J.: Adolescent mothers: how nurturant is their parenting? In McAnarney, E.R., editor: Premature adolescent pregnancy and parenthood, New York, 1983, Grune & Stratton.

Sorosky, A.D., and others: The adoption triangle: the effects of sealed records on adoptees, birth parents and adoptive parents, New York, 1978, Anchor Press.

Vernon, M.E.L., and others: Teenage pregnancy: a prospective study of self-esteem and other sociodemographic factors, Pediatrics 72:632, 1983.

World Health Organization: Pregnancy and abortion in adolescence, tech. series no. 583, Geneva, 1975, The Organization.

Zelnick, M.: Sexual activity among adolescents: perspectives of a decade. In McAnarney, E.R., editor: Premature adolescent pregnancy and parenthood, New York, 1983, Grune & Stratton.

Zuckerman, B., and others: Neonatal outcome: is adolescent pregnancy a risk factor? Pediatrics 71:489, 1983.

Bibliography

Alexander, S.J.: Suggested services and policies related to adolescent parenthood, Washington, D.C., 1981, National Association of State Boards of Education.

Baum, D.J.: Teenage pregnancy: a handbook for teachers, parents, counselors, and kids, New York, 1980, Beaufort Books.

Baumrind, D.: Clarification concerning birth rate among teenagers, Am. Psychol. 36:528, 1981.

Berek, J.S.: Helping a patient surrender her child for adoption, Contemp. Obstet. Gynecol. 22(12):29, 1983.

Blesky, J.: Child maltreatment: an ecological integration, Am. Psychol. 35:320, 1980.

Bolton, F.G., Jr.: The pregnant adolescent: problems of premature parenthood, Beverly Hills, Calif., 1980, Sage Publications.

Bolton, F.G., Jr., and others: Child maltreatment risk among adolescent mothers, Am. J. Orthopsychiatry 50:489, 1980.

Bracken, M.B., and others: Abortion, adoption or motherhood: an empirical study of decision-making during pregnancy, Am. J. Obstet. Gynecol. 130:251, 1978.

Broman, S.H.: Long-term development of children born to teenagers. In Scott, K.G., and others, editors: Teenage parents and their offspring, New York, 1981, Grune & Stratton.

Brown, A.: Adolescents and abortion: a theoretical framework for decision-making, J.O.G.N. Nurs. 12(4):241, 1983.

Bryan-Logan, B.N., and Dancy, B.L.: Unwed pregnant adolescents—their mothers' dilemma. Nurs. Clin. North Am. 9:57, March 1974.

Burbach, C.A.: Contraception and adolescent pregnancy, J.O.G.N. Nurs. 9(5):319, 1980.

Catano, J.W.: Teenage pregnancy: a resource kit, Halifax, Nova Scotia, 1979, The Prepared Childbirth Association of Nova Scotia.

Cates, W., Jr.: Adolescent abortions in the United States, J. Adolesc. Health Care 1:18, 1980.

Chilman, C.S.: Adolescent pregnancy and childbearing: findings from research, Washington, D.C., 1980 U.S. Department of Health and Human Services.

Christensen, M.L., and others: An interdisciplinary approach to preventing child abuse, M.C.N. 9:108, 1984.

Corkum, T.: Adolescent pregnancy outcomes in Halifax-Dartmouth since 1970. Paper presented at Sexuality and the Family Conference, Halifax, Novia Scotia, June 1979.

Cornely, D.A.: Title VI funding for adolescent pregnancy: what have we learned? In McAnarney, E.R., and Stickle, G., editors: Pregnancy and childbearing during adolescence, New York, 1981, Alan R. Liss.

Daniel, W.A., Jr.: Adolescents in health and disease, St. Louis, 1977, The C.V. Mosby Co.

Daniels, M., and Manning, D.: A clinic for pregnant teens, Am. J. Nurs. 83:68, 1983.

Edwards, L.E., and others: Adolescent pregnancy prevention services in high school clinics. In Furstenberg, F.F., Jr. and others, editors: Teenage sexuality, pregnancy, and childbearing, Philadelphia, 1981, The University of Pennsylvania Press.

Edwards, M.: Teenage parents, Seattle, 1978, The Pennypress.

Elster, A.B., and McAnarney, E.R.: Medical and psychosocial risks of pregnancy and childbearing during adolescence, Pediatr. Ann. 9:89, 1980.

Elster, A.B., and Panzarine, S.: Unwed teenage fathers: emotional and health educational needs, J. Adolesc. Health Care 1:116, 1980.

Enos, R., and Hisanaga, M.: Goal setting with pregnant teenagers, Child Welfare 58:541, 1979.

Foster, S.: The one girl in ten: a self-portrait of the teenage mother, Claremont, Calif., 1981, Arbor Press.

Gallas, H.B., special issue editor: Teenage parenting: social determinants and consequences, J. Soc. Issues 36:1, Winter 1980.

Green, J.W., and others: Childrearing attitudes, observed behavior, and perception of infant temperament in adolescent versus older mothers, Pediatr. Res. 15:442, 1981.

Greydanus, D.E.: Alternatives to adolescent pregnancy: a discussion of contraceptive literature from 1960 to 1980, Semin. Perinatol. 5(1):53, 1981.

Greydanus, D.E. The health system's responsibility toward the sexually active adolescent. In Wells, C.F., and Stuart, I.R., editors: Pregnancy in adolescence: needs, problems, and management, New York, 1982, Van Nostrand Reinhold Co.

Hardy, J.B., and others: Long-range outcome of adolescent pregnancy, Clin. Obstet. Gynecol. 21:1215, 1978.

Hardy, J.B., et al.: A comprehensive approach to adolescent pregnancy. In Scott, K.G., and others, editors: Teen parents and their offspring, New York, 1981, Grune & Stratton.

Hendricks, L.E.: Unwed adolescent fathers: problems they face and their sources of social support, Adolescence 60:861, 1980.

Hendricks, L.E., and others: Help-seeking behavior among select populations of black unmarried adolescent fathers: implications for human service agencies, Am. J. Public Health 71:733, 1981.

Hibbard, B.M.: The effectiveness of antenatal education, Health Educ. Q. 38:39, 1979.

Hingson, R., and others: Effects of maternal drinking and marijuana use on fetal growth and development, Pediatrics 70:539, 1982.

Hollingsworth, D.R., and Kreutner, A.K.K.: Teenage pregnancy: solutions are evolving, N. Engl. J. Med. 303:516, 1980.

Hutchins, F.L., Jr., and others: Experience with teenage pregnancy, Obstet. Gynecol. 54:1, July 1979.

JRB Associates: Final report on national study of teenage pregnancy (mimeographed), McLean, Va., 1981, JRB Associates.

Kerckhoff, A.C., and Parrow, A.A.: The effect of early marriage on the education attainment of young men, J. Marriage Fam. 41:97, 1979.

Kinard, E.M., and Klerman, L.V.: Teenage parenting and child abuse: are they related? Am. J. Orthopsychiatry 50:481, 1980.

Klaus, M.H., and Kennell, J.H.: Parent-infant bonding, ed. 2, St. Louis, 1982, The C.V. Mosby Co.

Kreipe, R.E.: Prevention of adolescent pergnancy. In McAnarney, editor: Premature adolescent pregnancy and parenthood, New York, 1983, Grune & Stratton.

Lamb, M.E.: The father's role in the facilitation of infant mental health, Infant Ment. Health J. 1:140, 1980.

Lamb, M.E.: The development of social expectations in the first year of life. In Lamb, M.E., and Sherrod, L.R., editors: Infant social cognition: empirical and theoretical considerations, Hillsdale, N.J., 1981, Lawrence Erlbaum Associates.

Lamb, M.E., and Easterbrooks, A.: Individual differences in parental sensitivity: origins, components, and consequences. In Lamb, M.E., and Sherrod, L.R., editors: Infant social cognition: empirical and theoretical considera-

tions, Hillsdale, N.J., 1981, Lawrence Erlbaum Associates.

Landy, S.: An investigation of teenage mothers, their infants, and the resulting mother-infant dyads, Doctoral dissertation, Regina, Saskatchewan, May 1981, University of Regina.

Lane, C., and Kemp, J.: Family planning needs of adolescents, J.O.G.N. Nurs. 13(2):61s, 1984.

March of Dimes—Birth Defects Foundation, Committee on Perinatal Health: Toward improving the outcome of pregnancy, White Plains, N.Y., 1979, The Foundation.

McAnarney, E.R., and Friedman, S.B.: Experience with an adolescent health care program, Public Health Rep. 90:412, 1975.

McAnarney, E., and Thiede, H.: Adolescent pregnancy and childbearing: what we learned in the 1970s and what remains to be learned in premature adolescent pregnancy and parenthood. In McAnarney, E., editor: Premature adolescent pregnancy and parenthood, New York, 1983, Grune & Stratton.

McAnarney, E.R., and others: Teenagers evaluate their own health care, Pediatrics 55:290, 1978.

McAnarney, E., and others: Adolescent mothers and their infants, Pediatrics 73:358, 1984.

McCarthy, J.: Social consequences of childbearing during adolescence. In McAnarney, E.R., and Stickle, G., editors: Pregnancy and childbearing during adolescence: research priorities for the 1980s, New York, 1981, Alan R. Liss.

Mercer, R.T.: Becoming a mother at sixteen, M.C.N. 1:44, 1976.

Mercer, R.T.: Teenage motherhood: the first year, J.O.G.N. Nurs. 9(1)16, 1980.

Mercer, R.T.: Assessing and counseling teenage mothers during the perinatal period, Nurs. Clin. North Am. 18(2):293, 1983.

Mercer, R.T.: Adolescent motherhood: comparison of outcome with older mothers, J. Adolesc. Health Care 5:7, Jan. 1984.

Moore, K.A.: Teenage childbirth and welfare dependency, Fam. Plann. Perspect. 10:233, 1978.

Parrains, J.: L'adolescent et ses pairs: élaboration d'un programme d'assistance, L'infirmiere Canadienne, 26:40, Aug. 1984.

Paul, E.W., and Schaap, P.: Legal rights and responsibilities of pregnant teenagers and their children. In Wells C.F., and Stuart, I.R., editors: Pregnancy in adolescence: needs, problems, and management, New York, 1982, Van Nostrand Reinhold Co.

Petrella, J.: Caring for the unwed adolescent, J.O.G.N. Nurs. 7(4):22, 1978.

Phipps-Yonas, S.: Teenage pregnancy and motherhood: a review of the literature, Am. J. Orthopsychiatry 50:403, 1980.

Rosen, R.H.: Adolescent pregnancy decision-making: are parents important? Adolescence 15(5):43, 1980.

Rotheberg, B., and Varga, P.: The relationship between age of mother, child health and development, Am. J. Public Health 81:810, 1981.

Sahler, O.J.: Adolescent parenting: potential for child abuse and neglect? Pediatr. Ann. 9:120, 1980.

Sung, K., and Rothcock, D.: An alternative school for pregnant teenagers and teenage mothers, Child Welfare 59:427, 1980.

Teenage childbearing and abortion patterns: U.S., 1977, M.M.W.R. 29(14):157, 1980.

Theirreu, M.E.: Evaluating empathy skill training for parents, Social Work 9:417, Sept. 1979.

Thompson, M.E., and Kramer, M.: Methodologic standards for controlled clinical trials of early contact and maternal infant behavior, Pediatrics 73:294, March 1984.

Thompson, R., and others: Neonatal behavior of infants of adolescent mothers, Dev. Med. Child Neurol. 21:474, 1979.

Trussell, J., and Abowd, J.: Teenage mothers, labor force participation and wage rates. In Menken, J., and others, editors: Sequelae to teenage childbearing: final report, Bethesda, Md., 1979, National Institute of Child Health and Human Development.

Urman, J., and Meginnis, S.K.: The process of problem pregnancy counseling, J. Am. Coll. Health Assoc. 28:308, 1980.

Velasquez, J., and others: Intensive services help prevent child abuse, M.C.N. 9(2):113, 1984.

Widmayer, S.M., and Field, T.M.: Effects of Brazelton demonstration on early interactions of preterm infants and their teenage mothers, Infant Behav. Dev. 3:79, 1980.

Wise, S., and Grossman, F.K.: Adolescent mothers and their infants: psychological factors in early attachment and interaction, Am. J. Orthopsychiatry 50:454, 1980.

Neonatal Conditions and Complications

Early identification and prompt management are imperative in treating newborns with complications. In this chapter, several conditions are described. General and specific care is discussed for the following compromising conditions of the newborn:

- Prematurity, dysmaturity, and postmaturity
- Birth trauma
- Hypoglycemia and hypocalcemia
- Hyperbilirubinemia and Rh isoimmunization
- Congenital anomalies
- Neonatal infection

Infants with Problems Related to Gestational Age and Weight

Infants born at risk for gestational age and weight problems exhibit physiologic and pathologic states related to the degree of maturity. Modern technology has contributed to the improved survival rate and overall health of preterm infants, but problems remain. These relate to the appearance of "new" diseases such as necrotizing enterocolitis (NEC) and the survival of very tiny babies whose expectancy of a "quality life" is questionable. The plan of care for the infant born prematurely must include an understanding of infant behavior. Nursing care emphasizes the need for parental support to give the infant his or her best chance for a healthy, happy life.

Classification. Classification of infants according to **gestational age** is as follows:

1. Preterm or premature: infants born before completion of 37 weeks' gestation regardless of birth weight.
2. Term: infants born between the beginning of the thirty-eighth week and the end of the forty-second week of gestation.
3. Postterm or postmature: infants born after completion of the forty-second week of gestation.

The **weight** of the infant has a normal range for each gestational week (Figs. 31.1 and 31.2). Variations in weight may occur in the preterm, term, or postterm. Classification of infants by **weight** is as follows:

1. Large for gestational age (LGA): the infant is said to be *large for gestational age* or *large for dates* if at any week the weight is above the 90th percentile (or two or more standard deviations above the norm).
2. Appropriate for gestational age (AGA). The infant is termed *appropriate for gestational age* if the weight falls between the 10th and 90th percentile for his or her age.
3. Small for gestational age (SGA). A baby is small for gestational age if the weight is below the 10th percentile (or two or more standard deviations below the norm).

Causes of variations in weight. Common causes of LGA newborns include gestational or true maternal diabetes mellitus, maternal overnutrition, and heredity. SGA newborns may be born to mothers who smoke or mothers with hypertensive states, maternal undernutrition, anemia, or nephritis. In addition, the birth of an SGA newborn may be associated with multiple gestation, a discordant twin pregnancy, or congenital anomalies. High altitude, rubella, or intrauterine infection may predispose a woman to the birth of an SGA newborn. Fetal malnutrition, intrauterine growth retardation, and chronic fetal distress are other processes that may result in the birth of babies who are SGA.

PRETERM INFANT

The preterm infant is at risk because of immaturity of physiologic functioning and lack of reserves. The morbidity and mortality rates occurring with preterm infants are higher by three to four times than those of older infants of comparable weight (Figs. 31.3 and

Fig. 31.1

Three babies of same gestational age, with weights of 600, 1400, and 2750 g, respectively, from left to right. Their weights are plotted in Fig. 31.2 at points *A, B,* and *C*. (From Korones, S.B.: High-risk newborn infants; the basis for intensive nursing care, ed. 4, St. Louis, 1986, The C.V. Mosby Co.)

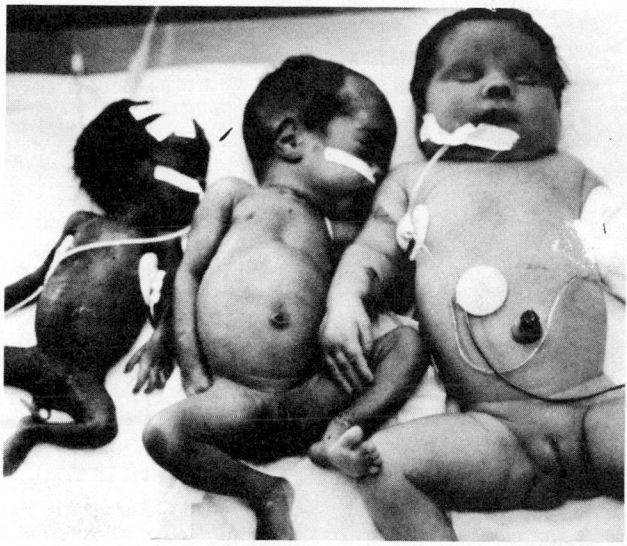

31.4). The potential problems of the preterm infant of 2000 g differ from those of the term or postterm infant of equal weight.

Potential problems. The clinical problems occuring in the preterm infant and their physiologic bases are summarized in Table 31.1.

Prognosis for preterm infants. Although it is impossible to predict with complete accuracy the growth and developmental potential of each premature newborn, some findings support an anticipated favorable outcome (Bennett, Robinson and Sells, 1983). The growth and development landmarks are corrected for gestational age.

The age of a preterm newborn is corrected by adding the gestational age and the postdelivery age. For example, if an infant was born at 32 weeks' gestation 4 weeks ago, the infant would be considered 36 weeks of age. Six months after the birth date, the child's corrected age is 4 months. Responses are evaluated against the norm expected for a 4-month-old infant.

Favorable findings that support the prediction of a growth and development pattern within the norm include the following:

1. At discharge from the hospital, which usually occurs between 37 and 40 weeks after the LMP the

Fig. 31.2

Intrauterine growth status for gestational age and according to appropriateness of growth. Weights of infants shown in Fig. 31.1 are plotted at points *A, B,* and *C*. (Courtesy Mead Johnson & Co., Evansville, Indiana. Modified from Battaglia, F.C., and Lubchenco, L.O.: J. Pediatr. 71:59, 1967.)

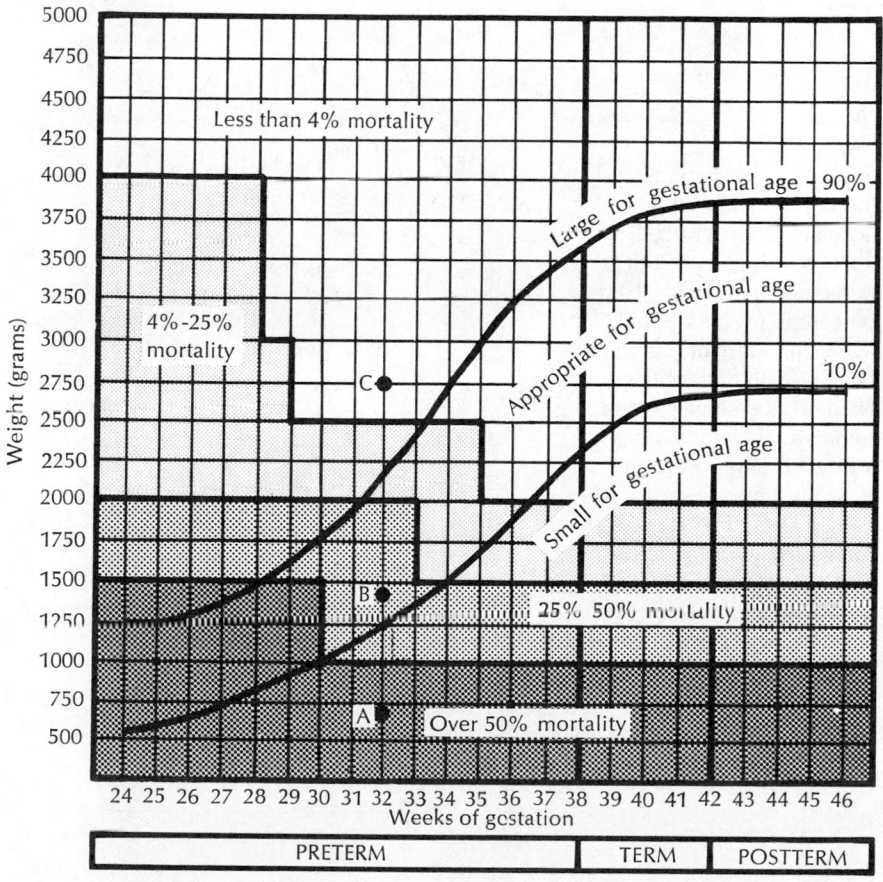

Fig. 31.3
Zones of mortality and morbidity in relation to both weight and gestation. (From Behrman, R.E., and Babson, S.G.: Am. J. Dis. Child. 121:486, 1971. Copyright 1971, American Medical Association.)

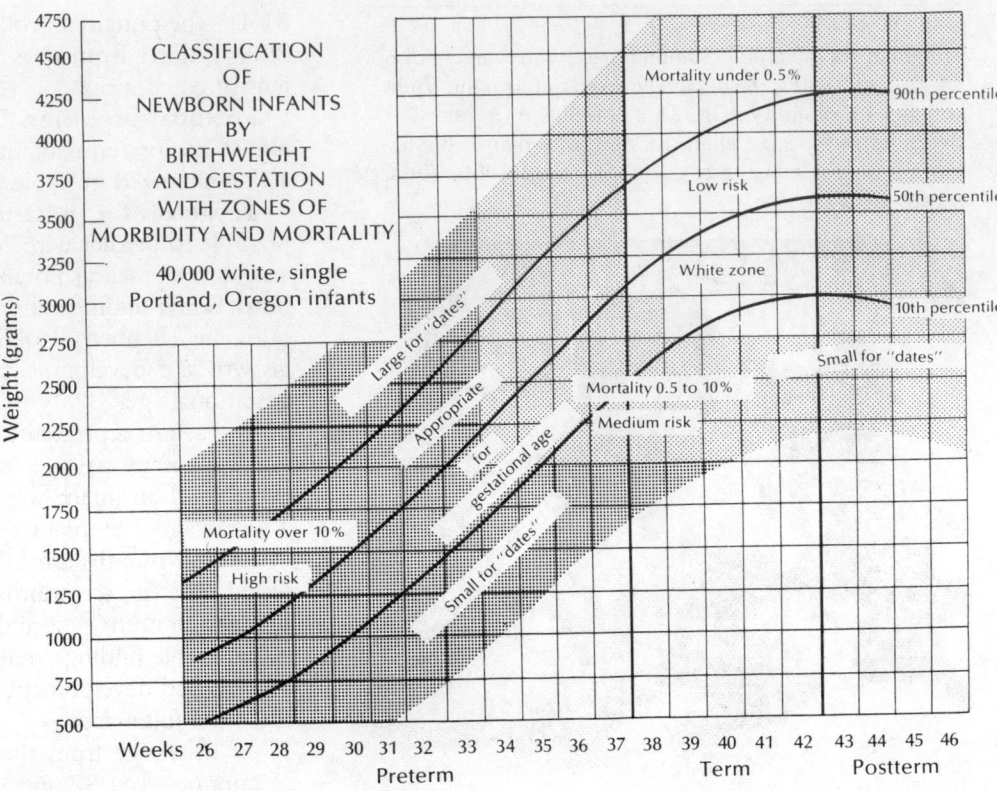

Fig. 31.4
Important associations and morbidity factors of accelerated or reduced fetal growth above 90th percentile and below 10th percentile for gestational age using Portland curves. Fetal growth data obtained from 40,000 single, white, middle-class infants born at sea level. (From Babson, S.G., and others: Diagnosis and management of the fetus and neonate at risk, ed. 4, St. Louis, 1980, The C.V. Mosby Co.)

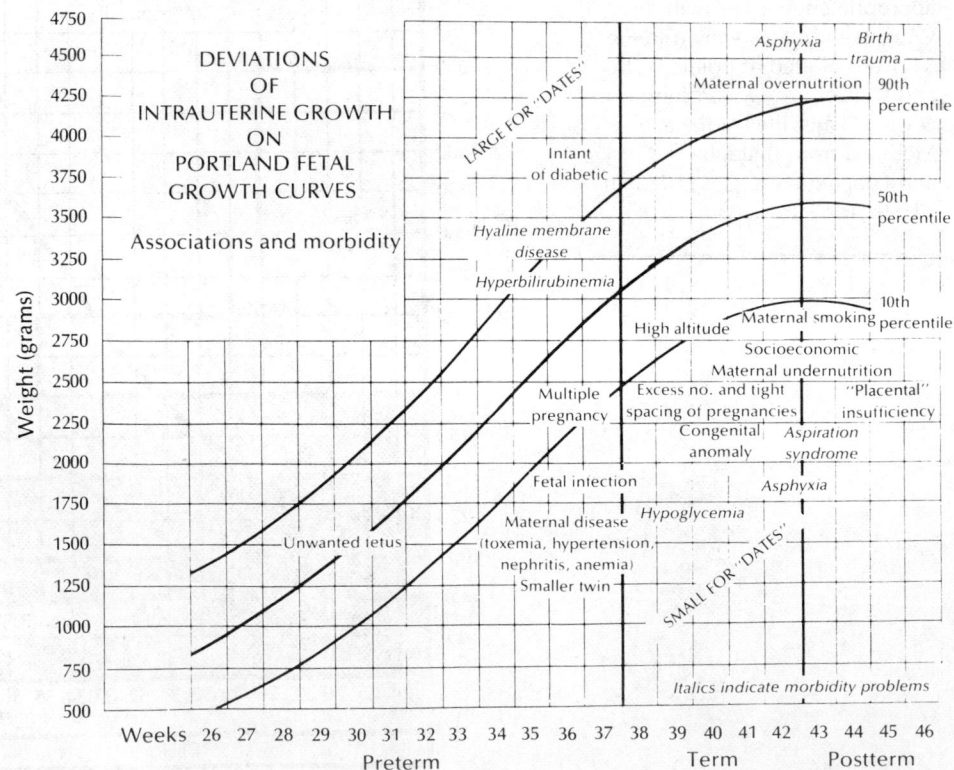

Table 31.1

Preterm Infant's Potential Problems and Their Physiologic Bases

Potential Problem	Physiologic Bases
Initiating and maintaining respirations	Paucity of functional alveoli; incomplete aeration of lungs caused by deficient surfactant Smaller lumen and greater collapsibility or obstruction of respiratory passages Weakness of respiratory musculature Insufficient calcification of bony thorax Absent or weak gag reflex Immature and friable capillaries in brain and lungs Few functional alveoli in infants less than 28 weeks' gestational age (usually nonviable); marginal function in infants at 29-30 weeks.
Maintaining body temperature	Large surface area in relation to body weight (mass) Absent or poor reflex control of skin capillaries (no shiver response) Small, inadequate muscle mass activity; absent or minimal flexion of extremities on body Meager insulating subcutaneous fat Friable capillaries and immature temperature regulating center in brain The smaller the infant, the more difficult it is for her or him to maintain normal body temperature.
Maintaining adequate nutrition	Mechanical feeding problems • Absent or weak sucking and swallow reflexes; unsynchronized • Absent or weak gag and cough reflexes • Small stomach capacity • Immature cardiac sphincter (stomach) • Lax abdominal musculature Absorption and assimilation problems • Paucity of stored nutrients: vitamins A and C; calcium, phosphorus, iron; loss of fat and fat-soluble vitamins in stool • Immature absorption, decreased amount of HCL • Impaired metabolism (enzyme systems) or enzyme pathology.
Maintaining CNS function	Birth trauma: damage to immature structures Fragile capillaries and impaired coagulation process; prolonged prothrombin time Recurrent anoxic episodes Tendency toward hypoglycemia
Maintaining renal function	Impaired renal clearance of metabolites and drugs Inability to maintain acid-base, fluid, and electrolyte homeostasis Impaired ability to concentrate urine
Resisting infection	Paucity of stored nutrients from mother Paucity of stored immunoglobulins from mother Impaired ability to synthesize antibodies Thin skin and fragile capillaries near surface Impaired ability to muster white blood cells
Resisting hematologic problems	Increased capillary friability and permeability Low plasma prothrombin levels (increased tendency to bleed) Relatively slowed erythropoietic activity in bone marrow Relatively increased rate of hemolysis Loss of blood for laboratory specimens
Maintaining musculoskeletal integrity	Weak, underdeveloped muscles Immature skeletal system (bones, joints) Meager subcutaneous fat with its cushioning effect
Maintaining retinal integrity	Immature vascular structures in retina Need for oxygen therapy

infant is assessed for the following characteristics:

a. When prone, the infant can raise the head and is able to hold the head parallel with the body when tested for head lag response. (When pulled up by the hands, the infant's head lags, but then the head and chest will be in line as the upright position is reached. This alignment will be held momentarily before the head falls forward [pull-to-sit or traction reflex]).

b. When the infant is hungry, he or she cries with vigor.

c. The growth grid shows appropriate weight gain and pattern of weight gain.

d. The neurologic examination reveals appropriate responses for corrected age. The retinas appear normal.

2. At 39 to 40 weeks the infant is able to focus on the examiner's or parent's face and is able to follow with her or his eyes.

3. At the corrected age of 6 and 12 months, the infant is assessed again for age-appropriate responses.

The infant may have continued problems if she or he displays any of the following behaviors:

- Was and continues to be a poor eater
- Is irritable
- Displays sensory, perceptual, intellectual, or motor deviations in development
- Displays or develops hypertonia or hypotonia

These behaviors must be interpreted with caution and the infant reevaluated by an interdisciplinary team at frequent intervals. Parents will need continued support and attention should these signs appear. Minor behavioral deviations are diagnosed also so that the parents can be assisted in their understanding and acceptance of the child. Deviations such as clumsiness, varying degrees of incoordination, slowness in reading and writing, and similar problems may be distressing to the child, parents, and other family members.

Parental adaptation to preterm infant. Parents who experience the premature birth of their infant have a totally different experience from parents giving birth to a full-term infant (Sammons and Lewis, 1985). Because of this difference, parental attachment and adaptation to the parental role will be different also. Table 31.2 summarizes the key differences in the two experiences.

Parental tasks. Parents face a number of psychologic tasks before effective relationships and parenting patterns can evolve. These tasks include:

1. *Anticipatory grief over the potential loss of an infant.* The parent grieves (see Chapter 26) in preparation for the infant's possible death, although the parent clings tenuously to the hope that the child will survive. This begins during labor and lasts until the infant dies or shows evidence of surviving.

2. *Acceptance by the mother of her failure to deliver a healthy, full-term infant.* Grief and depression typify this phase, which persists until the infant is out of danger and is expected to survive.

3. *Resumption of the process of relating to the infant.* As the baby begins to improve—gains weight, feeds by nipple, and is weaned from the incubator—the parent can begin the process of developing attachment to the infant that was interrupted by the infant's precarious condition at birth (Als and Brazelton, 1981; Goldberg, 1979).

4. *Learning how this baby differs in special needs and growth patterns.* Another parental task is to learn, understand, and accept this infant's caretaking needs and growth and development expectations (Sammons and Lewis, 1985).

5. *Adjusting the home environment to the needs of the*

Table 31.2

Differences in Experiences of Preterm and Term Delivery

Full-term Delivery	Premature Delivery
The parents have gone through the full developmental process of a 40-week pregnancy.	The parents have not completed the psychological and emotional growth of a 40-week-gestation pregnancy.
The infant is healthy and has the physiologic, motor, and state control and social capacities common to full-term infants.	The infant is small, immature, often physically unattractive, and sick.
The parents have an enormous surge of emotion postpartum, which is derived from a combination of feelings of achievement and pride in their own success and fulfilled expectations about the intactness and healthiness of their infant.	The parents are often overwhelmed by feelings of failure, loss, fear, and sadness.
Full-term infants in the first 1 to 2 hours after birth have a period of alert time during which they open their eyes, look around, nurse, and generally behave like or exceed most parent's fantasies of a little baby.	The infant has none of the cute, appealing behaviors of a full-term infant. He is not alert, does not suck, and may be too sick to be held at all.

From Sammons, W., and Lewis, J.: Premature babies: a different beginning, St. Louis, 1985, The C.V. Mosby Co.

Fig. 31.5

Mother interacting with her baby using touch. Oxygen hood and overhead warmer are being used in place of incubator.

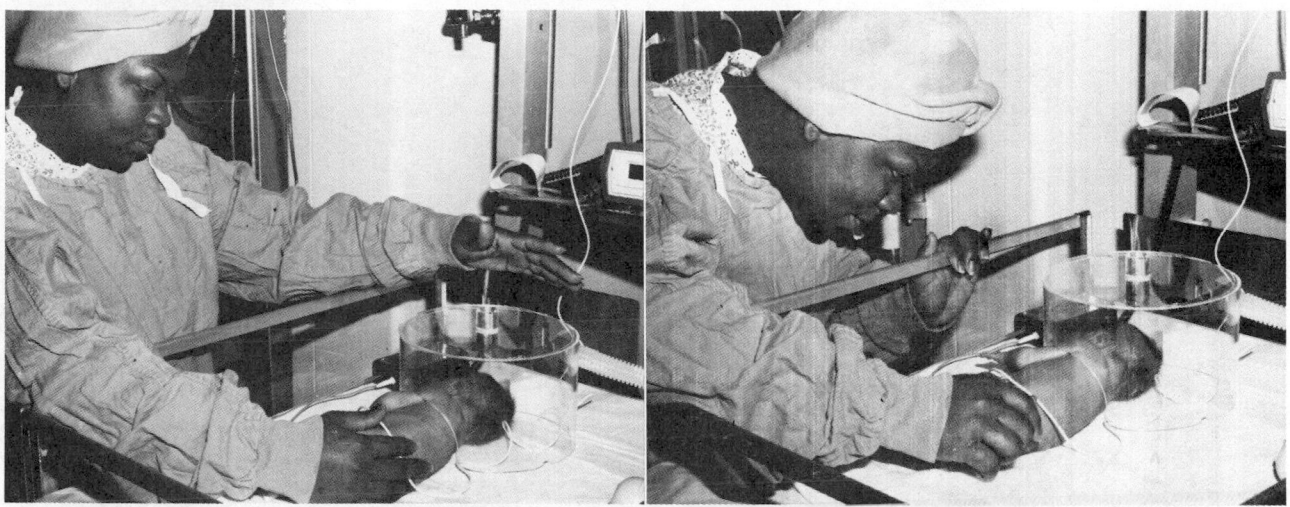

new infant. Grandparents and brothers and sisters also react to the birth of the preterm infant. Parents must reconcile the grief of grandparents and the bewilderment and anger of brothers and sisters at the disproportionate amount of parental time absorbed by the newborn.

Parental responses. Two different approaches noted by Newman (1980) are *coping through commitment and coping through distance.* With the first approach parents take each day as it comes, recognizing and accepting the lessened responses of their infant and noting the gradual progress in their child's condition. With the second approach the parents pull away from emotional attachment to the infant; they postpone becoming attached until the infant is in better health.

Parents have been observed to progress through stages as they spend more time with their infants. In the first stage they maintain an en face position, stroking and touching their infant (Figs. 31.5 and 31.6). In the second stage they assume some child care activities—feeding, bathing, changing the infant (Fig. 31.7). In the third stage the infant becomes a person and is seen as a whole child (Fig. 31.8) (Schraeder, 1980). Sosa and Grua (1982) reported a personal communication with Brazelton in which he correlated parental behaviors with the previously noted three stages. In the first stage parents ask about *chemical data,* such as "What is his bilirubin today?" In the second stage they note their baby yawning, sneezing, hiccoughing, *reflexes* that mark their infant as human. At this time the infant is still not "claimed." In later stages

Fig. 31.6

Father interacts with his baby. **A,** Stroking baby's back. **B,** Touching baby with fingertip.

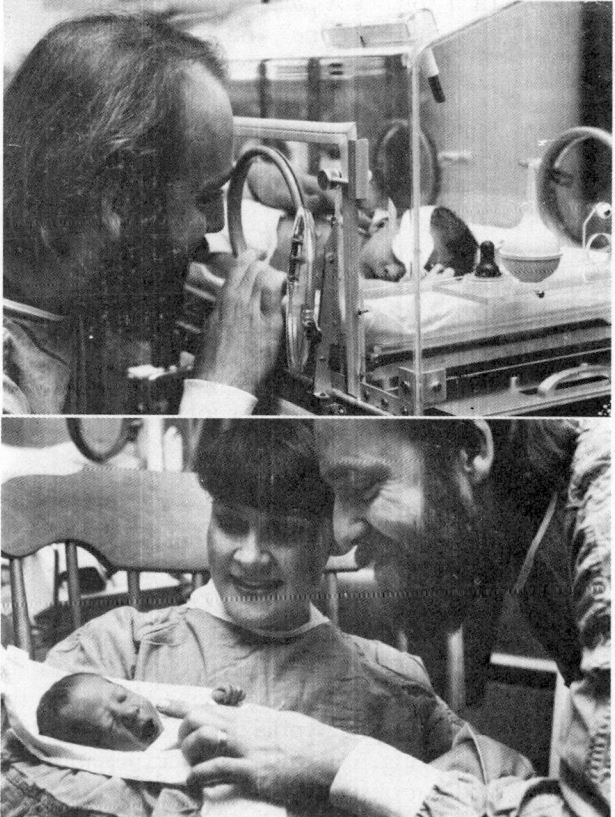

Fig. 31.7
Dressed for visitors; mother and father. Note hat (knitted by grandmother) to prevent heat loss through scalp.

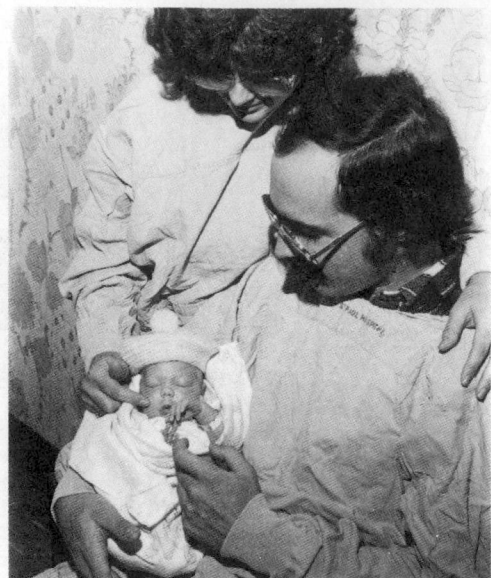

Fig. 31.8
Parents and child are united.

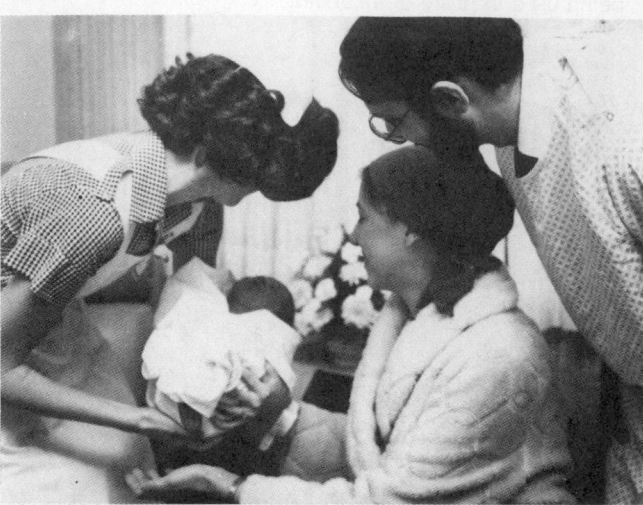

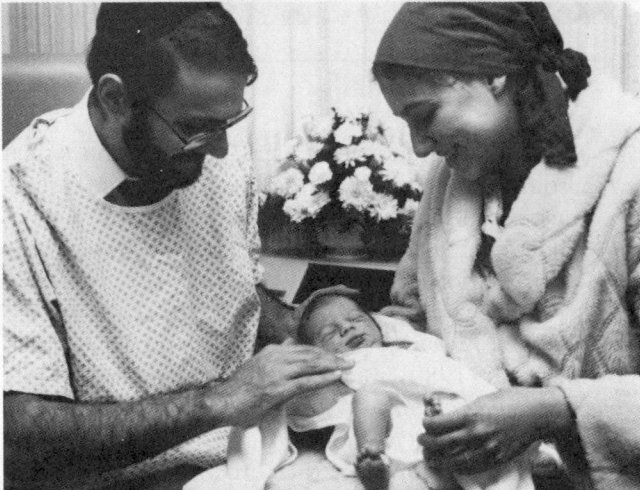

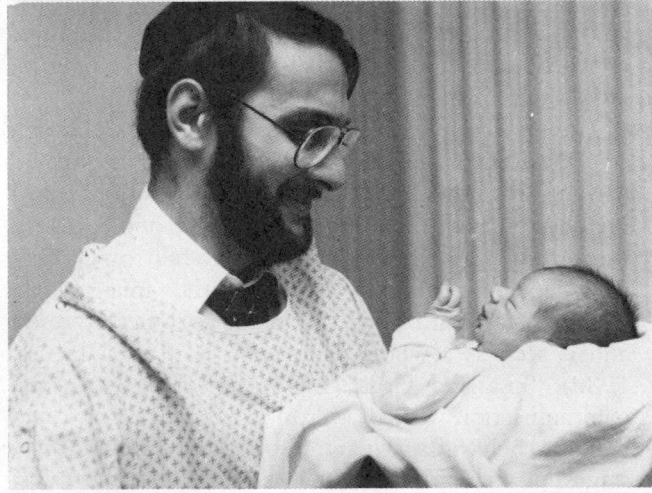

they note their infant's *responses* to them and begin to feel that "this child is mine" and part of our family. Parents take on the role of advocate for their child (Fig. 31.9).

Infant responsiveness. The preterm infant's states of consciousness are more labile than the term infant's. The quiet alert state is less evident and unpredictable. Field (1979) noted that if a mother concentrated her interactions on imitation of the infant's behavior, the infant was increasingly attentive and interested (Fig. 31.10). Too-active an involvment in child care tended to result in the infant's becoming disinterested and glancing away (gaze aversion). One young mother noted that "gentle stroking of her infant's head caused him to look at her." (She also reported that even at age 7 years, gentle head stroking calmed her child.)

Parenting disorders. The incidence of physical and emotional abuse is three times greater toward the infant who, by virtue of prematurity or illness, was separated from the mother for a period of time after birth (Fomufod, 1976). Physical abuse includes varying degrees of poor nutrition and poor hygiene. Emotional abuse ranges from subtle to outright dislike of the child. There may be preferential treatment for brothers and sisters, nagging, extremely high expectations of the child, and various other types of overt or covert negative responses by one or both parents.

Factors surrounding the birth may predispose par-

Fig. 31.9
A, Mother and father open their mouths in imitation of their infant; infant glances at them. **B,** Father and baby "yawn" together. **C,** Father and baby "purse" their mouths.

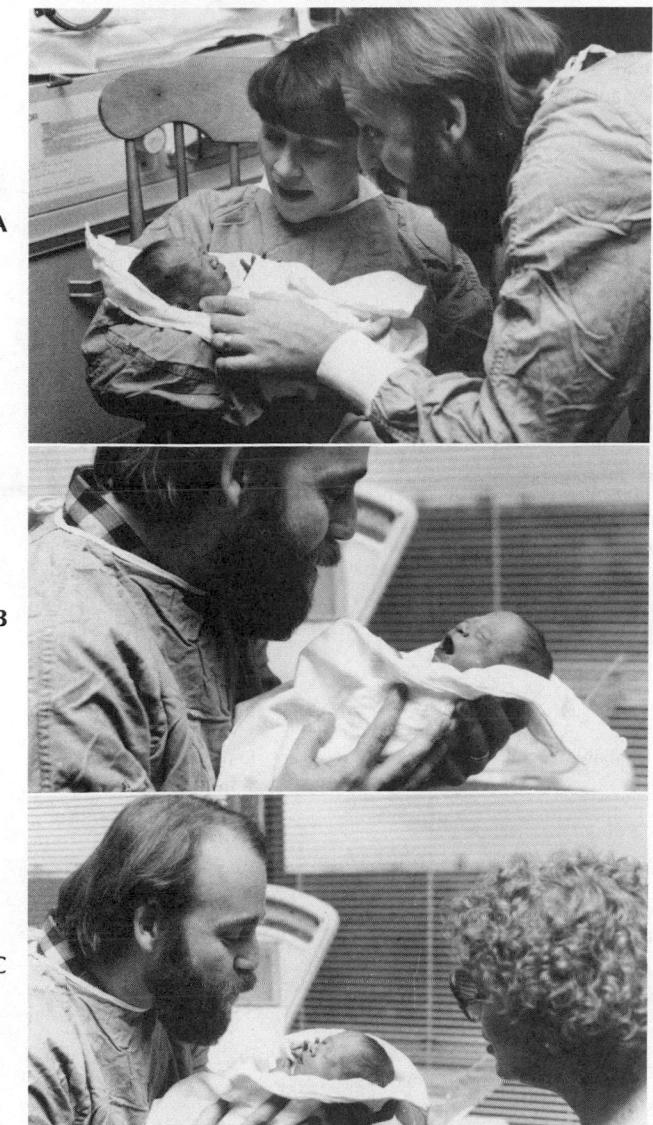

Fig. 31.10
Introduction of baby born 4 weeks prematurely to new sister and grandmother.

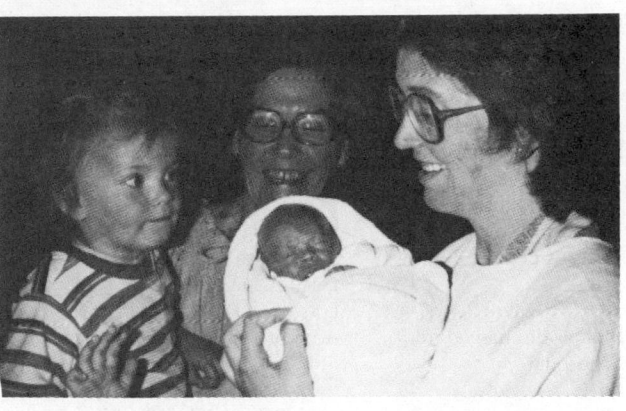

They parallel the stages in parental change with the change in medical care of the infant (Table 31.3).

Nursing care. The best environment for fetal growth and development is in the uterus of a healthy, well-nourished woman for 38 to 42 weeks. The extrauterine environment of the preterm newborn must approximate a healthy intrauterine environment for the normal sequence of growth and development to continue. The provision of such an environment is the basis for care of the preterm infant. Medical and nursing personnel and respiratory therapists work as a team to provide the intensive care needed. **The nurse acts as a constant in the infant's support system.**

Assessment. Nursing actions are based on knowledge of the *physiologic problems* (Table 31.1) *imposed on the preterm infant and on the need to conserve energy for repair, maintenance, and growth.* Assessment and reassessment of the infant's condition are prerequisites to nursing care.

Determination of gestational age. Premature infants are at a distinct disadvantage when they face the transition from intrauterine to extrauterine life. *The degree of disadvantage depends primarily on their level of maturity.* Physiologic disorders and anomalous malformations affect their response to treatment as well. In general, the closer they are to the normal term infant in gestational age and weight, the easier will be their adjustment to the external environment.

Determination of gestational age by physical examination. The procedures used today are based on the one devised by Dubowitz and associates (1970). Ideally the tests are performed between 2 and 8 hours of age. For the first hour the infant is recovering from the stress of birth, and this is reflected in muscle movements; for

ents to subconsciously or overtly reject the child. These factors might include parental pain and anxiety, a heavy financial burden for the infant's care, unresolved anticipatory grief, threat to self-esteem, or unwanted pregnancy. The goal of the helping professionals is to reduce the incidence of child abuse and neglect.

Growth in the parental role. Sammons and Lewis (1985) describe the steps in adaptation of the mother or father to the parenting role with a preterm infant.

Table 31.3
Parental and Medical Milestones

	Parent Milestones	Medical Milestones
Premature birth of baby Premature termination of pregnancy	Deprived of last trimester of pregnancy, a time of major adjustment during which the following are accomplished: 1. Resolution of issues of competency of parenting 2. Formulation of future hopes for the child 3. Change in couple's relationship as they approach parenthood	Hospital admission
Parents apart—different areas of hospital or different hospital Isolation Issues of fault	Reverse of caretaking role: father there first Initial time is a period of extreme disorganization 1. Loss of family and community supports 2. Long period before social interaction with baby (parents may need this) 3. Sense of distance from baby Death issue Loss of fantasy child dream	Transport Ventilator Multiple procedures Intravenous or arterial catheters
Mother discharged from hospital	Adaptation to NICU environment 1. Initial distance—uncertain where baby is 2. Numbers and machinery 3. Parents relate to different machine: breast pump	Baby physiologically unstable
Parents together	Observers of the nurse's role with the baby Begin to understand some of what the technicalities and the numbers mean Start to use the medical jargon on the telephone Start to see other people developing a relationship with the baby Dependent on relationships with nurse and physician	Getting better Nasogastric feedings Temperature instability Beginning of nursing and staff attachment to baby
Begin caretaking: adoption of the staff role	Competition with the staff Fathers start to perceive change in focus to mother-infant relationship Start to offer show of affection for the baby Signs Attachment to head "doughnut" support Toys Clothes	Baby off of major support systems Still on monitors Weight single focus of well-being
Attempts to read social cues of infant	Holding the baby; difficult to get to know the baby 1. Feeding problems 2. Caretaking but little attachment 3. Still feel like it is not "our baby" 4. Energy consumption: beginning to sense how to "help" the baby 5. Conflicting messages: "okay" but monitors just to make sure	Removal of last physical barriers Out of Isolette to bassinet
Changes in visiting patterns May visit separately	Need to form their own relationship—beginning of attachment 1. Subjective: not measureable by number of phone calls, duration of visits, etc. 2. What they want to do, not what they are told to do by staff Differentiation of mother and father roles 1. Different caretaking routines 2. Different visiting times 3. Competition over who had the "magic touch" at the last visit Reassessment of competency issues, parents' and infant's 1. Breast feeding: continuation or failure 2. Less competition over caretaking 3. Joy at increased awake time 4. Joy at increased response to inanimate stimulation	Off monitors Feeling that the baby has made it Parallel questions of whether the parents are ready Nursing detachment issues
Nesting behavior	Start forming identity of child 1. Push for discharge date, sometimes inappropriately soon before an emotional base established 2. Settle lingering medical and developmental concerns: apnea etc.; necessary for security to feel comfortable going home 3. Start to use name actively—not just she or he	
Start forming present role	Initial joy of predictable social response 1. Conflicting feelings of hope and risk 2. How do we form a relationship? Is it the same as for full-term infants? 3. Understanding child vs. understanding instructions, orders, and how to read behavior cues	

From Sammons, W., and Lewis, J.: Premature babies: a different beginning, St. Louis, 1985, The C.V. Mosby Co.

Table 31.3, cont'd
Parental and Medical Milestones

	Parent Milestones	Medical Milestones
Grandparents and friends visit (Fig. 31.10)	Need to reestablish community and family supports	
Discharge	Final home preparations	Medical discharge
	Often seem anxious—trying to adjust to facing new responsibilities	What to tell parents about high risk vs. recovery
	Frequent questions	Is the premie normal?
Coming home: learning to live together	New sense of isolation—need to be self-sufficient	
	Working out feeding and sleeping issues; new questions, uncertain answers	
	Increased sense of competence of the parent-infant response system	
	Predictability	
	New feelings of crisis and doubt	Visits to follow-up clinic
	Medical visits or illnesses	
	Grocery store at 6 months of age	
	Overprotection, doubt about the premie	
	Self-doubt	
Answering questions about the future	Increasing sense of who the child is	
	Independence vs. dependence issues	
	New milestones:	
	Smiles	
	Laughter	
	Talking	
	Elicit attention	
	Originate social games	
Feeling like the premie has made it	Personal time	
	Another child	
	Vacations	

example, the arm recoil is slower in a fatigued infant. After 48 hours some responses change significantly. The plantar creases on the soles of the feet appear to increase in number and become visible as the skin loses fluid and dries. See Figs. 31.11 to 31.15 and Tables 31.4 and 31.5 for the clinical estimation of gestational age. Fig. 31.16 is an example of the recording of the gestational age estimation. *Text continued on p. 982.*

Fig. 31.11
A, In prone position, premature infant lies with pelvis flat and legs splayed like a frog's.
B, Normal full-term infant lies with his limbs flexed, pelvis raised, and knees usually drawn under abdomen. (Courtesy Mead Johnson & Co., Evansville, Indiana.)

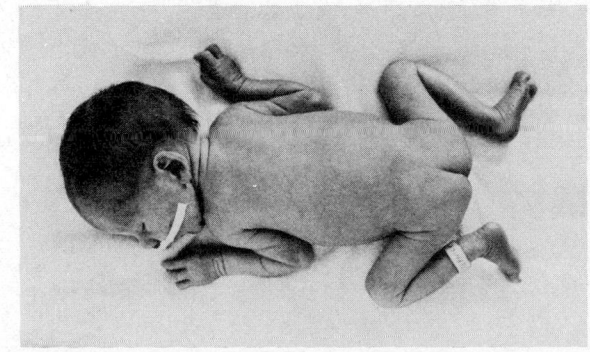
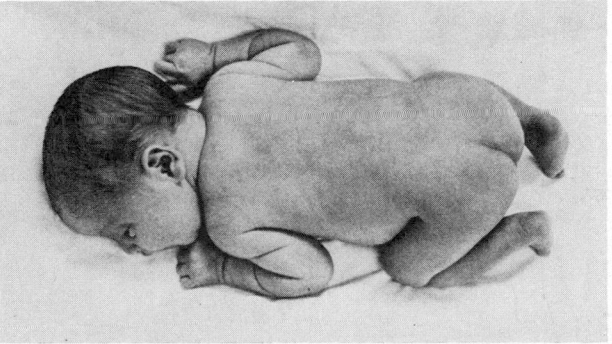

Fig. 31.12
A, Normal sole creases of full-term newborn. **B,** Sole of foot of premature infant. As infant loses interstitial fluid after birth, creases become apparent even in preterm infants. Therefore assessment needs to be done in first 2 hours after birth.

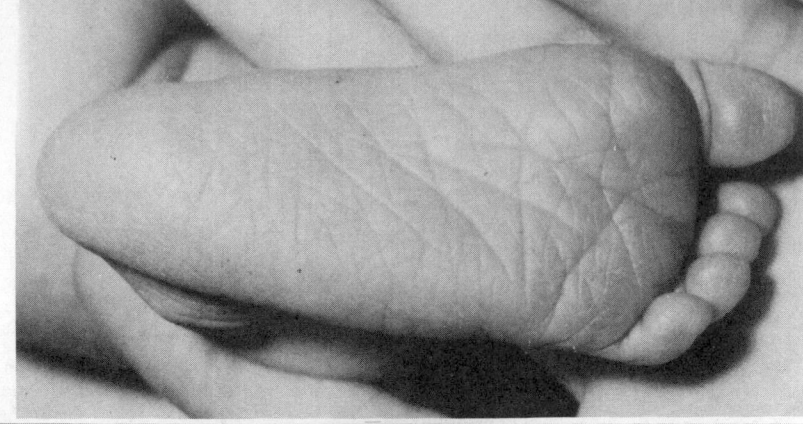

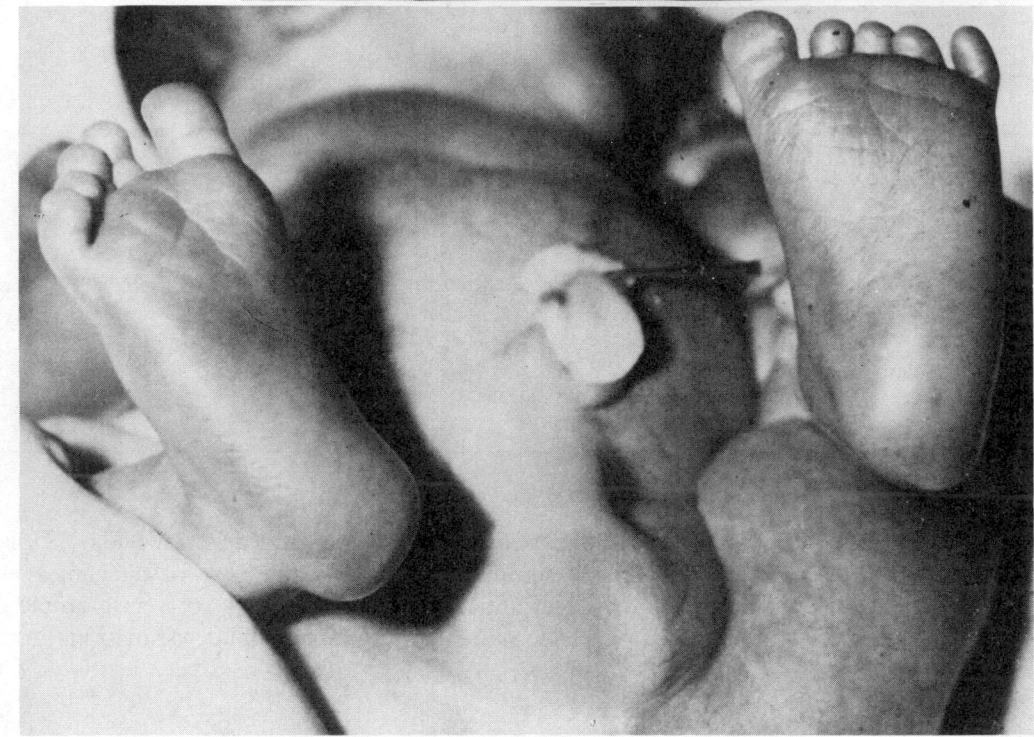

Fig. 31.13
Assessment of gestational age in term newborn, **A,** and preterm newborn, **B.**

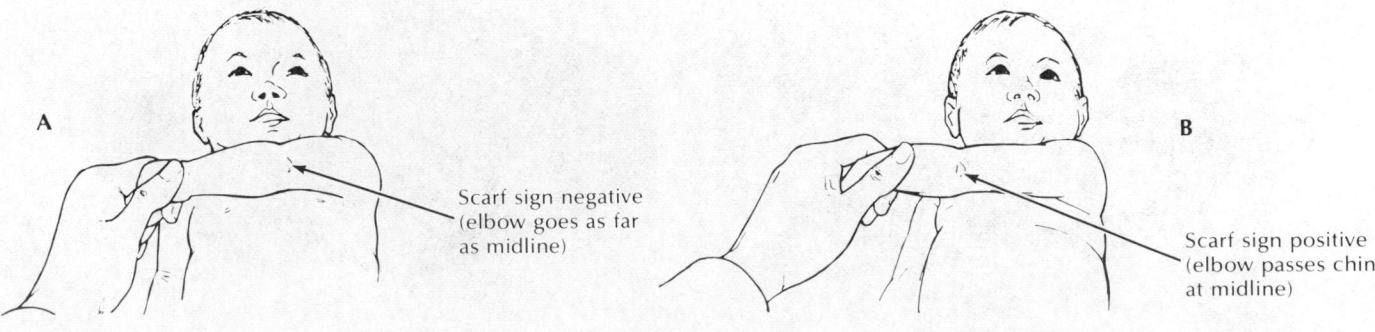

Scarf sign negative (elbow goes as far as midline)

Scarf sign positive (elbow passes chin at midline)

Fig. 31.14

Ankle dorsiflexion. **A,** Angle of 0 degrees in term newborn. **B,** Angle of 20 degrees in the preterm newborn.

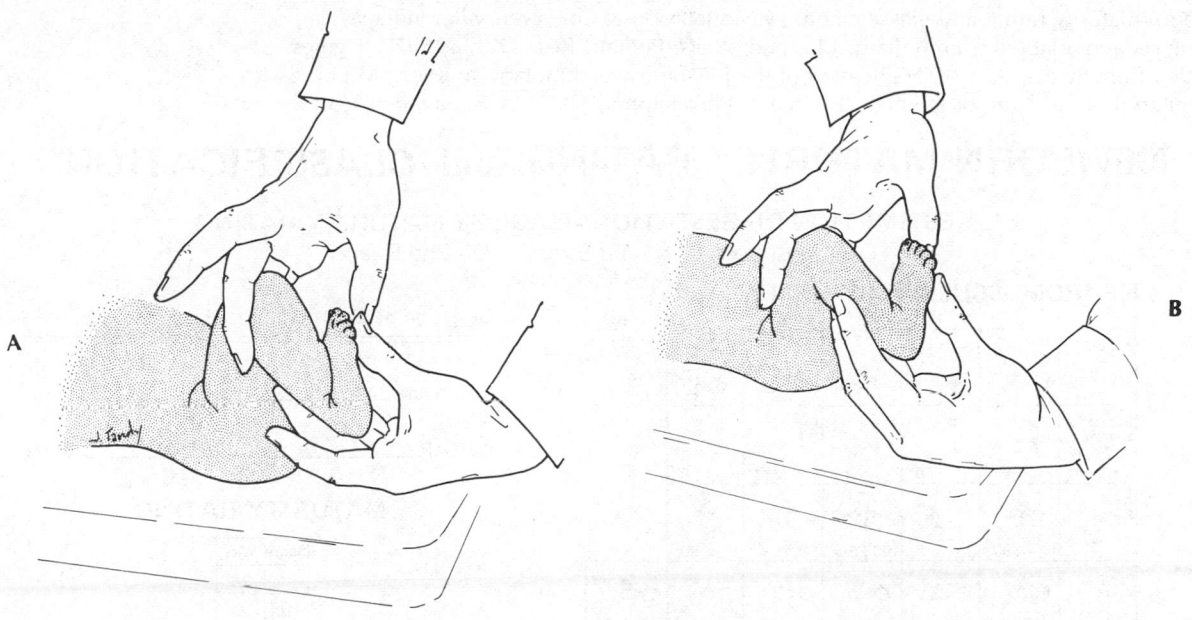

Fig. 31.15

A, Primitive grasp reflex present in all normal newborns usually weakens and disappears after 3 months. When palm is stimulated by finger, infant will grasp it. Full-term infant reinforces grip as finger is drawn upward. Dorsum of hand should not be touched, since this excites opposite reflex, and hand opens. **B,** Grasp reflex present in premature infant is distinct from that noted in term infant. Grip can be obtained and arm drawn upward, but when traction is applied, grip opens and there is much less muscle tension. **C,** Once grasp is obtained in term infant, grip is reinforced when the arm is drawn upward. There is progressive tensing of muscles until baby hangs momentarily. (**B** and **C** courtesy Mead Johnson & Co., Evansville, Indiana.)

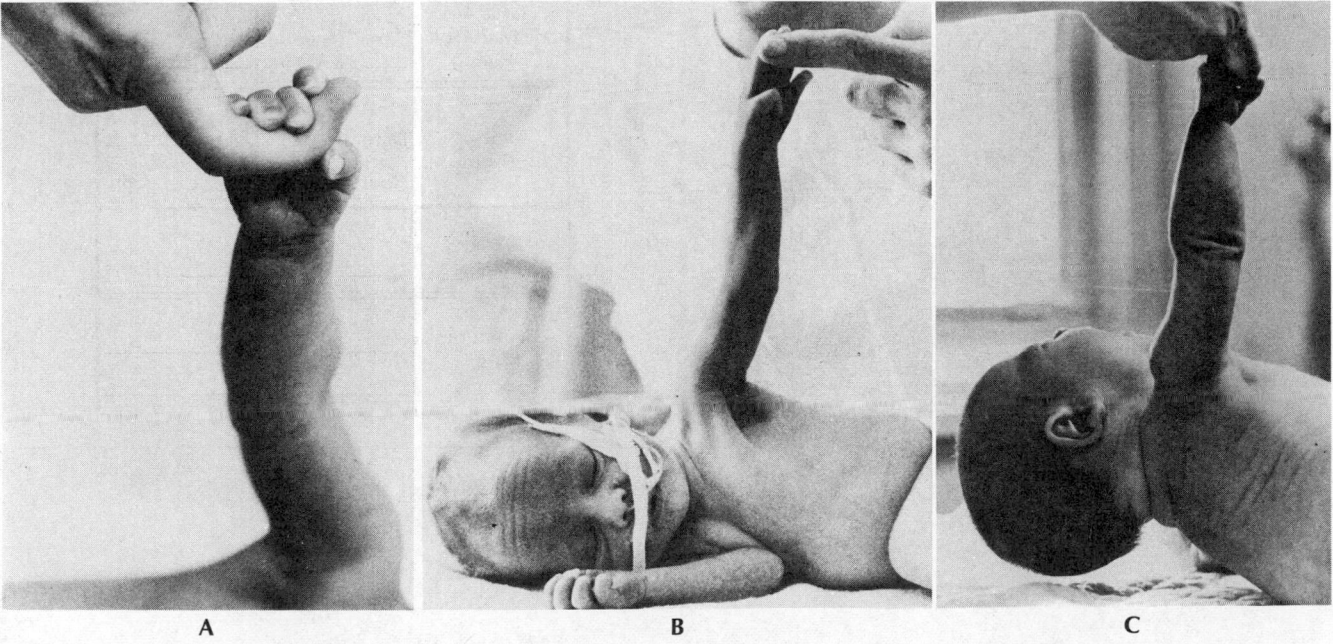

Fig. 31.16
Newborn maturity rating and classificaton. (Mead Johnson & Co., Evansville, Indiana.
Scoring section adapted from Ballard, J.L., and others: Pediatr. Res. 11:374, 1977. Figures
modified from Sweet, A.Y.: Classification of the low-birth-weight infant. In Klaus, M.H.,
and Fanaroff, A.A.: Care of the high-risk infant, Philadelphia, 1977, W.B. Saunders Co.)

NEWBORN MATURITY RATING and CLASSIFICATION

ESTIMATION OF GESTATIONAL AGE BY MATURITY RATING
Symbols: X - 1st Exam   O - 2nd Exam

NEUROMUSCULAR MATURITY

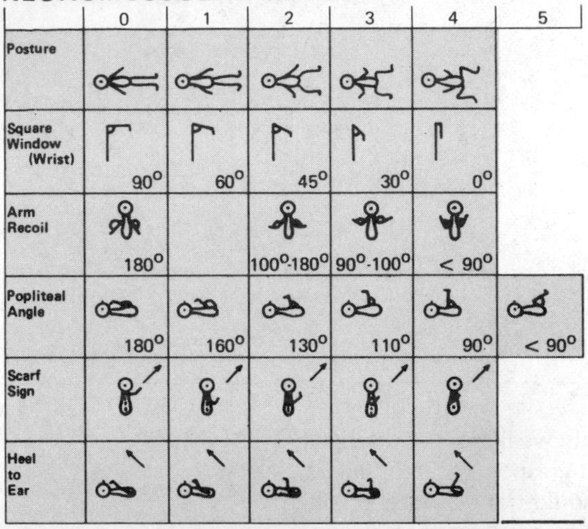

	0	1	2	3	4	5
Posture						
Square Window (Wrist)	90°	60°	45°	30°	0°	
Arm Recoil	180°		100°-180°	90°-100°	< 90°	
Popliteal Angle	180°	160°	130°	110°	90°	< 90°
Scarf Sign						
Heel to Ear						

PHYSICAL MATURITY

	0	1	2	3	4	5
SKIN	gelatinous red, transparent	smooth pink, visible veins	superficial peeling &/or rash, few veins	cracking pale area, rare veins	parchment, deep cracking, no vessels	leathery, cracked, wrinkled
LANUGO	none	abundant	thinning	bald areas	mostly bald	
PLANTAR CREASES	no crease	faint red marks	anterior transverse crease only	creases ant. 2/3	creases cover entire sole	
BREAST	barely percept.	flat areola, no bud	stippled areola, 1–2 mm bud	raised areola, 3–4 mm bud	full areola, 5–10 mm bud	
EAR	pinna flat, stays folded	sl. curved pinna, soft with slow recoil	well-curv. pinna, soft but ready recoil	formed & firm with instant recoil	thick cartilage, ear stiff	
GENITALS Male	scrotum empty, no rugae		testes descending, few rugae	testes down, good rugae	testes pendulous, deep rugae	
GENITALS Female	prominent clitoris & labia minora		majora & minora equally prominent	majora large, minora small	clitoris & minora completely covered	

Gestation by Dates _____ wks

Birth Date _____ Hour _____ am/pm

APGAR _____ 1 min _____ 5 min

MATURITY RATING

Score	Wks
5	26
10	28
15	30
20	32
25	34
30	36
35	38
40	40
45	42
50	44

SCORING SECTION

	1st Exam=X	2nd Exam=O
Estimating Gest Age by Maturity Rating	_____ Weeks	_____ Weeks
Time of Exam	Date _____ Hour _____ am/pm	Date _____ Hour _____ am/pm
Age at Exam	_____ Hours	_____ Hours
Signature of Examiner	_____ M.D.	_____ M.D.

Score is obtained by adding totals from Tables 31.4 and 31.5.

Table 31.4
Elaboration of Physical Maturity Scales

Criterion	Findings and Assigned Scores					Infant Score
	0	1	2	3	4	
Skin						
Edema	Edema evident over hands and feet; pitting seen over tibia	Pitting edema over tibia	No edema obvious	—	—	_____
Texture and opacity	Gelatinous, transparent; veins seen especially over abdomen	Visible, veins; thin, smooth	Few larger veins seen, especially over abdomen; medium-thick smooth skin	Veins rarely seen; some thickening superficial cracking	No vessels; parchmentlike, thick, cracking; if leathery, very cracked, and wrinkled, give score of 5	
Color	Dark red (infant is quiet for evaluation)	Pink	Pale pink	Pale; pink mainly over palms, soles, lips, and ears		
Lanugo	None	Abundant over body; long; thick	Thinning, especially over lumbosacral area	Bald areas; thinning over other areas	Mostly bald of lanugo; at least half of back bald	_____
Plantar creases	No creases seen	Faint red marks on upper half of sole	Red marks obvious over more than upper half; deeper lines over less than one third	Indentations noticeable over more than one third; lines seen over two thirds	Creases cover entire sole (Fig. 31.12)	_____
Breast	Nipple barely perceptible; no palpable breast tissue	Flat, smooth areola present around well-defined nipple; some breast tissue	Stippled areola but edge flat; 1-2 mm breast bud	Stippled areola with edges raised; 3-4 mm breast bud	Full areola; 5-10 mm breast bud; may have breast milk	_____
Ear Form Cartilage	Pinna flat, soft, easily folded	Slight incurving of pinna; soft, easily folded; slow recoil	Well-incurved pinna; soft; ready recoil	Upper pinna well curved; formed and firm to edge; instant recoil	Thick cartilage; ear stiff	_____
Genitals						
Male	No testes in scrotum and no rugae over scrotum	—	Testes descending; few rugations	Testes within scrotum good rugae	Scrotum pendulous with rugae covering scrotum	
Female	Prominent clitoris and labia minora; labia majora do not cover labia minora	—	Labia majora and labia minora equally prominent	Labia majora appear large; labia minora, small	Labia majora completely cover clitoris and labia minora	
					TOTAL	_____

Table 31.5
Elaboration of Neuromuscular Maturity Scales*

Criterion	Method of Assessment	0
Posture (Fig. 31.11)	Position: supine Activity: quiet Assessment: extension and flexion of arms, hips, legs	Complete extension
Square window (wrist)†	Position: supine Method: with thumb supporting back of arm below wrist, apply gentle pressure with index and third fingers on dorsum of hand; do not rotate infant's wrist Assessment: angle formed between hypothenar eminence and forearm	Very premature (<30 weeks) 90°
Arm recoil‡	Position: supine Method: flex forearms on upper arms for 5 s; pull on hands to full extension and release Assessment: degree of flexion	No recoil; arms remain extended 180°
Popliteal angle	Position: supine; pelvis on flat, firm surface Method: flex leg on thigh; then flex thigh on abdomen; holding knee with thumb and index finger, extend leg with index finger of other hand behind ankle Assessment: degree of angle behind knee	Complete extension; very premature 180°
Scarf sign (Fig. 31.13)	Position: supine Method: support head in midline with one hand; pull hand to opposite shoulder Assessment: position of elbow in relation to midline	Elbow to opposite arm like scarf around neck
Heel to ear	Position: supine, pelvis is kept flat on surface Method: pull foot up toward ear on same side; do not hold knee Assessment: distance of foot from ear and degree of extension of knee	Toes touch ear; leg completely extended (180°)

*Compare combined scores for physical and neuromuscular maturity to the "maturity rating" scores and read estimated weeks of gestational age. Estimate of
on appropriate graphs. All three measurements should fall within same approximate range, for example, all within SGA, LGA, or AGA. If one measurement is
†Counterpart: ankle dorsiflexion (see Fig. 31.14).
‡Counterpart: leg recoil.

Finding and Assigned Scores					Infant Score	
1	2	3	4	5	X	0
Extension of arms; slight flexion of hips, legs	Extension of arms	Slight flexion, arms full, with abduction of legs, hips	Complete flexion	—	_____	_____
Premature (30-35 weeks) 60°	Premature (30-35 weeks) 45°	Maturing (35-38 weeks) 30°	Term: hand lies flat on ventral surface of forearm 0°	—	_____	_____
—	Some recoil; sluggish response 100°-180°	Maturing (35-38 weeks) 90°-100°	Brisk recoil to complete flexion >90°	—	_____	_____
Premature (30-35 weeks) 160°	Premature (30-35 weeks) 130°	Maturing (35-38 weeks) 110°	Maturing (35-38 weeks) 90°	Extension is resisted >90°	_____	_____
Elbow beyond midline of thorax	Elbow just beyond midline	Elbow at midline	Elbow does not reach midline	—	_____	_____
Toes almost reach face (130°)	Knees flexed (110°)	Knees flexed (90°)	Knees flexed; popliteal angle is less than 90°	—		

NEUROMUSCULAR MATURITY TOTALS _____ _____

PHYSICAL MATURITY TOTALS _____ _____

(see Table 31.4)

COMBINED SCORE _____ _____

See Fig. 31.16 for Maturity Rating.

gestational age obtained is accurate only to plus or minus 2 weeks. After gestational age is estimated, infant's length, weight, and head circumference are entered excessively large (falling into LGA range) and other two fall into SGA range, growth deviation should be assessed. **X,** First examination; **O,** second examination.

Nursing diagnoses. To formulate nursing diagnoses, the nurse must analyze data obtained from continuous monitoring of the infant and from observation of and discussions with the parents. The diagnosis may be physical, cognitive, or psychological. Examples of such diagnoses are as follows:

1. Ineffective breathing patterns related to inadequate chest expansion, secondary to infant's assuming prone position.
2. Parental knowledge deficit related to feeding the infant.
3. Disturbance in maternal self-concept related to her feelings of inadequacy in caring for the infant.

Plan. The physiologic problems of immature body systems govern the plan of care of these infants. The infant is faced with many emergency treatments and procedures. Nursing care during this time of crisis is a critical factor in the infant's chances for survival and in the parents' eventual relationship with their child.

Goals. For the infant:
1. Initiate and maintain respirations.
2. Maintain body temperature.
3. Support CNS function.
4. Maintain renal function.
5. Maintain adequate nutrition.
6. Minimize hematologic problems.
7. Prevent infection.
8. Prevent retinal problems.
9. Prevent trauma to immature musculoskeletal system.
10. Promote parent-infant attachment.

For the parents:
1. Perceive the child as potentially normal (if this is medically substantiated).
2. Provide the child with realistic care comfortably.
3. Experience pride and satisfaction in the care of the child.
4. Organize time and energies to meet the love, attention, and care needs of the other members of the family and themselves as well.

Implementation. Nurses fulfill many roles in providing the intensive and extended care these infants require. Nurses' ability as skilled technicians is crucial. They must interpret data, make decisions, and initiate therapy in short periods of time. Their actions as support persons and teachers are a part of the first phase of the parents' adjustment to the birth of the preterm baby.

Admission to the intensive care nursery. Admission of a premature newborn to the intensive care nursery usually is an emergency situation. A rapid initial evaluation must be made to ascertain the need for lifesaving treatment. Resuscitative measures should be started in the delivery room. The newborn's need for warmth and oxygen must be ensured during transfer from the delivery room to the nursery.

Hospitals that are not staffed or equipped to care for high-risk infants arrange for their immediate transfer to specialized centers (see p. 720). During transport to a regional center the following are necessary to meet the infant's needs:

1. Prewarmed blankets, prewarmed incubator, or if incubator is not available, improvise: surround the infant with hot-water bottles at a distance of 5 to 10 cm from the infant's body.
2. Portable oxygen and suction apparatuses.
3. Bulb syringe or DeLee mucus-trap catheter.
4. Intravenous setup with a battery-powered infusion pump.
5. Medications as ordered by the physician.
6. Appropriate attendant or attendants.

Nurse/infant ratio. The preterm infant is classified according to the degree of supportive care required, and the staff is assigned to the infant on that basis:

- Class A: severely compromised infant—1 to 1 nurse/infant ratio.
- Class B: moderately compromised infant—1 to 2 nurse/infant ratio.
- Class C: recovery and progress—1 to 4 nurse/infant ratio satisfactory.
- Class D: ready for normal newborn nursery—1 to 8 nurse/infant ratio.

Nurse as technician. The nurse uses many modern technologic support systems to monitor body responses and maintain body function in the infant (Hansen, 1982). Gentle touch, concern for the traumatic effects of harsh lighting, and control of machinery noise are interwoven with the technical skill of the nurse in the intensive care nursery.

PHYSICAL CARE. The premature infant's environmental support consists of the following:
1. Incubator control for body temperature.
2. Air or oxygen administration, depending on the infant's color and respirations.
3. Electronic monitors as needed for the observation of respiratory and cardiac functions and blood gases

Metabolic support consists of measures such as the following:
1. Parenteral fluids to assist in supporting normal blood gas and acid-base homeostasis.
2. Parenteral fluids to facilitate antibiotic therapy if sepsis is a concern.
3. Blood specimen analyses to monitor blood gases, pH, hypoglycemia, and sepsis.

An overview of the technical support required for a preterm infant is presented on pp. 983-987.

Application of the Nursing Process

PRETERM INFANT

Shirley and Ron were expecting their first child. They were excited and pleased at the prospect of being parents. At 30 weeks' gestation Shirley had premature rupture of the membranes (PROM). She went into active labor. After 6 hours she delivered a male infant weighing 1530 g (3 lb 6 oz). The infant was transferred immediately to the intensive care nursery. The child exhibited the problems typical of a preterm infant (Table 31.1). Intensive care for a compromised infant was begun immediately.

FUNCTIONAL HEALTH PATTERN: ASSESSMENT	NURSING DIAGNOSIS	RATIONALE: PLAN/ IMPLEMENTATION	EVALUATION

ACTIVITY-EXERCISE
Respiratory function
■ Check respiration rate, depth, regularity; periodic breathing
■ Observe for apneic pauses: number? duration? whether accompanied by cyanosis?
  • Respiratory rate after apneic episode: same? increased or decreased?
■ Observe for seesaw respirations, expiratory grunt, chin tug, retractions, flaring of alae nasi,
  • Cry: feeble? whining? high pitched?
■ Check heart rate
■ Cyanosis: when it occurs? where (circumoral, generalized)? whether relieved by O_2? amount of O_2 needed? Accompanied by pallor?
■ Check reflexes: presence and condition of gag, swallow
■ Prebirth history:
  • Was mother treated with beta-methasone?
  • Preeclampsia (sedatives, magnesium sulfate, diuretics)?
	Alteration in respiratory function* related to warmth, positioning, feeding, oxygen need, and patency of airway	*To maintain adequate respirations:*
		■ Maintain warmth to decrease O_2 consumption and sequelae of cold stress.
		■ Suction as needed.
		■ Administer warmed and humidified compressed air at O_2 levels to relieve cyanosis and dyspnea
		■ Analyze O_2 concentration every 1-4 hours.
		■ Order and assist with procedures for blood gases and electrolytes. Record time, procedure, amount of blood drawn, and infant's response.
		■ Position infant to assist ventilatory effort (Chapter 20).
		■ Feed, using technique appropriate for this infant (see Chapters 21 and 25).
		■ Maintain respiratory monitor until infant weighs 1800 g (4 lb) or condition stabilizes; check rate every 1 or 2 hours and when necessary.
			Respirations of 40 breaths/min at birth without significant fluctuations.
			Respirations of 60/min after first hour of life, followed by no significant increase or decrease (e.g., ±15 breaths/min).
			Periods of periodic breathing must not exceed 10 seconds.
			Apneic episodes must not exceed 15 seconds.

Thermoregulation Check for variations in body temperature: ■ Thermistor probe on skin ■ Axillary temperature	Ineffective thermoregulation related to immaturity and convection loss	*To maintain adequate temperature (Chapter 20):* ■ Keep incubator away from windows, air conditioners. ■ Ensure warmth during all procedures: • Ambient warm air, draft-free	Skin: 36.5° C (97.6° F). Axillary: 36.5° C (97.6° F). Incubator: usually 33.5° to 35° C (92° to 95° F). Extremities should feel warm to touch.

*Diagnosis not included by NANDA, 1986.

Continued.

Application of the Nursing Process—cont'd

FUNCTIONAL HEALTH PATTERN: ASSESSMENT	NURSING DIAGNOSIS	RATIONALE: PLAN/ IMPLEMENTATION	EVALUATION
■ Rectal method (not recommended) ■ Extremities		• Warmed blankets and equipment • Blood transfusion warmed by passing tube through warm bath • Nurse's hands warm • Incubator lid and portholes closed • Warm air or O_2 to infant ■ Conserve infant's energy whenever possible; handle as little and as gently as possible.	
NUTRITIONAL-METABOLIC ■ Assess feeding behaviors: • Check reflex maturity: suck and swallow; gag and cough • Assess energy level: length of time needed to eat; degree of fatigability ■ Observe for the following: diarrhea, vomiting or regurgitation, gastric residual, color, amount, character of stools ■ Check for dehydration: • Early sign: loss of weight • Late signs: soft, sunken eyeball; depressed fontanel; poor skin tugor over abdomen, inner thigh ■ Assess absorption and assimilation ■ Observe for the following: • Steatorrhea (ordinarily not visible to naked eye) • Activity level: active or lethargic? • Color: pallor? • Symptoms of hypoglycemia ■ Test for hypoglycemia with Dextrostix (≤20 mg/dl blood for pre-	Alterations in nutrition: less than body requirements related to inability to feed or assimilate nutrients	*To institute appropriate feeding method for this infant:* ■ Select method: oral? gavage? (Nipple not used if respirations ≥60/min.) ■ Feed early: • To prevent depletion of reserves. • To support biochemical homeostasis. ■ Start feedings with sterile water, then proceed to glucose, then to formula if feeding by oral route. ■ Timing of feedings: • Infant under 1250 g (2 lb, 12 oz), feed every 2 hours. • Infant between 1500-1800 g (3½ to 4 lb), feed every 3 hours. • Infant in good condition and with active peristalsis, start first feeding between 6 and 12 hours after birth. • Infant with respiratory distress, give parenteral fluids. ■ Administer and record vitamins and minerals per physician order (vitamins A,C,D,E,iron). ■ Adjust formula, feeding method, etc. to infant's responses and changing needs.	Infant shows indication of "thriving": ■ Retains and assimilates nutrients. ■ Grows and develops. ■ Progresses from gavage to nipple feedings, breast or bottle.

Application of the Nursing Process—cont'd

FUNCTIONAL HEALTH PATTERN: ASSESSMENT	NURSING DIAGNOSIS	RATIONALE: PLAN/ IMPLEMENTATION	EVALUATION

term infant); may be otherwise asymptomatic
■ Assess for edema
■ Assess progress:
  • Weight gain, daily growth, weekly
  • Head circumference
  • Body length
		■ Plot daily weight on growth grid.
		  • Record measurements of head circumference, body length.	

COGNITIVE- PERCEPTUAL
■ Observe for symptoms of increased intracranial pressure (ICP)
■ Observe for convulsions:
  • Twitching and myoclonic jerks
  • Increased chewing movements
  • Eye rolling
■ Observe for behavior changes
	Potential sensory-perceptual alteration related to CNS damage	*To prevent dysfunction of CNS:*
		■ Maintain adequate oxygenation to relieve cyanosis.
		■ Maintain open airway.
		■ Prevent or promptly identify and relieve hypoglycemia, hypocalcemia.
			Infant does not exhibit symptoms of ICP or convulse.

HEALTH PERCEPTION– HEALTH MANAGEMENT
Infection
■ Check for variations in temperature
■ Note following:
  • Feeding behavior
  • Skin: irritations, rashes, jaundice
  • Drainage from eyes, umbilicus
  • Nasal congestion
  • Frequency of stools
  • Body temperature (unreliable)
  • Behavior change: "just not right," lethargic, listless
  • Respiratory rate increase or decrease (persistent) for 24 hours
■ Check prenatal record
  • Maternal temperature
  • Maternal infection
  • Premature rupture of membranes; length of time before delivery, color, odor, culture, amount of fluid
■ Check fluid intake and dehydration
	Alteration in thermoregulation related to infection, dehydration	*To prevent or minimize effects of infection:*
		■ Meticulous hand washing is imperative; check personnel's health.
		■ Use aseptic technique for anything puncturing skin and for umbilical catheterization.
		■ Prevent skin breakdown:
		  • Under monitor leads, tapes, restraints
		  • Over bony prominences (use flotation pad or sheepskin)
		  • By gentle insertion of orogastric or nasogastric tubes
		■ Supervise parents' hand washing and gowning when visiting.
		■ Monitor administration of medications.
		■ Restrict visitors, repairmen, equipment changes, etc.
		■ Maintain adequate fluid intake (prevent inanition fever).
			Temperature remains within normal limits.

Continued.

Application of the Nursing Process—cont'd

FUNCTIONAL HEALTH PATTERN: ASSESSMENT	NURSING DIAGNOSIS	RATIONALE: PLAN/ IMPLEMENTATION	EVALUATION
Fluid volume deficit; injury ■ Note presence of fragile capillaries ■ Note laboratory results: coagulation and prolonged prothrombin time ■ Note following: • Skin manifestations: ecchymoses, petechiae, jaundice, pallor • Increased bleeding or oozing around cord, injection sites, etc. • Symptoms of cerebral irritation (or increased intracranial pressure from hemorrhage)	Fluid volume deficit related to loss of blood Potential injury related to capillary fragility or immaturity	*To minimize tissue damage and hematologic problems:* ■ Protect fragile capillaries, restoring impaired coagulation process, reducing prolonged bleeding, and reduce hyperbilirubinemia. ■ Handle infant gently and as little as possible. ■ Give intramuscular injection of vitamin K (one dose) if infant not being given antibiotics that hamper its synthesis in gastrointestinal tract; if being given these antibiotics, more doses will be needed. ■ Reduce hyperbilirubinemia with phototherapy or assist with exchange transfusions. ■ Monitor amount of blood withdrawn for laboratory examinations and evaluations; assist with blood replacement as necessary.	Hemorrhage "bleeds" are controlled. Bilirubin levels remain within normal limits. Circumcision (if desired by parents) is delayed.
Injury ■ Molding of cranial bones ■ Note the following: • Unnatural rotation or extension of joints • Asymmetric contours of body • Muscle tone, muscle mass • Pressure area over bony prominences	Potential injury to immature musculoskeletal system related to positioning, support of body parts, too firm handling	*To prevent trauma to immature musculoskeletal system:* ■ Handle gently and move smoothly. ■ Position infant: • Change position frequently. • Place in correct body alignment; watch position of feet. ■ If diapers are used (infant under 1500 g [3 lb, 5 oz] should not be diapered), cut to size; pin or tape with posterior flap overlapping anterior flap. ■ Pad areas over bony prominences (sheepskin, bubble pads, other).	Injuries are not sustained. Molding of head is equalized.

Application of the Nursing Process—cont'd

FUNCTIONAL HEALTH PATTERN: ASSESSMENT	NURSING DIAGNOSIS	RATIONALE: PLAN/ IMPLEMENTATION	EVALUATION

COGNITIVE-PERCEPTUAL
■ Monitor the following:
  • Blood gas values
  • Oxygen concentration of inspired air
■ Note and record respiratory distress and amount and duration of oxygen therapy required to relieve distress
	Potential sensory-perceptual alteration caused by injury to retina related to prematurity and oxygen therapy	*To prevent retinal changes:*
		■ Monitor amount and duration of oxygen therapy to keep PaO$_2$ between 50 and 70 mm Hg or higher.
		■ Supervise collection of blood for study; method, time, amount.
			Retinopathy of prematurity does not occur.

ELIMINATION
■ Note the following:
  • Urinary output: diaper saturation; number of diapers each day; collect and measure urine, check specific gravity
  • Edema
  • Tachypnea
  • Vomiting
  • Abdominal distension
	Alteration in patterns of urinary elimination related to immature kidney function	*To assist kidney function by decreasing demands on that system:*
		■ Provide formula with right concentration of solute.
		■ Support respirations, normal body temperature, nutrition, fluid balance.
		■ Prevent infection.
		■ Prevent hypovolemia.
			Kidney function is maintained.

INFANT STIMULATION. Stimulation needs to be adjusted to the developmental level and tolerance of each infant (Gorski, Davison, and Brazelton, 1979). Infants in the early stages of development (less than 33 weeks) respond to stimulation with jerky limb extension, hyperflexion, and irregular vital signs. Stimulation for this group is kept to a minimum. They need to be handled with slow, sure motions. Their heads are supported and limbs held close to their body when changing position. This type of support reduces motor disorganization and stress. At age 34 to 36 weeks the infant will respond to visual and auditory stimuli in an alert state. At age 36 to 40 weeks infants are ready to respond to the caretaker's efforts to stimulate them.

INFANT FEEDING. The preterm infant may be fed by gavage, both bottle or breast, based on his developmental level (Chapter 25). Breast feeding is recommended if the infant is able. The criteria for breast feeding, developed by Boggs and Rau (1983) are as follows:

■ Weight at least 1500 g
■ Awake for short periods
■ Sucking, gagging, swallowing reflexes present

■ Gavage feedings well tolerated
■ Oxygen and ventilatory support not required

NONNUTRITIVE SUCKING. Nonnutritive sucking on a pacifier while gavage feeding has been demonstrated to have beneficial effects on preterm infants. The infants were ready for bottle feeding earlier, had better weight gain, were ready for discharge earlier, and suffered fewer complications (Field and others, 1982; Bernbaum and others, 1983). Makeshift pacifiers have been implicated in aspirations hazards (Milluncheck and McArtor, 1986). Ten deaths related to aspiration of baby bottle nipples were reported to the Consumer Product Safety Commission between 1975 and 1983. Nurseries and parents should buy only *one-piece pacifiers.*

CARDIOPULMONARY RESUSCITATION. Parents must be able to administer CPR to their infant before taking the child home (Chapter 20). Preterm infants are 8 to 10 times more likely than term infants to develop sudden infant death syndrome (SIDS). Further, infants discharged from a neonatal intensive care unit are about twice as likely to die unexpectedly during the first year of life as are infants in the general population

(Rehm, 1983). Parents need to know the phone number to be dialed in case of emergency, and the number should be posted near the phone.

Nurse as support person and teacher. The nurse as support person and teacher shapes the environment and makes the caregiving more responsive to the needs of parents and child. Nurses are instrumental in helping parents learn who their infant is and to recognize behavioral cues in his development.

As soon as possible the parents should see and touch the infant so they can begin to acknowledge the reality of the event and reaffirm the infant's true appearance and condition. They will need encouragement to begin working through the psychologic tasks imposed by the premature delivery.

A nurse or physician should be present when the parents visit the infant for the following reasons:
1. To help them "see" the infant rather than focus on the equipment. The significance and function of the apparatus that surround the infant should be explained to them.
2. To explain the characteristics normal for an infant of their baby's gestational age. In this way parents do not compare their child wih a full-term healthy infant.
3. To encourage the parents to express their feelings about the pregnancy, labor, and delivery.
4. To assess the parents' perceptions of the infant to determine the appropriate time for them (especially the mother) to become actively involved in care.

Parents who have negative feelings about the pregnancy or the infant at risk need support. Their feelings can be acknowledged as valid, including the burden they are experiencing financially and emotionally and their understandable feelings toward the infant.

Soon after delivery, the parents are given the opportunity to meet the infant in the en face position, to touch the infant, and to see his or her favorable characteristics. As soon as possible, depending primarily on her physical condition, the mother is allowed to visit the nursery at will and help with the infant's care. When she cannot be physically present, the staff devises appropriate methods to keep the family in almost constant touch with the newborn.

Some hospitals have instituted a parents' club for parents of infants in intensive care nurseries. These clubs encourage parents experiencing the same anxiety and grief to share their feelings. An "older" member often takes over a new member and provides additional support. Incorporating these actions into the infant's care plan acknowledges and supports nature's design by engaging and maintaining a bond between the mother and infant. This assures the infant the continued care she or he needs for physical and emotional survival at the optimal level.

Evaluation. Evaluation of the care given preterm infants and their families has to be multidimensional (Montgomery and Williams-Judge, 1986). In some families the infant dies despite all medical and nursing knowledge and skill (Kulkarmi, 1978). In other families the sequelae of prematurity result in infants who will face lifetime disability. For these families evaluation criteria relate to the concepts of loss, grief, and self-concept (see Chapter 26).

For many other infants and families the immediate threat to well-being is overcome by intensive neonatal care. The criteria for evaluation of the physical aspects of the care are the following:
1. Respirations are initiated and maintained.
2. Body temperature is maintained.
3. The infant is adequately nourished.
4. CNS trauma is prevented or minimized.
5. Infection is prevented.
6. Renal function is supported.
7. Hematologic problems are prevented or minimized.
8. Musculoskeletal problems are prevented or minimized.
9. Retinal damage is prevented or minimized.

The criteria for evaluation of the psychosocial aspects of care include the following:
1. The mother retains a positive self-concept as a woman, mother, and sexual being.
2. The mother, father, and family:
   a. Perceive the child as potentially normal (if this is medically substantiated).
   b. Provide the child with realistic care comfortably.
   c. Experience pride and satisfaction in the care of the child.
3. The parents are able to organize their time and energy to meet the needs for love, attention, and care of the other members of the family and themselves as well.

Complications of prematurity. Respiratory distress syndrome (RDS), retinopathy of prematurity (ROP) (formerly known as retrolental fibroplasia), and bronchopulmonary dysplasia (BPD) are seen almost exclusively in preterm newborns. RDS and BPD claim a significant number of lives. The impaired vision or blindness resulting from ROP places a serious burden on survivors and their families.

Respiratory distress syndrome

Incidence. RDS is a leading cause of morbidity and mortality among preterm infants, and it affects about 20,000 infants each year in North America. Generally the smaller the preterm infant, the higher the mortality. Occasionally a full-term newborn is affected.

Pathophysiology. The central problem in RDS is atelectasis, which results from the development of a hyaline membrane within the newborn's terminal bronchial tree, that is, within the alveolar ducts and the alveoli. It occurs within a few hours after birth. The *membrane* is composed in part of fibrin derived from the pulmonary circulation and is not the result of aspirated fluid or an irritant. Accompanying problems such as hypoxia, metabolic and respiratory acidosis, and pulmonary hypoperfusion with right-to-left shunting (i.e., persistent fetal circulation) are secondary to atelectasis.

Cause. The cause of RDS is still unknown. The role of surfactant in preventing alveolar collapse at the end of expiration has been established. A deficiency in surfactant production may be the basis for RDS.

Clinical problems. A deficiency in surfactant forces the infant to work to reexpand the lungs with each inspiration. The result is fatigue, depletion of energy reserves, hypoxia and hypercapnia, progressive atelectasis, and diminishing lung compliance (or increasing "stiffness"). Factors that impair the production of surfactant are hypoxia, acidosis, and reduced pulmonary blood circulation. Thus a vicious cycle is established. The normal newborn expends more calories and consumes more oxygen to breathe than does the adult. For the infant in respiratory distress this expenditure may be as much as six times that of the normal term newborn. The development of RDS may be expressed by the diagram shown in Fig. 31.17.

Onset. RDS may be apparent in the infant at birth. The newborn has a low Apgar score and frequently requires resuscitation and ventilatory assistance. Other symptoms generally appear within the first 6 hours. Initially expiratory grunting and nasal flaring are evident. As the disease progresses, tachypnea (60 breaths/min or more), retractions, and even cyanosis in room air may be noted. Hypotension and shock may be evident. Apneic pauses replace the expiratory grunting. An arterial PO_2 of 40 mm Hg or less in room air is a constant finding.

Diagnosis. The diagnosis is confirmed by x-ray films, blood tests for pH, serum nonprotein nitrogen (NPN), potassium, and phosphorus. Tests for arterial blood gases are also used as diagnostic indicators for RDS.

Prognosis. Formerly, if the infant with RDS survived the first 48 to 72 hours, the clinical condition improved slowly until recovery at about 10 to 12 days. Newer methods and equipment have sustained the severely affected infant beyond 72 hours. Because of the more serious effects of the disease, death still may occur several weeks after birth. Therefore, a guarded prognosis is given for several weeks.

Treatment. The following measures are important in the treatment of the infant with RDS:

1. A thermoneutral environment is provided so the

Fig. 31.17
Development of hyaline membrane disease. (Courtesy A. Hacket, Stanford University Medical Center, Stanford California, 1980.)

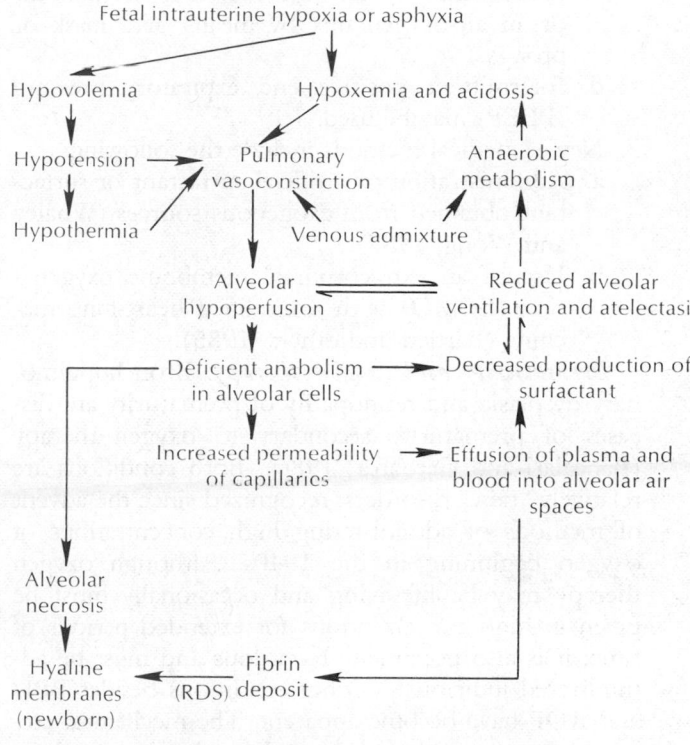

infant's body temperature is maintained at 36.5° C (97.6° F).

2. Gentle handling of the newborn is necessary. This infant is disturbed as little as possible.

3. Caloric intake is sufficient to prevent catabolism (40 kcal/kg/24 h or more).

4. Blood is replaced if an excessive amount is lost, usually as a result of samples taken for laboratory analysis.

5. Serum bilirubin levels are controlled by phototherapy, exchange transfusion, or both. Low serum albumin levels, hypoxia, and acidosis interfere with the albumin's binding to bilirubin and therefore subject these infants to kernicterus at low serum bilirubin levels (10 mg/dl or less; see Chapter 20 and discussion later in this Chapter).

6. Administer therapy, for example:
   a. Oxygen (60% or less) is administered by means of a hood (Fig. 31.5).
   b. Continuous positive airway pressure (CPAP) may be administered by means of an intratracheal tube, face mask, nasal prongs, or hood (see Chapter 25).

c. Continuous negative airway pressure (CNAP) may be needed. CNAP is a respirator that works in the same manner as CPAP but exerts negative pressure on the newborn's body while the head is exposed. The newborn may breathe room air or an air-oxygen mix by means of a mask or prongs.

d. Intermittent positive end expiratory pressure (PEEP) may be used.

7. Newer medical methods include the following:

a. Administration of artificial surfactant or surfactant obtained from exogenous sources (Whaley and Wong, 1987).

b. Use of an extracorporeal membrane oxygenation (ECMO) with a modified heart-lung machine (Bartlett and others, 1985).

Prematurity and oxygen therapy. Bronchopulmonary dysplasia and retinopathy of prematurity are diseases of prematurity secondary to oxygen therapy (Bancalari and Gerhardt, 1986). Both conditions are relatively "new" disorders, recognized since the advent of methods of administering high concentrations of oxygen beginning in the 1940s. Although oxygen therapy may be lifesaving and occasionally must be given in high concentrations for extended periods of time, it is also potentially hazardous and must be administered judiciously. Other conditions besides BPD and ROP have become apparent. The mechanical creation of positive pressure in the lungs has increased the incidence of "air leaks." Use of oxygen apparatus has also resulted in nasal, tracheal or pharyngeal perforation or inflammation (Whaley and Wong, 1987).

Bronchopulmonary dysplasia. Bronchopulmonary dysplasia is a pathologic process that may develop in the lungs of infants with lung disorders, primarily preterm infants. The cause is unknown, but the condition may develop as a sequela to the alveolar damage caused by lung disease, use of high oxygen concentrations and the prolonged use of CPAP or PEEP (Bancalari and Gerhardt, 1986).

Changes in the lung fields result in focal areas of emphysema. Symptoms of respiratory distress, tachypnea, and increased effort appear. It is difficult to wean the infant from the positive pressure ventilator. This finding may be the first indication of the disease process.

PROGNOSIS. The first sign that the infant is recovering from bronchopulmonary dysplasia is a decreasing dependence on oxygen therapy. Recovery may take several months. Mortality is between 30% and 50%; death may occur after the infant has been discharged from the hospital.

Retinopathy of prematurity. The retinal changes in retinopathy of prematurity were first described in 1942.

The condition has been related to the use of high levels of oxygen and prolonged oxygen therapy. Judicious use of oxygen therapy and monitoring of Pao_2 levels have reduced the incidence of ROP, but the disease has not been eradicated.

Pao_2 between 50 and 70 mm Hg may be within safe limits. (The recently developed transcutaneous oxygen tension monitor [$tcPo_2$] is a noninvasive device that provides continuous oxygen tension values.) The most crucial period for toxic levels to occur is during the recovery phase from RDS and other respiratory distress. The exact toxic level of arterial oxygen tension associated with retinopathy of prematurity is unknown.

Oxygen tensions that are too high for the level of retinal maturity initially result in vasoconstriction. After oxygen therapy is discontinued, neovascularization occurs in the retina and vitreous, with capillary hemorrhages, fibrotic resolution, and possible retinal detachment. Cicatricial (scar) tissue formation and consequent visual impairment may be mild or severe. The entire disease process in severe cases may take as long as 5 months to evolve. Examination by an ophthalmologist before discharge and a schedule for repeat examinations thereafter are recommended for the parents guidance.

Neonatal necrotizing enterocolitis. Necrotizing enterocolitis (NEC) is an inflammatory disease of the gastrointestinal mucosa, frequently complicated by perforation. This often fatal disease appears in about 5% of newborns in intensive care nurseries. Although its etiology is unknown, several possibilities are suspect:

1. Immaturity
2. Hypoxemia (postdelivery)
3. High-solute feedings
4. Excessive amounts of feedings
5. Perinatal asphyxia (frequently a historical antecedent)

Recent research suggests that reversal of asphyxia within 30 minutes may prevent gastrointestinal tract insult and so prevent the initiation of NEC pathophysiology. After 30 minutes, distribution of cardiac output tends to be directed more toward the heart and brain and away from the abdominal organs. Therefore, prompt delivery of the intrauterine asphyxiated fetus or ventilation of the asphyxiated newborn may be beneficial to the gastrointestinal tract as well as to other organs.

The onset is usually between 4 and 10 days. In the full-term infant the onset is almost always within the first 10 days. In the preterm infant the onset may be delayed up to 30 days. Signs of developing NEC are nonspecific, which is characteristic of many neonatal disease processes. Abdominal distention is probably the most frequent and regularly encountered sign. The infant's color is poor. Apneic periods increase in number. Frequently, there are gastric residuals of 2 ml or more before feedings. The stool may show occult blood (positive guaiac test). Diagnosis is confirmed by x-ray examination.

Treatment is supportive. Oral or tube feedings are discontinued to rest the gastrointestinal tract. Parenteral therapy (often by total parenteral nutrition [TPN]) is begun. NEC is an infectious disease, therefore control of infection is imperative. Antibiotic therapy may be instituted, and surgery is performed when necessary. Therapy may be prolonged, and recovery may be delayed by adhesions, complications of bowel resection (malabsorption), and intolerance of oral feedings.

SMALL-FOR-GESTATIONAL-AGE (DYSMATURE) INFANTS

Infants whose birth weight falls below the 10th percentile expected at term, for reasons other than heredity, are considered at high risk (mortality greater than 10%). Fetal growth retardation is attributable to the following possible causes:
- Deficient supply of nutrients (intrauterine malnutrition)
- Intrauterine infections
- Congenital malformations
- Heredity

Intrauterine growth retardation (IUGR) related to malnutrition will be discussed here. Two types of growth retardation are identified by the examination of cellular characteristics:
1. Hypoplasia or a deficient number of cells, although each cell has a normal amount of cytoplasm.
2. Diminished cell size resulting from a reduced amount of cytoplasm, although the total number of cells is unaffected.

Physical characteristics. Several physical findings are characteristic of the *growth-retarded neonate:*
1. Generally has normal skull, but reduced dimensions of rest of body make skull look inordinately large
2. Reduced subcutaneous fat
3. Loose and dry skin
4. Diminished muscle mass especially over buttocks and cheeks
5. Sunken abdomen (scaphoid) as opposed to being normally well rounded
6. Thin, yellowish, dry, and dull umbilical cord (normal cord is gray, glistening, round, and moist)
7. Sparse scalp hair
8. Wide skull sutures (inadequate bone growth)

Clinical problems. The infant who is SGA as a re-

sult of intrauterine nutritional growth retardation faces a number of physiologic problems. These include:
1. Initiation and maintenance of respirations
   a. Chronic intrauterine hypoxia, perinatal asphyxia
   b. Aspiration syndrome: ball-valve obstruction
2. Maintenance of adequate nutrition: chronic intrauterine malnutrition with meager stored fat and glycogen
3. Maintenance of body temperature
   a. Depleted subcutaneous fat and glycogen reserves
   b. Diminished muscle mass
   c. Large body surface compared to body weight
4. Prevention of CNS trauma
   a. Tendency to hypoglycemia
   b. Chronic intrauterine hypoxia, perinatal asphyxia
5. Prevention of infection
   a. Poor resistance to infection
   b. Growth retardation possibly caused totally or in part by exposure to intrauterine infection
6. Musculoskeletal system
   a. Inadequate bone growth: wide cranial suture
   b. Diminished muscle mass, especially over buttocks
   c. Meager subcutaneous fat lacks cushioning effect

Complications of dysmaturity
Perinatal asphyxia. Frequently, SGA infants have been exposed to chronic hypoxia for varying periods of time before labor and delivery. Labor is stressful to even a normal fetus and is more serious for one with growth retardation. The chronically hypoxic infant is severely compromised by even a normal labor and has difficulty compensating after birth. The alert, wide-eyed appearance of the newborn is attributed to prolonged prenatal hypoxia. Appropriate management and resuscitation are essential for the depressed infant.

The birth of SGA babies with perinatal asphyxia is often associated with a maternal history of heavy cigarette smoking, PIH, low socioeconomic status, multiple gestation, gestational infections such as rubella, cytomegalovirus, and toxoplasmosis, advanced diabetes mellitus, and cardiac problems. When a woman with this background arrives in labor, the nursing staff must be alerted to possible perinatal asphyxia.

Meconium aspiration syndrome. Two fetal responses to intrauterine hypoxia are the passage of meconium through a relaxed anal sphincter and reflex gasping. Gasping draws amniotic fluid and any particulate matter contained in the fluid deep into the bronchial tree. At birth, more aspiration may occur, and symptoms of respiratory distress often appear.

Hypoglycemia. Hypoglycemia is frequently encountered in SGA newborns, whether term or preterm. The incidence may be as high as 40%. Hypoglycemia in low-birth-weight infants is considered to be a glucose level of 20 mg/dl of blood or less. This disorder may occur anytime from birth until day 4 of life. If it is untreated, neurologic sequelae can be anticipated. Blood glucose levels are monitored by laboratory biochemical study and Dextrostix tests.

Heat loss. Diminution of subcutaneous fat and a large body surface compared to body weight subject the SGA newborn to problems in thermoregulation. Cold stress jeopardizes recovery from asphyxia. The meagerness of fat and glycogen reserves increases such an infant's vulnerability to cold and other stress.

Prognosis. Neonatal mortality is higher for the SGA term infant than for the infant of appropriate growth for gestational age (AGA) of the same age. Korones (1986) states: "Generally the immediate prognosis for survival and the long-term outlook for normal function seem to be better in small-for-dates infants than in those who are prematures and normally grown, yet neither of these groups fares as well as the normal-sized term infant."

Nursing care. Care of the SGA infant is based on the clinical problems present. The nursing care related to those problems is the same as for the preterm infant (pp. 983-987).

Evaluation. In assessing the effectiveness of nursing care the following evaluative criteria may be used:
1. Adequate ventilation is initiated and maintained.
2. Adequate nutritional state is achieved and maintained.
3. Body temperature is maintained.
4. CNS trauma is prevented or minimized.
5. Infection is prevented.
6. Musculoskeletal problems are prevented or minimized.
7. Positive parent-child relationships and socialization are begun.

POSTTERM INFANTS

Postterm, or *postdate,* refers to gestation prolonged beyond 42 *completed* weeks from the first day of the last menstrual cycle. *Postmaturity,* however, implies progressive placental insufficiency resulting in a dysmature (SGA) newborn. *Not all postterm newborns are postmature.*

Weights of postmature infants usually fall within the normal range for gestational age. However, the infant may be SGA because of deteriorating metabolic exchange in the aging placenta. Fetal malnutrition and hypoxia result in the wasted appearance of this dysmature infant.

These newborns have a higher incidence of fetal distress and perinatal death. The normal-appearing infants do well if fetopelvic disproportion (FPD) does not develop because of their increased size. A breakdown of perinatal deaths associated with prolonged pregnancy reveals that about one-third occurred during the prenatal period; approximately one-half occurred during the intranatal period; and about one-sixth during the postdelivery period.

Diagnosis. When a gravida is 2 weeks overdue, one of the following possibilities and its implications apply:
1. The pregnancy is not prolonged, and therefore, there is no threat to the fetus.
2. The pregnancy is prolonged, but the placenta continues to function efficiently and there is no threat to the fetus.
3. The pregnancy is prolonged, and there is acute placental failure with threat to the fetus.
4. The pregnancy is prolonged, there has been chronic placental insufficiency, and the threat to the fetus continues.

For safe delivery of the offspring, it becomes important to determine whether prolonged pregnancy actually has developed and if there is any evidence of fetal jeopardy. Data for determining fetal gestational age is obtained from several sources and correlated (Chapter 11).

Verification of the LMP or rejection of LMP as inaccurate is more important to the diagnosis of prolonged pregnancy. A correlation of the LMP with the estimated duration of pregnancy at two of the earliest obstetric examinations may lead to substantiation or recalculation of the EDC (see box, p. 254).

Gestational age. The gestational age of the fetus may be used to indicate the duration of pregnancy and the EDC. See Chapters 10 and 11 for details of the methods used in estimating gestational age.

If the dates are accurate but the uterus is larger than expected for the duration of pregnancy, hydramnios or multiple pregnancy may be the cause. If the dates seem correct but the size of the fetus is disparate, fetal compromise, such as intrauterine growth retardation (IUGR) may be the problem, particularly when it occurs in association with pregnancy-induced hypertension (PIH).

The woman's medical status is reappraised. Diabetic or gestational diabetic mothers have large babies, and this may confuse the estimate of gestational age. Amniocentesis to ascertain the true gestational age is also advised.

When the initial diagnosis of pregnancy is made at 20 weeks or less by physical examination, one or more of the *following observations* provide clinical confirmation of prolonged pregnancy.

1. Thirty-six weeks have elapsed since the recorded positive pregnancy test.
2. Thirty-two weeks have elapsed since the recorded FHT by Doppler instrument.
3. Twenty-four weeks have elapsed since recorded fetal movement.
4. Twenty-two weeks have elapsed since recorded FHR by auscultation.

Two serial *ultrasound examinations* and measurement of the *fetal biparietal diameter* should be accomplished 2 weeks apart after the twentieth week. This may confirm or reestablish the EDC. However, the EDC cannot be calculated when the initial biparietal diameter measures 9.5 cm or more (term size).

Other investigations may support the diagnosis of prolonged pregnancy; the following are examples:

1. Maternal weight loss in the last weeks of pregnancy (3 lb [1.3 kg] or more a week).
2. Reduced rate of uterine and fetal growth.
3. Palpation of a hard fetal head; lack of cephalic molding; high arrest of the fetal head.
4. Meconium staining of the amniotic fluid.
5. Oligohydramnios or decreased amniotic fluid (less than 300 ml).
6. Prolonged labor caused by uterine inertia or cephalopelvic disproportion (CPD).

Certain groups of mothers are especially prone to carry beyond term. These groups include nulliparas, high parity mothers (gravida 4 or greater), and mothers whose preceding pregnancy was postterm.

Physical characteristics. The majority of postterm and postmature infants are oversized but otherwise normal, with advanced development and bone age.

Some but not all postterm infants show the following physical characteristics:

1. Generally has normal skull, but reduced dimensions of rest of body make skull look inordinately large.
2. Dry, cracked skin (desquamating), parchmentlike at birth.
3. Nails of hard consistency extending beyond fingertips.
4. Profuse scalp hair.
5. Subcutaneous fat layers depleted, leaving skin loose and giving an "old person" appearance.
6. Long and thin body contour.
7. Absent vernix.
8. Often meconium staining (golden yellow to green) of skin, nails, and cord.
9. May have an alert, wide-eyed appearance symptomatic of chronic intrauterine hypoxia.

Possible perinatal hazards. Hazards to the fetus include the following:

1. The fetus may be exposed to the hazards of the oxytocin challenge test (OCT) (i.e., possible hypoxia)

and amniocentesis (i.e., possible infection, bleeding, direct trauma to infant).
2. The postterm fetus (AGA or SGA) may tolerate the stress of labor poorly. Indices of fetal jeopardy are late fetal heart rate deceleration patterns with a slow return to the baseline rate, meconium-stained amniotic fluid, oligohydramnios, and a fetal scalp blood pH of 7.2 or less. Cesarean delivery is frequently a necessity.
3. The oversized fetus may be exposed to excessive trauma such as fractures and intracranial hemorrhage and to asphyxia during dystocia (Chapter 29).

The mother is also exposed to possible hazards:

1. She often undergoes tests to evaluate placental sufficiency and fetal status (e.g., OCT, amniocentesis), and if indicated, labor is induced or cesarean delivery is performed.
2. Dystocia may accompany fetopelvic disproportion.
3. Emotional response of the woman can reflect feelings of fatigue, frustration, and anger as the pregnancy "never seems to end." She may experience negative feelings about her ability to cope and her "normalcy as a woman." Fears for the safety of her baby and the baby's future development can arise.

Management of postterm pregnancy. The management of an overly long pregnancy is as follows:

1. When the diagnosis of prolonged pregnancy is uncertain, additional information for or against the diagnosis is required. Expectant management with fetal monitoring should be carried out. The fetal monitoring will include fetal activity determination (FAD), weekly cervical assessment for dilatation and effacement, weekly estimate of fetal weight (EFW), nonstress test (NST), and serial estriol determinations.
2. When the diagnosis of prolonged pregnancy is established and there is a threat to the fetus, the woman should deliver. If induction is unsuccessful, if labor is unsatisfactory, or if fetal distress develops, cesarean delivery should be done.

Clinical problems. The postterm infant is at risk for many of the same physiologic problems as the preterm infant. These are related to the infant's ability for:

1. Initiation and maintenance of respirations
   a. Intrauterine hypoxia, perinatal asphyxia
   b. Meconium aspiration syndrome: ball-valve obstruction
2. Maintenance of body temperature
   a. Depleted subcutaneous fat and glycogen reserves
   b. Large body surface to body weight ratio
3. Maintenance of adequate nutrition
   a. Depleted fat and glycogen stores

b. Tendency to hypoglycemia
4. Prevention of CNS trauma
   a. Oversized infant: possible cephalopelvic disproportion and birth trauma
   b. Intrauterine hypoxia, perinatal asphyxia
   c. Tendency to hypoglycemia
5. Prevention of infection
   a. Diminished energy stores
   b. Skin dry, cracked, loose; vernix absent
   c. May have been exposed to infection during amniocentesis or application of internal fetal electrodes.

As a consequence, many of the same complications may result.
1. Respiratory function: altered blood gases and pH, asphyxia, aspiration pneumonia, atelectasis, pneumomediastinum, pneumothorax
2. Inadequate temperature maintenance: same as for the preterm infant
3. Nutrition
   a. Same as for the preterm infant
   b. Hypoglycemia with neurologic sequelae
4. CNS: same as for the preterm infant
5. Infection: same as for the preterm infant

Nursing care. The nursing care designed for the postterm infant will depend on the infant's size and condition. It may be similar to that needed for fetopelvic disproportion and prolonged labor (Chapter 29). If the infant is in distress, care similar to that prescribed for the preterm infant is instituted (Affonso, 1980).

Evaluation. Evaluation for the postterm infant occurs during the prenatal period, the intranatal period, and the early neonatal period. The following evaluative criteria are used:

Prenatal period
1. Maternal emotional stress with prolonged gestation and tests to evaluate fetoplacental status are minimized.
2. Evaluative tests such as OCT and amniocentesis are performed with no adverse sequelae.
3. Parents understand the situation.

Intranatal period
1. Outcome is physically safe for mother and fetus.
   a. Hypoxia is eliminated or minimized.
   b. Fetus suffers no birth trauma such as fractures, palsies, or intracranial hemorrhage.
   c. Dystocia, maternal infection, and bleeding are absent.
2. Parental fears are identified and minimized.

Early neonatal period
1. Asphyxia and birth trauma are averted or minimized.
2. There are no hypoglycemic episodes.
3. A positive parent-child relationship is initiated.

Infant Birth Trauma

Physical birth trauma may result from a number of factors:
1. The forces of labor, in combination with the fetal presentation and position.
2. The amount of resistance encountered during passage through the bony and soft birth canal.
3. The birth itself.

Many injuries are minor and readily resolve in the neonatal period without treatment. Other traumas require some degree of intervention. A few are serious enough to be fatal.

Classification of birth traumas. Birth traumas can be classified according to the following outline:
1. Soft tissue injuries
   a. Caput succedaneum
   b. Cephalhematoma
   c. Subcutaneous fat necrosis (pressure necrosis)
   d. Subconjunctival (scleral) hemorrhage
   e. Retinal hemorrhage
   f. Cyanosis, ecchymosis, and edema of buttocks and extremities
   g. Ecchymoses and petechiae of skin
   h. Hemorrhage into abdominal organs
2. Skeletal injuries
   a. Molding of fetal skull bones
   b. Fractures
      (1) Skull (depressed or linear)
      (2) Clavicle, humerus, or femur
3. Nervous system injury
   a. Peripheral nervous system
      (1) Brachial paralysis (Erb-Duchenne, Klumpke's)
      (2) Facial paralysis
      (3) Phrenic nerve injury (diaphragmatic paralysis)
   b. Central nervous system (intracranial hemorrhage, spinal cord injury)

The nurse's contributions to the welfare of the newborn begin with early observation and accurate recording. The prompt reporting of signs indicative of deviations from normal permits early initiation of appropriate therapy.

Goals for care. The overall goals for care of infants with birth trauma are as follows:

1. Anticipate and diagnose premonitory or early disease.
2. Minimize the effects of the disorder of avoid disability of the child.
3. Treat disease promptly and appropriately when possible.
4. Facilitate a positive parent-child relationship.

Soft tissue injuries

Caput succedaneum. Caput succedaneum is a localized edematous swelling of the scalp that persists for a few days after birth and then disappears. It has no pathologic significance (see Fig. 19.5, *A*).

Cephalhematoma. Cephalhematoma is a collection of blood from ruptured blood vessels between the periosteum and surface of the parietal bone (see Fig. 19.5, *B,* and discussion in Chapter 19). The swelling may appear unilaterally or bilaterally and disappears gradually in 2 to 3 weeks. Occasionally hyperbilirubinemia may result from breakdown of the accumulated blood.

Subcutaneous fat necrosis. Subcutaneous fat necrosis (pressure necrosis) results from pressure against the pelvis or from forceps. The lesion is clearly defined and is a firm mass (size varies) fixed to the overlying skin but movable over underlying tissue. Skin over the lesion may be reddish purple. These lesions usually resolve spontaneously in a few days.

Subconjunctival (scleral) and retinal hemorrhages. Subconjunctival and retinal hemorrhages result from rupture of capillaries from increased intracranial pressure during birth. They clear within 5 days after birth and usually present no problems. However, parents need reassurance about their presence.

Discoloration and petechiae. Cyanosis, ecchymosis, petechiae, and *edema* of buttocks and extremities may be present. Localized cyanosis may appear over presenting or dependent parts. Ecchymoses and edema appear as bruises anywhere on the body. They can appear on the presenting part from the application of forceps. They can result from manipulation of the infant's body during delivery. Petechiae, or pinpoint hemorrhagic areas, acquired during birth may extend over the upper trunk and face. These lesions are benign if they disappear within 2 days of birth and no new lesions appear. Ecchymoses and petechiae may be signs of a more serious disorder, such as thrombocytopenic purpura. If they do not disappear spontaneously in 2 days, the physician is notified.

To differentiate hemorrhagic areas from skin rashes and discolorations, the nurse blanches the skin with two fingers. Because extravasated blood remains within the tissues, petechiae and ecchymoses do not blanch.

Hemorrhage into abdominal organs. Hemorrhage into abdominal organs may occur following manipulation of the body during a difficult breech extraction. The liver is most susceptible to injury. The affected infant is pale, the liver enlarges progressively, and in some, a mass may be palpable. Rupture of the liver capsule occurs eventually, and the infant appears cyanotic and in shock. Surgical repair and blood transfusions are lifesaving.

Skeletal injuries

Molding. The shaping of the head as it passes through the bony pelvis during labor is discussed in Chapter 14. This is a normal process that facilitates descent of the head.

Skull fracture. The newborn's immature, flexible skull can withstand a great degree of deformation (molding) before fracture results. Considerable force is required to fracture the newborn's skull. Location of the fracture determines whether it is insignificant or fatal. If an artery lying in a groove on the undersurface of the skull is torn as a result of the fracture, increased intracranial pressure will ensue (pp. 997-998 and 1027). Unless a blood vessel is involved, linear fractures (which account for 70% of all fractures for this age group) heal without special treatment. The soft skull may become indented without laceration of either the skin or the dural membrane. These depressions, or "ping-pong ball" indentations, may occur during difficult deliveries from pressure of the head on the bony pelvis. They can also occur as a result of injudicious application of forceps.

Fracture of the clavicle. The clavicle is the bone most often fractured during delivery. Generally the break is in the middle third of the bone. Dystocia, particularly shoulder impaction, may be the predisposing problem. *Limitation of motion of the arm, crepitus of the bone, and no Moro's reflex on the affected side are diagnostic.* Except for use of gentle rather than vigorous handling, there is no accepted treatment for fractured clavicle. The figure-eight bandage appropriate for the older child should not be used for the newborn. The prognosis is good.

Fracture of the humerus or femur. The humerus and femur are other bones that may be fractured during a difficult delivery. Fractures in newborns generally heal rapidly. Immobilization is accomplished with slings, splints, swaddling, and other devices.

The parents need support in handling these infants because they are often fearful of hurting them. Parents are encouraged to practice handling, changing, and feeding the affected newborn in the nursery under the guidance of personnel. This will increase their confi-

Fig. 31.18
A, Erb-Duchenne paralysis in newborn infant. Right upper extremity failed to participate in Moro's reflex. Recovery was complete. **B,** Residual of Erb-Duchenne paralysis. Left arm was short; it could not be raised above level shown. (From Shirkey, H.C., editor: Pediatric therapy, ed. 6, St. Louis, 1975, The C.V. Mosby Co.)

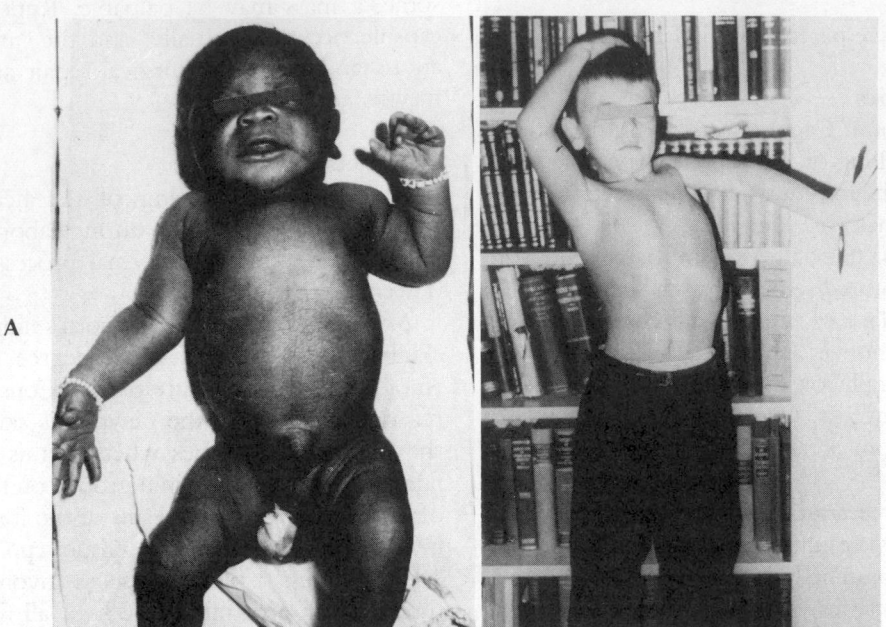

dence and knowledge and facilitate attachment. A plan for follow-up therapy is developed with the parents so that the times and arrangements for therapy are workable and acceptable to them.

Nervous system injuries
Peripheral nerves
Brachial paralysis: upper arm. Erb-Duchenne paralysis (upper arm brachial paralysis) is the most common type of paralysis associated with a difficult delivery (Fig. 31.18). Typical symptoms are a flaccid arm with the elbow extended and the hand rotated inward, negative Moro's reflex on the affected side, sensory loss over the lateral aspect of the arm, and an intact grasp reflex.

Treatment consists of intermittent immobilization, proper positioning, and exercise to maintain the range of motion of joints. Gentle manipulation and range-of-motion exercises are delayed until about the tenth day to prevent additional injury to the brachial plexus.

Immobilization may be accomplished with a brace or splint or by pinning the infant's sleeve to the mattress. The infant should be positioned for 2 or 3 hours at a time in the following manner: abduct the arm 90 degrees; externally rotate the shoulder; flex the elbow

Fig. 31.19
Recommended corrective positioning for treatment of Erb-Duchenne paralysis. Note abduction and external rotation at shoulder, flexion at elbow, supination of forearm, and slight dorsiflexion at wrist. (From Behrmann, R.E., editor: Neonatology: diseases of the fetus and infant, St. Louis, 1973, The C.V. Mosby Co.)

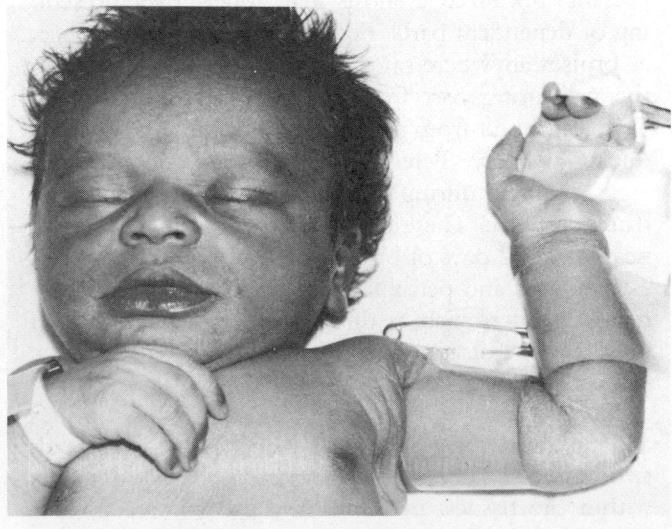

90 degrees; supinate the wrist with the palm directed slightly toward the face (Fig. 31.19). The arm should be freed periodically for good skin care. About the tenth day, gentle massage and range-of-motion exercises are begun to prevent contractures.

Brachial paralysis: lower arm. Damage to the lower plexus, Klumpke's palsy, is less common. With lower arm paralysis, the wrist and hand are flaccid, the grasp reflex is absent, deep tendon reflexes are present, and dependent edema and cyanosis may be apparent (in the affected hand). Treatment consists of placing the hand in a neutral position, padding the fist, and gently exercising the wrist and fingers.

Parents are taught to position and immobilize the arm or wrist or both. They can gently massage and manipulate the muscles to prevent contractures while the arm is healing. If edema or hemorrhage is responsible for the paralysis, the prognosis is good and recovery may be expected in a few weeks. If laceration of the nerves has occurred and healing does not result in return of function within a few months (3 to 6 months or 2 years at the most), surgery may be indicated; however, little or no function will develop.

Facial paralysis. Facial paralysis (Fig. 31.20) is generally caused by misapplication of forceps with pressure by one blade against the facial nerve during delivery. The face on the affected side is flattened and unresponsive to the grimace of crying or stimulation,

and the eye will remain open. Moreover, the forehead will not wrinkle. Often the condition is transitory, resolving within hours or days of birth. Permanent paralysis is rare.

Treatment involves careful, patient feeding, prevention of damage to the cornea of the open eye, and supportive care of the parents. Frequently the infant looks grotesque, especially when crying. Feeding may be prolonged, with the milk flowing out of the newborn's mouth around the nipple on the affected side. The mother will need understanding and sympathetic encouragement while learning how to feed and care for the infant, as well as how to hold and cuddle the baby.

Phrenic nerve injury. Phrenic nerve injury almost always occurs as a component of brachial plexus injury. Injury to the phrenic nerve results in diaphragmatic paralysis. Cyanosis and irregular thoracic respirations with no abdominal movement on inspiration are characteristic of paralysis of the diaphragm. Babies with diaphragmatic paralysis usually require mechanical ventilatory support, at least for the first few days after birth. Occasionally this support is essential for several weeks until corrective surgery can be performed.

Central nervous system

Intracranial hemorrhage. Intracranial hemorrhage as a result of birth trauma is more likely to occur in the full-term, large infant. The hemorrhage occurs into the

Fig. 31.20

A, Paralysis of right side of face 15 minutes after forceps delivery. Absence of movement on affected side is especially noticeable when infant cries. **B,** Same infant 24 hours later. (From Whaley, L.F., and Wong, D.L.: Nursing of infants and children, ed. 3, St. Louis, 1987, The C.V. Mosby Co.)

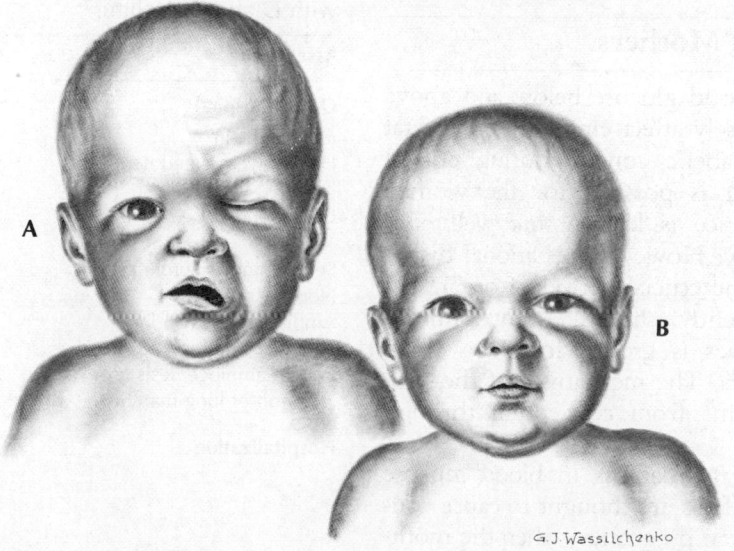

G.J. Wassilchenko

brain substance or as a subdural hematoma. The latter is the principal manifestation of intracranial hemorrhage. The diagnostic signs arise from **increased intracranial pressure** and are (1) **separation of the sutures** and (2) **bulging of the anterior fontanel.** Subdural hematoma is seen with relative infrequency today because of the remarkable improvements in obstetric care in the last decade.

Hypoxia and hypovolemia are the most common causes of intracranial hemorrhage. Hemorrhage from hypoxia occurs in the subarachnoid space or in the ventricles of the brain. *These intracranial hemorrhages, seen most frequently in premature infants, are not related to trauma.* The symptomatology varies. Abnormal respiration with cyanosis, hypotonia, reduced responsiveness (lethargy), irritability, a high-pitched, shrill cry, tense fontanel, twitching, or convulsions may be noted.

General treatment consists of elevation of the head several inches higher than the hips, warmth, oxygen to relieve cyanosis, and administration of intravenous fluids or other suitable means of meeting the neonate's food and fluid needs. Minimal handling to promote rest should guide nursing care.

The treatment of subdural hemorrhage is aspiration or surgical removal of the blood collection. Repeated subdural taps for the evacuation of subdural blood is indicated whether or not the head size is increasing and the fontanel is bulging.

Spinal cord injuries. Spinal cord injuries may occur during manipulation of the newborn's body during breech extraction. Injury occurs when considerable traction force is required to deliver the shoulders or head or both. This injury is rarely seen today as cesarean delivery is often used for delivery of a breech.

Infants of Diabetic Mothers

Wide fluctuations of blood glucose below and above the normal range adversely affect embryonic and fetal development. Good diabetic control during critical embryonic development is possible for the woman whose glucose intolerance is known *and* well controlled before pregnancy. However, gestational diabetes is diagnosed after the crucial period of organogenesis is over. Consequently, the risk of hydramnios and congenital anomalies is greater for the woman with gestational diabetes. The mechanism of the process leading to problems from conception through birth is as follows.

In early pregnancy, fluctuations in blood glucose and episodes of ketoacidosis are thought to cause congenital anomalies. Later in pregnancy, when the mother's pancreas cannot release sufficient insulin to meet increased demands, maternal hyperglycemia results. The high levels of glucose stimulate the fetal pancreas to release insulin. The combination of the increased supply of maternal glucose and fetal insulin results in excessive fetal growth called macrosomia. Hyperinsulinemia accounts for most of the problems seen. In addition, poor diabetic control or superimposed infection adversely affect the fetus. Normally, maternal blood has a more alkaline pH than does fetal blood (with its excess of CO_2). This phenomenon encourages exchange of O_2 and CO_2 across the placental membrane. When the maternal blood is more acidotic than the fetal blood, no CO_2 or O_2 exchange occurs at the level of the placenta. The fetus becomes asphyxiated and dies.

Management

Prepregnancy and prenatal period. There is some indication that some neonatal conditions—macrosomia, hypoglycemia, hypocalcemia, hyperbilirubinemia, and perhaps fetal lung immaturity—may be eliminated or the incidence decreased by maintaining control over maternal glucose levels within narrow limits (Fuhrmann and others, 1983). Table 31.6 lists a timetable for monitoring pregnancy complicated with diabetes mellitus.

Perinatal period. Perinatal management focuses on maternal hydration-calorie-insulin balance, adequate fetal perfusion and oxygenation, and prevention of maternal stress. Fetal hypoxia and acidosis can initiate or aggravate RDS. Careful assessment of labor identifies a dystotic labor early so that appropriate interventions

Table 31.6
Timetable: Monitoring Pregnancy Complicated with Diabetes Mellitus

Assessment	Gestational Age
Out of hospital	
α-Fetoprotein	10 weeks
Hb$_{Alc}$ (glycosylated hemoglobin)	Weekly
Ultrasound	18 and 28 weeks for fetal growth
Serial urine or serum estriols	Weekly starting at 32 weeks
Nonstress test	Weekly starting at 34 weeks
Amniocentesis (L/S ratio, phosphatidyl-glycerol)	36 weeks
Repeat amniocentesis for evaluation of lung maturity	If previous test showed immaturity
Hospitalization	Anytime for control of condition; at 36 weeks if good glucose/insulin control has not been achieved or if other risk develops

may be implemented for a safe vaginal or abdominal birth. Infusions given to the mother that contain dextrose require insulin to minimize the risk of fetal postnatal hypoglycemia and hyperbilirubinemia.

Postnatal period. No single physiologic or biochemical event can explain the diverse clinical manifestations seen in the infants of diabetic mothers (IDM) or infants of gestational diabetic mothers (IGDM). For the conditions described previously, and those listed and discussed below the same principles of management pertain, whether they occur in the IDM or any other newborn.

1. Macrosomia and birth trauma
2. Congenital anomalies
3. Hypoglycemia

4. Hypocalcemia
5. Lung immaturity—RDS
6. Hyperbilirubinemia
7. Polycythemia

Clinical picture of infants from pregnancies complicated by diabetes mellitus

Macrosomia. At birth the typical infant who is LGA has a round, cherubic, or cushingoid face, chubby body, and plethoric appearance (Fig. 31.21). This infant is **macrosomic.** The infant has enlarged viscera (hepatosplenomegaly, spanchnomegaly, cardiomegaly) and increased body fat. The placenta and umbilical cord are larger than average. The brain is the only organ that is not enlarged. With good prenatal care and control of diabetes mellitus, the incidence of macrosomia can be decreased.

The excessive size of these infants can and often does lead to dystocia because of fetopelvic disproportion. These infants, who may be born vaginally or by cesarean delivery after a trial of labor, may incur birth trauma.

Birth trauma and perinatal asphyxia. Birth trauma (secondary to macrosomia or to method of delivery)

Fig. 31.21
"During their first 24 or more extrauterine hours they lie on their backs, bloated and flushed, their legs flexed and abucted, their tightly closed hands on each side of their head, the abdomen prominent and their respiration sighing. They convey a distinct impression of having had so much food and fluid pressed upon them by an insistent hostess that they desire only peace so that they may recover from their excesses." (From Shirkey, H.C., editor: Pediatric therapy, ed. 6, St. Louis, 1980, The C.V. Mosby Co., Quotation from Whaley, L.F., and Wong, D.L.: Nursing care of infants and children, ed. 2, St. Louis, 1983, The C.V. Mosby Co.)

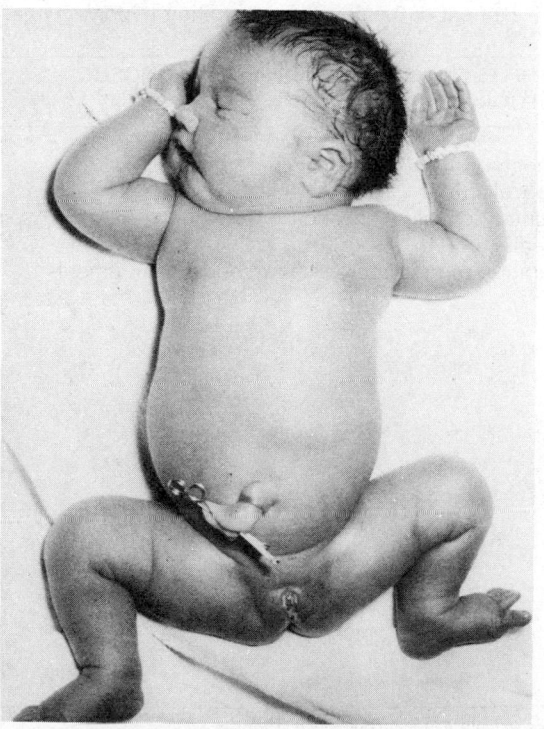

Fig. 31.22
Infant of diabetic mother with caudal regression syndrome (sacral agenesis). (From Fanaroff, A.A., and Martin, R.J., editors: Behrman's nenonatal-perinatal medicine: diseases of the fetus and infant, ed. 3, St. Louis, 1983, The C.V. Mosby Co.)

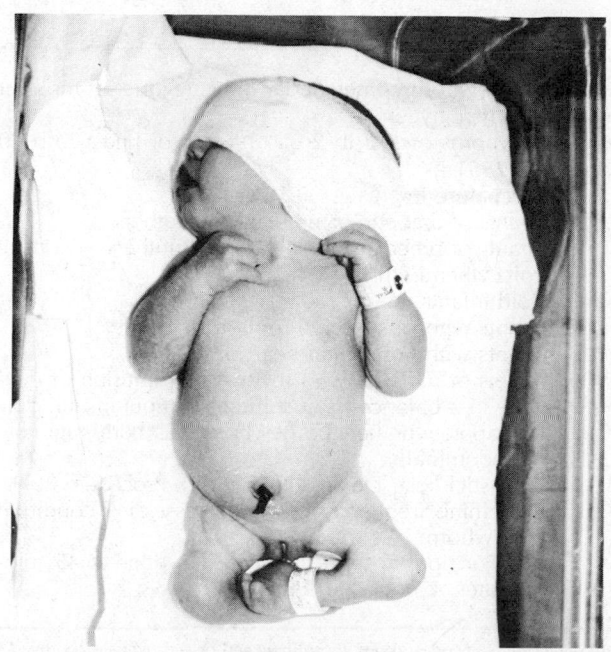

and perinatal asphyxia occur in 20% of IGDM and 35% of IDM. Examples of birth trauma include the following:

1. Cephalhematoma
2. Paralysis of the facial nerve (seventh cranial nerve)
3. Fracture of the clavicle
4. Brachial plexus paralysis, usually Erb-Duchenne (upper right arm) paralysis
5. Phrenic nerve paralysis, invariably associated with diaphragmatic paralysis

Congenital anomalies. Congenital anomalies occur in about 6% of IDM. The incidence is greatest among the SGA newborns. The most frequently occurring anomalies include the following:

1. CNS—anencephaly, encephalocele, meningomyelocele, hydrocephalus
2. Caudal regression syndrome—sacral agenesis with weakness or deformities of the lower extremities, malformation and fixation of the hip joints, and shortening or deformity of the femurs (Fig. 31.22)

3. Tracheoesophageal fistula
4. Congenital heart malformations

Hypoglycemia and hypocalcemia. Separation of the placenta interrupts the constant infusion of glucose. The high level of circulating glucose at the time the umbilical cord is severed falls rapidly in the presence of fetal hyperinsulinism. *Asymptomatic* or symptomatic hypoglycemia occurs within the first 1 to 3 hours after birth. Hypocalcemia occurs in 30% of IDM. In addition, hypocalcemia is associated with preterm delivery, birth trauma, and perinatal asphyxia. Symptoms of hypocalcemia, a prevalent finding in IDM and IGDM, are similar to those of hypoglycemia, but they occur between 24 and 36 hours of age. However, hypocalcemia must be considered if therapy for hypoglycemia is ineffective.

Summaries of nursing actions are presented for the following problems: (1) hypoglycemia, pp. 1000-1001, (2) hypocalcemia, pp. 1002-1003, (3) infant with hypocalcemia , hypoglycemia, or sepsis, p. 1004.

Summary of Nursing Actions

NEONATAL HYPOGLYCEMIA

GOAL

1. Prompt identification and treatment of hypoglycemia.

PRIORITIES

1. Identification of the newborn at risk.
2. Treatment of the newborn exhibiting hypoglycemia.

ASSESSMENT	EXAMPLES OF POTENTIAL NURSING DIAGNOSTIC CATEGORIES
A. Note if newborn comes under the categories of those at risk for hypoglycemia: 1. Newborns over 8 lb 2 oz (3969 g) or under 5 lb 10 oz (2551 g) 2. Dysmature infants 3. Infants of diabetic or prediabetic mothers 4. Infants of preeclamptic-eclamptic mothers 5. Polycythemic infants 6. Cold infants 7. Infants with severe erythroblastosis fetalis 8. Infants with congenital heart disease 9. Infants of mothers who received an infusion of dextrose in a balanced salt solution without insulin during labor, whether the newborn was born vaginally or abdominally. B. Do heel-stick test: Dextrostix, Clinistix Procedure 20.1 1. Determine frequency of test by assessing condition of newborn. a. For normal term infant, test is done at 45 minutes, 2 hours, and 6 hours of age.	Hypoglycemia† Hypocalcemia† Potential for injury secondary to hypoglycemia or hypocalcemia Alteration in nutrition: less than body requirements

*All diagnostic categories except those indicated by a dagger are approved by NANDA's seventh national conference (1986).
†Diagnosis not included by NANDA, 1986.

Summary of Nursing Actions—cont'd

ASSESSMENT	EXAMPLES OF POTENTIAL NURSING DIAGNOSTIC CATEGORIES

b. For infant at risk, do test at following intervals: 30 minutes at age, 1½ hours of age, 4 hours of age, 9 hours of age, 12 hours of age, 24 hours of age, and then once daily for 8 days.
2. Order blood sugar test by laboratory if tests reveal blood glucose concentration levels below 30 mg/dl during the first 72 hours of life or below 45 mg/dl after the first 3 days in the full-term infant (in premature newborns a blood sugar level below 20 mg/dl).
C. Observe for symptoms of hypoglycemia.
  1. Feeding difficulty, hunger
  2. Apnea
  3. Irregular respiratory effort
  4. Cyanosis
  5. Weak, high-pitched cry
  6. Jitteriness, twitching, eye rolling, convulsions
  7. Lethargy	

OUTCOME CRITERIA*	PLAN/IMPLEMENTATION
A. Newborn suffers no hypoglycemic episodes B. Newborn suffers no brain damage. C. Parents understand the condition and are able to establish a positive relationship with the newborn.	If suck-swallow reflex is well coordinated, feed the newborn according to hospital protocol. Term infants may be fed at 4 hours of age or earlier, as necessary. Small newborns or those born of diabetic mothers may need to be fed at 1 hour of age. Because newborns' stomach capacity is small, the amount should be small and the feedings frequent. Some pediatricians prefer early feedings of nonglucose carbohydrates, such as invert sugar or galactose. These preparations are less likely to overstimulate the newborn's pancreas to produce insulin (Whaley and Wong, 1987). If newborn cannot take fluids by mouth or if blood glucose is below 25 mg/dl, physician will administer 10% glucose in water intravenously.

EVALUATION The nurse can be assured that care was effective if the goals of care have been achieved.

*Outcome criteria direct the selection of nursing actions (**plan/implementation**) and measure their effectiveness (**evaluation**).

Summary of Nursing Actions

NEONATAL HYPOCALCEMIA

GOAL

1. Prevent neonatal hypocalcemia.

PRIORITIES

1. Prompt identification and treatment of neonatal hypocalcemia.

ASSESSMENT	EXAMPLES OF POTENTIAL NURSING DIAGNOSTIC CATEGORIES*

A. Identification of infants at risk:
  1. Infants receiving exchange transfusion of blood containing anticoagulant citrate. Citrate combines with calcium, thus depleting ionizable calcium needed for the coagulation process. To anticipate and replace this loss, 10% calcium gluconate is given.
  2. Other conditions that predispose an infant to hypocalcemia include the following:
    a. Perinatal asphyxia (33% of asphyxiated newborns)
    b. Use of bicarbonate to treat acidosis
    c. Diabetic mother (50% of newborns born to insulin-dependent mothers)
    d. Prematurity (33% of neonates born at 37 weeks' gestation or sooner regardless of birth weight)
    e. Preeclamptic-eclamptic mother treated before delivery with magnesium sulfate (a competitive antagonist to calcium)
  3. Tetany of the newborn was formerly a frequent occurrence, when 5- to 10-day-old infants were fed cow's milk.‡
B. Within the first 48 hours, hypocalcemia may be exhibited as edema, apnea, intermittent cyanosis, and abdominal distension, but classic symptoms of tetany are absent. Note that these symptoms are similar to those of other neonatal disorders, for example, hypoglycemia and sepsis. Therefore the infant's history must be taken to assist in the correct diagnosis.
	Hypocalcemia†
	Potential for injury

OUTCOME CRITERIA§	PLAN/IMPLEMENTATION
A. Newborn suffers no episodes of hypocalcemia. B. Newborn has no episodes to tetany. C. Parents understand the condition and are able to establish a positive relationship with the newborn	Medical therapy: acute care for hypocalcemia consists of calcium gluconate, 10% solution (100 to 150 mg/kg body weight) by intravenous infusion slowly; rapid infusion may cause flushing, vomiting, and circulatory collapse. Extravasation into surrounding tissue precipitates the calcium, causing necrosis and sloughing. Vitamin D_2 (ergocalciferol) every 24 hours for 2 or 3 weeks may be ordered. The nurse assists in medical management by monitoring the calcium gluconate infusion and the newborn's heart rate. If the heart rate is below 100 beats/min, the infusion is discontinued. A scalp vein is not used; the needle is taped securely at the site, and firm pressure is exerted over the site when the needle is removed to prevent seepage of the calcium gluconate into surrounding tissues.

*All diagnostic categories except those indicated by a dagger are approved by NANDA's seventh national conference (1986).
†Diagnosis not included by NANDA, 1986.
‡For a discussion of neonatal tetany from cow's milk, see Whaley and Wong (1987)
§Outcome criteria direct the selection of nursing actions (**plan/implementation**) and measure their effectivemenss (**evaluation**).

Summary of Nursing Actions—cont'd

OUTCOME CRITERIA	PLAN/IMPLEMENTATION
	The needle should be changed every 12 hours for the same reason. Supportive nursing care includes the following: ■ Maintenance of normal temperature, hydration, and oxygenation ■ Reduction of environmental stimuli (e.g., nursing care organized to minimize handling of infant) ■ Observation for and precautions against seizures ■ Keeping parents informed of care and progress; providing time for parents to express feelings; encouraging parents to visit frequently and to participate in care of infant.

EVALUATION The nurse can be assured that care was effective if the goals of care are met.

Lung immaturity. IDM or IGDM manifest a greater incidence of respiratory distress syndrome (RDS) than is found in normal infants of comparable gestational age. Synthesis of surfactant may be delayed because of the high fetal serum level of insulin. Fetal lung maturity as evidenced by a lecithin-sphingomyelin (L/S) ratio of 2 to 1 is not reassuring if the mother has diabetes mellitus or gestation-induced diabetes mellitus. For the infants of such mothers, an L/S ratio of 3 to 1 or more or the presence of **phosphatidylglycerol** in the amniotic fluid is more indicative of adequate lung maturity.

Hyperbilirubinemia. Fifty percent of newborns of 32 to 34 weeks' gestation develop hyperbilirubinemia; 15% of infants born at 37 weeks' gestation manifest this condition. Many newborns are plethoric because of polycythemia. *Polycythemia* increases blood viscosity and thereby impairs circulation. In addition, this increased number of red blood cells to be hemolyzed increases the potential bilirubin load that the newborn must clear. The excessive red blood cells are produced in extramedullary foci (liver and spleen) in addition to the usual sites in bone marrow. Therefore both liver function and bilirubin clearance may be adversely affected.

The summary of nursing actions for infants of diabetic mothers and infants of gestational diabetic mothers is presented on pp. 1004-1006.

Birth of large infants. Large-for-gestational-age (LGA) newborns may be preterm, term, or postterm; children of diabetic (or prediabetic) mothers; or postmature (see Figs. 31.1 and 31.2). Each of these categories has special concerns. Regardless of coexisting potential problems, the oversized infant is at risk by virtue of size alone. Birth trauma, especially associated with breech or shoulder presentation, is a serious hazard for the oversized neonate. Asphyxia or CNS injury or both may also occur.

An oversized infant traditionally has been one who weighs 4000 g (8 lb 13 oz) or more at birth. About 10% of newborns are of this weight, and about 2% weigh 4500 g (9 lb 15 oz) or more. Moreover, most of these newborns have other proportionately larger measurements. Many are delivered well after the estimated date of confinement (EDC).

A summary of nursing actions for large infants is presented on pp. 1006-1009.

Summary of Nursing Care of Infant with Hypocalcemia, Hypoglycemia, or Sepsis

Goals	Responsibilities
Recognize early signs of pathophysiologic state	Assess each system for signs and symptoms suggestive of each condition; correlate findings with general impression of progress of infant (feeding, weight gain, response to stimuli, and sleeping patterns).
Prevent or decrease potential side effects of medical intervention	
Hypocalcemia	Administer calcium gluconate slowly; if heart rate falls below 100 beats/min, stop infusion.
	Prevent extravasation of calcium gluconate into tissues:
	Avoid scalp vein.
	Ensure placement of needle before administering drug.
	Tape needle securely at site of insertion.
	Apply pressure to puncture site after removal of needle.
	Counsel mother regarding infant feeding (breast feeding or appropriate formulas).
Hypoglycemia	Begin oral feeding as soon as possible after birth.
	Administer glucose infusion carefully; avoid overloading the system by speeding up intravenous administration.
	Observe for signs of hyperglycemia (acidosis) and possible need for insulin.
	Decrease intravenous administration of glucose slowly to avoid hypoglycemia from physiologic hyperinsulinemia.
Sepsis	Observe for side effects of antibiotics.
	Regulate infusion carefully to allow for antibiotic to be administered within 1 hour.
	Use piggyback setup if main intravenous solution has added drugs.
Monitor environment to decrease factors that will complicate recovery from each condition	Maintain thermoregulation, hydration, and oxygenation of infant.
	Monitor vital signs and correlate with infant's progress.
Hypocalcemia	Reduce environmental stimuli
	Organize care to ensure minimal handling of infant.
	Discuss with parents reasons for minimal holding.
	Institute seizure precautions.
Sepsis	Institute appropriate isolation techniques.
Observe for complications of disease	
Hypocalcemia	Observe for tetany and convulsions.
Hypoglycemia	Check heel blood with Dextrostix.
	Check urine for glycosuria.
Sepsis	Observe for signs of meningitis, especially bulging anterior fontanel.
	Observe for pyarthrosis, usually evidenced by limited movement of affected joint.
	Observe for signs of shock, especially fall in blood pressure.
Provide emotional support for parents	Allow parents the opportunity to express their feelings.
	Keep parents informed of infant's progress.
	Encourage frequent visiting and participation in care to foster parent-child attachment.

From Whaley, L.F., and Wong, D.L.: Nursing care of infants and children, ed.2, St. Louis, 1983, The C.V. Mosby Co.

Summary of Nursing Actions

IDM AND IGDM

GOALS

1. For the mother: a physically safe and emotionally satisfying pregnancy and delivery.
2. For the fetus and newborn: a healthy intrauterine environment and transition to extrauterine existence.
3. For the family: an understanding of diabetes mellitus and willing compliance with management. If newborn exhibits a disorder or dies, the grieving process is initiated.

PRIORITIES

1. Maintenance of euglycemia throughout pregnancy.
2. Safe delivery of a live infant.
3. Prevention of or early identification and treatment of neonatal hypoglycemia and other conditions associated with maternal diabetes.
4. Initiation of a positive family-newborn attachment.

Summary of Nursing Actions—cont'd

ASSESSMENT	EXAMPLES OF POTENTIAL NURSING DIAGNOSTIC CATEGORIES*

A. Review prenatal records.
B. Assess the newborn frequently for the following associated clinical problems (in order of probably appearance):
  1. Respiratory distress and ventilatory adequacy.
  2. Congenital anomalies or disorders (incidence is 6% compared to 2% in all deliveries).
  3. Birth trauma (e.g., cephalhematoma, paralysis of the facial nerve, fracture of the clavicle).
  4. Meconium aspiration (if amniotic fluid was stained or if skin, nails, or cord is stained with meconium).
  5. Gestational age and degree of maturity (LGA, AGA, SGA).
  6. Hypoglycemia (within the first 3 hours).
  7. Polycythemia (by 6 hours of age).
  8. Hypocalcemia (within 24 to 36 hours).
  9. Hyperbilirubinemia (on day 2 or 3).
C. Weigh newborn soon after birth, then daily. Measure head and chest circumference.
D. Assess parent-newborn interaction.
	Infant
	Alteration in respiratory function†
	Ineffective airway clearance
	Ineffective breathing patterns
	Impaired gas exchange
	Alteration in nutrition: less or more than body requirements
	Ineffective thermoregulation related to immaturity, congenital disorder
	Potential for injury related to birth injury, hypoxia, kernicterus
	
	Parents
	Anxiety
	Fear
	Ineffective individual or family coping
	Alteration in family process
	Grieving
	Knowledge deficit
	Noncompliance
	Alteration in nutrition: less or more than body requirement
	Powerlessness
	Disturbance in self-concept
	Spiritual distress

OUTCOME CRITERIA‡	PLAN/IMPLEMENTATION

A. The newborn's airway remains patent, and respiratory distress is prevented or treated quickly.
B. The newborn does not experience cold stress, and the newborn's temperature stabilizes within 8 to 10 hours after birth.
C. The newborn experiences no hypoglycemic episodes (below 30 mg/dl), and blood glucose levels stabilize in the physiologic range (approximately between 45 and 130 mg/dl).
D. The newborn experiences no hypocalcemic episodes.
E. Bilirubin levels are maintained below toxic levels.
F. Fluid and electrolyte balance is maintained.
G. A positive relationship is established between parent and newborn.
H. Parents understand the care provided to the newborn.
I. Discharge planning is adequate:
  1. Parents feel ready to provide care to the newborn.
  2. Public health referral is made, if appropriate.
  3. Referral to other community resourses is made, if appropriate.
  4. Parents state motivation to carry out follow-up care.
	At birth
	Maintain equipment and ensure adequate oxygen and other supplies for resuscitative measures.
	Assist with resuscitation as necessary.
	Protect newborn against loss of body heat by drying, wrapping in warmed blankets, and positioning under a heat source.
	
	Subsequent care
	Position newborn on the side, with head slightly elevated and neck slightly extended.
	Observe, report, and record signs of respiratory distress.
	Treat as if infant is premature, regardless of weight, until gestational age and respiratory maturity are established.
	■ Place in incubator that has been set between 32° and 36° C (90° and 97° F) (depending on infant's maturity, size).
	■ Attach thermistor probe or take axillary temperature every 15 minutes until stabilized and then hourly. Temperature should stabilize at 36.5° C (97.6° F).
	■ Check respiratory rate every 15 minutes for 6 hours; place newborn on respiratory monitor if respirations are irregular.
	■ Have oxygen and resuscitative equipment available.
	Feed as necessary (glucose, calcium). Monitor parenteral fluid therapy. (See care of newborn with hypoglycemia, pp. 1000-1001.)

*All diagnostic categories except those indicated by a dagger are approved by NANDA's seventh national conference (1986).
†Diagnosis not included by NANDA, 1986.
‡Outcome criteria direct the selection of nursing actions (**plan/implementation**) and measure their effectiveness (**evaluation**).

Summary of Nursing Actions—cont'd

OUTCOME CRITERIA*	PLAN/IMPLEMENTATION
	Carry out orders for decreasing bilirubin levels. Promptly report and record any signs of anomalies, dysfunction, or disorder. Keep parents informed. Nurse is available to parents for their questions (e.g., explain that infant's condition is reflection of maternal condition rather than infant diabetes), discussion of feelings, and so on.

EVALUATION The nurse can be reasonably assured that nursing care has been effective if the goals of care have been met.

Summary of Nursing Actions

LARGE INFANTS

GOALS
1. For the mother: a satisfying birth.
2. For the newborn: a birth without trauma or injury and a neonatal period without hypoglycemia or hypocalcemia.
3. For the family: a positive birth experience.

PRIORITIES
1. Prevention of birth injuries by appropriate choice of delivery method.
2. Prompt identification and treatment of birth injuries.
3. Prompt identification and treatment of hypoglycemia or hypocalcemia.
4. Parental support.

ASSESSMENT	EXAMPLES OF POTENTIAL NURSING DIAGNOSTIC CATEGORIES*

A. Assess infant for hypoglycemia.
   1. Blood glucose level
   2. Symptoms
	Hypoglycemia†

B. Assess for gestational age.	Potential for compromised newborn†
C. After cesarean delivery: 1. Assess for pallor: usually caused by iatrogenic bleeding.	Ineffective airway clearance
2. If mother experienced prolonged labor prior to surgery, assess for anoxia, depressed skull fracture, possible paralyses; later assess for cephalhematoma.	Impaired gas exchange
3. If fetal distress had been noted, observe for aspiration.	Ineffective airway clearance
D. After vaginal delivery: 1. If fetal distress had been noted, observe for meconium aspiration	Impaired gas exchange

2. Note neurologic problems.
      a. Brachial paralysis: Erb-Duchenne type.
      Symptoms on affected side:
      (1) Arm: abducted and internally rotated
      (2) Wrist: flexed
      (3) Palm: limp, grasp reflex present
      (4) Moro's reflex: asymmetric
	Potential for injury

*All diagnostic categories except those indicated by a dagger are approved by NANDA's seventh national conference (1986).
†Diagnosis not included by NANDA, 1986.

Summary of Nursing Actions—cont'd

ASSESSMENT	EXAMPLES OF POTENTIAL NURSING DIAGNOSTIC CATEGORIES*
b. Paralysis of phrenic nerve (and usually diaphragmatic paralysis): (1) Color: cyanotic (2) Breath sounds: diminished (3) Respirations: on affected side labored, rapid (4) Abdomen: no rise with inspiration (5) Cry: weak or hoarse	Impaired gas exchange Alteration in respiratory function
c. Facial paralysis (symptoms on affected side): (1) Facial contour and movement: asymmetric (2) Cheek: flattened (3) Eye: open (4) Poor suck, drooling of formula on affected side	Potential for injury
d. Brain injury from anoxia, direct trauma, or both: (1) Convulsions: clonic, tonic, localized; apneic spells. Symptoms include altered respiratory pattern altered level of consciousness, abnormal eye movements, abnormal chewing movements (2) Evidence of increased intracranial pressure: bulging fontanel at rest; wide sutures; especially separation of the coronal and lambdoidal sutures (3) Muscle tone; hypotonic; hypertonic (4) Reflexes: hyperreflexic, difficult to elicit; absent; asymmetry of response	Impaired gas exchange Potential for injury
3. Orthopedic problems a. After vertex delivery: fractured clavicle; symptoms on affected side: (1) Arm: decreased or absent movement; pain response on passive movement (2) Deformity of clavicle over fracture site is sometimes seen and felt: distal part of clavicle is movable on palpation b. After breech delivery: fractured femur; symptoms on affected side: (1) Movement: absent; asymmetric Moro's reflex; pain response on passive movement (2) Deformity of femur is sometimes seen and felt	Potential for injury
4. Soft tissue trauma (a) Abrasions from bony pelvis or forceps (b) Ecchymoses from bony pelvis or forceps (c) Petechiae over traumatized area only from bony pelvis or forceps (d) After first or second day, cephalhematoma (e) Subconjunctival hemorrhage from rupture of scleral capillaries	Potential for injury
5. Miscellaneous (a) Long fingernails (b) Macerated dry, peeling skin	
E. Assess parental response.	Knowledge deficit Anxiety Fear Grieving Ineffective individual or family coping Spiritual distress

Continued.

Summary of Nursing Actions—cont'd

OUTCOME CRITERIA*	PLAN/IMPLEMENTATION

Hypoglycemia is prevented or identified and treated promptly.
Care appropriate to gestational age and needs is instituted.
 	
Injury is identified and treated promptly.
 	
Oxygen needs are met.
 	
Care appropriate for neurologic damage is instituted.
	A. Treat hypoglycemia.
	B. Evaluate for and institute appropriate nursing care based on gestational age.
	C. After cesarean delivery, record and report observations. Assist physician with treatments.
	  1. Possible transfusion.
	  2. Preoperative and postoperative care for reduction of depressed skull fracture; reemphasize to parents physician's explanation of cause and management of cephalhematoma, paralyses.
	  3. Administer oxygen position infant; medications as necessary.
	D. After vaginal delivery:
	  1. Facilitate respirations.
	  2. Note neurologic problems.
	    a. Brachial paralysis: No definitive treatment is given; usually self-limited; position neonate in good body alignment to aid healing; prevent further injury; prevent deformity.
	    b. Phrenic nerve paralysis: Position infant with head of mattress up. Place in optimum position to facilitate respiratory effort.
	    c. Facial paralysis: If eye stays open, keep moist; close eye and apply patch to protect it from corneal abrasions. Support infant in upright position during feeding. Take extra time to feed. Do not force, since this may cause aspiration.

Injury from convulsions is prevented.
Sepsis is prevented or identified and treated promptly.
Respirations are facilitated.
Nuturitional needs are met.
	d. Brain injury: Order and assist with laboratory tests for differential diagnosis to rule out other causes for convulsions.
	     (1) EEG, subdural tap, skull films
	     (2) Tests for sepsis; blood culture, urinalysis, lumbar puncture; chest x-ray film
	     (3) Tests for metabolic problems
	     (4) Tests for structural defects
	     (5) O_2 to relieve cyanosis
	    e. Position to facilitate respirations. Suction as necessary.
	    f. Nutrition: Use nipple with caution; can be fed intravenously.
	    g. Intravenous therapy: Administer medications, anticoagulants, antibiotics.
	    h. Minimize stimuli: auditory, visual, tactile.

Orthopedic injuries are identified and treated promptly.
 	
Soft tissue trauma is noted and treated if appropriate.
	3. Orthopedic problems: Maintain good body alignment to prevent deformity and further injury. Prevent pressure areas on skin.
	    a. Fractured clavicle: not treated actively.
	    b. Fractured femur: both legs placed in traction-suspension (Bryant's traction) with or without a spica cast for 3 or 4 weeks until adequate callus is formed.
	  4. Soft tissue trauma.
	    a. Prevent infection through broken skin.
	    b. Observe for hyperbilirubinemia as hemorrhagic areas are resolved.

*Outcome criteria direct the selection of nursing actions (**plan/implementation**) and measure their effectiveness (**evaluation**).

Summary of Nursing Actions—cont'd

OUTCOME CRITERIA*	PLAN/IMPLEMENTATION
c. Continue to observe and record changes in petechiae (e.g., progressive resolution vs. increase in number and distribution). Self-inflicted scratches are prevented. Parents' information and emotional needs are met.	5. Miscellaneous. a. Cover hands with mitts to prevent self-inflicted scratches. b. Dry, dead skin in bedding will not injure child. Small amounts of lotion may be used; avoid unnecessary bathing. 6. Parental response. a. Reinforce, simplify, or clarify physician's explanations of procedures, findings, and medical-surgical management. b. Initiate discussion and allow time for mother and father to express feelings about condition of infant, mode of delivery, prognosis, and so on. c. Encourage parents to visit, touch, and assist in care of infant when appropriate. Be available to assist parents at crib side. Help parents keep in touch with infant until his or her discharge.

EVALUATION The nurse can be assured that care was effective when the goals for care are met.

---

*Outcome criteria direct the selection of nursing actions (**plan/implementation**) and measure their effectiveness (**evaluation**).

Hyperbilirubinemia

Elevated serum levels, especially of unconjugated (indirect) bilirubin, pose a grave danger to the newborn. Physiologic hyperbilirubinemia may become pathologic and require diagnostic tests and vigorous treatment.

Physiologic hyperbilirubinemia is characterized by a progressive increase in serum levels of unconjugated bilirubin from 2 mg/dl in cord blood to a mean peak of 6 mg/dl by 72 hours of age, followed by a decline to 5 mg/dl by day 5, and not exceeding 12 mg/dl. These serum values are within the normal physiologic limitations of the healthy term newborn who was not exposed to perinatal complications (such as hypoxia). No bilirubin toxicity develops.

Pathologic hyperbilirubinemia cannot be defined solely in terms of serum concentrations of unconjugated bilirubin. Pathologic hyperbilirubinemia refers to that level of serum bilirubin at which a particular newborn will sustain lesions in the brain tissue (kernicterus), renal tubular cells, intestinal mucosa, and pancreatic cells. Hyperbilirubinemia may result from any of the following factors:

1. Physiologic limitations of the newborn, such as prematurity and low birth weight.
2. Presence of conditions associated with increased red blood cell (RBC) destruction such as Rh_0, ABO, or other RBC-antigen incompatibility or neonatal sepsis.
3. Maternal diabetes mellitus.
4. Superimposed perinatal risk factors such as hypoxia, asphyxia, acidosis, hypothermia, or hypoglycemia.

Laboratory reports that support the diagnosis of hyperbilirubinemia follow*:

1. Serum bilirubin levels increasing more than 5 mg/dl/24 h.
2. Full-term newborn: serum bilirubin level greater than 12 mg/dl, which represents the upper limit of peak concentration of physiologic jaundice (Chapter 20).
3. Low-birth-weight newborn: serum bilirubin levels of 10 to 12 mg/dl, even though the peak concentration of "physiologic jaundice" is 15 mg/dl.

---

*For the normal full-term newborn, serum bilirubin of 12 to 15 mg/dl is the cut-off point for phototherapy and 20 mg/dl for exchange transfusion. For sick or preterm newborns, it is best to prevent *any* rise in serum bilirubin altogether; no level can be regarded as "safe" in view of the possibility of opening the blood-brain barrier and the vulnerability of brain cells resulting from disease processes and inadequate energy reserves. For the sick or preterm newborn, phototherapy is advisable for visible jaundice, and exchange transfusion for serum bilirubin of 15 mg/dl (Wu, 1985).

4. Premature newborn: all visible jaundice, even with serum bilirubin levels as low as 5 mg/dl.

Transcutaneous bilirubinometry is a screening test for neonatal jaundice based on the relationship between the yellow color of the skin and total serum bilirubin level. This rapid, noninvasive transcutaneous procedure uses a spectrophotometric hand-held fiberoptic instrument that illuminates the skin and measures the intensity of its yellow color. The intensity of color is then displayed as a number that correlates with serum bilirubin concentration; it is *not* an absolute estimate of total bilirubin. This test screens for those jaundiced newborn infants with rising bilirubin levels whose condition may need further diagnostic investigation.

The small probe of the bilirubinometer is applied firmly against the newborn's skin over a bony surface of the forehead or the sternum. The photoprobe is held against the skin with enough pressure to blanch the skin. Then a pulse of light is transmitted through the skin to the subcutaneous tissues and the reflected color is recorded within a few seconds.

Skin pigmentation *does affect* the readings. Correlations between transcutaneous bilirubin index and serum bilirubin levels have been established for Japanese infants, American white infants, and American black infants at term. The different values for the preterm or low-birth-weight newborn of each racial group are not yet available. The instrument is not suitable for monitoring the newborn during or immediately following phototherapy or exchange transfusion.

No adverse effects on the newborn have been reported so far, and no short- or long-term effects are anticipated. The fiberoptic instrument releases a brief pulse of strong, cool, white light that does not harm underlying skin or tissues. The beam of light is absorbed mainly at the surface of the skin and underlying the subcutaneous tissue.

Kernicterus. Kernicterus refers to bilirubin encephalopathy that results from the deposit of bilirubin, especially within the brain stem and basal ganglia. The yellow staining (jaundice of the brain tissue) and necrosis of neurons results from unconjugated bilirubin. Unconjugated bilirubin is readily capable of crossing the bloodbrain barrier because of its high lipid solubility. Kernicterus may occur in certain newborns with no apparent clinical jaundice. Only one sequela in survivors is specific: **choreoathetoid cerebral palsy.** Other sequelae, such as mental retardation and serious sensory disabilities, may reflect hypoxic, vascular, or infectious injury that is often associated with kernicterus. About 70% of newborns who develop kernicterus die in the neonatal period.

The perinatal events that enhance the development of hyperbilirubinemia also increase the likelihood that kernicterus will develop, perhaps even in the presence of mild to moderate unconjugated hyperbilirubinemia. The perinatal events include hypoxia, asphyxia, acidosis, hypothermia, hypoglycemia, bacterial infection, certain medications, and hypoalbuminemia. These conditions interfere with conjugation or compete for albumin-binding sites.

Clinical manifestations of kernicterus commonly first appear between 2 and 6 days after birth. *Kernicterus is never present at birth.* Symptomatology changes as the disease process progresses. Four phases are recognized:

1. **Phase one:** the newborn is hypotonic and lethargic and exhibits a poor sucking reflex and depressed or absent Moro's reflex (some infants die during this phase).
2. **Phase two:** the newborn develops spasticity and hyperreflexia, often becomes opisthotonic, has a high-pitched cry, and may be hyperthermic. The newborn may convulse.
3. **Phase three:** at about 7 days of age, the newborn's spasticity lessens and may disappear.
4. **Phase four:** after the first month of life, the infant develops sequelae (e.g., spasticity, athetosis, partial or complete deafness, or mental retardation).

The summary of nursing actions related to newborns with hyperbilirubinemia is presented on p. 1011.

Isoimmune hemolytic disease of the newborn (erythroblastosis fetalis, Rh or ABO incompatibility)

RBC antigenicity. Isoimmune hemolytic disease of the newborn, or erythroblastosis fetalis, is a disorder of the blood and blood-forming organs of the fetus and newborn. It is characterized by hemolytic anemia and hyperbilirubinemia. A transfer of RBC-destroying antibodies from the mother to her fetus causes erythroblastosis. Once the mother is sensitized, this increasingly serious disease tends to develop in subsequent children who have a blood type or group that differs from hers.

ABO incompatibility. Fetal-maternal incompatibility of either ABO groups or the D factor of the Rh group may cause hemolytic disease. The blood type of a person who has RBCs without either the A antigen or the B antigen is designated as group O. Blood of group O individuals contains anti-A and anti-B antibodies. Therefore the group O mother who is carrying a fetus whose blood is A, B, or AB has anti-A and anti-B antibodies that are transferred across the placenta to her fetus. In this situation even the firstborn infant may be affected.

HYPERBILIRUBINEMIA

GOALS

1. For the mother: a satisfying birth.
2. For the newborn: a neonatal period uncomplicated by hyperbilirubinemia.
3. For the family: a positive birth experience.

PRIORITIES

1. Prevention of hyperbilirubinemia, or, prompt identification and treatment of hyperbilirubinemia.
2. Education and support of parents of newborn with hyperbilirubinemia.

ASSESSMENT

A. Review prenatal chart and intranatal record for presence of risk factors.
B. Assess for hyperbilirubinemia:
   1. If any predisposing factors are present, check to see that cord blood has been sent to laboratory for blood type, Rh, hemoglobin, hematocrit, Coombs test, or other values appropriate for that newborn. Obtain daily hemoglobin and hematocrit values until a stable state has been reached. Record results.
   2. Note appearance of jaundice during first 24 hours; and note degree of jaundice. Test for jaundice, preferably in daylight, because there is possible distortion of color from artificial lighting, reflection from nursery walls, and the like. (See also integument entry on p. 1010.)
      a. Blanch area over bony area (forehead) with thumb. Skin will look yellow before area is perfused again.
      b. Check conjunctival sacs and buccal mucosa in darker-skinned infants.
   3. Note infant's behavior:
      a. Changes in feeding and sleeping patterns,
      b. Color and consistency of stools; dark, concentrated urine.
      c. Pallor.
      d. Neurologic signs of kernicterus.
   4. Note laboratory reports on serum bilirubin levels.

EXAMPLES OF POTENTIAL NURSING DIAGNOSTIC CATEGORIES*

Hyperbilirubinemia in neonatal period†
Potential for injury related to hyperbilirubinemia
Impaired gas exchange related to anemia

OUTCOME CRITERIA‡

Perinatal risk factors are prevented.
Infection is prevented.
Early feedings are provided.
Hyperbilirubinemia and its sequela, kernicterus, are absent.
There are minimal or no sequelae from hyperbilirubinemia and its treatment.
Parents understand newborn's condition, therapies, and possible sequelae.

PLAN/IMPLEMENTATION

Record and report jaundice immediately for prompt diagnosis and initiation of treatment.
Maintain phototherapy (see p. 562).
Assist with exchange transfusion.
Support parents.
- Keep parents informed (see p. 564).
- Reinforce explanations of physiologic and pathologic hyperbilirubinemia. Explain need for adequate fluid intake for newborn (e.g., offer water between feedings).
- Reinforce physician's explanations regarding disease, its treatment, infant's condition, and possible prognosis.
- Especially if mother is discharged with infant soon after delivery, teach her how to identify jaundice and when to call physician.
- Involve parents with infant's care when possible.

EVALUATION The nurse can be assured that care was effective if the goals were met.

---

*All diagnostic categories except those indicated by a dagger are approved by NANDA's seventh national conference (1986).
IDiagnosis not included by NANDA, 1986.
‡Outcome criteria direct the selection of nursing actions (**plan/implementation**) and measure their effectiveness (**evaluation**).

Because fetal RBCs of groups A, B, or AB are not strongly antigenic, the maternal immune system is not stimulated to produce larger amounts of antibodies against the A and the B factors. The largest percentage of affected infants with ABO imcompatibility occurs with a mother of blood group O and an infant of blood type A_1. (Type A_1 has greater antigenicity than types A_2, A_3, or B.)

Although similar to Rh disease, the clinical manifestations of fetal-maternal ABO incompatibility are generally milder and of shorter duration. However, severe hemolysis, jaundice, and kernicterus are possible.

Other RBC antigen incompatibilities. Other, less common red blood cell antigens also capable of transplacental isoimmunization include Kell, Duffy, and Kidd. Fortunately, serious fetal damage from these factors is unlikely.

Rh incompatibility. The more severe forms of isoimmune hemolytic disease result from Rh_0D^u group incompatibility. This form of hemolytic disease of the newborn occurred in 0.5% to 1% of all mature pregnancies in North America before prophylactic $Rh_0(D)$ human immune globulin (RhoGAM) became available in the mid-1960s. Many children died or were seriously affected. Since immunization against this antigen began, the incidence of severe erythroblastosis has been drastically reduced.

Discovery of the Rh factor. During antibody studies in the 1940s, it was observed that the injection of RBCs of rhesus monkeys into rabbits caused the production of an antiserum that agglutinated the RBCs of these monkeys and of most humans as well. Consequently RBCs that could be agglutinated by this specific antiserum possessed the rhesus (Rh) antigen and were call **Rh positive.** Those RBCs that did not possess the Rh factor (antigen) could not be agglutinated and were called **Rh negative.** Subsequently it was discovered that the Rh factor is not a single antigen but a complex blood system with a number of variants.

Six common Rh (rhesus) antigens are identified as follows: C, D, E, c, d, e. Antibody formation results from the presence of one or more of these (and other less common) antigens. Because two chromosomes are present in every cell, one derived from each parent, the genetic constitution of an individual with reference to these antigens might be, for example, DD, dd, or Dd.

Different combinations allow eight Rh genotypes, each with a single Rh chromosome (e.g., CDE, cde, cDE). Actually, 36 different combinations (genotypes) are possible. The order of antigenicity potency of these antigens is D, C, E, c, e, and d.

Discovery of Rh isoimmunization. Soon after the Rh factor was reported, it was found that erythroblastosis fetalis, hydrops fetalis, and icterus gravis—variations of hemolytic disease of the newborn—were caused by the hemolysis of fetal RBCs by maternal antibodies. **Maternal isoimmunization (or sensitization) can result from a transfusion with Rh-positive blood.**

Identification of population at risk. Between 10% and 15% of marriages of white persons will involve Rh-incompatible partners. About 5% of black couples will be Rh incompatible. It is rare that an Oriental couple will be similarly affected.

Not all Rh-positive men are homozygous for the Rh factor, nor will all children of Rh-positive men married to Rh-negative women be Rh positive. About 50% of the progeny of Rh-positive men who are heterozygous will be Rh positive; the remainder will be Rh negative. Actually, approximately 65% of newborns of Rh-incompatible marriages are Rh positive.

The risk of maternal sensitization is less than expected. Some women have a greater antigenic (immune) response to the Rh factor. In the first pregnancy only 0.1% of mothers will be sensitized. In the second and third pregnancies 11% will be affected, and in the fourth or subsequent Rh-positive pregnancies, 15% will be affected. About 5% of Rh-incompatible matings produce affected infants.

Pathogenesis of hemolytic disease. Hemolytic disease of the newborn develops according to the following sequence (Fig. 31.23):
1. Isoimmunization of an Rh-negative woman (by the administration of Rh-positive blood or Rh-positive fetal RBCs) stimulates the production of anti-Rh antibodies.
2. Transplacental passage of the woman's anti-Rh antibodies to her fetus causes hemolysis of its RBCs together with other abnormal processes in utero and in neonatal life.

Sensitization during pregnancy. Sensitization of an Rh-negative woman must precede intrauterine transfer of antibodies and fetal damage. Hematopoiesis (formation and development of blood cells) begins in the embryo during the sixth week after conception (i.e., during the eighth week after the last menstrual period [LMP]). Therefore a woman who has experienced one or more abortions 2 months or more since her LMP or has given birth has received fetal transfusions generally at the time of placental separation.

Sensitization following blood transfusion. Sensitization of the mother occurs promptly after an incompatible blood transfusion (improperly typed [Rh-positive] blood) or after one or more pregnancies in which fetal erythrocytes have escaped into the maternal circulation.

Effects of sensitization on subsequent pregnancies. The placenta of the seriously affected fetus is larger

Fig. 31.23
Rh isoimmunization. **A,** Rh-negative woman before pregnancy. **B,** Pregnancy with Rh-positive fetus. Some Rh-positive blood passes into mother's blood. **C,** During separation of placenta, a massive inoculation of mother by Rh-positive red blood cells occurs. **D,** Approximately 72 hours after delivery, mother becomes sensitized to Rh-positive blood and develops anti–Rh-positive antibodies, shown as darkened squares. She now has titer, or positive Coombs test. **E,** During subsequent pregnancy with Rh-positive fetus, maternal anti–Rh-positive antibodies enter fetal circulation, attach to fetal Rh-positive red blood cells, and subject them to hemolysis.

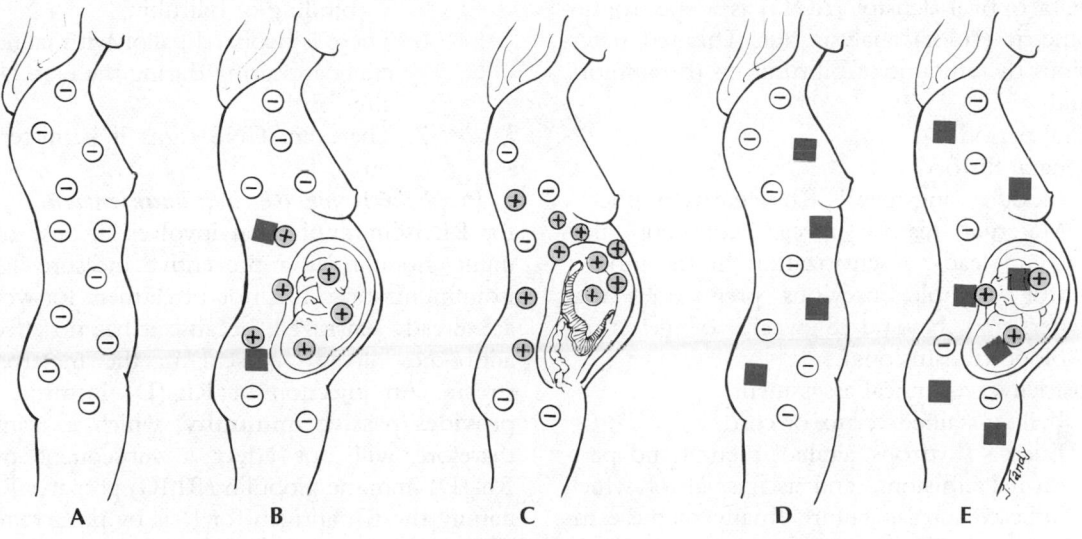

than normal. Increased villous size, persistence of Langerhans' cells, and foci of erythropoiesis are apparent. Frequently the amniotic fluid is yellowish, that is, pigment stained from the decomposition of bilirubin.

Severe Rh incompatibility results in marked fetal hemolytic anemia with erythroid hyperplasia of bone marrow and extramedullary (for example, spleen) hematopoiesis. The placenta clears the released blood pigments fairly well, however, so that only in extreme cases (such as, icterus gravis) is the fetus icteric (yellow, or jaundiced). The marked anemia leads to cardiac decompensation, cardiomegaly, hepatomegaly, and splenomegaly. Edema, ascites, and hydrothorax develop. Severe anemia may lead to hypoxia. Intrauterine or early neonatal death may occur.

Once delivery has occurred, the erythroblastotic newborn becomes icteric (in severe cases, within 30 minutes after birth) because it cannot excrete the considerable residue of RBC hemolysis. Yellowish pigmentation of cerebral basal nuclei, hippocampal cortex, and subthalamic nuclei often develops (kernicterus). Kernicterus occurs when the serum bilirubin rises to levels toxic to the newborn, and serious CNS abnormalities may develop and persist (such as, choreoathetoid cerebral palsy) if the infant survives. The most fre-

quent sequela of kernicterus in the neonatal period is death.

Prevention of Rh isoimmunization. The prevention of maternal Rh isoimmunization is primarily the responsibility of the physician. The nurse may assist with history-taking, obtaining blood specimens, and administering $Rh_0(D)$ immune globulin. Management related to the prevention of Rh isoimmunization follows.

Management: prenatal and neonatal periods
I. Prenatal period
   A. Rh (and ABO) typing should be done early in pregnancy.
   B. Hemantigen test. The diagnosis of hemolytic disease of the newborn of the woman sensitized to the $Rh_0(D)$ or other blood factors is likely when a Hemantigen test or its equivalent (cell pool containing antigens), done on maternal serum at about midpregnancy, is positive. If the test is negative initially, it should be repeated at 32 to 36 weeks.
   C. **Indirect Coombs' test.** In this test the **maternal blood** serum is mixed with RH_0-positive RBCs. The test is positive (maternal antibodies

are present) if Rh$_0$-positive RBCs agglutinate (clump). The dilution of the specimen of blood at which clumping occurs (if it does occur) determines the titer (level of maternal antibodies). The titer determines the degree of maternal sensitization (isoimmunization). If the titer reaches 1:16, an amniocentesis for delta optical density analysis is performed after 26 weeks' gestation.

D. Delta optical density (ΔOD) is a spectrophotometric (color) analysis test. This test determines the amount of bilirubin in the amniotic fluid.

II. Neonatal period

A. Prenatal history

1. Blood typing reveals Rh-negative mother.
2. Maternal history reveals condition that could lead to sensitization in the mother (for example, previous pregnancies that persisted beyond 8 weeks of gestation, blood transfusions).

B. Postdelivery physical assessment

1. Yellow-stained vernix or cord.
2. Edema (hydrops fetalis), pleural and pericardial effusions, and ascites, all of which indicate cardiac failure (many of these infants are stillborn).
3. Placental enlargement. There is an alteration of the average ratio of placental to fetal weight at term. The weight of the normal placenta is generally one sixth that of the fetus. With hemolytic disease of the newborn, the placenta may weigh as much as one half to three fourths the neonate's weight.
4. Hepatosplenomegaly.
5. Cord blood studies.
   a. Blood typing reveals an Rh-positive neonate. (Occasionally an Rh-positive infant is wrongly typed as Rh-negative because of so-called blocking antibodies covering the affected newborn's RBCs.)
   b. Positive **direct Coombs' test** is performed with **neonatal cord blood.** The neonate's RBCs are "washed" and mixed with Coombs' serum. The test is positive (maternal antibodies are present) if the infant's RBCs agglutinate (clump). The dilution of the specimen of blood at which clumping occurs (if it does occur) determines the titer of maternal antibodies in fetal serum. The titer determines the degree of maternal sensitization. If

the titer is 1:64, an exchange transfusion is performed.
   c. Hemolytic anemia of a progressive type is present, with increased erythropoiesis (many nucleated RBCs are seen).
   d. Hypoglycemia may be present.
   e. Indirect or occasionally direct serum bilirubin is present.
   f. There is a reduced capacity for albumin binding of bilirubin.
6. There is neonatal pallor with jaundice, generally appearing during the first 24 to 26 hr after birth.
7. There are CNS signs if kernicterus develops.

Prophylaxis for Rh isoimmunization. Prophylaxis for Rh isoimmunization involves the use of Rh immune globulin as a preventive measure against Rh isoimmunization. It is not a treatment for women who are already sensitized, because it has no effect against antibodies already present in the maternal bloodstream. An injection of **Rh$_0$(D) immune globulin provides passive immunity,** which is transient and therefore will not affect a subsequent pregnancy. Rh$_0$(D) immune globulin (RhIG) prepares RBCs containing the Rh antigen for lysis by phagocytes, before the recipient's immune system is activated to produce antibodies. **Production of one's own antibodies provides active immunity.**

Antibodies formed by an active immune response remain within the individual's bloodstream, presumably for life. RhIG is given to an Rh$_0$(D)-negative woman who is already sensitized would accomplish no purpose. Therefore it is recommended only for nonsensitized Rh-negative women at risk of developing Rh isoimmunization. Given to any Rh-positive person, an injection of RhIG would result in hemolysis of RBCs.

Antenatal administration of Rh$_0$(D) immune globulin (human). Rh sensitization is possible during pregnancy if the cellular layer separating fetal and maternal circulations is disrupted and fetal blood enters the maternal bloodstream. The cellular layer may be disrupted during amniocentesis or by placental abruption. For the woman who is Rh$_0$(D) negative D^u negative, and Coombs' negative, RhIG administered during the antenatal period at about 28 weeks' gestation and again within 72 hours following delivery can further reduce the incidence of maternal isoimmunization.

Postnatal administration of Rh$_0$(D) immune globulin (human). The United States Public Health Service recommendations are as follows:

1. Rh immunoglobulin (RhIG) is given only to a

woman after delivery or abortion who is $Rh_0(D)$ negative and D^u (allelomorph variant) negative and whose fetus is $Rh_0(D)$ positive or D^u positive. It is *never* given to an infant or father.

2. RhIG is not useful in a woman who has Rh antibodies.

3. RhIG should be given intramuscularly, not into fatty tissue or intravenously.

Prevention of isoimmunization of an Rh-negative woman to the Rh factor in her fetus is now possible in over 95% of cases. Prophylaxis is achieved by administering RhIG within 72 hours of evacuation of the uterus (by abortion or more advanced pregnancy).

Prognosis. In the United States Rh hemolytic disease of the newborn occurs once in approximately 150 to 200 full-term deliveries. At least 200,000 children are affected by Rh isoimmunization each year, of which 5000 are stillborn. If severe hemolytic disease of the newborn is untreated, about 10% of infants will develop kernicterus. With intrauterine (fetal) transfusions, about 40% of these children can be saved despite maternal and fetal hazards of the procedures. Amniocentesis studies, early delivery of affected fetuses, and exchange as well as replacement transfusions save many more.

Complete recovery may be expected in most infants who do not develop kernicterus. If hyperbilirubinemia is treated promptly and effectively, most infants recover without residua or sequelae.

Exchange transfusion. The nurse is alert to the fact that a significant risk for morbidity and a mortality risk of 0.1% to 1.0% exist with exchange transfusions. It is time consuming and expensive as well.

An exchange transfusion is accomplished by alternately removing a small amount of the infant's blood and replacing it with a like amount of donor blood. Depending on the infant's size, maturity, and condition, amounts of 5 to 20 ml at a time are slowly exchanged. The total amount of blood exchanged approximates 170 ml/kg of body weight (80 ml/lb) or 75% to 85% of the infant's total blood volume.

Intrauterine fetal transfusion. The transfusion is accomplished in the following manner: Ultrasonography is used to locate the placenta. Then a needle is passed transabdominally into the amniotic sac, and radiopaque dye is injected. The fetus swallows the amniotic fluid. The radiopaque dye in the fetal gastrointestinal tract can be visualized by x-ray film. Then the physician injects packed RBCs directly into the fetal peritoneal cavity. The packed RBCs (about 10 ml) are cross matched with maternal serum. The **blood type used is $Rh_0(D)$ negative and (usually) group 0.** The fetus is able to absorb these RBCs into the fetal circulation via the lymphatic vessels and great veins and to utilize them to counteract the anemia; cardiac decompensation is thus forestalled. Results of this procedure are encouraging. Transfusions may be required every 2 weeks until delivery.

Procedure 31.1

EXCHANGE TRANSFUSION

PURPOSE
1. Reduce serum bilirubin levels.
2. Remove red cells that are destined for hemolysis by circulating antibodies.
3. Correct the anemia.
4. Remove antibodies (or other causative agents) responsible for hemolysis.

EQUIPMENT
1. Disposable exchange transfusion set
2. Fresh donor's blood (under 3 days old and heparinized), two units on hand in case of error or contamination
3. Monitoring equipment
4. Transfusion record
5. Water bath (38° C [100° F]) to warm the blood
6. Medications: **calcium gluconate** in 5 ml syringe with no. 24 needle; 50% glucose solution in 10 ml syringe with no. 24 needle; sodium bicarbonate in 10 ml syringe with no. 24 needle
7. Sterile gowns, drapes, gloves, caps, and masks
8. Cleansing solution with sterile cotton pledgets or gauze sponges
9. Adequate lighting
10. Heat source to keep the infant warm

Continued.

Procedure 31.1—cont'd

NURSING ACTION	RATIONALE
1. Prepare and adjust heat lamps or overhead radiant heat shield; have warmed blankets available for infant.	1. Prevents cold stress.
2. Infant is given nothing orally for 3 or 4 hours, or stomach contents are aspirated by gastric tube.	2. Prevents aspiration.
3. Assemble resuscitative equipment: O₂ source, masks, breathing bag, airways, laryngoscope (extra batteries), endotracheal tube with obturator, suction, medication.	3. Is readily available if needed for immediate supportive therapy.
4. Position infant on back and restrain. Take and record vital signs	4. Facilitates treatment. Prevents dislodging catheter and tissue trauma. Provides base line to evaluate change.
5. Assemble electronic monitoring equipment or stethoscope. Attach electrodes, or keep stethoscope over apex of heart. Monitor and record results continuously during procedure.	5. Hazards of procedure include apnea, bradycardia (100 beats/min or less), cardiac arrhythmia or arrest.
6. Physician *and* nurse check donor blood: type, Rh, age, and free of sickle cell trait.	6. Minimizes chance of error. Provides donor RBCs that are not affected by maternal antibodies present in the fetal system. Acts as precaution against fatal intravascular sickling.
7. Run tubing from bottle (bag) through warm water bath to infant.	7. Avoids cold stress, ventricular fibrillation, vasospasm, or decrease in blood viscosity.
8. Before starting transfusion, assist physician as necessary.	8. Prevents microbial contamination.
a. Cleanse site of cutdown (jugular or femoral artery) or umbilical stump (umbilical vein).	
b. Drape.	
c. Put on gown and gloves.	
9. During transfusion:	9. During transfusion:
a. Physician measures central venous pressure (CVP) before initiating transfusion.	a. Acts as precaution against heart failure from volume overload. Change from 10 to 12 cm pressure is indication to stop and reassess infant's status.
b. Nurse notes and records time exchange is begun.	b. Maintains accurate record.
c. For *each* successive withdrawal of infant's blood *and* injection of donor's blood, nurse records time, amounts in and out, cumulative amounts in and out.	c. Maintains accurate, continuous record to assist with ongoing procedure and provides index of infant's response.
d. After 100 ml has been exchanged, physician gives **calcium gluconate;** nurse monitors heart and respiratory rates and records them.	d. Possibility of cardiac arrhythmias or arrest is minimized.
e. Nurse records pertinent comments.	e. Maintains accurate record.
f. Nurse records medications: time, type, amount, infant response.	f. Maintains accurate record.
10. After transfusion (catheter may be removed or left in place with dressing):	10. Infant is observed to prevent hemorrhage from site and to detect and treat promptly any complications of blood transfusion such as heart failure, hypocalcemia, acute hypercalcemia, hyperkalemia, hypernatremia, hypoglycemia and acidosis,* sepsis, shock thrombus formation, transfusion mismatch reaction.
a. Nurse finishes charting.	
b. Nurse continues to observe and record infant's behavior closely for 24 to 48 hours.	
(1) Vital signs: heart rate, respirations, temperatures, pedal pulses	
(2) Lethargy, jitteriness, convulsions	
(3) Dark urine	
(4) Edema	

*Red blood cells continue anaerobic glycolysis with production of acid metabolites after removal from donor. Blood stored for longer than 2 days is likely to contain potentially dangerous levels of potassium and to be more readily subjected to hemolysis.

Congenital Anomalies

Each year 250,000 infants are born with significant structural and functional disorders. The seriousness of this community health problem is reflected in the more than 6 million hospital days and $200 billion a year allocated to the care and treatment of these neonates. Prevention and detection procedures are being improved continuously. Methods of promoting the availability of these services to populations at risk challenge the community health care systems. An interdisciplinary team approach is imperative to provide holistic care: surgery, rehabilitation, and education of the child and social, psychologic, and financial assistance to the parents. Parental disappointment and disillusion and the nurses's own negative feelings toward (or stigmatization of) the infant's disorder add to the complexity of nursing care.

When studying and using this content, the student is asked to keep an open mind. New data are constantly being identified. Some of the appropriate procedures and treatments of the recent past are considered ineffective and even hazardous today. To support the goal of intact survival, therapy must be continuously reviewed and improved in light of progress.

Many congenital anomalies require intervention soon after birth. Careful assessment alerts the medical-nursing team to the infant's need for therapy.

Assessment of perinatal signs and factors. *Assessment for congenital anomalies* begins with a general assessment (see p. 464). Any deviations from normal are reported to the physician immediately.

Amount of amniotic fluid. An excessive amount of amniotic fluid, **hydramnios,** is frequently associated with congenital anomalies in the newborn. The infant should be examined closely at the earliest possible time. In the presence of hydramnios, any of the following may be suspected:

1. Cephalocaudal malformations, such as hydrocephalus, microcephaly, anencephaly, and spina bifida
2. Orogastrointestinal malformations, such as cleft palate, esophageal atresia with or without a tracheal fistula, pyloric stenosis, volvulus, and imperforate anus
3. Miscellaneous conditions, such as Down's syndrome, congenital heart disease, deformed extremities, and infants of diabetic or prediabetic mothers
4. Prematurity

Oligohydramnios (an insufficient amount of amniotic fluid) is primarily associated with those anomalies of the urinary tract that preclude normal micturition in utero. As a rule, renal agenesis or renal dysplasia is involved.

1. Urethral stenosis has also been reported to be associated with oligohydramnios.
2. Anomalies of the earlobes, rather than agenesis of the ear, are sometimes associated with renal abnormalities and are not direct results of oligohydramnios.
3. Potter's syndrome (renal agenesis) is the classic example of an association between oligohydramnios and renal anomalies. It includes a typical facies that involves abnormal earlobes.

Respiratory system. Screening for congenital anomalies of the respiratory tract is necessary even for the infant who is apparently normal at birth. Respiratory distress at birth or shortly thereafter may be the result of lung immaturity or anomalous development. Congenital laryngeal web and bilateral choanal atresia (Fig. 31.24) are readily apparent at birth. Both require emergency surgery.

Neurologic system. Neurologic signs may reflect hidden congenital anomalies as well as numerous other conditions. Many neonatal responses are nonspecific. Each sign, such as high-pitched cry, hypotonia, jitteriness, low-set ears, and microcephaly or hydrocephaly, must be evaluated carefully before appropriate therapy can be instituted.

Fig. 31.24
Choanal atresia. Posterior nares are obstructed by membrane or bone either bilaterally or unilaterally. Infant becomes cyanotic at rest. With crying, newborn's color improves. Nasal discharge is present. Snorting respirations are often observed with increased respiratory effort. Newborn may be unable to breathe and eat at same time. Diagnosis is made by noting inability to pass small feeding tube through one or both nares. (Courtesy Ross Laboratories, Columbus, Ohio)

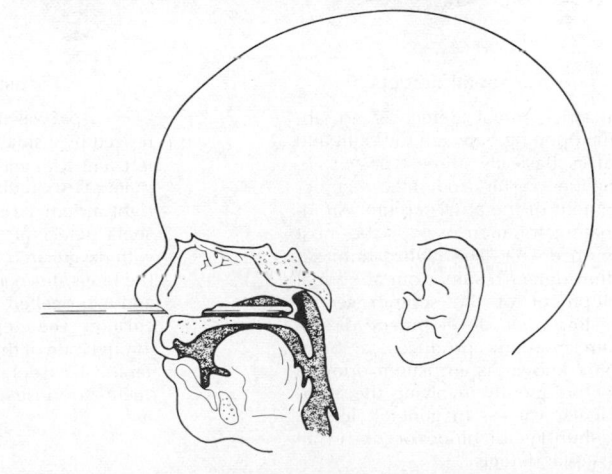

One of the therapeutic contributions the nurse can make is the identification of the neonate who is "just not right," even when there is a negative prenatal history or unreported laboratory or other data. This feeling that something may be wrong is the beginning of the statement of a hypothesis. The nurse thus alerted can mobilize and initiate further diagnostic procedures to institute corrective or palliative therapy.

Cardiovascular system. Severe congenital cardiovascular disorders often are evident immediately after birth, for example, severe cyanotic heart disease (Fig. 31.25). These infants usually are transferred directly to special nurseries or pediatric units. Some problems, such as a small patent ductus arteriosus or a minimal coarctation of the descending aorta, become apparent only as the infant is exposed to stresses such as growth

Fig. 31.25
Congenital heart abnormalities. (Courtesy Ross Laboratories, Columbus, Ohio)

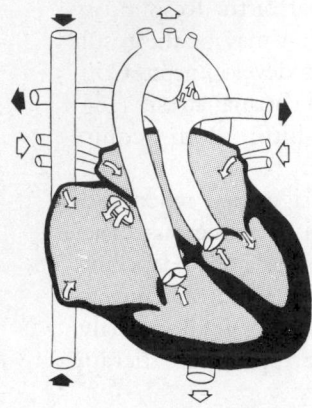

Complete transposition of great vessels

The anomaly is an embryologic defect caused by a straight division of the bulbar trunk without normal spiraling. As a result, the aorta originates from the right ventricle, and the pulmonary artery from the left ventricle. An abnormal communication between the two circulations must be present to sustain life.

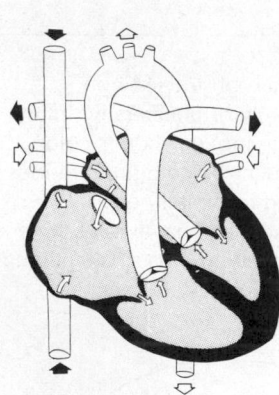

Atrial septal defects

An atrial septal defect is an abnormal opening between the right and left atria. Basically, three types of abnormalities result from incorrect development of the atrial septum. An incompetent foramen ovale is the most common defect. The high ostium secundum defect results from abnormal development of the septum secundum. Improper development of the septum primum produces a basal opening known as an ostium primum defect, frequently involving the atrioventricular valves. In general, left to right shunting of blood occurs in all atrial septal defects.

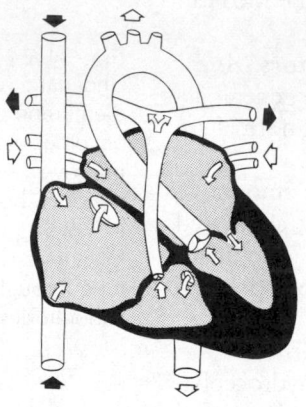

Tricuspid atresia

Tricuspid valvular atresia is characterized by a small right ventricle, large left ventricle, and usually a diminished pulmonary circulation. Blood from the right atrium passes through an atrial septal defect into the left atrium, mixes with oxygenated blood returning from the lungs, flows into the left ventricle, and is propelled into the systemic circulation. The lungs may receive blood through one of three routes: (1) a small ventricular septal defect, (2) patent ductus arteriosus, (3) bronchial vessels.

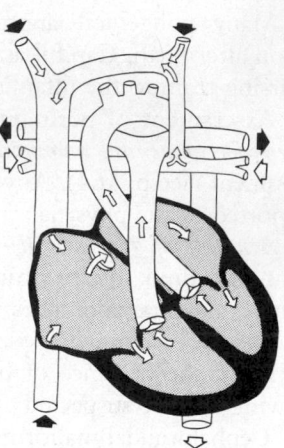

Anomalous venous return

Oxygenated blood returning from the lungs is carried abnormally to the right heart by one or more pulmonary veins emptying directly, or indirectly, through venous channels into the right atrium. Partial anomalous return of the pulmonary veins to the right atrium functions the same as an atrial septal defect. In complete anomalous return of the pulmonary veins, an interatrial communication is necessary for survival.

Fig. 31.25, cont'd.

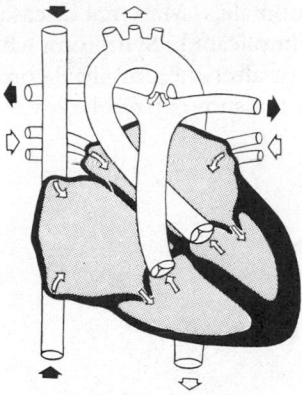

Patent ductus arteriosus

The patent ductus arteriosus is a vascular connection that, during fetal life, short circuits the pulmonary vascular bed and directs blood from the pulmonary artery to the aorta. Functional closure of the ductus normally occurs soon after birth. If the ductus remains patent after birth, the direction of blood flow in the ductus is reversed by the higher pressure in the aorta.

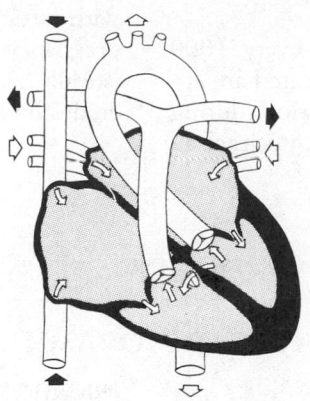

Ventricular septal defects

A ventricular septal defect is an abnormal opening between the right and left ventricle. Ventricular septal defects vary in size and may occur in either the membranous or muscular portion of the ventricular septum. Due to higher pressure in the left ventricle, a shunting of blood from the left to right ventricle occurs during systole. If pulmonary vascular resistance produces pulmonary hypertension, the shunt of blood is then reversed from the right to the left ventricle, with cyanosis resulting.

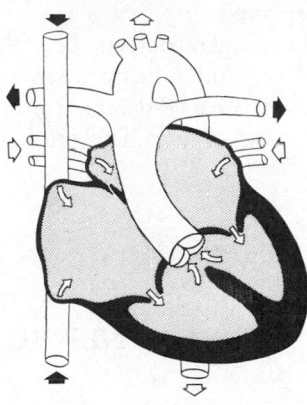

Truncus arteriosus

Truncus arteriosus is a retention of the embryologic bulbar trunk. It results from the failure of normal septation and division of this trunk into an aorta and pulmonary artery. This single arterial trunk overrides the ventricles and receives blood from them through a ventricular septal defect. The entire pulmonary and systemic circulation is supplied from this common arterial trunk.

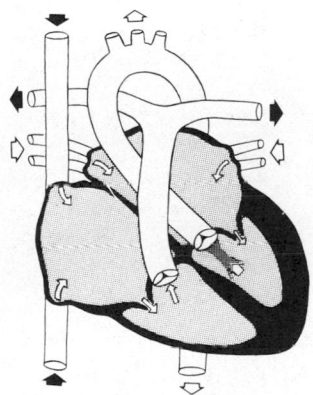

Subaortic stenosis

In many instances, the stenosis is valvular with thickening and fusion of the cusps. Subaortic stenosis is caused by a fibrous ring below the aortic valve in the outflow tract of the left ventricle. At times, both valvular and subaortic stenosis exist in combination. The obstruction presents an increased work load for the normal output of the left ventricular blood and results in left ventricular enlargement.

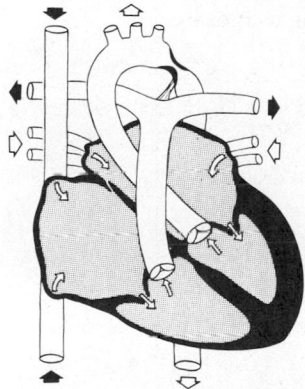

Coarctation of the aorta

Coarctation of the aorta is characterized by a narrowed aortic lumen. It exists as a preductal or postductal obstruction, depending on the position of the obstruction in relation to the ductus arteriosus. Coarctations exist with great variation in anatomic features. The lesion produces an obstruction to the flow of blood through the aorta causing an increased left ventricular pressure and work load.

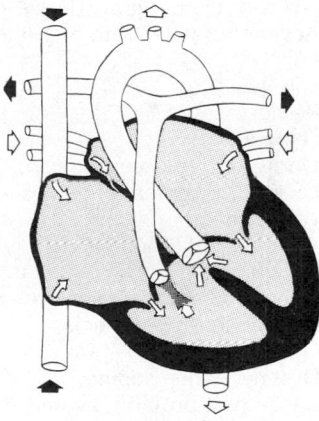

Tetralogy of Fallot

Tetralogy of Fallot is characterized by the combination of four defects: (1) pulmonary stenosis, (2) ventricular septal defect, (3) overriding aorta, (4) hypertrophy of right ventricle. It is the most common defect causing cyanosis in patients surviving beyond two years of age. The severity of symptoms depends on the degree of pulmonary stenosis, the size of the ventricular septal defect, and the degree to which the aorta overrides the septal defect.

demands of later infancy and early childhood, or infection. In about 75% of cases cardiovascular anomalies are unexpected.

Cardiovascular defects occur in 3 of every 1000 births. Congenital heart disease is implicated in approximately 50% of deaths from malformations during the first year of life. The etiology is still unclear, al-

though a familial tendency is evident in many cases. Coexisting congenital defects are frequent in newborns with cardiovascular anomalies. Maternal disease during pregnancy has been implicated. Symptoms characteristically are first evident after the umbilical cord is severed. Nursing actions are summarized below.

Summary of Nursing Actions

NEWBORN WITH CARDIOVASCULAR DISORDER

GOALS
1. For the mother: a satisfying birth.
2. For the newborn: a neonatal period in which the cardiovascular disorder is identified and treated promptly.
3. For the family: an experience for which they receive adequate education and support.

PRIORITIES
1. Prompt identification and treatment of cardiovascular disorders.
2. Education and support of parents of newborn with cardiovascular disorder.

ASSESSMENT	EXAMPLES OF POTENTIAL NURSING DIAGNOSTIC CATEGORIES*
A. Mother's previous and present obstetric histories; maternal and paternal medical histories	
B. Cry: weak and muffled, loud and breathless	
C. Color	Alteration in cardiac output
1. Cyanotic: usually generalized; increases in supine position; often unrelieved by oxygen†; usually deepens with crying; gray, dusky; mild, moderate, severe	Impaired gas exchange Alteration in tissue perfusion
2. Acyanotic: pale, with or without mottling with exertion	
D. Activity level	
1. Restless	
2. Lethargic	
3. Unresponsive except to pain	
4. Lack of movement of arms and legs when crying (severe distress)	
5. Arms flaccid when eating	
E. Posturing	
1. Hypotonic; flaccid even when sleeping	
2. Hyperextension of neck	
3. Opisthotonos	
4. Dyspnea when supine	
5. Knee-chest position favored	
F. Persistent bradycardia (120 beats/min or less) or persistent tachycardia (160 beats/min or more)	
G. Respirations: counted when newborn is sleeping to identify problem early	
1. Tachypnea (60 beats/min or more)	
2. Retractions with nasal flaring or tachypnea	
3. Dyspnea with diaphoresis‡ or grunting	
4. Gasping, followed in 2 or 3 minutes by respiratory arrest if not treated promptly	
5. Grunting with exertion such as crying or feeding by nipple	

*All diagnostic categories approved by NANDA's seventh national conference (1986).
†Suspect hematologic problem as well (e.g., methemoglobinemia).
‡Diaphoresis: uncommon response in normal newborn.

Summary of Nursing Actions—cont'd

ASSESSMENT	EXAMPLES OF POTENTIAL NURSING DIAGNOSTIC CATEGORIES*

H. Feeding behavior
  1. Anorexic
  2. Poor suck: from lack of energy or when unable to close mouth around nipple because of dyspnea
  3. Difficulty coordinating suck, swallow, breathing; pulls away from nipple to take breath
  4. Slow, with pauses to rest
  5. Unable to feed by nipple
	Alteration in nutrition: less than body requirements

OUTCOME CRITERIA‡	PLAN/IMPLEMENTATION

A. Adequate oxygenation of tissues is maintained.
B. The infant is protected from additional stress such as infection, inadequate nutrition, and cold.
C. Corrective or palliative surgery is perfomed.
D. Parents have an understanding and beginning acceptance of the problem and its treatment and any necessary continuing care after discharge.
E. Parents are able to initiate and maintain a positive parent-child relationship.
	A. General care: Support respiratory effort and decrease work of heart.
	  1. Administer O_2 to relieve cyanosis.
	  2. Suction.
	  3. Provide warmth.
	  4. Position for optimum respiratory effort.
	    a. Knee-chest, prone, side-lying
	    b. Upright over nurse's shoulder
	  5. Omit oral feedings until physician arrives. If oral feedings are ordered, offer small amounts more frequently to avoid overdistention of stomach and compromising respirations and to avoid fatigue.
	  6. If oral feedings are discontinued, prepare for gavage feeding or parenteral therapy.
	B. Record and report all findings to provide current data base for continuing therapy.
	  1. Degree and extent of cyanosis: palms, earlobes, scrotum (oral mucosa and tongue most reliable).
	  2. General body color: pale, grayish, cyanotic.
	  3. Muscle tone when active and when at rest.
	  4. Effect of O_2 on cyanosis; how much was needed to relieve symptoms; changes with change in activity level.
	  5. Heart rate; heart sounds: loudness, location.
	  6. Respirations.
	  7. Fatigability.
	C. Minimize distress. Painful procedures (e.g., venipuncture) increase distress, especially in cyanotic baby.
	  1. Place infant in prone position.
	  2. Administer O_2 by mask during procedure.
	  3. Keep infant warm.
	  4. Request technician to stop before infant begins to gasp.
	D. Prevent stress: infection, hypoglycemia.
	E. Medicate per physician order and observe infant response.
	  1. Digitalis preparation: When preparing digitalis dose, second nurse should double-check amount drawn into syringe. Take apical beat; **if heart rate is below 100 beats/min, report to physician before administering drug.**
	  2. Give diuretic.
	F. Support parents.

EVALUATION The nurse can be assured that care is effective if the goals of care are achieved.

‡Outcome criteria direct the selection of nursing actions (**plan/implementation**) and measure their effectiveness (**evaluation**).

Gastrointestinal system. Screening for gastrointestinal tract malformations is performed on a routine basis for all infants. Obstruction occurs in about 1 in 3,000 newborns. The following findings are reported immediately:

1. A scaphoid (sunken) abdomen usually indicates a diaphragmatic hernia.
2. Inability to pass a tube into the stomach suggests esophageal atresia.
3. Inability to pass a rectal thermometer or failure of meconium passage within the first 24 hours of life suggests imperforate anus or probable obstruction; with abdominal distention, probable meconium ileus.

The distended abdomen is particularly noteworthy in H-type tracheoesophageal fistula. These conditions require immediate surgery and are discussed later in this chapter.

Urogenital system. Careful notation of perinatal events and observations such as oligohydramnios and absence of voiding aids in the identification and confirmation of existing congenital anomalies. In cases of ambiguous genitalia, there is an urgent association between the parent-child relationship and the identification of the infant's sex. The identity of the newborn must be established as quickly as possible to facilitate initiation of a positive parent-child relationship.

General preoperative and postoperative care. The newborn withstands the stress of surgery surprisingly well, provided it is done as soon after birth as feasible and the facilities available for care are adequately equipped and staffed. The medical-nursing team must be specially trained to anticipate and meet the newborn's physiologic needs. The surgical team consists of the radiologist, surgeon, anesthesiologist, and nurse. Diagnostic studies are kept to a minimum, and consideration of the newborn's immaturity is kept in mind. Air may be used rather than standard radiopaque materials for diagnostic x-ray examinations to reduce the danger of regurgitation and aspiration. Microtechniques are utilized for the necessary blood chemistry studies (such as preoperative hemoglobin levels) to minimize blood loss.

The infant is transported to the operating room in an incubator with a self-contained power pack for the continuous provision of warmth. The infant is accompanied by an intensive care nursery nurse. Preanesthesia preparation includes hydration, administration of preoperative medications, usually minute amounts of atropine, insertion of an endotracheal tube, and gastric emptying.

During the operation, blood loss is constantly monitored. Blood is replaced milliliter for milliliter because the newborn's remarkable ability to maintain blood circulation through vasoconstriction means that vital signs remain unaltered until sudden and complete collapse occurs as the compensatory system is overtaxed. Temperature is maintained by positioning the infant on a thermal mattress and draping suitably.

Once the operation is completed, the infant is returned to the intensive care nursery. The first hour after the procedure is a crucial one; constant surveillance of recovery from the anesthesia is imperative. Body temperature is maintained between 36.1° and 36.7° C (97° and 98° F); optimal temperature is 36.5° C (97.6° F). An open airway is maintained by means of positioning of the head, suctioning, and use of high humidity. If the respiratory rate increases, suctioning is indicated. Oxygen dosage is prescribed on the basis of arterial blood gas values (such as Po_2). Fluid-electrolyte balance is monitored. Intravenous replacement is given as ordered. Postural drainage and percussion are ordered as necessary. The infant is turned from side to side to equalize pressure areas. An indwelling gastric catheter attached to intermittent suction removes gastric secretions. Removal of gastric contents prevents their possible aspiration because the infant's cough reflex is inadequate.

Most common surgical emergencies. The following five congenital anomalies account for more than 90% of surgical emergencies of the neonate:

1. Diaphragmatic hernia
2. Tracheoesophageal anomalies
3. Omphalocele

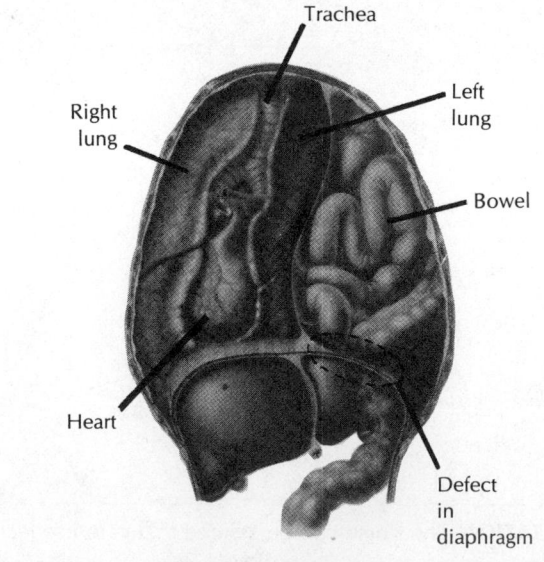

Fig. 31.26

Diaphragmatic hernia. (Courtesy Ross Laboratories, Columbus, Ohio.)

4. Intestinal obstruction
5. Imperforate anus

Diaphragmatic hernia. Diaphragmatic hernia is the most urgent of the neonatal emergencies. Incomplete embryonic development of the diaphragm allows herniation of abdominal viscera into the thoracic cavity (Fig. 31.26). The defect and herniation may be minimal and easily reparable or the defect may be so extensive that the viscera present in the thoracic cavity during embryonic life precluded the normal development of pulmonary tissue. Most cases involve a posterolateral defect, usually on the left. The extent of the defect and the severity and timing of the symptomatology determine the seriousness of the problem.

Signs that are suspicious of extensive diaphragmatic herniation can be assessed by the nurse. Signs include the following: constant respiratory distress from birth that becomes increasingly severe as bowels fill with air, large or asymmetric chest contour, dullness to percussion on affected side, bowel sounds heard in thoracic cavity, and diminished breath sounds.

Prompt surgical repair is imperative after correction of acidosis, insertion of a nasogastric tube and aspiration, and oxygen therapy. The prognosis depends largely on the degree of pulmonary development and the success of diaphragmatic closure. Prognosis in severe cases is guarded.

Tracheoesophageal anomalies. Esophageal atresia is an urgent congenital anomaly. Various types are recognized, depending on the presence or absence of an associated tracheoesophageal fistula, the site of the fistula, and the point and degree of esophageal obstruction (Fig. 31.27). The most common variety is associated with moderate hydramnios.

The following signs are suspicious for tracheoesophageal fistula: excessive oral secretions with drooling; progressive respiratory distress as unswallowed secretions spill over into trachea; and feeding intolerance. In feeding intolerance, choking, coughing, and cyanosis follow even a small amount of fluid taken by mouth. Soon after the first feeding is initiated, there is regurgitation of unaltered formula (unmixed with stomach secretions or bile).

Nursing actions are supportive. In the presence of excessive oral secretions and respiratory distress, **do not feed the infant orally** before consulting physician. In the presence of abdominal distension, place the neonate in semi-Fowler's position and raise the head 30

Fig. 31.27
Congenital atresia of esophagus and tracheoesophageal fistula. **A,** About 87%. Upper segment of esophagus ends in blind pouch; lower segment connects with trachea by small fistulous tract. **B,** About 8%. Upper and lower segments of esophagus end in blind sac. **C,** About 4%. Esophagus is continuous but connects by fistulous tract to trachea; known as *H-type.* **D,** Less than 1%. Both segments of esophagus connect by fistulous tracts to trachea. Infant may drown with first feeding. **E,** Less than 1%. Upper segment of esophagus ends in atresia and connects to trachea by fistulous tract. Infant may drown with first feeding.

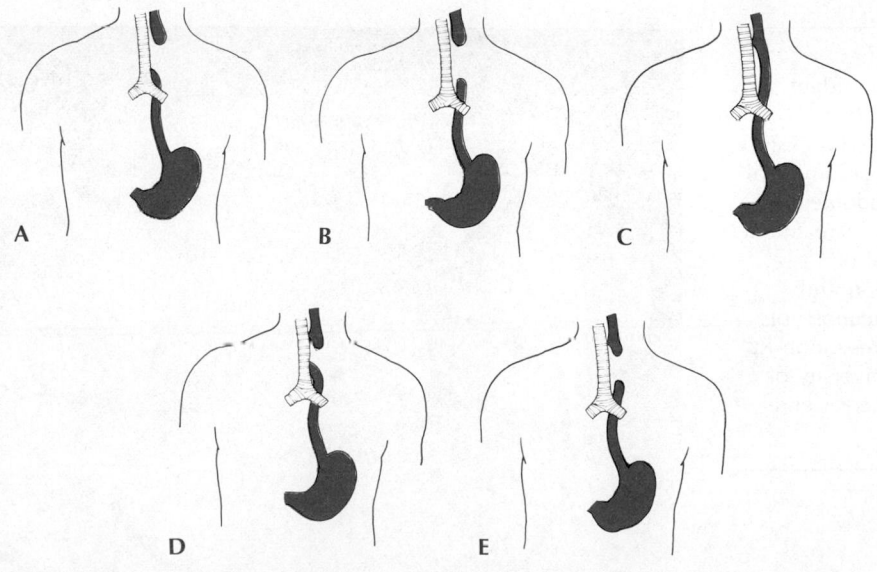

Fig. 31.28
Omphalocele containing liver. (Courtesy John R. Campbell, M.D., University of Oregon Health Sciences Center, Portland, Oregon.)

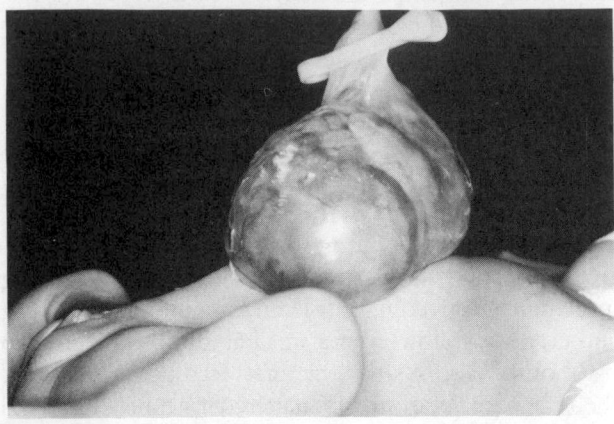

degrees or more (infant seat may be used). This position facilitates respiratory efforts and discourages reflux (spillage) of stomach secretions into the respiratory tree, with resultant chemical bronchitis and pneumonitis. On physician's order or per standing orders, insert a suction tube into the blind pouch. Connect the tube to low, intermittent suction.

Immediate surgical correction of the anomaly is mandatory. The prognosis depends on the degree of maturity of the newborn and the presence of a fistula or pneumonia. Cardiac and other gastrointestinal anomalies commonly are associated with esophageal atresia.

Omphalocele. Omphalocele is a herniation noted at birth in which part of the intestine protrudes through a defect in the abdominal wall at the umbilicus (Fig. 31.28). Failure of migration of the midgut in embryonic development probably is responsible for omphalocele. The protruding bowel is covered only by a thin, transparent membrane composed of amnion.

Prompt closure of defects of less than 5 cm in diameter usually is successful. Larger defects may require closure in stages. The general prognosis is related to associated anomalies.

There is usually only a short span of time between the infant's birth and surgical intervention. Planning for the provision of support to the parents is an essential aspect of nursing care. In addition to the usual preoperative orders, preparation of the infant for surgery includes protecting the defect from infection, rupture, and drying. The physician prescribes that the omphalocele be protected by one of the following:
1. Sterile towels or sponges kept moist with sterile saline solution that has been warmed to body temperature.
2. Protective sterile petrolatum dressings and a firm plastic or metal dome covering.

Intestinal obstruction. Congenital jejunal or ileal obstruction is suspected when distension and bile-stained or fecal vomiting occur in a newborn in the first 24 to 48 hours of life. Although this condition is uncommon, premature infants and those with other anomalies may be affected.

Nursing care is supportive: stop oral feedings and monitor intravenous therapy (see Procedure 25.5); prevent aspiration and suction gastric contents on physician's order (indwelling catheter to low, intermittent

Fig. 31.29
Meconium ileus with midgut volvulus. Meconium ileus is frequently associated with cystic fibrosis. Normal meconium stool is not passed, and abdomen distends progressively. Treatment is directed at removal of mechanical obstruction and prevention of complications of cystic fibrosis. (Courtesy John R. Campbell, M.D., University of Oregon Health Sciences Center, Portland, Oregon.)

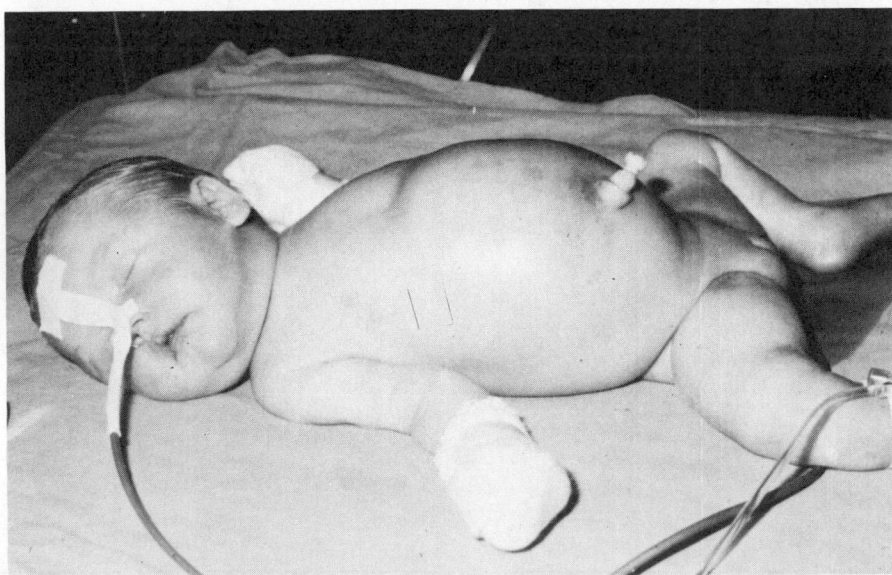

Fig. 31.30
Types of imperforate anus. Anal sphincter muscle may be present and intact. **A,** High lesion opening onto perineum through narrow fistulous tract. **B,** High lesion ending in fistulous tract to urinary tract. **C,** Low lesion in bowel passes through puborectal muscle. **D,** High lesion ending in fistulous tract to vagina.

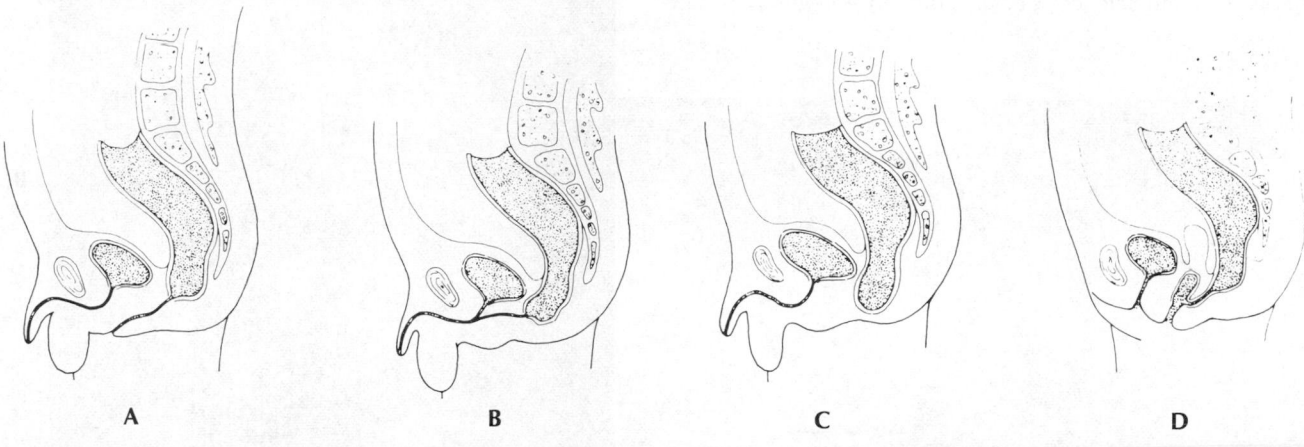

A   B   C   D

suction may be ordered); place infant in semi-Fowler's position to facilitate respiration.

X-ray films of the abdomen usually show a dilated small bowel without gas in the colon. A barium enema may be helpful in determining the cause of the obstruction. Hirschsprung's disease, ileus secondary to sepsis, meconium ileus, and volvulus must be considered in the differential diagnosis (Fig. 31.29). Prompt surgery usually provides good results.

Imperforate anus. Imperforate anus is a congenital disorder that is more common in infant boys than infant girls (Fig. 31.30). About 85% of affected girls will have developed a small fistula (Fig. 31.31), but this is rare in boys. The obstruction may be of the low type (anal membrane) or the high type (anal or rectal atresia). Because some anomalies are not apparent by direct visualization, initial insertion of a probe (thermometer) into the anal canal is done with *extra* caution until patency is established.

Since continence for a lifetime may be dependent on the proper corrective surgery, a pediatric surgeon is consulted at once. Surgery may be as simple as an incision of an anal membrane. With anorectal agenesis, a prompt colostomy will be necessary.

Survival is expected. Continence, on the other hand, is dependent on several factors, including sacral anomalies and proper surgery.

Common malformations
Meningomyelocele. **Meningomyelocele,** a neural tube defect, is a herniation of part of the meninges (containing cerebrospinal fluid [CSF] and CNS tissue) through a defect in the vertebral column or skull. The defect often occurs in the lower back (Fig. 31.32). In the accompanying spinal malformation, **spina bifida,** the meningomyelocele extrudes through the opening of the spinal column. The opening is the result of a congenital absence of one or more vertebral arches. Occasionally a familial history (5% recurrence rate) of this anomaly is identified. Most cases are of unknown (infectious?) origin. A **meningocele** is also a herniation of the meninges. A meningocele contains CSF but does not contain CNS tissue (cord or nerve roots).

Prenatal diagnosis of neural tube defects (meningomyelocele, meningocele, anencephaly) is now possible. Three methods are available:

1. Since the levels of **alpha-fetoprotein** in the maternal serum and amniotic fluid increase in the presence of neural tube defects, serum assays may be used for screening. Amniotic fluid determinations are needed for definitive diagnosis.
2. Ultrasound.
3. Amniography.

The couple may be advised of the existence of the defect and assisted in arriving at their own decision regarding the affected pregnancy. In utero surgery may be possible.

If the neonate is born with a large defect, the nurse aids in preventing its rupture and infection before surgery. Protection of the defect includes the following actions:

1. Position with care.

Fig. 31.31

A, Imperforate anus; fourchette fistula. Note meconium draining through fistula. Arrow indicates meconium exiting via fistulous tract. **B,** Imperforate anus with rectopectal penile fistula *(arrow)*. (Courtesy John R. Campbell, M.D., University of Oregon Health Sciences Center, Portland, Oregon.)

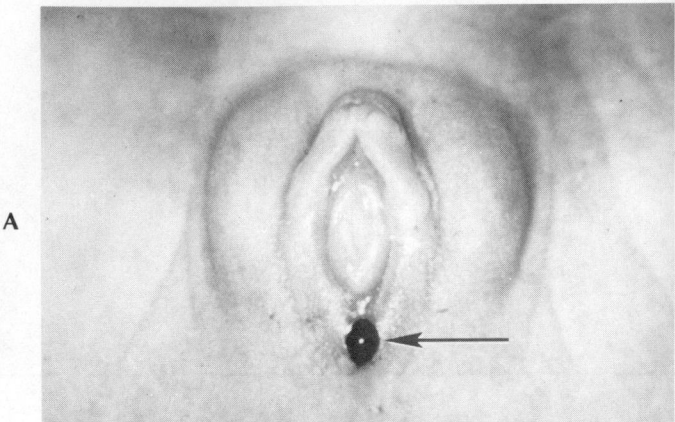

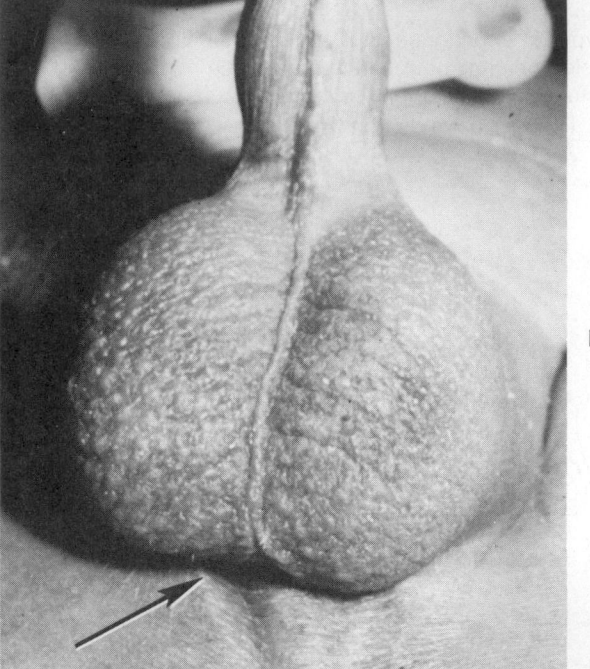

a. Position prone or side-lying with rolled towels to prevent pressure or injury to defect, thereby providing portal of entry for infectious agents.
b. Change position every hour to prevent pressure areas.
c. If physician permits infant to be held, exercise caution to avoid injury to defect.

Fig. 31.32

A, Myelomeningocele. **B,** Dermal sinus tract with dermoid cyst, often associated with spina bifida occulta. Note also tuft of hair. (Courtesy Ross Laboratories, Columbus, Ohio.)

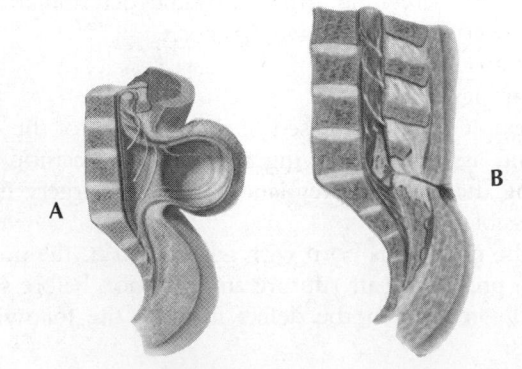

2. Provide skin care: skin around defect is cleansed and dried carefully to prevent breakdown, which would establish a portal of entry for infectious agents. Apply physician-ordered dressings, ointments, and so on.

The nurse assists in the diagnosis of a hidden defect. The nurse assesses neurologic function and notes the following:
1. Paralysis of lower extremities
2. Flaccidity and spasticity of muscles below defect
3. Sphincter control: character and number of voidings and stools; leakage of urine and stool

Surgical repair often can be done in the neonatal period. If other anomalies, such as hydrocephalus, are present, delayed correction may be elected. Permanent impairment of neuromuscular function below the level of the defect depends on the amount of CNS tissue involved. In severe cases, voluntary and involuntary functions are absent. The prognosis is guarded. Only about 60% of cases are operable. Many of these children die or achieve only partial function. Hydrocephalus ultimately develops in virtually all infants.

The parents will need considerable support and instruction regarding the infant's care. In some instances parents may require assistance in placing the child in a special care facility.

Congenital hydrocephalus. Congenital hydrocephalus is macrocephaly caused by abnormal enlargement of the cerebral ventricles and skull. Head enlargement is the result of increased intraventricular CSF pressure. This condition is accompanied by enlargement of the head, prominence of the forehead, "setting sun" sign of the eyes, atrophy of the brain, weakness, and convulsions as the condition worsens.

Congenital hydrocephalus is encountered in approximately 1 in 2000 fetuses (about 12% of all malformations). Several types are known.

External hydrocephalus is caused by an abnormal accumulation of fluid between the brain and the dura mater. Obstruction of the CSF anywhere along its course may be responsible. Maldevelopment, infection, hemorrhage, neoplasia, or unknown causes must be considered. A history of maternal (and possibly fetal) bacterial or viral infection may be elicited. The most common lesion is atresia of the aqueduct between the third and fourth ventricles (Arnold-Chiari syndrome).

In *internal hydrocephalus* an excessive amount of CSF accumulates in the ventricular system of the brain. Rarely, oversecretion of CSF by a choroid plexus papilloma, rather than an obstruction, may result in internal hydrocephalus.

The fetus with hydrocephalus frequently assumes the breech presentation in utero. Severe dystocia caused by cephalopelvic disproportion (CPD) is encountered; cesarean delivery is warranted. When vaginal delivery is attempted, puncture of the fetal head and drainage of the excess fluid may be necessary before the head can be delivered. Fetal mortality after this procedure is approximately three deaths out of every four deliveries. Regardless of the route of delivery, the experience is emotionally traumatic for the parents and family.

X-ray films should confirm widening of the fontanels and sutures. Intracranial calcifications caused by cytomegalic viral (CMV) inclusion disease or toxoplasmosis (a protozoal infection) may be revealed (see TORCH, Table 31.7 and box on p. 1036).

Subdural aspiration or transillumination of the head may disclose a subdural hematoma or tumor. The location and extent of obstruction usually can be identified by pneumoencephalography or ultrasonography.

Spina bifida occurs in approximately one-third of infants born with hydrocephalus.

Surgery is usually performed soon after birth. If surgical shunting is not accomplished, **increasing intracranial pressure,** evidenced by palpably widening fontanels and sutures, lethargy, irritability, or vomiting, results in irreversible neurologic damage. A period of observation is necessary to determine the type of operation required. Meanwhile, nursing care is individualized.

Assessment for hydrocephalus includes notations

describing the following typical signs:
1. Changes in head size every day
   a. Width of sutures
   b. Size and tension of anterior fontanel
   c. Head circumference
2. Facial appearance
   a. Flat, broad bridge of nose
   b. Bulging forehead
   c. "Setting-sun" effect as eyes are displaced downward by pressure from accumulating fluid
3. Neurologic signs
   a. High-pitched, shrill cry
   b. Irritability or restlessness
   c. Poor feeding or changes in feeding pattern from good to poor
   d. Behavior changes
   e. Spina bifida

Nursing actions appropriate to the needs of a newborn with hydrocephalus include the following:
1. Carefully note and report observations and changes.
2. Provide skin care to prevent infection.
   a. Prevent pressure areas. Use lamb's wool, sheepskin, flotation mattress, frequent position changes.
   b. Keep clean and dry.
3. Support head carefully when holding or turning infant.
4. Initiate feeding.
   a. Choose method, amount, and frequency of feeding to accommodate infant's tolerance and energy level.
   b. Be alert for vomiting and possible aspiration.
5. Meet infant's touching and cuddling needs.
6. Nurture parent: provide support and information regarding defect and treatment.

Damaged or destroyed brain tissue cannot be restored. Spontaneous arrest of hydrocephalus may occur, but often surgical shunting may be required to eliminate excess CSF. Despite arrest of the process, serious mental retardation and neurologic sequelae are common.

Anencephaly and microcephaly. Anencephaly and microcephaly are congenital fetal deformities in which the head is considerably smaller than normal. In anencephaly there is complete or partial absence of the brain and of the overlying skull. Because the pituitary gland is absent or vestigial, the adrenal cortex is diminutive (for lack of ACTH stimulation). About 70% of anencephalic infants are girls. This condition is frequently accompanied by hydramnios. The cause of anencephaly is unknown, but multiple environmental factors have been postulated. A 3% recurrence rate in familial histories has been noted.

Anencephaly is incompatible with life; warmth and fluid are provided until the neonate's death, which is usually before the end of the first 24 hours after birth. Microcephalic infants require specific nursing care and medical observation to appraise the extent of psychomotor retardation that almost always accompanies this abnormality. The nurse's supportive role with parents is considerable.

In microcephaly the head generally is well formed but small. X-ray exposure of the woman may result in fetal microcephaly. Rubella, cytomegalic inclusion disease (CMV), and perhaps other infectious processes are the causes in some cases.

Cleft-lip or palate. Cleft lip or palate is a common congenital midline fissure, or opening, in the lip or palate; one or both deformities may occur. The incidence is approximately 1 in 700 white neonates and 1 in 2000 black neonates. Polygenetic factors are causative in some cases, but fetal viral infection, maternal corticosteroid therapy, radiation, dietary influence, and hypoxia have been associated factors. The combination of cleft lip and palate affects more boy than girl infants.

Treatment requires special feeding techniques, for example, the use of uniquely designed nipples (Procedure 25.3). Cleft lip repair may be done soon after delivery if the neonate is free of infection, in good condition, and weighs 2500 g (5 lb, 9 oz). Cleft lip repair is best done with the infant weighs 4500 g (10 lb) or more since there is more tissue to work with. Advantages of earlier labial (lip) repair include facilitating a positive parent-child relationship and permitting the infant to learn to use and strengthen musculature around the mouth. Infants with palatolabial fissures often look grotesque and repulsive to the parents. After repair and with collaborative health team support, the mother frequently is able to assume responsibility for the newborn's care until palatal repair is feasible. Repair is done usually between 16 and 24 months of age (9 kg [20 lb] body weight or more). The plastic surgeon, pediatrician, orthodontist, hospital and community nurses, speech therapist, and social worker make up the collaborative health team that has made possible the effective treatment available today. Until repair of the palate is performed, a prosthesis is fitted to aid the infant's feeding and speech development and to reduce respiratory tract infections.

The grief reaction to having a child with this and other disorders and the nursing care involved are discussed in Chapter 26. Parents benefit from seeing before and after pictures of other babies born with this defect. Coupled with other verbal and nonverbal supportive care, this visual reassurance is effective. Parents can be referred to other parents (or organizations of parents such as the Cleft Palate Club) for continuing mutual support.

Musculoskeletal disorders. The two most common musculoskeletal deviations seen in the neonatal period are congenital dysplasia of the hip and congenital clubfoot. Both conditions are easily recognized. Early detection and definitive treatment are mandatory for successful correction. Delay makes repair more difficult and prognosis less favorable.

Congenital hip dysplasia (congenital dislocation of the hip). This often hereditary disorder occurs more commonly in infant girls (Fig. 31.33) because of the structure of

Fig. 31.33
Congenital dysplasia of hip. **A,** Normal gluteal and popliteal skin creases. **B,** Abnormal skin creases and asymmetry of skin folds. **C,** Apparent shortening of femur. Femur head is displaced. (Courtesy Ross Laboratories, Columbus, Ohio.)

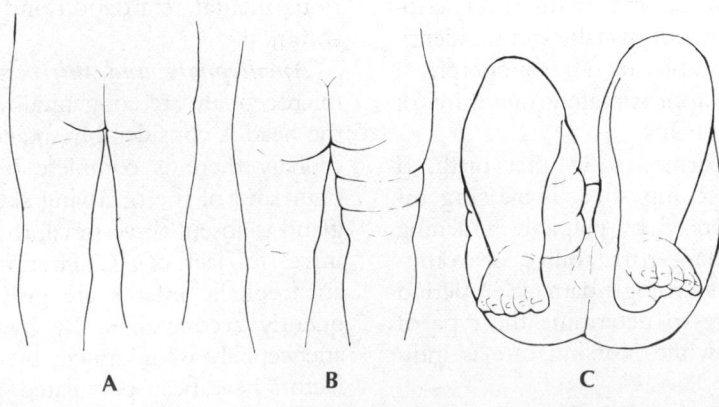

A   B   C

the pelvis. In this condition the acetabulum is abnormally shallow. The head of the femur becomes dislocated upward and backward to lie on the dorsal aspect of the ilium. The pressure of the displaced femoral head may form a false acetabulum on the ilium. A stretched joint capsule results, and ossification of the femoral head is delayed.

Before dislocation occurs, reduced movement, splinting of the affected hip, limited abduction, and asymmetry of the hip may be noted. After dislocation, all these signs will be present, together with the external rotation and shortening of the leg. A clicking sound may be noted on gentle forced abduction of the leg (Ortolani's sign), and a bulge of the femoral head is felt. X-ray films will reveal a deformity in congenital dysplasia of the hip.

Treatment involves pressing the femoral head into the acetabulum to form an adequate socket before ossification is complete. The following methods are possible:

1. Thick diapers to abduct and externally rotate leg and flex hip (pin anterior flaps of diapers under posterior flaps).
2. Frejka pillow (apply diapers and plastic pants, and then apply pillow). Later this appliance will be followed by a spica cast in most instances to maintain abduction, extension, and internal rotation, usually with the infant in a "frog-leg" position.

Talipes equinovarus. Talipes equinovarus, or clubfoot, is a congenital fixed postural deformity in which the foot is twisted out of shape or position. The heel is turned inward from the midline of the leg, the sole of the foot is flexed at the ankle joint, and the Achilles tendon is shortened.

Before the infant is 2 months old, often during the first days of life, successive plaster casts are applied first to correct the heel inversion and adduction of the forefoot and later, the equinus deformity. Special shoes with lower leg braces will be necessary when the child learns to walk. Surgery may even be required in childhood if correction is incomplete. The prognosis depends on the extent of the deformity and the response to progressive orthopedic treatment.

Phocomelia. Phocomelia, or "seal-like limbs," is a developmental anomaly typified by absence of the arms or legs, or both, or stunting of the extremities. In the early 1960s the drug **thalidomide** was implicated as the causative agent for the limb deformities of many thousands of infants, especially in Germany. As a result the United States Food and Drug Administration tightened its regulations governing drug approval. Painfully apparent was evidence that drugs ingested during pregnancy may have tragic implications for fetal development. Thalidomide (and perhaps imipra-

mine [Tofranil]) is a cause of this condition. Sporadic cases of congenital amputation or stunting are of unknown etiology.

The child born with these deformities requires special care as follows:

1. *Rehabilitative problems are often complex.* The prostheses require frequent refitting as the child grows. The child requires careful guidance and training in achieving the optimal level of functioning possible. Approximately 15 child amputee centers are located throughout the United States.

2. *Psychosocial developmental problems are significant.* The kinesthetic satisfaction derived from kicking the legs and waving the arms is not possible. The hand-to-mouth movement behavior pattern, necessary for self-gratification and exploration of one's environment, is missing. The child learns about the environment by pushing the trunk up by the arms; a pillow prop under the infant's chest will compensate somewhat. The child's concerns about body image and obvious differences from others will require attention in later years. Any child reflects the attitudes and sentiments of those around him or her. Positive attitudes help the child incorporate these into a positive self-concept.

3. *Supportive care of the parents must begin at the birth of the child and continue for years.* After the initial grief reaction, the parents need information regarding the rehabilitative and psychosocial components of their child's care.

Polydactyly. Extra digits on the hands or feet occur occasionally (Fig. 31.34). In some instances polydactyly is hereditary. If there is little or no bone involvement, the extra digit is tied with silk suture soon after

---

Fig. 31.34
Polydactyly: supernumerary digit of right hand. Most common congenital anomaly of upper extremity and is occasionally seen in conjunction with other congenital malformation. (Courtesy Mead Johnson & Co., Evansville, Indiana.)

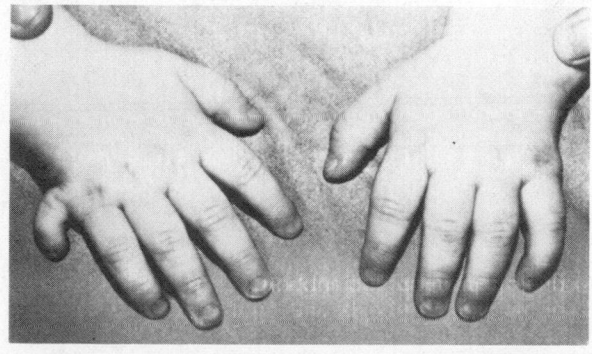

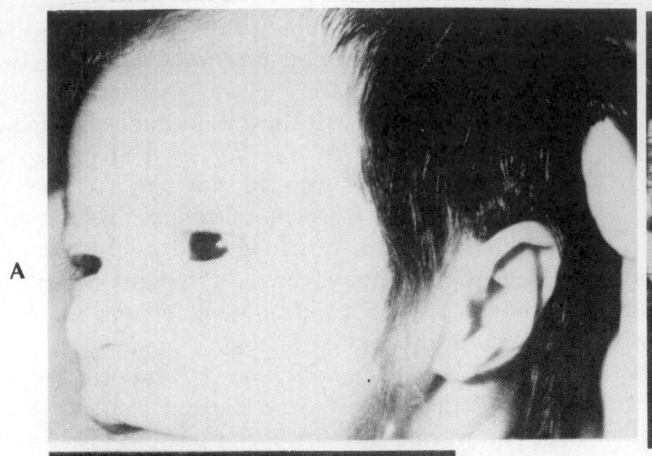

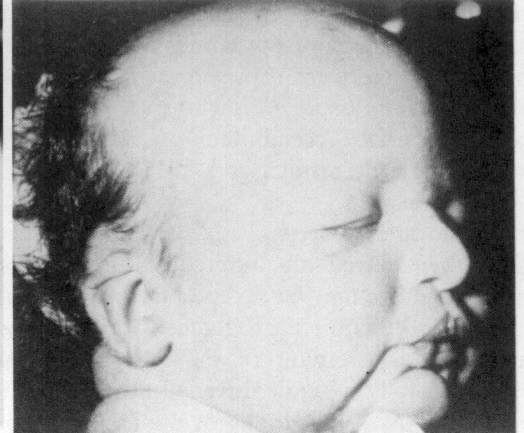

Fig. 31.35
Abnormally low-set ears characterize many syndromes and may indicate abnormality of internal organs, especially bilateral renal agenesis (Potter's syndrome). **A,** In normal infant, insertion of ear to scalp falls on extension of line drawn across inner and outer canthus of eye. **B,** If ear is twisted or rotated, it may give false impression of being low set. **C,** True low-set ear. (Courtesy Mead Johnson & Co., Evansville, Indiana.)

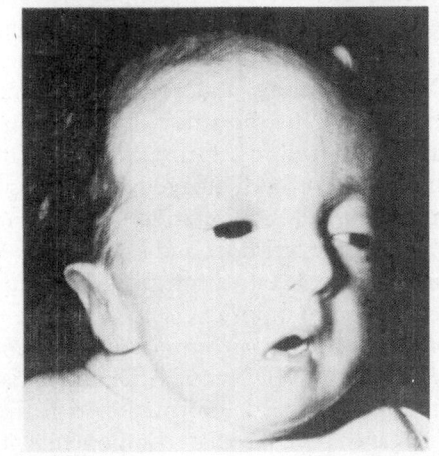

birth. The finger falls off within a few days, leaving a small scar. When there is bone involvement, surgical repair is indicated.

Genitourinary tract anomalies. Abnormally low-set or misshapen ears may indicate other, often genitourinary, anomalies (such as, renal agenesis) (Fig. 31.35).

Exstrophy of the bladder. Exstrophy of the bladder (Fig. 31.36) is a congenital anomaly of unknown etiology. With this anomaly a separation of the symphysis pubis and anterior abdominal wall structures results in exteriorization of the bladder trigone and surrounding mucosa. The exposed mucosa is deep red, has numerous folds, and is sensitive to touch. A direct passage of urine to the outside occurs. Associated anomalies, such as undescended testes, inguinal hernia, absence of the vagina, or bowel defects, should be sought. Surgical correction, often elimination of the bladder and construction of an ileal conduit, is rarely justified in the neonatal period. A prosthesis for collection of the urine and protection of the bladder may be employed.

Nursing management in the presence of exstrophy of the bladder involves the following:

Fig. 31.36
Exstrophy of bladder. (Courtesy Edward S. Tank, M.D., Division of Urology, University of Oregon Health Sciences Center, Portland, Oregon.)

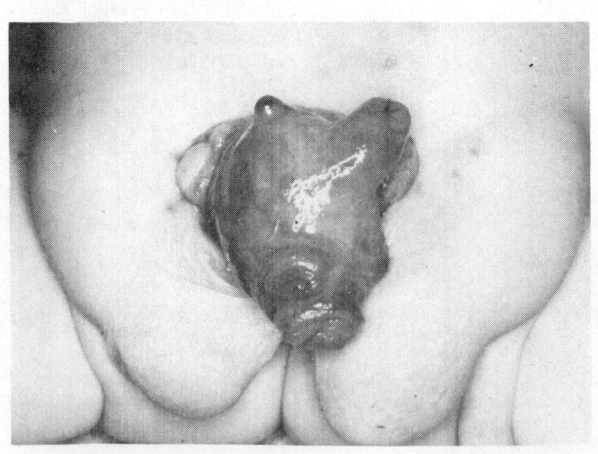

1. Prevent urinary tract infection.
2. Prevent ulceration of adjacent skin from the constant seepage of urine.
3. Meet the infant's touching and cuddling needs.
4. Support parents.
5. Teach parents to care for the defect if surgery is scheduled when the infant is several weeks or months of age.

Hypospadias and epispadias. Hypospadias in a developmental anomaly in which the urethral meatus is placed lower than normal. In an infant boy the meatus opens in the midline of the undersurface of the penis or on the perineum. In an infant girl the meatus opens into the vagina. This condition tends to be hereditary.

Epispadias, also occurring in both sexes but predominating in boys, is a congenital absence of the upper urethral wall. In girls it is often associated with exstrophy of the bladder. In boys the meatal opening is located anywhere along the dorsum (upper side) of the penis.

Most instances of hypospadias are minor and require no corrective surgery. Pronounced defects require extensive urethroplasty. If needed, surgery is completed before the boy enters school so that he can urinate from a standing position like other boys. The more serious defects often coexist with other, multiple anomalies.

Nursing management of the physical care of the infant with hypospadias is the same as that for the normal infant. Should urethroplasty be required, no circumcision is done, since the foreskin is used in the surgical procedure. The parents are taught how to care for the urethral meatus and foreskin to prevent infection and promote cleanliness.

Sexual ambiguity. Sexual ambiguity in the neonate (Fig. 31.37) often is discovered by the nurse, who is usually the first one to perform a physical assessment. The obstetrician is still concentrating on the mother during the third stage of labor.

Erroneous or abnormal sexual differentiation may be a genetic aberration (for example, congenital adrenal hypoplasia), or it may be caused by maternal problems (such as steroid sex hormone therapy for threatened abortion). It is imperative to establish the genetic sex and the sex of child rearing as soon as possible. Early identification is imperative to save embarrassment of reporting the birth of a (genetic) male who in fact is a female or the opposite. Early determination of genetic sex is important to permit the surgical correction of anomalies before an individual or social pattern is set. Prompt consultation with a surgeon who is experienced in the area of intersexuality should be arranged without delay. Meanwhile parents need supportive care as they await the decision.

Fig. 31.37
Ambiguous external genitals (e.g., structure can be an enlarged clitoral hood and clitoris or a malformed penis). (Courtesy Edward S. Tank, M.D., Division of Urology, University of Oregon Health Sciences Center, Portland, Oregon.)

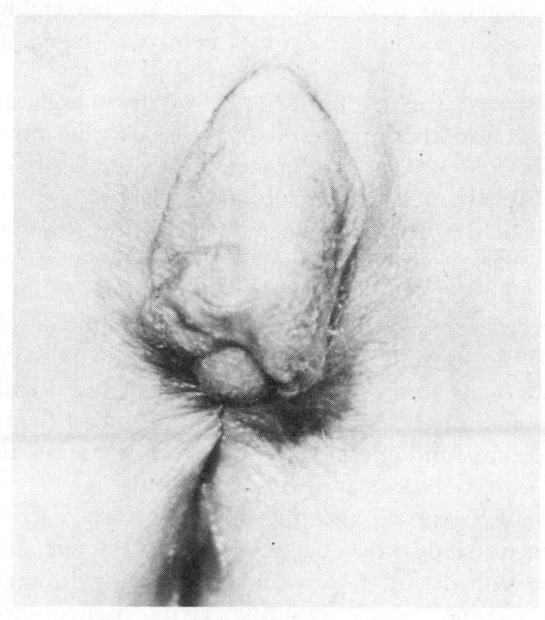

Teratoma. Teratoma, a solid or semisolid neoplasm, is composed of the three embryonal tissue types (ectoderm, mesoderm, entoderm). A teratoma in the newborn may occur in the skull, mediastinum, or abdomen. A solid or semisolid tumor in the sacral area also may prove to be a teratoma. It is protected by sterile dressings before surgical removal. Many teratomas diagnosed in the newborn are malignant. If the lesion cannot be removed entirely by surgery, x-ray therapy and chemotherapy are used. Long-term survival rate for infants with sacrococcygeal teratoma is 85% after surgical removal in the neonatal period. The survival rate is only 50% if surgery is delayed until the infant is more than 1 month old. Rectal and anal function can always be preserved.

Disorders not apparent at birth. Some disorders do not appear until some time after birth. The severity of the psychologic impact varies with the disorder and the time it appears. Together the parents and the affected child, if he is old enough, experience mourning, restructuring of self-image, and the reaction to stigmatization by society. Parents who had other children before the appearance of a disorder in an older child fear for the younger children. The middle-aged individual who develops Huntington's chorea, perhaps even after he has become a grandfather, fears for two generations of descendants. In many cases, affected individuals may experience anger and resentment toward the offending parents, just as parents of a child with a disorder feel resentment toward the child who "did this to us." If the mother unwittingly accepted therapy now shown to have adverse effects on her children (such as, DES), she may feel betrayed, angry, and afraid.

Diethylstilbestrol. Administration of diethylstilbestrol (DES) or another nonsteroidal estrogen to the mother may be followed by developmental or functional genital problems in both female and male progeny. The abnormalities are rare, when one considers the estimate that about 500,000 pregnant women received DES between 1940 and 1970. Single or multiple abnormalities may be noted. Some abnormalities develop or are recognized after puberty. Curiously, most individuals who were exposed prenatally appear to have been unaffected. Hence, an association rather than an actual cause-and-effect relationship is likely and a trigger factor or factors are being sought.

In DES-exposed girls the following developmental or functional disorders have been described: circumferential vaginal ridges; cervical deformity, for example, "cock's comb" cervix, hooding, clefts, pseudopolyps; hypoplastic or T-shaped uterus; constricting bands within the uterus; tubal anomalies; vaginal or cervical adenosis, dysplasia, or cervical incompetence. There appear to be an increased frequency of oligomenorrhea and a lower incidence of pregnancy in these women also. Most critical is the assessment that 3 or 4 out or 1000 women exposed to DES prenatally develop vaginal or cervical clear-cell carcinoma, usually during adolescence.

In DES-exposed males the most common gross lesions reported are epididymal cysts, hypotrophic testes, or testicular capsular thickening. In addition, sperm analyses have revealed low volume of ejaculate, oligospermia, diminished sperm density, and the lower motile sperm count per milliliter. No equivalent of female clear-cell carcinoma or increase in male genitourinary cancer has been noted, however.

Neonatal Infection

General considerations. Sepsis refers to a generalized infection in the bloodstream. Inadequate immunity accounts for the newborn's increased susceptibility. Inadequate immunity is expressed in diminished phagocytic response, delayed chemotaxis (response to chemical stimuli), absent or minimal IgA and IgM, and inadequate serum complement levels. Serum complement (C1 through C6) is involved in immunologic reactions, some of which act to kill or lyse bacteria and enhance phagocytosis. Sepsis of the newborn may begin in the prenatal or postdelivery period. Fulminating or persistent sepsis generally is apparent at birth. Other infections may be obscure and become manifest later.

Clinical findings. Clinical findings in sepsis may include lethargy, restlessness, or poor weight gain. Fever may be recorded. There may be leukocytosis. C-reactive protein may or may not be elevated. Vomiting, diarrhea, or CNS signs, such as convulsions, may be apparent. Examination usually reveals hyperbilirubinemia, hepatomegaly, or splenomegaly—notable after well-established sepsis. Hemorrhage may be an associated sign in sepsis.

Incidence. Sepsis occurs about twice as often in boys as it does in girls. Sepsis results in a higher mortality in boys. The incidence of sepsis for all newborns remains unchanged but is highest among those classified as high risk. Frequency increases with prematurity and in bottle-fed newborns.

Protective mechanisms exist in breast milk. Colostrum contains agglutinins that are active against gram-negative bacteria. Human milk contains iron-binding protein that exerts a bacteriostatic effect on *Escherichia coli.* Human milk also contains macrophages and lymphocytes. The vulnerability of infants to common mucosal pathogens such as respiratory syncytial virus (RSV) may be reduced by passive transfer of maternal immunity in colostrum and breast milk.

Prognosis. Before the advent of antibiotics, 90% of newborns with sepsis died. Antibiotic therapy decreased mortality to between 13% and 45% depending on the causative organism.

Sequelae. Sequelae to septicemia include meningitis, pyarthrosis, and septic shock. **Meningitis,** a frequent sequela, may be evidenced by a bulging anterior fontanel (see discussion of signs of increased intracranial pressure, pp. 998 and 1027). Systemic antibiotics may not diffuse into cerebrospinal fluid (CSF). Intrathecal infusion of a drug such as polymyxin may be initiated.

Pyarthrosis, which may affect any joint, usually localizes in the hips. Limitation in joint movement is one of the few signs of this condition.

Septic shock results from the toxins released into the bloodstream. The most common sign is a drop in blood pressure—a vital sign frequently overlooked in the care of the newborn. Other signs are rapid, irregular respirations and pulse (similar to septicemia in general).

Modes of transmission. Sepsis may occur by one or more modes of transmission. The mother, the newborn, and the newborn's environment are all sources

Routes of Maternal-Fetal Infection and Microorganisms

Transplacental Inoculation of Fetus	Ascending Infection from Vagina to Fetus in Utero; Infections Acquired Through Fetus's Direct Contact with Infected Birth Canal
Chlamydia trachomatis (?)	*Candida albicans*
Coxsackie B virus	*Chlamydia trachomatis* (?)
Cytomegalovirus (CMV—caused by one of the herpes viruses)	*Escherichia coli* and other enteric organisms (two thirds of infections)
Group B β-hemolytic streptococcus (bacterium) (*S. agalactiae*)	Gram-negative bacilli
Herpes simplex	Group B β-hemolytic streptococcus (*S. agalactiae*)
Listeria monocytogenes	Herpes simplex
Malaria (*Plasmodium falciparum,* a protozoan)	*Listeria monocytogenes*
Neisseria gonorrhoeae (bacterium)	*Mycoplasma hominis*
Rubella (virus)	*Neisseria gonorrhoeae*
Toxoplasmosis (protozoan)	Varicella
Treponema pallidum (syphilis) (spirochete)	*Vibrio* (bacterium)
Tuberculosis (rare)	Hepatitis B
Hepatitis B	AIDS
AIDS	

of infective agents. The fetus acquires the infection by (1) aspiration of infected amniotic fluid, (2) transplacental transmission, and (3) direct contact with an infected birth canal (see box above).

The newborn may acquire infections through (1) the umbilical stump, (2) skin and mucosa of the eye, ear, nose, and throat; and (3) body systems, such as respiratory, urinary, and gastrointestinal tracts and the CNS. The environment is an important source of infection. "Water bugs" thrive in humidifiers, sinks, and respiratory-assistance equipment. Direct contact with infected persons or their infected excrement or fomites is another environmental hazard.

General nursing care. Nursing care of infants with sepsis should follow these guidelines:

1. Actions to minimize or eliminate environmental sources of infectious agents include careful and through housecleaning, frequent replacement of used equipment (for example, changing intravenous tubing each day), **hand washing,** and disposal of excrement and linens in an appropriate manner.

2. Monitoring intravenous infusion rate and administering antibiotics are the nurse's responsbility. It is important to administer the prescribed dose of antibiotic within 1 hour after it is prepared to avoid loss of drug stability. If the intravenous fluid the infant is

Reminders: Prevention of Spread of Infection

Care of Specimens After Collection	Leaving Isolation Room
1. Place container on paper towel at bedside or sink area until after you have removed isolation gown and gloves.	1. Untie lower strings of gown.
2. Cleanse outside of container with alcohol swipe.	2. Remove gloves and discard in trash container; if gloves have not been used, wash hands.
3. Place container on paper towel on isolation cart.	3. Untie upper strings of gown, remove, place in laundry or trash container.
4. Affix addressographed sticker labeled "Isolation." (**Do not lick label!**)	4. Wash hands
5. Place specimen in a *single* plastic bag, marked "Isolation."	5. Use paper towel to turn off faucet and open door.
6. Attach requisition (also labeled "Isolation") with paper clip to outside of bag.	6. Remove mask and discard in trash container. **Mask shall not be worn around neck or reused.**
7. Send to appropriate laboratory.	7. If there are hand-washing facilities immediately outside of the door, wash hands there rather than in isolation room—use paper towel to turn faucet.
	8. Wash hands in utility room before continuing duties.

Table 31.7
TORCH Infections and AIDS in the Newborn

Infection	Mode of Transmission	Laboratory Diagnosis	Clinical Diagnosis	Isolation	Treatment
Toxoplasmosis (parasite)					
Most infants are asymptomatic at birth, but the prognosis is poor for infected infants: 10%-15% die; 85% have severe psychomotor problems or mental retardation by 2-4 years; 50% have visual problems by 1 year	Transplacental Congenital infection from primary maternal infection—usually from woman's handling raw meat, pork, or cat litter	Antitoxoplasma IgM antibodies in cord or baby's serum Maternal titer	Asymptomatic (60%-75%) Chorioretinitis, hydrocephalus, cerebral calcifications Prematurity, IUGR, microcephaly, hydrocephaly, convulsions, hepatosplenomegaly, anemia, purpura, DIC	*None* May breast feed	Pyrimethamine, which can depress hematopoiesis—counteract with folic acid Sulfadiazine, which can increase bilirubin These medications do not reverse neuro damage but do control progression
Other *Hepatitis B (virus)*					
25%-40% of all cases of viral hepatitis are B. Infants are most frequently infected during birth or in the first few days of life. Rate is highest when mother contracts virus immediately before delivery. Infants are at high risk of developing chronic hepatitis, cirrhosis of the liver, or liver cancer (NAA-COG, 1986)	Transplacental Serum to serum Contact with contaminated urine, feces, saliva, semen, or vaginal secretions during delivery Possibly through breast milk	Viral cultures of amniotic fluid Hepatitis B surface antigen IgM in cord or baby's serum	Asymptomatic Acute hepatitis with changes in liver function (few) (often fatal) Acute enteric hepatitis with chronic liver disease (rare) Acute and acute enteric hepatitis may appear years later in carriers of the virus	Acute A, B, non-A, non-B, unknown: *Enteric and blood* Chronic: *Blood* Asymptomatic carrier with HBsAg: *Blood* Hepatitis or non-A or B: *Blood* Clean baby thoroughly; may breast feed after prophylaxis	HBIG 0.5 ml IM within first 12 hours, or immune serum globulin. HBIG vaccine: a course of 3 doses induces antibodies in 90%. Second dose given at 1 month; third, at 6 months. The vaccine should protect the child for up to 9 years
Rubella (virus)					
90% of infected infants show signs of disease before 5 years: motor impairment and mental retardation. Anomalies are most severe if mother contracts virus during the first trimester	Transplacental Contact with contaminated urine or nasopharyngeal secretions	Viral cultures of amniotic fluid, placenta or baby's throat, urine or spinal fluid Rubella-specific IgM in cord or baby's serum HI antibody in blood CF antibodies in blood	Asymptomatic Small organs with fewer cells Cataracts, deafness, cardiac impairments IUGR, hepatosplenomegaly, adenopathy, encephalitis, retinopathy, interstitial pneumonia, severe prematurity, hepatitis, ITP, bony radiolucencies	Gown and gloves Isolate in Isolette or mother's room Exclude susceptible females from contact Breast feeding allowed; may shed virus up to 2 years	Symptomatic relief

Table 31.7, cont'd
TORCH Infections and AIDS in the Newborn

Infection	Mode of Transmission	Laboratory Diagnosis	Clinical Diagnosis	Isolation	Treatment
Cytomegalovirus (virus)					
Member of herpesvirus. Is most common cause of perinatal infections. Primary CMV infection during pregnancy transmits the virus to 50% of fetuses, of which 10%-12% will be born with CMV inclusion disease	Transplacental Contact with contaminated vaginal or nasopharyngeal secretions, urine or feces Blood transfusion Breast milk (have mother pump and discard while in acute CMV syndrome)	Viral cultures of amniotic fluid Anti-CMV IgM antibodies in cord or baby's serum CMV inclusion cells or CSF Viral cultures Maternal titer	Congenitally acquired asymptomatic form Systemic CMV inclusion disease, bone lesions, anemia, low birth weight, hepatomegaly, splenomegaly, jaundice, petechiae, heart disease, pneumonia, cataracts, chorioretinitis, microcephaly, obstructive hydrocephaly, intracranial calcifications, encephalitis	Gown and gloves Isolette or mother's room May breast feed unless mother has acute disease	Antimetabolites or antiviral agents may avert CNS destruction
Herpesvirus (virus) **Herpes simplex type II**					
30%-50% of contaminated births are infected; half of these babies die or are severely damaged. Positive cultures or active lesions last 2 weeks of pregnancy indicate cesarean delivery within 4 hours, if ROM	Transplacental Direct contact with lesion during birth	Herpes-specific IgM antibodies in cord or baby's serum Viral cultures of eyes, nose, throat, blood, urine, or CSF	More likely to be premature or of low birth weight. Mothers are more likely to be white, non-Hispanic, unmarried, and less than 20 years (NAACOG, 1986). Asymptomatic Localized lesions (eyes, throat, mouth, skin) Disseminated systemic infection (jaundice, purpura, respiratory distress, shock)	Gown and gloves Isolette or mother's room until cultures negative Secretion and blood precautions May breast feed if no lesions around breast	Gamma globulin Systemic antimetabolites Interferon stimulant Possibly poly 1C, idoxuridine, and vidarabine No known cure
AIDS					
Autoimmune deficiency syndrome (HTLV III: Human T cell lymphotropic virus)* Infants who contract AIDS: essentially 100% fatal Infants comprise 1% of AIDS victims in USA (Harris, 1986)	Unknown: mothers are IV drug users, have AIDS, or have had sexual partners who had or were at risk for AIDS	Test at-risk infants immediately after birth and at 1 year, for antibodies	Evidence of bacterial sepsis. Early symptoms usually nonspecific: failure to gain weight, lymphadenopathy, chronic diarrhea, hepatosplenomegaly, fever, cough, and respiratory distress (Boland and Gaskill, 1984)	Gown and gloves for persons likely to have direct contact with secretions Hand washing before and after contact with infected person Masks worn when infected person has a productive cough or when	Precautions to avoid infection if mother is from high-risk group: ■ No live vaccines against childhood diseases—measles, mumps, rubella ■ Monthly doses of immune globulin

*Renamed human immunodeficiency virus (HIV).

Continued.

Table 31.7, cont'd
TORCH Infections and AIDS in the Newborn

Infection	Mode of Transmission	Laboratory Diagnosis	Clinical Diagnosis	Isolation	Treatment
			Facial syndrome: smaller head circumference; a prominent, box-like forehead; slightly slanted eyes set far apart; a short, broad and flat nose; and large, loosely shaped lips with prominent triangular philtrum Mother is in the group at risk Mother exhibits symptomatology of AIDS	suctioning the intubated client Protective eyewear (goggles) should be worn when there is potential for splatter of blood, bloody secretions, or body fluids (Staff, Feb. 1986; Harris, 1986) Heavily soiled linens should be double-bagged and labeled infectious waste Contaminated needles and syringes: handle with exceptional care and dispose of into a puncture-resistant receptacle; mark full container "Contaminated" and send to incinerator (Loveman and others, 1986)	■ Circumcision in males is avoided ■ Umbilical cord stumps are cleaned meticulously every day

receiving contains electrolytes, vitamins, or other medications, *do not* add antibiotics. The antibiotic (or other medication) may be deactivated or may form a precipitate. Instead, piggyback another bottle of the prescribed fluid to be infused and attach its tubing with a three-way stopcock to the needle at the infusion site. Remember to include the number of milliliters of fluid used from the piggyback bottle when calculating the newborn's intake.

3. Follow isolation procedures according to hospital

Torch Infections that Affect the Fetus

T Toxoplasmosis
O Other: syphilis, varicella, group B β-hemolytic streptococcus, chlamydial infections, hepatitis B, AIDS
R Rubella
C Cytomegalovirus infections (CMV) or cytomegalic inclusion disease (CMID)
H Herpes simplex

---

policy as indicated. See p. 1033 for reminders about preventing the spread of infection.

TORCH infections. Many infections affect the newborn. The acronym for the most commonly encountered infections is TORCH. For maternal TORCH infections, see Tables 27.8 and 27.9. For TORCH infections affecting newborns, see the box at left and Table 31.7.

Toxoplasmosis. Toxoplasmosis is a multisystem disease caused by the protozoan *Toxoplasma gondii*. Cats who hunt infected mice harbor the parasite and excrete the infective oocysts in their feces. Human infection follows hand-to-mouth contact, such as after disposal of cat litter or following ingestion of rare cooked meat from cattle or sheep that grazed in contaminated fields.

About 30% of women who contract toxoplasmosis during gestation transmit the disease to their offspring. The diagnosis of toxoplasmosis in the newborn is supported by elevated cord blood serum IgM.

The clinical features of toxoplasmosis resemble cytomegalic inclusion disease in mother and infant. Both diseases are responsible for serious perinatal mortality and morbidity. Severe toxoplasmosis is associated with growth retardation, microcephalus or hydrocephalus, microphthalmia, chorioretinitis, CNS calcification, thrombocytopenia, jaundice, and fever.

Treatment of toxoplasmosis during pregnancy is problematic. Pyrimethamine currently is the first-choice drug against *T. gondii.* However, it may be teratogenic, especially during the first trimester. Sulfonamide therapy is effective, but the drug must be discontinued before delivery and even-exchange transfusion of the newborn may be necessary to avoid kernicterus. This may occur because sulfa drugs have a greater albumin-binding affinity than bilirubin, which may rise after delivery to critical levels. The newborn may be treated with pyrimethamine, but folinic acid supplement will be required to reduce the toxicity of the drug.

In congenital toxoplasmosis, maldevelopment or neurologic damage will not be affected by treatment. However, progression of the disease can be controlled by appropriate therapy. Regrettably, encysted (intramuscular) forms of *T. gondii* cannot be eradicated by any therapy and they may cause recurrence of the disease.

Gonorrhea. Gonorrheal infection (Table 27.8) other than ophthalmia neonatorum is an infrequent but significant cause of neonatal morbidity. Endocervical cultures for *Neisseria gonorrhoeae* should be obtained routinely during pregnancy and appropriate treatment instituted when necessary to prevent fetal-neonatal infection.

The newborn with a mild infection often recovers completely with appropriate treatment. Occasionally infants die in the early neonatal period from overwhelming infection or pneumonia.

Syphilis. Congenital and neonatal syphilis (Table 27.8) has reemerged in recent years as a significant health problem. Fetal infestation with the spirochete *Treponema pallidum* is blocked by Langhans' layer in the chorion until this layer begins to atrophy, namely, between 16 and 18 weeks' gestation. If spirochetemia is untreated, it will result in fetal death by midtrimester abortion or stillbirth in one out of four cases. All newborns in whom the infection occurs before 7 months' gestation are affected. Only 60% are affected if the infection occurs late in pregnancy. If maternal infection is adequately treated before the eighteenth week, newborns seldom demonstrate signs of the disease. Although treatment after the eighteenth week may cure fetal sphirochetemia, pathologic changes may not be prevented completely.

Because the fetus becomes infected after the period of organogenesis (first trimester), maldevelopment of organs does not result. Congenital syphilis may stimulate premature labor, but there is no evidence that it causes intrauterine growth retardation (IUGR). Stigmas of congenital syphilis (Fig. 31.38) may include inflammatory and destructive changes in the placenta, in organs such as the liver, spleen, kidneys, adrenal glands, and in bone covering and marrow. Disorders of the CNS, teeth, and cornea may not become evident until several months after birth.

Clinical findings. The most severely affected newborns may be **hydropic** (edematous) and **anemic,** with enlarged liver and spleen. Hepatosplenomegaly is probably secondary to extramedullary hematopoietic activity stimulated by the severe anemia.

In some cases signs of congenital syphilis do not appear until late in the neonatal period. In these newborns early signs, such as poor feeding, slight hyperthermia, and snuffles, may be nonspecific. **Snuffles** refers to the copious clear serosanguineous mucous discharge from the obstructed nose.*

By the end of the first week of life, in untreated cases, a copper-colored maculopapular **dermal rash** appears. The rash is characteristically first noticeable on the palms of the hands, soles of the feet, and diaper area, and around the mouth and anus. The maculopapular lesions may become vesicular and confluent and extend over the trunk and extremities. **Condylomas** (elevated wartlike lesions) may be seen around the anus. Rough, cracked mucocutaneous lesions of the lips heal to form circumoral radiating scars known as **rhagades.**

Other involvement results in exfoliation (separation, flaking) of nails and loss of hair. Iritis and choroiditis are characteristic of infection of the eyes. Nephrotic syndrome secondary to renal infection, hepatitis with **jaundice,** lymphadenopathy, inflammation of the pancreas, testes, and colon, and a pseudoparalysis of the extremites may be noted. Laboratory tests may show a pleocytosis (usually lymphocytosis) and elevated CSF protein levels.

By 3 months of age, in 90% of infants (treated or untreated), periostitis and metaphyseal osteochondritis may be demonstrated by roentgenography. These bone lesions generally disappear by 10 months of age whether or not the infant receives antibiotic treatment.

Diagnosis. After the physician determines that congenital syphilis is possible, the CSF (obtained by lumbar puncture) is examined with the FTA-ABS test (Chapter 27). If results are inconclusive, the physician will probably opt to treat the child as if the disease existed.

---

*NOTE: A mucopurulent discharge indicates secondary infection, usually by streptococci or staphylococci.

Fig. 31.38
Early congenital syphilis apparent at birth, which corresponds to secondary syphilis in the adult. (Late congenital syphilis, corresponding to tertiary syphilis, becomes apparent after 2 years of age.) **A,** Cutaneous lesions of congenital syphilis. Lines drawn on body indicate hepatosplenomegaly. No destruction of bridge of nose (common finding in congenital syphilis) is noted on this infant. **B,** Rhinitis (snuffles) resulting in rhagades and excoriation of upper lip. Red-colored rash is around mouth and on chin. (From Shirkey, H.C., editor: Pediatric therapy, ed. 6, St. Louis, 1980, The C.V. Mosby Co.)

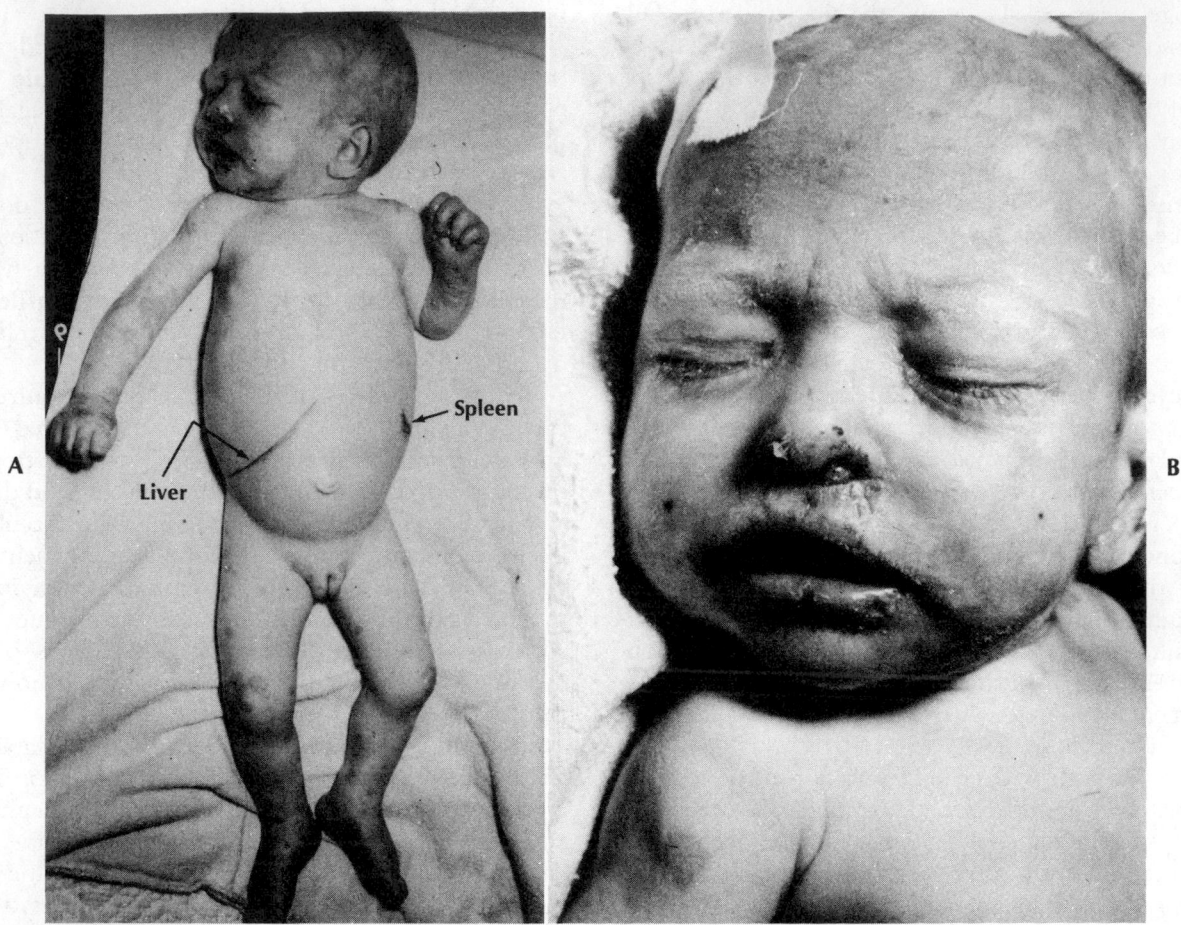

Medical management. If the mother had been adequately treated before delivery and serologic testing of the newborn does not show syphilis, generally the newborn is not treated with antibiotics. In this case the newborn is checked for antibody titer (received from the mother via the placenta) every 2 weeks for 3 months, at which time the test result should be negative. Some physicians recommended antibiotic therapy for asymptomatic or inconclusive cases.

For antibiotic treatment to be effective, an "adequate" blood level must be maintained for an "adequate" period of time. Suggested medication protocol in the presence of symptomatic systemic disease differs from author to author and physician to physician. After 12 hours of antibiotic therapy, the child is not considered contagious. It is generally accepted that erythromycin is the substitute antibiotic of choice for newborns sensitive to penicillin.

Prognosis and sequelae. In general, treatment of syphilis is more effective if it is begun early rather than late in the course of the disease. However, a recurrence rate of 5% can be expected. Even adequate treatment of congenital syphilis after birth does not always prevent late (5 to 15 years after initial infection) complications. Potential complications include neurosyphilis, deafness, Hutchinson's teeth (notched incisors), saber

Fig. 31.39
Newborn with congenital rubella syndrome, showing multiple purpuric lesions over face, trunk, and upper arm. (From Fanaroff, A.A., and Martin, R.J., editors: Behrman's neonatal-perinatal medicine: diseases of the fetus and infant. ed. 3, St. Louis, 1983, The C.V. Mosby Co.)

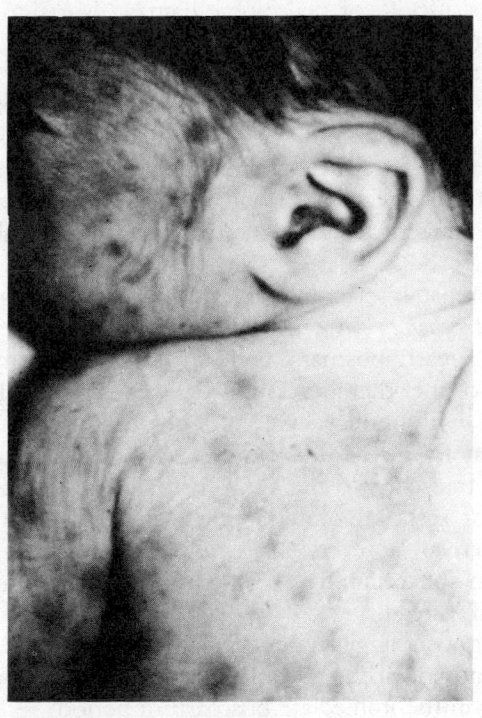

shins, joint involvement, saddle nose (depressed bridge), gummas (soft, gummy tumors) over the skin and other organs, and interstitial keratitis (inflammation of the cornea). The failure of therapy with the persistence of spirochetes in the eyes is not unusual. Antibiotics penetrate ocular tissue poorly. Mortality from congenital syphilis during early childhood is uncommon.

Rubella. Congenital rubella syndrome frequently results in spontaneous abortion, congenital cataract, microcephaly, nerve deafness, or cardiac anomalies when infection occurs between 5 and 10 weeks of pregnancy. Rubella acquired later in gestation may lead to intrauterine growth retardation or premature delivery (Tables 31.7 and 25.16).

Numerous infants whose mothers had rubella during gestation are born alive with active viral infection (Fig. 31.39). This so-called **extended rubella syndrome** is typified by one or more of the following disorders: encephalitis, ocular abnormalities, pneumonitis, cardiac maldevelopment, hepatosplenomegaly and hyperbilirubinemia, and thrombocytopenic purpura. A tendency for infants born with rubella syndrome to develop leukemia during childhood has been noted.

Although many babies with active rubella die in early infancy, others survive longer. The rubella virus has been cultured in babies for 1 to 1½ years after delivery. These infants are a serious source of infection to susceptible individuals, particularly potentially or actually pregnant women. Extended pediatric isolation is mandatory until the noncontagious stage of rubella has been reached. (Isolate newborn until pharyngeal mucus and urine are free of virus.)

For maternal vaccination in the puerperium, see Chapter 24.

Cytomegalic inclusion disease. Cytomegalic inclusion disease (CMID)* is a disorder caused by one or more of at least six strains of cytomegalovirus. Viremia during pregnancy may result in abortion, stillbirth, or congenital or neonatal CMID in a live-born infant. It is always a severely crippling disease of the infant.

Maternal infection with CMV may begin as a mononucleosis-like syndrome. However, in the majority of adults, the onset of the disease is uncertain. It may remain subclinical for years. Respiratory transmission is the major vector, but the virus has been recovered from semen and from bank blood. Maternal CMID may be diagnosed serologically. Many women, especially those in the lower socioeconomic classes, have antibody evidence of CMID.

The newborn with classic, full-blown CMID displays intrauterine growth retardation (IUGR) and has microcephaly. The newborn has a peticheal rash, jaundice, and hepatosplenomegaly. Anemia, thrombocytopenia, and hyperbilirubinemia are to be expected. Intracranial, periventricular calcification often will be noted on x-ray films. Inclusion bodies ("owl's eye" figures) in cells sedimented from freshly voided urine or in liver biopsy specimens are typical. The virus can be recovered from saliva or urine. Despite the extensive, endemic nature of the disease in women and men and its potential for havoc in perinatal life, critically affected newborns are only occasionally delivered. Milder forms of the disease may often result when the fetus is affected late in pregnancy. Severe mental and physical handicaps mark virtually all infants who survive CMID.

Elevated cord blood IgM, is suggestive evidence of disease. The virus may be isolated from urine or saliva of the newborn. Differential diagnosis includes other causes of jaundice, syphilis (positive VDRL), toxoplasmosis (positive Sabin-Feldman dye test), hemolytic disease of the newborn (positive Coombs' test), or coxsackie virus infection (culture).

---

*Also referred to as cytomegalovirus (CMV).

No reasonable prevention or specific therapy exists for mother or infant. Repeated pregnancies may be complicated by CMID.

Herpesvirus type 2 infection. Neonatal infection with herpesvirus type 2 is relatively rare. It occurs in an estimated 1 in 3500 to 1 in 30,000 live births. Infection is often fatal (Fig. 31.40). The newborn may acquire the virus by any of four modes of transmission:

- Transplacental infection
- Ascending infection by way of the birth canal
- Direct contamination during passage through an infected birth canal
- Direct transmission, from infected personnel or family

Fetal infection *may* be prevented if the following conditions are obtained: (1) Active cases of genital tract herpetic lesions are diagnosed before labor, and the mother delivers by cesarean birth. (2) Amniotic membranes remain intact. Genital herpes should be ruled out before artificial rupture of membranes or application of fetal scalp electrodes.

Fetal infection is almost certain if the mother has viremia. See Table 27.9. The nurse should note that

---

Fig. 31.40

Neonatal herpesvirus infection. (From Fanaroff, A.A., and Martin, R.J., editors: Behrman's neonatal-perinatal medicine: diseases of the fetus and infant, ed. 3, St. Louis, 1983, The C.V. Mosby Co.)

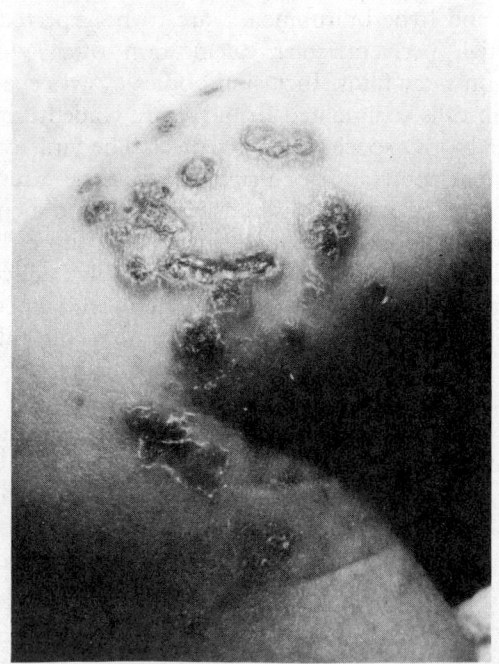

---

this disease is highly contagious. Although herpesvirus type 2 is responsible for herpetic infections primarily occurring in the genital area, the nurse's ungloved hands may pick up the virus through breaks in the skin when infected lesions are touched.

Prognosis is grave in severe herpesvirus type 2 infections. Ocular or neurologic damage is a significant sequela in survivors.

Chlamydial disease. *Chlamydia trachomatis* is an **intracellular bacterium** that causes **neonatal conjunctivitis** and **pneumonia.** The conjunctivitis is first noted about 3 or 4 days after birth. If chlamydial disease is not treated, chronic follicular conjunctivitis with conjunctival scarring and corneal neovascularization may result.

If prenatal screening reveals infection with *Chlamydia trachomatis,* treatment of the mother is deferred until the early postnatal period to avoid exposing the fetus to the therapy. After delivery the mother is treated with tetracycline, 500 mg orally four times each day for 7 to 14 days. The newborn is also treated with tetracycline, 6 mg/kg/24 h for 7 days, and ointment or solution of tetracycline is instilled into the conjunctival sac every 2 to 4 hours for 2 to 4 days. Sodium sulfacetamide (10%) drops or ointment may be used instead.

Prognosis is generally good. Ideally, the condition is diagnosed early, and both mother and newborn are treated in the immediate postpartum period.

Acquired immune deficiency syndrome (AIDS). Transmission of human immunodeficiency virus (HIV) occurs primarily through the exchange of body fluids, e.g., blood, semen. Severe depression of the cellular immune system characterizes AIDS (Chapter 5). Therefore the individual with AIDS is susceptible to a variety of other illnesses and "opportunistic" infections to which the normal population has resistance. Besides pneumocystosis and karposi's sarcoma, numerous other illnesses commonly are seen in this syndrome. They include disseminated fungal infections caused by *Mycobacterium avium* and *M. intracellulare* and *Candida albicans;* viral infections caused by the cytomegalovirus (CMV), hepatitis B, and herpes simplex; and immunologic manifestations such as thrombocytopenic purpura.

According to staff members in the AIDS unit at San Francisco General Hospital (Amer. Nurse, Feb. 1986), treatment precautions by health care providers are the same as those for the care of people with hepatitis B (Table 31.7). These precautions for health care providers and the nonpregnant people who come in contact with AIDS sufferers are as follows:

1. When handling needles and syringes, avoid accidental needle sticks.

2. Dispose of needles and syringes in puncture-proof containers.
3. Use meticulous hand washing at all times.
4. Use gown and gloves when in contact with blood, secretions, and enteric excretions.
5. Wear masks if the client has pneumocystosis and is coughing.
6. Wash washable surfaces and used equipment with a solution of sodium hypochlorite (household bleach) and water—1 cup of household bleach to 9 cups of water. Remove blood or other fluids before disinfection to avoid neutralizing the bleach solution.

About half of AIDs sufferers have elevated CMV titers. Because CMV inclusion disease poses a serious hazard to the fetus, **pregnant women are advised to avoid direct contact with AIDS sufferers.**

AIDS may be sexually transmitted among homosexual or bisexual males. Some AIDS cases have been reported among women whose sexual partners have AIDS or are from the group identified as high risk for AIDS (Centers for Disease Control, 1983). There have been some reports of infants born to women at risk for AIDS who have developed unexplained cellular immunodeficiencies and "opportunistic" infections, for example, CMV.

Oral thrush. Oral thrush, or mycotic stomatitis, is caused by *Candida albicans*. This infection results from direct contact with a contaminated birth canal, hands (mother's or others), feeding equipment, breast, or bedding. The appearance of white plaques on the oral mucosa, gums, and tongue is characteristic. The white patches are easily differentiated from milk curds; the patches cannot be removed and tend to bleed when touched. In most cases the infant does not seem to be discomforted by the infection. A few newborns seem to have some difficulty swallowing.

Infants who are sick, debilitated, or receiving anti-biotic therapy are more susceptible. Those with conditions such as cleft lip or palate, neoplasms, and hyperparathyroidism seem to be more vulnerable to mycotic infection.

The objectives of management are to eradicate the causative organism, control exposure to *Candida albicans,* and improve the infant's resistance. Interventions include the following:

1. Maintain scrupulous cleanliness to prevent reinfection (nursing personnel, parents, others).
   a. Use good hand-washing technique.
   b. Provide clean surfaces for newborns (newborn is never placed directly on sheets on which the mother has been sitting).
   c. Clean and store equipment well.
2. Support the compromised newborn's physiologic function (see Chapter 25).
3. Administer chemotherapy.
   a. Apply aqueous solution of gentian violet (1% to 2%) with swab to oral mucosa, gums, tongue. (Guard against permanent stain on skin, clothes, equipment. Warn parents about purple staining of baby's mouth.)
   b. Instill nystatin (Mycostatin) into mouth with a medicine dropper. Give infant sterile water to wash out milk before giving nystatin. Nystatin may also be swabbed over mucosa, gums, or tongue.

To give medication by medicine dropper, position the infant's head to the side or support the infant in a semi-Fowler position. Insert the dropper into the oral cavity so that the tip rests against the cheek, alongside the tongue. Wait until the infant begins to suck on the dropper, then squeeze the rubber end slowly until the dropper is empty.

A summary of nursing actions for newborns with infections is presented below.

Summary of Nursing Actions

NEONATAL INFECTION

GOALS

1. For the mother: a satisfying birth.
2. For the newborn: a neonatal period in which infection is identified and treated promptly, and if therapy is necessary, no harmful sequelae result.
3. For the family: a satisfying newborn period in which they receive information and support and family-newborn attachment occurs.

PRIORITIES

1. Prevent neonatal infection.
2. Identify and treat neonatal infection promptly.
3. Facilitate family-newborn attachment.

Continued.

Summary of Nursing Actions—cont'd

ASSESSMENT	EXAMPLES OF POTENTIAL NURSING DIAGNOSTIC CATEGORIES*
A. Review of prenatal record	Potential for infection
B. Age of onset	Hemorrhage†
C. Clinical manifestations	Alteration in bowel elimination: diarrhea
1. Nonspecific: "doesn't look right"; "not doing well"; "poor weight gain"	Alteration in comfort: pain
2. Organism-specific	Fluid volume deficit related to infection
a. *Pseudomonas aeruginosa:* purple necrotic skin lesions	Alteration in fluid volume: excess related to therapy for infection
b. Group B β-hemolytic streptococci:	Alteration in nutrition: less than body requirements
c. Herpesvirus type 2: fever, coryza, tachycardia, hemorrhage, often evidenced by hemoptysis, bloody stools	Alteration in oral mucous membrane
d. Gonorrhea: conjunctivitis, unstable temperature, hypotonia, poor feeding behavior	Alteration in respiratory function†
e. Syphilis; rash, lesions of skin and bone, rhinitis, hepatosplenomegaly	Ineffective airway clearance
3. Systemic signs	Ineffective breathing pattern
a. Respiratory system: apnea; irregular, grunting respirations with retractions	Impaired gas exchange
b. Gastrointestinal system: vomiting; bile-stained diarrhea; abdominal distension; paralytic ileus with no stools; poor suck	Impairment of skin integrity
c. Skin: cyanosis, pallor, mottling, jaundice, local lesions	Alteration in tissue perfusion
d. CNS: similar to signs of hypocalcemia, hypoglycemia; that is, lethargy, irritability, tremors, convulsions, coma (increased intracranial pressure if meningitis develops)	Alteration in patterns of urinary elimination
	Ineffective thermoregulation
e. Temperature: normal or low or unstable	Potential for injury
f. Hepatomegaly or splenomegaly: notable after well-established sepsis	
g. Hemorrhage	
D. Laboratory studies	
1. Cultures: blood, umbilical stump, naso-oropharynx, ear canals, skin, CSF, stool, urine	
2. Bilirubin: increased direct (conjugated) bilirubin level, especially if organism is gram negative	
3. Blood studies: for anemia, increased WBC, decreased RBC (an ominous sign)	
E. Drug side effects	
1. Penicillin: urticaria, skin rash, pruritus, vomiting, diarrhea, convulsions	
2. Kanamycin (Kantrex): WBCs, RBCs, protein in urine	
3. Polymyxin: proteinuria, irritability	
F. Signs of infection with antibiotic-resistant and fungal organisms	
G. Sequelae	
1. Meningitis	
2. Pyarthrosis	
3. Septic shock	
H. Family responses	Knowledge deficit
	Anxiety
	Fear
	Ineffective individual or family coping
	Alteration in family process

*All diagnostic categories except those indicated by a dagger are approved by NANDA's seventh national conference (1986).
†Diagnosis not included by NANDA, 1986.

Summary of Nursing Actions—cont'd

ASSESSMENT	EXAMPLES OF POTENTIAL NURSING DIAGNOSTIC CATEGORIES*
	Grieving Alteration in home maintenance Alteration in parenting Powerlessness Disturbance in self-concept Spiritual distress

OUTCOME CRITERIA*	PLAN/IMPLEMENTATION

A. Sepsis is prevented
B. Early signs of sepsis are recognized, and appropriate therapy is instituted.
C. If therapy is necessary, no harmful sequelae result.
D. Pathophysiologic sequelae to septicemia are avoided.
E. Parents are able to form attachment to newborn.
F. Parents' self-esteem is maintained.
G. Staff establishes caring relationship with parents to foster their trust and to encourage continuing, active, positive interactions of family with members of health care system.
	A. Medical management
	  1. Antibiotics
	    a. Penicillin, ampicillin, or kanamycin (Kantrex) for treatment of 90% of all organisms; treat for 10 days via intravenous infusion
	    b. Gentamicin: especially for gram-negative organisms, such as *Pseudomonas aeruginosa*
	  2. Support of physiologic systems
	    a. Oxygen
	    b. Fluids and electrolytes
	    c. Warmth
	  3. Isolation procedures according to hospital protocol
	B. Nursing management
	  1. Recognize signs
	  2. Institute preventive measures to block modes of transmission
	  3. Calculate dosage of medications accurately
	  4. Recognize side effects of medications
	  5. Monitor intravenous infusion rate, infusion site; change tubing and dressings at least every day
	  6. Monitor optimal thermal environment
	  7. Report symptoms of meningitis
	C. Facilitate parents' understanding of newborn's condition, medical and nursing management, expected results of therapies
	  1. Clarify misinterpretations or misinformation
	  2. Repeat explanations as often as needed
	  3. Prepare parents for possible prolonged hospitalization
	D. Care of parents (see Chapter 26)
	  1. Encourage parents to express feelings
	  2. Encourage parents to visit frequently and participate in newborn's care
	  3. Keep parents informed of newborn's progress
	E. Instruct parents about hygiene measures: hand washing, especially after voiding or defecating
	F. Give parents written instruction on the following:
	  1. Clinical manifestations
	  2. What to report and whom to call
	G. Teach use of and reading of thermometer, if necessary
	H. Support parents
	  1. Avoid blaming parents for infant's condition.
	  2. Educate parents regarding transmission, treatment, prevention.
	  3. Help parents communicate with pediatricians.

*Outcome criteria direct the selection of nursing actions **(plan/implementation)** and measure their effectiveness **(evaluation)**.

Summary of Nursing Actions—cont'd

OUTCOME CRITERIA*	PLAN/IMPLEMENTATION
	4. Involve parents with care if possible. Facilitate early and frequent parent-child contact. Acknowledge positive parent involvement (e.g., interest, cooperation, care of infant).
	5. If nurse feels unprepared or hesitant to provide necessary sexual counseling, as needed for sexually transmitted diseases, parents should be referred to someone else. Avoid critical attitude toward parents.

EVALUATION The nurse can be assured that care was effective if the goals of care are met.

Summary

The compromised newborn presents a challenge to the health care team. The nurse must have sound knowledge about conditions that place the newborn at risk, including problems related to gestational age and birth weight, birth trauma, maternal diabetes mellitus, hyperbilirubinemia, congenital disorders, and infection. Constant vigilance, prompt reporting, and timely therapy are necessary to prevent serious sequelae to the disorder and its therapy. The parents and other family members need a sensitive, thoughtful nurse to help them cope with the stress that arises from birth and care of a compromised newborn.

References

Preterm Infant

Als, H., and Brazelton, T.B.: A new model of assessing the behavioral organization in preterm and full term infants, J. Am. Acad. Child Psychiatry 20:239, 1981.

Bennett, F.C., Robinson, N.M., and Sells, C.J.: Growth and development of infants weighing less than 800 grams at birth, Pediatrics 71:319, 1983.

Benzyl alcohol may be toxic to newborns: FDA Drug Bull. 12:10, 1982.

Bernbaum, J.C., and others: Nonnutritive sucking during gavage feeding enhances growth and maturation in premature infants, Pediatrics 71:41, 1983.

Boggs, K.R., and Rau, P.K.: Breastfeeding the premature infant, Am J. Nurs. 83:1437, 1983.

Dubowitz, L.M.S., and others: Gestational age of the newborn, J. Pediatr. 77:1, 1970.

Field, T.M.: Interaction patterns of preterm and term infants. In Field, T.M., editor: Infants born at risk, Jamaica, N.Y., 1979, Spectrum Publications.

Field, T., and others: Nonnutritive sucking during tube feedings: effects on preterm neonates in an intesive care unit, Pediatrics 70:381, 1982.

Fomufod, A.K.: Low birthweight and early neonatal separation as factors in child abuse, J. Nat. Med. Assoc. 68:106, 1976.

Goldberg, S.: Premature birth: consequences of the parent-infant relationship, Am. Sci. 67:214, Mar./Apr., 1979.

Gorski, P.A., Davison, M.F., and Brazelton, T.B.: Stages of behavioral organization in the high-risk neonates: theoretical and clinical considerations, Semin. Perinatol. 3:61, 1979.

Hansen, F.H.: Nursing care in the neonatal intensive care unit, J.O.G.N. Nurs. 11:17, 1982.

Korones, S.: High-risk newborn infants: the basis for intensive nursing care, ed. 4, St. Louis, 1986, The C.V. Mosby Co.

Kulkarni, P., and others: Postneonatal infant mortality in infants admitted to a neonatal intensive care unit, Pediatrics 62:178, Aug. 1978.

Milluncheck, E., and McArtor, R.: Fatal aspiration of a make-shift pacifier, Pediatrics 77:369, March 1986.

Montgomery, L.A., and Williams-Judge, S.: An anticipatory support program for high-risk parents, Neonatal Network 5:33, Aug. 1986.

Newman, L.: Parent perceptions of their low birth weight infant, Pediatrician 9:182, 1980.

Rehm, R.: Teaching cardiopulmonary resuscitation to parents, MCN 8:411, Nov./Dec. 1983.

Sammons, W., and Lewis, J.: Premature babies: a different beginning, St. Louis, 1985, The C.V. Mosby Co.

Schraeder, B.D.: Attachment and parenting despite lengthy intensive care, MCN 5:37, 1980.

Sosa, R., and Grua, P.: Perinatal responses to normal and premature birth experiences, J. Calif. Perinat. Assoc. 2:36, 1982.

Complications of Prematurity and Postterm Birth

Affonso, D., and Harris, T.: Postterm pregnancy: implications for mother and infant, challenge for the nurse, J.O.G.N. Nurs. 9:139, 1980.

Bancalari, E., and Gerhardt, T.: Bronchopulmonary dysplasia, Pediatr. Clin. North Am. 33:1, 1986.

Bartlett, R.H., and others: Extracorporeal circulation in neonatal respiratory failure: a prospective randomized study, Pediatrics 76:479, 1985.

Korones, S.: High-risk newborn infants: the basis for intensive nursing care, ed. 4, St. Louis, 1986, The C.V. Mosby Co.

Whaley, L.F., and Wong, D.L.: Nursing care of infants and children, ed. 3, St. Louis, 1987, The C.V. Mosby Co.

Infants of Diabetic Mothers

Fuhrmann, K., and others: Prevention of congenital malformations in infants of insulin-dependent mothers, Diabetes Care 6:219, 1983.

Hyperbilirubinemia

Wu, P.Y., and others: Transcutaneous bilirubinometry: factors affecting the correlation of TcB index and serum bilirubin, J. Perinatol. 5:41, Summer 1985.

Infection

Boland, M., and Gaskill, T.B.: Managing AIDS in children, M.C.N. 9:384, Nov./Dec. 1984.

Center for Prevention Services, Centers for Disease Control, Atlanta, Ga. 30333. For Hepatitis: Hepatitis Branch, Epidemiology, Building 6, Room 154.

Centers for Disease Control: Morbidity and Mortality Weekly Report, Atlanta, July 14, 1983.

Harris, M.: S.F. Panel's Report: abortion urged in AIDS pregnancies, The San Francisco Chronicle, Jan. 4, 1986.

Klug, R.M.: AIDS beyond the hospital: part two of a CE feature—children with AIDS, Am. J. Nurs. 86(10):1126, 1986.

Loveman, A., Colburn, V., and Dobin, A.: AIDS in pregnancy, J.O.G.N. Nurs. 15:91, Mar./Apr. 1986.

Nurses Association of the American College of Obstetricians and Gynecologists: Neonatal herpes, NAACOG Newsletter 13:3, April 1986.

Nurses Association of the American College of Obstetricians and Gynecologists: Rubella/hepatitis B precautions advised, NAACOG Newsletter 13:3, April 1986.

Staff: AIDS unit at San Francisco General Hospital: infection control guidelines, Am. Nurse, Feb. 1986.

Whaley, L.F., and Wong, D.L.: Nursing care of infants and children, ed. 3, St. Louis, 1987, The C.V. Mosby Co.

Bibliography
Preterm Infant

Anderson, G.C., and others: Effects of time-controlled nonnutritive sucking opportunities, Nurs. Res. 31:63, 1982.

Barnard, K.E., and Bee, H.L.: The impact of temporally patterned stimulation on the development of preterm infants, Child Dev. 54:1156, 1983.

Beaton, J.L.: A systems model of premature birth: implications for neonatal intensive care, J.O.G.N. Nurs. 13:173, 1984.

Bergman, A.B., and others: Studies of the sudden infant death syndrome in King County, Washington, III. Epidemiology, Pediatrics 49:860, June 1972.

Bresadola, C.: Neonatal intensive care: one infant/one nurse/one objective: quality care, Denver General Hospital, Denver, Colo., M.C.N. 2:286, 1977.

Caplan, G., and others: Four studies of crisis in parents of prematures, Community Ment. Health J. 2:149, 1965.

Cole, C.H.: Prevention of prematurity: can we do it in America? Pediatrics 76:310, 1985.

Cole, J.G., and Frappier, P.A.: Infant stimulation reassessed. A new approach to providing care for the preterm infant, J.O.G.N. N. 14:471, 1985.

Dubowitz, L.M.S., and Dubowitz, V.: Gestational age of the newborn, Menlo Park, Calif., 1977, Addison-Wesley Publishing Co.

Eager, M.: Long-distance nurturing: the family bond, M.C.N. 2:293, 1977.

Eager, M., and Exoo, R.: Parents visiting parents for unequaled support, M.C.N. 5:35, 1980.

Erdman, D.: Parent-to-parent support: the best for those with sick newborns, M.C.N. 2:291, 1977.

Fanaroff, A., and others: Behrman's neonatal-perinatal medicine, St. Louis, 1983, The C.V. Mosby Co.

Ferrara, A., and Harin, A.: Emergency transfer of the high-risk neonate: a working manual for medical, nursing, and administrative personnel, St. Louis, 1980, The C.V. Mosby Co.

Field, T., and Goldson, E.: Pacifying effects of nonnutritive sucking on term and preterm neonates during heelstick procedures, Pediatrics 74:1012, 1984.

Fria, J.T.: Assessment of hearing, Pediatr. Clin. North Am. 28:757, 1981.

Gerhardt, T., and Bancalari, E.: Apnea of prematurity, I. Lung function and regulation of breathing, Pediatrics, 74:58, 1984.

Gerhardt, T., and Bancalari, E.: Apnea of prematurity. II. Respiratory reflexes, Pediatr. 74:63, 1984.

Gross, S.J., and Eckerman, C.O.: Normative early head growth in very-low-birth-weight infants, J. Pediatr. 103:946, 1983.

Hardgrove, C., and Warrick, L.H.: How shall we tell the children? Am. J. Nurs. 74:448, 1974.

Harvey, D., and others: Abilities of children who were small-for-gestational-age babies, Pediatrics 69:296, 1982.

Hawkins-Walsh, E.: Diminishing anxiety in parents of sick newborns, M.C.N. 5:30, 1980.

Henderson, K.J., and Newton, L.D.: Helping nursing mothers maintain lactation while separated from their infants, M.C.N. 3:352, 1978.

Hirata, T., and others: Survival and outcome of infants 501 to 750 gm: a six-year experience, J. Pediatr. 102:741, 1983.

Johnson, S.H.: High-risk parenting, Philadelphia, 1979, J.B. Lippincott Co.

Kuller, J.M., Lund, C., and Tobin, C.: Improved skin care for premature infants, M.C.N. 8:200, 1983.

Magyary, D.: Early social interactions: preterm infant-parent dyads, Issues Compr. Pediatr. Nurs. 7:233, 1984.

Mahan, C.K.: Care of the family of the critically ill neonate, Crit. Care Q. 4:89, 1981.

Mahan, C.K.: The family of the critically ill neonate, Crit. Care Update, 10(6):24, 1983.

Maloney, M., and others: A prospective controlled study of scheduled sibling visits to a newborn intensive care unit, J. Am. Acad. Child Psychiatry 22:565, 1983.

Manser, J.I.: Growth in the high-risk infant, Clin. Perinatol. 11:19, 1984.

Marino, B.L.: When nurses compete with parents, J.A.C.C.H. 8:94, 1980.

Miles, M.S., and Carter, M.C.: Assessing parental stress in intensive care units, M.C.N. 8:354, 1983.

Minde, K., and others: Mother-child relationships on the premature nursery: an observational study, Pediatrics 61:373, 1978.

Moore, T., and Resnic, R.: Special problems of VLBW infant, Contemp. OB/Gyn. 23(6):174, 1984.

Newman, L.: Parents' perceptions of their low birth weight infants, Pediatrician 9:182, 1980.

Perez, R.H.: Protocols for perinatal nursing practice, St. Louis, 1981, The C.V. Mosby Co.

Schraeder, B.D.: Attachment and parenting despite lengthy intensive care, M.C.N. 5:37, 1980.

Schwab, F., and others: Sibling visiting in a neonatal intensive care unit, Pediatrics, 71:835, 1983.

Sigman, M., and Parmalee, A.H.J.: Longitudinal evaluation of the preterm infant. In Field, T.M., editor: Infants born at risk, Jamaica, N.Y., 1979, Spectrum Publications.

Sosa, R., and Grua, P.: Perinatal responses to normal and premature birth experiences, J. Calif. Perinat. Assoc. 2:36, 1982.

Stengel, T.J.: Infant behavior, maternal psychological reactions, and mother-infant interactional issues associated with the crises of prematurity: a selected review of the literature, Phys. Occup. Ther. Pediatr. 2(2/3):3, 1982.

Whaley, L.F., and Wong, D.L.: Nursing care of infants and children, ed. 3, St. Louis, 1987, The C.V. Mosby Co.

Infants with Problems Related to Gestational Age and Weight

Avery, M.E.: The argument for prenatal administration of dexamethasone to prevent respiratory distress syndrome, J. Pediatr. 104:240, 1984.

Boros, S.J., and others: Using conventional infant ventilators at unconventional rates, Pediatrics 74:487, 1984.

Boynton, B.R., and others: Combined high-frequency oscillatory ventilation and intermittent mandatory ventilation in critically ill neonates, J. Pediatr. 105:297, 1984.

Brown, E.G., and Sweet, A.Y.: Neonatal necrotizing entercolitis, Pediatr. Clin. North Am. 29:1149, 1982.

Cassady, G.: Transcutaneous monitoring in the newborn infant, J. Pediatr. 103:837, 1983.

Cohen, M.A.: Transcutaneous oxygen monitoring for sick neonates, M.C.N. 9:324, 1984.

Committee on Fetus and Newborn: Vitamin E and the prevention of retinopathy of prematurity, Pediatrics 76:315, 1985.

Fuhrmann, K., and others: Prevention of congenital malformations in infants of insulin-dependent diabetic mothers, Diabetes Care 6:219, 1983.

Garn, S.M., and others: Effect of maternal cigarette smoking on Apgar scores, Am. J. Dis. Child, 135:503, 1981.

Fox, W.W., and Duara, S.: Persistent pulmonary hypertension in the neonate: diagnosis and management, J. Pediatr. 103:505, 1983.

Have ecmo, will travel: Am J. Nurs. 86:117, 1986.

Heldt, G.P., and others: Exercise performance of the survivors of hyaline membrane disease, J. Pediatr. 96:995, 1980.

Hodgman, J.E.: Bronchopulmonary dysplasia. In Gellils, S.S., and Kagan, B.M.: Current pediatric therapy, ed. 12, Philadelphia, 1986, W.B. Saunders Co.

Huch, A., and others: Experience with transcutaneous 0 (tcpO) monitoring of mother, fetus and newborn, J. Perinat. Med. 2:51, 1980.

Kaplow, R., and Fromme, L.R.: Nursing care plan for the patient receiving high-frequency jet ventilation, Crit. Care Nurs. 5:25, 1985.

Kirkpatrick, B.V., and others: Use of extracorporeal membrane oxygenation for respiratory failure in term infants, Pediatrics 72:872, 1983.

Kliegman, R.M., and Fanaroff, A.A.: Neonatal necrotizing enterocolitis: a 9-year experience. II. Outcome assessment, Am. J. Dis. Child, 135:608, 1981.

Levin, D.L.: Meconium inhalation syndrome. In Levin, D.L., Morriss, F.C., and Moore, G.C.: A practical guide to pediatric intensive care, St. Louis, 1984, The C.V. Mosby Co.

Lucey, J.F., and Dangman, B.: A reexamination of the role of oxygen in retrolental fibroplasia, Pediatrics 73:82,

1984. Mammel, M.D. and others: Comparison of high-frequency jet ventilation and conventional mechanical ventilation in a meconium aspiration model, J. Pediatr. 103:630, 1983.

Murphy, J.D., Vawter, G.F., and Reid, L.M.: Pulmonary vascular disease in fetal meconium aspiration, J. Pediatr. 104:785, 1984.

Plapp, P.R.: Nursing implications in the early recognition of necrotizing enterocolitis, Issues Compr. Pediatr. Nurs. 4(2):77, 1980.

Purohit, D.M., and others: Risk factors for retrolental fibroplasia experience with 3,025 premature infants, Pediatr. 76:339, 1985.

Shohat, M., and others: Retinopathy of prematurity: incidence and risk factors, Pediatrics 72:159, 1983.

Whiteman, L., Wuethrick, M., and Egan, E.: Infants who survive necrotizing enterocolitis, Matern, Child. Nurs. J. 14(3):123, 1985.

Wilson, R., and others: Age at onset of necrotizing enterocolitis: an epidemiologic analysis, Pediatr. Res. 16:82, Jan. 1982.

Wooten, B.: Death of an infant, M.C.N. 6:257, 1981.

Infants of diabetic mothers

Bohart, R.D., and others: Continuous insulin infusion during the peripartum period; maternal and neonatal outcome, J. Calif. Perinat. Assoc. 2(1):26, 1982.

Coustan, D.R., and Carpenter, M.W.: Detection and treatment of gestational diabetes, Clin. Obstet. Gynecol. 28:507, Sept. 1985.

Cowett, R.M., and Scshwartz, R.: The infant of the diabetic mother, Pediatr. Clin. North Am. 29:1213, 1982.

Golde, S., and Platt, L.: Antepartum testing in diabetes. Clin. Obstet. Gynecol. 28:516, Sept. 1985.

Hare, J.W.: Diabetes control to reduce congenital malformations, Contemp. OB/Gyn. 20:(2):85, 1982.

Miller, E.,and others: Elevated maternal Hb_{Alc} in early pregnancy and major congenital anomalies in infants of diabetic mothers, N. Engl. J. Med. 304:891, 1981.

Nurses Association of the American College of Ostetricians and Gynecologists: Care of the infant of the diabetic mother, N.A.A.C.O.G. Tech. Bull., No. 11, Sept. 1981.

Oh, W.: Heading off problems in the diabetic's baby, Contemp. OB/Gyn., 19:91, 1982.

Perlman, R.H.: The infant of the diabetic mother: pathophysiology and management, Primary Care 10:751, 1983.

Plauche, W.C., and others: Phosphatidylglycerol and lung maturity, Am. J. Obstet. Gynecol. 144:167, 1982.

Queenan, J.T.: Managing polyhydramnios, Contemp. OB/Gyn. 22:17, Aug. 1983.

Riblett, B.: Insuring a safe pregnancy for your diabetic patient, R.N. 46(2):50, 1983.

Teramo, K., and Hallman, M.: Ways to head off RDS in diabetics/ neonates, Contemp. OB/Gyn. 21(6):127, 1983.

Hyperbilirubinemia

Bowman, J.M., and Pollock, J.M.: Antenatal prophylaxis of Rh isoimmunization: 28 weeks' gestation service program, Can. Med. Assoc. J. 118:627, 1978.

Cashore, W.J.: Transcutaneous bilirubinometry, ICEA (International Childbirth Educators Association) News 20:3, 1983.

Cashore, W.J.: Transcutaneous bilirubinometry, NAACOG Newsletter, 11:4, 1984.

Hammer, R.M., and others: The prenatal use of Rh₀(D) immune globulin, M.C.N. 9(1):29, 1984.

Neonatal jaundice, ICEA News 22:3, 1983.

Lewis, H.M., and others: Use or abuse of phototherapy for physiological jaundice of newborn infants, Lancet 2:408, 1982.

Maisels, M.J., and Conrad, S.: Transcutaneous bilirubin measurements in full-term infants, Pediatricts 70:464, 1982.

Maisels, M.J., and Lee, C.: Transcutaneous bilirubin measurements: variations in meter response, Pediatrics 71:457, 1983.

Tovey, L.A., and Taverner, J.M.: a case for the antenatal administration and anti-D immunoglobulin to primigravidae, Lancet 2:878, 1981.

Congenital Anomalies

Chatterjee, M.S.: Parental age and Down's syndrome, Contemp. OB/Gyn. 21(5):171, 1983.

Inturrisi, M., Perry, S.E., and May, K.A.: Fetal surgery for congenital hydronephrosis, J.O.G.N.N. 14:271, July/Aug. 1985.

Niculescu, A.M.: Effects of *in utero* exposure to DES on male progeny, J.O.G.N.Nurs. 14:468, Nov./Dec. 1985.

Seeds, J.W., and Cefalo, R.C.: Anomalies with hydramnios: diagnostic role of ultrasound, Contemp. OB/Gyn. 23:32, 1984.

Smith, K.: Recognizing cardiac failure in neonates, M.C.N. 4:98, 1979.

Vintzileos, A.M., and others: Congenital defects: let ultrasound guide your delivery plan, Contemp. OB/Gyn. 24(2):46, 1984.

Neonatal Infection

Baker, D.A.: The dangers of varicella-zoster in pregnancy, Contemp. OB/Gyn. 20:71, 1982.

Bennett, J.: AIDS: What precautions do you take in the hospital? Am. J. Nurs. 86(8):952, 1986.

Bettoli, E.J.: Herpes: facts and fallacies, Am. J. Nurs. 82:924, 1982.

California Nurses Association: UC sets guide on AIDS, Calif. Nurse 79:1, July/Aug. 1983.

Campbell, C.E., and Herten, R.J.: VD to STD: redefining venereal disease, Am. J. Nurs. 81:1629, 1981.

Can AIDS be a threat to your patients? Contemp. OB/Gyn. 23:163, 1984.

Centers for Disease Control (CDC): Morbidity and Mortality Weekly Report, Atlanta, March 4, 1983.

Charles, D., and Larsen, B.: How pregnancy alters infection defenses, Contemp. OB/Gyn. 23(6):96, 1984.

Claypool, J.M.: Rubella protection for maternal child health care providers, M.C.N. 6:53, 1981.

Cohen, M., and Cohen, H.: Viral hepatitis during pregnancy, Contemp. OB/Gyn. 22:29, 1983.

Curran, James W., and others: Acquired immunodeficiency syndrome (AIDS) associated with transfusions, N. Engl. J. Med. 310:69, 1984.

Deresinski, S.C., and others: AIDS transmission via transfusion therapy, Lancet No. 8368, p. 102, Jan. 14, 1984.

Dilts, C.L.: Nursing management of mastitis due to breastfeeding, J.O.G.N. Nurs. 14:286, July/Aug. 1985.

Dowdle, Walter R.: The epidemiology of AIDS, Public Health Rep. 98:308, 1983.

Elder, J.M.: Genital herpes simplex virus infections during pregnancy, J. Calif. Perinatal Assoc. 2:90, 1982.

Fanaroff, A.A., and Martin, R.J., editors: Behrman's neonatal-perinatal medicine: diseases of the fetus and infant, ed. 3, St. Louis, 1983, The C.V. Mosby Co.

Freij, B.J., and Sever, J.L.: When is immunization in pregnancy really needed? Contemp. OB/G. 27:48, May 1986.

Gennoro, S.: Listerial infection: nursing care of mother and infant, M.C.N. 5:390, 1980.

Haggerty, L.: TORCH: a literature review and implications for practice, J.O.G.N. N. 14:124, Mar./Apr. 1985.

Hammerschlag, M.R., and others: Erythromycin ointment for ocular prophylaxis of neonatal chlamydial infections, JAMA 244:2291, 1981.

Martin, D.H., Prematurity and perinatal mortality in pregnancies complicated by maternal chlamydia trachomatis infections, JAMA 247:1585, 1982.

Miles, P.A.: Sexually transmitted diseases, J.O.G.N. Nurs. 13:102s, 1984.

Nurses Association of the American College of Obstetricians and Gynecologists: Erythromycin, tetracycline equally effective against chlamydia, NAACOG Newsletter 10:7, 1983.

Nurses Association of the American College of Obstetricians and Gynecologists: Toxoplasmosis during pregnancy threatens fetal health, NAACOG Newsletter 11:1, 1984.

Olsen, T.G.: Your pregnant patient's rash: is it PUPP syndrome? Contemp. OB/Gyn. 22:151, 1983.

Osborne, N.G., and Pratson, L.: Sexually transmitted diseases and pregnancy, J.O.G.N. Nurs. 13:9, 1984.

Perley, N., and Bills, B.J.: Herpes genitalis and the childbearing cycle, M.C.N. 8:213, 1983.

Pullan, C.R.: Breastfeeding and RSV infection, Br. Med. J. 281:1034, 1980.

Regan, J.A.: Maternal ABO blood group type B: a risk factor in the development of neonatal group B streptococcal disease, Pediatrics 62:504, 1978.

Renaud, M.T.: Effects of discontinuing cover gowns on a post-partal ward upon cord colonization of the newborn, J.O.G.N. Nurs. 12:399, 1983.

Ritter, S.E., and Vermund, S.H.: Congenital toxoplasmosis, J.O.G.N. Nurs. 14:435, Nov./Dec. 1985.

Romanowski, B., and Harris, J.R.: Sexually transmitted diseases, Ciba Clinical Symposia 36:1, 1984.

Schachter, J., and others: Erythromycin in the routine treatment of chlamydial infections in pregnancy, N. Engl. J. Med. 314:276, Jan. 30, 1986.

Shirkey, H.C., editor, Pediatric therapy, ed. 6, St. Louis, 1980, The C.V. Mosby Co.

Tafuro, P., and Gurevich, I.: Prevention and management of varicella in high-risk individuals, M.C.N. 9:314, Sept./Oct. 1984.

Toms, G.L., and others: Secretion of respiratory syncytial virus inhibitors and antibody in human milk throughout lactation, J. Med. Virol. 5:351, 1980.

Treating tuberculosis in pregnancy, Contemp. OB/Gyn. 20:23, 1982.

UCSF Task Force on AIDS: Report available from the office of Merle Sande, M.D., Chief of Medicine, San Francisco General Hospital, 1001 Potrero, Room 5H22, San Francisco, Calif. 94110.

USPHS AIDS information hotline: 800/342-AIDS.

Wager, G.P., and others: Puerperal infectious morbidity: relationship to route of delivery and to antepartum *Chlamydia trachomatis* infection, Am. J. Obstet. Gynecol. 7:1028, 1980.

When the pregnant patient has toxoplasmosis, Contemp. OB/Gyn. 20(2):23, 1982.

Witter, F.R.: Pharmacology: TB regimens during pregnancy, Contemp. OB/Gyn. 23:101, 1984.

General Bibliography

Behrman, R.E., editor: Neonatal-perinatal medicine: diseases of the fetus and infant, ed. 3, St. Louis, 1983, The C.V. Mosby Co.

Boynton, B.R., and Boynton, C.A.: Discharge planning for high-risk infants, J. Perinat. 5:44, Fall 1985.

Censullo, M.: Home care of the high-risk newborn, J.O.G.N. N. 15:146. Mar./Apr. 1986.

Consolvo, C.A.: Relieving parental anxiety in the care-by-parent unit, J.O.G.N. N. 15:154, Mar./Apr. 1986.

Gildea, J.: A crisis plan for pediatric code, Am. J. Nurs. 86:557, May 1986.

Jensen, M.D., and Bobak, I.M.: Maternity and gynecologic care: the nurse and the family, ed. 3, St. Louis, 1985, The C.V. Mosby Co.

Johnson, S.H.: Nursing assessment and strategies for the family at risk: high-risk parenting, ed. 2, Philadelphia, 1986, J.B. Lippincott Co.

Korones, S.B.: High-risk newborn infants: the basis for intensive nursing care, ed. 4, St. Louis, 1986, The C.V. Mosby Co.

Ledger, K.E., and Williams, D.L.: Parents at risk: an instructional program for perinatal assessment and preventive intervention, Victoria, B.C. Canada, 1981, Ministry of Health, Province of British Columbia, and Queen Alexandra Solarium for Crippled Children Society (Queen Alexandra Hospital, 2400 Arbutus Rd., Victoria, B.C., Canada V8N 1V7).

Merenstein, G.B., and Gardner, S.L.: Handbook of neonatal intensive care, St. Louis, 1985, The C.V. Mosby Co.

Raff, B.S.: The use of homemaker–home health aides' perinatal care of high-risk infants, J.O.G.N. N. 15:142, Mar./Apr. 1986.

Raff, B.S.: Nursing care of high-risk infants and their families—introduction. J.O.G.N. N. 15:141, Mar./Apr. 1986.

Segal, S., and others: The death of a child—parents' views of professional support, Can. Med. Assoc. J. 134:38, Jan. 1, 1986.

Appendixes

The Pregnant Patient's Bill of Rights

The Pregnant Patient has the right to participate in decisions involving her well-being and that of her unborn child, unless there is a clear-cut medical emergency that prevents her participation. In addition to the rights set forth in the American Hospital Association's "Patient's Bill of Rights" (which has also been adopted by the New York City Department of Health), the Pregnant Patient, because she represents *two* patients rather than one, should be recognized as having the additional rights listed below.

1. *The Pregnant Patient has the right,* prior to the administration of any drug or procedure, to be informed by the health professional caring for her of any potential direct or indirect effects, risks, or hazards to herself or her unborn or newborn infant which may result from the use of a drug or procedure prescribed for or administered to her during pregnancy, labor, birth or lactation.

2. *The Pregnant Patient has the right,* prior to the proposed therapy, to be informed, not only of the benefits, risks and hazards of the proposed therapy, but also of known alternative therapy, such as available childbirth education classes which could help to prepare the Pregnant Patient physically and mentally to cope with the discomfort or stress of pregnancy and the experience of childbirth, thereby reducing or eliminating her need for drugs and obstetric intervention. She should be offered such information early in her pregnancy in order that she may make a reasoned decision.

3. *The Pregnant Patient has the right,* prior to the administration of any drug, to be informed by the health professional who is prescribing or administering the drug to her that any drug which she receives during pregnancy, labor and birth, no matter how or when the drug is taken or administered, may adversely affect her unborn baby, directly or indirectly, and that there is no drug or chemical which has been proven safe for the unborn child.

4. *The Pregnant Patient has the right,* if cesarean section is anticipated, to be informed prior to administration of any drug, and preferably prior to her hospitalization, that minimizing her and, in turn, her baby's intake of nonessential preoperative medicine, will benefit her baby.

5. *The Pregnant Patient has the right,* prior to the administration of a drug or procedure, to be informed if there is *no* properly controlled follow-up research which has established the safety of the drug or procedure with regard to its direct and/or indirect effects on the physiological, mental and neurological development of the child exposed, via the mother, to the drug or procedure during pregnancy, labor, birth or lactation (this would apply to virtually all drugs and the vast majority of obstetric procedures).

6. *The Pregnant Patient has the right,* prior to the administration of any drug, to be informed of the brand name and generic name of the drug in order that she may advise the health professional of any past adverse reaction to the drug.

7. *The Pregnant Patient has the right* to determine for herself, without pressure from her attendant, whether she will accept the risks inherent in the proposed therapy or refuse a drug or procedure.

8. *The Pregnant Patient has the right* to know the name and qualifications of the individual administering a medication or procedure to her during labor or birth.

9. *The Pregnant Patient has the right* to be informed, prior to the administration of any procedure, whether that procedure is being administered to her for her or her baby's benefit (medically indicated) or as an elective procedure (for convenience or teaching purposes).

10. *The Pregnant Patient has the right to* be accompanied during the stress of labor and birth by someone she cares for, and to whom she looks for emotional comfort and encouragement.

11. *The Pregnant Patient has the right* after appropriate medical consultation to choose a position for labor and for birth which is least stressful to her baby and to herself.

12. *The Obstetric Patient has the right* to have her baby cared for at her bedside if her baby is normal, and to feed her baby according to her baby's needs rather than according to the hospital regimen.

13. *The Obstetric Patient has the right* to be informed in writing of the name of the person who actually delivered her baby and the professional qualifications of that person. This information should also be on the birth certificate.

14. *The Obstetric Patient has the right* to be informed if there is any known or indicated aspect of her or her baby's care or condition which may cause her or her baby later difficulty or problems.

15. *The Obstetric Patient has the right* to have her and her baby's hospital medical records complete, accurate and legible and to have their records, including Nurses' Notes, retained by the hospital until the child reaches at least the age of majority, or, alternatively, to have the records offered to her before they are destroyed.

16. *The Obstetric Patient,* both during and after her hos-

From Haire, D.B.: The Pregnant Patient's Bill of Rights, J. Nurs. Midwife. 20:29, Winter, 1975. This article is not reproduced here in its entirety.

pital stay, has the right to have access to her complete hospital medical records, including Nurses' Notes, and to receive a copy upon payment of a reasonable fee and without incurring the expense of retaining an attorney.

It is the obstetric patient and her baby, not the health professional, who must sustain any trauma or injury result-

ing from the use of a drug or obstetric procedure. The observation of the rights listed above will not only permit the obstetric patient to participate in the decisions involving her and her baby's health care, but will help to protect the health professional and the hospital against litigation arising from resentment or misunderstanding on the part of the mother.

Sources of Standards of
Care for Maternal-Child Nursing

American Academy of Pediatrics: Standards and recommendations for hospital care of newborn infants, Evanston, Ill., 1977, The Academy.

American College of Nurse-Midwives: Functions, standards, and qualifications, Washington, D.C., 1975, The College.

American College of Obstetricians and Gynecologists: Standards for obstetric-gynecologic services, Chicago, 1974, The College.

American Nurses' Association: Standards of maternal-child health nursing practice, 1973, The Association.

The American College of Obstetricians and Gynecologists and The Nurses Association of The American College of Obstetricians and Gynecologists: The obstetric-gynecologic nurse practitioner, Washington, D.C., 1979, The College.

Interprofessional Task Force on Health Care of Women and Children, The American College of Obstetricians and Gynecologists, The American College of Nurse-Midwives, and The Nurses Association of the American College of Obstetricians and Gynecologists: Joint position statement on the development of family-centered maternity/newborn care in hospitals, 1978.

Joint Commission on Accreditation of Hospitals: Accredita-

tion manual for hospitals, Chicago, 1976, The Commission.

NAACOG: The Organization for Obstetric, Gynecologic, and Neonatal Nurses. 600 Maryland Ave. S.W. Suite 200E Washington, DC 20024 (202) 638-0026.

The National Foundation-March of Dimes Committee on Perinatal Health: Toward improving the outcome of pregnancy: recommendations for the regional development of maternal and perinatal health services, White Plains, N.Y., 1976, The Foundation.

The Nurses Association of The American College of Obstetricians and Gynecologists: Guidelines for childbirth education, Washington, D.C., 1981, The Association.

The Nurses Association of The American College of Obstetricians and Gynecologists: Standards for obstetric, gynecologic, and neonatal nursing, ed. 3, Washington, D.C., 1986, The Association.

Planning and evaluating nursing care, Wakefield, Mass., 1974, Contemporary Publishing, Inc.

U.S. Department of Health, Education, and Welfare, Public Health Service, Health Services Administration: Guidelines for review of nursing care at the local level, Washington, D.C., 1976, The Department.

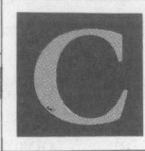

Community Resources

Alternative Birth Crisis Coalition
P.O. Box 48731
Chicago, IL 60648

American Academy of Husband-Coached Childbirth
P.O. Box 5224
Sherman Oaks, CA 91413
  Teaches Robert A. Bradley's method of "Husband-Coached Childbirth," an offshoot of Grantly Dick-Read's method.

American Academy of Pediatrics
P.O. Box 1034
Evanston, IL 60204
  Provides literature for families, parents, and health profession groups related to child health, illness, and welfare.

American Cancer Society
219 East 42nd St.
New York, NY 10017
  Provides brochures on Papanicolaou (Pap) smears, smoking during pregnancy, and breast self-examination.

American College of Nurse-Midwives
1012 14th St., N.W., Suite 801
Washington, DC 20005

American College of Obstetricians and Gynecologists
Suite 2700
Resource Center
1 East Wacker Dr.
Chicago, IL 60601
  Provides extensive lists of publications and resources.

American Society for Psychoprophylaxis in Obstetrics (ASPO)
1411 K St., N.W.
Washington, DC 20005
  Teaches Lamaze technique of prepared childbirth to interested couples; prepares qualified people for teaching this method. Offers brochures, publications, teaching materials, and audiovisual aids.

Association for the Aid of Crippled Children
345 East 46th St.
New York, NY 10017
  Devoted to the prevention of crippling diseases and conditions and to improvement in the care of disabled children and youth and their adjustment in society.

Association for Childbirth at Home, International
P.O. Box 1219
Cerritos, CA 90701

Boston Women's Health Book Collective, Inc.
Box 192
West Somerville, MA 02144
  Publishes books concerning women's health.

Center for Family Growth
555 Highland Ave.
Cotati, CA 94928

Cesarean Birth Council
1402 Nilde Ave.
Mt. View, CA 94040

Cesarean/Support, Education, and Concern (C/SEC)
66 Christopher Rd.
Waltham, MA 02154
  Provides informational pamphlets and slide presentations.

Channing L. Bete Co., Inc.
Greenfield, MA 01301
  Publishes material regarding childbearing in cartoon form.

Child Study Association of America
9 East 89th St.
New York, NY 10028
  Provides parent education materials.

Childbirth Without Pain Education Association
20134 Snowden
Detroit, MI 48235

Coalition for the Medical Rights of Women
4079A 24th St.
San Francisco, CA 94114
  Provides classes (1) for expectant and new mothers and parents, (2) on health concerns of middle-aged women, (3) on lesbian health issues and self-health, (4) on fertility awareness, and (5) on natural birth control.

Cooperative Birth Center Network
Box 1, Route 1
Perkiomenville, PA 18074

Council of Childbirth Education Specialists, Inc.
168 West 86th St.
New York, NY 10024

Cybele Society
Suite 414, Peyton Building
Spokane, WA 99201

Ed-U-Press
760 Ostrum Ave.
Syracuse, NY 13210
Offers series of excellent cartoon books for adolescents and parenting classes.

Educational and Scientific Plastics, Ltd.
76 Holmethorpe Ave.
Holmethorpe, Red Hill Surrey, RH1, 2PF, England
Offers numerous plastic models.

Feminist Women's Health Centers
112 Crenshaw Blvd.
Los Angeles, CA 90005
Provides information regarding women's health.

Florence Crittenton Association of America
608 South Dearborn St.
Chicago, IL 60605
Unites in forming an effective and continuing organization; develops and maintains standards of service; in general, assists in bringing about a greater understanding of factors relating to unmarried mothers and adolescent girls with other problems in adjustment.

Holistic Childbirth Institute
1627 Tenth Ave.
San Francisco, CA 94122
Sponsors an educational program for teaching about childbirth.

Home Oriented Maternity Experience (HOME)
511 New York Ave.
Takoma Park, MD 20012

International Childbirth Education Association (ICEA)
P.O. Box 20048
Milwaukee, WI 55420
Assists individuals and childbirth groups who are interested in family-centered maternity. ICEA is a worldwide organization. Has an excellent film and record directory. Provides books and pamphlets (e.g., *Bookmarks* is an annotated catalogue of resources available that is published several times a year and is available free of charge).

La Leche League International, Inc.
9615 Minneapolis Ave.
Franklin Park, IL 60131
Provides support and brochures for nursing mothers and pattern for making a baby carrier.

Maternity Center Association, Inc.
48 East 92nd St.
New York, NY 10028
Publishes free brochure describing their many publications and pattern for knitted uterus.

National Association of Childbirth Education, Inc. (NACE)
3940 Eleventh St.
Riverside, CA 92501

National Association of Parents and Professionals for Safe Alternatives in Childbirth (NAPSAC)
P.O. Box 1307
Chapel Hill, NC 27514

National Childbirth Trust
9 Queensborough Terrace
London, W2, England
Offers books, films, and other aids for use in classes or in labor.

National Conference of Catholic Charities
1346 Connecticut
Washington, DC 20036
Gives particular emphasis to service for children and youth; i.e., foster care, counseling (unmarried parents), adoption services (statewide), short-term counseling to families and youth, emergency material assistance.

National Women's Health Network
P.O. Box 24192
Washington, DC 20024
Provides information regarding women's health.

Nurses' Association of the American College of Obstetricians and Gynecologists
Suite 300, 60 Maryland Ave. S.W.
Washington, DC 20024
Provides numerous teaching aids and sponsors workshops for nurses.

Patient Counseling Library
Budlong Press Co.
5428 N. Virginia Ave.
Chicago, IL 60625
Provides videotapes (e.g., "A doctor discusses . . .") suitable for clinics or waiting rooms covering topics such as pregnancy, infant care, sexuality, breast feeding, and weight control.

Planned Parenthood Federation of America, Inc.
810 Seventh Ave.
New York, NY 10019
Provides leadership for universal acceptance of family planning as an essential element of responsible family life through education, service, and research.

Save the Children Federation, Inc.
345 East 46th St.
New York, NY 10017
  Helps eliminate the causes of poverty among children in
  the United States and overseas while maintaining efforts
  to ameliorate the effects of poverty in those areas where
  the needs are greatest.

SIECUS
Human Science Press
72 Fifth Ave.
New York, NY 10011
  Provides publications (e.g., "Sexual relations in
  pregnancy and postpartum") and teaching aids.

Trainex Corporation
Box 116
Garden Grove, CA 92642
  Provides audiovisual aids suitable for childbirth and
  parent education.

United States Government
  Children's Bureau
    U.S. Department of Health and Human Services
    Washington, DC 20402
  Consumer Product Safety Commission
    Washington, DC 20207
  Public Documents Distribution Center
    Consumer Information
    Pueblo, CO 81009
  U.S. Government Printing Office
    Washington, DC 20402
Provides information and publications on many aspects
related to pregnancy.

The Women's Health Forum (Healthright)
175 Fifth Ave.
New York, NY 10010

For genetics clinics and treatment centers in area,
contact the following organizations:

National Foundation/March of Dimes*
1275 Mamaroneck Ave.
White Plains, NY 10605

National Genetics Foundation, Inc.
250 West 57th St.
New York, NY 10019

Other resources include the following:
1. State Department of Public Health
2. Maternal and Child Health Services, Office of Economic
   Opportunity, Washington, D.C.
3. Local organizations: National Society for Crippled Children and Adults, Inc.; National Cystic Fibrosis Society;
   Muscular Dystrophy Association of America; organizations for parents of children with Tay-Sachs disease, sickle
   cell anemia, or crippling diseases; pediatric units in local
   hospitals and medical centers; city and county services
   (e.g., mental retardation).

---

*The National Foundation/March of Dimes publishes a directory of
genetic services. It is involved in professional education, as well as
research on genetic defects. The Foundation also sponsors programs
for purchase of teaching and disseminating information to the general public.

Expected Date of Confinement (EDC): Determination of Expected Date of Delivery from Last Menstrual Period

See page 1055.

Find the date of the last menstrual period in the top line (light-face type) of the pair of lines. The dark number (bold-face type) in the line below will be the expected day of delivery.

	1	2	3	4	5	6	7	8	9	10	11	12	13	14	15	16	17	18	19	20	21	22	23	24	25	26	27	28	29	30	31	
Jan.	1	2	3	4	5	6	7	8	9	10	11	12	13	14	15	16	17	18	19	20	21	22	23	24	25	26	27	28	29	30	31	
Oct.	**8**	**9**	**10**	**11**	**12**	**13**	**14**	**15**	**16**	**17**	**18**	**19**	**20**	**21**	**22**	**23**	**24**	**25**	**26**	**27**	**28**	**29**	**30**	**31**	**(1**	**2**	**3**	**4**	**5**	**6**	**7**	**Nov.**
Feb.	1	2	3	4	5	6	7	8	9	10	11	12	13	14	15	16	17	18	19	20	21	22	23	24	25	26	27	28				
Nov.	**8**	**9**	**10**	**11**	**12**	**13**	**14**	**15**	**16**	**17**	**18**	**19**	**20**	**21**	**22**	**23**	**24**	**25**	**26**	**27**	**28**	**29**	**30**	**(1**	**2**	**3**	**4**	**5**				**Dec.**
Mar.	1	2	3	4	5	6	7	8	9	10	11	12	13	14	15	16	17	18	19	20	21	22	23	24	25	26	27	28	29	30	31	
Dec.	**6**	**7**	**8**	**9**	**10**	**11**	**12**	**13**	**14**	**15**	**16**	**17**	**18**	**19**	**20**	**21**	**22**	**23**	**24**	**25**	**26**	**27**	**28**	**29**	**30**	**31**	**(1**	**2**	**3**	**4**	**5**	**Jan.**
April	1	2	3	4	5	6	7	8	9	10	11	12	13	14	15	16	17	18	19	20	21	22	23	24	25	26	27	28	29	30		
Jan.	**6**	**7**	**8**	**9**	**10**	**11**	**12**	**13**	**14**	**15**	**16**	**17**	**18**	**19**	**20**	**21**	**22**	**23**	**24**	**25**	**26**	**27**	**28**	**29**	**30**	**31**	**(1**	**2**	**3**	**4**		**Feb.**
May	1	2	3	4	5	6	7	8	9	10	11	12	13	14	15	16	17	18	19	20	21	22	23	24	25	26	27	28	29	30	31	
Feb.	**5**	**6**	**7**	**8**	**9**	**10**	**11**	**12**	**13**	**14**	**15**	**16**	**17**	**18**	**19**	**20**	**21**	**22**	**23**	**24**	**25**	**26**	**27**	**28**	**(1**	**2**	**3**	**4**	**5**	**6**	**7**	**Mar.**
June	1	2	3	4	5	6	7	8	9	10	11	12	13	14	15	16	17	18	19	20	21	22	23	24	25	26	27	28	29	30		
Mar.	**8**	**9**	**10**	**11**	**12**	**13**	**14**	**15**	**16**	**17**	**18**	**19**	**20**	**21**	**22**	**23**	**24**	**25**	**26**	**27**	**28**	**29**	**30**	**31**	**(1**	**2**	**3**	**4**	**5**	**6**		**April**
July	1	2	3	4	5	6	7	8	9	10	11	12	13	14	15	16	17	18	19	20	21	22	23	24	25	26	27	28	29	30	31	
April	**7**	**8**	**9**	**10**	**11**	**12**	**13**	**14**	**15**	**16**	**17**	**18**	**19**	**20**	**21**	**22**	**23**	**24**	**25**	**26**	**27**	**28**	**29**	**30**	**(1**	**2**	**3**	**4**	**5**	**6**	**7**	**May**
Aug.	1	2	3	4	5	6	7	8	9	10	11	12	13	14	15	16	17	18	19	20	21	22	23	24	25	26	27	28	29	30	31	
May	**8**	**9**	**10**	**11**	**12**	**13**	**14**	**15**	**16**	**17**	**18**	**19**	**20**	**21**	**22**	**23**	**24**	**25**	**26**	**27**	**28**	**29**	**30**	**31**	**(1**	**2**	**3**	**4**	**5**	**6**	**7**	**June**
Sept.	1	2	3	4	5	6	7	8	9	10	11	12	13	14	15	16	17	18	19	20	21	22	23	24	25	26	27	28	29	30		
June	**8**	**9**	**10**	**11**	**12**	**13**	**14**	**15**	**16**	**17**	**18**	**19**	**20**	**21**	**22**	**23**	**24**	**25**	**26**	**27**	**28**	**29**	**30**	**(1**	**2**	**3**	**4**	**5**	**6**	**7**		**July**
Oct.	1	2	3	4	5	6	7	8	9	10	11	12	13	14	15	16	17	18	19	20	21	22	23	24	25	26	27	28	29	30	31	
July	**8**	**9**	**10**	**11**	**12**	**13**	**14**	**15**	**16**	**17**	**18**	**19**	**20**	**21**	**22**	**23**	**24**	**25**	**26**	**27**	**28**	**29**	**30**	**31**	**(1**	**2**	**3**	**4**	**5**	**6**	**7**	**Aug.**
Nov.	1	2	3	4	5	6	7	8	9	10	11	12	13	14	15	16	17	18	19	20	21	22	23	24	25	26	27	28	29	30		
Aug.	**8**	**9**	**10**	**11**	**12**	**13**	**14**	**15**	**16**	**17**	**18**	**19**	**20**	**21**	**22**	**23**	**24**	**25**	**26**	**27**	**28**	**29**	**30**	**31**	**(1**	**2**	**3**	**4**	**5**	**6**		**Sept.**
Dec.	1	2	3	4	5	6	7	8	9	10	11	12	13	14	15	16	17	18	19	20	21	22	23	24	25	26	27	28	29	30	31	
Sept.	**7**	**8**	**9**	**10**	**11**	**12**	**13**	**14**	**15**	**16**	**17**	**18**	**19**	**20**	**21**	**22**	**23**	**24**	**25**	**26**	**27**	**28**	**29**	**30**	**(1**	**2**	**3**	**4**	**5**	**6**	**7**	**Oct.**

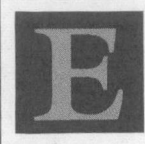

Standard Laboratory Values: Pregnant and Nonpregnant Women

	Nonpregnant	Pregnant
Hematologic values		
Complete blood count (CBC)		
Hemoglobin, g/dl	12-16*	10-14*
Hematocrit, PCV, %	37-47	32-42
Red cell volume, ml	1600	1900
Plasma volume, ml	2400	3700
Red blood cell count, million/mm^3	4-5.5	4-5.5
White blood cells, total per mm^3	4500-10,000	5000-15,000
Polymorphonuclear cells, %	54-62	60-85
Lymphocytes, %	38-46	15-40
Erythrocyte sedimentation rate, mm/h	≤20	30-90
MCHC, g/dl packed RBCs (mean corpuscular hemoglobin concentration)	30-36	No change
MCH/(mean corpuscular hemoglobin per picogram [less than a nanogram])	29-32	No change
MCV/µm^3 (mean corpuscular volume per cubic micrometer)	82-96	No change
Blood coagulation and fibrinolytic activity†		
Factors VII, VIII, IX, X		Increase in pregnancy, return to normal in early puerperium; factor VIII increases during and immediately after delivery
Factors XI, XIII		Decrease in pregnancy
Prothrombin time (protime)	60-70 s	Slight decrease in pregnancy
Partial thromboplastin time (PTT)	12-14 s	Slight decrease in pregnancy and again decrease during second and third stage of labor (indicates clotting at placental site)
Bleeding time	1-3 min (Duke) 2-4 min (Ivy)	No appreciable change
Coagulation time	6-10 min (Lee/White)	No appreciable change
Platelets	150,000 to 350,000/ mm^3	No significant change until 3-5 days after delivery, then marked increase (may predispose woman to thrombosis) and gradual return to normal
Fibrinolytic activity		Decreases in pregnancy, then abrupt return to normal (protection against thromboembolism)
Fibrinogen	250 mg/dl	400 mg/dl
Mineral/vitamin concentrations		
Serum iron, µg	75-150	65-120
Total iron-binding capacity, µg	250-450	300-500
Iron saturation, %	30-40	15-30
Vitamin B$_{12}$, folic acid, ascorbic acid	Normal	Moderate decrease
Serum proteins		
Total, g/dl	6.7-8.3	5.5-7.5
Albumin, g/dl	3.5-5.5	3.0-5.0
Globulin, total, g/dl	2.3-3.5	3.0-4.0

*At sea level. Permanent residents of higher levels (e.g., Denver) require higher levels of hemoglobin.
†Pregnancy represents a hypercoagulable state.

	Nonpregnant	Pregnant
Blood sugar		
Fasting, mg/dl	70-80	65
2-hour postprandial, mg/dl	60-110	Under 140 after a 100 g carbohydrate meal is considered normal
Cardiovascular determinations		
Blood pressure, mm Hg	120/80*	114/65
Peripheral resistance, dyne/s-cm^{-5}	120	100
Venous pressure, cm H_2O		
Femoral	9	24
Antecubital	8	8
Pulse, rate/min	70	80
Stroke volume, ml	65	75
Cardiac output, L/min	4.5	6
Circulation time (arm-tongue), s	15-16	12-14
Blood volume, ml		
Whole blood	4000	5600
Plasma	2400	3700
Red blood cells	1600	1900
Plasma renin, units/L	3-10	10-80
Chest x-ray studies		
Transverse diameter of heart	—	1-2 cm increase
Left border of heart	—	Straightened
Cardiac volume	—	70 ml increase
Electrocardiogram	—	15° left axis deviation
V_1 and V_2	—	Inverted T wave
V_4	—	Low T
III	—	Q + inverted T
aVr	—	Small Q
Hepatic values		
Bilirubin total	Not more than 1 mg/dl	Unchanged
Cephalin flocculation	Up to 2+ in 48 h	Positive in 10%
Serum cholesterol	110-300 mg/dl	↑60% from 16-32 weeks of pregnancy; remains at this level until after delivery
Thymol turbidity	0-4 units	Positive in 15%
Serum alkaline phosphatase	2-4.5 units (Bodansky)	↑ from week 12 of pregnancy to 6 weeks after delivery
Serum lactate dehydrogenase		Unchanged
Serum glutamic-oxaloacetic transaminase		Unchanged
Serum globulin albumin	1.5-3.0 g/dl	↑slight
	4.5-5.5 g/dl	↓3.0 g by late pregnancy
A/G ratio		Decreased
α$_2$-globulin		Increased
β-globulin		Increased
Serum cholinesterase		Decreased
Leucine aminopeptidase		Increased
Sulfobromophthalein (5 mg/kg)	5% dye or less in 45 min	Somewhat decreased
Renal values		
Bladder capacity	1300 ml	1500 ml
Renal plasma flow (RPF), ml/min	490-700	Increase by 25%, to 612-875
Glomerular filtration rate (GFR), ml/min	105-132	Increase by 50%, to 160-198
Nonprotein nitrogen (NPN), mg/dl	25-40	Decreases
Blood urea nitrogen (BUN), mg/dl	20-25	Decreases
Serum creatinine, mg/kg/24 h	20-22	Decreases
Serum uric acid, mg/kg/24/ h	257-750	Decreases
Urine glucose	Negative	Present in 20% of gravidas

*For the woman about 20 years of age
  10 years of age: 103/70.
  30 years of age: 123/82.
  40 years of age: 126/84.

Continued.

	Nonpregnant	Pregnant
Intravenous pyelogram (IVP)	Normal	Slight to moderate hydroureter and hydronephrosis; right kidney larger than left kidney
Miscellaneous laboratory values		
Total thyroxine concentration	5-12 µg/dl thyroxine	↑ 9-16 µg/dl thyroxine (however, unbound thyroxine not greatly increased)
Ionized calcium		Relatively unchanged
Aldosterone		↑ 1 mg/24 h by third trimester
Dehydroisoandrosterone	Plasma clearance 6-8 L/24 h	↑ plasma clearance tenfold to twentyfold

Commonly Used Drugs that Affect Urine Glucose Determinations

Drug	Clinitest	Testape, Keto-Diastix	Comments
Ascorbic acid (vitamin C)	False positive	False	Inhibits glucose-oxidase (Testape, Keto-Diastix); large doses produce false negative result with Clinitest
Cephalexin (Keflex)			
Cephaloridine (Loridine)	False positive		Confusing black-brown color
Cephalothin (Keflin)			
Chloral hydrate (Noctec)	False positive		Only with large doses
Chloramphenicol (Chloromycetin)	Flase positive*		
Isoniazid (INH)			False positive result with Benedict's; also has hyperglycemic activity and therefore may produce true glycosuria
Levodopa (L-dopa)(Dopar, Laro-dopa)			Small doses, either may result; doses 3.5-5 g, both result
Metaxalone (Skelaxin)	False negative		
Methyldopa (Aldomet)	False positive		One possible case reported
Nalidixic acid (NegGram)	False positive		
Probenecid (Benemid)	False positive		
Salicylates	False positive	False negative	Due to gentisic acid metabolite; occasional use of aspirin not likely to affect test significantly
Sulfonamides (Gantanol, Gantrisin, etc.)	False positive†		
Tetracycline	False positive		May be due to large amounts of ascorbic acid in parenteral product

From Jensen, M.D., and Bobak, I.M.: Handbook of maternity care: a guide for nursing practice, St. Louis, 1980, The C.V. Mosby Co.; data from Drug Intell. Clin. Pharm. 8(7):422-429, July 1974, and from Applied therapeutics for clinical pharmacists, 1975, pp. 229-232.
*Substantiating information not given.

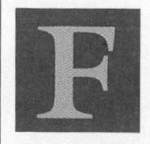

Standard and Deviations from Standard Weight (<85% and >120%) for 17- to 24-Year-Old Nonpregnant Women

Height		Underweight (<85%)		Standard Weight		Overweight (>120%)	
cm	in	kg	lb	kg	lb	kg	lb
140	52.2	38.0	84	45	99	53.8	118
142	56.0	39.0	86	46	101	55.0	121
144	56.7	40.0	88	47	103	56.4	124
146	57.5	40.7	90	48	105	57.6	127
148	58.3	41.8	92	49	108	59.0	130
150	59.1	42.8	94	50	110	60.4	133
152	60.0	43.8	96	51	112	61.8	136
154	60.7	44.6	98	52	115	63.0	139
156	61.5	45.6	100	53	117	64.4	142
158	62.2	46.6	103	55	121	65.8	145
160	63.0	47.7	105	56	123	67.4	148
162	63.8	49.0	108	57	126	69.1	152
164	64.6	50.0	110	58	129	70.6	155
166	65.4	51.0	112	59	131	72.1	159
168	66.2	52.0	114	61	134	73.6	162
170	66.9	53.4	118	63	138	75.4	166
172	67.7	54.6	120	64	141	77.2	170
174	68.5	56.0	124	66	145	79.1	174
176	69.3	57.5	127	68	149	81.2	179
178	70.1	59.1	130	69	152	83.4	184
180	70.9	60.6	134	71	157	85.6	189
182	71.7	61.9	137	73	161	87.4	193
184	72.4	63.2	139	74	163	89.3	197
186	73.2	64.5	142	76	167	91.1	201
188	74.0	65.7	145	78	171	92.8	205
190	74.8	66.7	147	79	173	94.2	208
192	75.6	67.7	149	80	175	95.6	211
194	76.4	68.7	152	81	179	97.0	214
196	77.2	69.5	153	82	180	98.2	217
198	78.0	70.4	155	83	182	99.4	219
200	78.7	71.2	157	84	185	100.6	222
202	79.5	72.0	159	85	107	101.6	224

Adapted from Task Force on Nutrition: Assessment of maternal nutrition, Chicago, 1978, The American College of Obstetricians and Gynecologists and the American Dietetic Association.

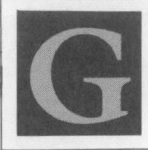

Human Fetotoxic Chemical Agents

Maternal Medication	Reported Effect on Fetus or Neonate
Analgesics	
Indomethacin (Indocin)	Prolongs gestation (monkey); in neonates, used to close patent ductus arteriosus
Narcotics	70% of maternal level; death, apnea, depression, bradycardia, hypothermia
Salicylates	Death in utero; hemorrhage, methemoglobinemia, ↓ albumin-binding capacity, salicylate intoxication, difficult delivery, ? prolonged gestation
Anesthesia	
Conduction	Indirect effect of maternal hypotension; direct effect—convulsions, death, acidosis, bradycardia, myocardial depression, fetal hypotension, methemoglobinemia
General	Apnea, depression (prolonged inhalation by gravid female), ? congenital malformations, chromosomal abnormality*; ether has direct narcotic effect on infant
Ether	
Halothane (Fluothane)	
Trichloroethylene (Trilene)	
Hypnosis	Indirect effect of maternal hyperventilation and excessive bearing down
Local	
Paracervical	Methemoglobinemia, fetal acidosis, bradycardia, neurologic depression, myocardial depression
Anticoagulants	
Coumarins	Fetal death, hemorrhage, calcifications
Anticonvulsant agents	
Barbiturates	Irritability and tremulousness 4-5 months after delivery; hemorrhage, enzyme inducer
Paramethadione (Paradione)	CHD, microphthalmia, mental retardation, abortion
Phenytoin and barbiturate	Congenital malformations, cleft lip and palate, congenital heart disease (CHD), CNS and skeletal anomalies, failure to thrive, enzyme inducer, hemorrhage
Trimethadione (Tridione)	
Antidiabetics	*See* hypoglycemic agents
Antimalarial	
Quinine	? Congenital anomalies of CNS and extremities, thrombocytopenia, hypoplastic optic nerve, congenital deafness
Antimicrobials	All antimicrobials cross placenta
Ampicillin	↓ Maternal urinary and plasma estriol levels
Cephaloridine	Blood levels maintained for hours after delivery; ? false positive direct Coombs' test
Chloramphenicol	Crosses placenta with no reported effect; interferes with biotransformation of tolbutamide, phenytoin, biohydroxycoumarin (i.e., hypoglycemia may occur if used in combination)
Chloroquine	Death, deafness, retinal hemorrhage
Erythromycin	Possible hepatic injury
Nitrofurantoin	Megaloblastic anemia, G6PD deficiency
Novobiocin	Hyperbilirubinemia
Quinine, quinidine	Possible ototoxicity, thrombocytopenia
Streptomycin	Therapeutic levels reached, nerve deafness
Sulfonamides	
Long and short acting	Icterus, hemolytic anemia, kernicterus, ? growth retardation, thrombocytopenia
Tetracycline	Placental transfer after 4 months' gestation; enamel hypoplasia, delay in bone growth, ? congenital cataract

Modified from Babson, S.G., and others: Diagnosis and management of the fetus and neonate at risk: a guide for team care, ed. 4, St. Louis, 1980, The C.V. Mosby Co., p. 26; and Perinatal pharmacology, Mead Johnson Symposium and Perinatal and Developmental Medicine (no. 5), Vail, Colo., June 9-13, 1974.
*Pregnant nurses working in operating rooms have shown a higher incidence of abortion, stillbirths, and congenital anomalies for unknown reasons.

Maternal Medication	Reported Effect on Fetus or Neonate
Antituberculosis	
Isoniazid	Toxic blood level in fetus; no reported effect; mother should be on pyridoxine supplement
Pyridoxine	*See* vitamins
Belladonna derivatives	
Atropine	Intrauterine tachycardia; dilated, nonreacting pupils
Scopolamine	? Delays labor, ? delays respiration, deleterious to premature infant
Cancer chemotherapeutic agents	
Aminopterin	Abortion, congenital anomalies (first trimester); combination of drugs detrimental to fetus; skeletal
Busulfan	and cranial malformations, hydrocephalus; questionable long-term effects = slow somatic
Cyclophosphamide	growth; ovarian agenesis; ↓ immune mechanisms
6-Mercaptopurine	
Methotrexate	
Cardiovascular agents	
Digitoxin	Placental transfer, no reported effect
Propranolol	Indirect effect of delay in cervical dilatation
Cholinesterase inhibitors	Myasthenia-like symptoms for 1 week; muscle weakness in 10% to 20% of infants
Cigarette smoking	Effect equal to number of cigarettes smoked; ↑ incidence of stillbirth; low birth weigth; ? effect on later somatic growth and mental development; reduction in O_2 transport to fetus
Diuretics	
Ammonium chloride	Maternal and fetal acidosis; thrombocytopenia, hemorrhage, hypoelectrolytemia, convulsions, respi-
Benzothiazides	ratory distress, death, hemolysis
Chlorothiazide	
Thiazide	
Diazoxide	Hypertrichosis lanuginosa, alopecia, ? hypoglycemia
Drugs of abuse (usually multiple drugs consumed)	
Alcohol	Blood level equal to mother's; convulsions, withdrawal syndrome, hyperactivity, crying, irritability, poor sucking reflex, low birth weight; cleft palate, ophthalmic malformation, malformation of extremities and heart; poor mental performance; microencephaly, small-for-dates, growth deficiency
Barbiturates	Withdrawal symptoms, convulsions, onset immediately after birth or at 2 weeks of age
Glutethimide	Small-for-dates, irritability
LSD (lysergic acid)	Chromosome breakage, limb and skeletal anomalies
Narcotics	Small-for-dates, 4% to 10% mortality, habituation, withdrawal symptoms, convulsions, sudden
Heroin	death, indirect effect of maternal complications (i.e., infection, hepatitis, venereal disease), ? per-
Methadone	manent effect on somatic growth
Fluorine	Placental transfer—utilized for growth and development of bones and teeth of fetus
Hormones	
Androgens	Labioscrotal fusion prior to week 12; after 12 weeks, phallic enlargement; ? other anomalies; ? ↑
Estrogens	bilirubin, vaginal cancer, cleft lip and palate; CHD; tracheoesophageal fistula; and atresia; cancer
Progestins	of prostate, testes, and bladder
Corticosteroids	Adrenal insufficiency, cleft palate, small-for-dates infant
Ovulatory agents	? Anencephaly, ? chromosomal abnormalities in abortus, multiple pregnancy
Hypoglycemic agents	
Chlorpropamide	Higher fetal mortality, prolonged hypoglycemia, competes for albumin-binding sites
Insulin	Insulin coma, ? increased fetal damage
Tolbutamide	? Potentiates hypoglycemia in newborn, thrombocytopenia
Hypotensive agents	
Hexamethonium	Paralytic ileus, perforation; death
Reserpine	1% to 15% of infants have symptoms; nasal stuffiness, bradycardia, respiratory distress, hypothermia, abnormal muscle tone (in mice, hyperactivity and increased emotionalism)
Insecticide and pesticides	
Organochlorine	Present in fetus, ? enzyme induction, ? premature labor
Intravenous alcohol	Hypoglycemia; abnormal bone marrow morphology in premature infant
Intravenous fluids	Excessive fluids—hyponatremia, seizures
Muscle relaxants	
Curare	Paralysis in utero (prolonged use), position deformities
Narcotic antagonist	
Nalorphine (Nalline)	Not effective unless large doses of narcotics administered to mother; act as respiratory depressant if
Levallorphan (Lorfan)	cause of depression is other than narcotic
Oxytocin	Thrombocytopenia, fetal bradycardia, water intoxication, ? ↑ bilirubin level; abortions (ergot)

Continued.

Maternal Medication	Reported Effect on Fetus or Neonate
Psychotropic drugs	
Antidepressants	
Aventyl	Withdrawal, coliclike syndrome, cyanosis, irritability, weight loss, hyperhydrosis, respiratory dis-
Chloropyramine	tress, craniofacial anomalies, CNS and skeletal anomalies; urinary retention
Imipramine	
Nortriptyline	
Diazepam (Valium)	High fetal levels; hypotonia, poor sucking reflex, hypothermia; ↑ low Apgar score; ↑ resuscitation, ↑ assisted deliveries; dose related
Lithium carbonate	Neonatal serum levels reach adult toxic range; lethargy, cyanosis for 10 days; teratogenic—dose related
Phenothiazine	? Effect on eyes; withdrawal; extrapyramidal dysfunction; delay in onset of respiration; maternal hypotension, ? prolongs labor, ↓ effective uterine contraction; ? chromosomal breakage; hypotonia, hyperactivity
Radiation	Microencephaly, mental retardation, many unknown effects; nondisjunction of chromosomes
Radiopaque media	Elevated parathyroid hormone inhibition (PHI), depressed ^{131}I uptake
Sedatives	
Barbiturate	Apnea, depression, depressed EEG, poor sucking reflex, slow weight gain; concentration of drug in brain; enzyme inducer = lower bilirubin level
Bromides	Growth failure, lethargy, dilated pupils, dermatitis, hypotonia, ? effect on mental development
Magnesium sulfate	Neonatal blood level does not correlate with clinical condition; respiratory depression, hypotonia, convulsions, death; exchange transfusion may be required
Paraldehyde	Apnea, depression
Thalidomide	Administered between days 34-50 of gestation causes phocomelia, malformation of cord, angiomas of face, CHD, intestinal stenosis, eye defects, absence of appendix
Thyroid medications	
Iodine	Normal or goitrous; euthyroid, hyperthyroid, or hypothyroid; respiratory distress due to tracheal
Thioureas	compression; thrombocytopenia
^{131}I	Uptake of fetal thyroid after 12 weeks' gestation; exophthalmos, arrest of brain development
Toxins	
Carbon monoxide	Stillbirth, brain damage equal to anoxia
Heavy metals	
Arsenic	Concentrated in brain
Lead	Abortion, growth retardation, congenital anomalies, sterility
Mercury	Cerebral palsy, mental retardation, convulsions, involuntary movements, defective vision; mother asymptomatic
Naphthalene	Hemolysis
Vitamins	
A and D	Congenital anomalies
K (water-soluble analogs)	Icterus, anemia, kernicterus
Pyridoxine	Withdrawal seizures

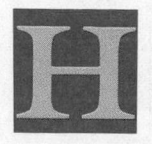

Conversion of Pounds and Ounces to Grams for Newborn Weights

						Ounces											
	0	**1**	**2**	**3**	**4**	**5**	**6**	**7**	**8**	**9**	**10**	**11**	**12**	**13**	**14**	**15**	
0	—	28	57	85	113	142	170	198	227	255	283	312	430	369	397	425	**0**
1	454	482	510	539	567	595	624	652	680	709	737	765	794	822	850	879	**1**
2	907	936	964	992	1021	1049	1077	1106	1134	1162	1191	1219	1247	1276	1304	1332	**2**
3	1361	1389	1417	1446	1474	1503	1531	1559	1588	1616	1644	1673	1701	1729	1758	1786	**3**
4	1814	1843	1871	1899	1928	1956	1984	2013	2041	2070	2098	2126	2155	2183	2211	2240	**4**
5	2268	2296	2325	2353	2381	2410	2438	2466	2495	2523	2551	2580	2608	2637	2665	2693	**5**
6	2722	2750	2778	2807	2835	2863	2892	2920	2948	2977	3005	3033	3062	3090	3118	3147	**6**
7	3175	3203	3232	3260	3289	3317	3345	3374	3402	3430	3459	3487	3515	3544	3572	3600	**7**
8	3629	3657	3685	3714	3742	3770	3799	3827	3856	3884	3912	3941	3969	3997	4026	4054	**8**
9	4082	4111	4139	4167	4196	4224	4252	4281	4309	4337	4366	4394	4423	4451	4479	4508	**9**
10	4536	4564	4593	4621	4649	4678	4706	4734	4763	4791	4819	4848	4876	4904	4933	4961	**10**
11	4990	5018	5046	5075	5103	5131	5160	5188	5216	5245	5273	5301	5330	5358	5386	5415	**11**
12	5443	5471	5500	5528	5557	5585	5613	5642	5670	5698	5727	5755	5783	5812	5840	5868	**12**
13	5897	5925	5953	5982	6010	6038	6067	6095	6123	6152	6180	6209	6237	6265	6294	6322	**13**
14	6350	6379	6407	6435	6464	6492	6520	6549	6577	6605	6634	6662	6690	6719	6747	6776	**14**
15	6804	6832	6860	6889	6917	6945	6973	7002	7030	7059	7087	7115	7144	7172	7201	7228	**15**
	0	**1**	**2**	**3**	**4**	**5**	**6**	**7**	**8**	**9**	**10**	**11**	**12**	**13**	**14**	**15**	

Pounds (left and right side labels); Ounces (top and bottom labels)

*To convert pounds and ounces to grams, multiply the pounds by 453.6 and the ounces by 28.35; add the totals.
To convert grams into pounds and decimals of a pound, multiply the grams by 0.0022.
To convert grams into ounces, divide the grams by 28.35 (16 oz = 1 lb).

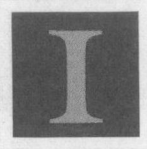

Standard Laboratory Values in the Neonatal Period

1. Hematologic values

	Neonatal
Clotting factors	
Activated clotting time (ACT)	2 min
Bleeding time (Ivy)	2 min
Clot retraction	1-8 min
Clotting time	Complete 1-4 h
2 tubes	5-8 min
3 tubes	5-15 min
Fibrinogen	150-300 mg/dl*
Fibrinolysin (plasminogen)	Lysis of clot
Partial thromboplastin time (PTT)	<90-120 s
Prothrombin time, one-stage (PT)	12-21 s
Thromboplastin generation test (TGT)	8-24 s in 6 min tube

	Term	Preterm
Hemoglobin (g/dl)	17-19	15-17
Hematocrit (%)	57-58	45-55
Sedimentation rate, erythrocytes (ESR) mm/h	0-2	1-5
Reticulocytes (%)	3-7	Up to 10
Fetal hemoglobin (% of total)	40-70	80-90
Nucleated RBC/mm³ (per 100 RBC)	200 (0.05)	(0.2)
Platelet count/mm³	100,000-300,000	120,000-180,000
WBC/mm³	15,000	10,000-20,000
Neutrophils (%)	45	47
Eosinophils and basophils (%)	3	
Lymphocytes (%)	30	33
Monocytes (%)	5	4
Immature WBC (%)	10	16

2. Biochemical values

		Neonatal
Ammonia		100-150 µg/dl
Amylase		0-1000 IU/h
Antistreptolysin O titer, group B		
Normal		12-100 Todd units
Recent streptococcal infection		200-2500 Todd units
Bilirubin, direct		0-1 mg/dl
Bilirubin, total	Cord:	<2 mg/dl
	Peripheral blood: 0-1 day	6 mg/dl
	1-2 day	8 mg/dl
	3-5 day	12 mg/dl
Blood gases	Arterial:	pH 7.31-7.45
		P_{CO_2} 33-48 mm Hg
		P_{O_2} 50-70 mm Hg
	Venous:	pH 7.28-7.42
		P_{CO_2} 38-52 mm Hg
		P_{O_2} 20-49 mm Hg

---

1 to 6 from Pierog, S.H., and Ferrara, A.: Medical care of the sick newborn, ed. 2, St. Louis, 1976, The C.V. Mosby Co.
*dl refers to deciliter (1 dl = 100 ml); this conforms to the SI system: international measurements that have been standardized.

Calcium, ionized	2.1-2.6 mEq/L
Calcium, total	4-7.0 mEq/L
Catecholamines (μg/24 h)	
Neonatal: norepinephrine, 2-12; epinephrine, 1-2	
Newborn: norepinephrine, 2-4; epinephrine, 0-1	
Ceruplasmin (p-phenylenediamine dihydrochloride, 37 C)	1-30 mg/dl
Chloride	95-110 mEq/L
Cholesterol, esters	42% to 71% of total
Cholesterol, total	45-170 mg/dl
Copper	20-70 μg/dl
Cortisol	
AM specimen	15-25 μg/dl
PM specimen	5-10 μg/dl
C-reactive protein (CRP)	0
Creatine	0.2-1 mg/dl (higher in females)
Creatine phosphokinase (CPK) (creatine phosphate, 30 C)	10-300 IU/L
Creatinine	0.3-1 mg/dl
Electrophoresis, total protein	Preterm: 4.3-7.6 g/dl
	Newborn: 4.6-7.4 g/dl

Preterm: albumin, 3.1-4.2; α_1-globulin, 0.1-0.5; α_2-globulin, 0.3-0.7; β-globulin, 0.3-1.2;
    γ-globulin, 0.3-1.4
Newborn: albumin, 3.6-5.4; α_1-globulin, 0.1-0.3; α_2-globulin, 0.2-0.5; β-globulin,
    0.2-0.6; γ-globulin, 0.2-1.2

Fatty acids, free	0.4-1 mg/L
α_1-fetoprotein	0
Fibrinogen	150-300 mg/dl
Glucose, fasting (FBS)	
Hepatitis-associated (Australia) antigen	0
Immunoglobulin levels, serum, newborn	660-1.439 mg/dl
IgG 645-1.244	
IgM 5-30	
IgA 0-11	
Iodine, butanol extractable (BEI)	3-13 μg/dl
Iodine, T_4-by-column (thyroxine)	3-12 μg/dl
Iodine, T_4 (competitive protein-binding thyroxine)	3-12 μg/dl
Iodine, total serum organic (PBI)	4-14 μg/dl
Iron	100-200 μg/dl
Iron-binding capacity (IBC)	60-175 μg/dl
17-Ketogenic steroids (17-KGS)	2.4 mg/24 h
17-Ketosteroids (17-KS)	0.5-2.5 mg/24 h
Lactic dehydrogenase (LDH) (pyruvate, 30 C)	300-1500 IU/L
Lipids, total	170-450 mg/dl
Lipoproteins, newborn (mg/dl)	
Alpha 70-180	
Beta 50-160	
Chylo 50-110	
Magnesium	1.4-2.9 mEq/L
Malate dehydrogenase (MDH) (oxaloacetic acid, 37 C)	41-68 IU/L
Phosphatase, acid	10.4-16.4 IU/L
Phosphatase, alkaline	50-275 IU/L
Phospholipids	75-170 mg/dl
Phosphorus	3.5-8.6 mg/dl
Potassium	4-7 mg/L
Pregnanediol	0 mg/24 h
Protein, total	4.3-7.6 g/dl
Sodium	140-160 mEq/L
Transaminases, serum	
Glutamic-oxaloacetic (SGOT) (aspartate, 30 C)	5-70 IU/L
Glutamic-pyruvic (SGPT)	5-50 IU/L
Triglycerides	5-40 mg/dl
Urea nitrogen (BUN)	5-15 mg/dl
Vanillylmandelic acid (VMA)	0-1 mg/24 h

Continued.

3. **Urinalysis**

Volume: 20-40 ml excreted daily in the first few days; by 1 week, 24 h urine volume close to 200 ml

Protein: may be present in first 2-4 days

Casts and WBCs: may be present in first 2-4 days

Osmolarity (mOsm/L): 100-600

pH: 5-7

Specific gravity: 1.001-1.020

4. **Cerebrospinal fluid**

Calcium	2-3 mg/L
Cell count	WBCs/mm^3 0-15
	RBCs/mm^3 0-500
Chloride	110-120 mg/L
Color	May be xanthochromic
Glucose	24-40 mg/dl
Lactate dehydrogenase (LDH)	5-80 IU/L
Magnesium	3-3.3 mg/dl
Pándy's test (for excess globulins)	Negative
pH (at 37° C)	7.33-7.42
Pressure	50-80 mm Hg
Protein, total	20-120 mg/dl
Sodium	130-165 mg/L
Specific gravity	1.007-1.009
Transaminase, glutamic-oxaloacetic (GOT)	2-10 IU/L
Volume	5 ml

5. **Cardiorespiratory determinations**

Blood pressure at birth

   Term: systolic, 78 mm Hg; diastolic, 42 mm Hg

   Preterm: systolic, 50-60 mm Hg; diastolic, 30 mm Hg

Respiratory rate: 30-60/min

Heart rate, fetus

   Baseline: 120-160/min

      Tachycardia: >160 beats/min (with maternal complication)

      Bradycardia: <120 beats/min (with maternal hypotension and hypoxia)

      Acceleration: tachycardia > 160 beats/min with uterine contraction—normal (usually)

   Beat-to-beat variability: disappears with fetal distress

   With uterine contraction

      Early deceleration: bradycardia with onset of contraction—benign

      Variable deceleration: bradycardia due to cord compression—usually benign

      Late deceleration: bradycardia after lag period due to fetal hypoxia—ominous sign

Heart rate, term infant: 140 ± 20 beats/min

6. **Urine screening tests for inborn errors of metabolism**

Benedict's test: for reducing substances in the urine—glucose, galactose, fructose, lactose; phenylketonuria, alkaptonuria, tyrosyluria, and tyrosinosis may give positive Benedict's test.

Ferric chloride test: an immediate, green color for phenylketonuria, histidinemia, and tyrosinuria; a gray to green color for presence of phenothiazines, isoniazid; red to purple color for presence of salicylates or ketone bodies.

Dinitrophenylhydrazine test: for phenylketonuria, maple syrup urine disease, Lowe's syndrome.

Cetyltrimethyl ammonium bromide test: for mucopolysaccharides: immediate positive reaction in gargoylism (Hurler's syndrome); delayed, moderately positive reaction for Marfan's, Morquio-Ullrich, and Murdoch syndromes.

Metachromatic stain (or urine sediment): Granules: (free or as inclusion bodies in cells) are seen in metachromatic leukodystrophy; may also be seen rarely in Tay-Sachs and other lipid diseases of the central nervous system.

Amino acid chromatography: Aminoaciduria may be normal in newborns; chromatography may be helpful to detect hypophosphatasia and argininosuccinicaciduria.

Diagnostic Tests
for Phenylketonuria

Test	Method	Use
Urine tests		
Diaper test	10% ferric chloride dropped on freshly wet diaper; green spot (postive): probable PKU	Inexpensive; useful in screening large groups of infants but not of value until infant is at least 6 weeks of age
Phenistix* test	Prepared test stick pressed against wet diaper or dipped in urine; green color reaction: probable PKU	Simple; more accurate than diaper test; useful in screening large groups of infants but not of value until after infant is 6 weeks of age
Dinitrophenyl-hydrazine (DNPH) test†	0.5-1 ml of urine placed in test tube, equal amount of DNPH solution added; immediate pale yellow-orange color reaction: negative; gradual change to opaque bright yellow: positive, indicates probable PKU	Inexpensive; accurate but more complicated than diaper test or Phenistix; most useful in clinical setting to confirm these tests
Blood serum phenylalanine tests		
Guthrie inhibition assay methods‡	Drops of blood placed on filter paper; laboratory uses bacterial growth inhibition test; phenylalanine level about 8 mg/dl blood; diagnostic of PKU	Effective in newborn period; used also to monitor PKU diet; blood easily obtained by heel or finger puncture; inexpensive; used for wide-scale screening
LaDu-Michael method§	5 ml of blood; serum separated and tested for phenylalanine; level 8 mg/dl blood: PKU; in persons with PKU, phenylalanine level above 8-12 mg/dl blood: loss of dietary control	Useful diagnostic tool and to monitor PKU diet; requires blood drawn from person; laboratory method difficult (test not available in many laboratories)
McCaman and Robins fluorometric method‖	5 ml of blood; serum separated and tested for phenylalanine; level above 8 mg; PKU or loss of dietary control	Diagnostic and diet monitoring tool; laboratory procedure more simple than LaDu-Michael method; test not available in many laboratories

From Williams, S.R.: Nutrition and diet therapy, ed. 2, St. Louis, 1973, The C.V. Mosby Co., p. 427.
*Manufactured by Ames Co., Elkhart, Ind.
†Centerwall, W., and Centerwall, S.: Phenylketonuria, U.S. Children's Bureau, pub. no. 338, Washington, D.C., 1961, U.S. Department of Health, Education, and Welfare.
‡Guthrie, R.: Blood screening for phenylketonuria, J.A.M.A. 178:863, 1961.
§LaDu, B., and Michael, P.: An enzymatic spectrophotometric method for the determination of phenylalanine in blood, J. Lab. Clin. Med. 55:491, 1960.
‖McCaman, M., and Robins, E.: Fluorometric method for the determination of phenylalanine in the serum, J. Lab. Clin. Med. 59:885, 1962.

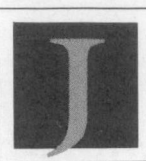

GIRLS: BIRTH TO 36 MONTHS
PHYSICAL GROWTH
NCHS PERCENTILES*

NAME _____ RECORD # _____

*Adapted from: Hamill PVV, Drizd TA, Johnson CL, Reed RB, Roche AF, Moore WM: Physical growth: National Center for Health Statistics percentiles. AM J CLIN NUTR 32:607-629,1979. Data from the Fels Research Institute, Wright State University School of Medicine, Yellow Springs, Ohio.

© 1980 ROSS LABORATORIES

DATE	AGE	LENGTH	WEIGHT	HEAD C.
	BIRTH			

DATE	AGE	LENGTH	WEIGHT	HEAD C.

Preferable to cow milk during the first year
SIMILAC® WITH IRON   **ADVANCE®**
Infant Formula   Nutritional Beverage

For milk-sensitivity
ISOMIL®
Soy Isolate Formula

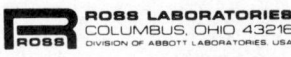

ROSS LABORATORIES
COLUMBUS, OHIO 43216
DIVISION OF ABBOTT LABORATORIES, USA

G106/January 1980

GIRLS: BIRTH TO 36 MONTHS
PHYSICAL GROWTH
NCHS PERCENTILES*

NAME _____

RECORD # _____

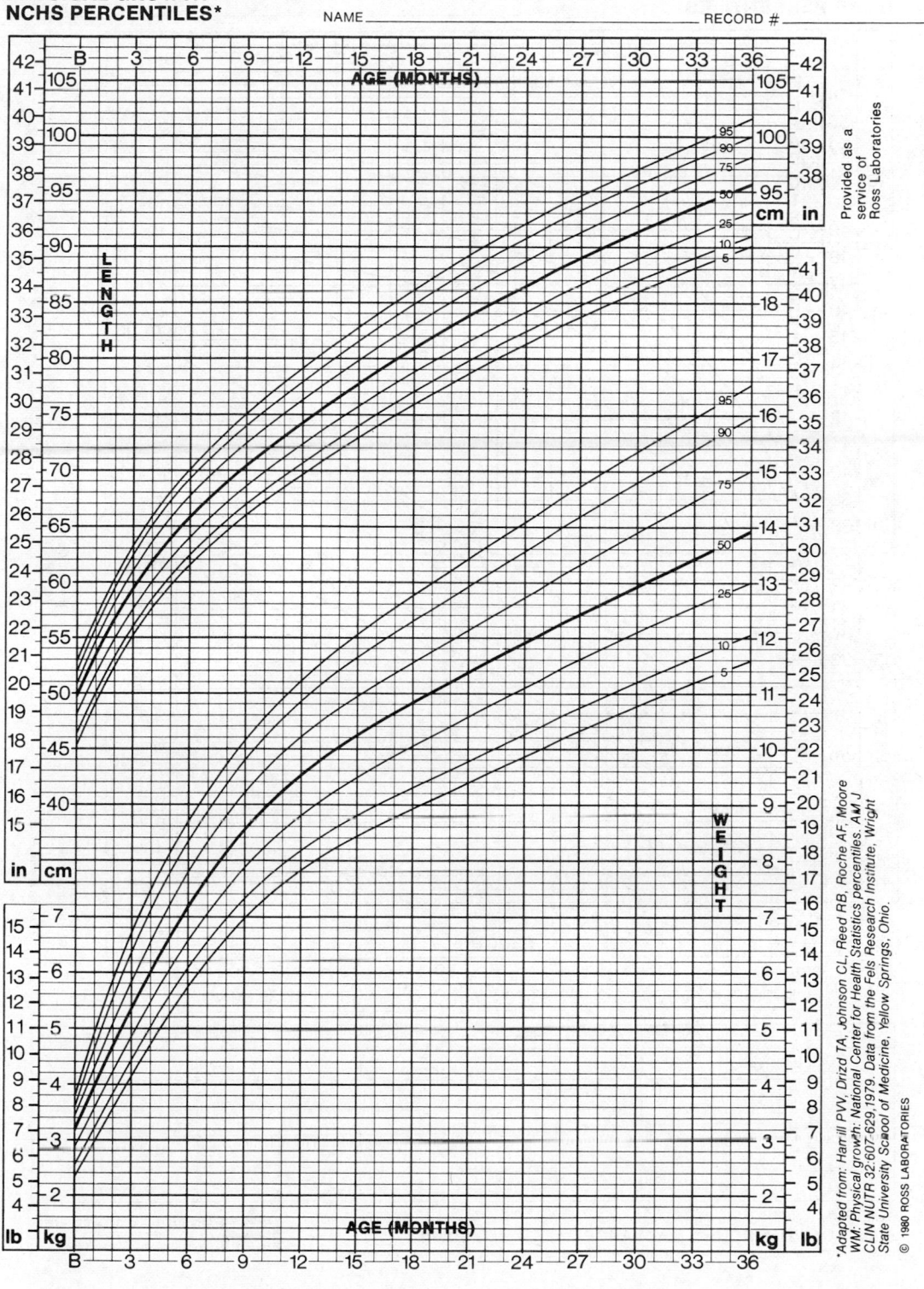

*Adapted from: Hamill PVV, Drizd TA, Johnson CL, Reed RB, Roche AF, Moore WM: Physical growth: National Center for Health Statistics percentiles. AM J CLIN NUTR 32:607-629,1979. Data from the Fels Research Institute, Wright State University School of Medicine, Yellow Springs, Ohio.

© 1980 ROSS LABORATORIES

BOYS: BIRTH TO 36 MONTHS
PHYSICAL GROWTH
NCHS PERCENTILES*

NAME _____   RECORD # _____

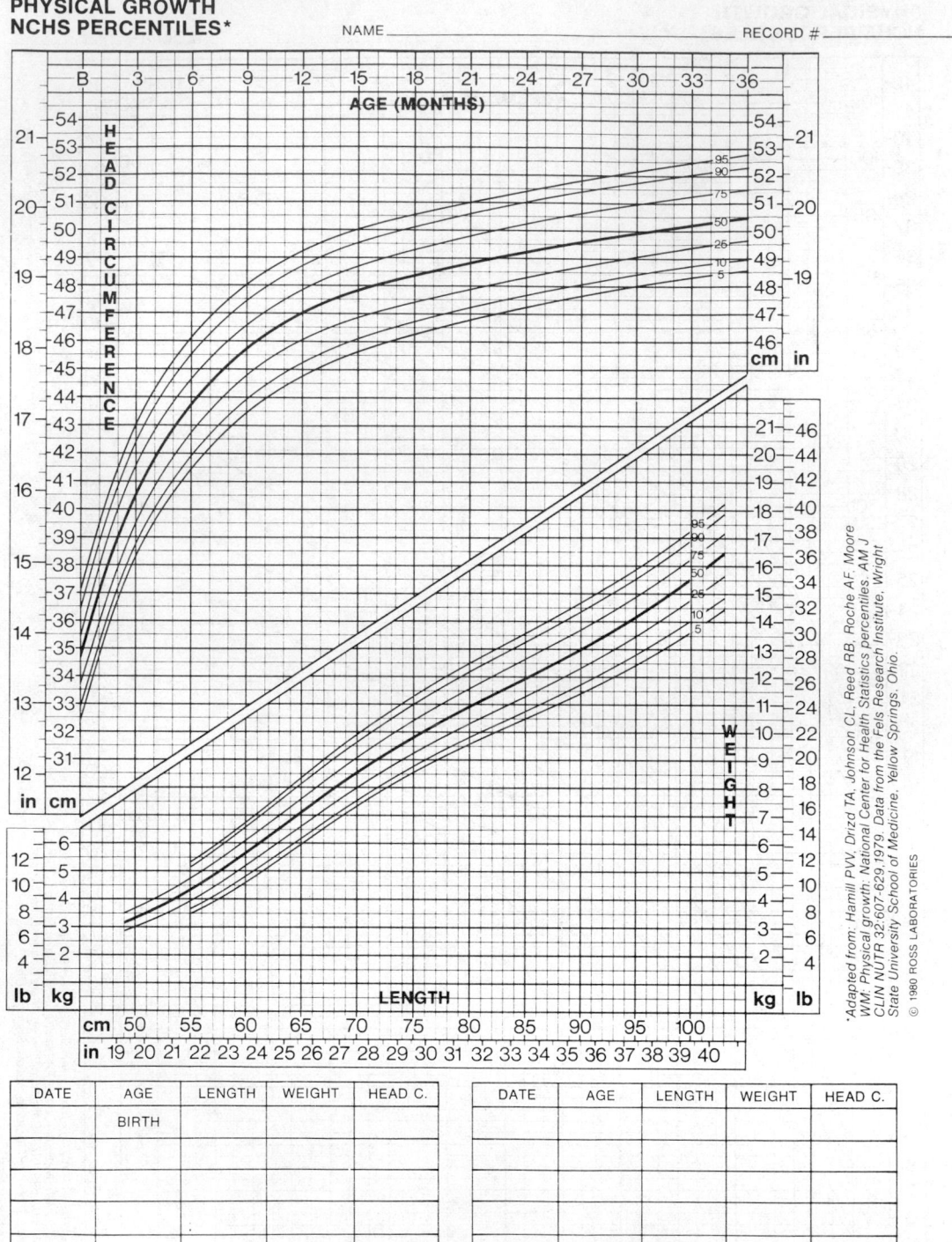

*Adapted from: Hamill PVV, Drizd TA, Johnson CL, Reed RB, Roche AF, Moore WM: Physical growth: National Center for Health Statistics percentiles. AM J CLIN NUTR 32:607-629,1979. Data from the Fels Research Institute. Wright State University School of Medicine. Yellow Springs, Ohio.
© 1980 ROSS LABORATORIES

DATE	AGE	LENGTH	WEIGHT	HEAD C.
	BIRTH			

DATE	AGE	LENGTH	WEIGHT	HEAD C.

BOYS: BIRTH TO 36 MONTHS
PHYSICAL GROWTH
NCHS PERCENTILES*

NAME _____   RECORD # _____

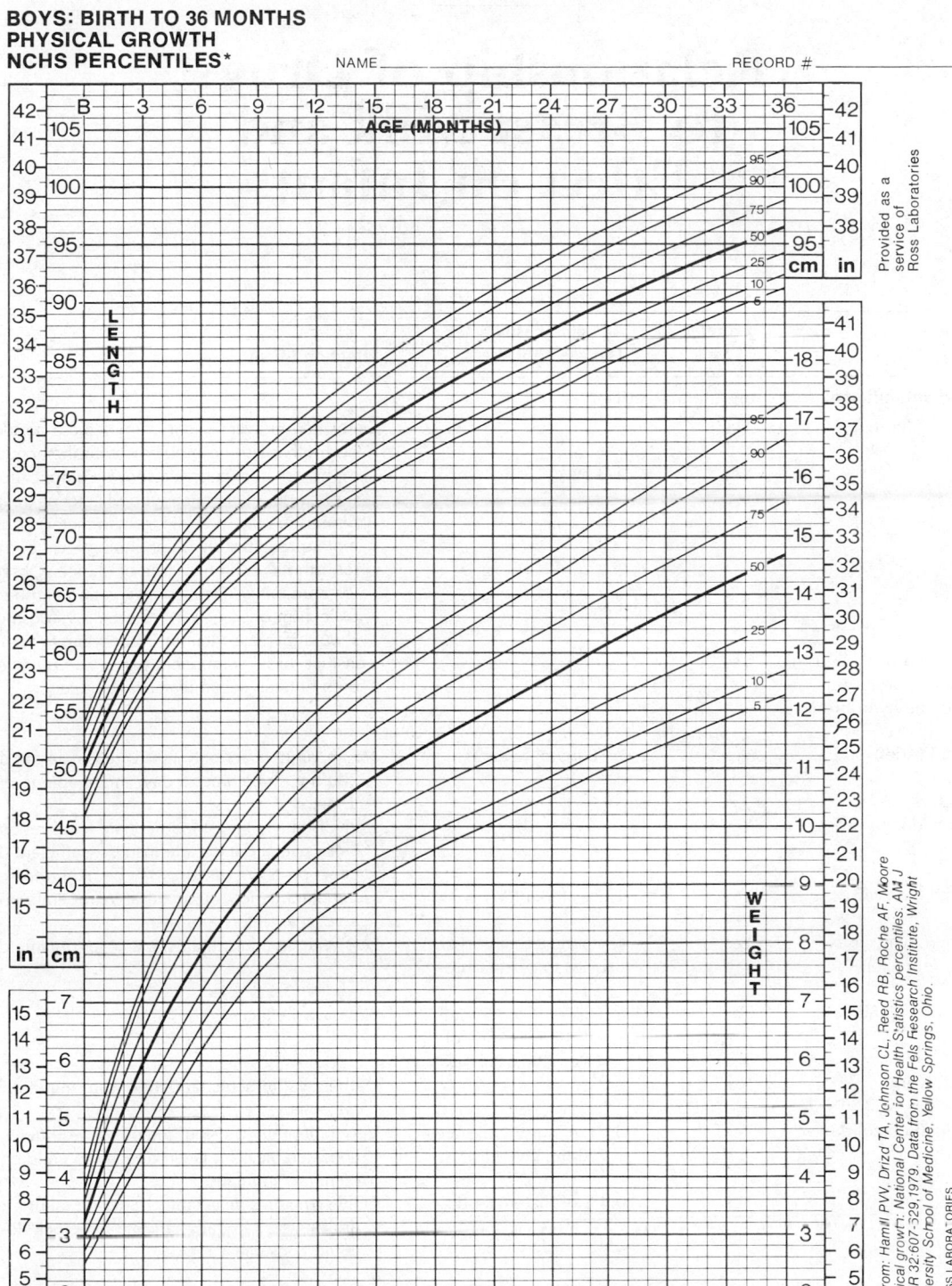

*Adapted from: Hamill PVV, Drizd TA, Johnson CL, Reed RB, Roche AF, Moore
WM: Physical growth: National Center for Health Statistics percentiles. AM J
CLIN NUTR 32:607-529,1979. Data from the Fels Research Institute, Wright
State University School of Medicine, Yellow Springs, Ohio.

© 1980 ROSS LABORATORIES

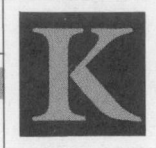

Relationship of Drugs to Breast Milk and Effect on Infant

Drug	Excreted in Milk	Amount in Milk After Therapeutic Dose	Effect on Infant
Analgesics and anti-inflammatory drugs (nonnarcotic)			
Acetaminophen (Datril, Tylenol)	Yes		Detoxified in liver. Avoid in immediate postdelivery period, otherwise no problems with therapeutic dose.
Aspirin	Yes	1-3 mg/dl*	Long history of experience shows complications rare. Can cause interference with platelet aggregation and diminished factor XII (Hageman factor) at birth. When mother requires high, continuing level of medication for arthritis, aspirin is drug of choice. Observe infant for bruisability. Platelet aggregation can be evaluated. Salicylism only seen in maternal overdosing. Mother should increase vitamin C and vitamin K intake.
Donnatal (phenobarbital, hyoscyamine sulfate, atropine sulfate, hyoscine hydrobromide)	Yes		Consider for its component parts. Can be given to children but can accumulate in neonate.
Flufenamic acid (Arlef)	Yes	0.50 µg/ml (mean)†	No apparent effect on infant when maternal dosage was 200 mg, three times a day. Infant able to excrete via urine.
Indomethacin (Indocin)	Yes		Convulsions in breast-fed neonate (case report). Used to close patent ductus arteriosus. Insufficient data as to effect on other vessels. May be nephrotoxic.
Mefenamic acid (Ponstel)	Yes	Trace amounts‡	No apparent effect on infant at therapeutic doses; infant able to excrete via urine.
Naproxen (Naproxyn, synaxyns, naprosine, naxen, proxen)	Yes	1% of maternal plasma; binds to plasma protein	Less toxic in adults than some other organic derivatives.
Oxyphenbutazone (Tandearil)	Yes	In milk of 2 of 55 mothers, 10% to 80% of maternal plasma level	No known effect.
Pentazocine (Talwin)	No		Withdrawal in neonatal period from ingestion during pregnancy.
Phenylbutazone (Butazolidin)	Yes	0.63 mg ml 90 min after 750 mg given IM	Very potent drug; risk to infant not well defined but considerable. Not given directly to children; may accumulate in infant.
Propoxyphene (Darvon)	Yes	0.4% of maternal§ dose	Only symptoms detectable would be failure to feed and drowsiness. On daily, around-the-clock dosage, infant could consume 1 mg/day.

Modified from Lawrence, R.A.: Breastfeeding: a guide for the medical profession, ed. 2, St. Louis, 1985, The C.V. Mosby Co., pp. 509-529.
*Plasma level was 1-5 mg/dl.
†Shown when mean maternal plasma level was 6.41 µg/ml. Mean level in infant's plasma was 0.12 µg/ml; In infant's urine, 0.08 µg/ml. (Maternal plasma level was 50 times that of infant).
‡0.91 µg/ml mean maternal plasma level showed 0.21 µg/ml mean milk level. Mean infant plasma level was 0.08 µg/ml and mean urine level, 9.8 µg/ml.
§Shown by animal experiments. Milk plasma ratio (M/P) = ½.

Drug	Excreted in Milk	Amount in Milk After Therapeutic Dose	Effect on Infant
Antibiotics			
Amantadine (Symmetrel)	Yes	Not defined	Vomiting, urinary retention, rash. Contraindicated.
Ampicillin (Polycillin, Amcill, Omnipen, Penbritin)	Yes	0.07 µg/ml	Sensitivity due to repeated exposure; diarrhea or secondary candidiasis.
Carbenicillin (Pyopen, Geopen)	Yes	0.265 µg/ml 1 h after 1 g given	Levels not significant. Drug is given to neonate.
Cefazolin (Ancef, Kefzol)	Yes	1.5 µg/ml (0.075% of dose)	Probably not significant.
Cephalexin (Keflex)	No		
Cephalothin (Keflin)	No		
Chloramphenicol (Chloromycetin)	Yes	Half blood level; 2.5 mg/dl	Gray syndrome. Infant does not excrete drug well, and small amounts may accumulate. Contraindicated. May be tolerated in older infant with mature glycuronide system.
Chloroquine (Aralen)	Yes	2.7 mg in 2 days*	Can be used to *treat* child under 6 months of age who is wholly breast fed.
Colistin (Colymycin)	Yes	0.05-0.09 mg/dl	Not absorbed orally.
Demeclocycline (Declomycin)	Yes	0.2-0.3 mg/dl	Not significant in therapeutic doses. Can be given to infants.
Erythromycin (Ilosone, E-Mycin, Erythrocin)	Yes	0.05-0.1 mg/dl; 3.6-6.2 µg/ml	Higher concentrations have been reported in milk than in plasma. Should not be given under 1 month of age because of risk of jaundice. Dose in milk higher when given IV to mother.
Gentamicin	Unknown		Not absorbed from gastrointestinal tract, may change gut flora. Drug is given to newborns directly.
Isoniazid (Nydrazid)	Yes	0.6-1.2 mg/dl†	Infant as risk for toxicity, but need for breast milk may outweigh risk.
Kanamycin (Kantrex)	Yes	18.4 µg/ml after 1 g given IM	Infant absorbs little from gastrointestinal tract. Infants can be given drug.
Lincomycin (Lincocin)	Yes	0.5-2.4 mg/dl	Not significant in therapeutic doses to affect child.
Mandelic acid	Yes	0.3 g/24 h after dose of 12 g/day	Not significant in therapeutic doses to affect child.
Methacycline (Rondomycin)	Yes	½ plasma level; 50-260 µg/dl	Same precautions as with tetracycline.
Methenamine (Hexamine)	Yes		Not significant in therapeutic doses to affect child.
Metronidazole (Flagyl)	Yes	Level comparable to serums‡	Caution should be exercised because of its high milk concentrations. Contraindicated when infant under 6 months may cause neurologic disorders and blood dyscrasia.
Nalidixic acid (Neggram)	Yes	0.4 mg/dl	Not significant in therapeutic doses beyond neonatal period. Hemolytic anemia in an infant attributed to nalidixic acid in G6PD deficiency or when mother has renal failure.
Nitrofurantoin (Furadantin)	Yes	Trace to 0.5 µg/ml	Not significant in therapeutic doses to affect child except in G6PD deficiency.
Novobiocin (Albamycin, cathomycin)	Yes	0.36-0.54 mg/dl	Infant can be given drug directly.
Nystatin (Mycostatin)	No	Not absorbed orally	Can be given to infant directly.
Oxacillin (Prostaphlin)	No		
Para-aminosalicylic acid	No		
Penethamate (Leocillin)	No	27-74 µg/dl	Animal study suggests it be avoided.
Penicillin G, benzathine (Bicillin)	Yes	10-12 units/dl	Clinical need should supersede possible allergic responses.
Penicillin G, potassium	Yes	Up to 6 units/dl; 1.2-3.6 µg/dl	Infant can be given penicillin directly. Parents should be told to inform physician that infant has been exposed to penicillin because of potential sensitivity.

*Peaks in 6 h.
†Same concentration in milk as in maternal serum.
‡Gives serum levels in infants of 0.05 to 0.4 µg/ml.

Continued.

Drug	Excreted in Milk	Amount in Milk After Therapeutic Dose	Effect on Infant
Antibiotics—cont'd			
Pyrimethamine (Daraprim)	Yes	0.3 mg/dl (3% of dose)	Significant in therapeutic doses when infant under 6 months and entirely breast-fed.
Quinine sulfate	Yes	0-0.1 mg/dl after maternal dose of 300-600 mg	In therapeutic doses, no effect on child except rare thrombocytopenia.
Sodium fusidate	Yes	0.2 μg/ml	Not significant in therapeutic doses to affect child.
Streptomycin	Yes	Present for long periods in slight amounts when given as dihydrostreptomycin	Not to be given more than 2 weeks. Ototoxic and nephrotoxic with long use. Is given to infants directly.
Sulfanilamide	Yes	9 mg/dl after dose of 2-4 g/24 h	Not significant in therapeutic doses; may cause a rash or hemolytic anemia. Should be avoided for first month after delivery.
Sulfapyridine	Yes	3-13 mg/dl after dose of 3 g/24 h	To be avoided; has caused skin rash.
Sulfathiazole	Yes	0.5 mg/dl after dose of 3 g/24 h	Not significant in therapeutic doses to affect child after 1 month of age.
Sulfisoxazole (Gantrisin)	Yes	Concentration similar to plasma level	To be avoided during first month after delivery; may cause kernicterus.
Tetracycline HC1 (Achromycin, Panmycin, Sumycin)	Yes	0.5-2.6 μg/ml after dose of 500 mg four times a day	Not enough to treat an infection in an infant. May cause discoloration of the teeth in the infant; the antibiotic, however, may be largely bound to the milk calcium. Do not give longer than 10 days or repeatedly.
Anticoagulants			
Coumarin derivatives Dicumarol (bishydroxycoumarin) Warfarin (Panwarfin)	Yes	Probably little but may be cumulative*	Monitor prothrombin time. Give vitamin K to infant. Discontinue if surgery or trauma occurs. Drug of choice if mother to continue nursing.
Ethyl biscoumacetate (Tromexan)	Yes	0-0.17 mg/dl†	Hemorrhage around umbilical stump and cephalhematoma reported. Prothrombin normal in infants with hemorrhage. Vitamin K has no effect. Contraindicated while nursing.
Heparin	No		Heparin ineffective orally.
Phenindione (Hedulin)(Dindevan)	Yes		Breast milk a major route of excretion. Reports of serious hemorrhage in infant. Prothrombin times prolonged in infant. Contraindicated while nursing.
Anticonvulsants and sedatives‡			
Barbital (Veronal)	Yes	8-10 mg/L after 500 mg dose	May produce sedation in infant, in general, barbiturates pass into milk but do not sedate infant. Watch for symptoms.
Carbamazepine (Tegretol)	Yes	60% of plasma levels§	Animal studies show lack of weight gain, unkempt appearance.
Chloral hydrate (Noctec, Somnos)	Yes	Up to 1.5 mg/dl	No significant symptoms, can be given to infants directly.
Phenytoin (Dilantin)	Yes	1.5 to 2.6 μg/ml after 300 mg/24 h dose	One case of hemolytic reaction reported. Other infants appear to tolerate the small doses. Therapeutic plasma level 10-20 μg/ml.
Mephenytoin (Mesantoin) (hydantoin homologue of mephobarbital)	Unknown		Detoxified in liver. No information.
Pentobarbital (Nembutal)	Yes		Depends on liver for detoxification so may accumulate in first week of life until infant is able to detoxify. No problem for older infant in usual doses.

*Reports conflict.
†No correlation with dosage, continues in milk after plasma clear.
‡All barbitals appear in breast milk.
§When plasma 13.0 μmole/L, 7.5 μmole/L in milk.

Drug	Excreted in Milk	Amount in Milk After Therapeutic Dose	Effect on Infant
Phenobarbital (Luminal)	Yes	0.1-0.5 mg when plasma level 0.6-1.8 mg	Sleepiness and decreased sucking possible. On usual analeptic doses infants alert and feed well. On hypnotic doses infant depressed and difficult to rouse.
Phensuximide (Milontin)			No specific data.
Primidone (Mysoline)	Yes		Causes drowsiness and decreased feeds. May cause bleeding due to hypoprothrombinemia. Infant needs vitamin K. Avoid drug during lactation.
Sodium bromide (Bromo-Seltzer and across-the-counter sleeping aids)	Yes	Up to 6.6 mg/dl	Drowsy, decreased crying, rash, decreased feeding.
Trimethadione (Tridione)			No specific data.
Antihistaminics	Yes	No specific data available. All pass into milk.	Drug is used in neonates. May cause sedation, decreased feeding, or may produce stimulation and tachycardia. Should avoid long-acting preparations, which may accumulate in infant. When combined with decongestants, may cause decrease in milk.
Brompheniramine (Dimetane)			
Diphenhydramine (Benadryl)			
Methdialzine (Tacaryl)			
Tripelennamine (Pyribenzamine)			
Autonomic drugs			
Atropine sulfate*	Yes	0.1 mg/dl	Hyperthermia, atropine toxicity, infants especially sensitive; also inhibits lactation. Infant dose 0.01 mg/kg.
Carisoprodol (Soma, Rela)	Yes	2-4 times maternal plasma level	Blocks interneuronal activity in descending reticular formation and spinal cord; drowsiness, hypotonia, poor feed.
Ergot (Cafergot)	Yes	Unknown	90% of infants had symptoms of ergotism: vomiting and diarrhea to weak pulse and unstable blood pressure. Short-term therapy for migraine should not exceed 6 mg. Cafergot also contains 100 mg caffeine.
Mepenzolate bromide (Cantil)	No		Postganglionic parasympathetic inhibitor used to diminish gastric acidity and decrease spasm of colon. Oral absorption low.
Methocarbamol (Robaxin)	Yes	Minimum	Too little in milk to produce effect.
Neostigmine	No		No known harm to infant.
Propantheline bromide (Pro-Banthine)	No	Uncontrolled data indicate no measurable levels.	Drug rapidly metabolized in maternal system to inactive metabolite. Mother should avoid long-acting preparations, however.
Scopolamine (hyoscine)	Yes		Usually given as single dose and of no problem to neonate. No data on repeated doses.
Cardiovascular drugs			
Diazoxide (Hyperstat)			Arteriolar dilators and antihypertensive, only given IV, not active orally.
Dibenzyline†			No data available.
Digoxin	Yes	0.96-0.61 ng/ml‡	Dixogin 20% bound to protein; infant receives <1/100 of dose. If mother at toxic level of 5 ng/ml, milk would have 4.4 ng/ml and infant would receive only 1/20 daily dose.
Guanethidine (Ismelin)§	Yes		Not significant in therapeutic doses to affect child.
Hydralazine (Apresoline)	Yes		Jaundice, thrombocytopenia, electrolyte disturbances possible.
Methyldopa (Aldomet)§	Yes		Galactorrhea. No specific data except as affects mother's milk production.
Propranolol (Inderal) ‖	Yes	40 ng/ml of maternal plasma¶	Insignificant amount. Infants reported had no symptoms noted. Should watch for hypoglycemia and/or "β-blocking" effects.

*Ingredient in many prescription and nonprescription drugs.
†α-blocking agent.
‡Peak level occurs 4-6 h after dose given. Maternal plasma level was higher, M/P = 0.9 and 0.8; Infant's plasma level was 0.
§Adrenergic blocking agent.
‖ β-blocking agent.
¶Total daily dose to infant via milk is 15-20 μg.

Continued.

Drug	Excreted in Milk	Amount in Milk After Therapeutic Dose	Effect on Infant
Cardiovascular drugs—cont'd			
Quinidine	Yes		Arrhythmia may occur.
Reserpine (Serpasil)*	Yes		May produce galactorrhea, lethargy, diarrhea, or nasal stuffiness.
Cathartics			
Aloin	Yes	Low	Occasionally caused colic and diarrhea in infant.
Anthraquinone laxatives such as dihydroxyanthraquinone (Dorbane and Dorbantyl)	Yes	High	Caused colic and diarrhea in infant.
Calomel	No	None	None.
Cascara	Yes	Low	Caused colic and diarrhea in infant.
Milk of magnesia	No	None	No effect.
Mineral oil	No	None	No effect.
Phenolphthalein	Unknown	Unknown†	Reported to cause symptoms in some.
Rhubarb	Unknown	None	None in syrup form. Fresh rhubarb may give symptoms of colic and diarrhea.
Saline cathartics	No	None	No effect.
Senna	No	None	None.
Stool softeners and bulk-forming laxatives	No	None	No effect.
Suppositories (for constipation)	No	None	Not absorbed.
Diagnostic materials and procedures			
Barium		No	Not absorbed.
Iopanoic acid (Telepaque)	Yes		Not sufficient to produce problem in infant on single dose. Does contain iodine radical.
Radioactive compounds			
Radioactive sodium	Yes	0.5% to 1.3% of dose/L‡	Diminished after 24 h; discontinue nursing 24 h
[^{67}Ga] citrate	Yes		Discontinue nursing until ^{67}Ga has cleared, usually 24 h.
^{125}I, ^{131}I	Yes	M/P = 0.13 μCi/0.002 μCi§	^{131}I content in milk proportional to amount of milk. Most excreted in 24 h. Discontinue nursing for 48 h or check milk prior to resuming feeding if under 48 h.
^{90}Sr	Yes	M/P = 1/10	Less than in cow's milk. Bottle infant doubles stores in 1 month.
^{99m}Tc	Yes		Reported to clear in 6-22 h. Discontinue breast feeding 24 h. ^{99m}Tc preferentially picked up by breast tissue.
Tuberculin test	No		Tuberculin-sensitive mothers can adoptively immunize their infants through breast milk, and that immunity may last several years.
X-ray films	No		No effect.
Diuretics			
Acetazolamide (Diamox)	Probable	No specific data available but probably similar to sulfonamide	Acts as enzyme inhibitor on carbonic anhydrase nonbacteriostatic sulfonamide. Observe only for dehydration and electrolyte loss by monitoring urine and turgor.
Furosemide (sulfamoylanthranilic acid) (Lasix)	No		Drug is given to children under medical management.
Mercurial diuretics (Dicurin, Thiomerin)	Yes		In addition to diuretic effect, there is risk of mercury deposition. However, drug not absorbed orally.
Spironolactone (Aldactone)	Yes	Canrenone, a metabolite, appears	Acts as antagonist of aldosterone; causes sodium excretion and potassium retention. The metabolite apparently has some activity.

*Adrenergic blocking agent.
†Reports differ.
‡Peak in 2 h; detectable for 96 h
§27% of dose in 48 h.

Drug	Excreted in Milk	Amount in Milk After Therapeutic Dose	Effect on Infant
Thiazides (Diuril, Enduron, Esidrix, Hydrodiuril, Oretic, Thiuretic tables)	Yes	>0.1 mg/dl*	Risk of dehydration and electrolyte imbalance, especially sodium loss, which would require monitoring. Watching weight and wet diapers and taking an occasional specific gravity reading of the urine and serum sodium would indicate status of infant. Risk, however, is extremely low. May suppress lactation due to dehydration in mother.
Environmental agents			
Aldrin	Yes	Varies by location	Not a reason to wean from breast. No need to test milk unless inordinate exposure.
Benzene hexachloride (BHC)	Yes	Varies by location	Not a reason to wean from breast. No need to test milk unless inordinate exposure.
Dichlorodiphenyltrichloroethane (DDT or DDE)	Yes	Varies by location	Not a reason to wean from breast. No need to test milk unless inordinate exposure.
Dieldrin	Yes	Varies by location	Also found in permanently mothproofed garments. Avoid these. Not a reason to wean.
Hexachlorobenzene (HCB)	Yes	Varies by location	Not a reason to wean from breast. No need to test milk unless inordinate exposure.
Heptachlorepoxide	Yes	Varies by location	Not a reason to wean from breast. No need to test milk unless inordinate exposure.
Methyl mercury	Yes	500-1,000 ng/ml†	Infant blood level 600 ng/ml in heavy exposure. Only in excessive exposure is testing and/or weaning necessary.
Polybrominated biphenyl (PBB)	Yes	Varies by location	If mother at high risk from the environment or the diet,
Polychlorinated biphenyl (PCB)	Yes	Varies by location	milk sample should be measured. If level in milk is high, then breast-feeding should be discontinued. Those at risk are (1) workers who handle PBB/PCB and (2) individuals who eat game fish from contaminated waters. Crash diets mobilize fats and should be avoided especially if PBB or PCB present.
^{90}Sr, ^{89}Sr (strontium)	Yes	1/10 of that in maternal diet	Cow's milk has six times as much as human milk. Cow's milk-fed infant doubles amount in body in 1 month.
Heavy metals			
Arsenic	Yes	Can be measured for given woman	Can accumulate. Check infant's blood level if there is reason to suspect exposure.
Copper	Yes		
Fluorine	Yes		Monitor for excessive dose.
Gold thiomalate (Myocrisin)	Yes	0.022 µg/ml when mother given 50 mg/week	No proteinuria or aminoaciduria observed.
Halothane	Yes	2 ppm	Nursing mothers who work in environment with halothane should be checked.
Iron	Yes		
Lead	Unknown		Nursing contraindicated if maternal serum 40 µg; conflicting reports, breast milk not always cause of lead poisoning in breast-fed infant.
Magnesium	Yes		Not sufficient to be toxic.
Mercury	Yes		Hazardous to infant.
Hormones and contraceptives			
Carbimazole (Neo-Mercazole)	Yes		Antithyroid effect may cause goiter.
Chlorotrianisene (Tace)	Yes		Has estrogenic effect although does not change consistency of milk. May have feminizing effect on infant.
Contraceptives (oral) Ethinyl estradiol Mestranol	Yes		May diminish milk supply. May decrease vitamins, protein, and fat in milk. One author showed no difference when mothers took norethindrone. Most signifi-

*Linear relationship between plasma and milk. In 1 L of milk at 0.1 mg/dl there would be 1 mg/24 h. Infant dose is 20 mg/kg/24 h.
†M/P = 8.6% in heavy exposure.

Continued.

Drug	Excreted in Milk	Amount in Milk After Therapeutic Dose	Effect on Infant
Hormones and contraceptives—cont'd			
19-Nortestosterone Norethindrone (Norlutin) Norethynodrel (Enovid)			cant concern is long-range impact of hormone on young infant, which is not certain. Reports of feminization of infant.
Corticotropin	Yes		Destroyed in gastrointestinal tract of infant. No effect.
Cortisone	Yes		Animal studies show 50% lower weight than controls and retarded sexual development and exophthalmos.
Dihydrotachysterol (Hytakerol)			May cause hypercalcemia; need monitoring of infant serum and urine calcium.
Epinephrine (Adrenalin)	Yes		Destroyed in GI tract of infant.
Estrogen	Yes	0.17 µg/dl after 1 g	Risks as with oral contraceptives.
Fluoxymesterone (Halotestin, Ora-Testryl, Ultrandren)	Yes		Suppress lactation; masculinizing
Insulin	Unknown		Destroyed in gastrointestinal tract.
Liothyronine (Cytomel)	No		Synthetic form of natural thyroid.
Medroxyprogesterone acetate (Provera)	No		
Phenformin HCl	Yes	Minimum	Not sufficient to cause symptoms in infant. Does not cause hypoglycemia in normal infants. No case reports available
Prednisone	Yes	0.07-0.23% dose/L after 5 mg dose*	Minimum amount not likely to cause effect on infant in short course.
Pregnanediol	Yes		Unknown risk as with other female hormones over a long period of time.
Tolbutamide (Orinase)	Yes		Not recommended in the childbearing years.
Narcotics			
Codeine		0 to trace after 32 mg every 4 h (6 doses)	No effect in therapeutic level and transient usage. Can accumulate. Individual variation. Watch for neonatal depression.
Heroin	Yes		13 of 22 infants had withdrawal. Historically breast feeding had been used to wean addict's infant. This is no longer recommended.
Marijuana (Cannabis)	Yes		Shown in laboratory animals to produce structural changes in nursling's brain cells; impairs DNA and RNA formation. Infant at risk of inhaling smoke during feeding or when held by person who is smoking.
Meperidine (Demerol)	Yes	>0.1 mg/dl†	Trace amounts may accumulate if drug taken around the clock when infant is neonate. Watch for drowsiness and poor feeding.
Methadone	Yes	0.03 µg/ml or 0.023-0.028 mg/24 h‡	When dosage not excessive, infant can be breast-fed if monitored for evidence of depression and failure to thrive.
Morphine	Yes	Trace	Single doses have minimum effect. Potential for accumulation. May be addicting to neonate. Breast feeding no longer considered appropriate means of weaning infant of an addict.
Percodan (oxycodone [derived from opiate thebaine] aspirin, phenacetin, caffeine)	Yes		Consider for its component parts. In neonatal period sleepiness and failure to feed, which increase maternal engorgement and neonatal weight loss, have been observed, probably caused by oxycodone.
Psychotropic and mood-changing drugs			
Alcohol	Yes	Similar to plasma level	Ordinarily no problem and can be therapeutic in moderation. Infants are more susceptible to effects. Chronic drinking reported to cause obesity in infant. Ethanol in

*0.16 µg/ml after 10 mg dose; 2.67 µg/ml after 2 h.
†Plasma 0.07-0.1 mg/dl.
‡Mother received 50 mg/24 h; M/P = 0.83. Peak level 4 h after oral dose. Results obscured if addict also taking the herbal root golden seal.

Drug	Excreted in Milk	Amount in Milk After Therapeutic Dose	Effect on Infant
			doses of 1-2 g/kg to mother causes depression of milk-ejection reflex (dose dependent). No acetaldehyde found in infants.
Amphetamine	Yes		Has caused stimulation in infants with jitteriness, irritability, sleeplessness. Long-acting preparations cumulative.
Benzodiazepines* Chlordiazepoxide HC1 (Librium)	Yes		Not sufficient to affect infant first week when glucuronyl system needed for detoxification. May accumulate. Older infant, no apparent problem.
Diazepam (Valium)	Yes	90 µg/L†	Detoxified in glucuronyl system. In first weeks of life may contribute to jaundice. Metabolite active. Effect on infant: hypoventilation, drowsiness, lethargy, and weight loss. Single doses over 10 mg contraindicated during nursing. Accumulation in infant possible.
Pineazepam	Yes	Metabolite, 5-11.2 ng/ml; pineazepam, >1.0 ng/ml‡	No data, probably similar to diazepam.
Haloperidol (Haldol)	Yes	Unknown	A butyrophenone antidepressant; animal studies in nurslings show behavior abnormalities.
Lithium carbonate (Eskalith, Lithane, Lithonate)	Yes	⅓-½ maternal plasma level§	Measurable lithium in infant's serum. Infant kidney can clear lithium; however, lithium inhibits adenosine 3':5:-cyclic monophosphate, significant for brain growth. Also affects amine metabolism. Real effects not measurable immediately. Report of cyanosis and poor muscle tone and ECG changes in nursing infant.
Monoamine oxidate (MAO) inhibitors (Eutonyl, Nardil)			Inhibits lactation.
Meprobamate (Miltown, Equanil)	Yes	2-4 times maternal plasma level	If therapy continued, infant should be followed closely.
Penfluridol ‖	Yes	Unknown	Animal studies show learning abnormalities in sucklings. This is a potent long-acting oral neuroleptic drug.
Phenothiazines Chlorpromazine (Thorazine)	Yes	⅓ plasma level¶	Can be safely nursed; minimum in milk. Increase maternal prolactin. No symptoms in infants reported; 5-year follow-up showed infants normal.
Mesoridazine (Serentil)	Yes	Minimum	
Piperacetazine (Quide)	Yes	Minimum	Probably no effect
Thioridazine (Mellaril)	Yes	No information	Thioridazine is less potent in general than other phenothiazines. Probably quite safe.
Trifluoperazine (Stelazine)	Yes	Minimum	
Tricyclic antidepressants			Apparently no accumulation. No infants that have been observed showed symptoms. Watch for depression or failure to feed. Increase maternal prolactin secretion.
Amitriptyline HC1 (Elavil)	Yes	Minimum amounts	
Desipramine HC1 (Norpramin, Pertofrane)	Yes	Minimum amounts	
Imipramine HC1 (Tofranil)	Yes	0.1 mg/dl#	
Stimulants			
Caffeine	Yes	1% of dose	Accumulates when intake moderate and continual. Causes jitteriness, wakefulness, and irritability. Caffeine present in may hot and cold drinks. Consider if infant very wakeful.

*Alcohol enhances effect of this group
†10 mg or less yields 45 mg of diazepam/ml and 85 ng of metabolite/ml. P/M ratio is variable. Mean P/M ratio of diazepam is 6.14; of metabolite is 3.64. Effect lasts about 4 days.
‡Both drug and active metabolite appear for about 4 days after dose.
§0.030 mmol/L in infant's serum, 0.57 mmole/L in infant's urine. Milk level was half of maternal serum level in one case report.
‖ Neuroleptic drug.
¶If dose<200 mg, milk contains bare trace. Dose of 1200 mg showed trace.
#Plasma level 0.2-1.3 mg/dl.

Continued.

Drug	Excreted in Milk	Amount in Milk After Therapeutic Dose	Effect on Infant
Stimulants—cont'd			
Theobromine	Yes	3.7-8.2 mg/L after 240 mg dose*	No adverse symptoms observed in the infants. Chocolate most common cause of exposure.
Theophylline	Yes	10% of maternal dose†	Irritability, fretfulness.
Thyroid and antithyroid medications			
Carbimazole (Neo-Mercazole)	Yes		May cause goiter.
Methimazole (Tapazole)	Yes	M/P > 1	Inhibits synthesis of thyroid hormone but does not inactivate existing thyroid. Can inhibit infant thyroid. ⅛ grain/day of thyroid can be given to infant simultaneously.
Potassium iodide	Yes	3 mg/dl‡	May alter thyroid function of infant; may cause goiter in infant.
Propylthiouracil	Yes	0.077% of dose	Risk of goiter and agranulocytosis. With present microtechniques for T_3, T_4 and TSH, close monitoring of infant is possible, as with methimazole.
Radioactive iodine ^{125}I, ^{131}I (as a treatment)	Yes	M/P > 1	*Treatment* doses are excreted via the breast for 1-3 weeks. Milk can be checked by Geiger counter if there is a question. Breast-feeding should be discontinued until milk is clear.
Thiouracil	Yes	9-12 mg/d§	Same as for propylthiouracil.
Thyroid and thyroxine	Yes		Does not produce adverse symptoms on long-range follow-up. Noted to improve milk supply of hypothyroid mothers. No contraindication.
Miscellaneous			
Cyclophosphamide	Yes	Present ‖	Antineoplastic agent. Any amounts contraindicated.
DPT	Yes	Minimum	Does not interfere with immunization schedule.
Methotrexate	Yes	Minor route of excretion: M/P = 0.08/1.0	Antimetabolite. Infant would receive 0.26 µg/dl, which researchers consider nontoxic for infant.
Nicotine	Yes	Mean 91 ppb (20-512 ppb)¶	Decreases milk production. No apparent effect on infant—perhaps a tolerance is developed in utero. Smoking may interfere with let-down reflex if smoking started before onset of a feeding.
Poliovirus vaccine	No		Live vaccine taken orally. Not necessary to withhold nursing 30 min before and after dose. Provide booster after infant no longer nursing.
Rh antibodies	Yes		Destroyed in gastrointestinal tract; not effective orally.
Rubella virus vaccine	Yes	Minimum	Will not confer passive immunity. Mother should not be given vaccine when at risk for pregnancy.
Smallpox vaccine	No		Exposure is by direct contact. Live virus. No longer given.

*113 g chocolate bar.
†M/P = 0.7.
‡Dose was 325-650 mg three times a day.
§Maternal plasma level was 3.4 mg/dl after a 1 g dose; M/P = 3.
‖ Single 500 mg IV dose in milk at 1,3,5, and 6 h after injection.
¶At ½-1½ packs/day. Large variation from single donor.

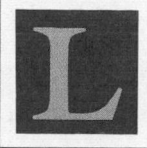

Recommended Schedule for Active Immunization of Normal Infants and Children

Recommended Age	Immunization(s)	Comments
2 months	DTP,[1] OPV[2]	Can be initiated as early as 2 weeks of age in areas of high endemicity or during epidemics
4 months	DTP,OPV	2-month interval desired for OPV to avoid interference from previous dose
6 months	DTP (OPV)	OPV is optional (may be given in areas with increased risk of polio exposure)
15 months	Measles, mumps, rubella, (MMR)[3]	MMR preferred to individual vaccines; tuberculin testing may be done
18 months	DTP,[4,5] OPV[5]	
24 months	HBPV[6]	
4-6 years[7]	DTP,OPV	At or before school entry
14-16 years	Td[8]	Repeat every 10 years throughout life

From American Academy of Pediatrics: Report of the Committee on Infectious Diseases, Ill., ed. 20, 1986. Copyright American Academy of Pediatrics, 1986.

[1]DTP—Diphtheria and tetanus toxoids with pertussis vaccine.
[2]OPV—Oral, poliovirus vaccine contains attenuated poliovirus types 1,2, and 3.
[3]MMR—Live measles, mumps, and rubella viruses in a combined vaccine.
[4]Should be given 6 to 12 months after the third dose.
[5]May be given simultaneously with MMR at 15 months of age.
[6]Haemophilus b polysaccharide vaccine.
[7]Up to the seventh birthday.
[8]Td—Adult tetanus toxoid (full dose) and diphtheria toxoid (reduced dose) in combination.

Glossary

abdominal Belonging or relating to the abdomen and its functions and disorders.

  a. delivery Birth of a child through a surgical incision made into the abdominal wall and uterus; cesarean delivery.

  a. gestation Implantation of a fertilized ovum outside the uterus but inside the peritoneal cavity.

  a. hysterectomy Surgical removal of the uterus through an abdominal wall incision.

  a. pregnancy See *abdominal gestation*.

ablatio placentae See *abruptio placentae*.

abortion Termination of pregnancy before the fetus is viable and capable of extrauterine existence, usually less than 21 to 22 weeks' gestation (or when the fetus weighs less than 600 g).

  complete a. Abortion in which fetus and all related tissue have been expelled from the uterus.

  criminal a. Termination of pregnancy performed by unqualified people usually under septic conditions. Women may resort to this if therapeutic abortions are unavailable.

  elective a. Termination of pregnancy chosen by the woman that is not required for her physical safety.

  habitual (recurrent) a. Loss of three or more successive pregnancies for no known cause.

  incomplete a. Loss of pregnancy in which some but not all the products of conception have been expelled from the uterus.

  induced a. Intentionally produced loss of pregnancy by woman or others.

  inevitable a. Threatened loss of pregnancy that cannot be prevented or stopped and is imminent.

  missed a. Loss of pregnancy in which the products of conception remain in the uterus after the fetus dies.

  septic a. Loss of pregnancy in which there is an infection of the products of conception and the uterine endometrial lining, usually resulting from attempted termination of early pregnancy.

  spontaneous a. Loss of pregnancy that occurs naturally without interference or known cause.

  therapeutic a. Pregnancy that has been intentionally terminated for medical reasons.

  threatened a. Possible loss of a pregnancy; early symptoms are present (e.g., the cervix begins to dilate).

  voluntary a. See *abortion, elective*.

abortus Fetus usually less than 21 weeks' gestational age and under 600 g.

abruptio placentae Partial or complete premature separation of a normally implanted placenta.

abstinence Refraining from sexual intercourse periodically or permanently.

accreta, placenta See *placenta accreta*.

acculturation Process of adopting the cultural traits or social patterns of another group.

acetonuria Presence of acetone and diacetic bodies in the urine.

acidosis Increase in hydrogen ion concentration resulting in a lowering of blood pH below 7.35.

  metabolic a. Increase in hydrogen ion concentration caused by increased acids from (1) abnormal metabolism (too many acids produced), (2) renal malfunction (acids not being excreted), or (3) excessive loss of base (diarrhea).

acini cells Milk-producing cells in the breast.

acme Highest point (e.g., of a contraction).

acrocyanosis Peripheral cyanosis; blue color of hands and feet in most infants at birth that may persist for 7 to 10 days.

acromion Projection of the spine of the scapula (forming the point of the shoulder); used to explain the presentation of the fetus.

adenomyoma Type of tumor affecting glandular and smooth muscle tissue, such as uterine musculature.

adnexa Adjacent or accessory parts of a structure.

  uterine a. Ovaries and fallopian tubes.

adult respiratory distress syndrome (ARDS) Set of symptoms including decreased compliance of lung tissue, pulmonary edema, and acute hypoxemia. The condition is similar to respiratory distress syndrome of the newborn.

afibrinogenemia Absence or decrease of fibrinogen in the blood such that the blood will not coagulate. In obstetrics, this condition occurs from complications of abruptio placentae or retention of a dead fetus.

afterbirth Lay term for the placenta and membranes expelled after the birth or delivery of the child.

afterpains Painful uterine cramps that occur intermittently for approximately 2 or 3 days after delivery and that result from contractile efforts of the uterus to return to its normal involuted condition.

AGA Appropriate (weight) for gestational age.

agalactia Absence or failure of milk secretion after childbirth.

agenesis Failure of an organ to develop.

alae nasi Nostrils.

albuminuria Presence of readily detectable amounts of albumin in the urine.

alkalosis Abnormal condition of body fluids characterized by a tendency toward an increased pH, as from an excess of alkaline bicarbonate or a deficiency of acid.

allantois Tubular diverticulum of the posterior part of the embryo's yolk sac that passes into the body stalk, accompanied by the allantoic blood vessels that develop and become the umbilical vein and paired umbilical arteries; later, after fusing with the chorion, it helps to form the placenta.

allele One of two or more alternative forms of a gene at the same site on a chromosome; alleles determine alternative characters in inheritance. Alleles that occur at the same position, or locus, on a chromosome pair may produce different effects during development.

alveoli, fetal Terminal pulmonary sacs that in fetal life are filled with fluid. This fluid is a transudate of fetal plasma.

ambient Surrounding; around.

amenorrhea Absence or suppression of menstruation.

amnesia Loss of memory.

amnii, liquor See *liquor amnii*.

amniocentesis Procedure in which a needle is inserted through the abdominal and uterine walls into the amniotic fluid; used for assessment of fetal health and maturity and for therapeutic abortion.

amniography Procedure used primarily to detect placenta previa by x-ray examination, entailing injection of radiopaque dye into amniotic fluid.

amnion Inner membrane of two fetal membranes that form the sac and contain the fetus and the fluid that surrounds it in utero.

amnionitis Inflammation of the amnion, occurring most frequently after early rupture of membranes.

amniotic Pertaining or relating to the amnion.

   a. fluid Fluid surrounding fetus derived primarily from maternal serum and fetal urine.

   a. sac Membrane ''bag'' that contains the fetus before delivery.

amniotomy Artificial rupture of the fetal membranes (AROM).

anaerobic catabolism In the absence of free oxygen, the breakdown of organized substances into simpler compounds, with the resultant release of energy.

analgesia Lack of pain without loss of consciousness.

analgesic Any drug or agent that will relieve pain.

androgen Substance that produces masculinizing effects (e.g., testosterone).

androgynous personality Having some characteristics of both sexes.

android pelvis Male type of pelvis.

anencephaly Congenital deformity characterized by the absence of cerebrum, cerebellum, and flat bones of skull.

anesthesia Partial or complete absence of sensation with or without loss of consciousness.

anomaly Organ or structure that is malformed or in some way abnormal with reference to form, structure, or position.

anorexia nervosa Psychoneurotic disorder characterized by a prolonged refusal to eat, resulting in emaciation, amenorrhea, emotional disturbance concerning body image, and an abnormal fear of becoming obese.

anovular menstrual period Cyclic uterine bleeding not accompanied by the production and discharge of an ovum.

anovulatory Failure of the ovaries to produce, mature, or release eggs.

anoxia Absence of oxygen.

antenatal Occurring before or formed before birth.

antepartal Before labor.

anterior Pertaining to the front.

   a. fontanel See *fontanel, anterior*.

anteroposterior repair Operation in which the upper and lower walls of the vagina are reconstructed to correct relaxed tissue.

anthropoid pelvis Pelvis in which the anteroposterior diameter is equal to or greater than the transverse diameter.

antibody Specific protein substance developed by the body that exerts restrictive or destructive action on specific antigens, such as bacteria, toxins, or Rh factor.

anticipatory grief Grief that predates the loss of a beloved object.

antigen Protein foreign to the body that causes the body to develop antibodies. Examples: bacteria, dust, Rh factor.

Apgar score Numeric expression of the condition of a newborn obtained by rapid assessment at 1, 5, and 15 minutes of age; developed by Dr. Virginia Apgar.

apnea Cessation of respirations for more than 10 seconds associated with generalized cyanosis.

Apt test Differentiation of maternal and fetal blood when there is vaginal bleeding. It is performed as follows: Add 0.5 ml blood to 4.5 ml distilled water. Shake. Add 1 ml 0.25N sodium hydroxide. Fetal and cord blood remains pink for 1 or 2 minutes. Maternal blood becomes brown in 30 seconds.

areola Pigmented ring of tissue surrounding the nipple.

   secondary a. During the fifth month of pregnancy, a second faint ring of pigmentation seen around the original areola.

arthralgia Any pain that affects a joint.

articulation Fastening together or connection of the various bones of the skeleton; a joint. The articulations of the bones are classified as (1) immovable (synarthrosis), (2) slightly immovable (amphiarthrosis), and (3) freely movable (diarthrosis).

artificial insemination Introduction of semen by instrument injection into the vagina or uterus for impregnation.

Aschheim-Zondek test Pregnancy determination in which a woman's urine is injected into a mouse. After 5 days the animal is killed and its ovaries are examined. Enlarged ovaries and maturing follicles indicate pregnancy.

asphyxia Decreased oxygen and/or excess of carbon dioxide in the body.

   fetal a. Condition occurring in utero, with the following biochemical changes: hypoxemia (lowering of Po_2), hypercapnia (increase in Pco_2), and respiratory and metabolic acidosis (reduction of blood pH).

   a. livida Condition in which the infant's skin is characteristically pale, pulse is weak and slow, and reflexes are depressed or absent; also known as *blue asphyxia*.

   a. pallida Condition in which the infant appears pale and limp and suffers from bradycardia (80 beats/min or less) and apnea.

aspiration pneumonia Inflammatory condition of the lungs and bronchi caused by the inhalation of vomitus containing acid gastric contents.

aspiration syndrome See *meconium aspiration syndrome*.

asynclitism Oblique presentation of the fetal head at the superior strait of the pelvis; the pelvic planes and those of the fetal head are not parallel.

ataractic Drug capable of promoting tranquility; a tranquilizer.

atelectasis Pulmonary pathosis involving alveolar collapse.

atherosclerosis Common arterial disorder characterized by yellowish plaques of cholesterol, lipids, and cellular debris in the inner layers of the walls of large and medium-sized arteries, resulting in reduced circulation in organs and areas normally supplied by the artery.

athetosis Neuromuscular condition characterized by slow, writhing, continuous, and involuntary movement of the extremities, as seen in some forms of cerebral palsy and in motor disorders resulting from lesions in the basal ganglia.

atony Absence of muscle tone.

atresia Absence of a normally present passageway.

   biliary a. Absence of the bile duct.

   choanal a. Complete obstruction of the posterior nares, which open into the nasopharynx, with membranous or bony tissue.

   esophageal a. Congenital anomaly in which the esophagus ends in a blind pouch or narrows into a thin cord, thus failing to form a continuous passageway to the stomach.

attachment Relationship between two persons (e.g., a parent and a child).

attitude Body posture or position.

   fetal a. Relation of fetal parts to each other in the uterus (e.g., all parts flexed, all parts flexed except neck is extended, etc.).

auscultation Process of listening for sounds produced within the body.

autoimmunization Development of antibodies against constituents of one's own tissues (e.g., a man may develop antibodies against his own sperm).

autosomes Any of the paired chromosomes other than the sex (X and Y) chromosomes.

axis Line, real or imaginary, about which a part revolves or that runs through the center of a body.

  pelvic a. Imaginary curved line that passes through the centers of all the anteroposterior diameters of the pelvis.

azoospermia Absence of sperm in the semen.

bacteremic shock Shock that occurs in septicemia when endotoxins are released from certain bacteria in the bloodstream.

bag of waters Lay term for the sac containing amniotic fluid and fetus.

ballottement (1) Movability of a floating object (e.g., fetus). (2) Diagnostic technique using palpation: a floating object, when tapped or pushed, moves away and then returns to touch the examiner's hand.

Bandl's ring Abnormally thickened ridge of uterine musculature between the upper and lower segments that follows a mechanically obstructed labor, with the lower segment thinning abnormally.

Barr body (sex chromatin) Chromatin mass located against the inner surface of the nucleus in females, possibly representing the inactive X chromosome.

Bartholin's glands Two small glands situated on either side of the vaginal orifice that secrete small amounts of mucus during coitus and that are homologous to the bulbourethral glands in the male.

basalis, decidua See *decidua basalis*.

Bell's palsy See *palsy, Bell's*.

bicornuate uterus Anomalous uterus that may be either a double or single organ with two horns.

biliary atresia See *atresia, biliary*.

bilirubin Yellow or orange pigment that is a breakdown product of hemoglobin. It is carried by the blood to the liver, where it is chemically changed and excreted in the bile or is conjugated and excreted by the kidneys.

Billings method See *ovulation method*.

bimanual Performed with both hands.

  b. palpation Examination of a woman's pelvic organs done by placing one hand on the abdomen and one or two fingers of the other hand in the vagina.

biopsy Removal of a small piece of tissue for microscopic examination and diagnosis.

birthing chair Chair used in labor and delivery to promote the comfort of the mother and the efficiency of parturition. The chair may be specially designed, having many technical features, or it may be a simple three-legged stool with a high, slanted back and a circular seat with a large central hole in it.

blastoderm Germinal membrane of the ovum.

  b. vesicle Stage in the development of a mammalian embryo that consists of an outer layer, or trophoblast, and a hollow sphere of cells enclosing a cavity.

bleeding diathesis See *diathesis, bleeding*.

blood-brain barrier Obstruction that prevents passage of certain substances from blood into brain tissue.

bloody show Vaginal discharge that originates in the cervix and consists of blood and mucus; increases as cervix dilates during labor.

body image Person's subjective concept of his or her physical appearance.

bonding See *attachment*.

born out of asepsis (BOA) Pertaining to birth without the use of sterile technique.

Bradley method Preparation for parenthood with active participation of father and mother.

Braxton Hicks sign Mild, intermittent, painless uterine contractions that occur during pregnancy. These contractions occur more frequently as pregnancy advances but do not represent true labor.

Braxton Hicks version One of several types of maneuvers designed to turn the fetus from an undesirable position to a more acceptable one to facilitate delivery.

Brazelton assessment Criteria for assessing the interactional behavior of a newborn.

breakthrough bleeding Escape of blood occurring between menstrual periods; may be noted by women using chemical contraception (birth control pill).

breast milk jaundice See *jaundice, breast milk*.

breech presentation Presentation in which buttocks and/or feet are nearest the cervical opening and are born first; occurs in approximately 3% of all deliveries.

  complete b. p. Simultaneous presentation of buttocks, legs, and feet.

  footling (incomplete) b.p. Presentation of one or both feet.

  frank b. p. Presentation of buttocks, with hips flexed so that thighs are against abdomen.

bregma Point of junction of the coronal and sagittal sutures of the skull; the area of the anterior fontanel of the fetus.

brim Edge of the superior strait of the true pelvis; the inlet.

bronchopulmonary dysplasia Emphysematous changes caused by oxygen toxicity.

brown fat Source of heat unique to neonates that is capable of greater thermogenic activity than ordinary fat. Deposits are found around the adrenals, kidneys, and neck, between the scapulas, and behind the sternum for several weeks after birth.

bruit, uterine Sound of passage of blood through uterine blood vessels, synchronous with fetal heart rate.

cachexia Severe generalized weakness, malnutrition, and emaciation.

caked breast See *engorgement*.

calcemia See *hypercalcemia*.

Candida vaginitis Vaginal, fungal infection; moniliasis.

capsularis, decidua See *decidua capsularis*.

caput Occiput of fetal head appearing at the vaginal introitus preceding delivery of the head.

  c. succedaneum Swelling of the tissue over the presenting part of the fetal head caused by pressure during labor.

carrier Individual who carries a gene that does not exhibit itself in physical or chemical characteristics but that can be transmitted to children (e.g., a female carrying the trait for hemophilia, which is expressed in male offspring).

catamenia Menses.

caudal anesthesia Type of regional anesthesia used in childbirth in which the anesthetic agent is injected into the caudal area of the spinal canal through the sacral hiatus, affecting the caudal nerve roots and thereby anesthetizing the cervix, vagina, and perineum. Medication does not mix with cerebrospinal fluid (CSF).

caul Hood of fetal membranes covering fetal head during delivery.

cautery Method of destroying tissue by the use of heat, electricity, or chemicals.

centesis suffix pertaining to a surgical puncture or perforation.

cephalhematoma Extravasation of blood from ruptured vessels between a skull bone and its external covering, the periosteum. Swelling is limited by the margins of the cranial bone affected (usually parietals).

cephalic Pertaining to the head.

  c. presentation Presentation of any part of the fetal head.

cephalopelvic disproportion (CPD) Condition in which the infant's head is of such a shape, size, or position that it cannot pass through the mother's pelvis.

cervical amputation Removal of the neck of the uterus.

cervical cap (custom) Individually fitted contraceptive covering for the cervix.

cervical cauterization Destruction (usually by heat or electric current) of the superficial tissue of the cervix.

cervical conization Excision of a cone-shaped section of tissue from the endocervix.

cervical erosion Alteration of the epithelium of the cervix caused by chronic irritation or infection.

cervical mucus method See *ovulation method*.

cervical os "Mouth" or opening to the cervix.

cervical polyp Small tumor on a stem (pedicle) attached inside the cervix.

cervical stenosis Narrowing of the canal between the body of the uterus and the cervical os.

cervicitis Cervical infection.

cervix Lowest and narrow end of the uterus; the "neck." The cervix is situated between the external os and the body or corpus of the uterus, and its lower end extends into the vagina.

cesarean delivery Birth of a fetus by an incision through the abdominal wall and uterus.

cesarean hysterectomy Removal of the uterus immediately after the cesarean delivery of an infant.

Chadwick's sign Violet color of mucous membrane that is visible from about the fourth week of pregnancy; caused by increased vascularity of the vagina.

change of life See *climacteric*.

chemotaxis Response involving movement that is positive (toward) or negative (away from) to a chemical stimulus.

chloasma Increased pigmentation over bridge of nose and cheeks of pregnant women and some women taking oral contraceptives; also known as *mask of pregnancy*.

choanal atresia See *atresia, choanal*.

cholecystitis Acute or chronic inflammation of the gallbladder.

cholelithiasis Presence of gallstones in the gallbladder.

choreoathetoid cerebral palsy Condition characterized by both choreiform (jerky, ticlike twitching) and athetoid (slow, writhing) movements.

chorioamnionitis Stimulated by organisms in the amniotic fluid, which then become infiltrated with polymorphonuclear leukocytes.

chorioepithelioma Carcinoma of the chorion; rapid malignant proliferation of the epithelium of the chorionic villi.

chorion Fetal membrane closest to the intrauterine wall that gives rise to the placenta and continues as the outer membrane surrounding the amnion.

chorionic villi See *villi, chorionic*.

chromosome Element within the cell nucleus carrying genes and composed of DNA and proteins.

circumcision Excision of the male's prepuce (foreskin).

cleft lip Incomplete closure of the lip; harelip.

cleft palate Incomplete closure of the palate or roof of mouth; a congenital fissure.

climacteric (change of life) Period when the human body undergoes significant psychologic and physiologic changes, such as the termination of reproductive function in the woman.

clitoris Female organ analogous to male penis; a small, ovoid body of erectile tissue situated at the anterior junction of the vulva.

　prepuce of the c. see *prepuce of the clitoris*.

coccyx Small bone at the base of the spinal column.

coitus Penile-vaginal intercourse.

　c. interruptus Intercourse during which penis is withdrawn from vagina before ejaculation.

colostrum Yellow secretion from the breast containing mainly serum and white blood corpuscles preceding the onset of true lactation 2 or 3 days after delivery.

colpectomy Surgical excision of the vagina.

colporrhaphy (1) Procedure of suturing the vagina. (2) Procedure whereby the vagina is denuded and sutured for the purpose of narrowing the vagina.

colpotomy Any surgical incision into the wall of the vagina.

communicating hydrocephalus See *hydrocephalus, communicating*.

complement Naturally occurring blood component that is a factor in the destruction of bacteria.

complementary feeding Supplemental feeding given to the infant if he is still hungry after breast feeding.

complete abortion See *abortion, complete*

complete breech presentation See *breech presentation, complete*.

compliance, lung Degree of distensibility of the lung's elastic tissue.

conception Union of the sperm and ovum resulting in fertilization; formation of the one-celled zygote.

conceptional age In fetal development, the number of completed weeks since the moment of conception. Because the moment of conception is almost impossible to determine, conceptional age is estimated at 2 weeks less than gestational age.

conceptus Embryo or fetus, fetal membranes, amniotic fluid, and the fetal portion of the placenta.

concurrent sterilization Method of preparing formula in which all the ingredients and equipment are sterilized prior to mixing.

condom Mechanical barrier worn on the penis for contraception; "rubber."

condyloma Wartlike growth on the skin usually seen near the anus or external genitals. There is a pointed type, and there is the flat, broad, moist papule of secondary syphilis.

confinement Period of childbirth and early puerperium.

congenital Present or existing before birth as a result of either heredity or prenatal environmental factors.

conjoined twins See *twins, conjoined*.

conjugate

　diagonal c. Radiographic measurement of distance from *inferior border* of SP to sacral promontory; may be obtained by vaginal examination; 12.5 to 13 cm.

　true c. (c. vera) Radiographic measurement of distance from *upper margin* of symphysis pubis (SP) to sacral promontory; 1.5 to 2 cm less than diagonal conjugate.

conjunctivitis Inflammation of the mucous membrane that lines the eyelids and that is reflected onto the eyeball.

consanguinity Existing blood relationship between persons.

contraception Prevention of impregnation or conception.

contraction ring See *Bandl's ring*.

Coombs' test Indirect: determination of Rh-positive antibodies in maternal blood; direct: determination of maternal Rh-positive antibodies in fetal cord blood. A positive test result indicates the presence of antibodies or titer.

coping mechanism Any effort directed at stress management. It can be task oriented and involve direct problem-solving efforts to cope with the threat itself or be intrapsychic or ego defense oriented with the goal of regulating one's emotional distress.

copulation Coitus; sexual intercourse.

corpus Discrete mass of material.

c. cavernosum Term referring to one of two cylinders of spongy tissue within the penis or tissue within the clitoris that engorges with blood during sexual excitement resulting in erection.

c. luteum Yellow body. After rupture of the graafian follicle at ovulation, the follicle develops into a yellow structure that secretes progesterone in the second half of the menstrual cycle, atrophying about 3 days before sloughing of the endometrium in menstrual flow. If impregnation occurs, this structure continues to produce progesterone until the placenta can take over this function.

c. spongiosum One of the spongy cylinders of tissue within the penis; has a protective function.

cotyledon One of the 15 to 28 visible segments of the placenta on the maternal surface, each made up of fetal vessels, chorionic villi, and an intervillous space.

couvade Custom whereby the husband goes through mock labor while his wife is giving birth.

Couvelaire uterus See *uterus, Couvelaire*.

CPAP Continuous positive airway pressure.

cradle cap Common seborrheic dermatitis of infants consisting of thick, yellow, greasy scales on the scalp.

craniotabes Localized softening of cranial bones.

creatinine Substance found in blood and muscle; measurement of levels in maternal urine correlates with amount of fetal muscle mass and therefore fetal size.

Crede's method Obsolete method by which the placenta is expelled by downward manual pressure on the uterus through the abdominal wall. The thumb is placed on the posterior surface of the fundus of the uterus and the flat of the hand on the anterior surface. Pressure is applied in the direction of the birth canal.

Crede's prophylaxis Instillation of 1% silver nitrate solution into the conjunctivas of newborn infants immediately after birth to prevent ophthalmia neonatorum, particularly that caused by gonorrheal organisms.

crepitus (1) Noise produced when pressure is applied to tissues containing abnormal amounts of air. (2) Grating sound heard when broken bone ends are moved. (3) Noise of gas being expelled from the intestines.

crib death Unexpected and sudden death of an apparently normal and healthy infant that occurs during sleep and with no physical or autopsic evidence of disease. Also referred to as sudden infant death syndrome (SIDS).

cri-du-chat syndrome Rare congenital disorder recognized at birth by a kittenlike cry, which may prevail for weeks, then disappear. Other characteristics include low birth weight, microcephaly, "moon face," wide-set eyes, strabismus, and low-set misshaped ears. Infants are hypotonic; heart defects and mental and physical retardation are common. Also called cat-cry syndrome.

crowning Stage of delivery when the top of the fetal head can be seen at the vaginal orifice.

cryo- Prefix meaning cold, freezing.

cryosurgery Local freezing and removal of tissue without injury to adacent tissue and with minimum blood loss, done with special equipment.

cryptochidism Failure of one or both of the testicles to descend into the scrotum. Also called undescended testis.

cul-de-sac of Douglas Pouch formed by a fold of the peritoneum dipping down between the anterior wall of the rectum and the posterior wall of the uterus; also called *Douglas' cul-de-sac, pouch of Douglas,* and *rectouterine pouch.*

culdocentesis Use of needle puncture or incision to remove intraperitoneal fluid (blood, purulent material) by way of the vagina.

culdotomy Incision or needle puncture of the cul-de-sac of Douglas by way of the vagina.

Cullen's sign Faint, irregularly formed, hemorrhagic patches on the skin around the umbilicus. The discolored skin is blue-black and becomes greenish brown or yellow. Cullen's sign may appear 1 to 2 days after the onset of anorexia and the severe, poorly localized abdominal pains characteristic of acute pancreatitis. Cullen's sign is also present in massive upper gastrointestinal hemorrhage, ruptured ectopic pregnancy.

culture The total learned way of life of a society.

curettage Scraping of the endometrium lining of the uterus with a curet to remove the contents of the uterus (as is done after an inevitable or incomplete abortion) or to obtain specimens for diagnostic purposes.

cutis marmorata Transient vasomotor phenomenon occurring primarily over extremities when the infant is exposed to chilling. It appears as a pink or faint purple capillary outline on the skin. Occasionally it is seen if the infant is in respiratory distress.

cyesis Pregnancy.

cystocele Bladder hernia; injury to the vesicovaginal fascia during labor and delivery may allow herniation of the bladder into the vagina.

cytogenics Branch of genetics concerned primarily with the study of chromosomes and correlations with associated gene behavior.

cytology The study of cells, including their formation, origin, structure, function, biochemical activities, and pathology.

death Cessation of life.

fetal d. Intrauterine death. Death of a fetus weighing 500 g or more of 20 weeks' gestation or more.

infant d. Death during the first year of life.

maternal d. Death of a woman during the childbearing cycle.

neonatal d. Death of a newborn within the first 28 days after birth.

perinatal d. Death of a fetus of 20 weeks' gestation or older or death of a neonate 28 days old or younger.

decidua Mucous membrane, lining of uterus, or endometrium of pregnancy that is shed after giving birth.

d. basalis Maternal aspect of the placenta made up of uterine blood vessels, endometrial stroma, and glands. It is shed in lochial discharge after delivery.

d. capsularis That part of the decidual membranes surrounding the chorionic sac.

d. vera Nonplacental decidual lining of the uterus.

decrement Decrease or stage of decline, as of a contraction.

deletion Loss of a piece of a chromosome that has broken off.

delivery Expulsion of the child with placenta and membranes by the mother or their extraction by the obstetric practitioner.

abdominal d. See *abdominal delivery.*

ΔOD$_{450}$ (read delta OD$_{450}$) Delta optical density (or absorbance) at 450 nm, obtained by spectral analysis of amniotic fluid. This prenatal test is used to measure the degree of hemolytic activity in the fetus and to evaluate fetal status in women sensitized to Rh(D).

deoxyribonucleic acid (DNA) Intracellular complex protein that carries genetic information, consisting of two purines (adenine and guanine) and two pyrimidines (thymine and cytosine).

dermatoglyphics Study of skin ridge patterns on fingers, toes, palms of hands, and soles of feet.

DES Diethylstilbestrol, used in treating menopausal symptoms. Exposure of female fetus predisposes her to reproductive tract malformations and (later) dysplasia.

desquamation Shedding of epithelial cells of the skin and mucous membranes.

developmental crisis Severe, usually transient, stress that occurs when a person is unable to complete the tasks of a psychosocial stage of development and is therefore unable to move on to the next stage.

developmental task Physical or cognitive skill that a child must accomplish during a particular age period in order to continue developing, as walking, which precedes the development of sense of autonomy in the toddler period.

diaphragmatic hernia Congenital malformation of diaphragm that allows displacement of the abdominal organs into the thoracic cavity.

diastasis recti abdominis Separation of the two rectus muscles along the median line of the abdominal wall. This is often seen in women with repeated childbirths or with a multiple gestation (triplets, etc.). In the newborn it is usually due to incomplete development.

diathesis Hereditary condition, tendency, or susceptibility of an individual to some abnormality or disease.

  bleeding d. Predisposition to abnormal blood clotting.

DIC Disseminated intravascular coagulation.

Dick-Read method An approach to childbirth based on the premise that fear of pain produces muscular tension, producing pain and greater fear. The method includes teaching physiological processes of labor, exercise to improve muscle tone, and techniques to assist in relaxation and prevent the fear-tension-pain mechanism.

dilatation of cervix Stretching of the external os from an opening a few millimeters in size to an opening large enough to allow the passage of the infant.

dilatation and curettage (D and C) Vaginal operation in which the cervical canal is stretched enough to admit passage of an instrument called a *curet*. The endometrium of the uterus is scraped with the curet to empty the uterine contents or to obtain tissue for examination.

discordance Discrepancy in size (or other indicator) between twins.

disparate twins See *twins, disparate*.

disseminated lupus erythematosus Chronic inflammatory disease affecting many systems of the body. The pathophysiology of the disease includes severe vasculitis, renal involvement, and lesions of the skin and nervous system. The primary cause of the disease has not been determined; viral infection or dysfunction of the immune system has been suggested. Also called systemic lupus erythematosus (SLE).

diverticulum Pouch-like herniation through muscular wall of a tubular organ. A diverticulum may be present in the stomach, small intestine, or, most commonly, in the colon.

dizygotic Related to or proceeding from two zygotes (fertilized ova).

dizygous twins See *twins, dizygous*.

Döderlein's bacillus Gram-positive bacterium occurring in normal vaginal secretions.

dominant trait Gene that is expressed whenever it is present in the heterozygous gene state (e.g., brown eyes are dominant over blue).

Douglas' cul-de-sac See *cul-de-sac of Douglas*.

Down's syndrome Abnormality involving the occurrence of a third chromosome, rather than the normal pair (trisomy 21), that characteristically results in a typical picture of mental retardation and altered physical appearance. This condition was formerly called *mongolism* or *mongoloid idiocy*.

dry labor Lay term referring to labor in which amniotic fluid has already escaped. A "dry birth" does not exist.

Dubowitz assessment Estimation of gestational age of a newborn, based on criteria developed for that purpose.

ductus arteriosus In fetal circulation, an anatomic shunt between the pulmonary artery and arch of the aorta. It is obliterated after birth by a rising Po_2 and change in intravascular pressures in the presence of normal pulmonary function. It normally becomes a ligament after birth but in some instances remains patent.

ductus venosus In fetal circulation, a blood vessel carrying oxygenated blood between the umbilical vein and the inferior vena cava, bypassing the liver. It is obliterated and becomes a ligament after birth.

Duncan's mechanism Delivery of placenta with the maternal surface presenting, rather than the shiny fetal surface.

dura (dura mater) Outermost, toughest of the three meninges covering the brain and spinal cord.

dynamic ileus Spastic ileus; intestinal obstruction characterized by recurrent and continuous spasms (sudden muscular contractions).

dys- Prefix meaning abnormal, difficult, painful, faulty.

dyscrasia Incompatible mixture (e.g., fetal and maternal blood incompatibility).

dysfunction, placental See *placental dysfunction*.

dysfunctional uterine bleeding Abnormal bleeding from the uterus for reasons that are not readily established.

dysmaturity See *intrauterine growth retardation (IUGR)*.

dysmenorrhea Difficult or painful menstruation.

dysmorphogenesis Development of ill-shaped or malformed structures.

dyspareunia Painful sexual intercourse.

dystocia Prolonged, painful, or otherwise difficult delivery or birth because of mechanical factors produced by either the passenger (the fetus) or the passage (the pelvis of the mother) or because of inadequate powers (uterine and other muscular activity).

  placental d. Difficulty in the delivery of the placenta.

ecchymosis Bruise; bleeding into tissue caused by direct trauma, serious infection, or bleeding diathesis.

eclampsia Severe complication of pregnancy of unknown cause and occurring more often in the primigravida; characterized by tonic and clonic convulsions, coma, high blood pressure, albuminuria, and oliguria occurring during pregnancy or shortly after delivery.

ectoderm Outer layer of embryonic tissue giving rise to skin, nails, and hair.

ectopic Out of normal place.

  e. pregnancy Implantation of the fertilized ovum outside of its normal place in the uterine cavity. Locations include the abdomen, fallopian tubes, and ovaries.

EDC Expected date of confinement; "due date."

effacement Thinning and shortening or obliteration of the cervix that occurs during late pregnancy or labor or both.

effleurage Gentle stroking used in massage.

ejaculation Sudden expulsion of semen from the male urethra.

elective abortion See *abortion, elective*.

electroshock (therapy) Induction of a brief convulsion by passing an electric current through the brain for the treatment of affective disorders, especially in clients resistant to psychoactive drug therapy. Also called electroconvulsive therapy (ECT).

embolus Any undissolved matter (solid, liquid, or gaseous) that is carried by the blood to another part of the body and obstructs a blood vessel.

embryo Conceptus from the second or third week of development until about the eighth week after conception, when mineralization (ossification) of the skeleton begins. This period is characterized by cellular differentiation and predominantly hyperplastic growth.

empathy Projection of one's own consciousness and awareness onto that of another so as to obtain an objective awareness of and insight into the emotions, feelings, and behavior of another person and their meaning and significance. Empathy may be distinguished from sympathy in that sympathy is usually nonobjective and noncritical, whereas the state of empathy includes relative freedom from emotional involvement.

endocervical Pertaining to the interior of the canal of the cervix of the uterus.

endocrine glands Ductless glands that secrete hormones into the blood or lymph.

endometriosis Tissue closely resembling endometrial tissue but aberrantly located outside the uterus in the pelvic cavity. Symptomatology may include pelvic pain or pressure, dysmenorrhea, dyspareunia, abnormal bleeding from the uterus or rectum, and sterility.

endometrium Inner lining of the uterus that undergoes changes caused by hormones during the menstrual cycle and pregnancy; decidua.

engagement In obstetrics, the entrance of the fetal presenting part into the superior pelvic strait and the beginning of the descent through the pelvic canal.

engorgement Distention or vascular congestion. In obstetrics, the process of swelling of the breast tissue brought about by an increase in blood and lymph supply to the breast, which precedes true lactation. It lasts about 48 hours and usually reaches a peak between the third and fifth postdelivery days.

engrossment Sustained involvement of a parent with an infant.

entoderm Inner layer of embryonic tissue giving rise to internal organs such as the intestine.

entrainment Phenomenon observed in the microanalysis of sound films in which the speaker moves several parts of the body and the listener responds to the sounds by moving in ways that are coordinated with the rhythm of the sounds. Infants have been observed to move in time to the rhythms of adult speech but not to random noises or disconnected words or vowels. Entrainment is thought to be an essential factor in the process of maternal-infant bonding.

epicanthus Fold of skin covering the inner canthus and caruncle that extends from the root of the nose to the median end of the eyebrow; characteristically found in certain races but may occur as a congenital anomaly.

episiotomy Surgical incision of the perineum at the end of the second stage of labor to facilitate delivery and to avoid laceration of the perineum. (See also *perineotomy*.)

epispadias Defect in which the urethral canal terminates on dorsum of penis or above the clitoris (rare).

Epstein's pearls Small, white blebs found along the gum margins and at the junction of the soft and hard palates. They are a normal manifestation and are commonly seen in the newborn. Similar to Bohn's nodules.

epulis Tumorlike benign lesion of the gingiva seen in pregnant women.

equilibrium A state of balance or rest owing to the equal action of opposing forces, as calcium and phosphorus in the body. In psychiatry, a state of mental or emotional balance.

Erb-Duchenne paralysis Paralysis caused by traumatic injury to the upper brachial plexus, occurring most commonly in childbirth from forcible traction during delivery. The signs of Erb's paralysis include loss of sensation in the arm and paralysis and atrophy of the deltoid, the biceps, and the branchialis muscles. Also called Erb's palsy.

ergot Drug obtained from *Claviceps purpurea*, a fungus, which stimulates the smooth muscles of blood vessels and the uterus, causing vasoconstriction and uterine contractions.

erythema toxicum Innocuous pink papular neonatal rash of unknown cause, with superimposed vesicles appearing within 24 to 48 hours after birth and resolving spontaneously within a few days.

erythroblastosis fetalis Hemolytic disease of the newborn usually caused by isoimmunization resulting from Rh incompatibility or ABO incompatibility.

erythropoiesis Erythrocyte (RBC) production, which involves the maturation of a nucleated precursor into a hemoglobin-filled, nucleus-free erythrocyte regulated by erythropoietin, a hormone produced by the kidney.

escutcheon Pattern of distribution of pubic hair.

esophageal atresia See *atresia, esophageal.*

estradiol An estrogen.

estrangement, psychologic Reaction to the birth of and subsequent separation from a sick and/or premature infant, whereby the mother is diverted from establishing a normal relationship with her baby.

estriol Major metabolite of estrogen that increases during the second half of pregnancy with an intact fetoplacental unit (normal placenta, normal fetal liver and adrenals) and normal maternal renal function.

estrogen Female sex hormone produced by the ovaries and placenta

estrus Cyclic period of sexual activity in mammals other than primates; state of being in heat.

ethnocentrism Belief in the inherent superiority of the race or group to which one belongs. Also a proclivity to consider other ethnic groups in terms of one's own racial origins.

eu- Prefix meaning normal, good, well, easy.

eugenics Science that deals with the improvement of the human race through control of hereditary (genetic) factors by voluntary social action.

euthenics Science that deals with the improvement of the human race through the control of environmental factors (pollution, drug abuse, malnutrition, and disease).

eutocia Normal or natural labor or birth.

exchange transfusion Replacement of 75% to 85% of circulating blood by withdrawing the recipient's blood and injecting a donor's blood in equal amounts, the purposes of which are to prevent an accumulation of bilirubin in the blood above a dangerous level, to prevent the accumulation of other by-products of hemolysis in hemolytic disease, and to correct anemia.

exocervix Outer layer of the portion of the cervix that protrudes into the vagina; ectocervix.

exostosis Benign cartilage-covered hump on the surface of a bone, often resulting from chronic irritation.

expulsive Having the tendency to drive out or expel.

    e. contractions Labor contractions that are characteristic of the second stage of labor.

exstrophy Eversion; the turning inside out of a part.

extension Straightening of a body part; opposite of flexion.

extraperitoneal Occurring or located outside the peritoneal cavity.

extrauterine Occurring outside the uterus.

  e. pregnancy Ectopic pregnancy in which the fertilized ovum implants itself outside the uterus.

facies Pertaining to the appearance or expression of the face; certain congenital syndromes typically present with a specific facial appearance.

FAD Fetal activity determination.

failure to thrive Condition in which neonate's or infant's growth and development patterns are below the norms for age.

fallopian tubes Two canals or oviducts extending laterally from each side of the uterus through which the ovum travels, after ovulation, to the uterus.

false labor Uterine contractions that do not result in cervical dilatation, are irregular, are felt more in front, often do not last more than 20 seconds, and do not become longer or stronger.

false pelvis The part of the pelvis superior to a plane passing through the linea terminalis.

familial Pertaining to a condition present in more members of a family than would be expected by chance.

fecundation Act of fertilization or impregnation.

fecundity Ability to bear children frequently and in large numbers.

Ferguson's reflex Reflex contractions of the uterus after stimulation of the cervix.

ferning (arborization) test The appearance of a fernlike pattern in dried smears of uterine cervical mucus, indicating the presence of estrogen.

  ovulation f. t. Test in which cervical mucus, placed on a slide, dries in a branching pattern in the presence of high estrogen levels at the time of ovulation.

  pregnancy f. t. Test in which cervical mucus, placed on a slide, does not dry in a branching pattern because of high levels of progesterone along with estrogen.

fertility Quality of being able to reproduce.

fertility rate Number of births per 1000 women aged 15 through 44 years.

fertilization Union of an ovum and a sperm.

fetal Pertaining or relating to the fetus.

  f. alcholol syndrome Congenital abnormality or anomaly resulting from maternal alcohol intake above 3 oz. of absolute alcohol per day. It is characterized by typical craniofacial and limb defects, cardiovascular defects, intrauterine growth retardation, and developmental delay.

  f. alveoli See *alveoli, fetal.*

  f. attitude See *attitude, fetal.*

  f. asphyxia See *asphyxia, fetal.*

  f. death See *death, fetal.*

  f. distress Evidence such as a change in the fetal heartbeat pattern or activity indicating that the fetus is in jeopardy.

  f. lie Relation of the fetal spine to the maternal spine; i. e., in vertical lie, maternal and fetal spines are parallel and the fetal head or breech presents; in transverse lie, fetal spine is perpendicular to the maternal spine and the fetal shoulder presents.

  f. presentation The part of the fetus that presents at the cervical os.

fetofetal transfusion See *parabiotic syndrome.*

α-fetoprotein (AFP) Fetal antigen; elevated levels in amniotic fluid associated with neural tube defects.

fetotoxic Poisonous or destructive to the fetus.

fetus Child in utero from about the eighth week after conception, until birth.

fibroid Fibrous, encapsulated connective tissue tumor, especially of the uterus.

fimbria Structure resembling a fringe, particularly the fringelike end of the fallopian tube.

FiO₂ (fraction of inspired oxygen) Percentage of oxygen a person is receiving.

fissure Groove or open crack in tissue.

fistula Abormal tubelike passage that forms between two normal cavities, possibly congenital or caused by trauma, abscesses, or inflammatory processes.

flaccid Having relaxed, flabby, or absent muscle tone.

flaring of nostrils Widening of nostrils (alae nasi) during inspiration in the presence of air hunger; sign of respiratory distress.

flexion In obstetrics, resistance to the descent of the baby down the birth canal causes the head to flex, or bend, so that the chin approaches the chest. Thus the smallest diameter (suboccipitobregmatic) of the vertex presents.

fluid, amniotic See *amniotic fluid.*

folic acid deficiency anemia Anemia caused by lack of folic acid in the diet.

follicle Small secretory cavity or sac.

  graafian f. Mature, fully developed ovarian cyst containing the ripe ovum. The follicle secretes estrogens, and after ovulation, the corpus luteum develops within the ruptured graafian follicle and secretes estrogen and progesterone.

follicle-stimulating hormone (FSH) Hormone produced by the anterior pituitary during the first half of the menstrual cycle. Stimulates development of the graafian follicle.

fomites Nonliving material on which disease-producing organisms may be conveyed (e.g., bed linen).

fontanel Broad area, or soft spot, consisting of a strong band of connective tissue contiguous with cranial bones and located at the junctions of the bones.

  anterior f. Diamond-shaped area between the frontal and two parietal bones just above the baby's forehead at the junction of the coronal and sagittal sutures.

  mastoid f. Posterolateral fontanel usually not palpable.

  posterior f. Small, triangular area between the occipital and parietal bones at the junction of the lambdoidal and sagittal sutures.

  sagittal f. Soft area located in the sagittal suture, halfway between the anterior and posterior fontanels; may be found in normal newborns and in some neonates with Down's syndrome.

  sphenoid f. Anterolateral fontanel usually not palpable.

footling (incomplete) breech presentation See *breech presentation, footling.*

foramen ovale Septal opening between the atria of the fetal heart. The opening normally closes shortly after birth, but if it remains patent, surgical repair usually is necessary.

foreskin Prepuce, or loose fold of skin covering the glans penis.

fornix Any structure with an arched or vaultlike shape.

  f. of the vagina Anterior and posterior spaces, formed by the protrusion of the cervix into the vagina, into which the upper vagina is divided.

fossa Shallow depression.

fourchet Tense band of mucous membranes at the posterior angle of the vagina connecting the posterior ends of the labia minora.

Fowler's position Posture assumed by client when head of bed is raised 18 or 20 inches and individual's knees are elevated.

frank breech presentation See *breech presentation, frank.*

fraternal twins Nonidentical twins that come from two separate fertilized ova.

frenulum Thin ridge of tissue in midline of undersurface of tongue extending from its base to varying distances from the tip of the tongue.

Friedman's curve Labor curve; pattern of descent of presenting part and of dilatation of cervix; partogram.

Friedman's test Modification of the Aschheim-Zondek pregnancy test: the urine of a woman suspected of pregnancy is injected into a mature, unmated female rabbit. If at the end of 2 days of these injections, the ovaries of the rabbit contain fresh corpora lutea or hemorrhagic corpora, the test is positive, signifying that the woman is pregnant.

frigidity Archaic term designating a woman's inability to achieve orgasm; orgasmic dysfunction.

FSH See *follicle-stimulating hormone.*

fulguration Destruction of tissue by means of electricity.

fundus Dome-shaped upper portion of the uterus between the points of insertion of the fallopian tubes.

funic souffle See *souffle, funic.*

funis Cordlike structure, especially the umbilical cord.

galacto-, galact- Combining form denoting milk.

galactorrhea Excessive flow or secretion of milk.

galactosemia Inherited, autosomal recessive disorder of galactose metabolism, characterized by a deficiency of the enzyme galactose-l-phosphate uridyl transferase.

gamete Mature male or female germ cell; the mature sperm or ovum.

gastroschisis Abdominal wall defect at base of umbilical stalk.

gastrostomy Surgical creation of an artificial opening into the stomach through the abdominal wall, performed to feed a client when oral feeding is not possible.

gastrula Early embryonic stage of development that follows the blastula.

gate control theory Proposed in 1965 by Melzack and Wall, this theory explains the neurophysical mechanism underlying the perception of pain.

gavage Feeding by means of a tube passed to the stomach.

gender identity The sense or awareness of knowing to which sex one belongs. The process begins in infancy, continues throughout childhood, and is reinforced during adolescence.

gene Factor on a chromosome responsible for hereditary characteristics of offspring.

generative Capable of reproduction.

genetic Dependent of the genes. A genetic disorder may or may not be apparent at birth.

genetic counseling Process of determining the occurrence or risk of occurrence of a genetic disorder within a family and of providing appropriate information and advice about the courses of action that are available, whether care of a child already affected, prenatal diagnosis, termination of a pregnancy, sterilization, or artificial insemination is involved.

genetics Biologic science that deals with the genetic transmission of physical and chemical characteristics from parents to offspring, as well as the influence of environmental agents on genes and genetic expression.

genitalia Organs of reproduction.

genotype Hereditary combinations in an individual determining his physical and chemical characteristics. Some genotypes are not expressed until later in life (e.g., Huntington's chorea); some hide recessive genes, which can be expressed in offspring; and others are expressed only under the proper environmental conditions (e.g., diabetes mellitus appearing under the stress of obesity or pregnancy).

gestation Period of intrauterine fetal development from conception through birth; the period of pregnancy.

abdominal g. See *abdominal gestation.*

gestational age In fetal development, the number of completed weeks counting from the first day of the last normal menstrual cycle.

glabella Bony prominence above the nose and between the eyebrows.

glans penis Smooth, round head of the penis, analogous to the female glans clitoris.

glomerulonephritis Noninfectious disease of the glomerulus of the kidney, characterized by proteinuria, hematuria, decreased urine production, and edema.

glycosuria Presence of glucose (a sugar) in the urine.

gonad Gamete-producing, or sex, gland; the ovary or testis.

gonadotropic hormone Hormone that stimulates the gonads.

Goodell's sign Softening of the cervix, a probable sign of pregnancy, occurring during the second month.

gossypol Oral contraceptive produced from cotton plants; currently in experimental stage of use by males in the United States.

graafian follicle (vesicle) See *follicle, graafian.*

gravid Pregnant.

grieving process A complex of somatic and psychological symptoms associated with some extreme sorrow or loss, specifically the death of a loved one.

grunt, expiratory Sign of respiratory distress (hyaline membrane disease [respiratory distress syndrome, or RDS] or advanced pneumonia) indicative of the body's attempt to hold air in the alveoli for better gaseous exchange.

gynecoid pelvis Pelvis in which the inlet is round instead of oval or blunt; heart shaped. Typical female pelvis.

gynecology Study of the diseases of the female, especially of the genital, urinary, and rectal organs.

habitual (recurrent) abortion See *abortion, habitual.*

habituation An acquired tolerance from repeated exposure to a particular stimulus. Also called negative adaptation; a decline and eventual elimination of a conditioned response by repetition of the conditioned stimulus.

habitus Indications in appearance of tendency or disposition to disease or abormal conditions.

harlequin sign Rare color change of no pathologic significance occurring between the longitudinal halves of the neonate's body. When infant is placed on one side, the dependent half is noticeably pinker than the superior half.

Hegar's sign Softening of the lower uterine segment that is classified as a probable sign of pregnancy and that may be present during the second and third months of pregnancy and is palpated during bimanual examination.

hematocrit Volume of red blood cells per deciliter (dl) of circulating blood; packed cell volume (PCV).

hematoma Collection of blood in a tissue; a bruise or blood tumor.

hemoconcentration Increase in the number of red blood cells resulting from either a decrease in plasma volume or increased erythropoiesis.

hemoglobin Component of red blood cells consisting of globin, a protein, and hematin, an organic iron compound.

h. electrophoresis Test to diagnose sickle cell disease in newborns. Cord blood is used.

hemorrhagic disease of newborn Bleeding disorder during first few days of life based on a deficiency of vitamin K.

hereditary Pertaining to a trait or characteristic transmitted from parent to offspring by way of the genes; used synonymously with *genetic.*

hermaphrodite Person having genital and sexual characteristics of both sexes.

heterologous insemination Artificial insemination in which the semen specimen is provided by an anonymous donor. The procedure is used primarily in cases where the husband is sterile. Also called artificial insemination donor (AID).

heterozygous Having two dissimilar genes at the same site, or locus, on paired chromosomes (e.g., at the sites for eye color, one chromosome carrying the gene for brown, the other for blue).

high risk An increased possibility of suffering harm, damage, loss, or death.

hirsutism Condition characterized by the excessive growth of hair or the growth of hair in unusual places.

Homans' sign Early sign of phlebothrombosis of the deep veins of the calf in which there are complaints of pain when the leg is in extension and the foot is dorsiflexed.

homoiothermic Referring to the ability of warm-blooded animals to maintain internal temperature at a specified level regardless of the environmental temperature. This ability is not fully developed in the human neonate.

homologous Similar in structure or origin but not necessarily in function.

homologous insemination Artificial insemination in which the semen specimen is provided by the husband. The procedure is used primarily in cases of impotence or when the husband is incapable of sexual intercourse because of some physical disability. Also called artificial insemination husband (AIH).

homozygous Having two similar genes at the same locus, or site, on paired chromosomes.

hormone Chemical substance produced in an organ or gland that is conveyed through the blood to another organ or part of the body, stimulating it to increased functional activity or secretion. See specific hormones.

hour-glass uterus Uterus in which a segment of circular muscle fibers contracts during labor. The resultant "constriction ring" dystocia is characterized by lack of progress in spite of adequate contractions; by pain experienced prior to palpation of a uterine contraction and persisting after the observer feels the contraction end; and by recession of the presenting part during a contraction, instead of descent of the presenting part.

human chorionic gonadotropin (HCG) See *prolan*.

human chorionic somatomammotropin (HCS) Another term for human placental lactogen (HPL) and placental growth hormone.

hyaline membrane disease (HMD) Disease characterized by interference with ventilation at the alveolar level, theoretically caused by the presence of fibrinoid deposits lining alveolar ducts. Membrane formation is related to prematurity (especially with fetal asphyxia) and insufficient surfactant production (L/S ratio less than 2:1). Otherwise known as *respiratory distress syndrome (RDS)*.

hydatidiform mole Abnormal pregnancy characterized by a degenerative process in the chorionic villi that produces high levels of human chorionic gonadotropin (HCG), multiple cysts, and rapid growth of the uterus with hemorrhage. Signs and symptoms include vaginal bleeding, the discharge containing grapelike vesicles. Sequela may be chorioadenoma, a highly malignant neoplasm.

hydramnios (polyhydramnios) Amniotic fluid in excess of 1.5L; often indicative of fetal anomaly and frequently seen in poorly controlled, insulin-dependent, diabetic pregnant women even if there is not coexisting fetal anomaly.

hydremia Excess of watery fluid in the blood.

hydrocele Collection of fluid in a saclike cavity, especially in the sac that surrounds the testis, causing the scrotum to swell.

hydrocephalus Excessive accumulation of cerebrospinal fluid within the ventricles of the brain resulting from interference with normal circulation and absorption of the cerebrospinal fluid and especially from the destruction of the foramens of Magendie and Luschka because of congenital anomaly, infection, injury, or brain tumor. In infants, the increased head diameter is possible because the sutures of the skull have not closed.

    communicating h. Hydrocephalus in which normal communication between the fourth ventricle and the subarachnoid space is maintained, allowing cerebral fluid to circulate into the lumbar thecal space.

    noncommunicating h. Failure of the ventricular fluid to empty into the lumbar thecal space because of an obstruction.

hydropic Dropsical or pertaining to dropsy; abnormal accumulation of serous fluid in the body tissues and cavities.

hydrops fetalis Most severe expression of fetal hemolytic disorder, a possible sequela to maternal Rh isoimmunization; infants exhibit gross edema (anasarca), cardiac decompensation, and profound pallor from anemia and seldom survive.

hymen Membranous fold that normally partially covers the entrance to the vagina in the virgin.

hymenal caruncles Small, irregular bits of tissue that are remnants of the hymen.

hymenal tag Normally occurring redundant hymenal tissue protruding from the floor of the vagina that disappears spontaneously in a few weeks after birth.

hymenotomy Surgical incision of the hymen.

hyperbilirubinemia Elevation of unconjugated serum bilirubin concentrations.

hypercalcemia Excess of calcium in the blood.

hypercapnia Excessive arterial Pco_2 caused by inadequate ventilation. In greater degrees it acts as a respiratory depressant.

hypercarbia Greater than normal amounts of carbon dioxide in the blood. Also called hypercapnia.

hyperemesis gravidarum Abnormal condition of pregnancy characterized by protracted vomiting, weight loss, and fluid and electrolyte imbalance.

hyperesthesia Unusual sensibility to sensory stimuli, such as pain or touch.

hyperlipidemia Excessive amount of fats in the blood.

hypermagnesemia Excessive amount of serum magnesium; in obstetrics, it occurs in the mother or fetus or both after the mother is treated with magnesium sulfate for preeclampsia-eclampsia.

hyperplasia Increase in number of cells; formation of new tissue.

hyperreflexia Increased action of the reflexes.

hypertrophy Enlargement, or increase in size, of existing cells.

hyperventilation Rapid, shallow (or prolonged, deep) respirations resulting in respiratory alkalosis: a decrease in H^+ concentration and Pco_2 and an increase in the blood pH and the ratio of $NaHCO_3$ to H_2CO_3. Symptoms may include faintness, palpitations, and carpopedal (hands and feet) muscular spasms. Relief may result from rebreathing in a paper bag or into one's cupped hands to replace the CO_2 "blown off" during hyperventilation.

hypocalcemia Deficiency of calcium in the serum that may be caused by hypoparathyroidism, vitamin D deficiency, kidney failure, acute pancreatitis, or inadequate plasma magnesium and protein.

hypochlorhydria Diminished secretion of hydrochloric acid.

hypofibrinogenemia Deficient level of a blood clotting factor, fibrinogen, in the blood; in obstetrics, it occurs following complications of abruptio placentae or retention of a dead fetus.

hypogastric Pertaining to the lower middle of the abdomen or hypogastrium.

hypogastric arteries Branches of the right and left iliac arteries carrying deoxygenated blood from the fetus through the umbilical cord, where they are known as *umbilical arteries,* to the placenta.

hypoglycemia Less-than-normal amount of glucose in the blood, usually caused by administration of too much insulin, excessive secretion of insulin by the islet cells of the pancreas, or by dietary deficiency.

hypospadias Anomalous positioning of urinary meatus on undersurface of penis or close to or just inside the vagina.

hypotensive drugs Drugs that lower the blood pressure.

hypothalamus Portion of the diencephalon of the brain forming the floor and part of the lateral wall of the third ventricle. It activates, controls, and integrates the peripheral autonomic nervous system, endocrine processes, and many somatic functions, as body temperature, sleep, and appetite.

hypothenar Fleshy elevation on the ulnar (little finger) side of the palm of the hand. Also called *hypothenar eminence.*

hypotonia Reduced tension; relaxation of arteries. Also, loss of tonicity of the muscles or intraocular pressure.

hypoxemia Reduction in arterial Po_2 resulting in metabolic acidosis by forcing anaerobic glycolysis, pulmonary vasoconstriction, and direct cellular damage.

hypoxia Insufficient availability of oxygen to meet the metabolic needs of body tissue.

hysterectomy Surgical removal of the uterus.

 abdominal h. See *abdominal hysterectomy.*

 panhysterectomy Removal of entire uterus, but ovaries and tubes remain.

 subtotal h. Removal of fundus and body of the uterus, but the cervical stump remains.

 total h. Removal of entire uterus, including the cervix, but the ovaries and tubes remain.

hysterosalpingography Recording by x-ray of the uterus and uterine tubes after injecting them with radiopaque material.

hysterotomy Surgical incision into the uterus.

iatrogenic Caused by a physician's words, actions, or treatment.

icterus gravis Acute yellow atrophy of the liver with cerebral disorders.

icterus neonatorum Jaundice in the newborn.

idiopathic respiratory distress syndrome (hyaline membrane disease) Severe respiratory condition found almost exclusively in premature infants and in some infants of diabetic mothers regardless of gestational age. See also *hyaline membrane disease (HMD).*

IDM Infant of a diabetic mother.

IgA Primary immunoglobulin in colostrum

IgG Transplacentally acquired immunoglobulin that confers passive immunity against the infections to which the mother is immune.

IgM Immunoglobulin neonate can manufacture soon after birth. Fetus produces it in the presence of amnionitis.

iliopectineal line Bony ridge on the inner surface of the ilium and pubic bones that divides the true and false pelvises; the brim of the true pelvic cavity; the inlet.

immature baby Infant usually weighing less than 1134 g (2½ lb) and who is considerably underdeveloped at birth.

implantation Embedding of the fertilized ovum in the uterine mucosa; nidation.

impotence Archaic term designating a man's inability, partial or complete, to perform sexual intercourse or to achieve orgasm; erectile dysfunction.

impregnate To fertilize, or make pregnant.

inanition Pathophysiologic condition of the body resulting from lack of food and water; starvation.

inborn error of metabolism Hereditary deficiency of a specific enzyme needed for normal metabolism of specific chemicals (e.g. deficiency of phenylalanine hydroxylase results in phenylketonuria [PKU]; a deficiency of hexosaminidase results in Tay-Sachs disease).

incompetent cervix Cervix that is unable to remain closed until a pregnancy reaches term, because of a mechanical defect in the cervix resulting in dilatation and effacement usually during the second or early third trimester of pregnancy.

incomplete abortion See *abortion, incomplete.*

increment An increase, or buildup, as of a contraction.

incubator Apparatus used for an infant in which the temperature may be regulated.

induced abortion See *abortion, induced.*

induction Artificial stimulation or augmentation of labor.

inertia Sluggishness or inactivity; in obstetrics, refers to the absence or weakness of uterine contractions during labor.

inevitable abortion See *abortion, inevitable.*

infant A child who is under 1 year of age.

infantile uterus Uterus that has failed to attain adult characteristics.

infertility Decreased capacity to conceive.

infiltration Process by which a substance such as a local anesthetic drug is deposited within the tissue.

inhalation analgesia Reduction of pain by administration of anesthetic gas. Occasionally given during the second stage of labor. Consciousness is retained to allow the woman to follow instructions and to avoid the adverse effects of general anesthesia.

inlet Passage leading into a cavity.

 pelvic i. Upper brim of the pelvic cavity.

innominate Without a name.

 i. bone The hip bone.

internal os Inside mouth or opening.

interstitial cell–stimulating hormone (ICSH) Hormone that stimulates production of testosterone; analogous to LH in the female.

intertuberous diameter Distance between ischial tuberosities. Measured to determine dimension of pelvic outlet.

intervillous space Irregular space in the maternal portion of the placenta, filled with maternal blood and serving as the site of maternal-fetal gas, nutrient, and waste exchange.

intrapartum During labor and delivery.

intrathecal Within the subarachnoid space.

intrauterine device (IUD) Small plastic or metal form placed in the uterus to prevent implantation of a fertilized ovum.

intrauterine growth retardation (IUGR) Fetal undergrowth of any etiology, such as deficient nutrient supply or intrauterine infection, or associated with congenital malformation.

introitus Entrance into a canal or cavity such at the vagina.

intromission Insertion of one part or object into another (e.g., introduction of penis into vagina).

intussusception Prolapse of one segment of bowel into the lumen of the adjacent segment.

in utero Within or inside the uterus.

in vitro fertilization Fertilization in a culture dish or test tube.

inversion Turning end for end, upside down, or inside out.

 i. of the uterus Condition in which the uterus is turned inside out so that the fundus intrudes into the cervix or vagina, caused by a too vigorous removal of the placenta before it is detached by the natural process of labor.

involution (1) Rolling or turning inward. (2) Reduction in size of the uterus after delivery and its return to its normal size and condition.

iontophoretic pilocarpine test Sweat test, usually a diagnostic test for cystic fibrosis (mucoviscidosis).

ischium Lower lateral two fifths of the acetabulum and the short, stout column of bone that supports it.

isoimmune hemolytic disease Breakdown (hemolysis) of fetal/neonatal Rh-positive RBCs because of Rh antigens formed by an Rh-negative mother who had been previously exposed to Rh-positive RBCs.

isoimmunization Development of antibodies in a species of animal with antigens from the same species (e.g., development of anti-Rh antibodies in an Rh-negative person).

ITP Abbreviation for idiopathic thrombocytopenic purpura.

jaundice Yellow discoloration of the body tissues caused by the deposit of bile pigments (unconjugated bilirubin); icterus.

    breast milk j. Yellowing of infant's skin from pregnanediol (in mother's milk) inhibition of enzyme (glucuronyl transferase) necessary for conjugation of bilirubin.

    pathologic j. Jaundice noticeable within 24 hours after birth; caused by some abnormal condition such as an Rh or ABO incompatibility and resulting in bilirubin toxicity (e.g., kernicterus)

    physiologic j. Jaundice usually occurring 48 hours or later after birth, reaching a peak at 5 to 7 days, gradually disappearing by the seventh to tenth day, and caused by the normal reduction in the number of red blood cells. The infant is otherwise well.

Kahn test Precipitation or flocculation test for the diagnosis of syphilis.

kalemia Presence of potassium in the serum.

karyotype Schematic arrangement of the chromosomes within a cell to demonstrate their numbers and morphology.

Kegel exercises Excises to stengthen the pubococcygeal muscles.

kernicterus Bilirubin encephalopathy involving the deposit of unconjugated bilirubin in brain cells, resulting in death or impaired intellectual, perceptive, or motor function, and adaptive behavior.

Kernig's sign Stiffness of the back; nuchal rigidity.

ketoacidosis Acidosis accompanied by an accumulation of ketones in the body, resulting from faulty carbohydrate metabolism.

ketonemia Acetone bodies in the blood, causing the characteristic fruity breath odor of ketoacidosis.

ketosis Increase in ketone bodies (acetone) from incomplete metabolism of fatty acids.

kin group People related by blood or marriage.

Klumpke's palsy Atrophic paralysis of forearm.

labia Lips or liplike structures.

    l. majora Two folds of skin containing fat and covered with hair that lie on either side of the vaginal opening and from each side of the vulva.

    l. minora Two thin folds of delicate, hairless skin inside the labia majora.

labor Series of processes by which the fetus is expelled from the uterus; parturition; childbirth.

laceration Irregular tear of wound tissue; in obstetrics, it usually refers to a tear in the perineum, vagina, or cervix caused by childbirth.

lactase Enzyme necessary for the digestion of lactose.

lactation Function of secreting milk or period during which milk is secreted.

lactogen Drug or other substance that enhances the production and secretion of milk.

lactogenic Stimulating the production of milk.

    l. hormone Gonadotropin produced by anterior pituitary and responsible for promoting growth of breast tissue and lactation; prolaction; luteotropin.

lactose intolerance Inherited absence of the enzyme lactose.

lactosuria Presence of lactose in the urine during late pregnacy and during lactation. Must be differentiated from glycosuria.

Lamaze method Method of psychophysical preparation for childbirth developed in the 1950s by a French obstetrician, Fernand Lamaze. It requires classes, practice at home, and coaching during labor and delivery.

lambdoid Having the shape of the Greek letter lambda.

    l. suture Suture line extending across the posterior third of the skull, separating the occipital bone from the two parietal bones, and forming the base of the triangular posterior fontanel.

laminaria tent Cone of dried seaweed that swells as it absorbs moisture. Used to dilate the cervix nontraumatically in preparation for an induced abortion or in preparation for induction of labor.

lanugo Downy, fine hair characteristic of the fetus between 20 weeks' gestation and birth that is most noticeable over the shoulder, forehead, and cheeks but is found on nearly all parts of the body except the palms of the hands, soles of the feet, and the scalp.

laparoscopy Examination of the interior of the abdomen by inserting a small telescope through the anterior abdominal wall.

laparotomy Incision into the abdominal cavity.

large for dates (large for gestational age [LGA]) Exhibiting excessive growth for gestational age.

lavage Washing out of a cavity such as the stomach.

lecithin A phospholipid that decreases surface tension; surfactant.

lecithin/sphingomyelin ratio Ratio of lecithin to sphingomyelin in the amniotic fluid. This is used to assess maturity of the fetal lung.

Leopold's maneuver Four maneuvers for diagnosing the fetal position by external palpation of the mother's abdomen.

let-down reflex Oxytocin-induced flow of milk from the alveoli of the breasts into the milk ducts.

leukorrhea White or yellowish mucous discharge from the cervical canal or the vagina that may be normal physiologically or caused by pathologic states of the vagina and endocervix (e.g., *Trichomonas vaginalis* infections).

LH See *luteinizing hormone (LH)*.

libido Sexual drive.

lie Relationship existing between the long axis of the fetus and the long axis of the mother. In a longitudinal lie, the fetus is lying lengthwise or vertically, whereas in a transverse lie the fetus is lying crosswise or horizontally in the mother's uterus.

ligation Act of suturing, sewing, or otherwise tying shut.

    tubal l. Abdominal operation in which the fallopian tubes are tied off and a section is removed to interrupt tubal continuity and thus sterilize the woman.

lightening Sensation of decreased abdominal distention produced by uterine descent into the pelvic cavity as the fetal presenting part settles into the pelvis. It usually occurs 2 weeks before the onset of labor in nulliparas.

linea nigra Line of darker pigmentation seen in some women during the latter part of pregnancy that appears on the middle of the abdomen and extends from the symphysis pubis toward the umbilicus.

linea terminalis Line dividing the upper (false) pelvis from the lower (true) pelvis.

lingua Tongue or tonguelike structure.

    l. frenata Tongue with a very short frenulum, resulting in tongue-tie, an extremely rare condition.

liquor Any fluid liquid.

    l. amnii Amniotic fluid that surrounds the fetus within the amniotic sac.

lithotomy position Position in which the woman lies on her back with her knees flexed and abducted thighs drawn up toward her chest.

live birth Birth in which the neonate, regardless of gestational age, manifests any heartbeat, breathes, or displays voluntary movement.

livida, asphyxia See *asphyxia livida*.

lochia Vaginal discharge during the puerperium consisting of blood, tissue, and mucus.

    l. alba Thin, yellowish to white, vaginal discharge that follows lochia serosa on about the tenth postdelivery day and that may last from the end of the third to the sixth postdelivery week.

    l. rubra Red, distinctly blood-tinged vaginal flow that follows delivery and lasts 2 to 4 days after delivery.

    l. serosa Serous, pinkish brown, watery vaginal discharge that follows lochia ruba until about the tenth postdelivery day.

L/S ratio (lecithin/sphingomyelin ratio) Test for fetal lung maturity.

lunar month Four weeks (28 days).

lutein Yellow pigment derived from the corpus luteum, egg yolk, and fat cells.

    l. cells Ovarian cells involved in the formation of the corpus luteum and that contain a yellow pigment.

luteinizing hormone (LH) Hormone produced by the anterior pituitary that stimulates ovulation and the development of the corpus luteum.

luteotropin (LTH) Lactogenic hormone; prolactin; an adenohypophyseal hormone.

lysis of adhesions Operation to free adhesions (bands of scar tissue) that have caused organs to be abnormally drawn or tied to each other.

lysozyme Enzyme with antiseptic qualities that destroys foreign organisms and that is found in blood cells of the granulocytic and monocytic series and is also normally present in saliva, sweat, tears, and breast milk.

maceration (1) Process of softening a solid by soaking it in a fluid. (2) Softening and breaking down of fetal skin from prolonged exposure to amniotic fluid as seen in a postterm infant. Also seen in a dead fetus.

macroglossia Hypertrophy of tongue or tongue large for oral cavity; seen in some preterm neonates and in neonates with Down's syndrome.

macrophage Any phagocytic cell of the reticuloendothelial system including Kupffer cell in the liver, splenocyte in the spleen, and histocyte in the loose connective tissue.

macrosomia Large body size as seen in neonates of diabetic or prediabetic mothers; macrosomatia.

magnesemia Presence of serum magnesium.

malpractice Professional negligence that is the proximate cause of injury or harm to a client, resulting from a lack of professional knowledge, experience, or skill that can be expected in others in the profession or from a failure to exercise reasonable care or judgment in the application of professional knowledge, experience, or skill.

mammary gland Compound gland of the female breast that is made up of lobes and lobules that secrete milk for nourishment of the young. Rudimentary mammary glands exist in the male.

manic depressive psychosis Major affective disorder characterized by episodes of mania and depression. One or the other phase may be predominant at any given time; one phase may appear alternately with the other; or elements of both phases may be present simultaneously. Also called bipolar disorder.

mask of pregnancy See *chloasma*.

mastalgia Breast soreness or tenderness.

mastectomy Excision, or removal, of the breast.

mastitis Inflammation of mammary tissue of the breasts.

maternal mortality Death of a woman related to childbearing.

maturation (1) Process of attaining maximum development. (2) In biology, a process of cell division during which the number of chromosomes in the germ cells (sperm or ova) is reduced to one half the number (haploid) characteristic of the species.

maturational crisis Crisis that arises during normal growth and development, e.g., puberty.

meatus Opening from an internal structure to the outside (e.g., urethral meatus).

mechanism Instrument or process by which something is done, results, or comes into being; in obstetrics, labor and delivery.

meconium First stools of infant: viscid, sticky; dark greenish brown, almost black; sterile; odorless

    m. aspiration syndrome Function of fetal hypoxia: with hypoxia, the anal sphincter relaxes and meconium is released; reflex gasping movements draw meconium and other particulate matter in the amniotic fluid into the infant's bronchial tree, obstructing the air flow after birth.

    m. ileus Lower intestinal obstruction by thick, puttylike, inspissated meconium that may be the result of deficiency of trypsin production in the newborn with cystic fibrosis.

    m.-stained fluid In response to hypoxia, fetal intestinal activity increases and anal sphincter relaxes, resulting in the passage of meconium, which imparts a greenish coloration.

megaloblastic anemia Hematologic disorder characterized by the production and peripheral proliferation of immature, large, and dysfunctional erythrocytes.

meiosis Process by which germ cells divide and decrease their chromosomal number by one half.

-melia Pertaining to a limb or part of a limb or extremity, as in amelia (absence of a limb) or phocomelia (absence of part of arms or legs).

membrane Thin, pliable layer of tissue that lines a cavity or tube, separates structures, or covers an organ or structure; in obstetrics, the amnion and chorion surrounding the fetus.

membrane rupture Tearing of the fetal membranes (amnion and chorion) with the release of amniotic fluid.

menarche Onset, or beginning, of menstrual function.

meningomyelocele Saclike protrusion of the spinal cord through a congenital defect in the vertebral column.

menopause From the Greek word *men* (month) and *pausis* (to stop), the actual permanent cessation of menstrual cycles.

menorrhagia Abnormally profuse or excessive menstrual flow.

menses (menstruation) Periodic vaginal discharge of bloody fluid from the nonpregnant uterus that occurs from the age of puberty to menopause.

mentum Chin, a fetal reference point in designating position (e.g., "Left mentum anterior" [LMA], meaning that the fetal chin is presenting in the left anterior quadrant of the maternal pelvis).

mesoderm Embryonic middle layer of germ cells giving rise to all types of muscles, connective tissue, bone marrow, blood, lymphoid tissue, and all epithelial tissue.

metabolic acidosis See *acidosis, metabolic*.

metritis Inflammation of the endometrium and myometrium.

metrorrhagia Abnormal bleeding from the uterus, particularly when it occurs at any time other than the menstrual period.

microcephaly Congenital anomaly characterized by abnormal smallness of the head in relation to the rest of the body and by underdevelopment of the brain, resulting in some degree of mental retardation.

micrognathia Abnormal smallness of mandible or chin.

midwife One who practices the art of helping and aiding a woman to give birth.

migration In obstetrics, the passage of the ovum from the ovary into the fallopian tubes and thence into the uterus.

milia Unopened sebaceous glands appearing as tiny, white, pinpoint papules on forehead, nose, cheeks, and chin of a neonate that disappear spontaneously in a few days or weeks.

milk-leg See *phlegmasia alba dolens*.

miscarriage Spontaneous abortion; lay term usually referring specifically to the loss of the fetus between the fourth month and viability.

missed abortion See *abortion, missed*.

mitleiden Suffering along with.

mitochondria Slender microscopic filaments or rods found in the cell cytoplasm; the principal sites of oxidative reactions by which the cell is provided with energy.

mitosis Process of somatic cell division in which a single cell divides, but both of the new cells have the same number of chromosomes as the first.

mittelschmerz Abdominal pain in the region of an ovary during ovulation, which usually occurs midway through the menstrual cycle. Present in many women, mittelschmerz is useful for identifying ovulation, thus pinpointing the fertile period of the cycle.

molding Overlapping of cranial bones or shaping of the fetal head to accommodate and conform to the bony and soft parts of the mother's birth canal during labor.

mongolian spot Bluish gray or dark nonelevated pigmented area usually found over the lower back and buttocks present at birth in some infants, primarily nonwhite. The spot fades by school age in black or Oriental infants and within the first year or two of life in other infants.

mongolism, See *Down's syndrome*.

moniliasis Infection of the skin or mucous membrane by a yeastlike fungus, *Candida albicans*. see *thrush*.

monitrice One trained in psychoprophylactic methods and who supports women during labor.

monosomy Chromosomal aberration characterized by the absence of one chromosome from the normal diploid complement.

monozygotic Originating or coming from a single fertilized ovum, such as identical twins.

monozygous twins See *twins, monozygous*.

mons veneris Pad of fatty tissue and coarse skin that overlies the symphysis pubis in the woman and that, after puberty, is covered with short curly hair.

Montgomery's glands tubercles Small, nodular prominences (sebaceous glands) on the areolas around the nipples of the breasts that enlarge during pregnancy and lactation.

morbidity (1) Condition of being diseased. (2) Number of cases of disease or sick persons in relationship to a specific population; incidence.

morning sickness Nausea and vomiting that affect some women during the first few months of their pregnancy; may occur at any time of day.

Moro's reflex Normal, generalized reflex in a young infant elicited by a sudden loud noise or by striking the table next to the child, resulting in flexion of the legs, an embracing posture of the arms, and usually a brief cry. Also called startle reflex.

mortality (1) Quality or state of being subject to death. (2) Number of deaths in relation to a specific population; incidence.

   fetal m. Number of fetal deaths per 1000 births (or per live births). See also *death, fetal*.

   infant m. Number of deaths per 1000 children 1 year of age or younger.

   maternal m. Number of maternal deaths per 100,000 births.

   neonatal m. Number of neonatal deaths per 1000 births (or per live births). See also *death, neonatal*.

   perinatal m. Combined fetal and neonatal mortality. See also *death, perinatal*.

morula Developmental stage of the fertilized ovum in which there is a solid mass of cells resembling a mulberry.

mosaicism Condition in which some somatic cells are normal, whereas others show chromosomal aberrations.

muscous membrane Specialized thin layer of tissue lining certain cavities and passages that is kept moist by the secretion of mucus.

mucous-trap suction apparatus Device consisting of a catheter with a mucous trap that prevents mucus aspirated from the newborn infant's nasopharynx and trachea from being sucked or drawn into the operator's mouth.

mucus Viscid fluid secreted by the mucous membranes.

multigravida Woman who has been pregnant two or more times.

multipara Woman who has carried two or more pregnancies to viability, whether they ended in live infants or stillbirths.

multiple pregnancy Pregnancy in which there is more than one fetus in the uterus at the same time.

multiple sclerosis (MS) Progressive disease characterized by disseminated demyelination of nerve fibers of the brain and spinal cord.

mutation Change in a gene or chromosome in gametes that may be transmitted to offspring.

myasthenia gravis Abnormal condition characterized by the chronic fatigability and weakness of muscles, especially in the face and throat, as a result of a defect in the conduction of nerve impulses at the myoneural junction.

Naegele's rule Method for calculating the estimated date of confinement (EDC), or "due date."

natal Relating or pertaining to birth.

navel Depression in the center of the abdomen, where the umbilical cord was attached to the fetus; umbilicus.

necrotizing bronchitis Pathologic death of cells within the bronchi.

necrotizing enterocolitis (NEC) Acute inflammatory bowel disorder that occurs primarily in preterm or low-birth-weight neonates. It is charcterized by ischemic necrosis (death) of the gastrointestinal mucosa that may lead to perforation and peritonitis.

negligence Commission of an act that a prudent person would not have done or the omission of a duty that prudent person would have fulfilled, resulting in injury or harm to another person. In particular, in a malpractice suit a professional person is negligent if harm to a client results from such an act or such a failure to act, but it must be proved that other prudent persons of the same profession would ordinarily have acted differently under the same circumstances.

neonatal hypovolemic shock Cardiovascular collapse due to a diminished volume of circulating fluid in the cardiovascular system.

neonatal mortality Statistical rate of infant death during the first 28 days after live birth, expressed as the number of such deaths per 1,000 live births in a specific geographic area or institution in a given period of time.

neonatology Study of the neonate.

nephroureterolithiasis Stones in the kidneys and ureters.

neurofibromatosis Congenital condition transmitted as an autosomal dominant trait, characterized by numerous neurofibromas of the nerves and skin, by cafe-au-lait spots on the skin, and, in some cases, by developmental anomalies of the muscles, bones, and viscera.

neutral temperature range That grouping of environmental conditions in which the neonate's oxygen consumption is at a minimum and his temperature is within normal limits.

nevus Natural blemish or mark; a congenital circumscribed deposit of pigmentation in the skin; mole.

    n. flammeus Port-wine stain; reddish, usually flat, discoloration of the face or neck. Because of its large size and color, it is considered a serious deformity.

    n. vasculosus (strawberry hemangioma) Elevated lesion of immature capillaries and endothelial cells that regresses over a period of years.

nidation Implantation of the fertilized ovum in the endometrium, or lining, of the uterus.

nondisjunction Failure of homologous pairs of chromosomes to separate during the first meiotic division or of the two chromatids of a chromosome to split during anaphase of mitosis or the second meiotic division. The result is an abnormal number of chromosomes in the daughter cells.

nonshivering thermogenesis Infant's method of producing heat by increasing his metabolic rate.

nonstress test (NST) Evaluation of fetal response (fetal heart rate) to natural contractile uterine activity or to an increase in fetal activity.

nosocomial Pertaining to a hospital.

nucleotide Single segment of helical strand of DNA.

nulligravida Woman who has never been pregnant.

nullipara Woman who has not yet carried a pregnancy to viability.

nursing practitioner Registered nurse who has additional education to practice nursing in an expanded role.

nystagmus Constant, involuntary, rhythmic oscillation of the eyeball. The movements may be in any direction.

obstetrix Midwife; from *obstare*, to stand before.

occipitobregmatic Pertaining to the occiput (the back part of the skull) and the bregma (junction of the coronal and sagittal sutures) or anterior fontanel; the smallest diameter of the fetal head.

occiput Back part of the head or skull.

oligohydramnios Abnormally small amount or absence of amniotic fluid; often indicative of fetal urinary tract defect.

oliguria Diminished secretion of urine by the kidneys.

omphalic Concerning or pertaining to the umbilicus.

omphalitis Inflammation of the umbilical stump characterized by redness, edema, and purulent exudate in severe infections.

omphalocele Congenital defect resulting from failure of closure of the abdominal wall or muscles and leading to hernia of abdominal contents through the navel.

oocyesis Ectopic ovarian pregnancy.

oocyte Primordial or incompletely developed ovum.

oophorectomy Excision or removal of an ovary.

operculum Plug of mucus that fills the cervical canal during pregnancy.

ophthalmia neonatorum Infection in the neonate's eyes usually resulting from gonorrheal or other infection contracted when the fetus passes through the birth canal (vagina).

opisthotonos Tetanic spasm resulting in an arched, hyperextended position of the body.

oral GTT Test for blood sugar following oral ingestion of a concentrated sugar solution.

orchitis Inflammation of one or both of the testes, characterized by swelling and pain, often caused by mumps, syphilis, or tuberculosis.

orgasmic platform Congestion of the lower vagina during sexual intercourse.

orifice Normal mouth, entrance, or opening, to any aperture.

os Mouth, or opening.

    external o. (o. externum) External opening of the cervical canal.

    internal o. (o. internum) Internal opening of the cervical canal.

    o. uteri Mouth, or opening, of the uterus.

ossification Mineralization of fetal bones.

-otomy Combining form meaning cutting, incision, section.

outlet Opening by which something can exit.

    pelvic o. Inferior aperture, or opening, of the true pelvis.

ovary One of two glands in the female situated on either side of the pelvic cavity that produces the female reproductive cell, the ovum, and two known hormones, estrogen and progesterone.

ovulation Periodic ripening and discharge of the unimpregnated ovum from the ovary, usually 14 days prior to the onset of menstrual flow.

    o. method Evaluation of cervical mucus throughout the menstrual cycle; ovulation occurs just after the appearance of the peak mucus sign; Billings method.

ovum Female germ, or reproductive cell, produced by the ovary; egg.

oxygen toxicity Oxygen overdosage that results in pathologic tissue changes (e.g., retrolental fibroplasia, bronchopulmonary dysplasia).

oxytocics Drugs that stimulate uterine contractions, thus accelerating childbirth and preventing postdelivery hemorrhage. They may be used to increase the let-down reflex during lactation.

oxytocin Hormone produced by the posterior pituitary that stimulates uterine contractions and the release of milk in the mammary gland (let-down reflex).

    o. challenge test (OCT) Evaluation of fetal response (fetal heart rate) to contractile activity of the uterus stimulated by exogenous oxytocin (Pitocin).

PaCO$_2$ Partial pressure of carbon dioxide in arterial blood.

pallida, asphyxia See *asphyxia pallida*.

palpation Examination performed by touching the external surface of the body with the fingers or palmar surface of the hand.

    bimanual p. See *bimanual palpation*.

palsy Permanent or temporary loss of sensation or ability to move and control movement; paralysis.

　Bell's p. Peripheral facial paralysis of the facial nerve (cranial nerve VII), causing the muscles of the unaffected side of the face to pull the face into a distorted position.

　Erb's p. See *Erb-Duchenne paralysis*.

panhysterectomy See *hysterectomy*.

PaO₂ Partial pressure of oxygen in arterial blood.

Papanicolaou (Pap) smear Microscopic examination using scrapings from the cervix, endocervix, or other mucous membranes that will reveal, with a high degree of accuracy, the presence of premalignant or malignant cells.

para Term used to refer to past pregnancies that reached viability regardless of whether the infant was dead or alive at birth.

parabiotic syndrome Fetofetal blood transfer caused by placental vascular anastomoses occurring in a small plethoric twin (polycythemia) and one pale twin (anemia).

parametritis Inflamed condition of the cellular tissue or parmetrium of the uterus; pelvic cellulitis.

parametrium Flat, smooth muscle, and loose connective tissue lying around the uterus and extending laterally between the layers of the broad ligaments.

parenteral Administration or injection of nutrients, fluids, or drugs into the body by any way other than the digestive tract.

parity Number of pregnancies that reached viability.

parovarian Pertaining to the residual structure in the broad ligament between the fallopian tubes and the ovary.

parturient Woman giving birth.

parturition Process or act of giving birth.

patent Open.

pathogen Substance or organism capable of producing disease.

pathognomonic Characteristic or distinctive symptom or sign of a disease that facilitates recognition or differentiation from other conditions.

pathologic hyperbilirubinemia High (toxic) levels of serum bilirubin due to a disease process causing hemolysis (e.g., Rh incompatibility); jaundice apparent within first 24 hours.

pathologic jaundice See *jaundice, pathologic*.

pathosis A disease condition.

patulous Open or spread apart.

peak mucus sign Lubricative, cloudy-to-clear-egg white cervical mucus occurring under high estrogen levels close to time of ovulation; ferns; good spinnbarkeit.

pedigree Shorthand method of depicting family lines of individuals who manifest a physical or chemical disorder.

pelvic Pertaining or relating to the pelvis.

　p. axis See *axis, pelvic*.

　p. inlet See *inlet, pelvic*.

　p. outlet See *outlet, pelvic*.

pelvimeter Device for measuring the diameters and capacity of the pelvis.

pelvimetry Measurement of dimensions and proportions of the pelvis to determine its capacity and ability to allow the passage of the fetus through the birth canal.

pelvis Bony structure formed by the sacrum, coccyx, innominate bones, and symphysis pubis, and the ligaments that unite them.

　android p. See *android pelvis*.

　anthropoid p. See *anthropoid pelvis*.

　false p. Pelvis above the linea terminalis and symphysis pubis.

　gynecoid p. See *gynecoid pelvis*.

　platypelloid p. See *platypelloid pelvis*.

　true p. Pelvis below the linea terminalis.

pemphigus An uncommon, serious disease of the skin and mucous membranes, characterized by thin-walled bullae arising from apparently normal skin or mucous membrane. The bullae rupture easily, leaving raw patches. The person loses weight, becomes weak, and is subject to major infections.

pemphigus neonatorum Neonatal impetigo.

penis Male organ used for urination and copulation.

perforation of the uterus Accidental puncture of the uterus, usually with a curet and occasionally by an intrauterine device (IUD).

peridural anesthesia Injection of anesthetic outside the dura mater (anesthetic does not mix with spinal fluid); epidural anesthesia.

perinatal Of or pertaining to the time and process of giving birth or being born.

perinatal period Period extending from the twentieth or twenty-eighth week of gestation through the end of the twenty-eighth day after birth.

perinatologist Physician who specializes in fetal and neonatal care.

perineorrhaphy Suture or operation used in repairing a laceration of the perineum, usually following labor.

perineotomy Surgical incision into the perineum. In obstetrics the perineotomy is usually called an *episiotomy* and is done at the end of the second stage of labor to avoid laceration of the perineum and to facilitate delivery. (See also *episiotomy*.)

perineum Area between the vagina and rectum in the female and between the scrotum and rectum in the male.

periodic breathing Sporadic episodes of cessation of respirations for periods of 10 seconds or less not associated with cyanosis commonly noted in premature infants.

peritoneum Strong serous membrane reflected over the viscera and lining the abdominal cavity.

pessary Device placed inside the vagina to function as a supportive structure for the uterus or a contraceptive device.

petechiae Pinpoint hemorrhagic areas caused by numerous disease states involving infection and thrombocytopenia and occasionally found over the face and trunk of the newborn because of increased intravascular pressure in the capillaries during delivery.

pH Hydrogen ion concentration.

phenotype Expression of certain physical or chemical characteristics in an individual resulting from interaction between genotype and environmental factors.

phenylketonuria (PKU) Recessive hereditary disease that results in a defect in the metabolism of the amino acid phenylalanine caused by the lack of an enzyme, phenylalanine hydroxylase, that is necessary for the conversion of the amino acid phenylalanine into tyrosine. If PKU is not treated, brain damage may occur, causing severe mental retardation.

phimosis Tightness of the prepuce, or foreskin, of the penis.

phlebitis Inflammation of a vein with symptoms of pain and tenderness along the course of the vein, inflammatory swelling and acute edema below the obstruction, and discoloration of the skin because of injury or bruise to the vein, possibly occurring in acute or chronic infections or after operations or childbirth.

phlebothrombosis Formation of a clot or thrombus in the vein; inflammation of the vein with secondary clotting.

phlebotomy Incision of a vein for the letting of blood, as in collecting blood from a donor.

phlegmasia alba dolens Phlebitis of the femoral vein with thrombosis leading to a venous obstruction, causing acute edema of the leg, and occurring occasionally after delivery; also called *milk-leg*.

phocomelia Developmental anomaly characterized by the absence of the upper portion of one or more limbs so that the feet or hands or both are attached to the trunk of the body by short, irregularly shaped stumps, resembling the fins of a seal.

phototherapy Utilization of lights to reduce serum bilirubin levels by oxidation of bilirubin into water-soluble compounds that are then processed in the liver and excreted in bile and urine.

physiologic hyperbilirubinemia Hemolysis of excessive fetal RBCs in the early neonatal period; jaundice not apparent during first 24 hours. Levels are nontoxic to the individual.

physiologic jaundice See *jaundice, physiologic*.

pica Unusual craving during pregnancy (e.g., of laundry starch, dirt, red clay).

pinna Ear cartilage.

placenta Latin, flat cake; afterbirth; specialized vascular disc-shaped organ for maternal-fetal gas and nutrient exchange. Normally it implants in the thick muscular wall of the upper uterine segment.

    abruptio p. See *abruptio placentae*.

    battledore p. Umbilical cord insertion into the margin of the placenta.

    circumvallate p. Placenta having a raised white ring at its edge.

    p. accreta Invasion of the uterine muscle by the placenta, thus making separation from the muscle difficult if not impossible.

    p. previa Placenta that is abnormally implanted in the thin, lower uterine segment and that is typed according to proximity to cervical os: total—completely occludes os; partial—does not occlude os completely; and marginal—placenta encroaches on margin of internal cervical os.

    p. succenturiata Accessory placenta.

placental Pertaining or relating to the placenta.

    p. dysfunction Failure of placenta to meet fetal needs and requirements; placental insufficiency.

    p. dystocia See *dystocia, placental*.

    p. infarct Localized, ischemic, hard area on the fetal or maternal side of the placenta.

    p. souffle See *souffle, placental*.

platypelloid pelvis Broad pelvis with a shortened anteroposterior diameter and a flattened, oval, transverse shape.

plethora Deep beefy red coloration (''boiled lobster'' hue) of a newborn caused by an increased number of blood cells (polycythemia) per volume of blood.

pneumomediastinum Accumulation of air around the heart and vena cava.

pneumothorax Escaped air from affected lung into the pleural space, displacing the heart and mediastinum toward the unaffected side of the chest.

podalic Concerning or pertaining to the feet.

    p. version Shifting of the position of the fetus so as to bring the feet to the outlet during labor.

polycythemia Increased number of erythrocytes per volume of blood, which may be caused by large placental transfusion, fetofetal transfusion, or maternal-fetal transfusion, or it may be due to hypovolemia resulting from movement of fluid out of vascular into interstitial compartment.

polydactyly Excessive number of digits (fingers or toes).

polygenic Pertaining to the combined action of several different genes.

polyhydramnios See *hydramnios*.

polyuria Excessive secretion and discharge of urine by the kidneys.

position Relationship of an arbitrarily chosen fetal reference point, such as the occiput, sacrum, chin, or scapula on the presenting part of the fetus to its location in the front, back, or sides of the maternal pelvis.

positive sign of pregnancy Definite indication of pregnancy (e.g., hearing the fetal heartbeat, visualization and palpation of fetal movement by the examiner, sonographic examination).

posterior Pertaining to the back.

    p. fontanel See *fontanel, posterior*.

postmature infant Infant born at or after the beginning of week 43 of gestation or later and exhibiting signs of dysmaturity.

postnatal Happening or occurring after birth.

postpartum Happening or occurring after birth.

Potter's syndrome Silicosis.

precipitate delivery Rapid or sudden labor of less than 3 hours' duration beginning from onset of cervical changes to completed birth of neonate.

preeclampsia Disease encountered during pregnancy or early in the puerperium characterized by increasing hypertension, albuminuria, and generalized edema; pregnancy-induced hypertension (PIH): toxemia.

pregnancy Period between conception through complete delivery of the products of conception. The usual duration of pregnancy in the human is 280 days, 9 calendar months, or 10 lunar months.

    abdominal p. See *abdominal gestation*.

    ectopic p. See *ectopic pregnancy*.

    extrauterine p. See *extrauterine pregnancy*.

premature infant Infant born before completing week 37 of gestation, irrespective of birth weight; preterm infant.

premenstrual syndrome Syndrome of nervous tension, irritability, weight gain, edema, headache, mastalgia, dysphoria, and lack of coordination occurring during the last few days of the menstrual cycle preceding the onset of menstruation.

premonitory Serving as an early symptom or warning.

prenatal Occurring or happening before birth.

prepartum Before delivery; prior to giving birth.

prepuce Fold of skin, or foreskin, covering the glans penis of the male.

    p. of the clitoris Fold of the labia minora that the glans clitoris.

presentation That part of the fetus which first enters the pelvis and lies over the inlet: may be head, face, breech, or shoulder.

    breech p. See *breech presentation*.

    cephalic p. See *cephalic presentation*.

presenting part That part of the fetus which lies closest to the internal os of the cervix.

pressure edema Edema of the lower extremities caused by pressure of the heavy pregnant uterus against the large veins; edema of fetal scalp after cephalic presentation (caput succedaneum).

presumptive signs Manifestations that suggest pregnancy but that are not absolutely positive. These include the cessation of menses, Chadwick's sign, morning sickness, and quickening.

preterm infant See *premature infant*.

previa, placenta See *placenta previa*.

priapism Continous erection of the penis, not usually accompanied by sexual feeling, which may appear in conjunction with leukemia, renal calculi, and spinal cord lesions.

primigravida Woman who is pregnant for the first time.

primipara Woman who has carried a pregnancy to viability without regard to the child's being dead or alive at the time of birth.

primordial Existing first or existing in the simplest or most primitive form.

probable signs Manifestations or evidence which indicates that there is a definite likelihood of pregnancy. Among the probable signs are enlargement of abdomen, Goodell's sign, Hegar's sign, Braxton Hicks' sign, and positive hormonal tests for pregnancy.

proband Individual in a family who comes to the attention of a genetic investigator because of the occurrence of a trait; the index case, or propositus.

prodromal Serving as an early symptom or warning of the approach of a disease or condition (e.g., prodromal labor).

progesterone Hormone produced by the corpus luteum and placenta whose function is to prepare the endometrium of the uterus for implantation of the fertilized ovum, develop the mammary glands, and maintain the pregnancy.

projectile vomiting Extremely forceful, expulsive vomiting.

prolactin See *lactogenic hormone*.

prolan Hormone produced by chorionic villi, now called *human chorionic gonadotropin (HCG),* that is found in the serum and urine of pregnant women and forms the basis of the biologic and immunologic pregnancy tests.

prolapsed cord Protrusion of the umbilical cord in advance of the presenting part.

proliferative phase of menstrual cycle Preovulatory, follicular, or estrogen phase of the menstrual cycle.

promontory of the sacrum Superior projecting portion of the sacrum at the junction of the sacrum and the L-5.

prophylactic Pertaining to prevention or warding off of disease or certain conditions; condom, or ''rubber.''

propositus See *proband*.

prostaglandin (PG) Substance present in many body tissues; has a role in many reproductive tract functions.

proteinuria Excretion of protein into urine.

pruritus Itching.

pruritus gravidarum Itching of the skin caused by pregnancy.

pseudocyesis Condition in which the woman has all the usual signs of pregnancy, such as enlargement of the abdomen, cessation of menses, weight gain, and morning sickness, but is not pregnant; phantom or false pregnancy.

pseudopregnancy See *pseudocyesis*.

pseudoprematurity See *intrauterine growth retardation (IUGR)*.

psychologic miscarriage Absence or lack of love for one's infant.

psychoprophylaxis Mental and physical education of the parents in preparation for childbirth, with the goal of minimizing the fear and pain and promoting positive family relationships.

ptyalism Excessive salivation.

puberty Period in life in which the reproductive organs mature and one becomes functionally capable of reproduction.

pubic Pertaining to the pubis.

pubis Pubic bone forming the front of the pelvis.

pudendal block Injection of a local anesthetizing drug at the pudendal nerve root in order to produce numbness of the genital and perianal region.

pudendum External genitalia of either sex; Latin, ''that of which one should be ashamed.''

puerperal sepsis Infection of the pelvic organs during the postdelivery period; childbed fever.

puerperium Period of time following the third stage of labor and lasting until involution of the uterus takes place, usually about 3 to 6 weeks.

pulse pressure Difference between systolic and diastolic blood pressure.

pyloric stenosis Narrowing of the pyloric sphincter at the outlet of the stomach, causing an obstruction that blocks the flow of food into the small intestine.

quickening Maternal perception of fetal movement; usually occurs between weeks 16 and 20 of gestation.

rabbit test See *Friedman's test*.

radium insertion Introduction of metallic element radium (Ra) into the uterus or cervix to treat cancer.

rales Crackling sounds heard as air passes through the fluid present within the terminal bronchioles and alveoli.

raphe A line of union of the halves of various symmetrical parts, as the abdominal raphe of the linea alba or the raphe penis, which appears as a narrow, dark streak on the inferior surface of the penis.

RDS See *respiratory distress syndrome (RDS)*.

recessive trait Genetically determined characteristic that is expressed only when present in the homozygotic state.

rectocele Herniation or protrusion of the rectum into the posterior vaginal wall.

rectovaginal ligament A posterior ligament.

reflex Automatic response built into the nervous system that does not need the intervention of conscious thought (e.g., in the newborn, rooting, gagging, grasp).

regional block anesthesia Anesthesia of an area of the body by injecting a local anesthetic to block a group of sensory nerve fibers.

regurgitate Vomiting or spitting up of solids or fluids.

residual urine Urine that remains in the bladder after urination.

respiratory distress syndrome (RDS) Condition resulting from decreased pulmonary gas exchange, leading to retention of carbon dioxide (increase in arterial Pco_2). Most common neonatal causes are prematurity, perinatal asphyxia, and maternal diabetes mellitus; hyaline membrane disease (HMD).

restitution In obstetrics, the turning of the fetal head to the left or right after it has completely emerged from the introitus as it assumes a normal alignment with the infant's shoulders.

resuscitation Restoration of consciousness or life in one who is apparently dead or whose respirations or cardiac function or both have ceased.

retained placenta Retention of all or part of the placenta in the uterus after delivery.

reticulocytosis Increase in number of reticulocytes in circulating blood.

retraction (1) Drawing in or sucking in of soft tissues of chest, indicative of an obstruction at any level of the respiratory tract from the oropharynx to the alveoli. (2) Retraction of uterine muscle fiber. After contracting, the muscle fiber does not return to its original length but remains slightly shortened, a unique attribute of uterine muscle that aids in preventing postdelivery hemorrhage and results in involution.

retroflexion Bending backward.

   r. of the uterus Condition in which the body of the womb is bent backward at an angle with the cervix, whose position usually remains unchanged.

retrolental fibroplasia (RLF) Retinopathy of prematurity associated with hyperoxemia, resulting in eye injury and blindness.

retroversion Turning or a state of being turned back.

   r. of the uterus Displacement of the uterus; the body of the uterus is tipped backward with the cervix pointing forward toward the symphysis pubis.

Rh factor Inherited antigen present on erythrocytes. The individual with the factor is known as *positive* for the factor.

rhonchi Coarse, snorelike sounds produced as air passes through the fluid in the large bronchi, frequently heard after aspiration of oral secretions or feedings.

rhythm method Contraceptive method in which a woman abstains from sexual intercourse during the ovulatory phase of her menstrual cycle and at least 3 days before and 1 day after the ovulation date.

ribonucleic acid (RNA) Element responsible for transferring genetic information within a cell; a template, or pattern.

risk factors Factors that cause a person or a group of people to be particularly vulnerable to an unwanted, unpleasant, or unhealthful event.

Ritgen maneuver Procedure used to control the delivery of the head.

role playing Psychotherapeutic technique in which a person acts out a real or simulated situation as a means of understanding intrapsychic conflicts.

rooming-in unit Maternity unit designed so that the newborn's crib is at the mother's bedside or in a nursery adjacent to the mother's room.

rooting reflex Normal response in newborns when the cheek is touched or stroked along the side of the mouth to turn the head toward the stimulated side, to open the mouth, and to begin to suck. The reflex disappears by 3 to 4 months of age but in some infants may persist until 12 months.

rotation In obstetrics, the turning of the fetal head as it follows the curves of the birth canal downward.

Rubin's test Transuterine insufflation of the fallopian tubes with carbon dioxide to test their patency.

rugae Folds of vaginal mucosa.

sac, amniotic See *amniotic sac*.

sacroiliac Of or pertaining to the sacrum and ilium.

sacrum Triangular bone composed of five united vertebras and situated between L-5 and the coccyx; forms the posterior boundary of the true pelvis.

saddle block anesthesia Type of regional anesthesia produced by injection of a local anesthetic solution into the cerebrospinal fluid intrathecal (subarachnoid) space in the spinal canal.

sagittal suture Band of connective tissue separating the parietal bones, extending from the anterior to the posterior fontanel.

salpingo-oophorectomy Removal of a fallopian tube and an ovary.

scaphoid abdomen Abdomen with a sunken interior wall.

schizophrenia Any one of a large group of psychotic disorders characterized by gross distortion of reality, disturbances of language and communication, withdrawal from social interaction, and the disorganization and fragmentation of thought, perception, and emotional reaction.

Schultze's mechanism Delivery of the placenta with the fetal surfaces (shiny in appearance) presenting (archaic).

sclerema Hardening of skin and subcutaneous tissue that develops in association with such life threatening disorders as severe cold stress, septicemia, and shock.

scrotum Pouch of skin containing the testes and parts of the spermatic cords.

sebaceous glands Oil-secreting glands found in the skin.

secondary areola See *areola, secondary*.

secretory phase of menstrual cycle Postovulatory, luteal, progestational, premenstrual phase of menstrual cycle; 14 days in length.

secundines Fetal membranes and placenta expelled after childbirth; afterbirth.

segmentation Process of cleavage or division by which the fertilized ovum multiplies before differentiating into layers.

semen Thick, white, viscid secretion discharged from the urethra of the male at orgasm; the transporting medium of the sperm.

sensitization Development of antibodies to a specific antigen.

septic abortion See *abortion, septic*.

shake test "Foam" test for lung maturity of fetus; more rapid than determination of L/S ratio.

Sims' position Position in which the client lies on the left side with the right knee and thigh drawn upward toward the chest.

singleton Pregnancy with a single fetus.

situational crisis Crisis that arises suddenly in response to an external event or a conflict concerning a specific circumstance. The symptoms are transient, and the episode is usually brief.

Skene's glands Paraurethral glands situated on each side of urethral meatus.

small for dates (small for gestational age [SGA]) Refers to inadequate growth for gestational age.

smegma Whitish secretion around labia minora.

socioeconomic status Combined social and economic level of individuals or groups.

souffle Soft, blowing sound or murmur heard by auscultation.
  funic s. Soft, muffled, blowing sound produced by blood rushing through the umbilical vessels and synchronous with the fetal heart sounds.
  placental s. Soft, blowing murmur caused by the blood current in the placenta and synchronous with the maternal pulse.
  uterine s. Soft, blowing sound made by the blood in the arteries of the pregnant uterus and synchronous with the maternal pulse.

sperm Male sex cell. Also called spermatozoon.

spermatic cord Structure supporting the testis and containing blood vessels, nerves, muscle fibers, and the vas deferens.

spermatogenesis Process by which mature spermatozoa are formed, during which the diploid chromosome number (46) is reduced by half (haploid, 23).

spermicide Chemical substance that kills sperm by reducing their surface tension, causing the cell wall to break down by a bactericidal effect or by creating a highly acidic environment. Also called spermatocide.

spina bifida occulta Congenital malformation of the spine in which the posterior portion of laminas of the vertebras fails to close but there is no herniation or protrusion of the spinal cord or meninges through the defect. The newborn may have a dimple in the skin or growth of hair over the malformed vertebras.

spinnbarkeit Formation of a stretchable thread of cervical mucus under estrogen influence at time of ovulation.

splanchnic engorgement Excessive filling or pooling of blood within the visceral vasculature that occurs following the removal of pressure from the abdomen, e.g., birth of a child, removal of an excess of urine from bladder (1000 ml), removal of large tumor.

spontaneous abortion See *abortion, spontaneous*.

square window Angle of wrist between hypothenar prominence and forearm; one criterion for estimating gestational age of neonate.

station Relationship of the presenting fetal part to an imaginary line drawn between the ischial spines of the pelvis.

sterility (1) State of being free from living microorganisms. (2) Complete inability to reproduce offspring.

sterilization Process or act that renders a person unable to produce children.

stillborn Born dead.

striae gravidarum ("stretch marks") Shining reddish lines caused by stretching of the skin, often found on the abdomen, thighs, and breasts during pregnancy. These streaks turn to a fine pinkish white or silver tone in time in fair-skinned women and brownish in darker-skinned women.

stroma Supporting tissue.

subculture Group having social, economic, ethnic, or other traits distinctive enough to distinguish it from others within the same culture or society.

subinvolution Failure of a part (e.g., the uterus) to reduce to its normal size and condition after enlargement from functional activity (e.g., pregnancy).

subluxation Incomplete dislocation.

subtotal hysterectomy See *hysterectomy, subtotal.*

succedaneum See *caput succedaneum.*

superfecundation Successive fertilization of two or more ova formed during the same menstrual cycle by the sperm of the same father or different fathers.

superfetation Fertilization of an ovum when the woman is already pregnant.

supernumerary nipples Excessive number of nipples varying in size from small pink spots to the size of normal nipples and usually not associated with underlying glandular tissue.

supine hypotension Shock; fall in blood pressure caused by impaired venous return when gravid uterus presses on ascending vena cava, when woman is lying flat on her back; vena caval syndrome.

suppuration Process by which pus is formed.

surfactant Phosphoprotein necessary for normal respiratory function that prevents the alveolar collapse (atelectasis). See also *lecithin* and *L/S ratio.*

suture (1) Junction of the adjoining bones of the skull. (2) Operation uniting parts by sewing them together.

symphysis pubis Fibrocartilaginous union of the bodies of the pubic bones in the midline.

syndactyly Malformation of digits, commonly seen as a fusion of two or more toes to form one structure.

synostosis Articulation by osseous tissue of adjacent bones; union of separate bones by osseous tissue.

taboo Proscribed (forbidden) by society as improper and unacceptable.

tachypnea Excessively rapid respiratory rate (e.g., in neonates, respiratory rate of 60 breaths/min or more).

talipes equinovarus Deformity in which the foot is extended and the person walks on the toes.

telangiectasia Permanent dilatation of groups of superficial capillaries and venules.

telangiectatic nevi ("stork bites") Clusters of small, red, localized areas of capillary dilatation commonly seen in neonates at the nape of the neck or lower occiput, upper eyelids, and nasal bridge that can be blanched with pressure of a finger.

teratogenic agent Any drug, virus, or irradiation, the exposure to which can cause malformation of the fetus.

teratogens Nongenetic factors that cause malformations and disease syndromes in utero.

teratoma Tumor composed of different kinds of tissue, none of which normally occur together or at the site of the tumor.

term infant Live infant born between weeks 38 and 42 of completed gestation.

testis One of the glands contained in the male scrotum that produces the male reproductive cell, or sperm, and the male hormone testosterone; testicle.

tetany, uterine Extremely prolonged uterine contractions.

tetralogy of Fallot Congenital cardiac malformation consisting of pulmonary stenosis, intraventricular septal defect, dextroposed aorta that receives blood from both ventricles, and hypertrophy of the right ventricle.

thalassemia Hemolytic anemia characterized by microcytic, hypochromic, and short-lived red blood cells (RBCs) caused by deficient hemoglobin synthesis. It is an autosomal recessive, genetically transmitted disease occurring in two forms.

t. major (homozygous form) evident in infancy, it is recognized by anemia, fever, failure to thrive, and splenomegaly and confirmed by characteristic changes in the RBCs on microscopic examination.

t. minor (heterozygous form) it is characterized only by a mild anemia and minimal RBC changes.

therapeutic abortion See *abortion, therapeutic.*

thermogenesis Creation or production of heat, especially in the body.

thermoneutral environment Environment that enables the neonate to maintain a body temperature of 36.5° C (97.7° F) with minimum use of oxygen and energy.

threatened abortion See *abortion, threatened.*

thrombocytopenia Abnormal hematologic condition in which the number of platelets is reduced, usually by destruction of erythroid tissue in bone marrow owing to certain neoplastic diseases or to an immune response to a drug.

thrombocytopenic purpura Hematologic disorder characterized by prolonged bleeding time, decreased number of platelets, increased cell fragility, and purpura, which result in hemorrhages into the skin, mucous membranes, organs, and other tissue.

thromboembolism Obstruction of a blood vessel by a clot that has become detached from its site of formation.

thrombophlebitis Inflammation of a vein with secondary clot formation.

thrombus Blood clot obstructing a blood vessel that remains at the place it was formed.

thrush Fungal infection of the mouth or throat characterized by the formation of white patches on a red, moist, inflamed mucous membrane and is caused by *Candida albicans.*

toco- (toko-) Combining form that means childbirth or labor.

tocolytic drug Drug used to suppress premature labor.

tocotransducer Electronic device for measuring uterine contractions.

tongue-tie Congenital shortening of the frenulum, which, if servere, may interfere with sucking and articulation; a rare condition.

TORCH organisms Organisms that damage the embryo or fetus; acronym for *toxoplasmosis, o*ther (e.g., syphilis), *ru*bella, *c*ytomegalovirus, and *h*erpes simplex.

torticollis Congenital or acquired stiff neck caused by shortening or spasmodic contraction of the neck (sternocleidomastoid) muscles that draws the head to one side with the chin pointing in the other direction; wryneck.

total hysterectomy See *hysterectomy, total.*

toxemia Term previously used for disorders occurring during pregnancy or early puerperium, known as *preeclampsia-eclampsia,* that are characterized by one or all of the following: edema, hypertension, proteinuria, and, in severe cases, convulsion and coma; pregnancy-induced hypertension (PIH).

tracheoesophageal fistula Congenital malformation in which there is an abnormal tubelike passage between the trachea and esophagus.

transition Last phase of first stage of labor; 8 to 10 cm dilatation.

translocation Condition in which a chromosome breaks and all or part of that chromosome is transferred to a different part of the same chromosome or to another chromosome.

trauma Physical or psychic injury.

Trichomonas vaginitis Inflammation of the vagina caused by *Trichomonas vaginalis*, a parasitic protozoon and characterized by persistent burning and itching of the vulvar tissue and a profuse, frothy, white discharge.

trimester Time period of 3 months.

trisomy Condition whereby any given chromosome exists in triplicate instead of the normal duplicate pattern.

trophectoderm See *trophoblast*.

trophoblast Outer layer of cells of the developing blastodermic vesicle that develops the trophoderm or feeding layer which will establish the nutrient relationships with the uterine endometrium.

tubal ligation See *ligation, tubal*.

tubercles of Montgomery Small papillae on surface of nipples and areolae that secrete a fatty substance that lubricates the nipples.

twins Two neonates from the same impregnation developed within the same uterus at the same time.

  conjoined t. Twins who are physically united; Siamese twins.

  disparate t. Twins who are different (e.g., in weight) and distinct from one another.

  dizygous t. Twins developed from two separate ova fertilized by two separate sperm at the same time; fraternal twins.

  monozygous twins. Twins developed from a single fertilized ovum; identical twins.

ultrasonography High frequency sound waves to discern fetal heart rate or placental location or body parts.

umbilical cord (funis) Structure connecting the placenta and fetus and containing two arteries and one vein encased in a tissue called *Wharton's jelly*. The cord is ligated at birth and severed; the stump falls off in 4 to 10 days.

umbilical vasculitis Inflammation of the umbilical cord and its blood vessels.

umbilicus Navel, or depressed point in the middle of the abdomen that marks the attachment of the umbilical cord during fetal life.

urachus Epithelial tube connecting the apex of the urinary bladder with the allantois. Its connective tissue forms the median umbilical ligament.

urethra Small tubular structure that drains urine from the bladder.

urinary frequency Need to void often or at close intervals.

urinary meatus Opening, or mouth, of the urethra.

uterine Referring or pertaining to the uterus.

  u. adnexa See *adnexa, uterine*.

  u. bruit Abnormal sound or murmur heard while auscultating the uterus.

  u. ischemia Decreased blood supply to the uterus.

  u. prolapse Falling, sinking, or sliding of the uterus from its normal location in the body.

  u. souffle See *souffle, uterine*.

uterus Hollow muscular organ in the female designed for the implantation, containment, and nourishment of the fetus during its development until birth.

  Couvelaire u. Interstitial myometrial hemorrhage following premature separation (abruptio) of placenta. A purplish-bluish discoloration of the uterus and boardlike rigidity of the uterus are noted.

  inversion of the u. See *inversion of the uterus*.

  retroflexion of the u. See *retroflexion of the uterus*.

  retroversion of the u. See *retroversion of the uterus*.

vagina Normally collapsed musculomembranous tube that forms the passageway between the uterus and the entrance to the vagina.

vaginismus Intense, painful spasm of the muscles surrounding the vagina.

varices (varicose veins) Swollen, distended, and twisted veins that may develop in almost any part of the body but are most commonly seen in the legs, caused by pregnancy, obesity, congenital defective venous valves, and occupations requiring much standing.

vasectomy Ligation or removal of a segment of the vas deferens, usually done bilaterally to produce sterility in the male.

VDRL test Abbreviation for Venereal Disease Research Laboratory test, a serological flocculation test for syphilis.

venous Pertaining or relating to the veins.

vera, decidua See *decidua vera*.

vernix caseosa Protective gray-white fatty substance of cheesy consistency covering the fetal skin.

version Act of turning the fetus in the uterus to change the presenting part and facilitate delivery.

  podalic v. See *podalic version*.

vertex Crown or top of the head.

  v. presentation Presentation in which the fetal skull is nearest the cervical opening and born first.

vesicle Tiny blister; a small, thin-walled raised skin lesion containing clear fluid.

vesicle, blastoderm See *blastoderm vesicle*.

vestibule Area at the entrance to another structure.

  v. of vagina Space between the labia minora where the urinary meatus and vaginal introitus are lcoated.

viable Capable of living, such as a fetus that has reached a stage of development, usually 24 to 28 weeks, which will permit it to live outside the uterus.

villi Short, vascular processes or protrusions growing on certain membranous surfaces.

  chorionic v. Tiny vascular protrusions on the chorionic surface that project into the maternal blood sinuses of the uterus and that help to form the placenta and secrete HCG.

voluntary abortion See *abortion, elective*.

volvulus Twisting of the bowel on itself, causing intestinal obstruction.

vulva External genitalia of the female that consist of the labia majora, labia minora, clitoris, urinary meatus, and vaginal introitus.

vulvectomy Removal of the external genitalia of the female.

well-baby clinics Clinics that offer medical supervision and services to healthy infants.

Wharton's jelly White, gelatinous material surrounding the umbilical vessels within the cord.

witch's milk Secretion of a whitish fluid for about a week after birth from enlarged mammary tissue in the neonate, presumably resulting from maternal hormonal influences.

womb See *uterus*.

X chromosome Sex chromosome in humans existing in dupicate in the normal female and singly in the normal male.

X linkage Genes located on the X-chromosome.

Y chromosome Sex chromosome in the human male necessary for the development of the male gonads.

zero fluid balance Equality of amount of intake and amount of output.

zero population growth In a given year, live births equal to total number of deaths (i.e., no population increase for that year).

zona pellucida Inner, thick, membranous envelope of the ovum.

zygote Cell formed by the union of two reproductive cells or gametes; the fertilized ovum resulting from the union of a sperm and an ovum.

Index

Exercise
  diabetes mellitus and, 856
  flying, 272, 273
  Kegel's, 260-261, 679, 682
  postpartum, 679, 680
  pregnant woman and, 259, 260
Exhibitionism, 121-122
Expected date of confinement, 369
Expulsion, 361
Exstrophy of bladder, 1030-1031
Extended rubella syndrome, 1039
Extension in labor, 361
  in vertex presentation, 364
External rotation, 361
  in vertex presentation, 364
Extracorporeal membrane oxygenation
      (ECMO) for infant with respiratory
      distress syndrome, 990
Extraction, vacuum, 922
Extremities of neonate, assessment of, 530
Extrusion reflex, diminishing of, 594
Eye(s)
  fetal abnormalities of, and maternal
      alcohol consumption, 886
  neonatal
    assessment of, 525
    fetal alcohol syndrome and, 888
Eye contact
  attachment process and, 643-644
  compensating for, by blind parent, 654
  ethnic practices and, 507
  in neonate, 507
  in nonverbal communication, 54
Eye prophylaxis, 465, 467, 468, 469
Eyelids as immune defense mechanism, 105

F

Face, paralysis of, 994, 997
Facial asymmetry in neonate, 517
Facial nerve, paralysis of, in infant of
      diabetic mother, 1000
Facies of neonate, assessment of, 526
Factor VIII deficiency, 838, 839
Factor IX deficiency, 838
FAD; see Fetal activity determination
Failure to thrive in breast-feeding infant,
      613, 615
Faintness, prevention and treatment of, 268
Fallopian tube, cancer of, 883-884
Fallot, tetralogy of, 1019
Falope ring for sterilization, 168
False labor, 370
Family, 2-14
  adaptation of, to pregnancy, 224-241
  adaptive and maladaptive behaviors of,
      687
  adjustment of, during postpartum period,
      640-659
  of adolescent mother, 950
  adolescent's emancipation from, 124
  American, 12
  assessing, 60
  biologic functions of, 3
  blended, 7

Family—cont'd
  boundaries and, 4
  channels in, 4
  communal, 6
  coping behaviors of, 3
  crises in, 9-10
  cultural context of, 10-12
  culture patterning and, 3
  and death of infant, 761
  defined, 2-3
  development of communication in, 4
  developmental tasks of, 8
  divorce and separation in, 7
  dynamics of, 3, 4
    assessing, 59
  economic functions of, 3
  educational functions of, 3
  equilibrium of, 5
  extended, 6
  gene transmission in, 184
  grieving, assessment of, 765
  health of, 3
  hierarchies in, 4
  homosexual, 7
  identification of, 59
  identifying strengths of, 60
  informed choice of, about childbirth, 342
  internal relationships of, 7
  interview of, 243
  and larger social system, 7
  maturational crises in, 9
  nuclear, 5-6
  nursing care of, 44-62
    after maternal death, 774
  nursing process with (example), 61
  nurturing role of, 4
  power in, 4
  preparation of, for home birth, 346
  and preparation for childbirth, 330-347;
      see also Childbirth education
  problem-solving in, 4
  psychologic functions of, 3-4
  reciprocal relationships of, 7
  response of
    to birth of compromised neonate, 773
    to maternal death, 773-775
  role changes in, 9
  roles in, 4
  as semiclosed system, 8
  single-parent, 7
  socialization role of, 4
  sociocultural functions of, 4
  stress in, 9
  theories of; see Family theories
  during third stage of labor, 461
  values and attitudes of, 4
Family care plan, 57-61
  assessment in, 57-60
  evaluation of, 60-61
  implementation of, 60
  nursing diagnosis in, 60
  setting goals in, 60
Family history, 243, 248
Family life cycle, 8

Family planning; see also Contraception;
      Contraceptive methods;
      Contraceptives
  for diabetic mother, 858
  "natural," 151
  third world attitudes toward, 149-150
Family theories, 4-9
  developmental, 7-8
  interactional, 8-9
  Malinowski's, 5
  structural-functional, 5-7
Family unit, adult in, 2
Fascia, cremaster, 96
Fasting blood sugar test, 855, 856
Fat
  body; see Body fat
  brown, in neonate, 505
  deposition of, in breasts, 85
  infant requirement for, 596
  subcutaneous, in neonate, 503
Father
  acceptance of pregnancy by, 233-234
  adaptation of, to pregnancy, 233-237
  adjustment of, in postpartum period,
      648-649
  adolescent, 961-962
  anticipation of labor by, 236-237
  cultural influences on participation in birth
      process, 405
  emotional responses of, to pregnancy,
      234-235
  engrossment of, 648
  identification of, with fatherhood role,
      235
  involvement styles of, 234-235
  involving, in labor process, 403-405
  preparing for labor, 275
  relationship of, with wife, 235-236
  role of
    in childbirth, 333
    during early pregnancy, 18
    strategies to support and promote, 690
  stress of, during labor, 387
Fatigue, 271
  in postpartum period, 647
  in pregnancy, 200, 214
Federal right-to-know law, 257
Feedback, positive, in attachment process,
      641
Feedback, relaxation during labor, 398
Feeding
  bottle; see Bottle feeding
  with cleft lip or palate, 1028
  on demand, 621
  developmental readiness for, 593-594
  difficulties in, from fetal alcohol syndrome,
      887
  early
    of compromised neonate, 747
    and serum bilirubin levels, 501
  formula; see Formula feeding
  frequency of, 621
  gavage; see Gavage feeding
  of high-risk infant, 749-757

Netrazine paper test, 374, 375, 380
Neural crest, 197
Neural plate, 197
Neural tube, 197
Neural tube defects, 1025
Neurofibromatosis, 877
Neurologic disorders during pregnancy, 877-878
Neurologic system
    changes in
        during postpartum period, 638
        during pregnancy, 217
    congenital anomalies of, screening for, 1017-1018
    discomforts of, prevention and treatment of, 270-271
    fetal, 197-198
    during labor, 366
Neuromuscular behavior of fetus, 197
Neuromuscular development in infant, implications of, for feeding, 595
Neuromuscular maturity, assessment of, in newborn, 980-981
Neuromuscular system of infant, 499, 594
Neuroocular lesions, oral contraceptives and, 160
Neutrophils, 112-113
Nevus flammeus, 503, 504, 505
Nevus vasculosus, 503, 504
New York Heart Association, heart disease classification of, 868-869
Newborn; see Infant; Neonate
Niacin, infant requirement for, 597
Nicotine in breast milk, A-32
NICUs; see Neonatal intensive care units
Nidation, 90, 185, 187-188
Night sweats; see Diaphoresis
Nightingale, Florence, 330
Nipple(s), 86
    changes in, during pregnancy, 211
    for infant with cleft palate, 751
    sore, 610
        nursing intervention for, 626-627
    stimulated, 265
    teaching new mother to assess, 668
Nipple cups, 266
Nipple erection reflex, breast feeding and, 598
Nipple formation, pinch test of, 266
Nipple rolling, 266
Nipple stretching, 266
Nisentil; see Alphaprodine hydrochloride
Nitrofurantoin (Furadantin)
    in breast milk, A-25
    effect of, on fetus or neonate, A-12
Nodes, lymph, 107
Nodules in breast, 88
Nonoxynol, 9, 155
Nonpitting edema, 778
Nonstress test, 432, 737-739
    clinical significance of results of, 739
    indications for, 737-738
    interpretation of, 738
    in pregnancy complicated by diabetes, 998
    in prolonged pregnancy, 993

Nonverbal communication; see Communication, nonverbal
Norethindrone (Norlutin) in breast milk, A-30
Norethynodrel (Enovid) in breast milk, A-30
Norlutin; see Norethindrone
19-Nortestosterone in breast milk, A-30
Nortriptyline, effect of, on fetus or neonate, A-14
Nose
    of neonate
        assessment of, 525
        fetal alcohol syndrome and, 888
    removing mucus from, 551
Novobiocin
    in breast milk, A-25
    effect of, on fetus or neonate, A-12
NST; see Nonstress test
Nuchal cord, 456
Nuclear family, 5-6
Nulligravida, 206
Nullipara, 206
    abdominal, cervical, and vulval changes in, during pregnancy, 211, 212
    cervix of, 210
Numbness, prevention and treatment of, 271
Nurse
    attitude of, toward sex, 122-123, 128
    and client education, 26-28; see also Client teaching
    duty of, 32, 33-34
    and family choices about childbirth, 342
    liability of, 34
    personal characteristics of, 49
    reaction of, to client's pain, sociocultural basis of, 400
    response of, to fetal or neonatal death, 767-768
    as sex educator, 126, 128
    as support person, 255-256
    as teacher/counselor/advocate, 256-275
Nurse Practice Act, 33
Nurse practitioner, obstetric-gynecologic, 19-20
Nurse-client relationships, 46-57
    and client compliance, 47, 48
    and client dependency, 48
    closeness and, 48
    communication in, 50-54
    confidentiality and, 48
    decision making and, 49-50
    and nurse's personal characteristics, 49
    personal values and, 54
    during prenatal period, 255-256
    as process, 46-49
    quality of, 36
    self-awareness and, 54-57
    self-concept and, 55-56
    termination phase of, 48-49
    values clarification and, 56-57
Nurse/infant ratio for care of preterm infants, 982
Nurse-midwife, 344, 345; see also Midwife

Nursery
    intensive care, admitting preterm infant to, 982
    newborn, standards for, 544
    special care, 759
Nurses' Association of the American College of Obstetrics and Gynecologists, 341, A-5
    guidelines for childbirth education, 330
    position paper on abortion client, 172
Nursing
    ANA definition of, 33
    as decision-making process, 330
    family and, 3
    independent practice of, legally defined, 34
    maternal-child, sources of standards of care for, A-3
    risk management and, 34-38
Nursing actions
    in elective abortion, 174-175
    with infertile client, 147-148
    in newborn nutrition, 622-625
    for nutrition education, 324
    in Pap smear procedure, 280
    during pelvic examination, 276
    in pharmacologic control of discomfort, 425-427
    in response to client's pain, 401, 403
    selecting, 23, 25
    for sterilization, 169-170
    in treating vasovagal syncope, 281
Nursing brassiere, 608
Nursing care
    of childbearing family, 44-62
    client compliance with, 47
    contract for, 47
    during first stage of labor, 407-410
    during fourth stage of labor, 486-491
    goals of, 254-255
        physiologic, 255
        psychosocial, 255
    implementation of, 25
    maternal and fetal nutrition and, 325-327
    of normal neonate, 515-592
        summary of, 578-591
    during postpartum period, 660-715
        summary of, 696-711
    during pregnancy, 242-301
    standard of; see Standard of care
    supportive, 255-256
Nursing diagnosis, 23
    in adolescent pregnancy, 957
    in family care plan, 60
    of family's emotional needs, 688
    during fourth stage of labor, 476, 480
    and functional health patterns, 24
    of grieving family, 765
    of heart disease, 870, 871
    of infant with respiratory distress, 742
    during labor, 387
    and learning objectives, 28
    for neonate, 544
        in third stage of labor, 464

MAGNESIUM SULFATE (INJECTION)

Rx

Category: anticonvulsant

Brand Names:
Magnesium Sulfate (various)

Dosage Forms:
injection (IM/IV): 10%, 12.5%, 50%

Action/Use: Anticonvulsant activity due to inhibition of peripheral neuromuscular transmission.
- Anticonvulsant for seizures associated c̄ epilepsy and pregnancy-induced hypertension (PIH)
- Treatment of Mg deficiency

Pharmacokinetics:

	Onset	Duration	Excretion
IV	immediate	30m	via urine
IM	1h	3-4h	via urine

Dosage:
(Parenteral)
Anticonvulsant Adult
Dose range of 1-40g/d; IM: 1-5g in 25-50% solution as needed; IV: 1-4g in 10-20% solution; Infusion: 4g in 250ml 5% dextrose at 3ml or less/m

Pediatric
IM: 20-40mg/kg in a 20% solution prn

Cerebral edema
Up to 2.5g IV

Magnesium deficiency
Usual IM adult dose:1g q 6h for 4 doses; for severe cases up to 250mg/kg IV over 4h period; hyperalimentation for adults is 8-24mEq/d

Contraindications: heart block or myocardial damage (parenteral), severe renal impairment

Adverse Effects:
CNS: depression of deep tendon reflexes
CV: hypotension, depressed cardiac function, circulatory collapse
GI: diarrhea
INT: sweating, flushing
OTHER: respiratory depression

ERGONOVINE MALEATE

Rx

Category: oxytoxic

Brand Names:
Ergotrate Maleate (Lilly)

Dosage Forms:
injection (IM/IV): 0.2mg/ml
tablets: 0.2mg

Action/Use: Oxytoxic effect due to direct stimulation of uterine smooth muscle resulting in intense contractions followed by periods of relaxation. There is an ↑ in uterine tone which ↓ postpartum uterine bleeding. Occasionally produces severe hypertensive episodes esp. in toxemic pts.
- Treatment or prevention of postpartum & postpartal hemorrhage due to uterine atony

Pharmacokinetics:

	Onset	Duration	Elimination
PO	10m	up to	via feces
IM	2-5m	3h or	via feces
IV	immediate	more	via feces

Dosage:
PO 0.2mg usually administered parenterally; followed by 0.2-0.4mg PO q 6-12h until danger of atony is over (approximately 48 h)

IM 0.2mg; may be repeated for severe hemorrhage

IV Should be restricted to excessive hemorrhage because of higher rate of side effects, esp. nausea & vomiting

Contraindications: hypersensitivity, induction of labor, threatened spontaneous abortion

Adverse Effects:
CNS: headache   GI: nausea, vomiting
CV: hypertension, particularly when administered IV   OTHER: possible symptoms of ergot poisoning

Drug Interactions:
Concurrent or sequential use c̄ vasoconstrictors or regional anesthesia may ↑ BP

MEPERIDINE HYDROCHLORIDE

Rx C-II

Category: narcotic: synthetic opiate

Brand Names:
Demerol HCl (Winthrop-Breon)

Dosage Forms:
injection (IM/IV/SCl): 50mg/ml, 100mg/ml (multiple dose vials);
25mg/, 50mg/, 75mg/, 100mg/dose (UniNest amps & Carpujects)
syrup: 50mg/5ml   tablets: 50mg, 100mg

Pethadol (Halsey)   tablets: 50mg, 100mg

Combination Products:
Mepergan (Wyeth)   meperidine HCl 25mg/promethazine HCl 25mg/ml injection
Demerol APAP (Winthrop-Breon)   meperidine HCl 50mg/acetaminophen 300mg/tablet

Action/Use: Produces analgesia, euphoria, & sedation. Equianalgesic doses of meperidine & morphine produce the same amount of euphoria, respiratory depression & sedation, & have about the same addiction liability. PO administration is significantly less effective. A parenteral dose of 70mg is clinically equivalent to 10mg of morphine.
- Relief of moderate to severe pain • Pre-op sedation, post-op analgesic, obstetrical analgesia, anesthesia support

Pharmacokinetics:

	Onset	Peak	Duration	Protein Binding	Half-Life	Excretion
PO	15-20m	60m	2-4h	60-70%	4-8h	Renal-as
IM	10m	40-60m	2-4h	60-70%	4-8h	metabolites
SC	10m	30-50m	2-4h	60-70%	4-8h	5% is unchanged

Dosage:
Analgesic
Pediatric PO, IM, SC 0.5-0.8mg/lb q 3-4h prn
Adult PO, IM, SC 50-150mg q 3-4h prn
OB 50-100mg when pain is regular. May be repeated at 1-3h intervals.
Anesthesia Titrated against patient needs by IV, injection, or continuous infusion.

Pre-op
IM, SC: 0.5-1mg/lb 30-90m before anesthesia
IM, SC: 50-100mg 30-90m before anesthesia

ERYTHROMYCIN OPHTHALMIC OINTMENT

Rx

Category: antibiotic: macrolide antibiotic

Brand Names:
Ak-Mycin (Akorn)

Ilotycin (Dista)

Dosage Forms:
ophthalmic ointment: 0.5%
(5mg/g)
(same as Ak-Mycin)

Action/Use: Bacteriostatic activity due to inhibition of ribosomal protein synthesis in susceptible microorganisms. Topical ophthalmic application has limited tissue penetration; may fail to protect against gonococcal PPNG strains.
- Treatment of ophthalmic infections due to susceptible organisms
- Prophylaxis of gonococcal & /or chlamydial ophthalmia neonatorum

Dosage:
Ophthalmic Infection: Apply a ribbon (approximately 1cm) to infected eye(s), usually in conjunctival sac 1 or more times/d

Ophthalmia Neonatorum: Apply a ribbon of ointment 0.5-1cm in length in each conjunctival sac after delivery & NOT later than 1h after delivery

Contraindication: hypersensitivity

Adverse Effects:
EENT:Local ophthalmic irritation
OTHER: possible overgrowth of non-susceptible organisms, sensitivity rx

NURSING MANAGEMENT:
Administration:
- Avoid contamination of ointment tube tip • Use new tube of ointment for each neonate • Apply thin strip into each lower conjunctival sac after delivery • Do NOT flush from eye after administration • Avoid excessive heat & light in storage; do NOT freeze

Drug Interactions:
Use c̄ CNS depressants may ↑ effect
Use c̄ great caution in digitalized pt

NURSING MANAGEMENT:
Administration:
• IM--do NOT exceed a 50% solution for adults; 1% procaine may be added to ↓ injection pain; DEEP gluteal injection • IV--do NOT exceed a 20% solution or a rate of 150mg/m • Assess patellar reflex (knee jerk); hold dose until (↑) response obtained • Assess respirations; do NOT administer if < 16/m • Institute seizure precautions • Do NOT administer discolored/precipitated solutions • Do NOT leave pt unattended • Place pt in left lateral position • Assess urinary output (> 25ml/h) • Have emergency supportive equipment available • Avoid abrupt withdrawal • Provide emotional support

Evaluation:
• Monitor: CV & renal status; BP continuously; serum Mg levels; respirations (toxicity: < 16/m); urinary output
• Observe for seizure activity; record details (duration, characteristics, pt response) • Assess: patellar reflex; neonate for Mg toxicity; for absence of convulsive activity • Therapeutic serum Mg concentration: 4-6mEq/L

Education:
• Explain procedure & rationale to pt/family • Safety precautions • Comfort measures

Overdose Management:
Symptoms: hypotension, ↓ respirations or respiratory paralysis, absence of deep tendon reflexes, ↓ FHR
Treatment: administer IV 10ml 10% aqueous solution calcium gluconate in 3m period; WARNING: do NOT give to digitalized pts (arrhythmias may occur)
Emergency artificial ventilation may be necessary

Contraindications: Hypersensitivity, during MAO-1 therapy, nursing mothers

Adverse Effects:
CNS: sedation, lightheadedness, euphoria, dysphoria, weakness, tremor, disorientation, transient hallucination
CV: hypotension, palpitation, flushing of face, phlebitis following IV administration
GI: nausea, vomiting, dry mouth, biliary tract spasm, constipation
GU: urine retention INT: sweating, pruritus, urticaria OTHER: respiratory depression, addiction

Drug Interactions: Use c̄ alcohol, antihistamines, barbiturates, benzodiazepines, methotrimeprazine, phenothiazines, & depressants can produce additive CNS depression. Dosage reductions may be required

NURSING MANAGEMENT:
Administration: • Store under double lock & key; document use accurately • Check compatibility chart for mixing pre-op IM preparations • Do NOT administer if respirations are <12/m • IM--inject DEEP into muscle; rotate sites • IV--dilute; administer SLOWLY • Have narcotic antagonist & supportive measures available • Avoid in cases of suspected head injury • Administer BEFORE patient experiences intense pain • Utilize power of suggestion • Avoid abrupt withdrawal

Evaluation:
• Monitor respirations & circulatory function • Assess: bowel function, abdominal distension, renal function, urinary retention • Check for signs of dependence • Assess for potentiation of CNS depressant effect; signs of overdosage (coma, pin-point pupils, respiratory depression); relief of pain

Education:
• Avoid: changing positions (lying-sitting-standing) rapidly; excessive sensory stimulation; engaging in potentially hazardous activities; smoking; use of alcohol & other CNS depressants • Keep bed-rails up when non-ambulatory • Obtain assistance as needed when ambulatory • Turn, cough & deep-breathe following surgery
• Constipation may occur; ↑ fluids & bulk-containing foods • Indiscriminate use may lead to severe dependence

Overdose Management:
Principal symptoms: respiratory depression & stupor or coma **Treatment:** naloxone HCl 0.01mg/kg IV; maintain respiration, remove drug by gastric lavage, & administer IV to maintain adequate blood pressure.

NURSING MANAGEMENT:
Administration:
• NOT routinely used prior to delivery • Assess: BP; serum calcium - IV calcium gluconate if hypocalcemic • PO--avoid excessive moisture in storage • INJECTION--store in cold place (<46°F); do NOT exceed 60d at normal room temperature • Do NOT administer discolored/precipitated solutions • IV--use infusion control device; administer SLOWLY • Have emergency supportive equipment available • Provide emotional support

Evaluation:
• Monitor: BP & pulse; uterine contractions--stop if prolonged; serum calcium • Fetal monitoring (heart rate, intra-uterine pressure) • Observe for signs of ergotism (nausea, vomiting, dizziness, cramps, headache, confusion)
• POSTPARTUM--monitor fundal height and tone; assess amount & character of lochia • Assess for: ↑ in BUN, urine aminolevulinic acid, proteins, & porphyrins; ↓ serum prolactin concentration; ↑ uterine contractions / ↑ uterine bleeding

Education:
• Explain procedure & rationale to pt/family • Occurrence of contractions • Relaxation techniques • Comfort measures • Store in well-closed container • Avoid smoking • Notify physician if infection or signs of ergotism occur (cramps, vomiting, thirst, weakness, tingling in extremities)

Evaluation:
• Observe for signs of local hypersensitivity; notify physician if present • Assess for absence of conjunctivitis & ocular infection

Education:
• Explain procedure & rationale to family • Report signs of local hypersensitivity (redness, tearing, irritation) immediately

NALOXONE HYDROCHLORIDE

Rx
Preg Cat B

Category: narcotic antagonist

Brand Names:
Narcan (DuPont)

Dosage Forms:
injection (IM/IV/SC): 0.4mg/ml
neonatal injection (IM/IV/SC): 0.02mg/ml

Action/Use: Narcotic antagonism primarily due to competition c̄ narcotics for CNS receptor sites
- Induces complete or partial reversal of narcotic depression (incl respiratory) induced by natural or synthetic narcotics, propoxyphene, & the narcotic-antagonists nalbuphine, pentazocine, & butorphanol
- Diagnosis of suspected acute opioid overdosage

Pharmacokinetics:

	Onset	Half-Life*	Elimination**
IM	2-5m	60-90m	via urine
SC	2-5m	60-90m	via urine
IV	1-2m	60-90m	via urine

*longer for infants   **primarily as metabolites

Dosage:
(IM/IV/SC)

		Usual Dose
Adult	Overdose	0.4-2mg IV; repeat at 2-3m intervals to the desired degree of reversal
	Post-op	0.1-0.2mg/kg IV; repeat at 2-3m intervals to the desired degree of reversal
Pediatric	Overdose	0.01mg/kg IV; subsequent dose of 0.1mg/kg may be given IV if needed
	Post-op	0.005-0.01mg/kg IV; repeat at 2-3m intervals to the desired degree of reversal
Neonate		0.01mg/kg IM/IV/SC; repeat at 2-3m intervals to the desired degree of reversal

---

Rho (D) IMMUNE GLOBULIN (HUMAN)

Rx
Preg Cat C

Category: immunosuppressant: biological

Brand Names:
Gamulin Rh (Armour)
HypRho-D (Cutter)
HypoRho-D Mini-Dose (Cutter)
Mini-Gamulin Rh (Armour)
MICRhoGAM (Ortho)
RhoGAM (Ortho)

Dosage Forms:
300mcg
300mcg
50mcg
50mcg
50mcg
300mcg

Action/Use: Suppresses immune response of non-sensitized Rho_o (D)-negative, D^U-negative individuals who receive Rho_o (D)-positive or D^U-positive blood as the result of a fetomaternal hemorrhage or a transfusion accident.
- Used to suppress antibody formation in Rho_o (D)-negative, D^U-negative mothers after delivering an Rho (D)-positive or D^U-positive infant
- Abortion of an Rh-positive fetus
- Transfusion accident where Rho_o (D)-positive blood used in an Rho_o (D)-negative recipient

Dosage:
IM injection of the total contents of a single dose vial (50mcg or 300mcg) in a non-sensitized individual w/in 72h or less after Rh-incompatible delivery, terminated incomplete pregnancies or blood transfusions

Spontaneous or induced abortion up to 12 wks gestation; ectopic pregnancy, amniocentesis — 50mcg
Spontaneous or induced abortion after 12 wks gestation — 300mcg
Antepartum prophylaxis at 26 to 28 wks gestation — 300mcg
Postpartum, if infant is Rh positive, w/in 72h of delivery — 300mcg
Additional vials may be necessary following transfusions of more than 15 ml of packed red cells or in the case of unusually large fetomaternal hemorrhage

---

OXYTOCIN

Rx

Category: oxytoxic
Brand Names:
Pitocin (Parke-Davis)
Syntocinon (Sandoz)

Dosage Forms:
injection (IM/IV): 5U/0.5ml, 10U/ml
injection (IM/IV): 10U/ml
nasal spray: 40U/ml (2 & 5ml bottles)

Action/Use: Oxytoxic effect due to ↑ sodium ion permeability in uterine smooth muscle cells which ↑ the number of contracting myofibrils & enables the uterus to contract. Uterine sensitivity to oxytocin gradually ↑ during pregnancy reaching a peak before parturition.
- Antepartum—initiation or augmentation of uterine contractions
- Produce uterine contractions during 3-d stage of labor & control of postpartum hemorrhage
- Initiate milk let-down reflex (spray)

Pharmacokinetics:

	Absorption	Onset	Duration	Excretion
IM	excellent	3-5m	2-3h	via urine primarily as metabolites

Dosage:
Antepartum — Start c̄ an infusion rate of 1-2mU/m; slowly ↑ until contractions reach desired rate & intensity

Postpartum — 10-40U n 1000ml, infused at sufficient rate to control uterine atony or 3-10U/m after delivery of placenta

Nasal Spray — One spray in one or both nostrils 2-3m before nursing or pumping of breasts

Contraindications: hypersensitivity, cephalopelvic disproportion, unfavorable fetal position, obstetrical emergencies that favor surgical intervention, fetal distress when delivery is not imminent, multiple pregnancy, prolonged use in uterine inertia or severe toxemia, hypertonic uterine patterns, when vaginal delivery is contraindicated

---

RITODRINE HYDROCHLORIDE

Rx
Preg Cat B

Category: sympathomimetic: beta$_2$-adrenergic, uterine relaxant

Brand Names:
Yutopar (Astra)

Dosage Forms:
injection (IV): 10-15mg/ml
tablet: 10mg

Action/Use: Sympathomimetic activity is selective for beta receptors, esp. beta$_2$-adrenoreceptors of the bronchial tree, peripheral vascular beds, & uterus. Predominant betamimetic effect is on the uterine smooth muscle which ↓ the intensity & frequency of contraction. Placental drug transfer occurs & limited beta$_1$ activity results in transitory ↑ in maternal & fetal heart rates.
- Management of preterm labor in suitable patients

Pharmacokinetics:

PO Availability	Peak	Half-Life	Protein Binding	Excretion
30%	30-60m	1.3-20h	32%	via urine as unchanged drug & metabolites

Dosage:
IV infusion — Usual starting dose: 50-100ug/m; & ↑ q 10m by 50ug/m until desired effect is obtained. Usual effective range is 150-350ug/m; treatment should continue for at least 12h after uterine contractions cease

PO maintenance — 10mg 30m before termination of IV therapy: usual dosage for the 1st 24h is 10mg q 2h; usual maintenance dose is 10-20mg q 4-6h; do NOT exceed 120mg/d

Contraindications: Before 20th wk of pregnancy & conditions in which continuation of pregnancy is hazardous incl:
- Antepartum hemorrhage requiring immediate delivery ● Chorioamnionitis ● Eclampsia & severe preeclampsia
- Intrauterine fetal death ● Maternal cardiac disease, hyperthyroidism, or uncontrolled diabetes ● Pulmonary hypertension

Contraindications: hypersensitivity, in Rho (D)-positive or Du-positive individuals, in Rho (D)-negative & Du-negative & have been previously sensitized to the Rho (D) antigen, for genetic amniocentesis at 15-18 wks gestation or antepartum prophylaxis at 28 wks gestation

Adverse Effects:
limited allergic rxs incl anaphylaxis

NURSING MANAGEMENT:
Administration:
● Assess for hx of allergy ● Pre-administration criteria (type & cross-match neonate's cord blood): ● Mother must be Rho (D)-negative & Du-negative ● Mother should NOT have been previously sensitized to the Rho (D) factor ● Infant must be Rho (D)-positive or Du-positive & direct Coombs' negative ● Verify that lot numbers are the same for cross-match solution & preparation to be administered ● Cross-match a 5% suspension of the mother's RBCs c̄ 2 gtt of the cross-match solution ● Administer w/in 72h after Rh-incompatible delivery, terminated incomplete pregnancies or blood transfusions ● Administer IM (deltoid) ● Check preparation c̄ another nurse ● Do NOT administer to an infant ● Do NOT administer discolored/precipitated solutions ● Store in refrigerator
● Provide emotional support

Evaluation:
● Assess for: signs of tenderness at injection site; ↑ body temperature; lethargy & myalgia if > 1 dose administered; passive immunity / absence of future Rh-incompatibility rxs

Education:
● Explain procedure & rationale to pt/family ● Importance of screening both parents for Rh-incompatibility

---

Preexisting maternal medical conditions that would be seriously affected by ritodrine betamimetic activity which incl:

● Asthma already treated c̄ beta adrenergics or steroids ● Cardiac arrhythmias associated c̄ tachycardia or drug toxicity ● Hypovolemia ● Pheochromocytoma ● Ritodrine hypersensitivity ● Uncontrolled hypertension

Adverse Effects:
CNS: nervousness, anxiety, emotional upset, tremor, headache
CV: dose-related changes in maternal BP & maternal-fetal heart rates: pulmonary edema
GI: nausea, vomiting, epigastric distress, diarrhea, constipation
OTHER: rash, dyspnea, hyperventilation, lactic acidosis
FETAL: hypoglycemia, ileus

Drug Interactions:
Use c̄ corticosteroids can produce pulmonary edema
Use c̄ beta blockers will antagonize therapeutic effects
Use c̄ anesthetics can produce exaggerated hypotensive effects
Use c̄ sympathomimetics will produce additive effects

NURSING MANAGEMENT:
Administration:
● Assess VS ● Do NOT use saline diluents unless dextrose is undesirable (diabetics) ● Use solution w/in 48h of preparation ● Do NOT administer discolored/precipitated solution ● Place pt in left lateral position ● IV--use infusion control device ● Restrict fluids ● Store parenteral form at room temperature; do NOT freeze ● Provide emotional support

Evaluation:
● Monitor; I & O; VS, esp. BP; uterine contractions & fetal heart rate ● Observe for occurrence of pulmonary edema; stop if present ● Assess for: ↑ serum glucose, esp. diabetics; ↑ uterine contractions

Education:
● Explain procedure & rationale to pt/family ● Relaxation techniques ● Comfort measures ● Check c̄ physician before using OTC preparations ● Notify physician if contractions occur or H_2O breaks

---

Contraindications: hypersensitivity

Adverse Effects:
GI: nausea & vomiting (rare) c̄ high doses in post-op pt

NURSING MANAGEMENT:
Administration:
● Mix c̄ sterile H_2O for injection if needed ● Do NOT leave pt unattended ● Have emergency supportive equipment available ● Store in original container; avoid excessive light

Evaluation:
● Monitor VS, esp. respirations ● Observe for: ↓ in respiration after treatment; signs of narcotic withdrawal (restlessness, muscle spasms, ↑ VS,lacrimation) ● Assess: for ↑ PTT; ABGs; for reversal of narcotic overdosage

Education:
● Explain procedure & rationale to pt/family ● Safety precautions ● Comfort measures

---

Adverse Effects:
CV: cardiac arrhythmia, postpartum hemorrhage, fetal bradycardia
GI: nausea, vomiting
GU: pelvic hematoma; uterine hypertonicity, spasms, tetanic contractions, & rupture

Drug Interactions:
Use c̄ vasopressors can produce severe hypertension

NURSING MANAGEMENT:
Administration:
● Fetal monitoring; assess fetal maturity & position ● Administer by only ONE route, NOT simultaneous routes ● IV--use infusion pump ● Place pt in left lateral position ● Do NOT leave pt unattended ● Have emergency supportive equipment available ● Avoid overstimulation of uterus ● Do NOT administer discolored/precipitated solutions ● PARENTERAL--store in original container, avoid freezing

Evaluation:
● Monitor: BP & pulse q 15m; uterine contractions--stop if prolonged (< q 2m);↓ &O--assess hydration status (continuous infusion & PO fluids can lead to H_2O intoxication) ● Fetal monitoring (heart rate, intrauterine pressure) ● Assess for: uterine rupture or fetal distress; ↑ uterine contractions ●POSTPARTUM--monitor fundal height and tone

Education:
● Explain procedure & rationale to pt/family ●Occurrence of contractions ●Relaxation techniques ●Comfort measures ●Procedure for use of nasal spray